a **LANGE** medical book

W9-AUM-671

CURRENT
Medical Diagnosis
& Treatment

Thirty-third Edition

Edited By

Lawrence M. Tierney, Jr., MD
Professor of Medicine
University of California, San Francisco
Assistant Chief of Medical Services
Veterans Affairs Medical Center, San Francisco

Stephen J. McPhee, MD
Professor of Medicine
Division of General Internal Medicine
University of California, San Francisco

Maxine A. Papadakis, MD
Professor of Clinical Medicine and Epidemiology
Director of Student Programs, Internal Medicine
University of California, San Francisco

With Associate Authors

APPLETON & LANGE
Norwalk, Connecticut

Notice: The authors and the publisher of this volume have taken care to
make certain that the doses of drugs and schedules of treatment are correct
and compatible with the standards generally accepted at the time of
publication. Nevertheless, as new information becomes available, changes in
treatment and in the use of drugs become necessary. The reader is advised to
carefully consult the instruction and information material included in the
package insert of each drug or therapeutic agent before administration.
This advice is especially important when using new or infrequently used drugs.
The publisher disclaims any liability, loss, injury, or damage incurred as
a consequence, directly or indirectly, of the use and application of any of
the contents of this volume.

Prentice Hall International (UK) Limited, *London*
Prentice Hall of Australia Pty. Limited, *Sydney*
Prentice Hall Canada, Inc., *Toronto*
Prentice Hall Hispanoamericana, S.A., *Mexico*
Prentice Hall of India Private Limited, *New Delhi*
Prentice Hall of Japan, Inc., *Tokyo*
Simon & Schuster Asia Pte. Ltd., *Singapore*
Editora Prentice Hall do Brasil Ltda., *Rio de Janeiro*
Prentice Hall, *Englewood Cliffs, New Jersey*

ISSN: 0092–8682

Acquisitions Editor: Shelley Reinhardt
Production Editor: Christine Langan
Designer: Penny Kindzierski

ISBN 0-8385-1375-1

9 780838 513750

90000

PRINTED IN THE UNITED STATES OF AMERICA

Table of Contents

Preface

Current Medical Diagnosis & Treatment 1994 is the 33rd annual volume of a general medical text designed as a single-source reference for practitioners in both hospital and ambulatory settings. *CMDT* covers all fields of internal medicine plus important other topics of concern to the primary care physician and to all specialists who provide generalist care. It emphasizes the practical features of diagnosis and patient management. Appropriate biochemical and pathophysiologic background information is provided as necessary to facilitate understanding of concepts.

OUTSTANDING FEATURES

- Reissued annually in January to incorporate current advances.
- Coverage of all aspects of internal medicine plus gynecology/obstetrics, dermatology, ophthalmology, otolaryngology, psychiatry, neurology, imaging procedures, and other topics relevant to generalist care.
- Concise, readable format, affording efficient use in various practice settings.
- More than 1000 diseases and disorders.
- Only book of its kind to include an annual update on HIV infection.
- Brevity, conciseness, and easy accessibility of key information.
- Quick reference index to common presenting problems on inside front cover.
- Emphasis on prevention and cost-consciousness.
- Handy access to drug dosages.
- Inexpensively priced.

INTENDED AUDIENCE

House officers and medical students will find the concise, up-to-date descriptions of diagnostic and therapeutic procedures, with citations to the current literature, of daily usefulness in the immediate management of patients.

Internists, family physicians, and other specialists who provide generalist care will appreciate *CMDT* as a useful ready reference and refresher text.

Physicians in other specialties, surgeons, and dentists will find the book useful as a basic internal medicine reference.

Nurses and other health practitioners will welcome the concise format and broad scope of the book as a means of enhancing their understanding of diagnostic principles and therapeutic procedures.

ORGANIZATION

CMDT is developed and organized chiefly by organ system. Chapter 1 presents general information on patient care, including health maintenance and disease prevention and management of pain and other common symptoms. Chapter 2 discusses laboratory tests and the diagnostic process. Chapter 3 summarizes the available imaging procedures, with estimates of their costs. Chapter 4 addresses special problems of the older patient. Chapter 5 discusses medical management of cancer. Chapters 6–27 describe diseases and disorders and their treatment, including the principles of genetics as applied to medical disorders. Chapter 28 sets forth the basic concepts of nutrition in modern medical practice. Chapters 29–37 cover infectious diseases and antimicrobial therapy. Chapters 38 and 39 cover disorders due to physical agents and poisoning. The Appendix provides reference ranges for the commonly used laboratory tests.

NEW TO THIS EDITION

- Drug information and bibliographies updated through June, 1993.
- A new chapter on use of laboratory tests and diagnostic decision making.
- An up-to-date chapter on HIV Infection and information on AIDS in other chapters.
- An update on antibiotics.
- Major revisions in the chapters on the Alimentary Tract; Liver, Gallbladder, and Pancreas; Gynecology and Obstetrics; Endocrinology; and Genitourinary Disorders.

ACKNOWLEDGMENTS

We wish to thank our associate authors for participating once again in the annual updating of this important book. Many students and physicians have contributed useful suggestions to this and previous editions, and we are grateful. We continue to welcome comments and recommendations for future editions.

Lawrence M. Tierney, Jr., MD
Stephen J. McPhee, MD
Maxine A. Papadakis, MD

San Francisco
September 1993

Authors

Daniel C. Adelman, MD
Director, Clinical Programs in Allergy and Immunology, University of California, San Francisco
Allergic & Immunologic Disorders

Michael J. Aminoff, MD, FRCP
Professor of Neurology, University of California, San Francisco
Nervous System

Robert B. Baron, MD, MS
Associate Professor of Clinical Medicine; Director of Primary Care Internal Medicine Residency Program; and Director of Continuing Medical Education, Department of Medicine, University of California, San Francisco
Nutrition

James J. Brophy, MD
Associate Clinical Professor of Psychiatry, University of California, San Diego
Psychiatric Disorders

Warren S. Browner, MD, MPH
Associate Professor of Epidemiology and Biostatistics, Medicine, and Anesthesia, University of California, San Francisco
Evaluation & Treatment of Lipid Abnormalities

Peter R. Carroll, MD
Associate Professor Department of Urology, University of California, San Francisco
Genitourinary Tract

Henry F. Chambers, MD
Associate Professor of Medicine and Chief, Division of Infectious Diseases, San Francisco General Hospital and University of California, San Francisco
Infectious Diseases: Bacterial & Chlamydial

Richard Cohen, MD, MPH
Associate Clinical Professor, Division of Occupational and Environmental Medicine, University of California, San Francisco
Disorders Due to Physical Agents

William M. Detmer, MD
Assistant Clinical Professor of Medicine, University of California, San Francisco; Postdoctoral Fellow, Section on Medical Informatics, Stanford University School of Medicine, Stanford, California.
Diagnostic Testing & Medical Decision Making

Arthur T. Evans, MD
Associate Professor of Obstetrics and Gynecology and Chief, Division of Maternal-Fetal Medicine, Eastern Virginia Medical School, Norfolk, Virginia
Gynecology & Obstetrics

Paul A. Fitzgerald, MD
Associate Clinical Professor of Medicine, Department of Medicine and Metabolic Research Unit, University of California, San Francisco
Endocrine Disorders

Richard M. Freeman, MD
Professor of Medicine and Vice Chairman, Department of Medicine, University of California, San Francisco; Chief, Medical Service, Veterans Affairs Medical Center, Fresno
Genitourinary Tract

Lawrence S. Friedman, MD
Associate Physician, Gastrointestinal Unit Massachusetts General Hospital and Department of Medicine, Harvard Medical School, Boston
Liver, Biliary Tract, & Pancreas

Eva Patricia Gill, MD
Fellow in Infectious Diseases, Baylor College of Medicine, Houston
Infectious Diseases: Viral & Rickettsial

Armando E. Giuliano, MD
Clinical Professor of Surgery, University of California, Los Angeles; Chief of Surgical Oncology and Director, Joyce Eisenberg Keefer Breast Center, John Wayne Cancer Institute, Saint John's Hospital and Health Center, Santa Monica, California
Breast

Robert S. Goldsmith, MD, MPH, DTM&H
Professor of Tropical Medicine and Epidemiology, University of California, San Francisco
Infectious Diseases: Protozoal; Infectious Diseases: Helminthic

Sanford M. Goldstein, MD
Associate Clinical Professor of Dermatology, University of California, San Francisco
Skin & Appendages

David B. Hellmann, MD
Associate Professor of Medicine and Deputy Director, Department of Medicine, The Johns Hopkins Hopsital, Baltimore
Arthritis & Musculoskeletal Disorders

Harry Hollander, MD
Associate Professor of Clinical Medicine and Director, AIDS Clinic, University of California, San Francisco
HIV Infection; Infectious Diseases: Mycotic

Robert K. Jackler, MD
Associate Professor of Otolaryngology and Neurological Surgery, University of California, San Francisco
Ear, Nose, & Throat

Richard A. Jacobs, MD, PhD
Clinical Professor of Medicine and Clinical Pharmacy, University of California, San Francisco
General Problems in Infectious Diseases; Infectious Diseases: Spirochetal; Anti-infective Chemotherapeutic & Antibiotic Agents

Michael J. Kaplan, MD
Associate Professor, Department of Otolaryngology-Head and Neck Surgery, University of California, San Francisco; and Chief, Department of Otolaryngology-Head and Neck Surgery, Veterans Affairs Medical Center, San Francisco
Ear, Nose, & Throat

John H. Karam, MD
Professor of Medicine, Metabolic Research Unit and Diabetes Center, University of California, San Francisco
Diabetes Mellitus & Hypoglycemia

Mitchell H. Katz, MD
Director, AIDS Office, San Francisco Department of Public Health, San Francisco; Assistant Clinical Professor of Medicine and Epidemiology and Biostatistics, University of California, San Francisco
HIV Infection

C. Michael Knauer, MD
Chief of Division of Gastroenterology, Santa Clara Valley Medical Center, San Jose, California; and Clinical Professor of Medicine, Stanford University School of Medicine, Stanford, California
Alimentary Tract; Liver, Biliary Tract, & Pancreas

Charles A. Linker, MD
Professor of Medicine, University of California, San Francisco; Director, Adult Leukemia and Bone Marrow Transplant Program, San Francisco
Blood

H. Trent MacKay, MD, MPH
Associate Clinical Professor, Department of Obstetrics & Gynecology, University of California, Davis
Gynecology & Obstetrics

Barry M. Massie, MD
Professor of Medicine, University of California, San Francisco; Director, Coronary Care Unit, and Chief, Hypertension Unit, Veterans Affairs Medical Center, San Francisco
Cardiovascular Diseases; Systemic Hypertension

Stephen J. McPhee, MD
Professor of Medicine, Division of General Internal Medicine, Department of Medicine, University of California, San Francisco
General Approach to the Patient; Health Maintenance & Disease Prevention; & Common Symptoms

Kenneth R. McQuaid
Assistant Clinical Professor of Medicine, University of California, San Francisco
Alimentary Tract

Diana Nicoll, MD, PhD
Clinical Professor and Vice Chair, Department of Laboratory Medicine, University of California, San Francisco; Chief, Laboratory Medicine Service, Veterans Affairs Medical Center, San Francisco
Diagnostic Testing & Medical Decision Making; Laboratory Reference Ranges

Richard B. Odom, MD
Clinical Professor of Dermatology, University of California, San Francisco
Skin & Appendages

Kent R. Olson, MD
Medical Director, San Francisco Bay Area Regional Poison Control Center; Associate Clinical Professor of Medicine and Lecturer in Pharmacy, University of California, San Francisco
Poisoning

Maxine A. Papadakis, MD
Professor of Clinical Medicine and Epidemiology and Director of Student Programs, Department of Medicine, University of California, San Francisco
Fluid & Electrolyte Disorders

Joseph C. Presti, Jr., MD
Assistant Professor, Department of Urology, University of California, San Francisco
Genitourinary Tract

Reed E. Pyeritz, MD, PhD
Professor of Medicine and Pediatrics, Medical College of Pennsylvania; Chair, Department of Human Genetics, Allegheny-Singer Research Institute; Director, Center for Medical Genetics, Allegheny Health, Education and Research Foundation, Pittsburgh
Medical Genetics

Neil M. Resnick, MD
Chief of Gerontology, Brigham and Women's Hospital, Harvard Medical School, Boston
Geriatric Medicine & the Elderly Patient

Paul Riordan-Eva, FRCS, FCOphth
Senior Registrar in Ophthalmology, National Hospital for Neurology and Neurosurgery, London
Eye

Hope S. Rugo, MD
Assistant Clinical Professor of Medicine, Division of Hematology and Oncology, University of California, San Francisco
Cancer

Steven A. Schroeder, MD
President, Robert Wood Johnson Foundation, Princeton, New Jersey; Clinical Professor of Medicine, University of Medicine & Dentistry of New Jersey, Robert Wood Johnson Medical School, New Brunswick, New Jersey
General Approach to the Patient; Health Maintenance & Disease Prevention; & Common Symptoms

Wayne X. Shandera, MD
Assistant Professor of Internal Medicine, Baylor College of Medicine, Houston
Infectious Diseases: Viral & Rickettsial

John L. Stauffer, MD
Professor of Medicine, College of Medicine, The Pennsylvania State University; and Attending Physician, The Milton S. Hershey Medical Center, Hershey, Pennsylvania
Pulmonary Diseases

Marshall L. Stoller, MD
Assistant Professor of Urology and Director, Endourology and Lithotripsy, University of California, San Francisco.
Genitourinary Tract

Abba Terr, MD
Clinical Professor of Medicine, Stanford University School of Medicine, Stanford, California
Allergic & Immunologic Disorders

Lawrence M. Tierney, Jr., MD
Professor of Medicine, University of California, San Francisco; and Assistant Chief of Medical Services, Veterans Affairs Medical Center, San Francisco
Blood Vessels & Lymphatics

Daniel G. Vaughan, MD
Clinical Professor of Ophthalmology, University of California, San Francisco; and Governor, Francis I. Proctor Foundation for Research in Ophthalmology, San Francisco
Eye

Susan D. Wall, MD
Associate Professor of Radiology, University of California, San Francisco; and Assistant Chief of Radiology, Veterans Affairs Medical Center, San Francisco
Imaging

From inability to let alone; from too much zeal for the new and contempt for what is old; from putting knowledge before wisdom, and science before art and cleverness before common sense; from treating patients as cases; and from making the cure of the disease more grievous than the endurance of the same, Good Lord, deliver us.

—Sir Robert Hutchinson

General Approach to the Patient; Health Maintenance & Disease Prevention; & Common Symptoms

1

Steven A. Schroeder, MD, & Stephen J. McPhee, MD

GENERAL APPROACH TO THE PATIENT

This book is a reservoir—replenished annually—of instructions and guidelines for medical practitioners. The successful practitioner, however, needs more than the facts that make up the body of knowledge called medicine. Successful diagnosis and treatment demands that the practitioner consider the often complex personal, familial, and economic circumstances of the patient and establish and maintain a supportive and open relationship with each one.

The approach to diagnosis begins with the history and pertinent physical examination, each of which is susceptible to errors of omission and commission. Patient satisfaction may be increased by discussion of psychosocial issues and by lack of physician dominance of the encounter. If diagnostic procedures are indicated, they must be based on principles of diagnostic test selection, which in turn depend upon principles of test characteristics (sensitivity and specificity), disease incidence and prevalence, the potential risk to the patient, and the cost:benefit profile of the test determined by reference to the indications for it. Successful treatment—particularly management of patients with chronic illnesses—must be tailored to the circumstances of the individual patient and reinforced by a well-established doctor-patient relationship. For many illnesses, treatment depends on fundamental behavioral changes—including alterations in diet, exercise, smoking, and drinking—that may be difficult even for motivated patients. Compliance with prescribed drug regimens is a problem in every practice, with up to 50% of patients failing to achieve full compliance and a third never taking their medicines at all. Patient compliance is improved when strong and trusting doctor-patient relationships have been established. Physicians can improve patient compliance by inquiring specifically about the be-

havior in question and by reinforcement through key family members. When confronted directly, many patients will admit to noncompliance with medication regimens or with exhortations about cigarette smoking cessation or safe sex techniques. Other ways of detecting noncompliance include pill counts, comparing dates on prescription labels with the number of pills remaining, monitoring serum levels of drugs such as digoxin, or assessing predictable drug side effects such as hypokalemia from thiazide diuretics.

Fundamental ethical principles must also undergird a successful approach to diagnosis and treatment: honesty, beneficence, justice, avoidance of conflict of interest, and the pledge to do no harm. Increasingly, Western medicine has involved patients in important decisions about medical care, including how far to proceed with treatment of patients who have terminal illnesses.

Finally, the physician's role does not end with diagnosis and the prescribing of a treatment regimen. The importance of the empathic physician in helping patients and their families bear the burden of serious illness and death cannot be overemphasized. "To cure sometimes, to relieve often, and to comfort always" is a French saying as apt today as it was five centuries ago—as is Francis Peabody's admonition: "The secret of the care of the patient is in caring for the patient."

Bertakis KD et al: The relationship of physician medical interview style to patient satisfaction. J Fam Pract 1991;32:175. (Meeting both the biomedical and emotional needs of the patient may increase patient compliance and satisfaction.)

Fletcher RH, Fletcher SW: Has medicine outgrown physical diagnosis? (Editorial.) Ann Intern Med 1992;117:786. (Limitations of physical diagnosis and the hazards of overusing diagnostic tests.)

Peterson MC et al: Contributions of the history, physical examination, and laboratory investigation in making medical diagnoses. West J Med 1992;156:163. (Affirms primacy of patient history.)

HEALTH MAINTENANCE & DISEASE PREVENTION

Preventing disease is more important than treating it. Preventive medicine is categorized as primary, secondary, or tertiary. Primary prevention aims to remove or reduce disease risk factors (eg, by immunization to prevent hepatitis B infection and its sequelae, or by giving up or not starting smoking to reduce the incidence of lung carcinoma). Secondary prevention techniques are designed to promote early detection of disease or precursor states (eg, routine cervical Papanicolaou screening to detect invasive carcinoma or carcinoma in situ of the cervix, or chemoprophylaxis for positive tuberculin reactors). Tertiary prevention measures are aimed at limiting the impact of established disease (eg, partial mastectomy and radiation therapy to remove and control localized breast cancer). Primary prevention is by far the most effective and economical of all methods of disease control, but most physicians are deficient in their counseling practices concerning preventable conditions.

Table 1–1 lists the five leading causes of death in

Table 1–1. The five leading causes of death in the USA and associated modifiable risk factors.[1]

Cause of Death	Risk Factors
1. Cardiovascular disease	Tobacco use Elevated serum cholesterol High blood pressure Obesity Diabetes mellitus Sedentary life-style
2. Cancer	Tobacco use Improper diet Alcohol Occupational and environmental exposures
3. Cerebrovascular disease	High blood pressure Tobacco use Elevated serum cholesterol
4. Accidental injuries	Safety belt noncompliance Cycle helmet noncompliance Alcohol and substance abuse Reckless driving Occupational hazards Guns in the home Stress and fatigue
5. Chronic lung disease	Tobacco use Occupational and environmental exposures

[1]Adapted from National Center for Health Statistics/U.S. Department of Health and Human Services: *Health United States: 1986.* DHHS Pub. No. (PHS) 87–1232, 1987.

the USA, along with important risk factors linked to these causes. Physicians can have a major role in reducing almost all of these risk factors. Table 1–2 estimates the years of potential life lost from the nine leading causes of death, as well as the percentage of those deaths attributable to substance abuse.

Health maintenance and disease prevention usually begin with the office or clinic encounter. Table 1–3 compares and contrasts recommendations for periodic health examinations as developed by the United States Preventive Services Task Force, the American College of Physicians, and the Canadian Task Force on the Periodic Health Examination. Although there is emerging consensus on many of the preventive services recommended, controversy persists for many others. Recently, there has been a shift away from recommendations based solely on patients' age and sex to recommendations based on their additional risk factors.

Hayward RSA et al: Preventive care guidelines: 1991. Ann Intern Med 1991;114:758. (Recommendations for history taking and physical examination, laboratory tests, adult immunization and chemoprophylaxis, and preventive counseling maneuvers.)

Lewis CE et al: The counseling practices of internists. Ann Intern Med 1991;114:54. (Counseling efforts of internists fell far short of desired levels.)

Report of the US Preventive Services Task Force: Guide to Clinical Preventive Services. Williams & Wilkins, 1989. (Evidence for efficacy of prevention strategies.)

INFECTIOUS DISEASES

The impressive 20th century accomplishments in immunization and antibiotic therapy notwithstanding, much of the decline in the incidence and fatality rates of infectious diseases is attributable to improved social conditions and public health measures—especially improved sanitation, better nutrition, and greater prosperity.

Immunization remains the best means of preventing many infectious diseases, including tetanus, diphtheria, poliomyelitis, measles, mumps, rubella, hepatitis B, yellow fever, influenza, and pneumococcal pneumonia. Recommended immunization schedules for children and adults are set forth in Table 29–4. Persons traveling to countries where infections are endemic should take special precautions, as described in Chapter 29.

Skin testing for tuberculosis and then treating selected skin-positive patients with prophylactic isoniazid reduces the risk of reactivation tuberculosis (see Table 9–9). Patients with HIV infection are at an especially high risk for reactivation of tuberculosis. The prophylaxis and treatment of tuberculosis in HIV-infected patients is discussed in Chapter 30, as is the emerging concern about multidrug-resistant tuberculosis.

Table 1-2. Nine leading causes of potential life lost, with proportion attributable to substance abuse, United States.[1]

Cause of Death	Years of Potential Life Lost, 1989	Percentage of Deaths Attributed to Substance Abuse
Cancer	4,397,072	32
Heart disease	3,619,749	20
Accidents and trauma	2,951,036	47
Suicide	972,512	28
Homicide	966,957	46
HIV infection	776,957	>50(?)
Cerebrovascular disease	578,439	25
Chronic lung disease	435,517	76
Liver disease	419,630	>68

[1]Reproduced, with permission, from Schroeder SA: The importance of relating medicine and public health. Am J Med Sci 1992;303:355.

AIDS is now the major infectious disease problem in the Western world. Since sexual contact is the usual mode of transmission, prevention must rely on safe sexual practices, although increasingly cases of HIV infection are transmitted by use of intravenous drugs. Antibody testing for infection with HIV is now widely available and highly sensitive and specific. However, in patients with no risk factors, a positive test is still likely to be falsely positive. Furthermore, serum conversion after infection can take as long as 6 months, and perhaps even longer, so false-negatives can also occur. Most clinicians now favor elective testing for those at high risk. Detection of asymptomatic persons with HIV infection is important for preventive strategies and allows these persons to consider treatments that may prolong life (see Chapter 30).

Although live virus vaccines (such as measles, mumps and rubella [MMR] vaccines) are not generally recommended for immunocompromised patients, *asymptomatic* HIV-infected patients have generally not shown adverse consequences when given them. Thus, these individuals should receive MMR and influenza vaccinations as well as tetanus and pneumococcal vaccinations. However, if poliomyelitis immunization is required, the inactivated poliomyelitis vaccine should be used. *Symptomatic* HIV-infected patients should be given annual influenza vaccination, but live virus vaccines such as MMR should be used cautiously.

Recently, the CDC has published a new strategy to eliminate hepatitis B virus transmission at all stages of life. These recommendations include prenatal testing of all pregnant women for HBsAg to identify

Table 1-3. Expert recommendations for preventive care for asymptomatic, low-risk adults.

Preventive Service	United States Preventive Services Task Force			American College of Physicians			Canadian Task Force on the Periodic Health Examination		
	Sex	Age	Minimum Frequency	Sex	Age	Minimum Frequency	Sex	Age	Minimum Frequency
Physical examination									
Blood pressure	MF	18+	q 2 yrs	MF	18+	q 2 yrs	MF	25-64	q 5 yrs
							MF	65+	q 2 yrs
Clinical breast examination	F	40+	Annually	F	40+	Annually	F	40+	Annually
Laboratory tests									
Papanicolaou smear	F	18[1]-65	q 3 yrs	F	20[1]-65	q 3 yrs	F	18[1]-35	q 3 yrs[2]
								36-74	q 5 yrs
Stool for occult blood	NR	NR	NR	MF	50+	Annually	NR	NR	NR
Sigmoidoscopy	NR	NR	NR	MF	50+	q 3-5 yrs	NR	NR	NR
Mammography	F	50-75	Annually	F	50+	Annually	F	50+	Annually
Cholesterol	M	18+	q 5 yrs	MF	18-70	q 5 yrs	M	30-59	q 5 yrs
Immunizations									
Tetanus-diphtheria booster	MF	18+	q 10 yrs	MF	18+	q 10 yrs	MF	18+	q 10 yrs
Influenza vaccination	MF	65+	Annually	MF	65+	Annually	MF	65+	Annually
Pneumococcal vaccination	MF	65+	Once	MF	65+	Once	NR	NR	NR
Counseling[3]	MF	18+	At routine visits	MF	18+	At routine visits	MF	18+	At routine visits

NR = no recommendation.
[1]Or following onset of sexual activity.
[2]After two normal smears.
[3]Regarding tobacco use, nutrition, exercise, sexual behavior, substance abuse, injury prevention, and dental care.

Table 1-4. Some immediate consequences of smoking cessation.[1]

1. Improve ability to breathe.
2. Regain sense of smell and taste.
3. Reduce passive exposure of family and others.
4. Save money.
5. Require less sleep.
6. Increase energy.
7. Fresh breath.
8. Odor-free environment.
9. No ashtrays to empty.
10. No burn holes.
11. Cut risk of death by fire 50%.
12. Alleviate tobacco stains on teeth, fingers.
13. Decrease risks of passive smoking for family and co-workers.
14. More employable.
15. Better insurance risk and cheaper insurance premiums.
16. Improve lung cleansing through ability to cough and improved ciliary activity.
17. Improve coronary and peripheral circulation.
18. Decrease heart rate.
19. Reduce blood carbon monoxide levels.
20. Reduce perspiration.
21. Improve exercise tolerance.
22. Improve ability to perform physical work.
23. Lower grocery bills.
24. Extra time.
25. Decrease social pressure.

[1]Reproduced, with permission from Green HL, Goldberg RJ, Ockene JK: Cigarette smoking: The physician's role in cessation and maintenance. J Gen Intern Med 1983;3:75.

newborns who require immunoprophylaxis at birth with hepatitis B immune globulin followed by hepatitis B vaccination and to identify household contacts who should be vaccinated; routine vaccination of all children not previously vaccinated at well-child visits; vaccination of adolescents in communities where intravenous drug use, teenage pregnancy, or sexually transmitted diseases are common; and vaccination of adults at high risk of infection. The latter include persons with occupational risk; clients and staff of institutions for the developmentally disabled; hemodialysis patients; recipients of clotting factor concentrates; household contacts and sex partners of HBV carriers; adoptees from countries where HBV infection is endemic; international travelers; injecting drug users; sexually active homosexual and bisexual men; sexually active heterosexual men and women, particularly those with recent sexually transmitted diseases; and inmates of long-term correctional facilities.

It appears that 1991 was the final year for new reports of poliomyelitis cases in the Western Hemisphere. A goal has been established of worldwide eradication of poliomyelitis by the year 2000; if successful, its eradication will follow that of smallpox (1978) and guinea worm disease (anticipated in 1996).

Centers for Disease Control: General recommendations on immunization. Ann Intern Med 1989;111:133. (Published also in two parts in JAMA 1989;262:22, 187.)
Hepatitis B virus: A comprehensive strategy for eliminating transmission in the United States through universal childhood vaccination. Recommendations of the Immunization Practices Advisory Committee (ACIP). MMWR Morb Mortal Wkly Rep 1991;40(RR 13):1.
Ramsbottom MT: Who should get a shot in the arm? The latest recommendations for adult vaccinations. J Gen Intern Med 1991;6:247.
Rhame FS, Maki DG: The case for wider use of testing for HIV infection. N Engl J Med 1989;320:1248.

CARDIOVASCULAR & CEREBROVASCULAR DISEASES

Impressive declines in age-specific mortality rates from heart disease and stroke have been achieved in all age groups in North America during the past 2 decades. The chief reason for this favorable trend appears to be a modification of risk factors, especially cigarette smoking and hypercholesterolemia, plus more aggressive detection and treatment of hypertension.

Cigarette Smoking

Cigarette smoking remains the most important cause of preventable morbidity and early demise in developed countries. Tobacco dependence may have a genetic component. Smokers die 5–8 years earlier than nonsmokers; have twice the risk of fatal heart disease; ten times the risk of lung cancer and several times the risk of cancers of the mouth, throat, esophagus, pancreas, kidney, bladder, and cervix; have a two- to threefold higher incidence of peptic ulcers (which heal less well than in nonsmokers); a two- to fourfold greater risk of fractures of the hip, wrist, and vertebrae; and a twofold increase in the risk of developing cataracts. Olfaction and taste are impaired in smokers, and facial wrinkles are increased. Diabetic patients who smoke may have an increased risk of proteinuria. Patients with head and neck cancer who continue to smoke during radiation therapy have lower rates of response than those who do not smoke. Smoking cessation lessens the risk of death and myocardial infarction in both men and women with coronary artery disease; lessens the risk of stroke; slows the rate of progression of carotid atherosclerosis; and is associated with reversal of chronic bronchitis and improved pulmonary function. Smoking cessation can improve life expectancy even for those who stop after the age of 65.

The children of patients who smoke have lower birth weights, more frequent respiratory infections, less efficient pulmonary function, and a higher incidence of chronic ear infections than children of nonsmokers and are more likely to become smokers themselves. In addition, passive smoking by adults has been shown to increase the risk of cervical cancer, lung cancer, and heart disease and to promote endothelial damage and platelet aggregation.

There has recently been an encouraging national trend away from smoking. In 1991, 29% of adults in the USA were smokers. Smoking was slightly more common in men than in women (30.6% versus 27.2%). One-fourth of United States adults are former smokers.

The clinician should adopt a five-step smoking cessation strategy: (1) Ask the patient about interest in quitting. (2) Motivate the patient to stop. (3) Set a date to stop entirely. (4) Consider drug treatment for withdrawal. (5) Follow up. A recent survey showed that only 44% of smokers who had seen a physician in the previous year had been advised to quit. Depressed smokers may have more difficulty quitting than nondepressed smokers, and when depressed individuals do quit, their depression may worsen. Table 1–4 lists immediate benefits from smoking cessation that the physician can call to the attention of smokers.

Nicotine polacrilex 2 mg gum can reduce tobacco withdrawal symptoms and has led in some studies to improved quit rates, especially for those who are most addicted. However, some patients are unable to chew the gum without developing unwanted side effects such as hiccups, oral discomfort, heartburn, nausea and gastrointestinal upset. Contraindications to the use of nicotine gum are pregnancy or nursing, inability to chew, recent myocardial infarction, and life-threatening arrhythmias. Recently, a transdermal patch has been developed to provide a continuous, controlled release of nicotine. A single morning application of a 15 cm^2 patch may provide up to 24 hours of relief from nicotine withdrawal symptoms. The patch is easy to apply, eliminates oral discomfort, and minimizes gastrointestinal side effects. It comes in different doses (eg, 21 mg, 14 mg, or 7 mg per 24 hours). It is common to start with the higher-dose patch for about 3 weeks and to use the lower-dose patches to taper the patient off nicotine gradually over a period of at least 3 additional weeks. (The optimal duration is unknown.) A 21-mg patch costs about $3.00. Early reports on the use of the nicotine patch show significantly higher rates of smoking cessation than for groups using a placebo. Pharmacologic therapy with gum or patch must be combined with some form of counseling, either in group therapy or by individual providers, to be maximally effective. Nicotine inhalation may emerge as a substitute or supplement to the gum and patch. Clonidine may reduce withdrawal symptoms in patients trying to quit. Its role in smoking cessation is still controversial.

Some weight gain occurs in most patients following smoking cessation, and for some patients (10–14%) major weight gain (over 29 lb) may occur.

Clinicians should avoid appearing to disapprove of patients who are unable to stop smoking. Concerned exhortation, family or social pressures, or the opportunity presented by intercurrent illness may eventually enable even the most addicted chronic smoker to give up the habit or at least to cut back. Even under the most pessimistic assumptions, such counseling is more cost-effective than treating hypertension or hypercholesterolemia. The physician's role in smoking cessation is summarized in Table 1–5.

Corelli D et al: Genetic influence on smoking: A study of male twins. N Engl J Med 1992;327:829. (Moderate genetic influences.)

Fiore MC et al: Tobacco dependence and the nicotine patch. JAMA 1992;268:2687.

Peto R et al: Mortality from tobacco in developed countries: Indirect estimation from national vital statistics. Lancet 1992;339:1268. (If current smoking patterns continue, over 20% of persons now living in developed countries will die because of tobacco.)

Tonnesen P et al: A double-blind trial of a 16-hour transdermal nicotine patch in smoking cessation. N Engl J Med 1991;325:311. (Abstinence was significantly higher for patch than for placebo. The side effects were minimal.)

Hypercholesterolemia

Lowering elevated LDL cholesterol concentrations reduces the risk from coronary heart disease. Calculated gain in life expectancy from modest decreases in blood cholesterol is low, especially in patients without other risk factors such as cigarette smoking and hypertension. However, for high-risk patients,

---

Table 1–5. The physician's role in smoking cessation.

I. For the patient[1]

Ask all patients about smoking.
Advise all smokers to stop.
   State your advice clearly, eg, "As your physician, I must advise you to stop smoking now."
Assist patients who want to stop now.
   Help the patient select a quit date.
   Provide self-help materials.
   Consider providing nicotine gum or transdermal nicotine patches, especially for highly addicted patients.
Arrange follow-up visits.
   Schedule a follow-up visit within 1–2 weeks after the quit date.
   Have a member of the office staff call or write the patient within 7 days after the initial visit, reinforcing the decision to stop and reminding the patient of the quit date.
   Schedule a second follow-up visit in 1–2 months.

II. For society[2]

Set a personal example.
Become involved in the legislative process.
Be an adviser to industry.
Work through public health and school health programs to keep young people from starting to smoke.
Work with voluntary agencies: American Heart Association, American Cancer Society, American Lung Association, etc.
Work toward a smoke-free society.

---

[1]Modified, with permission, from Manley M et al: Clinical interventions in tobacco control: A National Cancer Institute Training Program for Physicians. JAMA 1991;266:3172. Copyright © 1991 by the American Medical Association.
[2]Modified, with permission, from Green HL, Goldberg RJ, Ockene JK: Cigarette smoking: The physician's role in cessation and maintenance. J Gen Intern Med 1988;3:75.

such as those who have had a myocardial infarction, benefits from lowering cholesterol levels may be great.

Specific guidelines for therapy, which include diet, weight reduction, exercise, and drugs, are discussed in Chapter 27.

Hypertension

Over 50 million adults in the USA have hypertension. In every adult age group, higher values of systolic and diastolic blood pressure carry greater risks of stroke and congestive heart failure. Even so, clinicians must be able to apply specific blood pressure criteria as a means of deciding at what levels treatment should be considered in individual cases. Table 11–1 presents a classification of hypertension based on blood pressures that was proposed in 1993. Fifty-five percent of hypertensive patients in the United States are now adequately controlled, compared with only 16% in 1972 (see Chapter 11).

The Fifth Report of the Joint National Committee on Detection, Evaluation, and Treatment of High Blood Pressure (JNC V). Arch Intern Med 1993;153:154.

CANCER

Primary Prevention

Cigarette smoking is the most important preventable cause of cancer. Primary prevention of skin cancer consists of restricting exposure to ultraviolet light by wearing appropriate clothing and use of sunscreens. In the past 2 decades, there has been a three-fold increase in the incidence of squamous cell carcinoma and a fourfold increase in melanoma in the United States. Prevention of occupationally induced cancers involves minimizing exposure to carcinogenic substances such as asbestos, ionizing radiation, and benzene compounds.

Secondary Prevention

Generally accepted techniques exist for secondary prevention of cancers of the breast, colon, and cervix through cancer screening procedures. Note that Table 1–6, derived from American Cancer Society guidelines, differs in many instances from the recommendations of other authorities as shown previously in Table 1–3, which take a more conservative view of the efficacy of cancer screening maneuvers. Screen-

Table 1–6. Screening for cancer: American Cancer Society (1993) guidelines for the early detection of cancer in people without symptoms.[1]

Test or Procedure	Sex	Age	Frequency
Sigmoidoscopy, preferably flexible	MF	50 and over	Every 3–5 years.
Stool test for occult blood	MF	50 and over	Every year.
Digital rectal examination	MF	40 and over	Every year.
Prostate examination[2]	M	50 and over	Every year.
Papanicolaou test	F	Women who are or have been sexually active or have reached 18 years.	Annually until at least 3 consecutive satisfactory normal examinations, then less often at discretion of physician.
Pelvic examination	F	18–40	Every 1–3 years with Papanicolaou test.
		Over 40	Every year.
Endometrial tissue sample	F	At menopause; women at high risk.[3]	At menopause and thereafter at the discretion of the physician.
Breast self-examination	F	20 and over	Every month.
Breast physical examination	F	20–40	Every 3 years.
		Over 40	Every year.
Mammography[4]	F	40–50	Every 1 or 2 years.
		Over 50	Every year.
Health counseling and cancer checkup[5]	MF	Over 20	Every 3 years.
		Over 40	Every year.
Chest x-ray		Not recommended.	
Sputum cytologic examination		Not recommended.	

[1]From Update January 1992: The American Cancer Society Guidelines for the Cancer-Related Check-Up. CA 1992;42(1):44; and from Mettlin C et al: Defining and updating the American Cancer Society's Guidelines for the cancer-related checkup: Prostate and endometrial cancers. CA 1993;43:42.
[2]Digital rectal examination and serum prostate-specific antigen; if either is abnormal, further evaluation by transrectal ultrasound and biopsy as indicated.
[3]History of infertility, obesity, failure of ovulation, abnormal uterine bleeding, or unopposed estrogen or tamoxifen therapy.
[4]Screening mammography should begin by age 40.
[5]To include examination for cancers of the thyroid, testicles, ovaries, lymph nodes, oral region, and skin.

ing for other cancers in normal asymptomatic or even high-risk segments of the population is not recommended because adequate screening tests are not available.

Levin B: Screening sigmoidoscopy for colorectal cancer. (Editorial.) N Engl J Med 1992;326:700. (Recommends 5-year interval screening with flexible sigmoidoscopy if performed at low cost. For those with a positive family history of colorectal cancer, screening colonoscopy is recommended between ages 40 and 50, especially if the family cancer occurred in a relative under the age of 55.)

Littrup PJ, Lee F, Mettlin C: Prostate cancer screening: Current trends and future implications. CA 1992;42:198. (Positive predictive values of combinations of transrectal ultrasound, digital rectal examination, and prostate-specific antigen.)

Oesterling JE: Prostate-specific antigen: Improving its ability to diagnose early prostate cancer. JAMA 1992;267: 2236. (Recommends routine use along with digital rectal examination in men over age 55.)

Selby JV et al: A case-control study of screening sigmoidoscopy and mortality from colorectal cancer. N Engl J Med 1992;326:653. (Suggests that screening once every 10 years may be nearly as efficacious as more frequent screening.)

Thun MJ et al: Aspirin use and reduced risk of fatal colon cancer. N Engl J Med 1991;325:1593. (Death rates from colon cancer were 40% lower than among those who took no aspirin regularly.)

ACCIDENTS & VIOLENCE

Accidents remain the most important cause of loss of potential years of life before age 65, followed by cancer, heart disease, and suicide and homicide. Despite incontrovertible evidence that seat belt use protects against serious injury and death in motor vehicle accidents, at least one-fourth of adults do not use seat belts routinely. It is estimated that fewer than 20% of bicycle and motorcycle riders use safety helmets, a simple protective device that can greatly reduce the risk of head and brain injuries following an accident. As part of routine medical care, physicians should try to educate their patients about seat belts, safety helmets, drinking and driving, and the risks of having guns in the home. Males aged 16–35 are at especially high risk for serious injury and death from accidents and violence, with blacks at particularly high risk for violent death.

Kaplan BH, Cowley RA: Seatbelt effectiveness and cost of noncompliance among drivers admitted to a trauma center. Am J Emerg Med 1991;9:4. (Evidence for benefits from seatbelts is impressive and incontrovertible.)

Thompson RS, Rivara FP, Thompson DC: A case-control study of the effectiveness of bicycle safety helmets. N Engl J Med 1989;320:1361. (Helmets reduce the risk of head injury by 85%.)

SUBSTANCE ABUSE
(See also Chapter 24.)

Substance abuse—including alcohol and illicit drugs—is a major public health problem in the United States and is estimated to be a factor in half of highway fatality accidents. Alcohol abuse affects both adolescents and adults. Approximately two-thirds of high school seniors are regular users of alcohol, and the lifetime prevalence of alcoholism is estimated to be between 12% and 16%. Underdiagnosis of alcoholism is substantial, both because of patient denial and lack of physician alertness to historical and physical clues of the condition. The fact that alcohol-related traffic fatalities declined almost 10% in 1991 testifies to the success of recent pressures to limit drinking and driving. There appears, however, to be an increase in binge drinking among college students. There is some evidence that, as with cigarette use, physician identification and counseling about alcoholism may improve the chance of recovery. Although about 10% of all adults seen in medical practices are problem drinkers, that fact is seldom recognized. The CAGE test (see Table 1–7) is a simple screening test that is both sensitive and specific. Alternatively, asking the two questions: "Have you ever had a drinking problem?" and "When did you have your last drink?"—positive if in the past 24 hours—yields a 91% sensitivity for alcoholism but is obviously less specific than the CAGE test. Treatment of alcoholism and its complications is discussed in Chapter 24. Choice of therapy remains controversial.

Despite a steady recent decline in the numbers of Americans using illegal drugs—including cocaine—either sporadically or episodically, the use of such drugs remains an important problem. Many drug users are employed, and many use drugs during pregnancy. As with alcohol abuse, the recognition of drug abuse presents special problems and requires that the physician actively consider the diagnosis. Clinical aspects of substance abuse and treatment issues are discussed in Chapter 24.

Bradley KA: Screening and diagnosis of alcoholism in the primary care setting. West J Med 1992;156:166. (Risk

Table 1–7. CAGE screening test for alcoholism.[1]

Have you ever felt the need to	**Cut down** on drinking?
Have you ever felt	**Annoyed** by criticism of your drinking?
Have you ever felt	**Guilty** about your drinking?
Have you ever taken a morning	**Eye opener?**

INTERPRETATION: Two "yes" answers are considered a positive screen. One "yes" answer should raise a suspicion of alcohol abuse.

[1]Modified from Mayfield D et al: The CAGE questionnaire: Validation of a new alcoholism screening instrument. Am J Psychiatry 1974;131;1121.

factors, screening criteria, and how to communicate diagnosis to the patient.)

Bradley KA: Management of alcoholism in the primary care setting. West J Med 1992;156:273. (Treatment options and evidence of their efficacy.)

Klatsky AL et al: Alcohol and mortality. Ann Intern Med 1992;117:646. (Women and younger persons at greater risk.)

Magarian GJ et al: Clinical significance in alcoholic patients of commonly encountered laboratory test results. West J Med 1992;156:287. (The AST-to-ALT ratio is approximately 1.5:1 or 2:1 in alcoholic liver disease even when neither level is elevated.)

Walsh DC et al: The impact of a physician's warning on recovery after alcoholism treatment. JAMA 1992;267:663. (Among 200 problem drinkers in a large firm, 74% saw a physician during the year, but only 24% recalled being warned about alcohol by the physician. Two years later, those warned were more likely to be abstaining and sober and were less impaired.)

COMMON SYMPTOMS

PAIN*

Approach to the Patient

Pain is the most common symptom causing patients to seek medical attention. It can provide the clinician with important diagnostic information. Information about the timing, nature, location, severity, and radiation is crucial for proper treatment; the same is true for aggravating or alleviating factors.

Many emotional and cultural factors influence the perception of pain. The primary cause (eg, trauma, infection), pathogenesis (eg, inflammation, ischemia), and contributory factors (eg, recent changes in life situation, symbolic attributes of pain) must all be sought.

Administration of a systemic analgesic is the usual method of pain management, but many other nonpharmacologic methods are useful. Examples include graded physical activity, simple reassurance, support groups, and biofeedback training. For severe chronic nerve pain, such as occurs in metastatic cancer or neuropathic conditions, therapies such as nerve block, radiation, and even rhizotomy may be useful in selected patients. More liberal use of short-term opioid analgesics is a promising approach to sickle cell pain crises and may have applications for other episodic pain syndromes. It is doubtful whether transcutaneous electrical nerve stimulation provides effective relief for chronic pain.

---

*Management of chronic pain is discussed in Chapter 24.

1. DRUGS FOR SEVERE PAIN

Opioid narcotic analgesics are indicated for severe pain that cannot be relieved with less effective agents. Examples include the pain of severe trauma, myocardial infarction, ureteral stone, and postoperative pain. Patients can achieve more reliable plasma opioid levels through the self-administration of small, repeated intravenous doses. Such **patient-controlled analgesia** (PCA) permits repeated dosing of fixed amounts of analgesic drugs when the patient requires pain relief. The amount of medication is limited by preestablished dosing intervals and maximum doses within a defined period. Alternatively, continuous or basal delivery is also possible. Treatment starts with a bolus dose followed by a basal continuous rate to achieve desired baseline levels and to permit sleep. Additional doses are available on demand, within the limits established by the physician. A recent study concluded that routine use of a continuous morphine infusion in combination with a standard PCA regimen did not improve pain control when compared to PCA alone. Thus, the conventional intermittent dosing regimen is probably preferred, with a continuous infusion to be used only if pain relief is unsatisfactory. Adverse side effects occur less than half as often with PCA as with conventional therapy. Problems with the intravenous catheter can occur but are infrequent. Those who have experienced patient-controlled analgesia overwhelmingly prefer it to conventional pain control.

Table 1–8 lists opioid narcotic analgesics with some of their characteristics. These drugs have pharmacologic similarities to opium. They are employed principally for the control of severe pain, but they also act to suppress cough and gastrointestinal motility. All can produce **physical dependence,** but to varying degrees and after varying periods of use. The risk of addiction or habituation should not prevent their appropriate use, especially in the management of terminal illness.

A common error in management of pain from cancer is to prescribe insufficient doses "prn" rather than adequate doses around-the-clock at staged intervals. In such cases, the major goal of management should be patient comfort.

The effects of all opioid narcotics are reversed by naloxone. Continued narcotic use produces tolerance, so that increasing doses are needed to produce the same analgesic effect.

Contraindications

The opioid narcotic drugs are relatively contraindicated in some acute illnesses. In the acute abdomen, for example, the pattern of pain may provide important diagnostic clues. However, some analgesia may be necessary in order to perform an adequate physical examination for diagnostic purposes. In acute head

Table 1–8. Useful opioid analgesics.

	Approximate Equivalent Dose and Route	Duration of Analgesia (hours)	Maximum Efficacy	Addiction/Abuse Liability
Morphine	10 mg IM	4–5	High	High
Hidromorphone (Dilaudid)	1.5 mg IM	4–5	High	High
Oxymorphone (Numorphan)	1.5 mg IM	3–4	High	High
Methadone (Dolophine)	10 mg IM	4–6	High	High
Meperidine (Demerol)	75–100 mg IM	2–4	High	High
Codeine	30–60 mg PO[1]	3–4	Low	Medium
Oxycodone (Percodan)[2]	4.5 mg PO[1]	3–4	Moderate	Low to medium
Hydrocodone (Vicodin, others)[3]	5 mg PO[1]	3–5	Moderate	Medium to high

[1]Analgesic efficacy at this oral dose not equivalent to 10 mg of morphine.
[2]Available only in tablets containing aspirin 325 mg (Percodan) or acetaminophen 325 mg (Percocet).
[3]In tablets or capsules with acetaminophen 500 mg (Vicodin) or aspirin.

injuries, these drugs interfere with clinical interpretation of neurologic changes.

Adverse Effects

The drugs in this category have the potential adverse effects listed below. Patients with hypothyroidism, adrenal insufficiency, hypopituitarism, acute intermittent porphyria, reduced blood volume, and severe debility are particularly apt to suffer adverse effects from opioid narcotic analgesics.

(1) Opioid narcotics should be given with great caution to patients with pulmonary insufficiency, because of dose-dependent respiratory depression.

(2) Central nervous system effects include sedation, euphoria, nausea, and vomiting. Antidepressants, antihistamines, phenothiazines, hypnotics, and alcohol can potentiate these effects.

(3) Cardiovascular effects include hypotension. This is less common than hypoventilation, however.

(4) Gastrointestinal effects are chiefly decreased bowel motility and consequent constipation.

(5) Genitourinary effects include bladder spasm and urinary retention.

(6) Enhanced sensitivity to the drugs occurs in patients with hepatic impairment; biliary spasm may cause severe biliary colic.

(7) Allergic manifestations also occur, but rarely.

Frequently Used Opioid Narcotic Analgesics

A. Morphine sulfate, 8–15 mg subcutaneously or intramuscularly in adults, is an effective drug for control of severe pain. The effects last 4–5 hours. In acute myocardial infarction or in acute pulmonary edema due to left ventricular failure, 2–6 mg may be injected slowly intravenously in 5 mL of saline solution. Long-acting, sustained-release oral morphine preparations (MS Contin, Roxanol SR) are available and allow less frequent dosing. Patient-controlled administration is discussed above.

B. Morphine congeners give effects equivalent to 10 mg of morphine sulfate but have no specific advantages—eg, hydromorphone or oxymorphone, 2–4 mg of either orally every 4 hours, or 1–3 mg of either subcutaneously every 4 hours.

C. Meperidine (Demerol), 50–150 mg orally or intramuscularly every 3–4 hours, provides analgesia similar to that achieved with morphine. Its indications and side effects are similar to those of morphine.

D. Methadone, 15–20 mg orally every 6–8 hours, is most often used for treatment of addiction based on its long duration of action. Its side effects are similar to those of morphine, but tolerance and physical dependence are slower to develop.

E. Codeine (sulfate or phosphate), 15–60 mg orally or subcutaneously every 4–6 hours, is somewhat less effective than morphine but also less habit-forming. It is often given together with aspirin or acetaminophen for enhanced analgesic effect. Codeine is a powerful cough suppressant in a dose of 15–30 mg orally every 4 hours, but is constipating.

F. Oxycodone and hydrocodone are given orally and prescribed with another analgesic. The dosage is 5 mg every 4–6 hours in tablets that contain aspirin 325 mg (Percodan) or acetaminophen 325 mg (Percocet) or 500 mg (Vicodin).

2. DRUGS FOR MODERATE OR MILD PAIN

Most people can manage their minor aches and pains with OTC analgesics available at drugstores and food stores, which now stock ibuprofen in 200 mg dosage. Drugs such as codeine, oxyco and pentazocine, listed above as "addictive ics," are sometimes used for moderate p cylates or acetaminophen in higher highly visible class of NSAIDs (

salicylates) are often better for this purpose. (See Table 1–9.)

The activity—both anti-inflammatory and analgesic—of aspirin and other NSAIDs is mediated through inhibition of the biosynthesis of prostaglandins. All of these drugs to varying degrees inhibit platelet aggregation and may cause gastric irritation (the risk of associated upper gastrointestinal bleeding is about one and one-half times normal, and may be considerably higher in elderly patients), kidney damage (including acute renal failure, decreased glomerular filtration, nephrotic syndrome, and type IV renal tubular acidosis), bone marrow suppression, rashes, anorexia, and nausea. Kidney damage is more apt to

Table 1–9. Useful nonsteroidal anti-inflammatory drugs.

Generic Name	Proprietary Name	Dosage Range	Costs for 30 Days' Treatment[1] (based on average dosage)	Comments[2]
Aspirin		325–650 mg 4–6 times daily	$4.00	Available also in enteric-coated form that is more expensive and less well absorbed.
Diclofenac	Voltaren	50–75 mg 2 or 3 times daily	$78.00	May impose higher risk of hepatotoxicity.
Etodolac	Lodine	200–300 mg 3 times daily	$87.00	Perhaps less gastrointestinal toxicity.
Fenoprofen	Nalfon	300–600 mg 2–4 times daily	$42.00	Perhaps more side effects than others, including tubulointerstitial nephritis.
Flurbiprofen	Ansaid	50–100 mg 3 or 4 times daily	$62.00	Adverse gastrointestinal side effects may be more common among elderly.
Ibuprofen	Advil (OTC), Motrin, etc	200–600 mg 3 or 4 times daily	$17.00	Now available without prescription; relatively well tolerated.
Indomethacin	Indameth, Indocin, etc	25–50 mg 2–4 times daily	$17.00	Higher incidence of dose-related toxic effects, especially gastrointestinal and bone marrow effects.
Ketoprofen	Orudis	50–75 mg 2–4 times daily	$99.00	Lower doses for elderly.
Ketorolac (parenteral)	Toradol	30 mg IM 3 or 4 times daily	$615.00	Intramuscular NSAID as alternative to opioid.
Ketorolac (oral tablets)	Toradol	10 mg 4–6 times daily	$128.00	Not intended for long-term use.
Meclofenamate sodium	Meclomen	100 mg 2–4 times daily	$41.00	Diarrhea relatively more common.
Nabumetone	Relafen	500–1000 mg once daily	$54.00	First of a new class of NSAIDs (naphthylalkones).
Naproxen	Anaprox, Naprosyn	250–500 mg 2 or 3 times daily	$53.00	Generally well-tolerated. Lower doses for elderly.
Oxaprozin	Daypro	600–1200 mg once daily	$67.50	Similar to ibuprofen. May cause rash, pruritus, photosensitivity.
Piroxicam	Feldene	20 mg daily	$61.00	Single daily dosage convenient; may cause higher rate of gastrointestinal bleeding.
Sulindac	Clinoril	150–200 mg twice daily	$53.00	May cause higher rate of gastrointestinal bleeding; less nephrotoxic potential.
Tolmetin	Tolectin	200–600 mg 4 times daily	$111.00	Perhaps more side effects than others, including anaphylactic reactions.
Acetaminophen		325–650 mg 4–6 times daily	$6.00	Not an NSAID because it lacks anti-inflammatory effects. Equivalent to aspirin as analgesic and antipyretic agent.

[1] Cost to pharmacist (average wholesale price) for 30 days' treatment based on average dosage (generic when possible). When estimating daily costs for medications, dosage frequency must be taken into account.

[2] Adverse effects of headache, tinnitus, dizziness, confusion, rashes, anorexia, nausea, vomiting, gastrointestinal bleeding, nephrotoxicity, visual disturbances, etc, can occur with any of the drugs that have been available for shorter periods. Toxicity and efficacy are subject to great individual variations among patients.

occur in old men, diuretic users, and patients with heart disease. The principal advantages of the newer NSAIDs over aspirin are the longer duration of action—permitting less frequent dosing and better compliance—and the decreased frequency of gastrointestinal side effects. For most patients, however, aspirin remains the preferred (and much less expensive) drug—though the risk of gastrointestinal bleeding is higher with aspirin than with the other NSAIDs. All NSAIDs are analgesic, antipyretic, and anti-inflammatory in dose-dependent fashion. However, they may activate quiescent inflammatory bowel disease. Their principal uses are in the control of moderate pain of various musculoskeletal disorders, menstrual cramps, and other—mainly self-limited—conditions, including moderate postoperative discomfort. Suicide attempts with overdoses of the other NSAIDs are less serious and less often successful than attempts with aspirin.

Table 1–9 lists the most commonly used NSAIDs along with dosages and pertinent comments. The most widely used agents for these purposes are aspirin and acetaminophen.

Aspirin is the drug of first choice for management of mild to moderate pain and is an effective antipyretic and anti-inflammatory agent. Analgesia is achieved with much lower doses and blood levels than are needed for anti-inflammatory action. Aspirin is available in many forms for oral administration in a single 325 mg unit dose, as well as smaller (eg, 60 mg) and larger (eg, 500 mg) doses. The usual dose is 1–2 tablets (325–650 mg) every 4 hours as needed, taken with fluid. Gastrointestinal irritation can be reduced by ingestion with food or with an antacid. Enteric-coated aspirin, which is more expensive (Ecotrin; many others), can be used to avoid gastric irritation, but absorption is delayed.

The main untoward effect of aspirin—especially in large doses or when taken chronically—is gastric irritation and microscopic blood loss from the gut. Rarely, there may be massive gastrointestinal hemorrhage, most commonly in heavy drinkers or patients with a history of peptic ulcer disease. Gastrointestinal symptoms do not correlate with the amount of blood lost.

Aspirin allergy occurs infrequently and may be manifested as rhinorrhea, nasal polyps, asthma, and—very rarely—anaphylaxis. The incidence is less than 0.1%. Aspirin in high doses may produce a vitamin K-responsive prolongation of the prothrombin time.

Because of a possible association with Reye's syndrome, salicylates are best avoided by children and teenagers with febrile viral illnesses such as influenza and chickenpox.

Acetaminophen in the same dosage as aspirin (650 mg orally every 4 hours) has comparable analgesic and antipyretic effects but lacks the anti-inflammatory property of aspirin. It is useful for peo-

ple who cannot tolerate aspirin, for those with bleeding disorders, and for those at risk for Reye's syndrome. In very large doses (eg, > 4 g/d chronically, > 7 g/d acutely), acetaminophen can be hepatotoxic, manifested by appreciable hepatic necrosis with very high serum aminotransferase levels, often in the thousands. Toxicity may occur at considerably lower doses in the chronic alcoholic.

See Chapter 39 for further details on salicylate and acetaminophen overdosage.

Babb RR: Gastrointestinal complications of nonsteroidal anti-inflammatory drugs. West J Med 1992;157:444. (Ulcerations, hemorrhage, perforation, stricture, and exacerbation of inflammatory bowel disease.)
Camp JF: Patient-controlled analgesia. Am Fam Physician 1991;44:2145. (Earlier ambulation, decreased overall narcotic use, improved postoperative pulmonary function, shorter hospital stays, and reduced health care costs.)
Gabriel SE et al: Risk for serious gastrointestinal complications related to use of nonsteroidal anti-inflammatory drugs: A meta-analysis. Ann Intern Med 1991;115:787. (Patients at increased risk include elderly persons, concomitant corticosteroid users, and NSAID users in the first 3 months of therapy.)
Parker RK et al: Patient-controlled analgesia: Does a concurrent opioid infusion improve patient management after surgery? JAMA 1991;266:1947. (No.)
Sandler DP et al: Nonsteroidal anti-inflammatory drugs and the risk for chronic renal disease. Ann Intern Med 1991;115:165. (Specific groups at greater risk.)
Shankel SW et al: Acute renal failure and glomerulopathy caused by nonsteroidal anti-inflammatory drugs. Arch Intern Med 1992;152:986.

FEVER & HYPERTHERMIA

The average normal oral body temperature is 36.7 °C (range 36–37.4 °C), or 98 °F (range 96.8–99.3 °F). These ranges include 2 SD and thus encompass 95% of a normal population, measured in mid-morning. The normal rectal or vaginal temperature is 0.5 °C (1 °F) higher than the oral temperature, and the normal axillary temperature is correspondingly lower. Rectal temperature is more reliable than oral temperature, particularly in the case of patients who are mouth-breathers or who are tachypneic.

The normal diurnal temperature variation may be as much as 1 °C, being lowest in the early morning and highest in the late afternoon. There is a slight sustained temperature rise following ovulation during the menstrual cycle and in the first trimester of pregnancy.

Fever is a regulated rise to a new "set poir body temperature. When proper stimuli act c priate monocyte-macrophages, these cel' one of several pyrogenic cytokines, wh vation of the set point through effects amus. These cytokines include interleukin-1 (IL-1), tumor necrosis factor (TNF), interferon-gamma, and interleukin-6 (IL-6). The elevation in temperature may result from either increased heat production (eg, shivering) or decreased heat loss (eg, peripheral vasoconstriction). Body temperature in interleukin-1 induced fever seldom exceeds 41.1°C (106 °F) unless there is structural damage in the hypothalamus.

Hyperthermia—not mediated by cytokines—occurs when body metabolic heat production or environmental heat load exceeds normal heat loss capacity or when there is impaired heat loss; heat stroke is an example. Body temperature may rise to alarming levels (> 41.1 °C [106 °F]) capable of producing irreversible brain damage; no diurnal variation is observed.

Neuroleptic malignant syndrome is a rare and potentially lethal idiosyncratic reaction to major tranquilizers, particularly haloperidol and fluphenazine. The syndrome, which may be a variant of malignant hyperthermia of anesthesia, consists of hyperthermia, muscular rigidity, autonomic dysfunction, and altered consciousness occurring after therapeutic doses of the medication; it is not dose- or duration-related. Some benefit has been reported from the use of amantadine, bromocriptine, and dantrolene (see Hyperthermia, Chapter 39).

Effect of Elevated Body Temperature

Fever as a symptom should generally be regarded with appropriate concern. The body temperature may provide important information about the presence of illness, particularly infections, and about changes in the clinical status of the patient. The fever pattern, however, is of rather limited use for specific diagnosis. Furthermore, the degree of temperature elevation does not necessarily correspond to the severity of the illness. In general, the febrile response tends to be greater in children than in adults; in elderly persons and neonates, the febrile response is less marked or absent, even in the face of bacteremia.

Markedly elevated body temperature may result in profound metabolic disturbances. High temperature during the first trimester of pregnancy may cause birth defects, such as anencephaly. Fever may increase insulin requirements and also alter the metabolism and disposition of drugs used for the treatment of the diverse diseases associated with fever.

Diagnostic Considerations

The outline below illustrates the wide variety of clinical disorders that may cause fever. Most febrile illnesses are due to common infections, are short-lived, and are relatively easy to diagnose. In certain instances, however, the origin of the fever may remain obscure ("fever of undetermined origin," FUO) lengthy diagnostic examination. The term FUO litionally been reserved for cases of fever of

over 38.3 °C (101 °F) for three weeks in patients whose diagnosis is not apparent after 1 week or more of studies (see FUO, Chapter 32). In the United States, fever of unknown origin associated with HIV and HIV-related infections is becoming increasingly important.

In a prospective case series of 199 consecutive cases of FUO patients from the 1980s, infections—especially tuberculosis, cytomegalovirus, and abscesses—accounted for 23% of cases; multisystem illnesses—such as giant cell arteritis and Still's disease—for 22%; malignant tumors—hematologic and solid—for 7%; drug-related fever for 3%; factitious fever for 4%; habitual hyperthermia for 3%; and miscellaneous causes—such as pulmonary embolism and Crohn's disease—for 15%. No diagnosis could be firmly established in 26% of cases. Diagnostic ultrasound and CT scans led to specific diagnoses in 8% and 15% of cases, respectively.

Important Causes of Fever & Hyperthermia (With Examples)

A. Infections: Bacterial, viral, rickettsial, fungal, parasitic.

B. Autoimmune Diseases: Systemic lupus erythematosus, polyarteritis nodosa, rheumatic fever, polymyalgia rheumatica, giant cell arteritis, Still's disease, Wegener's granulomatosis, relapsing polychondritis; less prominent in dermatomyositis, adult rheumatoid arthritis.

C. Central Nervous System Disease: Cerebral hemorrhage, head injuries, brain and spinal cord tumors, degenerative central nervous system disease (eg, multiple sclerosis), spinal cord injuries. (This category represents interference with the thermal regulatory process rather than true "fever.")

D. Malignant Neoplastic Disease: Primary neoplasms (eg, colon and rectum, liver, kidney, neuroblastoma), tumors metastatic to the liver.

E. Hematologic Disease: Lymphomas, leukemias, hemolytic anemias.

F. Cardiovascular Disease: Myocardial infarction, pulmonary embolism.

G. Gastrointestinal Disease: Inflammatory bowel disease, liver abscess, alcoholic hepatitis, granulomatous hepatitis.

H. Endocrine Disease: Hyperthyroidism, pheochromocytoma may raise temperature because of altered thermoregulation.

I. Diseases Due to Chemical Agents: Drug reactions (including serum sickness), neuroleptic malignant syndrome, malignant hyperthermia of anesthesia.

J. Miscellaneous Diseases: Sarcoidosis, familial Mediterranean fever.

K. Factitious, or "false," fever.

Treatment

Most fever is well tolerated. When the temperature

is greater than 40 °C (104 °F), particularly if prolonged, symptomatic treatment may be required. *Temperature over 41 °C (105.8 °F) is a medical emergency.* (See Heat Stroke, Chapter 38.)

A. Measures for Removal of Heat: Alcohol sponges, cold sponges, ice bags, ice-water enemas, and ice baths will lower body temperature and provide physical comfort for patients who complain of feeling hot.

B. Antipyretic Drugs: In most instances, antipyretic therapy by itself is not needed except for reasons of comfort or in patients with fragile hemodynamic status. Aspirin or acetaminophen, 0.325–0.65 g every 4 hours, is quite effective in reducing fever. If given, these drugs are best administered continuously rather than as needed, since "prn" dosing results in periodic chills and sweats due to varying levels of drug.

C. Fluid Replacement: Oral or parenteral fluids must be administered to compensate for increased insensible fluid and electrolyte losses as well as those from perspiration.

Durack DT, Street AC: Fever of unknown origin: Reexamined and redefined. Curr Clin Top Infect Dis 1991;11:35. (Four-part categorization: classic, neutropenic, nosocomial, and HIV-related.)

Knockaert D et al: Fever of unknown origin in the 1980s: An update of the diagnostic spectrum. Arch Intern Med 1992;152:51.

Mackowiak PA et al: A critical appraisal of 98.6 °F, the upper limit of the normal body temperature, and other legacies of Carl Reinhold August Wunderlich. JAMA 1992;268:1578.

Rosenberg MR, Green M: Neuroleptic malignant syndrome: Review of response to therapy. Arch Intern Med 1989;149:1927. (Supports use of dantrolene or bromocriptine.)

WEIGHT LOSS

Marked unexplained weight loss is often an indication of serious physical or psychologic illness. It should be distinguished from voluntary weight loss. Significant weight loss may be due to a wide variety of disease processes of any organ system as well as psychiatric disorders.

When the patient complains of weight loss but appears to be adequately nourished, inquiry should be made about exact weight changes (with approximate dates) and about changes in clothing size. Family members may provide confirmation of weight loss, as may old documents such as driver's licenses.

Once it has been established that the patient has marked weight loss, further laboratory and radiologic investigation may be indicated, such as chest x-ray, complete blood count, serum chemistries, urinalysis, and upper gastrointestinal series radiograph. Involuntary weight loss is rarely due to "occult disease." Almost all physical causes are clinically evident during the initial evaluation of the patient. Marked weight loss can sometimes occur in the absence of serious physical illness. Psychiatric consultation should be considered when there is evidence of depression, dementia, anorexia nervosa, or other psychologic problems.

A mild, gradual weight loss occurs in some elderly persons. It is due to physiologic changes in body composition, including loss of height and lean body mass and lower basal metabolic rate, which leads to decreased energy requirements. However, rapid unintentional weight loss is highly predictive of morbidity and mortality in the elderly population. Causes include loss of teeth and consequent difficulty chewing, alcoholism, and social isolation in addition to various disease states.

Involuntary weight loss is a frequent complication of AIDS. Wasting, indicative of severe protein-calorie malnutrition (HIV wasting syndrome), is one element of the CDC's AIDS case definition (Table 30–1). Malnutrition in HIV-infected patients may further compromise immune function and contribute to the progression of AIDS. The mechanism of weight loss in AIDS patients is most probably multifactorial, including decreased caloric intake, malabsorption, and altered energy expenditures caused by hormonal or metabolic abnormalities. In some cases, weight loss is reversible with treatment of opportunistic infections or other identifiable abnormalities. Megestrol acetate, a synthetic progestational agent, has proved effective in stimulating appetite and weight gain of up to 0.5 kg per week in some patients with HIV-related cachexia. The drug is administered orally; the usual dose is 80 mg four times daily.

Fischer J et al: Low body weight and weight loss in the aged. J Am Diet Assoc 1990;90:1697. (Physical illness probably accounts for most cases; however, psychiatric disorders may also cause severe nutritional deficiencies.)

Marton KI, Sox HC Jr, Krupp JR: Involuntary weight loss: Diagnostic and prognostic significance. Ann Intern Med 1981;95:568. (Best article on diagnostic approach to weight loss.)

Von Roenn JH et al: HIV-related cachexia: Potential mechanisms and treatment. Oncology 1992;49(Suppl 2):50.

Wannamethee G et al: Weight change, perceived health status and mortality in middle-aged British men. Postgrad Med J 1990;66:910. (Significant weight loss was associated with deaths from cancer regardless of self-assessment of health status.)

FATIGUE

Fatigue is one of the most common symptoms confronting the office practitioner. In primary care settings, fatigue as an isolated symptom or diagnosis accounts for 1–3% of visits to generalists. The symptoms of fatigue may be less well defined and explained by patients than symptoms associated with specific functions, such as fever or dyspnea. Fatigue or lassitude and the closely related complaints of weakness, tiredness, and lethargy are most often readily explained by common factors such as overexertion, poor physical conditioning, inadequate rest, obesity, undernutrition, stress, and emotional problems. Taking a history of the patient's daily living and working habits may obviate the need for extensive and unproductive diagnostic studies.

Important diseases that can cause fatigue include endocrine disorders such as hyperthyroidism and hypothyroidism, cardiac disease (congestive heart failure), infections (endocarditis, hepatitis), respiratory disorders (COPD, sleep-associated breathing disorders), anemia, the arthritides and related disorders, cancer, alcoholism, drug side effects such as from sedatives and beta-blockers, and psychologic conditions such as depression and somatization disorder. However, a recent study suggests that psychiatric disorders may be pathogenic in less than 50% of cases.

Chronic Fatigue Syndrome

A syndrome of chronic fatigue has received much recent attention. A working case definition of chronic fatigue syndrome was developed in 1988 (Table 1–10). Chronic fatigue syndrome is not a homogeneous abnormality, and there is no single pathogenic mechanism. No physical finding or laboratory test can be used to confirm the diagnosis of chronic fatigue syndrome.

One recent study raises the question whether some cases of chronic fatigue syndrome may be caused by a chronic immunologically mediated inflammatory process of the central nervous system. The study found CD4:CD8 T cell ratios higher than among matched controls; more frequent brain MRI findings of punctate, subcortical areas of high signal intensity, suggesting edema or demyelination; and more frequent lymphocyte cell cultures showing active replication of human herpesvirus-6. However, the finding of active replication of HHV-6 probably represents reactivation of latent infection rather than primary infection.

This syndrome does not appear to be related to chronic infection with Epstein-Barr virus (see Chap-

Table 1–10. Definition of chronic fatigue syndrome (CFS).[1]

A case of chronic fatigue syndrome must fulfill both of the major criteria listed and, of the minor criteria listed, either 6 or more of the 11 symptom criteria and 2 or more of the 3 physical examination criteria or 8 or more of the 11 symptom criteria.

MAJOR CRITERIA FOR CFS

1. **Fatigue of at least 6 months' duration.** New onset of persistent or relapsing debilitating fatigue or easy fatigability in a person with no previous history of similar symptoms that does not resolve with bed rest and that is severe enough to reduce or impair average daily activity below 50% of the patient's premorbid activity level for a period of at least 6 months.

2. **Exclusion of other causes of chronic fatigue.** Other clinical conditions that may produce similar symptoms must be excluded by thorough evaluation based on history, physical examination, and appropriate laboratory investigations. These conditions include malignancy, autoimmune diseases, infections, chronic psychiatric disease, neuromuscular disease, endocrine disease, drug dependency, or other known or defined chronic pulmonary, cardiac, gastrointestinal, hepatic, renal, or hematologic disease.

MINOR CRITERIA FOR CFS

Symptom criteria: The symptoms must have begun at or after the time of onset of increased fatigability and must have persisted or occurred over a period of at least 6 months.
 1. Mild fever (oral temperature between 37.5 and 38.6 °C measured by the patient).
 2. Sore throat.
 3. Painful cervical or axillary lymph nodes.
 4. Unexplained general muscle weakness.
 5. Myalgia.
 6. Prolonged (> 24 hours) generalized fatigue (after levels of exercise that would have been easily tolerated in the patient's premorbid state).
 7. Generalized headaches (of a type, severity, or pattern that is different from headaches the patient may have had in the premorbid state).
 8. Migratory arthralgias, without swelling or erythema.
 9. Neuropsychologic complaints (photophobia, transient scotoma, forgetfulness, excessive irritability, confusion, difficulty thinking, inability to concentrate, depression).
 10. Sleep disturbance (hypersomnia or insomnia).
 11. Description of the main symptom complex as initially developing over a few hours to a few days.

Physical examination criteria: These must be documented by a physician on at least two occasions at least 1 month apart.
 1. Low-grade fever (oral temperature 37.6–38.6 °C).
 2. Nonexudative pharyngitis.
 3. Palpable or tender cervical or axillary lymph nodes (< 2 cm in diameter).

[1]Reproduced, with permission, from Holmes GP et al: Chronic fatigue syndrome: A working case definition. Ann Intern Med 1988;108:387.

ter 31) or to chronic yeast infection; some cases of Lyme disease may be clinically similar.

A 1991 NIH panel recommended a standard panel of laboratory tests for initial patient examination, including complete blood count with differential, erythrocyte sedimentation rate, serum chemistries (electrolytes, blood urea nitrogen, glucose, creatinine, calcium, thyroid function tests), antinuclear antibody, urinalysis, and tuberculin skin test, and screening questionnaires for psychiatric disorders. Other tests to be performed as clinically indicated are serum cortisol, rheumatoid factor, immunoglobulin levels, Lyme serology in endemic areas, and tests for HIV antibody. This seems a more reasonable diagnostic strategy than the more extensive testing others have recommended. Antibody to EBV is not helpful in evaluation of patients with chronic fatigue.

A variety of treatments have been tried. Acyclovir does not appear to improve symptoms, nor does oral or vaginal nystatin. There is a greater prevalence of past and current psychiatric diagnoses in patients with this syndrome. Affective disorders are especially common. In all cases, patients should be encouraged to exercise and engage in life's activities to the extent possible and to be reassured that full recovery is eventually possible in most cases.

Buchwald D et al: A chronic illness characterized by fatigue, neurologic and immunologic disorders, and active human herpesvirus type 6 infection. Ann Intern Med 1992;116:103. (Immunologic and central nervous system imaging findings.)

Cathebras PJ et al: Fatigue in primary care: Prevalence, psychiatric comorbidity, illness behavior, and outcome. J Gen Intern Med 1992;7:276. (Depression was the most common psychiatric cause.)

Levine PH et al: Clinical, epidemiologic, and virologic studies in four clusters of the chronic fatigue syndrome. Arch Intern Med 1992;152:1611. (After 3 years, almost all subjects were able to return to pre-illness activity.)

Schluerderberg A et al: Chronic fatigue syndrome research: Definition and medical outcome assessment. Ann Intern Med 1992;117:325. (Refinement of definition.)

Shafran SD: The chronic fatigue syndrome. Am J Med 1991;90:730. (Prolonged duration and considerable morbidity, though no mortality.)

2 Diagnostic Testing & Medical Decision Making

William M. Detmer, MD, & Diana Nicoll, MD, PhD

The clinician's main task is to make reasoned decisions about patient care despite imperfect clinical information and uncertainty about clinical outcomes. Information from the history and physical examination is often imprecise and ambiguous, and treatment must often be started before the diagnosis is confirmed. Under these conditions, clinicians often turn to diagnostic tests or procedures for help.

BENEFITS; COSTS & RISKS

When used appropriately by the clinician, diagnostic tests can be of great assistance to the clinician. Tests can help rule a diagnosis in or out, screen for specific diseases, guide the management of an established disease, and help formulate a prognosis.

Diagnostic tests are not without disadvantages, however. Their benefit is often outweighed by their financial cost, risks to the patient's health, discomfort associated with the procedure, and consequences for further care. Expenditures for diagnostic tests are a significant portion of health care costs. The risk of complications or death is a significant drawback of some diagnostic tests. The severity of potential complications and the degree of risk should always be weighed against the benefits of testing. Patient discomfort is another significant cost of diagnostic tests. Although some tests cause little pain (eg, electrocardiography, ultrasound), many cause significant discomfort (eg, barium enema, sigmoidoscopy). Finally, the result of a diagnostic test often has implications for further care in that a test result may mandate further testing or frequent follow-up. For instance, if a test is falsely positive, the patient may incur significant cost and risk during follow-up testing.

USES OF DIAGNOSTIC TESTS

Screening
Screening tests are used to identify risk factors for disease and to detect occult disease in asymptomatic persons. Identification of risk factors may allow early intervention to prevent disease occurrence, and early detection of occult disease may reduce disease morbidity and mortality through early treatment. Optimal screening tests meet the criteria listed in Table 2–1.

Diagnosis
Diagnostic tests are used to help establish or exclude the presence of disease in symptomatic persons. Some tests assist in early diagnosis after onset of symptoms and signs; others assist in differential diagnosis of various possible diseases. Still others help determine the stage or activity of disease.

Management
Tests used in patient management may enable the clinician to (1) evaluate the severity of disease, (2) estimate prognosis, (3) monitor the course of disease (progression, stability, or resolution), (4) detect disease recurrence, (5) select drugs and adjust dosages, and (6) monitor the response to treatment. An example of tests used in patient management is therapeutic drug monitoring (see below).

PERFORMANCE OF DIAGNOSTIC TESTS

PREPARATION FOR TESTS

Test results are only as good as the specimen sent for testing.

16

Table 2–1. Criteria for use of screening procedures.

Characteristics of population
Sufficiently high prevalence of disease.
Likely to be compliant with subsequent tests and treatments.

Characteristics of disease
Significant morbidity and mortality.
Effective and acceptable treatment available.
Presymptomatic period when disease is detectable.
Improved outcome from early treatment.

Characteristics of test
High sensitivity and specificity.
Low cost and risk.
Confirmatory test available and practical.

Patient Preparation

The preparation of the patient is important for certain tests. For example, a fasting state is needed for glucose and triglyceride measurements. Controlled conditions are frequently needed for endocrinology testing (eg, dietary sodium and posture must be controlled for aldosterone studies). Drug ingestion may affect test results—eg, alcohol increases γ-glutamyl transpeptidase, and diuretics may affect electrolyte measurements.

Specimen Collection

Careful attention must be paid to patient identification and specimen labeling, since the most common problem in the clinical laboratory is specimen mislabeling. The phlebotomy site should not be immediately above an intravenous line.

Diagnostic tests require the use of specific specimen containers. Table 2–2 lists the commonly used specimen collection tubes. Certain test specimens may require special handling or storage (eg, blood gas specimens must be sent to the laboratory on ice). Lysis of cells during blood specimen collection will result in spuriously increased serum levels of substances concentrated in cells (eg, lactate dehydrogenase and potassium). Delay in delivery of some spec-

imens to the laboratory can result in ongoing cellular metabolism and therefore spurious results (eg, low glucose and high lactate levels).

TEST CHARACTERISTICS

Table 2–3 lists the characteristics of all diagnostic tests.

Accuracy
The accuracy of a laboratory test is its correspondence with the true value. An inaccurate test is one that consistently differs from the true value even though the results may be reproducible.

Precision
Test precision is a measure of a test's reproducibility when repeated on the same sample. An imprecise test is one that yields widely varying results on repeated measurements. The precision of diagnostic tests must be high enough to distinguish clinically relevant changes in a patient's status from the analytic variability of the test.

Reference Ranges
Patient test results are interpreted by comparing them with published reference ranges. These reference ranges are method- and laboratory-specific. In practice, reference ranges often represent test results found in 95% of a small sample population presumed to be healthy (Figure 2–1). It is important to consider whether published reference ranges are appropriate for the patient being evaluated and to interpret slightly abnormal results in a critical fashion. For instance, a healthy person subjected to 20 independent tests has a 64% probability of having at least one abnormal test result (Table 2–4). The Appendix to this book contains the reference ranges for commonly used serum and urine chemistry and hematology tests.

Table 2–2. Commonly used specimen collection tubes.

Tube Color	Tube Contents	Typically Used In
Lavender	EDTA	Complete blood count
Marbled	Serum separator	Serum chemistry tests
Red	None	Blood banking (serum)
Blue	Citrate	Coagulation studies
Gray	Inhibitor of glycolysis (sodium fluoride)	Lactic acid
Green	Heparin	Plasma studies
Yellow	Acid citrate	HLA typing
Navy	Trace metal free	Trace metals (eg, lead)

Table 2–3. Properties of useful diagnostic tests.

- Test methodology has been described in detail so that it can be accurately and reliably reproduced.
- Test accuracy and precision have been determined.
- The reference range has been established appropriately.
- Sensitivity and specificity have been reliably established by comparison with a gold standard. The evaluation has used a range of patients, including those who have different but commonly confused disorders and those with a spectrum of mild and severe, treated and untreated disease. The patient selection process has been adequately described, so that results will not be generalized inappropriately.
- Independent contribution to overall performance of a test panel has been confirmed if a test is advocated as part of a panel of tests.

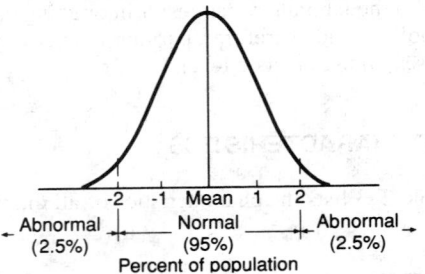

Figure 2–1. The normal range is usually defined as within 2 SD of the mean (shown as –2 and 2) on a plot of a frequency distribution of laboratory test results in healthy volunteers.

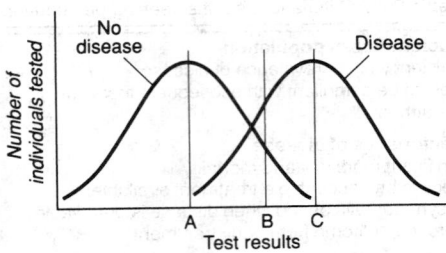

Figure 2–2. Hypothetical distribution of test results for healthy and diseased individuals (eg, serum uric acid values in men without and with gouty arthritis). Because no test unfailingly distinguishes between healthy and ill persons, the distribution of test results overlaps as shown. Defining the "cut-off point" between "normal" and "abnormal" (or "negative" and "positive") test results determines the relationship between test sensitivity and specificity. For example, if "A" is chosen as the cutoff point and all patients with values to the right of "A" are said to have "abnormal" or "positive" results, the test will have 100% sensitivity but low specificity. This would be an appropriate cutoff point if the test were being used to screen for or to exclude a disease. However, if "C" is chosen as the cut-off point and all patients with values to the right of "C" are said to have " abnormal" results, the test would have 100% specificity but low sensitivity. This would be an appropriate cutoff point if the test were being used to confirm a suspected diagnosis. For most tests, the cutoff point is usually somewhere between points "A" and "C" at a point "B." Exactly where to fix point "B" depends on why the test is usually performed and the relative importance of false-positive and false-negative results. (Modified, with permission, from Griner PF et al: Selection and interpretation of diagnostic tests and procedures: Principles and applications. Ann Intern Med 1981;84[4 Part 2]:453.)

Sensitivity & Specificity

A test's **sensitivity** is the probability that an abnormal result will occur if the patient has the disease. If all patients with a given disease have a positive test, then the test sensitivity is 100%. A test with high sensitivity is useful to "rule out" a diagnosis, because a highly sensitive test will give few results that are falsely negative.

A test's **specificity** is the probability that a normal test result will occur if the patient does not have the disease. If all patients who do not have a given disease have negative tests, then the test specificity is 100%. A test with high specificity is useful to "rule in" a diagnosis because a highly specific test will have few results that are falsely positive.

To determine test sensitivity and specificity for a particular disease, the test must be compared against a "gold standard," a procedure that defines the true disease state of the patient. However, for many disease states, such a gold standard either does not exist or is very difficult to apply. Therefore, reliable estimates of test sensitivity and specificity may be difficult to obtain. In addition to comparison with a gold standard, test sensitivity and specificity can be profoundly affected by the cutoff point above which a test is interpreted as positive (Figure 2–2).

Predictive Value

In a particular clinical situation, the value of a diagnostic test depends not only on the test sensitivity and specificity but also on the probability that the patient has the disease before the test is performed (**pretest probability**).

Perhaps the best measure of a test's value in a particular clinical context is the predictive value, which can be calculated using sensitivity, specificity, and pretest probability (Figure 2–3). The **positive predictive value** is the probability that a patient has the disease if the test result is positive. The **negative predictive value** is the probability that a patient is free of the disease if the test result is negative.

The pretest probability of disease has a profound effect on the predictive value of a test. As demonstrated in Table 2–5, the positive predictive value of a test with 90% sensitivity and specificity varies from 1% to 99% depending on the pretest probability of disease. Furthermore, as the pretest probability of disease decreases, it becomes less likely that someone with a positive test actually has the disease and more likely that the result is falsely positive.

The usefulness of a test in a given clinical situation thus depends both on the pretest probability and on

Table 2–4. Relationship between the number of tests and the probability that a healthy person will have one or more abnormal results.

Number of Tests	Probability That One or More Results Will Be Abnormal
1	5%
6	26%
12	46%
20	64%

		Disease	
		Present	Absent
Test result	Positive (abnormal)	TP	FP
	Negative (normal)	FN	TN

$$\text{Sensitivity} = \frac{\text{Number of diseased patients with positive test}}{\text{Number of diseased patients}} = \frac{TP}{TP + FN}$$

$$\text{Specificity} = \frac{\text{Number of nondiseased patients with negative test}}{\text{Number of nondiseased patients}} = \frac{TN}{TN + FP}$$

$$\text{Positive predictive value} = \text{Probability of disease if test positive} = \frac{TP}{TP + FP}$$

$$= \frac{(\text{sensitivity}) \, (\text{pretest probability})}{(\text{sensitivity}) \, (\text{pretest probability}) + (1 - \text{specificity})(1 - \text{pretest probability})}$$

Figure 2–3. Calculation of sensitivity, specificity, and positive predictive value. (TP, true positive; FP, false positive; FN, false negative; TN, true negative.)

the sensitivity and specificity of the test. For example, suppose the clinician estimates that a newly hypertensive patient has a low probability (2%) of having renovascular hypertension. If a test for this disease has a sensitivity of 95% and a specificity of 95%, the predictive value of a positive test is only 28%—ie, even though the test is positive, there is still a 72% chance that the patient does not have renovascular hypertension (Figure 2–4A). In contrast, if the pretest probability is 50%, the positive predictive value of the same test is 95% (Figure 2–4B). This example illustrates that tests are most likely to be useful when the diagnosis is truly uncertain (pretest probability about 50%); diagnostic tests add little when the diagnosis is either extremely unlikely or almost certain.

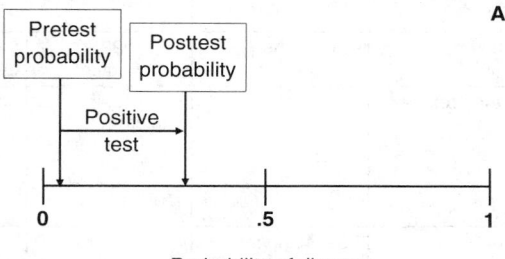

A.

Probability of disease

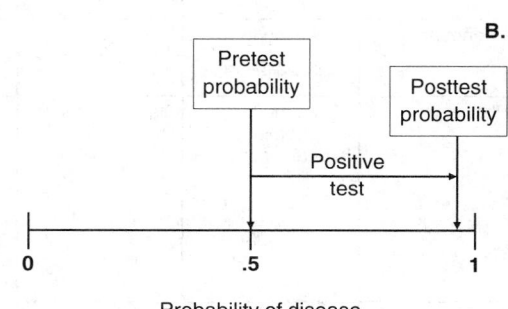

B.

Probability of disease

Figure 2–4. Effect of a test with 95% sensitivity and 95% specificity on the probability of disease (see text for explanation.)

Table 2–5. The predictive value of a test with 90% sensitivity and 90% specificity at various pretest probabilities of disease.

Pretest Probability	Positive Predictive Value
0.001	0.01
0.01	0.08
0.05	0.32
0.50	0.90
0.95	0.994
0.99	0.999

Table 2–6. Therapeutic drug monitoring.[1]

Drug	Effective Concentration	Half-Life (hours)	Dosage Adjustment	Comments
Amikacin	Peak: 20–30 mg/L Trough: <30 mg/L	1–25 ↑ in uremia	↓ in renal dysfunction	Concomitant kanamycin or tobramycin therapy may give falsely elevated amikacin results by immunoassay.
Amitriptyline	160–240 ng/mL	9–161		Drug is highly protein-bound. Patient-specific decrease in protein binding may invalidate quoted range of effective concentration.
Carbamazepine	4–8 mg/L	10–30		Induces its own metabolism. Metabolite 10,11-epoxide exhibits 13% cross-reactivity by immunoassay.
Desipramine	>225 ng/mL	13–23		Drug is highly protein-bound. Patient-specific decrease in protein binding may invalidate quoted range of effective concentration.
Digoxin	0.8–2.0 ng/mL	42 ↑ in uremia, CHF, hypothyroidism; ↓ in hyperthyroidism	↓ in renal dysfunction, CHF	Bioavailability of digoxin tablets is 50–90%. Specimen must not be drawn within 6 hours of dose. Dialysis does not remove a significant amount. Hypokalemia potentiates toxicity. Digitalis toxicity is a clinical and *not* a laboratory diagnosis. Digibind (digoxin-specific antibody) therapy of digoxin overdose interferes with measurement of digoxin levels. Elimination reduced by quinidine, amiodarone, and verapamil.
Gentamicin	Peak: 4–8 mg/L Trough: <2 mg/L	2–5 ↑ in uremia (7.3 during dialysis)	↓ in renal dysfunction	Draw peak specimen 30 minutes after end of infusion. Draw trough just before next dose. In uremic patients, carbenicillin may ↓ gentamicin half-life from 46 to 22 hours.
Imipramine	>225 ng/mL	10–16		Drug is highly protein-bound. Patient-specific decrease in protein binding may invalidate quoted range of effective concentration.
Lidocaine	1–5 mg/L	1.8 ↔ in uremia, CHF; ↑ in cirrhosis	↓ in CHF, liver disease	Levels increased with cimetidine therapy. CNS toxicity common in the elderly.
Lithium	0.5–1.5 meq/L	22 ↑ in uremia	↓ in renal dysfunction	Thiazides and loop diuretics may increase serum lithium levels.
Methotrexate		8.4 ↑ in uremia	↓ in renal dysfunction	7-Hydroxymethotrexate cross-reacts 1.5% in immunoassay. To minimize toxicity, leucovorin should be continued if methotrexate level is >0.1 μmol/L at 48 hours after start of therapy. Methotrexate >1 μmol/L at >48 hours requires an increase in leucovorin rescue therapy.
Nortriptyline	50–140 ng/mL	18–44		Drug is highly protein-bound. Patient-specific decrease in protein binding may invalidate quoted range of effective concentration.
Phenobarbital	10–40 mg/L	86 ↑ in cirrhosis	↓ in liver disease	Metabolized primarily by the hepatic microsomal enzyme system. Many drug-drug interactions.
Phenytoin	10–20 mg/L ↓ in uremia, hypoalbuminemia	Dose-dependent		Metabolite cross-reacts 10% in immunoassay. Metabolism is capacity-limited. Increase dose *cautiously* when level approaches therapeutic range, since new steady-state level may be disproportionately higher. Drug is very highly protein-bound and when protein binding is decreased in uremia and hypoalbuminemia, usual therapeutic range does not apply. In this situation, use a reference range of 5–10 mg/L.
Primidone	5–10 mg/L	8		Phenobarbital cross-reacts 0.5%. Metabolized to phenobarbital. Primidone:phenobarbital ratio >1:2 suggests poor compliance.

(continued)

Table 2–6. (cont) Therapeutic drug monitoring.

Drug	Effective Concentration	Half-Life (hours)	Dosage Adjustment	Comments
Procainamide	4–8 mg/L	3 ↑ in uremia	↓ in renal dysfunction	30% of patients with plasma levels of 12–16 mg/L have electrocardiographic changes; 40% of patients with plasma levels of 16 mg/L have severe toxicity. Metabolite N-acetylprocainamide is active.
Quinidine	1–4 mg/L	7 ↔ in CHF; ↑ in liver disease	↓ in liver disease, CHF	Effective concentration is lower in chronic liver disease and nephrosis where binding is decreased. Inflammation can increase binding and total concentration.
Salicylate	150–300 mg/L	Dose-dependent		
Theophylline	10–20 mg/L	9	↓ in CHF, cirrhosis, and with cimetidine	Caffeine cross-reacts 10%. Elimination is increased 1½–2 times in smokers. 1,3-Dimethyl uric acid metabolite ↑ in uremia and because of cross-reactivity may cause an apparent slight ↑ in serum theophylline.
Tobramycin	Peak: 5–10 mg/L Trough: <2 mg/L	2 ↑ in uremia	↓ in renal dysfunction	Tobramycin, kanamycin, and amikacin may cross-react in immunoassay.
Valproic acid	55–100 mg/L	8–19		95% protein-bound. ↓ binding in uremia and cirrhosis.
Vancomycin	Trough: 5–15 mg/L	6 ↑ in uremia	↓ in renal dysfunction	Toxicity in uremic patients leads to irreversible deafness. Keep peak level <30–40 mg/L to avoid toxicity.

[1]Modified and reproduced, with permission, from Detmer WM et al: *Pocket Guide to Diagnostic Tests.* Appleton & Lange, 1992.
Key:
↔ = unchanged; ↑ = increase(d); ↓ = decrease(d); CHF = congestive heart failure

Likelihood Ratio

Another way to characterize the discriminatory power of a test is the likelihood ratio (LR):

$$LR = \frac{\text{Probability of result in diseased persons}}{\text{Probability of result in nondiseased persons}}$$

Every test has two likelihood ratios, one corresponding to a positive test (LR^+) and one to a negative test (LR^-).

$$LR^+ = \frac{\text{Probability that test is positive in diseased persons}}{\text{Probability that test is positive in nondiseased persons}}$$
$$= \frac{\text{Sensitivity}}{1-\text{specificity}}$$

$$LR^- = \frac{\text{Probability that test is negative in diseased persons}}{\text{Probability that test is negative in nondiseased persons}}$$
$$= \frac{1-\text{sensitivity}}{\text{Specificity}}$$

Likelihood ratios can be used to make quick estimates of the usefulness of a contemplated diagnostic test in a particular clinical situation. When using the likelihood ratio, it is helpful to use an "odds" formulation of probability, where the odds of having a disease are expressed as the chance of having the disease divided by the chance of not having the disease. For instance, a probability of 0.75 is the same as 3:1 odds.

To estimate the potential benefit of a diagnostic test, the clinician first estimates the pretest odds of disease given all available clinical information and then multiplies the pretest odds by the positive and negative likelihood ratios. The results are the posttest odds, or the chance of having the disease if the test is positive or negative. The general form for this relationship is expressed as follows:

Pretest odds × **Likelihood ratio** = **Posttest odds**

For example, if the clinician believes that the patient has a 60% chance of having a myocardial infarction (pretest odds of 3:2) and the creatine kinase MB test result is elevated ($LR^+ = 32$), then the posttest chance of having a myocardial infarction is

$$3{:}2 \times 32 = 96{:}2 \text{ or } 48{:}1 \text{ odds} \left(\frac{48}{49} = 98\% \text{ probability}\right)$$

THERAPEUTIC DRUG MONITORING

The basic assumption underlying therapeutic drug monitoring is that there is variability in drug metabolism from patient to patient and that the serum level of a drug is more closely related to the drug's therapeutic effect or toxicity than is the dosage.

Drug Monitoring Useful

Indications for therapeutic drug monitoring include the following:

(1) Drugs with a **narrow therapeutic index** (therapeutic drug levels do not differ greatly from levels associated with serious toxicity) should be monitored. *Example:* Lithium.

(2) Patients who have **impaired clearance** of a drug with a narrow therapeutic index are candidates for drug monitoring. The clearance mechanism of the drug involved must be known. *Example:* Patients with renal failure have decreased clearance of gentamicin and therefore are at a higher risk for gentamicin toxicity.

(3) Drugs whose **toxicity is difficult to distinguish from a patient's underlying disease** may require monitoring. *Example:* Theophylline in patients with chronic obstructive pulmonary disease.

(4) Drugs whose **efficacy is difficult to establish clinically** may require monitoring of plasma levels. *Example:* Phenytoin.

Drug Monitoring Perhaps Not Useful

Situations in which therapeutic drug monitoring may not be useful include the following:

(1) Drugs that can be given in extremely high doses before toxicity is apparent are not candidates for monitoring. *Example:* Penicillin.

(2) If there are better means of assessing drug effects, drug level monitoring may not be appropriate. *Example:* Warfarin is monitored by prothrombin time determinations, not by serum levels of warfarin.

(3) Drug level monitoring to assess compliance is unreliable, since poor compliance cannot be distinguished from rapid metabolism without direct inpatient scrutiny of drug administration. *Example:* Phenytoin.

(4) Drug toxicity cannot be diagnosed with drug levels alone; it is a clinical diagnosis. Drug levels within the usual therapeutic range do not rule out drug toxicity in a given patient. *Example:* Digoxin, where other physiologic variables (eg, hypokalemia) affect drug toxicity.

Specimen Collection for Drug Monitoring

In general, a therapeutic drug level specimen should be drawn after the steady state plasma drug level has been reached (at least three or four drug half-lives after a dosage adjustment) and just before the next dose (trough level). For some drugs, peak and trough levels may be indicated, eg, to evaluate the dosage of drugs whose half-lives are much shorter than the dosing interval (eg, gentamicin).

Table 2–6 lists therapeutic drug monitoring information for commonly used drugs.

REFERENCES

Detmer WM et al: *Pocket Guide to Diagnostic Tests.* Appleton & Lange, 1992.

Eddy DM (editor): *Common Screening Tests.* American College of Physicians, 1991.

Sox HC (editor): *Common Diagnostic Tests: Use and Interpretation,* 2nd ed. American College of Physicians, 1991.

Sox HC et al: Sensitivities and specificities of diagnostic tests. In: *Medical Decision Making.* Butterworths, 1988.

Winter M: *Basic Clinical Pharmacokinetics,* 2nd ed. Applied Therapeutics, 1988.

Imaging

3

Susan D. Wall, MD

Selection of the proper radiographic examination is becoming increasingly difficult with the numerous new techniques available today. Complex and often overlapping examinations that have been developed in the past decade offer sophisticated diagnostic tools to today's clinicians. Physicians can best use this complex armamentarium of radiographic examinations by having a clear awareness of their indications and limitations. The "study of choice" for many presumptive diagnoses depends on several factors, some of which are discussed here. Indications for computerized tomography (CT), magnetic resonance imaging (MRI), ultrasound (US), gastrointestinal and urologic radiography, and radionuclide imaging (nuclear medicine) are summarized, along with a discussion of pertinent risks and contraindications for each examination. Patient preparation is included as well as approximate total costs (hospital plus physician charges). The limitations of radiology often are overlooked or not recognized, and so they are listed in some detail. Alternative examinations are suggested, and the advantages of each method are discussed.

I. CROSS-SECTIONAL IMAGING

It is important to recognize that local expertise and the availability of equipment are fundamental to the selection of imaging examinations. Clear and direct communication with the radiologist allows him or her to modify each examination as needed in order to answer the specific question referable to each patient. No study is "routine." The radiologist should be consulted regarding which studies to do, when, and in what order. The information below provides a guideline for the nonradiologist physician.

COMPUTED TOMOGRAPHY (CT)

Indications
   A. Head: Although MRI is the technique of choice for imaging of most pathologic processes in-

volving the head, a few entities are better evaluated with CT. Examples are acute cranial-facial trauma and acute (< 72 hours neurologic dysfunction. Stroke, which is manifested by low-density edema or mass effect, can sometimes be detected as early as 2–3 hours following the onset of symptoms. Suspected subarachnoid or intracranial hemorrhage, especially within the first 24–48 hours, also is better evaluated with CT. When the hematocrit is normal, the density of blood initially is greater than brain tissue, and it decreases with age. Hence, a chronic subdural hematoma will be hypodense relative to brain, and a fresh bleed can be isodense in a patient with a low hematocrit. CT of the sinuses is useful for evaluation of ostia and sinus drainage. Temporal bone CT is useful except for evaluation of asymmetric sensorineural hearing loss. CT is useful also for further characterization of some intracranial lesions identified by MRI (eg, presence or absence of calcium, evaluation of bony extension). Because artifacts from bone may interfere with detection of disease at the skull base and in the posterior fossa, MRI is preferable to CT in that location.
   B. Spine: Indicated for patients in whom MRI is contraindicated and for evaluation of a few specific limitations of MRI such as defining calcification of the posterior longitudinal ligament, tumoral calcification, osteophytic spurring, retropulsed bone fragments following trauma.
   C. Chest: Indicated for differentiation of mediastinal and hilar lymphadenopathy from vascular structures; staging of some lung cancers; characterization of possibly calcified nodules; differentiation of interstitial lung disease as well as bronchiectasis with thin section images (1.5 mm); differentiation of parenchymal versus pleural processes; staging of some tumors involving the esophageal wall.
   D. Abdomen and Pelvis: Indicated for morphologic evaluation of all abdominal and pelvic organs; differentiation of intraperitoneal versus retroperitoneal disorders; abscess; mesenteric and retroperitoneal lymphadenopathy; bowel wall thickening; site of gastrointestinal obstruction; aortoenteric fistula with perigraft abscess in patient with reconstructed aorta; abdominal aortic aneurysm; appendicitis and diverticulitis when diagnosis is unclear or when there is a question of extraluminal dis-

ease; acalculous acute cholecystitis; staging of some carcinomas of the gastrointestinal tract; site of partial or complete small or large bowel obstruction; anastomotic breakdown (leak); staging of hypernephroma; obstructive biliary disease; splenic infarction; course of ureters; trauma; spontaneous retroperitoneal hemorrhage; response to chemotherapy; pancreatitis and its complications; pancreatic cancer; liver metastasis with bolus of intravenous contrast and fast ("dynamic") imaging. *Note:* Increased sensitivity can be achieved with delayed imaging (4–6 hours after intravenous contrast study) and especially with CT arterial portography (CTAP). The latter is performed with a rapid bolus of intravenous contrast medium administered via catheter placed previously in the superior mesenteric artery (in angiography). Although offering greater sensitivity, it also is more invasive and less specific, and so it is used selectively.

Risks & Contraindications

Intravenous contrast material imposes a hazard of allergic reaction, resulting in death in 1:40,000–1:30,000 examinations; accumulating data suggest reduced risk with nonionic contrast medium, which increases the cost of any study approximately $270.00–360.00. Blood urea nitrogen and serum creatinine may be permanently increased in patients with diabetes mellitus and multiple myeloma but returns to normal in others. (See Chapter 21 regarding intravenous contrast medium-induced renal failure.) There is a risk of bleeding with percutaneous fine-needle aspiration, especially with abnormal clotting parameters.

Patient Preparation

Normal hydration; sedation in agitated patients. The gastrointestinal tract must be filled with an opacifying oral contrast agent in order to differentiate gut from abscess, tumor, and lymphadenopathy. One to 2 liters of very dilute (1–2%) water-soluble iodinated contrast medium or 1–2% barium should be ingested by the patient during the 1–2 hours prior to the study, or it can be administered slowly via a nasogastric tube.

Limitations

Availability; generally limited to transaxial images and therefore lacks the advantage of MRI and ultrasound regarding multiplanar imaging, which may be necessary to clarify confusing findings; limited differentiation of cystic versus solid lesions; bowel opacification important; dense barium or Hypaque from prior fluoroscopic study causes a severe artifact that precludes a diagnostic study; patient must be able to hold still and to hold his or her breath on inspiration; surgical clips and metallic prostheses cause artifacts and degrade images; cachexia limits the diagnostic quality of images because of the paucity of fat. *Note:* Increasingly, patients are being asked to give written informed consent for injection of intravenous contrast material.

Usual Billed Amount

Brain, $670.00–850.00.
Chest, abdomen, pelvis (each), $900.00–1250.00.

Alternatives

Ultrasound (often complementary) and sometimes MRI.

Advantages

Rapid; superb spatial resolution; not limited by overlying bowel, as in ultrasound; can guide percutaneous fine-needle aspiration of possible tumor or abscess; can evaluate success of prior drainage procedures and determine catheter course and tip position. Multiple organ systems can be evaluated simultaneously.

ULTRASOUND (US)

Indications

A. Abdomen and Pelvis: Intraperitoneal fluid; cystic versus solid lesions of liver and kidneys; intra- and extrahepatic biliary dilatation; hydronephrosis; pancreatic morphology; peripancreatic fluid collections and pseudocyst; aortic aneurysm; size of prostate and volume of residual urine; intraperitoneal abscess; primary and metastatic liver tumor; intrahepatic versus subhepatic lesion; cholelithiasis; gallbladder wall thickness; perigallbladder fluid; appendicitis; possible pregnancy; fetal assessment; pelvic inflammatory disease.

B. Chest: Pleural fluid; supra- versus infradiaphragmatic fluid; paralyzed diaphragm.

C. Neck: Parathyroid adenoma; thyroid for localization of a palpable nodule and to determine the number of nodules—also to assess response to suppressive therapy; lymphadenopathy versus vessels; patency of carotid arteries.

D. Vascular: Doppler flow of arteries and veins.

Risks & Contraindications

None.

Patient Preparation

Preferably NPO for 6 hours; full urinary bladder for pelvic studies.

Limitations

Abdominal and pelvic organs may be obscured by overlying bowel; somewhat operator-dependent (less so with newer equipment); presence of barium impairs sound waves.

Usual Billed Amount

$275.00–375.00. Intraoperative, $600.00.

Alternatives

Computed tomography (often complementary).

Advantages

No radiation; can be portable; imaging in all planes; endovaginal and endorectal probes enhance pelvic imaging; can guide percutaneous fine-needle aspiration of possible tumor or abscess; less expensive than CT or MRI. Can guide drainage of biliary tree, gallbladder, abscess, and other fluid collections.

MAGNETIC RESONANCE IMAGING (MRI)

Indications

A. Head: Essentially all intracranial pathologic processes except those listed above for CT; especially good for the brain stem and posterior fossa.

B. Neck: Evaluation of the upper aerodigestive tract; staging of neck masses, including suspected vascular tumors; better than CT for differentiation of lymphadenopathy from blood vessels as well as supra- and infraglottic extension of laryngeal tumors; suspected abscess.

C. Chest: Mediastinal and hilar lymphadenopathy; tumor staging with respect to invasion of vessels or pericardium; aortic dissection; aortic aneurysm; congenital anomalies of the heart (especially pulmonary atresia) when echocardiography is inconclusive.

D. Abdomen: Clarification of CT findings when surgical clip artifacts degrade images; follow-up liver metastasis (or hepatoma) after partial hepatectomy (because of less clip artifact compared with CT); retroperitoneal lymphadenopathy when CT cannot differentiate blood vessels or diaphragmatic crus; preoperative staging of large hypernephroma; differentiation of benign nonhyperfunctioning adrenal adenoma from malignant adrenal mass; complementary to CT in evaluation of liver lesions, especially regarding metastatic disease and possible tumor invasion of hepatic or portal veins; differentiation of cavernous hemangioma of the liver from cancer.

E. Pelvis: Staging of cancers of the uterus, cervix, and prostate; complementary to CT for staging of cancer of the urinary bladder and prostate; recurrent rectal cancer following abdominal-perineal resection.

F. Musculoskeletal System: Joints (except where a prosthesis is in place), especially knees and hips; shoulders for rotator cuff tear and instability; wrists for carpal tunnel syndrome; temporomandibular joint; extent of primary or malignant tumor (bone and soft tissue); aseptic necrosis of the femoral head or elsewhere; infections of bone and soft tissue; marrow disorders and contusions; stress fractures.

G. Spine: MRI is the best examination to begin the workup of most abnormalities of the spine and cord, especially disk disease; spinal stenosis; partial or complete block; metastatic or primary tumor; syringohydromyelia; most arteriovenous malformations (see limitations, below); myelitis.

Risks & Contraindications

Cardiac pacemaker; intraocular metallic foreign body; intracranial aneurysm clips; cochlear implants; some artificial cardiac valves; life support devices.

Patient Preparation

Sedation for patients unable to lie still. Screening CT of orbits to rule out metallic foreign body in eye if history uncertain. For examination of the abdomen and pelvis, the colon should be clean, the patient should be NPO for 6 hours, and glucagon should be given during the study in order to ablate gastrointestinal peristalsis and reduce motion artifact.

Limitations

Sensitivity to motion artifacts; need for intravenous contrast (such as gadolinium DTPA) for subarachnoid lesions and for small extra-axial masses; gastrointestinal opacification not yet readily available; claustrophobia; detection of calcification; dural-based or perimedullary arteriovenous malformations are easily missed because of their small size (supine myelography better); detection of loose bodies; osseous encroachment of the spinal canal and neural foramina can be exaggerated by patient movement; cerebrospinal fluid pulsation artifacts may mimic flow void associated with arteriovenous malformation; contraindications include mechanical life support equipment. Inferior to CT in the setting of acute trauma because it is insensitive to acute hemorrhage, incompatible with life support and traction devices, and inferior in detection of bony injury and foreign bodies and because it requires longer imaging time.

Usual Billed Amount

$1400.00–2000.00.

Alternatives

CT scan.

Advantages

No beam-hardening artifacts; exquisite sensitivity to lesions; multiplanar capability; no ionizing radiation; can demonstrate flowing blood; intracranial cryptic vascular malformations can be detected.

II. GENERAL RADIOLOGY & NUCLEAR MEDICINE

INFLAMMATORY & NEOPLASTIC IMAGING

LEUKOCYTE SCAN

Radiopharmaceuticals
111 In oxine-labeled leukocytes

Indications
Fever of unknown origin, postoperative patient, suspected abscess, pyelonephritis, osteomyelitis.

Risks & Contraindications
High radiation dose to spleen. Sterile handling of leukocytes necessary. Contraindicated in pregnancy because of the hazard of ionizing radiation to the fetus.

Patient Preparation
Patients must be able to hold still during relatively long acquisition times (5–10 minutes). Venous blood is drawn and the patient's leukocytes are harvested and labeled in vitro prior to reinjection. Process requires 1–2 hours. Scanning takes place 24 hours later. Homologous donor leukocytes should be used in neutropenic patients.

Limitations
Twenty-four-hour delayed imaging may be contraindicated in critically ill patients. Imaging may be performed as early as 4 hours at the expense of lower sensitivity for detection of infection (can detect 30–50% of those abscesses detected at 24 hours). False-negative scan possible in theory as a consequence of antibiotic administration or in chronic infection. Perihepatic or splenic infection foci can be missed as a result of normal leukocyte accumulation in these organs; liver and spleen scan is a necessary adjunct in this situation. Many causes of false-positive scans such as swallowed leukocytes, bleeding, indwelling tubes and catheters, surgical skin wound uptake, bowel activity due to inflammatory processes. Leukocytes may also accumulate in tumors in the absence of infection. Pulmonary uptake is nonspecific and has low predictive value for infection.

Usual Billed Amount
$725.00–900.00.

Alternatives
Ultrasound or CT for assessment of suspected abscess, particularly in critically ill patient, where 24-hour delayed imaging is undesirable. Bone scan and gallium scan often complementary in assessment of osteomyelitis.

Advantages
Although false-positive causes of uptake exist, the leukocyte scan is highly sensitive (98%) for infection—in contrast to gallium. Sensitivity for detection of abdominal source of infection is higher with indium, since leukocytes do not normally accumulate in abdominal organs other than liver and spleen. In patients with fever of unknown origin, total body imaging is advantageous compared to CT scan or ultrasound. Preliminary imaging as early as 4 hours is possible but less sensitive. Especially helpful prior to CT when that study is limited by patient's inability to ingest oral contrast for opacification of the gastrointestinal tract, which is necessary for an abscess search on CT. A positive leukocyte scan can guide such a CT study.

GALLIUM SCAN

Radiopharmaceuticals
67 Ga citrate

Indications
Fever of unknown origin, infection (particularly chronic), inflammatory processes (most useful in lung), tumor (largely replaced by CT).

Risks & Contraindications
Not advisable in pregnancy because of the risk of ionizing radiation to the fetus. Patient must be reliable to return for imaging 72 hours after injection.

Patient Preparation
Gallium dose is injected 72 hours prior to imaging.

Limitations
Long time (2–3 days) necessary for clearance of background activity prior to imaging. Normal accumulation in bowel and reticuloendothelial system may obscure detection of abdominal abscess. Early accumulation of activity in kidneys (< 24 hours) may impair evaluation. Because of the poor imaging characteristics of gallium, resolution may be insufficient for detection of lesions less than 2 cm in lung, brain, and bone. Even larger lesions may be missed in the abdomen and pelvis, where background activity is high.

Usual Billed Amount
$725.00–925.00.

Alternatives

Leukocyte scan more specific for infection. Radionuclide bone scan often complementary in evaluation of osteomyelitis. CT has largely replaced gallium in evaluation of cancer. Plain chest radiograph or CT for evaluation of pulmonary disease.

Advantages

Gallium more sensitive than CT or chest x-ray in detection of pulmonary disease such as *Pneumocystis carinii* pneumonia, sarcoidosis, and other inflammatory processes. Gallium may be more helpful than leukocyte scan in assessment of chronic infection.

NERVOUS SYSTEM

SPINE MRI

Indications

Diseases involving the spine and cord except where CT is superior (see above).

Risks & Contraindications

Contraindicated in patients with cardiac pacemakers, intraocular metallic foreign bodies, intracranial aneurysm clips, cochlear implants, some artificial heart valves, and life support devices.

Patient Preparation

Sedation of agitated patients; screening CT of orbits if history suggests possible metallic foreign body in the eye.

Limitations

Less useful in detection of calcification, small spinal vascular malformations, acute spinal trauma (because of longer acquisition time, incompatibility with life support devices and inferior detection of bony injury). Subject to motion artifacts.

Usual Billed Amount

$1300.00–2000.00.

Alternatives

CT, bone scan.

Advantages

Provides exquisite spatial resolution; multiplanar imaging capability; no beam-hardening artifacts, as can sometimes occur with bone on CT; no ionizing radiation.

SPINE CT

Indications

Evaluation of structures that are not well visualized on MRI, such as ossification of the posterior longitudinal ligament, tumoral calcification, osteophytic spurring, and retropulsed bone fragments after trauma.

Risks & Contraindications

Contraindicated in pregnancy because of the potential harm of ionizing radiation to the fetus. Use of contrast agents for CT myelography is associated with infrequent but substantial risks, such as those associated with intravenous contrast administration.

Patient Preparation

Normal hydration; sedation of agitated patients.

Limitations

MRI is unequivocally superior in evaluation of the spine and cord except for conditions mentioned in Indications (above). Artifacts from metal prostheses degrade images. Generally limited to transaxial views.

Usual Billed Amount

$850.00–1250.00. With myelographic contrast, add $450.00–500.00.

Alternatives

MRI.

Advantages

Can guide percutaneous fine-needle aspiration of possible tumor or abscess; rapid; superb spatial resolution.

BRAIN SCAN

Radiopharmaceuticals

99m Tc pertechnetate (TcO_4)
99m Tc diethylenetriamine pentaacetic acid (DTPA)
99m Tc glucoheptonate
SPECT agents (single photon emission computed tomography)
123 I iodoamphetamine (IMP)
99m Tc hexamethyl-propyleneamine oxime (HMPAO)

Indications

Establishment of brain death, suspected herpes simplex encephalitis, seizures, neuropsychiatric disorders. SPECT imaging: Alzheimer's dementia and stroke.

Risks & Contraindications

Caution in pregnancy is advised because of the risk of ionizing radiation to the fetus.

Patient Preparation

Sedation in agitated patients. Premedication with potassium perchlorate when using TcO_4 in order to block choroid plexus uptake.

Limitations

Limited resolution. Delayed imaging (1–4 hours) often required. Regional blood flow with SPECT reflects relative distribution; one cannot extrapolate to absolute flow measurement, as with positron emission tomography (PET).

Usual Billed Amount

$450.00–950.00.

Alternatives

CT, MRI.

Advantages

Functional information. Portable capability of brain scan can be valuable in ICU for assessment of brain death. Earlier detection of stroke (compared with CT and MRI) because of focal hypoperfusion with SPECT agents.

CISTERNOGRAPHY

Radiopharmaceuticals

111 In DTPA

Indications

Hydrocephalus (particularly normal pressure), shunt patency, cerebrospinal fluid rhinorrhea or otorrhea.

Risks & Contraindications

Strict sterile precautions for intrathecal injection. Caution in pregnancy is advised because of the risk of ionizing radiation to the fetus.

Patient Preparation

For suspected cerebrospinal fluid leak, the patient's nose or ears should be packed with cotton pledgets prior to administration of dose. Sedation of agitated patients. Must follow strict sterile precautions for intrathecal injection.

Limitations

Availability of 111 indium. Patients must be able to hold still. Requires multiple delayed imaging sessions up to 48–72 hours after injection.

Usual Billed Amount

$550.00–700.00.

Alternatives

CT often complementary.

Advantages

Functional information, particularly in distinguishing normal pressure hydrocephalus from senile atrophy in elderly patients. Very sensitive in detecting cerebrospinal fluid leaks.

CARDIOVASCULAR SYSTEM

MYOCARDIAL PERFUSION

Radiopharmaceuticals

201 thallium chloride
Tc-99m isonitro compounds (sestamibi)
Tc-99m teboroxime

Indications

Evaluation of atypical chest pain. Detection of presence, location, and extent of myocardial ischemia. Determine functional significance of coronary artery stenosis demonstrated by angiography.

Risks & Contraindications

Recent infarct. Risk of arrhythmia, ischemia, infarct, and, rarely, death. Testing during exercise on a treadmill is optimal, but, in cases of peripheral vascular disease or of neurovascular or musculoskeletal disorders, pharmacologic stress can be induced with dipyridamole. Dependence on aminophylline (inhibitor of dipyridamole) is a contraindication to the use of dipyridamole. Patient must be able to hold still for single photon emission computed tomography (SPECT). Caution in pregnancy because of the risk of ionizing radiation to the fetus.

Patient Preparation

Exercise and thallium administration should be performed in fasting state. Patients optimally should remain fasting between stress and redistribution. Dipyridamole may be administered orally or intravenously prior to thallium, though intravenous route is greatly preferred. Both stress and rest tests are performed. Stress is induced with exercise or when exercise is not possible (or safe) by pharmacologic vasodilators such as dipyridamole or adenosine.

Limitations

The patient must be carefully monitored during stress on treadmill or pharmacologic stress—optimally, under the supervision of a cardiologist. Submaximal stress decreases sensitivity for ischemia. Imaging must begin immediately following stress to prevent early redistribution. Patients should not eat heavily or exercise between stress and redistribution images. Patients must return for redistribution images 4 hours following stress. SPECT, which increases sensitivity, may not be available at some institutions. Interpretation of study may be difficult in severe three-vessel coronary artery disease.

Usual Billed Amount
$575.00–1300.00.

Alternatives
Radionuclide ventriculography often complementary. Coronary angiography is "gold standard."

Advantages
Highly sensitive for detection of physiologically significant coronary stenosis. Noninvasive.

MYOCARDIAL INFARCT SCANNING

Radiopharmaceuticals
99m Tc pyrophosphate
111 In-labeled antimyosin monoclonal antibody

Indications
For determination of localization and extent of acute myocardial infarction.

Risks & Contraindications
Patient must be able to hold still. Caution in pregnancy because of the risk of ionizing radiation to the fetus.

Patient Preparation
Sedation of agitated patients.

Limitations
Pyrophosphate scan most sensitive at 48–72 hours. Sensitivity of pyrophosphate lower for nontransmural infarcts. Location of infarct also affects sensitivity (highest for anterior wall; lowest for inferior wall). Patients with unstable angina may have falsely positive thallium scan. Pyrophosphate scan may be positive in patients who have undergone recent cardioversion. Pyrophosphate scan may be persistently positive in up to 20% of patients with remote histories of infarct.

Usual Billed Amount
$500.00–750.00.

Alternatives
Myocardial isoenzymes and electrocardiographic evaluation. Radionuclide ventriculography often complementary. Coronary angiography for identification of occluded vessels.

Advantages
Pyrophosphate imaging identifies acutely infarcted myocardium—in contrast to thallium and coronary angiography. Also helpful in the evaluation of perioperative infarcts in patients who have undergone recent cardiac surgery where creatine kinase and electrocardiographic findings may be misleading. Utility optimal at 3–4 days when enzymes are no longer elevated.

RADIONUCLIDE VENTRICULOGRAPHY

Radiopharmaceuticals
99m Tc-labeled red blood cells

Indications
Evaluation of patients with ischemic heart disease, other cardiomyopathies, response to pharmacologic therapy of heart disease, effects of cardiotoxic drugs.

Risks & Contraindications
Recent infarct is a contraindication to exercise ventriculography, as arrhythmia, ischemia, infarct, and, rarely, death can occur with exercise. Caution advised in pregnancy because of the risk of ionizing radiation to the fetus. Sterile technique required in handling of red cells.

Limitations
Requires labeling and reinjection of red cells if in vitro labeling is used; in vivo labeling is done without withdrawing any of the patient's blood. Gated data acquisition may be difficult in patients with severe arrhythmias, in which case "list mode" acquisition sometimes is possible (after gate acquisition). Limited to resting study in patients who are unable to exercise on a supine bicycle. Right ventricle less reliably isolated at equilibrium than left ventricle. Valvular function better evaluated by echocardiography.

Usual Billed Amount
$500.00–1200.00.

Alternatives
Thallium perfusion scan often complementary. Cardiac echogram. Cardiac catheterization ventriculography. Gated magnetic resonance imaging.

Advantages
Noninvasive. Resting ejection fraction is a reproducible index that can be used for prognosis as well as to follow the course of disease and the response to therapy. More reproducible and comprehensive survey of both resting global (percent ejection fraction) and regional (segmental) myocardial contractility than echocardiography. First-pass studies can estimate left-to-right shunt fraction.

VASCULAR ULTRASOUND

Indications

Evaluation of deep venous thrombosis; extremity vascular grafts; patency of inferior vena cava, portal vein, and hepatic veins. Carotid Doppler indicated for symptomatic carotid bruit, atypical transient ischemic attack, monitoring after endarterectomy, and baseline prior to major vascular surgery.

Risks & Contraindications

None

Patient Preparation

None

Limitations

Technique is very operator-dependent; not sensitive to ulcerated plaque; may be difficult to diagnose tight stenoses versus occlusion and to distinguish acute from chronic deep venous thrombosis.

Usual Billed Amount

$300.00–475.00.

Alternatives

Angiography

Advantages

Noninvasive; no ionizing radiation; imaging in all planes; can be portable.

CHEST

CHEST RADIOGRAPH

Indications

Evaluation of pleural and parenchymal pulmonary disease, mediastinal disease, cardiogenic and noncardiogenic pulmonary edema, congenital and acquired cardiac disease. Screening for traumatic aortic rupture (though angiography is the standard). Evaluation of possible pneumothorax (expiratory upright film) or free-flowing pleural effusion (decubitus views).

Risks & Contraindications

Caution in pregnancy because of the potential harm of ionizing radiation to the fetus.

Patient Preparation

None

Limitations

Difficult to distinguish between causes of hilar enlargement (ie, vasculature versus lymphadenopathy); less sensitive than CT regarding small parenchymal nodules, mild mediastinal lymphadenopathy, bronchiectasis, and early interstitial lung disease. Also, the latter can be better characterized with CT.

Usual Billed Amount

$130.00–165.00. Portable, add $60.00–75.00.

Alternatives

Computed tomography

Advantages

Inexpensive, widely available.

VENTILATION-PERFUSION SCAN

Radiopharmaceuticals

99m Tc macroaggregated albumin (MAA, perfusion)
133 xenon (ventilation)
99m Tc DTPA aerosol (ventilation)

Indications

Pulmonary embolism, preoperative evaluation of patients with COPD or those who are candidates for pneumonectomy, burn inhalation injury.

Risks & Contraindications

The number of particles injected should be reduced in patients with severe pulmonary artery hypertension. Patients must be able to cooperate for ventilation portion of examination. However, an isolated ventilation study can be helpful, since a normal examination effectively rules out pulmonary embolus. Caution advised in pregnancy because of the risk of ionizing radiation to the fetus.

Patient Preparation

Current chest radiograph is essential.

Limitations

Adequate means of trapping xenon. When ventilation with xenon is performed prior to perfusion scan, identification of ventilation-perfusion mismatch may be limited by single posterior ventilation image. Correlation with chest radiograph is mandatory for interpretation. High proportion of indeterminate studies in patients with underlying lung disease. Low probability scan still has an up to 10% possibility of pulmonary embolus.

Usual Billed Amount

$550.00–600.00 (ventilation or perfusion)

Alternatives
Pulmonary angiography.

Advantages
Noninvasive. Functional information in preoperative assessment.

GASTROINTESTINAL SYSTEM

UPPER GASTROINTESTINAL STUDY

Indications
Air-contrast technique demonstrates esophageal, gastric, and duodenal mucosa for evaluation of inflammatory disease and other subtle mucosal abnormalities. This technique requires patient cooperation and mobility, since thick barium is used to coat the mucosa following gaseous distention with ingested CO_2 particles. To accomplish this, the patient must be able to roll over (360 degrees) on the x-ray table (multiple times), hold on inspiration, and follow directions. Single-contrast technique is less demanding of the patient, uses thin barium, and is suitable for evaluation of possible outlet obstruction, peristalsis, gastroesophageal reflux and hiatal hernia, esophageal cancer, esophageal varices. Water-soluble contrast (Gastrografin) is suitable for evaluation of anastomotic leak or gastrointestinal perforation, but can be dangerous (see below).

Risks & Contraindications
Aspiration of water-soluble contrast material incites severe pulmonary edema and may be lethal, but aspiration of barium generally is well tolerated; perforation with barium can cause a granulomatous inflammatory reaction; insensitive to limited or contained perforation. Caution in pregnancy because of hazards of exposure of fetus to x-rays.

Patient Preparation
Patient *must* be NPO for 8 hours.

Limitations
Identification of a lesion does not prove it to be the site of blood loss in patients with gastrointestinal bleeding; endoscopy is required, and the presence of barium delays both endoscopy (because it will obliterate the findings and can ruin the endoscope) and body CT examination (because it will cause severe artifact); retained gastric secretions prevent mucosal coating with barium; patient cooperation and ability to move about is required.

Usual Billed Amount
$400.00–500.00.

Alternatives
Endoscopy.

Advantages
Mucosal evaluation with double-contrast examination; no sedation required; less expensive than endoscopy.

ENTEROCLYSIS

Indications
Location of site of intermittent partial small bowel obstruction; extent of Crohn's disease; small bowel disease in patients with persistent gastrointestinal bleeding who have normal upper gastrointestinal and colonic evaluations; metastatic disease to small bowel.

Risks & Contraindications
Because radiation exposure is substantial during the lengthy fluoroscopic examination required, this modality should be used sparingly in children and women of childbearing age. *Must not be used if the patient might be pregnant.*

Patient Preparation
Colonic cleansing and 24 hours of clear liquid diet. (The latter is the more important part of the preparation and is crucial in order to cleanse the small bowel of particulate matter.)

Limitations
Requires nasogastric or orogastric intubation and manipulation of tube to position it beyond the ligament of Treitz; "biphasic" examination is then performed with barium (for "single contrast") followed by methylcellulose (for "double contrast") introduced by means of a hemodialysis pump at a controlled rate; often cannot optimally evaluate the first loop of jejunum (because of catheter position) or terminal ileum (because of overlapping opacified bowel).

Usual Billed Amount
$600.00–675.00.

Alternatives
Dedicated small bowel examination with oral ingestion of barium and frequent fluoroscopic imaging; CT of abdomen and pelvis.

Advantages
Clarification of possible lesions noted on more traditional barium examination of the small bowel; best means of establishing small bowel as normal; con-

trolled high rate of flow of barium can elicit dilatation at site of intermittent partial obstruction.

PERORAL PNEUMOCOLON

Indications

The best means of evaluation of the terminal ileum by means of insufflation of air per rectum after orally ingested barium has reached the cecum.

Risks & Contraindications

Contraindicated in patients with toxic megacolon (because of air enema and risk of perforation).

Patient Preparation

The patient should take a clear liquid diet for 24 hours as well as colon cleansing.

Limitations

Undigested food in the small bowel interferes with the evaluation.

Usual Billed Amount

Adds about $50.00–75.00 to the cost of upper gastrointestinal series.

Alternatives

CT for wall thickening.

Advantages

Best evaluation of terminal ileum; can be performed concurrently with upper gastrointestinal series.

BARIUM ENEMA

Indications

Double-contrast technique (air and thick barium; also called "pneumocolon") for evaluation of colonic mucosa in patients with suspected inflammatory or neoplastic disease; single-contrast technique (thin barium) for investigation of possible fistulous tracts or bowel obstruction, large or palpable masses in the abdomen, diverticulitis, and for debilitated patients, who cannot maneuver adequately for the double-contrast technique.

Risks & Contraindications

Contraindicated in patients with toxic megacolon because of risk of perforation.

Patient Preparation

Colon cleansing with enemas, cathartic, and clear liquid diet (1 day in young patients; may take 2 days in older patients); possible use of intravenous glucagon (which inhibits peristalsis) for spasm versus mass lesion during the study.

Limitations

Retained fecal material; requires patient cooperation and movement; marked diverticulosis precludes evaluation of possible neoplastic lesion in that area; evaluation of right colon occasionally incomplete or limited by reflux of barium across ileocecal valve as well as overlapping opacified small bowel; presence of barium delays colonoscopy and body CT; abnormal finding may still require colonoscopy for diagnostic confirmation by visual inspection or biopsy.

Usual Billed Amount

Double-contrast ("pneumocolon"), $525.00–575.00

Single-contrast, $375.00–425.00.

Alternatives

Colonoscopy, abdominopelvic CT for possible wall thickening.

Advantages

Mucosal evaluation; no sedation required; less risky and less expensive than colonoscopy.

HYPAQUE (DIATRIZOATE) ENEMA

Indications

Evaluation of sigmoid or cecal volvulus; anastomotic leak or other type of perforation; differentiation of colonic versus distal small bowel obstruction; therapeutic for obstipation.

Risks & Contraindications

Contraindicated in patients with toxic megacolon because of risk of perforation.

Patient Preparation

Colonic cleansing is desirable but not always necessary.

Limitations

Demonstrates only colonic morphologic features and not mucosal abnormalities.

Usual Billed Amount

About $400.00–425.00.

Alternatives

Colonoscopy.

Advantages

Water-soluble contrast medium is evacuated much faster than barium (because it does not adhere to the mucosa), so it can be followed immediately or within several hours by oral ingestion of barium for evaluation of possible distal small bowel obstruction.

ABDOMINAL PLAIN RADIOGRAPH (KUB [Kidneys, Ureters, Bladder])

Indications

Assessment of bowel gas pattern (eg, gastric outlet obstruction, ileus, small bowel obstruction, etc), pneumoperitoneum, pneumatosis intestinalis (intramural air). Good screening test for renal calculi (90% are radiopaque) but not for gallstones (only 15% are radiopaque).

Risks & Contraindications

Caution in pregnancy because of the risk of ionizing radiation to the fetus.

Patient Preparation

None.

Limitations

Supine film alone is inadequate to rule out pneumoperitoneum (see alternatives). Obstipation may obscure lesions. Subtle gut abnormalities may not be detected.

Usual Billed Amount

$150.00–230.00. Portable, add $60.00–75.00.

Alternatives

Upright chest radiograph with KUB best for possible pneumoperitoneum; left lateral (down) decubitus KUB for pneumoperitoneum in patients who cannot stand; CT for gut wall air or thickening as well as the site and cause of obstruction; barium fluoroscopic evaluation for intermittent small bowel obstruction (preferably enteroclysis).

Advantages

Inexpensive, widely available, easy to perform.

GASTROINTESTINAL BLEEDING SCAN

Radiopharmaceuticals

99m Tc-labeled red cells
99m Tc sulfur colloid

Indications

Evaluation of upper or lower gastrointestinal blood loss.

Risks & Contraindications

Caution advised in pregnancy because of the risk of ionizing radiation to the fetus. Sterile technique required in handling of red cells if in vitro labeling is used.

Patient Preparation

None.

Limitations

Bleeding must be active during time of imaging. Sulfur colloid imaging positive only if bleeding is active within 10–15 minutes of injection, whereas labeled red cells demonstrate intermittent bleeding for up to 24 hours. When sulfur colloid is used, upper gastrointestinal bleeding can be obscured by liver and spleen activity. Longer imaging time required for labeled red cells because of higher background activity. The presence of free pertechnetate (poor labeling efficiency) can lead to gastric, kidney, and bladder activity that can be misinterpreted as sites of bleeding. Penile radioactivity is often present with both labeled red cells and sulfur colloid and may mimic rectal bleeding.

Usual Billed Amount

$625.00–850.00.

Alternatives

Angiography.

Advantages

Noninvasive compared to angiography. Longer period of imaging possible, which aids in detection of intermittent bleeding. Both labeled red cells and sulfur colloid can detect bleeding rates of as little as 0.05–0.10 mL/min (angiography requires active bleeding of about 0.5 mL/min). However, while there is greater potential for false-positive interpretation of labeled red cell scan, this method has been shown to be more sensitive than sulfur colloid for detection of gastrointestinal bleeding.

GASTRIC EMPTYING

Radiopharmaceuticals

99m Tc sulfur colloid in solid portion of meal
111 In DTPA in liquid portion of meal

Indications

Dumping syndrome, vagotomy, gastric outlet obstruction due to inflammatory or neoplastic disease, effects of drugs, diabetes mellitus, and other causes of gastroparesis.

Risks & Contraindications

Not advisable in pregnancy due to risk of ionizing radiation to fetus.

Patient Preparation

Fasting for 4–6 hours. Must be able to eat a 300-g meal consisting of liquids and solids.

Limitations

Meaningful data requires adherence to standard protocol and establishment of normal values.

Usual Billed Amount
$380.00–575.00.

Alternatives
Gastrointestinal endoscopy. Barium fluoroscopic examination for upper gastrointestinal series demonstrates peristalsis but cannot quantitate emptying.

Advantages
Gives functional information not available by other means of evaluation.

ESOPHAGEAL REFLUX

Radiopharmaceuticals
99m Tc sulfur colloid in 300 mL liquid

Indications
Evaluation of heartburn, regurgitation, and recurrent aspiration pneumonia.

Risks & Contraindications
Not advisable in pregnancy because of the risk of ionizing radiation to the fetus.

Patient Preparation
Fasting for 4–6 hours. Must be able to consume 300 mL of liquid.

Limitations
Incomplete emptying of esophagus may mimic reflux. Use of abdominal binder to increase lower esophageal pressure may not be tolerated in patients who have undergone recent abdominal surgery.

Usual Billed Amount
$470.00–650.00.

Alternatives
Barium fluoroscopy, endoscopy, lower esophageal sphincter pressure measurements, acid reflux study.

Advantages
Noninvasive and well tolerated. More sensitive than fluoroscopy, endoscopy, and measurement of lower esophageal sphincter pressure. Similar to acid reflux test in sensitivity. Permits quantitation of reflux. Can also evaluate aspiration into lung.

GALLBLADDER, PANCREAS, LIVER, & SPLEEN

LIVER & SPLEEN SCAN

Radiopharmaceuticals
99m Tc sulfur colloid
99m Tc heat-damaged red blood cells (spleen)

Indications
Metastatic or primary tumor, inflammatory process, palpable mass, organomegaly, elevated hepatic enzymes, alcoholic liver disease, thrombocytopenia, search for accessory spleen, suspected subphrenic abscess.

Risks & Contraindications
Caution in pregnancy advised because of the risk of ionizing radiation to the fetus.

Patient Preparation
None.

Limitations
Diminished sensitivity for small (< 2 cm), deep lesions. SPECT increases sensitivity; can detect 1–1.5 cm lesions. Nonspecific; unable to distinguish solid from cystic or inflammatory or neoplastic tissue. Lower sensitivity for diffuse hepatic tumor; may be difficult to distinguish from liver disease due to other causes. Artifacts can be caused by dense foreign body within gastrointestinal tract (eg, barium).

Usual Billed Amount
$575.00–775.00.

Alternatives
Ultrasound for evaluation of solid or cystic mass. CT more sensitive than scintigraphy and ultrasound, particularly for detection of deep lesions. MRI offers the advantage of improved tissue specificity.

Advantages
Better sampling and more sensitive than ultrasound. May detect lesions missed by CT as a result of isodensity. Reproducible means of following response to chemotherapy.

HEPATOBILIARY SCAN

Radiopharmaceuticals
99m Tc N-substituted iminodiacetic acids (IDA)

Indications

Suspected acute cholecystitis or common bile duct obstruction. Functional status of hepatocytes and biliary excretion. Hepatocellular dysfunction, obstruction from stone, tumor or infection, biliary atresia. Assessment of biliary bypass patency.

Risks & Contraindications

Caution in pregnancy because of the risk of ionizing radiation to the fetus.

Patient Preparation

Fasting 4–6 hours.

Limitations

Does not demonstrate cause of obstruction (ie, tumor or gallstones). Sensitivity my be lower for acalculous cholecystitis. May not be able to evaluate biliary excretion if hepatocellular function is severely impaired. May require delayed imaging (up to 24 hours) to distinguish acute from chronic cholecystitis. Visualization may be expedited by use of intravenous morphine sulfate. Nonvisualization or delayed visualization (false-positive) can occur in hyperalimentation, nonfasting, prolonged fasting, acute pancreatitis, severe hepatocellular disease.

Usual Billed Amount

$475.00–575.00.

Alternatives

Oral cholecystogram, ultrasonography, CT for acute cholecystitis (especially acalculous).

Advantages

Hepatobiliary functional information. Not dependent on intestinal absorption, as in oral cholecystography. Can be performed in patients with elevated bilirubin (up to 10–20 mg/dL). Does not expose patients to risk of iodinated contrast media. Normal gallbladder visualization effectively excludes acute cholecystitis (sensitivity approximately 95%).

GALLBLADDER ULTRASOUND

Indications

Demonstrates cholelithiasis (95% sensitive), gallbladder wall thickening, pericholecystic fluid, intra- and extrahepatic biliary dilatation.

Risks & Contraindications

None.

Patient Preparation

Preferably NPO for 6 hours to optimize gallbladder distension and thereby enhance its visualization.

Limitations

Difficult in obese patients; presence of barium obscures sound waves; examination is very operator-dependent.

Usual Billed Amount

$200.00–250.00.
For complete abdomen, $375.00–425.00.

Alternatives

Computed tomography, oral cholecystography.

Advantages

Noninvasive; no ionizing radiation; can be portable; imaging in all planes; can guide fine-needle aspiration, percutaneous transhepatic cholangiography, and biliary drainage procedures.

ORAL CHOLECYSTOGRAM

Indications

Fluoroscopic evaluation of suspected cholelithiasis when clinical symptoms are highly suggestive but the ultrasound is normal or equivocal. Can assess gallbladder function and possible chronic cholecystitis.

Risks & Contraindications

Cannot be performed in patients with elevated bilirubin (> 3 mg/dL). Contraindicated in pregnancy because of the potential harm of ionizing radiation to the fetus.

Patient Preparation

Iopanoic acid (Telepaque) or tyropanoate sodium (Bilopaque) is taken orally the night before the examination. Both are excreted via the biliary system, and so the gallbladder becomes opacified with dense bile. To avoid contraction and emptying of the gallbladder, the patient is kept NPO. Test may be repeated in 24 hours for "double-dose" examination if gallbladder is not visualized initially.

Limitations

Less sensitive for cholelithiasis than ultrasound. Test sensitivity depends on intestinal absorption and liver function. Many reasons for false-negative results, as nonvisualization of the gallbladder can be caused by other factors besides obstruction of the cystic duct (eg, tablets were not absorbed by the gut).

Usual Billed Amount

$250.00–300.00.

Alternatives

Ultrasound (much more sensitive for cholelithiasis).

Advantages

Compliments ultrasound.

ENDOSCOPIC RETROGRADE CHOLANGIOPANCREATOGRAPHY (ERCP)

Indications

Primary sclerosing cholangitis, AIDS cholangitis, cholangiocarcinoma. Demonstrates cause, location, and extent of extrahepatic biliary obstruction (eg, choledocholithiasis). Can diagnose pancreatic carcinoma as well as chronic pancreatitis. Assessment of possible pancreatic ductal communication with persistent pseudocyst.

Risks & Contraindications

May cause pancreatitis (1%), cholangitis (< 1%), duodenal perforation and peritonitis or hemorrhage (especially if sphincterotomy is performed), and death (rare). Risk of procedure-induced pancreatitis higher in patients with concurrent or recent (< 6 weeks) acute pancreatitis; possible infection of communicating pancreatic pseudocyst; contraindicated in pregnancy because of potential harm of ionizing radiation to the fetus.

Patient Preparation

NPO for 6 hours. Sedation is required, and patient must be monitored by a registered nurse during the examination.

Limitations

Requires endoscopy.

Usual Billed Amount

$700.00–750.00.

Alternatives

Transhepatic cholangiography.

Advantages

Can sometimes preclude surgery. If stone is suspected, ERCP offers therapeutic potential (sphincterotomy and extraction of common bile duct stone). Finds gallstones in up to 14% of patients with symptoms but negative ultrasound and oral cholecystogram.

LIVER ULTRASOUND

Indications

Differentiation of cystic versus solid intrahepatic lesions; screening for primary and metastatic liver tumors; surgical staging of some liver tumors by assessment of vascular contiguity or invasion; color Doppler sonography for Budd-Chiari syndrome to assess patency of hepatic veins and intrahepatic inferior vena cava as well as patency of portal vein; evaluation of intra- and extrahepatic biliary dilatation; ascites.

Risks & Contraindications

None.

Patient Preparation

None.

Limitations

Technique is very operator-dependent; more difficult in obese patients.

Usual Billed Amount

$200.00–250.00.
For complete abdomen, $375.00–425.00.

Alternatives

CT, MRI, liver-spleen scan.

Advantages

Noninvasive; no radiation; can be portable; imaging in all planes; can guide fine-needle aspiration and percutaneous biliary drainage procedures.

LIVER CT

Indications

Metastatic disease, hepatoma, abscess, biliary dilatation, acute cholecystitis (especially acalculous). Imaging is optimized by rapid (2 mL/s) bolus injection of intravenous contrast medium and dynamic imaging (complete entire liver within 2 minutes). Sensitivity for vascular lesions increased with delayed imaging (4–6 hours after intravenous contrast) because of hepatocyte uptake of iodine in normal tissue but not tumors). Sensitivity for small lesions increased with computed tomography arterial portography (CTAP). The latter is performed with dynamic imaging during intravenous contrast infusion via a catheter placed in the superior mesenteric artery during angiography.

Risks & Contraindications

Contraindicated in pregnancy because of the potential harm of ionizing radiation to the fetus; use of intravenous contrast is associated with infrequent but substantial risk (see above); CTAP has associated risk inherent in angiography and catheterization of the superior mesenteric artery.

Patient Preparation

Normal hydration, preferably NPO 4–6 hours. Optimal study is performed after opacification of the gastrointestinal tract in order to perform a complete abdominal examination, but this is not necessary if the study is isolated to the liver.

Limitations

Patient must be able to hold on inspiration to suspend diaphragmatic motion during image acquisition. Intravenous contrast is necessary for most examinations. Cannot differentiate malignant from inflammatory or other benign processes without tissue sampling; cannot image in multiple planes to clarify sometimes confusing findings.

Usual Billed Amount

$900.00–1250.00. For nonionic contrast, add $270.00–360.00.

Alternatives

US, MRI, liver-spleen scan.

Advantages

Best first study for liver metastases; can evaluate entire abdomen (and pelvis) in same setting; rapid; readily available; can guide percutaneous fine-needle aspiration biopsy and drainage procedures; CTAP most sensitive modality for metastatic disease (but has more false-positives).

PANCREAS CT

Indications

Pancreatic carcinoma for staging as well as diagnosis; acute pancreatitis for diagnosis as well as possible complications and follow-up of pseudocysts; chronic pancreatitis; evaluation of biliary obstruction; endocrine tumors of pancreas.

Risks & Contraindications

Contraindicated in pregnancy because of the potential harm of ionizing radiation to the fetus; use of intravenous contrast media is associated with infrequent but substantial risks (see above).

Patient Preparation

Normal hydration, preferably NPO 4–6 hours. Opacification of the gastrointestinal tract in order to differentiate adjacent bowel loops from pancreas.

Limitations

Cannot always differentiate malignant from inflammatory mass of the pancreas, and tissue sampling is necessary for definitive diagnosis of carcinoma. Cannot diagnose hemorrhagic component of pancreatitis. Intravenous contrast is necessary for detection of carcinoma and for staging of acute pancreatitis, especially regarding tissue necrosis in the latter. Optimal imaging requires scanner capable of contiguous thin (0.5 cm) sections and dynamic imaging. Patient must be able to hold on inspiration in order to suspend diaphragmatic motion.

Usual Billed Amount

$900.00–1250.00. For nonionic contrast, add $270.00–360.00.

Alternatives

Ultrasound (less sensitive because of overlying bowel gas); ERCP (evaluates pancreatic duct by not organ morphology).

Advantages

Superb spatial resolution and sensitivity to morphologic abnormality due to malignant and inflammatory disease; best means of imaging the pancreas; can diagnosis early necrosis in acute pancreatitis; can guide percutaneous fine-needle aspiration biopsy for possible carcinoma as well as catheter placement for drainage of peripancreatic fluid collections in acute pancreatitis.

PANCREAS ULTRASOUND

Indications

Identification of peripancreatic fluid collections, pseudocysts, and pancreatic ductal dilatation. Intraoperative US good for detection of small endocrine tumors of pancreas.

Risks & Contraindications

None.

Patient Preparation

Preferably NPO for 46 hours.

Limitations

Pancreas may be obscured by overlying bowel gas; presence of barium in the gastrointestinal tract obscures sound waves; technique very operator-dependent; cannot detect areas of early necrosis in acute pancreatitis as can CT.

Usual Billed Amount

$200.00–250.00.
For complete abdomen, $375.00–425.00.

Alternatives

Computed tomography; ERCP for evaluation of pancreatic duct.

Advantages

Noninvasive; no ionizing radiation; can be portable; imaging in all planes; good for evaluation of splenic and portal vein patency; intraoperative ultrasound best means of identifying isolated or multiple small endocrine tumors of pancreas.

GENITOURINARY SYSTEM

INTRAVENOUS PYELOGRAPHY (IVP)

Indications

Uroepithelial neoplasm, calculus, papillary necrosis and medullary sponge kidney; screening for urinary system injury following trauma.

Risks & Contraindications

Intravenous contrast material imposes a hazard of allergic reactions, resulting in death in 1:40,000–1:30,000 examinations (see Chapter 18); increasing data suggest reduced risk with nonionic contrast medium, which increases the cost approximately $250.00–270.00. Blood urea nitrogen and serum creatinine may be permanently increased in patients with diabetes mellitus and multiple myeloma but return to normal in others.

Patient Preparations

Adequate hydration; colon cleansing is not essential but is preferred.

Limitations

Optimal evaluation of the collecting system only; suboptimal evaluation of the renal parenchyma; does not adequately evaluate cause of ureteral deviation.

Usual Billed Amount

$400.00–875.00.

Alternatives

Ultrasound, CT, MRI.

Advantages

Better at evaluation of collecting system than alternative techniques listed above.

RENAL SCAN

Radiopharmaceuticals

99m Tc diethylenetriamine pentaacetic acid (DTPA, glomerular filtration rate agent)
131 I orthoiodohippurate (Hippuran, tubular agent)
99m Tc dimercaptosuccinic acid (DMSA, parenchymal agent)
99m Tc glucoheptonate (parenchymal agent)
99m Tc mercaptoacetyltriglycerine (MAG3, tubular and glomerular agent)

Indications

Evaluation of renal blood flow and function in acute or chronic renal failure. Evaluation of both medical and surgical complications of renal transplant. Estimation of glomerular filtration rate (GFR) and effective renal plasma flow (ERPF). Determination of relative function prior to nephrectomy. Parenchymal agents useful in assessment of obstruction. Captopril used in suspected renovascular hypertension.

Risks & Contraindications

Relatively high radiation dose with 131 I Hippuran. Good hydration and frequent bladder emptying advised in order to minimize radiation exposure to bladder mucosa. Caution in pregnancy because of the risk of ionizing radiation to the fetus.

Patient Preparation

None—though best results are obtained with patient well hydrated.

Limitations

Findings of poor renal blood flow and function are nonspecific as to etiology. High background activity with extremely poor renal function limits usefulness in evaluation of other factors such as obstruction, relative function, cortical lesions. Estimation of GFR and ERPF are based on anatomic presumptions that often introduce error. One- to 4-hour delayed images necessary with parenchymal agents. Parenchymal agents are nonspecific and do not give information about solid versus cystic nature of lesions.

Usual Billed Amount

$570.00–775.00.

Alternatives

Intravenous pyelography, ultrasound, CT.

Advantages

Functional information available without risk of iodinated contrast used in IVP. Provides quantitative information not available by other means. Renal scan before and after captopril challenge provides relatively noninvasive screen for renal vascular hypertension with better sensitivity than does unilateral renal scan alone.

ENDOCRINE SYSTEM

THYROID UPTAKE & SCAN

Radiopharmaceuticals

99m TcO_4
123 I sodium iodide
131 I sodium iodide

Indications

Uptake indicated for evaluation of clinical hypothyroidism, hyperthyroidism, and thyroiditis and for calculation of therapeutic dosage. Uptake also used to assess effect of thyroid-stimulating and suppressing medications. Thyroid scanning indicated for evaluation of palpable nodules, mediastinal mass, hyperthyroidism, and in patients with history of head and neck irradiation. Total body scanning used for evaluation of metastatic thyroid cancer.

Risks & Contraindications

Not advised in pregnancy because of the risk of ionizing radiation to the fetus (iodides cross placenta and concentrate in fetal thyroid). Because of possible adjacent radiation exposure with therapeutic ^{131}I, patients should be instructed by nuclear medicine personnel regarding precautionary measures.

Patient Preparation

Administration of dose in the fasting state—nothing by mouth for 4–6 hours—aids absorption.

Substances that interfere with thyroid uptake should be withheld for days to several weeks depending on substance (prior TcO_4 scan, iodides in vitamins and medicines, radiographic procedures using iodinated contrast, thyroid replacement medications, antithyroid drugs).

Limitations

Many common substances interfere with thyroid uptake and scanning (see substances to withhold, above). Small size of the thyroid gland requires use of a pinhole collimator. This technique does not distinguish solid from cystic masses. Poor resolution with 131 I limits use to uptake and total body scanning. Delayed imaging is required with iodides (123 I, 6 hours; 131 I total body, 72 hours).

Usual Billed Amount

$375.00–725.00.

Alternatives

Ultrasound often complementary.

Advantages

Functional information as well as morphology. Identification of "cold" nodules that have a greater risk of malignancy. Identification of ectopic thyroid tissue. Imaging of total body with one dose (131 I).

PARATHYROID SCAN

Radiopharmaceuticals
201 thallium chloride
99m TcO_4 subtraction

Indications

Suspected parathyroid adenoma.

Risks & Contraindications

Patient must be able to hold still. Caution in pregnancy is advised because of the risk of ionizing radiation to the fetus. Use of agents that block thyroid uptake of TcO_4 (see above).

Patient Preparation

None required.

Limitations

Pinhole collimator recommended by some. Computer subtraction requires strict patient immobility between administration of radiopharmaceuticals. Small adenomas may not be detected (< 5–10 mm).

Usual Billed Amount

$425.00–525.00.

Alternatives

Ultrasound often complementary.

Advantages

Identification of hyperfunctioning tissue, particularly when planning surgery.

ADRENAL MEDULLARY IMAGING

Radiopharmaceuticals
123 I metaiodobenzylguanidine (MIBG)

Indications

Suspected pheochromocytoma, especially when CT is negative or equivocal and when multiple or extra-adrenal tumor is suspected.

Risks & Contraindications

Contraindicated in pregnancy because of the risk of ionizing radiation to the fetus. Because of the relatively high dose of 131 I, patients must be instructed regarding precautionary measures by nuclear medicine personnel.

Patient Preparation

Administration of Lugol's iodine solution (to block thyroid uptake) prior to and following administration of dose. Patient must be compliant (return for imaging on 1–3 consecutive days).

Limitations

High radiation dose to adrenal gland. High cost and limited availability of radiopharmaceutical (MIBG). Delayed imaging (1–3 days) necessitates return of patient.

Usual Billed Amount
$1000.00–1400.00.

Alternatives
CT, MRI.

Advantages
Test is useful for localization of pheochromocytomas—particularly those found in extra-adrenal tissue—and for multiple lesions.

MUSCULOSKELETAL SYSTEM

BONE SCAN

Radiopharmaceuticals
99m Tc phosphate compounds (methylene diphosphonate—MDP most widely used)

Indications
Primary or metastatic neoplasm, infection, arthritis, metabolic disorders, trauma, avascular necrosis, joint prosthesis.

Risks & Contraindications
Caution in pregnancy because of the risk of ionizing radiation to the fetus.

Patient Preparation
None.

Limitations
Nonspecific. Correlation with plain film radiographs often necessary. Two- to 3-hour delayed images necessary. In patients with poor renal function, image quality may be poor because of high background activity. Resolution often insufficient for localization of disease in distal extremities, head, and spine; in these instances, SPECT is often useful. In evaluation of infection, it may be difficult to distinguish osteomyelitis from cellulitis or septic joint. Dual imaging with gallium or with indium-labeled leukocytes can be helpful but not always definitive. Diagnosis of infection also limited by surgery or fracture. In avascular necrosis, bone scan may be hot, cold, or normal, depending on the stage. Bone scan may be negative within the first 24 hours after trauma.

Usual Billed Amount
$625.00–800.00.

Alternatives
Plain film radiography, MRI for tumor or infection. Leukocyte or gallium scan often complementary for infection.

Advantages
Entire body is surveyed. Highly sensitive compared to plain film radiography for detection of bone neoplasm. Best screening examination for skeletal metastases. Bone scan may be positive much earlier in osteomyelitis (24 hours) compared to plain film (10–14 days).

Geriatric Medicine & the Elderly Patient

4

Neil M. Resnick, MD

Of all the people who have ever lived to age 65, more than two-thirds are currently alive. Although the implications of this startling statistic are usually viewed in demographic and economic terms, the impact of age on medical care is also substantial and requires significant alterations in the approach to the older patient.

GENERAL PRINCIPLES OF GERIATRIC MEDICINE

Human aging is best characterized as the progressive constriction of each organ system's homeostatic reserve. This decline, often referred to as "homeostenosis," begins in the third decade and is gradual, linear, and variable among individuals. Each organ system's decline (Table 4–1) is independent of changes in other organ systems and is influenced by diet, environment, and personal habits.

Several principles follow from these facts: Individuals become more dissimilar as they age, belying any stereotype of aging; an abrupt decline in any system or function is always due to disease and not to "normal aging"; "normal aging" can be attenuated to some extent by modification of risk factors (eg, increased blood pressure, smoking, sedentary lifestyle); and "healthy old age" is not an oxymoron. In the absence of disease, the decline in homeostatic reserve should cause no symptoms and impose no restrictions on activities of daily living regardless of age. In short, "old people are sick because they are sick, not because they are old."

Appreciation of these facts may make it easier to understand the striking increases that have occurred in longevity. Average life expectancy is now 17 years at age 65, 11 years at age 75, 6 years at age 85, 4 years at age 90, and 2 years at age 100. Moreover, the bulk of those years is characterized by a lack of significant impairment—only 35% of people over age 85 are impaired in any activity required for daily living, and only 20% reside in a nursing home. These striking and often unappreciated figures have substantial implications for disease screening, patient counseling, and medical decision making.

On the other hand, as individuals age they are more likely to suffer from disease, disability, and drug side effects. Combined with the decrease in physiologic reserve, these added burdens (if present) make the older person more vulnerable to any additional environmental, pathologic, or pharmacologic insult. Understanding the implications of these facts is crucial if one is to provide optimal care to older patients, especially those over age 75–80.

The following principles underlie the remainder of the chapter:

(1) First, the onset of a new disease in the elderly generally affects the organ system rendered most vulnerable by prior physiologic and pathologic change. Because the most vulnerable organ system often differs from the newly diseased organ system, disease presentation is often atypical in the elderly. For example, less than one-fourth of older patients with hyperthyroidism present with the classic triad of goiter, tremor, and exophthalmos; more likely are atrial fibrillation, confusion, depression, syncope, and weakness. Significantly, because the "weakest link" is so often the brain, the lower urinary tract, or the cardiovascular or musculoskeletal system, a limited number of presenting symptoms predominate—acute confusion, depression, falling, incontinence, and syncope—no matter what the underlying disease. *Thus, regardless of the presenting symptom in older people, the differential diagnosis is often largely the same.The corollary is equally important: the organ system usually associated with a particular symptom is less likely to be the source of that symptom in older individuals than in younger ones.* Thus, compared with middle-aged individuals, acute confusion in older patients is less often due to a new brain lesion, incontinence to a bladder disorder, falling to a neuropathy, or syncope to heart disease.

(2) Second, because of their impaired compensatory mechanisms, disease in older patients often presents at an earlier stage. Heart failure may be precipitated by only mild hyperthyroidism, significant cognitive dysfunction by only mild Alzheimer's disease, urinary retention by only mild prostatic enlargement, and nonketotic hyperosmolar coma by only mild glucose intolerance. Thus, paradoxically,

Table 4–1. Selected age-related changes and their consequences.[1]

Organ or System	Age-Related Physiologic Change[2]	Caused by Age-Related Physiologic Change	Caused by Disease, Not Age
General	↑ Body fat ↓ Total body water	↑ Volume of distribution for fat-soluble drugs ↓ Volume of distribution for water-soluble drugs	Obesity Anorexia
Eyes and ears	Presbyopia Lens opacification ↓ High-frequency acuity	↓ Accommodation ↑ Susceptibility to glare Difficulty discriminating words if background noise is present	Blindness Deafness
Endocrine	Impaired glucose ↓ Thyroxine clearance (and production) ↑ ADH, ↓ renin, and ↑ aldosterone ↓ Testosterone ↓ Vitamin D absorption and activation	↑ Glucose level in response to acute illness ↓ T_4 dose required in hypothyroidism Osteopenia	Diabetes mellitus Thyroid dysfunction ↓ Na^+, ↑ K^+ Impotence Osteoporosis, osteomalacia
Respiratory	↓ Lung elasticity and ↑ chest wall stiffness	Ventilation-perfusion mismatch and ↓ PaO_2	Dyspnea, hypoxia
Cardiovascular	↓ Arterial compliance and ↑ systolic BP → LVH ↓ β-Adrenergic responsiveness ↓ Baroreceptor sensitivity and ↓ SA note automaticity	Hypotensive response to ↑ HR, volume depletion, or loss of atrial contraction ↓ Cardiac output and HR response to stress not standing, volume depletion Impaired blood pressure response to standing, volume depletion	Syncope Heart failure Heart block
Gastrointestinal	↓ Hepatic function ↓ Gastric acidity ↓ Colonic motility ↓ Anorectal function	Delayed metabolism of some drugs ↓ Ca^{2+} absorption on empty stomach Constipation	Cirrhosis Osteoporosis, B_{12} deficiency Fecal impaction Fecal incontinence
Hematologic and immune systems	↓ Bone marrow reserve (?) ↓ T cell function ↑ Autoantibodies	False-negative PPD response False-positive rheumatoid factor, antinuclear antibody	Anemia Autoimmune disease
Renal	↓ GFR ↓ Urine concentration-dilution (see also Endocrine, above)	Impaired excretion of some drugs Delayed response to salt or fluid restriction or overload; nocturia	↑ Serum creatinine ↓ or ↑ Na^+
Genitourinary	Vaginal or urethral mucosal atrophy Prostate enlargement	Dsypareunia, bacteriuria ↑ Residual urine volume	Symptomatic UTI Urinary incontinence; urinary retention
Musculoskeletal	↓ Lean body mass, muscle ↓ Bone density	Osteopenia	Functional impairment Hip fracture
Nervous system	Brain atrophy ↓ Brain catechol synthesis ↓ Brain dopaminergic synthesis ↓ Righting reflexes ↓ Stage 4 sleep	Benign senescent forgetfulness Stiffer gait ↑ Body sway Early awakening, insomnia	Dementia, delirium Depression Parkinson's disease Falls Sleep apnea

[1]From Resnick NM: Geriatric medicine. In: *Harrison's Principles of Internal Medicine,* 13th ed. Isselbacher K et al (editors). McGraw-Hill, 1994.
[2]Changes generally observed in healthy elderly subjects free of symptoms and detectable disease in the organ system studied. The changes are usually important only when the system is stressed or other factors are added (eg, drugs, disease, or environmental challenge); they rarely result in symptoms otherwise.

treatment of the underlying disease may be easier in the elderly because it is less advanced at the time of presentation. Another ramification of this principle is that drug side effects can occur even with low doses of drugs that usually produce no side effects in younger people. For instance a mild anticholinergic agent (eg, diphenhydramine) may cause confusion, diuretics may precipitate urinary incontinence, digoxin

may induce depression even with normal serum levels, and over-the-counter sympathomimetics may precipitate urinary retention in older men with mild prostatic obstruction.

(3) Third, since many homeostatic mechanisms are often compromised concurrently, there are usually multiple abnormalities amenable to treatment, and small improvements in each may yield dramatic benefits overall. For instance, cognitive impairment in patients with Alzheimer's disease may be exacerbated by hearing or visual impairment, depression, heart failure, electrolyte imbalance, and anemia. Similarly, urinary incontinence is often worsened by fecal impaction, medications, excess urinary output, and arthritis. In each case, substantial functional improvement can result from treating the contributing factors even if—as in Alzheimer's disease—specific treatment of the underlying condition is not possible.

(4) Fourth, many findings that are abnormal in younger patients are relatively common in older people and may not be responsible for a particular symptom. Such findings include bacteriuria, premature ventricular contractions, low bone mineral density, impaired glucose tolerance, and uninhibited bladder contractions. Instead, they may be only incidental findings that result in missed diagnoses and misdirected therapy. For instance, finding bacteriuria should not end the search for a source of fever in an acutely ill older patient, nor should an elevated random blood sugar—especially in an acutely ill patient—be incriminated as the cause of neuropathy. On the other hand, other abnormalities must not be dismissed as due to old age—eg, there is no anemia, impotence, depression, or confusion of old age (Table 4–1).

(5) Fifth, because symptoms in older people are often due to multiple causes, the diagnostic "law of parsimony" often does not apply. For instance, fever, anemia, retinal embolus, and a heart murmur prompt almost a reflex diagnosis of endocarditis in a younger patient but are more apt to reflect aspirin-induced blood loss, a cholesterol embolus, insignificant aortic sclerosis, and a viral illness in an older patient. "Never think of one diagnosis when three will do" is a useful maxim.

Moreover, even when the diagnosis is correct, treatment of a single disease in an older patient is unlikely to result in cure. For instance, in a younger patient, incontinence due to uninhibitable bladder contractions is treated effectively with a bladder relaxant medication. However, in an older patient whose incontinence is also associated with fecal impaction, who is taking medications that cloud the sensorium, and who has impaired mobility and manual dexterity due to arthritis, treatment of the bladder abnormality alone is unlikely to restore continence. On the other hand, disimpaction, discontinuation of the offending medications, and treatment of the arthritis are likely to restore continence without the need for a bladder relaxant. Failure to recognize these principles often leads to prescribing "ineffective" therapy and unjustified therapeutic nihilism towards older patients.

(6) Sixth, because the older patient is more likely than a younger one to suffer the adverse consequences of disease, treatment—and even prevention—may be equally or even more effective. For instance, the benefits to survival of exercise as well as thrombolysis and beta-blocker therapy after a myocardial infarction, appear to be at least as impressive in older patients as in younger ones; and treatment of hypertension, as well as immunization against influenza and pneumococcal pneumonia, is even more effective in older patients than in younger ones. In addition, prevention in older patients often must be seen in a broader context. For instance, although efforts to increase bone density may be futile in older patients, fracture may still be prevented by interventions that improve balance, strengthen legs, treat contributing medical conditions, replete nutritional deficits, remove adverse medications, and reduce environmental hazards.

In summary, optimal treatment of the older person usually requires treating much more than the organ system usually associated with the disease—and often even permits ignoring that organ system entirely.

These principles guide the remainder of the discussion, which focuses on their specific implications for the evaluation and treatment of geriatric patients.

HISTORY TAKING WITH ELDERLY PATIENTS

It must not be assumed that an older patient is unable to provide a reliable medical history. However, obtaining a history often takes longer than in younger patients since there is often a multitude of complaints (rather than a "chief" complaint), and adequate time must be allotted. At the initial interview, the examiner should note any impairment of hearing or speech, mood disturbance, or apparent difficulty with thought processes, any of which may interfere with history taking. If the patient is unable to comprehend or communicate, data should be sought from family and friends. If the patient has a hearing aid, it should be working properly. It is important to note any differences between the patient's chief complaint and that of the family; both need to be attended to.

Drug History

It is essential to review *all* drugs the patient has been taking, because 75% of the elderly take over-the-counter medications which often cause or contribute to symptoms and interact with other medication. Since many older patients do not consider these "drugs" worth mentioning to a physician, the patient or family should bring in both prescribed and nonprescribed drugs. Each should be reviewed, inquiring about the reason for taking the drug, its prescribed dosage and actual frequency of administration, its expiration date, and any adverse side effects the patient may attribute to the drug.

In addition, it is important to realize that drug abuse and alcoholism are more common in the elderly than is generally recognized, especially in depressed patients. Moreover, because of enhanced susceptibility to the side effects of these agents and decreased metabolism, relatively small amounts can yield adverse consequences.

Dietary History

Many elderly patients have limited nutritional intake of not only calories and protein but also iron, calcium, and vitamin D. In addition to concurrent medical illness, reasons include inadequate income, problems with shopping or preparing meals, eating habits, impaired senses of taste and smell, difficulties with dentures, cognitive impairment, or depression. On the other hand, some elderly people take excess vitamins, many of which (eg, vitamins A and D) may accumulate and cause toxicity. Thus, especially for the older patient with weight loss, the differential diagnosis must go well beyond the usual list of medical causes.

Falls History

One-third of community-dwelling elderly and a higher proportion of institutionalized elderly fall annually. Aside from the serious injuries that may result, a debilitating "fear of falling" may also ensue, leading many elderly people to restrict their activities and social life. Since the causes are disparate, often serious, and usually treatable, falls are important to ask about.

Incontinence History

Close to 50% of women and 25% of men over age 80 residing in the community have some urinary incontinence, but only 10–30% of primary care physicians are aware of the extent of this treatable problem. Many patients are too embarrassed to mention this distressing symptom, which can have serious psychologic and social impact and increase the risk of institutionalization; for these reasons, it is important to ask about incontinence.

Psychiatric History

Depression and anxiety are relatively common in the elderly. Although the prevalence of depression does not change with age, the highest incidence of suicide in the USA is in white men over age 75. Psychiatric illness in old people can often be successfully treated. Once medical and pharmacologic causes have been excluded, psychiatric consultation should be recommended without hesitation if the history arouses concern about the patient's emotional status.

Questions about sexual feelings or problems should not be avoided. Such problems are often treatable, and elderly patients may welcome an opportunity to discuss such matters.

A careful history is essential in any elderly patient who has recently become confused. To assume that confusion is a manifestation of dementia without having inquired into factors such as other illnesses, new medications, or increased doses of drugs that may produce delirium may overlook an easily correctable and serious condition. To make matters worse, if delirium is overlooked and assumed to be dementia with behavioral abnormalities, tranquilizers or psychotropic agents may be prescribed (especially in the nursing home or hospital) that may then further aggravate the delirium.

Advance Directives

All patients should be asked whether they have drafted advance directives, and, if they have, a copy should be placed in the record. Such directives may consist of (1) a health care proxy or durable power of attorney for health care, in which patients designate a surrogate decision-maker who makes health care decisions if the patient cannot; (2) a living will or medical directive, in which patients specify their desires for treatment in specific situations if they cannot communicate at the critical time; or (3) a combination of the two. Different forms are legally binding in different states, and most can be completed by the patient and proxy with witnesses, without the need for legal counsel.

Whether or not the patient has formally drafted these directives, it is useful to indicate in the record who should make health care decisions if the patient is no longer able to do so. Patients should then be encouraged to discuss with the physician as well as the designated proxy their feelings about resuscitation, intubation, feeding tubes, hospitalization, etc, in their current state of health and possible future declining states of health. Although the list of possibilities is potentially endless, it is often possible to predict the situations that might arise, such as intubation for a patient with COPD or a feeding tube in the event of a major stroke for a patient with atrial fibrillation. In addition, such conversations can and should take place over time. The early elicitation of a patient's preferences and values can often help both physicians and families in subsequent difficult decisions by giving all surrogate decision-makers the sense that they are doing "as the patient would have wanted."

Annas GJ: The health care proxy and the living will. N Engl J Med 1991;324:1210.

Emanuel LL, Emanuel EJ: The medical directive: A new comprehensive advance care document. JAMA 1989; 261;3288.

Pellegrino ED: Ethics. JAMA 1992;268:354. (Brief but excellent review of advance directives.)

Sachs GA, Siegler M: Guidelines for decision making when the patient is incompetent. J Crit Ill 1991;6:348.

PHYSICAL EXAMINATION

For patients being seen for routine evaluation, it is useful to screen for conditions that could impair function; a simple inventory is shown in Table 4–2. For the remainder of patients, because of the multiple interacting and contributing causes of dysfunction in the elderly, a complete physical examination is essential, including pelvic examination in women and rectal examination in both sexes. Certain features of the examination should receive special attention, depending in part on clues from the history. Weight and postural blood pressure should be measured at each visit. Vision and hearing should also be checked; if hearing is impaired, excess cerumen should be removed from the external auditory canals. Denture fit should be assessed. The oral cavity should be inspected with the dentures removed, remembering that malignant lesions of the mouth are more often red than white. Although thyroid disease becomes more common with age, because the sensitivity and specificity of related findings are substantially lower than

Table 4–2. Procedure for functional assessment screening in the elderly.

Target Area	Assessment Procedure	Abnormal Result	Suggested Intervention
Vision	Test each eye with Jaeger card while patient wears corrective lenses (if applicable).	Inability to read greater than 20/40.	Refer to ophthalmologist.
Hearing	Whisper a short, easily answered question such as "What is your name?" in each ear while the examiner's face is out of direct view.	Inability to answer question.	Examine auditory canals for cerumen and clean if necessary. Repeat test; if still abnormal in either ear, refer for audiometry and possible prosthesis.
Arm	Proximal: "Touch the back of your head with both hands." Distal: "Pick up the spoon."	Inability to do task.	Examine the arm fully (muscle, joint, and nerve), paying attention to pain, weakness, limited range of motion. Consider referral for physical therapy.
Leg	Observe the patient after instructing as follows: "Rise from your chair, walk 10 feet, return, and sit down."	Inability to walk or transfer out of chair.	Do full neurologic and musculoskeletal evaluation, paying attention to strength, pain, range of motion, balance, and traditional assessment of gait. Consider referral for physical therapy.
Continence of urine	Ask, "Do you ever lose your urine and get wet?"	"Yes."	Ascertain frequency and amount. Search for remediable causes, including local irritations, polyuric states, and medications. Consider urologic referral.
Nutrition	Weigh the patient. Measure height.	Weight is below acceptable range for height.	Do appropriate medical evaluation.
Mental status	Instruct as follows: "I am going to name three objects (pencil, truck, book). I will ask you to repeat their names now and then again a few minutes from now." [See text discussion.]	Inability to recall all three objects after 1 minute.	Administer Folstein Mini-Mental Status Examination. If score is less than 24, search for causes of cognitive impairment. Ascertain onset, duration, and fluctuation of overt symptoms. Review medications. Assess consciousness and affect. Do appropriate laboratory tests.
Depression	Ask: "Do you often feel sad or depressed?" or "How are your spirits?"	"Yes" or "Not very good, I guess."	Administer Geriatric Depression Scale. If positive (normal score, 0–10), check for antihypertensive, psychotropic, or other pertinent medications. Consider appropriate pharmaceutical or psychiatric treatment.
ADL-IADL[2]	Ask, "Can you get out of bed yourself?" "Can you dress yourself?" "Can you make your own meals?" "Can you do your own shopping?"	"No" to any question.	Corroborate responses with patient's appearance; question family members if accuracy is uncertain. Determine reasons for the inability (motivation compared with physical limitation). Institute appropriate medical, social, or environmental interventions.
Home environment	Ask, "Do you have trouble with stairs inside or outside of your home?" Ask about potential hazards inside the home with bathtubs, rugs, or lighting.	"Yes."	Evaluate home safety and institute appropriate countermeasures.
Social support	Ask, "Who would be able to help you in case of illness or emergency?"	. . .	List identified persons in the medical record. Become familiar with available resources for the elderly in the community.

[1]Modified from Lachs MS et al: A simple procedure for general screening for functional disability in elderly patients. Ann Intern Med 1990;112:699.
[2]Activities of daily living–instrumental activities of daily living.

in younger individuals, the physical examination can rarely corroborate or exclude the possibility of thyroid dysfunction in older patients. The breast examination should not be overlooked, since older women are more likely to have breast cancer and less likely to do breast self-examination than younger women. In auscultating the chest, the physician must recall that the systolic murmur of aortic sclerosis is a common finding and may be difficult to differentiate from aortic stenosis, especially since the presence of a fourth heart sound in an elderly patient does not imply clinically significant cardiac disease, and the carotid upstroke normally increases due to age-related arterial stiffening.

In inactive patients and those with fecal or urinary incontinence, one should check for fecal impaction. In patients with urinary incontinence—especially men—a distended bladder must be sought, since it may be the only finding in urinary retention; perineal sensation and the bulbocavernosus reflex also should be tested. Patients who fall should be observed standing up from a chair, walking 10 feet, turning, returning, and sitting again; abnormalities of gait and steadiness on standing should be evaluated, with the patient's eyes open and closed and in response to a sternal push. Careful examination of the feet and assessment of shoe fit are also important in the patient with gait disturbance. If the patient uses a cane or walker, one should make certain it is the correct length or height (ie, equal to the distance from the wrist crease to the ground) and has a good grip. If the patient is chair-bound or bed-bound, the skin should be examined for reddening or evidence of early ulceration over pressure points. Finally, it should be appreciated that "frontal release signs" (eg, "snout," "glabellar," or palmomental reflexes), as well as absent ankle jerks and vibratory sense in the feet, may be found in elderly patients with no other evidence of neurologic disease.

MENTAL STATUS EXAMINATION

In addition to evaluating mood and affect, some form of cognitive testing is desirable with all elderly patients, even if it involves only checking different components of the history for consistency; for instance, patients may say that they eat well and enjoy fish but later describe a shopping list that includes no fish and only a limited quantity of other items. Remember that patients with mild degrees of dementia may mask intellectual impairment by a cheerful and cooperative manner. Thus, the examiner should always probe for content. For patients who follow the news, ask what stories they're particularly interested in and why; the same applies to reading, social events—even the "soap operas" on television.

If there is any suspicion of a cognitive deficit after this kind of conversational probing, the physician should explain that a mental status evaluation is part of every complete examination, so that the patient will not feel singled out and insulted. An examination that tests only orientation as to person, place, and time is not sufficient to detect mild or moderate intellectual impairment. As a quick screen, simply assessing orientation and asking the patient to draw a clock with the hands at a set time (eg, 10 minutes before 2:00) can be very informative regarding cognitive status, visuospatial deficits, ability to comprehend and execute instructions in logical sequence, and presence or absence of perseveration. For slightly more detailed examinations, many practical mental status tests are available, but the one most widely used is the Mini-Mental Status Examination of Folstein, which provides a numerical score that can be of great value as a baseline test and can be completed in 5–10 minutes. However, regardless of the test employed, the total score is much less useful diagnostically than is knowledge of the specific domain of the deficit. As a general rule, disproportionate difficulty with recent memory suggests dementia, while predominant difficulty with immediate recall (eg, a list of three items) suggests depression. For patients with deficits of attention—recognized by inability to spell "world" backwards, repeat five digits, or recite the months of the year backwards—delirium is probably present and the accuracy of the remainder of the test is dubious. However, the test can only be interpreted accurately in the context of a comprehensive evaluation, and no single question or task can establish or rule out cognitive impairment. Moreover, these are only screening tests, which must be interpreted in the context of the patient's baseline intellectual function; a few incorrect responses has different connotations in a previously gifted individual: An engineer concerned about recent intellectual mistakes should not be reassured by a perfect score on a screening test.

Kane RA, Kane RL: *Assessing the Elderly: A Practical Guide to Measurement.* Lexington Books, 1981.

Siu A: Screening for dementia and assessing its causes. Ann Intern Med 1991;115:122. (Usefulness of mental status screening tests. Although laboratory diagnostic tests are also reviewed, the critique's utility is limited by the absence of available data and by cost-benefit considerations.)

EVALUATION OF FUNCTIONAL CAPACITY IN THE ELDERLY

Simply taking a history, performing a physical examination, and listing medical diagnoses are not sufficient for elderly patients, particularly those who are frail and at high risk for institutional care; a problem list that includes past stroke, metastatic prostatic cancer, and osteoporosis could describe a Supreme Court Justice as well as a bed-bound nursing home patient.

Thus, a clear description of the patient's degree of fitness or functional incapacity based on both medical and psychosocial problems is essential. In addition to the physician, the assessment may include input from the following professionals as necessary:

(1) Medical, psychiatric, and surgical specialists.

(2) A neuropsychologist, for more thorough testing for organicity and localization of deficits as well as evidence of affective or psychotic disorders. In difficult cases, neuropsychologic testing can be helpful in differentiating the causes of cognitive impairment, including depression, Alzheimer's disease, stroke, delirium, and Korsakoff's syndrome. In addition, such testing can identify areas of preserved cognitive function even when the cause of cognitive impairment is known. Such knowledge can be helpful in structuring the patient's environment to optimize function.

(3) A social worker, who assesses the ability of the family, friends, and community agencies to provide those supports that will allow the patient to remain at home. Financial and family problems are often elucidated by the social worker.

(4) An occupational therapist, who assesses the patient's ability to perform the basic activities of daily living (ADLs), which are those activities needed for self-care. Patients who are less incapacitated should be evaluated for their ability to perform more complex functions that require both physical and cognitive ability. These include bathing, dressing, toileting, feeding, getting in and out of bed and chairs, and walking. These tasks are called instrumental activities of daily living (IADLs) and include shopping, cooking, money management, housework, using a telephone, and traveling outside the home. Assessment of these functions and careful consideration of what steps can be taken to help the patient become more independent are often the most important contributions the health team can make in improving the patient's quality of life and preventing or delaying institutionalization.

A home visit is of great value in assessing the patient's ability to function in his or her own environment. It may provide a very different perception from what is gained from the history regarding the patient's ability to cope, eg, a refrigerator and cupboards with little or no staples, rotting food, burned pots, major disarray. Practical advice can be given to the patient or family on how to decrease risks of accidents in the home. These may include installation of handrails, grab bars, better lighting, and smoke alarms as well as elimination of slippery throw rugs or long and loose extension cords.

Many patients on waiting lists for nursing home care can remain in their homes if a comprehensive functional assessment is carried out and appropriate recommendations implemented.

Lachs MS et al: A simple procedure for general screening for functional disability in elderly patients. Ann Intern Med 1990;112:699. (Quick screening device.)

Podsialo D, Richardson S: The timed "up and go": A test of basic functional mobility for frail elderly persons. J Am Geriatr Soc 1991;39:142. (Quick, practical assessment of mobility.)

Wasson JH et al: The prescription of assistive devices for the elderly. J Gen Intern Med 1990;5:46. (Practical suggestions every physician should heed.)

LABORATORY EXAMINATIONS & IMAGING

With few exceptions, standard normal laboratory values are the same for the elderly as for younger adults. Arterial PO_2 declines as a result of age-associated small airway collapse, which is most marked in the dependent portions of the lung; since these are also the best-perfused areas, ventilation-perfusion mismatch results. The resting PaO_2 can be estimated by the following equation:

$$Pao_2 = \left(\begin{array}{c} 104 - 0.42\ \text{supine} \\ \text{or} \\ 104 - 0.27\ \text{sitting} \end{array} \right) \times \text{Age (yrs)}$$

The sedimentation rate rises somewhat with age, but the range of suggested normal values is large and its utility in older patients is poorly established. The fasting blood glucose is not significantly altered by age, but the 2- and 3-hour postprandial blood glucose may be higher than for younger adults. Hemoglobin A_{1c} is useful in managing the elderly diabetic; however, one must keep in mind that there may be a slight increase in levels in nondiabetic elderly patients. Although glomerular filtration rate declines by an average of 40% with age, the variability among individuals—like that of other physiologic parameters—is great, and healthy elderly persons without hypertension may experience little decline. However, in the absence of renal disease, even patients with an age-related decrease in GFR do not have an increased serum creatinine because creatinine production decreases owing to the decline in lean body mass.

THE FRAIL ELDERLY & THE FIVE I'S

Diseases more common in the elderly are listed in Table 4–3 and covered elsewhere in the text. A number of medical problems, however, do not usually present as clear-cut organ-specific diagnoses. These problems are most common in the frail elderly, especially those over 80 years of age, and are often re-

Table 4–3. Diseases more common with aging.

Atherosclerotic cardiovascular and cerebrovascular diseases with resultant myocardial infarction, strokes, multi-infarct dementia, and abdominal aortic aneurysms and peripheral vascular disease (see Chapters 10, 12, and 23).
Cardiac conduction system disease leading to conduction block (see Chapter 10).
Senile dementia of the Alzheimer type (see text).
Polymyalgia rheumatica (see Chapter 19).
Type II diabetes mellitus and nonketototic hyperglycemic coma (see Chapter 26).
Cancer, especially of the colon, prostate, lung, breast, and skin (see Chapter 5).
Pressure ulcers (see Chapter 6).
Tuberculosis (see Chapter 9).
Macular degeneration, cataract, and glaucoma (see Chapter 7).
Deafness (see Chapter 8).
Multiple myeloma, myelodysplasia, and myelofibrosis (see Chapter 13).
Constipation, fecal impaction, and fecal incontinence (see Chapter 14).
Osteoarthritis, spinal stenosis, osteoporosis, hip fracture, crystal disease, and Paget's disease (see Chapter 19).
Parkinson's disease (see Chapter 23).
Depression and suicide (the latter most common in elderly white men) (see Chapter 24).
Chronic obstructive pulmonary disease (see Chapter 9).
Benign prostatic hypertrophy (see Chapter 2).
Diverticulitis and angiodysplasia (see Chapter 14).
Herpes zoster (see Chapters 6 and 31).
Systemic hypothermia (see Chapter 38).

ferred to as the "five I's": (1) intellectual impairment, (2) immobility, (3) instability, (4) incontinence, and (5) iatrogenic drug reactions.

INTELLECTUAL IMPAIRMENT

Dementia is defined as an acquired persistent and progressive impairment of intellectual function with compromise in experience at least two of the following spheres of mental activity: language, memory, visuospatial skills, emotional behavior or personality, and cognition (calculation, abstraction, judgment, etc). It is probably the most feared condition among the aging population. It is important to reassure elderly patients who may have some degree of benign forgetfulness that senile dementia is not inevitable. Clinically significant intellectual impairment affects an estimated 5–10% of people over age 65 and only 20% of people over age 80, though recent estimates are as high as 47% for people over 85. Approximately 60–70% of cases of senile dementia are of the Alzheimer type, and 15–20% are vascular dementias, usually called multi-infarct dementias. These include (1) multiple cortical infarcts, (2) Binswanger's disease (subcortical arteriosclerotic encephalopathy), and (3) lacunar infarcts. Another 15–20% of patients show evidence of both Alzheimer's disease and vascular dementia.

Clinical Features

The earliest manifestation of dementia is usually forgetfulness in the absence of depression and inattentiveness. Many patients with dementia maintain their social graces even in the face of significant cognitive impairment; thus, a clinical impression of preserved intellectual function without mental status testing may miss the diagnosis. As the disease progresses, there is loss of computational ability, word-finding and concentration problems, difficulty with ordinary activities such as dressing, cooking, and balancing the checkbook, then severe memory loss and, ultimately, complete disorientation and social withdrawal. Senile dementia of the Alzheimer type has an insidious onset and is steadily progressive. Multi-infarct dementia is more common in men, associated with hypertension with or without a history of transient ischemic attacks or strokes, and is more likely to progress in a series of recognizably distinct steps. The modified Hachinski Ischemia score (see Table 4–4) is commonly used in making the clinical diagnosis, with a total of four or more suggestive of multi-infarct dementia (Siu reference, above in the section on mental status examination). Although Alzheimer's disease may coexist with multi-infarct dementia, it is important that it be detected since its progression may be slowed by antihypertensive therapy, aspirin therapy, treatment of atrial fibrillation, and smoking cessation.

Diagnosis

Diagnosis is based on the history and on the physical and mental status examinations—supplemented by careful review of the medication list and alcohol intake—and by laboratory investigations to exclude other causes of cognitive impairment. Useful tests include serum electrolytes, calcium, glucose, TSH, vitamin B_{12}, and drug levels; urinalysis; arterial oxygen if hypoxemia is suspected; and MRI or CT scan. These tests should be done in most cases when there are signs of early dementia of relatively short duration (months to 1–2 years). After that time, they should be ordered only upon specific indications.

Table 4–4. Factors suggesting multi-infarct dementia: modified Hachinski Ischemia Score.[1]

Characteristic	Point Score[2]
Abrupt onset	2
Stepwise deterioration	1
Somatic complaints	1
Emotional incontinence	1
History or presence of hypertension	1
History of strokes	2
Focal neurologic symptoms	2
Focal neurologic signs	2

[1]Fischer P, Jellinger K, Gatterer G, Danielczyk W. J Neurol, Neurosing and Psychiatry 1991;54:580.

Neither MRI nor CT scan is diagnostic of Alzheimer's disease, but both are useful in ruling out subdural hematoma, frontal lobe tumor, hydrocephalus, stroke or hemorrhage, and multi-infarct dementia, all of which may mimic dementia of the Alzheimer type. However, an MRI or CT scan "consistent with Alzheimer's" is not diagnostic and may be found in cognitively normal elderly patients and thus should not keep the physician from doing other tests to rule out "treatable dementias."

The significance of the rather frequent diagnosis of Binswanger's disease (subcortical arteriosclerotic encephalopathy) by CT scan or MRI remains to be elucidated, since the finding of periventricular white matter hypodensity may be present in normal as well as in demented patients.

Normal-pressure hydrocephalus should be considered in the mildly demented patient who also has a gait disturbance and urinary incontinence. Surgical procedures for cerebrospinal diversion may be helpful, but it is difficult to predict which patients will show clinical improvement. A short duration of symptoms with early gait disturbance and a specific cause correlate best with surgical benefit. Moderately to severely demented patients are seldom helped by surgery.

Creutzfeldt-Jakob disease is characterized by a rapidly progressive course of dementia, behavioral changes, myoclonus, and rigidity, with periodic triphasic waves on the EEG. This disease has no specific treatment and is uniformly fatal, usually within 1–2 years.

A very small percentage of patients prove to have a condition whose treatment reverses the dementia. *However, regardless of whether a "reversible" dementia is present, cognitive function can often be improved significantly by discontinuation of medications that exacerbate confusion and by detection and treatment of contributing disorders such as heart failure, hypoxia, thyroid disease, anemia, and depression.*

Differential Diagnosis

One of the most important tasks of the physician dealing with older people is to differentiate dementia from depression and from delirium (see Table 4–5). Delirium is a confusional state characterized by inattention, rapid onset, and fluctuating course that may persist for months if untreated. Delirium in the hospitalized elderly patient is easily missed and may be mistaken for dementia. It occurs most commonly in individuals over age 80 with preexisting cognitive impairment. It has multiple causes, the commonest of which are severe illness, drugs, abnormal (either high or low) serum sodium levels, fever, and azotemia. The following other common causes of confusional states may be missed if not specifically looked for.

A. Drugs: A wide variety of agents, including over-the-counter medications, may cause confusion

Table 4–5. *DSM-IIIR* diagnostic criteria for delirium.

A. Reduced ability to maintain attention to external stimuli (eg, questions must be repeated because attention wanders) and to appropriately shift attention to new external stimuli (eg, perseverates answer to a previous question).
B. Disorganized thinking, as indicated by rambling, irrelevant, or incoherent speech.
C. At least 2 of the following:
  (1) Reduced level of consciousness, eg, difficulty keeping awake during examination.
  (2) Perceptual disturbances: misinterpretations, illusions, or hallucinations.
  (3) Disturbance of sleep-wake cycle with insomnia or daytime sleepiness.
  (4) Increased or decreased psychomotor activity.
  (5) Disorientation to time, place, or person.
  (6) Memory impairment, eg, inability to learn new material, such as the names of several unrelated objects, after 5 minutes, or to remember past events, such as history of current episode of illness.
D. Clinical features develop over a short period of time (usually hours to days) and tend to fluctuate over the course of a day.
E. Either (1) or (2):
  (1) Evidence from the history, physical examination, or laboratory tests of a specific organic factor (or factors) judged to be etiologically related to the disturbance.
  (2) In the absence of such evidence, an etiologic organic factor can be presumed if the disturbance cannot be accounted for by any nonorganic mental disorder, eg, manic episode accounting for agitation and sleep disturbance.

in the elderly. The most common are sedatives, hypnotics, H_2 blockers, digoxin, neuroleptics, antidepressants, anticholinergics, antihypertensives, chronic heavy salicylate use, and nonsteroidal anti-inflammatory drugs. If, as sometimes happens, the patient is receiving the same drug under different brand names, there is an increased likelihood of drug-induced confusion.

Chronic alcoholism can occur in the elderly. It is the third most common cause of mental disorder (after dementia and anxiety and phobic disorders) in elderly men but is frequently undiagnosed.

B. Depression: (See Psychiatric History, above; and Management of Depression, below. See also Chapter 24.) Depression of significant degree probably occurs in 5–10% of community-dwelling elderly but is often overlooked. The diagnosis requires the presence of a depressed mood for at least two consecutive weeks plus at least four of eight "vegetative" signs, including *S*leep disturbance, lack of *I*nterest, feelings of *G*uilt, decreased *E*nergy, decreased *C*oncentration, decreased *A*ppetite, *P*sychomotor agitation/retardation, and *S*uicidal ideation. These can be recalled using the mnemonic *SIG E CAPS* (as if prescribing energy capsules). Also helpful diagnostically is a personal or family history of depression, past response to an antidepressant, and the presence of anhedonia. Depression may be superimposed on mild dementia or may even mimic dementia, since decreased attention span, loss of sense of humor, irritability, and poor performance on mental status testing may occur in both conditions. One helpful diagnostic clue is that the depressed patient is more likely to complain of difficulty in answering mental status questions, whereas the demented patient usually is oblivious to the incorrect answers except in the early stages of the disease. Nonetheless, differentiation may be difficult and may warrant a therapeutic trial of antidepressant drugs or psychiatric consultation.

C. Other Psychiatric Problems: Confusion may result from the anxiety and disorienting effect of being in a hospital or other unfamiliar surroundings. Severe anxiety over normal forgetfulness or psychotic behavior may be misdiagnosed as dementia. Sleep deprivation may result in confusion.

D. Sensory Loss: Hearing loss not only leads to social isolation but results in inappropriate answers that may be misinterpreted as evidence of dementia. Behavior resulting from abnormalities of perception in patients with lesions of the nondominant parietal lobe may be mistaken for dementia.

E. Metabolic Disturbances: Hyponatremia is a common cause of confusional state in hospitalized elderly people because of the age-related increase in antidiuretic hormone (ADH) responsiveness to stress (eg, hypovolemia, morphine, trauma) and the syndrome of inappropriate antidiuretic hormone (SIADH) secretion, many of whose causes are common in the elderly (eg, tuberculosis, carcinoma of the lung, head injury, brain tumor, and drugs [phenothiazines, chlorpropamide, carbamazepine, and opiates]). Other metabolic derangements such as hypo- or hyperglycemia, liver failure, renal failure, and cardiopulmonary failure can also cause metabolic confusional states. Confusion due to hypercalcemia is particularly apt to occur in bone disorders that are more often seen in elderly patients (eg, Paget's disease, multiple myeloma, metastatic carcinoma).

F. Endocrine Abnormalities: Thyroid disorders and rarely hyperparathyroidism may cause confusion and be interpreted as senile dementia.

G. Bladder and Bowel Disorders: Acute urinary retention and fecal impaction are easily treated causes of delirium, especially in hospitalized elderly patients. These causes are especially important to identify before initiating neuroleptic therapy, which not only may be unnecessary in such cases but may in fact exacerbate them.

H. Nutritional Deficiencies: Cognitive impairment can be produced by vitamin B_{12}, niacin, riboflavin, and thiamin deficiencies. Many factors including poor appetite, loss of taste and smell, poorly fitting dentures, and difficulty in shopping for and preparing meals as well as alcoholism increase the likelihood of nutritional problems.

I. Trauma: Subdural hematoma must always be considered as a possible cause of confusion, since brain size decreases with age while the venous sinuses are fixed to the dura, predisposing them to rupture with minimal trauma. Falls with head injury may be forgotten or not reported by the patient and unknown to the family, and headache is often absent in chronic subdural hematoma.

J. Brain Tumor: Metastatic lesions and gliomas are the most common brain tumors in old people, but in published reports they are rare as a cause of dementia.

K. Infections: Acute infection in the elderly may cause confusion even in the absence of fever. Chronic infections of lung, bone, kidneys, skin (associated with pressure sores), and the central nervous system (including AIDS) may also present as dementia. Central nervous system syphilis is now a rare cause of dementia.

L. Cardiovascular or Cerebrovascular Accidents: Acute myocardial infarction, acute congestive heart failure, or pulmonary embolism may present as an acute confusional state. Strokes that involve the nondominant parietal lobe or that result in fluent or receptive aphasias are often mistaken for dementia.

Treatment

A. General Measures: The most important first step in management of a "demented" elderly patient is the search for and correction of treatable factors contributing to cognitive impairment (see above).

Until recently, specific therapy for Alzheimer's disease did not exist, including ergoloid mesylates. However, several recent short-term randomized trials have established the efficacy of tacrine and have led to its approval by the FDA. Nonetheless, only about one-third of patients respond. Moreover, response is more significant statistically than clinically; the costs are high; the need for weekly monitoring of liver function is strict; and the long-term efficacy of treatment with tacrine is unknown. Thus, tacrine appears to be useful, if at all, only in the healthy patient with mild to moderate cognitive impairment who is able to comply with close monitoring.

However, the limited efficacy of specific therapy does not mean that the physician has no role in treating the patient and family.

1. Discontinue nonessential medications, particularly sedatives and hypnotics.

2. Treat coexisting medical and psychiatric problems such as heart failure, anemia, depression, malnutrition, thyroid dysfunction, and infections. Improvement in these conditions may result in striking amelioration of behavioral and functional disturbances, although the maximum benefit may not be achieved for weeks or even months.

3. After underlying causes are excluded and environmental manipulation maximized, disruptive behavior should be treated pharmacologically as outlined in Chapter 24, albeit generally with lower doses.

4. Help the patient's family cope with this devastating condition. Legal counsel should be sought regarding plans for ongoing management and ultimate disposition of assets. The family should be told that any abrupt change in the patient's function is due to drugs or disease, not to dementia, and the physician should be alerted. They should be urged to read The Thirty-Six-Hour Day, by Mace and Rabins (Johns Hopkins University Press, 1981) or one of the many other useful guides. Support groups such as the Alzheimer's Association often are of great value to the family and help to anticipate problems. Day care centers also involve the patient and provide a family respite. Watch for signs of elder abuse by an overstressed caregiver.

5. If an advance directive has not been drafted (see above), that should be done as early in the course of the dementia as possible to allow the patient to participate in the difficult ethical decisions that may have to be made in future.

B. Management of Depression: For the hospitalized patient in whom acute depression is delaying recovery or rehabilitation—when correction of medical and pharmacologic contributing factors is ineffective and when there is no prior history of mania or major depression—methylphenidate, 5–10 mg at 8 AM and noon (to avoid insomnia), is often very effective, with benefits discernible in just a few days.

For the remainder of patients with major depression, there is no ideal antidepressant drug. All are about equally effective, but there are significant differences in side effects (see Chapter 24) that must be considered. Rather than memorizing a list of medications, however, one should become comfortable using one or two agents for depressed patients with psychomotor retardation (eg, desipramine, fluoxetine) or agitation (eg, nortriptyline, trazodone); because of its potent anticholinergic and orthostatic side effects, amitriptyline should be avoided whenever possible in older patients. Initial dosage should be low, and dosage increases should be made slowly to avoid serious side effects; low doses of each medication (eg, doxepin, 10–20 mg daily; desipramine, 25–75 mg daily) are often effective in the elderly. Careful follow-up supervision is required in order to anticipate and minimize anticholinergic side effects, orthostatic hypotension, sedating effects, confusion, bizarre mental symptoms, cardiovascular complications, and drug overdose with suicidal intent. Adverse drug reactions should not be assumed to be due to the aging process.

Experience with the tetracyclic agents and other new antidepressants in the elderly has been limited. The monoamine oxidase inhibitors are sometimes of benefit when other antidepressants are ineffective. However, they commonly cause or exacerbate orthostatic hypotension (peak risk at 4–5 weeks) and thus should be used with additional caution in the elderly; they should not be used in combination with the cyclic compounds. Electroconvulsive therapy has been successfully used and is usually well tolerated by elderly patients who remain severely depressed despite drug treatment; however, the addition of maintenance pharmacotherapy is usually required.

Foley JM et al: NIH Consensus Conference: Differential diagnosis of dementing diseases. JAMA 1987;258:3411.

Francis J: Delirium in older patients. J Am Geriatr Soc 1992;40:829.

Howell T, Watts DT: Behavioral complications of dementia: A clinical approach for the general internist. J Gen Intern Med 1990;5:431.

Katzman R, Jackson JE: Alzheimer's disease: Basic and clinical advances. J Am Geriatr Soc 1991;39:516.

NIH Consensus Development Panel. Diagnosis and treatment of depression in late life. JAMA 1992;268:1018.

IMMOBILITY
(Chair- or Bed-Bound)

The main causes of immobility in the elderly are weakness, stiffness, pain, imbalance, and psychologic problems. Weakness may result from disuse of muscles, malnutrition, electrolyte disturbances, anemia, neurologic disorders, or myopathies. The commonest cause of stiffness in the elderly is osteoarthritis, but Parkinson's disease, rheumatoid arthritis, gout, and pseudogout also occur in this age group, and drugs such as haloperidol may also contribute. Polymyalgia rheumatica should not be overlooked in the elderly patient with pain and stiffness, particularly of the pelvic and shoulder girdle, and with associated systemic symptoms (see Chapter 19).

Pain, whether from bone (eg, osteoporosis, osteomalacia, Paget's disease, metastatic bone cancer, trauma), joints (eg, osteoarthritis, rheumatoid arthritis, gout), bursa, or muscle (eg, polymyalgia rheumatica, intermittent claudication or "pseudoclaudication"), may immobilize the patient. Foot problems are common and include plantar warts, ulceration, bunions, corns, and ingrown and overgrown toenails. Poorly fitting shoes are a frequent cause of these disorders.

Imbalance and fear of falling are major causes of immobilization. Imbalance may result from general debility, neurologic causes (eg, stroke; loss of postural reflexes; peripheral neuropathy due to diabetes, alcohol, or malnutrition; vestibulocerebellar abnormalities), anxiety, orthostatic or postprandial hypotension, or drugs (eg, diuretics, antihypertensives, neuroleptics, and antidepressants) or may occur following prolonged bed rest (see Instability, below).

Psychologic conditions such as severe anxiety or depression may produce or contribute to immobilization.

Treatment

A. Consequences: The hazards of bed rest in the elderly are multiple, serious, quick to develop, and slow to reverse. Deconditioning of the cardiovascular system occurs within days and involves fluid shifts, fluid loss, decreased cardiac output, decreased peak oxygen uptake, and increased resting heart rate. Perhaps more striking changes occur in skeletal muscle. At the cellular level, there are decrements in intracellular ATP and glycogen concentrations, increased rates of protein degradation, and loss of contractile velocity and strength, while at the whole muscle level, atrophy, weakness, and shortening are seen. Pressure sores are a third serious complication; mechanical pressure, moisture, friction, and shearing forces all predispose to their development. Thrombophlebitis and pulmonary embolus are additional risks. As a result, within days after being confined to bed, the risk of postural hypotension, falls, skin breakdown, and pulmonary embolus rises rapidly in the older patient. Moreover, recovery from these changes usually takes weeks to months.

B. Management: The most important step is preventive—to avoid bed rest whenever possible. When it cannot be avoided, several measures can be employed to minimize its consequences. Adequate nutrition should be ensured, and the skin over pressure points should be inspected frequently. To minimize cardiovascular deconditioning, patients should be positioned as close to the upright position as possible several times daily. To reduce the risks of contracture and weakness, range of motion exercises should begin immediately and isometric and isotonic exercises should be performed while the patient is in bed. Whenever possible, patients should assist with their own positioning, transferring, and self-care. For individuals confined to a wheelchair, ring-shaped devices ("donuts") should not be used to prevent pressure ulcers, since they cause venous congestion and edema and may actually increase the risk. As long as the patient remains immobilized, pharmacologic (eg, low-dose heparin) or nonpharmacologic means (eg, graduated compression stockings) should be employed to reduce the risk of thrombosis. As mobility becomes feasible, graduated ambulation should begin.

If a pressure ulcer develops, the multiplicity of topical therapies underscores the fact that no single one is clearly more effective than others. Surgical debridement may be required for severely undermined lesions. A special mattress (eg, foam or static air mattress) or air-fluidized bed or water bed may be required for the very debilitated patient.

In addition to treating all identified factors that contribute to immobility, consultation with a physical therapist should be sought. Installing handrails, lowering the bed, and providing chairs of proper height with arms and rubber skid guards may allow the patient to be safely mobile in the home. A properly fitted cane or walker may be helpful. Podiatric care is often essential.

In treating arthritis in the elderly, it must be re-membered that nonsteroidal anti-inflammatory drugs, especially indomethacin, may cause more serious gastrointestinal bleeding than in younger individuals, as well as central nervous system side effects with resultant confusion or even hallucinations. Aspirin remains a useful and inexpensive drug, although chronic use can lead to salicylism. Enteric-coated aspirin may be used for patients with upper gastrointestinal problems. For osteoarthritis, acetaminophen may be as effective as an NSAID.

Allman RM: Pressure ulcers among the elderly. N Engl J Med 1989;320:850.

Bradley JD et al: Comparison of an anti-inflammatory dose of ibuprofen, an analgesic dose of ibuprofen, and acetaminophen in the treatment of patients with osteoarthritis of the knee. N Engl J Med 1991;325:87.

Goldhaber SZ, Morpurgo M, for the WHO/ISFC Task Force on Pulmonary Embolism: Diagnosis, treatment, and prevention of pulmonary embolism. JAMA 1992; 268:1727.

Hoenig HM, Rubenstein LZ: Hospital-associated deconditioning and dysfunction. J Am Geriatr Soc 1991;39:220.

Pressure Ulcer Guideline Panel: Pressure ulcers in adults: Prediction and prevention. AHCPR Publication No. 92–0047. Rockville, MD, 1992.

INSTABILITY
(Physical Instability, Falls, Unstable Gait)

Falls are a major problem for elderly people, especially women. Thirty percent of people over the age of 65 in the community fall each year; and one out of four of those who fall have serious injuries, including 6% who have fractures. Falls are the sixth leading cause of death for older people and a contributing factor in 40% of admissions to nursing homes. Resultant hip problems and fear of falls are major causes of loss of independence. Nonetheless, they must not be viewed as accidental, inevitable, or untreatable.

Causes of Falls

Balance and ambulation require a complex interplay of cognitive, neuromuscular, and cardiovascular function, and the ability to adapt rapidly to an environmental challenge. Balance becomes impaired, and sway increases with age. The resulting vulnerability predisposes the older person to a fall when challenged by an additional insult to *any* of these systems. Thus, a seemingly minor fall may be due to a serious problem, such as pneumonia or myocardial infarction. Much more commonly, however, falls are due to the complex interaction between a variably impaired patient and an environmental challenge. While a warped floorboard may pose little problem for a vigorous, unmedicated, cognitively intact person, it may be sufficient to precipitate a fall and hip fracture in the patient with altered balance, muscle tone, and cognition. Thus, falls in older people are rarely due to a single cause, and effective intervention entails a comprehensive assessment of the patient's intrinsic deficits (usually diseases and medications), the activity engaged in at the time of the fall, and environmental obstacles.

Intrinsic deficits are those that impair sensory input, judgment, blood pressure regulation, reaction time, and balance and gait (Table 4–6). Although some of these may not be treatable, most are, and since the risk of falling is directly related to the number and severity of abnormalities, correction or amelioration of even a few contributory conditions may decrease the risk significantly. As for most geriatric conditions, medications and alcohol use are among the most common, significant, and reversible causes of falling. Other often overlooked but treatable contributors include postprandial hypotension (which peaks 30–60 minutes after a meal), insomnia, urinary urgency, and peripheral edema (which can burden impaired leg strength and gait with an additional 5–10 lb).

Environmental obstacles are listed in Table 4–7 (this list is also useful to give to patients). Since most falls occur in or around the home, a home visit by a visiting nurse, physical therapist, or physician often reaps substantial dividends and is generally reimbursed by third-party payers, including Medicare. Insufficient lighting is an underappreciated factor in many cases. In addition to the number and location of lamps, noting their wattage is also important since—because of a loss of contrast sensitivity—older people often need twice the wattage to maximize acuity; replacement of 60-watt bulbs with 100-watt bulbs may be quite cost-effective.

Complications of Falls

The most common fractures resulting from falls are of the wrist, hip, and vertebrae. There is a high mortality rate (approximately 20% in 1 year) in elderly women with hip fractures, particularly if they were debilitated prior to the time of the fracture.

Fear of falling again is a common but treatable factor in the elderly person's loss of confidence and independence. Referral to a physical therapist for gait training with special devices is often all that is re-

Table 4–6. Intrinsic risk factors for falling and possible interventions.[1]

Risk Factor	Intervention	
	Medical	**Rehabilitative or Environmental**
Reduced visual acuity, dark adaptation, and perception	Refraction; cataract extraction	Home safety assessment
Reduced hearing	Removal of cerumen; audiologic evaluation	Hearing aid if appropriate (with training); reduction in background noise
Vestibular dysfunction	Avoidance of drugs affecting the vestibular system; neurologic or ear, nose, and throat evaluation, if indicated	Habituation exercises
Proprioceptive dysfunction, cervical degenerative disorders, and peripheral neuropathy	Screening for vitamin B_{12} deficiency and cervical spondylosis	Balance exercises; appropriate walking aid; correctly sized footwear with firm soles; home safety assessment
Dementia	Detection of reversible causes; avoidance of sedative or centrally acting drugs	Supervised exercise and ambulation; home safety assessment
Musculoskeletal disorders	Appropriate diagnostic evaluation	Balance-and-gait training; muscle-strengthening exercises; appropriate walking aid; home safety assessment
Foot disorders (calluses, bunions, deformities, edema)	Shaving of calluses; bunionectomy; treatment of edema	Trimming of nails; appropriate footwear
Postural hypotension	Assessment of medications; rehydration; possible alteration in situational factors (eg, meals, change of position)	Dorsiflexion exercises; pressure-graded stockings; elevation of head of bed; use of tilt table if condition is severe
Use of medications (sedatives: benzodiazepines, phenothiazines, antidepressants; antihypertensives; others: antiarrhythmics, anticonvulsants, diuretics, alcohol)	Steps to be taken: 1. Attempted reduction in the total number of medications taken 2. Assessment of risks and benefits of each medication 3. Selection of medication, if needed, that is least centrally acting, least associated with postural hypotension, and has shortest action 4. Prescription of lowest effective dose 5. Frequent reassessment of risks and benefits	

[1]Modified slightly from Tinetti ME, Speechley M: Prevention of falls among the elderly. N Engl J Med 1989;320:1055.

Table 4–7. Environmental factors affecting the risks of falling in the home.[1]

Environmental Area or Factor	Objective and Recommendations
All areas Lighting	Absence of glare and shadows; accessible switches at room entrances; night light in bedroom, hall bathroom
Floors	Nonskid backing for throw rugs; carpet edges tacked down; carpets with shallow pile; nonskid wax on floors; cords out of walking path; small objects (eg, clothes, shoes) off floor
Stairs	Lighting sufficient, with switches at top and bottom of stairs; securely fastened bilateral handrails that stand out from wall; top and bottom steps marked with bright, contrasting tape; stair rises of no more than 6 inches; steps in good repair; no objects stored on steps
Kitchen	Items stored so that reaching up and bending over are not necessary; secure step stool available if climbing is necessary; firm, nonmovable table
Bathroom	Grab bars for tub, shower, and toilet; nonskid decals or rubber mat in tub or shower; shower chair with handheld shower; nonskid rugs; raised toilet seat; door locks removed to ensure access in an emergency
Yard and entrances	Repair of cracks in pavement, holes in lawn; removal of rocks, tools, and other tripping hazards; well-lit walkways, free of ice and wet leaves; stairs and steps as above
Institutions	All the above; bed at proper height (not too high or low); spills on floor cleaned up promptly; appropriate use of walking aids and wheelchairs.
Footwear	Shoes with firm, nonskid, nonfriction soles; low heels (unless person is accustomed to high heels); avoidance of walking in stocking feet or loose slippers

[1]From Tinetti ME, Speechley M: Prevention of falls among the elderly. N Engl J Med 1989;320:1055.

quired. Patients are often reassured by the availability of phones at floor level, a portable phone, or a lightweight radio call system.

Subdural hematoma is a treatable but easily overlooked complication of falls that must be considered in any elderly patient presenting with new neurologic signs, including confusion.

Dehydration, electrolyte imbalance, pressure sores, and hypothermia may all occur and endanger the patient's life following a fall.

Prevention & Management

The risk of falling and consequent injury, disability, and potential institutionalization can be reduced by modifying those factors outlined in Tables 4–6 and 4–7.

Grisso JA et al: Risk factors for falls as a cause of hip fracture in women. N Engl J Med 1991;324:1326.

Hindmarsh JJ, Estes H Jr: Falls in older persons: Causes and interventions. Arch Int Med 1989;149:2217. (US Preventive Task Force report.)

Tinetti ME, Speechley M: Prevention of falls among the elderly. N Engl J Med 1989;320:1055.

Rubenstein LZ et al: The value of assessing falls in an elderly population. Ann Intern Med 1990;113:308. (Assessment resulted in fewer falls, deaths, hospitalizations, and hospital days among residents of a long-term care facility.)

Sudarsky L: Gait disorders in the elderly. N Engl J Med 1990;322:1441.

URINARY INCONTINENCE

Loss of bladder control has a major psychologic and social impact and often contributes to institutionalization. Too often, the patient is simply labeled "incontinent of urine," and no attempt is made to discern the type of urinary incontinence, to determine if it is transient or chronic, or to provide proper treatment.

Classification
(Table 4–8)

A. Transient Causes: Because continence requires adequate mobility, mentation, motivation, and manual dexterity—in addition to integrated control of the lower urinary tract—problems outside the bladder can result in incontinence. Although known as causes of transient incontinence, the following common conditions may give rise to prolonged incontinence if not identified and treated. Moreover, since they are associated with morbidity that goes beyond urinary incontinence, each should be carefully sought in the incontinent patient.

1. Delirium—A clouded sensorium impedes recognition of both the need to void and the location of the nearest toilet. Delirium is the most common cause

Table 4–8. Classification of geriatric incontinence.

Transient
  Delirium/confusional state
  Infection, urinary (symptomatic)
  Atrophic urethritis/vaginitis
  Pharmaceuticals
  Psychologic, especially depression
  Excessive urine output (eg, congestive heart failure, hyperglycemia)
  Restricted mobility
  Stool impaction

Established
  Detrusor overactivity
  Detrusor underactivity
  Urethral obstruction
  Urethral incompetence

of incontinence in hospitalized patients; once it clears, incontinence resolves.

2. Infection–Symptomatic urinary tract infection commonly causes or contributes to incontinence; asymptomatic infection does not.

3. Atrophic urethritis/vaginitis–Because it usually coexists with atrophic vaginitis, atrophic urethritis can be established presumptively by the presence of vaginal mucosal telangiectasia, petechiae, erosions, erythema, or friability. Urethral inflammation, which often extends to the trigone, commonly contributes to incontinence in women and responds to a short course of low-dose estrogen (eg, 0.3–0.6 mg conjugated estrogens by mouth; topical administration is much more expensive and uncomfortable).

4. Pharmaceuticals–Drugs are one of the most common causes of transient incontinence. The most common agents and their mechanisms are listed in Table 4–9.

5. Psychologic–Especially depression or psychosis.

6. Excess urine output–Excess urine output may overwhelm the ability of the older person to reach a toilet in time. In addition to diuretics, common causes of nocturnal incontinence include excess fluid intake (many people believe that 8–12 glasses of fluid per day are necessary for good health); metabolic abnormalities (eg, hyperglycemia, hypercalcemia, diabetes insipidus); disorders associated with peripheral edema (heart failure, venous insufficiency, drugs [eg, calcium channel blockers, NSAIDs]; and low albumin states (eg, malnutrition, cirrhosis).

7. Restricted mobility–(See immobility and instability sections, above.) If mobility cannot be im-

proved, access to a urinal or commode may restore continence.

8. Stool impaction–This is a common cause of urinary incontinence, especially in hospitalized or immobile patients. Although the mechanism is still unknown, a clinical clue to its presence is the onset of both urinary and fecal incontinence. Disimpaction restores continence.

B. Established Causes: The established causes should be addressed only after the transient causes have been remedied.

1. Detrusor overactivity–Detrusor overactivity is diagnosed when uninhibitable bladder contractions cause leakage that reproduces the patient's symptoms. It is the most common cause of established geriatric incontinence, accounting for two-thirds of cases, regardless of whether patients are demented. Detrusor overactivity can be diagnosed presumptively in a woman (without urodynamic testing) when leakage occurs in the absence of stress maneuvers and urinary retention and is preceded by the precipitant onset of an intense urge to urinate that cannot be forestalled. In men, the symptoms are similar, but since detrusor overactivity may be due to coexisting urethral obstruction, urodynamic testing should be done if prescription of a bladder relaxant is planned. Because detrusor overactivity also may be due to bladder stones or tumor, the abrupt onset of otherwise unexplained urge incontinence—especially if accompanied by perineal/suprapubic discomfort or sterile hematuria—should prompt cystoscopy and cytologic examination.

2. Stress incontinence–The second most common cause of established incontinence in older

Table 4–9. Medications that can potentially affect continence.

Type of Medication	Examples	Potential Effects on Continence
Potent diuretics	Furosemide	Polyuria, frequency, urgency
Anticholinergics	Antihistamines, trihexyphenidyl, benztropine, dicyclomine, disopyramide	Urinary retention, overflow incontinence, delirium, impaction
Psychotropics		
Antidepressants	Amitriptyline, desipramine	Anticholinergic actions, sedation
Antipsychotics	Thioridazine, haloperidol	Anticholinergic actions, sedation, rigidity, immobility
Sedative-hypnotics	Diazepam, flurazepam	Sedation, delirium, immobility
Narcotic analgesics		Urinary retention, fecal impaction, sedation, delirium
α-Adrenergic blockers	Prazosin, terazosin	Urethral relaxation (stress incontinence in women)
α-Adrenergic agonists	Decongestants	Urinary retention in men
ACE inhibitors	Captopril, enalapril	Stess incontinence (if drug produces coughing)
Calcium channel blockers	All	Urinary retention
Alcohol		Polyuria, frequency, urgency, sedation, delirium, immobility
Vincristine		Urinary retention

women (it is rare in men), stress incontinence is characterized by *instantaneous* leakage of urine in response to a stress maneuver. Leakage is worse or occurs only during the day unless another abnormality (eg, detrusor overactivity) is also present. To test for stress incontinence, have the patient relax her perineum and cough vigorously (a single cough) while standing with a full bladder. Instantaneous leakage strongly suggests stress incontinence, especially if it reproduces symptoms and urinary retention has been excluded by a postvoiding residual determination (PVR). A delay of several seconds suggests that leakage is instead caused by an uninhibited bladder contraction induced by coughing.

3. Urethral obstruction–Rarely present in women, urethral obstruction (due to prostatic enlargement, urethral stricture, bladder neck contracture, or prostatic cancer) is the second most common cause of established incontinence in older men. It can present as dribbling incontinence after voiding; urge incontinence due to detrusor overactivity, which coexists in approximately two-thirds of cases; or overflow incontinence due to urinary retention. Renal ultrasound is required to exclude hydronephrosis in men whose PVR exceeds 100 mL; in older men for whom surgery is planned, urodynamic confirmation of obstruction is usually required in addition to cystoscopy.

4. Detrusor underactivity–Detrusor underactivity is the least common cause of incontinence. It may be idiopathic or due to sacral lower motor nerve dysfunction. When it causes incontinence, detrusor underactivity is associated with urinary frequency, nocturia, and frequent leakage of small amounts. The elevated postvoiding residual (generally over 450 mL) distinguishes it from detrusor overactivity and stress incontinence, but only urodynamic testing (rather than cystoscopy or intravenous urography) differentiates it from urethral obstruction in men; such testing usually is not required in women, in whom obstruction is rarely present.

Treatment

A. Transient Causes: Each identified transient cause should be treated regardless of whether an established cause coexists. For patients with urinary retention induced by an antidepressant or neuroleptic medication, several options are possible. First, since remission is common in both depression (in 6–12 months) and agitation (within days after an underlying illness resolves), discontinuation of the drug should be considered. If this is not feasible, other approaches should be tried, such as psychotherapy or ECT for depression and environmental modification, reorientation, and treatment of precipitants (eg, arthritis, adhesive capsulitis) for agitation. If medication is still required, substituting a nonanticholinergic agent or one with less anticholinergic effect may be useful (eg, fluoxetine, trazodone, or an MAO inhibi-

tor for depression; haloperidol or a benzodiazepine for agitation). Finally, bethanechol (10–25 mg three times daily) may be helpful but only if the anticholinergic drug must be continued.

B. Established Causes:

1. Detrusor overactivity–The cornerstone of treatment is behavioral therapy. Instruct cooperative patients to void every 1–2 hours while awake. Once daytime continence is restored, increase the interval by 30 minutes, in an iterative process, until the interval reaches 4–5 hours; most patients who become continent during the day on this regimen become continent at night as well.

For patients who are unable to cooperate, caregivers should ask whether they need to void at intervals designed to preempt incontinence. When drugs are necessary, they should be added to these regimens, selected on the basis of side effects, and monitored to avoid inducing urinary retention. Because each drug except the calcium channel blockers has anticholinergic side effects, each should be used at the lowest effective dose. Oxybutynin (2.5–5 mg three or four times daily) has a rapid onset of action, which also makes it useful for episodic use. Imipramine (25–100 mg at bedtime) and doxepin (25–100 mg at bedtime) have a slower onset of action but require less frequent dosing and are useful if the patient is also depressed; orthostatic hypotension must be watched for. Calcium channel blockers (in doses used for cardiac disease) may be useful for patients with delayed diastolic relaxation, angina, or hypertension. Flavoxate has not yet proved effective. Propantheline, which has the most potent anticholinergic side effects, should be avoided in frail or confused older patients.

In refractory cases, where intermittent catheterization is feasible, the physician may choose intentionally to induce urinary retention with a bladder relaxant and have the patient empty the bladder three or four times daily. Clean but not sterile technique is required.

If all measures fail, an external collection device or protective pad or undergarment may be required. A comprehensive, illustrated catalogue of these aids is available (write HIP, PO Box 544, Union, SC 29379).

2. Stress incontinence–Surgery is the most effective treatment for stress incontinence, resulting in a cure rate of approximately 85% even in older women. For women who wish to avoid surgery and who can comply indefinitely, pelvic muscle exercises are effective for mild to moderate stress incontinence. If not contraindicated, an alpha-adrenergic agonist such as phenylpropanolamine (25–50 mg twice daily) is also useful (but rarely curative) for mild to moderate stress incontinence, especially if combined with estrogen (eg, conjugated estrogens, 0.3–0.6 mg daily). Occasionally, a pessary or even a tampon (for women with vaginal stenosis) provides some relief, especially for frail women.

3. Urethral obstruction–Surgical decompression is the most effective treatment for obstruction, especially in the setting of urinary retention; a variety of newer, less invasive techniques make decompression feasible even for frail men. For a nonoperative candidate, intermittent or indwelling catheterization is used; a condom catheter is contraindicated when urinary retention is present. However, for a man with prostatic obstruction who is not in retention and who either wishes to defer surgery or is not a surgical candidate, treatment with an alpha-adrenergic antagonist (eg, prazosin, 1–2 mg two to four times daily) may relieve symptoms; the 5α-reductase inhibitor finasteride may partially relieve obstruction in one-third of patients, but the onset of effect requires nearly a year.

4. Detrusor underactivity–For the patient with a poorly contractile bladder, augmented voiding techniques (eg, double voiding, or adding suprapubic pressure) often prove effective; pharmacologic agents (eg, bethanechol) rarely work. If further emptying is needed, or for the patient with an acontractile bladder, intermittent or indwelling catheterization is the only option. Antibiotics should be used only for symptomatic upper tract infection or as prophylaxis for recurrent symptomatic infections in a patient using intermittent catheterization; they should not be used as prophylaxis with an indwelling catheter.

DuBeau CE, Resnick NM: Controversies in the diagnosis and management of benign prostatic hypertrophy. Adv Intern Med 1992;37:55.

Resnick NM, Ouslander JG (editors): National Institutes of Health Consensus Development Conference on Urinary Incontinence. J Am Geriatr Soc 1990;38:263.

Urinary Incontinence Guidelines Panel: Urinary incontinence in adults: Clinical practice guideline. AHCPR Publication No. 92–0038. Rockville, MD, 1992.

"IATROGENIC" DRUG REACTIONS

Older patients are two or three times more likely than young to middle-aged adults to have adverse drug reactions, for a number of reasons. Changes in absorption, even with achlorhydria, are usually not of clinical significance, but drug clearance is often markedly reduced. This is due to a decrease in renal plasma flow and glomerular filtration rate as well as reduced hepatic clearance. The latter is due to a decrease in activity of the drug-metabolizing microsomal enzymes as well as an overall decrease in blood flow to the liver with aging. The volume of distribution of drugs also is affected, since the elderly have a decrease in total body water and a relative increase in body fat. Thus, water-soluble drugs become more concentrated, and fat-soluble drugs have longer half-lives. In addition, serum albumin levels decrease, especially in sick patients, so that there is some decrease in protein binding of some drugs (eg, warfarin, phenytoin), leaving more free (active) drug available.

In addition to impaired drug clearance, which results in altered pharmacokinetics, older patients have altered responses to similar serum drug levels, a phenomenon known as altered pharmacodynamics. Thus, they are more sensitive to some drugs (eg, opiates) and less sensitive to others (eg, beta-adrenergic agents).

Finally, the older patient with multiple chronic conditions is likely to be receiving many drugs. Thus, adverse drug reactions and dosage errors are more likely to occur, especially if the patient has visual, hearing, or memory deficits.

Precautions in Administering Drugs

To avoid drug toxicity in the elderly, the following should be kept in mind:

A. Drug Selection and Administration:

1. Ensure that the symptom requiring treatment is not itself due to another drug.

2. Use drug therapy only after nonpharmacologic means have been considered or tried and only when the benefit clearly outweighs the risk.

3. Start with less than the usual adult dosage, and increase the dosage slowly, consistent with its pharmacokinetics in older patients. However, age-related changes in drug distribution and clearance are variable among individuals, and some patients require full doses. Determine acceptable measures of success and toxicity, and increase the dose until encountering one or the other.

4. Keep the dosage schedule as simple and the number of pills as low as possible.

5. Have the patient or a family member bring in all medications at frequent intervals for reinforcing instructions regarding reasons for drug use, dosage, frequency of administration, and possible adverse effects.

6. Serum drug levels are useful for monitoring certain potentially toxic drugs with narrow therapeutic indices such as phenytoin, theophylline, quinidine, aminoglycosides, lithium, and some other psychotropic drugs (eg, nortriptyline). However, one must realize that toxicity can occur even with "normal" therapeutic levels of some drugs (eg, digoxin, phenytoin).

7. Instruct the pharmacist not to use safety cap containers unless the patient is confused or at high risk for suicide or is living with small grandchildren, since it may be difficult or impossible for the patient to open them.

B. Over-the-Counter Drugs: Adverse drug reactions may result from taking over-the-counter drugs or drugs prescribed for others in the household in addition to those prescribed for the patient. Have the patient or a family member bring in for review all over-the-counter drugs as well as prescription drugs the patient may be taking. All over-the-counter hypnotics and most cold pills contain antihistamines that can produce drowsiness or confusion as well as anticholinergic side effects (eg, dryness of mouth, blurring of vision, confusion, urinary hesitancy or retention). In addition, ibuprofen is now available without prescription and may cause renal or central nervous system side effects.

C. Sedative-Hypnotics: Remember that the effects of sedative-hypnotics persist much longer in the elderly and may produce confusional states. Avoid this class of drugs whenever possible. Even the shortest-acting benzodiazepines may have adverse effects. If nonpharmacologic treatment of insomnia is unsuccessful, short-term use of an intermediate-acting agent whose metabolism is not affected by age (eg, oxazepam, 10–30 mg) may be useful.

D. Antibiotics: Serum creatinine is not a good index of renal function in old people. Concentrations of toxic agents excreted by the kidney should be measured directly. (See Laboratory Examinations & Imaging, above.)

E. Cardiac Drugs: Digitalis, procainamide, and quinidine have prolonged half-lives in older patients and have narrow therapeutic windows, so toxicity is common at the usual dosages. In addition, digoxin toxicity—especially anorexia, confusion, or depression—can occur with therapeutic digoxin levels.

F. H_2 Receptor Blockers: Cimetidine and ranitidine interfere with hepatic drug metabolism, resulting in a higher incidence of toxicity of drugs metabolized mainly in the liver (eg, propranolol, lidocaine, warfarin, theophylline, phenytoin). In addition, all of the H_2 blockers can produce confusion in the elderly; none is less likely than another.

G. Antidepressants and Antipsychotics: Antidepressants and antipsychotics are very likely to produce anticholinergic side effects in old people (eg, confusion, urinary retention, constipation, dry mouth). This can be minimized by switching to a nonanticholinergic agent or one with less anticholinergic effect (see section on depression, above). Moreover, since both depression and agitation usually remit, consider cautious discontinuation of these agents.

H. Glaucoma Medications: Not only can topical beta-blockers cause systemic side effects, but so too can oral carbonic anhydrase inhibitors. The latter commonly cause malaise and anorexia and can even lead to symptoms suggestive of metastatic cancer. Such symptoms may occur independently of the induced metabolic acidosis.

I. Anticoagulants: Recent data show that elderly patients benefit from anticoagulation as much as younger individuals. However, since they are more vulnerable to anticoagulant side effects, more careful monitoring and less aggressive anticoagulation are advisable.

J. Avoid Overtreatment: Drugs are not necessarily indicated in some common clinical situations:

1. Asymptomatic bacteriuria–Antibiotics need not be given unless associated with obstructive uropathy, other anatomic abnormalities, or stones.

2. Ankle edema–Often due to venous insufficiency, drugs (eg, NSAIDs or some calcium antagonists), or even inactivity in chair-bound patients; diuretics are usually not indicated unless edema is associated with heart failure. Fitted pressure-gradient stocking are often helpful.

3. Sleep pattern changes–Avoid prescribing hypnotics until nonpharmacologic interventions have been tried (Chapter 24).

Everitt DE, Avorn J: Systemic effects of drugs used to treat glaucoma. Ann Intern Med 1990;112:120.

Gurwitz JH, Avorn J: The ambiguous relationship between aging and adverse drug reactions. Ann Intern Med 1991;114:956.

Larson EB at al: Adverse drug reactions with global cognitive impairment in elderly persons. Ann Intern Med 1987;107:169.

Montamat SC et al: Management of drug therapy in the elderly. N Engl J Med 1989;321:303.

SUMMARY

Special Considerations in Treating the Elderly

A. Always Ascribe Dysfunction to Disease Rather Than Aging: Remember that 80% of patients over age 80 function well and relatively independently in the community and should not be assumed to be demented, helpless, untreatable, or hopeless. Remember also that the average 75-year-old man can expect to live to age 84 and the average 85-year-old woman to age 92. When deciding on the advisability of various interventions, including surgery, age alone should almost never be a contraindication.

B. Prevention: Much can be done to prevent the progression and even the onset of disease in older people. For a summary of suggested screening tests and counseling practices, see Chapter 1. Some points should be emphasized, however. Dietary inadequacies should be repleted; for the patient with inadequate sun exposure and intake of vitamin D, a daily multivitamin capsule is recommended. Tobacco and alcohol use should be minimized, since the benefits of discontinuing these accrue even to individuals over age 65. The importance of reviewing all of a patient's medications and discontinuing them whenever feasible cannot be overemphasized.

Recent studies have now conclusively documented the benefits to ambulatory elderly patients of treating combined systolic and diastolic hypertension as well as isolated systolic hypertension. Treatment of either one *substantially* reduces the risk of stroke as well as the risk of death due to cardiovascular causes in this group. It is important to realize that conclusive results were achieved using *low* doses of a thiazide or thiazide-like diuretic (eg, chlorthalidone 12.5–25 mg) as the first step and adding *low-dose* reserpine (0.05–0.1 mg) or atenolol (25–50 mg) daily only as needed. Side effects were minimal, cost was trivial, and concerns about potential toxicity were not borne out. Thus, as opposed to more costly and theoretically preferable agents, the benefits of these inexpensive, time-honored agents have now been established in the elderly, and they should be considered the drugs of choice when initiating therapy.

Glaucoma should be detected, though perhaps best by an ophthalmologist, and visual and auditory impairment corrected. Dentures should be assessed for their fit, and oral lesions beneath them should be detected.

A Papanicolaou test should be done in the 15–25% of women who deny having had one in the past decade. Immunizations (for influenza, pneumococcal pneumonia, tetanus) should be current. PPD testing should be done on residents of chronic care facilities and on those at high risk of tuberculosis; if negative, the test should be repeated at 1 week to identify the remainder of exposed patients, and those who have recently converted (not compared with the previous week) should probably be treated.

Screening mammography is indicated every 1–2 years until at least age 75; insufficient data are available for a recommendation above this age, though a recent decision analysis supports its use. The relative risks and benefits of low-dose aspirin and (for women) estrogen replacement therapy have not yet been elucidated sufficiently to warrant their use as a routine practice, but these agents should be considered on an individual basis.

Exercise should be encouraged not only because of its beneficial effects on blood pressure, cardiovascular conditioning, glucose homeostasis, bone density, and even longevity but also because it may improve mood, insomnia, and constipation and prevent falls; spinal flexion exercises should be avoided in patients with osteopenia, and consultation with a physical therapist may be helpful.

Measures should be taken to prevent falling, as outlined in Tables 4–6 and 4–7. Counseling about driving, especially for patients with cognitive impairment, remains problematic. All older people should be advised of the availability of a "refresher" driving course offered inexpensively through AARP. In those with a recent history of accidents or cognitive impairment, professional evaluation (eg, through the Department of Motor Vehicles or a local rehabilitation facility) should be recommended until better criteria become available.

But perhaps the most valuable procedure for prevention of disease in old people is to take a careful history, focusing not only on the "chief complaint" but also on common and often hidden conditions such as falls, confusion, sexual dysfunction, and incontinence. In addition, one should always identify the complications that the specific patient is at risk for and take steps to avert them. For instance, a patient with cognitive impairment who smokes is at risk not only for lung cancer but also for starting a fire, and a patient who requires narcotics is at risk for fecal impaction, delirium, and confusion.

C. Provide Prompt Medical Care: Because of impaired homeostatic reserve, older people may present with only nonspecific symptoms or a decline in function, even when a serious acute illness is present (eg, confusion, falls, or incontinence–without fever or cough in a patient with pneumonia). Thus, even mild changes in function in the frail elderly mandate *prompt* medical attention.

D. Attend to Psychosocial Problems: Early attention to social and psychologic problems may be critical factors in the patient's ability to remain independent.

E. Encourage Home Care: Every attempt should be made to allow the patient to stay at home. Some community resources that may be of value include the following: Home Health Care, Day Health Care, Respite Beds (families who care for elderly relatives at home often require periods of relief from that burden if they are to be able to continue to keep the patient at home), Meals on Wheels, Home Health Aides, Transportation Services for the Disabled, and Visiting Nurses. Daily telephone contact, emergency radio systems, and communal and sheltered living arrangements all have obvious advantages in overall management of old people needing care and attention. Keep in mind the burden that maintaining the patient at home may impose on the family's primary caregiver. This person will need a great deal of support.

F. Advance Directives: See above.

G. Assess Feasibility of Surgery: Age alone should never be the sole criterion for deciding whether a surgical procedure should be done. Survival following surgery in the elderly has increased dramatically in recent years. Premorbid health status and the patient's wishes are far more important than age in making this decision.

H. Assist the Family: If the patient has dementia or other complex medical and psychosocial problems, the family often needs the physician's support even more than the patient.

Amery A, Schaepdryver AD: Introduction: The European Working Party on High Blood Pressure in the Elderly (EWPHE). Am J Med 1991;90(Suppl 3A):3.

Hayward RSA et al: Preventive care guidelines: 1991. Ann Intern Med 1991;114:758. (Evaluates recommendations of most prior task forces; includes summary tables.)

LaCroix AZ et al: Smoking and mortality among older men and women in three communities. N Engl J Med 1991;324:1619. (Corroborates benefit of smoking cessation for cardiovascular, cancer, and all-cause mortality among people over 65 and probably over 75 as well.)

Shepard RJ: The scientific basis of exercise prescribing for the very old. J Am Geriatr Soc 1990;38:62.

SHEP Cooperative Research Group: Prevention of stroke by antihypertensive drug treatment in older persons with isolated systolic hypertension. Final results of the Systolic Hypertension in the Elderly Program (SHEP). JAMA 1991;265:3255.

Steel K: Home care for the elderly: The new institution. Arch Intern Med 1991;151:439.

Woolf SH et al: The periodic health examination of older adults: The recommendations of the US Preventive Services Task Force. Part II: Screening tests. J Am Geriatr Soc 1990;38:933.

Identification of the "High-Risk" Elderly

The following patients are at greater risk of rapid deterioration and institutionalization than others and should be monitored more closely:

(1) Those over age 80.
(2) Those who live alone.
(3) Those who are bereaved or depressed.
(4) Those who are intellectually impaired.
(5) Those who have fallen several times.
(6) Those with incontinence.
(7) Those who have not coped well in the past.

REFERENCES

Balducci L et al: Breast cancer of the older women: An annotated review. J Am Geriatr Soc 1991;39:1113.

Fabiszewski KJ, Volicer B, Volicer L: Effect of antibiotic treatment outcome of fevers in institutionalized Alzheimer's patients. JAMA 1990;263:3168.

Ferrell BA: Pain management in elderly people. J Am Geriatr Soc 1991;39:64.

Greenspan SL, Resnick NM: Geriatric endocrinology. In: *Basic and Clinical Endocrinology*, 4th ed. Greenspan FS (editor). Appleton & Lange, 1993.

Harris J: The treatment of cancer in an aging population. JAMA 1992;268:96.

Harper CM, Lyles YM: Physiology and complications of bed rest. J Am Geriatr Soc 1988;36:1047.

Health and Public Policy Committee, American College of Physicians: Financing long-term care. Ann Intern Med 1988;108:279.

Libow LS, Starer P: Care of the nursing home patient. N Engl J Med 1989;321:93.

Lipsitz LA: Orthostatic hypotension in the elderly. N Engl J Med 1989;321:952.

Madoff RD et al: Fecal incontinence. N Engl J Med 1992;326:1002.

Mansour A, Lipschitz DA: Myeloplastic syndrome in the elderly. J Am Geriatr Soc 1992;40:386.

Morley JE et al: Nutrition in the elderly: UCLA conference. Ann Intern Med 1988;109:890.

National Institutes of Health Consensus Development Conference Statement: Geriatric assessment methods for clinical decision-making. J Am Geriatr Soc 1988;36:342.

Ouslander JG: Medical care in the nursing home. JAMA 1989;262:2582.

Palmore E, Nowlin J, Wang M: Predictors of function among the old-old: A 10-year follow-up. J Gerontol 1985;40:244.

Prinz PN et al: Sleep disorders and aging. N Engl J Med 1990;323:520.

Resnick NM, Greenspan SL: Senile osteoporosis reconsidered. JAMA 1989;261:1025. (Critical review of geriatric issues.)

Salzman C: *Clinical Geriatric Psychopharmacology,* 2nd ed. Williams & Wilkins, 1992.

Schneider E, Reed JD Jr: Life extension. N Engl J Med 1985;312:1159.

Schwab R, Walters CA, Weksler ME: Host defense mechanisms and aging. Semin Oncol 1989;16:20.

Shamburek RD, Farrare JT: Disorders of the digestive system in the elderly. N Engl J Med 1990;322:438.

Thompson MP, Morris LK: Unexplained weight loss in the ambulatory elderly. J Am Geriatr Soc 1991;39:497.

Wrenn K: Fecal impaction. N Engl J Med 1989;321:658.

Yoshikawa TT: Tuberculosis in aging adults. J Am Geriatr Soc 1992;40:178.

Cancer

Hope S. Rugo, MD

INCIDENCE & ETIOLOGY

Cancer is the second most common cause of death in the United States, accounting for almost 25% of all deaths in 1989. There are over 1 million new cases of cancer in the USA each year and 500,000 deaths. An additional 700,000 new cases of nonmelanomatous skin cancer and 100,000 new cases of carcinoma in situ are diagnosed every year. Table 5–1 summarizes current United States incidence figures for the ten leading types of cancer as well as for all sites combined. Although prostate and breast cancers are the most common malignancies in men and women, respectively, the most common cause of cancer death is still lung cancer. Inasmuch as the single most important recognized carcinogen is tobacco and since tobacco-related cancers account for one-third of all fatal forms of cancer, smoking cessation is an important area for continued education and prevention efforts. Strategies for helping patients give up the smoking habit are described in Chapter 1.

Although the cause of most cancers remains unknown, recent research has led to significant advances in understanding the molecular basis of the malignant proliferation of cells. Mutation in DNA sequences leading to amplification or increased expression of "oncogenes" or deletion of "tumor suppressor genes"—or both processes—have been linked to abnormal proliferation and malignant conversion. Oncogenes are usually normal genes that encode for cellular growth factor receptors, growth factors, or elements of the proliferative machinery of the cancer cell. Tumor suppressor genes encode for regulatory proteins that normally suppress cellular proliferation. The consequence of these and other mutations that may be due to environmental exposure, genetic susceptibility, infectious agents, and other unknown factors is the disease process called cancer. Most tumors exhibit one or several chromosomal abnormalities such as deletions, inversions, translocations, or duplications. Although many of these abnormalities appear to be nonspecific, certain genetic alterations are strongly associated with specific malignancies. Determination of the abnormal chromosome may aid in diagnosis as well as prognostic assessment. An example of a specific chromosomal translocation is seen in Burkitt's lymphoma, where the c-*myc* oncogene is activated by translocation of genetic material from chromosome 8 to chromosome 14. A high number of genetic alterations ("allelic deletions") in colon cancer is associated with a poor prognosis.

Exposure to carcinogens probably accounts for a much larger percentage of cancer than is currently recognized. It is difficult to trace exposures to the development of cancer in an individual since the latency period tends to be long and the degree and nature of exposure unclear or poorly documented. General classes of environmental carcinogens include chemical carcinogens such as benzene and asbestos, oncogenic viruses such as the human papillomavirus and the Epstein-Barr virus, and physical causes such as exposure to ionizing radiation and ultraviolet light. There appears to be a hereditary predisposition to specific forms of cancer that have been linked to specific molecular events within a gene (eg, hereditary retinoblastoma and familial adenomatous polyposis). Infection with the human immunodeficiency virus has been associated with an increased risk of cancer, especially non-Hodgkin's lymphoma, Kaposi's sarcoma, and cervical cancer. The human papillomavirus has also been implicated in the development of cervical carcinoma. Specific types of this virus are associated with high- or low-risk lesions.

Gallie BL et al: The genetics of retinoblastoma: Relevance to the patient. Pediatr Clin North Am 1991;38:299. (Use of genetics for counseling and prenatal diagnosis.)

Koeffler HP et al: Molecular mechanisms of cancer. West J Med 1991;155:505. (Oncogenes, tumor suppressor genes, and evaluation in specific malignancies.)

Slebos RJC et al: K-*ras* oncogene activation as a prognostic marker in adenocarcinoma of the lung. N Engl J Med 1990;323:561. (Activation of an oncogene appears to correlate with poor prognosis.)

Tops CMJ et al: Presymptomatic diagnosis of familial adenomatous polyposis by bridging DNA markers. Lancet 1989;2:1361. (A molecular technique to aid in the diagnosis of asymptomatic family members for cancer prevention.)

CHEMOPREVENTION

Chemoprevention is an exciting new area of cancer research and a major strategy for cancer prevention.

Table 5–1. Incidence of the ten most common cancers in the USA in males and females (all races).

Rank	Males	Rate[1]	Females	Rate[1]
1	Prostate	109	Breast	105
2	Lung	80	Colorectal	40
3	Colorectal	58	Lung	39
4	Bladder	29	Endometrium	21
5	Lymphoma	20	Ovary	15
6	Oropharyngeal	16	Lymphoma	13
7	Melanoma	13	Melanoma	9
8	Leukemia	13	Cervix	9
9	Kidney	12	Pancreas	8
10	Stomach	12	Leukemia	8
	All sites	362	All sites	267

[1]Rates are per 100,000 in 1989 and rounded to the nearest whole number and age-adjusted to the 1970 United States standard population. Both Hodgkin's disease and non-Hodgkin's lymphoma are included under lymphoma. Data from National Cancer Institute's SEER Program.

Instead of screening for disease that is often extensive at the time of initial detection, chemoprevention focuses on the prevention of cancer by administering chemical compounds that interfere with the multi-staged carcinogenic process. Recent progress in understanding of the biochemical and molecular mechanisms of carcinogenesis has allowed the identification of potential chemopreventive agents. Four risk groups have been identified for intervention: (1) previous cancer patients (to prevent second malignancies); (2) patients with preneoplastic lesions; (3) patients at high risk for malignancy (family history, life-style, occupation); and (4) the general population.

Two important factors have influenced the development of clinical trials. First, the chemicals used in chemoprevention must be nontoxic and well-tolerated by this otherwise asymptomatic population. Second, there must be a method of following the potential efficacy of chemopreventive agents other than waiting for the development of tumors (a time-consuming and expensive end point). Attention has been focused on determining effective intermediate biomarkers (defined as molecular and histologic changes occurring early in the carcinogenic process—eg, during the preinvasive stage of intraepithelial neoplasia—that can be used as surrogates for reduction in cancer incidence). These biomarkers either identify patients at high risk for developing cancer or serve as surrogates for cancer. Examples of such biomarkers include leukoplakia and colonic polyps.

Several potential sources of anticarcinogens are currently under investigation. These include factors present within the diet (eg, vitamins), nonsteroidal anti-inflammatory drugs, and hormone suppressing agents (eg, tamoxifen). Retinoids, the natural derivatives and synthetic analogues of vitamin A, are the best-studied chemopreventive agents. Data from epidemiologic investigations, studies in vitro and in animals, and now clinical trials support the role of these agents as cytostatic agents in the prevention of epithelial carcinogenesis. Retinoids are modulators of epithelial cell differentiation in vivo and in vitro that are thought to act by regulation of gene expression (nuclear tumor suppression).

Clinical trials have focused on suppressing carcinogenesis in the epithelial tissues of the aerodigestive tract. Isotretinoin (13-cis-retinoic acid) has been shown to suppress leukoplakia, a premalignant lesion that is felt to indicate the presence of field carcinogenesis throughout the aerodigestive tract. Although the high doses (1.5 mg/kg/d) used in the initial trial are not well tolerated, a recent study has demonstrated the effectiveness and tolerability of low doses (0.5 mg/kg/d) of isotretinoin. Only patients with a demonstrated response to high-dose induction were placed on low dose maintenance therapy. The disease progression rate on maintenance was only 8% compared with a rate of 55% in a separate group taking beta-carotene. In addition, the use of high doses of isotretinoin has prevented the development of second primary tumors in patients with early squamous cell carcinoma of the head and neck. Only 4% of patients in the isotretinoin group developed second primary tumors, compared with 24% in the placebo group with a follow-up period 32 months.

Current large clinical trials are attempting to substantiate these data and are investigating the use of isotretinoin in preventing both second primary lung cancers and second primary head and neck cancers in patients with prior low-stage malignancy.

In addition to preventing second cancers, isotretinoin may also decrease the risk of primary epithelial malignancy. The beta-carotene and retinol efficacy trial (CARET) is a multicenter two-armed double-blind randomized trial designed to test the hypothesis that the combination of an antioxidant (beta-carotene) and a tumor suppressor (isotretinoin) will decrease the risk of lung cancer in high-risk populations. The high-risk population includes heavy smokers and asbestos-exposed workers who have smoked. Over 8000 participants have been randomized, and efficacy results are expected in 1998.

The major toxicity of isotretinoin is at higher doses and includes severe skin dryness, cheilitis, hypertriglyceridemia, and conjunctivitis. These toxicities may require dose reduction or temporary discontinuation of the drug. In the case of leukoplakia, the suppressive effect is reversed when the medication is discontinued.

NSAIDs are another group of drugs now under widespread investigation for chemoprevention of cancer. Aspirin and other NSAIDs inhibit prostaglandin synthesis and tumor growth in experimental systems. Such therapy can reduce both the size and the number of tumors in the colon induced by chemicals or radiation in rats. A large prospective mortality trial collected information on aspirin use and death rates from colon cancer. Other risk factors were evaluated in a multivariate analysis which concluded that regular aspirin use at low doses (16 or more uses per month for at least 1 year) might reduce the risk of fatal colon cancer. A follow-up study concluded that low-dose aspirin may protect not only against colon cancer but also against cancers of the esophagus, stomach, and rectum. The effect of possible increased screening in this population is not clear.

A recent randomized, double-blind, placebo-controlled study evaluated the use of sulindac versus placebo in patients with familial adenomatous polyposis. Both the number and the size of colorectal adenomas were reduced; however, the effect was incomplete without complete regression of all polyps in any patient. After the sulindac was discontinued, both polyp size and number increased. Although the drug was well tolerated, it is unlikely to replace colectomy in this high-risk group. The effect on polyp regression is intriguing, however, and a large trial is now investigating the use of aspirin in the prevention of polyps in patients previously diagnosed with early stage colon cancer.

Tamoxifen is an antiestrogen that has become a potential chemopreventive agent as well as continuing to be an important part of adjuvant and metastatic breast cancer treatment. The Tamoxifen Trial is based on preclinical data in animals that showed a reduced rate of breast cancer in the group receiving this drug. In addition, several adjuvant trials of women with unilateral breast cancer taking tamoxifen have shown a 30–40% reduction in the risk of developing a second primary breast cancer in the opposite breast. In the present prospective, double-blind, placebo-controlled nationwide trial, 16,000 women will be randomized to receive 5 years of daily tamoxifen or placebo. Women 35 years of age or older with high risk factors and all women over the age of 60 years are eligible. Three end points will be evaluated. First is the development of breast cancer or death from breast cancer. Tamoxifen is also an agonist for bone mineral content and cholesterol metabolism, so the second and third end points are fractures due to osteoporosis and myocardial infarction.

Other large ongoing chemoprevention trials include the use of finasteride to prevent the development of prostate cancer in men with a normal digital rectal examination but an elevated prostate specific antigen concentration. Finasteride is a drug used for benign prostatic hypertrophy that suppresses the local effects of testosterone. Eighteen thousand men will be randomized in this 5-year study. The long-term randomized, prospective Physician's Health Study is evaluating whether beta-carotene reduces the incidence of cancer.

Results of these and other studies should be available over the next decade. Chemoprevention is an exciting new strategy for cancer control that may play a significant role in the future management of high-risk populations.

Bollag W et al: Retinoids in cancer prevention and therapy. Ann Oncol 1992;3:513. (Rationale and use.)
Giardiello FM et al: Treatment of colonic and rectal adenomas with sulindac in familial adenomatous polyposis. N Engl J Med 1993;328:1313. (Randomized study in a high-risk population.)
Hong WK et al: Prevention of second primary tumors with isotretinoin in squamous-cell carcinoma of the head and neck. N Engl J Med 1990;323:795. (The first randomized, prospective trial using retinoic acid to prevent second primary tumors.)
Lippman SM et al: Comparison of low-dose isotretinoin with beta carotene to prevent oral carcinogenesis. N Engl J Med 1993;328:15. (The most recent randomized trial using retinoic acid to suppress oral leukoplakia.)
Omenn GS: CARET, the beta-carotene and retinol efficacy trial to prevent lung cancer in high-risk populations. Pub Health Rev 1991–92;19:205.
Thun MJ et al: Aspirin use and the risk of fatal cancer. Cancer Res 1993;53:1322. (Correlating aspirin use as assessed by questionnaire with the subsequent risk of fatal cancer.)

PREVENTION & EARLY DETECTION

Prevention of cancer due to specific known causes is an important goal of medicine. Unfortunately, effective prevention can only be achieved for a minority of malignancies given the inadequacy of current knowledge concerning cause and effect. Other than patient education regarding known carcinogens such as tobacco, ultraviolet light, and ionizing radiation, the most effective intervention possible by the physician is early diagnosis. Early diagnosis can improve the cure rate of certain malignancies and can be enhanced by standardized screening tests (eg, Papanicolaou smears and routine mammography). (See Screening for Early Detection of Cancer in Chapter 1.) For most cancers, stage at presentation is related to curability, with the highest cure rates reported when the tumor is small and there is no evidence of metastasis. However, for some tumors (eg, lung or ovarian cancer), distant metastases occur even from a small primary before it can be detected. More sensitive detection methods such as tumor markers are being developed for many forms of cancer, but it is still uncertain if they will be useful as screening tools for detection of less common cancers.

DeVita VT Jr, Hellman S, Rosenberg SA (editors): *Principles and Practice of Oncology*, 3rd ed. Lippincott, 1989.
Yandell DW et al: Oncogenic point mutations in the human retinoblastoma gene: Their application to genetic counseling. N Engl J Med 1989;321:1689.

STAGING OF CANCER

Standardized staging for tumor burden at the time of diagnosis is extremely valuable and important both for determining prognosis and for making decisions about treatment in individual cases. The American Joint Committee on Cancer (AJCC) has developed a simple classification scheme that can be incorporated into a form for staging and universally applied. This scheme is designed to encompass the life history of a tumor and is referred to as the TNM system. The untreated primary tumor (T) will gradually increase in size, leading to regional lymph node involvement (N) and, finally, distant metastases (M). The tumor is usually not clinically evident until local invasion or even spread to regional draining lymph nodes has occurred.

TNM staging is used clinically to indicate the extension of cancer before definitive therapy begins. The manner in which staging is accomplished—eg, by clinical examination or pathologic examination of a surgical specimen—must be carefully documented. Certain types of tumors, such as lymphomas and Hodgkin's disease, are usually staged by a different classification scheme that reflects the natural history of this type of tumor spread and helps to direct treatment decisions.

The TNM system allows a numerical assessment of the extent of primary tumor (T), the absence or presence and extent of regional lymph node metastases (N), and the absence or presence of distant metastases (M). For a detailed example of cancer staging using the TNM system applied to a specific disease, see the discussion of staging of breast cancer in Chapter 14.

Traditional staging does not take into account the biology or aggressiveness of a particular tumor and may not allow differentiation of prognostic risk groups. For this reason, specific pathologic characteristics are added into the prognostic evaluation for certain tumors (eg, estrogen and progesterone receptors or proliferative index for breast cancer; histologic grade for sarcoma). As these characteristics become standardized and better understood, they may allow us to identify patients with a poorer prognosis early in the course of disease when the patient might benefit from more aggressive therapy.

This chapter primarily covers the clinical aspects of cancer: (1) primary cancer treatment, including (a) surgery and radiation therapy, (b) systemic cancer therapy, (c) adjuvant chemotherapy for micrometastases, and (d) toxicity and dose modifications of chemotherapeutic agents; (2) diagnosis and management of emergent cancer complications; and (3) paraneoplastic syndromes that may aid in diagnosis and influence management. Specific cancers are discussed in the appropriate organ system chapters of this book. Further information may be obtained by calling the NCI Cancer Information Service at 1–800–4CANCER.

Beahrs OH et al (editors): *Manual for Staging of Cancer,* 3rd ed. Lippincott, 1988. (The bible of TNM staging.)

PRIMARY CANCER TREATMENT

SURGERY & RADIATION THERAPY

Most cancers present initially as localized tumor nodules and cause local symptoms. Depending on the type of cancer, initial therapy may be directed locally in the form of surgery or radiation therapy. Surgical excision or local radiation (or both) is the treatment of choice for a variety of potentially curable cancers, including most gastrointestinal and genitourinary cancers, central nervous system tumors, and cancers arising from the breast, thyroid, or skin as well as most sarcomas.

In other circumstances, surgery may be used for palliation of noncurable cases or for reconstruction and rehabilitation.

Surgery at presentation has both diagnostic and therapeutic effectiveness, since it permits pathologic staging of the extent of local and regional invasion as well as an opportunity for removal of the primary neoplasm. CT scanning and MRI play an increasing role in noninvasive tumor staging. However, it is usually necessary for the surgeon to identify patients intraoperatively whose disease can perhaps be cured by local treatment alone.

For certain tumor sites, complete surgical removal of the tumor can be disfiguring, disabling, or unachievable. Under those circumstances, primary local therapy with ionizing radiation may prove to be the treatment of choice. In other instances, surgery and radiation therapy are used in sequence.

Radiation therapy is usually delivered as brachytherapy or teletherapy. In brachytherapy, the radiation source is placed close to the tumor. This intracavitary approach is used for many gynecologic or oral neoplasms. In teletherapy, supervoltage radiotherapy is usually delivered with a linear accelerator, as this instrument permits more precise beam localization and avoids the complication of skin radiation toxicity. Various beam-modifying wedges, rotational techniques, and other specific approaches are used to increase the radiation dosage to the tumor bed while minimizing toxicity to adjacent normal tissues.

Well-oxygenated tumors are more radiosensitive than hypoxic tumors. Hypoxic tumors are often bulky, implying a potential synergistic role of surgical debulking prior to radiotherapy. Radiation therapy is normally delivered in a fractionated fashion, this method appearing to have radiobiologic superiority by permitting time for recovery of normal host tissues (but not the tumor) from sublethal damage during the period of treatment. Various normal tissues (particularly the skin, mucosal surfaces, spinal cord, bone marrow, and lymphoid system) can exhibit early or late toxicity from radiation therapy and limit radiation dosage. Fractionated radiation doses are usually administered for 5 days per week until the desired total dose has been delivered, usually over the course of 4–6 weeks.

For most tumor types, there is a sigmoid curve of increasing rate of control of the local tumor with increasing radiation dose. Radiosensitive tumors usually exhibit radiosensitivity over the dose range of 3500–5000 cGy.

Currently, more than 50% of all patients with cancer receive radiation therapy during the course of their illness. Radiation therapy is frequently the sole agent used with curative intent for tumors of the larynx (permitting cure without loss of the voice), oral cavity, pharynx, esophagus, uterine cervix, vagina, prostate, skin, Hodgkin's disease, and some tumors of the brain and spinal cord. For more extensive cancers, radiation is combined with surgery (eg, cancer of the breast, ovary, uterus, urinary bladder, rectum, lung, soft tissue sarcomas, and seminoma of the testis). Radiation is used as an adjuvant to chemotherapy for some patients with lymphoma or lung cancer and for several cancers in children. Occasionally, chemotherapy may be used to sensitize tumor cells to the toxic effects of radiation. Radiation therapy for palliation of pain or dysfunction may significantly improve the quality of life of patients suffering from incurable malignancies.

Radiation therapy has both acute and late toxicity. Acute toxicity may include generalized fatigue and malaise, anorexia, nausea and vomiting, local skin changes, diarrhea, and mucosal ulceration of the irradiated area. Radiation of large areas, especially the pelvis and proximal long bones, may result in significant bone marrow suppression. Radiation of the lungs, heart, and gastrointestinal tract must be approached with caution and with appropriate shielding to avoid severe toxicity. Long-term toxicity can include hyperpigmentation of the involved skin, decreased function of the irradiated organ, myelopathy, bone necrosis, and secondary malignancies. These toxicities may be minimized or avoided by careful shielding and fractionation. Both acute and long-term toxicity are dose-related.

Increasingly, the primary local therapy of cancer is integrated with systemic therapy, an approach that has proved to be superior for apparently localized tumor types with a high propensity for early metastatic spread and for which anticancer drugs are available. Locoregional hyperthermia (40–42 °C) is a modality that is of value as an adjunct to ionizing irradiation for some tumor sites. Hyperthermia's greatest use to date has been in superficial or easily implantable tumors as well as in relatively bulky hypovascular tumors with some degree of hypoxia.

Bagshaw MA et al: Prostate cancer: Radiation therapy for localized disease. Cancer 1993;71(3 Suppl):939. (Effective treatment for highly localized prostate cancer.)

Krishnan L et al: Early stage breast cancer: Local control after conservative surgery and radiation therapy with immediate interstitial boost. Radiology 1993;187:95. (Combining surgery and radiation therapy to preserve anatomy.)

Overgaard J: The current and potential role of hyperthermia in radiotherapy. Int J Radiat Oncol Biol Phys 1989; 16:535.

Patchell RA et al: A randomized trial of surgery in the treatment of single metastasis to the brain. N Engl J Med 1990;322:494.

SYSTEMIC CANCER THERAPY

Use of cytotoxic drugs, hormones, antihormones, and biologic agents has become a highly specialized and increasingly effective means of treating cancer. Therapy is usually administered by a medical oncologist. Selection of specific drugs or protocols for various types of cancer has traditionally been based on results of prior clinical trials. Many patients are treated on protocols to provide optimal therapy for refractory or poorly responsive malignancies. Treatment may be inadequate or ineffective because of drug resistance of the tumor cells. This has been attributed to spontaneous genetic mutations in subpopulations of cancer cells prior to exposure to chemotherapy. After chemotherapy has eliminated the sensitive cells, the resistant subpopulation grows to become the predominant cell type (Goldie-Coldman hypothesis). This has been the basis of alternating non-cross-resistant chemotherapy regimens.

Molecular mechanisms of drug resistance are now the subject of intense study. In many instances, specific drug resistance results from an amplification in the number of gene copies for an enzyme inhibited by a specific chemotherapeutic agent. A more general form of "multidrug resistance" has been described in association with expression of a gene (MDR1) encoding a transmembrane glycoprotein of MW 170 (P-glycoprotein) on tumor cells. This protein is an energy-dependent transport pump that facilitates drug efflux from tumor cells and promotes resistance to a broad spectrum of unrelated cancer drugs. Acquired multidrug resistance in multiple myeloma and lymphoma has been reversed clinically by adding the calcium channel blocker verapamil to chemotherapy regimens. Unfortunately, the doses of verapamil required to overcome drug resistance are associated with significant cardiovascular side effects. High doses of cyclosporine appear to increase the cytotoxicity of etoposide both in vitro and in vivo, probably by inhibiting the function of P-glycoprotein. The use of cyclosporine to enhance the effect of etoposide in purging resistant tumor cells in vitro from autologous bone marrow is under investigation. Cyclosporine has also been shown to enhance the cytotoxic effect of multi-agent chemotherapy on resistant multiple myeloma. Other novel immunosuppressant drugs may also be useful to reverse multidrug resistance.

Chemotherapy is used to cure a small percentage of malignancies, as adjuvant therapy to decrease the rate of relapse or improve the disease-free interval, and to palliate symptoms in some patients with incurable malignancies. In addition, chemotherapy may play a role as preoperative or "neoadjuvant" therapy to reduce the size and extent of the primary tumor, thereby allowing complete excision at the time of surgery. Chemotherapy was first shown to be curative in the treatment of advanced stages of choriocarcinoma in women. In addition, it is usually curative in Hodgkin's disease, diffuse large-cell and some high-grade lymphomas (including Burkitt's), carcinoma of the testis, some cases of acute leukemia, and embryonal rhabdomyosarcoma. When combined with initial surgery—and in some instances with irradiation—chemotherapy also increases the cure rate in Wilms's tumor and may increase the rate of long-term control and cure of breast cancer, colon cancer, rectal cancer, and osteogenic sarcomas. Combination chemotherapy provides significant palliation and prolongation of survival in adults with Hodgkin's disease, non-Hodgkin's lymphoma, mycosis fungoides, multiple myeloma and macroglobulinemia, acute and chronic leukemias, and breast, ovary, and small-cell lung carcinoma as well as carcinoid. Childhood cancers, including Ewing's sarcoma, retinoblastoma, and acute leukemia, may be cured or obtain significant palliation from chemotherapy. The results of currently available treatments are largely unsuccessful in squamous cell cancer of the lung, metastatic malignant melanoma, and extensive adenocarcinoma of the pancreas, kidney, gallbladder, colon, and liver. Patients with incurable tumors who desire aggressive treatment should be referred for experimental protocol therapy. Newer trials are available utilizing the biologic agents interleukin-2, alpha interferon, and others (especially in children).

Very high doses of chemotherapeutic agents followed by bone marrow transplantation has been shown to be curative in the therapy of various types of leukemia and high-risk lymphoma. Allogeneic or autologous bone marrow with or without ex vivo purging is used depending on the disease. In addition, dose-intense chemotherapy regimens with autologous bone marrow or peripheral blood progenitor cell rescue are currently being investigated in the high-risk adjuvant or early relapse setting for patients with carcinoma of the breast, testis, and ovaries (see Adjuvant Therapy for Micrometastases, below).

While most anticancer drugs are used systemically, there are selected indications for local or regional administration. Regional administration involves direct infusion of active chemotherapeutic agents into the tumor site (eg, intravesical therapy, intraperitoneal therapy, hepatic artery infusion with or without embolization of the main blood supply of the tumor). These treatments can result in significant palliation and improved survival.

A summary of the types of cancer responsive to chemotherapy and the current treatment of choice is offered in Table 5–2. In some instances (eg, Hodgkin's disease), optimal therapy may require a combination of therapeutic resources, eg, radiation plus chemotherapy rather than either modality alone. Patients with stage I, II, and IIIA Hodgkin's disease are often treated with radiation alone, thereby avoiding the potential toxicity of systemic chemotherapy. A small percentage of these patients may go on to require chemotherapy in the future for disease recurrence.

Table 5–3 sets forth the currently used dosage schedules and toxicities of the most commonly used cancer chemotherapeutic agents. The dosage schedules given are for single-agent therapy. Combination therapy is used for many diseases, including advanced-stage Hodgkin's disease, non-Hodgkin's lymphoma, and testicular carcinoma. This aggressive treatment may result in significant hematologic toxicity requiring dosage reductions or delay in treatment cycles. This may significantly limit the therapeutic effectiveness of the chemotherapy. It is possible to avoid the need for dose reductions or delay in therapy by using granulocyte colony-stimulating factor (G-CSF; filgastrim) or granulocyte-macrophage colony-stimulating factor (GM-CSF; sargramostim) (see below). Combination therapy should be attempted only by oncologic specialists who have adequate supportive services available (see below).

Hormonal therapy also plays an important role in cancer management. Hormonal therapy or ablation is important in treatment and palliation of breast and prostatic carcinoma, while added progestins are useful in suppression of endometrial carcinoma. Women with metastatic breast cancer who show objective improvement with hormonal therapy have tumors that contain cytoplasmic estrogen and progesterone receptors. Patients whose tumors lack these receptor proteins may be unresponsive to hormonal management but frequently respond to cytotoxic chemotherapy. Antiestrogens (eg, tamoxifen) and aromatase inhibitors (eg, aminoglutethimide) that block peripheral conversion of adrenal androgens into estrogens have substantial additive effects to or may avoid the need for oophorectomy in premenopausal women whose tumors are estrogen- or progesterone receptor-positive. Thus, estrogen and progesterone receptor status should be assessed on all breast cancers at the time of mastectomy and on biopsy material (if avail-

Table 5–2. Treatment choices for cancers responsive to systemic agents.

Diagnosis	Current Treatment of Choice	Other Valuable Agents and Procedures
Acute lymphocytic leukemia	**Induction:** Combination chemotherapy. *Adults:* Vincristine, prednisone, and daunorubicin with or without asparaginase. *Children:* Vincristine, prednisone with or without asparaginase. **Remission maintenance:** Methotrexate, thioguanine. CNS prophylaxis mandatory. Consolidation with multiagent protocols for young adults or allogeneic bone marrow transplantation.	Doxorubicin, cytarabine, cyclophosphamide, etoposide, teniposide (VM-26),[1] allopurinol[2]
Acute myelocytic and myelomonocytic leukemia	**Induction:** Combination chemotherapy with cytarabine and daunorubicin. **Consolidation:** For young adults, autologous (with or without purging) or allogeneic bone marrow transplantation.	Mitoxantrone, idarubicin, etoposide, mercaptopurine, thioguanine, azacitidine,[1] amsacrine,[1] methotrexate, doxorubicin, tretinoin, allopurinol,[2] leukapheresis, prednisone
Chronic myelocytic leukemia	Hydroxyurea with or without alpha interferon. Allogeneic bone marrow transplantation for young patients.	Busulfan, mercaptopurine, thioguanine, cytarabine, plicamycin, melphalan, autologous bone marrow transplantation
Chronic lymphocytic leukemia	Chlorambucil and prednisone or fludarabine (if treatment is indicated)	Vincristine, cyclophosphamide, doxorubicin, cladribine (2-chlorodeoxyadenosine; CdA), androgens,[2] allopurinol[2]
Hairy cell leukemia	Alpha interferon or cladribine (2-chlorodeoxyadenosine; CdA)	Pentostatin (deoxycoformycin)
Hodgkin's disease (stages III and IV)	**Combination chemotherapy:** doxorubicin (Adriamycin), bleomycin, vinblastine, dacarbazine (ABVD) or mechlorethamine, vincristine, prednisone, procarbazine (MOPP) or alternating MOPP/ABVD or MOPP/ABV	Carmustine, lomustine, etoposide, thiotepa, autologous bone marrow transplantation
Non-Hodgkin's lymphoma	**Combination therapy** depending on histologic classification but usually including cyclophosphamide, vincristine, doxorubicin, and prednisone with or without other agents	Bleomycin, methotrexate, etoposide, chlorambucil, fludarabine, lomustine, carmustine, cytarabine, thiotepa, amsacrine, mitoxantrone, autologous or allogeneic bone marrow transplantation
Multiple myeloma	**Combination chemotherapy:** melphalan and prednisone or melphalan, cyclophosphamide, carmustine, vincristine, and prednisone. Allogeneic bone marrow transplantation for high-risk young patients.	Alpha interferon, doxorubicin, dexamethasone, autologous bone marrow transplantation
Waldenström's macroglobulinemia	Chlorambucil versus combination chemotherapy: cyclophosphamide, vincristine, prednisone. Allogeneic bone marrow transplantation for high-risk young patients.	Alpha interferon, doxorubicin, dexamethasone, plasmapheresis, autologous bone marrow transplantation
Polycythemia vera	Hydroxyurea, phlebotomy	Busulfan, chlorambucil, cyclophosphamide, alpha interferon, radiophosphorus ^{32}P
Carcinoma of lung Small cell	**Combination chemotherapy:** cisplatin and etoposide. Palliative radiation therapy.	Cyclophosphamide, doxorubicin, vincristine
Non-small cell[3]	**Combination chemotherapy:** cisplatin, mitomycin, vinblastine	Doxorubicin, vindesine,[1] etoposide
Carcinoma of the head and neck[3]	**Combination chemotherapy:** cisplatin and fluorouracil	Methotrexate, bleomycin, hydroxyurea, doxorubicin, vinblastine
Carcinoma of the esophagus[3]	**Combination chemotherapy:** fluorouracil, cisplatin, mitomycin	Methotrexate, bleomycin, doxorubicin
Carcinoma of the stomach and pancreas[3]	**Stomach:** Combination chemotherapy: fluorouracil, doxorubicin, methotrexate; or doxorubicin, etoposide, cisplatin. **Pancreas:** fluorouracil	Carmustine, mitomycin, lomustine. Etoposide, leucovorin,[2] fluorouracil for stomach.
Carcinoma of the colon and rectum[3]	**Colon:** fluorouracil plus levamisole (adjuvant) or with leucovorin.[2] **Rectum:** fluorouracil with radiation therapy (adjuvant)	Mitomycin, carmustine, cisplatin, floxuridine
Carcinoma of the kidney[3]	Vinblastine, IL-2 with or without LAK cells (see text)	Alpha interferon

(*continued*)

Table 5–2. Treatment choices for cancers responsive to systemic agents.[1] (continued)

Diagnosis	Current Treatment of Choice	Other Valuable Agents and Procedures
Carcinoma of the bladder[3]	Intravesical BCG or thiotepa. Combination chemotherapy: methotrexate, vinblastine, doxorubicin (Adriamycin), cisplatin (M-VAC)	Cyclophosphamide, fluorouracil
Carcinoma of the testis[3]	**Combination chemotherapy:** etoposide and cisplatin	Bleomycin, vinblastine, ifosfamide, mesna,[2] carmustine, carboplatin, autologous bone marrow transplantation
Carcinoma of the prostate[3]	Estrogens or LHRH analogue (leuprolide) plus an antiandrogen (flutamide)	Ketoconazole, doxorubicin, aminoglutethimide, progestins, cyclophosphamide, cisplatin, suramin[1]
Carcinoma of the uterus[3]	Progestins or tamoxifen	Doxorubicin, cisplatin, fluorouracil, ifosfamide
Carcinoma of the ovary[3]	**Combination chemotherapy:** cyclophosphamide and cisplatin (or carboplatin)	Doxorubicin, melphalan, fluorouracil, altretamine (hexamethylamine), paclitaxel (Taxol), ?autologous bone marrow transplantation
Carcinoma of the cervix[3]	**Combination chemotherapy:** methotrexate, doxorubicin, cisplatin, and vinblastine; or mitomycin, bleomycin, vincristine, and cisplatin	Carboplatin, ifosfamide, lomustine
Carcinoma of the breast[3]	**Combination chemotherapy:** cyclophosphamide, doxorubicin, fluorouracil. Tamoxifen for estrogen/progesterone receptor-positive tumors. Adjuvant therapy for high-risk patients: ?dose intensification or autologous bone marrow transplantation.	Mitoxantrone, vinblastine, leucovorin,[2] thiotepa, vincristine, carboplatin, mitomycin, prednisone, progestins, androgens, aminoglutethimide, hydrocortisone, ?autologous bone marrow transplantation
Choriocarcinoma (trophoblastic neoplasms)[3]	Methotrexate or dactinomycin (or both) plus chlorambucil	Vinblastine, cisplatin, mercaptopurine, doxorubicin, bleomycin, etoposide
Carcinoma of the thyroid gland[3]	Radioiodine (^{131}I)	Doxorubicin, cisplatin, bleomycin, melphalan
Carcinoma of the adrenal gland[3]	Mitotane	Doxorubicin, suramin[1]
Carcinoid[3]	Fluorouracil plus streptozocin with or without alpha interferon	Doxorubicin, cyclophosphamide, octreotide, cyproheptadine,[2] methysergide[2]
Osteogenic sarcoma[3]	High-dose methotrexate, doxorubicin, vincristine	Cyclophosphamide, ifosfamide, bleomycin, dacarbazine, cisplatin, dactinomycin
Soft tissue sarcoma[3]	Doxorubicin, dacarbazine	Ifosfamide, cyclophosphamide, etoposide, cisplatin, high-dose methotrexate, vincristine
Melanoma[3]	Dacarbazine, alpha interferon, IL-2 with or without LAK cells (see text)	Carmustine, lomustine, melphalan, thiotepa, cisplatin, paclitaxel (Taxol),[1] tamoxifen, vincristine
Kaposi's sarcoma	Vincristine alternating with vinblastine or vincristine alone. Palliative radiation therapy.	Alpha interferon, bleomycin, etoposide, doxorubicin
Wilms's tumor (in children)[3]	**Combination chemotherapy** with vincristine and dactinomycin with or without doxorubicin after surgery and radiation therapy	Cyclophosphamide, methotrexate, etoposide, cisplatin
Neuroblastoma[3]	**Combination chemotherapy** with variations of cyclophosphamide, cisplatin, vincristine, doxorubicin, dacarbazine	Melphalan, ifosfamide, autologous or allogeneic bone marrow transplantation

[1]Investigational agent. Treatment is available through qualified investigators and centers authorized by the National Cancer Institute and Cooperative Oncology Groups.

[2]Supportive agent; not oncolytic.

[3]These tumors are generally managed initially with surgery with or without radiation therapy with or without adjuvant chemotherapy. For metastatic disease, the role of palliative radiation therapy is as important as that of chemotherapy.

Table 5–3. Single-agent dosage and toxicity of anticancer drugs.

Drug	Dosage	Acute Toxicity	Delayed Toxicity
Alkylating agents			
Mechlorethamine	6–10 mg/m² IV every 3 weeks	Severe vesicant; severe nausea and vomiting	Moderate suppression of blood counts. Melphalan effect may be delayed 4–6 weeks. Excessive doses produce severe bone marrow suppression with leukopenia, thrombocytopenia, and bleeding. Alopecia and hemorrhagic cystitis occur with cyclophosphamide, while busulfan can cause hyperpigmentation, pulmonary fibrosis, and weakness (see text). Ifosfamide is always given with mesna to prevent cystitis. Acute leukemia may develop in 5–10% of patients receiving prolonged therapy with melphalan, mechlorethamine, or chlorambucil; all alkylators probably increase the risk of secondary malignancies with prolonged use. Most cause either temporary or permanent aspermia/amenorrhea.
Chlorambucil	0.1–0.2 mg/kg/d orally (6–12 mg/d) or 0.4 mg/kg pulse every 4 weeks	None	
Cyclophosphamide	100 mg/m²/d orally for 14 days; 400 mg/m² orally for 5 days; 1–1.5 g/m² IV every 3–4 weeks	Nausea and vomiting with higher doses	
Ifosfamide	1.2 g/m²/d IV for 5 days every 3 weeks with mesna	Nausea and vomiting with higher doses	
Melphalan	0.25 mg/kg/d orally for 4 days every 6 weeks	None	
Busulfan	2–8 mg/d orally; 150–250 mg/course	None	
Carmustine (BCNU)	200 mg/m² IV every 6 weeks	Local irritant	Prolonged leukopenia and thrombocytopenia. Rarely hepatitis. Acute leukemia has been observed to occur in some patients receiving nitrosoureas. Nitrosoureas can cause delayed pulmonary fibrosis with prolonged use.
Lomustine (CCNU)	100–130 mg orally every 6–8 weeks	Nausea and vomiting	
Procarbazine	100 mg/m²/d orally for 14 days every 4 weeks	Nausea and vomiting	Bone marrow suppression, mental suppression, MAO inhibition, disulfiram-like effect.
Dacarbazine	250 mg/m²/d IV for 5 days every 3 weeks; 1500 mg/m² IV as single dose	Severe nausea and vomiting; anorexia	Bone marrow suppression; flu-like syndrome.
Cisplatin	50–100 mg/m² IV every 3 weeks; 20 mg/m² IV for 5 days every 4 weeks	Severe nausea and vomiting	Nephrotoxicity, mild otic and bone marrow toxicity, neurotoxicity.
Carboplatin	360 mg/m² IV every 4 weeks	Severe nausea and vomiting	Bone marrow suppression, prolonged anemia; same as cisplatin but milder.
Structural analogues or antimetabolites			
Methotrexate	2.5–5 mg/d orally; 20–25 mg IM twice weekly; high-dose: 500–1000 mg/m² IV every 2–3 weeks; 12–15 mg intrathecally every week for 4–6 doses	None	Bone marrow suppression, oral and gastrointestinal ulceration, acute renal failure; hepatotoxicity, rash, increased toxicity when effusions are present. **Note:** Citrovorum factor (leucovorin) rescue for doses over 100 mg/m².
Mercaptopurine	2.5 mg/kg/d orally; 100 mg/m²/d orally for 5 days for induction	None	Well tolerated. Larger doses cause bone marrow suppression.
Thioguanine	2 mg/kg/d orally; 100 mg/m²/d IV for 7 days for induction	Mild nausea, diarrhea	Well tolerated. Larger doses cause bone marrow suppression.
Fluorouracil	15 mg/kg/d IV for 3–5 days every 3 weeks; 15 mg/kg weekly as tolerated; 500–1000 mg/m² IV every 4 weeks	None	Nausea, diarrhea, oral and gastrointestinal ulceration, bone marrow suppression, dacryocystitis.
Cytarabine	100–200 mg/m²/d for 5–10 days by continuous IV infusion; 2–3 g/m² IV every 12 hours for 3–7 days; 20 mg/m² SC daily in divided doses	High-dose: nausea, vomiting, anorexia	Nausea and vomiting; severe bone marrow suppression; megaloblastosis; CNS toxicity with high-dose cytarabine.
Hormonal agents			
Testosterone propionate	100 mg IM 3 times weekly	None	Fluid retention, masculinization, leg cramps. Cholestatic jaundice in some patients receiving fluoxymesterone.
Fluoxymesterone	20–40 mg/d orally	None	

(continued)

Table 5–3. Single-agent dosage and toxicity of anticancer drugs. (continued)

Drug	Dosage	Acute Toxicity	Delayed Toxicity
Hormonal agents (cont'd)			
Flutamide	250 mg 3 times a day orally	None	Gynecomastia, hot flushes, decreased libido, mild gastrointestinal side effects.
Diethylstilbestrol	1–5 mg/d orally in divided doses	Occasional nausea and vomiting	Fluid retention, feminization, uterine bleeding, exacerbation of cardiovascular disease, painful gynecomastia, thromboembolic disease.
Ethinyl estradiol	3 mg/d orally	None	
Tamoxifen	20 mg/d orally in 2 divided doses	Transient flare of bone pain	?Increased risk of venous thrombosis; anovulation.
Hydroxyprogesterone caproate	1 g IM twice weekly	None	Occasional fluid retention; rare thrombosis.
Medroxyprogesterone	100–200 mg/d orally; 200–600 mg orally twice weekly	None	
Megestrol acetate	40 mg 4 times a day orally	None	
Adrenocorticosteroid			
Prednisone	20–100 mg/d orally or 50–100 mg every other day orally with systemic chemotherapy	Alteration in mood	Fluid retention, hypertension, diabetes, increased susceptibility to infection, "moon facies," osteoporosis, electrolyte abnormalities, gastritis.
Aromatase inhibitor			
Aminoglutethimide	500 mg/d orally, along with hydrocortisone, 40 mg/d orally	Initial drowsiness	Transient skin rash, which usually subsides with continued therapy; weight gain, fluid retention, leg cramps; cholestatic jaundice.
GnRH analogues			
Leuprolide	7.5 mg IM (depot) once a month; 1 mg/d SC	Local irritation, transient flare of symptoms	Hot flushes, decreased libido, impotence, gynecomastia, mild gastrointestinal side effects.
Goserelin acetate	3.6 mg SC monthly	Transient flare of symptoms	
Biologic response modifiers			
Interferon alfa-2a Interferon alfa-2b	3–5 million units SC 3 times weekly or daily	Fever, chills, fatigue, anorexia	General malaise, weight loss, confusion.
Aldesleukin (IL-2)	600,000 IU/kg IV over 15 minutes every 8 hours for 14 doses, repeated after 9-day rest period. Some doses may be withheld or interrupted because of toxicity. *Caution:* High doses must be administered in an ICU setting by experienced personnel.	Hypotension, fever, chills, rigors, diarrhea, nausea, vomiting, pruritus, liver, kidney, and CNS toxicity, capillary leak (primarily at high doses), pruritic skin rash, infections (can be severe).	Hypothyroidism, anemia.
Peptide hormone inhibitor			
Octreotide acetate	100–600 µg/d SC in 2 divided doses	Local irritant; nausea and vomiting	Diarrhea, abdominal pain, hypoglycemia.
Natural products and miscellaneous agents			
Vinblastine	0.1–0.2 mg/kg or 6 mg/m^2 IV weekly	Mild nausea and vomiting; severe vesicant	Alopecia, loss of reflexes, bone marrow suppression, constipation, SIADH.
Vincristine	1.5 mg/m^2 (maximum: 2 mg weekly)	Severe vesicant	Areflexia, muscle weakness, peripheral neuritis, paralytic ileus, alopecia (see text), SIADH.
Paclitaxel (Taxol)	135 mg/m^2 by continuous infusion over 24 hours every 3 weeks	Hypersensitivity reaction, severe bone marrow suppression	Peripheral neuropathy
Dactinomycin	0.04 mg/kg IV weekly	Nausea and vomiting; severe vesicant	Alopecia, stomatitis, diarrhea, bone marrow suppression.

(continued)

Table 5–3. Single-agent dosage and toxicity of anticancer drugs. (continued)

Drug	Dosage	Acute Toxicity	Delayed Toxicity
Natural products and miscellaneous agents (cont'd)			
Daunorubicin	30–60 mg/m² daily IV for 3 days, or 30–60 mg/m² IV weekly	Nausea, fever, red urine (not hematuria); severe vesicant; acute cardiotoxicity	Alopecia, stomatitis, bone marrow suppression, late cardiotoxicity. Risk of cardiotoxicity increases with radiation, cyclophosphamide.
Idarubicin	12 mg/m² daily IV for 3 days		
Doxorubicin	60 mg/m² IV every 3 weeks to a maximum total dose of 550 mg/m²		
Etoposide	100 mg/m²/d IV for 5 days or 50–150 mg/d orally	Nausea and vomiting; occasionally hypotension	Alopecia, bone marrow suppression.
Plicamycin (mithramycin)	25–50 µg/kg IV every other day for up to 8 doses	Nausea and vomiting	Thrombocytopenia, diarrhea, hepatotoxicity, nephrotoxicity, stomatitis.
Mitomycin	10–20 mg/m² every 6–8 weeks	Severe vesicant; nausea	Prolonged bone marrow suppression, rare hemolytic-uremic syndrome.
Mitoxantrone	12–15 mg/m²/d IV for 3 days with cytarabine; 8–12 mg/m² IV every 3 weeks	Mild nausea and vomiting	Alopecia, mild mucositis, bone marrow suppression.
Bleomycin	Up to 15 units/m² IM, IV, or SC twice weekly to a total dose of 200 units/m²	Allergic reactions, fever, hypotension	Fever, dermatitis, pulmonary fibrosis.
Hydroxyurea	500–1500 mg/d orally	Mild nausea and vomiting	Hyperpigmentation, bone marrow suppression.
Mitotane	6–12 g/d orally	Nausea and vomiting	Dermatitis, diarrhea, mental suppression, muscle tremors.
Fludarabine	25 mg/m²/d IV for 5 days every 4 weeks	Nausea and vomiting	Bone marrow suppression, diarrhea, mild hepatotoxicity.
Supportive agents Allopurinol	300–900 mg/d orally for prevention or relief of hyperuricemia	None	Rash, Stevens-Johnson syndrome; enhances effects and toxicity of mercaptopurine when used in combination.
Mesna	20% of ifosfamide dosage at the time of ifosfamide administration, then 4 and 8 hours after each dose of chemotherapy to prevent hemorrhagic cystitis	Nausea, vomiting, diarrhea	None
Leucovorin	10 mg/m² every 6 hours IV or orally until serum methotrexate levels are below 5×10⁻⁸ mol/L with hydration and urinary alkalinization (about 72 hours)	None	Enhances toxic effects of fluorouracil.
Epoetin alfa (erythropoietin)	50–300 units/kg IV or SC 3 times a week	Skin irritation or pain at injection site	Hypertension, headache, seizures in patients on dialysis (rare).
Filgastrim (G-CSF)	5 µg/kg/d SC or IV	Mild to moderate bone pain, mild hypotension (rare), irritation at injection sites (rare)	?Unknown risk of tumor cell stimulation.
Sargramostim (GM-CSF)	250 µg/kg/d as a 2-hour IV infusion (can be given SC)	Fluid retention, dyspnea, capillary leak (rare), supraventricular tachycardia (rare), mild to moderate bone pain, irritation at injection sites	

able) from patients with metastatic breast cancer. This requires fresh, unfixed tissue. Although the assessment of estrogen and progesterone receptors in breast cancer is crucial to the therapy of this disease, androgen receptors remain difficult to measure in prostate cancer. In addition to estrogen therapy, new hormonal approaches are also available to treat prostate cancer. These include the use of gonadotropin-releasing hormone agonists (eg, leuprolide), aromatase inhibitors (eg, aminoglutethimide), and anti-androgens (eg, flutamide). The use of leuprolide plus flutamide can be considered as an alternative to orchiectomy but also causes impotence. High-dose ketoconazole has been used to rapidly suppress adrenal production of steroids in crises such as cord compression. Use of this agent requires cortisone supplementation.

Several recombinant growth factors have been shown to be effective in the treatment of malignancy. Recombinant alpha interferon has marked antitumor effects in hairy cell leukemia and chronic myelogenous leukemia, moderate effects in lymphomas, the epidemic form of Kaposi's sarcoma (AIDS-associated), and multiple myeloma. Interferon has some utility also in metastatic melanoma, renal cell carcinoma, and carcinoid syndrome. The use of alpha interferon together with other methods of treatment will probably increase significantly in the coming years. For example, the addition of alpha interferon to systemic chemotherapy for multiple myeloma appears to significantly increase the degree of cytoreduction achieved as compared with chemotherapy alone. Unfortunately, this therapy can be quite toxic and may adversely affect the quality of life. Use of alpha interferon for myeloma following chemotherapy has significantly prolonged remission duration. Patients with chronic myelogenous leukemia may benefit from treatment with alpha interferon and achieve both a hematologic and cytogenetic remission. The effect on overall survival, however, is still unknown. Another cytokine, interleukin-2 (IL-2), when administered alone or in combination with lymphocyte-activated killer (LAK) cells or tumor-infiltrating lymphocytes (TILs), exhibits marked antitumor activity in a minority of patients with melanoma or renal cancer, although its use is associated with significant toxicities. Aldesleukin has received regulatory approval in the USA for treatment of metastatic renal cancer in adults. The use of genetic engineering to transduce cytokine genes into TIL cells or into the tumors cells themselves in order to enhance tumor cell death is an exciting new area of research in cytokine cancer therapy.

In addition to cytokines, other agents have recently been shown to be efficacious in the treatment of some tumors. For chronic lymphocytic leukemia and low-grade lymphomas, fludarabine phosphate, cladribine (2-chlorodeoxyadenosine; CdA), and pentostatin (2-deoxycoformycin) are effective. Studies using cladribine to treat hairy cell leukemia have resulted in a high remission rate that is durable with tolerable toxicities after a 1-week course of therapy. This has revolutionized the previous at least year-long and probably less effective treatment of choice with alpha interferon. Pentostatin has recently been approved for use in hairy cell leukemia that is refractory to alpha interferon. Paclitaxel (Taxol) is a novel agent isolated from the Pacific yew tree that has been found to be effective in reducing tumor size in 20-30% of patients with refractory metastatic ovarian cancer. These results are from uncontrolled studies, and the drug's impact on survival has not been determined. Approval of paclitaxel is limited to its use in refractory ovarian cancer; however, trials are under way to determine whether it is effective treatment for other cancers. Preliminary activity has been shown in refractory metastatic carcinoma of the breast as well as in other cancers.

Chan HSL et al: Immunohistochemical detection of P-glycoprotein: Prognostic correlation in soft tissue sarcoma of childhood. J Clin Oncol 1990;8:689.

Dillman RO et al: Continuous interleukin-2 and lymphokine-activated killer cells for advanced cancer: A National Biotherapy Study Group trial. J Clin Oncol 1991;9:1233. (One of many studies using IL-2 in treatment of cancer.)

Eddy DM: High-dose chemotherapy with autologous bone marrow transplantation for the treatment of metastatic breast cancer. J Clin Oncol 1992;1);657. (Analysis of current published data.)

Eilber FR, Rosen G: Adjuvant chemotherapy of osteosarcoma. Semin Oncol 1989;16:312. (Includes evaluation of prognostic factors and staging.)

Fisher RI et al: Comparison of a standard regimen (CHOP) with three intensive chemotherapy regimens for advanced non-Hodgkin's lymphoma. N Engl J Med 1993; 328:1002. (CHOP is as effective as more complicated treatment.)

Foon KA, Rai KR, Gale RP: Chronic lymphocytic leukemia: New insights into biology and therapy. 1990;113; 525.

Hu XF et al: Combined use of cyclosporin A and verapamil in modulating multidrug resistance in human leukemia cell lines. Cancer Res 1990;50:2953.

Lum BL et al: Alteration of etoposide pharmacokinetics and pharmacodynamics by cyclosporine in a phase I trial to modulate multidrug resistance. J Clin Oncol 1992; 10:1635. (Evaluates drug levels of etoposide with and without concurrent cyclosporine administration.)

McMillan AK, Goldstone AH: Autologous bone marrow transplantation for non-Hodgkin's lymphoma. Eur J Haematol 1991;46:129.

Miller TP et al: P-glycoprotein expression in malignant lymphoma and reversal of clinical drug resistance with chemotherapy plus high-dose verapamil. J Clin Oncol 1990;9:17.

Prosnitz LR, Roberts KB: Combined chemotherapy and radiotherapy for Hodgkin's disease. Oncology 1992;6:113.

Redman JR et al: Phase II trial of fludarabine phosphate in lymphoma: An effective new agent in low-grade lymphoma. J Clin Oncol 1992;10:790.

Rosenberg SA: Gene therapy for cancer. JAMA 1992; 268:2416. (Genetic engineering and TIL cells.)

Rowinsky EK et al: Taxol: A novel investigational anti-microtubule agent. J Natl Cancer Inst 1990;82:1247. (Phase II trial demonstrating effectiveness of paclitaxel in refractory ovarian cancer.)

Salmon SE et al: Multidrug-resistant melanoma: Laboratory and clinical effects of verapamil as a chemosensitizer. Blood 1991;78:44.

Saven A, Piro LD: Treatment of hairy cell leukemia. Blood 1992;79:1111. (Current and investigational treatments of hairy cell leukemia, including interferon, deoxycoformycin, and cladribine.)

Stagg RJ et al: Alternating hepatic intra-arterial floxuridine and fluorouracil: A less toxic regimen for treatment of liver metastases from colorectal cancer. J Natl Cancer Inst 1991;83:424.

Venook AP et al: Chemoembolization for hepatocellular carcinoma. J Clin Oncol 1990;8:1108. (Significant activity demonstrated.)

ADJUVANT CHEMOTHERAPY FOR MICROMETASTASES

One of the most important roles of cancer chemotherapy is as "adjuvant" therapy to eradicate or suppress minimal residual disease after "primary field" treatment with surgery or irradiation. Failure of primary field therapy to eradicate tumor is due principally to occult micrometastases of tumor stem cells outside the primary field. These distant micrometastases are more likely to be present in patients with positive lymph nodes at the time of surgery (eg, breast cancer), in patients with tumors known to have a propensity for early hematogenous spread (eg, osteogenic sarcoma, Wilms's tumor), and in patients with certain pathologic or molecular risk factors (eg, high proliferative index, vascular invasion, oncogene amplification). Given specific risk factors, the risk of recurrent or metastatic disease can be extremely high (> 80%). Only systemic therapy can adequately prevent micrometastases. Chemotherapeutic regimens that have been shown to be effective in inducing regression of advanced cancers may be curative when combined with surgery for high-risk "early" cancer. Initial studies in experimental animals showed that chemotherapy could eradicate small numbers of residual cancer cells after surgery. In other instances, micrometastases may be suppressed though not eradicated, as may be the case when antiestrogen therapy is used for breast cancer.

The efficacy of adjuvant chemotherapy is well established in pediatric neoplasms, including Wilms's tumor, rhabdomyosarcoma, and osteosarcoma. In this case, adjuvant therapy has resulted in substantial improvement in survival rates. In adults, more data are now available to support the use of adjuvant therapy in several neoplasms. Recent studies have shown significant prolongation in survival for women with breast cancer and positive or negative axillary lymph nodes (stage I, II, and III) from combination chemotherapy following surgical resection. Several useful combination chemotherapy regimens for adjuvant therapy include CA (cyclophosphamide and Adriamycin [doxorubicin]), alone or with the addition of fluorouracil (CAF), and CMF (cyclophosphamide, methotrexate, and fluorouracil), alone or with prednisone (CMFP). Node-negative patients are treated with CMF or variants, whereas high-risk, node-positive patients are generally treated with regimens that include doxorubicin. Neoadjuvant (preoperative) and perioperative chemotherapy is used in some settings and may improve surgical resectability or time to disease progression. The antiestrogen tamoxifen is used routinely either with or without antecedent chemotherapy if receptors for estrogen and progesterone are present. In postmenopausal women, tamoxifen alone may be used. The main challenge in treating women with node-negative (stage I) breast cancer is to identify prognostic factors to determine which patients are at higher risk and therefore more likely to benefit from adjuvant therapy.

Adjuvant chemotherapy with fluorouracil plus levamisole is now indicated in Dukes C (node-positive) colon cancer and has been shown to reduce the risk of cancer recurrence. Early clinical trials suggested a benefit from adjuvant therapy of Dukes B and C rectal cancer with radiation therapy combined with fluorouracil and semustine (methyl-CCNU). Unfortunately, use of semustine appeared to result in an increased risk of both leukemia and renal insufficiency. Recent preliminary data have shown that the omission of semustine still results in enhanced cure rates with decreased local and overall tumor recurrence.

Other tumors that have been shown to respond to adjuvant therapy include osteogenic sarcoma and ovarian cancer. Adjuvant therapy remains investigational and unproved for a number of common tumors, including non-small-cell lung cancer and pancreatic cancer. Patients with Hodgkin's disease or testicular carcinoma do not benefit from adjuvant therapy, as the cure rates with chemotherapy for advanced or recurrent disease remain high and the toxicity of early treatment far outweighs the potential benefit.

Although adjuvant therapy has been shown to reduce the rate of recurrence for some cancers, there is still a significant failure rate (up to 80% in high-risk breast cancer despite adjuvant therapy). In most cases, tumor recurrence signifies incurability. There is clear evidence of a dose-response effect of adjuvant chemotherapy; however, doses have been limited by bone marrow toxicity. Current studies are investigating the use of dose-intense chemotherapy regimens with or without autologous bone marrow or peripheral blood progenitor cell rescue in the high-risk adjuvant setting for patients with carcinoma of the breast, testis, and ovaries. Early studies suggest significant efficacy with tolerable side effects of high-dose chemotherapy with stem cell support in the setting of high-risk breast cancer (more than ten positive lymph nodes). Young patients with high-risk malignancies should be considered for entry into clinical trials investigating this aggressive, potentially curable therapy.

Bonadonna G: Evolving concepts in the systemic adjuvant treatment of breast cancer. Cancer Res 1992;52:2127.

Fisher B et al: A randomized clinical trial evaluating sequential methotrexate and fluorouracil in the treatment of patients with node-negative breast cancer who have estrogen receptor-negative tumors. N Engl J Med 1989; 320:473.

Fisher B et al: A randomized clinical trial evaluating tamoxifen in the treatment of patients with node-negative breast cancer who have estrogen receptor-positive tumors. N Engl J Med 1989;320:479.

Gradishar WJ et al: The impact on survival by adjuvant chemotherapy and radiation therapy in stage II non-small cell lung cancer. Am J Clin Oncol 1992;15:405. (Improved survival with chemotherapy.)

Henderson IC et al: Effects of adjuvant tamoxifen and of cytotoxic therapy on mortality in early breast cancer: An overview of 61 randomized trials among 28,896 women. N Engl J Med 1988;319:1681.

Kwak LW et al: Prognostic significance of actual dose intensity in diffuse large-cell lymphoma: Result of a tree-structured survival analysis. J Clin Oncol 1990;8:963. (Dose intensity is critical to outcome.)

Mansour EG et al: Efficacy of adjuvant chemotherapy in high-risk node-negative breast cancer. N Engl J Med 1989;320:485.

Moertel CG et al: Levamisole and fluorouracil for adjuvant therapy of resected colon carcinoma. N Engl J Med 1990:322:352.

Neville AM et al: Factors predicting responsiveness and prognosis in node-negative breast cancer. The International (Ludwig) Breast Cancer Study Group. J Clin Oncol 1992;10:696.

Salmon SE (editor): Adjuvant Therapy of Cancer VI. Saunders, 1990.

Sigurdsson H et al: Indicators of prognosis in node-negative breast cancer. N Engl J Med 1990;322:1045.

Tandon AK et al: Cathepsin D and prognosis in breast cancer. N Engl J Med 1990;322:297.

Young RC et al: Adjuvant therapy in stage I and II epithelial ovarian cancer. N Engl J Med 1990;322:1021.

TOXICITY & DOSE MODIFICATION OF CHEMOTHERAPEUTIC AGENTS

A number of cancer chemotherapeutic agents have cytotoxic effects on rapidly proliferating normal cells in bone marrow, mucosa, and skin. Still other drugs such as the *Vinca* alkaloids produce neuropathy, and the hormones often have psychic effects. Acute and chronic toxicities of the various drugs are summarized in Table 5–3. Appropriate dose modification usually minimizes these side effects, so that therapy can be continued with relative safety.

Bone Marrow Toxicity

Depression of bone marrow is usually the most significant limiting toxicity of cancer chemotherapy. Autologous bone marrow or peripheral blood progenitor cell transplantation or rescue can reduce the myelosuppressive toxicity of high-dose chemotherapy; however, cost and toxicity limit its general use. Growth factors that stimulate myeloid proliferation (eg, granulocyte colony-stimulating factor [G-CSF; filgastrim] and granulocyte-macrophage stimulating factor [GM-CSF; sargramostim]) or erythroid proliferation (erythropoietin [epoetin alfa]) are now used to ameliorate bone marrow toxicity. G-CSF and GM-CSF have been shown to shorten the period of neutropenia following both standard and high-dose chemotherapy. Mucosal toxicity is also reduced, allowing shorter hospital stays. The myeloid growth factors are also used to stimulate circulation of progenitor cells in the peripheral blood either at steady state or during white blood cell recovery following myelosuppressive chemotherapy. These cells are then harvested using an apheresis machine (this can be done in the outpatient setting) and frozen for later use. When "stimulated" peripheral blood progenitor cells (PBPCs) such as these are used instead of or in conjunction with bone marrow for autologous transplantation following high-dose chemotherapy and radiotherapy, recovery of both neutrophils and platelets may be hastened by as much as 7–10 days over the use of bone marrow alone. This results in significantly shortened hospital stays, decreased toxicity, and decreased cost.

Epoetin alfa (erythropoietin) has been shown to improve anemia associated with malignancy. Patients must have adequate iron stores to respond to this agent, and even patients with marrow infiltration with tumor may benefit. Higher doses may be necessary for patients with cancer compared to the doses used for patients with renal failure. Although quality of life may be improved and frequency of red cell transfusions may be reduced, these benefits must be weighed against the cost of this growth factor.

Thrombocytopenia remains a problem with high doses of or prolonged exposure to chemotherapeutic agents and may limit therapy. Several agents currently under investigation may help with this problem. Interleukin-3 (IL-3) stimulates myeloid growth and, to a lesser extent, platelet recovery. In order to enhance both of these effects, a fusion molecule has been created that produces a GM-CSF/IL-3 hybrid protein (PIXY321). Early trials suggest that this molecule may be effective in stimulating both myeloid and platelet recovery following chemotherapy.

Commonly used short-acting drugs that affect the bone marrow are the alkylating agents (eg, cyclophosphamide, melphalan, chlorambucil), procarbazine, mercaptopurine, methotrexate, vinblastine, flu-orouracil, dactinomycin, and doxorubicin. In general, it is preferable to use alkylating agents in intensive "pulse" courses every 3–4 weeks rather than to administer the drugs in continuous daily schedules. This allows for complete hematologic (and immunologic) recovery between courses rather than continuously suppressing the bone marrow with a cytotoxic agent. Pulse therapy reduces side effects to some degree but does not reduce therapeutic efficacy. The standard dosage schedules required to produce tumor responses with these agents often induce bone marrow depression. Patients must be carefully monitored and may require dose reductions or even discontinuation of the offending drug. Continuing some drugs in the face of falling blood counts may result in severe bone marrow aplasia with pancytopenia, bleeding, or infection. Simple guidelines for treatment and follow-up can usually prevent severe marrow depression.

White blood cell and differential counts, hematocrit or hemoglobin, and platelet counts should be obtained frequently. With long-term chemotherapy, counts should be obtained initially at weekly intervals; the frequency of counts may be reduced only after the patient's sensitivity to the drug can be well predicted (eg, 3–4 months) and cumulative toxicity excluded.

In patients with normal blood counts as well as normal liver and kidney function, drugs should be started at full doses. Dosage modifications may be required for future cycles. Toxicity to the bone marrow is cumulative over time, and this must be anticipated during follow-up. Patients with bone marrow involvement may tolerate chemotherapy poorly initially, with improved counts on future cycles as the tumor burden is reduced. Dose escalation is currently being studied for the treatment of some malignancies.

Drug dosage can usually be modified as a function of the peripheral white blood count or platelet count (or both). These modifications assume that the blood counts are checked shortly before the next course of chemotherapy is to be administered. In this fashion, smooth control of drug administration and peripheral blood counts can usually be attained for oral alkylating agents or antimetabolites. A scheme for dose modifications is shown in Table 5–4. Alternatively, the interval between drug courses can be lengthened, thereby permitting more complete hematologic recovery and repetition of full-dose chemotherapy. Both dose modification and delay of chemotherapy significantly limit the efficacy of treatment. The current availability of myeloid growth factors has eliminated the need for both maneuvers in most cases. Thrombocytopenia remains a problem, as mentioned above.

Drugs with delayed hematologic toxicities do not always fit into such a simple scheme, and in general they should be administered by specialists familiar with the specific toxicities. Drugs requiring special

Table 5–4. A common scheme for dose modification of cancer chemotherapeutic agents.

Granulocyte Count (/μL)	Platelet Count (/μL)	Suggested Drug Dosage (% of full dose)
>3000	>100,000	100%
2000–3000	75,000–100,000	50%
<2000	<50,000	0%

precautions with respect to toxicity include doxo-rubicin, mitomycin, busulfan, cytarabine, bleomycin, plicamycin (mithramycin), carmustine, lomustine, semustine, and daunorubicin.

Lieschke GJ et al: Granulocyte colony-stimulating factor and granulocyte-macrophage colony-stimulating factor. N Engl J Med 1992;327:28.

Spivak JL: The application of recombinant erythropoietin in anemic patients with cancer. Semin Oncol 1992;19:25. (Good review of the uses of erythropoietin in various types of malignancies.)

Chemotherapy-Induced Nausea & Vomiting

A number of cytotoxic anticancer drugs induce nausea and vomiting as side effects. In general, these symptoms are thought to originate in the central nervous system rather than peripherally. Parenteral administration of agents such as doxorubicin, etoposide, or cyclophosphamide frequently is associated with mild to moderate nausea and vomiting, whereas nitrosoureas, dacarbazine, and particularly cisplatin usually cause severe symptoms. These symptoms can limit patient tolerance and acceptance of chemotherapy. Combination chemotherapy with agents including those listed above can also cause severe symptoms. Antiemetics clearly reduce and often eliminate nausea and vomiting associated with these drugs and are especially useful in conjunction with cisplatin.

Metoclopramide is a particularly useful agent, especially when administered parenterally at a dosage of 1–2 mg/kg both 30 minutes before and again 30 minutes after the administration of chemotherapy. Extrapyramidal signs may be induced with this drug but frequently can be suppressed with 25–50 mg of oral or parenteral diphenhydramine. Dexamethasone has antiemetic effects when administered at a dosage of 6–10 mg either as a single dose prior to or prior to and every 6 hours following the administration of chemotherapy for two to four total doses. Both of these drugs are significantly more potent than conventional agents such as prochlorperazine, diphenhydramine, and thiethylperazine. Prochlorperazine is given at a dose of 10 mg by mouth or intravenously every 6 hours. The total dose given over 24 hours should not exceed 40 mg. A 25 mg rectal suppository is available and may be useful for patients who are too nauseated to swallow pills without experiencing further emesis. Unfortunately, all phenothiazines can induce extrapyramidal side effects that range from muscle spasms and anxiety to a true parkinsonism-like syndrome. These side effects must be watched for carefully and can be treated with diphenhydramine, but they may preclude further use of this class of drugs. Diphenhydramine is usually used in conjunction with other antiemetics and may prevent extrapyramidal side effects as well as help to control emesis. It is given at a dose of 25–50 mg every 6 hours either by mouth or parenterally. Thiethylperazine is given at a dose of 10 mg every 8 hours by mouth and is also available at the same dose in a rectal suppository. Lorazepam has both antiemetic and sedating effects and is administered at a dose of 0.5–1 mg every 4–6 hours by the sublingual route, making it particularly useful in the outpatient setting. Older patients may have intolerable psychologic side effects. Combinations of antiemetics (eg, metoclopramide with dexamethasone and lorazepam) are often more effective than maximal doses of any one agent for blocking cisplatin-induced vomiting. An example of a common antiemetic regimen for intermediate-dose to high-dose cisplatin or other highly emetogenic chemotherapy regimens might be as follows: 30 minutes prior to starting cisplatin, 10 mg of dexamethasone (oral), 50 mg of diphenhydramine (oral), 1–2 mg/kg of metoclopramide (parenteral), and 0.5–1 mg of lorazepam (sublingual) are given. Repeated doses of metoclopramide combined with diphenhydramine at a lower dose such as 25 mg are given every 3–4 hours for three doses following administration of chemotherapeutic agents. Lorazepam or prochlorperazine is then given for persistent nausea at home. For less emetogenic regimens, attenuated doses and schedules of these drugs are used.

Ondansetron may now replace high-dose metoclopramide in the treatment and prevention of emesis induced by cisplatin and other high-dose agents. A new and very potent antiemetic, ondansetron is a serotonin receptor-blocking agent that has few side effects. Several studies have shown that it is both more effective and less toxic than metoclopramide in cisplatin-treated patients. It is also effective against radiation-induced and postanesthetic vomiting as well as for patients with refractory nausea and vomiting following other chemotherapeutic agents. Ondansetron is administered by the parenteral route at a dose of 0.15 mg/kg for three doses. The first dose is given 30 minutes before the start of chemotherapy; subsequent doses are given 4 and 8 hours after the first dose. A typical antiemetic regimen might include ondansetron combined with lorazepam and dexamethasone, omitting both metoclopramide and diphenhydramine. Although ondansetron is very expensive, the total cost of this regimen is about $1\frac{1}{2}$ times to twice the cost of the traditional combination regimen described above and has fewer side effects as well as perhaps higher efficacy. For less emeto-

genic regimens, ondansetron alone may be no more effective than metoclopramide and dexamethasone.

Dronabinol (Δ^9-tetrahydrocannabinol) is effective in some patients at a dose of 5 mg/m^2 prior to and then every 2–4 hours following chemotherapy for a total of four to six doses a day. Dronabinol may cause undesirable side effects such as dysphoria, and it is available only for oral administration. A patient receiving potent antiemetics along with chemotherapy on an outpatient basis must be escorted to and from the clinic, since the antiemetics often induce marked sedation and transient impairment of balance and reflexes.

Hesketh PJ, Gandara DR: Serotonin antagonists: A new class of antiemetic agents. J Natl Cancer Inst 1991; 83:613.

Levitt M et al: Ondansetron compared with dexamethasone and metoclopramide as antiemetics in the chemotherapy of breast cancer with cyclophosphamide, methotrexate, and fluorouracil. N Engl J Med 1993;328:1081. (The two regimens appear equal in this widely used but only moderately emetogenic chemotherapy.)

Marty M et al: Comparison of the 5-hydroxytryptamine$_3$ (serotonin) antagonist ondansetron with high dose metoclopramide in the control of cisplatin-induced emesis. N Engl J Med 1990;322:816.

Roila R et al: Prevention of cisplatin-induced emesis: A double-blind multicenter randomized crossover study comparing ondansetron and ondansetron plus dexamethasone. J Clin Oncol 1991;9:675. (Ondansetron with dexamethasone appears to be more effective than ondansetron alone.)

Pisters KM, Kris MG: Management of nausea and vomiting caused by anticancer drugs: State of the art. Oncology 1992;6(2 Suppl):99.

Gastrointestinal & Skin Toxicity

Since antimetabolites such as methotrexate and fluorouracil act only on rapidly proliferating cells, they damage the cells of mucosal surfaces such as the gastrointestinal tract. Methotrexate has similar effects on the skin. These toxicities are at times more significant than bone marrow suppression, and they should be looked for routinely when these agents are used.

Erythema of the buccal mucosa is an early sign of mucosal toxicity. If therapy is continued beyond this point, oral ulceration will develop. In general, it is wise to discontinue therapy at the time of appearance of early oral ulceration. This finding usually heralds the appearance of similar but potentially more serious ulceration at other sites lower in the gastrointestinal tract. Therapy can usually be reinstituted when the oral ulcer heals (1 week to 10 days). The dose of drug used may need to be modified downward at this point, with titration to an acceptable level of mucosal toxicity. Adequate mouth care with antimicrobial mouthwashes and attention to dental hygiene are essential and may prevent significant toxicity. Common mouthwashes include the microbicidal oral rinse chlorhexidine and a mixture of salt and bicarbonate of soda in warm water, which aids in debridement of dead mucosa. A prophylactic antifungal mouthwash such as nystatin oral suspension may also be used. High doses of methotrexate require special consideration, as noted in the following section.

Miscellaneous Drug-Specific Toxicities

The toxicities of individual drugs have been summarized in Table 5–3. Several of these warrant additional mention, since they occur with commonly administered agents, and special preventive measures are often indicated.

A. Hemorrhagic Cystitis Induced by Cyclophosphamide or Ifosfamide: Metabolic products of cyclophosphamide that retain cytotoxic activity are excreted into the urine. Some patients appear to metabolize more of the drug to these active excretory products. If their urine is concentrated, the toxic metabolite may cause severe bladder damage. Patients receiving cyclophosphamide must be advised to maintain a high fluid intake. Early symptoms of bladder toxicity include dysuria and frequency despite the absence of bacteriuria. Such symptoms develop in about 20% of patients who receive the drug chronically. If microscopic hematuria develops, it is advisable to stop the drug temporarily or switch to a different alkylating agent, increase fluid intake, and administer a urinary analgesic such as phenazopyridine. With severe cystitis, large segments of bladder mucosa may be shed and the patient may have prolonged gross hematuria. Such patients should be observed for signs of urinary obstruction and may require cystoscopy for removal of obstructing blood clots. The risk of developing hemorrhagic cystitis is dose-related. For high doses of cyclophosphamide, preventive continuous bladder irrigation with normal saline solution is used during the period of drug administration and for the following 24 hours.

The cyclophosphamide analogue ifosfamide, which was recently approved by the FDA, can cause severe hemorrhagic cystitis when used alone. However, when it is used in conjunction with a series of doses of the neutralizing agent mesna, bladder toxicity can be prevented. Mesna can also be used to prevent cystitis in patients receiving cyclophosphamide in high doses.

B. Vincristine-Induced Neuropathy: Neuropathy is a toxic side effect that is peculiar to the *Vinca* alkaloid drugs, especially vincristine. The peripheral neuropathy can be sensory, motor, autonomic, or a combination of these effects. In its mildest form, it consists of paresthesias ("pins and needles") of the fingers and toes. Occasional patients develop acute jaw or throat pain after vincristine therapy. This may be a form of trigeminal or glossopharyngeal neuralgia. With continued vincristine therapy, the paresthesias may extend to the proximal interphalangeal joints, hyporeflexia can appear in the lower extremi-

ties, and significant weakness may develop in the quadriceps muscle group. At this point, it is wise to discontinue vincristine therapy until the neuropathy has subsided. A useful means of judging whether peripheral motor neuropathy is significant enough to warrant stopping treatment is to have the patient attempt to do deep knee bends or get up out of a chair without using their arm muscles.

Constipation is the most common symptom of autonomic neuropathy associated with vincristine therapy. Patients receiving vincristine should be started on stool softeners and mild cathartics when therapy is begun; otherwise, severe impaction may result along with an atonic bowel.

More serious autonomic involvement can lead to acute intestinal ileus with signs indistinguishable from those of an acute abdomen. Bladder neuropathies are uncommon but may be severe. These two complications are absolute contraindications to continued vincristine therapy. The majority of symptoms from vincristine are mild and will resolve slowly after therapy has been completed.

C. Methotrexate Toxicity and "Citrovorum Rescue": In addition to standard uses of methotrexate for chemotherapy, this drug is also used in very high doses that could lead to fatal bone marrow toxicity if given without an antidote. High-dose methotrexate therapy with citrovorum factor rescue is routinely used to treat osteogenic sarcoma, acute lymphocytic leukemia, and some cases of non-Hodgkin's lymphoma.

The bone marrow and mucosal toxicity of methotrexate can be prevented by early administration of citrovorum factor (folinic acid; leucovorin). Serum levels of methotrexate are usually monitored and doses of citrovorum factor adjusted accordingly. Rescue is required for methotrexate doses over 80 mg/m^2 and is usually begun within 4 hours after completing treatment. Up to 100 mg/m^2 of citrovorum factor is given initially every 6 hours, with further doses adjusted for the serum methotrexate level. Rescue is usually continued orally for 3 days or longer until the serum methotrexate level is below 0.05 μmol/L. If an overdose of methotrexate is administered accidentally, folinic acid therapy should be initiated as soon as possible, preferably within 1 hour. Intravenous infusion should be employed for larger overdosages to ensure adequate drug delivery. It is generally advisable to give citrovorum factor repeatedly in this situation.

Vigorous hydration and bicarbonate loading also appear to be important in preventing crystallization of high-dose methotrexate in the renal tubular epithelium. Serum creatinine must be monitored before beginning therapy and daily thereafter, since methotrexate excretion is slowed by renal insufficiency and the toxicity will be enhanced. In high doses, methotrexate can itself cause renal injury. Methotrexate doses are routinely reduced for renal insufficiency.

Concomitant use of certain drugs will slow methotrexate excretion, and it is mandatory that they be avoided during therapy. These drugs include aspirin, nonsteroidal anti-inflammatory agents, penicillins, sulfonamides, and probenecid.

D. Busulfan Toxicity: The alkylating agent busulfan, frequently used for the treatment of chronic myelogenous leukemia, has curious delayed toxicities, including increased skin pigmentation, a wasting syndrome similar to that seen in adrenal insufficiency, and progressive pulmonary fibrosis. Patients who develop either of the latter two problems should be switched to a different drug (eg, melphalan) when further therapy is needed. The pigmentary changes are innocuous and will usually regress slowly after treatment is discontinued.

E. Bleomycin Toxicity: This antibiotic has found increasing application in cancer chemotherapy in view of its activity in squamous cell carcinomas, Hodgkin's disease, non-Hodgkin's lymphomas, and testicular tumors. Bleomycin can produce edema of the interphalangeal joints and hardening of the palmar and plantar skin. More serious toxicities include an anaphylactic or serum sickness-like reaction and a serious, potentially fatal pulmonary fibrotic reaction (seen especially in elderly patients receiving a total dose of over 300 units). If a nonproductive cough, dyspnea, and pulmonary infiltrates develop, the drug is discontinued, and high-dose corticosteroids are instituted as well as empiric antibiotics pending cultures. Fever alone or with chills is an occasional complication of bleomycin treatment and is not an absolute contraindication to continued treatment. The fever may be avoided by hydrocortisone administration just prior to the injection. Fever alone is not predictive of pulmonary toxicity. About 1% of patients (especially those with lymphoma) may have a severe or even fatal hypotensive reaction after the initial dose of bleomycin. In order to identify such patients, it is wise to administer a test dose of 5 units of bleomycin first and to have adequate monitoring and emergency facilities available in case they are needed. Patients exhibiting a hypotensive reaction should not receive further bleomycin therapy.

F. Doxorubicin-Induced Cardiomyopathy: The anthracycline antibiotics doxorubicin and daunomycin both have acute and delayed cardiac toxicity. The problem is greater with doxorubicin because it has a major role and is used in repeated doses in the treatment of sarcomas, breast cancer, lymphomas, acute leukemia, and certain other solid tumors. Studies of left ventricular function and endomyocardial biopsies indicate that some changes in cardiac dynamics occur in most patients by the time they have received 300 mg/m^2 of doxorubicin. The *multiple-gated* ("MUGA") radionuclide cardiac scan appears to be the most useful noninvasive test for assessing toxicity. Doxorubicin should not be used in elderly patients with significant intrinsic cardiac disease. The risk of cardiomyopathy is usually dose-dependent. In general, patients should not receive a total dose in excess of 550 mg/m^2, and 1–10% of patients who receive this dose develop cardiomyopathy. Patients who have had prior chest or mediastinal radiotherapy may develop doxorubicin heart disease at lower total doses. The appearance of a high resting pulse may herald the appearance of overt cardiac toxicity. Unfortunately, the toxicity may be irreversible and frequently fatal at dosage levels above 550 mg/m^2. At lower doses (eg, 350 mg/m^2), the symptoms and signs of cardiac failure generally respond well to digitalis, diuretics, and cessation of doxorubicin therapy. Recent evidence suggests that cardiac toxicity can be correlated with high peak plasma levels obtained with intermittent high-dose bolus therapy (eg, every 3–4 weeks). Use of weekly injections or low-dose continuous infusion schedules appears to delay the occurrence of cardiac toxicity. Current laboratory studies suggest that cardiac toxicity may be due to a mechanism involving the formation of intracellular free radicals in cardiac muscle. Pretreatment with ICRF-187, an iron chelator that decreases free radical formation, may protect the myocardium from anthracycline-induced injury. This agent is investigational and in clinical trials. Newer anthracycline analogues include idarubicin, which has shown efficacy against acute nonlymphocytic leukemia and breast cancer and may have less cardiotoxicity than doxorubicin.

G. Cisplatin Nephrotoxicity and Neurotoxicity: Cisplatin is effective in the treatment of testicular, bladder, and ovarian cancer as well as in several other types of tumor. Nausea and vomiting are common, but nephrotoxicity and neurotoxicity are more serious. Vigorous hydration with or without mannitol diuresis may substantially reduce nephrotoxicity. Renal function must be carefully monitored during cisplatin therapy. Ototoxicity is a potentially serious neurotoxicity that can result in deafness. The neurotoxicity of this drug is delayed and is more common after a total dose of 300 mg/m^2 has been administered. Other manifestations include peripheral neuropathy of mixed sensorimotor type that may be associated with painful paresthesias. The neuropathy may be secondary to hypomagnesemia, which can be induced by cisplatin. Therefore, the serum magnesium should be measured and replaced routinely. If neuropathy develops, treatment with parenteral magnesium sulfate should be tried. These supportive measures do not appear to reduce the therapeutic effectiveness of cisplatin. The second-generation platinum analogue carboplatin is now available and has been shown to be as effective as cisplatin in ovarian cancer. Carboplatin is less nephrotoxic and causes less severe nausea or vomiting, but it does induce myelosuppression. A recent report suggests that an experimental ACTH(4–9) analogue (referred to as Org-2766) or a heavy metal chelating agent (diethyldithiocarbamate; DDTC) may be useful in preventing cisplatin neurotoxicity.

H. Alpha Interferon Toxicities: While alpha interferon is generally well tolerated in the standard doses listed in Table 5–3, it has increasing toxicity with increasing doses and is more toxic in elderly patients. Even standard doses may be intolerable to some patients. Fever and chills are initial side effects but are infrequent after continued treatment. These symptoms may be ameliorated or prevented by premedication with acetaminophen and bedtime dosing. However, anorexia, fatigue, and weight loss can be cumulative and with time become severe. These symptoms may be dose- or treatment-limiting. In some patients, central nervous system symptoms develop, usually manifested as confusion or somnolence. Reduction in peripheral blood counts can develop, but this abnormality is usually not clinically important and may even be a desired effect in the treatment of chronic myelogenous leukemia. These interferon-induced side effects can sometimes be confused with the symptoms of progressive cancer. Fortunately, the side effects usually clear within 1 week after cessation of interferon therapy.

Berry JM et al: Modification of cisplatin toxicity with diethyldithiocarbamate. J Clin Oncol 1990;8:1585. (A study using a metal chelator to modify cisplatin neurotoxicity.)

Chabner BA (editor): *Cancer Chemotherapy: Principles and Practice.* Lippincott, 1990.

Greene MH et al: Melphalan may be a more potent leukemogen than cyclophosphamide. Ann Intern Med 1986; 105:360.

Kaldor JM et al: Leukemia following chemotherapy for ovarian cancer. N Engl J Med 1990;322:1.

Kaldor JM et al: Leukemia following Hodgkin's disease. N Engl J Med 1990;322:7.

Tucker MA et al: Risk of second cancers after treatment for Hodgkin's disease. N Engl J Med 1988;318:76.

van der Hoop RG et al: Prevention of cisplatin neurotoxicity with an ACTH(4–9) analog in patients with ovarian cancer. N Engl J Med 1990;322:89.

EVALUATION OF TUMOR RESPONSE

Inasmuch as cancer chemotherapy can induce clinical improvement, significant toxicity, or both, it is important to critically assess the beneficial effects of treatment in patients with advanced cancer to determine that the net effect is favorable. The most valuable signs to follow during therapy include the following:

TUMOR SIZE

Shrinkage in tumor size can be demonstrated by physical examination, chest film or other x-ray, sonography, or a radionuclide scanning procedure such as bone scanning (breast, lung, prostate cancer). CT scanning is important for the accurate evaluation of tumor size and location and the extent of distant spread for a wide variety of tumors and sites. MRI is now the best noninvasive means of evaluating posterior fossa brain tumors, spinal cord tumors, spinal cord compression, and pelvic disease, but CT scanning remains useful and may provide additional information. Sonography is also particularly helpful in the evaluation of pelvic neoplasms. A partial response (PR) is defined as a 50% or greater reduction in the original tumor mass. A complete response (CR) refers to the complete disappearance of detectable tumor. Progression is an increase of more than 25% in the size of the tumor or the appearance of any new lesions. Careful staging is required to accurately determine the response.

TUMOR MARKERS

A significant decrease in the quantity of a tumor product or marker substance reflects a reduced amount of tumor in the body. Examples of such markers include paraproteins (abnormal immunoglobulins) in multiple myeloma and macroglobulinemia, human chorionic gonadotropin (hCG) in choriocarcinoma and testicular tumors, prostatic acid phosphatase and prostate-specific antigen (PSA) in prostatic cancer, urinary steroids in adrenal carcinoma and paraneoplastic Cushing's syndrome, and 5-HIAA in carcinoid syndrome.

Tumor-secreted fetal antigens are becoming of increasing importance. These include $alpha_1$-fetoprotein (AFP) in hepatoma, in teratoembryonal carcinoma, and in occasional cases of gastric carcinoma; ovarian tumor antigen (CA 125) in ovarian cancer; and carcinoembryonic antigen (CEA) in carcinomas of the colon, lungs, and pancreas. A newly described fetal antigen, CA 15:3, may become important in detecting early recurrence of breast cancer. Monoclonal antibodies are now used for measurement of a number of tumor markers and offer the potential of delineating a number of additional markers for diagnostic purposes.

Tumor markers may play an important role in the early detection of some common tumors when combined with good physical examinations. PSA, an immunogenic glycoprotein produced solely by the prostate, is currently the only tumor marker with widespread use in cancer screening. Although PSA was initially used only to indicate tumor bulk and disease progression, it has recently been found to be an effective screening tool when paired with the digital rectal examination. The American Cancer Society National Prostate Cancer Detection Project is a multi-center study evaluating the use of PSA, rectal examination, and transrectal ultrasound in a large cohort of healthy men. In this and other studies, the combination of a monoclonal PSA greater than 4 ng/mL or an abnormal digital rectal examination were felt to produce cost-effective early detection of prostate cancer. Annual screening is recommended beginning at age 40 in men with a family history of prostate cancer and in black men, and beginning at age 50 for all others. An abnormal PSA or digital examination requires further evaluation by transrectal ultrasound and possible biopsy. The increase in screening for prostate cancer over the last few years has markedly increased the reported incidence of this disease, though the true incidence is probably stable. (See Table 5–1. The 1988 estimated rate was 103 versus 109 for the 1989 estimated rate.) The PSA may be falsely elevated in benign prostatic hypertrophy. Unfortunately, most other tumor markers are not specific or sensitive enough to be useful as screening tools owing to their frequent elevation in benign disease and absence in some cases of malignancy.

GENERAL WELL-BEING & PERFORMANCE STATUS

The functional status of the cancer patient at diagnosis (or at the start of treatment) is a major prognostic factor and determinant of outcome with or without tumor-directed therapy. It is therefore important to assess functional status as well as tumor burden and symptoms before deciding on possible anticancer therapy. Functional status or performance status evaluates the patient's ability to carry on activities of daily living and is clearly related to tumor burden, tumor site, and the patient's underlying physical condition.

Two scales are commonly used to measure PS. The Karnofsky scale ranges from 100% (asymptomatic and fully functional) through 0% (dead) in steps of 10%. For example, a Karnofsky performance status of 40% implies a patient who is disabled and requires special care and assistance. This patient would be unable to work but able to live at home with special assistance. The more commonly used Eastern Cooperative Oncology Group (ECOG) scale is a five-point system that is simpler and easier to apply to clinical practice. The ECOG scoring system ranges for 0 to 4 as follows: 0, entirely asymptomatic; 1, symptomatic but fully ambulatory; 2, symptomatic and in bed less than 50% of the day; 3, symptomatic and in bed more than 50% of the day but not bedridden; and 4, bedridden. These two scoring systems are the basis for clinical decisions in many situations when treatment options are considered despite their obvious lack of precision. They are also useful in assessing the impact of therapy and disease progression on the patient.

The measures assessing functional status described above do not adequately assess quality of life, a major goal of cancer chemotherapy. Performance status is only one component of quality of life, which is a combination of subjective and objective factors and may in some cases be partly a placebo effect. Factors included in the assessment of general well-being include improved appetite and weight gain and decreased pain as well as improved performance status. It is only by completely evaluating all of the factors described above that the physician is able to judge whether the net effect of chemotherapy is worthwhile palliation. In addition, a thorough evaluation will identify cancer patients who are candidates for aggressive rehabilitation.

Bates SE: Clinical applications of serum tumor markers. Ann Intern Med 1991;115:623.

Catalona W et al: Measurement of prostate-specific antigen in serum as a screening test for prostate cancer. N Engl J Med 1991;324:1156.

Conill C, Verger E, Salamero M: Performance status assessment in cancer patients. Cancer 1990;65:1864. (Patients are useful and reliable in self-evaluation of performance status.)

Cupp MR et al: Prostate-specific antigen, digital rectal examination, and transrectal ultrasonography: Their roles in diagnosing early prostate cancer. Mayo Clin Proc 1993;68:297. (Includes a useful algorithm for prostate screening.)

Littrup PJ et al: Prostate cancer screening: Current trends and future implications. CA 1992;42:198. (Modalities used for prostate cancer screening.)

Roila F et al: Intra- and interobserver variability in cancer patients' performance status assessed according to Karnofsky and ECOG scales. Ann Oncol 1991;2:437. (Evaluation of the scales in the selection of patients for inclusion in clinical trials.)

CANCER COMPLICATIONS: DIAGNOSIS & MANAGEMENT

ONCOLOGIC EMERGENCIES

Cancer is a chronic disease, but acute emergencies may occur as a consequence of local involvement (spinal cord compression, superior vena cava syndrome, malignant effusions, etc) or generalized systemic effects (hypercalcemia, opportunistic infections, hypercoagulability, hyperuricemia, etc). These complications may be the presenting manifestation of neoplasia and are important to understand and recognize. Two relatively common complications covered elsewhere will not be discussed here: superior vena cava syndrome (Chapter 12) and hypercoagulability (Chapter 13).

Berger NA (guest editor): Oncologic emergencies. Semin Oncol 1989;16:461.

1. SPINAL CORD COMPRESSION

Spinal cord compression by tumor mass is manifested by back pain, progressive weakness, and sensory loss (usually in the lower extremities). Less commonly, spinal cord disease may present as chest or abdominal pain or as signs of nerve root compression due to the epidural location of the tumor. Bowel and bladder dysfunction are late findings. Spinal cord compression may occur as a complication of metastatic solid tumor, lymphoma, or myeloma. Back pain at the level of the spinal cord lesion occurs in over 80% of cases and may be aggravated by lying down, weight-bearing, sneezing, or coughing. Because back pain may precede the development of neurologic symptoms or signs, it is important to investigate this complaint thoroughly in any patient with cancer.

Prompt diagnosis and early therapy of impending spinal cord compression are essential. The neurologic defects present at diagnosis are usually irreversible, though treatment immediately after symptoms develop may result in partial recovery. Neurologic impairment can progress overnight, and patients must be followed very carefully. Treatment of early lesions may completely avoid significant compromise. Although patients who present with paralysis may not recover function, they should still be treated for pain relief and to limit the extent of further progression. In addition, patients may respond to systemic therapy depending on the specific tumor type.

The diagnosis of spinal cord compression has traditionally been made by CT scanning in conjunction with myelography. MRI now provides a noninvasive and extremely sensitive alternative to myelography. It is possible to obtain detailed views of the area in question as well as sagittal images of the entire spinal cord and vertebral canal. This detailed examination is important for detection and treatment of multiple lesions. Bone radiographs and bone scans are useful for detecting vertebral metastases but do not aid in assessing spinal cord compromise.

Emergency Treatment

Radiation therapy to the area of spinal cord compression and two adjacent vertebrae above and below the lesion is the treatment of choice. High doses of glucocorticoids (usually dexamethasone, 10–100 mg intravenously) are administered on an emergency basis as soon as the diagnosis is strongly suspected or confirmed to decrease swelling at the tumor site. A lower dose (eg, 4–6 mg every 6 hours intravenously or orally) is continued throughout the course of radi-

ation therapy and tapered at or near the end of treatment.

Emergency surgery is indicated (1) for spinal cord compression in the absence of a diagnosis of malignancy, (2) for patients who have already received maximal doses of radiation to the involved area of the spine, and (3) for patients who develop progressive neurologic deficits during radiation whose prognosis warrants aggressive therapy. Chemotherapy is useful in treating lymphomas and multiple myeloma in conjunction with or following completion of radiation therapy.

Wilson JKV, Masaryk TJ: Neurologic emergencies in the cancer patient. Semin Oncol 1989;16:490.

2. HYPERCALCEMIA

Hypercalcemia secondary to cancer is a fairly common medical emergency, occurring in 10–20% of patients with cancer. Common causes include breast, lung, kidney, and head and neck carcinomas as well as multiple myeloma. Although the majority of cancers associated with hypercalcemia metastasize to the bones, approximately 20% of cases are not associated with bony lesions. Hypercalcemia may be of humoral origin or may be due to direct bony destruction, as discussed above under paraneoplastic syndromes. The recent identification of a novel protein called parathyroid hormone-related protein (PTHrP) has revised some previous thoughts regarding the pathogenesis of hypercalcemia. Radioimmunoassays have identified this peptide in the serum of approximately two-thirds of cancer patients with hypercalcemia. High levels have been found in patients with hypercalcemia previously thought to be due solely to local osteolysis. PTHrP may become a useful tumor marker in normocalcemic patients. In addition, antibodies to PTHrP may be useful as treatment.

The symptoms of hypercalcemia include nausea, vomiting, constipation, polyuria, muscular weakness and hyporeflexia, confusion, psychosis, tremor, and lethargy. Some patients may be asymptomatic. Electrocardiography often shows a shortening of the QT interval. When the serum calcium rises above 12 mg/dL, sudden death may occur due to cardiac arrhythmia or asystole. The presence of hypercalcemia does not invariably indicate a dismal prognosis, especially in breast or prostate cancer and multiple myeloma. In the absence of signs or symptoms of hypercalcemia, a laboratory finding of elevated serum calcium should be rechecked immediately to exclude the possibility of error.

Emergency Treatment

A. Hydration: Emergency treatment consists of aggressive intravenous hydration with 3–4 L/d of saline followed by diuresis with furosemide. It is essential that the patient be well hydrated before beginning diuretic therapy and that hydration be maintained after diuresis is initiated. Although hydration alone is effective at slowly reducing the calcium level, it is rarely sufficient treatment and can lead to problems with fluid overload.

B. Drug Therapy: There are now several options for the emergent treatment of hypercalcemia used in conjunction with aggressive hydration.

1. Bisphosphonates–The bisphosphonate etidronate, which acts by decreasing bone resorption, must be administered initially by the intravenous route. It is given in doses of 7.5 mg/kg/d over 2 or more hours for 3 consecutive days. Care must be taken when using this drug in patients with renal insufficiency. Emergent therapy is usually followed by chronic oral therapy, though this is seldom effective for continued control of hypercalcemia. A new bisphosphonate compound, pamidronate disodium, is now available for the treatment of hypercalcemia of malignancy. Pamidronate is the most potent bisphosphonate available and has been demonstrated to have efficacy superior to that of etidronate in a randomized double-blind trial. A single 24-hour intravenous infusion of 60–90 mg with adequate hydration produced complete normalization of serum calcium by day 7 in 70–100% of patients. The most commonly reported side effects have been transient fever and an infusion site reaction. The low toxicity profile and high effectiveness of this agent may significantly improve therapy for hypercalcemia.

2. Calcitonin–Synthetic salmon calcitonin works immediately to inhibit bone resorption, whereas etidronate may take 3–5 days to achieve its maximum effect. Calcitonin alone is usually not effective at lowering serum calcium levels but can be added to etidronate to achieve normal calcium levels within a few days in most cases. Repeated treatment with calcitonin is usually not as effective.

3. Gallium nitrate–This agent has only recently been approved by the FDA for treatment of hypercalcemia. It is given by continuous intravenous infusion at a dose of 100–200 mg/m^2/d for 5 days. In a double-blind randomized trial comparing calcitonin to this new agent, gallium nitrate was found to be far superior both in reducing calcium levels acutely and in keeping the levels low after treatment was completed. Renal function must be carefully monitored.

4. Other drugs–Prednisone has not been shown to be effective as a single agent to treat hypercalcemia, though it can be used in diseases that are responsive to steroids such as multiple myeloma. Refractory hypercalcemia may be treated with intravenous plicamycin (mithramycin), 25 µg/kg/d for 3 or 4 days. Although often effective, its effect may be short-lived, and repeated use is associated with significant hepatic, renal, and bone marrow toxicity.

C. Chemotherapy: Once the acute episode has been treated, chemotherapy may be considered. Pa-

tients with breast cancer may develop hypercalcemia as a "flare" associated with bone pain after initiation of estrogen or antiestrogen therapy. These patients will often achieve excellent tumor response with continued therapy. Tumors may respond to chemotherapy or radiation therapy, leading to resolution of hypercalcemia. If chronic hypercalcemia persists and is refractory to chemotherapy, oral etidronate, phosphates, low-dose prednisone, and aggressive oral hydration may be tried but are unfortunately rarely effective for long. When the more potent bisphosphonates become available in oral formulations, the management of chronic hypercalcemia may improve.

Coleman RE: Bisphosphonate treatment of bone metastases and hypercalcemia of malignancy. Oncology 1991;5:55.

Gucalp R et al: Comparative study of pamidronate disodium and etidronate disodium in the treatment of cancer-related hypercalcemia. J Clin Oncol 1992;10:134. (A multicenter randomized trial.)

Hall TG et al: Update on the medical treatment of hypercalcemia of malignancy. Clin Pharm 1993;12:117. (Old and new therapies and their relative merits.)

Theriault RL: Hypercalcemia of malignancy: Pathophysiology and implications for treatment. Oncology 1993;7:47.

Warrell RP et al: Gallium nitrate for acute treatment of cancer-related hypercalcemia. Ann Intern Med 1988;108:669.

Yarbro JW (editor): Advances in hypercalcemia of malignancy. Semin Oncol 1990;17(Suppl 5):1.

3. HYPERURICEMIA & ACUTE URATE NEPHROPATHY

Hyperuricemia can occur both as a complication of rapidly proliferating malignancies or with treatment-associated tumor lysis of hematologic malignancies such as leukemia, lymphoma, and multiple myeloma. Neoplasms with a high nucleic acid turnover such as acute leukemia and lymphoma may present with an elevated serum uric acid and associated renal insufficiency. This problem may be compounded by use of thiazide diuretics, which decrease urate excretion. If a patient presents with hyperuricemia, care must be taken to reduce the uric acid as much as possible before institution of cancer therapy. Patients at risk for tumor lysis syndrome should be followed carefully with twice-daily measurements of uric acid, phosphate, calcium, and creatinine for the first 2 to 3 days following initiation of chemotherapy. Rapid elevation of the serum uric acid concentration presents the danger of acute urate nephropathy caused by uric acid crystallization in the distal tubules, collecting ducts, and renal parenchyma. A serum urate concentration above 15 mg/dL is associated with a high risk of developing uric acid nephropathy. Gouty arthritis is usually a problem only in patients with a history of gout.

Prophylactic therapy consists of decreasing the

production and increasing the renal excretion of uric acid. Allopurinol is a competitive inhibitor of xanthine oxidase and prevents conversion of highly soluble hypoxanthine and xanthine to the relatively insoluble uric acid. Twelve to 24 hours before beginning therapy, a dose of 600 mg is given, followed by 300 mg/d during the period of high risk. Higher doses (up to 900–1200 mg/d) are used when severe hyperuricemia is anticipated following chemotherapy. Patients receiving the purine antagonists mercaptopurine or azathioprine should be given only 25–35% of the calculated dose of chemotherapy if they are also receiving allopurinol, since the latter drug will potentiate both the therapeutic effects and the toxicity of these agents. Renal excretion of uric acid is enhanced by maintaining a high urine flow and by alkalinizing the urine to prevent uric acid crystallization (occurs at acid pH). Alkaline diuresis to maintain a urine pH near 7.0 is required only for prophylaxis in patients expected to have a rapid tumor response with marked hyperuricemia.

Emergency Treatment

Emergency therapy for established severe hyperuricemia consists of (1) hydration with 2–4 L of fluid per day; (2) alkalinization of the urine with 6–8 g of sodium bicarbonate per day; (3) allopurinol, 900–1200 mg/d; and (4) in severe cases, emergency hemodialysis. When severe hyperuricemia is present, adequate therapy may be impossible because of associated renal insufficiency and inadequate urine output. Intravenous allopurinol has recently been approved for use in patients unable to tolerate the oral form of this drug.

Patients suffering from hyperuricemia are usually responding to chemotherapy and have a good prognosis. Therefore, aggressive prophylaxis is indicated to avoid renal damage. Even if renal failure occurs and dialysis is required, renal function may return to normal after the acute tumor lysis has resolved.

4. MALIGNANT CARCINOID SYNDROME

Although tumors of argentaffin cells are uncommon, they are important because they secrete a variety of vasoactive materials. These include serotonin, histamine, catecholamines, prostaglandins, and vasoactive peptides. Carcinoid syndrome is usually associated with carcinoid tumors of the small bowel and less commonly with primary carcinoid tumors in other sites, such as the lung or stomach. These tumors tend to metastasize early but have a relatively indolent course, making control of the syndrome important. Related syndromes occur in patients with pancreatic tumors secreting vasoactive peptides, which can cause severe watery diarrhea (pancreatic cholera).

The manifestations of carcinoid syndrome include facial flushing, edema of the head and neck (especially with bronchial carcinoid), abdominal cramps and diarrhea, bronchospasm, cardiac lesions (tricuspid or pulmonary stenosis or regurgitation), telangiectasias, and increased urinary 5-hydroxyindoleacetic acid (5-HIAA). The most common symptoms are flushing and diarrhea. The diagnosis is made by finding elevated levels of 5-HIAA in a 24-hour urine collection. Patients with symptomatic carcinoid usually excrete more than 25 mg of 5-HIAA per day in the urine. Ideally, all drugs and serotonin-rich foods such as bananas should be withheld for several days before beginning the urine collection.

Emergency Treatment

Emergency therapy for patients with symptomatic bronchial carcinoid includes prednisone, 15–30 mg/d. The associated abdominal cramping and diarrhea of intestinal carcinoids can often be managed by hydration and diphenoxylate with atropine. For severe diarrhea, the H_1 histamine receptor antagonist cyproheptadine or an antiserotonin agent such as methysergide maleate may be effective. Other useful agents include the H_2 receptor blocker cimetidine and the phenothiazines.

A new synthetic peptide somatostatin agonist, octreotide acetate, is the most effective agent for reducing symptoms due to the carcinoid syndrome in association with achieving a significant reduction in levels of urinary 5-HIAA. Octreotide is also effective in the treatment of symptoms related to vasointestinal peptide-secreting pancreatic tumors (VIPomas), markedly reducing the watery diarrhea syndrome associated with this neoplasm.

Surgery is important in the treatment of localized carcinoid. Chemotherapy is used for patients with progressive advanced-stage disease. Active agents include fluorouracil, streptozocin, dacarbazine, cisplatin, doxorubicin, and alpha interferon.

Feldman JM: Carcinoid tumors and the syndrome. Semin Oncol 1987;14:235.

Vinik AI et al: Clinical features of carcinoid syndrome and the use of somatostatin analogue in its management. Acta Oncol 1989;28:389.

Wynick D, Bloom SR: Clinical review 23: The use of the long-acting somatostatin analog octreotide in the treatment of gut neuroendocrine tumors. J Clin Endocrinol Metab 1991;73:1.

OTHER COMPLICATIONS

1. MALIGNANT EFFUSIONS

The development of effusions in the pleural, pericardial, and peritoneal spaces may be the presenting sign of some tumors or may cause diagnostic and therapeutic problems in patients with advanced neo-plasms. Although the differential diagnosis of a malignant effusion can be difficult in a newly diagnosed asymptomatic patient, it is rarely difficult in the patient with advanced cancer. Approximately half of undiagnosed effusions in patients not known to have cancer will be malignant. The differential diagnosis includes congestive heart failure, pulmonary embolism, trauma, and infections such as tuberculosis. Direct involvement of the serous surface of the involved space with tumor appears to be the most frequent initiating factor, though many other mechanisms such as lymphatic drainage that control the flow of fluid in the pleural space may play a role.

Most patients with a pleural or pericardial effusion are symptomatic at presentation with chest pain, shortness of breath, or cough. The diagnosis is made by tapping the involved space. Pericardial effusions are aspirated under fluoroscopic guidance. The fluid should be heparinized and sent for cell count and differential, protein content, lactic dehydrogenase level, and cytologic study. The gross appearance of the fluid is often helpful as well. Bloody effusions are usually due to cancer but occasionally are due to pulmonary embolism, tuberculosis, or trauma. Chylous effusions may be associated with thoracic duct obstruction or may result from enlarged mediastinal lymph nodes in lymphoma. The presence of an effusion is suggestive of malignancy, and the diagnosis is often confirmed by cytologic examination. If the cytologic smear is negative on two occasions but the suspicion of tumor is still high, closed pleural biopsy may be helpful.

The management of effusions should be appropriate to the severity of involvement. Treatment of the underlying neoplasm would be ideal but is often not effective in controlling local effusions. Treatment may result in significant palliation and improve short-term survival when there is significant pulmonary or cardiac compromise. Diuretics are used as initial treatment for small to moderate-sized peritoneal effusions and as an adjunct to local drainage of large effusions to minimize the possibility of reexpansion pulmonary edema that can occur after thoracentesis. Small or loculated effusions may require ultrasonographic localization, but drainage of a large pleural or peritoneal effusion can be accomplished rapidly using an intravenous catheter and phlebotomy tubing connected to a vacuum bottle. Thoracentesis alone controls less than 10% of effusions but may be useful in conjunction with systemic chemotherapy for sensitive tumors (eg, lymphoma, small-cell lung cancer, breast cancer). Pleural effusions may occasionally be managed by closed water-seal drainage with a chest tube for 3–4 days, though this procedure is usually performed in conjunction with chemosclerosis (see below). The aim of this procedure is to allow the pleural surfaces to come into close contact and become adherent.

Recurrent symptomatic effusions can often be controlled by drainage followed by chemosclerosis. In this procedure, a chemotherapeutic or nonchemotherapeutic agent is instilled into the involved space with lidocaine to prevent local pain. The intended effect is local inflammation and sclerosis to encourage adherence of the serosal surfaces. Many drugs used for this purpose have been abandoned because of severe local pain or systemic toxicity, including myelosuppression. Agents commonly used include bleomycin, tetracycline, talc, and the anthracenedione compound mitoxantrone. Despite its high cost, a recent prospective trial has shown bleomycin to be more effective at controlling pleural effusions than tetracycline, with almost double the recurrence rate 90 days after sclerosis when tetracycline was used rather than bleomycin, with similar side effects. At the present time, tetracycline is no longer manufactured for intracavitary instillation and is not available for this indication. The major side effects of bleomycin are pain, fever, and hypersensitivity reactions. Mitoxantrone has been reported to be effective in controlling malignant pleural effusions causing minimal fever and local pain. However, one recent prospective, randomized trial evaluated the effectiveness of mitoxantrone alone versus pleural tube alone and found no statistically significant differences in response or in duration of response. The authors suggest that the instillation of sclerosing agents be reserved for patients who fail pleural tube drainage alone. Talc poudrage has been used successfully to control malignant pleural effusions and appears to be relatively painless. In addition, intrapleural chemotherapy has been used both to control the effusion and to treat the underlying malignancy with variable results. Sclerosis is generally less useful for the management of malignant ascites, but success has been reported using bleomycin, doxorubicin, thiotepa, and other agents.

Before instilling the sclerosing agent, it is important that the space be drained as thoroughly as possible. For pleural effusions, a small-bore chest tube or pigtail catheter is usually placed and fluid is removed by negative suction until the drainage is under 100 mL per 24 hours and the lung has expanded. Sclerotherapy is ineffective if there is a large residual effusion. The patient is then premedicated with a narcotic, and 60 units of bleomycin or 30 mg of mitoxantrone in 50–100 mL of normal saline is instilled directly into the chest tube. The chest tube is then clamped, and the patient is placed in different positions every 15 minutes for 4 hours to distribute the agent equally within the pleural space. At the end of this 4-hour period, the clamp is removed and the chest tube is allowed to drain with suction. After 24 hours, the chest tube is removed from suction, and when the drainage is minimal, the tube is removed. The whole process can take anywhere from 3 to 5 days. Occasionally, repeated doses of the sclerosing agent may be required to stop persistent reaccumulation of the effusion. Talc has been insufflated into the pleural space via a thoracoscope or instilled in a 5 g slurry with iodide via a chest tube.

Surgery is infrequently used for patients with pleural or pericardial effusions who have failed sclerosis and who continue to have an expected survival of at least 1 year. Pleuroperitoneal shunting may have limited value in selected patients with high performance status who can participate actively in pumping the shunt the 100 times on five separate occasions each day required for adequate shunt function and fluid drainage. Pleurectomy has a high complication rate but offers excellent control of effusion in carefully selected patients. A pericardial window or stripping also offers good control with a lower complication rate and may also be performed for constrictive pericarditis following radiation therapy to the chest.

Aelony Y, King R, Boutin C: Thoracoscopic talc poudrage pleurodesis for chronic recurrent pleural effusions. Ann Intern Med 1991;115:778. (Prospective evaluation of the efficacy for both malignant and benign effusions.)

Buzaid AC, Garewal HS, Greenberg BR: Managing malignant pericardial effusion. West J Med 1989;150:174.

Groth G et al: Intrapleural palliative treatment of malignant pleural effusions with mitoxantrone versus placebo (pleural tube alone). Ann Oncol 1991;2:213. (No differences in response or response duration.)

Moores DW: Malignant pleural effusion. Semin Oncol 1991;18(1 Suppl 2):59. (Treatment options.)

Parker LA, Charnock GC, Delany DJ: Small bore catheter drainage and sclerotherapy for malignant pleural effusions. Cancer 1989;64:1218. (Efficacy of pigtail catheters versus large-bore chest tubes.)

Ruckdeschel JC: Management of malignant pleural effusion: An overview. Semin Oncol 1988;15:24.

Ruckdeschel JC et al: Intrapleural therapy for malignant pleural effusions: A randomized comparison of bleomycin and tetracycline. Chest 1991;100:1528.

Rusch VW et al: Intrapleural cisplatin and cytarabine in the management of malignant pleural effusions: A Lung Cancer Study Group trial. J Clin Oncol 1991;9:313. (Intrapleural chemotherapy to treat pleural effusion from a variety of solid tumors.)

2. INFECTIOUS COMPLICATIONS

Many patients with cancer have increased susceptibility to both bacterial and opportunistic infections. This may result from impaired host defense mechanisms (eg, Hodgkin's or non-Hodgkin's lymphoma, chronic lymphocytic leukemia, multiple myeloma, acute leukemia or preleukemia) or from the myelosuppressive and immunosuppressive effects of cancer chemotherapy. Impaired host defense mechanisms include defects in neutrophil function, abnormalities in antibody production, depressed cell-mediated immune function, impairment of mechanical barriers by indwelling intravenous catheters, and impairment of mucosal integrity. At least half of infections seen in neutropenic patients are felt to be endogenous.

The bacterial organisms accounting for the majority of infections in cancer patients include Enterobacteriaceae (*Klebsiella, Enterobacter, Serratia, Escherichia coli*), *Pseudomonas, Staphylococcus,* and *Streptococcus*. Other important pathogens include *Corynebacterium, Clostridium, Mycobacterium,* and *Legionella*. Patients with prolonged neutropenia or following bone marrow transplantation are at risk for fungal infections such as *Candida* and *Aspergillus*, viral infections such as herpes zoster and cytomegalovirus, and *Pneumocystis carinii*. The incidence of bacteremia rises dramatically when the white count is less than $600/\mu L$ or when there are fewer than 200 granulocytes per microliter. In patients with neutropenia, hematologic malignancies, or following bone marrow transplantation, infection is a medical emergency and must be treated emergently and empirically. Although fever may be due to multiple causes, including mucositis, drugs, and the malignancy itself, infection must be the greatest suspect. Infection may be present even in the absence of fever, especially in patients who are receiving glucocorticoids as part of their treatment regimen. Appropriate cultures of the blood, urine, sputum, and cerebrospinal fluid as indicated should always be obtained before starting therapy. Negative cultures in febrile neutropenic patients do not rule out infection, and treatment should be instituted immediately without waiting for culture results to become available. If an indwelling line is present, blood cultures should be drawn from the periphery as well as through the line itself.

Treatment

Infection management has been aimed at treatment of gram-negative bacterial sepsis, the most rapidly lethal infection. Current concepts have been broadened to include prophylaxis and prevention of the most common infections, including those caused by gram-negative, gram-positive, and fungal pathogens. Until recently, empiric therapy of fever consisted of two- or three-drug combinations, including an aminoglycoside and an antipseudomonal penicillin, with resolution of fever and bacteremia in about 70% of patients. Current results using initial monotherapy with ceftazidime or combination β-lactam appear to yield similar results. Vancomycin or amphotericin B may be added on the basis of clinical suspicion, culture results, or prolonged fever in the absence of positive cultures. Adding aminoglycosides or changing ceftazidime to a different antibiotic with broad-spectrum gram-negative activity (eg, imipenem) is also indicated for prolonged fever or clinical deterioration.

Prevention

Prophylaxis of infections in high-risk or neutropenic patients can prevent the complications of sepsis. Oral norfloxacin or parenteral ciprofloxacin has been shown to be effective in suppressing gram-negative infections arising from the gastrointestinal tract in neutropenic patients with leukemia or after autologous bone marrow transplantation. Ciprofloxacin may also prevent infections in neutropenic outpatients but can lead to the selection of resistant bacterial strains. Patients undergoing bone marrow transplantation have long-term indwelling catheters and are at high risk for gram-positive bacterial infections. Vancomycin, when given throughout the period of neutropenia as prophylaxis, has been shown to effectively reduce the incidence of gram-positive infections as well as infection morbidity and the number of days of fever following bone marrow transplantation. Trimethoprim-sulfamethoxazole (TMP-SMZ) has been used as prophylaxis in neutropenic patients with variable results. TMP-SMZ is given routinely to prevent infections by *Pneumocystis* in patients with lymphocytic malignancies, AIDS (see Chapter 30), and following bone marrow transplantation. Other active agents to prevent *Pneumocystis* infection include pentamidine and dapsone. Low-dose amphotericin B and the less toxic triazole fluconazole have been used to prevent fungal infections in immunocompromised patients, though only high-dose amphotericin B is effective against *Aspergillus*. Patients at high risk for fungal infections include those with prolonged granulocytopenia, those with indwelling catheters, those taking broad-spectrum antibiotics over long periods, and those receiving parenteral nutrition. Viral prophylaxis with acyclovir is usually given only to patients undergoing bone marrow transplantation or those with mucosal ulcerations.

In patients who are severely immunocompromised, some bacterial infections may be prevented with intravenous immune globulin. This is important in patients with chronic lymphocytic leukemia, multiple myeloma, and following bone marrow transplantation who have associated immunoglobulin deficiencies.

The recent availability of recombinant bone marrow growth factors has helped to reduce the morbidity and mortality of infections in immunocompromised hosts. Granulocyte colony-stimulating factor (G-CSF; filgastrim) and granulocyte-macrophage colony-stimulating factor (GM-CSF; sargramostim) have been shown to be effective at reducing the duration of neutropenia and the frequency and severity of infection after myelosuppressive chemotherapy or autologous bone marrow transplantation for nonmyeloid malignancies. Trials are under way to study the use of these and other growth factors to improve bone marrow tolerance of escalating doses of chemotherapy. GM-CSF and G-CSF have been used to stimulate bone marrow stem cell production in both the circulating blood and in bone marrow cell populations collected for autologous transplantation. Administration of growth factors may improve survival after the failure of autologous or allogeneic bone marrow grafts. These growth factors are currently being used experimentally to stimulate the growth of refractory myeloid malignancies and thus perhaps enhance cell killing by cytotoxic agents.

Attal M et al: Prevention of gram-positive infections after bone marrow transplantation by systemic vancomycin: A prospective, randomized trial. J Clin Oncol 1991;9:865. (Efficacy in neutropenic patients with indwelling central venous catheters.)

Gabrilove JL et al: Effect of granulocyte colony-stimulating factor on neutropenia and associated morbidity due to chemotherapy for transitional-cell carcinoma of the urothelium. N Engl J Med 1988;318:1414.

Herrmann F et al: Hematopoietic responses in patients with advanced malignancy treated with recombinant human granulocyte-macrophage colony-stimulating factor. J Clin Oncol 1989;7:159.

Lazarus HM et al: Infectious emergencies in oncology patients. Semin Oncol 1989;16:543.

Morstyn G et al: Effect of granulocyte colony stimulating factor on neutropenia induced by cytotoxic chemotherapy. Lancet 1988;1:667.

Nemunaitis J et al: Recombinant granulocyte-macrophage colony-stimulating factor after autologous bone marrow transplantation for lymphoid cancer. N Engl J Med 1991;324:1773. (GM-CSF significantly reduces morbidity.)

Sanders JW, Powe NR, Moore RD: Ceftazidime monotherapy for empiric treatment of febrile neutropenic patients: A meta-analysis. J Infect Dis 1991;164:907. (Efficacy of monotherapy versus combination regimens.)

Winston DJ et al: Beta-lactam antibiotic therapy in febrile granulocytopenic patients. A randomized trial comparing cefoperazone plus piperacillin, ceftazidime plus piperacillin, and imipenem alone. Ann Intern Med 1991;115;849. (Combination versus single β-lactam therapy as empiric therapy for febrile neutropenic patients.)

THE PARANEOPLASTIC SYNDROMES

The clinical manifestations of cancer are usually nonspecific—eg, anorexia, malaise, weight loss, fever—or are due to local effects of tumor growth, either in the primary site or at a distant site. The term "paraneoplasia" has been coined to denote the remote effects of malignancy that cannot be attributed either to direct invasion or metastatic lesions. These syndromes may be the first sign of a malignancy and may affect up to 15% of patients with cancer.

The paraneoplastic syndromes are of considerable clinical importance for the following reasons:

(1) They may accompany relatively limited neoplastic growth and provide an early clue to the presence of certain types of cancer.

(2) The course of the paraneoplastic syndrome usually parallels the course of the tumor. Therefore, effective treatment should be accompanied by resolution of the syndrome, and, conversely, recurrence of the cancer may be heralded by return of systemic symptoms.

(3) The metabolic or toxic effects of the syndrome may constitute a more urgent hazard to life than the underlying cancer (eg, hypercalcemia, hyponatremia).

The paraneoplastic syndromes are often considered to be due to aberrant hormonal or metabolic effects not associated with a cancer's normal tissue equivalent. Clinical findings may resemble those of primary endocrine, metabolic, hematologic, or neuromuscular disorders. The mechanisms for such remote effects can be classified into three groups: (1) effects initiated by a tumor product (eg, carcinoid syndrome), (2) effects due to the destruction of normal tissues by tumor (eg, hypercalcemia due to osteolytic skeletal metastases), and (3) effects due to unknown mechanisms such as unidentified tumor products or circulating immune complexes stimulated by the tumor (eg, osteoarthropathy due to bronchogenic carcinoma). Even such nonspecific symptoms as fever and weight loss are truly paraneoplastic and probably are due to the production of specific factors (eg, tumor necrosis factor) by the tumor itself.

Paraneoplastic syndromes associated with ectopic hormone production are among the most common and best understood. Tumor tissue secretes a hormone or prohormone that may be of a higher or lower molecular weight than hormones secreted by the more differentiated normal endocrine cell. This ectopic hormone production by cancer cells is believed to result from activation of genes in malignant cells that are normally suppressed in most somatic cells. Neoplastic cells may secrete growth factors that play an autocrine role for tumor growth and also result in paraneoplastic syndromes. A single syndrome such as hypercalcemia may be due to any one or more than one of a variety of causes. These can include (1) secretion of humoral factors such as parathyroid hormone precursors or homologues (parathyroid hormone-related protein [PTHrP]), osteoclast-activating factor (lymphotoxin), transforming growth factor alpha, or prostaglandins; or (2) direct destruction of bone, as in the bony metastases of breast cancer. Effective antitumor treatment usually results in return of the serum calcium to normal, though additional therapy is often required (see Hypercalcemia, below). In occasional cases, a rapid response to cytotoxic chemotherapy may briefly increase the severity of the paraneoplastic syndrome in association with tumor lysis (eg, hyponatremia with inappropriate antidiuretic hormone excretion).

The most common cancer associated with para-

Table 5–5. Paraneoplastic syndromes and certain endocrine secretions associated with cancer.

Hormone Excess or Syndrome	Bronchogenic Carcinoma	Breast Carcinoma	Renal Carcinoma	Adrenal Carcinoma	Hepatoma	Multiple Myeloma	Lymphoma	Thymoma	Prostatic Carcinoma	Pancreatic Carcinoma	Choriocarcinoma	Sarcoma
Hypercalcemia	++	++++	++	++	+	++++	+	+	++	+	+	+
Cushing's syndrome	+++		+	+++				++	+	++		
Inappropriate ADH secretion	+++						+			+		
Hypoglycemia				+	++		+					+++
Gonadotropins	+				+						++++	
Thyrotropin											+++	
Polycythemia			+++	+	++							
Erythroid aplasia								++				
Fever			+++		++		+++	++		+		+
Neuromyopathy	++	+						++	+	+		
Dermatomyositis	++	+								+		
Coagulopathy	+	++			+	+			+++	+++		
Thrombophlebitis			+						+	+++		
Humoral immune deficits						+++	+++	+++				

neoplastic syndromes is small-cell cancer of the lung. This is thought to be due to its neuroectodermal origin. Common paraneoplastic syndromes and associated malignancies are summarized in Table 5–5.

Brooks PM: Rheumatic manifestations of neoplasia. Curr Opin Rheumatol 1992;4;90.

Daughaday WH et al: Synthesis and secretion of insulinlike growth factor II by a leiomyosarcoma with associated hypoglycemia. N Engl J Med 1988;319:1434.

Patel A et al: Paraneoplastic syndromes associated with lung cancer. Mayo Clin Proc 1993;68:278. (Potential mechanisms, diagnosis, and treatment.)

Poole S et al: Cutaneous markers of internal malignancy: I. Malignant involvement of the skin and genodermatoses. J Am Acad Dermatol 1993;28:1.

Posner JB: Paraneoplastic syndromes. Neurol Clin 1991;9:919. (Neuromuscular complications of cancer.)

Richardson GE, Johnson BE: Paraneoplastic syndromes in thoracic malignancies. Curr Opin Oncol 1991;3:320. (Emphasis on recent advances in our understanding of underlying molecular and immunologic mechanisms.)

Skin & Appendages

Sanford M. Goldstein, MD, & Richard B. Odom, MD

DIAGNOSIS OF SKIN DISORDERS

Morphology

A dermatologic differential diagnosis is based on one feature: the appearance—or morphology—of the skin lesion. While it is true that skin diseases can present in myriad ways, it is also generally true that specific diseases cause characteristic lesions. All lesions need not have the characteristic feature, but identifying lesions as pustules, vesicles, or scaly plaques will guide the clinician to the right *group* of diseases to be considered further. This chapter will group and discuss diseases according to the types of lesions they cause and guide the reader through appropriate features of the history, physical findings, and laboratory tests that discriminate among the differential diagnoses. If one cannot make a firm diagnosis using these principles, then either referral to a dermatologist, skin biopsy, or in some cases empiric therapy is indicated.

History

A detailed history is important when done in the context of the differential diagnosis. For example, a history of a change in a pigmented lesion is important in evaluating moles. A history of exposure to specific allergens is vital when assessing lesions thought to represent contact allergic dermatitis. A personal or family history of allergic disease can be helpful in assessing a rash thought to be atopic dermatitis. However, in general, when choosing between conclusions suggested by the history and by one's own observations—with regard to skin cancer or moles (nevi), for example—the physical examination takes precedence. Important components of a thorough history include assessing the role of systemic disorders, inquiring about prescription or OTC systemic and topical medications, and questioning about recent or unusual exposure to physical and chemical agents in the home and work environments. The history is also very important in assessing therapeutic failure. In dermatology, this part of the history includes detailing exactly how the patient is using topical medications.

Physical Examination

If possible, it is best to examine the entire skin surface, including the nails, scalp, palms, soles, and mucous membranes, in good (preferably natural) light. For some diseases, such as psoriasis, examination of these areas is vital in establishing the diagnosis. This total skin examination is not necessary for diagnosis of most conditions but will be most important in identifying malignant melanoma in its earliest and most curable stages by nondermatologist clinicians, who see most of these patients. In examining the faces of older individuals at risk for nonmelanoma skin cancer, pay special attention to the lid margins, nose, ears, and lips.

PRINCIPLES OF DERMATOLOGIC THERAPY

Planning Topical Treatment

Many topical agents are available for the treatment of dermatologic disorders. In general, it is better to be thoroughly familiar with a few drugs and treatment methods than to attempt to use a great many. In addition, not all generic topical medications are equivalent to their brand-name counterparts, either in potency or in the formulation of inert components. This should be kept in mind when assessing unexpected side effects or lack of efficacy. When in doubt about the proper method of treatment, one should *undertreat* rather than overtreat: Inappropriate chronic use of a potent topical corticosteroid without supervision may cause irreversible side effects.

Complications of Topical Dermatologic Therapy

Complications of topical therapy can be largely avoided by proper management. They fall into several categories:

A. Allergy: Of the topical antibiotics, neomycin has the greatest potential for sensitization. Diphenhydramine, benzocaine, and ethylenediamine are potential sensitizers in topical medications.

B. Irritation: Preparations of retinoic acid, benzoyl peroxide, and other acne medications should be used appropriately and with instruction. Repeated use of lindane (Kwell, etc) and antiseptic soaps can be irritating. Podophyllum resin can be very irritating.

Sunscreens with high sun protection factors may irritate the skin of some patients.

C. Absorption: Drugs may be absorbed through the skin, especially near mucous membranes, through broken or inflamed skin, or from under occlusive dressings. On average, the systemic dose absorbed by children is three times that of adults. One should ask if a patient is pregnant before using podophyllum resin. Lindane should probably not be used in babies, children, or pregnant women, and it should be replaced by permethrin 5% cream (Elimite) in children or with permethrin or precipitated sulfur in pregnant women. Agents containing phenol are contraindicated on open skin or mucous membranes of neonates. Injudicious use of topical corticosteroids in large amounts or over prolonged periods, especially with occlusive plastic wrapping, can result in significant systemic absorption of steroids, resulting rarely in hypothalamic pituitary adrenal axis suppression and aseptic bone necrosis.

D. Overuse: Fluorinated topical corticosteroids may induce acne-like processes on the face (steroid rosacea) and atrophic striae in body folds.

Frequently Employed Treatment Measures

A. General Measures: Soaps and detergents should be used only in the axillae and groin and on the feet by persons with dry or irritated skin. Unless their occupations expose them to oils or soot, most people do not need soaping over all body surfaces, and when so informed they will comply with this restriction rather than with a total ban on soap. Baths containing a small amount of bath oil may be used but are less effective than application of oils to the skin after bathing (see below).

B. Local Measures:

1. Corticosteroids–Representative topical corticosteroid creams, lotions, ointments, gels, and sprays are presented in the following list. They are useful only when treating inflammatory pruritic dermatoses. Dispensing should be guided by the following general rule: It takes an average of 20–30 g to cover the body surface area of an adult once.

a. Lowest potency–Hydrocortisone (Hytone, others), desonide (DesOwen, Tridesilon), alclometasone dipropionate (Aclovate). Best for chronic use and for the face, groin, and body folds. However, chronic unsupervised use of desonide may result in side effects in some patients.

b. Mid potency–Flurandrenolide (Cordran), fluocinolone (Synalar), triamcinolone (Aristocort, Kenalog), hydrocortisone valerate (Westcort), hydrocortisone butyrate (Locoid), betamethasone valerate (Valisone), etc.

c. High potency–Desoximetasone (Topicort), amcinonide (Cyclocort), halcinonide (Halog), fluocinonide (Lidex), betamethasone dipropionate (Diprosone), etc.

d. Highest potency–Betamethasone dipropionate in optimized vehicle (Diprolene), diflorasone (Psorcon), clobetasol (Temovate), and halobetasol (Ultravate). These should be used for brief periods only, on limited areas, and, like mid- and high-potency steroids, not on the face, breasts, or genitalia or in body folds.

2. Potentiation of topical corticosteroid creams–By covering selected lesions of psoriasis, lichen planus, and localized eczemas each night, first with the corticosteroid and then with a thin light plastic pliable film (eg, Saran Wrap), the potency of a topical steroid will be increased. In some rare cases, an appreciable amount of the medicament may be systemically absorbed. For erythrodermic psoriatics or atopics with generalized involvement, the use of a plastic occlusive suit may be most helpful. Complications include miliaria, striae, pyoderma, local skin atrophy, malodor, fungal infections, urticarial erythema, and, rarely, adrenocortical suppression when extensive areas of body surface are occluded. Clobetasol and halobetasol should not be used with occlusion.

3. Emollients for dry skin–(Petrolatum or mineral oil, Aquaphor, or Eucerin cream.) If the skin is too dry, wet it, as in a bath (to hydrate the keratin), and after patting dry, apply petrolatum immediately to the hydrated skin to trap the moisture. Mineral oil should be applied while the skin is still wet. Do not rub up and down against the hair but in one direction with the "grain" of the hair to avoid folliculitis. If the skin is too greasy after application, pat dry again with the damp towel.

Five percent lactic acid in petrolatum or a lotion vehicle may relieve the pruritus and the improve the appearance of dry skin and ichthyosis. A 12% lactate lotion is useful (Lac-Hydrin lotion). In some cases, lotions such as Lubriderm, Nutraderm, and Eucerin or moisture may be useful and are not as greasy as the creams and ointments listed above.

4. Drying agent for weepy dermatoses–If the skin is weepy from infection or inflammation, drying agents may afford relief. The best drying agent is water, and repeated compresses, with or without such agents as aluminum salts (Burow's solution, Domeboro tablets; follow package instructions) or colloidal oatmeal (Aveeno; dispense one box) are a good first step. Shake lotions (eg, starch or calamine lotions) and powders (especially if the process is acute) may be useful but at times result in messy crusts.

5. Nonspecific antipruritics–Lotions that contain 0.5% each of camphor, menthol, and phenol (Sarna) are effective for mild pruritic dermatoses. Pramoxine hydrochloride, 1% (Prax) cream or lotion, or pramoxine hydrochloride, 1%, with 0.5% menthol (Pramagel), as a surface anesthetic may be an effective antipruritic agent. Hydrocortisone, 1% or 2.5%, may be incorporated for its anti-inflammatory effect (Pramosone cream, lotion, or ointment).

6. Systemic antipruritic drugs—

a. Antihistamines—In general, H_1 blockers are the agents of choice for pruritus when due to histamine, such as in urticaria. The antipruritic effect of antihistamines otherwise appears to correlate with their sedating effects, and it is unclear that they affect pruritus not due to histamine except by sedating the patient. Different classes of antihistamines differ in their sedating properties, and it appears that the less sedating second-generation antihistamines are not very effective as antipruritics.

Traditional H_1 antihistamines are usually grouped into six classes. Alkylamines (chlorpheniramine and dexchlorpheniramine) are the least sedating. Ethanolamines (diphenhydramine) are very sedating, as are phenothiazines (promethazine). Piperidines (cyproheptadine), piperazines (hydroxyzine), and ethylenediamines (tripelennamine) cause less sedation. Some tricyclic antidepressants, such as doxepin, have antihistaminic activity and are useful in urticaria.

b. Psychotropic medications—Various antianxiety, antidepressant, and other psychotropic medications may be quite useful in pruritic dermatologic disorders but often require monitoring and special expertise.

c. Systemic corticosteroids—(See Chapter 25.) Corticosteroids have multiple in vitro and in vivo effects, but it is not clear which are responsible for their efficacy in skin disorders such as allergic contact dermatitis, pemphigus, pemphigoid, atopic dermatitis, or pressure urticaria.

Lowitt MH, Bernhard JD: Pruritus. Semin Neurol 1992;12:374.
Phillips WG: Pruritus: What to do when the itching won't stop. Postgrad Med 1992;92:34, 39, 43.

Sunscreens

Excessive exposure of fair skin to sun radiation is a major cancer risk factor. Inculcation of informed attitudes about sunbathing and development of measures to counteract the adverse effects of sun damage are important public health objectives. Sunlight on fair complexions can induce actinic (solar) keratoses, nevi, basal and squamous cell carcinoma, and melanoma. The best protection is shelter, but protective clothing, avoidance of direct sun exposure during the 5 peak hours of the day, and the assiduous use of commercially available chemical sunscreens or sunshades are helpful. Estimates are that if fair children were to use such sunscreens regularly, their lifetime incidence of skin cancer might be reduced by 75%.

A number of highly effective sunscreens are available. Fair-complexioned persons should not use a sunscreen with a rating less than SPF (sun protective factor) 15. For those who are sensitive to PABA (*p*-aminobenzoic acid), Neutrogena PABA-free sunscreen SPF 15, Solbar SPF 15 PABA-free cream, TI-Screen SPF 15, or PreSun 29 may be used. Solbar PF (PABA-free) cream with an SPF rating of 50 is available. Photoplex Broad Spectrum Sunscreen Lotion as well as sunscreens with high SPF values (> 25) afford some protection against UVA as well as UVB light exposure and may be helpful in managing photosensitivity disorders. Many cosmetics, such as Oil of Olay daily UV protectant, contain a SPF 15 sunscreen in a nongreasy base suitable for daily use.

The sunshades include those containing opaque materials such as titanium dioxide and zinc oxide. Zinc oxide alone is a surprisingly poor sunscreen.

Kaye ET et al: Efficiency of opaque photoprotective agents in the visible light range. Arch Dermatol 1991;127:351.

I. COMMON DERMATOSES

Dermatologic diseases will be classified and discussed here, when possible, according to the types of lesions they cause. Therefore, in order to make a diagnosis, it is best to (1) focus on the type of individual lesion the patient presents, (2) choose the morphologic category the lesions seem to fit, and then (3) determine the specifics of the history, physical examination, and laboratory tests that distinguish among the diseases in the differential diagnosis.

The major morphologic types of skin lesion—and pruritic lesions—are listed in Table 6–1 along with the disorders with which they are most prominently associated. Miscellaneous skin, hair, and nail disorders and drug eruptions are discussed at the end of the chapter.

PIGMENTED LESIONS

Malignant melanoma accounts for the greatest number of deaths due to skin disease, and such deaths might be prevented by early diagnosis followed by excision. The nondermatologist physician is not expected to make the final diagnosis of all the pigmented lesions mentioned below but must be able to recognize when a lesion is typical and when a pigmented lesion is atypical and needs referral for evaluation. The most relevant question is, "Is this mole *suspicious*?" Most of the lesions referred to dermatologists will be determined to be benign, but if the physician is to avoid overlooking some malignant melanomas, many benign lesions will be properly referred as well. Therefore, clinicians should examine

Table 6–1. Morphologic categorization of skin lesions and diseases.

Pigmented	Freckle, lentigo, seborrheic keratosis, nevus, blue nevus, halo nevus, dysplastic nevus, melanoma
Scaly	Psoriasis, dermatitis (atopic, stasis, seborrheic, chronic contact or allergic contact irritant, nummular), xerosis (dry skin), lichen simplex chronicus, tinea, tinea versicolor, secondary syphilis, pityriasis rosea, discoid lupus erythematosus, exfoliative dermatitis, actinic keratoses, Bowen's disease, Paget's disease, intertrigo
Vesicular	Herpes simplex, varicella, herpes zoster, dyshidrosis (vesicular dermatitis of palms and soles), vesicular tinea, dermatophytid, dermatitis herpetiformis, miliaria, scabies, photosensitivity
Weepy or encrusted	Impetigo, acute contact allergic dermatitis, any vesicular dermatitis
Pustular	Acne vulgaris, acne rosacea, folliculitis, candidiasis, miliaria, any vesicular dermatitis
Figurate(-shaped) erythema	Urticaria, erythema multiforme, erythema chronicum migrans, cellulitis, erysipelas, erysipeloid, arthropod bites
Bullous	Impetigo, blistering dactylitis, pemphigus, pemphigoid, porphyria cutanea tarda, drug eruptions, erythema multiforme, toxic epidermal necrolysis
Papular	Hyperkeratotic: warts, corns, seborrheic keratoses Purple/violet: lichen planus, drug eruptions, Kaposi's sarcoma Flesh-colored, umbilicated: molluscum contagiosum Pearly: basal cell carcinoma, intradermal nevi Small, red, inflammatory: acne, miliaria, candidiasis, intertrigo, scabies, folliculitis
Pruritus[1]	Xerosis, scabies, pediculosis, bites, systemic causes, anogenital pruritus
Nodular, cystic	Erythema nodosum, furuncle, cystic acne, follicular (epidermal) inclusion cyst
Photodermatitis (photodistributed rashes)	Drug, polymorphic light eruption, lupus erythematosus
Maculopapular	Drug, viral, secondary syphilis
Erosive	Any vesicular dermatitis, impetigo, aphthae, lichen planus, erythema multiforme; oral erosions
Ulcerated	Decubiti, herpes simplex, skin cancers, parasitic infections, syphilis (chancre), chancroid, vasculitis, stasis, arterial disease

[1]Not a morphologic class but included because it is one of the most common dermatologic presentations.

all patients with an eye to spotting the "funny-looking" mole.

In general, a **benign mole** is a small (< 5 mm), well-circumscribed lesion with a well-defined border and a single shade of pigment from light brown to dark brown. Most or all of the individual patient's moles often are similar to each other with respect to size and color, or there may be two different types of moles on the same patient. The physical examination takes precedence over the history, though a reliable history that a lesion has been present without change for decades is obviously a comfort.

Suspicious moles have an irregular and asymmetric or fuzzy border where the pigment appears to be leaking into the normal surrounding skin; the topography may be irregular, ie, partly raised and partly flat. Color variegation is disturbing, and colors such as pink, blue, gray, white, and black are indications for referral. Bleeding and ulceration are ominous signs. A mole that stands out from the patient's other moles deserves special scrutiny. A patient with a large number of moles deserves careful examination, particularly if the lesions are atypical.

The history of a changing mole is the single most important historical reason for close evaluation and possible referral. Referral of suspicious pigmented lesions is always appropriate.

Moles have their own natural history. In the first decade of life, moles often appear as flat, small, brown lesions. They are called **junctional nevi** because the nevus cells are at the junction of the epidermis and dermis. Over the next 2 decades, these moles grow in size and often become raised, reflecting the appearance of a dermal component, giving rise to **compound nevi.** Moles may darken and grow during pregnancy. As Caucasian patients enter their seventh and eighth decades, most moles have lost their junctional component and dark pigmentation, and many become even more raised as they undergo fibrosis or other degenerative changes. Still, at every stage of life, normal moles should be well-demarcated, symmetric, and uniform in contour and color.

CONGENITAL NEVI

The management of small congenital nevi—less than a few centimeters in diameter—is controversial. The vast majority (perhaps > 97%) will never become malignant, but some experts feel that the risk of melanoma in these lesions may be somewhat increased. Since 1% of Caucasians are born with these lesions, management should be conservative and excision advised only for lesions in cosmetically nonsensitive areas where the patient cannot easily see the lesion and note any suspicious changes. Excision should be considered for congenital nevi whose contour (bumpiness, nodularity) or color (different shades) makes it difficult for examiners to note early signs of malignant change. Giant congenital melanocytic nevi are at greater risk for development of melanoma, and surgical removal in stages is often recommended.

DYSPLASTIC NEVI

Dysplastic nevi are another area of controversy in dermatology. These lesions are large (> 5 mm) and pigmented, with irregular borders and reddish colors mixed with brown. The biopsy shows characteristic features, but pathologists may differ about the degree of histologic atypia of any one lesion. The nondermatologist should regard dysplastic nevi as suspicious lesions calling for referral.

A patient may have many or only one such lesion. While there are well-characterized families with multiple melanomas in which such lesions are melanoma precursors, the significance of a single dysplastic mole in an individual with no personal or family history of melanoma is far less clear, and the risk of melanoma is probably small. However, a conservative approach is to refer patients with such moles for total body examination, excision of lesions suspected to be melanoma, and examination of family members as indicated. Patients with moles that are quite atypical deserve close follow-up, which is often aided by photography. All patients with dysplastic nevi deserve periodic follow-up for life. Again, the goal of the nondermatologist is not to determine whether these are dysplastic moles or melanoma but to identify all suspicious lesions for referral.

Barnhill RL: Current status of the dysplastic melanocytic nevus. J Cutan Pathol 1991;18:147.

BLUE NEVI

Blue nevi are small, slightly elevated, and blue-black lesions. They are common in persons of Asian descent, and an individual patient may have several of them. If present without change for many years, they may be considered benign. However, blue-black papules and nodules that are new or growing must be further evaluated to rule out nodular melanoma.

FRECKLES & LENTIGINES

Freckles (ephelides) and lentigines are flat brown spots. Freckles first appear in young children, darken with ultraviolet exposure despite use of sunscreens, and fade with cessation of sun exposure (in the winter). Freckles were previously thought to represent normal numbers of melanocytes producing extra amounts of pigment, but some lesions appear to have increased numbers of melanocytes. In older children and adults, depending on the fairness of the complexion, flat brown spots (lentigines), often with smooth borders, gradually appear in sun-exposed areas, particularly the dorsa of the hands. These lesions have increased numbers of melanocytes. They tend not to fade with cessation of sun exposure. They should be evaluated like all pigmented lesions: If the pigmentation is homogeneous and they are symmetric and flat, they are most likely benign.

SEBORRHEIC KERATOSES

Seborrheic keratoses consist of benign overgrowths of epithelium that have a pigmented velvety or warty surface. They are relatively common—especially in the elderly—both on exposed and covered parts and are commonly mistaken for melanomas or other types of cutaneous neoplasms. They range in color from beige to very dark brown.

MALIGNANT MELANOMA

Essentials of Diagnosis

- May be flat or raised.
- Should be suspected in any pigmented skin lesion with recent change in appearance.
- Examination with good light shows varying colors, including red, white black, and bluish.
- Borders typically irregular.

General Considerations

Malignant melanoma is the leading cause of death from skin disease. It is estimated that 27,300 cases of melanoma occurred in the USA in 1988, causing melanoma to be ranked as the ninth most common cancer, with over 6000 deaths in 1989. Although melanomas are more frequently recognized at earlier and more curable stages, the overall death rate for Caucasian men has risen from 2.2 to 3.3 per 100,000 population during the period 1973–1988, and that of Caucasian women from 1.4 to 1.7 per 100,000. Overall survival for melanomas diagnosed from 1981 to 1987 were 77% for men and 88% for women.

Depth of invasion (or tumor thickness) is the single most important prognostic factor. Five-year survival rates—related to thickness in millimeters—are as follows: < 0.76 mm, 99%; 0.76–1.49 mm, 95%; 1.5–2.49 mm, 84%; 2.5–3.99 mm, 70%; and > 4 mm, 44%. With lymph node involvement, the 5-year survival rate is 30%; and with distant metastases, it is less than 10%.

Deaths from malignant melanoma are increasing at a faster rate than death from any other malignant neoplastic disease except lung cancer. The mean age of those dying from melanomas is less than that of those dying from other skin cancers. There is a trend toward a younger age incidence each year. However, because of increased awareness, most melanomas are being diagnosed at a much earlier stage.

Clinical Findings

Primary malignant melanomas may be classified into various clinicohistologic types, including lentigo maligna melanoma; superficial spreading malignant melanoma (the most common type, occurring in two-thirds of individuals developing melanoma); nodular malignant melanoma; acral-lentiginous melanomas; malignant melanomas on mucous membranes; and miscellaneous forms such as amelanotic (nonpigmented) melanoma arising from blue nevi (rare) and congenital and giant nevocytic nevi.

While superficial spreading melanoma is largely a disease of Caucasians, persons of other races are at risk for other types of melanoma, particularly acral lentiginous melanoma. These occur as dark, sometimes irregularly shaped lesions on the palms and soles and as new, often broad and solitary, darkly pigmented longitudinal streaks in the nails. Acral lentiginous melanoma is a difficult diagnosis in view of the much more common occurrence of benign pigmented lesions of the hands, feet, and nails of more darkly pigmented persons and the clinician's hesitation to biopsy the palms and especially the soles and nail beds. As a result, the diagnosis is often delayed until the tumor has spread. Clinicians should give special attention to new or changing lesions in these areas.

True melanomas vary from macules to nodules, with a surprising play of colors from flesh tints to pitch black and a frequent admixture of white, blue, purple, and red. The border tends to be irregular, and growth may be rapid or indolent. Again, the best approach is to recognize lesions that are suspicious because of their variegation and asymmetry or because of their behavior and to refer these lesions at an early stage.

Treatment

Treatment of melanoma consists of excision. After histologic diagnosis, the area is usually reexcised with margins dictated by the thickness of the tumor. Large margins (radius $\geq$ 5 cm) are rarely indicated. Thin low-risk and intermediate-risk tumors require only conservative margins of 1–3 cm. More specifically, surgical margins of 0.5 cm for melanoma in situ and 1 cm for lesions less than 1 mm in thickness are common.

Elective lymph node dissection in the absence of clinical involvement is an area of great controversy. Until definitive data from large prospective studies are available, lymph node dissection is often dictated by the clinician's personal interpretation of the data. In general, lymph node dissection is indicated only for tumors of intermediate thickness with one draining chain of lymph nodes. Elective regional lymph node dissection is not recommended for melanomas less than 1 mm thick.

Friedman RJ, Rigel DS, Kopf AW: Early detection of malignant melanoma: The role of physician examination and self-examination of the skin. CA (May-June) 1985; 35:130.

Koh HK: Cutaneous melanoma. N Engl J Med 1991; 325:171.

Sober AJ et al: Epidemiology of cutaneous melanoma: An update. Dermatol Clin 1991;9:617. (UV light appears to play some role in melanoma pathogenesis, but it is still unclear how this occurs.)

SCALING DISORDERS

ATOPIC DERMATITIS (Eczema)

Essentials of Diagnosis

- Pruritic, exudative, or lichenified eruption on face, neck, upper trunk, wrists, and hands and in the folds of knees and elbows.
- Personal or family history of allergic manifestations (eg, asthma, allergic rhinitis, eczema).
- Tendency to recur, with remission from adolescence to age 20.

General Considerations

Atopic dermatitis looks different at different ages and in people of different races. Because most patients have scaly dry skin at some point, this disease is being discussed under scaly dermatoses. However, acute flares may present with red dermatitic patches and plaques and papules. Diagnostic criteria for atopic dermatitis must include pruritus, typical morphology and distribution (flexural lichenification in adults; facial and extensor involvement in infants), and a tendency toward chronic or chronically relapsing dermatitis. Also helpful are (1) a personal or family history of atopic disease (asthma, allergic rhinitis, atopic dermatitis), (2) xerosis-ichthyosis-hyperlinear palms, (3) facial pallor with infraorbital darkening, (4) elevated serum IgE, (5) a tendency toward nonspecific hand dermatitis, and (6) a tendency toward repeated skin infections.

Clinical Findings

A. Symptoms and Signs: Itching may be extremely severe and prolonged, leading often to emotional disturbances, which have been erroneously interpreted by some as being causative. It is difficult to describe the exact appearance of acute but non-weeping dermatitis, but it represents inflammation of the epidermis. Thus, dermatitis presents with erythema but not with the smooth surface of dermal inflammation that characterizes hives. The epidermal inflammation of acute dermatitis results in rough, red patches without the thickening and discrete demarcation of a proliferative epidermal disorder such as psoriasis. The distribution of the lesions is characteristic, with involvement of the face, neck, and upper trunk ("monk's cowl"). The bends of the elbows and knees are involved. In infants, the eruption usually begins on the cheeks and is often vesicular and exudative. In children (and later) it is dry, leathery, and lichenified, though intraepidermal vesicles are occasionally present histologically. Black children tend to present with a papular eruption instead of scaly patches seen in Caucasians. Adults generally have dry, leathery, hyperpigmented or hypopigmented lesions in typical distribution. In black patients with severe disease, pigmentation may be lost in lichenified areas around the wrists and ankles.

The role of food allergy in atopic dermatitis is debatable but is probably significant in about 30% of cases. There may be a subset of patients with atopic dermatitis and food sensitivities, with implicated foods causing the release of a histamine releasing factor for basophils. Other patients may be sensitive to dust mites and other antigens.

B. Laboratory Findings: Laboratory findings, including scratch and intradermal tests, do not correlate with exacerbating factors. Eosinophilia and increased serum IgE levels may be present but are usually not needed for diagnosis.

Differential Diagnosis

In infants, atopic dermatitis must be distinguished from seborrheic dermatitis (frequent scalp and face involvement, greasy and scaly lesions, and quick response to therapy). Contact dermatitis and impetigo may be in the differential, especially for hyperacute, weepy flares of atopic dermatitis (although typically these diseases do not have a chronic course and characteristic distribution). Atopic individuals are much more likely to be colonized with *Staphylococcus aureus,* and impetiginization of atopic skin should be considered when the patient presents with weepy areas or small erosions that should not be confused with more linear excoriations.

Treatment

Treatment is not difficult, but the patient must be instructed about many aspects of skin care and specific ways to use medications.

A. General Measures: These patients should be thought of as having hyperirritable skin, so one must first explain to the patient or parents that anything that dries or irritates the skin will be a problem. Atopic individuals are sensitive to low humidity and often get worse in the winter, when the air is dry. A

reasonable approach is not to let children or adults bathe more than once daily, not to let children sit in soapy water, and not to permit use of bubble bath unless it is shown not to irritate the skin of that child. Soap should be confined to the armpits, groin, and feet and should be used only just before rinsing and ending the bath. Washcloths and brushes should not be used. Soaps should not be drying, and Dove, Eucerin, Aveeno, Basis, Alpha Keri, Emulave, Purpose, and other soaps or cleansers, such as Cetaphil or Aquanil, may be recommended. A recently introduced skin cleanser containing 30% petrolatum, Prothera, is also useful for patients with dry skin. After rinsing, the skin should be patted dry (not rubbed) and then immediately—before it dries completely—covered with a thin film of an emollient, such as Aquaphor, Eucerin, Vaseline, mineral oil, or a corticosteroid as needed. Atopic patients may be irritated by scratchy fabrics, including wools and acrylics, and should wear clothing that can breathe. Cottons often are preferable, but synthetic blends also are well tolerated. Since some children begin their cycle of itching and scratching with perspiration, one should do what is possible to avoid overheating. Some patients cannot use ointments because they are more occlusive than creams and cause itching. Very hot baths may exacerbate the itching of some patients. Some patients do not tolerate animal danders well, and the etiologic role of pets should be considered.

To determine the potential effect of foods, the parent may eliminate one food at a time that is thought to induce flares. Foods that are a problem typically cause itching within minutes to a few hours after eating.

B. Local Treatment: Corticosteroids in lotion, cream, or ointment form have almost completely supplanted other topical medications. They should be applied sparingly twice daily. Their potency should be determined by the severity of the dermatitis. In general, one should use weaker corticosteroids in young children. It is vital that patients taper corticosteroids and substitute emollients when the dermatitis clears to avoid both tachyphylaxis and the side effects of corticosteroids. Tapering is important to avoid rebound flares of the dermatitis that may follow their abrupt cessation.

Treatment is dictated by the stage of the dermatitis.

1. Acute weeping lesions–Use saline, bicarbonate, aluminum subacetate solution (Domeboro tablets, one in a pint of cool water), or colloidal oatmeal (Aveeno; dispense one box, and use as directed on box) as soothing or astringent soaks, baths, or wet dressings for 10–30 minutes two to four times daily. Lesions on extremities particularly may be bandaged for protection at night without letting tape touch the skin. Steroid lotions or creams are preferred to ointments for this stage. Adults may use high-potency corticosteroids and children mid-potency steroids, used after bathing and sparing the face and body folds.

2. Subacute or scaly lesions–At this stage, the lesions are dry but still red and pruritic. Compresses are not needed, but mid- to high-potency steroids in ointment form if tolerated—creams if not—should be continued until scaling and elevated skin lesions are cleared and itching is decreased substantially. At that point, patients should begin a 2- to 4-week taper from twice-daily to daily to alternate-day dosing with topical steroids to reliance on emollients, with occasional use of steroids on specific itchy areas. Instead of tapering the frequency of usage of a more potent steroid, it may be preferable in children to switch to a low-potency steroid such as hydrocortisone cream (Hytone 1% or other available OTC) or aclometasone (Aclovate). Another approach to avoiding tachyphylaxis is to apply a potent corticosteroid twice daily for 2 days, alternating with 2 days of less potent steroid preparations, coal tar products, or emollients.

3. Chronic, dry, lichenified lesions thickened and usually well-demarcated. They are best treated with high-potency to highest-potency ointments, sometimes under occlusion for 2–6 weeks as a start. Occasionally, tar preparations such as LCD (liquor carbonis detergens) 5% in Aquaphor, or Fototar cream, may be beneficial if corticosteroids are not sufficient.

C. Systemic and Adjuvant Therapy: Systemic corticosteroids are indicated only in extensive and more severe cases. Oral prednisone dosages should be high enough to suppress the dermatitis quickly, usually starting with 60 mg daily for adults. The dosage is then tapered to nil over a period of 2–4 weeks. Triamcinolone acetonide suspension, 40–60 mg intramuscularly for adults, used occasionally—but not more frequently than every 4–6 weeks (or less often)—may exert control but is not a good form of maintenance therapy. Antihistamines may be used to aid in the relief of severe pruritus. Hydroxyzine, brompheniramine, or doxepin may be useful, but the dosage must be increased gradually to avoid drowsiness. There is increased IgE binding to *S aureus*. Interaction of staphylococcal antigen and specific antistaphylococcal antibodies may induce mast cell release, causing itching and aggravation of the dermatitis. Fissures, crusts, erosions, or pustules indicate staphylococcal infection clinically. Therefore, antibiotics given systemically—such as erythromycin or dicloxacillin—may be helpful in management and are often used during flares. Phototherapy can be an important adjunct for severely affected patients, and the properly selected patient with recalcitrant disease may benefit greatly from UVB therapy with or without coal tar, or from PUVA therapy.

Complications of Treatment

Patients are at risk of side effects of improperly used corticosteroids, and the physician should monitor for skin atrophy. **Eczema herpeticum,** a generalized herpes simplex infection superimposed on atopic dermatitis or other extensive eczematous processes, is usually treated successfully with oral acyclovir, 400 mg five times daily for adults, or intravenous acyclovir in a dose of 1500 mg/m^2/d.

Prognosis

The disease runs a chronic course, often with a tendency to disappear only to recur. Many children outgrow generalized involvement at puberty but develop hand dermatitis as adults. Poor prognostic factors for eventual complete remission in atopic dermatitis include onset early in childhood, early generalized disease, and asthma. Only 40–60% of these patients have lasting remissions.

Hanifin JM: Atopic dermatitis. J Am Acad Dermatol 1991;24:1097.

LICHEN SIMPLEX CHRONICUS (Circumscribed Neurodermatitis)

Essentials of Diagnosis

- Chronic itching associated with pigmented lichenified skin lesions.
- Lichenified lesions exhibit exaggerated skin lines overlying a thickened, well-circumscribed scaly plaque.
- Predilection for nape of neck, wrists, external surfaces of forearms, inner thighs, lower legs, popliteal and antecubital areas.

General Considerations

A traditional explanation for lichen simplex chronicus (circumscribed neurodermatitis) is that it represents a self-perpetuating scratch-itch cycle, but there is no evidence that this is solely initiated by the patient's behavior. Hypertrophic nerve fibers have been found in lichenified, thickened lesions of long standing, but it is not known if these are of pathogenetic significance. Patients with very chronic recalcitrant lesions may be depressed or have other psychologic symptoms.

Clinical Findings

Intermittent itching incites the patient to manipulate the lesions. Itching may be so intense as to interfere with sleep. Dry, leathery, hypertrophic, lichenified plaques appear on the neck, wrists, perineum, thighs, or almost anywhere. The patches are well-localized and rectangular, with sharp borders, and are thickened and pigmented. The lines of the skin are exaggerated and divide the lesion into rectangular plaques.

Differential Diagnosis

This disorder may be confused with plaque-like lesions such as those of psoriasis, which is commonly manifested by redder lesions having tighter and whiter scales on the elbows, knees, and scalp and with nail findings; with lichen planus, manifested by violaceous, usually smaller polygonal papules; and with nummular (coin-shaped) dermatitis. Skin biopsy can distinguish among these presentations when necessary, but all respond to high-potency topical steroids.

Treatment

Topical corticosteroids give relief. Clobetasol (Temovate), halobetasol (Ultravate), diflorasone (Psorcon), and betamethasone dipropionate in augmented vehicle (Diprolene) are effective without occlusion and are used twice daily for several weeks. These superpotent steroids are probably the treatment of choice but must be used with careful follow-up to avoid local and systemic side effects. The injection of triamcinolone acetonide suspension (5–10 mg/mL) into the lesions may occasionally be curative. Use of tars, such as LCD (coal tar, liquor carbonis detergens, Fototar) or anthralin, or continuous occlusion with DuoDerm (occlusive flexible hydrocolloid dressing) for 7 days at a time for 1–2 months, may also be helpful. Tar gels (Estargel, Psorigel) may also be used alone or with a steroid; they are rarely curative alone. The area should be protected and the patient encouraged to become aware of when he or she is scratching and to avoid stressful and emotionally charged situations if these induce itching.

Prognosis

The disease tends to remit during treatment but may recur, or another site may develop.

Bernhard JD: Itching in the nineties. International Symposium on Itch: Basic and Clinical Aspects. Stockholm, Sweden 1990. J Am Acad Dermatol 1991;24:309.

PSORIASIS

Essentials of Diagnosis

- Silvery scales on bright red plaques, usually on the knees, elbows, and scalp.
- Nail findings including pitting and onycholysis (separation of the nail plate from the bed).
- Mild itching unless psoriasis is eruptive or occurs in body folds.
- May be associated with psoriatic arthritis.
- Specific histopathologic features, though biopsy is usually unnecessary.

General Considerations

Psoriasis is a common benign, acute or chronic inflammatory skin disease that appears based upon a genetic predisposition. For the relationship of psoriasis to histocompatibility (HLA) antigens, see Chapter 18. Polyamines, proteases, cAMP, growth factors such as TGFα, and the leukotrienes have been proposed as mediators. The beneficial effect of cyclosporine has raised the possibility that psoriasis may be immunologically mediated. Injury or irritation of psoriatic skin tends to provoke lesions of psoriasis in the site in some patients (Koebner's phenomenon). Psoriasis has several variants—the most common is the plaque type. Eruptive (guttate) psoriasis occurs occasionally in periods of stress or after streptococcal pharyngitis. Grave, occasionally life-threatening forms (generalized pustular and erythrodermic psoriasis) may rarely occur. Plaque type or extensive erythrodermic psoriasis with abrupt onset may accompany AIDS.

Clinical Findings

There are usually no symptoms. Eruptive psoriasis may itch, and psoriasis in body folds may itch severely ("inverse psoriasis"). One should examine the scalp, elbows, knees, palms and soles, and nails. The lesions are red, sharply outlined plaques covered with silvery scales. The elbows, knees, and scalp are the most common sites. The glans penis and vulva may be affected. Fine stippling ("pitting") in the nails is highly suggestive of psoriasis. Psoriatics are said to often have a pink or red line in the intergluteal fold. Not all patients have findings in all locations, but the occurrence of a few may be diagnostic. Some patients present mainly with hand dermatitis and only minimal findings elsewhere, posing a difficult diagnostic problem even for experts. There may be associated arthritis that resembles the rheumatoid variety but with a negative rheumatoid factor; distal interphalangeal joints are frequently involved.

Differential Diagnosis

The combination of red plaques with silvery scales on elbows and knees, with scaliness in the scalp or nail findings, is diagnostic. Psoriasis lesions are well demarcated and affect extensor surfaces—in contrast to atopic dermatitis, with poorly demarcated plaques in flexural distribution. In the scalp, psoriasis is distinguished from seborrheic dermatitis by well-demarcated red plaques with thick scales, in contrast to diffuse or patchy redness and scaling of seborrheic dermatitis; in body folds, scraping and culture for *Candida* and examination of scalp and nails will distinguish psoriasis from intertrigo and candidiasis. Onycholysis may simulate onychomycosis, but again, the general examination combined with a fungal culture will be valuable in diagnosis. The cutaneous features of Reiter's syndrome may mimic psoriasis.

Treatment

There are many therapeutic options in psoriasis, to

be chosen according to the extent and severity of disease and with a clear understanding of the risks and benefits of therapy.

A. Limited Disease: For many patients with disease limited to the scalp or to the elbows and knees, the easiest regimen is to use a high-potency to highest-potency topical steroid cream or ointment. It is best to restrict the highest-potency steroids to 2–3 weeks of twice-daily use and then switch to a less potent (but still high-potency) corticosteroid and apply a tar, such as Fototar, LCD (coal tar; liquor carbonis detergens), 10% in Nutraderm lotion, or mixed directly with triamcinolone 0.1% cream; it is messier to use than a steroid alone. Tar gels (Estargel, Psorigel) may also be used alone or with a steroid; they are rarely curative alone. Steroids rarely induce a lasting remission, and some clinicians feel that steroids may make psoriasis more difficult to treat by other measures. One must avoid tachyphylaxis and atrophy from chronic use and abrupt withdrawal with subsequent rebound. Occlusion alone has been shown to clear some isolated plaques in some patients. Patches of occlusive dressings such as Duoderm are placed on the lesions and left undisturbed for as long as possible (a minimum of 5 days, up to 7 days) and then replaced. Responses may be seen within several weeks. Perhaps 30–40% of patients respond to this therapy. Anthralin is another agent available for localized disease, but it must be used properly, is irritating, and may stain the skin. All tar preparations stain clothing and bedding.

For the scalp, start with a tar shampoo (Neutrogena T/Gel or Ionil T Plus), used daily if possible, or Nizoral shampoo (used twice weekly). For thick scales, use Keralyt gel, P & S solution, or Dermasmoothe under a shower cap at night, and shampoo in the morning. In order of increasing potency, triamcinolone or fluocinolone, betamethasone dipropionate, fluocinonide or amcinonide, and clobetasol are available in solution form for use on the scalp twice daily. For psoriasis in the body folds, treatment is much more difficult, since potent steroids cannot be used. One may try hydrocortisone or desonide steroid creams.

B. Generalized Disease: If psoriasis involves more than 30% of the body surface, it is difficult to treat with topical agents. The treatment of choice is outpatient UVB light exposure three times weekly. Clearing occurs in an average of 7 weeks, and maintenance is needed since relapses are frequent. Severe psoriasis calls for treatment in the hospital or a day care center with the Goeckerman regimen. Hospitalization may be required for Goeckerman treatment, which involves use of crude coal tar for many hours and exposure to UVB light. Such treatment may offer the best chance for prolonged remissions.

PUVA (psoralen plus ultraviolet A, ie, ultraviolet light in the 320- to 400-nm wavelength range; same as black light) tends to be a long-term form of treatment, since maintenance therapy is usually required. The relapse rate is about 63% in 1–6 months. The ultraviolet dose is cumulative, and the total safe dose is unknown. The incidence of skin cancer is increased mainly in persons of very fair skin or those who have received previous x-ray radiation or have received the highest dosages of UVA light, with an increased number of squamous cell carcinomas. Epidermal dystrophy by light microscopy is seen in 50% of patients treated with PUVA, and atypical lentigines are common. There can be rapid aging of the skin in fair individuals. Cataracts are a threat but have not been reported with proper use of sunglasses, and there may be a rare conversion to a positive ANA and the even rarer appearance of localized discoid lupus lesions. PUVA should typically not be used alone but in combination with other therapy, such as a few weeks of etretinate or methotrexate administration.

Parenteral corticosteroids should not be used except in the most severe cases, because of the possibility of induction of pustular lesions. Methotrexate is available and very effective for severe psoriasis in doses up to 25 mg once weekly or in divided doses every 12 hours for three doses once a week. Liver biopsy is performed at or around the time of initiation of methotrexate and yearly during chronic use. Often the initial biopsy is delayed until the patient is shown to tolerate and respond to the drug.

Etretinate (Tegison), a synthetic retinoid, may also be used for psoriasis, but it is most effective for pustular psoriasis, followed by the erythrodermic and plaque types, and for psoriatic arthritis. Liver enzymes and serum lipids must be checked periodically. The drug has a prolonged half-life. Diffuse idiopathic skeletal hyperostosis (DISH syndrome) has been reported from long-term, high-dose therapy, but its clinical significance is unclear. Only under extraordinary circumstances should the drug be given to women of childbearing age. Acitretin (etretin), the active form of etretinate, has a much shorter half-life, and it is expected that this compound will soon be available in the United States. However, small amounts of the prodrug etretinate have been found in the blood of patients treated only with acetretin, particularly in patients who consume ethanol. Thus, it is still unclear when it will be absolutely safe to conceive after taking acetretin. The retinoids should, in general, not be used alone as single agents.

Cyclosporine has shown much promise in the treatment of severe psoriasis, but relapses are the rule after cessation of therapy, and the long-term safety of the drug and the incidence of lymphoma have not been established. Sulfasalazine in dosages of 1 g three times daily markedly improved 8 of 23 patients in a double-blinded study. Thus, sulfasalazine may be considered for patients who are not candidates for— or who cannot tolerate—more toxic drugs.

The treatment of psoriasis in patients with AIDS is somewhat controversial because of in vitro studies suggesting that HIV virus may be activated by UVB and UVA—despite reported successes of several centers in using UVB. In general, psoriasis in AIDS patients that is resistant to topical therapy may be treated with etretinate, 25–50 mg/d, with the addition of UVB as needed. PUVA and methotrexate are not usually recommended.

Prognosis

The course tends to be chronic and unpredictable, and the disease may be refractory to treatment.

Arnett FC, Reveille JD, Duvic M: Psoriasis and psoriatic arthritis associated with human immunodeficiency virus infection. Rheum Dis Clin North Am 1991;17:59. (Psoriasis-like and Reiter's-like rashes are not uncommon in HIV infection and may respond to zidovudine.)

Grossier DS et al: A review and update of the clinical uses of cyclosporine in dermatology. Dermatol Clin 1991;9: 805.

Meola T Jr, Soter NA, Lim HW: Are topical steroids useful adjunctive therapy for the treatment of psoriasis with ultraviolet radiation? A review of the literature. Arch Dermatol 1991;127:1708. (Topical corticosteroids with PUVA therapy may increase the rate of clearing and decrease total UV exposure but may cause a higher relapse rate. Most studies fail to show an additive effect of corticosteroids and UVB.)

Tung JP, Maibach HI: The practical use of methotrexate in psoriasis. Drugs 1990;40:697. (Reviews proper use of the drug.)

Lowe NJ, Lazarus V, Matt L: Systemic retinoid therapy for psoriasis. J Am Acad Dermatol 1988;19:186.

PITYRIASIS ROSEA

Essentials of Diagnosis

- Oval, fawn-colored, scaly eruption following cleavage lines of trunk.
- Herald patch commonly precedes eruption by 1–2 weeks.
- Occasional pruritus.

General Considerations

This is a common mild, acute inflammatory disease which is 50% more common in females. Young adults are principally affected, mostly in the spring or fall. Concurrent household cases have been reported, and recurrences may take place over a period of years. The cause is unknown, but it is speculated that a picornavirus may be causative. The attack rate in married couples is less than 2%, so whatever the cause, it is not highly infectious.

Clinical Findings

Occasionally, there is severe itching. The diagnosis is made by finding one or more classic lesions. The lesions consist of oval, fawn-colored macules 4–5 mm in diameter. The centers of the lesions have a crinkled or "cigarette paper" appearance or a collar-

ette scale, ie, a thin bit of scale that is bound at the periphery and free in the center. Lesions follow cleavage lines on the trunk (so-called Christmas tree pattern), and the proximal portions of the extremities are often involved. Variants that affect the flexures (axillae and groin), so called inverse pityriasis rosea, and papular variants, especially in black patients, also occur. An initial lesion ("herald patch") that is often larger than the later lesions usually precedes the general eruption by 1–2 weeks. Attacks usually last 4–8 weeks.

Differential Diagnosis

If at least a few perfectly typical lesions are not present, if the rash does not itch, and especially if there are palmar and plantar or mucous membrane lesions that are suggestive of secondary syphilis, a serologic test for syphilis should be performed. For the nonexpert, an RPR test in all cases is not unreasonable. Tinea corporis may present with red, slightly scaly plaques, but rarely are there more than a few lesions of tinea corporis compared to the many lesions of pityriasis rosea. A scraping of scale for a KOH test will rapidly make the diagnosis. Seborrheic dermatitis on occasion presents on the body with large patches over the sternum, in the pubic area, and in the axillae. The classic lesions of pityriasis rosea are not present. Tinea versicolor lesions, viral exanthems, and drug eruptions may simulate pityriasis rosea.

Treatment

Pityriasis rosea often requires no treatment. The most effective management consists of daily UVB treatments for a week, or prednisone as used for contact dermatitis. Topical steroids of medium strength (triamcinolone 0.1%) may also be used if pruritus is bothersome. Nonspecific antipruritics may be used (pramoxine, Sarna as described above), but these are rarely satisfactory. Antihistamines may be tried but often cause sedation.

Prognosis

Pityriasis rosea is usually an acute self-limiting illness that disappears in about 6 weeks.

Ginsberg CM: Pityriasis rosea. Pediatr Infect Dis J 1991;10:858.

SEBORRHEIC DERMATITIS & DANDRUFF

Essentials of Diagnosis

- Dry scales and underlying erythema.
- Scalp, central face, presternal, interscapular areas, umbilicus, and body folds.

General Considerations

Seborrheic dermatitis is an acute or chronic papulosquamous dermatitis. It is based upon a genetic predisposition mediated by an interplay of such factors as hormones, nutrition, infection, and emotional stress. The response of seborrheic dermatitis to the antifungal ketoconazole has raised the possibility that seborrheic dermatitis represents an inflammatory reaction to *Pityrosporum ovale* yeasts present on the scalp of all humans. However, the effect of ketoconazole in this disease may not be due to its antifungal properties alone.

Clinical Findings

Pruritus may be present but is an inconstant finding. The scalp, face, chest, back, umbilicus, and body folds may be oily or dry, with dry scales or oily yellowish scurf. Eyelid margins (seborrheic blepharitis) may be involved in the process. Erythema, fissuring, and secondary infection may be present. Patients with Parkinson's disease frequently develop moderately severe seborrheic dermatitis, as do elderly patients who become acutely ill and are hospitalized for a variety of reasons.

Differential Diagnosis

There is often a clinical spectrum ranging from simple dandruff to seborrheic dermatitis to scalp psoriasis, and there is no single specific test for each entity. Patients with psoriasis often have moderate to extensive seborrheic dermatitis. On the scalp, the presence of well-demarcated red plaques usually is termed psoriasis, and general erythema without tight, thick, silvery scale is usually called seborrheic dermatitis. The presence of mild scaling without any erythema is often termed simple dandruff. The treatment of all three conditions is determined by the severity. Extensive seborrheic dermatitis may simulate intertrigo in flexural areas, but scalp, face, and sternal involvement suggests seborrheic dermatitis. As long as *Candida* infection is absent, mild corticosteroids will help both conditions. Fungal infections, unlike seborrheic dermatitis, rarely involve the brows, the scalp behind the ear, and the nasal folds. Scaling of the scalp due to tinea capitis may simulate dandruff or seborrheic dermatitis, and scrapings should be taken for KOH examination and fungal culture.

Treatment

A. Seborrhea of the Scalp: For mild to moderate seborrhea, the clinician should suggest several shampoos, so that the patient can use the one that proves most acceptable, as this will likely become a chronic if intermittent treatment. Shampoos that contain tar, zinc pyrithione, or selenium are used daily if possible, while ketoconazole shampoo is used twice weekly. Topical corticosteroid solutions or lotions (dispense 60 mL) are then added if necessary, and are used twice daily intermittently to avoid tachyphylaxis. Atrophy of the scalp is uncommon except in patients with alopecia. For very resistant cases, selenium sulfide 2.5% suspension (Exsel, Selsun) may be used once a week as a shampoo. The patient should be instructed to shampoo vigorously once and then shampoo again, leaving the second shampoo on for 5–10 minutes to loosen the scales.

B. Facial Seborrhea: Mild soaps are usually used as described under atopic dermatitis so as not to further irritate the skin. Treatment of the scalp, if involved, is thought to decrease facial involvement. The mainstay of therapy is a mild corticosteroid used intermittently and not near the eyes. Potent fluorinated corticosteroids used regularly on the face may produce steroid rosacea or atrophy and telangiectasia. These are rarely indicated for seborrheic dermatitis. If the disorder has not cleared after a few weeks, ketoconazole (Nizoral) 2% cream is prescribed, and the patient should be told that improvement will often take 4 more weeks.

C. Seborrhea of Nonhairy Areas: Low-potency steroid creams—ie, 1% or 2.5% hydrocortisone, desonide, or alclometasone dipropionate—are highly effective.

D. Seborrhea of Intertriginous Areas: Avoid greasy ointments. Apply low-potency steroid lotions or creams twice daily for 5–7 days and then once or twice weekly for maintenance as necessary. Ketoconazole shampoo may be a useful adjunct.

E. Involvement of Eyelid Margins: "Marginal blepharitis" usually responds to gentle cleaning of the lid margins nightly as needed, with undiluted Johnson and Johnson Baby Shampoo using a cotton swab.

Prognosis

The tendency is to lifelong recurrences. Individual outbreaks may last weeks, months, or years.

Bergbrant IM, Faergemann J: The role of *Pityrosporum ovale* in seborrheic dermatitis. Semin Dermatol 1990;9:262.

Cockerell CJ: Seborrheic dermatitis-like and atopic dermatitis-like eruptions in HIV infected patients. Clin Dermatol 1991;9:49.

FUNGAL INFECTIONS OF THE SKIN

Mycotic infections are traditionally divided into two principal groups—superficial and deep. In this chapter, we will discuss only the superficial infections: tinea capitis, tinea corporis, and tinea cruris; dermatophytosis of the feet and dermatophytid of the hands; tinea unguium (onychomycosis); and tinea versicolor.

The diagnosis of fungal infections of the skin is usually based on the location and characteristics of the lesions and on the first two of the following laboratory examinations: (1) Direct demonstration of fungi in 10% potassium hydroxide (KOH) in water or 20% KOH in DMSO preparations of scrapings from suspected lesions. "If it's scaly, scrape it" is a time-honored maxim. (2) Cultures of organisms. Dermatophytes responsive to griseofulvin are easily detectable, with color change from yellow to red on dermatophyte test medium (DTM); or one may use a microculture slide that produces color change and allows for direct microscopic identification. (3) Examination with Wood's light (an ultraviolet light with a special filter), which causes hairs to fluoresce a brilliant green when they are infected by *Microsporum* organisms, used to be a valuable test. However, because most infections of the scalp are not caused by *Microsporum* organisms, this test is rarely positive, and a negative test is meaningless. (4) Histologic sections stained with periodic acid-Schiff (Hotchkiss-McManus) technique. Fungal elements stain red and are easily found. Serologic and skin tests are of no value in the diagnosis of superficial fungal infections.

Principles of Treatment

In general, treatment follows a diagnosis confirmed by KOH preparation or culture, especially if systemic antifungal therapy is to be used. Many other diseases cause scaling, and use of an antifungal agent without a firm diagnosis makes subsequent diagnosis by a dermatologist more difficult. In general, fungal infections are treated topically except for those involving the scalp or nails or those deep in hair follicles on the face or body.

The systemic agent of choice is still griseofulvin, but this may change soon. For patients who cannot tolerate griseofulvin or who are unresponsive to that drug in adequate doses, the azoles, itraconazole, fluconazole, and ketoconazole may be used. Ketoconazole is now approved for treatment of all candidal infections, coccidioidomycosis, histoplasmosis, chromoblastomycosis, and paracoccidioidomycosis. It is also indicated for the treatment of patients with severe recalcitrant cutaneous dermatophyte infections who have not responded to topical therapy or oral griseofulvin or who are unable to take griseofulvin. Chief concerns with ketoconazole are abnormal levels of liver enzymes, gynecomastia, nausea, and urticaria.

One person in 10,000–15,000 may have drug-associated, occasionally fatal hepatitis after ketoconazole. It is critical to warn patients to stop the drug at onset of nausea, indigestion, dark urine, clay-colored stools, or jaundice, though this may not stop progression of hepatitis. Hepatitis can occur as early as 2 weeks after starting the drug. Liver function tests often return rapidly to normal when ketoconazole is stopped. Many patients show mild abnormalities of liver chemistries and do not develop clinical hepatitis; thus, it is preferable to follow symptoms and signs. Gynecomastia can be avoided by giving the

total dose once daily. It is best to avoid giving more than 200 mg/d (one tablet) if possible. In general, the use of ketoconazole for benign disease, despite the low risk of hepatitis, should be determined by the severity of the disease and the availability of other safer therapeutic alternatives.

Itraconazole, another axole antifungal, has recently been approved for use in the USA only for treatment of histoplasmosis and blastomycosis. However, there is ample evidence that this drug is quite effective against dermatophytes and in particular against onychomycosis, as it rapidly accumulates in the nail plate from the matrix and nail bed and persists for months after oral administration is discontinued. Like ketoconazole, itraconazole has been associated with idiosyncratic hepatotoxicity.

Fluconazole is another axole antifungal that is effective in treating cutaneous and mucous membrane candidiasis. However, it is usually not necessary to use this agent in cutaneous infections. Experience with fluconazole in dermatophyte infections is too limited to recommend its use.

General Measures & Prevention

The skin should be kept dry, since moist skin favors the growth of fungi. Dry the skin carefully after bathing or after perspiring heavily, and let it dry for 10–15 minutes before dressing, or use a hair dryer on low setting. Loose-fitting underwear is advisable. Socks and other clothing should be changed frequently. Sandals or open-toed shoes should be worn if possible. Skin secretions should be controlled with talc or other drying powders or with drying soaks. The use of topical corticosteroids for other diseases may be complicated by intercurrent tinea or candidal infection, and topical antifungals are often used in intertriginous areas with steroids to prevent this.

Benfield P, Clissold SP: Sulconazole: A review of its antimicrobial activity and therapeutic use in superficial dermatomycoses. Drugs 1988;35:143.

Knight TE et al: Ketoconazole-induced fulminant hepatitis necessitating liver transplantation. J Am Acad Dermatol 1991;25:398. (Fatalities due to ketoconazole-induced hepatitis.)

Lambert DR et al: Griseofulvin and ketoconazole in the treatment of dermatophyte infections. Int J Dermatol 1989;28:300.

1. TINEA CAPITIS (Ringworm of Scalp)

Essentials of Diagnosis

- Round, gray, scaly "bald" patches on the scalp or generalized scaling with patchy alopecia
- Usually in prepubertal children.
- Microscopic examination or culture identifies the fungus.

General Considerations

This persistent, contagious, and sometimes epidemic infection occurs almost exclusively in children and disappears spontaneously at puberty. Two general species (*Microsporum* and *Trichophyton*) cause ringworm infections of the scalp. *Microsporum* accounts for a small percentage of the infections, and hairs infected with this genus fluoresce brilliantly under Wood's light. *Trichophyton tonsurans* is the most common cause of tinea capitis in the USA today and does not fluoresce. *Trichophyton* species account for some of the very resistant infections, which may persist into adulthood.

Clinical Findings

A. Symptoms and Signs: There are usually no symptoms with noninflammatory tinea capitis, though there may be slight itching. The lesions are round, gray, scaly, apparently bald patches on the scalp. (The hairs are broken off, and the patches are not actually bald.) "Black dot" ringworm caused primarily by *T tonsurans* presents as multiple areas of alopecia studded with black dots representing infected hairs broken off at or below the surface of the scalp. At times, scalp ringworm presents as a localized spot accompanied by pronounced swelling and develops into boggy and indurated areas exuding pus known as kerion celsi. Regional lymphadenopathy is frequently associated.

B. Laboratory Findings: Microscopic or culture demonstration of the organisms in the hairs is necessary. This can be easily accomplished by rubbing a small disposable toothbrush into the scalp and then pressing it onto a fungal culture plate. The KOH examination should be done on the scales and—very importantly—on the small black dystrophic hairs, looking for spores within the hair shaft.

Differential Diagnosis

The KOH examination and fungal culture are essential for diagnosis. Pediculosis capitis will show adherent nits on hairs and moving lice that can be further examined in oil under a coverslip. Yellow crusts and weepiness may represent primary or secondary impetigo, and bacterial culture is indicated. Alopecia areata is marked by bald, often salmon-colored patches with short, thin hairs but minimal scaliness, by hairs with white bulbs easily dislodged on slight tugging at the periphery of the lesion, and by negative fungal studies. Trichotillomania (voluntary pulling out of one's own hair) is not associated with scaling and presents with bizarre patterns of hair loss with variable lengths of the hairs remaining.

Prevention

Exchange of headgear must be avoided, and infected individuals or household pets must be vigorously treated and scrupulously reexamined to verify cure. The scalp should be washed after haircuts.

Complications

Kerion (a nodular, exudative pustule), possibly followed by scarring, is the only complication. Since it represents an inflammatory reaction to the infection, it is treated with prednisone, 1 mg/kg daily for 10–14 days, combined with systemic antifungal therapy.

Treatment

Microcrystalline griseofulvin (tablets or suspension) may be given orally for 8 weeks or more until there are no clinical and microbiologic signs of infection: for children weighing 3–50 lb, 0.125–0.25 g/d; for children weighing 50–90 lb, 0.2–0.5 g/d; and for children and adolescents weighing over 90 lb and for adults, 0.5–1 g/d. (Or one may give griseofulvin ultramicrosize, 15–20 mg/kg orally.) The drug is best taken with the midday meal. Selenium sulfide shampoo is recommended to reduce spore shedding. Parents of infected children should be examined also and treated if necessary. Future studies will define the role of itraconazole in the treatment of tinea capitis in children.

Prognosis

Tinea capitis may be persistent but usually clears spontaneously by puberty, except for infections caused by certain resistant organisms such as *T tonsurans*. Kerion responds promptly to short-term prednisone therapy. Treatment of parents, where warranted, may decrease recurrences.

Hall JH, Lesher JL: Superficial fungal infections. Pediatrician 1991;18:224.

Pariser DM: Superficial fungal infections: A practical guide for primary care physicians. Postgrad Med 1990;87:205.

2. TINEA CORPORIS OR TINEA CIRCINATA (Body Ringworm)

Essentials of Diagnosis

- Ring-shaped lesions with an advancing scaly border and central clearing or scaly patches with a distinct border.
- On exposed skin surfaces.
- Laboratory examination by microscope or culture confirms diagnosis.

General Considerations

The lesions are often on exposed areas of the body such as the face and arms. A history of exposure to an infected cat may occasionally be obtained. All species of dermatophytes may cause this disease, but some are more common causes than others.

Clinical Findings

A. Symptoms and Signs: Itching is often present. Rings of erythema have an advancing scaly border and central clearing, occasionally with hyper-pigmentation, usually on an exposed surface. Tinea corporis may lack this ring shape and present with scaly patches of 1 to many centimeters.

B. Laboratory Findings: Hyphae can be demonstrated by removing peripheral scale and examining it microscopically using KOH. The diagnosis may be confirmed by culture.

Material can be obtained for culture on Sabouraud's medium by thoroughly rubbing a cotton swab over the lesion and then rotating the swab while thoroughly rubbing it on the medium; this technique is just as accurate as scraping the lesions with a scalpel or curette.

Differential Diagnosis

Positive fungal studies distinguish tinea corporis from other skin lesions with annular configuration, such as the annular lesions of psoriasis, lupus erythematosus, syphilis, erythema multiforme, and pityriasis rosea. Psoriasis has typical lesions on elbows, knees, scalp, and nails. Secondary syphilis is often manifested by characteristic palmar, plantar, and mucous membrane lesions. Erythema multiforme rarely does not have peripheral scale, is mostly acral in distribution, and is often associated with recent herpes simplex infection. Tinea corporis rarely has the large number of lesions seen in pityriasis rosea.

Complications

Complications include extension of the disease to the scalp, hair, or nails (in which case it becomes much more difficult to cure), pyoderma, and dermatophytid.

Prevention

Avoid contact with infected household pets and exchange of clothing without adequate laundering.

Treatment

A. Local Measures: The following applied topically are effective against dermatophyte infections other than those of the nails: miconazole, 2% cream; clotrimazole, 1% liquid, cream, or lotion; ketoconazole, 2% cream; econazole, 1% cream; sulconazole, 1% cream; oxiconazole, 1% cream; ciclopirox, 1% cream; naftifine, 1% cream; and terbinafine, 1% cream. Have the patient continue treatment for 1–2 weeks after clinical clearing. Tolnaftate, 1% solution or cream, and haloprogin, 1% solution or cream, are older second-line remedies. Betamethasone dipropionate with clotrimazole (Lotrisone) applied twice daily for 3–5 days may be beneficial for acutely inflamed tinea lesions. After the inflammation subsides, switch to a topical antifungal without a steroid component. In general, short-term use of Lotrisone (betamethasone-clotrimazole) does not justify the expense, and chronic improper use may result in side effects from the high-potency steroid component, es-

pecially in body folds. Cases of tinea that are clinically resistant to this combination have been reported.

B. Systemic Measures: Griseofulvin (microcrystalline) may be given to children as described for tinea capitis and griseofulvin (ultramicrosize) at 250–500 mg twice daily is used for adults. Typically, only 2–4 weeks of therapy are required. Ketoconazole is also indicated for the treatment of patients with severe recalcitrant cutaneous dermatophyte infections, starting at doses of 200 mg/d.

Prognosis

Body ringworm usually responds promptly to conservative topical therapy within 4 weeks or to griseofulvin by mouth.

3. TINEA CRURIS
(Jock Itch)

Essentials of Diagnosis

- Marked itching in intertriginous areas, often sparing the scrotum.
- Peripherally spreading, sharply demarcated, centrally clearing erythematous macular lesions.
- May have associated tinea infection of feet.
- Laboratory examination with microscope or culture confirms diagnosis.

General Considerations

Tinea cruris lesions are confined to the groin and gluteal cleft and are as a rule more indolent than those of tinea corporis and tinea circinata. The scrotum is generally spared. The disease often occurs in athletes as well as in persons who are obese or who perspire a great deal. Any of the dermatophytes may cause tinea cruris, and it may be transmitted to the groin from active dermatophytosis of the foot. Intractable pruritus ani may occasionally be caused by a tinea infection.

Clinical Findings

A. Symptoms and Signs: Itching may be severe, or the rash may be generally asymptomatic. The lesions consist of erythematous macules with sharp margins, cleared centers, and active, spreading scaly peripheries in intertriginous areas. There rarely may be vesicle formation at the borders, and satellite vesicular lesions are rarely present. Follicular pustules are sometimes encountered.

B. Laboratory Findings: Hyphae can be demonstrated microscopically in 10% potassium hydroxide preparations. The organism may be cultured readily. The area may be hyperpigmented on resolution.

Differential Diagnosis

Tinea cruris must be distinguished from other lesions involving the intertriginous areas, such as candidiasis, tinea versicolor, seborrheic dermatitis, intertrigo, psoriasis of body folds ("inverse psoriasis"), and erythrasma. Candidiasis is generally bright red and marked by satellite papules and pustules outside of the main border of the lesion. Tinea versicolor can be distinguished by the KOH preparation, since the causative organisms are morphologically distinguishable. Seborrheic dermatitis of the inguinal area also often involves the face, sternum, and axillae. Intertrigo tends to be more red, less scaly, and present in obese individuals in moist body folds. The KOH preparation is negative. Inverse psoriasis may itch more than tinea cruris. Other areas of typical psoriatic involvement should be checked, and the KOH examination will be negative. Erythrasma is best diagnosed with Wood's light—a brilliant coral-red fluorescence is seen.

Treatment

A. General Measures: Drying powder should be dusted into the involved area two or three times a day, especially when perspiration is excessive. Keep the area clean and dry but avoid overbathing. Prevent intertrigo or chafing by avoiding overtreatment, which predisposes to further infection and complications. Underwear should be loose-fitting. Rough-textured clothing should be avoided.

B. Local Fungistatic Measures: Any of the preparations listed in the section on tinea corporis may be used. There is great variation in expense, with miconazole and clotrimazole available OTC and usually at a lower price. Ketoconazole and sulconazole cream may be used daily instead of twice daily.

C. Systemic Measures: Griseofulvin ultramicrosize is indicated for severe cases. Give 250–500 mg orally twice daily for 1–2 weeks.

Prognosis

Tinea cruris usually responds promptly to topical or systemic treatment.

4. TINEA MANUUM & TINEA PEDIS (Dermatophytosis, Tinea of Palms & Soles, "Athlete's Foot")

Essentials of Diagnosis

- Itching, burning, and stinging of interdigital webs, palms, and soles; deep vesicles in inflammatory cases.
- Scaling, fissuring, and maceration in subacute or chronic stages.
- Skin scrapings examined microscopically or by culture may reveal fungus.

General Considerations

Tinea of the feet is an extremely common acute or chronic dermatosis. Certain individuals appear to be more susceptible than others. Most infections are caused by *Trichophyton* and *Epidermophyton* species.

Clinical Findings

A. Symptoms and Signs: The presenting symptom is usually itching. However, there may be burning, stinging, and other sensations, or frank pain from secondary infection with complicating cellulitis, lymphangitis, and lymphadenitis. Tinea pedis has several presentations that vary with the location. On the sole and heel, tinea may appear as chronic noninflammatory scaling, occasionally with thickening and cracking of the epidermis. The KOH preparation is usually positive. Tinea pedis often appears as fissuring of the toe webs, perhaps with denudation and sodden maceration. As the web spaces become more macerated, the KOH preparation and fungal culture are less often positive because bacterial species then begin to dominate. There may also be grouped vesicles distributed anywhere on the soles or palms, generalized exfoliation of the skin of the soles, or destructive nail involvement in the form of discoloration and thickening and crumbling of the nail substance. Acute reddened, weeping vesicular lesions are occasionally seen on the skin in cases marked by inflammation.

B. Laboratory Findings: Hyphae can often be demonstrated microscopically in skin scales treated with 10% potassium hydroxide. Culture with Sabouraud's medium is simple and often informative but does not always demonstrate pathogenic fungi. Microbiologic procedures are more often positive when the infection is dry and scaly and less often when macerated (as between the toes).

Differential Diagnosis

Differentiate from other skin conditions involving the same areas, such as interdigital erythrasma (use Wood's light), candidiasis (culture), and intertrigo in the interdigital webs. Intertrigo is diagnosed by negative fungal studies, no response to therapy, and response to agents as described below. Psoriasis may be a cause of chronic scaling on the soles and may cause nail changes. Repeated fungal cultures should be negative, and the condition will not respond to antifungal therapy. Contact dermatitis (from shoes, powders, nail polish) will often involve the dorsal surfaces and will respond to topical or systemic corticosteroids. Vesicular lesions should be differentiated from dyshidrosis and scabies by proper scraping of the vesicles. Rarely, gram-negative organisms may cause toe web infections in the setting of prior tinea or in its absence. Culture is not very specific, because gram-negative organisms can be cultured from normal toe webs. Treatment of gram-negative organisms is with aluminum salts (see below) and imidazole antifungal agents or ciclopirox.

Prevention

The essential factor in prevention is personal hygiene. Rubber or wooden sandals should be used in community showers and bathing places, though the effectiveness of this practice has not been studied. Careful drying between the toes after showering is recommended. A hair dryer used on low setting may be recommended before dressing. Socks should be changed frequently. Apply dusting and drying powders as necessary. The use of powders containing antifungal agents (eg, Zeasorb-AF) may prevent recurrences of systemically cured tinea pedis.

Treatment

A. Local Measures: *Caution:* Do not overtreat.

1. Macerated stage–Treat with aluminum subacetate (Domeboro) solution soaks for 20 minutes two or three times daily. If secondary infection is present, use 1:10,000 potassium permanganate. If secondary infection is severe or complicated, treat as described on decubitus ulcers. Toe web intertrigo may respond better to 30% aqueous aluminum chloride or to carbolfuchsin paint (this is messy) than to antifungal agents. Broad-spectrum antifungal creams and solutions (containing imidazoles or ciclopirox) instead of tolnaftate and haloprogin will help combat diphtheroids and other gram-positive organisms present at this stage and alone may be adequate therapy.

2. Dry and scaly stage–Use any of the agents listed in the section on tinea capitis. Older methods of treatment are (1) sulfur-salicylic acid ointment or cream; (2) Whitfield's ointment, one-fourth to one-half strength; (3) alcoholic Whitfield's solution; and (4) compound undecylenic acid ointment applied twice daily.

B. Systemic Measures: Griseofulvin should be used only for severe cases or those that are recalcitrant to topical therapy. If the infection is cleared by systemic therapy, the patient should be encouraged to begin maintenance with topical therapy.

Ketoconazole, 200 mg daily by mouth, is an effective agent for griseofulvin-resistant dermatophytosis, though relapse may occur after discontinuing therapy. The drug is usually well tolerated, though hepatotoxicity has been reported from its use (see above).

Itraconazole, a new oral antifungal, is effective for relief of recalcitrant dermatophyte infections, but it is expensive and may not prevent recurrences. The dosage is 100 mg daily for 1–3 months.

Prognosis

For many individuals, tinea pedis becomes a chronic affliction, temporarily cleared by systemic therapy only to recur. Treatment of toenail fungal infections is quite difficult, and in some patients the nails serve as reservoirs for fungal organisms.

Bergstresser MD et al: Topical terbinafine and clotrimazole in interdigital tinea pedis: A multicenter comparison of cure and relapse rates with 1- and 4-week treatment regimens. J Am Acad Dermatol 1993;28:6480. (Terbinafine superior to clotrimazole.)

Roth RR, James WD: Microbiology of the skin: Resident flora, ecology, infection. J Am Acad Dermatol 1989; 20:367.

5. TINEA VERSICOLOR (Pityriasis Versicolor)

Essentials of Diagnosis

- Pale macules that will not tan, or hyperpigmented macules.
- Velvety, tan, pink, whitish, or brown macules that scale with scraping.
- Trunk distribution the most frequent site.
- Fungus observed on microscopic examination of scales.

General Considerations

Tinea versicolor is a mild, superficial *Pityrosporum orbiculare (Malassezia furfur)* infection of the skin (usually of the trunk). This organism is a colonizer of all humans. It is not understood why some patients manifest the spore and hyphal form of the organism and the clinical disease. However, the colonization of humans probably accounts for the high recurrence rate after treatment and initial cure. The eruption is often called to Caucasian patients' attention by the fact that the involved areas will not tan, and the resulting pseudoachromia may be mistaken for vitiligo. A hyperpigmented form is not uncommon. The disease is not particularly contagious and is apt to occur more frequently in those who wear heavy clothing and who perspire a great deal.

Clinical Findings

A. Symptoms and Signs: There may be mild itching. The lesions are velvety, tan, pink, whitish, or brown macules that vary from 4–5 mm in diameter to large confluent areas. The lesions initially do not look scaly, but scales may be readily obtained by scraping the area. Lesions may appear on the trunk, upper arms, neck, face, and groin.

B. Laboratory Findings: Large, blunt hyphae and thick-walled budding spores ("spaghetti and meatballs") may be seen under the low-power objective when skin scales have been cleared in 10% KOH. Fungal culture is not useful, as *P orbiculare* and *P ovale* require special conditions and are commonly present on the skin of unaffected individuals.

Differential Diagnosis

Hypopigmented lesions can be distinguished from vitiligo on basis of appearance. Vitiligo usually presents with periorificial lesions or lesions on the tips of the fingers. Vitiligo (and not tinea versicolor) is characterized by total depigmentation, not just a lessening of pigmentation. Differentiate pink and red-brown lesions on the chest also from seborrheic dermatitis of the same areas by the KOH preparation.

Treatment & Prognosis

Topical treatments include selenium sulfide lotion (Exsel, Selsun), which may be applied from neck to waist daily and left on for 5–15 minutes for 7 days; this treatment is repeated weekly for a month and then monthly for maintenance. Ketoconazole shampoo may also be used for maintenance. One must stress to the patient that the raised and scaly aspects of the rash are being treated; the alterations in pigmentation may take months to fade or fill in. One may also use equal parts of propylene glycol and water topically, diluting with water if there is irritation. Other choices are 3% salicylic acid in rubbing alcohol and Tinver lotion (contains sodium thiosulfate). Irritation and odor from these agents are common complaints from patients. Relapses are common.

Sulfur-salicylic acid soap or shampoo (Sebulex) used on a continuing basis may be effective.

Ketoconazole, 200 mg daily orally for 1 week or 400 mg as a single oral dose, apparently results in short-term cure of 90% of cases. The single dose may not work in more hot and humid areas of the USA, and more protracted therapy carries a small but finite risk of drug-induced hepatitis for a completely benign disease. Without maintenance therapy, recurrences will occur in over 80% of "cured" cases over the subsequent 2 years. Patients should be instructed not to shower for 12–18 hours after taking ketoconazole, because it is delivered in sweat to the skin.

Newer imidazole creams, solutions, and lotions are quite effective for localized areas but are too expensive for use over large areas such as the chest and back.

Borelli D et al: Tinea versicolor: Epidemiologic, clinical, and therapeutic aspects. J Am Acad Dermatol 1991; 25:300.

CHRONIC DISCOID LUPUS ERYTHEMATOSUS (Chronic Cutaneous Lupus Erythematosus)

Essentials of Diagnosis

- Red, asymptomatic, localized plaques, usually on the face, often in butterfly distribution.
- Scaling, follicular plugging, atrophy, and telangiectasia of involved areas.
- Histology distinctive.
- May be photosensitive.

General Considerations

This type of lupus erythematosus is a localized dis-coid inflammation of the skin occurring most frequently in areas exposed to solar or ultraviolet irradiation. The cause is not known. Systemic lupus erythematosus is discussed in Chapter 19.

Clinical Findings

A. Symptoms and Signs: There are usually no symptoms. The lesions consist of dusky red, well-localized, single or multiple plaques, 5–20 mm in diameter, usually on the face. The scalp, external ears, and oral mucous membranes may be involved. There is atrophy, telangiectasia, and follicular plugging. The lesion is usually covered by dry, horny, adherent scales.

B. Laboratory Findings: If ANA is positive in high titer or when the clinical picture suggests systemic involvement, antibody to double-stranded DNA and hypocomplementemia suggest the diagnosis of systemic lupus erythematosus. Rare patients with marked photosensitivity and a picture otherwise suggestive of lupus have negative ANA tests but are positive for antibodies against Ro/SSA. A direct immunofluorescence test reveals basement membrane antibody but may be falsely positive in sun-exposed skin.

Differential Diagnosis

The diagnosis is based on the clinical appearance combined with skin biopsy in the majority of cases. The scales are dry and "tack-like" and can thus be distinguished from those of seborrheic dermatitis and psoriasis. Older lesions that have left scarring (classically in the concha of the ear) or areas of hair loss will also differentiate lupus from these diseases. Solitary lesions may rarely appear similar to the very rare type of sclerosing basal cell epithelioma. A skin biopsy will be diagnostic. Discoid lupus differs from the rarely seen lupus vulgaris by the absence of nodules and ulceration. Ten percent of patients with systemic lupus erythematosus have discoid type lesions.

Complications

Lesions may be widespread, resulting in dyspigmentation, permanent alopecia, and scarring.

Treatment

A. General Measures: Provide protection from sunlight in photosensitive patients. *Caution:* Do not use any form of radiation therapy. Avoid using drugs that are potentially photosensitizing (eg, thiazides, piroxicam) where possible.

B. Local Treatment: The following should be tried before systemic therapy: high-potency corticosteroid creams applied each night and covered with airtight, thin, pliable plastic film (eg, Saran Wrap); or halobetasol propionate (Ultravate) or clobetasol propionate (Temovate) cream or ointment applied twice daily without occlusion.

C. Local Infiltration: Triamcinolone acetonide

suspension, 2.5–10 mg/mL, may be injected into the lesions once a month. This should be tried before systemic therapy.

D. Systemic Treatment:

1. Antimalarials–*Caution:* These drugs should be used only when the diagnosis is secure, because they have been associated with flares of psoriasis, which may be in the clinical diagnosis. They may also cause serious eye changes, and ophthalmologic evaluation is required before beginning treatment and repeated every 3 months. The use of antimalarials in children is controversial. Baseline G6PD levels must be obtained prior to use of antimalarials.

a. Hydroxychloroquine sulfate, 0.2–0.4 g orally daily for several weeks, may be effective and is often used prior to chloroquine. A 3-month trial is recommended.

b. Chloroquine sulfate, 250 mg daily, may be effective in some cases where hydroxychloroquine is not.

c. Quinacrine (Atabrine), 100 mg daily, may be the safest of the antimalarials, since eye damage has not been reported. It colors the skin yellow and is therefore not acceptable to some patients.

2. Dapsone–Dapsone, 50 mg/d orally, may be helpful.

3. Isotretinoin–In a limited open study, isotretinoin, 80 mg/d, was effective in returning the skin and laboratory findings to normal in chronic or subacute cutaneous lupus erythematosus. Because of teratogenicity, the drug cannot be used in women of childbearing age without the use of effective contraception and informed consent as well as a pregnancy test before therapy is started.

Prognosis

The disease is persistent but not life-endangering unless systemic lupus intervenes, which is uncommon. Treatment with antimalarials is effective in perhaps 60% of cases. Although the only morbidity may be cosmetic, this can be of overwhelming significance in more darkly pigmented patients with widespread disease. Scarring alopecia can be prevented or lessened with close attention and aggressive therapy.

Callen JP: Treatment of cutaneous lesions in patients with lupus erythematosus. Dermatol Clin 1990;8:355. (An approach for treatment of mild to severe disease, including sunscreens, intralesional steroids, antimalarials, azathioprine, retinoids, and other medications.)
Hymes SR, Jordan RE: Chronic cutaneous lupus erythematosus. Med Clin North Am 1989;73:1055.
Sontheimer RD: Subacute cutaneous lupus erythematosus: A decade's perspective. Med Clin North Am 1989;73:1073.

EXFOLIATIVE DERMATITIS
(Exfoliative Erythroderma)

Essentials of Diagnosis

- Scaling and erythema over large area of body.
- Itching, malaise, fever, chills, weight loss.
- Primary disease or exposure to toxic agent (contact, oral, parenteral) may be evident.

General Considerations

A preexisting dermatosis may be found as the cause in approximately 40% of cases, including psoriasis, atopic dermatitis, contact dermatitis, pityriasis rubra pilaris, and seborrheic dermatitis. Many adult patients with exfoliative dermatitis have psoriasis. Reactions to external and internal drugs account for perhaps one-fourth of cases and cancer (cutaneous T cell lymphoma, Sézary syndrome) for 10%. Causation of the remainder is indeterminable. At the time of acute presentation, without a clear-cut prior history of skin disease or drug exposure, it is often impossible to make a specific diagnosis of the underlying condition even with skin biopsy, and diagnosis may require follow-up with time.

Clinical Findings

A. Symptoms and Signs: Symptoms may include itching, weakness, malaise, fever, and weight loss. Chills are prominent. Exfoliation may be generalized or universal and sometimes includes loss of hair and nails. Generalized lymphadenopathy may be due to lymphoma or leukemia or may be part of the clinical picture of the skin disease (dermatopathic lymphadenitis). Mucosal sloughs are uncommon.

B. Laboratory Findings: A complete blood count is indicated in all patients with this problem, and skin biopsy may show changes of a specific inflammatory dermatitis or cutaneous T cell lymphoma or leukemia.

Differential Diagnosis

It is often impossible to identify the cause of exfoliative dermatitis early in the course of the disease, so careful follow-up is necessary. Psoriasis, lichen planus, severe seborrheic dermatitis, and drug eruptions may themselves develop into exfoliative dermatitis.

Complications

Debility (protein loss) and dehydration may develop in patients with generalized inflammatory erythroderma; associated bacteriuria may also occur.

Treatment

A. Topical Therapy: Home treatment is with cool to tepid baths and application of mid-potency steroids under wet dressings or with the use of an occlusive plastic suit (Simmons Co., Chattanooga, Tennessee; or Sleep Sauna, Lower Bwynedd, Pennsylvania). Topical anti-infective drugs may be used when necessary. If the erythroderma becomes chronic and is not manageable in an outpatient setting, hospitalize the patient. Keep the room at a constant warm temperature and provide the same topical treatment as for an outpatient.

B. Specific Measures: Stop all drugs, if possible. Systemic corticosteroids may provide spectacular improvement in severe or fulminant exfoliative dermatitis, but long-term therapy should be avoided (see Chapter 25). In addition, systemic corticosteroids must be used with caution because some patients with erythroderma have psoriasis and could develop pustular psoriasis. For recalcitrant cases of psoriatic erythroderma and pityriasis rubra pilaris, either isotretinoin, etretinate, or methotrexate—or isotretinoin and methotrexate in combination—may be indicated. Erythroderma secondary to lymphoma or leukemia requires specific topical or systemic chemotherapy combined with radiation therapy. Suitable antibiotic drugs should be given when there is evidence of bacterial infection; pyoderma is a possible complication of exfoliative dermatitis.

Prognosis

Most patients recover completely or improve greatly over time but may require chronic therapy. Deaths have been reported but are rare unless there is underlying cancer. A minority of patients will suffer from undiminished erythroderma for indefinite periods.

Wieselthier JG, Koh HK: Sézary syndrome: Diagnosis, prognosis and critical review of treatment options. J Am Acad Dermatol 1990;22:381.

MISCELLANEOUS SCALING DERMATOSES

Isolated scaly patches may represent actinic (solar) keratoses, nonpigmented seborrheic keratoses, or Bowen's or Paget's disease.

Actinic Keratoses

Actinic keratoses are flesh-colored to pink and feel like small patches of sandpaper when the finger is drawn over them. They occur on exposed parts of the body in persons of fair complexion. Nonactinic keratoses may be provoked by exposure to arsenic systemically or occupational irritants such as tars. In keratoses, the cells are atypical and similar to those seen in squamous cell epitheliomas, but there is no invasion into the dermis. Approximately 1:1000 lesions per year progress to become squamous cell carcinomas.

Application of liquid nitrogen is a rapid and effective method of eradication. The lesions are frozen for a few seconds with a cotton-tipped applicator that has been dipped in liquid nitrogen or with a spraying unit containing liquid nitrogen. The lesions crust and dis-

appear in 5–10 days. An alternative treatment is the use of 1–5% fluorouracil cream. This agent may be rubbed into the lesions morning and night until they become first red and sore and then crusted and eroded (usually 1–3 weeks), and then stopped. Similarly, 5%fluorouracil solution may be used two times a day on one or two consecutive days weekly for 7–10 weeks without causing pain and crusting. The eyes and mouth should be avoided. Any lesions that persist may then be biopsied for histologic examination.

A new agent, masoprocol, available as 10% cream (Actinex), has been approved for treatment of actinic keratoses. While it seems to cause less inflammation, it also appears to be far less effective in totally clearing actinic keratoses compared to fluorouracil.

Pearlman DL: Weekly pulse dosing: Effective and comfortable topical 5-fluorouracil treatment of multiple facial actinic keratoses. J Am Acad Dermatol 1991;25:665.

Bowen's Disease & Paget's Disease

Bowen's disease (intraepidermal squamous cell carcinoma) is relatively uncommon, occurring either on sun-exposed or sun-protected cutaneous surfaces. The lesion is a small (1–3 cm), well-demarcated, slightly raised, pink to red, scaly plaque and may resemble psoriasis. The course is relatively benign, but since these lesions may progress to invasive squamous cell carcinoma, excision or other definitive treatment is indicated.

Paget's disease, considered by some to be a manifestation of apocrine sweat gland carcinoma, may occur around the nipple, resembling chronic eczema, or may involve apocrine areas such as the genitalia (extramammary Paget's disease). There seems to be less likelihood of an underlying sweat gland carcinoma if the lesions are on the vulva than if they are on the nipple or perianal area.

INTERTRIGO

Intertrigo is caused by the macerating effect of heat, moisture, and friction. It is especially likely to occur in obese persons and in humid climates. Poor hygiene is an important etiologic factor. There is often a history of seborrheic dermatitis. The symptoms are itching, stinging, and burning. The body folds develop fissures, erythema, and sodden epidermis, with superficial denudation. Urine and blood examination may reveal diabetes mellitus, and the skin examination may reveal candidiasis. A direct smear may show abundant cocci. "Inverse psoriasis," tinea cruris, erythrasma, and candidiasis must be ruled out.

Maintain hygiene in the area, and keep it dry. Compresses may be useful acutely. If there is evidence of colonization of yeasts or bacteria, apply a topical antifungal or antibacterial solution, lotion, or powder. A mild topical steroid and antifungal agent to suppress fungal overgrowth is effective. Recurrences are common.

VESICULAR DERMATOSES

HERPES SIMPLEX
(Cold or Fever Sore)

Essentials of Diagnosis

- Recurrent small grouped vesicles on an erythematous base, especially around oral and genital areas.
- May follow minor infections, trauma, stress, or sun exposure; regional lymph nodes may be swollen and tender.
- Tzanck smear is positive for large multinucleated epithelial giant cells; viral cultures, ELISA tests, and slide immunofluorescence tests are positive.

General Considerations

Although approximately 90% of the population acquire herpes simplex infection before the age of 4 or 5 years (based on antibody studies), it is generally type 1 infection, following which the virus establishes latency in the regional ganglia for life. The disease may manifest itself as severe gingivostomatitis in small children, or the initial infection may be subclinical. Thereafter, the subject may have recurrent self-limited attacks, provoked by fever, a viral infection, fatigue, menstruation, and other triggering factors such as sun and wind. In AIDS and rarely in patients with normal immune status, herpes simplex type 1 causes sporadic encephalitis.

Herpes simplex type 2 causes lesions of similar morphology and natural history on the genitalia of both sexes. The infection is initially acquired by sexual contact. A recent study of monogamous heterosexual couples in which one partner had herpes simplex type 2 infection demonstrated seroconversion of the noninfected partner in 10% of couples over a 1-year period. Up to 70% of such infections appeared to be acquired during asymptomatic periods. Uninfected female partners were at greater risk than males, especially if they were seronegative for herpes simplex type 1 antibodies as well. Transverse myelitis, neuropathic pain in the sacral distribution, and encephalitis are rare complications.

Clinical Findings

A. Symptoms and Signs: The principal symptoms are burning and stinging. Neuralgia may precede and accompany attacks. The lesions consist of small, grouped vesicles that can occur anywhere but which most often occur on the lips, mouth, and buttocks. Regional lymph nodes may be swollen and tender. The lesions eventually crust and become noninfectious when all crusts fall off. It has been demonstrated that patients can be educated to recognize attacks that they previously did not identify as recurrences of herpes simplex. Herpesviruses may also cause chronic painful, perianal ulcerations in patients with AIDS.

B. Laboratory Findings: Lesions clinically diagnosed as chancroid, syphilis, pyoderma, or trauma have been found to be herpes simplex virus infections on culture. Viral culture, although not highly sensitive, is most helpful in confirming the clinical diagnosis. Other methods rely on detection of viral antigen by immunologic methods (immunoperoxidase or immunofluorescence) or demonstration of multinucleated cells. The latter is the least sensitive but is readily available, positive for herpes simplex and for varicella zoster virus, and easy to perform.

Complications

Complications include pyoderma, eczema herpeticum, herpetic whitlow, herpes gladiatorum (epidemic herpes in wrestlers transmitted by contact), esophagitis, transplacental fetal infection, keratitis, and a severe encephalitis.

Prevention:

Prophylactic use of oral acyclovir may prevent some but not all predictable recurrences due to sunlight or menstrual periods. Acyclovir should be started at a dosage of 200 mg five times daily beginning 24 hours prior to ultraviolet light exposure. Sunscreens may also be useful adjuncts in preventing sun-induced recurrences.

Treatment

A. Systemic Therapy: Acyclovir is effective systemically (intravenously or orally), and when properly administered it is practically nontoxic. With episodes of primary genital herpes simplex, the period of viral shedding, pain, crusting, and other symptoms can be shortened and healing can be hastened by giving acyclovir, 200 mg orally five times daily, 400 mg three times daily, or 800 mg twice daily—for 10 days. Acyclovir is effective in preventing frequent subsequent genital recurrences if suppressive dosages of 200 mg three times daily are maintained. If recurrences are infrequent (every 3–6 months), episodic treatment employing 200 mg orally five times daily or 800 mg twice daily is effective in shortening the duration of the recurrence and viral shedding by a few days if initiated at the first sign or symptom of recurrence. Long-term acyclovir therapy appears to be effective and safe. Acyclovir has no effect on asymptomatic cervical or oral shedding.

B. Local Measures: Topical therapy is not particularly effective. It is strongly urged that 5% acyclovir ointment (Zovirax), if used at all, be limited to the restricted indications for which it has been approved, ie, initial herpes genitalis and mucocutaneous herpes simplex infections in immunocompromised patients, because of promotion of resistant strains of the virus and the possible mutagenicity of the drug. The effectiveness of other topicals is anecdotal. Cloths used in compresses may contain infectious virus for some hours while wet and should be kept separate from other family members.

Prognosis

Aside from the complications described above, recurrent attacks last several days, and patients recover without sequelae.

Guinan ME: Oral acyclovir for treatment and suppression of genital herpes simplex virus infection: A review. JAMA 1986;255:1747.

Mertz GJ et al: Risk factors for the sexual transmission of genital herpes. Ann Intern Med 1992;116:197.

Solomon AA: New diagnostic tests for herpes simplex and varicella zoster infections. J Am Acad Dermatol 1988;18:218.

HERPES ZOSTER
(Shingles)

Essentials of Diagnosis

- Pain along the course of a nerve followed by painful grouped vesicular lesions.
- Involvement is unilateral; some lesions may occur outside the affected dermatome.
- Lesions are usually on face and trunk.
- Swelling of regional lymph nodes (inconstant).
- Tzanck smear may be positive, especially in early lesions.

General Considerations

Herpes zoster is an acute vesicular eruption due to a virus that is morphologically identical with the virus of varicella. It usually occurs in adults. With rare exceptions, patients suffer only one attack of zoster. In immunocompromised patients, generalized, life-threatening dissemination may occur. In patients at risk for HIV infection, development of zoster may be one sign that precedes marked depression of cellular immunity associated with AIDS or ARC.

Clinical Findings

Pain usually precedes the eruption by 48 hours or more and may persist and actually increase in intensity after the lesions have disappeared. The lesions consist of grouped, tense, deep-seated vesicles distributed unilaterally along the neural pathways of the trunk. The commonest distributions are on the trunk or face. Regional lymph glands may be tender and swollen.

Dermatomal herpes zoster does not imply the presence of a visceral malignancy; generalized disease, however, raises the suspicion of an associated immunosuppressive disorder such as AIDS or Hodgkin's disease.

Differential Diagnosis

Since poison oak and poison ivy dermatitis may be produced unilaterally and in a streak by a single brush with the plant, it must be differentiated at times from herpes zoster. Linear vesicles are more typical of contact allergic dermatitis, grouped vesicles of viral infection. One must differentiate herpes zoster also from similar lesions of herpes simplex, which may be less painful. The main reason to differentiate between HSV and VZV infection is the dose of acyclovir used to treat the condition and the chance of subsequent recurrence. The pain of preeruptive herpes zoster may lead the clinician to diagnose migraine, myocardial infarction, acute abdomen, herniated nucleus pulposus, etc, depending on the dermatome involved.

Complications

Persistent neuralgia, anesthesia or scarring of the affected area following healing, facial or other nerve paralysis, and encephalitis may occur. Postherpetic neuralgia is most common after involvement of the trigeminal region, in patients over the age of 60, and in immunocompromised individuals. Zoster ophthalmicus may result in visual loss.

Treatment

A. General Measures: Attacks of shingles in the immunocompetent host can be ameliorated by acyclovir. Both intravenous and high-dose oral acyclovir (800 mg five times daily for 7 days) have been reported to accelerate healing and reduce acute pain if started within 48–72 hours. Patients should maintain good hydration, and elderly patients with reduced renal function should be followed closely. One study showed an effect on postherpetic neuralgia over the first few months after an attack, when treatment lasted for 10 days. However, patients in this study had mild pain, and none had pain that lasted more than 6 months. Narcotic analgesics may be used but often cause constipation in the elderly. Nerve blocks may be important in the management of initial severe pain. A single intragluteal injection of 40 mg of triamcinolone acetonide suspension has been reported (anecdotally) to give prompt relief. Steroid therapy may decrease the incidence of postherpetic neuralgia, but this is controversial, with some studies documenting benefit and others not. It is probably safe if patients with cancer, lymphoma, leukemia, or other causes of immunodeficiency are not so treated and if acyclovir is used at the same time. Doses of 40–60 mg/d of prednisone tapering over 3 weeks should be used. Ophthalmologic consultation is vital for involvement of the first branch of the trigeminal nerve.

Varicella-zoster immune globulin is not effective

in established zoster but is important in immunocompromised patients without prior varicella who are then exposed to varicella.

The goal of herpes zoster therapy for immunocompromised patients is prevention of possibly life-threatening viral spread. Both intravenous acyclovir and vidarabine will prevent progression in this patient population. However, special caution and follow-up is necessary for patients with HIV infection and low helper T cell counts, or with malabsorption or lymphoma, or for patients receiving immunosuppressive drugs. Progression of disease may necessitate intravenous therapy. Adverse effects include decreased renal function from crystallization, nausea and vomiting, and abdominal pain. One may give acyclovir, 7.5 mg/kg of ideal body weight intravenously, three times daily for 7 days. May patients, however, may be managed with oral acyclovir depending on their immune status.

B. Local Measures: Calamine or starch shake lotions may be of some help.

C. Postzoster Neuralgia: Topical capsaicin (Zostrix) appears to help about half of patients with neuralgia. Chronic postherpetic neuralgia is usually not relieved by regional blocks (stellate ganglion, epidural, local infiltration, or peripheral nerve) with bupivacaine hydrochloride, with or without corticosteroids added to the injections. Amitriptyline, 25 mg orally three times daily, perphenazine, 4 mg orally three times daily, and fluphenazine, 1 mg four times daily, have also been suggested. Doxepin, 25–50 mg three times daily, has also been reported to be helpful. Somnolence may occur with the drugs.

Prognosis

The eruption persists 2–3 weeks and does not recur. It is said that the total duration of the eruption may be predicted by the number of days over which new vesicular lesions continue to appear. Motor involvement in 2–3% may lead to temporary palsy. No age group is exempt from the possibility of postzoster neuralgia persisting for a year or more, but the likelihood is greater in the 60- to 69-year age group (20%) and in those over 70 (30%). Ocular involvement may lead to blindness. Documented recurrences of zoster are rare and often are really herpes simplex on culture.

Balfour HH Jr: Acyclovir therapy for herpes zoster: Advantages and adverse effects. JAMA 1986;255:387.

Hernandez E et al: Acute renal failure induced by oral acyclovir. (Letter.) Clin Nephrol 1991;36:155.

Huff JC et al: Therapy of herpes zoster with oral acyclovir. Am J Med 1988;85(Suppl 2A):84.

Peikert A et al: Topical 0.025% capsaicin in chronic postherpetic neuralgia: Efficacy, predictors of response and long-term course. J Neurol 1991;348:452. (Many patients improved, but some discontinued therapy due to burning sensation or mastitis.)

Watson C et al: Amitriptyline vs placebo in postherpetic neuralgia. Neurology 1982;32:671.

DYSHIDROSIS
(Dyshidrotic Eczema, Pompholyx)

Essentials of Diagnosis

- "Tapioca" vesicles of 1–2 mm on the palms, soles, and sides of fingers, associated with pruritus.
- Vesicles may coalesce to form multiloculated blisters.
- Scaling and fissuring may follow drying of the blisters.
- Appearance in the third decade, with lifelong recurrences.

General Considerations

Dyshidrosis is a misnomer, suggesting that the vesicles of this condition are related to eccrine sweat ducts and sweating, which they are not. This is an extremely common form of hand dermatitis, called also pompholyx (Gr "bubble") or vesicular dermatitis of the palms and soles. Patients often seem to have an atopic background and report flares with stress. In Scandinavia, women with contact allergy to nickel and dyshidrotic eczema appear to flare when given oral challenges with nickel. Nickel-free diets have given variable results. The chelator disulfiram has been reported to cause a 25% improvement in one controlled study, and oral cromolyn sodium has also been shown to be of benefit. Some patients treated with oral urushiol, the poison ivy and oak antigen, in order to induce tolerance have also reported pompholyx-like eruptions. Therefore, it has been suggested that this condition represents some form of hypersensitivity or allergy.

Clinical Findings

Small clear vesicles stud the skin at the sides of the fingers and on the palms or soles. They look like the round grains in tapioca. They may be associated with intense itching. Later, the vesicles dry and the area desquamates. Marked vesiculation is associated with greater scaling and fissuring. Areas that are scaly and fissured are prone to irritant dermatitis and fissuring.

Differential Diagnosis

Unroofing the vesicles and scraping the underside of the roof will reveal hyphae in cases of vesicular tinea. Rarely, blisters extending onto the dorsum of the hands represent true contact allergic dermatitis, and the culprit must be sought by patch testing. Patients with inflammatory tinea pedis may have a vesicular dermatophytid of the palms, but this is relatively unusual. Rare patients with HIV infection have HSV lesions on the palms that may mimic coalescent vesicles of dyshidrosis.

Prevention

There is no known way to prevent attacks.

Treatment

Dyshidrotic eczema is often not a very steroid-sensitive dermatitis, though topical and systemic corticosteroids help some patients dramatically. Since this is a chronic problem, systemic steroids are generally not appropriate therapy. A high-potency topical steroid used early in the attack may help abort the flare and ameliorate pruritus. Topical steroids are also important in treating the scaling and fissuring that are seen after the vesicular phase. It is essential that patients avoid anything that irritates the skin; they should wear cotton gloves inside latex or vinyl gloves when doing dishes or other wet chores, use long-handled brushes instead of sponges, and use a hand cream after washing the hands. If a history of nickel allergy (rashes with costume jewelry or from watchbands) is obtained, disulfiram therapy in patients not allergic to thiurams may be attempted, as may oral cromolyn therapy. Nickel-free diets should be tried only as a last resort. Patients may also slowly respond to PUVA therapy using topical psoralen and special UVA light sources designed to treat hands and feet, or to UVA alone.

Prognosis

For most patients, the disease is an inconvenience. Even with moderate to severe disease, flares can be controlled with scrupulous care. For some, dyshidrosis can be incapacitating.

Epstein WL, Byers VS, Frankart W: Induction of antigen specific hyposensitization to poison oak in sensitized adults. Arch Dermatol 1982;118:630.

Fisher AA: Possible role of diet in pompholyx and nickel dermatitis: A critical survey. Cutis 1978;22:412.

Grettan CE et al: Comparison of topical PUVA with UVA for chronic vesicular hand eczema. Acta Derm Venereol 1991;71:118.

Pigatto PD et al: Disodium cromoglycate versus diet in the treatment and prevention of nickel-positive pompholyx. Contact Dermatitis 1990;22:27. (Improvement with high-dose cromolyn sodium.)

DERMATOPHYTID
(Allergy or Sensitivity to Fungi)

Essentials of Diagnosis

- Pruritic, grouped vesicular lesions involving the sides and flexor aspects of the fingers and the palms.
- Fungal infection elsewhere on the body, usually the feet.
- No fungus demonstrable in lesions.

General Considerations

Dermatophytid is a rare disorder that must be considered in the differential diagnosis of vesicles on the hands and feet. It is a sensitivity reaction to an active focus of inflammatory dermatophytosis elsewhere on the body, usually the feet. Fungi are present in the primary lesions but are not present in the lesions of dermatophytid. The hands are most often affected, but dermatophytid may occur on other areas also.

Clinical Findings

A. Symptoms and Signs: Itching is the only symptom. The lesions consist of grouped vesicles, often involving the thenar and hypothenar eminences. Lesions occasionally involve the backs of the hands or may even be generalized.

B. Laboratory Findings: This entity is best diagnosed morphologically and by response to treatment. The trichophytin skin test is positive, but it may also be positive with other disorders. A negative trichophytin test rules out dermatophytid. Culture from the primary site tends to reveal *Trichophyton mentagrophytes* organisms rather than *Trichophyton rubrum.*

Differential Diagnosis

Dermatophytid must be distinguished from all diseases causing vesicular eruptions of the hands—especially contact dermatitis, dyshidrosis, and photosensitive drug eruptions and "id" reactions due to inflammatory rashes, such as poison oak or other causes of contact dermatitis elsewhere on the body.

Treatment

The lesions should be treated according to type of dermatitis. The primary focus of tinea should be treated with griseofulvin or by local measures as described for dermatophytosis (see above). A single injection of triamcinolone acetonide suspension, 40 mg intragluteally, may suppress the eruption until the causative focus is controlled.

Prognosis

Dermatophytid may occur in an explosive series of episodes, and recurrences are not uncommon; however, it clears with adequate treatment of the primary infection elsewhere on the body.

DERMATITIS HERPETIFORMIS

Dermatitis herpetiformis is an uncommon disease manifested by pruritic papules, vesicles, and papulovesicles mainly on the elbows, knees, buttocks, posterior neck, and scalp. It appears to have its highest prevalence in Scandinavia and is associated with transplantation antigens HLA-B8, -DR3, and -DQw2. The diagnosis is made by light microscopy, which demonstrates neutrophils at the dermal papillary tips and occasionally eosinophils and a mild perivascular lymphohistiocytic infiltrate. Direct immunofluorescence studies show granular deposits of IgA along the dermal papillae and occasionally C3. One must distinguish this pattern of deposition of IgA from linear deposition of IgA seen in linear IgA bullous dermatosis, an unrelated disease. Circulating anti-endomysium antibodies can be detected in all cases, but this test may not be widely available. Patients have gluten-sensitive enteropathy, but for the great majority it is subclinical. However, ingestion of gluten plays a role in the exacerbation of skin lesions, and strict long-term avoidance of dietary gluten has been shown to decrease the dose of dapsone required to control the disease and may can even eliminate the need for drug treatment. Although adherence to a gluten-free diet is difficult, the availability of many gluten-free foods now makes this easier to accomplish. Some patients with dermatitis herpetiformis may develop gastrointestinal lymphoma, although this association is related to the enteropathy rather than the dermopathy.

Fry L: Fine points in the management of dermatitis herpetiformis. Semin Dermatol 1988;7:206.
Hall RP: Dermatitis herpetiformis. J Invest Dermatol 1992;99:873.

WEEPING OR ENCRUSTED LESIONS

IMPETIGO

Impetigo is a contagious and autoinoculable infection of the skin caused by staphylococci or streptococci (or both). Classically, two forms have been recognized: (1) a vesiculopustular type, with thick golden-crusted lesions caused by group A β-hemolytic *Streptococcus* or coagulase-positive *Staphylococcus aureus*; and (2) a bullous type, generally associated with phage group II *S aureus*. However, most cases of impetigo of either presentation now appear to be due to staphylococci.

Clinical Findings

A. Symptoms and Signs: Itching is the only symptom. The lesions consist of macules, vesicles, bullae, pustules, and honey-colored gummy crusts that when removed leave denuded red areas. The face and other exposed parts are most often involved. **Ecthyma** is a deeper form of impetigo caused by streptococci, with ulceration and scarring. It occurs frequently on the legs and other covered areas, often as a complication of debility and local cutaneous trauma.

B. Laboratory Findings: Gram stain and culture offer the best means of confirming the diagnosis.

Differential Diagnosis

The main differential diagnosis is between impetigo and acute contact allergic dermatitis. Contact dermatitis may be suggested by the history or by linear distribution of the lesions, and culture should be negative for staphylococci and streptococci. Herpes simplex infection usually presents with grouped vesicles or discrete erosions and may be associated with a history of recurrences. Viral culture and smears of the lesions will be positive.

Treatment

It appears unlikely that topical antibiotics could be as effective as systemic antibiotics, except for 2% mupirocin ointment (Bactroban), dispensed as 15 g and used three times daily for 10 days. If the affected area is large or if there is fever or toxicity—or if there is any concern over the possibility that a nephritogenic strain of *Streptococcus* may be causative—systemic antibiotics should be given. Dicloxacillin, 1 g daily, is usually effective, or one may use cephalexin, 50 mg/kg/24 h. Erythromycin is a reasonable alternative depending on the prevalence of erythromycin-resistant staphylococci in the community.

Crusts and weepy areas may be treated with compresses, and washcloths and towels must be segregated and washed separately.

Coskey RJ, Coskey LA: Diagnosis and treatment of impetigo. J Am Acad Dermatol 1987;17:62.
Grossman KL, Rasmussen JE: Recent advances in pediatric infectious disease and their impact on dermatology. J Am Acad Dermatol 1991;24:379. (Exanthem subitum, erythema infectiosum, cat scratch disease, congenital syphilis, and impetigo.)
Rice TD et al: Cost-effectiveness of erythromycin versus mupirocin for the treatment of impetigo in children. Pediatrics 1992;89:210. (Equal efficacy but a small increase in cost with mupirocin.)

CONTACT ALLERGIC DERMATITIS

Essentials of Diagnosis

- Erythema and edema, with pruritus, often followed by vesicles and bullae in an area of contact with a suspected agent.
- Later, weeping, crusting, or secondary infection.
- Often a history of previous reaction to suspected contactant.
- Patch test with agent usually positive.

General Considerations

Contact dermatitis is an acute or chronic dermatitis that results from direct skin contact with chemicals or allergens. Lesions are most often on exposed parts. Four-fifths of such disturbances are due to excessive exposure to or additive effects of primary or universal irritants (eg, soaps, detergents, organic solvents) and are called contact irritant dermatitis. Others are due to actual contact allergy such as poison ivy or poison oak. The most common dermatologic compounds causing allergic rashes include antimicrobials (especially neomycin), topical antihistamines, anesthetics (benzocaine), hair dyes, and preservatives, eg, parabens. Occupational exposure is an important cause of contact allergic dermatitis. Weeping and crusting are typically due to allergic and not irritant dermatitis, which often appears red and scaly. With widespread precautions being taken against HIV infection, contact dermatitis due to latex rubber in gloves and condoms is being seen more frequently.

Clinical Findings

A. Symptoms and Signs: The acute phase is characterized by tiny vesicles and weepy and encrusted lesions, whereas resolving or chronic contact dermatitis will present with scaling, erythema, and possibly thickened skin. Itching, burning, and stinging may be severe. The lesions, distributed on exposed parts or in bizarre asymmetric patterns, consist of erythematous macules, papules, and vesicles. The affected area is often hot and swollen, with exudation and crusting, simulating and at times complicated by infection. The pattern of the eruption may be diagnostic (eg, typical linear streaked vesicles on the extremities in poison oak or ivy dermatitis). The location will often suggest the cause: Scalp involvement suggests hair tints, sprays, or tonics; face involvement, creams, cosmetics, soaps, shaving materials, nail polish; neck involvement, jewelry, hair dyes, etc.

B. Laboratory Findings: Gram stain and culture will rule out impetigo or secondary infection (impetiginization). If itching is generalized and impetiginized scabies is considered, a scraping for mites should be done. During the acute episode, patch testing cannot be used, often because the back is involved or because the primary rash will cause many false-positive reactions. After the episode has cleared, the patch test may be useful, but not all potential allergens are available for testing. In the event of a positive reaction, the clinical relevance of the chemical agent and the dermatitis must be determined. In suspected photosensitivity contact dermatitis—involvement of face, "V" of the upper chest, and hands, sparing the skin under the nose, chin, and inner upper eyelid—photopatch tests may be done by exposing the traditional patch test site to ultraviolet light after 24 hours.

Differential Diagnosis

Asymmetric distribution, blotchy erythema around the face, linear lesions, and a history of contact help distinguish contact dermatitis from other skin lesions. The most commonly confused diagnosis is impetigo. Differentiation may be difficult if the area of involvement is consistent with that seen in other types of skin disorders such as scabies, dermatophytid, atopic dermatitis, dyshidrotic eczema, and other eczemas.

Prevention

Prompt and thorough removal of allergens by prolonged washing with water or by dousing with solvents such as isopropyl alcohol or other chemical agents may be effective if done very shortly after exposure to poison oak or ivy. Recently, several barrier creams (Stokogard, Ivy Shield) have been introduced that may offer some protection to patients at high risk for poison oak and ivy dermatitis. Otherwise, barrier creams are typically not useful for other types of contact dermatitis. Ingestion of *Rhus* antigen is of limited clinical value for the induction of tolerance.

The mainstay of prevention is identification of agents causing the dermatitis and avoidance of exposure or use of protective clothing and gloves. In industry-related cases, prevention may be accomplished by moving the worker to another part of the workplace with different responsibilities.

Treatment

A. Overview: While local measures are important, severe or widespread involvement is difficult to manage without systemic corticosteroids because even the highest-potency topical steroids seem not to work well on vesicular and weepy skin. Localized involvement (except on the face) can often be managed solely with topical agents. An age-old remedy for itching disorders is repeated exposure to hot water, as in a shower, without soap; this treatment may have the effect of prolonging and aggravating any underlying disorder (eg, atopic or nummular dermatitis). Contact irritant dermatitis is treated by protection from the irritant and use of topical steroids as for atopic dermatitis (described above). The treatment of contact allergic dermatitis is detailed below.

B. Local Measures:

1. Acute weeping dermatitis–Compresses are most often used. It is unwise to scrub lesions with soap and water. Calamine or starch shake lotions may sometimes be used instead of wet dressings or in intervals between wet dressings, especially for involvement of intertriginous areas or when oozing is not marked. Lesions on the extremities may be bandaged with wet dressings for 30–60 minutes several times a day. Potent topical corticosteroids in gel or cream form may help suppress acute contact dermatitis and relieve itching. In cases where weeping is marked or in intertriginous areas, ointments will make the skin even more macerated and should be avoided. Suggested preparations are Lidex gel, 0.05%, used two or three times daily with compresses, or Temovate or Ultravate cream, used twice daily for a maximum of 2 weeks—for adults only and not in body folds or on the face. This should be followed by tapering of the number of applications per day or use of a mid-potency steroid such as triamcinolone 0.1% cream to prevent rebound of the dermatitis. A soothing formulation is 0.1% triamcinolone acetonide in Sarna lotion (0.5% camphor, 0.5% menthol, 0.5% phenol). Frequent continued use may induce tachyphylaxis.

2. Subacute dermatitis (subsiding)—Mid-potency (triamcinolone 0.1%) to high-potency steroids (Cyclocort, Lidex, Topicort) are the mainstays of therapy.

3. Chronic dermatitis (dry and lichenified)—High- to highest-potency steroids are used in ointment form if acceptable to the patient; creams if not. In some cases, tars (Fototar, or LCD 10%) are useful, often combined with a moderate-strength corticosteroid (eg, 0.1% triamcinolone).

C. Systemic Therapy: For acute severe cases, one may give prednisone orally for 12–14 days. Clinicians use many regimens, and prednisone, 60 mg for 4 days, 40 mg for 5 days, and 20 mg for 5 days without a further taper is one useful regimen. Another is to dispense seventy-eight 5 mg pills to be taken 12 the first day, 11 the second day, and so on in diminishing dosage. The key is to use enough corticosteroid (and as early as possible) to achieve a clinical effect and to taper slowly enough to avoid rebound. A Medrol Dosepak (methylprednisolone) with 5 days of medication is inappropriate on both counts. Triamcinolone acetonide (Kenalog-40), 40–60 mg once intragluteally. with 0.5–1 mL of betamethasone for rapid onset of action, may be used instead. (See Chapter 25.)

Prognosis

Contact allergic dermatitis is self-limited if reexposure is prevented but often takes 2–3 weeks for full resolution. Spontaneous desensitization may occur. Increasing sensitivity to industrial contactants may necessitate a change of occupation.

Adams RM: Recent advances in contact dermatitis. Ann Allergy 1991;67:552.

Dunkel FG et al: Contact allergies to topical corticosteroids: Ten cases of contact dermatitis. Contact Dermatitis 1991;25:97. (An important possibility to consider when patients worsen on treatment.)

Fisher AA: Management of allergic contact dermatitis due to rubber gloves in health and hospital personnel. Cutis 1991;47:301.

Grevelink SA, Murrell DF, Olsen EA: Effectiveness of various barrier preparations in preventing and/or ameliorating experimentally produced *Toxicodendron* dermatitis. J Am Acad Dermatol 1992;27:182. (Stokogard, Hollister moisture barrier, and Hydropel were most effective.)

PUSTULAR DISORDERS

ACNE VULGARIS

Essentials of Diagnosis

- Pimples (papules or pustules) over the face, back, and shoulders.
- Occurs often at puberty, though onset may be delayed into the third or fourth decade.
- Open and closed comedones. Cyst formation with slow resolution, scarring.
- The most common of all skin conditions.

General Considerations

Acne vulgaris is discussed under pustular diseases, but it is polymorphic. Open and closed comedones, papules, pustules, and cysts are commonly found. Acne vulgaris is one of the most common diseases of humans. It is of unknown cause and is apparently activated by androgens in those who are genetically predisposed. Eunuchs are spared. Similar involvement may occur in identical twins. Acne can present in the neonatal period and may last for weeks to a few months.

The disease is more common and more severe in males. Contrary to popular belief, it does not always clear spontaneously when maturity is reached. If untreated, it may persist into the fourth, fifth, or even sixth decade of life. The skin lesions follow sebaceous overactivity, plugging of the infundibulum of the follicles, retention of sebum, overgrowth of the acne bacillus (*Propionibacterium acnes*) in incarcerated sebum with resultant release of and irritation by accumulated fatty acids, and foreign body reaction to extrafollicular sebum. The mechanism of antibiotics in controlling acne is not clearly understood, but they may work because of their antianabolic effect on the sebaceous gland or antibacterial or anti-inflammatory properties.

When a resistant case of acne is encountered in a woman, hyperandrogenism may be suspected. This may or may not be accompanied by hirsutism, irregular menses, or other signs of virilism.

Clinical Findings

There may be mild soreness, pain, or itching. The lesions occur mainly over the face, neck, upper chest, back, and shoulders. Comedones are common, and these are the hallmark of acne vulgaris. Closed comedones are tiny, flesh-colored, noninflamed bumps that give the skin a rough texture or appearance. Open comedones typically are a bit larger and have black material in them. Inflammatory papules, pustules, ectatic pores, acne cysts, and scarring are also seen.

Acne may have different presentations at different

ages. Preteens often present with comedones as their first lesions. Some patients have primarily comedones, with few inflammatory lesions. Inflammatory lesions in young teenagers are often found in the middle of the face, extending outward as the patient becomes older. Women in their third and fourth decades (often with no prior history of acne) commonly present with papular lesions on the chin and around the mouth—so-called perioral dermatitis.

Differential Diagnosis

Other diseases that cause papules and pustules on the face are relatively uncommon compared to acne vulgaris. In adults, acne rosacea will present with papules and pustules in the middle third of the face, but telangiectasia, flushing, and perhaps rhinophyma distinguish this disease from acne vulgaris. Primary bacterial folliculitis of the face is uncommon, but a pustular flare on the face in patients receiving antibiotics or with otitis externa should be investigated with culture to rule out an uncommon gram-negative folliculitis. Patients who use systemic steroids or topical fluorinated steroids on the face may develop acne, but comedones are often absent. Acne may be exacerbated or caused by irritating creams or oils, such as coconut oil. The acneiform lesions caused by bromides, iodides, steroids, and contact with chlorinated naphthalenes and diphenyls occur quite rarely. Fluorinated toothpaste may be associated with perioral dermatitis. Pustules on the face can also—not commonly—be caused by tinea infections. Lesions on the back are more problematic. When they occur alone, one should suspect staphylococcal folliculitis, miliaria, or, uncommonly, *Pityrosporum* folliculitis. Bacterial culture, trial of an antistaphylococcal antibiotic, and observing the response to therapy, will help in the differential diagnosis. In patients with HIV infection, folliculitis is common and severe and may be due to staphylococcal folliculitis or to eosinophilic folliculitis—the latter a poorly understood entity.

Complications

Cyst formation, pigmentary changes in darkly pigmented patients, severe scarring, and psychologic problems may result.

Treatment

A. General Measures:
1. Education of the patient–When scarring seems out of proportion to the severity of the lesions, one must suspect that the patient is manipulating the lesions. It is essential that the patient be educated in a supportive way about this complication. Although there are exceptions, it is wise to let the patient know that at least 4–6 weeks will be required to see improvement and that old lesions may take months to fade. Therefore, improvement will be judged according to the number of new lesions forming after 6

weeks of therapy. Additional time will be required to see improvement on the back and chest, as these areas are slowest to respond.

2. Diet–Specific dietary factors are less important than formerly thought in causing acne. If the patient feels that a particular food is exacerbating acne, the food should be avoided for 4–6 weeks and then reintroduced.

3. Avoid topical exposure to oils and greases.

B. Comedonal Acne: Treatment of acne is based on the type and severity of lesions. Comedones require treatment different from that of papules, and papules are treated differently from severe cystic lesions. In assessing severity, one must also take the sequelae of the lesions into account. Therefore, one must treat a more darkly pigmented individual who gets only two new lesions per month that scar or leave postinflammatory hyperpigmentation much more aggressively than a comparable patient whose lesions clear without sequelae. Soaps play little role in acne treatment today, and unless the patient's skin is exceptionally oily, a mild soap should be used to avoid irritation that will limit the usefulness of other topicals, all of which are themselves somewhat irritating.

1. Tretinoin (retinoic acid, Retin-A)–Tretinoin is very effective for comedonal acne or for treatment of the comedonal component of more severe acne, but its usefulness is limited by irritation. Start with 0.025% cream (not gel or liquid) and have the patient use it at first in a test area twice weekly at night, then build up to treat all areas of the face that develop acne as often as nightly. A few patients cannot use even this low-strength preparation more than three times weekly, but even that may cause improvement. A pea-sized amount is sufficient to cover almost half the entire face. It should be put on the skin when dry; to avoid irritation, have the patient wait 10 minutes after washing to let the skin dry. Patients whose skin has become red and irritated from the product will rarely be willing to try it again, so prevention of irritation is essential. Although the absorption of tretinoin is minimal and some authorities use it during pregnancy, its use in pregnancy has not be extensively studied. Some patients report photosensitivity with tretinoin. Patients should be warned that they may flare in the first 2 weeks of treatment.

2. Benzoyl peroxide is also somewhat effective for comedonal acne. Commercial preparations include Fostex cream and cake; Acne-Dome cleanser, cream, and lotion; Benzac W gel and wash; Desquam-X gel and wash; Brevoxyl, Benzagel, Persa-Gel, Clear By Design; and Xerac BP. All of these gels contain benzoyl peroxide. Benzoyl peroxide products are available in concentrations of 2.5%, 5%, and 10%, but it appears that 2.5% is as effective as 10% and less irritating. In general, water-based and not alcohol-based gels should be used to decrease irritation. Benzoyl peroxide washes such as Desquam-X wash or Benzac W wash may also be used but should be stopped or limited if they are irritating.

3. Antibiotics–Use of topical antibiotics (see below) has demonstrated a decrease in comedonal lesions in controlled studies.

4. Comedo extraction–Open and closed comedones may be removed with a comedo extractor but will recur if not prevented by tretinoin or perhaps benzoyl peroxide.

C. Papular Inflammatory Acne: Antibiotics are the mainstay for treatment of inflammatory acne. They may be used topically or orally. The oral antibiotics of choice are tetracycline, erythromycin, and finally (because of its cost) minocycline. Doxycycline is effective, but commonly causes photosensitivity. Rarely, other antibiotics such as trimethoprim-sulfamethoxazole may be tried. Topical clindamycin phosphate and erythromycin are also used. Topicals are probably the equivalent of about 500 mg/d of tetracycline given orally, which is half the usual starting dose. Topical antibiotics are used in three situations: for mild papular acne that can be controlled by topicals alone, for patients who refuse or cannot tolerate oral antibiotics, or to wean patients under good control from oral to topical preparations. There are no studies that have evaluated the usefulness of topical antibiotics while a patient is taking systemic antibiotics, though this is common practice, and there is no study establishing which topical antibiotic to use with each systemic antibiotic.

1. Mild acne–Either clindamycin (Cleocin T lotion, gel, or solution, in order of least to most drying) twice daily or one of many brands of topical erythromycin is effective. The separate use of tretinoin at night may be additive, as it works via a different mechanism. Instead of using two separate products, erythromycin with benzoyl peroxide (Benzamycin) topical gel is an effective combination product, but it should be kept refrigerated to prevent loss of activity over a 1-month period. For patient compliance, a small amount may be stored in a separate jar for 7–10 days at room temperature in the bathroom without significant loss of activity.

2. Moderate acne–Tetracycline, 500 mg twice daily, erythromycin, 500 mg twice daily, and minocycline, 50–100 mg twice daily, are all effective though minocycline is very expensive. Plan a return visit in 6 weeks and at 3–4 months after that. If the patient's skin is quite clear, instructions should be given for tapering the dose by 250 mg for tetracycline and erythromycin or by 50 mg for minocycline every 6–8 weeks—while treating with topicals—to arrive at the lowest systemic dose needed to maintain clearing. In general, lowering the dose to zero without other therapy results in prompt recurrence of acne. Tetracycline is contraindicated in pregnancy or renal failure and in young children, since it may discolor growing teeth. Minocycline may cause vertigo if started at high doses. Gram-negative folliculitis developing from acne during broad-spectrum antibiotic therapy will respond to oral isotretinoin.

3. Severe acne–

a. Isotretinoin (Accutane) is a vitamin A analogue for treatment of severe cystic acne that has not responded to conventional therapy. Informed consent should be obtained before its use in women of childbearing age. A dosage of 0.5–1 mg/kg/d for 4–5 months is usually adequate for severe cystic acne. The drug is *absolutely contraindicated during pregnancy* because of its teratogenicity; serum pregnancy tests should be obtained before starting the drug in a female and every month thereafter. Sufficient medication for only 1 month should be dispensed at each monthly visit. Effective contraception—some authorities say in two forms—must be used. Therapeutic abortion is an alternative for the patient who becomes pregnant during therapy, and the patient's feelings about this option should be discussed before starting therapy. Side effects occur in most patients, usually related to dry skin and mucous membranes (dry lips, nosebleed, and dry eyes). If headache occurs, pseudotumor cerebri must be considered. Depression has been reported. At higher dosage levels, about 25% of patients will develop hypertriglyceridemia, 15% hypercholesterolemia, and 5% a lowering of high-density lipoproteins. Some patients develop reversible fatty infiltration of the liver, with minor elevation of transaminase levels. Fasting blood sugar may be elevated. Miscellaneous adverse reactions, usually not seen with doses of 0.5 mg/kg/d, include decreased night vision, musculoskeletal or bowel symptoms, rash, thinning of hair, exuberant granulation tissue in lesions, and bony hyperostoses (seen only with very high doses or with long duration of therapy). Moderate to severe myalgias necessitate decreasing the dosage or stopping the drug. Laboratory tests to be performed regularly in all patients include cholesterol, triglycerides, and liver function studies.

Isotretinoin—in contrast to its prototype, vitamin A (retinol)—is not stored in the liver, and few significant laboratory abnormalities other than noted above have been reported. At doses of 1 mg/kg/d, even elevations of serum triglycerides have rarely been high enough to be of concern. Elevations of liver enzymes and triglycerides return to normal upon conclusion of therapy. The drug may induce long-term remissions, or acne may recur that is more easily controlled with conventional therapy. Occasionally, acne does not respond or promptly recurs after therapy.

b. Intralesional injection–In otherwise moderate acne, intralesional injection of dilute suspensions of triamcinolone acetonide (2.5 mg/mL, 0.05 mL per lesion), will often hasten the resolution of deeper papules and occasional cysts.

c. Dermabrasion–Cosmetic improvement may be achieved by excision and punch-grafting of deep scars and by abrasion of inactive acne lesions, particularly flat, superficial scars. The skin is first frozen and anesthetized with ethyl chloride or Freon and then carefully abraded with fine sandpaper, special motor-driven abrasive brushes, or diamond fraises. The technique is not without untoward effects, since hyperpigmentation, hypopigmentation, grooving, and scarring have been known to occur. Dark-skinned individuals do poorly. Dermabrasion within 18 months after isotretinoin therapy may not be advisable.

Prognosis

Untreated acne vulgaris eventually remits spontaneously, but when this will occur cannot be predicted. The condition may persist throughout adulthood and may lead to severe scarring if left untreated. Patients treated with antibiotics continue to improve for the first 3–6 months of therapy. The disease is chronic and tends to flare intermittently in spite of treatment. Remissions following systemic treatment with isotretinoin may be lasting in some cases.

American Academy of Dermatology: Guidelines of care for acne vulgaris. J Am Acad Dermatol 1990;22:676.

Winston MH, Shalita AA: Acne vulgaris: Pathogenesis and treatment. Pediatr Clin North Am 1991;38:889.

ROSACEA

Essentials of Diagnosis

- A chronic facial disorder of middle-aged and older people.
- A large vascular component (erythema and telangiectasis) and a tendency to flush easily.
- A glandular aspect accompanied by hyperplasia of the soft tissue of the nose (rhinophyma).
- An acneiform component (papules, pustules, and oily skin) may also be present.

General Considerations

No single factor adequately explains the pathogenesis of this disorder. A statistically significant incidence of migraine headaches accompanying rosacea has been reported.

Potent topical steroids can change trivial dermatoses of the face into recognizable entities called **perioral dermatitis** and **steroid rosacea.** These occur predominantly in young women and may be confused with acne rosacea.

Clinical Findings

The cheeks, nose, and chin—at times the entire face—may have a rosy hue. One sees few or no comedones. Inflammatory papules are prominent, and there may be pustules. Associated seborrhea may be found. The patient often complains of burning or stinging with episodes of flushing. It is not uncommon for patients to have associated ophthalmic disease, including blepharitis and keratitis. This often requires systemic antibiotic therapy.

Differential Diagnosis

Rosacea is distinguished from acne by age, the presence of the vascular component, and the absence of comedones. Bromoderma and iododerma are similar but uncommon. The rosy hue of rosacea is due to inflammation and telangiectases and generally will pinpoint the diagnosis.

Treatment

Medical management is aimed only at the inflammatory papules and pustules and the erythema that surrounds them. The only satisfactory treatment for the telangiectasias is a yellow light laser, eg, pulsed dye or copper vapor laser. Rhinophyma responds only to surgical therapy.

A. Local Therapy: Metronidazole, 0.75% gel (MetroGel) applied twice daily, is probably the topical treatment of choice. Occasionally, a mild topical steroid such as 1% hydrocortisone or aclometasone dipropionate 0.05% (Aclovate) may be used in the early weeks of treatment. If metronidazole is not tolerated, topical clindamycin or erythromycin as described above may be helpful (see Acne Vulgaris). Five to 8 weeks of treatment are needed for significant response.

B. Systemic Therapy: Tetracycline or erythromycin, 250 or 500 mg orally twice daily on an empty stomach, should be used when topical therapy is inadequate.

Isotretinoin (13-cis-retinoic acid; Accutane) may succeed where other measures fail. A dosage of 0.5–1 mg/kg/d orally for 12–28 weeks is recommended.

Metronidazole, 250 mg twice daily for 3 weeks, may be worth trying but is seldom required. Side effects are few, though it may have a disulfiram-like effect when the patient uses alcohol.

Prognosis

Rosacea tends to be a stubborn and persistent process. With the regimens described above, it can usually be controlled adequately.

Bleicher PA, Charles JH, Sober AJ: Topical metronidazole therapy for rosacea. Arch Dermatol 1987;123:609.

Lowe NJ et al: Flash lamp pumped dye laser for rosacea-associated telangiectasia and erythema. J Dermatol Surg Oncol 1991;17:522.

FOLLICULITIS
(Including Sycosis)

Essentials of Diagnosis

- Itching and burning in hairy areas.
- Pustules in the hair follicles.
- In sycosis, inflammation of surrounding skin area.

General Considerations

Folliculitis has multiple causes. It may be caused by staphylococcal infection and may be more common in the diabetic. When the lesion is deep-seated, chronic, and recalcitrant, it is called sycosis. Sycosis is usually propagated by the autoinoculation and trauma of shaving. The upper lip is particularly susceptible to involvement in men with chronic nasal discharge from sinusitis or hay fever.

Gram-negative folliculitis, which may develop during antibiotic treatment of acne, may present as a flare of acne. A range of gram-negative organisms has been implicated as the cause.

"Hot tub folliculitis," caused by *Pseudomonas aeruginosa,* is characterized by pruritic follicular, maculopapular, vesicular, or pustular lesions occurring within 1–4 days after bathing in a hot tub, whirlpool, or public swimming pool. Rarely, systemic infections may result.

Nonbacterial folliculitis may also be caused by oils that are irritating to the follicle, and these may be encountered in the workplace (machinists) or at home (various cosmetics and cocoa butter or coconut oils).

Folliculitis may also be caused by occlusion, perspiration, and rubbing, such as that resulting from tight jeans and other heavy fabrics on the upper legs.

Folliculitis that looks like acne but does not respond to acne therapy may be caused by the yeast *Pityrosporum orbiculare.* This infection may require biopsy for diagnosis and is treated with oral ketoconazole or topical 2.5% selenium sulfide.

Folliculitis—so called "steroid acne"—may be seen in the first week of systemic steroid therapy or on tapering of the dose.

A form of sterile folliculitis with prominent eosinophilic infiltration has been reported in patients with AIDS.

Pseudofolliculitis is caused by ingrowing hairs in the beard area and on the nape. In this entity, the papules and pustules are located at the side of and not in follicles. It may be treated by growing a beard or by using chemical depilatories or various proprietary shaving systems (eg, Moore Technique Shaving System).

Clinical Findings

The symptoms are slight burning and itching and pain on manipulation of the hair. The lesions consist of pustules of hair follicles. In sycosis, the surrounding skin becomes involved also and so resembles eczema, with redness and crusting.

Differential Diagnosis

It is important to differentiate bacterial from nonbacterial folliculitis. The history is important for pinpointing the causes of nonbacterial folliculitis, and a Gram stain and culture is indispensable. One must differentiate folliculitis from acne vulgaris or pustular miliaria (heat rash) and from infections of the skin such as impetigo or fungal infections. Gram-negative folliculitis is often suggested by the history of hot tub use. Eosinophilic folliculitis in AIDS often requires biopsy.

Complications

Abscess formation is the major complication of bacterial folliculitis. If the process involves the upper lip, nose, and eyes, a rare complication is cavernous sinus thrombosis.

Prevention

Correct any predisposing local causes (eg, irritations of a mechanical or chemical nature, discharges). Control of blood glucose in diabetes may reduce the number of these infections. Be sure that the water in hot tubs and spas is treated properly with chlorine. If staphylococcal folliculitis is persistent, diagnosis and treatment of nasal or perineal carriage with dicloxacillin, 250 mg four times daily for 14 days, with rifampin, 300 mg twice daily for 5 days during this time, or with topical mupirocin ointment twice daily for 5 days, may help. the latter may cause stinging in some patients. Clindamycin, 100 mg/d, has also been shown to be effective.

Treatment

A. Local Measures: Cleanse the area gently with chlorhexidine (Hibiclens) and apply saline or aluminum subacetate soaks or compresses to the involved area for 15 minutes twice daily.

Anhydrous ethyl alcohol containing 6.25% aluminum chloride (Xerac AC), applied to lesions and environs and followed by an antibiotic ointment (see above), may be very helpful. It is especially useful for chronic folliculitis of the buttocks.

B. Specific Measures: For bacterial folliculitis, topical 2% mupirocin (Bactroban) is extremely effective in achieving clinical cure, bringing about improvement in primary and secondary skin infections and eliminating infecting organisms. It should be applied three times daily for 10 days and protected if possible by dressings; soaks should be applied during the day.

Sulfonamides should not be used topically, since this practice may sensitize the patient to sulfonamides.

Systemic antibiotics may be tried if the skin infection is resistant to local treatment, if it is extensive or severe and accompanied by a febrile reaction, if it is complicated, or if it involves the nose or upper lip. Extended periods of treatment (4 weeks or more) with antistaphylococcal antibiotics are required in some cases.

Hot tub *Pseudomonas* folliculitis often is self-remitting but may be treated in adults with ciprofloxacin.

Gram-negative folliculitis in acne patients may be treated with isotretinoin (Accutane) in compliance with all precautions discussed above (see Acne Vulgaris).

Irritant folliculitis is best treated by protection from the offending substance and use of drying agents such benzoyl peroxide or Xerac-AC.

Eosinophilic folliculitis is difficult to treat. Some anecdotal success has been reported with use of the antihistamine astemizole and with UVB therapy.

Prognosis

Bacterial folliculitis is occasionally stubborn and persistent, lasting for months and even years. Irritant folliculitis will reflect exposure to the irritant. Steroid folliculitis is treatable by acne therapy and resolves as steroids are discontinued.

Breitenbach AA: *Pseudomonas* folliculitis from a health club whirlpool. Postgrad Med 1991;90:169.

Rosenthal D et al: Human immunodeficiency virus-associated eosinophilic folliculitis: A unique dermatosis associated with advanced human immunodeficiency virus infection. Arch Dermatol 1991;127:206.

MILIARIA
(Heat Rash)

Essentials of Diagnosis

- Burning, itching, superficial aggregated small vesicles, papules, or pustules on covered areas of the skin.
- More common in hot, moist climates.
- Rare forms associated with fever and even heat prostration.

General Considerations

Miliaria is an acute dermatitis that occurs most commonly on the upper extremities, trunk, and intertriginous areas. A hot, moist environment is the most frequent cause, but individual susceptibility is important, and obese persons are most often affected. Bedridden febrile patients are also susceptible. Plugging of the ostia of sweat ducts occurs, with consequent ballooning and ultimate rupture of the sweat duct, producing an irritating, stinging reaction. Increase in numbers of resident aerobes, notably cocci, apparently plays a role.

Clinical Findings

The usual symptoms are burning and itching. In severe cases, fever, heat prostration, and even death may result. The lesions consist of small, superficial, reddened, thin-walled, discrete but closely aggregated vesicles, papules, vesicopapules, or pustules. The reaction occurs most commonly on covered areas of the skin.

Differential Diagnosis

Miliaria is to be distinguished from similar skin manifestations occurring in drug rash and folliculitis.

Prevention

Avoidance of overbathing and strong, irritating soaps may be helpful. Use of an antibacterial preparation such as chlorhexidine prior to exposure to heat and humidity may help prevent the condition. Susceptible persons should avoid exposure to hot, humid environments.

Treatment

Triamcinolone acetonide, 0.1% in Sarna lotion, or a mid-potency corticosteroid in a lotion or cream—but not ointment—base, should be applied two to four times daily. Alternative measures that have been employed with varying success are drying shake lotions and antipruritic powders or other dusting powders. Secondary infections (superficial pyoderma) are treated with erythromycin or dicloxacillin, 250 mg four times daily by mouth. Anticholinergic drugs given by mouth may be very helpful in severe cases, eg, glycopyrrolate, 1 mg twice daily.

Prognosis

Miliaria is usually a mild disorder, but death may occur with the severe forms (tropical anhidrosis and asthenia) as a result of interference with the heat-regulating mechanism. The process of the severe form may also be irreversible to some extent, requiring permanent removal of the individual from the humid or hot climate.

MUCOCUTANEOUS CANDIDIASIS

Essentials of Diagnosis

- Severe pruritus of vulva, anus, or body folds.
- Superficial denuded, beefy-red areas with or without satellite vesicopustules.
- Whitish curd-like concretions on the oral and vaginal mucous membranes.
- Fungus on microscopic examination of scales or curd.

General Considerations

Mucocutaneous candidiasis is a superficial fungal infection that may involve almost any cutaneous or mucous surface of the body. It is particularly likely to occur in diabetics, during pregnancy, and in obese persons who perspire freely. Antibiotics and oral contraceptive agents may be contributory. Oral candidiasis may be the first sign of HIV infection. Esophageal candidiasis can be detected by endoscopy in many patients with AIDS and oral candidiasis.

Clinical Findings
A. Symptoms and Signs: Itching may be in-

tense. Burning sensations are sometimes reported, particularly around the vulva and anus. The lesions consist of superficially denuded, beefy-red areas in the depths of the body folds such as in the groin and the intergluteal cleft, beneath the breasts, at the angles of the mouth, and in the umbilicus. The peripheries of these denuded lesions are superficially undermined, and there may be satellite vesicopustules. Whitish, curd-like concretions may be present on the surface of the lesions (particularly in the oral and vaginal mucous membranes). Paronychia and interdigital erosions may occur.

B. Laboratory Findings: Clusters of budding cells and short hyphae can be seen under the high-power lens when skin scales or curd-like lesions have been cleared in 10% KOH. The organism may be isolated on Sabouraud's medium. Tests for diabetes should be ordered when indicated.

Differential Diagnosis

Intertrigo, seborrheic dermatitis, tinea cruris, "inverse psoriasis," and erythrasma involving the same areas may mimic mucocutaneous candidiasis.

Complications

Systemic invasive candidiasis with candidemia may be seen with immunosuppression and in patients receiving broad-spectrum antibiotic and hypertonic glucose solutions, as in hyperalimentation. There may or may not be clinically evident mucocutaneous candidiasis.

Treatment

A. General Measures: Affected parts should be kept dry and exposed to air as much as possible. If possible, discontinue systemic antibiotics; otherwise, give nystatin by mouth concomitantly in a dose of 1.5 million units three times daily. Fluconazole at a dosage of 50 mg/d or as a single oral dose of 150 mg is very effective and may be the treatment of choice for mucocutaneous candidiasis. Ketoconazole, 200 mg daily by mouth, will also eradicate lesions with minimal side effects except for rare instances of liver damage. Liver function must be monitored. Recurrences follow discontinuance of therapy. For treatment of systemic invasive candidiasis, see Chapter 36.

B. Local Measures:

1. Nails and skin–Apply 1% ciclopirox cream, nystatin cream, 100,000 units/g, or miconazole, ketoconazole, or clotrimazole cream or lotion three or four times daily. Gentian violet, 1%, or carbolfuchsin paint (Castellani's paint) may be applied once or twice weekly as an alternative.

2. Vulvar and anal mucous membranes–For vaginal candidiasis, use miconazole cream (Monistat 7), one applicatorful vaginally at bedtime for 7 days; clotrimazole (Gyne-Lotrimin, Mycelex-G), one suppository vaginally per day for 7 days; terconazole

vaginal cream (Terazol 7) or suppositories (Terazol 3); or nystatin, one tablet (100,000 units) vaginally twice daily for 7 days. Topical agents may not be as effective in women with recurrent vaginal candidiasis, and these "intractable" cases may require chronic suppressive therapy. The availability of fluconazole has added new treatment options. Single-dose fluconazole (150 mg) is as effective as ketoconazole, 200 mg twice daily for 5 days.

Prognosis

Cutaneous candidiasis may be intractable and prolonged, particularly in children, in whom the disturbance may take the form of a granuloma.

Hay RJ: Overview of studies of fluconazole in oropharyngeal candidiasis. Rev Infect Dis 1990;12(Suppl 3):5334.
Ro BI: Chronic mucocutaneous candidosis. Int J Dermatol 1988;27:457.

FIGURATE ERYTHEMAS

URTICARIA & ANGIOEDEMA

Essentials of Diagnosis

- Eruptions of evanescent wheals or hives.
- Itching is usually intense but may on rare occasions be absent.
- Special forms of urticaria have special features (dermographism, cholinergic urticaria, solar urticaria, or cold urticaria).
- Most incidents are acute and self-limited over a period of 1–2 weeks.
- Chronic urticaria (episodes lasting > 6 weeks) may defy the best efforts of the clinician to find and eliminate the cause.

General Considerations

Urticaria can result from many different stimuli. The pathogenetic mechanism may be either immunologic or nonimmunologic. The most common immunologic mechanism is hypersensitivity mediated by IgE; another involves activation of the complement cascade, which produces anaphylatoxins. These in turn can release histamine. Finally, some patients demonstrate autoantibodies directed against mast cell epitopes, with histamine-releasing activity. Whether the pathogenesis is allergic or nonallergic, modulating factors act on mast cells and basophils to release mediators capable of increasing vascular permeability, producing wheals.

Clinical Findings

A. Symptoms and Signs: Lesions are itchy red

swellings of a few millimeters to many centimeters. For most types of urticaria, the erythema and the wheal are the same size. The morphology of the lesions may vary over a period of minutes to hours, resulting in geographic or bizarre patterns. With involvement of deeper vessels, there may be swelling of the lips, tongue, eyelids, larynx, palms, soles, and genitalia in association with more typical lesions. For cholinergic urticaria, associated with hot showers or a rise in core body temperature after exercise, there is often a wheal 2–3 mm in diameter with a large surrounding red flare.

B. Laboratory Findings: Laboratory studies are not likely to be helpful in the evaluation of acute or chronic urticaria unless there are suggestive findings in the history and physical examination. The most common causes of acute urticaria are foods, viral and parasitic infections, and medications. The cause of chronic urticaria is rarely found. In patients with individual lesions that persist past 24 hours, a skin biopsy may help exclude the uncommon entity urticarial vasculitis. Quantitative immunoglobulins, cryoglobulins, cryofibrinogens, and antinuclear antibodies are indicated in cold urticaria. Liver function tests may be of interest, since a serum sickness-like prodrome, with urticaria, may be associated with hepatitis B.

Differential Diagnosis

Papular urticaria resulting from insect bites may persist for long periods. Bite reactions can be very severe histologically and may occasionally be mistaken for lymphoma or leukemia cutis. A central punctum can usually be seen, as with flea or gnat bites. Streaked urticarial lesions may be seen in acute allergic plant dermatitis, eg, poison ivy, oak, or sumac. Contact urticaria may be caused by a host of substances varying from chemicals to foods to medications and may be one type of reaction to latex gloves. Contact urticaria is limited to areas exposed to the contactant. Urticarial response to heat, sun, water, and pressure are quite rare. Urticaria may be seen as part of serum sickness, associated with fever and arthralgia, with or without hepatitis B.

In familial angioedema, there is generally a positive family history of angioedema of the extremities and gastrointestinal or respiratory symptoms, but urticaria is not part of the syndrome. Instead, these patients may demonstrate a rapidly expanding annular lesion with an urticarial border.

Treatment

A. General Measures: A detailed search for a cause of acute urticaria should be undertaken, and treatment may then be tailored to include the provocative condition. The chief nonallergic causes are drugs, eg, atropine, pilocarpine, morphine, and codeine; arthropod bites, eg, insect bites and bee stings (though the latter may cause anaphylaxis as well as angioedema); physical factors such as heat, cold, sunlight, injury, and pressure; and, presumably, neurogenic factors such as in cholinergic urticaria induced by exercise, excitement, hot showers, etc.

Allergic causes may include penicillin, aspirin, and other medications; inhalants such as feathers and animal danders; ingestion of shellfish or strawberries; injections of sera and vaccines; external contactants, including various chemicals and cosmetics; and infections such as hepatitis.

B. Systemic Treatment: Epinephrine 1:1000, 0.3 mL subcutaneously, is indicated for rapidly progressing urticaria. Sus-Phrine (epinephrine 1:200 suspension), 0.1–0.3 mL, may be injected subcutaneously for more prolonged action for acute urticaria. However, both medications often give only temporary relief and must be used with caution in elderly patients and those taking beta-blockers.

The mainstay of treatment initially includes H_1 antihistamines (see above). Hydroxyzine, 10 mg twice daily to 25 mg three times daily to even 100 mg three times daily, may be very useful if tolerated. Giving hydroxyzine as one dose of 50–75 mg at night may reduce sedation and other side effects. Antihistamines from different classes should be systematically tried, and doses should be increased weekly to tolerance. Combinations of different antihistamines are often effective, though they have not been systematically investigated. Cyproheptadine, 4 mg four times daily, may be especially useful for cold urticaria. Terfenadine (Seldane), a nonsedating antihistamine, has been reported to be effective in chronic idiopathic urticaria. The dosage is 60 mg twice daily. Cardiac arrhythmias and perhaps death may result from interactions with erythromycin and related antibiotics or with ketoconazole and related azoles; from dosages exceeding 60 mg twice daily; or from use in patients with liver disease. The drug is considerably more expensive than other antihistamines. Its use is not recommended during pregnancy and lactation. Another nonsedating antihistamine—astemizole—has been reported to be effective in a majority of patients with seasonal allergic rhinitis and chronic idiopathic urticaria. The recommended dosage is 10 mg/d, and larger doses may be associated with cardiac arrhythmias. The long half-life of astemizole is a major disadvantage if skin prick testing is needed or if a patient becomes pregnant while on the drug. The third less-sedating antihistamine approved for use is loratadine in a dosage of 10 mg/d. It has a shorter half-life than astemizole and is similar to the other H_1 antihistamines in effectiveness.

Doxepin (a tricyclic antidepressant), 25 mg three times daily or, more commonly, 25–75 mg or more at bedtime, appears to be effective in some cases of chronic urticaria. It should be used with caution because of its anticholinergic side effects and promotion of cardiac arrhythmias. Blood levels of doxepin and nordoxepin should be obtained when the dose reaches 75–100 mg at bedtime.

H_2 antihistamines may be effective if used in combination with H_1 blockers, but these are expensive medications, and cimetidine may interact with doxepin and other medications.

Some clinicians feel that it is necessary to give a course of oral prednisone in a dose of 40 mg/d for 10 days. This may be satisfactory if only a short course is required, but it often results in chronic administration of prednisone without adequate antihistamine trials. Other agents with some promise as adjuvants include calcium channel blockers (used for at least 4 weeks), terbutaline, colchicine, and attenuated androgens such as danazol. Plasmapheresis and sulfasalazine may help selected patients with chronic urticaria, but these treatments require further study. A few patients with chronic urticaria may respond to a salicylate- and tartrazine-free diet. Although salicylates are ubiquitous in nature, drugs and foods are the most obvious sources. One group has reported curing over 60% of chronic urticaria patients with an allergen elimination diet over a 3-month period. This diet proscribes milk products; beer, wine, and cider; mushrooms, soy sauce, canned tomatoes, pickled and smoked meats, shellfish, vinegar, soured breads, melon, dried fruit, diet soda, chocolate, nuts, peanut products, and strawberries. The treatment of chronic urticaria continues to be frustrating because only a few treatment options are available.

C. Local Treatment: Local treatment is rarely rewarding. Starch baths twice daily or Aveeno baths may be useful, prepared by adding one cupful of finely refined cornstarch or a packet of Aveeno to a comfortably warm bath. Alternatively, one may use a lotion containing 0.5% camphor, 0.5% menthol, and 0.5% phenol (Sarna) topically or in addition to the bathing.

Prognosis

Acute urticaria usually lasts only a few days to 6 weeks. Half of patients whose urticaria persists for more than 6 weeks will have it for years.

Armenaka M, Lehach J, Rosenstreich DL: Successful management of chronic urticaria. Clin Rev Allergy 1992;10:371. (Review of management, including a detailed allergen elimination diet.)

Cooper KD: Urticaria and angioedema: Diagnosis and evaluation. J Am Acad Dermatol 1991;25:166.

Kennard CD, Ellis CN: Pharmacologic therapy for urticaria. J Am Acad Dermatol 1991;25:176. (Reviews various treatments.)

Soter NA: Acute and chronic urticaria and angioedema. J Am Acad Dermatol 1991;25:146. (Laboratory workup not useful. Twenty percent of patients have a very chronic course.)

ERYTHEMA MULTIFORME

Essentials of Diagnosis

- Sudden onset of symmetric erythematous skin lesions with history of recurrence.
- May be macular, papular, urticarial, bullous, or purpuric.
- "Target" lesions with clear centers and concentric erythematous rings or "iris" lesions may be noted.
- Mostly on extensor surfaces, palms, soles, or mucous membranes.
- Herpes simplex, systemic infection or disease, and drug reactions may be associated.

General Considerations

Erythema multiforme is an acute inflammatory, polymorphic skin disease due to multiple causes or of undetermined origin. It may represent several diseases with different presentations, and pathogenetic mechanisms. Erythema multiforme is usually divided clinically into minor and major types based on the clinical findings. Approximately 90% of cases of erythema multiforme minor follow outbreaks of herpes simplex and are marked by cutaneous involvement. A few may follow infections caused by *Mycoplasma pneumoniae*. Erythema multiforme major (Stevens-Johnson syndrome), a disease in the differential diagnosis of blisters, is marked by toxicity and involvement of usually two mucosal surfaces (often oral and conjunctival) and is most often associated with drugs, especially sulfonamides, nonsteroidal anti-inflammatory drugs, and anticonvulsants such as phenytoin. Erythema multiforme may also present as a variant that presents as recurring oral ulceration, with skin lesions present in only half of the cases, and is diagnosed by oral biopsy. The list of conditions and agents associated with erythema multiforme is very long. Since erythema multiforme may have its own prodrome, many medications taken for such symptoms have been implicated in its pathogenesis without definitive proof. As in all drug eruptions, the exposure to drugs associated with erythema multiforme may be systemic or topical; any agent should be considered a potential offender.

Clinical Findings

A. Symptoms and Signs: The clinical hallmark of erythema multiforme is the target or bulls-eye lesion, which is most often found acrally on the hands and feet. Not all lesions will have this appearance, and there may be fixed erythematous papules and wheals, some of which evolve into blisters or target lesions. In erythema multiforme major, mucous membrane ulcerations are frequent, causing pain on eating, swallowing, and urination.

B. Laboratory Findings: Blood tests are not useful for diagnosis. In cases lacking the classic target or bulls-eye lesions, skin biopsy is indicated. On biopsy, the characteristic change is keratinocyte necrosis. There is also a prominent perivascular lymphocytic infiltrate in the upper dermis. Edema of the papillary dermis leading to the formation of a subepidermal blister is characteristic of bullous lesions. Direct immunofluorescence may show vascular deposits of IgM and C3, but this is not diagnostic.

Differential Diagnosis

Urticaria and drug eruptions are the chief entities that must be differentiated from erythema multiforme minor. Individual lesions of true urticaria should come and go within 24 hours, are usually responsive to antihistamines, and do not affect the mucosa. In erythema multiforme major, the main differential diagnosis is toxic epidermal necrolysis, and some investigators regard these entities as variants of the same disease. The presence of blisters is always worrisome and should suggest the need for consultation. The differential diagnosis includes pemphigus, pemphigoid, and bullous drug eruptions. Again, skin biopsy is the mainstay of diagnosis.

Complications

Visceral lesions are rare complications (eg, pneumonitis, myocarditis, nephritis). The tracheobronchial mucosa and conjunctiva may be involved in severe cases (Stevens-Johnson variant).

Treatment

A. General Measures: Erythema multiforme major (Stevens-Johnson syndrome) may present with extensive denudation of skin and is best treated in a burn unit. Otherwise, patients need not be admitted unless mucosal involvement interferes with hydration and nutrition.

B. Specific Measures: Although there are no good data to support the use of corticosteroids, they are still often prescribed. There are data showing that children with erythema multiforme treated with large doses of corticosteroids actually have a poorer outcome because of the complications of therapy. If corticosteroids are to be tried in more severe cases, they should be used early in moderate doses (prednisone, 40–80 mg) and stopped within days if there is no dramatic response. Oral and topical corticosteroids are useful in the oral variant of erythema multiforme. Oral acyclovir prophylaxis of herpes simplex infections may be effective in preventing recurrent herpes-associated erythema multiforme. Antistaphylococcal antibiotics are used for secondary infection.

C. Local Measures: Topical therapy is not very effective in this disease. For oral lesions, 1% diphenhydramine elixir mixed with Kaopectate or with 1% dyclonine may be used as a mouth rinse several times daily.

Prognosis

Erythema multiforme minor usually lasts 2–6 weeks and may recur. Stevens-Johnson syndrome, in which visceral involvement may occur, may be serious or even fatal in the most severe cases.

Bastuji-Garin S et al: Clinical classification of cases of toxic epidermal necrolysis, Stevens-Johnson syndrome, and erythema multiforme. Arch Dermatol 1993;129:92.
Huff JC Therapy and prevention of erythema multiforme with acyclovir. Semin Dermatol 1988;7:212.

ERYTHEMA CHRONICUM MIGRANS
(See also Chapter 33.)

Erythema chronicum migrans is a unique cutaneous eruption that characterizes the localized or generalized early stage of Lyme disease. Three to 32 days (median: 7 days) after a tick bite, there is gradual expansion of redness around the papule representing the bite site. The advancing border is usually slightly raised, warm, red to bluish-red, and free of any scale. Centrally, the site of the bite may clear, leaving only a rim of peripheral erythema, or it may become indurated, vesicular, or necrotic. The annular erythema usually grows to a median diameter of 15 cm (range: 3–68 cm). It is accompanied by a burning sensation in half of patients; rarely, it is pruritic or painful. Twenty-five to 50 percent of patients will develop multiple secondary annular lesions similar in appearance to the primary lesion but without indurated centers and generally of smaller size.

Without treatment, erythema chronicum migrans and the secondary lesions fade in a median of 28 days, though some may persist for months. Ten percent of untreated patients experience recurrences over the ensuing months. Treatment is necessary to prevent systemic involvement. However, only 60–70% of those with systemic involvement experience erythema chronicum migrans.

Berger BW, Lesser RL: Lyme disease. Dermatol Clin 1992;10:763.
Malane MS et al: Diagnosis of Lyme disease on dermatologic manifestations. Ann Intern Med 1991;114:490.

ERYSIPELAS

Essentials of Diagnosis

- Edematous, spreading, circumscribed, hot, erythematous area, with or without vesicle or bulla formation.
- Face frequently involved.
- Pain, chills, fever, and systemic toxicity may be striking.

General Considerations

Erysipelas is a superficial form of cellulitis that occurs classically on the cheek, caused by β-hemolytic streptococci.

Clinical Findings

A. Symptoms and Signs: The symptoms are pain, malaise, chills, and moderate fever. A bright red spot appears first, very often near a fissure at the angle of the nose. This spreads to form a tense, sharply demarcated, glistening, smooth, hot area. The margin characteristically makes noticeable advances from day to day. The patch is somewhat edematous and can be pitted slightly with the finger. Vesicles or bullae occasionally develop on the surface. The patch does not usually become pustular or gangrenous and heals without scar formation. The disease may complicate any break in the skin that provides a portal of entry for the organism.

B. Laboratory Findings: Leukocytosis and an increased sedimentation rate are almost invariably present but are not specific; blood cultures may be positive.

Differential Diagnosis

Cellulitis is characterized by a less definite margin and involvement of deeper tissues; erysipeloid is a benign bacillary infection producing redness of the skin of the fingers or the backs of the hands in fishermen and meat handlers.

Complications

Unless erysipelas is promptly treated, death may result from extension of the process and systemic toxicity, particularly in the very young and in the aged.

Treatment

Place the patient at bed rest with the head of the bed elevated, apply hot packs, and give aspirin for pain and fever. Penicillin is specific for β-hemolytic streptococcal infections. Erythromycin is a good alternative in penicillin-allergic patients.

Prognosis

Erysipelas formerly was a life-threatening infection. It can now usually be quickly controlled with systemic penicillin or erythromycin therapy.

CELLULITIS

Cellulitis, a diffuse spreading infection of the skin, involves deeper tissues than erysipelas and may be due to one of several organisms, usually gram-positive cocci, though gram-negative rods such as *Escherichia coli* may also be responsible. The lesion is hot and red but has a more diffuse border than does erysipelas. Cellulitis usually occurs after a break in the skin. Recurrent attacks may sometimes affect lymphatic vessels, producing a permanent swelling called "solid edema."

The response to systemic anti-infective measures (penicillin or broad-spectrum antibiotics) is usually prompt and satisfactory.

ERYSIPELOID

Erysipelothrix insidiosa infection must be differentiated from erysipelas and cellulitis. It is usually a benign infection, common in fishermen and meat handlers, and characterized by purplish erythema of the skin, most often of a finger or the back of the hand, which gradually extends over a period of several days. Systemic involvement occurs rarely; endocarditis may occur.

Penicillin is usually promptly curative. Broad-spectrum antibiotics may be used instead if the patient appears toxic and the diagnosis is uncertain.

BLISTERING DISEASES

PEMPHIGUS

Essentials of Diagnosis

- Relapsing crops of bullae appearing on normal skin.
- Often preceded by mucous membrane bullae, erosions, and ulcerations.
- Superficial detachment of the skin after pressure or trauma variably present (Nikolsky's sign).
- Acantholysis on biopsy.
- Immunofluorescence studies are confirmatory.

General Considerations

Pemphigus is an uncommon intraepidermal blistering disease occurring on skin and mucous membranes and caused by autoantibodies to adhesion molecules in the cadherin family (in pemphigus vulgaris) and to a complex containing desmosomal proteins, including desmoglein I (in pemphigus foliaceus), expressed in skin and mucous membranes. These autoantibodies cause acantholysis, the separation of epidermal cells from each other. The cause is unknown, and the condition, if untreated, is usually fatal within 2 months to 5 years. The bullae appear spontaneously and are relatively asymptomatic, but the lesions become extensive and the complications of the disease lead to great toxicity and debility. The disease occurs almost exclusively in middle-aged or older adults of all races and ethnic groups. Drug-induced autoimmune pemphigus from penicillamine and captopril has been reported. The pathogenetic role of IgG antibodies has been proved by passive transfer of antibodies to neonatal mice, reproducing the disease, and acantholysis can develop in a culture of normal human skin tissue when pemphigus serum is added. There is an association with HLA-A10 antigen. In addition, more than 95% of patients with pemphigus vulgaris are positive for HLA-DR4/DQw3 or HLA-

DRw6/DQw1, and in one series of 13 patients, all of whom were DQw1-positive, all had a single DQ_β allele designated $PV6_\beta$. Pemphigus may present with atypical features, and repeated reevaluation of clinical findings and changes shown by immunofluorescence and histopathologic studies may be necessary.

There are two forms of pemphigus: **pemphigus vulgaris** and its variant, **pemphigus vegetans;** and **pemphigus foliaceus** and its variant, **pemphigus erythematosus.** Both forms may occur at any age but most commonly in middle age. The vulgaris form begins in the mouth in over 50% of cases. The foliaceus form is especially apt to be associated with other autoimmune diseases, or it may be drug-induced, eg, by exposure to penicillamine.

Clinical Findings

A. Symptoms and Signs: Pemphigus is characterized by an insidious onset of flaccid bullae in crops or waves. The lesions often appear first on the oral mucous membranes, and these rapidly become erosive. In some cases, erosions and crusts predominate over blisters. The scalp is another site of early involvement. Toxemia and a "mousy" odor may develop rapidly. Rubbing a cotton swab or finger laterally on the surface of uninvolved skin may cause easy separation of the epidermis (**Nikolsky's sign**).

B. Laboratory Findings: The diagnosis is made by light microscopy and by direct and indirect immunofluorescence microscopy. Microscopically, acantholysis is the hallmark of pemphigus, but in some patients there may be eosinophilic spongiosis initially. Immunofluorescence microscopy shows deposits of IgG intercellularly in the epidermis, forming a honeycomb pattern. C3 and other immunoglobulins and complement components may be present on occasion. Indirect immunofluorescence microscopy uses the patient's serum and an animal source of tissue to detect circulating pemphigus antibodies. This is not necessary for the diagnosis, but titers in some patients may correspond with disease activity and might help in management. While a biopsy is diagnostic, less definitive information may be more rapidly gained if necessary from a smear taken from the base of a bulla and stained with Giemsa's stain (**Tzanck test**), which will show an almost unique histologic picture of disruption of the epidermal intercellular connections called **acantholysis.** This is seldom necessary.

Differential Diagnosis

Blistering diseases include erythema multiforme, drug eruptions, bullous impetigo, contact dermatitis, dermatitis herpetiformis, and bullous pemphigoid, but flaccid blisters are not typical of these diseases, and acantholysis is not seen. In the early stages, pemphigus tends to be treated as impetigo, but bacterial cultures and clinical suspicion leading to early biopsy will clarify the diagnosis. All of these diseases have gross clinical characteristics and different immunofluorescence test results that distinguish them from pemphigus. Transient acantholytic dermatosis (a harmless disease) may show some foci of acantholysis, but the clinical picture and immunofluorescence tests distinguish this disease easily.

Complications

Secondary infection commonly occurs; this is a major cause of morbidity and mortality. Disturbances of electrolyte balance are also common due to fluid losses through the involved skin in severe cases.

Treatment

A. General Measures: When the disease is severe, hospitalize the patient at bed rest and provide antibiotics and intravenous feedings as indicated. Anesthetic troches used before eating ease painful oral lesions.

B. Systemic Measures: Pemphigus requires systemic therapy as early in its course as possible. However, the main morbidity in this disease today is generally due to the side effects of such therapy. Although high doses of prednisone have been advocated—180–360 mg/d for 6–10 weeks—most clinicians use doses of 80–120 mg to start and increase the dose for rapid progression of the disease or lack of response within a few weeks. Azathioprine, 100–150 mg/d, is often given concurrently with prednisone. Some clinicians use methotrexate, 25 mg/wk, instead of azathioprine. When control is achieved, the prednisone is slowly tapered. Plasmapheresis combined with cyclophosphamide or azathioprine may be of use, as well as dapsone, 100 mg or less daily, in resistant cases associated with low circulating antibody titers. Gold sodium thiomalate, given as for rheumatoid arthritis, is said to be effective following initial prednisone, but it has been less well studied. Many investigators feel that by initiating and carefully monitoring treatment with concomitant use of methotrexate or azathioprine or with gold and corticosteroids, it is possible to reduce the dosage of steroids gradually with fewer of the hazards of long-term steroid therapy.

C. Local Measures: Skin and mucous membrane lesions should be treated as for vesicular, bullous, and ulcerative lesions due to any cause. Complicating infection requires appropriate systemic and local antibiotic therapy.

Prognosis

The course tends to be chronic in most patients, though some appear to experience remission. Infection is the most frequent cause of death, usually from *Staphylococcus aureus* septicemia. Signs and symptoms are often masked by high-dose corticosteroids, suggesting caution in their use.

Aagai M, Klaus-Kovtun V, Stanley JR: Autoantibodies against a novel epithelial cadherin in pemphigus vulgaris, a disease of cell adhesion. Cell 1991;67:869.

Bystryn JC: Therapy of pemphigus. Semin Dermatol 1988;7:186.

Korman NJ: Pemphigus. Dermatol Clin 1990;8:689.

Koulu L, Stanley JR: Clinical, histologic, and immunopathologic comparison of pemphigus vulgaris and pemphigus foliaceus. Semin Dermatol 1988;7:82.

OTHER BLISTERING DISEASES

Many other skin disorders are characterized by formation of bullae, or blisters. These include bullous pemphigoid, cicatricial pemphigoid, dermatitis herpetiformis, herpes gestationis, and other less common bullous disorders, including the mechanobullous diseases grouped under epidermolysis bullosa, which are due to defects in epidermal keratin synthesis.

Bullous Pemphigoid

Bullous pemphigoid is a relatively benign pruritic disease characterized by tense blisters in flexural areas, typically in elderly individuals, usually remitting in 5 or 6 years, with a course characterized by exacerbations and remissions. Oral lesions are present in about one-third of affected persons. Rarely, young people may be affected. The disease may occur in various forms, including localized, vesicular, vegetating, erythematous, erythrodermic, and nodular. There is no statistical association with internal malignant disease.

The diagnosis is made by biopsy followed by light and immunofluorescence microscopy. Light microscopy shows a subepidermal blister. With direct immunofluorescence, IgG and C3 are commonly found, at times with other immunoglobulins and complement components. Immunoelectronmicroscopy, though rarely required for the diagnosis, has localized the deposits of IgG and C3 to the lamina lucida of the basement membrane. Circulating basement membrane antibodies can be found in the sera of patients in about 70% of cases.

Corticosteroids are the treatment of choice. Some authorities add methotrexate, azathioprine, or cyclophosphamide. In a few cases, sulfapyridine or dapsone may be adequate. Although slower in onset of action, tetracycline or erythromycin, 1–1.5 g/d, combined with nicotinamide—*not nicotinic acid!*—(up to 1.5 g/d), if tolerated, may control the disease in patients who cannot use corticosteroids. Topical steroids of high potency may control localized early lesions.

Herpes Gestationis

Herpes gestationis occurs in about one in 50,000–60,000 pregnancies. The bullae often appear first in periumbilical distribution, and there may be erythematous papules and plaques, vesicles, and large bullae. It usually begins in the fifth or sixth month of pregnancy, or the onset may be delayed to the postpartum period. The disease is self-limited, but it may recur in subsequent pregnancies. Use of estrogens or progesterone or the onset of menses may trigger flare-ups. The risks to mother and fetus appear to be less significant than was formerly thought. Blisters are subepidermal, with eosinophils present. Direct immunofluorescence shows C3 at the basement membrane zone in most cases. IgG is found less often. Herpes gestationis factor is an avid complement-fixing IgG antibody found in the serum but rarely in the basement membrane zone.

Corticosteroids are the treatment of choice and are sometimes effective when used topically only.

Morrison LH, Anhalt GJ: Herpes gestationis. J Autoimmun 1991;4:37.

Ruocco V, Sacerdoti G: Pemphigus and bullous pemphigoid due to drugs. Int J Dermatol 1991;30:307.

Thomas I, Khorenian S, Arbesfeld DM: Treatment of generalized bullous pemphigoid with oral tetracycline. J Am Acad Dermatol 1993;28:74.

PAPULES

WARTS

Essentials of Diagnosis

- Warty elevation anywhere on skin or mucous membranes, usually no larger than 0.5 cm in diameter.
- Prolonged incubation period (average 2–18 months). Spontaneous "cures" are frequent (50%), but warts are often unresponsive to any form of treatment.
- "Recurrences" (new lesions) are frequent.

General Considerations

Over 40 different subtypes of human papillomaviruses have been identified by serologic typing of viral proteins, molecular hybridization of viral DNA, and monoclonal antibody assays, using immunoperoxidase staining. Most common warts are associated with this virus. In addition, about 25% of abnormal Papanicolaou smears are associated with the presence of human papillomaviruses, and 80% of cases of carcinoma of the cervix have similar associations, indicating that wart viruses may be more important than herpes simplex virus.

Cervical warts may be transmitted to the newborn via passage through the infected birth canal. Colposcopy with application of 3% acetic acid to suspicious lesions on the cervix may detect premalignant flat warts. A number of children with laryngeal papillomas (types 11 and 6) treated with x-rays have developed squamous cell carcinoma of the larynx.

Clinical Findings

There are usually no symptoms. Tenderness on pressure occurs with plantar warts; itching occurs with anogenital warts. Occasionally a wart will produce mechanical obstruction (eg, nostril, ear canal, urethra).

Warts vary widely in shape, size, and appearance. Flat warts are most evident under oblique illumination. Subungual warts may be dry, fissured, and hyperkeratotic and may resemble hangnails or other nonspecific changes. Plantar warts resemble plantar corns or calluses.

Differential Diagnosis

Large chronic warts in older individuals should be biopsied to rule out the emergence of squamous cell carcinoma in the wart. Some warty-looking lesions in sun-damaged skin are actually hypertrophic actinic keratoses or squamous cell carcinomas. Some venereal warty lesions may be due to secondary syphilis. The lesions of molluscum contagiosum may be mistaken for warts, especially when they are very large in immunocompromised persons. Seborrheic keratosis may also be confused with warts. In AIDS, wart-like lesions may be caused by varicella-zoster virus.

Prevention

Prevention consists of avoiding contact with warts. A person with flat warts should be educated about the infectivity of warts and advised not to scratch or traumatize the areas. Using an electric shaver will in occasional cases prevent the spread of warts in razor scratches. Anogenital warts may be transmitted sexually.

Treatment

Treatment is aimed at inducing "wart-free" intervals for as long as possible without scarring, since no treatment can guarantee a remission or prevent recurrences. In immunocompromised patients, the goal is probably even more modest, ie, to control the size and number of lesions present.

A. Removal: For common warts of the hands, patients are usually offered liquid nitrogen or keratolytic agents. The former may work in fewer treatments but requires office visits and is painful. Keratolytic agents are irritating but effective and usually painless if used correctly. They can be used at home but must be applied almost daily for 8–12 weeks for maximum effect.

1. Liquid nitrogen applied for 5–15 seconds for two freeze-thaw cycles may be used every 2 weeks for several visits. Scarring will occur if it is used incorrectly or too aggressively. For example, the face,

dorsal hands, and legs are more sensitive than the palms. Improper use along the sides of the fingers has been reported to cause nerve damage and paresthesias. Liquid nitrogen may cause permanent depigmentation in darkly pigmented individuals. It is useful on dry penile warts and on filiform warts involving the face and body. While liquid nitrogen is used by some on the feet, its use on the soles and other pressure areas can result in painful and temporarily debilitating blisters. Liquid nitrogen may be used in condylomas, but snipping of perianal lesions followed by light electrodesiccation may be more effective.

2. Keratolytic agents–Any of the following salicylic acid products may be used against common warts or plantar warts: Occlusal, Occlusal-HP, Trans-Ver-Sal, Duofilm, Duoplant, and Viranol. Plantar warts may be treated by applying a 40% salicylic acid plaster after paring. The plaster may be left on for 5–6 days, then removed, the lesion pared down, and another plaster applied. Although in this way it may take weeks or months to eradicate the wart, the method is safe and effective with almost no side effects.

3. Podophyllum resin–Anogenital warts are initially best treated by painting them weekly with 25% podophyllum resin (podophyllin) in compound tincture of benzoin if they are moist and occluded by apposing skin surfaces. Normal skin may be protected with petrolatum and by dusting the treated area with cornstarch or talc. Pregnant patients should not be so treated. Recently, the purified active component of the resin, podofilox (Condylox), has been introduced for use at home twice daily three times a week for cycles of 4–6 weeks. It is indicated for genital warts on nonmucosal surfaces. After a single 4-week cycle, 45% of patients were wart-free; but of these, 60% relapsed at 6 weeks. Thus, multiple cycles of treatment are often necessary.

4. Operative removal–Plantar warts may be removed by blunt dissection. Local anesthetic is injected into the base, and the wart is then removed with a dermal curette or scissors or by shaving off at the base of the wart with a scalpel. Trichloroacetic acid or Monsel's solution on a tightly wound cotton-tipped applicator may be painted on the wound, or light electrocautery may be used. Excision of warts, however, may result in a permanent painful scar on the foot and is not recommended.

5. Laser therapy–The CO_2 laser is particularly effective for treating recurrent warts, periungual warts, plantar warts, and condylomata acuminata. The wart tissue is vaporized under magnified vision in a bloodless procedure without damage to surrounding areas. The plume of vaporization has been shown to contain wart virus particles.

6. Other agents–Application of **cantharidin** (Cantharone, Cantharone Plus) is also effective in managing plantar warts. It is applied to the wart after it is pared, allowed to dry, and covered by tape. The area may be sensitive or slightly painful for 2 or 3 days. It should be debrided in 10–14 days and the treatment repeated. A test wart should be treated first, as pigmentary changes or scarring may result.

Bleomycin diluted to 0.1% with physiologic saline may be injected under warts, not exceeding 0.1 mL per puncture; with multiple punctures, it has been shown to have a high cure rate for plantar and common warts. It may cause loss of nails and symptoms similar to those of Raynaud's syndrome when used for periungual warts.

Intralesional recombinant **interferon alfa-2a** is more effective than placebo in clearing a single condyloma when used three times a week for 3 weeks, but plantar warts do not respond. This treatment is of research interest but has no place in routine management of warts.

B. Immunotherapy: Dinitrochlorobenzene (DNCB) may be effective for resistant warts but is difficult to use.

Persistent conservative application of topical irritants may cure warts by nonspecific boosting of wart antibodies. Specific wart antibodies (especially IgG) have been found in the serum of individuals with regressing warts.

C. Retinoids: Tretinoin (Retin-A) cream or gel applied topically twice daily may be effective (anecdotally) for facial or beard area warts. Extensive warts have been reported to disappear when etretinate was given by mouth for a month. Oral isotretinoin may cure some warts (see Acne Vulgaris).

Prognosis

There is a striking tendency to the development of new lesions. Warts may disappear spontaneously or may be unresponsive to treatment.

Beutner KR et al: Epidemiology of human papillomavirus infections. Dermatol Clin 1991;9;211.

Beutner KR, von Krogh G: Current status of podophyllotoxin for the treatment of genital warts. Semin Dermatol 1990;9:148. (A review of this drug and the development of podofilox for home use.)

CALLOSITIES & CORNS OF FEET OR TOES

Callosities and corns are caused by pressure and friction due to faulty weight-bearing, orthopedic deformities, improperly fitting shoes, or neuropathies such as occur in diabetes mellitus. Some persons are hereditarily predisposed to excessive and abnormal callus formation. It is crucial to provide optimal foot care for diabetics and those with insensitive extremities.

Tenderness on pressure and "after-pain" are the only symptoms. The hyperkeratotic well-localized overgrowths always occur at pressure points. On paring, a glassy core is found (which differentiates these disorders from plantar warts, which have multiple capillary bleeding points or black dots when pared). A soft corn often occurs laterally on the proximal portion of the fourth toe as a result of pressure against the bony structure of the interphalangeal joint of the fifth toe.

Treatment consists of correcting mechanical abnormalities that cause friction and pressure. Shoes must be properly fitted and orthopedic deformities corrected. Callosities may be removed by careful paring of the callus after a warm water soak or with keratolytic agents, eg, Keralyt gel, which contains 6% salicylic acid. It is applied locally to the callus every night, covered with a polyethylene plastic film (Saran Wrap), and removed in the morning. Treatments are repeated until the corn or callus is removed.

Extensive and severe palmar and plantar hyperkeratosis can be treated successfully by using 20% urea (Carmol 20) nightly and a pumice stone after soaking in water; by applying equal parts of propylene glycol and water nightly and covering with thin polyethylene plastic film (Baggies); or by soaking in 3% acetic acid solution.

Women who tend to form calluses and corns should not wear confining footgear and high-heeled shoes.

MOLLUSCUM CONTAGIOSUM

Molluscum contagiosum is characterized by single or multiple rounded, dome-shaped, waxy papules 2–5 mm in diameter that are umbilicated and contain a caseous plug. Lesions at first are firm, solid, and flesh-colored but upon reaching maturity become softened, whitish, or pearly gray and may suppurate. The principal sites of involvement are the face, hands, and lower abdomen and genitals, but the papules are commonly found on other parts of the skin and at times are widely distributed.

The lesions are probably spread by autoinoculation. In sexually active individuals, they may be confined to such genital areas as the penis, pubis, and inner thighs. Molluscum contagiosum is one of the common viral infections seen in patients with AIDS, and in adults sensitive inquiries should be made about risk factors for HIV infection.

These individuals tend to develop extensive lesions over the face and neck as well as the genital area.

The diagnosis is easily established in most instances because of the distinctive central umbilication of the dome-shaped lesion. The best treatment is by curettage or applications of liquid nitrogen as for warts—but more briefly, since molluscum contagiosum is more responsive to therapy than warts. Other forms of treatment include light electrosurgery with a fine needle. Applications of cantharidin without occlusion are appropriate for children, but test areas and light application are advised to avoid scarring or dyspigmentation. Lesions tend to resolve spontaneously, and it has been estimated that individual lesions persist for about 2 months. They are difficult to eradicate in patients with HIV infection.

Berger TG et al: Dermatologic manifestations of HIV infection. Am Fam Physician 1990;41:1729.
Williams LR, Webster G: Warts and molluscum contagiosum. Clin Dermatol 1991;9:87.

BASAL CELL CARCINOMA

Basal cell carcinoma occurs mostly on sun-exposed skin. These lesions grow slowly, attaining a size of 1–2 cm in diameter, often after years of growth. There is a waxy, "pearly" appearance, with telangiectatic vessels easily visible, though these may be present in adjacent "normal" skin as well. Metastases almost never occur, but neglected lesions may ulcerate and produce great destruction, ultimately invading vital structures and rarely invading the brain, ultimately killing the patient. Excision and suturing may be used, or one may shave the entire growth, following which the base of the wound is treated with curettage and electrodesiccation.

Miller SJ: Biology of basal cell carcinoma. (Two parts.) J Am Acad Dermatol 1991;24:1, 161.

SQUAMOUS CELL CARCINOMA

Squamous cell carcinoma usually occurs on exposed parts in fair-skinned individuals who sunburn easily and tan poorly. It may arise out of actinic keratoses and tends to develop slowly in the course of a few months. The lesions appear as small red, conical, hard nodules that occasionally ulcerate. They are not as distinctive as basal cell carcinomas and are more easily misdiagnosed clinically. The frequency of metastasis is not precisely known, though metastatic spread is said to be less likely with squamous cell carcinoma arising out of actinic keratoses than with those that arise de novo. In actinically induced squamous cell cancers, rates of metastasis are estimated from retrospective studies to be 3–7%. Squamous cell carcinomas of the lip, oral cavity, tongue, and genitalia deserve special care and management.

Keratoacanthomas most often act in benign fashion but resemble squamous cell carcinoma histologically and for all practical purposes should be treated as though they were skin cancers.

The preferred treatment of squamous cell carcinoma is excision. Electrodesiccation and curettage and x-ray radiation may be used instead, and fresh tissue microscopically controlled excision (Mohs) is excellent treatment also. Some keratoacanthomas respond to intralesional injection of fluorouracil or methotrexate, but they must be excised if they do not. Patients with squamous cell carcinoma deserve frequent careful follow-up.

Kwa RE et al: Biology of cutaneous squamous cell carcinoma. J Am Acad Dermatol 1992;26;1.

VIOLACEOUS TO PURPLE PAPULES & NODULES

LICHEN PLANUS

Essentials of Diagnosis

- Pruritic, violaceous, flat-topped papules with fine white streaks and symmetric distribution.
- Commonly seen along linear scratch marks (Koebner phenomenon) on anterior wrists, sacral region, penis, legs, mucous membranes.
- Histopathologic examination is diagnostic.

General Considerations

Lichen planus is an inflammatory pruritic disease of the skin and mucous membranes, characterized by distinctive papules with a predilection for the flexor surfaces and trunk. It may be an "allergic" reaction pattern, particularly following exposure to dyes, color film developers, and gold. The three cardinal findings are typical skin lesions, histopathologic features of band-like infiltration of lymphocytes, histiocytes, and melanophages in the dermis, and fluorescence with clumps of IgM subepidermally. Direct immunofluorescence testing is helpful but not usually required for diagnosis. Links have been seen with bullous pemphigoid, alopecia areata, vitiligo, chronic ulcerative colitis, hypogammaglobulinemia, and graft-versus-host reactions. Drugs associated with lichen planus-like drug reactions include gold, demeclocycline, streptomycin, tetracycline, arsenic, iodides, chloroquine, quinacrine, quinidine, and paraphenylenediamine. Antimony, phenothiazines, aminosalicylic acid, chlorothiazide, hydrochlorothiazide, and amiphenazole have also been incriminated.

Clinical Findings

Itching is mild to severe. The lesions are violaceous, flat-topped, angulated papules, 1–4 mm in diameter, discrete or in clusters, with white streaks on the surface (Wickham's striae) on the flexor surfaces of the wrists and on the penis, lips, tongue, and buccal and vaginal mucous membranes. Mucosal lichen planus has been reported in the genital and anorectal areas, the gastrointestinal tract, the bladder, the larynx, and the conjunctiva. The papules may become bullous or ulcerated. The disease may be generalized. Mucous membrane lesions have a lacy white network overlying them that is often confused with leukoplakia. The Koebner phenomenon (appearance of lesions in areas of trauma) may be seen.

A special form of lichen planus is the erosive variety. On palms and soles, it can be disabling. It is a major problem in the mouth, and squamous cell carcinoma may develop.

Differential Diagnosis

Lichen planus must be distinguished from similar lesions produced by quinacrine or bismuth sensitivity and other papular lesions such as psoriasis, lichen simplex chronicus, and syphilis. Lichen planus on the mucous membranes must be differentiated from leukoplakia. Histologic examination may make the distinction from graft-versus-host disease and in some cases from lichen planus-like drug eruptions.

Treatment

A. Topical Therapy: Intralesional injection of triamcinolone acetonide is useful for localized forms. Corticosteroid cream or ointment may be used nightly under thin pliable plastic film. Betamethasone dipropionate (Diprolene), diflorasone diacetate (Psorcon), clobetasol propionate (Temovate), and halobetasol propionate (Ultravate) ointments applied twice daily are most helpful.

Application of tretinoin cream (retinoic acid; vitamin A acid), 0.05%, to mucosal lichen planus, followed by a corticosteroid ointment, may be helpful. For disabling hypertrophic lichen planus of the soles, tretinoin cream applied and covered with thin, pliable polyethylene film nightly is said to be effective.

B. Systemic Therapy: Corticosteroids (see Chapter 25) may be required in severe cases, or where the most rapid response to treatment is desired.

Psoralens plus long-wave ultraviolet light (PUVA) may be effective treatment for lichen planus, and maintenance therapy apparently is not required.

Isotretinoin (Accutane) and etretinate (Tegison) by mouth appear to be effective for oral and cutaneous lichen planus, though this is not a labeled indication for these drugs. Some clinicians, however, believe that isotretinoin may be the treatment of choice for widespread disease.

After testing for the presence of glucose-6-phosphate dehydrogenase, erosive lichen planus may be treated with dapsone, 50 mg/d; this may be given over a period of many weeks, if necessary, with appropriate clinical and laboratory monitoring. Anecdotal reports suggest that metronidazole, 250 mg three times daily, may help both mucous membrane and cutaneous lichen planus in selected patients with intestinal or bladder infections.

Prognosis

Lichen planus is a benign disease, but it may persist for months or years and may be recurrent. Hypertrophic lichen planus and oral lesions tend to be especially persistent, and neoplastic degeneration has been described in chronically eroded lesions. The oral retinoids appear to induce remissions and facilitate healing of erosive lesions in some patients.

KAPOSI'S SARCOMA

Until recently in the USA, this rare malignant skin lesion was seen mostly in elderly white men, had a chronic clinical course, and was rarely fatal. Kaposi's sarcoma occurs endemically in an often aggressive form in young black men of equatorial Africa, but it is rare in American blacks. However, epidemic clusters of Kaposi's sarcoma, predominantly in homosexual men who were infected early in the AIDS epidemic, have been found in large cities of the USA. Systemic symptoms associated with red, purple, or dark plaques or nodules on cutaneous or mucosal surfaces should alert the clinician to the possibility of the disease. Kaposi lesions in this patient population commonly involve the lung and gastrointestinal tract, as well as the skin. For reasons which remain obscure, the incidence of AIDS-associated Kaposi's sarcoma appears to be diminishing.

Management of AIDS-associated Kaposi's sarcoma consists of observation and supportive care for slowly progressive disease; cryotherapy, vinblastine (0.1–0.5 mg/mL), and alpha interferon intralesionally for cosmetically objectionable lesions; radiation therapy for accessible and space-occupying lesions; laser surgery for certain intraoral and pharyngeal lesions; and, for progressive disease, intravenous chemotherapy.

Boudreaus AA et al: Intralesional vinblastine for cutaneous Kaposi's sarcoma associated with acquired immunodeficiency syndrome: A clinical trial to evaluate efficacy and discomfort associated with injection. J Am Acad Dermatol 1993;28:61.

Tappero JW et al: Kaposi's sarcoma. J Am Acad Dermatol 1993;28:371.

PRURITUS (Itching)

Pruritus is a disagreeable sensation that provokes a desire to scratch. It is a primary sensory impulse carried on unmyelinated C fibers in the spinothalamic tract. It is modulated by central factors, including cortical ones. Not all cases of pruritus are mediated by histamine, though several mediators—bradykinin, neurotensin, secretin, and substance P—release histamine.

Although most cases of generalized pruritus can be attributed to dry skin—whether naturally occurring and precipitated or aggravated by climatic conditions or arising from disease states—there are many other causes: scabies, dermatitis herpetiformis, atopic dermatitis, pruritus vulvae et ani, miliaria, insect bites, pediculosis, contact dermatitis, drug reactions, urticaria, urticarial eruptions of pregnancy, psoriasis, lichen planus, lichen simplex chronicus, exfoliative dermatitis, folliculitis, sunburn, bullous pemphigoid, and fiberglass dermatitis.

Perhaps the commonest cause of pruritus associated with systemic disease is uremia in conjunction with hemodialysis. Both this condition and the pruritus of obstructive biliary disease may be helped by irradiation with ultraviolet B. Endocrine disorders, psychiatric disturbances, lymphoma, leukemia, and other internal malignant disorders, iron deficiency anemia, and certain neurologic disorders may also be manifested by pruritus.

Burning or itching involving the face, scalp, and genitalia may be manifestations of primary depression and treatable with antidepressant drugs such as amitriptyline, imipramine, or doxepin.

Prognosis

Elimination of external factors and irritating agents is often successful in giving complete relief from pruritus. Pruritus accompanying specific skin disease will subside when the disease is controlled. Idiopathic pruritus and that accompanying serious internal disease may not respond to any type of therapy.

Bergasa NV, Jones EA: Management of the pruritus of cholestasis: Potential role of opiate antagonists. Am J Gastroenterol 1991;86:1404.

Buchness MR, Sanchez M: HIV-associated pruritus. Clin Dermatol 1991;9:111.

Gupta M et al: Psychotropic drugs in dermatology: A review and guidelines for use. J Am Acad Dermatol 1986;14:633.

Lowitt MH, Bernhard JD: Pruritus. Semin Neurol 1992;12(4):374.

Phillips WG: Pruritus: What to do when the itching won't stop. Postgrad Med 1992;92:34.

ANOGENITAL PRURITUS

Essentials of Diagnosis

- Itching, chiefly nocturnal, of the anogenital area.
- Examination is highly variable, ranging from no skin reactions to excoriations and inflammation of any degree, including lichenification.

General Considerations

Most cases have no obvious cause, but multiple specific causes have been identified. Anogenital pruritus may have the same causes as intertrigo, lichen simplex chronicus, or seborrheic or contact dermatitis (from soaps, colognes, douches, contraceptives), or it may be due to irritating secretions, as in diarrhea, leukorrhea, or trichomoniasis, or to local disease (candidiasis, dermatophytosis, erythrasma). Psoriasis or seborrheic dermatitis may be present. Uncleanliness may be at fault. It has been postulated that fecal bacterial endopeptidases play a causative role in pruritus ani.

Many women experience pruritus vulvae. In women, pruritus ani by itself is rare, and pruritus vulvae does not usually involve the anal area, though anal itching will usually spread to the vulva. In men, pruritus of the scrotum is less common than pruritus ani. When all possible known causes have been ruled out, the condition is diagnosed as idiopathic or essential pruritus—by no means rare.

Proctosigmoidoscopic examination is seldom helpful. Oxyuriasis (pinworm) is rarely a cause in adults. Psychologic abnormalities are usually not evident. Lichen sclerosus et atrophicus may at times be the cause, but gross pathologic changes are evident in this disorder. The disease is probably more common than currently thought, especially in young girls. Erythrasma is easily diagnosed by demonstration of coral-red fluorescence with Wood's light; it is easily cured with erythromycin orally and topically.

Clinical Findings

A. Symptoms and Signs: The only symptom is itching, which is chiefly nocturnal. Physical findings are usually not present, but there may be erythema, fissuring, maceration, lichenification, excoriations, or changes suggestive of candidiasis or tinea.

B. Laboratory Findings: Urinalysis and blood glucose testing may lead to a diagnosis of diabetes mellitus. Microscopic examination or culture of tissue scrapings may reveal yeasts, fungi, or parasites. Stool examination may show intestinal parasites.

Differential Diagnosis

The etiologic differential diagnosis consists of *Candida* infection, parasitosis, local irritation from contact with drugs and irritants, and other primary skin disorders of the genital area such as psoriasis, seborrhea, intertrigo, or lichen sclerosus et atrophicus.

Prevention

Instruct the patient in proper anogenital hygiene after treating systemic or local conditions.

Treatment

A. General Measures: Treating constipation, preferably with high-fiber management (psyllium

[Metamucil; many others]), may help. Instruct the patient to use very soft or moistened tissue or cotton after bowel movements and to clean the perianal area thoroughly with cool water if possible. Women should use similar precautions after urinating. Instruct the patient regarding the harmful and pruritus-inducing effects of scratching.

B. Local Measures: Pramoxine (Prax) cream or lotion or hydrocortisone-pramoxine (Pramosone), 1% or 2.5% cream, lotion, or ointment, is helpful in managing pruritus in the anogenital area. Iodochlorhydroxyquin-hydrocortisone creams are useful also but may stain underwear. Potent fluorinated topical corticosteroids may lead to atrophy and striae if used for more than a few days. Sitz baths twice daily using silver nitrate, 1:10,000–1:200; potassium permanganate, 1:10,000; or aluminum subacetate solution, 1:20, are of value if the area is acutely inflamed and oozing. Underclothing should be changed daily. Affected areas may be painted with Castellani's solution. Balneol Perianal Cleansing Lotion or Tucks premoistened pads, ointment, or cream (all Tucks preparations contain witch hazel) may be very useful for pruritus ani.

Prognosis

Although benign, anogenital pruritus may be persistent and recurrent.

Eusebio EB et al: Treatment of intractable pruritus ani. Dis Colon Rectum 1990;33:770. (Conservative therapy and therapy directed to underlying disease is usually effective. One intracutaneous injection of 0.5% methylene blue was effective in intractable cases.)

Hanno R, Purphy P: Pruritus ani: Classification and management. Dermatol Clin 1987;5:811.

Helm KF, Gibson LE, Miller SA: Lichen sclerosus et atrophicus in children and young adults. Pediatr Dermatol 1991;8:97.

SCABIES

Essentials of Diagnosis

- Generalized itching, worse at night.
- Pruritic vesicles and pustules in "runs" or "galleries," especially on the sides of the fingers and the heels of the palms.
- Mites, ova, and brown dots of feces visible microscopically.
- Red papules or nodules on the penile glans and shaft are pathognomonic.

General Considerations

Scabies is a common dermatitis caused by infestation with *Sarcoptes scabiei*. The entire family may be affected. The infestation usually spares the head and neck (though even these areas may be involved in infants). The mite may be barely visible with the naked eye as a white dot. Scabies is usually acquired by sleeping with or in the bedding of an infested individual or by other close contact.

Clinical Findings

A. Symptoms and Signs: Itching occurs almost exclusively at night. The lesions consist of more or less generalized excoriations with small pruritic vesicles, pustules, and "runs" or "burrows" on the sides of the fingers and the heels of the palms, wrists, elbows, and around the axillae. The run or gallery appears as a short irregular mark, perhaps 2–3 mm long and the width of a hair. Characteristic lesions may occur on the nipples in females and as pruritic papules on the scrotum or penis in males. Pruritic papules may be seen over the buttocks. Pyoderma is often the presenting sign.

B. Laboratory Findings: The diagnosis should be confirmed by microscopic demonstration of the organism, ova, or feces in a mounted specimen in glycerin, mineral oil, or immersion oil. The success of this procedure depends on choosing the best unexcoriated lesions from interdigital webs, wrists, elbows, beltline, etc. A bit of immersion oil is placed on the lesion and a No. 15 blade is used to scrape the lesion until it is flat. Pinpoint bleeding may result from the scraping. The diagnosis can also be confirmed in most cases with the burrow ink test. Apply ink to the burrow and then do a very superficial shave biopsy by sawing off the burrow with a No. 15 blade, painlessly and bloodlessly. The mite, ova, and feces can be seen under the light microscope.

Differential Diagnosis

Scabies must be distinguished from the various forms of pediculosis and from other causes of pruritus.

Treatment & Prognosis

Bedding and clothing should be laundered or cleaned. Unless the lesions are complicated by severe secondary pyoderma, treatment consists primarily of disinfestation. If secondary pyoderma is present, it should be treated with systemic and topical antibiotics. Unless treatment is aimed at all infected persons in a family or institutionalized group, reinfestations will probably occur. Cases apparently "resistant" to lindane and crotamiton are not uncommon, but resistance to 5% permethrin cream (Elimite) is uncommon.

Disinfestation with lindane (gamma benzene hexachloride), 1% in cream or lotion base, applied from the neck down overnight, is a popular treatment for adults. A warning has been issued by the FDA regarding potential neurotoxicity, and any use in infants and pregnant women, as well as overuse in adults, is discouraged. This preparation can be used before secondary infection is controlled.

Permethrin 5% dermal cream is highly effective

and safe in the management of scabies. Treatment consists of a single application. The drug has been used safely in infants aged 2 months to 5 years and is the treatment of choice in children. An alternative drug is crotamiton (Eurax) cream or lotion, which may be applied in the same way as lindane but is used nightly for 5 nights. It is far less effective.

Pregnant patients should be treated only if they have documented scabies themselves, and permethrin 5% cream is probably the drug of choice.

The old-fashioned medication consisting of 5% or 6% sulfur in petrolatum may still be used for pregnant patients, applying it nightly from the collarbones down, for 3 nights, but one must be prepared to treat irritant dermatitis.

Benzyl benzoate may be compounded as a lotion or emulsion in strengths from 20% to 35% and used as generalized applications (from collarbones down) overnight for two treatments 1 week apart. The NF XIV formula is 275 mL benzyl benzoate (containing 5 g of triethanolamine and 20 g of oleic acid) in water to make 1000 mL. It is cosmetically acceptable, clean, and not overly irritating.

Persistent pruritic postscabietic papules may be treated with mid- to high-potency steroids or with intralesional triamcinolone acetonide (2.5–5 mg/mL).

Orkin M, Maibach HI (editors): *Cutaneous Infestations and Insect Bites.* Marcel Dekker, 1985.

Taplin D et al: Community control of scabies: A model based on use of permethrin cream. Lancet 1991;337: 1016.

PEDICULOSIS

Essentials of Diagnosis

- Pruritus with excoriation.
- Nits on hair shafts; lice on skin or clothes.
- Occasionally, sky-blue macules (maculae ceruleae) on the inner thighs or lower abdomen in pubic louse infestation.

General Considerations

Pediculosis is a parasitic infestation of the skin of the scalp, trunk, or pubic areas. It usually occurs among people who live in overcrowded dwellings with inadequate hygiene facilities, though pubic lice may be acquired by sexual transmission. Head louse infestations may be transmitted by shared use of hats or combs and may be spread quickly among children in school.

There are three different varieties: (1) pediculosis pubis, caused by *Pthirus pubis* (pubic louse, "crabs"); (2) pediculosis corporis, by *Pediculus humanus* var *corporis* (body louse); and (3) pediculosis capitis, by *Pediculus humanus* var *capitis* (head louse).

Head and body lice are similar in appearance and are 3–4 mm long. The body louse can seldom be found on the body, because the insect comes onto the skin only to feed and must be looked for in the seams of the underclothing. Trench fever, relapsing fever, and typhus are transmitted by the body louse in countries where those diseases are endemic.

Clinical Findings

Itching may be very intense in body louse infestations, and scratching may result in deep excoriations over the affected area. In some cases, only itching is present, with few excoriations seen. Pyoderma may be the presenting sign in any of these infestations. Head lice can be found on the scalp or may be manifested as small nits resembling pussy willow buds on the scalp hairs close to the skin. They are easiest to see above the ears and at the nape of the neck. Body lice may deposit visible nits on vellus hair. Pubic louse infestations are occasionally generalized, particularly in hairy individuals; the lice may even be found on the eyelashes and in the scalp.

Differential Diagnosis

Head louse infestation may resemble seborrheic dermatitis, body louse infestation from scabies, and pubic louse infestation from anogenital pruritus and eczema.

Treatment

For all types of pediculosis, lindane lotion (Kwell, Scabene) is used extensively. A thin layer is applied to the infested and adjacent hairy areas. It is removed after 12 hours by thorough washing. Remaining nits may be removed with a fine-toothed comb or forceps. Sexual contacts should be treated.

Permethrin 1% cream rinse (Nix) is a topical OTC pediculicide and ovicide for the treatment of head lice and eggs. It is applied to the scalp and hair and left on for 10 minutes before being rinsed off with water. Treatment should be repeated in 1 week. Permethrin 1% cream is more effective than synergized pyrethrins (A-200 Pyrinate, Pyrinyl, Rid), OTC products that are applied undiluted until the infested areas are entirely wet. After 10 minutes, the areas are washed thoroughly with warm water and soap and then dried. Nits may be treated as indicated above. For involvement of eyelashes, petrolatum is applied thickly twice daily for 8 days, and remaining nits are then plucked off.

Buntin DM et al: Sexually transmitted diseases: Viruses and ectoparasites: Committee on Sexually Transmitted disease of the American Academy of Dermatology. J Am Acad Dermatol 1991;25:527.

Burns DA: the treatment of human ectoparasite infection. Br J Dermatol 1991;125:89.

Elgart ML: Pediculosis. Dermatol Clin 1990;8:219.

SKIN LESIONS DUE TO OTHER ARTHROPODS

Essentials of Diagnosis

- Localized rash with pruritus.
- Furuncle-like lesions containing live arthropods.
- Tender erythematous patches that migrate ("larva migrans").
- Generalized urticaria or erythema multiforme in some patients.

General Considerations

Some arthropods (eg, most pest mosquitoes and biting flies) are readily detected as they bite. Many others are not, eg, because they are too small, because there is no immediate reaction, or because they bite during sleep. Reactions may be delayed for many hours; many are allergic. Patients are most apt to consult a physician when the lesions are multiple and pruritus is intense.

Many persons will react severely only to their earliest contacts with an arthropod, thus presenting pruritic lesions when traveling, moving into new quarters, etc. Body lice, fleas, bedbugs, and local mosquitoes should be considered. Spiders are often incorrectly believed to be the source of bites; they rarely attack humans, though the brown spider (*Loxosceles laeta, Loxosceles reclusa*) may cause severe necrotic reactions and death due to intravascular hemolysis, and the black widow spider (*Latrodectus mactans*) may cause severe systemic symptoms and death.

In addition to arthropod bites, the most common lesions are venomous stings (wasps, hornets, bees, ants, scorpions) or bites (centipedes), furuncle-like lesions due to fly maggots or sand fleas in the skin, and a linear creeping eruption due to a migrating larva.

Clinical Findings

The diagnosis may be difficult when the patient has not noticed the initial attack but suffers a delayed reaction. Individual bites are often in clusters and tend to occur either on exposed parts (eg, midges and gnats) or under clothing, especially around the waist or at flexures (eg, small mites or insects in bedding or clothing). The reaction is often delayed for 1–24 hours or more. Pruritus is almost always present and may be all but intolerable once the patient starts to scratch. Secondary infection may follow scratching. Urticarial wheals, are common. Papules may become vesicular. The diagnosis is aided by searching for exposure to arthropods and by considering the patient's occupation and recent activities.

The principal arthropods are as follows:

(1) Bedbugs: In crevices of beds or furniture; bites tend to occur in lines or clusters. Papular urticaria is a characteristic lesion of bedbug bites. It is thought that *Cimex lectularius* (bedbug) could play a role in the transmission of hepatitis B. The closely related kissing bug (conenose) has been reported with increasing frequency as attacking humans.

(2) Fleas: Fleas are bloodsucking ectoparasites that feed on dogs, cats, humans, and other species. Flea saliva produces papular urticaria in sensitized individuals. *Ctenocephalides felis* and *Ctenocephalides canis* are the most common species found on cats and dogs, and both species attack humans. The human flea, *Pulex irritans,* is not commonly recognized by veterinarians as a pet animal problem.

To break the life cycle of the flea, one must treat the home, pets, and outside environment, using quick-kill insecticides, residual insecticides, and a growth regulator. Obviously, this is a repetitive job for the exterminator. Home foggers and flea collars are not always adequate. Birds and fish are especially sensitive and must be protected during disinfestation.

(3) Ticks: Usually picked up by brushing against low vegetation. Larval ticks may attack in large numbers; in Africa and India, they have been confused with chiggers. Ascending paralysis may occasionally be traced to a tick bite, and removal of the embedded tick results in clearing of symptoms. Ticks may transmit Rocky Mountain spotted fever, Lyme disease, and relapsing fever.

(4) Chiggers or red bugs are larvae of trombiculid mites. A few species confined to particular countries and usually to restricted and locally recognized habitats (eg, berry patches, woodland edges, lawns, brush turkey mounds in Australia, poultry farms) attack humans, often around the waist, on the ankles, or in flexures, raising intensely itching erythematous papules after a delay of many hours. The red chiggers may sometimes be seen in the center of papules that have not yet been scratched. Chiggers are the commonest cause of multiple lesions associated with arthropods.

(5) Bird mites: Larger than chiggers, bird mites infest pigeon lofts or nests of birds in eaves. Bites are multiple anywhere on the body, although poultry handlers are most often attacked on the hands and forearms. Room air conditioning units may suck in bird mites and infest the inhabitants of the room. Rodent mites from mice or rats may cause similar effects.

The diagnosis of bird mites, rodent mites, or carpet mites may easily be overlooked and the patient treated for other dermatoses.

(6) Mites in stored products: These are white and almost invisible and infest products such as copra, vanilla pods, sugar, straw, cottonseeds, and cereals. Persons who handle these products may be attacked, especially on the hands and forearms and sometimes on the feet. Infested bedding may occasionally lead to generalized dermatitis.

(7) Caterpillars of moths with urticating hairs: The hairs are blown from cocoons or carried by emergent moths, causing severe and often seasonally recurrent outbreaks after mass emergence, eg, in some southern states of the USA.

(8) Tungiasis is due to the burrowing flea known as *Tunga penetrans* and is found in Africa, the West Indies, and South America. The female burrows under the skin, sucks blood, swells to 0.5 cm, and then ejects her eggs onto the ground. Ulceration, lymphangitis, gangrene, and septicemia may result, in some cases with lethal effect. Ethyl chloride spray will kill the insect when applied to the lesion, and disinfestation may be accomplished with insecticide applied to the terrain.

Differential Diagnosis

Arthropods should be considered in the differential diagnosis of skin lesions showing any of the above symptoms.

Prevention

Arthropod infestations are best prevented by avoidance of contaminated areas, personal cleanliness, and disinfection of clothing, bedclothes, and furniture as indicated. Lice, chiggers, red bugs, and mites can be killed by lindane (Gammexane, Kwell, Scabene) applied to the head and clothing. (It is not necessary to remove clothing.) Benzyl benzoate and dimethylphthalate are excellent acaricides; clothing should be impregnated by spray or by dipping in a soapy emulsion.

Treatment

Living arthropods should be removed carefully with tweezers after application of alcohol and preserved in alcohol for identification. In endemic Rocky Mountain spotted fever areas, ticks should not be removed with the bare fingers, because infection may occur.

Corticosteroid lotions or creams are helpful. Crotamiton (Eurax) cream or lotion may be used; it is a miticide as well as an antipruritic. Calamine lotion or a cool wet dressing is always appropriate. Antibiotic creams, lotions, or powders may be applied if secondary infection is suspected.

Localized persistent lesions may be treated with intralesional corticosteroids. Creams containing local anesthetics are not very effective and may be sensitizing.

Stings produced by many arthropods may be alleviated by applying papain powder (Adolph's Meat Tenderizer) mixed with water, or aluminum chloride hexahydrate (Xerac AC).

Extracts from venom sacs of bees, wasps, yellow jackets, and hornets are now available for immunotherapy of patients at risk for anaphylaxis, but they are expensive. Treatment is advisable, however, as there are 50–100 deaths yearly is the USA due to this problem. Approximately 5% of patients fail to respond.

Muller U et al: Emergency treatment of allergic reactions to Hymenoptera stings. Clin Exp Allergy 1991;21:281.

Wilson DC, King LE Jr: Spiders and spider bites. Dermatol Clin 1990;8:277. (Brown recluse and black widow spiders cause most of the significant reactions in the USA.)

INFLAMMATORY NODULES

ERYTHEMA NODOSUM

Essentials of Diagnosis

- Painful red nodules without ulceration on anterior aspects of legs.
- Slow regression over several weeks to resemble contusions.
- Some cases associated with infection or drug sensitivity; women are predominantly affected.

General Considerations

Erythema nodosum is a symptom complex characterized by tender, erythematous nodules that appear most commonly on the extensor surfaces of the legs. It usually lasts about 6 weeks and may recur. The disease may be associated with various infections (streptococcosis, primary coccidioidomycosis, other deep fungal infections, primary tuberculosis, hepatitis B, or syphilis) or may be due to drug sensitivity (penicillin, progestins). It may accompany leukemia, sarcoidosis, rheumatic fever, and ulcerative colitis. Infections with unusual organisms such as *Pasteurella (Yersinia) pseudotuberculosis* and *Yersinia enterocolitica* may be responsible. Erythema nodosum may be associated with pregnancy or with use of oral contraceptives.

Clinical Findings

A. Symptoms and Signs: The swellings are exquisitely tender and are usually preceded by fever, malaise, and arthralgia. They are most often located on the anterior surfaces of the legs below the knees but may occur (rarely) on the arms, trunk, and face. The lesions, 1–10 cm in diameter, are at first pink to red; with regression, all the various hues seen in a contusion can be observed. The nodules occasionally become fluctuant, but they do not suppurate.

B. Laboratory Findings: The histologic finding of septal panniculitis is characteristic of erythema nodosum. Otherwise, the findings are those of the associated illness.

Differential Diagnosis

Erythema induratum is seen on the posterior surfaces of the legs and shows ulceration. Nodular vasculitis is usually on the calves and is associated with phlebitis. Erythema multiforme occurs in generalized distribution. Lupus panniculitis presents as tender nodules on the buttocks and trunk that heal with depressed scars. In the late stages, erythema nodosum must be distinguished from simple bruises and contusions.

Treatment

A. General Measures: One must first identify and treat the underlying cause, eg, systemic infection or exogenous toxin. Primary therapy is with nonsteroidal anti-inflammatory agents in usual doses. Saturated solution of potassium iodide, 5–15 drops three times daily, may result in prompt involution in many cases. Side effects of potassium iodide include salivation, swelling of salivary glands, and headache. Complete bed rest may be advisable if the lesions are very painful. Systemic therapy directed against the lesions themselves may include corticosteroid therapy (see Chapter 25) unless contraindicated by associated infection; salicylates are helpful for several days during the acute painful stage.

B. Local Treatment: This is usually not necessary. Hot or cold compresses may help.

Prognosis

The lesions usually disappear after about 6 weeks, but they may recur.

FURUNCULOSIS (BOILS) & CARBUNCLES

Essentials of Diagnosis

- Extremely painful inflammatory swelling of a hair follicle that forms an abscess.
- Primary predisposing disease, especially diabetes, sometimes present.
- Coagulase-positive *Staphylococcus aureus* is the causative organism.

General Considerations

A furuncle (boil) is a deep-seated infection (abscess) involving the entire hair follicle and adjacent subcutaneous tissue. The most common sites of occurrence are the hairy parts exposed to irritation and friction, pressure, or moisture or to the plugging action of petroleum products. Because the lesions are autoinoculable, they are often multiple. Thorough investigation usually fails to uncover a predisposing cause, though an occasional patient may have unsuspected diabetes mellitus.

A carbuncle consists of several furuncles developing in adjoining hair follicles and coalescing to form a conglomerate, deeply situated mass with multiple drainage points.

Clinical Findings

A. Symptoms and Signs: Pain and tenderness may be prominent, and more severe with carbuncles than with furuncles. The follicular abscess is either rounded or conical. It gradually enlarges, becomes fluctuant, and then softens and opens spontaneously after a few days to 1–2 weeks to discharge a core of necrotic tissue and pus. The inflammation occasionally subsides before necrosis occurs. Infection of the soft tissue around the nails (paronychia) is usually due to staphylococci when it is acute. This is a variant of furuncle. Other organisms may be involved, including *Pseudomonas* and herpes simplex (herpetic whitlow).

B. Laboratory Findings: There may be slight leukocytosis, but a white blood cell count is rarely required. The same is true for culture, since *S aureus* is nearly always the cause.

Differential Diagnosis

The most common entity in the differential is an inflamed epidermal inclusion cyst that suddenly becomes red, tender, and expands greatly in size over one to a few days. The history of a prior small cyst in the same location, the presence of a clearly visible cyst orifice, and the extrusion of cheesy rather than purulent material helps in the diagnosis. Furuncle is also to be distinguished from deep mycotic infections such as sporotrichosis (often in gardeners) and blastomycosis, from other bacterial infections such as anthrax and tularemia (rare), and from acne cysts. Hidradenitis suppurativa, a disease of apocrine glands, presents with tender sterile abscesses in the axillae, groin, on the buttocks, or below the breasts. The presence of old scars or sinus tracts plus negative cultures suggests this diagnosis.

Complications

Serious and sometimes fatal cavernous sinus thrombosis may occur as a complication of a manipulated furuncle on the central portion of the upper lip or near the nasolabial folds. Perinephric abscess, osteomyelitis, and even endocarditis may also occur from manipulation of any furuncle.

Treatment

A. Specific Measures: Systemic anti-infective agents are indicated (chosen on the basis of cultures and sensitivity tests if possible). Sodium cloxacillin, 1 g daily in divided doses by mouth for 10 days, is usually effective. Cephalexin is an effective alternative drug. Ciprofloxacin is effective against strains of staphylococci resistant to other antibiotics. Erythromycin may be used in penicillin-allergic individuals in communities with low populations of erythromycin-resistant staphylococci or if the particular isolate is sensitive.

Recurrent furunculosis may be effectively treated with a combination of dicloxacillin, 250–500 mg four times daily for 2–4 weeks, and rifampin, 300 mg twice daily for 5 days during this period. Family members and intimate contacts may need evaluation for staphylococcal carrier state and perhaps concomitant treatment. Applications of topical 2% mupirocin (Bactroban) to the nares, axillae, and anogenital areas three times daily for 5–7 days eliminates the staphylococcal carrier state. However, in its current formulation, mupirocin may be irritating inside the nose.

B. Local Measures: Immobilize the part and avoid overmanipulation of inflamed areas. Use moist heat to help larger lesions "localize." Use surgical incision and debridement *after* the lesions are "mature." Do not incise deeply. Apply anti-infective ointment and bandage the area loosely during drainage. It is not necessary to incise and drain an acute staphylococcal paronychia. Inserting a flat metal spatula or sharpened hardwood stick into the nail fold where it adjoins the nail will release pus from a mature lesion.

Inflamed epidermal cysts are best treated in the initial stages with intralesional injections of triamcinolone acetonide (10 mg/mL) into the borders of the lesions, attempting not to puncture the cyst itself. At times, these may require drainage if very fluctuant.

Prognosis

Recurrent crops may harass the patient for months or years. Carbunculosis is more severe and more hazardous than furunculosis.

Aly R: The pathogenic staphylococci. Semin Dermatol 1990;9:292.

PHOTODERMATITIS

Essentials of Diagnosis

- Painful erythema, edema, and vesiculation on sun-exposed surfaces: the face, neck, hands, and "V" of the chest.
- Inner upper eyelids spared, as is the area under the chin.

General Considerations

Photodermatitis is an acute or chronic inflammatory skin reaction due to overexposure or hypersensitivity to sunlight or other sources of actinic rays, photosensitization of the skin by certain drugs, or idiosyncrasy to actinic light as seen in some constitutional disorders including the porphyrias and many hereditary disorders (phenylketonuria, xeroderma pigmentosum, and others). Contact photosensitivity may occur with perfumes, antiseptics, and other chemicals.

Photodermatitis is manifested most commonly as photosensitivity—a tendency for the individual to sunburn more easily than usual—or, more rarely, as photoallergy, a true immunologic reaction that often presents with papular or vesicular lesions.

Clinical Findings

A. Symptoms and Signs: The acute inflammatory skin reaction, if severe enough, is accompanied by pain, fever, gastrointestinal symptoms, malaise, and even prostration, but this is not common. Signs include erythema, edema, and possibly vesiculation and oozing on exposed surfaces. Peeling of the epidermis and pigmentary changes often result. The key to diagnosis is localization of the rash to photoexposed areas, though these eruptions may become generalized with time to involve even photoprotected areas. The lips are commonly involved in polymorphous light eruption, a disorder seen in persons of South American descent.

B. Laboratory Findings: Blood and urine tests are not helpful in diagnosis unless porphyria cutanea tarda is suggested by the presence of blistering, scarring, milia (white cysts 1–2 mm in diameter) and skin fragility of the dorsal hands, and hirsutism. Testing for photosensitivity may be necessary to define the wavelengths of light (long and medium wavelength ultraviolet light or visible light) responsible.

Differential Diagnosis

The differential diagnosis is long. If a clear history of use of a topical or systemic photosensitizer is not available and if the eruption is persistent, then a workup including biopsy and light testing may be required. Photodermatitis must be differentiated from contact dermatitis that may develop from one of the many substances in suntan lotions and oils, as these may often have a similar distribution. This may sometimes be accomplished without photopatch testing by cautiously reapplying the agent to the forearm or back daily for 1–2 weeks and avoiding sun exposure. Sensitivity to actinic rays may also be part of a more serious condition such as porphyria cutanea tarda, variegate porphyria, or lupus erythematosus. These disorders are diagnosed by appropriate blood or urine tests. Erythropoietic protoporphyria is a rare childhood disorder, and pellagra is not commonly seen in the United States. Phenothiazines, sulfones, chlorothiazides, griseofulvin, oral antidiabetic agents, nonsteroidal anti-inflammatory agents, and antibiotics (eg, some tetracyclines) may photosensitize the skin. Polymorphous light eruption appears to be a very common idiopathic photodermatitis that affects both sexes equally and often has its onset in the third to fourth decades except in Native Americans, in whom it commonly presents in childhood. Polymorphous light eruption is chronic in nature but shows diminishing sunlight sensitivity over the long term. Transitory periods of spontaneous remission do occur, and the risk of developing systemic lupus erythematosus and perhaps other autoimmune disorders is negligible. The action spectrum often lies in both long (320–400 nm) and short (below 320 nm) ultraviolet wavelengths. Contact photodermatitis may be caused by halogenated salicylanilides (weak antiseptics in soaps, creams, etc).

Complications

Delayed cumulative effects in fair-skinned people include keratoses and skin cancers. Some individuals continue to be chronic light reactors even when they apparently are no longer exposed to photosensitizing or phototoxic drugs.

Prevention

While sunscreeens are useful agents in general and should be used by persons with photosensitivity, those patients typically react to such low amounts of energy that sunscreens alone may not be sufficient. Protective sunscreening agents (eg, those containing PABA and oxybenzone or dioxybenzone) may be applied before exposure, though PABA and benzophenones themselves may uncommonly cause photosensitivity or contact allergic dermatitis. There are several PABA-free sunscreens of great efficacy, but sunscreens in general provide the best protection against middle-wavelength "burning" UVB rays and not against long-wavelength "tanning" UVA rays that cause most cases of drug-associated phototoxicity. For UVA-associated photodermatitis, Photoplex sunscreen not only provides protection from UVB radiation but also offer absorbent protection from UVA rays and may be somewhat beneficial. Sunscreens with an SPF of at least 15 should be used, and SPFs greater than 15 are needed for photosensitive patients.

Treatment

A. Specific Measures: It is of primary importance to identify and avoid the offending topical or systemic agent. Drugs should be suspected in cases of photoallergy even if the particular medication (such as hydrochlorothiazide) has been used for months.

B. Local Measures: Treatment is similar to that of any acute dermatitis, first using cooling and soothing wet dressings with saline, bicarbonate, or aluminum subacetate solutions and following with calamine or starch lotions. Because of the occlusive effect, ointments should be avoided while the lesions are still vesicular or weeping.

Sunscreens should be used as described above under prevention. Mid-potency to high-potency topical steroids are of limited benefit in phototoxic reactions but may help in polymorphous light eruption and, photoallergic reactions. Since the face is often involved, close monitoring every 2 weeks is necessary to avoid side effects of potent steroids.

C. Systemic Measures: Aspirin may have some value for fever and pain, as prostaglandins appear to play a pathogenetic role in acute sunburn.

Systemic corticosteroids in doses as described for acute contact dermatitis may be required for severe reactions. Phlebotomy, letting 500 mL of blood every 2 weeks, is first-choice therapy for porphyria cutanea tarda but may be complicated by anemia or hypotension. Antimalarial drugs such as chloroquine and hydroxychloroquine in very low doses twice weekly are effective alternatives in treating porphyria cutanea tarda but must be used cautiously to avoid hepatotoxicity. Liver toxins, including alcohol, should be interdicted.

Triamcinolone acetonide suspension, 40 mg, may be injected deeply into the gluteal muscle intermittently for flare-ups of polymorphous light eruption.

PUVA (psoralen plus UVA light) therapy can actually be a very important therapy for polymorphous light eruption and other idiopathic photosensitive conditions, perhaps by altering immune function in the skin. This is usually administered under strict supervision, using a photosensitizer (psoralen) and artificial light sources or sunlight, and systemic steroids are not uncommonly required to control initial flares. The eyes must be examined prior to treatment, and protective eyewear must be worn while outdoors for 24 hours after psoralen ingestion.

Patients with severe photosensitivity may require immunosuppressives, such as azathioprine, in the range of 50–150 mg/d.

Prognosis

The most common phototoxic sunburn reactions are usually benign and self-limiting except when the burn is severe or when it occurs as an associated finding in a more serious disorder. Polymorphous light eruption and some cases of photoallergy can persist for years.

Dromgoole SH, Maibach MI: Sunscreening agent tolerance: Contact and photocontact sensitization and contact urticaria. J Am Acad Dermatol 1990;22:1068.

Hawk JL: Photosensitivity in the elderly. Br J Dermatol 1990;35:29. (Describes the causes, including drugs, of photodermatoses in elderly patients.)

Norris PG, Hawk JL: The acute idiopathic photodermatoses. Semin Dermatol 1990;9:32.

Stern RS, Weinstein MC, Baker SG: Risk reduction for nonmelanoma skin cancer with childhood sunscreen use. Arch Dermatol 1986;122:537.

ULCERS

DECUBITUS ULCERS
(Bedsores, Pressure Sores)

Bedsores (pressure sores) are a special type of ulcer caused by impaired blood supply and tissue nutrition resulting from prolonged pressure over bony or cartilaginous prominences. The skin overlying the sacrum and hips is most commonly involved, but bedsores may also be seen over the occiput, ears, elbows, heels, and ankles. They occur most readily in aged, paralyzed, debilitated, and unconscious patients. Low-grade infection may occur as a complication.

Differential Diagnosis

Herpes simplex virus should be suspected in ulcers in immunocompromised patients, particularly if there is a scalloped border, representing the erosions of herpetic vesicles. Rarely, ulcerated lesions in the perianal area represent actual skin cancers. Rapidly expanding ulcers may also represent pyoderma gangrenosum associated with inflammatory bowel disease in some patients. Ecthyma gangrenosum is an ulcerating lesion associated with sepsis, commonly due to *Pseudomonas*, and observed in debilitated patients. All ulcerative lesions should be biopsied and cultured if suspicious or if they do not heal properly

Prevention

Good nursing care and nutrition and maintenance of skin hygiene are important preventive measures. The skin and the bed linens should be kept clean and dry. Bedfast, paralyzed, moribund, or listless patients who are candidates for the development of decubiti must be turned *frequently* (at least every hour) and must be examined at pressure points for the appearance of small areas of redness and tenderness. Water-filled mattresses, rubber pillows, alternating-pressure mattresses, and thick papillated foam pads are useful in prevention and in the treatment of lesions.

Treatment

A large number of treatments and protocols exist for management of decubiti. Early lesions should be treated with topical antibiotic powders and adhesive absorbent bandage (Gelfoam). Once clean, they may be treated with hydrocolloid dressings such as Duo-Derm. Established lesions require surgical consultation and care. A spongy foam pad placed under the patient may work best in some cases. It must be laundered often. A continuous dressing of 1% iodochlorhydroxyquin (Vioform) in Lassar's paste may be effective.

Deep infections are commonly present in pressure sores, often requiring systemic antibiotics.

Parish LC, Witkowski JA, Crissey JT: *The Decubitus Ulcer.* Masson, 1983.
Sugarman B: Infection and pressure sores. Arch Phys Med Rehabil 1985;66:177.

LEG ULCERS SECONDARY TO VENOUS INSUFFICIENCY

Essentials of Diagnosis

- Past history of varicosities, thrombophlebitis, or postphlebitic syndrome.
- Irregular ulceration, often on the medial aspect of the lower legs above the malleolus.
- Edema of the legs, varicosities, hyperpigmentation, and red and scaly areas (stasis dermatitis) and scars from old ulcers support the diagnosis.

General Considerations

Patients at risk have a history of venous insufficiency, either with obvious varicosities or with a past history of thrombophlebitis, or with immobility of the calf muscle group (paraplegics, etc). Red, pruritic patches of stasis dermatitis often precede ulceration. Venous hypertension, edema, and extravasation of high-molecular-weight proteins such as fibrinogen are thought to impair oxygenation and nutrient flow into tissues. White blood cell injury to venous capillary endothelium may further increase tissue damage.

Clinical Findings

A. Symptoms and Signs: The patient usually has a long history of venous insufficiency. Chronic edema is followed by a dermatitis, which is often pruritic. These changes are followed by hyperpigmentation, skin breakdown, and eventually sclerosis of the skin of the lower leg. The ulcer base may be clean, but it often has a yellow fibrin eschar that would appear easy to debride by using compresses but often requires surgical treatment. Ulcers that are not accompanied by stasis changes or that appear on the feet, toes, or above the knees should be approached with other diagnoses in mind.

B. Laboratory Findings: Thorough evaluation of the patient's vascular system is essential and includes a Doppler examination for venous insufficiency. Recently, light rheography has been introduced to measure venous capillary refill time.

Differential Diagnosis

The differential includes vasculitis, pyoderma gangrenosum, arterial ulcerations, infection, trauma, insect bites (spiders) and sickle cell anemia. When the diagnosis is in doubt, a punch biopsy from the border (not base) of the lesion may be helpful.

Prevention

Compression stockings to reduce edema are the most important means of prevention. Compression should achieve a pressure of 30 mm Hg below the knee and 40 mm Hg at the ankle. The stockings should not be used in patients with arterial insufficiency with an ankle-brachial pressure index less than 0.7. Pneumatic sequential compression devices may be of great benefit.

Treatment

Leg ulcers can be chronic and debilitating lesions. While many respond to standard therapy, new methods of evaluation and treatment offer hope for more effective management in the near future.

A. Local Measures: Institution of compression therapy is begun with cleaning of the ulcer. The patient is instructed to clean the base with saline or cleansers such as Saf-clens or Cara-klenz daily. A curette or small scissors can be used to remove the yellow fibrin eschar, under local anesthesia if the areas are very tender.

Once the base is clean, the ulcer is treated with metronidazole gel (MetroGel) to reduce gram-negative bacterial growth and odor. Any red dermatitic skin is treated with a medium- to high-potency steroid ointment. The ulcer is then covered with an occlusive hydroactive dressing (Duoderm or Cutinova) or a polyurethan foam (Allevyn) followed by an Unna zinc paste boot. This is changed weekly. The ulcer should begin to heal within weeks, and healing should be complete within 2–3 months. Some ulcerations require grafting. Full- or split-thickness grafts often do not take, and pinch grafts (small shaves of skin laid onto the bed) may be more effective. The new technique of cultured epidermal cell grafts, while expensive, has been effective in some cases that had failed all other therapy.

B. Systemic Therapy: If cellulitis accompanies the ulcer, systemic antibiotics are recommended: both dicloxacillin, 250 mg orally four times a day, and ciprofloxacin, 500 mg orally twice a day, are effective.

Prognosis

The combination of compression stockings and newer dressings enables venous stasis ulcers to heal within weeks or months. Newer modalities appear to be effective in recalcitrant cases. Control of edema is essential to prevent recurrent ulceration.

Phillips TJ, Dover JS: Leg ulcers. J Am Acad Dermatol 1991;25:965.

II. MISCELLANEOUS DERMATOLOGIC DISORDERS*

PIGMENTARY DISORDERS

Melanin is formed in the melanocytes in the basal layer of the epidermis. Its precursor, the amino acid tyrosine, is slowly converted to dihydroxyphenylalanine (dopa) by tyrosinase, and there are many further chemical steps to the ultimate formation of melanin. This system may be affected by external influences such as exposure to heat, trauma, solar or ionizing radiation, heavy metals, and changes in oxygen potential. These influences may result in hyperpigmentation, hypopigmentation, or both. Local trauma may destroy melanocytes temporarily or permanently, causing hypopigmentation—sometimes with surrounding hyperpigmentation, as in eczema and dermatitis. Hypermelanosis appears to be associated with increased plasma immunoreactive β-MSH (melanocyte-stimulating hormone from the pituitary) only in Addison's disease. Melatonin, a pineal hormone, regulates pigment dispersion and aggregation.

Other pigmentary disorders include those resulting from exposure to exogenous pigments such as carotenemia, argyria, deposition of other metals (such as gold when given chronically for rheumatoid arthritis), and tattooing. Other endogenous pigmentary disorders are attributable to metabolic substances—including hemosiderin (iron)—in purpuric processes and in hemochromatosis; or homogentisic acid in ochronosis; bile pigments; and carotenes.

Classification

One should first determine whether the disorder is hyper- or hypopigmentation. Each may be considered to be primary or to be secondary to other disorders.

A. Primary Pigmentary Disorders:

1. Hyperpigmentation–The disorders in this category are nevoid, congenital or acquired, and include pigmented nevi, mongolian spots, incontinentia pigmenti, ephelides (juvenile freckles), and lentigines (senile freckles). Hyperpigmentation occurs also in arsenical melanosis or in association with Addison's disease (due to lack of the inhibitory influence of hydrocortisone on the production of MSH by the pituitary gland). Axillary freckling and café au lait spots may be seen in neurofibromatosis.

2. Hypopigmentation and depigmentation–The disorders in this category are vitiligo, albinism, and piebaldism. In vitiligo, pigment cells (melanocytes) are destroyed. The greater the pigment loss, the

---

*Hirsutism is discussed in Chapter 25.

fewer the number of melanocytes. Vitiligo, present in approximately 1% of the population, may be associated with hyperthyroidism and hypothyroidism, pernicious anemia, diabetes mellitus, addisonism, and carcinoma of the stomach. Albinism represents a number of different genetically determined traits, with different phenotypes. These may be autosomal dominant or recessive and often affect the eye and vision. Piebaldism, a localized hypomelanosis manifested by a white forelock, is an autosomal dominant trait that in some cases may be associated with neurologic abnormalities. Hypopigmented ash leaf spots may be seen in tuberous sclerosis. Hypopigmented halos are common around nevi and may occur rarely around melanomas. Loss of pigment surrounding nevi and in melanomas may represent immune responses.

B. Secondary Pigmentary Disorders: Any damage to the skin (irritation, allergy, infection, excoriation, burns, or dermatologic therapy such as curettage, dermabrasion, chemical peels, freezing with liquid nitrogen) may result in hyper- or hypopigmentation. Several disorders of clinical importance are as described below:

1. Hyperpigmentation–The most common type of secondary hyperpigmentation occurs after another dermatologic condition, such as acne, and is most commonly seen in dark-skinned persons. It is called postinflammatory hyperpigmentation. **Melasma** occurs as patterned hyperpigmentation of the face. The localized pigmentation of **chloasma** may be a direct effect of certain steroid hormones, estrogens, and progesterones in predisposed clones of melanocytes. It occurs not only during pregnancy but also in 30–50% of women taking oral contraceptives.

Berloque hyperpigmentation is the pigmentation left behind by phototoxicity from essential oils in perfumes. Similar hyperpigmentation has been seen in phototoxic reactions to chemicals in the rinds of limes and other citrus fruits and to celery. Pigmentation may be produced by certain drugs, eg, chloroquine, chlorpromazine, minocycline, and amiodarone. Irritation from benzoyl peroxide and tretinoin can result in hyperpigmentation, as may topical fluorouracil. Fixed drug eruptions to phenolphthalein in laxatives, to barbiturates, and to tetracyclines, for example, are further causes.

2. Hypopigmentation–Leukoderma may complicate atopic dermatitis, lichen planus, psoriasis, alopecia areata, discoid lupus erythematosus, lichen simplex chronicus, and such systemic conditions as myxedema, thyrotoxicosis, and syphilis. It may follow local skin trauma of various sorts or may complicate dermatitis due to exposure to gold or arsenic. Antioxidants in rubber goods, such as monobenzyl ether of hydroquinone, cause leukoderma from the wearing of gauntlet gloves, rubber pads in brassieres, etc. This is most likely to occur in blacks. Physicians must exercise special care in using liquid nitrogen on black skin, since this often results in hypopigmentation or depigmentation, at times permanent. Intralesional or intra-articular injections of high concentrations of corticosteroids may also cause localized temporary hypopigmentation.

Differential Diagnosis

One must distinguish true lack of pigment from pseudoachromia, such as occurs in tinea versicolor, pityriasis simplex, and seborrheic dermatitis. It may be difficult to differentiate true vitiligo from leukoderma and even from partial albinism, but distribution of lesions is often helpful. The evaluation of pigmentary disorders in Caucasians is helped by Wood's light, which accentuates epidermal pigmentation and highlights hypopigmentation.

Complications

Actinic keratoses and epitheliomas are more likely to develop in persons with vitiligo and albinism. Vitiligo tends to cause pruritus in anogenital folds. There may be severe emotional trauma in extensive vitiligo and other types of hypo- and hyperpigmentation, particularly when they occur in naturally dark-skinned persons.

Treatment & Prognosis

A. Hyperpigmentation: Bleaching preparations generally contain hydroquinone or its derivatives. This is not without hazard, and it is best to start with the weakest preparation offered by the manufacturer. The use of this kind of agent may result in unexpected hypopigmentation, hyperpigmentation, or even secondary ochronosis and pigmented milia, particularly with prolonged use.

The role of exposure to ultraviolet light cannot be overstressed as a factor promoting or contributing to most disorders of hyperpigmentation, and such exposure should be minimized. Melasma, ephelides, and postinflammatory hyperpigmentation may be treated with varying success with 3–4% hydroquinone cream, gel (Eldoquin forte) or solution (Melanex) and a sunscreen with a SPF of 15. Solaquin forte contains both hydroquinone and a sunscreen. Tretinoin cream, 0.025–0.05%, may be added. The superficial melasma responds well, but if there is predominantly dermal deposition of pigment, the prognosis is poor. Response to therapy takes months and will not occur if sunlight is not avoided. Hyperpigmentation often recurs after treatment if the skin is exposed to ultraviolet light without potent sunscreens. Solar lentigines are resistant to topicals but respond to liquid nitrogen application or to newer green light lasers.

B. Hypopigmentation: The pigment dilution is stable in various forms of albinism; spontaneous return of pigment is rare in vitiligo; in secondary hypopigmentation, repigmentation may occur spontaneously. Therapy of vitiligo is long and tedious. Cosmetics such as Covermark and Dermablend are highly effective for concealing disfiguring patches. The patient must be strongly motivated. If less than 20% of the skin is involved (most cases), topical methoxsalen, 0.1% in ethanol and propylene glycol or in Acid Mantle cream or Unibase, is used, with cautious exposure to long-wavelength ultraviolet light (UVA), followed by thorough washing and application of an SPF 15 sunscreen. With 20–25% involvement, oral methoxsalen, 0.6 mg/kg 2 hours before UVA exposure, is best. Severe phototoxic response (sunburn) may occur with topical or oral psoralens plus UVA. New techniques of using epidermal autografts and cultured epidermis combined with PUVA therapy give hope for surgical correction of vitiligo with a very low risk of scarring. Potent topical corticosteroids have been advocated for treatment of vitiligo, with daily use for 10 days followed by 10 days of rest, then repetition. However, this strategy is often not successful, and on the face it may result in thinning of the skin and other changes. Freezing small areas lightly with liquid nitrogen followed by fluorouracil may be of occasional benefit. In rare cases of near-total depigmentation refractory to repigmentation, the use of 20% monobenzyl ether of hydroquinone has been reported to depigment the remaining unaffected skin.

Antoniou C, Katsambas A: Guideline for the treatment of vitiligo. Drugs 1992;43:490.
Hatchcome N et al: Therapeutic success of epidermal grafting in generalized vitiligo is limited by the Koebner phenomenon. J Am Acad Dermatol 1990;22:87.
Wildfang IL, Jacobsen FK, Thestrup-Pedersen K: PUVA treatment of vitiligo: A retrospective study of 59 patients. Acta Derm-Venereol 1992;72:305.

BALDNESS
(Alopecia)

Baldness Due to Scarring

Cicatricial baldness may occur following chemical or physical trauma, lichen planopilaris, severe bacterial or fungal infections, severe herpes zoster, chronic discoid lupus erythematosus, scleroderma, and excessive ionizing radiation. The specific cause is often suggested by the history, the distribution of hair loss, and the appearance of the skin, as in lupus erythematosus and other infections. Biopsy may be necessary to differentiate lupus from the others.

Scarring alopecias are irreversible and permanent. There is no treatment except for surgical hair transplants. It is important to diagnose and treat the scarring process as early in its course as possible.

Baldness Not Due to Scarring

Nonscarring alopecia may occur in association with various systemic diseases such as systemic lupus erythematosus, secondary syphilis, hyper- or hypothyroidism, and pituitary insufficiency. The only treatment necessary is prompt and adequate control of the underlying disorder, in which case hair loss may be reversible.

Male pattern baldness, the most common form of alopecia, is of genetic predetermination. The earliest changes occur at the anterior portions of the calvarium on either side of the "widow's peak." Associated seborrhea may be evident as excessive oiliness and erythema of the scalp, with scaling. The extent of hair loss is variable and unpredictable. Extensive studies with minoxidil applied topically have shown good results in the treatment of androgenetic (male pattern) alopecia of the vertex of the scalp. The commercial product, Rogaine, is a solution containing 20 mg/mL of minoxidil. The best results are achieved in patients under 50 years of age and in those with recent onset (< 5 years) and smaller diameters of alopecia. Approximately 40% of patients treated twice daily for a year will have moderate to dense regrowth of the vertex. Seborrhea may be treated as described in that section, but it is not likely to affect androgenetic hair loss.

Hair loss or thinning of the hair in women results from the same cause as common baldness in men (androgenetic alopecia); thus, it occurs most often postmenopausally. Minoxidil (Rogaine) is the treatment of choice for women with androgenetic alopecia after an adequate endocrinologic workup, which in premenopausal women includes determination of testosterone, DHEAS, androstenedione, and T_3, T_4, and TSH levels. Spironolactone, a synthetic steroidal aldosterone antagonist, has been used successfully for the treatment of diffuse hair loss in women (androgenetic alopecia) in a dose of 25 mg daily by mouth. This is not a listed indication for the drug, which has been shown to be a tumorigen in long-term toxicity studies in rats. Oral corticosteroids have been recommended to suppress adrenal androgen production, but these drugs are likely to result in osteoporosis and have additional important toxicity. Topical estrogens are of occasional value.

Women who complain of thin hair but show little evidence of alopecia need follow-up, because 20% of the scalp hair can be lost before the clinician can perceive it.

Telogen effluvium is a cause of temporary hair loss in some patients. A transitory increase occurs in the number of hairs in the telogen (resting) phase of the hair growth cycle. This may occur spontaneously, may appear at the termination of pregnancy, may be precipitated by "crash dieting," high fever, stress from surgery or shock, or malnutrition, or may be provoked by hormonal contraceptives. Whatever the cause, telogen effluvium usually has a latent period of 2–4 months. The prognosis is generally good. The condition is diagnosed by the presence of large numbers of hairs with white bulbs coming out upon gentle tugging of the hair—or more than six such hairs if the patient has shampooed that morning. Counts of hairs lost by the patient on combing or shampooing often exceed 150 per day, compared to an average of 70–100. In one study, a major cause of telogen effluvium was found to be iron deficiency, and the hair counts bore a clear relationship to serum iron levels.

Alopecia areata is of unknown cause but is believed to be an immunologic process. Typically, there are salmon-colored patches that are perfectly smooth and without scarring. Tiny hairs 2–3 mm in length, called "exclamation hairs," may be seen. Telogen hairs are easily dislodged from the periphery of active lesions. The beard, brows, and lashes may be involved. Involvement may extend to all of the scalp hair (alopecia totalis) or to all hair, including hairs inside the nose (alopecia universalis). Histopathologically, there are numerous small anagen hairs and a lymphocytic infiltrate. Severe forms may be treated by systemic corticosteroid therapy, although systemic therapy is rarely justified unless the disease is of serious emotional or economic significance. Alopecia areata is occasionally associated with Hashimoto's thyroiditis, pernicious anemia, Addison's disease, and vitiligo.

Anthralin, 0.5% ointment applied daily, may provoke hair growth. Intralesional corticosteroids are frequently effective. Triamcinolone acetonide in a concentration of 10 mg/mL is injected in aliquots of 0.1 mL at approximately 1- to 2-cm intervals, not exceeding a total dose of 50 mg per month for adults. Alopecia areata is usually self-limiting, with complete regrowth of hair in 80% of patients, but some mild cases are resistant, as are the extensive totalis and universalis types. Topical minoxidil (Rogaine) is effective in some patients. Both topical dinitrochlorobenzene (DNCB) and an experimental topical allergen, squaric acid dibutyl ester, have been used to treat persistent alopecia areata. The principle is to sensitize the skin, then intermittently apply weaker concentrations to produce and maintain a slight dermatitis. Hair regrowth in 3–6 months in some patients has been reported to be remarkable. Long-term safety and efficacy have not been established. Support groups for patients with extensive alopecia areata have been very beneficial for some patients. In **trichotillomania** (the pulling out of one's own hair), the patches of hair loss are irregular and growing hairs are always present, since they cannot be pulled out until they are long enough. The patches are often unilateral, occurring on the same side as the patient's dominant hand. The patient may be unaware of the habit.

Drug-induced alopecia is becoming increasingly important. Such drugs include thallium, excessive and prolonged use of vitamin A, retinoids, antimitotic agents, anticoagulants, clofibrate (rarely), antithyroid drugs, oral contraceptives, trimethadione, allopurinol, propranolol, indomethacin, amphetamines, salicylates, gentamicin, and levodopa.

Bergfeld WF, Redmond GP: Androgenetic alopecia. Dermatol Clin 1987;5:491.

Nelson DA, Spielvogel RL: Alopecia areata: A review. Int J Dermatol 1985;24:26.

Stern RS: Topical minoxidil: A survey of use and complications. Arch Dermatol 1987;123:62.

NAIL DISORDERS

Nail changes are generally not diagnostic of a specific systemic or cutaneous disease. All of the nail manifestations of systemic disorders may be seen also in the absence of any systemic illness.

Classification

Nail disorders may be classified as (1) local, (2) congenital or genetic, and (3) those associated with systemic or generalized skin diseases.

A. Local Nail Disorders:

1. Onycholysis (distal separation of the nail plate from the nail bed, usually of the fingers) is caused by excessive exposure to water, soaps, detergents, alkalies, and industrial keratolytic agents. Candidal infection of the nail folds and subungual area, nail hardeners, and demeclocycline-induced photosensitivity may cause onycholysis, as may hyper- and hypothyroidism.

2. Distortion of the nail occurs as a result of chronic inflammation of the nail matrix underlying the eponychial fold. Such changes may also be caused by warts, tumors, nevi, synovial and mucous cysts, etc, impinging on the nail matrix.

3. Discoloration and crumbly thickened nails are noted in dermatophyte infection.

4. Allergic reactions (to formaldehyde and resins in undercoats and polishes or to nail glues) are characterized by onycholysis or by grossly distorted, hypertrophic, and misshapen nails.

B. Congenital and Genetic Nail Disorders:

1. A longitudinal single nail groove may occur as a result of a genetic or traumatic defect in the nail matrix underlying the eponychial fold.

2. Nail atrophy may be congenital.

3. Clubbed fingers may be congenital.

C. Nail Changes Associated With Systemic or Generalized Skin Diseases:

1. Beau's lines (transverse furrows) may follow any serious systemic illness.

2. Atrophy of the nails may be related to trauma or to vascular or neurologic disease.

3. Clubbed fingers may be due to the prolonged hypoxemia associated with cardiopulmonary disorders.

4. Spoon nails may be seen in anemic patients.

5. Stippling or pitting of the nails is seen in psoriasis, alopecia areata, and pompholyx.

6. Nail hyperpigmentation may be caused by zidovudine, doxorubicin, cyclophosphamide, methotrexate, bleomycin, dacarbazine, daunorubicin, fluorouracil, hydroxyurea, melphalan, mechlorethamine, and nitrosoureas.

Differential Diagnosis

It is important to distinguish congenital and genetic disorders from those caused by trauma and environmental disorders. Nail changes due to dermatophyte fungi (see below) may be difficult to differentiate from those due to *Candida* infections. Direct microscopic examination of a specimen cleared with 10% potassium hydroxide—or culture on Sabouraud's medium—may be diagnostic. Onychomycosis may be closely similar to the changes seen in psoriasis and lichen planus, in which case careful observation of more characteristic lesions elsewhere on the body is essential to the diagnosis of the nail disorders. Cancer should be suspected (eg, Bowen's disease or squamous cell carcinoma) as the cause of any persistent solitary subungual or periungual lesion.

Complications

Secondary bacterial infection occasionally occurs in onychodystrophies and leads to considerable pain and disability and more serious consequences if circulation or innervation is impaired. Toenail changes may lead to an ingrown nail—in turn often complicated by bacterial infection and occasionally by exuberant granulation tissue. Poor manicuring and poorly fitting shoes may contribute to this complication. Cellulitis may result.

Treatment & Prognosis

Treatment consists usually of careful debridement and manicuring and, above all, reduction of exposure to irritants (soaps, detergents, alkali, bleaches, solvents, etc). Antifungal measures may be used in the case of onychomycosis and candidal onychia. Congenital or genetic nail disorders are usually uncorrectable. Longitudinal grooving due to temporary lesions of the matrix, such as warts, synovial cysts, and other impingements, may be cured by removal of the offending lesion. Intradermal triamcinolone acetonide suspension, 2.5 mg/mL, may be injected in the area of the nail matrix at intervals of 2–4 weeks for the successful management of various types of nail dystrophies (psoriasis, lichen planus) but is painful.

If it is necessary to remove dystrophic nails for any reason (eg, fungal nails or severe psoriasis), a nonsurgical method is to apply urea 40%, anhydrous lanolin 20%, white wax 5%, white petrolatum 25%, and silica gel type H. The nail folds are painted with compound tincture of benzoin and covered with cloth adhesive tape. The urea ointment is applied generously to the nail surface and covered with plastic film, and then adhesive tape. The ointment is left on for 5–10 days; then the nail plate may be lifted off. Medication can then be applied that is appropriate for the condition being treated.

Tinea Unguium Onychomycosis

Tinea unguium is a destructive *Trichophyton* infection of one or more (but rarely all) fingernails or toenails. The species most commonly found are *Trichophyton mentagrophytes* and *Trichophyton rubrum. Candida albicans* causes candidal onychomycosis. "Saprophytic" fungi may cause onychomycosis.

There are usually no symptoms. The nails are lusterless, brittle, and hypertrophic, and the substance of the nail is friable and even pithy. Irregular segments of the diseased nail may be broken. Laboratory diagnosis is mandatory. Portions of the nail should be cleared with 10% potassium hydroxide and examined under the microscope for branching hyphae or collections of spores. Fungi may also be cultured, using Sabouraud's medium. Periodic acid-Schiff stain of a histologic section will also demonstrate the fungus readily.

Onychomycosis is difficult to treat because of the long duration of therapy required and the frequency of recurrences. Fingernails respond in general more readily than toenails. For toenails, it is often best to discourage therapy in many patients and to control discomfort by having a podiatrist pare the thickened nail plate.

Griseofulvin ultramicrosize, 1–1.5 g/d, has been the initial treatment of choice. For toenail infections, 12–18 months of treatment may be required. Ketoconazole, 200 mg/d, is sometimes used for onychomycosis, though it is not approved for that indication. Increasing ketoconazole to 400 mg/d will substantially increase the cure rate of onychomycosis, but the side effects of ketoconazole (liver abnormalities, effects on the adrenal cortex, and antiandrogenic activity) must be taken into account. Although it is not approved for this indication, the use of itraconazole, 200 mg twice daily for 1 week per month for 4 months, may be an alternative treatment for toenail infection that takes advantage of the persistence of this drug in the nail plate after therapy is discontinued. It is likely that other dosing schedules will be proposed and that oral terbinafine, when available, will change how onychomycosis is treated.

The nails should be sandpapered or filed daily (down to the nail bed if necessary). Ciclopirox (Loprox) is a topical fungicidal cream that contains a pyridone-ethanolamine salt and seems to penetrate nails better than other topical agents. To date, no topical agent has been very effective. However, agents in new vehicles are currently being tested.

Even when the nails clear after months of treatment, recurrences can be expected shortly after discontinuance of systemic therapy. Topical therapy should be used as maintenance after systemic therapy has been completed.

Table 6–2. Skin reactions due to systemic drugs.

Reaction	Appearance	Distribution and Comments	Common Offenders
Toxic erythema	Morbilliform, maculopapular, exanthematous reactions.	The commonest skin reaction to drugs. Often more pronounced on the trunk than on the extremities. In previously exposed patients, the rash may start in 2–3 days. In the first course of treatment, the eruption often appears about the seventh to ninth days. Fever may be present.	Antibiotics (especially ampicillin and trimethoprimsulfamethoxazole), sulfonamides and related compounds (including thiazide diuretics, furosemide, and sulfonylurea hypoglycemic agents), and barbiturates.
Erythema multiforme major	Target-like lesions. Bullae may occur. Mucosal involvement.	Mainly on the extensor aspects of the limbs.	Sulfonamides, penicillamine, barbiturates, sulindac, and fenoprofen.
Erythema nodosum	Inflammatory cutaneous nodules.	Usually limited to the extensor aspects of the legs. May be accompanied by fever, arthralgias, and pain.	Oral contraceptives.
Allergic vasculitis	Inflammatory changes may present as urticaria that lasts over 24 hours, hemorrhagic papules ("palpable purpura"), vesicles, bullae, or necrotic ulcers.	Most severe around veins and venules.	Sulfonamides, indomethacin, phenytoin, allopurinol, and ibuprofen.
Purpura	Itchy, petechial macular rash.	Dependent areas. Results most typically from thrombocytopenia.	Thiazides, sulfonamides, sulfonylureas, barbiturates, quinine, and sulindac.
Eczema	Similar to contact dermatitis.	A rare epidermal reaction in patients previously sensitized by external exposure who are given the same or a related substance systemically.	Penicillin, neomycin, phenothiazines, and local anesthetics.
Exfoliative dermatitis and erythroderma	Red and scaly.	Entire skin surface.	Allopurinol, sulfonamides, isoniazid, gold, or carbamazepine.
Photosensitivity: Increased sensitivity to light, often of ultraviolet A wavelengths, but may be due to UVB or visible light as well	Sunburn, vesicles, papules in photodistributed pattern.	Exposed skin of the face, the neck, and the backs of the hands and, in women, the lower legs. Exaggerated response to ultraviolet light. On occasion, ultraviolet emission from fluorescent lighting may be sufficient.	Sulfonamides and sulfonamide-related compounds (thiazide diuretics, furosemide, sulfonylureas), tetracyclines (especially demeclocycline), phenothiazines, sulindac, amiodarone, piroxicam, and indomethacin.
Drug-related lupus erythematosus	May present with a photosensitive rash accompanied by fever, polyarthritis, myalgia, and serositis.	Less severe than systemic lupus erythematosus, sparing the kidneys and central nervous system. Recovery often follows drug withdrawal.	Most commonly hydralazine and procainamide; less often, isoniazid and phenytoin.
Lichenoid and lichen planus-like eruptions	Pruritic, erythematous to violaceous polygonal papules that coalesce or expand to form plaques.	May be in photo- or nonphotodistributed pattern.	Bismuth, carbamazepine, chlordiazepoxide, chloroquine, chlorpropamide, dapsone, ethambutol, furosemide, gold salts, hydroxychloroquine, levamisole, meprobamate, methyldopa, paraphenylenediamine salts, penicillamine, phenothiazines, pindolol, propranolol, quinidine, quinine, quinacrine, streptomycin, sulfonylureas, tetracyclines, thiazides, and triprolidine.
Fixed drug eruptions	Single or multiple demarcated, round, erythematous plaques that often become hyperpigmented.	Recur at the same site when the drug is repeated. Hyperpigmentation, if present, remains after healing.	Numerous drugs, including antimicrobials, analgesics, barbiturates, cardiovascular drugs, heavy metals, antiparasitic agents, antihistamines, phenolphthalein, ibuprofen, and naproxen.

(continued)

Table 6–2. Skin reactions due to systemic drugs. (continued)

Reaction	Appearance	Distribution and Comments	Common Offenders
Toxic epidermal necrolysis	Large sheets of erythema, followed by separation, which looks like scalded skin.	Rare.	In adults, the eruption has occurred after administration of many classes of drugs, particularly barbiturates, phenytoin, sulfonamides, and NSAIDs.
Urticaria	Red, itchy wheals that vary in size from < 1 cm to many centimeters. May be accompanied by angioedema.	Chronic urticaria is rarely caused by drugs.	Acute urticaria: penicillins, NSAIDs, sulfonamides, opiates, and salicylates. Angioedema is common in patients receiving ACE inhibitors.
Pruritus	Itchy skin without rash.		Pruritus ani may be due to overgrowth of *Candida* after systemic antibiotic treatment. Contraceptive pills, phenothiazines, and rifampin cause pruritus by producing cholestatic jaundice.
Hair loss		Hair loss most often involves the scalp, but other sites may be affected.	A predictable side effect of cytotoxic agents and oral contraceptives. Diffuse hair loss also occurs unpredictably with a wide variety of other drugs, including anticoagulants, antithyroid drugs, newer antimicrobials, cholesterol-lowering agents, heavy metals, corticosteroids, androgens, NSAIDs, retinoids (isotretinoin, etretinate), and beta-blockers.
Pigmentary changes	Flat hyperpigmented areas.	Forehead and cheeks (chloasma, melasma). The most common pigmentary disorder associated with drug ingestion. Improvement is slow despite stopping the drug.	Oral contraceptives are the usual cause.
	Blue-gray discoloration.	Light-exposed areas.	Chlorpromazine and related phenothiazines.
	Brown or blue-gray pigmentation.	Generalized.	Heavy metals (silver, gold, bismuth, and arsenic). Arsenic, silver, and bismuth are not used therapeutically, but patients who receive gold for rheumatoid arthritis may show this reaction.
	Yellow color.	Generalized.	Usually quinacrine.
	Blue-black patches on the shins.		Minocycline.
	Blue-black pigmentation of the nails and palate and depigmentation of the hair.		Chloroquine.
	Slate-gray color.	Primarily in photoexposed areas.	Amiodarone.
	Brown discoloration of the nails.	Especially in more darkly pigmented patients.	Zidovudine (azidothymidine; AZT).
Psoriasiform eruptions	Scaly red plaques.	May be located on trunk and extremities. Palms and soles may be hyperkeratotic. May cause psoriasiform eruption or worsen psoriasis.	Amodiaquine, chloroquine, debrisoquin, lithium, oxprenolol, pindolol, propranolol, quinacrine, and sulfonamides.
Pityriasis rosea-like eruptions	Oval, red, slightly raised patches with central scale.	Mainly on the trunk.	Barbiturates, bismuth, captopril, clonidine, gold salts, methopromazine, metoprolol, metronidazole, and tripelennamine.
Seborrheic dermatitis-like eruptions	Diffuse redness and loose scale.	On scalp, face, mid chest, axillae, groin.	Cimetidine, gold salts, and methyldopa.
Bullous eruptions	Tense blisters > 1 cm.	Hands, feet, genital areas common; other sites possible.	Aspirin, barbiturates, bromides, chlorpromazine, warfarin, phenytoin, sulfonamides and related compounds, and promethazine.

Scher RK: Differential diagnosis and treatment of onychomycosis. Curr Concepts Skin Disorders 1985;6:4.

Willemsen M et al: Post treatment itraconazole levels in the nail: New implications for treatment in onychomycosis. J Am Acad Dermatol 1992;26:731.

DERMATITIS MEDICAMENTOSA
(Drug Eruption)

Essentials of Diagnosis

- Usually, abrupt onset of widespread, symmetric erythematous eruption.
- May mimic any inflammatory skin condition.
- Constitutional symptoms (malaise, arthralgia, headache, and fever) may be present.

General Considerations

As is well recognized, only a minority of cutaneous drug reactions result from allergy. True allergic drug reactions involve prior exposure, an "incubation" period, reactions to doses far below the therapeutic range, manifestations different from the usual pharmacologic effects of the drug, involvement of only a small portion of the population at risk, restriction to a limited number of syndromes (anaphylactic and anaphylactoid, urticarial, vasculitic, etc), and reproducibility.

Rashes are among the most common adverse reactions to drugs and occur in 2–3% of hospitalized patients. Amoxicillin, trimethoprim-sulfamethoxazole, and ampicillin or penicillin are the commonest causes of urticarial and maculopapular reactions. Toxic epidermal necrolysis and Stevens-Johnson syndrome are most commonly produced by sulfonamides and anticonvulsants. Phenolphthalein, pyrazolone derivatives, tetracyclines, and barbiturates are the major causes of fixed drug eruptions.

Clinical Findings

A. Symptoms and Signs: The onset is usually abrupt, with bright erythema and often severe itching, but may be delayed. Fever and other constitutional symptoms may be present. The skin reaction usually occurs in symmetric distribution. In a given situation, the physician may suspect one specific drug (or one of several) and must therefore inquire specifically about whether it has been used.

Table 6–2 summarizes the types of skin reactions, their appearance and distribution, and the common offenders in each case.

B. Laboratory Findings: Routinely ordered blood work is of no value in the diagnosis of drug eruptions. However, skin biopsies may be helpful in making the diagnosis.

Differential Diagnosis

Observation after discontinuation, which may be a slow process, helps establish the diagnosis. Rechallenge, though of theoretical value, may pose a danger to the patient and is best avoided.

Complications

All drugs with dermatologic side effects also have toxicity affecting other organ systems, and each agent exhibits its own profile.

Treatment

A. General Measures: Systemic manifestations are treated as they arise (eg, anemia, icterus, purpura). Antihistamines may be of value in urticarial and angioneurotic reactions, but epinephrine 1:1000, 0.5–1 mL intravenously or subcutaneously, should be used as an emergency measure. Corticosteroids may be used as for acute contact dermatitis in severe cases.

B. Local Measures: The varieties and stages of dermatitis are treated according to the major dermatitis simulated. Extensive blistering eruptions resulting in erosions and superficial ulcerations demand hospitalization and nursing care as for burn patients.

Prognosis

Drug rash usually disappears upon withdrawal of the drug and proper treatment.

Bigby M, Stern R: Cutaneous reactions to nonsteroidal anti-inflammatory drugs: A review. J Am Acad Dermatol 1985;12:866.

Bigby M et al: Drug-induced cutaneous reactions. JAMA 1986;256:3358.

Bork K: Cutaneous Side Effects of Drugs. Saunders, 1988.

Shear NH: Diagnosing cutaneous adverse reactions to drugs. Arch Dermatol 1990;126:94.

Wintroub BU, Stern R: Cutaneous drug reactions: Pathogenesis and clinical classification. J Am Acad Dermatol 1985;13:167.

REFERENCES

Arnold HL Jr, Odom RB, James WD: Andrews' Diseases of the Skin, 8th ed. Saunders, 1990.

Ely H, Thiers BH (editors): Dermatologic therapy II. (Symposium.) Dermatol Clin 1989;7:1. [Entire issue.]

Fitzpatrick TB et al: Dermatology in General Medicine, 3rd ed. McGraw-Hill, 1987.

Lever WF, Schaumberg-Lever G: Histopathology of the Skin, 7th ed. Lippincott, 1990.

Moschella SL, Hurley HJ: *Dermatology,* 2nd ed. 2 vols. Saunders, 1985.

Phillips TJ, Dover JS: Recent advances in dermatology. (Medical Progress.) N Engl J Med 1992;326:167.

Pinkus H, Mehregan AH: *A Guide to Dermatohistopathology,* 4th ed. Appleton-Century-Crofts, 1986.

Sande MA, Volberding PA: *The Medical Management of AIDS,* 2nd ed. Saunders, 1990.

Shelley WP, Shelley ED: *Advanced Dermatologic Therapy.* Saunders, 1987.

7

Eye

Paul Riordan-Eva, FRCS, FCOphth, & Daniel G. Vaughan, MD

SYMPTOMS OF OCULAR DISEASE

Redness

Redness is the most frequently encountered symptom of ocular disorders. It is due to hyperemia of the conjunctival, episcleral, or ciliary vessels; erythema of the eyelids; or subconjunctival hemorrhage. The major differential diagnoses are conjunctivitis, corneal disorders, acute glaucoma, and acute uveitis (Table 7–1).

Ocular Discomfort

Ocular pain may be caused by trauma (chemical, mechanical, or physical), infection, inflammation, or sudden increase in intraocular pressure.

Foreign body sensation is most commonly due to corneal or conjunctival foreign bodies. Other causes are disturbances of the corneal epithelium and rubbing of eyelashes against the cornea (trichiasis).

Photophobia is commonly due to corneal inflammation, aphakia, iritis, or albinism. A less common cause is fever associated with viral infections.

Itching is characteristically associated with allergic eye disease.

Scratching and burning due to dryness of the eyes are common complaints of older people but may occur at any age. Deficiency of tear film components may be due to dry environment, local ocular disease, systemic disorders, or drugs (eg, atropine-like agents).

Watering is usually due to inadequate tear drainage through obstruction of the lacrimal drainage system or malposition of the lower lid. Reflex tearing occurs with any disturbance of the corneal epithelium.

"Eyestrain" & Headache

Eyestrain is a common complaint that usually means discomfort associated with prolonged reading or close work. Significant refractive error, presbyopia, inadequate illumination, and phoria (usually exophoria with poor convergence) should be ruled out. Headache is only occasionally due to ocular disorders, but these same conditions should be considered, as well as corneal inflammation, iritis, and acute glaucoma. Headache with scalp tenderness is a major feature of giant cell arteritis, which should always be considered in older patients.

Conjunctival Discharge

Purulent discharge usually indicates bacterial infection of the conjunctiva, cornea, or lacrimal sac. Viral conjunctivitis or keratitis produces watery discharge. Allergic conjunctivitis usually causes tearing and ropy discharge associated with itching.

Visual Loss

The most important causes of blurred vision are refractive error, cataract, macular degeneration, diabetic retinopathy, vitreous hemorrhage, retinal detachment involving the macula, central retinal vein occlusion, central retinal artery occlusion, corneal opacities, and optic nerve disorders.

Monocular field loss indicates disease of the retina or optic nerve. Important causes are retinal detachment, chronic glaucoma, branch retinal artery or vein occlusion, optic neuritis, and anterior ischemic optic neuropathy. (All these conditions may of course produce bilateral visual field loss.) Lesions of the optic chiasm due to pituitary tumors characteristically produce bitemporal field loss. Retrochiasmal lesions cause contralateral homonymous field defects. The more posterior the lesion in the visual pathway, the more congruous (similar in size, shape, and location) are the defects in the two eyes. Cerebrovascular disease and tumors are responsible for most lesions of the retrochiasmal visual pathways.

Visual Impairment & Blindness

An individual may be considered to be visually impaired if the best corrected distant visual acuity in the better eye is 20/80 or less or if visual fields are significantly restricted. Legal blindness (partial) in the USA is defined for practical purposes as visual acuity for distant vision of 20/200 or less in the better eye with best correction or widest diameter of the visual field subtending an angle of less than 20 degrees. There are approximately 500,000 legally blind people in the USA; about half are over the age of 65. The leading causes of blindness are glaucoma, diabetic retinopathy, and age-related macular degeneration.

Table 7–1. The inflamed eye: Differential diagnosis of common causes.

	Acute Conjunctivitis	Acute Uveitis	Acute Glaucoma[1]	Corneal Trauma or Infection
Incidence	Extremely common	Common	Uncommon	Common
Discharge	Moderate to copious	None	None	Watery or purulent
Vision	No effect on vision	Often blurred	Markedly blurred	Usually blurred
Pain	Mild	Moderate	Severe	Moderate to severe
Conjunctival injection	Diffuse; more toward fornices	Mainly circumcorneal	Mainly circumcorneal	Mainly circumcorneal
Cornea	Clear	Usually clear	Steamy	Clarify change related to cause
Pupil size	Normal	Small	Moderately dilated and fixed	Normal
Pupillary light response	Normal	Poor	None	Normal
Intraocular pressure	Normal	Commonly low but may be elevated	Elevated	Normal
Smear	Causative organisms	No organisms	No organisms	Organisms found only in corneal ulcers due to infection

[1]Angle-closure glaucoma.

The visual requirements for obtaining a driver's license in the USA vary from state to state. Most states require best corrected visual acuity with both eyes of 20/40 for a license with no restrictions. Licenses with specific restrictions may be available for those with poorer acuity. Some states also stipulate minimum visual field requirements. The Department of Motor Vehicles in each state will provide details of the visual requirements for licensing.

WHO estimates that at least 28 million of the world's population have vision of 10/200 or less, and millions more have loss of sight sufficient to interfere with normal living. The most frequent causes of blindness worldwide are cataract, trachoma, leprosy, onchocerciasis, and xerophthalmia.

Diplopia

Double vision usually results from extraocular muscle imbalance. This may be caused by disturbance of third, fourth, or sixth cranial nerve function by head injury, vascular disturbance, intracranial tumors, or intraorbital lesions; disease of the neuromuscular junction due to myasthenia; direct involvement of muscle as in dysthyroid eye disease; or entrapment as a result of orbital blowout fracture. Decompensation of a phoria (latent deviation) to a manifest deviation may also be responsible. Monocular diplopia, which persists when the fellow eye is covered, is usually due to lens opacities.

"Spots Before the Eyes" & "Flashing Lights"

Spots before the eyes (floaters) are usually caused by vitreous opacities that have no significance. However, they may also be caused by posterior vitreous detachment, vitreous hemorrhage, or posterior uveitis. Sudden onset of floaters, particularly when associated with flashing lights (photopsia), necessitates dilated fundal examination to exclude a retinal tear or detachment.

OCULAR EXAMINATION

Visual Acuity (VA)

Corrected distant visual acuity should be tested for each eye in turn, using a standardized chart such as the Snellen chart. If appropriate refractive correction is not available, a pinhole will overcome most refractive errors. The Snellen chart is annotated according to the distance at which each line can be read by a normal individual. Visual acuity is expressed as a fraction—the test distance over the figure assigned to the lowest line the patient can read. If the patient is unable to read the top line of the chart, acuity is recorded as counting fingers (CF), hand movements (HM), perception of light (PL), or no light perception (NLP). Distant acuity is usually measured at 20 feet. A corrected acuity of less than 20/30 is abnormal.

If assessment of distant visual acuity is not possible, near acuity should be tested with a reduced Snellen chart or standardized reading test types. The patient must be wearing an appropriate reading correction.

Visual Fields

Confrontation field testing is extremely valuable for rapid assessment of field defects. Use of a red target enhances the detection of neurologic field defects. Amsler charts are the easiest method of detecting central field abnormalities due to macular disease.

Pupils

The pupils should be examined for absolute and relative size and reactions to both light and accommodation. A large, poorly reacting pupil may be due to third nerve palsy, iris damage caused by acute glaucoma, or pharmacologic mydriasis. A small, poorly reacting pupil may be due to Horner's syndrome (oculosympathetic paralysis), inflammatory adhesions between iris and lens (posterior synechiae), or neurosyphilis (Argyll Robertson pupils). Physiologic anisocoria is a common cause of unequal pupils that react normally.

A relative afferent pupillary defect, in which the pupillary light reaction is of reduced intensity when light is shined into the affected eye compared to when light is shined into the normal eye, is an important objective sign that usually indicates optic nerve disease. It is most easily detected with the "swinging light test," in which the pupillary light reactions are compared as a bright light is moved from one eye to the other. It is only necessary to observe the pupillary reactions of one eye to detect the presence of a relative afferent pupillary defect.

Extraocular Movements

Examination of extraocular movements begins with the detection of any manifest deviation. (Manifest deviation is any deviation present when both eyes are open. Latent deviation is any additional deviation that then becomes apparent when one eye is covered.) This can be quickly achieved by comparing the relative positions of the corneal light reflexes. More accurate assessment requires a cover test in which the deviated eye moves to take up fixation when the other eye is occluded. This correctional movement is in a direction opposite to that of the original manifest deviation. (This movement may not occur if the deviated eye is poorly sighted.)

Horizontal diplopia indicates dysfunction of horizontally acting muscles (medial and lateral recti), and vertical diplopia indicates dysfunction of vertically acting muscles (superior and inferior recti and the obliques). The false outer image arises from the affected eye. If a muscle is underacting, the image separation will be greatest in its normal direction of action. If a muscle is prevented from relaxing, image separation will be greatest in the direction opposite to its normal action. For example, a paretic lateral rectus or a tethered medial rectus of the right eye will cause maximal image separation on looking to the right.

Minor degrees of nystagmus at the extremes of gaze are normal. Other forms of physiologic nystagmus include optokinetic nystagmus and those induced by rotation or caloric stimulation. Exaggerated gaze-evoked nystagmus may be due to drugs or posterior fossa disease. Nystagmus in the primary position is always abnormal. Certain acquired forms specifically localize lesions within the nervous system.

Congenital nystagmus may be a benign isolated anomaly or associated with poor vision.

Proptosis (Exophthalmos)

Proptosis may be suspected by observing widening of the palpebral aperture, with exposure of sclera both superiorly and inferiorly. (Eyelid retraction generally causes more exposure superiorly than inferiorly.) By viewing the patient from above, while the patient is asked to look down and the upper lids are lifted by the examiner, a further estimate of the degree of proptosis can be made. Exophthalmometry should be performed for objective assessment. In nonaxial proptosis, there is also horizontal or vertical displacement of the globe, indicating the presence of a mass lesion outside the extraocular muscle cone.

The most frequent cause of proptosis in adults is dysthyroid eye disease. Other causes of (usually unilateral) proptosis include cellulitis, tumors, and pseudotumor of the orbit.

Ptosis

Neurologic causes of ptosis include third nerve palsy and Horner's syndrome, which are differentiated by pupil size. Local causes include congenital and acquired disorders of the levator muscle complex and tumors and infections of the eyelid. Myasthenia should always be considered.

Anterior Segment Examination

Although slit lamp examination is recommended for accurate documentation of anterior segment abnormalities, examination with a flashlight and loupe usually provides sufficient information for initial diagnosis. Patterns of redness indicate the site of the underlying problem. Conjunctivitis produces redness that extends diffusely across the globe and the inner surface of the lids. Keratitis, intraocular inflammation, and acute glaucoma produce predominantly circumcorneal injection. Episcleritis and scleritis cause localized or diffuse deep injection, which in the case of scleritis is associated with blue discoloration.

Focal lesions of the cornea due to infection or trauma can be differentiated from the diffuse corneal haze of acute glaucoma and from the cloudiness of the anterior chamber and perhaps hypopyon (accumulation of white cells within the anterior chamber) of iritis. Instillation of fluorescein and examination with a blue light aids in detection of corneal epithelial defects. Palpation of the globe will reveal the stony hardness of acute glaucoma.

Direct Ophthalmoscopy

Direct ophthalmoscopy is principally used for examining the retina, but much other useful information can also be gained. Assessment of the red reflex and clarity of fundal details indicates the degree of media opacity. Abnormalities may then be localized to the cornea, lens, or vitreous by variations of focus of the ophthalmoscope and use of parallax.

The optic disk should be examined for swelling, pallor, and glaucomatous cupping. Macular lesions causing poor central vision are usually apparent. The retinal vessels are examined for caliber and wall changes. Retinal hemorrhages, exudates, and cotton-wool spots should be noted.

Dilation of the pupil aids direct ophthalmoscopy but should be done with caution in patients with shallow anterior chambers.

OPHTHALMOLOGIC REFERRALS

Sudden loss of vision is a serious symptom requiring urgent or emergency ophthalmologic consultation. The most important causes of sudden visual loss in an uninflamed eye are vitreous hemorrhage, retinal detachment, exudative age-related macular degeneration, retinal vein occlusions, retinal artery occlusions, anterior ischemic optic neuropathy, and optic neuritis. Sudden visual loss in an inflamed eye may be due to acute anterior uveitis, acute glaucoma, or corneal ulcer. Other ophthalmologic emergencies include orbital cellulitis, gonococcal keratoconjunctivitis, and major ocular trauma.

Any patient developing gradual loss of vision should be referred for ophthalmologic assessment. Important causes include cataract, atrophic age-related macular degeneration, chronic glaucoma, chronic uveitis, and intraorbital and intracranial tumors.

Patients with diabetes mellitus must undergo regular fundus examination through dilated pupils. Myopic patients should be warned of the increased risk of retinal detachment and made aware of the importance of reporting relevant symptoms. Close relatives of patients with chronic glaucoma should be encouraged to undergo annual glaucoma screening once they have reached adulthood.

REFRACTIVE ERRORS

Refractive errors are the most common cause of blurred vision. In **emmetropia** (the normal state), objects at infinity are seen clearly with the unaccommodated eye. Objects nearer than infinity are seen with the aid of accommodation, which increases the refractive power of the lens. In **hyperopia,** objects at infinity are not seen clearly unless accommodation is used, and near objects may not be seen because accommodative capacity is finite. Hyperopia is corrected with plus (convex) lenses. In **myopia,** the unaccommodated eye brings to a focus images of objects closer than infinity, the distance of such objects from the patient becoming shorter and shorter with increasing myopia. (Thus, the high myope is

able to focus on very near objects without glasses.) However, objects beyond this distance cannot be seen without the aid of corrective (minus, concave) lenses. In **astigmatism,** the refractive errors in the horizontal and vertical axes differ. Various surgical techniques are available for the correction of refractive errors, particularly myopia. Photorefractive keratectomy, in which the excimer laser is used to reshape the anterior cornea, is becoming the most widely used. **Presbyopia** is the natural loss of accommodative capacity with age. Emmetropes usually notice inability to focus on objects at a normal reading distance at about age 45. Hyperopes experience symptoms at an earlier age. Presbyopia is corrected with plus lenses for near work.

Use of a pinhole will overcome most refractive errors and thus allows their exclusion as a cause of visual loss. Transient refractive errors occur in diabetes—often when diabetic control is erratic—and may be the presenting feature. Autoinoculation of scopolamine from seasickness patches or atropine from vials for parenteral use leads to pupillary dilatation and loss of accommodation.

Bechara SJ, Thompson KP, Waring GO: Surgical correction of nearsightedness. Br Med J 1992;305:813.

Gartry DS, Kerr Muir MG, Marshall J: Excimer laser photorefractive keratectomy: 18-month follow-up. Ophthalmology 1992;99:1209.

Gartry DS et al: The effect of topical corticosteroids on refractive outcome and corneal haze after photorefractive keratectomy: A prospective, randomized, double-blind study. Arch Ophthalmol 1992;110:944.

(Two studies from the group with the longest published follow-up of the procedure.)

Contact Lenses

Contact lenses are increasingly being used for correction of refractive errors (cosmetic contact lenses) in addition to their well-established but much less frequent use in the management of diseases of the cornea, conjunctiva, or lids (therapeutic contact lenses). It has been estimated that in 1987 there were 18 million contact lens wearers in the USA.

The various types of contact lenses are hard lenses made of polymethylmethacrylate (PMMA), rigid gas-permeable lenses made of cellulose acetate butyrate (CAB) or silicone acrylates, and soft or hydrogel lenses based on hydroxyethylmethacrylate (HEMA). Hard lenses are much more durable and easy to care for than soft lenses but are more difficult to tolerate. Rigid gas-permeable lenses are an effective compromise.

Contact lens care includes cleaning and sterilization whenever the lenses are removed and removal of protein deposits as required. Contact lens sterilization may involve thermal or chemical methods. For individuals developing reactions to preservatives in contact lens solutions, various preservative-free systems are available. All contact lenses can be used on a daily-wear basis, ie, they are inserted in the morning and removed at night. Soft lenses are also available for extended wear (ie, overnight). Disposable soft lenses to avoid the necessity for lens cleaning and sterilization are available for daily wear or extended wear.

The major risk from contact lens wear is corneal ulceration, which is potentially a blinding condition. Among the contact lens wearers in the USA, there are an estimated 12,000 corneal ulcers per year. Soft lenses present the major hazard, particularly with extended wear, for which there is an approximately ten-fold greater risk of corneal ulceration compared with daily wear. The increased risk from extended wear begins with the first night of overnight wear and increases progressively thereafter. Disposable lenses do not overcome the risk of corneal ulceration. Preservative-free cleaning systems particularly predispose to *Acanthamoeba* keratitis.

It is essential that cosmetic contact lens wearers be made aware of the risks they face and ways to minimize them, such as avoiding extended-wear soft lenses and maintaining meticulous lens hygiene. Whenever there is ocular discomfort or redness, contact lenses should be removed. If symptoms do not resolve, immediate ophthalmologic care should be sought.

Dart JKG: Diseases and risks associated with contact lenses. Br J Ophthalmol 1993;77:49.

Poggio EC et al: The incidence of ulcerative keratitis among users of daily-wear and extended-wear soft contact lenses. N Engl J Med 1989;321:779.

Schein OD et al: The relative risk of ulcerative keratitis among users of daily-wear and extended-wear soft contact lenses: A case-control study. N Engl J Med 1989; 321:773.

(Three articles from the USA and England detailing the risks of corneal ulceration in contact lens wearers.)

DISORDERS OF THE LIDS & LACRIMAL APPARATUS

Hordeolum

Hordeolum is a common staphylococcal abscess that is characterized by a localized red, swollen, acutely tender area on the upper or lower lid. Internal hordeolum is a meibomian gland abscess that points onto the conjunctival surface of the lid; external hordeolum or sty (infection of the glands of Moll or Zeis) is smaller and on the margin. The chief symptom is pain of an intensity directly related to the amount of swelling.

Warm compresses are helpful. Incision is indicated if resolution does not begin within 48 hours. An antibiotic ointment (bacitracin or erythromycin) instilled into the conjunctival sac every 3 hours may be beneficial during the acute stage. Internal hordeolum may lead to generalized cellulitis of the lid.

Chalazion

Chalazion is a common granulomatous inflammation of a meibomian gland that may follow an internal hordeolum. It is characterized by a hard, nontender swelling on the upper or lower lid. The conjunctiva in the region of the chalazion is red and elevated. If the chalazion is large enough to impress the cornea, vision will be distorted.

Incision and curettage is done by an ophthalmologist.

Tumors

Verrucae and papillomas of the skin of the lids can often be excised by the general physician if they do not involve the lid margin; otherwise, surgery should be performed by an ophthalmologist so as to avoid permanent notching of the lid. Cancer—including basal cell carcinoma, squamous cell carcinoma, meibomian gland carcinoma, and malignant melanoma—should be ruled out by microscopic examination of the excised material.

Blepharitis

Blepharitis is a common chronic bilateral inflammation of the lid margins. Anterior blepharitis involves the eyelid skin, eyelashes, and associated glands. It may be ulcerative, because of infection by staphylococci; or seborrheic, which is almost always associated with seborrhea of the scalp, brows, and ears. Both types are commonly present. Posterior blepharitis is inflammation of the eyelids secondary to dysfunction of the meibomian glands. There may be bacterial infection, particularly with staphylococci, or a primary glandular dysfunction, in which there is a strong association with acne rosacea.

Symptoms are irritation, burning, and itching. In anterior blepharitis, the eyes are "red-rimmed," and scales or "granulations" can be seen clinging to the lashes. In the staphylococcal type, the scales are dry, the lid margins are red and ulcerated, and the lashes tend to fall out; in the seborrheic type, the scales are greasy, ulceration is absent, and the margins are less red. In the more common mixed, type, both dry and greasy scales are present and the lid margins are red and may be ulcerated. In posterior blepharitis, the lid margins are hyperemic with telangiectasias; the meibomian glands and their orifices are inflamed, with dilation of the glands, plugging of the orifices, and abnormal secretions. The lid margin is frequently rolled inward to produce a mild entropion, and the tears may be frothy or abnormally greasy.

Both anterior and, more particularly, posterior blepharitis may be complicated by hordeola, chalazions; abnormal lid or lash positions, producing trichiasis; recurrent conjunctivitis, epithelial keratitis of the lower third of the cornea, marginal corneal infiltrates, and inferior corneal vascularization and thinning.

In anterior blepharitis, cleanliness of the scalp,

eyebrows, and lid margins is essential to effective local therapy. Scales must be removed from the lids daily with a damp cotton applicator and baby shampoo. An antistaphylococcal antibiotic eye ointment such as bacitracin or erythromycin is applied daily to the lid margins with a cotton-tipped applicator. Antibiotic sensitivity studies may be required in severe staphylococcal blepharitis.

In mild posterior blepharitis, regular meibomian gland expression may be sufficient to control symptoms. Inflammation of the conjunctiva and cornea indicates a need for more active treatment, including long-term low-dose systemic antibiotic therapy, usually with tetracycline (250 mg twice daily) or erythromycin (250 mg three times daily), and short-term topical steroids, eg, prednisolone, 0.125% twice daily. Topical therapy with antibiotics may be helpful but should be restricted to short courses because of the risk of toxicity reactions.

Entropion & Ectropion

Entropion (inward turning of usually the lower lid) occurs occasionally in older people as a result of degeneration of the lid fascia, or may follow extensive scarring of the conjunctiva and tarsus. Surgery is indicated if the lashes rub on the cornea.

Ectropion (outward turning of the lower lid) is fairly common in elderly people. Surgery is indicated if ectropion causes excessive tearing, exposure keratitis, or a cosmetic problem.

Dacryocystitis

Dacryocystitis is infection of the lacrimal sac due to obstruction of the nasolacrimal system. It may be acute or chronic and occurs most often in infants and in persons over 40. It is usually unilateral.

In acute dacryocystitis, the usual infectious organisms are S aureus and β-hemolytic streptococci; in chronic dacryocystitis, Streptococcus pneumoniae (rarely, Candida albicans). Mixed infections do not occur.

Acute dacryocystitis is characterized by pain, swelling, tenderness, and redness in the tear sac area; purulent material may be expressed. In chronic dacryocystitis, tearing and discharge are the principal signs. Mucus or pus may be expressed from the tear sac.

Acute dacryocystitis responds well to systemic antibiotic therapy, but recurrences are common if the obstruction is not surgically removed. The chronic form may be kept latent by using antibiotic drugs, but surgical relief of the obstruction is the only cure.

CONJUNCTIVITIS

Conjunctivitis is the most common eye disease. It may be acute or chronic. Most cases are due to bacterial (including chlamydial) or viral infection. Other causes include keratoconjunctivitis sicca, allergy, and chemical irritants. The mode of transmission of infectious conjunctivitis is usually direct contact via fingers, towels, handkerchiefs, etc, to the fellow eye or to other persons.

Conjunctivitis must be differentiated from acute uveitis, acute glaucoma, and corneal disorders (Table 7–1).

Bacterial Conjunctivitis

The organisms found most commonly in bacterial conjunctivitis are staphylococci, streptococci (particularly S pneumoniae), Haemophilus spp, Pseudomonas spp, and Moraxella spp. All may produce a copious purulent discharge. There is no blurring of vision and only mild discomfort. In severe cases, examination of stained conjunctival scrapings and culture studies are recommended.

The disease is usually self-limited, lasting about 10–14 days if untreated. A sulfonamide (eg, sulfacetamide, 10% ophthalmic solution or ointment) instilled locally three times daily will usually clear the infection in 2–3 days.

Gonococcal Conjunctivitis

Gonococcal conjunctivitis, usually acquired through contact with infected genital secretions, is manifested by a copious purulent discharge. It is an ophthalmologic emergency because corneal involvement may rapidly lead to perforation. The diagnosis should be confirmed by stained smear and culture of the discharge. If the cornea is not involved, a single intramuscular dose of ceftriaxone, 1 g, is effective. When the cornea is involved, a 5-day course of parenteral ceftriaxone, 1–2 g daily, is required. Topical treatment should include frequent saline lavage. Topical antibiotics, such as erythromycin and bacitracin, may also be used, particularly if the cornea is involved. All patients should be screened for other sexually transmitted diseases, including chlamydiosis, syphilis, and HIV infection.

Haimovici R, Roussel TJ: Treatment of gonococcal conjunctivitis with single-dose intramuscular ceftriaxone. Am J Ophthalmol 1989;107:511. (Clinical and microbiologic cure in patients without corneal involvement.)

Chlamydial Keratoconjunctivitis

A. Trachoma: Trachoma is a major cause of blindness worldwide. Recurrent episodes of infection in childhood are manifest as bilateral follicular conjunctivitis, epithelial keratitis, and corneal vascularization (pannus). Cicatrization of the tarsal conjunctiva leads to entropion and trichiasis in adulthood, with secondary central corneal scarring.

The specific diagnosis can be made in Giemsa-stained conjunctival scrapings. Treatment should be started on the basis of clinical findings without waiting for laboratory confirmation. Oral tetracycline or erythromycin, 250 mg six times a day, or doxycycline, 100 mg twice a day, is given for 3–5 weeks. Local treatment is not necessary. *Caution:* Tetracyclines are contraindicated during pregnancy and in young children. Surgical treatment includes correction of eyelid deformities and corneal transplantation.

B. Inclusion Conjunctivitis: The agent of inclusion conjunctivitis is a common cause of genital tract disease in adults. The eye is usually involved following accidental contact with genital secretions. Adult inclusion conjunctivitis thus occurs most frequently in sexually active young adults. The disease starts with acute redness, discharge, and irritation. The eye findings consist of follicular conjunctivitis with mild keratitis. A nontender preauricular lymph node can often be palpated. Healing usually leaves no sequelae. Cytologic examination of conjunctival scrapings shows a picture similar to that of trachoma. Treatment is with oral tetracycline or erythromycin, 250–500 mg four times a day, or doxycycline, 300 mg initially followed by 100 mg once a day, for 2 weeks. Before treatment, all cases should be appropriately assessed for genital tract infection so that management can be adjusted accordingly.

Viral Conjunctivitis

One of the most common causes of viral conjunctivitis is adenovirus type 3. Conjunctivitis due to this agent is usually associated with pharyngitis, fever, malaise, and preauricular adenopathy (pharyngoconjunctival fever). Locally, the palpebral conjunctiva is red, and there is a copious watery discharge and scanty exudate. Children are more often affected than adults, and contaminated swimming pools are sometimes the source of infection. Epidemic keratoconjunctivitis is caused by adenovirus types 8 and 19. It is more likely to be complicated by visual loss due to corneal subepithelial infiltrates. There is no specific treatment for viral conjunctivitis, though local sulfonamide therapy may prevent secondary bacterial infection, hot compresses reduce the discomfort of the associated lid edema, and weak topical steroids (eg, prednisolone, 0.125% four times daily), may be necessary to treat the corneal infiltrates. The disease usually lasts at least 2 weeks.

Keratoconjunctivitis Sicca

This is a common disorder, particularly in elderly women. A wide range of conditions predispose to or are characterized by dry eyes. Hypofunction of the lacrimal glands, causing loss of the aqueous component of tears, may be due to aging, hereditary disorders, systemic disease (eg, rheumatoid arthritis and other autoimmune disorders), or systemic and topical drugs. Excessive evaporation of tears may be due to environmental factors (eg, a hot, dry, or windy climate) or abnormalities of the lipid component of the tear film, as in blepharitis. Mucin deficiency may be due to malnutrition, infection, burns, or drugs.

The patient complains of dryness, redness, or a scratchy feeling of the eyes. In severe cases there is persistent marked discomfort, with photophobia, difficulty in moving the eyelids, and often excessive mucus secretion. In many cases, gross examination reveals no abnormality, but on slit lamp examination there are subtle abnormalities of tear film stability and reduced volume of the tear film meniscus along the lower lid. In more severe cases, damaged corneal and conjunctival cells stain with 1% rose bengal. (Rose bengal staining should be avoided in severe cases because of the intense pain it may cause.) In the most severe cases there is marked conjunctival injection, loss of the normal conjunctival and corneal luster, epithelial keratitis that may progress to frank ulceration, and mucous strands. Schirmer's test, which measures the rate of production of the aqueous component of tears by the amount of wetting of filter paper strips during a 5-minute period, may be helpful when the diagnosis is in doubt, but false-positive and false-negative results are frequent.

Treatment depends upon the cause. In most early cases, the corneal and conjunctival epithelial changes are reversible. Aqueous deficiency can be treated by replacement of the aqueous component of tears with various types of artificial tears. The simplest preparations are physiologic (0.9%) or hypo-osmotic (0.45%) solutions of sodium chloride. Balanced salt solution is a more physiologic but also more expensive preparation. All these drop preparations can be used as frequently as every half-hour but in most cases are needed only three or four times a day. More prolonged duration of action can be achieved with drop preparations containing methylcellulose (eg, Isopto Plain) or polyvinyl alcohol (eg, Liquifilm Tears or Hypo Tears) or by using petrolatum ointment (Lacri-Lube). Such mucomimetics are particularly indicated when there is mucin deficiency. Artificial tear preparations are generally very safe and without side effects. However, the preservatives necessary to maintain their sterility are potentially toxic and allergenic and may cause keratitis and cicatrizing conjunctivitis in frequent users. Furthermore, the development of such reactions may be misinterpreted by both the patient and the doctor as a worsening of the dry eye state requiring more frequent use of the artificial tears and leading in turn to further deterioration, rather than being recognized as a need to change to a preservative-free preparation. If the mucus is tenacious, mucolytic agents (eg, acetylcysteine, 20% six times a day) may provide some relief. Blepharitis should be treated appropriately (see above).

Allergic Eye Disease

Allergic eye disease takes a number of different forms, but all are expressions of an atopic diathesis, which may also be manifested as atopic asthma, atopic dermatitis, or allergic rhinitis. Symptoms include itching, tearing, redness, stringy discharge, and, in the more severe forms, photophobia and visual loss.

Allergic conjunctivitis is a benign disease, occurring usually in late childhood and early adulthood. It may be seasonal (hay fever conjunctivitis), developing usually during the spring or summer, or perennial. Clinical signs are limited to conjunctival hyperemia and edema (chemosis), the latter occasionally being so marked and sudden in onset as to cause alarm. Vernal keratoconjunctivitis also tends to occur in late childhood and early adulthood. It is usually seasonal, with a predilection for the spring. The conjunctivitis is characterized by large "cobblestone" papillae on the upper tarsal conjunctiva. There may be lymphoid follicles at the limbus. Atopic keratoconjunctivitis is a more chronic disorder of adulthood. Both the upper and the lower tarsal conjunctiva exhibit a fine papillary conjunctivitis with fibrosis, resulting in forniceal shortening and entropion with trichiasis. Staphylococcal blepharitis is a frequent complicating factor. Corneal involvement, including refractory ulceration, is frequent during acute exacerbations of both vernal and atopic keratoconjunctivitis. They are also commonly complicated by herpes simplex keratitis.

Topical cromolyn sodium four times a day is the mainstay of treatment in allergic eye disease, being both safe and effective. It is best used continuously while the disease is likely to develop and not just as treatment for acute episodes. Topical vasoconstrictors and antihistamines are advocated in hay fever conjunctivitis but are of limited efficacy and may produce rebound hyperemia. Systemic antihistamines may be useful in atopic keratoconjunctivitis when the prolonged, severe nature of the disease justifies the systemic side effects. Topical corticosteroids are essential to the control of acute exacerbations of both vernal and atopic keratoconjunctivitis. Steroid-induced side effects, including cataracts, glaucoma, and exacerbation of herpes simplex keratitis, are major problems. Whether topical corticosteroid therapy is justifiable in allergic conjunctivitis is debatable. Systemic steroid therapy and even plasmapharesis may be required in severe atopic keratoconjunctivitis. In allergic conjunctivitis specific allergens may be identifiable and thus avoidable. In vernal keratoconjunctivitis, a cooler climate often provides significant benefit.

Foster CS: The Cromolyn Sodium Collaborative Study Group: Evaluation of topical cromolyn sodium in the treatment of vernal keratoconjunctivitis. Ophthalmology 1988;95:194. (Clinical efficacy and minimal side effects of cromolyn sodium)
Foster CS, Calonge M: Atopic keratoconjunctivitis. Ophthalmology 1990;97:992. (Potentially serious nature of the disease.)
Friedlaender MH: Immunologic aspects of diseases of the eye. JAMA 1992;268:2869. (Pathogenesis and manifestations of all forms of immunologic disease affecting the eye.)

PINGUECULA & PTERYGIUM

Pinguecula is a yellow elevated nodule on either side of the cornea (more commonly on the nasal side) in the area of the palpebral fissure. It is common in persons over age 35.

Pterygium is a fleshy, triangular encroachment of the conjunctiva onto the nasal side of the cornea and is usually associated with constant exposure to wind, sun, sand, and dust. Pterygium may be either unilateral or bilateral. There may be a genetic predisposition, but no hereditary pattern has been described. Pterygium is fairly common in the southwestern USA.

Histologically, pinguecula and pterygium show similar features of which the most important is elastoid degeneration of the conjunctival substantia propria.

Pingueculae rarely grow, but inflammation (pingueculitis) may occur. No treatment is indicated.

Excision of a pterygium is indicated if the growth threatens to interfere with vision by approaching the visual axis. Recurrences are frequent and often more aggressive than the primary lesion. Various forms of treatment are available to reduce the frequency of recurrence.

MacKenzie FD et al: Recurrence rate and complications after beta irradiation for pterygia. Ophthalmology 1991;98:1776.
Rubinfeld RS et al: Serious complications of topical mitomycin-C after pterygium surgery. Ophthalmology 1992;99;1647.
Singh G, Wilson MR, Foster CS: Long-term follow-up study of mitomycin eye drops as adjunctive treatment for pterygia and its comparison with conjunctival autograft transplantation. Cornea 1990;9:331.
(A series of articles outlining the main methods of reducing the recurrence rate after pterygium surgery and their respective complications.)

CORNEAL ULCER

Corneal ulcers are most commonly due to infection, which may involve bacteria, viruses, fungi, or amebas. Noninfectious causes—all of which may be complicated by infection—include neurotrophic keratitis (resulting from loss of corneal sensation), exposure keratitis (due to inadequate eyelid closure), severe dry eyes, severe allergic eye disease, and various inflammatory disorders, that may be purely ocular or part of a systemic vasculitis. These noninfectious conditions will not be discussed further.

Delayed or ineffective treatment of corneal infection may lead to devastating consequences through intraocular infection or corneal scarring. Prompt effective treatment is essential, and for that reason patients must be referred immediately to an ophthalmologist.

Patients present with pain, photophobia, tearing, and reduced vision. The eye is red, with predominantly circumcorneal injection, and there may be purulent or watery discharge. The corneal appearance varies according to the organisms involved, of which the major types will be discussed.

Bacterial Keratitis

Bacterial keratitis tends to pursue an aggressive course. Precipitating factors include contact lens wear, especially soft contact lenses worn overnight, and corneal trauma. The pathogens most commonly isolated are *Pseudomonas aeruginosa,* pneumococcus, *Moraxella* sp, and staphylococci. The cornea is hazy, with a central ulcer and adjacent stromal abscess. Sterile hypopyon is often present. The ulcer should be scraped to recover material for Gram's stain and culture prior to starting treatment with high-concentration (fortified) topical antibiotics, given at least every hour night and day for the first 24 hours. The initial choice of antibiotics is based on the Gram stain result. For example, gram-positive cocci are treated with a cephalosporin, such as cefazolin, 50 mg/mL; and gram-negative bacilli are treated with an aminoglycoside, such as gentamicin, 10 mg/mL. If no organisms are seen, these two agents are used in parallel.

Herpes Simplex Keratitis

Herpes simplex keratitis is an important cause of ocular morbidity, particularly in adults of working age. The ability of the virus to colonize the trigeminal ganglion leads to recurrences that may be precipitated by specifically identifiable forms of stress such as fever and excessive exposure to sunlight.

The dendritic (branching) ulcer is the most characteristic manifestation of epithelial keratitis due to the herpes simplex virus. More extensive ("geographic") ulcers may also occur, particularly if topical corticosteroids have been used. These ulcers are most easily seen after instillation of sterile fluorescein and examination with a blue light. Epithelial disease in itself does not lead to corneal scarring. It responds well to simple debridement and patching. More rapid healing can be achieved by the addition of topical antivirals. Trifluridine drops or idoxuridine drops or ointment are used every 2 hours during the day. Acyclovir ophthalmic ointment is still not commercially available in the USA. Topical corticosteroids must not be used.

Stromal herpes simplex keratitis produces increasingly severe corneal opacity and irregularity with each recurrence. Topical corticosteroids are frequently used in combination with topical antivirals to control stromal disease, but steroid dependence is a common consequence. Corticosteroids may also enhance viral replication, leading to severe epithelial disease. Whether topical antivirals alone are sufficient to fully control stromal disease has yet to be demonstrated. Oral acyclovir, 200–400 mg five times

a day, may be effective for the treatment of severe herpetic keratitis and for prophylaxis against recurrences, particularly in atopic individuals who are prone to severe herpetic keratitis. *Caution:* For patients with known or possible herpetic disease, topical corticosteroids should be prescribed only under strict ophthalmologic supervision.

Margolis TP, Ostler HB: Treatment of ocular disease in eczema herpeticum. Am J Ophthalmol 1990;110:274. (Management in atopes.)

Porter SM, Patterson A, Kho P: A comparison of local and systemic acyclovir in the management of herpetic disciform keratitis. Br J Ophthalmol 1990;74:283.

Schwab IR: Oral acyclovir in the management of herpes simplex ocular infections. Ophthalmology 1988;95:423. (Two studies showing useful effects from oral acyclovir in recalcitrant herpes simplex infections of the cornea.)

Fungal Keratitis

Fungal keratitis tends to occur after corneal injury involving plant material or in an agricultural setting and in immunocompromised patients. There is often an indolent course. The cornea characteristically has multiple stromal abscesses with relatively little epithelial loss. Intraocular infection is common. Corneal scrapings must be cultured on media suitable for fungi whenever the history or corneal appearance is suggestive of fungal disease.

Acanthamoeba Keratitis

Acanthamoeba has recently become a more commonly recognized cause of suppurative keratitis in contact lens wearers, particularly those who use homemade saline solutions. Although severe pain and perineural and ring infiltrates in the corneal stroma are characteristic features, earlier forms of the disease with changes confined to the corneal epithelium are being recognized. Culture requires specialized media. Treatment is severely hampered by the organism's ability to encyst within the corneal stroma. Various agents have been used, including the investigational agent propamidine isethionate, neomycin-polymyxin-gramicidin, and various oral and topical imidazoles such as ketoconazole, miconazole, and itraconazole. Epithelial debridement may be useful in early infections. Corneal grafting may be required in the acute stage to arrest the progression of infection or after resolution of the infection to restore vision.

Berger ST et al: Successful medical management of *Acanthamoeba* keratitis. Am J Ophthalmol 1990;110:395. (Six out of seven patients cured with prolonged and intensive triple antiamebic therapy.)

Lindquist TD, Sher NA, Doughman DJ: Clinical signs and medical therapy of early *Acanthamoeba* keratitis. Arch Ophthalmol 1988;106:73.

Herpes Zoster Ophthalmicus

Herpes zoster frequently involves the ophthalmic division of the trigeminal nerve. It presents with malaise, fever, headache, and burning and itching in the periorbital region. The rash is initially vesicular, quickly becoming pustular and then crusting. Involvement of the tip of the nose or the lid margins indicates a high likelihood of intraocular involvement. Ocular signs include conjunctivitis, keratitis, episcleritis, and anterior uveitis, often with elevated intraocular pressure. Recurrent anterior segment inflammation, neurotrophic keratitis, and posterior subcapsular cataract are possible long-term effects. Optic neuropathy, cranial nerve palsies, acute retinal necrosis, and cerebral angiitis are infrequent complications of the acute stage.

Treatment with high-dose oral acyclovir (800 mg five times a day for 10 days, started within 72 hours after eruption of the rash) reduces the incidence of ocular complications but not of postherpetic neuralgia. Anterior uveitis requires topical steroids and cycloplegics.

Liesegang TJ: Diagnosis and therapy of herpes zoster ophthalmicus. Ophthalmology 1991;98:1216. (Emphasis on pathogenesis.)

ACUTE (ANGLE-CLOSURE) GLAUCOMA

Essentials of Diagnosis

- Rapid onset in older age groups, particularly hyperopes and Asians.
- Severe pain and profound visual loss.
- Red eye, steamy cornea, dilated pupil.
- Hard eye.

General Considerations

Primary acute angle-closure glaucoma can occur only with closure of a preexisting narrow anterior chamber angle, as is found in elderly persons (owing to physiologic enlargement of the lens), hyperopes, and Asians. About 1% of people over age 35 have narrow anterior chamber angles, but many of these never develop acute glaucoma; thus, the condition is uncommon. Angle closure is associated with pupillary dilation and thus might occur with sitting in a darkened movie theater, at times of stress (owing to increased circulating epinephrine), and with pharmacologic mydriasis for ophthalmoscopic examination or incidentally with systemic anticholinergic medications such as atropine (eg, preoperative medication). Dilation of the pupil should be undertaken with caution if the anterior chamber is shallow (readily determined by oblique illumination of the anterior segment of the eye).

Acute angle-closure glaucoma may also occur secondary to long-standing anterior uveitis or dislocation of the lens. Symptoms are the same as in primary acute angle-closure glaucoma, but differentiation is important because of differences in management.

Clinical Findings

Patients with acute glaucoma usually seek treatment immediately because of extreme pain and blurred vision, though there are subacute cases in which presentation is delayed. The blurred vision is characteristically associated with halos around lights. Nausea and even abdominal pain may occur, and for this reason acute glaucoma must be remembered in the differential diagnosis of abdominal pain and vomiting in elderly patients. The eye is red, the cornea steamy, and the pupil moderately dilated and nonreactive to light. Tonometry (or palpation of the globe) reveals elevated intraocular pressure.

Differential Diagnosis

Acute glaucoma must be differentiated from conjunctivitis, acute uveitis, and corneal disorders (Table 7–1).

Treatment

A. Primary: In primary acute angle-closure glaucoma, laser peripheral iridectomy will usually result in permanent cure. Intraocular pressure must be lowered preoperatively. A single 500 mg intravenous dose of acetazolamide, followed by 250 mg orally four times a day, is usually sufficient. Osmotic diuretics, such as oral glycerol and intravenous urea or mannitol—the dosage of all three being 1–2 g/kg—can be used if necessary. Once the intraocular pressure has started to fall, topical 4% pilocarpine, 1 drop every 15 minutes for 1 hour and then four times a day, is used to treat the underlying angle closure. The fellow eye should be dealt with by prophylactic iridectomy.

B. Secondary: In secondary acute angle-closure glaucoma, systemic acetazolamide is also used, with or without osmotic agents, to control intraocular pressure. Further treatment is determined by the underlying pathogenesis.

Prognosis

Untreated acute glaucoma results in severe and permanent visual loss within 2–5 days after onset of symptoms.

OPEN-ANGLE GLAUCOMA

Essentials of Diagnosis

- Insidious onset in older age groups.
- No symptoms in early stages.
- Gradual loss of peripheral vision over a period of years, resulting in tunnel vision.
- Persistent elevation of intraocular pressure associated with pathologic cupping of the optic disks.

- "Halos around lights" are not present unless the intraocular tension is markedly elevated.

General Considerations

In open-angle glaucoma, the intraocular pressure is consistently elevated. Over a period of months or years, this results in optic atrophy with loss of vision varying from slight constriction of the upper nasal peripheral fields to complete blindness.

The cause of the decreased rate of aqueous outflow in open-angle glaucoma has not been clearly established. The disease is bilateral and is genetically determined, multifactorial, with no clear inheritance pattern. Glaucoma occurs at an earlier age and more frequently in blacks and may result in more severe optic nerve damage. There is increasing evidence that factors other than the level of intraocular pressure—particularly vascular abnormalities—may play a role in certain individuals in the pathogenesis of glaucomatous optic nerve damage.

In the USA, it is estimated that 1–2% of people over 40 have glaucoma; about 25% of these cases are undetected. About 90% of all cases of glaucoma are of the open-angle type.

Clinical Findings

Patients with open-angle glaucoma have no symptoms initially. On examination, there may be slight cupping of the optic disk observed as an absolute increase—or an asymmetry between the two eyes—of the ratio of the diameter of the optic cup to the diameter of the whole optic disk (cup-to-disk ratio). Changes in the retinal nerve fiber layer may be observed as an earlier finding in some patients. The visual fields gradually constrict, but central vision remains good until late in the disease.

Tonometry, ophthalmoscopic visualization of the optic nerve, and central visual field testing are the three prime tests for the diagnosis and continued evaluation of glaucoma. The normal intraocular pressure is about 10–21 mm Hg. Except in acute glaucoma, however, the diagnosis is never made on the basis of one tonometric measurement, since various factors can influence the pressure (eg, diurnal variation). Transient elevations of intraocular pressure do not constitute glaucoma (for the same reason that periodic or intermittent elevations of blood pressure do not constitute hypertensive disease). Field testing may prove unreliable in some patients.

Prevention

All persons over age 40, particularly blacks, should have tonometric and ophthalmoscopic examinations every 3–5 years. If there is a family history of glaucoma, more frequent examination is indicated.

Treatment

Timolol, a β-adrenergic blocking agent, is an effective antiglaucoma agent in a dosage of 1 drop of 0.25% or 0.5% solution every 12 hours. Alternative agents are levobunolol, 0.5%, and metipranolol, 0.1–0.6%, each used twice daily. They should not be used in patients with reactive airway disease or heart failure. Betaxolol, 0.25% or 0.5%, a β_1-receptor selective blocking agent, may be safer in patients with reactive airway disease. Epinephrine eye drops, 0.5–1%, or the prodrug dipivefrin, 0.1%, may be used twice a day either alone or in combination with betaxolol (to overcome the reduction in effect of betaxolol compared to the nonselective beta-blocking agents). Pilocarpine, which has been the standard drug for a century, is still used in 1–4% concentrations three or four times a day. Because of the induced myopia in younger patients and the pupillary constriction that compromises vision in patients with cataract, it is most often employed when additional therapy to either a beta-blocking agent, epinephrine, or dipivefrin is required. Carbonic anhydrase inhibitors (eg, acetazolamide) are used until surgery or laser treatment can be performed when topical therapy is inadequate or causes too many side effects, or may be used long-term if these options are not available. Laser trabeculoplasty is used increasingly as an adjunct to topical therapy to postpone the need for surgery. It has also been advocated as primary treatment. Surgical trabeculectomy is necessary for patients whose intraocular pressure remains elevated despite medical and laser therapy and may be used as primary treatment in some individuals. Adjunctive treatment with subconjunctival fluorouracil or mitomycin at the time of surgery is being used increasingly in difficult cases to increase the chances of success of trabeculectomy.

Prognosis

Untreated chronic glaucoma that begins at age 40–45 will probably cause complete blindness by age 60–65. Early diagnosis and treatment will preserve useful vision throughout life in most cases.

Tielsch JM et al: Racial variations in the prevalence of primary open angle glaucoma. The Baltimore Eye Survey. JAMA 1991;266:369. (Four to five times greater prevalence in black Americans.)

Drance SM: Glaucoma: Changing concepts. (Bowman Lecture.) Eye 1992;6:337.

Van Buskirk EM, Cioffi GA: Glaucomatous optic neuropathy. Am J Ophthalmol 1992;113:448.

(Two reviews of the potentially multifactorial origin of glaucomatous optic nerve damage.)

Spaeth GL, Baes KA: Argon laser trabeculoplasty controls one-third of cases of progressive, uncontrolled, open angle glaucoma for 5 years. Arch Ophthalmol 1992; 110:491.

Migdal C: Rational choice of therapy in established open angle glaucoma. Eye 1992;6:346.

(Two articles in the continuing debate over the appropriate timimg of laser and surgical treatment for primary open-angle glaucoma.)

Palmer SS: Mitomycin as adjunct chemotherapy with trabeculectomy. Ophthalmology 1991;98:317.

Herschler J: Long-term results of trabeculectomy with collagen sponge implant containing low-dose antimetabolite. Ophthalmology 1992;99:666.

(Two studies using the increasingly popular application of an antimetabolite at the time of trabeculectomy to increase the chances of success.)

UVEITIS

Uveitis means inflammation of the uveal tract, which is formed by the iris (iritis), ciliary body (cyclitis), and choroid (choroiditis). Inflammatory eye disease may, however, also originate primarily in the retina (retinitis) or retinal blood vessels (retinal vasculitis).

Intraocular inflammation is classified as anterior uveitis, posterior uveitis, or panuveitis according to whether inflammatory signs are predominantly present in the anterior or posterior segment of the eye or equally distributed between the two. Uveitis may also be categorized as acute or chronic and granulomatous or nongranulomatous.

Clinical Findings

Anterior uveitis is characterized by inflammatory cells and flare within the aqueous. Cells may also be seen on the corneal endothelium as keratic precipitates (KPs). In granulomatous uveitis, these are large "mutton-fat" KPs, and iris nodules may be seen. In nongranulomatous uveitis, the KPs are smaller and iris nodules are not seen. Occasionally, granulomatous uveitis may initially masquerade as nongranulomatous disease. In severe anterior uveitis, there may be hypopyon (layered collection of white cells) and fibrin within the anterior chamber. In virtually all forms of anterior uveitis, the pupil is small, and with the development of posterior synechiae (adhesions between the iris and anterior lens capsule), it also becomes irregular.

Nongranulomatous anterior uveitis tends to present acutely with unilateral pain, redness, photophobia, and visual loss. Granulomatous anterior uveitis is more likely to present less acutely with blurred vision in a mildly inflamed eye.

In posterior uveitis, there are cells in the vitreous. Inflammatory lesions may be present in the retina or choroid. Fresh lesions are yellow, with indistinct margins, whereas older lesions have more definite margins and are commonly pigmented. Retinal vessel sheathing may occur adjacent to such lesions or more diffusely. In severe cases, vitreous opacity precludes visualization of retinal details.

Posterior uveitis tends to present with gradual visual loss in a relatively quiet eye. Bilateral involvement is common. Visual loss may be due to vitreous haze and opacities, inflammatory lesions involving the macula, macular edema, retinal vein occlusion, or, rarely, associated optic neuropathy.

Etiology

The systemic disorders associated with acute nongranulomatous anterior uveitis are the HLA-B27-related conditions sacroiliitis, ankylosing spondylitis, Reiter's syndrome, psoriasis, ulcerative colitis, and Crohn's disease. Behçet's syndrome produces both anterior uveitis with recurrent hypopyon and posterior uveitis with marked retinal vascular changes. Both herpes simplex and herpes zoster infections may cause nongranulomatous anterior uveitis.

Diseases producing granulomatous anterior uveitis also tend to be causes of posterior uveitis. These include sarcoidosis, which is commonly bilateral; tuberculosis; syphilis; toxoplasmosis; Vogt-Koyanagi-Harada syndrome (bilateral uveitis associated with alopecia, poliosis, vitiligo, and learning deficits); and sympathetic ophthalmia. Syphilis produces a characteristic "salt and pepper" fundus, often with surprisingly little visual loss unless there is also primary syphilitic optic atrophy. In congenital toxoplasmosis, there is usually evidence of previous episodes of retinochoroiditis.

Autoimmune retinal vasculitis and pars planitis (intermediate uveitis) are idiopathic conditions that produce posterior uveitis.

Retinal detachment, intraocular tumors, and central nervous system lymphoma may all masquerade as uveitis.

Evaluation & Treatment

Besides the history and physical examination, investigations may include erythrocyte sedimentation rate, VDRL and FTA-ABS tests, serum angiotensin-converting enzyme, and chest x-ray. PPD skin test and x-rays of sacroiliac joints may also be indicated.

Anterior uveitis will usually respond to topical corticosteroids. Occasionally, periocular steroid injections or even systemic steroids may be required. Dilation of the pupil is important to relieve discomfort and prevent posterior synechiae.

Posterior uveitis more commonly requires systemic corticosteroid therapy and occasionally systemic immunosuppression with azathioprine or cyclosporine. Pupillary dilation is not usually necessary.

In all cases if an infective cause is identified, specific chemotherapy may be indicated. In general, the prognosis for anterior uveitis, particularly the nongranulomatous type, is better than that for posterior uveitis.

Management of patients with uveitis must remain primarily in the hands of an ophthalmologist, but the cooperation of other physicians is essential for determining causes and in assisting in the administration of antimicrobials, high-dose systemic corticosteroids, and systemic immunosuppressants.

Rosenbaum JT, Robertson JE, Watzke RC: Retinal vasculitis: A primer. West J Med 1991;154:182.

Smith RE, Nozik RM: *Uveitis: A Clinical Approach to Diagnosis and Management,* 2nd ed. Williams & Wilkins, 1988.

CATARACT

Essentials of Diagnosis

- Blurred vision, progressive over months or years.
- No pain or redness.
- Lens opacities (may be grossly visible).

General Considerations

A cataract is a lens opacity. Cataracts are usually bilateral. They may be congenital (owing to intrauterine infections such as rubella and cytomegalovirus, inborn errors of metabolism such as galactosemia, or as yet unidentified hereditary factors); traumatic; or secondary to systemic disease (diabetes, myotonic dystrophy, atopic dermatitis), systemic corticosteroid treatment, or uveitis. Senile cataract is by far the most common type; most persons over age 60 have some degree of lens opacity. Cigarette smoking increases the risk of cataract formation.

Clinical Findings

Even in its early stages, a cataract can be seen through a dilated pupil with an ophthalmoscope, a slit lamp, or an ordinary hand illuminator. As the cataract matures, the retina will become increasingly more difficult to visualize, until finally the fundus reflection is absent and the pupil is white.

The degree of visual loss corresponds to the density of the cataract.

Treatment

Functional visual impairment is the prime criterion for surgery. The cataract is usually removed by one of the techniques in which the delicate posterior lens capsule remains (extracapsular). It is now possible to perform cataract surgery through a smaller incision, thus reducing the postoperative complication rate and accelerating the patient's visual rehabilitation.

It is routine practice to implant an intraocular lens at the time of surgery. This dispenses with the need for heavy cataract glasses or contact lenses. With modern techniques and improved intraocular lenses, the success rate is high.

Prognosis

If surgery is indicated, lens extraction improves visual acuity in 95% of cases. The remainder either have preexisting retinal damage or develop postoperative complications such as glaucoma, hemorrhage, retinal detachment, or infection.

Christen WG et al: A prospective study of cigarette smoking and risk of cataract in men. JAMA 1992;268:989.

Hankinson SE et al: A prospective study of cigarette smoking and risk of cataract in women. JAMA 1992;268:994.
(Two studies of male physicians and registered nurses, respectively, demonstrating an association between cigarette smoking and cataract formation, particularly posterior subcapsular cataract.)

Javitt JC et al: National outcomes of cataract extraction. Endophthalmitis following inpatient surgery. Arch Ophthalmol 1991;109:1085. (Small but significant risk of serious intraocular infection after cataract surgery.)

Javitt JC et al: National outcomes of cataract surgery: I. Retinal detachment after inpatient surgery. Ophthalmology 1991;98:895. (Retinal detachment in 1% of eyes following cataract surgery.)

RETINAL DETACHMENT

Essentials of Diagnosis

- Blurred vision in one eye becoming progressively worse. ("A curtain came down over my eye.")
- No pain or redness.
- Detachment seen by ophthalmoscopy.

General Considerations

Detachment of the retina is usually spontaneous but may be secondary to trauma. Spontaneous detachment occurs most frequently in persons over 50 years of age. Cataract extraction and myopia are the two most common predisposing causes.

Clinical Findings

As soon as the retina is torn, fluid vitreous is able to pass through the tear and lodge behind the sensory retina. This, combined with vitreous traction and the pull of gravity, results in progressive detachment. The superior temporal area is the most common site of detachment. The area of detachment rapidly increases, causing corresponding progressive visual loss. Central vision remains intact until the macula becomes detached.

On ophthalmoscopic examination, the retina is seen hanging in the vitreous like a gray cloud. One or more retinal tears, usually crescent-shaped and red or orange, are usually present and can be seen by an experienced examiner.

Treatment

All cases of retinal detachment should be referred immediately to an ophthalmologist. During transportation, the patient's head should be positioned so that the detached portion of the retina will fall back with the aid of gravity.

Treatment is directed primarily at closing the retinal tears. A permanent adhesion between the neurosensory retina, the retinal pigment epithelium, and the choroid is produced in the region of the tears by applying cryotherapy to the sclera or laser photocoagulation to the retina. In order to achieve apposition of the neurosensory retina to the retinal pigment epithelium whilst this adhesion is developing, an indentation may be made in the sclera with a silicone sponge or buckle, the fluid between the neurosensory retina and the retinal pigment epithelium (subretinal fluid) may be drained via an incision in the sclera, and an expansile gas may be injected into the vitreous cavity. Certain types of uncomplicated retinal detachment may be treated by the technique of pneumatic retinopexy, in which an expansile gas is initially injected into the vitreous cavity followed by careful positioning of the patient's head to facilitate reattachment of the retina. Once the retina is repositioned, the retinal tear is sealed by laser photocoagulation or cryotherapy. All the stages of pneumatic retinopexy can be performed under local anesthesia as an office procedure. The last stage is the same as is used to seal retinal tears without associated detachment as prophylaxis against detachment.

In complicated retinal detachments—particularly those in which fibroproliferative tissue has developed on the surface of the retina or within the vitreous cavity—retinal reattachment can only be accomplished by removal of the vitreous, direct manipulation of the retina, and internal tamponade of the retina with air, expansile gases, or even silicone oil. (The presence of an expansile gas within the eye is a contraindication to air travel. Such gases may persist in the globe for weeks after surgery.)

Prognosis

About 80% of uncomplicated cases can be cured with one operation; an additional 15% will need repeated operations; and the remainder never reattach. The prognosis is worse if the macula is detached or if the detachment is of long duration. Without treatment, retinal detachment often becomes total within 6 months. Spontaneous detachments are ultimately bilateral in 2–25% of cases.

American Academy of Ophthalmology: The repair of rhegmatogenous retinal detachments. Ophthalmology 1990;97:1562. (Evaluation of current techniques.)
Tornambe PE et al: Pneumatic retinopexy. A two-year follow-up study of the multicenter clinical trial comparing pneumatic retinopexy with scleral buckling. Ophthalmology 1991;98:1115. (Favorable results at 2 years in carefully selected cases.)

VITREOUS HEMORRHAGE

Patients with vitreous hemorrhage complain of sudden visual loss, sudden onset of floaters that may progressively increase in severity, or, occasionally,

"bleeding within the eye." Visual acuity ranges from 20/20 to light perception only. The eye is not inflamed, and the clue to diagnosis is the inability to see fundal details clearly despite the presence of a clear lens. Causes of vitreous hemorrhage include diabetic retinopathy, retinal tears (with or without retinal detachment), retinal vein occlusions, exudative age-related macular degeneration, blood dyscrasias, and trauma. In all cases, examination by an ophthalmologist is essential. Retinal tears and detachments necessitate urgent treatment (see above).

O'Malley C: Vitreous. In: *General Ophthalmology*, 13th ed. Vaughan D, Asbury T, Riordan-Eva P (editors). Appleton & Lange, 1992. (Many helpful illustrations.)

AGE-RELATED MACULAR DEGENERATION

Age-related macular degeneration is the leading cause of permanent visual loss in the elderly. The exact cause is unknown, but the incidence increases with each decade over age 50 (to almost 30% by age 75). Other associations besides age include race (usually white), sex (slight female predominance), family history, and a history of cigarette smoking.

Age-related macular degeneration includes a broad spectrum of clinical and pathologic findings that can be classified into two groups: atrophic ("dry") and exudative ("wet"). Although both types are progressive and usually bilateral, they differ in manifestations, prognosis, and management.

Atrophic degeneration is characterized by gradually progressive bilateral visual loss of moderate severity due to atrophy and degeneration of the outer retina, retinal pigment epithelium, Bruch's membrane, and choriocapillaris. In exudative degeneration, visual loss is of more rapid onset and greater severity, and the two eyes are usually affected sequentially over a period of a few years. The exudative form accounts for about 90% of all cases of legal blindness due to this disorder. Impairment of the barrier function of Bruch's membrane (between the retinal pigment epithelium and the choriocapillaris) allows serous fluid or blood to leak into the retina to produce elevation of the retinal pigment epithelium from Bruch's membrane (retinal pigment epithelial detachment) or separation of the neurosensory retina from the retinal pigment epithelium (serous retinal detachment). These changes may resolve spontaneously, with variable visual outcome, but are often associated with neovascularization arising from the choroidal vessels and extending between the retinal pigment epithelium and Bruch's membrane (subretinal neovascular membrane). This membrane produces permanent progressive visual loss.

Sudden visual loss in patients with exudative age-related macular degeneration occurs at the time of pigment epithelial or sensory retinal detachment or hemorrhage from a subretinal neovascular membrane. All these changes may occur in previously undiagnosed patients, in patients known to have atrophic changes, and in the other eye of patients with exudative disease. Laser photocoagulation of subretinal neovascular membranes may delay the onset of permanent visual loss but only when the membrane is far enough away from the fovea to permit such treatment. The value of laser photocoagulation in reducing the progression of visual loss in patients with disease at the fovea at the time of presentation is still being determined. Elderly patients developing sudden visual loss due to macular disease—particularly paracentral distortion or scotoma with preservation of central acuity—should be referred urgently to an ophthalmologist for assessment.

There is no specific treatment for atrophic age-related macular degeneration, but—as with the exudative form—patients often benefit from carefully prescribed low vision aids. It is important to reassure all patients that the disorder results in loss of central vision only. Peripheral fields and hence navigational vision are always maintained, though these may become impaired by cataract formation for which surgery may well be helpful.

Bressler NM, Bressler SB, Fine SL: Age-related macular degeneration. Surv Ophthalmol 1988;32:375. (Clinical manifestations and management.)

Macular Photocoagulation Study Group: Argon laser photocoagulation for neovascular maculopathy: Five-year results from randomized clinical trials. Arch Ophthalmol 1991;109:1109.

Macular Photocoagulation Study Group: Laser photocoagulation of subfoveal neovascular lesions in age-related macular degeneration: Results of a randomized clinical trial. Arch Ophthalmol 1991;109:1220. (Preliminary evidence of benefit.)

CENTRAL & BRANCH RETINAL VEIN OCCLUSIONS

The severity of visual loss in central retinal vein occlusion is variable. Younger patients may present with near-normal acuity. Older patients present with acuities ranging from 20/40 to hand movements only. The visual impairment is commonly first noticed upon waking in the morning. Ophthalmoscopic signs include disk swelling, venous dilatation and tortuosity, retinal hemorrhages, and cotton-wool spots.

In those with initially good acuity (20/60 or better), the visual prognosis is good. In those with poor initial acuity (20/200 or worse), extensive hemorrhages and multiple cotton-wool spots indicate widespread retinal ischemia, which can be confirmed by demonstrating extensive areas of capillary closure on fluorescein angiography. These eyes are at high risk of developing neovascular (rubeotic) glaucoma, typically within

3 months after venous occlusion, and should be considered for prophylactic laser panretinal photocoagulation. The visual prognosis in these cases is poor.

Branch retinal vein occlusions may present in a variety of ways. Sudden loss of vision may occur at the time of occlusion if the fovea is involved or some time afterward from vitreous hemorrhage due to retinal new vessels. More gradual visual loss may occur with development of macular edema or exudate. In a significant proportion, the occlusion is noted incidentally in patients with glaucoma, systemic hypertension, diabetes mellitus, or uveitis.

In acute branch retinal vein occlusion there are signs similar to those of central retinal vein occlusion but affecting only the retina drained by the obstructed vein. There is no specific treatment, but if retinal neovascularization develops, the area of retina affected by the initial occlusion should be laser-photocoagulated. Macular edema may also respond to laser treatment.

All patients with retinal vein occlusion should be referred urgently to an ophthalmologist for confirmation of the diagnosis and further management. It is important to look for glaucoma, systemic hypertension, diabetes mellitus, and hyperlipidemia. In younger patients, deficiency of the anticoagulant plasma proteins protein C, protein S, and antithrombin III should be excluded. Hyperviscosity syndromes and other hematologic abnormalities are only rarely associated with retinal vein occlusions but may worsen their prognosis. Branch retinal vein occlusion is an important feature of Behçet's syndrome.

Clarkson JG: Photocoagulation for ischemic central retinal vein occlusion: Central vein occlusion study. (Editorial.) Arch Ophthalmol 1991;109:1218.

Elman MJ et al: The risk for systemic vascular diseases and mortality in patients with central retinal vein occlusion. Ophthalmology 1990;97:1543. (Need to exclude systemic hypertension and diabetes mellitus.)

Hayreh SS et al: Differentiation of ischemic from non-ischemic central retinal vein occlusion during the early acute phase: Graefe's Arch Clin Exp Ophthalmol 1990;228:201. (A determination of indicators of retinal ischemia.)

CENTRAL & BRANCH RETINAL ARTERY OCCLUSIONS

Central retinal artery occlusion presents as sudden profound visual loss. Visual acuity is reduced to counting fingers or worse, and visual field is commonly restricted to an island of vision in the temporal field. Ophthalmoscopy reveals pallid swelling of the retina, most obvious in the posterior segment, with a cherry-red spot at the fovea. The retinal arteries are attenuated, and "box-car" segmentation of blood in the veins may be seen. Occasionally, emboli are seen in the central retinal artery or its branches. The retinal swelling subsides over a period of 4–6 weeks, leaving a relatively normal retinal appearance but a pale optic disk and attenuated arterioles.

The patient should be referred as an emergency to an ophthalmologist. If seen within a few hours after onset, emergency treatment—including laying the patient flat, ocular massage, high concentrations of inhaled oxygen, intravenous acetazolamide, and anterior chamber paracentesis—may influence the visual outcome. Thrombolytic therapy is currently being evaluated.

The main management problem is identifying any treatable underlying disorder. Giant cell arteritis must be excluded in all older patients, especially because of the risk—highest in the first few days—of involvement of the other eye. If giant cell arteritis is diagnosed, either on the basis of associated symptoms (especially headache or polymyalgia), clinical signs, or a high erythrocyte sedimentation rate, one should give methylprednisolone, 250–500 mg intravenously four times daily for 3 days), starting within 24 hours after onset, followed by high-dose systemic corticosteroids (60–80 mg prednisolone per day); this may produce recovery of vision in arteritic central retinal artery occlusion. Temporal artery biopsy should be obtained within 5–7 days after starting steroid therapy. Carotid and cardiac sources of emboli must be identified and appropriate treatment given to reduce the risk of stroke.

Branch retinal artery occlusion may also present with sudden loss of vision if the fovea is involved, but more commonly sudden loss of visual field is the presenting complaint. Fundal signs of retinal swelling and adjacent cotton-wool spots are limited to the area of retina supplied by the occluded vessel. Embolic causes are proportionately more common than in central retinal artery occlusion. Migraine, oral contraceptives, and vasculitis must also be considered. Antiphospholipid antibodies have been associated with branch and central retinal artery occlusions in younger patients. Patients with branch retinal artery occlusions should be referred urgently to an ophthalmologist.

Matzkin DC et al: Visual recovery in two patients after intravenous methylprednisolone treatment of central retinal artery occlusion secondary to giant-cell arteritis. Ophthalmology 1992;99:68.
Schmidt D, Schumacher M, Wakhloo AK: Microcatheter urokinase infusion in central retinal artery occlusion. Am J Ophthalmol 1992;113:429. (Good visual recovery in a small proportion of patients.)

AMAUROSIS FUGAX

Amaurosis fugax ("fleeting blindness") is characteristically caused by retinal emboli from ipsilateral carotid disease. The visual loss is usually described as a curtain passing vertically across the visual field with complete monocular visual loss lasting a few minutes and a similar curtain effect as the episode passes. In order to reduce the risk of stroke, patients with high-grade stenosis (70–99%) of the ipsilateral internal carotid artery should be considered for carotid endarterectomy. Patients with low-grade stenosis (0–29%) are better treated medically with aspirin or other antiplatelet drugs. The optimal treatment for patients with medium-grade stenosis has not been determined. The initial assessment of carotid stenosis, particularly the identification of low-grade stenosis, can be undertaken with carotid Doppler studies. But angiography is essential for determining the suitability for surgery of higher grade stenosis. Emboli from cardiac sources may also be responsible for amaurosis fugax. Echocardiography should be undertaken in young patients, in any patient with clinical evidence of a potential cardiac source of emboli, and in all patients being considered for carotid endarterectomy. Early ophthalmologic consultation is advisable to ratify the diagnosis.

Similar obscurations of vision may occur with poor ocular perfusion due to severe occlusive carotid disease. More transient obscurations (lasting only a few seconds to 1 minute) affecting both eyes occur in patients with raised intracranial pressure. In young patients, amaurosis fugax is not usually due to carotid or cardiac disease but is often a manifestation of migraine.

Barnett HJM, Barnes RW, Robertson JT: The uncertainties surrounding carotid endarterectomy. JAMA 1992;268:3120.
Brown MM, Humphrey PRD: Carotid endarterectomy: recommendations for management of transient ischaemic attack and ischaemic stroke. Br Med J 1992;305:1071.
Crouse JR: Assessment and management of carotid disease. Ann Rev Med 1992;43:301. (Three perspectives on the value of surgery for carotid artery disease.)
European Carotid Surgery Trialists' Collaborative Group: MRC European carotid surgery trial: Interim results for symptomatic patients with severe (70–99%) or with mild (0–29%) carotid stenosis. Lancet 1991;337:1235.
North American Symptomatic Carotid Endarterectomy Trial Collaborators: Beneficial effect of carotid endarterectomy in symptomatic patients with high-grade carotid stenosis. N Engl J Med 1991;325:445. (Two papers establishing the optimal management of patients with amaurosis fugax.)
O'Sullivan F, Rossor M, Elston JS: Amaurosis fugax in young people. Br J Ophthalmol 1992;76:660. (Thought to be due to migraine.)

RETINAL DISORDERS ASSOCIATED WITH SYSTEMIC DISEASES

Many systemic diseases are associated with retinal manifestations. These include diabetes mellitus, essential hypertension, preeclampsia-eclampsia of pregnancy, blood dyscrasias, and AIDS. The retinal changes caused by these disorders can be easily observed with the aid of the ophthalmoscope.

Diabetic Retinopathy

Diabetic retinopathy is the leading cause of new blindness among US adults aged 20–65. It is broadly classified as proliferative and nonproliferative.

Nonproliferative retinopathy is characterized by dilatation of veins, microaneurysms, retinal hemorrhages, retinal edema, and hard exudates. A major subgroup are those patients in which visual loss develops owing to edema, ischemia, or exudates at the macula (diabetic maculopathy). This is the most common cause of legal blindness in maturity-onset diabetes.

Proliferative retinopathy is characterized by neovascularization, arising either from the optic disk or the major vascular arcades. Vitreous hemorrhage is a common sequela. Proliferation into the vitreous of blood vessels, with their associated fibrous component, leads to tractional retinal detachment. Without treatment, the visual prognosis with proliferative retinopathy is generally much worse than that with nonproliferative retinopathy. Severe proliferative retinopathy is often complicated by maculopathy.

Nonproliferative retinopathy is present at the time of diagnosis in a significant number of maturity-onset diabetics and may be the presenting feature. Treatment is focused on optimizing control of blood glucose and any associated systemic hypertension. Regular assessment of visual acuity and fundal examination are essential for the detection of macular changes. As soon as there is a decline in acuity or the fovea is seen to be threatened by exudates, the patient should be referred to an ophthalmologist. Laser photocoagulation is helpful in treating macular exudates. Maculopathy due to ischemia or edema is assessed by fluorescein angiography. Laser treatment may be helpful.

It is essential that proliferative retinopathy be recognized early and treated by panretinal laser photocoagulation to prevent blindness. Unfortunately, the presence of neovascularization is all too often diagnosed only at the time of vitreous hemorrhage. In some patients, a "preproliferative" retinopathy—characterized as nonproliferative retinopathy complicated by multiple cotton-wool spots and gross venous abnormalities—may be identified. Whether panretinal laser photocoagulation should be undertaken at this time is determined by the degree of retinal ischemia as assessed by fluorescein angiography.

Surgical treatment (vitrectomy) is being used increasingly in the treatment of severe proliferative retinopathy, either to remove vitreous hemorrhage or to deal with retinal detachments involving the macula.

Patients with diabetes mellitus should have at least yearly ophthalmoscopic examination through dilated pupils. Examination by an ophthalmologist is usually advisable in juvenile-onset diabetes of more than 5 years' duration; at the time of diagnosis in maturity-onset diabetes; if ocular symptoms develop; or if there are suspicious findings of retinopathy, especially neovascularization or macular exudates. Failure to diagnose diabetic retinopathy by ophthalmoscopic examination is common, particularly if the pupils are not dilated. Many clinicians believe that the severity of diabetic retinopathy can be lessened by careful control of blood glucose levels. It is probable that good diabetic control is most important in preventing the development of retinopathy rather than influencing its subsequent course.

Ai E: Current management of diabetic retinopathy. West J Med 1992;157:67.
Raskin P, Arauz-Pacheco C: The treatment of diabetic retinopathy: A view for the internist. Ann Int Med 1992;117:226.
Singer DE et al: Screening for diabetic retinopathy. Ann Int Med 1992;116:660.
(Three articles providing an overall view of the management of diabetic retinopathy.)

Hypertensive Retinopathy

One method of classifying hypertensive retinopathy (modified after Keith and Wagener) is shown in Table 7–2.

Preeclampsia-eclampsia is manifested in the retina as rapidly progressive hypertensive retinopathy, and extensive permanent retinal damage may occur if the pregnancy is not terminated. Occasionally, the choroidal circulation is mainly affected, leading to infarction of the retinal pigment epithelium.

Table 7–2. A classification of hypertensive retinopathy. (Modified after Keith and Wagener.)

Stage	Ophthalmoscopic Appearance	Clinical Classification
I	Minimal narrowing or sclerosis of arterioles.	"Essential" hypertension (chronic, benign, "arteriosclerotic")
II	Thickening and dulling of vessel reflection (copper wire appearance). Localized and generalized narrowing of arterioles. Changes at arteriovenous crossings (A-V nicking). Scattered tiny round or flame-shaped hemorrhages. Vascular occlusion may be present.	
III	Sclerotic changes may not be marked. "Angiospastic retinopathy": localized arteriolar spasm, hemorrhages, exudates, "cotton-wool patches," retinal edema.	Malignant hypertensive retinopathy.
IV	Same as III, plus optic disk swelling.	

Blood Dyscrasias

In blood dyscrasias characterized by thrombocytopenia and severe anemia, various types of hemorrhages are present in both the retina and choroid and may lead to visual loss. If the underlying dyscrasia is successfully treated and macular hemorrhages have not occurred, it is possible to regain normal vision.

Proliferative retinopathy (sickle cell retinopathy) is particularly common in hemoglobin SC disease but may also occur with other hemoglobin S variants. Severe visual loss is rare, and retinal photocoagulation, though it reverses the retinal abnormalities and reduces the frequency of vitreous hemorrhage, does not affect the long-term visual outcome. Surgery is occasionally needed for unresolving vitreous hemorrhage or tractional retinal detachment.

AIDS

Cotton-wool spots, retinal hemorrhages, and microaneurysms are the most common ophthalmic abnormalities in AIDS patients. These microvascular changes may arise from direct retinal infection by HIV or from deposition of circulating immune complexes. Cotton-wool spots are more commonly seen in patients with AIDS than in those with asymptomatic HIV infections, but the significance of this observation is not known.

Cytomegalovirus retinitis occurs in many AIDS patients. It is characterized by progressively enlarging yellowish-white patches of retinal opacification, which are accompanied by retinal hemorrhages; they usually begin adjacent to the major retinal vascular arcades. Patients are often asymptomatic until there is involvement of the fovea or optic nerve or until retinal detachment develops.

Ganciclovir has been shown to be useful in the management of cytomegalovirus retinitis in patients with AIDS. Induction therapy is with 5 mg/kg twice a day for 10–14 days; maintenance therapy is 5 mg/kg daily. Unfortunately, progression of the disease is common even when maintenance therapy is used. Systemic ganciclovir must be administered intravenously and commonly causes bone marrow suppression, which is particularly a problem if zidovudine therapy is being undertaken. Intravitreal ganciclovir has been used as an alternative. Systemic foscarnet, 60 mg/kg three times a day for 14 days followed by 90 mg/kg/d as maintenance therapy, is as effective against cytomegalovirus retinitis as systemic ganciclovir but less well tolerated. Foscarnet is associated with improved patient survival, but this may be due to coincidental treatment with zidovudine. Retinal detachments generally require vitrectomy and often intravitreal silicone oil.

Other opportunistic ophthalmic infections occurring in AIDS patients include herpes simplex retinitis, toxoplasmic and candidal chorioretinitis, and herpes zoster ophthalmicus. Kaposi's sarcoma of the conjunctiva and orbital lymphoma may also be seen.

Central nervous system involvement by primary HIV infection, opportunistic infections, and intracranial neoplasms may produce a variety of neuro-ophthalmologic abnormalities.

Cantrill HL et al: Treatment of cytomegalovirus retinitis with intravitreal ganciclovir: Long-term results. Ophthalmology 1989;96:367.

Jabs DA: Treatment of cytomegalovirus retinitis—1992. (Editorial.) Arch Ophthalmol 1992;110:185.

Studies of Ocular Complications of AIDS Research Group: Mortality in patients with the acquired immunodeficiency syndrome treated with either foscarnet or ganciclovir for cytomegalovirus retinitis. N Engl J Med 1992;326:213. (Three articles describing the various aspects of treating cytomegalovirus retinitis in AIDS patients.)

Holland GN: Acquired immunodeficiency syndrome and ophthalmology: The first decade. Am J Ophthalmol 1992;114:86. (A thorough review of the ophthalmic consequences of AIDS and their management.)

ANTERIOR ISCHEMIC OPTIC NEUROPATHY

Anterior ischemic optic neuropathy—due to occlusion of the posterior ciliary arteries that supply the anterior portion of the optic nerve—produces sudden visual loss, usually with an altitudinal field defect, and optic disk swelling. In older patients, it is often caused by giant cell arteritis. In all other patients, systemic hypertension, arteriosclerosis, systemic lupus erythematosus, and polyarteritis nodosa should be considered. Urgent ophthalmologic consultation should be arranged. There is a significant risk of subsequent involvement of the fellow eye. In the uncommon progressive form of nonarteritic anterior ischemic optic neuropathy, characterized by increasing visual loss during the first 6 weeks after onset, optic nerve sheath fenestration (also known as optic nerve sheath decompression) should be considered.

Hayreh SS: Anterior ischaemic optic neuropathy: Differentiation of arteritis from non-arteritis type and its management. Eye 1990;4:25.

Kelman SE, Elman MJ: Optic nerve sheath decompression for nonarteritic ischemic optic neuropathy improves multiple visual function measurements. Arch Ophthalmol 1991;109:667. (Seven patients improved.)

OPTIC NEURITIS

Optic neuritis is characterized by unilateral loss of vision which usually develops suddenly and may increase during the following few days. At its worst, the level of vision may vary from 20/30 to no perception of light. Visual acuity often then improves within 2–3 weeks and frequently returns to normal. Commonly there is pain in the region of the eye, particularly on eye movements. Field loss is usually a central scotoma, but a wide range of monocular field defects are possible. There is marked loss of color vision and a relative afferent pupillary defect. The optic disk may be swollen, with occasional flame-shaped peripapillary hemorrhages. (In retrobulbar optic neuritis, the optic disk is normal.) In all forms of optic neuritis, optic atrophy subsequently develops if there has been destruction of sufficient optic nerve fibers.

Optic neuritis is particularly associated with demyelinative disease, occurring in patients known to have multiple sclerosis and as a first manifestation of the disease in others. In patients with clinically isolated optic neuritis, as many as 75% will have developed multiple sclerosis within 15 years. Consideration should thus be given to whether such patients should be informed of the possibility of subsequently developing multiple sclerosis. MRI of the brain, which frequently reveals multiple white matter lesions similar to those seen in multiple sclerosis, cerebrospinal fluid analysis, and brain stem and somatosensory evoked potentials may provide more specific information on the likelihood of developing multiple sclerosis.

Optic neuritis may also occur in association with viral infections—including measles, mumps, influenza, and those caused by the varicella-zoster virus—in association with various autoimmune disorders, particularly systemic lupus erythematosus, and by spread of inflammation from meninges, orbital tissues, or paranasal sinuses.

It has now been shown that oral prednisolone alone has no beneficial effect on the rate of recovery or visual outcome in acute demyelinative optic neuritis and that it may increase the risk of recurrent disease. Intravenous methylprednisolone (250 mg every 6 hours for 3 days) followed by oral prednisolone (1 mg/kg for 11 days, then tapered off over 4 days) accelerates visual recovery and minimally improves certain parameters of visual outcome other than visual acuity, but with a small risk of systemic side effects. Whether such therapy is to be used in an individual patient should be determined by the degree of visual loss, the state of the fellow eye, the patient's visual requirements, and the patient's susceptibility to systemic side effects from steroid therapy. Optic neuritis due to herpes zoster or systemic lupus erythematosus generally has a poorer prognosis than other forms of optic neuritis and requires megadose intravenous steroid therapy. All patients with optic neuritis should be referred urgently for neuro-ophthalmologic assessment. Any patient with a clinical diagnosis of isolated optic neuritis in which visual recovery does not occur requires further investigation, particularly to exclude a compressive lesion or an intrinsic optic nerve tumor.

Beck RW et al: A randomized, controlled trial of corticosteroids in the treatment of acute optic neuritis. N Engl J Med 1992;326:581.

McDonald WI, Barnes D: The ocular manifestations of multiple sclerosis: 1. Abnormalities of the afferent visual system. J Neurol Neurosurg Psychiatry 1992;55:747. (Optic neuritis and its relationship to multiple sclerosis.)

Slamovits TL et al: What to tell the patient with optic neuritis about multiple sclerosis. Surv Ophthalmol 1991;36: 47.

OPTIC DISK SWELLING

Optic disk swelling may result from intraocular disease, orbital and optic nerve lesions, systemic hypertension (grade IV retinopathy), or raised intracranial pressure. Intraocular causes include central retinal vein occlusion, posterior uveitis, and posterior scleritis. Optic nerve lesions causing disk swelling include optic neuritis, anterior ischemic optic neuropathy; optic disk drusen (pseudopapilledema); optic nerve sheath meningioma; and optic nerve infiltration by sarcoidosis, leukemia, or lymphoma. Any orbital lesion causing optic nerve compression may produce disk swelling.

Papilledema (optic disk swelling due to raised intracranial pressure) is usually bilateral and most commonly produces enlargement of the blind spot without loss of acuity. Chronic papilledema, as occurs in idiopathic intracranial hypertension (previously known as benign intracranial hypertension) and dural venous sinus occlusion, may be associated with progressive visual field loss and occasionally profound loss of acuity. All patients with chronic papilledema must be monitored carefully, especially their visual fields, and optic nerve sheath fenestration (also known as optic nerve sheath decompression) should be considered in those with progressive visual failure not controlled by medical therapy (weight loss where appropriate and acetazolamide). Optic neuritis causes visual loss, usually with a central scotoma; loss of color vision; and a relative afferent pupillary defect. Anterior ischemic optic neuropathy is usually associated with an altitudinal field defect.

Optic disk drusen are a major source of confusion. Recognizing their presence may avoid much needless investigation. Optic disk drusen should be considered when disk swelling is not associated with any visual disturbance or symptoms of raised intracranial pressure. Exposed optic disk drusen may be obvious clinically or can be demonstrated by their autofluorescence. Buried or exposed drusen are best detected by CT scanning. Other family members may be similarly affected.

Horton JC et al: Decompression of the optic nerve sheath for vision-threatening papilledema caused by dural sinus occlusion. Neurosurgery 1992;31:203.

Spoor TC et al: Treatment of pseudotumor cerebri by pri-

mary and secondary optic nerve sheath decompression. Am J Ophthalmol 1991;112:177.
(Two papers documenting the value of optic nerve sheath fenestration in controlling progressive visual loss in patients with chronic papilledema.)

Wall M, George D: Idiopathic intracranial hypertension: A prospective study of 50 patients. Brain 1991;114:155. (Clearly demonstrates the risk to vision.)

OCULAR MOTOR PALSIES

In complete third nerve paralysis, there is complete ptosis and the eye is divergent and slightly depressed. Extraocular movements are restricted in all directions except laterally (preserved lateral rectus function). Intact fourth nerve (superior oblique) function is detected by the presence of inward rotation on attempted depression of the eye.

Pupillary involvement (dilated pupil that does not react to accommodation or to light shined in either eye) is an important sign differentiating "surgical" from "medical" causes of isolated third nerve palsy. (Compressive lesions of the third nerve, such as aneurysm of the posterior communicating artery and uncal herniation due to a supratentorial mass lesion, characteristically have pupillary involvement.) It is crucial that patients presenting with isolated third nerve palsy with pupillary involvement be assumed to have a posterior communicating artery aneurysm until this has been excluded by cerebral arteriography—and thus they should be referred immediately for neuro-ophthalmologic assessment. Medical causes of isolated third nerve palsy include diabetes, systemic hypertension, syphilis, and giant cell arteritis.

Fourth nerve paralysis causes upward deviation of the eye with failure of depression on adduction. There is vertical diplopia that becomes most apparent on attempted reading and descending stairs. Many cases of isolated fourth nerve palsy are due to decompensation of a congenital lesion. Trauma is a major cause of acquired—particularly bilateral—fourth nerve palsy, but cerebral neoplasms and medical causes such as in third nerve palsies should also be considered.

Sixth nerve paralysis causes convergent squint in the primary position with failure of abduction of the affected eye, producing horizontal diplopia that increases on gaze to the affected side and on looking into the distance. It is an important sign of raised intracranial pressure, particularly in children. Sixth nerve palsy may also be due to trauma, neoplasms, brain stem lesions, or medical causes (see above).

Any patient presenting with an isolated ocular motor palsy should be investigated with CT or MRI to exclude an intracranial or intraorbital mass lesion. In all patients with isolated ocular motor nerve palsies presumed to be due to medical causes, such investigations must be performed if recovery has not begun within 3 months.

Ocular motor nerve palsies occurring in association with other neurologic signs may be due to lesions in the brain stem, around the cavernous sinus, or in the orbit. Lesions around the cavernous sinus involve the upper divisions of the trigeminal nerve, the ocular motor nerves, and occasionally the optic chiasm. Orbital apex lesions involve the optic nerve and the ocular motor nerves.

Myasthenia and dysthyroid eye disease must always be considered in the differential diagnosis of disordered extraocular movements.

Levi L: Ocular motor nerves and the pupil. Curr Opin Ophthalmol 1991;2:544. (Recent changes in the investigation of ocular motor nerve palsies.)

Richards BW, Jones FR, Younge BR: Causes and prognosis in 4,278 cases of paralysis of the oculomotor, trochlear, and abducens cranial nerves. Am J Ophthalmology 1992;113:489.

DYSTHYROID EYE DISEASE

Dysthyroid eye disease is a clinical syndrome caused by deposition of mucopolysaccharides and infiltration with chronic inflammatory cells of the orbital tissues, particularly the extraocular muscles. Patients may have clinical or laboratory evidence of thyroid dysfunction, elevated thyroid autoantibodies, or no detectable abnormality outside the orbit.

The primary clinical features are proptosis, lid retraction and lid lag, conjunctival chemosis and episcleral inflammation, and extraocular muscle abnormalities due to restriction of their actions. Resulting symptoms are cosmetic abnormalities, surface irritation, which usually responds to artificial tears, and diplopia, which should be treated conservatively (eg, with prisms) in the active stages of the disease and only by surgery when the disease has been static for at least 6 months.

The important complications are corneal exposure and optic nerve compression, both of which may lead to profound visual loss. Treatment is by urgent orbital decompression, either medically, with high-dose systemic steroids (prednisolone 80–100 mg/d)—although this is often of only short-term benefit—by radiotherapy, or, most effectively, by surgery, usually consisting of extensive removal of bone from the medial wall and floor of the orbit.

Surgical decompression of the orbit is also being used for unsightly proptosis, but at the risk of visual loss and of inducing extraocular muscle abnormalities. Lateral tarsorrhaphy may be used for moderately severe corneal exposure. Other lid procedures are particularly useful for correcting lid retraction but should not be undertaken until the orbital disease is quiescent and orbital decompression or extraocular muscle surgery has been undertaken if necessary.

Carter JA, Utiger RD: The ophthalmopathy of Graves' disease. Ann Rev Med 1992;43:487. (Pathogenesis of dysthyroid ophthalmopathy together with an outline for management.)

Carter KD et al: Long-term efficacy of orbital decompression for compressive optic neuropathy of Graves' disease. Ophthalmology 1991;98:1435.

Kazim M, Trokel S, Moore S: Treatment of Graves orbitopathy. Ophthalmology 1991;98:1443.

(Two retrospective reviews covering the various modalities of treatment for compressive optic neuropathy in dysthyroid eye disease.)

Fells P: Management of dysthyroid eye disease. Br J Ophthalmol 1991;75:245.

ORBITAL CELLULITIS

Orbital cellulitis is manifested by an abrupt onset of fever, proptosis, restriction of extraocular movements, and swelling and redness of the lids, usually in a child. Infection of the paranasal sinuses is the usual underlying cause. Immediate treatment with intravenous antibiotics is necessary to prevent optic nerve damage and spread of infection to the cavernous sinuses—manifested as increased restriction of extraocular movements, impaired visual acuity, diminished pupillary reflexes, and papilledema, all of which may be bilateral—meninges, and brain. The response to antibiotics is usually excellent, but abscess formation may necessitate surgical drainage.

Jones DB, Steinkuller PG: Strategies for the initial management of acute preseptal and orbital cellulitis. Trans Am Ophthalmol Soc 1988;86:94. (Algorithm for management.)

OCULAR TRAUMA

Conjunctival & Corneal Foreign Bodies

If a patient complains of "something in my eye" and gives a consistent history, a foreign body is usually present on the cornea or under the upper lid even though it may not be readily visible. Visual acuity should be tested before treatment is instituted, as a basis for comparison in the event of complications.

After a local anesthetic (eg, proparacaine, 0.5%) is instilled, the eye is examined with the aid of a hand flashlight, using oblique illumination, and loupe. Corneal foreign bodies may be made more apparent by the instillation of sterile fluorescein. They are then removed with a sterile wet cotton-tipped applicator. Polymyxin-bacitracin ophthalmic ointment should be instilled. It is not necessary to patch the eye, but the patient must be examined 24 hours later for secondary infection of the crater. If a corneal foreign body

cannot be removed in this manner, the patient should be referred to an ophthalmologist.

Steel foreign bodies usually leave a diffuse rust ring. This requires excision of the affected tissue and is best done under local anesthesia using a slit lamp. **Caution:** Anesthetic drops should not be given to the patient for self-administration.

If there is no infection, a layer of corneal epithelial cells will line the crater within 24 hours. It should be emphasized that the intact corneal epithelium forms an effective barrier to infection, but once it is disturbed it becomes extremely susceptible to infection. Early infection is manifested by a white necrotic area around the crater and a small amount of gray exudate. These patients should be referred immediately to an ophthalmologist, since untreated corneal infection may lead to severe corneal ulceration, panophthalmitis, and loss of the eye.

In the case of a foreign body under the upper lid, a local anesthetic is instilled and the lid is everted by grasping the lashes gently and exerting pressure on the mid portion of the outer surface of the upper lid with an applicator. If a foreign body is present, it can easily be removed by passing a wet sterile cotton-tipped applicator across the conjunctival surface.

Intraocular Foreign Body

Intraocular foreign body requires emergency treatment by an ophthalmologist. Patients giving a history of "something hitting the eye"—particularly if it happens while hammering on metal or using grinding equipment—must be carefully assessed for the possibility of an intraocular foreign body, especially when no corneal foreign body is seen, a corneal or scleral wound is apparent, or there is marked visual loss or media opacity. Such patients must be treated as for corneal laceration (see below) and referred without delay to an ophthalmologist. Intraocular foreign bodies significantly increase the risk of intraocular infection.

Mieler WF et al: Retained intraocular foreign bodies and endophthalmitis. Ophthalmology 1990;97:1532. (Aggressive policy of early removal together with topical, subconjunctival, and in certain cases intravitreal prophylactic antibiotics.)

Corneal Abrasions

A patient with a corneal abrasion complains of severe pain and photophobia. There is often a history of trauma to the eye, commonly involving a fingernail, piece of paper, or contact lens. Visual acuity is recorded, and the cornea and conjunctiva are examined with a light and loupe to rule out a foreign body. If an abrasion is suspected but cannot be seen, sterile fluorescein is instilled into the conjunctival sac: the area of corneal abrasion will stain a deeper green than the surrounding cornea.

Treatment includes polymyxin-bacitracin ophthalmic ointment and application of a bandage with firm pressure to prevent movement of the lid. The patient should rest at home, keeping the fellow eye closed, and should be observed the following day to be certain the cornea has healed. Recurrent corneal erosion may follow corneal abrasions.

Contusions

Contusion injuries of the eye and surrounding structures may cause ecchymosis ("black eye"), subconjunctival hemorrhage, edema or rupture of the cornea, hemorrhage into the anterior chamber (hyphema), rupture of the root of the iris (iridodialysis), paralysis of the pupillary sphincter, paralysis of the muscles of accommodation, cataract, subluxation or luxation of the lens, vitreous hemorrhage, retinal hemorrhage and edema (most common in the macular area), detachment of the retina, rupture of the choroid, fracture of the orbital floor ("blowout fracture"), or optic nerve injury. Many of these injuries are immediately obvious; others may not become apparent for days or weeks. Patients with moderate to severe contusions should be seen by an ophthalmologist.

Any injury severe enough to cause hyphema involves the danger of secondary hemorrhage, which may cause intractable glaucoma with permanent visual loss. Any patient with traumatic hyphema should be advised to rest quietly until complete resolution has occurred. Daily ophthalmologic assessment is essential. Aspirin and related drugs increase the risk of secondary hemorrhage and must be avoided.

Dutton JJ et al: Management of blow-out fractures of the orbital floor. Surv Ophthalmol 1991;35:279.

Schein OD et al: The spectrum and burden of ocular injury. Ophthalmology 1988;95:300. (Epidemiologic survey in an urban setting.)

Lacerations

A. Lids: If the lid margin is lacerated, the patient should be referred for specialized care, since permanent notching may result. Lacerations of the lower eyelid near the inner canthus often sever the lower canaliculus. Lid lacerations not involving the margin may be sutured just like any other skin laceration.

B. Conjunctiva: In superficial lacerations of the conjunctiva, sutures are not necessary. In order to prevent infection, sulfonamides or other antibiotics are instilled into the eye until the laceration is healed.

C. Cornea or Sclera: Patients with suspected corneal or scleral lacerations must be seen by an ophthalmologist as soon as possible. Manipulation is kept to a minimum, since pressure may result in extrusion of the intraocular contents. The eye is bandaged lightly and covered with a metal shield that rests on the orbital bones above and below. The patient should be instructed not to squeeze the eye shut and to remain as quiet as possible. The eye is routinely studied radiographically to exclude the presence of metallic foreign bodies.

Reifler DM: Management of canalicular laceration. Surv Ophthalmol 1991;36:113.

Ultraviolet Keratitis (Actinic Keratitis)

Ultraviolet burns of the cornea are usually caused by use of a sunlamp without eye protection, exposure to a welding arc, or exposure to the sun when skiing ("snow blindness"). There are no immediate symptoms, but about 6–12 hours later the patient complains of agonizing pain and severe photophobia. Slit lamp examination after instillation of sterile fluorescein shows diffuse punctate staining of both corneas.

Treatment consists of binocular patching and instillation of 1–2 drops of 1% cyclopentolate (to relieve the discomfort of ciliary spasm). All patients recover within 24–48 hours without complications. Local anesthetics should not be prescribed.

Chemical Conjunctivitis & Keratitis

Chemical burns are treated by irrigation of the eyes with saline solution or plain water as soon as possible after exposure. Neutralization of an acid with an alkali or vice versa generates heat and may cause further damage. Alkali injuries are more serious and require prolonged irrigation, since alkalies are not precipitated by the proteins of the eye as are acids. It is important to remove any retained particulate matter such as is typically present in injuries involving cement and building plaster. This may require double eversion of the upper lid. The pupil should be dilated with 0.2% scopolamine or 2% atropine, 1 drop twice a day, to relieve discomfort and prophylactic topical antibiotics should be started. In moderate to severe injuries, intensive topical corticosteroids and topical and systemic vitamin C are also necessary. Complications include mucus deficiency, scarring of the cornea and conjunctiva, symblepharon (adhesions between the tarsal and bulbar conjunctiva), tear duct obstruction, and secondary infection.

PRINCIPLES OF TREATMENT OF OCULAR INFECTIONS

Before one can determine the drug of choice, the causative organisms must be identified, but in most instances empirical treatment, based on clinical experience, is used in the first instance. In the treatment of conjunctivitis and for prophylaxis against ocular infection, it is preferable to use a drug that is not given systemically. Of the available local antibacterial agents, the sulfonamides are effective and inexpensive. Two reliable sulfonamides for ophthalmic use are sulfisoxazole and sodium sulfacetamide. The sulfonamides have the added advantages of low allergenicity and effectiveness against the chlamydial group of organisms. They are available in ointment or solution form. Combined bacitracin-polymyxin ointment is often used prophylactically after corneal foreign body removal for the protection it affords against both gram-positive and gram-negative organisms.

Among the most effective broad-spectrum antibiotics for ophthalmic use are gentamicin, tobramycin, and neomycin. These drugs have some effect against gram-negative as well as gram-positive organisms but are generally not effective against the pneumococcus. Allergic reactions to neomycin are common. Other antibiotics frequently used are erythromycin, the tetracyclines, and the cephalosporins.

Method of Administration

Most ocular anti-infective drugs are administered locally. Ointments have greater therapeutic effectiveness than solutions, since contact can be maintained longer. However, they do cause blurring of vision; if this must be avoided, solutions should be used.

Systemic administration is required for all intraocular infections, orbital cellulitis, dacryocystitis, gonococcal keratoconjunctivitis, inclusion conjunctivitis, and severe external infection that does not respond to local treatment.

TECHNIQUES USED IN THE TREATMENT OF OCULAR DISORDERS

Instilling Medications

The patient is placed in a chair with head tilted back, both eyes open, and looking up. The lower lid is retracted slightly, and 2 drops of liquid are instilled into the lower cul-de-sac. The patient looks down while finger contact is maintained, so that the eyes are not squeezed shut. Ointments are instilled in the same general manner.

For self-medication, the same techniques are used except that medications are usually better instilled with the patient lying down.

Eye Bandage

Most eye bandages should be applied firmly enough to hold the lid securely against the cornea. An ordinary patch consisting of gauze-covered cotton is usually sufficient. Tape is applied from the cheek to the forehead.

PRECAUTIONS IN MANAGEMENT OF OCULAR DISORDERS

Use of Local Anesthetics

Unsupervised self-administration of local anesthetics is dangerous because the patient may further injure an anesthetized eye without knowing it. The

drug may also interfere with the normal healing process.

Rosenwaller GOD et al: Topical anesthetic abuse. Ophthalmology 1990;97:967. (Six patients with severe ocular disease.)

Pupillary Dilation

Dilating the pupil can very occasionally precipitate an acute glaucoma attack if the patient has a narrow anterior chamber angle. Dilation of the pupil should still be undertaken, but with caution if the anterior chamber is obviously shallow (readily determined by oblique illumination of the anterior segment of the eye). A short-acting mydriatic such as tropicamide should be used and the patient warned to report immediately if ocular discomfort or redness develops. Angle closure is probably more likely to occur if pilocarpine is used to overcome pupillary dilatation than if the pupil is allowed to constrict naturally.

Local Corticosteroid Therapy

Repeated use of local corticosteroids presents several hazards: herpes simplex (dendritic) keratitis, fungal infection, open-angle glaucoma, and cataract formation. Furthermore, perforation of the cornea may occur when the corticosteroids are used for herpes simplex keratitis.

Contaminated Eye Medications

Ophthalmic solutions are prepared with the same degree of care as fluids intended for intravenous administration, but once bottles are opened there is always a risk of contamination, particularly with solutions of tetracaine, proparacaine, fluorescein, and any preservative-free preparations. The most dangerous is fluorescein, as this solution is frequently contaminated with *P aeruginosa,* an organism that can rapidly destroy the eye. Sterile fluorescein filter paper strips are now available and are recommended for use in place of fluorescein solutions.

Whether in plastic or glass containers, eye solutions should not remain in use for long periods after the bottle is opened. Four weeks after opening is an absolute maximal time to use a solution containing preservatives before discarding. Preservative-free preparations should be kept refrigerated and discarded within 1 week after opening. Any solution should of course be checked for signs of bacterial contamination prior to use.

If the eye has been injured accidentally or by surgical trauma, it is of the greatest importance to use freshly opened bottles of sterile medications or single-use eyedropper units.

Toxic & Hypersensitivity Reactions to Topical Therapy

Patients receiving long-term topical therapy may develop local toxic or hypersensitivity reactions to

Table 7–3. Adverse ocular effects of systemic drugs.

Drug	Possible Side Effects
Respiratory drugs	
Oxygen	Retinopathy of prematurity.
Cardiovascular system drugs	
Digitalis	Disturbances of color vision, scotomas.
Quinidine	Optic neuritis (rare).
Thiazides (Diuril, etc)	Xanthopsia (yellow vision), myopia.
Carbonic anhydrase inhibitors (acetazolamide)	Ocular hypotony, transient myopia.
Amiodarone	Corneal deposits.
Oxyprenolol	Photophobia, ocular irritation.
Gastrointestinal drugs	
Anticholinergic agents	Risk of angle-closure glaucoma due to mydriasis. Blurring of vision due to cycloplegia (occasional).
Central nervous system drugs	
Barbiturates	Extraocular muscle palsies with diplopia, ptosis, cortical blindness.
Chloral hydrate	Diplopia, ptosis, miosis.
Phenothiazines	Deposits of pigment in conjunctiva, cornea, lens, and retina. Oculogyric crises.
Amphetamines	Widening of palpebral fissure. Dilatation of pupil, paralysis of ciliary muscle with loss of accommodation.
Monoamine oxidase inhibitors	Nystagmus, extraocular muscle palsies, optic atrophy.
Tricyclic agents	Dilatation of pupil (risk of angle-closure glaucoma), cycloplegia.
Phenytoin	Nystagmus, diplopia, ptosis, slight blurring of vision (rare).
Neostigmine	Nystagmus, miosis.
Morphine	Miosis.
Haloperidol	Capsular cataract.
Lithium carbonate	Exophthalmos, oculogyric crisis.
Diazepam	Nystagmus.
Hormones	
Corticosteroids	Cataract (posterior subcapsular), local immunologic suppression, causing susceptibility to viral (herpes simplex), bacterial, and fungal infections; steroid-induced glaucoma.
Female sex hormones	Retinal artery occlusion, retinal vein occlusion, papilledema, ocular palsies with diplopia, nystagmus, optic neuropathy, retinal vasculitis, scotomas, migraine, mydriasis and cycloplegia, and macular edema.
Antibiotics	
Chloramphenicol	Optic neuritis and atrophy.
Streptomycin	Optic neuritis.
Tetracycline	Pseudotumor cerebri, transient myopia.
Antimalarial agents	
Chloroquine, etc	Macular changes, central scotomas, pigmentary degeneration of the retina, chloroquine keratopathy, ocular palsies, ptosis, ERG depression.
Amebicides	
Iodochlorhydroxyquin	Optic atrophy.
Chemotherapeutic agents	
Sulfonamides	Stevens-Johnson syndrome.
Ethambutol	Optic neuritis and atrophy.
Isoniazid	Optic neuritis and atrophy.
Heavy metals	
Gold salts	Deposits in the cornea and conjunctiva.
Lead compounds	Optic atrophy, papilledema, ocular palsies.
Chelating agents	
Penicillamine	Ocular pemphigoid, optic neuritis, ocular myasthenia.
Oral hypoglycemic agents	
Chlorpropamide	Transient change in refractive error, diplopia, Stevens-Johnson syndrome.
Vitamins	
Vitamin A	Papilledema, retinal hemorrhages, loss of eyebrows and eyelashes, nystagmus, diplopia, blurring of vision.
Vitamin D	Band-shaped keratopathy.
Antirheumatic agents	
Salicylates	Nystagmus, retinal hemorrhages, cortical blindness (rare).
Indomethacin	Corneal deposits.
Phenylbutazone	Retinal hemorrhages.

the active agent or preservatives, especially if there is inadequate tear secretion. Preservatives in contact lens cleaning solutions may produce similar problems. Burning and soreness are exacerbated by drop instillation or contact lens insertion; occasionally, fibrosis and scarring of the conjunctiva and cornea may occur.

An antibiotic instilled into the eye can sensitize the patient to that drug and cause a hypersensitivity reaction upon subsequent systemic administration.

Schwab IR, Abbott RL: Toxic ulcerative keratopathy: An unrecognized problem. Ophthalmology 1989;96:1187. (Self-inflicted and iatrogenic.)

Systemic Effects of Ocular Drugs

The systemic absorption of certain topical drugs (through the conjunctival vessels and lacrimal drainage system) must be considered when there is a systemic medical contraindication to the use of the drug. Ophthalmic solutions of the nonselective beta-blockers timolol, levobunolol, and metipranolol, may worsen patients with cardiac failure or asthma. Atro-

pine ointment should be prescribed for children rather than the drops, since absorption of the 1% topical solution may be toxic. Phenylephrine eye drops can precipitate hypertensive crises and angina. Also to be considered are adverse interactions between systemically administered and ocular drugs. Using only 1 or 2 drops at a time and a few minutes of nasolacrimal occlusion or eyelid closure ensure maximum efficacy and decrease systemic side effects of topical agents.

ADVERSE OCULAR EFFECTS OF SYSTEMIC DRUGS

Systemically administered drugs produce a wide variety of adverse effects on the visual system. Table 7–3 lists the major examples.

Fraunfelder FT, Mayer SM: Ocular and systemic side effects of drugs. In: *General Ophthalmology,* 13th ed. Vaughan D, Asbury T, Riordan-Eva P (editors). Appleton & Lange, 1992.

REFERENCE

Vaughan D, Asbury T, Riordan-Eva P (editors): *General Ophthalmology,* 13th ed. Appleton & Lange, 1992.

Ear, Nose, & Throat

8

Robert K. Jackler, MD, & Michael J. Kaplan, MD

DISEASES OF THE EAR

HEARING LOSS

Classification

A. Conductive Hearing Loss: Conductive hearing loss results from dysfunction of the external or middle ear. There are four mechanisms, each resulting in impairment of the passage of sound vibrations to the inner ear: (1) obstruction (eg, cerumen impaction), (2) mass loading (eg, middle ear effusion), (3) stiffness effect (eg, otosclerosis), and (4) discontinuity (eg, ossicular disruption). Conductive hearing loss is generally correctable with medical or surgical therapy—or in some cases both.

B. Sensory Hearing Loss: Sensory hearing loss results from deterioration of the cochlea, usually due to loss of hair cells from the organ of Corti. Among the many common causes are noise trauma, ototoxicity, and aging (presbycusis). Sensory hearing loss is not correctable with medical or surgical therapy but often may be prevented or stabilized.

C. Neural Hearing Loss: Neural hearing loss occurs with lesions involving the eighth nerve, auditory nuclei, ascending tracts, or auditory cortex. It is the least common clinically recognized cause of hearing loss. Examples include acoustic neuroma, multiple sclerosis, and cerebrovascular disease.

Epidemiology of Hearing Loss

Conductive losses in adults are most commonly due to cerumen impaction or transient auditory tube dysfunction associated with upper respiratory tract infection. Persistent conductive losses usually result from chronic ear infection, trauma, or otosclerosis.

Sensorineural losses in adults are common. A gradually progressive, predominantly high-frequency loss with advancing age is typical though not invariable. Other than aging effects, common causes of sensorineural loss include excessive noise exposure, head trauma, and systemic diseases such as diabetes mellitus.

Evaluation of Hearing (Audiology)

In a quiet room, the hearing level may be estimated by having the patient repeat aloud words presented in a soft whisper, a normal spoken voice, or a shout. Tuning forks are useful in differentiating conductive from sensorineural losses. A 512-Hz tuning fork is employed, since frequencies below this level elicit a tactile response. In the **Weber test,** the tuning fork is placed on the forehead or front teeth. In conductive losses, the sound appears louder in the poorer-hearing ear, whereas in sensorineural losses it radiates to the better side. In the **Rinne test,** the tuning fork is placed alternately on the mastoid bone and in front of the ear canal. In conductive losses, bone conduction exceeds air conduction; in sensorineural losses, the opposite is true.

Formal audiometric studies are performed by an audiologist in a soundproofed room. Pure-tone thresholds in decibels (dB) are obtained over the range of 250–8000 Hz (the main speech frequencies are between 500 and 3000 Hz) for both air and bone conduction. Conductive losses create a gap between the air and bone thresholds, whereas in sensorineural losses both air and bone conduction are equally diminished. The threshold of normal hearing is from 0 to 20 dB, which corresponds to the loudness of a soft whisper. Mild hearing loss is indicated by a threshold of 20–40 dB (soft spoken voice), moderate loss by a threshold of 40–60 dB (normal spoken voice), severe loss by a threshold of 60–80 dB (loud spoken voice), and profound loss by a threshold of 80 dB (shout). The clarity of hearing is often impaired in sensorineural hearing loss. This is evaluated by speech discrimination testing, which is reported as percentage correct (90–100% is normal). The site of the lesion responsible for sensorineural loss—in the cochlea or in the central auditory system—may be determined with auditory brain stem-evoked responses.

Every patient who complains of a hearing loss should be referred for audiologic evaluation unless the cause is easily remediable (eg, cerumen impaction) or is expected to be of short duration (eg, acute otitis media). Audiologic screening is not recommended for adults with apparently normal hearing unless they are exposed to potentially injurious levels of noise or have reached the age of 65, after which screening evaluations should be done every few years.

Martin FN: *Introduction to Audiology.* Prentice-Hall, 1991.
Schow RL: Considerations in selecting and validating an adult/elderly hearing screening protocol. Ear Hear 1991; 12:337.
Sutherland JE, Campbell K: Immitance audiometry. Prim Care 1990;17:233.

Hearing Rehabilitation

Patients with hearing loss not correctable by medical therapy may benefit from hearing amplification. Contemporary hearing aids are comparatively free of distortion and have been miniaturized to the point where they often may be contained entirely within the ear canal. To optimize the benefit, a hearing aid must be carefully selected to conform to the nature of the hearing loss. Digitally programmable hearing aids are now becoming available that promise substantial improvements in speech intelligibility, especially under difficult listening circumstances.

Aside from hearing aids, many assistive devices are available to improve comprehension in individual and group settings, to help with hearing television and radio programs, and for telephone communication. In individuals with profound sensory deafness, the cochlear implant—an electronic device that is surgically implanted to stimulate the auditory nerve—offers socially beneficial auditory rehabilitation to most adults with acquired deafness.

Berger KW: Introduction to three current hearing aid fitting methods. Am J Otol 1991;12:40.
Loeb GE: Cochlear prosthetics. Ann Rev Neuroscience 1990;13:357.
Waltzman SB et al: Benefits of cochlear implantation in the geriatric population. Otolaryngol Head Neck Surg 1993;108:329. (Improved auditory performance and quality of life.)

DISEASES OF THE AURICLE

Disorders of the external ear are for the most part dermatologic. Skin cancers due to actinic exposure are common and may be treated with standard techniques. Traumatic auricular hematoma must be recognized and drained to prevent significant cosmetic deformity (cauliflower ear) resulting from dissolution of supporting cartilage. Similarly, cellulitis of the auricle must be treated promptly to prevent development of perichondritis and its resultant deformity. Relapsing polychondritis is a systemic disorder often associated with recurrent, frequently bilateral, painful episodes of auricular erythema and edema. Treatment with corticosteroids may help forestall cartilage dissolution. Respiratory compromise may occur as a result of progressive involvement of the tracheobronchial tree. Chondritis and perichondritis may be dif- ferentiated from auricular cellulitis by sparing of involvement of the lobule, which does not contain cartilage.

Vuyk HD, Bakkers EJM: Absorbable mattress sutures in the management of auricular hematoma. Laryngoscope 1991;101:1124. (A simple technique to prevent reaccumulation of blood.)

DISEASES OF THE EAR CANAL

1. CERUMEN IMPACTION

Cerumen is a protective secretion produced by the outer portion of the ear canal. In most individuals, the ear canal is self-cleansing. Recommended hygiene consists of cleaning the external opening with a washcloth over the index finger without entering the canal itself. In most cases, cerumen impaction is self-induced through ill-advised attempts at cleaning the ear. It may be relieved with detergent ear drops (eg, 3% hydrogen peroxide; 6.5% carbamide peroxide), mechanical removal, suction, or irrigation. Irrigation is performed with water at body temperature to avoid a vestibular caloric response. The stream should be directed at the ear canal wall adjacent to the cerumen plug. Irrigation should be performed only when the tympanic membrane is known to be intact.

Use of jet irrigators designed for cleaning teeth (eg, WaterPik) for wax removal should be avoided since they may result in tympanic membrane perforations. Following irrigation, the ear canal should be thoroughly dried (eg, by instilling isopropyl alcohol or using a hair blow drier on low-power setting) to reduce the likelihood of inducing external otitis. Specialty referral for cleaning under microscopic guidance is indicated when the impaction has not responded to routine measures or if the patient has a history of chronic otitis media or tympanic membrane perforation.

Dinsdale RC et al: Catastrophic otologic injury from oral jet irrigation of the external auditory canal. Laryngoscope 1991;101:75. (Cautions against use.)
Sharp JF et al: Ear wax removal: A survey of current practice. Br Med J 1990;301:1251. (A survey of 289 general practitioners in Scotland. Complications requiring specialty referral occurred in 1:1000 syringed ears.)

2. FOREIGN BODIES

Foreign bodies in the ear canal are more frequent in children than in adults. Firm materials may be removed with a loop or a hook, taking care not to displace the object medially toward the tympanic membrane. Aqueous irrigation should not be performed for organic foreign bodies (eg, beans, insects), because water may cause them to swell. Living insects are best immobilized before removal by filling the ear canal with lidocaine. When practical, foreign bodies of the ear canal are best removed under microscopic guidance.

Bressler K Shelton C: Ear foreign-body removal: A review of 98 consecutive cases. Laryngoscope 1993;103:367. (Ear canal lacerationwhen removal was performed without microscopic guidance.)

3. EXTERNAL OTITIS

External otitis, commonly known as swimmer's ear, presents with otalgia, frequently accompanied by pruritus and purulent discharge. There is often a history of recent water exposure or mechanical trauma (eg, scratching, cotton applicators). External otitis is usually caused by gram-negative rods (eg, *Pseudomonas, Proteus*) or fungi (eg, *Aspergillus*), which grow in the presence of excessive moisture.

Examination reveals erythema and edema of the ear canal skin, often with a purulent exudate. Manipulation of the auricle often elicits pain. Because the lateral surface of the tympanic membrane is ear canal skin, it is often erythematous. However, in contrast to acute otitis media, it moves normally with pneumatic otoscopy. When the canal skin is very edematous, it may be impossible to visualize the tympanic membrane. Fundamental to the treatment of external otitis is protection of the ear from additional moisture and avoidance of further mechanical injury by scratching. Otic drops containing a mixture of aminoglycoside antibiotic and anti-inflammatory corticosteroid in an acid vehicle are generally very effective (eg, neomycin sulfate, polymyxin B sulfate, and hydrocortisone). Purulent debris filling the ear canal should be gently removed to permit entry of the topical medication. Drops should be used abundantly (5 or more drops), since too much is harmless and too little will fail to penetrate the depths of the canal. When substantial edema of the canal wall prevents entry of drops into the ear canal, a wick is placed to facilitate entry of the medication.

Brook I, Frazier EH, Thompson DH: Aerobic and anaerobic microbiology of external otitis. Clin Infect Dis 1992; 15:955.

4. PRURITUS

Pruritus of the external auditory canal, particularly at the meatus, is a common problem. While it may be associated with external otitis or with dermatologic conditions such as seborrheic dermatitis and psoriasis, most cases are self-induced either from excoriation or by overly zealous ear cleaning. To permit regeneration of the protective cerumen blanket, patients should be instructed to avoid use of soap and water or cotton swabs in the ear canal. Patients with excessively dry canal skin may benefit from application of mineral oil, which helps to counteract dryness and repel moisture. When an inflammatory component is present, topical application of a corticosteroid (eg, 0.1% triamcinolone) may be beneficial. It is axiomatic in persistent pruritus that the patient must cease scratching the ear. In stubborn cases, the fingernails must be kept short and the patient may need to wear cotton gloves at night to avoid manipulation during sleep. Symptomatic reduction of pruritus may be obtained by use of oral antihistamines (eg, diphenhydramine, 25 mg orally at bedtime). Topical application of isopropyl alcohol promptly relieves ear canal pruritus in many patients.

5. MALIGNANT EXTERNAL OTITIS

Persistent external otitis in the diabetic or immunocompromised patient may evolve into osteomyelitis of the skull base, often called malignant external otitis. Usually caused by *Pseudomonas aeruginosa,* osteomyelitis begins in the floor of the ear canal and may extend into the middle fossa floor, the clivus, and even the contralateral skull base. The patient usually presents with persistent foul aural discharge, granulations in the ear canal, deep otalgia, and progressive cranial nerve palsies involving nerves VI, VII, IX, X, XI, or XII. Diagnosis is confirmed by the demonstration of osseous erosion on CT and radionuclide scanning.

Treatment is chiefly medical, requiring prolonged antipseudomonal antibiotic administration, often for several months. Although intravenous therapy is often required, selected patients may be managed with the oral agent ciprofloxacin (500–1000 mg orally twice daily), which has proved effective against many of the causative *Pseudomonas* strains. To avoid relapse, antibiotic therapy should be continued, even in the asymptomatic patient, until gallium scanning indicates a marked reduction in the inflammatory process. Surgical debridement of infected bone is reserved for cases of deterioration despite medical therapy.

Giamarellou H: Malignant otitis externa: The therapeutic evolution of a lethal infection. J Antimicrob Chemother 1992;30:745. (Increasing role of fluroquinolones.)
Johnson MP, Ramphal R: Malignant external otitis: Report on therapy with ceftazidime and review of therapy and prognosis. Rev Infect Dis 1990;12:173.

6. EXOSTOSES & OSTEOMAS

Bony overgrowths of the ear canal are a frequent incidental finding and occasionally have clinical significance. Clinically, they present as skin-covered mounds in the medial ear canal obscuring the tympanic membrane to a variable degree. Solitary osteomas are of no significance as long as they do not cause obstruction or infection. Multiple exostoses, which are generally acquired from repeated exposure to cold water, often progress and require surgical removal.

7. NEOPLASIA

The most common neoplasm of the ear canal is squamous cell carcinoma. Clinically, this tumor may simulate persistent external otitis. When an apparent otitis externa does not resolve on therapy, early biopsy is warranted. This disease carries a very high 5-year mortality rate and must be treated with wide surgical resection and radiation therapy. Adenomatous tumors, originating from the ceruminous glands, generally follow a more indolent course.

Arriaga M et al: Squamous cell carcinoma of the external auditory meatus (canal). Otolaryngol Head Neck Surg 1989;101:330.

DISEASES OF THE AUDITORY (EUSTACHIAN) TUBE

1. AUDITORY TUBE DYSFUNCTION

The tube that connects the middle ear to the nasopharynx—the auditory tube, or eustachian tube—provides ventilation and drainage for the middle ear cleft. It is normally closed, opening only during the act of swallowing or yawning. When auditory tube function is compromised, air trapped within the middle ear becomes absorbed and negative pressure results. The most common causes of auditory tube dysfunction are diseases associated with edema of the tubal lining, such as viral upper respiratory tract infections and allergy. The patient usually reports a sense of fullness in the ear and mild to moderate impairment of hearing. When the tube is only partially blocked, swallowing or yawning may elicit a popping or crackling sound. Examination reveals retraction of the tympanic membrane and decreased mobility on pneumatic otoscopy. Following a viral illness, this disorder is usually transient, lasting days to weeks. Treatment with systemic and intranasal decongestants (eg, pseudoephedrine, 60 mg orally every 4 hours; oxymetazoline, 0.05% spray every 8–12 hours) combined with autoinflation by forced exhalation against closed nostrils may hasten relief. Air travel, rapid altitudinal change, and underwater diving should be avoided. Autoinflation should not be recommended to patients with active intranasal infection, since this maneuver may precipitate middle ear infection. Allergic patients may also benefit from desensitization or intranasal corticosteroids (eg, beclomethasone dipropionate, two sprays in each nostril twice daily for 2–6 weeks).

An overly patent auditory tube is a relatively uncommon problem that may be quite distressing. Typical complaints include fullness in the ear and autophony, an exaggerated ability to hear oneself breath and speak. A patulous auditory tube may develop during rapid weight loss, or it may commence without a discernible cause. In contrast to a hypofunctioning auditory tube, the aural pressure is often made worse by exertion and may diminish during an upper respiratory tract infection. Although physical examination is usually normal, respiratory excursions of the tympanic membrane may occasionally be detected during vigorous breathing. Treatment includes avoidance of decongestant products, insertion of a ventilating tube to reduce the outward stretch of the ear drum during phonation, and surgical narrowing of the auditory tube (rarely).

Bluestone CD, Doyle WJ: Anatomy and physiology of eustachian tube and middle ear related to otitis media. J Allergy Clin Immunol 1988;81:997.
Dyer RK, McElveen JT: The patulous eustachian tube: Management options. Otolaryngol Head Neck Surg 1991;105:832. (Medical and surgical.)

2. SEROUS OTITIS MEDIA

When the auditory tube remains blocked for a prolonged period, the resultant negative pressure will result in transudation of fluid. This condition, known as serous otitis media, is especially common in children because their auditory tubes are narrower and more horizontal in orientation than adults. It is less common in adults, in whom it usually follows an upper respiratory tract infection or barotrauma. In an adult with persistent unilateral serous otitis media, nasopharyngeal carcinoma must be excluded. The tympanic membrane in serous otitis media is dull and hypomobile, occasionally accompanied by air bubbles in the middle ear and conductive hearing loss. The treatment of serous otitis media is similar to that for auditory tube dysfunction. A short course of oral corticosteroids (eg, prednisone, 40 mg/d for 7 days) has been advocated by some in the management of serous otitis media, as have oral antibiotics (eg, amoxicillin, 250 mg orally three times daily for 7 days)—or even a combination of the two. The role of these regimens remains controversial, but they are probably of little lasting benefit.

When medication fails to bring relief after several months, a ventilating tube placed through the tympanic membrane may restore hearing and alleviate the sense of aural fullness. Recent evidence suggests that adenoidectomy modifies the underlying pathology of serous otitis media in young children and constitutes effective therapy regardless of whether the adenoids are of normal size or enlarged.

Gacek RR: A differential diagnosis of unilateral serous otitis media. Laryngoscope 1992;102:461. (In the adult may indicate the presence of a serious underlying pathologic process.)

Gates GA et al: Adenoidectomy and otitis media. Ann Otol Rhinol Laryngol 1992;101:24. (Adenoidectomy should be considered for primary treatment of serous otitis media in children over 4 years of age.)

Kinney SE: Violence and the ear and temporal bone. Arch Otolaryngol 1992;118,581.

Sham JST: Serous otitis media: An opportunity for early recognition of nasopharyngeal carcinoma. Arch Otolaryngol 1992;118, 794. (More than 40% initially presented with serous otitis.)

Stangerup SE et al: Autoinflation as treatment of secretory otitis media: A randomized controlled study. Arch Otolaryngol 1992;118:149. (Improvement utilizing autoinflation compared with controls.)

3. BAROTRAUMA

Individuals with auditory tube dysfunction due either to congenital narrowness or to acquired mucosal edema may be unable to equalize the barometric stress exerted on the middle ear by air travel, rapid altitudinal change, or underwater diving. The problem is generally most acute during airplane descent, since the negative middle ear pressure tends to collapse and lock the auditory tube. Several measures are useful to enhance auditory tube function and avoid otic barotrauma. The patient should be advised to swallow, yawn, and autoinflate frequently during descent. Systemic decongestants (eg, pseudoephedrine, 30–60 mg) should be taken several hours before anticipated arrival time so that they will be maximally effective during descent. Topical decongestants such as 1% phenylephrine nasal spray should be administered 1 hour before arrival. It is important that the susceptible individual not sleep during the descent phase, since one may awaken with severe pain and markedly negative pressure from a collapsed auditory tube. Infants are especially prone to barotrauma and should be given a bottle to suck during descent.

The treatment of acute negative middle ear pressure that persists on the ground is with decongestants and attempts at autoinflation. Myringotomy provides immediate relief and is appropriate in the setting of severe otalgia and hearing loss. Repeated episodes of barotrauma in persons who must fly frequently may be alleviated by insertion of ventilating tubes.

Underwater diving represents even a greater barometric stress to the ear than flying. The problem occurs most commonly during the descent phase, when pain develops within the first 15 feet if inflation of the middle ear via the auditory tube has not occurred. Divers must descend slowly and equilibrate in stages to avoid the development of severely negative pressures in the tympanum that may result in hemorrhage (hemotympanum) or perilymphatic fistulization. In the latter, the oval or round window ruptures, resulting in sensory hearing loss and acute vertigo. Emesis due to acute labyrinthine dysfunction can be very dangerous during an underwater dive. Sensory hearing loss or vertigo, which develops during the ascent phase of a saturation dive, may be the first (or only) symptom of decompression sickness. Immediate recompression will return intravascular gas bubbles to solution and restore the inner ear microcirculation. Patients should be warned to avoid diving when they have upper respiratory infections or episodes of nasal allergy. Tympanic membrane perforation is an absolute contraindication to diving, as the patient will experience an unbalanced thermal stimulus to the semicircular canals and may experience vertigo, disorientation, and even emesis. Finally, individuals with only one hearing ear should be discouraged from diving because of the significant risk of otologic injury.

Shupak A et al: Diving-related inner ear injuries. Laryngoscope 1991;101:173.

DISEASES OF THE MIDDLE EAR

1. ACUTE OTITIS MEDIA

Acute otitis media is a bacterial infection of the mucosally lined air-containing spaces of the temporal bone. Purulent material forms not only within the middle ear cleft but also within the mastoid air cells and petrous apex when they are pneumatized. Acute otitis media is usually precipitated by a viral upper respiratory tract infection that causes auditory tube edema. This results in accumulation of fluid and mucus, which becomes secondarily infected by bacteria. The most common pathogens both in adults and in children are *Streptococcus pneumoniae, Haemophilus influenzae,* and *Streptococcus pyogenes.*

Acute otitis media is most common in infants and children, though it may occur at any age. The patient presents with otalgia, aural pressure, decreased hearing, and often fever. The typical physical findings are erythema and decreased mobility of the tympanic membrane. Occasionally, bullae will be seen on the tympanic membrane. Although it is commonly taught that this represents infection with *Mycoplasma pneu-*

moniae, most cases involve more common pathogens.

Rarely, when middle ear empyema is severe, the tympanic membrane can be seen to bulge outward. In such cases, tympanic membrane rupture is imminent. Rupture is accompanied by a sudden decrease in pain, followed by the onset of otorrhea. With appropriate therapy, spontaneous healing of the tympanic membrane occurs in most cases. When perforation persists, chronic otitis media frequently evolves. Mastoid tenderness often accompanies acute otitis media and is due to the presence of pus within the mastoid air cells. At this stage, this does not indicate suppurative (surgical) mastoiditis.

The treatment of acute otitis media is specific antibiotic therapy, often combined with nasal decongestants. The first-choice antibiotic treatment is either amoxicillin (20–40 mg/kg/d) or erythromycin (50 mg/kg/d) plus sulfonamide (150 mg/kg/d) for 10 days. Alternatives useful in resistant cases are cefaclor (20–40 mg/kg/d) or amoxicillin-clavulanate (20–40 mg/kg/d) combinations.

Tympanocentesis for bacterial (aerobic and anaerobic) and fungal culture may be performed by any experienced physician. A 20-gauge spinal needle bent 90 degrees to the hub of a 3 mL syringe should be inserted atraumatically through the inferior portion of the tympanic membrane. Interposition of a pliable connecting tube between the needle and syringe permits an assistant to aspirate without inducing movement of the needle. Tympanocentesis is useful for otitis media in immunocompromised patients; in neonates, in whom gram-negative organisms are common; and in cases of persistent infection despite multiple courses of antibiotics.

Surgical drainage of the middle ear (myringotomy) is reserved for patients with severe otalgia or when complications of otitis (eg, mastoiditis, meningitis) have occurred.

Recurrent acute otitis media may be managed with long-term antibiotic prophylaxis. Single daily doses of sulfamethoxazole (500 mg) or amoxicillin (250 or 500 mg) are given over a period of 1–3 months. Failure of this regimen to control infection is an indication for insertion of ventilating tubes.

Giebink GS: Otitis media update: Pathogenesis and treatment. Ann Otol Rhinol Laryngol 1992;101:21.

Goldenberg RA: Hydroxyapatite ossicular replacement prostheses: Results in 157 consecutive cases. Laryngoscope 1992;102:1091. (Favorable results in patients with chronic otitis media.)

Heald MM et al: Pressure equalization (PE) tubes in the treatment of otitis media: National survey of otolaryngologists. Otolaryngol Head Neck Surg 1990;102:334. (Indications for tympanostomy tube insertion.)

Lalwani AK, Sooy CD: Otologic and neurotologic manifestations of acquired immunodeficiency syndrome. Otolaryngol Clin North Am 1992;25:1183.

Paradise JL: Antimicrobial prophylaxis for recurrent otitis
media. Ann Otol Rhinol Laryngol 1992;101:33. (Advocates prophylaxis as the first approach.)

Sade J, Luntz M: Adenoidectomy in otitis media: A review. Ann Otol Rhinol Laryngol 1991:100:226. (Reduces the relapse rate in acute and serious otitis media by a factor of two.)

2. CHRONIC OTITIS MEDIA & CHOLESTEATOMA

Chronic infection of the middle ear and mastoid generally develops as a consequence of recurrent acute otitis media, although it may follow other diseases and trauma. Perforation of the tympanic membrane is usually present. This may be accompanied by mucosal changes such as polypoid degeneration and granulation tissue and osseous changes such as osteitis and sclerosis. The bacteriology of chronic otitis media differs from that of acute otitis media. Common organisms include *P aeruginosa, Proteus* sp, *Staphylococcus aureus,* and mixed anaerobic infections. The clinical hallmark of chronic otitis media is purulent aural discharge. Drainage may be continuous or intermittent, with increased severity during upper respiratory tract infection or following water exposure. Pain is uncommon except during acute exacerbations. Conductive hearing loss results from destruction of the tympanic membrane and ossicular chain. The medical treatment of chronic otitis media includes regular removal of infected debris, use of earplugs to protect against water exposure, and topical antibiotic drops for exacerbations. Ciprofloxacin, an antipseudomonal agent, may help to dry a chronically discharging ear when given in a dosage of 500 mg orally twice a day for 1–6 weeks.

The definitive management of chronic otitis media is surgical in most cases. Tympanic membrane repair may be accomplished with temporalis muscle fascia or with homograft middle ear structures. Successful reconstruction of the tympanic membrane may be achieved in about 90% of cases, often with elimination of infection and significant improvement in hearing. When the mastoid air cells are involved by irreversible infection, they should be exenterated through mastoidectomy.

Cholesteatoma is a special variety of chronic otitis media. The most common cause is prolonged auditory tube dysfunction, with resultant chronic negative middle ear pressure that draws inward the upper flaccid portion of the tympanic membrane. This creates a squamous epithelium-lined sac, which—when its neck becomes obstructed—fills with desquamated keratin and becomes chronically infected. Cholesteatomas typically erode bone, with early penetration of the mastoid and destruction of the ossicular chain. Over time, they may erode the inner ear or facial nerve and on rare occasions may spread intracranially. Physical examination reveals an epitympanic retraction pocket or marginal tympanic membrane perforation that exudes keratin debris. The treatment of cholesteatoma is surgical marsupialization of the sac or its complete removal. This often requires creation of a "mastoid bowl" in which the ear canal and mastoid are joined into a large common cavity that must be periodically cleaned.

Kimmelman CP: Office management of the draining ear. Otolaryngol Clin North Am 1992;25:739.
Scularati N, Bluestone CD: Pathogenesis of cholesteatoma. Otolaryngol Clin North Am 1989;22:859.
Sheehy JL: Acquired cholesteatoma in adults. Otolaryngol Clin North Am 1989;22:967.

3. COMPLICATIONS OF OTITIS MEDIA

Mastoiditis

Acute suppurative mastoiditis usually evolves following several weeks of inadequately treated acute otitis media. It is characterized by postauricular pain and erythema accompanied by a spiking fever. Radiography reveals coalescence of the mastoid air cells due to destruction of their bony septa. Initial treatment consists of intravenous antibiotics and myringotomy for culture and drainage. Failure of medical therapy indicates the need for surgical drainage (mastoidectomy).

Petrous Apicitis

The medial portion of the petrous bone between the inner ear and clivus may become a site of persistent infection when the drainage of its pneumatic cell tracts becomes blocked. This may cause foul discharge, deep ear and retro-orbital pain, and sixth nerve palsy (Gradenigo's syndrome). Treatment is with prolonged antibiotic therapy (based on culture results) and surgical drainage via petrous apicectomy.

Otogenic Skull Base Osteomyelitis

Infections originating in the external or middle ear may result in osteomyelitis of the skull base, usually due to *P aeruginosa*. The diagnosis and management of this disease are discussed in the section on external otitis.

Beneke JE: Management of osteomyelitis of the skull base. Laryngoscope 1989;99:1220.

Facial Paralysis

Facial palsy may be associated with either acute or chronic otitis media. In the acute setting, it results from inflammation of the nerve in its middle ear segment, perhaps mediated through bacterially secreted neurotoxins. Treatment consists of myringotomy for drainage and culture, followed by intravenous antibi-

otics (based on culture results). The use of corticosteroids is controversial. The prognosis is excellent, with complete recovery in the vast majority of cases.

Facial palsy associated with chronic otitis media usually evolves slowly due to chronic pressure on the nerve in the middle ear or mastoid by cholesteatoma. Treatment requires surgical correction of the underlying disease. The prognosis is less favorable than for facial palsy associated with acute otitis media.

Engstrom M et al: Facial nerve enhancement in Bell's palsy demonstrated by different gadolinium-enhanced magnetic resonance imaging techniques. Arch Otolaryngol Head Neck Surg 1993;119:221. (Ipsilateral enhancement was detected in 12 of 21 patients. Within 4 months, it had resolved in 10 patients.)
Moore GF: Facial nerve paralysis. Prim Care 1990;17:437. (Differential diagnosis and management.)
Selesnick SH, Jackler RK: Facial paralysis in suppurative ear disease. Oper Techniques Otolaryngol Head Neck Surg 1992;3:61. (Pathophysiology, diagnosis, and management.)

Sigmoid Sinus Thrombosis

Trapped infection within the mastoid air cells adjacent to the sigmoid sinus may cause septic thrombophlebitis. This is heralded by signs of systemic sepsis (spiking fevers, chills), at times accompanied by signs of increased intracranial pressure (headache, lethargy, nausea and vomiting, papilledema). If not recognized early, it may lead to widespread septic embolization and death. Treatment is with intravenous antibiotics (based on culture results), surgical drainage, and—when emboli are suspected—ligation of the internal jugular vein in the neck.

Kelly KE et al: Diagnosis of septic sigmoid sinus thrombosis with magnetic resonance imaging. Otolaryngol Head Neck Surg 1991;105:617. (Includes management strategies.)

Central Nervous System Infection

Otogenic meningitis is by far the most common intracranial complication of ear infection. In the setting of acute suppurative otitis media, it arises from hematogenous spread of bacteria, most commonly *H influenzae* and *S pneumoniae*. In chronic otitis media, it results either from passage of infections along preformed pathways such as the petrosquamous suture line or from direct extension of disease through the dural plates of the petrous pyramid.

Epidural abscesses arise from direct extension of disease in the setting of chronic infection. They are usually asymptomatic but may present with deep local pain, headache, and low-grade fever. They are often discovered as an incidental finding at surgery. Intraparenchymal brain abscesses may arise in the temporal lobe or cerebellum. They most commonly evolve from retrograde thrombophlebitis adjacent to an epidural abscess. The predominant causative organisms are *S aureus, S pyogenes,* and *S pneumoniae.* Rupture into the subarachnoid space results in catastrophic meningitis and often rapid death.

Friedman EM et al: Central nervous system complications associated with acute otitis media in children. Laryngoscope 1990;100:149.

4. OTOSCLEROSIS

Otosclerosis is a progressive disease with a marked familial tendency that affects bone surrounding the inner ear. Lesions involving the footplate of the stapes result in increased impedance to the passage of sound through the ossicular chain, producing conductive hearing loss. This may be corrected through surgical replacement of the stapes with a prosthesis (stapedectomy). When otosclerotic lesions impinge on the cochlea, permanent sensory hearing loss occurs. Some evidence suggests that this level of hearing loss may be stabilized by treatment with oral sodium fluoride over prolonged periods of time (Florical—8.3 mg sodium fluoride and 364 mg calcium carbonate—two tablets orally each morning). Fluorides have minimal adverse effects other than occasional mild gastric irritation, which may be eliminated by ingesting the drug with meals.

Langman AW et al: Stapedectomy: Long term hearing results. Laryngoscope 1991;101:810. (Avoidance of the need for hearing amplification in the majority of cases.)

5. TRAUMA TO THE MIDDLE EAR

Tympanic membrane perforation may result from impact injury or explosive acoustic trauma. Spontaneous healing occurs in the great majority of cases. Persistent perforation may result from secondary infection brought on by exposure to water. Patients should be advised to wear earplugs while swimming or bathing during the healing period. Hemorrhage behind an intact tympanic membrane (hemotympanum) may follow blunt trauma or extreme barotrauma. Spontaneous resolution over several weeks is the usual course. When a conductive hearing loss greater than 30 dB persists for more than 3 months following trauma, disruption of the ossicular chain should be suspected. Middle ear exploration with reconstruction of the ossicular chain, combined with repair of the tympanic membrane when required, will usually restore hearing.

Kronenberg J, Ben-Shoshan J, Wolf M: Perforated tympanic membrane after blast injury. Am J Otol 1993; 14:92. (Intervention not recommended unless the perforation remains open longer than 10 months.)

6. MIDDLE EAR NEOPLASIA

Primary middle ear tumors are rare. Glomus tumors arise either in the middle ear (glomus tympanicum) or in the jugular bulb with upward erosion into the hypotympanum (glomus jugulare). They present clinically with pulsatile tinnitus and hearing loss. A vascular mass may be visible behind an intact tympanic membrane. Large glomus jugulare tumors are often associated with multiple cranial neuropathies, especially involving nerves VII, IX, X, XI, and XII. Treatment may require surgery, radiotherapy, or both.

EARACHE

External otitis and acute otitis media are both painful conditions. In external otitis, there is often a recent history of swimming, Q-tip use, or physical trauma, while in acute otitis media there is usually an antecedent or concurrent upper respiratory infection. The physical findings also differ. In external otitis, the ear canal skin is erythematous, while in acute otitis media this generally occurs only if the tympanic membrane has ruptured, spilling purulent material into the ear canal. Also, in external otitis the tympanic membrane may be erythematous, but it retains its mobility owing to the normal aeration of the middle ear cavity. Acute severe pain out of proportion to the physical findings may be due to herpes zoster oticus, especially when vesicles appear in the ear canal or concha. Chronic otitis media is usually not painful except during acute exacerbations. Persistent pain and discharge from the ear suggest osteomyelitis of the skull base or cancer.

The sensory innervation of the ear is derived from the trigeminal, facial, glossopharyngeal, vagal, and upper cervical nerves. Because of this rich innervation, referred otalgia is quite frequent. Temporomandibular joint dysfunction is a common cause of ear pain. It is often made worse by chewing or psychogenic grinding of the teeth (bruxism) and may be associated with dental malocclusion. Management includes soft diet, local heat to the masticatory muscles, massage, analgesics, and dental referral. Repeated episodes of severe lancinating otalgia may occur in glossopharyngeal neuralgia. Treatment with carbamazepine (100–300 mg orally every 8 hours) often confers substantial symptomatic relief. Severe glossopharyngeal neuralgia, which is refractory to medical management, may respond to microvascular decompression of the ninth nerve. Infections and neoplasia that involve the oropharynx, hypopharynx, and larynx frequently cause otalgia. Persistent earache demands specialty referral to exclude cancer of the upper aerodigestive tract.

McDonald JS, Pensak ML, Phero JC: Differential diagnosis of chronic facial, head, and neck pain conditions. Am J Otol 1990;11:299. (Wide variety of disease processes.)

Yanagisawa K, Kveton JF: Referred otalgia. Am J Otolaryngol 1992;13:323. (Nonotologic causes.)

DISEASES OF THE INNER EAR

1. SENSORY HEARING LOSS

Diseases of the cochlea result in sensory hearing loss, a condition that is usually irreversible. Most cochlear diseases result in bilateral symmetric hearing loss. The presence of unilateral or asymmetric sensorineural hearing loss suggests a lesion proximal to the cochlea. Lesions affecting the eighth nerve and central auditory system are discussed in the section on neural hearing loss. The primary goals in the management of sensory hearing loss are prevention of further losses and functional improvement with amplification and auditory rehabilitation.

Presbycusis

Presbycusis is the progressive, predominantly high-frequency symmetric hearing loss of advancing age. It is difficult to separate the various etiologic factors (eg, noise trauma) that may contribute to presbycusis, but genetic predisposition appears to play a role. Most patients notice a loss of speech discrimination that is especially pronounced in noisy environments. About 25% of people between the ages of 65 and 75 years and almost 50% of those over 75 experience hearing difficulties.

Gates GA et al: Presbycusis. Otolaryngol Head Neck Surg 1989;100:266.

Noise Trauma

Noise trauma is the second most common cause of sensory hearing loss. Sounds exceeding 85 dB are potentially injurious to the cochlea, especially with prolonged exposures. The loss typically begins in the high frequencies (especially 4000 Hz) and progresses to involve the speech frequencies with continuing exposure. Among the more common sources of injurious noise are industrial machinery, weapons, and excessively loud music. In recent years, monitoring of noise levels in the workplace by regulatory agencies has led to preventive programs that have reduced the frequency of occupational losses. Individuals of all ages, especially those with existing hearing losses, should wear earplugs when exposed to moderately loud noises and specially designed earmuffs when exposed to explosive noises such as gunfire.

Consensus conference: Noise and hearing loss. JAMA 1990;263:3185.

Dancer AL et al (editors): *Noise-Induced Hearing Loss.* Mosby Year Book, 1992.

Sataloff RT: Hearing loss in musicians. Am J Otol 1991; 12:122. (Rock musicians and other professional performers.)

Physical Trauma

Head trauma has effects on the inner ear similar to those of severe acoustic trauma. Some degree of sensory hearing loss may occur following simple concussion and is frequent after skull fracture.

Ototoxicity

Ototoxic substances may affect both the auditory and vestibular systems. The most common ototoxic medications are salicylates, aminoglycosides, loop diuretics, and several antineoplastic agents, notably cisplatin. The latter three categories may cause irreversible hearing loss even when administered in therapeutic doses. When using these medications, it is important to identify high-risk patients such as those with preexisting hearing losses or renal insufficiency. Patients simultaneously receiving multiple ototoxic agents are at particular risk owing to ototoxic synergy. Useful measures to reduce the risk of ototoxic injury include serial audiometry and monitoring of serum peak and trough levels and substitution of equivalent nonototoxic drugs whenever possible.

Boettcher FA, Salvi RJ: Salicylate ototoxicity: Review and synthesis. Am J Otolaryngol 1991;12:33.

de Oliveira JAA: *Audiovestibular Toxicity of Drugs.* CRC Press, 1989. (Encyclopedic reference source for the ototoxic potential of drugs.)

Govaerts PJ et al: Aminoglycoside-induced ototoxicity. Toxicol Lett 1990;52:227. (The most important class of iatrogenic ototoxins.)

Hughes G, Schuring AG: Medicolegal aspects of ototoxicity. Am J Otol 1992;13:95.

Sudden Sensory Hearing Loss

Sudden loss of hearing in one ear may occur at any age but is more common in the elderly. It most probably is the result of sudden vascular occlusion of the internal auditory artery or of a viral inner ear infection. Prognosis is mixed, with many patients suffering permanent deafness in the involved ear while others have complete recovery. Oral corticosteroids are felt by many to improve the odds of recovery. A common regimen is prednisone, 80 mg/d, followed by a tapering dose over a 10-day period.

Grandis JR et al: Treatment of idiopathic sudden sensorineural hearing loss. Am J Otology 1993;14:183. (Medical therapy does not alter the natural history.)

Other Causes of Sensory Hearing Loss

There are numerous less common causes of sensory hearing loss. Metabolic derangements (eg, diabetes, hypothyroidism, hyperlipidemia, and renal failure), infections (eg, measles, mumps, syphilis), autoimmune disorders (eg, polyarteritis, lupus erythematosus), physical factors (eg, radiation therapy) and hereditary syndromes are some of the chief examples. Identification of metabolic, infectious, or autoimmune sensory hearing losses is especially important, as these may occasionally be reversible with medical therapy. Meniere's syndrome and labyrinthitis are discussed in the section on vestibular disorders.

2. TINNITUS

Tinnitus is the perception of abnormal ear or head noises. Persistent tinnitus usually indicates the presence of sensory hearing loss. Intermittent periods of mild, high-pitched tinnitus lasting for several minutes are common in normal-hearing persons. When severe and persistent, tinnitus may interfere with sleep and the ability to concentrate, resulting in considerable psychologic distress.

The most important treatment of tinnitus is avoidance of exposure to excessive noise, ototoxic agents, and other factors that may cause cochlear damage. Masking the tinnitus with music or through amplification of normal sounds with a hearing aid may also bring some relief. Although pharmacologic treatment with antiarrhythmic drugs has been advocated, recent evidence suggests no benefit with available oral regimens. Among the numerous drugs that have been used in attempts to suppress tinnitus, oral antidepressants (eg, nortriptyline at an initial dosage of 50 mg orally at bedtime) have proved to be the most efficacious.

Pulsatile tinnitus should be distinguished from tonal tinnitus. Pulsations most often result from conductive hearing loss, which renders transmitted carotid pulsations more apparent. However, it may also indicate a vascular abnormality such as glomus tumor, carotid vaso-occlusive disease, arteriovenous malformation, or aneurysm. CT scan and vascular studies are often necessary to establish a definitive diagnosis.

Jungreis CA: Pulsatile tinnitus from a dural arteriovenous malformation. Ann Otol Rhinol Laryngol 1991;100:951. (Radiographic evaluation.)

Murai K: Review of the pharmacologic treatment of tinnitus. Am J Otol 199;213:454.

Shulman A et al (editors): *Tinnitus: Diagnosis/Treatment.* Lea & Febiger, 1991.

3. VERTIGO
(Table 8–1)

Vertigo is the cardinal symptom of vestibular disease. It is either a sensation of motion when there is no motion or an exaggerated sense of motion in response to a given bodily movement. Thus, vertigo is not just "spinning" but may present, for example, as a sense of tumbling, of falling forward or backward, or of the ground rolling beneath one's feet ("earthquake-like"). It should be distinguished from imbalance, light-headedness, and syncope, all of which are usually nonvestibular in origin. The vertigo that results from peripheral vestibulopathy is usually of sudden onset, may be so severe that the patient is unable to walk or stand, and is frequently accompanied by nausea and vomiting. Tinnitus and hearing loss may be associated and provide strong support for a peripheral origin.

A minimal physical examination of the patient with vertigo includes the Romberg test, an evaluation of gait, and observation for the presence of nystagmus. In peripheral lesions, nystagmus is usually horizontal with a rotatory component; the fast phase usually beats away from the diseased side. Visual fixation tends to inhibit nystagmus except in very acute peripheral lesions or with central nervous system disease. The Nylen-Bárány maneuvers are intended to induce positioning nystagmus but are of limited use when the patient is able to visually fixate. This objection may be overcome either by placing +2-diopter lenses (Fresnel glasses) over the eyes or by making observations in the dark by means of electronystagmographic recording. The Fukuda test, in which the patient marches in place with eyes closed, is useful for detecting subtle defects. A positive response is observed when the patient rotates, usually

Table 8–1. Common vestibular disorders: Differential diagnosis based on classic presentations.

Duration of Typical Vertiginous Episodes	Auditory Symptoms Present	Auditory Symptoms Absent
Seconds	Perilymphatic fistula	Positioning vertigo (cupulolithiasis), vertebrobasilar insufficiency, cervical vertigo
Hours	Endolymphatic hydrops (Meniere's syndrome), syphilis	Recurrent vestibulopathy, vestibular migraine
Days	Labyrinthitis, labyrinthine concussion	Vestibular neuronitis
Months	Acoustic neuroma, ototoxicity	Multiple sclerosis, cerebellar degeneration

toward the side of the diseased labyrinth. Vertigo arising from central lesions tends to develop gradually and then become progressively more severe and debilitating. Nystagmus is not always present but can occur in any direction and may be dissociated in the two eyes. The associated nystagmus is often nonfatigable, vertical rather than horizontal in orientation, without latency, and unsuppressed by visual fixation. Electronystagmography is useful in documenting these characteristics. The evaluation of central audiovestibular dysfunction usually requires imaging of the brain with CT scans or, particularly, MRI.

Episodic vertigo can occur in patients with diplopia from external ophthalmoplegia and is maximal when the patient looks in the direction where the separation of images is greatest. Cerebral lesions involving the temporal cortex may also produce vertigo, which is sometimes the initial symptom of a seizure. Finally, vertigo may be a feature of a number of systemic disorders and can occur as a side effect of certain anticonvulsant, antibiotic, hypnotic, analgesic, and tranquilizing drugs or of alcohol.

Laboratory investigations such as audiologic evaluation, caloric stimulation, electronystagmography, CT scan, and brain stem auditory evoked potential studies are indicated in patients with persistent vertigo or when central nervous system disease is suspected. These studies will help to distinguish between central and peripheral lesions and to identify causes requiring specific therapy. Electronystagmography consists of objective recording of the nystagmus induced by head and body movements, gaze, and caloric stimulation. It is helpful in quantifying the degree of vestibular hypofunction and may help with the differentiation between peripheral and central lesions. Computer-driven rotatory chairs and posturography platforms offer improved diagnostic abilities but are not widely available.

Vertigo Syndromes Due to Peripheral Lesions

A. Endolymphatic Hydrops (Meniere's Syndrome): Meniere's syndrome results from distention of the endolymphatic compartment of the inner ear. The primary lesion appears to be in the endolymphatic sac, which is thought to be responsible for endolymph filtration and excretion. Although a precise cause of hydrops cannot be established in most cases, two known causes are syphilis and head trauma. The classic syndrome consists of episodic vertigo, usually lasting 1–8 hours; low-frequency sensorineural hearing loss, often fluctuating; tinnitus, usually low-tone and "blowing" in quality; and a sensation of aural pressure. Symptoms wax and wane as the endolymphatic pressure rises and falls. Caloric testing commonly reveals loss or impairment of thermally induced nystagmus on the involved side.

Specific treatment is intended to lower endolymphatic pressure. A low-salt diet (< 2 g sodium daily), at times supplemented by diuretics, adequately controls symptoms in the great majority of patients. A typical diuretic regimen is hydrochlorothiazide, 50–100 mg daily. In those who have failed medical therapy and remain disabled by their vertigo, surgical decompression of the endolymphatic sac may bring relief.

Episodic vertigo resembling that of Meniere's syndrome but without accompanying auditory symptoms is known as recurrent vestibulopathy. The pathogenic mechanism of this symptom complex is unknown in most cases, though a few patients suffer from a variant of migraine whereas others go on to develop the classic syndrome of endolymphatic hydrops.

B. Labyrinthitis: Patients with labyrinthitis suffer from continuous, usually severe vertigo lasting several days to a week, accompanied by hearing loss and tinnitus. During a recovery period that lasts for several weeks, rapid head movements may bring on transient vertigo. Hearing may return to normal or remain permanently impaired in the involved ear. The cause of labyrinthitis is unknown, although it frequently follows an upper respiratory tract infection. For this reason, it is generally known as "viral" or "infectious" labyrinthitis.

C. Vestibular Neuronitis: In vestibular neuronitis, a paroxysmal, usually single attack of vertigo occurs without accompanying impairment of auditory function and may persist for several days to weeks before clearing. Examination reveals nystagmus and absent responses to caloric stimulation on one or both sides. The cause of the disorder is unclear. Viral mononeuritis has been suggested as the cause. Treatment is symptomatic.

D. Traumatic Vertigo: The most common cause of vertigo following head injury is labyrinthine concussion. Symptoms generally diminish within several days but may linger for a month or more. Basilar skull fractures that traverse the inner ear usually result in severe vertigo lasting several days to a week and deafness in the involved ear. Chronic posttraumatic vertigo may result from cupulolithiasis. This occurs when traumatically detached statoconia (otoconia) settle on the ampulla of the posterior semicircular canal and cause an excessive degree of cupular deflection in response to head motion. Clinically, this presents as episodic positioning vertigo. A less common source of posttraumatic vertigo is disruption of the oval or round window with leakage of perilymph into the middle ear. Perilymphatic fistulization may follow physical or barometric trauma or may result from erosion of the inner ear by cholesteatoma or neoplasm. Symptomatic fistulas are usually associated with both vertigo and hearing loss. Surgical repair may be necessary.

E. Positioning Vertigo: This form of vertigo is usually peripheral in origin, though it occasionally occurs with central lesions. Transient vertigo following changes in head position is a frequent complaint. The term "positioning vertigo" is more accurate than "positional vertigo" because it is provoked by changes in head position rather than by the maintenance of a particular posture. Use of the term "benign position*al* vertigo" is discouraged except for cases known to be unassociated with central nervous system disorders. True positional vertigo suggests either vertebrobasilar insufficiency or dysfunction of the cervical spine.

The typical symptoms of positioning vertigo occur in clusters that persist for several days. Typically with peripheral lesions, there is a latency period of several seconds following a head movement before symptoms develop, and they subside within 10–60 seconds. Constant repetition of the positional change leads to habituation. In central lesions, there is no latent period, fatigability, or habituation of the sign and symptoms.

F. Acoustic Neuromas: These tumors, which are schwannomas of the vestibular nerve, typically are associated with chronic vestibular symptoms in the form of unsteadiness and imbalance. Less commonly, they are manifested by repeated episodes of true vertigo. Unilateral hearing loss with relatively poor speech discrimination and tinnitus is common.

Vertigo Syndromes Due to Central Lesions

Central nervous system causes of vertigo include brain stem vascular disease, arteriovenous malformations, tumor of the brain stem and cerebellum, multiple sclerosis, and vertebrobasilar migraine. Vertigo of central origin often becomes unremitting and disabling. There are commonly other signs of brain stem dysfunction (eg, cranial nerve palsies; motor, sensory, or cerebellar deficits in the limbs) or of increased intracranial pressure. Auditory function is generally spared. The underlying cause should be treated.

Management of the Patient With Vertigo

Unfortunately, few specific treatments for labyrinthine disorders have been designed to reverse a known pathogenic mechanism. Examples include low-salt diet and diuretics in Meniere's disease, antibiotic treatment of infectious diseases, and surgical repair of perilymphatic fistulas.

Symptomatic treatment is useful in the vertiginous patient to lessen the abnormal sensation and to alleviate vegetative symptoms such as nausea and vomiting. The most common drug classes employed are the antihistamines, anticholinergics, and sedative-hypnotics. Ample evidence exists that vestibular suppressant medications adversely affect the process of central compensation following acute vestibular disease. For this reason, these drugs should be used only for brief periods. Generally, they are best admin-

istered to patients with prominent vegetative symptoms and are best tapered and halted when symptoms are resolved, usually within 1–2 weeks.

In acute severe vertigo, diazepam, 2.5–5 mg intravenously, may abate an attack. Relief from nausea and vomiting usually requires an antiemetic delivered intramuscularly or by rectal suppository (eg, prochlorperazine, 10 mg intramuscularly, or 25 mg rectally every 6 hours). Less severe vertigo may often be successfully alleviated with antihistamines such as meclizine, 25 mg, or cyclizine or dimenhydrinate, 25–50 mg, orally every 6 hours. Scopolamine, administered in low dosage transdermally (0.5 mg/d), has proved beneficial to many patients with recurrent vertigo, although side effects (dry mouth, blurred vision, urinary obstruction) often limit its utility. Sometimes employing one-half or even one-fourth of a patch may allow therapeutic effect without the usual adverse consequences. A combination of drugs sometimes helps when the response to one drug is disappointing.

Bed rest may reduce the severity of acute vertigo. In chronic or recurrent vertigo, one of the most important therapies is exercise. Physical activity substantially enhances the central nervous system's ability to compensate for labyrinthine dysfunction and should be encouraged once nausea and vomiting have resolved. In general, the patient should be instructed to repeatedly perform maneuvers that provoke vertigo—up to the point of nausea or fatigue—in an effort to habituate them. Patients with vertigo and imbalance refractory to conventional therapy may benefit from a formal rehabilitation program under the guidance of a physical therapist. Substantial success has been reported in such patients through use of customized habituation protocols and specialized equipment, including tilt tables.

Surgical remedies are reserved for those who remain substantially disabled despite a prolonged and varied trial of medical therapy and exercises. Selective section of the vestibular portion of the eighth nerve brings relief of vertigo in over 90% of such patients. Surgical removal of the semicircular canals (labyrinthectomy) is also highly effective but is appropriate only for patients with little or no hearing in the involved ear.

Brackmann DE: Surgical treatment of vertigo. J Laryngol Otol 1990;104:849. (Indications reviewed.)

Dickins JR, Graham SS: Meniere's disease—1983–1989. Am J Otol 1990;11:51.

Herdman SJ et al: Single treatment approaches to benign paroxysmal positional vertigo. Arch Otolaryngol Head Neck Surg 1993;119:450. (Vertigo was improved in 70% of 60 patients who underwent a single physical therapy session.)

McIntosh S et al: Outcome of an integrated approach to the investigation of dizziness, falls and syncope in elderly patients referred to a "syncope" clinic. Age Ageing

1993;22:53. (A wide variety of cardiac and vascular causes.)

Olsky M, Murray J: Dizziness and fainting in the elderly. Emerg Med Clin North Am 1990;8:295. (Causes of falls and instability in the aged.)

Shepard NT et al: Vestibular and balance rehabilitation therapy. Ann Otol Rhinol Laryngol 1993;102:198. (A customized program of habituation and balance rehabilitation reduced symptoms and disability scores in over 80%.)

Smith-Wheelock M et al: Physical therapy program for vestibular rehabilitation. Am J Otol 1991;12:218. (An 85% improvement rate, with complete symptomatic relief in 30%.)

DISEASES OF THE CENTRAL AUDITORY & VESTIBULAR SYSTEMS (Table 8–1)

Lesions of the eighth cranial nerve and central audiovestibular pathways produce neural hearing loss and vertigo. One characteristic of neural hearing loss is deterioration of speech discrimination out of proportion to the decrease in pure tone thresholds. Another is auditory adaptation, wherein a steady tone appears to the listener to decay and eventually disappear. Auditory evoked responses are useful in distinguishing cochlear from neural losses and may give insight into the site of lesion within the central pathways.

Vertigo arising from central lesions tends to be more chronic and debilitating than that seen in labyrinthine disease. The associated nystagmus is often nonfatigable, vertical rather than horizontal in orientation, without latency, and unsuppressed by visual fixation. Electronystagmography is useful in documenting these characteristics. The evaluation of central audiovestibular dysfunction usually requires imaging of the brain with CT scans or MRI. The paramagnetic contrast agent gadolinium-DTPA, when used with MRI scanning, substantially improves diagnostic sensitivity in the detection of central audiovestibular lesions.

Kumar A, Dobben GD: Central auditory and vestibular pathology. Otolaryngol Clin North Am 1988;21:377. (Imaging modalities in diagnosis.)

1. VESTIBULAR SCHWANNOMA (Acoustic Neuroma)

Tumors of the cerebellopontine angle, most notably acoustic neuroma, cause central audiovestibular symptoms. Acoustic neuromas are among the most common intracranial neoplasms. These schwannomas generally arise from the vestibular division of the eighth nerve. When small, they may occasionally be excised, with preservation of hearing. Large tumors can also be safely removed in most cases, but cranial nerve palsies—especially facial paralysis and deafness—are common sequelae.

Flexon PB et al: Bilateral acoustic neurofibromatosis (NF 2): A disorder distinct from von Recklinghausen's neurofibromatosis (NF 1). Ann Otol Rhinol Laryngol 1991; 100:830.

Jackler RK, Pitts LP: Selection of surgical approach to acoustic neuroma. Otolaryngol Clin North Am 1992; 25:361.

Selesnick SH et al: The changing clinical presentation of acoustic tumors in the MRI era. Laryngoscope 1993; 103:431. (Refined diagnoses with gadolinium MRI.)

2. VASCULAR COMPROMISE

Vertebrobasilar insufficiency is a common cause of vertigo in the elderly. It is often triggered by changes in posture or extension of the neck. Empirical treatment is with vasodilators, aspirin, and exercise.

Migraine may cause vertiginous attacks. The diagnosis is obvious when vertigo accompanies a typical headache pattern, but this is not always the case. In patients with a history of both migraine headaches and recurrent vertigo, a therapeutic trial of β-adrenergic blocking drugs (propranolol, 80–240 mg orally every 12–24 hours) and ergots (ergotamine, 1 mg orally every 4–6 hours) is reasonable.

Vascular loops that impinge upon the brain stem root entry zone of cranial nerves have been shown to cause dysfunction. Widely recognized examples are hemifacial spasm and tic douloureux. It has been suggested that hearing loss, tinnitus, and disabling positioning vertigo may result from such a loop abutting the eighth nerve.

Olsson JE: Neurotologic findings in basilar migraine. Laryngoscope 1991;101(No. 1 Part 2 Suppl 52):1.

Parker W: Migraine and the vestibular system. Am J Otol 1991;12:25. (Sixteen patients and review of the literature.)

3. MULTIPLE SCLEROSIS

Most patients with multiple sclerosis suffer from episodic vertigo and chronic imbalance. Hearing loss in this disease is most commonly unilateral and of rapid onset. Spontaneous recovery may occur.

Cure JK et al: Auditory dysfunction caused by multiple sclerosis: Detection with MR imaging. AJNR 1990; 11:817. (T2-weighted MRI scans.)

DISEASES OF THE NOSE & PARANASAL SINUSES

INFECTIONS OF THE NOSE & PARANASAL SINUSES

1. VIRAL RHINITIS (Common Cold)

The nonspecific symptoms of the ubiquitous common cold are present in the early phases of many diseases that affect the upper aerodigestive tract. Because there are numerous serologic types of rhinoviruses, adenoviruses, and other viruses, patients remain susceptible throughout life. Headache, nasal congestion, watery rhinorrhea, sneezing, and a scratchy throat accompanied by general malaise are typical in viral infections. Nasal examination usually shows reddened, edematous mucosa and a watery discharge. The presence of purulent nasal discharge suggests bacterial infection.

There is no proved specific treatment for a cold, but supportive measures such as decongestants (pseudoephedrine, 30 mg every 4 hours, or 120 mg twice daily) may provide some relief of rhinorrhea and nasal obstruction. Nasal sprays such as oxymetazolone or phenylephrine are rapidly effective. They should not be used for more than a few days at a time, since chronic use leads to a rebound congestion that is often worse than the original symptoms. This chronic nasal stuffiness is known as rhinitis medicamentosa. Treatment requires complete cessation of the sprays. This triggers a period of severe nasal congestion that usually lasts 1–2 weeks. Topical intranasal corticosteroids (flunisolide), two sprays in each nostril twice daily) or a short tapering course of oral prednisone may help during the process of withdrawal.

Other than transient middle ear effusion, complications of viral rhinitis are unusual. Secondary bacterial infection may occur and is suggested by a change in color of the rhinorrhea from clear and watery to mucoid and yellow or green. In such cases, nasal cultures may help treatment. The most common pathogens are the same as those responsible for acute otitis media, ie, *Streptococcus pneumoniae,* other streptococci, *Haemophilus influenzae, Staphylococcus aureus,* and *Moraxella catarrhalis.*

2. ACUTE SINUSITIS

Acute sinus infections are uncommon compared to viral rhinitis. Because sinusitis usually has followed an acute respiratory infection and because media advertisements often use the term "sinusitis" when "rhinitis" would be more accurate, it is understandable that patients and physicians alike sometimes confuse these entities. In addition to the symptoms of rhinitis, the diagnosis of sinusitis requires clinical signs and symptoms that indicate involvement of the affected sinus or sinuses such as pain and tenderness over the involved sinus.

Sinusitis occurs when an undrained collection of pus accumulates in a sinus. Diseases that swell the nasal mucous membrane, such as viral or allergic rhinitis, are usually the underlying cause. Edematous mucosa causes obstruction of a sinus drainage tract, resulting in the accumulation of mucous secretion in the sinus cavity that becomes secondarily infected by bacteria. The typical pathogens of bacterial sinusitis are the same as those that cause acute otitis media: *S pneumoniae,* other streptococci, *H influenzae,* and, less commonly, *S aureus* and *Moraxella catarrhalis.*

Clinical Findings

A. Symptoms and Signs: Because the maxillary sinus is the largest of the paranasal sinuses and its ostia into the nose is superiorly placed, thereby failing to take advantage of gravity, it is the most commonly affected sinus. Pain and pressure over the cheek are the usual symptoms. Pain may refer to the upper incisor and canine teeth via branches of the trigeminal nerve, which traverse the floor of the sinus. It is not uncommon for maxillary sinusitis to result from dental infection, and teeth that are tender should be carefully examined for signs of abscess. Discolored nasal discharge and poor response to decongestants may also suggest sinusitis. Other possible causes for facial pain, such as trigeminal neuralgia and optic neuritis, should be kept in mind as well.

Acute ethmoiditis in adults is usually accompanied by maxillary sinusitis. In such cases, the symptoms of maxillary sinusitis generally predominate. Ethmoidal infection presents with pain and pressure over the high lateral wall of the nose that may radiate to the orbit. Periorbital cellulitis may be present.

Sphenoid sinusitis is usually seen in the setting of pansinusitis. The patient may complain of a headache "in the middle of the head" and often points to the vertex. Sixth nerve palsy may occur as the abducens nerve courses just lateral to the sinus.

Acute frontal sinusitis usually causes pain and tenderness of the forehead. This is most easily elicited by palpation of the orbital roof just below the medial end of the eyebrow. Palpation here is more accurate than percussion of the supraorbital area or forehead.

B. Imaging: Although it is often possible to make the diagnosis of sinusitis on clinical grounds alone, radiologic confirmation allows a more definitive diagnosis and is an objective monitor of the course of infection. Transillumination may aid in diagnosis, but variations in soft tissue thickness and technique often make interpretation difficult. The authors have not found it particularly helpful in practice.

The standard set of conventional sinus films and the sinus best seen in each view are Caldwell (frontal), Waters (maxillary), lateral (sphenoid), and submentovertical (ethmoid). Opacification without bone destruction is a typical feature of sinusitis. An air-fluid level may be seen if the films are taken with the patient upright rather than supine. The frontal sinus may occasionally appear normal even in the face of clinically compelling evidence of sinusitis. Limited coronal CT scans have in many medical centers replaced sinus films in screening sinusitis. They are no more expensive than conventional films and are more sensitive to both inflammatory changes and bone destruction (which would lead one to suspect a tumor). In recurrent sinusitis, CT scanning may help delineate anatomic blockage of the osteomeatal complex and thus suggest a role for functional endoscopic sinus surgery. If, however, malignancy is suspected (eg, because of unilateral cranial neuropathy or a nasoantral mass), then MRI with gadolinium should be ordered. MRI will distinguish tumor from inflammation and inspissated mucus far better than CT.

Treatment

In uncomplicated sinusitis with mild symptoms, outpatient management is usually successful. Oral decongestants (eg, pseudoephedrine, 60–120 mg orally three or four times daily), nasal decongestant sprays (eg, oxymetazoline, 0.05%, one or two sprays each nostril every 6–8 hours for up to 3 days; xylometazoline, 0.05–0.1%, one or two sprays each nostril every 6–8 hours for up to 3 days), and appropriate oral antibiotics are recommended. If purulent discharge is seen in the nose, it should be cultured. Maxillary sinus puncture and aspiration frequently provides a sample for culture; endoscopic sinus lavage may accomplish the same purpose. This is especially important when there is reason to suspect that the pathogen may not be typical, such as in nosocomial sinusitis in an intensive care unit. Although radiologic sinus findings are common, sinusitis in an ICU is rarely the sole source of fever in this setting. Interestingly, the bacterial spectrum seen in sinusitis in AIDS is similar to that in more common settings; but aspiration for cytology may lead to a diagnosis of lymphoma, a not uncommon finding in apparent "sinusitis" in AIDS patients.

Because amoxicillin (250 mg orally three times a day) achieves better sinus penetration than ampicillin, it is an appropriate first choice. Alternatives include trimethoprim-sulfamethoxazole (4 mg/kg TMP and 20 mg/kg SMZ twice daily; available as tablets containing 80 or 160 TMP and 160 or 800 SMZ); cephalexin (250–500 mg orally daily); cefuroxime (250 mg orally twice daily); and cefaclor (250 mg orally three times a day). Cefixime (400 mg orally daily) is recommended by some on a cost basis, though it fails to cover common β-lactamase-producing organisms. Antibiotic treatment for sinusitis should be continued for 2 weeks, with longer courses sometimes required to prevent relapses.

Failure of sinusitis to resolve after an adequate course of oral antibiotics may necessitate hospital admission for intravenous antibiotics and possible surgical drainage. Frontal sinusitis that does not promptly respond to outpatient care should be managed aggressively, because the posterior sinus wall is adjacent to the dura and because undertreated infection may lead to intracranial extension. If intravenous antibiotics fail to ameliorate symptoms, a frontal sinus trephine may be necessary to drain and irrigate the sinus. Persistent maxillary empyema may be cultured and relieved with a needle inserted through the lateral wall of the nose or anterior wall of the antrum through the gingivobuccal sulcus.

Complications

Local complications of sinusitis include osteomyelitis and mucocele. Mucoceles, a consequence of long-standing ductal obstruction, are more common in the supraorbital ethmoids and frontal sinuses and may become secondarily infected. They appear radiologically as a smoothly expanded sinus filled with homogeneous soft tissue density. Treatment is surgical, requiring either drainage of the mucocele intranasally or its complete excision with fat ablation of the sinus cavity.

Osteomyelitis requires prolonged antibiotics as well as removal of necrotic bone. The frontal sinus is most commonly affected, with bone involvement suggested by a tender puffy swelling of the forehead. Following treatment, secondary cosmetic reconstructive procedures may be necessary.

Intracranial complications of sinusitis occur either through hematogenous spread, as in cavernous sinus thrombosis and meningitis, or by direct extension, as in epidural and intraparenchymal brain abscesses. Fortunately, they are rare today. Cavernous sinus thrombosis is heralded by ophthalmoplegia, chemosis, and visual loss. Frontal epidural abscess is usually quiescent. It may be detected on CT scan, a study recommended in all cases of atypical or complicated sinusitis.

It should always be kept in mind that paranasal sinus cancer is in the differential diagnosis of sinusitis. The presence of bone destruction radiologically, cranial neuropathies (especially V_2), persistent pain, epistaxis, or a prolonged clinical course should raise the suspicion of possible cancer.

Bamberger DM: Antimicrobial treatment of sinusitis. Semin Respir Infect 1991;6(2):77. (Antimicrobial choices in common and uncommon circumstances.)

Borman KR et al: Occult fever in surgical intensive care

unit patients is seldom caused by sinusitis. Am J Surg 1992;164:415.

Kennedy DW (ed): First line management of sinusitis: A national problem. Otolaryngol Head Neck Surg 1990; 103(No. 5, Part 2):845. (Pathophysiology, radiology, and medical and surgical approaches, with a special section on the primary care perspective.)

Mandel S: Facial pain: Why does my face hurt, doctor? Postgrad Med 1990;87:77. (A discussion of neuralgias, with selected references.)

Richtsmeier WJ: Medical and surgical management of sinusitis in adults. Ann Otol Rhinol Laryngol 1992;155 (Suppl):46.

Wald ER: Antimicrobial therapy of pediatric patients with sinusitis. J Allergy Clin Immunol 1992;90(3 Part 2):469.

Williams JW Jr et al: Clinical evaluation for sinusitis: Making the diagnosis by history and physical examination. Ann Intern Med 1992;117:705.

3. NASAL VESTIBULITIS

Inflammation at the nasal vestibule commonly results from folliculitis of the hairs that line this orifice. Systemic antibiotics effective against *S aureus* (such as dicloxacillin, 250 mg orally four times daily) are indicated. Topical mupirocin (applied two or three times daily) may be a helpful addition. If recurrent, it is possible that the addition of rifampin (10 mg/kg orally twice daily for the last 4 days of treatment) may eliminate the *S aureus* carrier state. If a furuncle exists, it should be incised and drained, preferably intranasally. Adequate treatment of these infections is important to prevent retrograde spread of infection through valveless veins into the cavernous sinus and intracranial contents.

4. RHINOCEREBRAL MUCORMYCOSIS

Although mucormycosis is rare, any physician seeing patients in a primary care setting must be aware of its presenting signs and symptoms. The fungus (*Mucor, Absidia, Rhizopus*) spreads rapidly through vascular channels and may be lethal if not detected early. Patients with mucormycosis almost invariably have an underlying disease, often diabetes mellitus or uremia. The initial symptoms may be similar to those of bacterial sinusitis, although facial pain is often more severe. Examination of the nasal mucosa is likely to show black, necrotic eschar adherent to the inferior turbinate. Cranial neuropathies and black necrotic skin overlying the ethmoid sinuses are advanced signs. Diagnosis requires biopsy, which reveals broad nonseptate hyphae within tissues.

Mucormycosis represents a medical and surgical emergency. Once recognized, prompt wide surgical debridement and amphotericin B by intravenous infusion are indicated. Close management of the underlying disease is also of great importance. Even with early diagnosis and immediate appropriate intervention, the prognosis is guarded. In diabetics, the mortality rate is about 20%; in patients with renal failure, the mortality rate is over 50%.

Goering P, Berlinger NT, Weisdorf DJ: Aggressive combined modality treatment of progressive sinonasal fungal infections in immunocompromised patients. Am J Med 1988;85:619.

Karam F, Chmel H: Rhino-orbital cerebral mucormycosis. Ear Nose Throat J 1990;69:187.

Parfrey NA: Improved diagnosis and prognosis of mucormycosis: A clinicopathologic study of 33 cases. Medicine 1986;65:113.

Sugar AM: Mucormycosis. Clin Infect Dis 1992;14(Suppl 1):S126.

ALLERGIC RHINITIS

The symptoms of "hay fever" are similar to those of viral rhinitis but are usually more persistent and show seasonal variation. Nasal symptoms are often accompanied by eye irritation, which causes pruritus, erythema, and excessive tearing. Numerous allergens may cause these symptoms: pollens are most common in the spring, grasses in the summer, and ragweed in the fall. Dust and household mites may produce year-round symptoms.

On physical examination, the mucosa of the turbinates is usually pale or violaceous because of venous engorgement—in contrast to the erythema of viral rhinitis. Nasal polyps, which are yellowish boggy masses of hypertrophic mucosa, may be seen.

Treatment is symptomatic in most cases. Oral decongestants alone (eg, pseudoephedrine, 60–120 mg orally three or four times daily) are usually helpful, although antihistamines more specifically counteract allergic mechanisms. Numerous over-the-counter preparations are available. Common antihistamines include brompheniramine or chlorpheniramine (4 mg orally every 6–8 hours, or 8–12 mg orally every 8–12 hours as a sustained-release tablet) and clemastine (1.34–2.68 mg orally twice daily). Nonsedating long-acting antihistamines such as astemizole (10 mg orally daily), loratidine (10 mg orally daily), and terfenadine (60 mg orally twice daily), though expensive and by prescription, are especially helpful in patients intolerant of the drowsiness associated with many other classes of antihistamines.

Astemizole and terfenadine have been associated with sudden death from presumed QT prolongation, especially in patients receiving erythromycin or ketoconazole concomitantly.

Nasal corticosteroid sprays such as beclomethasone (42 μg/spray) and flunisolide (25 μg/spray) are often remarkably effective if used appropriately. These sprays should be administered as two activations into each nostril twice daily for 1 month. Compliance is poor unless patients know that improvement usually does not begin until 1–2 weeks after starting therapy. Intranasal steroids have a role in seasonal allergies in shrinking nasal polyps, often eliminating the need for surgery. Intranasal cromolyn may be useful, especially when administered before expected contact with an offending allergen.

Maintaining an allergen-free environment by covering pillows and mattresses with plastic covers, substituting synthetic materials (foam mattress, acrylics) for animal products (wool, horsehair), and removing dust-collecting household fixtures (carpets, drapes, bedspreads, wicker) is worth the attempt to help more troubled patients. Air purifiers and dust filters (such as Bionair models) may also aid in maintaining an allergen-free environment. When symptoms are extremely bothersome, a search for offending allergens may prove helpful. This can either be done by skin testing or by serum RAST testing. Desensitization by gradually increasing subdermal exposure to identified allergens may be tried in selected patients, with variable results.

Badhwar AK, Druce HM: Allergic rhinitis. Med Clin North Am 1992;76(4):789. (History, laboratory findings, and therapeutic alternatives.)

Mabry RL: Topical pharmacotherapy for allergic rhinitis: New agents. South Med J 1992;85:149. (New topical preparations, including antihistamines, anti-inflammatory agents, anticholinergics, and IgE pentapeptide.)

Naclerio RM: Allergic rhinitis. N Engl J Med 1991; 325:860.

White MV, Kaliner MA: Mediators of allergic rhinitis. J Allergy Clin Immunol 1992;90(4 Part 2):699. (As histamine is not the sole mediator, antihistamines alone are often insufficient for symptomatic relief.)

Ziering RW, Klein GL: Allergic rhinitis: Measures to control the misery. Postgrad Med 1992;91:225,231.

OLFACTORY DYSFUNCTION

The physiology of olfaction is less well understood than that of the other special senses. Odorous molecules must traverse the nasal vault to reach the cribriform area and become soluble in the mucus overlying the exposed dendrites of receptor cells. Anatomic lack of access to the receptor cells of the first cranial nerve is the most common cause of olfactory dysfunction (hyposmia or anosmia). Polyps, septal deformities, and nasal tumors may all contribute to this inability of air to reach the area of the cribriform plate high in the nose where these receptors are located. Transient olfactory dysfunction often accompanies the common cold, nasal allergies, and perennial rhinitis. About 20% of impaired olfactory function is idiopathic, although it often follows a viral illness. Some have suggested administering large doses of vitamin A and zinc to such patients, although little evidence supports their use. Central nervous system neoplasms, especially those that involve the olfactory

groove or temporal lobe, may affect olfaction. Head trauma accounts for less then 5% of cases of hyposmia. Absent, diminished, or distorted smell or taste has been reported in a wide variety of endocrine, nutritional, and nervous disorders. A great many medications have also been implicated.

Evaluation of olfactory dysfunction should include a thorough history of systemic illnesses and medication use as well as a physical examination focusing on the nose and nervous system. Most clinical offices are not set up to test olfaction, but such feats may at times be worthwhile if only to assess whether a patient possesses any sense of smell at all. Odor threshold should be tested in increasing concentrations. For example, use n-butyl alcohol (1-butanolol) in concentrations up to 4% in deionized water. Serial 3:1 dilutions in 12 steps produce an initial test of 46 ppb (v/v) and the maximum of 3055 ppm (at 4%). Odor identification can be tested using standardized choices (see references). In permanent hyposmia, counseling should be offered about seasoning foods with spices (eg, pepper) that stimulate the trigeminal as well as olfactory chemoreceptors and safety issues such as the use of smoke alarms and electric rather than gas home appliances.

Cain WS: Testing olfaction in a clinical setting. Ear Nose Throat J 1989;68:316. (Taste and smell disorders. See also articles by Frank et al and by Scott.)

Leopold DA: Physiology of olfaction. In: Otolaryngology: Head and Neck Surgery, 3rd ed. Cummings CW, Frederickson J (editors). Mosby, 1992.

Wright HN: Characterization of olfactory dysfunction. Arch Otolaryngol Head Neck Surg 1987;113:163. (Qualitative analysis of available tests.)

EPISTAXIS

Bleeding from Kiesselbach's plexus, a vascular plexus on the anterior nasal septum, is by far the most common type of epistaxis encountered. Predisposing factors include nasal trauma (nose picking, foreign bodies, forceful nose blowing), rhinitis, drying of the nasal mucosa from low humidity, and deviation of the nasal septum. Most cases of anterior epistaxis may be successfully treated by direct pressure on the bleeding site. The nasal alae should be firmly compressed for at least 10 minutes. Venous pressure is reduced in the sitting position, and leaning forward lessens the swallowing of blood. Short-acting topical nasal decongestants (eg, phenylephrine, 0.125–1% solution, one or two sprays), which act as vasoconstrictors, may also be helpful. When the bleeding does not readily subside, the nose should be examined, using good illumination and suction, in an attempt to locate the bleeding site. Topical 4% cocaine applied either as a spray or on a cotton strip serves both as an anesthetic and as a vasoconstricting agent.

When visible, the bleeding site may be cauterized with silver nitrate, diathermy, or electrocautery. A supplemental patch of Surgicel or Gelfoam may be helpful.

Occasionally, a site of bleeding may be inaccessible to direct control, or attempts at direct control may be unsuccessful. In such cases, nasal packing is necessary. A properly placed anterior pack requires several feet of half-inch iodoform packing lubricated with bacitracin or petroleum ointment. The packing is carefully and systematically placed along the floor and then the vault of the nose. If the equipment necessary to place a pack is not available, various manufactured nasal balloons may serve as either a temporizing or definitive solution.

About 5% of nasal bleeding originates in the posterior nasal cavity. This requires placement of a pack to occlude the choana before placement of a pack anteriorly. Because this is uncomfortable for the patient and because it requires oxygen supplementation to prevent hypoxia, hospitalization for several days is indicated. Narcotic analgesics are needed to reduce the considerable discomfort and elevated blood pressure caused by a posterior pack. Immediate ligation of the nasal arterial supply (internal maxillary artery and ethmoid arteries) is a reasonable alternative to posterior nasal packing. This surgery is certainly necessary when packing fails to control life-threatening hemorrhage. On rare occasions, selective arterial embolization or ligation of the external carotid artery may be necessary.

After control of epistaxis, the patient is advised to avoid vigorous exercise for several days. Avoidance of hot or spicy foods and tobacco is also advisable, as they may cause vasodilation. Avoiding nasal trauma is an obvious necessity and may require trimming children's nails. Lubrication with petroleum jelly or bacitracin ointment and increasing home humidity may be useful ancillary measures.

It is important in all patients with epistaxis to consider underlying causes of the bleeding. A check of the PT, PTT, platelet count, and bleeding time may be indicated, especially in recurrent cases. Other causes of recurrent epistaxis, such as hereditary hemorrhagic telangiectasia (Osler-Weber-Rendu syndrome), should also be considered. Similarly, once the acute episode has passed, careful examination of the nose and paranasal sinuses to rule out neoplasia is wise.

Jackson KR, Jackson RT: Factors associated with active, refractory epistaxis. Arch Otolaryngol Head Neck Surg 1988;114:862. (Hypertension, alcohol, and aspirin were common.)

Josephson GD, Codley FA, Stierna P: Practical management of epistaxis. Med Clin North Am 1991;75(6):1311.

Randall DA, Freeman SB: Management of anterior and posterior epistaxis. Am Fam Phys 1991;43(6):2007. (Finding the site influences both management and referral.)

Singh B: Combined internal maxillary and anterior ethmoidal arterial occlusion: The treatment of choice in intractable epistaxis. J Laryngol Otol 1992;106:507. (Surgical ligation was usually successful when packs failed.)

Vitek J: Idiopathic intractable epistaxis: Endovascular therapy. Radiology 1991;181:113. (Embolization of the internal maxillary artery is often a good alternative, where available, to surgical ligation).

NASAL TRAUMA

The nasal pyramid is the most frequently fractured bone in the body. Fracture is suggested by crepitance or palpably mobile bony segments. Epistaxis and pain are common, as are soft tissue hematomas ("black eye"). It is important to make certain that there is no palpable step-off of the infraorbital rim, which would indicate the presence of a zygomatic complex fracture. Radiologic confirmation may at times be helpful but is not necessary in uncomplicated nasal fractures.

Treatment is aimed at maintaining long-term nasal airway patency and nasal aesthetics. Closed reduction, using topical 4% cocaine and locally injected 1% lidocaine, should be attempted within 1 week of injury. In the presence of marked nasal swelling, it is best to wait several days for the edema to subside before undertaking reduction. Persistent functional or cosmetic defects may be repaired by delayed reconstructive nasal surgery.

Intranasal examination should be performed in all cases to rule out septal hematoma, which appears as a widening of the anterior septum, visible just posterior to the columella. The septal cartilage receives its only nutrition from its closely adherent mucoperichondrium. An untreated subperichondrial hematoma will result in loss of the nasal cartilage with resultant saddlenose deformity. Undrained septal hematomas may become infected, with S aureus the predominant organism. Treatment consists of incision and drainage via an intranasal septal mucosal incision. It is important to be sure that both sides of the septal cartilage are adequately drained. A small Penrose drain sutured in place is helpful. Antibiotics should be given and the drained fluid sent for culture.

Owen GO, Parker AJ, Watson DJ: Fractured-nose reduction under local anaesthesia: Is it acceptable to the patient? Rhinology 1992;30:89. (Yes.)

Pollock RA: Nasal trauma: Pathomechanics and surgical management of acute injuries. Clin Plast Surg 1992; 19(1):133. (Biomechanical forces.)

Verwoerd CD: Present day treatment of nasal fractures: Closed versus open reduction. Facial Plast Surg 1992; 8:220.

TUMORS & GRANULOMATOUS DISEASE

1. BENIGN NASAL TUMORS

Nasal Polyps

Nasal polyps are pale, edematous, mucosally covered masses commonly seen in patients with allergic rhinitis. They may result in chronic nasal obstruction and a diminished sense of smell. In patients with nasal polyps and a history of asthma, aspirin should be avoided, as it may precipitate a severe episode of bronchospasm. The presence of polyps in children should alert the physician to the possibility of cystic fibrosis.

Medical treatment with topical nasal steroid sprays (such as beclomethasone, 42 μg/spray), is usually successful for small polyps. A short course of oral corticosteroids (eg, prednisone, 6-day course using twenty-one 5 mg tablets: 30 mg on day 1 and tapering by 5 mg each day) may also be of benefit. When medical management is unsuccessful, polyps should be removed surgically. In healthy persons, this is a minor outpatient procedure. When frequent recurrence is likely or when surgery itself is associated with increased risk (such as in asthmatics), a more complete procedure, such as ethmoidectomy, may be advisable initially. In recurrent polyposis, it may be necessary to remove polyps from the ethmoid, sphenoid, and maxillary sinuses to provide longer-lasting relief. This may be done intranasally, endoscopically, via an anterior transantral route through the gingivolabial sulcus (Caldwell-Luc), or through an external skin incision depending on the extent of disease.

Perkins JA, Blakeslee DB, Andrade P: Nasal polyps: A manifestation of allergy? Otolaryngol Head Neck Surg 1989;101:641. (Etiology of nasal polyps.)

Levine HL: Functional endoscopic sinus surgery: Evaluation, surgery, and follow-up of 250 patients. Laryngoscope 1990;100:79. (High success rate in properly selected patients. Serious potential complications.)

Inverted Papilloma

Inverted papillomas are benign tumors that usually arise from the lateral wall of the nose. They present with unilateral nasal obstruction and occasionally hemorrhage. Because squamous cell carcinomas are seen in 5–10% of inverted papillomas, complete excision is necessary. All excised tissue (not just a sampling) should be carefully reviewed by the pathologist to be sure no carcinoma is present.

Dolgin SR et al: Different options for treatment of inverting papilloma of the nose and paranasal sinuses: A report of 41 cases. Laryngoscope 1992;102:917. (External approach recommended.)

Pelausa EO, Fortier MA: Schneiderian papilloma of the nose and paranasal sinuses: The University of Ottawa experience. J Otolaryngol 1992;21:9. (Lateral rhinotomy resulted in the lowest recurrence rate.)

Waitz G, Wigand ME: Results of endoscopic sinus surgery for the treatment of inverted papillomas. Laryngoscope 1992;102(8):917. (Although the authors report comparable recurrence rates of about 20% using the endoscopic route, most surgeons prefer an extranasal procedure because of its presumed wider exposure and subsequent lower recurrence rate.)

Juvenile Angiofibroma

These highly vascular tumors arise in the nasopharynx, typically in adolescent males. Initially, they cause nasal obstruction and hemorrhage. Any adolescent male with recurrent epistaxis should be checked to be sure he is not harboring an angiofibroma. Though benign, these tumors expand locally from the nasopharynx to involve the nasal cavity, the sphenoid and other paranasal sinuses, the clivus, and the intracranial structures.

Gullane PJ et al: Juvenile angiofibroma: A review of the literature and a case series report. Laryngoscope 1992; 102:928. (Overview of Toronto experience.)

Kaplan MJ: Angiofibroma. In: *Current Therapy in Otolaryngology–Head and Neck Surgery.* Gates GA (editor). Mosby, 1993. (Overview of experience at the University of California, San Francisco.)

2. MALIGNANT NASOPHARYNGEAL & PARANASAL SINUS TUMORS

Unfortunately, malignant tumors of the nose, nasopharynx, and paranasal sinuses tend to remain asymptomatic until late in their course. In general, the prognosis is poor. Early symptoms are nonspecific, mimicking those of rhinitis or sinusitis. Unilateral nasal obstruction and discharge are common, with pain and recurrent hemorrhage often clues to the diagnosis of cancer. Any patient with unilateral or persistent nasal symptoms should be thoroughly evaluated. A high index of suspicion remains a key to the earlier diagnosis of these tumors. Patients often present with advanced symptoms such as proptosis, expansion of a cheek, or ill-fitting maxillary dentures. Malar hypesthesia, due to involvement of the infraorbital nerve, is common in maxillary sinus tumors. Biopsy is necessary for definitive diagnosis, and MRI or CT scan will usually delineate the extent of disease.

Squamous cell carcinoma is the most common cancer seen in this anatomic region. It is especially common in the nasopharynx, where it obstructs the auditory tube and results in serous otitis media. Nasopharyngeal carcinoma (poorly differentiated squamous cell carcinoma, nonkeratinizing squamous cell carcinoma, or lymphoepithelioma) is usually associated with elevated IgA antibody to the viral capsid antigen of the Epstein-Barr virus. It is particularly common in patients of southern Chinese descent but is seen in all populations. Any adult with persistent serous otitis media, especially when unilateral, requires careful evaluation of the nasopharynx. Adenocarcinomas, mucosal melanomas, sarcomas, and non-Hodgkin's lymphomas are less commonly encountered neoplasms of this area.

Treatment depends on the tumor type and the extent of disease. Nasopharyngeal carcinoma may be treated, with considerable success, by radiotherapy alone. Other squamous cell carcinomas are best treated—when resectable—with a combination of surgery and irradiation. Numerous protocols investigating the role of chemotherapy are under evaluation.

Carrau RL, Myers EM, Johnson JT: Paranasal sinus carcinoma: Diagnosis, treatment, and prognosis. Oncology (Huntingt) 1992;6:43, 55.

Johns ME, Kaplan MJ: Advances in the management of paranasal sinus tumors. In: *Head and Neck Oncology.* Wolf GT (editor). Martinus Nijhoff, 1984. (Evaluation, histology, and treatment.)

MacNab TI, Flores AD, Anderson DW: Treatment of paranasal sinus malignancy: The BCCA experience. J Otolaryngol 1992;21:244. (Reviews 119 cases over 17 years in British Columbia.)

3. WEGENER'S GRANULOMATOSIS, POLYMORPHIC RETICULOSIS, & SARCOIDOSIS

The nose and paranasal sinuses are involved in over 90% of cases of Wegener's granulomatosis. It is often not realized that involvement at these sites is more common than involvement of lungs or kidneys. Examination shows bloodstained crusts and friable mucosa. Biopsy classically shows necrotizing granulomas and vasculitis, but in practice the differential diagnosis may be more difficult. Sarcoidosis also commonly presents in the paranasal sinuses and is clinically similar. Biopsy shows nonnecrotic granulomas. Polymorphic reticulosis (midline malignant reticulosis, idiopathic midline destructive disease, lethal midline granuloma), as the multitude of apt descriptive terms suggest, is not well understood. In contrast to Wegener's granulomatosis, involvement is limited to the mid face, and there may be extensive bone destruction. Its progression in time to a T cell lymphoma is being described with increasing frequency, and recent studies suggest clonal T cell proliferation. Histologically, there is a dense infiltrate of mature lymphocytes, histiocytes, and immunoblasts. Even with appropriate immunohistochemical stains, differentiation from lymphoma may be difficult.

Unlike Wegener's granulomatosis, which is treated with drugs such as steroids and cyclophosphamide, polymorphic reticulosis is usually best managed by local irradiation and sustained vigilance for the development of lymphoma.

Fauci AS et al: Wegener's granulomatosis: Prospective clinical and therapeutic experience with 85 patients for 21 years. Ann Intern Med 1983;98:76.

Maeda H et al: Malignant lymphomas and related conditions involving nasal cavity and paranasal sinuses: A clinicopathologic study of forty-two cases with emphasis on prognostic factors. Eur J Surg Oncol 1988;14:9.

Murty GE: Wegener's granulomatosis: Otorhinolaryngological manifestations. Clin Otolaryngol 1990;15:385.

O'Connor JC, Robinson RA: Review of diseases presenting as "midline granuloma": Clinical implications for the appropriate workup of patients with midline granuloma syndrome with emphasis on recent diagnostic advances in lymphoid neoplasms that present as midline destructive lesions. Acta Otolaryngol Suppl 1988;439:1.

DISEASES OF THE ORAL CAVITY & PHARYNX

LEUKOPLAKIA, ERYTHROPLAKIA & ORAL CANCER

Leukoplakia is any white lesion that, unlike oral candidiasis, cannot be removed by simply rubbing the mucosal surface. These areas are usually small but may be several centimeters in diameter. Histologically, they may be simple hyperkeratoses occurring in response to chronic irritation (eg, from dentures, tobacco); about 2–6%, however, represent either dysplasia or early invasive squamous cell carcinoma.

Erythroplakia is similar to leukoplakia except that it has a definite erythematous component. The distinction is important, since about 90% of cases of erythroplakia are either dysplasia or carcinoma. Squamous cell carcinoma accounts for 90% of oral cancer. Alcohol and tobacco are the major epidemiologic factors. The differential diagnosis may include oral candidiasis, necrotizing sialometaplasia, pseudoepitheliomatous hyperplasia, median rhomboid glossitis, and vesiculoerosive inflammatory disease such as erosive lichen planus. This should not be confused with the brown-black gingival melanin pigmentation—diffuse or speckled—common in nonwhites, blue-black embedded fragments of dental amalgam, or other systemic disorders associated with general pigmentation (neurofibromatosis, familial polyposis, Addison's disease). Intraoral melanoma is extremely rare.

Any erythroplakic or enlarging leukoplakic area should have an incisional biopsy or an exfoliative cytologic examination done by the clinician who will direct management of a cancer if one is discovered. Specialty referral should be sought early both for diagnosis and treatment. Intraoral staining with 1% toluidine blue may aid in selection of the most suspicious biopsy site. A systematic intraoral examination—including the lateral tongue, floor of the mouth, gingiva, buccal area, palate, and tonsillar fossae—and palpation of the neck for enlarged lymph nodes should be part of any general physical examination, especially in patients over 45 who smoke tobacco or drink immoderately. Indirect or fiberoptic examination of the nasopharynx, oropharynx, hypopharynx, and larynx should also be done by an otolaryngologist–head and neck surgeon or radiation oncologist. Fine-needle aspiration biopsy may be indicated if an enlarged lymph node is found.

Early detection of squamous cell carcinoma is the key to successful management. Lesions less than 4 mm in depth have a low propensity to metastasize. Most patients in whom the tumor is detected before it is 2 cm in diameter are cured. Small lesions are best treated with surgical excision, often with a laser. Radiation is an alternative but is associated with xerostomia, osteonecrosis of the mandible, and inability to use a curative dose again in the treatment field. Large tumors nevertheless are usually treated with a combination of resection and irradiation. Reconstruction, if required, is done at the time of resection and can involve the use of myocutaneous flaps or vascularized free flaps without bone.

Silverman S Jr: *Oral Cancer,* 3rd ed. American Cancer Society, 1990. (Epidemiology, early recognition, prognosis. Color photographs.)

CANDIDIASIS

Oral candidiasis (thrush) is usually painful and looks like creamy-white curd-like patches overlying erythematous mucosa. Because these white areas are easily rubbed off (eg, by a tongue depressor)—unlike leukoplakia or lichen planus—only the underlying irregular erythema may be seen. Oral candidiasis is commonly encountered among denture wearers; in debilitation, diabetes, and anemia; in those undergoing chemotherapy or local irradiation; and in patients receiving corticosteroids or broad-spectrum antibiotics. Candidiasis is often seen prior to other manifestations of HIV infection in high-risk groups. Angular cheilitis is also a manifestation of candidiasis, though it is also seen in nutritional deficiencies.

The diagnosis is usually not difficult—painful intraoral white patches on an erythematous base in a patient at risk for candidiasis. A wet preparation of a smear with potassium hydroxide will confirm spores and may show nonseptate mycelia. Biopsy will show intraepithelial pseudomycelia of *Candida albicans.*

Effective antifungal therapy may be achieved with any of the following: fluconazole (100 mg daily for 7–14 days), ketoconazole (200–400 mg with breakfast [requires acidic gastric environment for absorption] for 7–14 days), clotrimazole troches (10 mg dis-

solved orally five times daily), or nystatin vaginal troches (100,000 units dissolved orally five times daily) or mouth rinses (500,000 units [5 mL of 100,000 units/mL] held in the mouth before swallowing three times daily). Shorter-duration therapy has also proved effective in many cases, using, for instance, fluconazole. In addition, 0.12% chlorhexidine or half-strength hydrogen peroxide mouth rinses may provide local relief. Nystatin powder (100,000 units/g) applied to dentures three or four times daily for several weeks may help denture wearers.

Epstein JB: Antifungal therapy in oropharyngeal mycotic infections. Oral Surg Oral Med Oral Pathol 1990;69:32.
Samaranayke LP: Superficial oral fungal infections. Curr Opin Dent (Aug) 1991;1:415.

GLOSSITIS & GLOSSODYNIA

Inflammation of the tongue with loss of filiform papillae leads to a red, smooth-surfaced tongue (glossitis). Rarely painful, it may be secondary to nutritional deficiencies (eg, niacin, riboflavin, or vitamin E), drug reactions, dehydration, irritants, and possibly autoimmune reactions or psoriasis. Cultures may occasionally be helpful. If the primary cause cannot be identified and corrected, empiric nutritional replacement therapy may be of diagnostic value.

Glossodynia is burning and pain of the tongue; it may occur with or without glossitis. It has been associated with diabetes, drugs (eg, diuretics), tobacco, xerostomia, and candidiasis as well as the sometimes obscure causes of glossitis. Periodontal disease is not apt to be a factor. Treating possible underlying causes, changing chronic medications to alternative ones, and smoking cessation may resolve symptoms. Reassurance that there is no infection or tumor is likely to be appreciated.

Drinka PJ et al: Nutritional correlates of atrophic glossitis: Possible role of vitamin E in papillary atrophy. J Am Coll Nutr 1993;12:14.
Gorsky M, Silverman S Jr, Chinn H: Burning mouth syndrome: A review of 98 cases. J Oral Med 1987;42:7.

NECROTIZING ULCERATIVE GINGIVITIS (Trench Mouth, Vincent's Infection)

Necrotizing ulcerative gingivitis, often caused by an infection of both spirochetes and fusiform bacilli, is common in young adults under stress (classically at examination time). Underlying systemic diseases may also predispose to this disorder. Clinically, there is painful acute gingival inflammation and necrosis, often with bleeding, halitosis, fever, and cervical lymphadenopathy. In addition to altering or removing, if possible, underlying factors and correcting dietary inadequacies, warm half-strength peroxide rinses and oral penicillin *(250 mg three times daily for 10 days)* may help. Dental gingival curettage may prove necessary.

Melnick SL et al: Epidemiology of acute necrotizing ulcerative gingivitis. Epidemiol Rev 1988;10:191.

APHTHOUS ULCER
(Canker Sore, Ulcerative Stomatitis)

Aphthous ulcers are very common and easy to recognize. Their cause remains uncertain. Found on non-keratinized mucosa (eg, buccal and labial mucosa and not gingiva or palate), they may be single or multiple, are usually recurrent, and appear as painful small (usually 1–2 mm, but sometimes 1–2 cm) round ulcerations with yellow-gray fibrinoid centers surrounded by red halos. The painful stage lasts 7–10 days; healing is completed in 1–3 weeks.

Treatment is nonspecific. Fluocinonide ointment, 0.05%, in an adhesive base (Orabase), 1:1, does appear to provide symptomatic relief. A 1-week tapering course of prednisone (beginning with 20–60 m/d) has been advocated by some.

Large or persistent areas of ulcerative stomatitis may be secondary to erythema multiforme or drug allergies, acute herpes simplex, pemphigus, pemphigoid, or bullous lichen planus. Squamous cell carcinoma may occasionally present in this fashion. When the diagnosis is not clear, incisional biopsy is indicated.

HERPETIC STOMATITIS

Primary herpetic gingivostomatitis, usually a disease of childhood, may be so mild as to go unrecognized. Clinically, there initially is burning, followed by typical small viral vesicles that rupture and then form scabs. Differential diagnosis includes erythema multiforme, syphilitic chancre, and carcinoma. Acyclovir (200 mg five times daily for 7–14 days) may shorten the course and reduce postherpetic pain. In children under age 6, the yellow-gray ulcerations of stomatitis should be distinguished from the gray-white tonsillar or palatal ulcers of Coxsackie-caused herpangina or the buccal and lip ulcers of Coxsackie-caused hand-foot-and-mouth disease. This is especially helpful in immunocompromised individuals, in whom frequent and severe herpes simplex virus reactivation may occur.

Mattingly G, Rodu B: Differential diagnosis of oral mucosal ulcerations. Compendium 1993;14:136, 138, 140 passim.
Molinari JA, Merchant VA: Herpesviruses: Manifestations and transmission. J Calif Dent Assoc 1989;17:24.

Rodu B, Mattingly G: Oral mucosal ulcers: Diagnosis and management. J Am Dent Assoc 1992;123:83.
Scully C: Orofacial herpes simplex virus infections: Current concepts in the epidemiology, pathogenesis, and treatment, and disorders in which the virus may be implicated. Oral Surg Oral Med Oral Pathol 1989;68:701.

PHARYNGITIS & TONSILLITIS

As common as respiratory tract infections are—and they account for over 10% of all office visits to primary care physicians and 50% of outpatient antibiotics used—one would think the most appropriate management would be a matter of agreement among physicians. However, the issues are deceptively complex. Controversy exists over when to culture an inflamed throat and how long to treat confirmed group A β-hemolytic streptococcal pharyngitis—and with what. Numerous well-conceived and well-controlled studies in the past few years as well as the recent availability of rapid laboratory tests for detection of streptococci (eliminating the delay caused by culturing) appear to make a rational approach possible.

The clinical features suggestive of group A β-hemolytic streptococcal pharyngitis include fever, anterior cervical adenopathy, and a pharyngotonsillar exudate. The sore throat may be severe, with odynophagia, tender adenopathy, and a scarlatiniform rash. An elevated white blood count and left shift are consistent with group A β-hemolytic streptococcal pharyngitis. Hoarseness, cough, and coryza are not suggestive of this disease. Marked lymphadenopathy and a shaggy white-purple tonsillar exudate, often extending into the nasopharynx, suggest mononucleosis, especially if present in a young adult. Hepatosplenomegaly and a positive heterophil agglutination test or elevated anti-EBV titer of course are corroborative. It should be kept in mind that about one-third of patients with infectious mononucleosis have secondary streptococcal tonsillitis, requiring treatment. (Ampicillin should be avoided if mononucleosis is suspected because it induces a rash in such patients.) Diphtheria (extremely rare today but described in the alcoholic population) presents with high fever in an ill patient with a gray tonsillar pseudomembrane; it should be distinguished from the more common acute necrotizing ulcerative gingivitis and herpangina.

The most common pathogens other than group A β-hemolytic streptococci in the differential diagnosis of "sore throat" are viruses, *Neisseria gonorrhoeae*, *Mycoplasma*, and *Chlamydia trachomatis*. Rhinorrhea would suggest a virus, as would lack of an exudate, but in practice the most reasonable assumption is that it is not possible to distinguish viral upper respiratory infection from group A β-hemolytic streptococcal infection on clinical grounds alone. Infections with *Corynebacterium diphtheriae*, anaerobic streptococci, and *Corynebacterium haemolyticum* (which responds better to erythromycin than penicillin) may also mimic pharyngitis due to group A β-hemolytic streptococci.

Treatment strategies for a sore throat range from "treat all comers" to "culture all comers, reserving treatment for positive cultures." At issue are the reliability of cultures and rapid tests for streptococci such as latex agglutination (LA) antigen tests and solid-phase enzyme immunoassays (ELISA), the incidence of pharyngitis not due to group A β-hemolytic streptococci, patient follow-up and reliability, and cost. The advantage of the "treat all" approach is the apparent initial short-term cost and prevention of most streptococcal complications, but such an approach necessarily causes the highest rate of penicillin reactions and therefore overall the highest cost. At the other extreme is the "culture all" approach, which is associated with the fewest penicillin reactions but is more costly than an "antigen test and culture" approach and is also dependent on the excellent follow-up not routinely available in some busy city health clinics. With current sensitivity of LA tests between 55% and 75%, the strategy of treating patients with positive antigen test results while culturing (and waiting for results) patients with negative test results appears to be best. If the sensitivity of newer LA tests or ELISA proves to exceed 90%, then the fourth strategy of relying solely on such antigen tests to decide whether to treat would become increasingly more attractive. Individual decisions need to be based on the prevalence of streptococcal infection (seasonally and locally); patient allergic history, reliability, and compliance; availability of LA tests; and reliability of available bacteriology laboratories.

Thirty years ago, a single injection of benzathine penicillin or procaine penicillin was standard antibiotic treatment. Penicillin remains effective even though the injections are painful; if compliance is an issue, it may be the best choice. Oral treatment, however, is also effective. The controversy over choice of preparation revolves around reducing the already low (10–20%) incidence of treatment failures (positive culture after treatment despite symptomatic resolution) and recurrences. A review of recent controlled studies suggests that penicillin V potassium (250 mg orally three times daily—not once or twice daily—for 10 days) or cefuroxime axetil (125 mg orally twice daily for 10 days in children, 250 mg orally twice daily for 10 days in adults) are both effective. A full 10-day antibiotic course (not less) is necessary. Erythromycin (active against *Mycoplasma*) is a reasonable alternative to penicillin. Several cephalosporins in their usual dosage schedules are also effective.

Adequate antibiotic treatment usually avoids the streptococcal complications of scarlet fever, glomerulonephritis, rheumatic myocarditis, and local abscess formation. About 10% of the time, repeat cultures show persistent presence of group A streptococci.

Antibiotic choices for treatment failures are also somewhat controversial. Perhaps surprisingly, penicillin-tolerant strains are not necessarily isolated more frequently in those who fail to improve with treatment than in those treated successfully with penicillin. The reasons for failure appear to be complex, and a second course of treatment with the same drug is therefore not necessarily unreasonable. Alternatives to penicillin include cefuroxime and certain other cephalosporins, dicloxacillin (which is β-lactamase-resistant), and amoxicillin with clavulanate. In penicillin-allergic patients, the usual alternatives should be used, such as erythromycin and cephalosporins. When there is a history of possible penicillin allergy, the usual alternatives should be used, such as erythromycin or cephalosporin. In cases of prior severe penicillin reaction, however, cephalosporins should probably be avoided as the cross-reaction is felt to be higher than the overall 8% rate.

Ancillary treatment of pharyngitis includes appropriate analgesics and anti-inflammatory agents, such as aspirin or acetaminophen. Some patients find that salt water gargling is soothing. In severe cases, anesthetic gargles and lozenges (eg, benzocaine) may provide additional symptomatic relief. Occasionally, odynophagia is so intense that hospitalization for intravenous hydration and antibiotics is warranted.

Dippel DW, Touw-Otten F, Habbema JD: Management of children with acute pharyngitis: A decision analysis. J Fam Pract 1992;34:149. (Applicable to adults as well.)

Lieu TA, Fleisher GR, Schwartz JS: Cost effectiveness of rapid latex agglutination testing and throat cultures for streptococcal pharyngitis. Pediatrics 1990;85:246.

Paradise JL: Etiology and management of pharyngitis and pharyngotonsillitis in children: A current review. Ann Otol Rhinol Laryngol 1992;155(Suppl):51.

Perlman PE, Ginn DR: Respiratory infections in ambulatory adults. Postgrad Med 1990;87:175.

Pichichero ME: Explanations and therapies for penicillin failure in streptococcal pharyngitis. Clin Pediatr 1992; 31:642. (Options such as cephalosporins, amoxicillin-clavulanate, and newer macrolide antibiotics.)

Timon CI et al: Changes in tonsillar bacteriology of recurrent acute tonsillitis: 1980 vs. 1989. Respiratory Med 1990;84:395. (Increased incidence of *H influenzae*, with almost half β-lactamase-producing; *S aureus*—all β-lactamase-producing; and mixed flora. Anaerobes rarely grew.)

Tunik MG et al: Latex agglutination for the rapid diagnosis of streptococcal pharyngitis: Use by house staff in a pediatric emergency service. Pediatr Emerg Care 1990; 6:93. (Many patients receive unnecessary treatment.)

Wegner DL, Witte DL, Schrantz RD: Insensitivity of rapid antigen detection methods and single blood agar plate culture for diagnosing streptococcal pharyngitis. JAMA 1992;267:695. (Recommends two-plate culture method.)

PERITONSILLAR ABSCESS & CELLULITIS

When infection penetrates the tonsillar capsule and involves the surrounding tissues, peritonsillar cellulitis results. Peritonsillar abscess and cellulitis present with severe sore throat, odynophagia, trismus, medial deviation of the soft palate and peritonsillar fold, and a "hot potato" voice. Following therapy, peritonsillar cellulitis usually either resolves over several days or evolves into peritonsillar abscess. The existence of an abscess may be confirmed by aspirating pus from the peritonsillar fold just superior and medial to the upper pole of the tonsil. A No. 19 or No. 21 needle should be passed no deeper than 1 cm, because the internal carotid artery passes posterior and deep to the tonsillar fossa. There is controversy about the best way to treat peritonsillar abscesses. Some incise and drain the area and continue with parenteral antibiotics, whereas others aspirate only and follow as an outpatient. At times it is appropriate to consider immediate tonsillectomy (quinsy tonsillectomy) both to drain the abscess and to avoid recurrence. Both approaches are rational and have support in the literature. Whichever approach is taken, one must be sure the abscess is adequately drained, since complications such as extension to the retropharyngeal, deep neck, and posterior mediastinal spaces are possible. Pus may also be aspirated into the lungs, resulting in pneumonia. While there is controversy about whether a single abscess is sufficient indication for tonsillectomy, most would agree that patients with recurrent abscesses should have their tonsils removed.

Epperly TD, Wood TC: New trends in the management of peritonsillar abscess. Am Fam Phys 1990;42:102.
Ophir D et al: Peritonsillar abscess: A prospective evaluation of outpatient management by needle aspiration. Arch Otolaryngol Head Neck Surg 1988;114:661.
Petruzzelli GJ, Johnson JT: Peritonsillar abscess: Why aggressive management is appropriate. Postgrad Med 1990;88:99.
Stringer SP, Schaefer SD, Close LG: A randomized trial for outpatient management of peritonsillar abscess. Arch Otolaryngol Head Neck Surg 1988;114:296.
(The randomized studies by Ophir and Stringer suggest that needle aspiration on an outpatient basis is a viable alternative to incision and drainage in uncomplicated peritonsillar abscesses.)

TONSILLECTOMY

Despite the frequency with which tonsillectomy is performed, the indications for the procedure remain controversial. Most would agree that airway obstruction causing sleep apnea or cor pulmonale is an absolute indication for tonsillectomy. Similarly, persistent marked tonsillar asymmetry should prompt an excisional biopsy to rule out lymphoma. Relative indications include recurrent streptococcal tonsillitis, causing considerable loss of time from school or work, recurrent peritonsillar abscess, and chronic tonsillitis.

Tonsillectomy is not an entirely benign procedure. Postoperative bleeding occurs in 2–8% of cases and on rare occasions can lead to laryngospasm and airway obstruction. Pain may be considerable, especially in the adult. The pros and cons of the procedure need to be discussed with each prospective patient. In addition, there is increasing economic pressure for these procedures to be done as outpatient surgery. Hemorrhage, protracted emesis, or fever appears to occur in about 1% of cases, and such immediate complications usually appear within 6 hours but continue to occur later within the once frequent 24-hour period of hospitalized observation. This topic will continue to receive attention; at present it seems clear that outpatient tonsillectomy is usually safe when followed by a 6-hour period of uneventful observation, but each decision rests on individual circumstances.

Although reports in the 1970s suggested an association of tonsillectomy with Hodgkin's disease, careful review of this literature reveals no causative association whatever.

Bluestone CD: Current indications for tonsillectomy and adenoidectomy. Ann Otol Rhinol Laryngol 1992;155 (Suppl):58.
Colclasure JB, Graham SS: Complications of outpatient tonsillectomy and adenoidectomy: A review of 3340 cases. Ear Nose Throat J 1990;69:155. (A reminder of the hazards.)
Guida RA, Mattucci KF: Tonsillectomy and adenoidectomy: An inpatient or outpatient procedure? Laryngoscope 1990;100:491. (Discharge home to a reliable environment after uneventful monitoring for several hours is safe.)
Kornblut AD (editor): The tonsils and adenoids. Otolaryngol Clin North Am 1987;20:207. (Entire issue.) (A good starting point for further reading about immunology, controversies, misconceptions, and management.)
Rosenfeld RM, Green RP: Tonsillectomy and adenoidectomy: Changing trends. Ann Otol Rhinol Laryngol 1990;99(No. 3 Part 1):187. (Although infection remains the most common indication, by 1986 almost 20% of the procedures were done for obstructive sleep apnea.)

DEEP NECK INFECTIONS

Deep neck abscesses usually present with marked neck pain and swelling in a toxic febrile patient. They are emergencies because they may rapidly compromise the airway. They may also spread to the mediastinum or cause septicemia. Most commonly, they originate from odontogenic infections. Other causes include suppurative lymphadenitis, direct spread of pharyngeal infection, penetrating trauma, pharyngoesophageal foreign bodies, and intravenous injection of the internal jugular vein, especially in drug abusers. Fundamentals of treatment include securing the airway, intravenous antibiotics, and incision and drainage. The airway may be secured either by intubation or tracheostomy. Tracheostomy is preferable in the patients with substantial pharyngeal edema, since attempts at intubation may precipitate acute airway obstruction. CT scan may be helpful in defining the extent of the abscess. Bleeding in association with a deep neck abscess suggests the possibility of carotid artery or internal jugular vein involvement and requires prompt neck exploration both for drainage of pus and for vascular ligation.

Ludwig's angina is the most commonly encountered neck space infection. It is a cellulitis of the sublingual and submaxillary spaces, often arising from infection of the tooth roots that extend below the mylohyoid line of the mandible. Clinically, there is edema and erythema of the upper neck under the chin and often of the floor of the mouth. The tongue may be displaced upward and backward by the posterior spread of cellulitis. This may lead to occlusion of the airway and necessitate tracheostomy. Hospitalization and intravenous antibiotics effective against streptococci and staphylococci (such as nafcillin, 4–6 g/d intravenously in divided doses, until cultures and sensitivities become available) are necessary. Dental consultation is advisable. External drainage via bilateral submental incisions is required immediately if the airway is threatened and when medical therapy has not reversed the process.

Stiernberg CM: Deep-neck space infections. Arch Otolaryngol Head Neck Surg 1986;112:1274.

DISEASES OF THE SALIVARY GLANDS

The salivary glands are divided into the two large parotid glands, two submandibular glands, several sublingual glands, and 600–1000 minor salivary glands located throughout the upper aerodigestive tract.

ACUTE INFLAMMATORY SALIVARY GLAND DISORDERS

1. SIALADENITIS

Acute bacterial sialadenitis in the adult most commonly affects either the parotid or submandibular gland. It typically presents with acute swelling of the gland, increased pain and swelling with meals, and tenderness and erythema of the duct opening. Pus often can be massaged from the duct. Sialadenitis often occurs in the setting of dehydration or in association with chronic illness. Underlying Sjögren's syndrome also predisposes. The pathogenesis is ductal obstruction, often by an inspissated mucous plug, followed by salivary stasis and secondary infection. The most common organism recovered from purulent draining saliva is *S aureus*. Treatment consists of intravenous antibiotics such as nafcillin (1 g intravenously every 4–6 hours) and measures to increase salivary flow, including hydration, warm compresses, sialagogues (eg, lemon drops), and massage of the gland. Failure of the process to resolve on this regimen suggests abscess formation, ductal stricture, stone, or tumor causing obstruction. Ultrasound or CT scan may be helpful in establishing the diagnosis. Sialography is best avoided in acute cases.

Brook I: Diagnosis and management of parotitis. Arch Otolaryngol Head Neck Surg 1992;118:469.
Sreebny LM, Valdini A, Yu A: Xerostomias: Relationship to non-oral symptoms, drugs, and diseases. Oral Med Oral Pathol 1989;68(Part II):419.

2. SIALOLITHIASIS

Calculus formation is more common in Wharton's duct (draining the submandibular glands) than in Stensen's duct (draining the parotid glands). Clinically, a patient may note postprandial pain and local swelling, often with a history of recurrent acute sialadenitis. Stones in Wharton's duct are usually large and radiopaque, whereas those in Stensen's duct are usually radiolucent and smaller. Those very close to the orifice of Wharton's duct may be palpated manually in the anterior floor of the mouth and removed intraorally by dilating or incising the distal duct. The duct proximal to the stone must be temporarily clamped (using, for instance, a single throw of a suture) to keep manipulation of the stone from pushing it back toward the submandibular gland. Those more than 1.5–2 cm from the duct are too close to the lingual nerve to be removed safely in this manner. Similarly, dilation of Stensen's duct, located on the buccal surface opposite the second maxillary molar, may relieve distal stricture or allow a small stone to pass. The location of the facial nerve makes intraoral retrieval of more proximal parotid stones unsafe.

Repeated episodes of sialadenitis invariably lead to stricture and chronic infection. If the obstruction cannot be safely removed or dilated, excision of the gland may be necessary. In selected cases, piezoelectric shock wave lithotripsy may be successful.

Iro H et al: Shockwave lithotripsy of salivary duct stones. Lancet 1992;339:1333.

CHRONIC INFLAMMATORY & INFILTRATIVE DISORDERS OF THE SALIVARY GLANDS

Numerous infiltrative disorders may cause unilateral or bilateral parotid gland enlargement. Sjögren's disease and sarcoidosis are examples of lymphoepithelial and granulomatous diseases that may affect the salivary glands. Metabolic disorders, including alcoholism, diabetes mellitus, and vitamin deficiencies, may also cause diffuse enlargement. Several drugs have been associated with parotid enlargement, including thioureas, iodine, and drugs with cholinergic effects (eg, phenothiazines), which stimulate flow and cause more viscous saliva.

SALIVARY GLAND TUMORS

Approximately 80% of salivary gland tumors occur in the parotid gland. In adults, about 80% of these are benign. In the submandibular triangle, it is sometimes difficult to distinguish a primary submandibular gland tumor from a metastatic submandibular space node. Only 50–60% of primary submandibular tumors are benign. Tumors of the minor salivary glands are most likely to be malignant, with adenoid cystic carcinoma predominating.

Most parotid tumors present as an asymptomatic mass in the superficial part of the gland. Their presence may have been noted by the patient for months or years. Facial nerve involvement correlates strongly with malignancy. Tumors may extend deep to the plane of the facial nerve or may originate in the parapharyngeal space. In such cases, medial deviation of the soft palate is visible on intraoral examination. MRI and CT scans have largely replaced sialography in defining the extent of tumor.

Although the accuracy of fine-needle aspiration is improving, superficial parotidectomy with facial nerve dissection is required for both diagnosis and treatment of most primary tumors. Similarly, submandibular gland masses generally require excision of the gland. In benign and small low-grade malignant tumors, no additional treatment is needed. Postoperative irradiation is required for larger and high-grade cancers.

Kaplan MJ, Johns ME: Malignant neoplasms (of the salivary glands): In: *Otolaryngology-Head and Neck Surgery,* 2nd ed. Cummings CW, Frederickson J (editors). Mosby, 1992. Prognostic factors, treatment recommendations, and new developments in imaging and treatment.)

DISEASES OF THE LARYNX

HOARSENESS & STRIDOR

The primary symptoms of laryngeal disease are hoarseness and stridor. Hoarseness is caused by an abnormal flow of air past the vocal cords. The voice is "breathy" when too much air passes incompletely apposed vocal cords, as in unilateral vocal cord paralysis. The voice is harsh when turbulence is created by irregularity of the vocal cords, as in laryngitis or a mass lesion. Stridor, a high-pitched sound, is produced by lesions that narrow the airway. Airway impairment above the vocal cords produces predominantly inspiratory stridor. Lesions below the vocal cord level produce either expiratory or mixed stridor.

INFECTIONS OF THE LARYNX

1. EPIGLOTTITIS

Epiglottitis in adults should be suspected when odynophagia seems out of proportion to pharyngeal findings. It may be viral or bacterial in origin. Unlike the case of children, indirect laryngoscopy is generally safe and may demonstrate the swollen, erythematous epiglottis. Initial treatment is hospitalization for intravenous antibiotics (eg, ceftizoxime, 1–2 g intravenously every 8–12 hours; or cefuroxime, 750–1500 mg intravenously every 8 hours); and dexamethasone, usually 4–10 mg as initial bolus, then 4 mg intravenously every 6 hours) and observation of the airway. When adult epiglottitis is recognized early, it is usually possible to avoid intubation. In such cases, it would seem prudent to monitor oxyhemoglobin saturation with continuous pulse oximetry.

Fontanarosa PB, Polsky SS, Goldman GE: Adult epiglottitis. J Emerg Med 1989;7:223. (Less severe than in children.)

Mayo-Smith MF et al: Acute epiglottitis in adults. An eight-year experience in the state of Rhode Island. N Engl J Med 1986;314:1133. (In contrast to other articles, emphasizes that epiglottitis in adults can be fulminant. Biased toward severe cases, however.)

Rivron RP, Murray JA: Adult epiglottitis: Is there a consensus on diagnosis and treatment? Clin Otolaryngol 1991;16:338.

Shapiro J, Eavey RD, Baker AS: Adult supraglottitis: A prospective analysis. JAMA 1988;259:563. (Non-*H influenzae* infection can, if recognized early, follow a more benign course than epiglottitis in children.)

Wolf M et al: Conservative management of adult epiglottitis. Laryngoscope 1990;100:183. (Management without intubation. Ampicillin was associated with 27% abscess rate. In 1994, other antibiotics would be first choice. See text.)

Wurtelle P: Acute epiglottitis in children and adults: A large-scale incidence study. Otolaryngol Head Neck Surg 1990;103:902. (About 25% of cases occur in adults; the incidence in adults is about 1:100,000.)

2. LARYNGEAL PAPILLOMAS

Papillomas, thought to be caused by human papovavirus, are common lesions of the larynx in both children and adults. Patients present with hoarseness that progresses to stridor over weeks to months. Repeated laser excisions are often needed to control the disease. Tracheostomy should be avoided, as this may lead to seeding of papillomas in the tracheobronchial tree, a potentially lethal complication.

3. VIRAL LARYNGITIS

Viral laryngitis is probably the most common cause of hoarseness, which may persist for a week or so after other symptoms of upper respiratory infection have cleared. The patient should be warned to avoid vigorous use of the voice (singing, shouting) while laryngitis is present, since this may foster the formation of vocal nodules.

4. GASTROESOPHAGEAL REFLUX & HOARSENESS

Gastroesophageal reflux leading to posterior laryngitis should be considered a possible cause of chronic hoarseness. As less than half of patients with documented reflux have typical symptoms of heartburn and regurgitation, the lack of such symptoms should not be construed as eliminating this cause. Management should initially exclude more serious laryngeal disease. Twenty-four-hour pH monitoring is the diagnostic tool that best documents reflux. Alternatively, a month-long clinical trial of appropriate antireflux measures and antacids may be tried first.

Koufam JA: The otolaryngologic manifestations of gastroesophageal reflux disease (GERD): A clinical investigation of 225 patients using ambulatory 24-hour pH monitoring and an experimental investigation of the role of acid and pepsin in the development of laryngeal injury. Laryngoscope 1991;101(4 Part 2 Suppl 53):1.

Wiener GJ et al: Chronic hoarseness secondary to gastroesophageal reflux disease: Documentation with 24-hour ambulatory pH monitoring. Am J Gastroenterol 1989;84:1503.

TUMORS OF THE LARYNX

1. BENIGN TUMORS OF THE LARYNX

Vocal cord nodules are smooth, paired lesions that form at the junction of the anterior one-third and posterior two-thirds of the vocal cords. They are a common cause of hoarseness resulting from vocal abuse. In adults, they are referred to as "singer's nodules"; in children, "screamer's nodules." Treatment requires modification of voice habits, and referral to a speech therapist is indicated. Recalcitrant nodules may require surgical excision.

Polypoid changes in the vocal cords may result from vocal abuse, smoking, or chemical industrial irritants or may be seen in hypothyroidism. Attention to the underlying problem may resolve the polypoid changes. Inhaled steroid spray (eg, beclomethasone, 42 μg/spray, or dexamethasone, 84 μg/spray, two or three times a day) may hasten resolution. At times, removal of the hyperplastic vocal cord mucosa may be indicated.

A common but often unrecognized cause of hoarseness is contact ulcers on the vocal processes of the arytenoid cartilages secondary to esophageal reflux. Treatment of the underlying reflux with antacids or H_2-receptor blockers (eg, cimetidine, 800 mg orally daily or 300–600 mg orally every 6 hours; or ranitidine, 300 mg orally daily or 150 mg orally twice daily) and elevation of the head of the bed is often curative. Intubation granulomas may also be seen posteriorly between the vocal processes.

2. LARYNGEAL LEUKOPLAKIA

Leukoplakia is a frequent cause of hoarseness, most commonly arising in smokers. Direct laryngoscopy with biopsy is advised. Histologic examination usually demonstrates mild, moderate, or severe dysplasia. Cessation of smoking may reverse dysplastic changes. A certain percentage of patients—estimated to be less than 5% of those with mild dysplasia and about 35–60% of those with severe dysplasia—will subsequently develop squamous cell carcinoma. In some cases, invasive squamous cell carcinoma is present in the initial biopsy.

3. SQUAMOUS CELL CARCINOMA OF THE LARYNX

Squamous cell carcinoma is the most common cancer seen in the larynx. It occurs predominantly in heavy smokers, with alcohol an apparent cocarcinogen. It is most common between ages 50 and 70. Hoarseness is the usual presenting symptom. Any patient with hoarseness that has persisted beyond 2–3 weeks should be evaluated by indirect laryngoscopy. Odynophagia, hemoptysis, weight loss, referred otalgia, vocal cord immobility, and cervical adenopathy suggest more advanced disease.

Early squamous cell carcinoma is best treated with radiation, with cure rates in excess of 85–95%. Conservation surgery or total laryngectomy is necessary for radiation failures and for more advanced disease. Today, the use of tracheoesophageal valves following total laryngectomy restores useful speech for most laryngectomy patients.

VOCAL CORD PARALYSIS

Most cases of vocal cord paralysis result from lesions of the recurrent laryngeal nerve. In the adult, unilateral vocal cord paralysis generally presents as hoarseness with a breathy character. The most common cause is thyroid surgery. In left vocal cord paralysis, it is important to eliminate a mediastinal or pulmonary apical lesion (Pancoast's tumor) as the causative factor. Involvement of the vagus nerve by tumors involving the jugular foramen may cause vocal cord paralysis that is usually accompanied by additional cranial neuropathies (IX, XI). When no cause can be found, function may return spontaneously within 1 year. Hoarseness secondary to unilateral vocal cord paralysis may be improved by injecting Teflon or other substances into the paralyzed cord in order to medialize it, or by laryngoplastic phonosurgery (medialization laryngoplasty or thyroplasty).

Bilateral vocal cord paralysis usually causes stridor. If sudden in onset, the stridor will be inspiratory and expiratory, causing sufficient airway compromise to warrant emergency cricothyrotomy. If insidious in onset, it may (curiously) be asymptomatic at rest. The voice may be quite good, as the cords are apposed in the midline. Thyroid surgery, neck trauma, and tumor invasion from anaplastic thyroid or esophageal carcinoma are among the more common causes. Immobility of the vocal cords may also result from cricoarytenoid arthritis, as seen in advanced rheumatoid arthritis. When airway obstruction is severe, tracheostomy is indicated. Various procedures, which open the glottis by lateralizing a vocal cord, have been used in order to remove the tracheostomy. A less powerful, breathy voice often accompanies these procedures.

Dedo HH: Injection and removal of Teflon for unilateral vocal cord paralysis. Ann Otol Rhinol Laryngol 1992;101:81. (The standard with which the long-term results of newer techniques must be compared.)

Koufman JA, Isaacson G: Laryngoplastic phonosurgery. Otolaryngol Clin North Am 1991;24:1151. (Laryngeal framework techniques to improve phonation in unilateral vocal cord paralysis.)

Rontal E, Rontal M: Vocal cord injection techniques. Otolaryngol Clin North Am 1991;24:1141. (Options for injection to improve phonation in unilateral vocal cord paralysis.)

TRACHEOSTOMY & CRICOTHYROTOMY

There are two primary indications for tracheostomy: airway obstruction at or above the level of the larynx and respiratory failure requiring prolonged mechanical ventilation. In an acute emergency, cricothyrotomy secures an airway more rapidly than tracheostomy, with fewer potential immediate complications such as pneumothorax and hemorrhage. A percutaneous minitracheotomy approach is also being evaluated as an alternative to cricothyrotomy. In order to reduce the chance of subglottic stenosis, cricothyrotomy should be converted to tracheostomy as soon as the patient is stable.

The most common indication for elective tracheostomy is the need for prolonged mechanical ventilation. There is no firm rule about how many days a patient must be intubated before conversion to tracheostomy should be advised. The incidence of serious complications such as subglottic stenosis increases with extended endotracheal intubation. As soon as it is apparent that the patient will require protracted ventilatory support, tracheostomy should replace the endotracheal tube. Less frequent indications for tracheostomy are life-threatening aspiration pneumonia, the need to improve pulmonary toilet to correct problems related to insufficient clearing of tracheobronchial secretions, and sleep apnea.

Posttracheostomy care requires humidified air to prevent secretions from crusting and occluding the inner cannula of the tracheostomy tube. The tracheostomy tube should be cleaned several times daily. The most frequent early complication of tracheostomy is dislodgment of the tracheostomy tube. Surgical creation of an inferiorly based tracheal flap sutured to the inferior neck skin may make reinsertion of a dislodged tube easier. It should be recalled that the act of swallowing requires elevation of the larynx, which is prevented by tracheostomy. Therefore, frequent tracheal and bronchial suctioning is often required to clear the aspirated saliva as well as the increased tracheobronchial secretions. Care of the skin around the stoma is important to prevent maceration and secondary infection.

Astrachan DI, Kirchner JC, Goodwin WJ Jr: Prolonged intubation vs. tracheotomy: Complications, practical and psychological considerations. Laryngoscope 1988;98:

1165. (Tracheostomy is far superior: fewer complications, ability to speak, comfort, ease of care.)

DeCarle B: Tracheostomy care. Nursing Times (Oct 2) 1985;81:50. (If a tracheostomy care protocol is unavailable at your institution, this article represents one reasonable approach.)

Kuriloff DB et al: Laryngotracheal injury following cricothyroidotomy. Laryngoscope 1989;99:125. (Cricothyrotomy should be used only in a true emergency and should be replaced with conventional tracheostomy as soon as convenient.)

Myers EN, Carrau RL: Early complications of tracheotomy: Incidence and management. Clin Chest Med 1991; 12:589. (Bleeding, dislodgment of the tube, subcutaneous emphysema, and pneumothorax.)

Nash M: Swallowing problems in the tracheotomized patient. Otolaryngol Clin North Am 1988;21:701. (Some common misunderstandings of the effect of tracheostomy on swallowing and aspiration.)

Wenig BL, Applebaum EL: Indications for and techniques of tracheotomy. Clin Chest Med 1991;12:545. (One of many sources offering a review of the technique.)

FOREIGN BODIES IN THE UPPER AERODIGESTIVE TRACT

FOREIGN BODIES OF THE TRACHEA & BRONCHI

Aspiration of foreign bodies occurs less frequently in adults than in children. The elderly and denture wearers appear to be at greatest risk. Wider familiarity with the Heimlich maneuver has reduced deaths. If the maneuver is unsuccessful, cricothyrotomy may be necessary. Plain chest radiographs may reveal a radiopaque foreign body. Detection of radiolucent foreign bodies may be aided by inspiration-expiration films that demonstrate air trapping distal to the obstructed segment. Atelectasis and pneumonia may occur later.

Tracheal and bronchial foreign bodies should be removed under general anesthesia by a skilled endoscopist working with an experienced anesthesiologist.

Kitay G, Shafer N: Cafe coronary: Recognition, treatment and prevention. Nurse Pract (Jun) 1989;14:35.

ESOPHAGEAL FOREIGN BODIES

Foreign bodies in the esophagus create urgent but not life-threatening situations as long as the airway is not compromised. It is a useful diagnostic sign of complete obstruction if the patient is drooling or cannot handle secretions. There is probably time to con-

sult an experienced clinician for management. Patients are likely to have difficulty handling secretions and may be spitting out their saliva. They may often point to the exact level of the obstruction. Indirect laryngoscopy often shows pooling of saliva at the esophageal inlet. Plain films may detect radiopaque foreign bodies such as chicken bones. Coins tend to align in the coronal plane in the esophagus and sagittally in the trachea. If a foreign body is suspected but not certainly known to be present, barium swallow may help make the diagnosis or establish that a foreign body is not (or is no longer) present.

Although some have suggested that a Foley catheter may be used to remove an esophageal foreign body, this method risks displacing it into the larynx with resultant airway obstruction. Endoscopic removal with conscious sedation or under general anaesthesia is safest. Highly selected patients with a prior history of food impaction may be treated with a likelihood of success by spasmolytic drugs, such as intravenous glucagon.

Brady PG: Esophageal foreign bodies. Gastroenterol Clin North Am 1991;20:691.

Taylor RB: Esophageal foreign bodies. Emerg Med Clin North Am 1987;5:301. (Includes an algorithmic approach to management by the emergency physician.)

Tibbling L, Stenquist M: Foreign bodies in the esophagus: A study of causative factors. Dysphagia 1991;6:224. (Selected patients may be treated with spasmolytic agents.)

Webb WA: Management of foreign bodies of the upper gastrointestinal tract. Gastroenterol 1988;94:216.

DISEASES PRESENTING AS NECK MASSES

The differential diagnosis of neck masses is heavily dependent on the location in the neck, the age of the patient, and the presence of associated disease processes. Rapid growth and tenderness suggest an inflammatory process, while firm, painless, and slowly enlarging masses are often neoplastic. In children, most neck masses are benign: congenital problems (eg, branchial cleft cysts, lymphangioma, hemangioma) or infection. In HIV-negative adults, cancer is the most common cause of persistent neck mass. A metastasis from squamous cell carcinoma arising within the mouth, pharynx, larynx, or upper esophagus should be suspected, especially if there is a history of tobacco or significant alcohol use. Among patients younger than 30 or older than 70, more consideration of a lymphoma should be given. Most important is a comprehensive otolaryngologic examination. Cytologic evaluation of the neck mass via fine-needle aspiration biopsy is likely to be the next step if an obvious primary tumor is not visible or palpable on physical examination.

CONGENITAL LESIONS PRESENTING AS NECK MASSES IN ADULTS

1. BRANCHIAL CLEFT CYSTS

Branchial cleft cysts usually present as a soft cystic mass along the anterior border of the sternocleidomastoid muscle. These lesions are usually recognized in the second or third decades of life, often when they suddenly swell or become infected. To prevent recurrent infection and possible carcinoma, they should be completely excised, along with their fistulous tracts.

First branchial cleft cysts present high in the neck, sometimes just below the ear. A fistulous connection with the floor of the external auditory canal may be present. Second cleft cysts, which are far more common, may communicate with the tonsillar fossa. Third cleft cysts, which may communicate with the piriform sinus, are rare.

2. THYROGLOSSAL DUCT CYST

Thyroglossal duct cysts are remnants occurring along the embryologic course of the thyroid's descent from the tuberculum impar of the tongue base to its usual position in the low neck. Although they may occur at any age, they are commonest before age 20. They present as a midline neck mass, often just below the hyoid bone, that moves with swallowing. Surgical excision is recommended to prevent recurrent infection. This requires removal of the entire fistulous tract along with the middle portion of the hyoid bone.

INFECTIOUS & INFLAMMATORY NECK MASSES

1. REACTIVE CERVICAL LYMPHADENOPATHY

The normal cervical lymphatic chain is not palpable. Infections involving the pharynx, salivary glands, and scalp often cause tender enlargement of neck nodes. Enlarged nodes are common in HIV-infected persons. Except for the occasional node that suppurates and requires incision and drainage, treatment is directed against the underlying infection. An enlarged lymph node that persists may warrant fine-needle aspiration biopsy in order to confirm that it is reactive and allay concern about malignancy. An en-

larging node unassociated with infection must be further evaluated.

2. NECK INFECTIONS WITH ATYPICAL MYCOBACTERIA (Scrofula)

Granulomatous neck masses are not uncommon. The differential diagnosis includes cat-scratch disease (probably more common than realized), sarcoidosis, and, especially in children, mycobacterial adenitis. Atypical mycobacterial adenitis (scrofula) usually presents as persistent adenopathy and can become fixed to the skin and drain externally. Although fine-needle aspiration may suggest a granulomatous origin, demonstration of mycobacteria by acid-fast staining (of material taken by fine-needle aspiration or open excisional biopsy) or culture is necessary to confirm this diagnosis. Treatment of scrofula is most successful with total excision of the involved nodes and appropriate antituberculous antibiotics for at least 9 months. The antibiotics used will depend on sensitivity studies but are likely to include isoniazid, rifampin, and, for at least the first 2 months, ethambutol in standard doses (see Table 9–10). When total excision might pose formidable surgical risks (eg, facial nerve proximity), a trial of needle aspiration or incision and drainage (along with antituberculosis medication) is worthwhile.

Mycobacterial lymphadenitis among HIV-positive patients is on the rise.

Alessi DP, Dudley JP: Atypical mycobacteria-induced cervical adenitis: Treatment by needle aspiration. Arch Otolaryngol Head Neck Surg 1988;114:664. (An acceptable alternative to excision.)

Cheung WL, Siu KF, Ng A: Tuberculosis cervical abscess: Comparing the results of total excision against simple incision and drainage. Br J Surg 1988;75:563. (Total excision cured 94%, versus 77% for incision and drainage.)

Lau SK et al: Source of tubercle bacilli in cervical lymph nodes: A prospective study. J Laryngol Otol 1991; 105:558.

Shikhani AF et al: Mycobacterial cervical lymphadenitis. Ear Nose Throat J 1989;68:662. (Two typical presentations with cervical involvement.)

Shriner KA, Mathisen GE, Goetz MB: Comparison of mycobacterial lymphadenitis among persons infected with human immunodeficiency virus and seronegative controls. Clin Infect Dis 1992;15:601.

3. LYME DISEASE

Lyme disease, caused by the spirochete *Borrelia burgdorferi* and transmitted by an *Ixodes ricinus* tick, may have protean manifestation, but over 75% of patients have symptoms involving the head and neck. Facial paralysis, dysesthesias, dysgeusia, dysesthesias, or other cranial neuropathies are most common. Headache, pain, and cervical lymphadenopathy may occur. See Chapter 33 for a more through discussion.

Lesser TH, Dort JC, Simmen DP: Ear, nose, and throat manifestations of Lyme disease. J Laryngol Otol 1990;104:301.

Moscatello AL et al: Otolaryngologic aspects of Lyme disease. Laryngoscope 1991;101(6 Part 1):592.

Sigal LH: Current recommendations for the treatment of Lyme disease. Drugs 1992;43:683.

TUMOR METASTASES

In older adults, 80% of firm, persistent, and enlarging neck masses are metastatic in origin. The great majority of these arise from squamous cell carcinoma of the upper aerodigestive tract. A complete head and neck examination may reveal the tumor of origin, but examination under anesthesia with direct laryngoscopy, esophagoscopy, and bronchoscopy is usually required to fully evaluate the tumor and exclude second primaries.

It is often helpful to obtain a cytologic diagnosis if initial head and neck examination fails to reveal the primary tumor. An open biopsy should be done only if physical examination fails to detect the primary tumor and fine-needle aspiration biopsy has also failed to yield a diagnosis.

Other than thyroid carcinoma, non-squamous cell metastases to the neck are infrequent. While tumors not involving the head and neck seldom metastasize to the middle or upper neck, the supraclavicular region is quite often involved by lung and breast tumors. Infradiaphragmatic tumors, with the exception of renal carcinoma, rarely metastasize to the neck.

LYMPHOMA

About 10% of lymphomas present in the head and neck. Multiple rubbery nodes, especially in the young adult, are suggestive of this disease. A thorough physical examination may demonstrate other sites of nodal or organ involvement. Needle aspiration may be diagnostic, but open biopsy is often required.

OTOLARYNGOLOGIC MANIFESTATIONS OF HIV INFECTION (See also Chapter 30.)

ORAL CAVITY & PHARYNX

Severe gingivitis and stomatitis are frequent presenting symptoms in HIV-infected patients. Candidiasis is common and may require prolonged treatment with fluconazole (100 mg daily) or ketoconazole (200–400 mg daily) for control, with clotrimazole or topical nystatin less effective. Giant intraoral ulcers have been seen in some patients. Hairy leukoplakia occurring on the lateral border of the tongue is often an early finding. It may develop quickly and appears as slightly raised leukoplakic areas with a corrugated or "hairy" surface. Histologically, parakeratosis and koilocytes are seen with little or no underlying inflammation. Among HIV-positive patients with oral lesions, hairy leukoplakia was seen in 19% in one study. Although clinical response following administration of, zidovudine or acyclovir has been reported, the success of treatment or even the need for treatment is under active investigation. The greater significance of the appearance of hairy leukoplakia among seropositive patients is that it may correlate positively with subsequent more ominous manifestations of AIDS.

Kaposi's sarcoma is most common on the hard palate but may be seen anywhere in the oral cavity and pharynx. It usually appears as a raised violaceous lesion beneath an intact mucosa, although it may be ulcerated, erythematous, and bleeding. Radiation therapy may control the tumor. A brisk mucositis can be expected following radiation therapy.

In addition to Kaposi's sarcoma, an increased incidence of non-Hodgkin's lymphoma is seen in AIDS. An increase in squamous cell carcinoma is also seen in the homosexual population, perhaps related to HIV infection.

Greenspan D, Greenspan JS: Significance of oral hairy leukoplakia. Oral Surg Oral Med Oral Pathol 1992;73:151. (In seropositive individuals, usually a harbinger of rapid progression to AIDS. May rarely be seen in non-HIV immunosuppressed patients.)

McCarthy GM: Host factors associated with HIV-related oral candidiasis: A review. Oral Surg Oral Med Oral Pathol 1992;73:181. (Xerostomia and low CD4 counts correlate with increased candidiasis.)

Samaranayade LP: Oral mycoses in HIV infection. Oral Surg Oral Med Oral Pathol 1992;73:171. (Oral candidiasis is a premonitory sign of HIV infection in a patient without local risk factor.)

Scully C, McCarthy G: Management of oral health in persons with HIV infection. Oral Surg Oral Med Oral Pathol 1992;73:215. (Reviews Candida, hairy leukoplakia, non-

HIV viral infections, and treatment of common problems such as bleeding and xerostomia.)

THE NECK

Persistent generalized lymphadenopathy is extremely common in HIV infection. In this setting, a tender or growing node may represent secondary infection, lymphoma, or other tumor. Fine-needle aspiration for culture and cytology is the best initial diagnostic step. Open biopsy will often be needed if granulomatous disease or lymphoma is suspected, though fine-needle aspiration biopsy may be diagnostic of *M tuberculosis* infection in seropositive patients.

Burton F, Patete ML, Goodwin WJ Jr: Indications for open cervical node biopsy in HIV-positive patients. Otolaryngol Head Neck Surg 1992;107:367. (Fine-needle aspiration is often sufficient to diagnose tuberculosis. Nontender or nonenlarging nodes do not require open biopsy.)

PARANASAL SINUSES

Sinusitis is common in HIV infection and the causative organisms are diverse, but the same pathogens encountered in nonimmunocompromised patients remain the most common. Early sinus irrigation, with aspirates sent for cytologic examination as well as fungal, viral, *Legionella,* and aerobic and anaerobic cultures is warranted. Initial antibiotic coverage should be based on the aspirate smear. If antibiotics fail to resolve the infection, functional endoscopic surgery to provide sinus drainage is often helpful. Guaifenesin (600 mg orally four times daily), a mucolytic agent, may offer some symptomatic relief.

Rubin JS, Honigberg R: Sinusitis in patients with the acquired immunodeficiency syndrome. Ear Nose Throat J 1990;69:460.

EAR

Given the common neurologic manifestations in AIDS, it is not surprising that there is a higher incidence of sensorineural hearing loss and auditory brain stem response abnormalities in AIDS patients than in the general population. Kaposi's sarcoma of the auricle is not uncommon. Seborrheic dermatitis, more common in AIDS, may be more difficult to treat in the external auditory canal.

General References for Otolaryngologic Manifestations of HIV Infection

Corey JP, Seligman I: Otolaryngology problems in the immune-compromised patient: An evolving natural history. Otolaryngol Head Neck Surg 1991;104:196.

Lucente FE: Otolaryngologic aspects of acquired immunodeficiency syndrome. Med Clin North Am 1991; 75:1389.

Rothstein SG et al: Emergencies in AIDS patients: The otolaryngologic perspective. Otolaryngol Head Neck Surg 1991;104:545.

REFERENCES

Alberti PW, Ruben RJ (editors): *Otologic Medicine and Surgery.* Churchill Livingstone, 1988.

Cummings CW, Frederickson J: *Otolaryngology–Head and Neck Surgery,* 2nd ed. Mosby, 1992.

Gates GA: *Current Therapy in Otolaryngology–Head and Neck Surgery,* 3rd ed. Mosby, 1993.

Kaplan MJ, Jackler RK: Drugs used in ear, nose and throat disorders. In: *Drug Therapy,* 2nd ed. Katzung BG (editor). Appleton & Lange, 1991.

Meyerhoff WL, Rice DH (editors): *Otolaryngology–Head and Neck Surgery.* Saunders, 1992.

Paparella MM et al (editors): *Otolaryngology,* 4 vols. Saunders, 1991.

Sande MA, Volberding PA: *The Medical Management of AIDS.* Saunders, 1988.

Vogt HB: Disorders of the ear, nose, and throat. Prim Care 1990;17:213.

Pulmonary Diseases

9

John L. Stauffer, MD

DIAGNOSTIC METHODS

SYMPTOMS OF PULMONARY DISEASES

Dyspnea is the sensation of breathlessness that is excessive for any given level of physical activity. The physician should record the level of activity that induces dyspnea, to serve as a basis for assessing the results of therapy. Dyspnea of pulmonary origin may be due to disorders of the airway, lung parenchyma, pleura, respiratory muscles, or chest wall. Extrapulmonary disorders causing dyspnea include heart disease, shock, anemia, hypermetabolic states, and anxiety. **Paroxysmal nocturnal dyspnea** (inappropriate breathlessness at night) and orthopnea (dyspnea on recumbency) usually are caused by left ventricular dysfunction but may also be observed in asthma, aspiration, and chronic obstructive pulmonary disease.

Platypnea, the opposite of orthopnea, is dyspnea in the upright position relieved by recumbency. This rare symptom is usually caused by right-to-left intracardiac or pulmonary vascular shunting of venous blood.

Persistent cough should always be considered abnormal. The cough reflex may be triggered by stimulation of receptors located in the tracheobronchial tree, the upper airway, and in other sites such as the sinuses, auditory canal, pleura, pericardium, esophagus, stomach, and diaphragm. Chronic, persistent cough is often caused by cigarette smoking, asthma, or chronic obstructive pulmonary disease. Cough may also be caused by drugs (angiotensin-converting enzyme inhibitors), cardiac disease, occupational agents, and psychogenic factors. However, the physician may encounter patients with this complaint in whom the history, physical examination, chest x-ray, and pulmonary function tests do not suggest a specific cause. In such cases, the cough is usually found to be caused by postnasal drip from sinusitis, occult asthma, gastroesophageal reflux, bronchitis, or bronchiectasis. Complications of severe cough include

worsening of bronchospasm, vomiting, rib fractures, urinary incontinence, and, occasionally, syncope.

Stridor is a crowing sound during breathing caused by turbulent airflow through a narrowed upper airway. Inspiratory stridor suggests extrathoracic variable airway obstruction, while expiratory stridor indicates intrathoracic variable airway obstruction. Inspiratory and expiratory stridor occurring together suggest fixed obstruction anywhere in the upper airway. Snoring is an inspiratory sound due to vibration in the pharynx during sleep.

Wheezes are continuous musical or whistling noises caused by turbulent airflow through narrowed intrathoracic airways. Most, but not all, complaints of wheezing are due to asthma. Wheezing may be accompanied by a sensation of chest tightness, a nonspecific feeling of labored breathing that implies bronchoconstriction.

Hemoptysis—the expectoration of blood or blood-tinged sputum—is often the first indication of serious bronchopulmonary disease; the history usually distinguishes it from hematemesis and from nasopharyngeal bleeding. Bright red, frothy blood implies a bronchopulmonary origin of bleeding. Though bronchitis and bronchiectasis are more common causes of hemoptysis, carcinoma must always be excluded. Massive hemoptysis, defined arbitrarily as the coughing up of more than 200–600 mL of blood in 24 hours, is often caused by bronchiectasis, tuberculosis (particularly from a Rasmussen aneurysm in cavitary disease), mycetomas, and other chronic suppurative parenchymal diseases. Self-limited minimal hemoptysis occasionally occurs with vigorous coughing accompanying upper or lower respiratory tract infection.

Irwin RS, Curley FJ, French CL: Chronic cough. The spectrum and frequency of causes, key components of the diagnostic evaluation, and outcome of specific therapy. Am Rev Respir Dis 1990;141:640. (Cough can be effectively treated in nearly all cases after identification of a specific cause.)

Tobin MJ: Dyspnea: Pathophysiologic basis, clinical presentation, and management. Arch Intern Med 1990; 150:1604. (Pathophysiologic basis for the sensation of dyspnea.)

SIGNS OF PULMONARY DISEASES

Tachypnea, or rapid, shallow breathing, may be defined arbitrarily as a respiratory rate in excess of 18/min, though some would set the limit of normal at 16, 20, or 25 breaths per minute. A sudden onset or persistence of tachypnea is particularly alarming. **Hyperpnea** is rapid, deep breathing. **Hyperventilation** is an increase in the amount of air entering the alveoli, causing hypocapnia (defined as arterial PCO_2 < 40 mm Hg).

The thorax is normally symmetric, and both sides expand equally on inspiration. Asymmetry at rest is observed in scoliosis, chest wall deformity, severe fibrothorax, and conditions with unilateral loss of lung volume. Symmetrically reduced chest expansion during deep inspiration is seen in such conditions as neuromuscular disease, emphysema, and ankylosis of the spine. Asymmetric chest expansion during inspiration suggests unilateral airway obstruction, pleural or pulmonary fibrosis, or splinting due to chest pain. Expansion of the chest but collapse of the abdomen on inspiration indicates weakness or paralysis of the diaphragm. If the chest collapses and the abdomen rises on inspiration, airway obstruction, intercostal muscle paralysis, or a flail deformity of the chest wall may be present.

The arterial blood pressure normally falls about 5 mm Hg on inspiration. **Paradoxic pulse,** an exaggeration of the normal response, is defined as a fall in systolic arterial blood pressure of 10 mm Hg or more on inspiration. This occurs in severe asthma or emphysema, upper airway obstruction, pulmonary embolism, pericardial constriction or tamponade, and restrictive cardiomyopathy.

Cyanosis is a bluish discoloration of skin or mucous membranes caused by increased amounts (> 5 g/dL) of unsaturated hemoglobin in the blood. Anemia may preclude detection of cyanosis in a hypoxemic patient. **Central cyanosis,** which is usually caused by hypoxemia from respiratory failure or a right-to-left intracardiac or intrapulmonary shunt, is apparent on inspection of the oral mucous membranes; **peripheral cyanosis** is more likely due to nonrespiratory causes such as reduced cardiac output and vasoconstriction.

Digital clubbing is present when the anteroposterior thickness of the index finger at the base of the fingernail exceeds the thickness of the distal interphalangeal joint. Nail bed sponginess, rounding of the nail plate, and flattening of the angle between the nail plate and proximal nail skin fold are helpful clues to clubbing. Symmetric clubbing occurs in lung cancer, bronchiectasis, lung abscess, pulmonary arteriovenous malformation, idiopathic pulmonary fibrosis, and cystic fibrosis. It is rarely seen in chronic obstructive pulmonary disease and asthma. Nonpulmonary causes of symmetric clubbing include cyanotic congenital heart disease, infective endocar-

ditic, cirrhosis, and inflammatory bowel disease. Clubbing may be congenital.

Hyperresonance to percussion occurs in diseases accompanied by hyperinflation (asthma, emphysema) and in pneumothorax. **Dullness** to percussion is observed in thickening of the chest wall or pleura, pleural effusion, atelectasis, parenchymal infiltration or consolidation, elevation of the diaphragm, or displacement of abdominal contents into the thorax.

Vesicular breath sounds are normal soft, low-pitched sounds heard at the periphery of the lung. The finding of harsh **bronchial (tracheal) breath sounds** in areas where vesicular sounds are normally heard implies consolidation, compression, or infiltration of the lung with a patent bronchus. **Bronchovesicular breath sounds** are intermediate in tone quality between vesicular and bronchial sounds. Diminished breath sounds imply inspiratory obstruction to airflow in large airways, pleural disease (especially effusion), pneumothorax, or low tidal volumes.

Adventitious sounds are abnormal sounds on auscultation and may be classified as continuous **(wheezes, rhonchi)** or discontinuous **(crackles, crepitations, or rales).** High-pitched wheezes result from bronchospasm, bronchial or bronchiolar mucosal edema, or airway obstruction by mucus, tumors, or foreign bodies. Low-pitched rhonchi are often caused by sputum in large airways and frequently clear after cough. Crackles are probably generated by the snapping open of small airways during inspiration. Fine crackles are heard in interstitial diseases and in early pneumonia or congestive heart failure. Coarse crackles are heard late in the course of pulmonary edema or pneumonia.

Tactile (vocal) fremitus denotes palpable voice vibrations on the chest wall. This is a normal finding. Localized reduction in fremitus occurs in pleural effusion, pneumothorax, or thickening of the chest wall. Increased fremitus suggests lung consolidation. **Rhonchal fremitus** means palpable coarse vibrations on the chest wall in patients with loud rhonchi.

Bronchophony refers to increased intensity and clarity of the spoken word during auscultation; it is heard over areas of consolidation or lung compression. **Whispered pectoriloquy** is an extreme form of bronchophony in which softly spoken words are readily heard by auscultation. **Egophony** refers to auscultation of an "a" sound when the patient speaks an "e" sound. It is demonstrated over compressed lung above a pleural effusion, and in consolidation.

DIAGNOSTIC TESTS: PULMONARY FUNCTION TESTS, PULMONARY EXERCISE STRESS TESTING, & BRONCHOSCOPY

Pulmonary Function Tests

Pulmonary function tests objectively measure the ability of the respiratory system to perform gas exchange by assessing its ventilation, diffusion, and mechanical properties. Indications for pulmonary function testing include the following:

(1) Evaluation of the type and degree of pulmonary dysfunction.

(2) Evaluation of dyspnea, cough, and other symptoms.

(3) Early detection of lung dysfunction.

(4) Surveillance in occupational settings.

(5) Follow-up of response to therapy.

(6) Preoperative evaluation.

(7) Disability assessment.

Relative contraindications to pulmonary function testing include severe acute asthma or respiratory distress, chest pain aggravated by testing, pneumothorax, brisk hemoptysis, and active tuberculosis. Most of the tests depend on the efforts of the patient; some patients may be too impaired to make an optimal effort. Pulmonary function tests derived from **spirometry** (the measurement of airflow rates and forced vital capacity) and measurement of lung volumes are defined in Table 9–1.

Spirometry and measurement of lung volumes allow determination of the presence and severity of *obstructive* and *restrictive* pulmonary dysfunction.

The hallmark of obstructive pulmonary dysfunction is reduction in airflow rates. Causes include asthma, chronic bronchitis, emphysema, small airway dysfunction, bronchiolitis, bronchiectasis, cystic fibrosis, and upper airway obstruction. Some advanced chronic interstitial lung diseases such as sarcoidosis may also cause obstructive dysfunction. Restrictive pulmonary dysfunction is characterized by reduction in lung volumes. Pulmonary infiltrates, lung resection, pleural diseases, chest wall disorders, reduced diaphragm movement, and neuromuscular disease may be responsible. Pulmonary function alterations in obstructive and restrictive disorders are summarized in Table 9–2. The changes in airflow rates and lung volumes in the restrictive category vary according to the specific cause of the disorder.

Obstructive dysfunction is graded according to the reduction in the ratio of forced expiratory volume in 1 second (FEV_1) to forced vital capacity (FVC). Restrictive dysfunction is graded by reduction in the FVC or total lung capacity, comparing observed with predicted values. Predicted values are derived from studies of normals and in general vary with gender, age, and height. Spirometry provides a **spirogram** that displays time (x-axis) versus expired volume (y-axis) and an expiratory **flow-volume curve** (first derivative of the spirogram) that plots expiratory volume (x-axis) versus expiratory airflow rate (positive y-axis) (Figure 9–1). The **flow-volume loop** combines the expiratory and inspiratory flow-volume curves and is especially helpful for determining intrathoracic and extrathoracic airway dynamics and the site of airway obstruction.

Spirometry (cost approximately $90.00–125.00) is

Table 9–1. Definitions of selected pulmonary function tests.

Tests	Definition
Tests derived from spirometry	
Forced vital capacity (FVC)	The volume of gas that can be forcefully expelled from the lungs after maximal inspiration.
Forced expiratory volume in 1 second (FEV_1)	The volume of gas expelled in the first second of the FVC maneuver.
Forced expiratory flow from 25% to 75% of the forced vital capacity (FEF_{25-75})	The maximal midexpiratory airflow rate.
Peak expiratory flow rate (PEFR)	The maximal airflow rate achieved in the FVC maneuver.
Maximum voluntary ventilation (MVV)	The maximum volume of gas that can be breathed in 1 minute (usually measured for 15 seconds and multipled by 4).
Lung volumes	
Slow vital capacity (SVC)	The volume of gas that can be slowly exhaled after maximal inspiration.
Total lung capacity (TLC)	The volume of gas in the lungs after a maximal inspiration.
Functional residual capacity (FRC)	The volume of gas in the lungs at the end of a normal tidal expiration.
Residual volume (RV)	The volume of gas remaining in the lungs after maximal expiration.
Expiratory reserve volume (ERV)	The volume of gas representing the difference between functional residual capacity and residual volume.

Table 9–2. Results of pulmonary function tests in obstructive and restrictive pulmonary dysfunction.[1]

Tests	Obstructive[2]	Restrictive[2]
Spirometry		
FVC (liters)	N or ↓	↓
FEV$_1$ (liters)	↓	N or ↓
FEV$_1$/FVC (%)	↓	N or ↑
FEF$_{25-75}$ (L/s)	↓	N or ↓
PEFR (L/s)	↓	N or ↑
MVV (L/min)	↓	N or ↓
Lung volumes		
SVC (liters)	N or ↓	↓
TLC (liters)	N or ↑	↓
FRC (liters)	↑	N or ↓
ERV (liters)	N or ↓	N or ↓
RV (liters)	↑	N, ↓, or ↑
RV/TLC ratio	↑	N or ↑

[1]See Table 9–1 for definitions of tests.
[2]N = normal; ↓ = less than predicted; ↑ = greater than predicted.

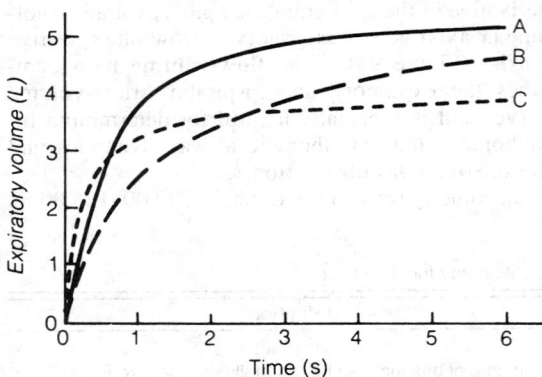

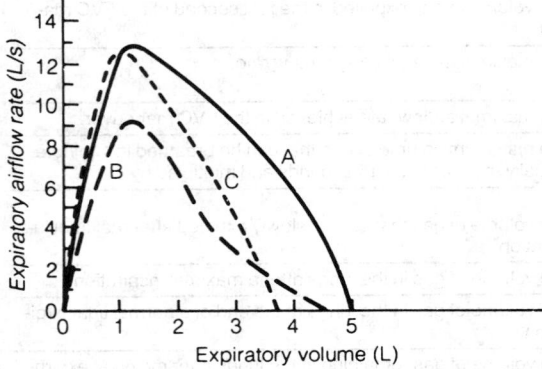

Figure 9–1. Representative spirograms (upper panel) and expiratory flow-volume curves (lower panel) for normal (A), obstructive (B), and restrictive (C) patterns.

adequate for evaluation of most patients with suspected respiratory disease. If airflow obstruction is evident, spirometry is repeated 10–20 minutes after an inhaled bronchodilator is administered. This doubles the cost of the study. The absence of improvement in spirometry after inhaled bronchodilator in the pulmonary function laboratory does not preclude a successful clinical response to bronchodilator therapy. Measurements of lung volumes and diffusing capacity are useful in selected patients, but these tests double the cost of pulmonary function testing and should not be ordered routinely.

Measurement of the single-breath **diffusing capacity** for carbon monoxide (D$_L$CO), which reflects the ability of the lung to transfer gas across the alveolar/capillary interface, is particularly helpful in evaluation of patients with diffuse infiltrative lung disease or emphysema. The total pulmonary diffusing capacity (D$_L$) depends upon the diffusion capacity of the alveolar-capillary membrane and the volume of hemoglobin occupying the pulmonary capillaries. A diffusing capacity less than 80% of predicted value, after correction for the blood hemoglobin level,* is abnormally low. Reporting the ratio of measured diffusing capacity to alveolar volume (D$_L$CO/V$_A$) is helpful, because a diminished diffusing capacity may only reflect a reduction in lung volume. In patients with emphysema, the diffusing capacity is characteristically low, the alveolar volume normal or increased, and the D$_L$CO/V$_A$ ratio is low. In patients with diffuse infiltrative lung disease, both the diffusing capacity and the alveolar volume are characteristically reduced, and the D$_L$CO/V$_A$ ratio is normal or near normal.

In patients with AIDS, D$_L$CO is a highly sensitive screening test for the presence of pulmonary disease, especially *Pneumocystis carinii* pneumonia, but it lacks specificity. A normal D$_L$CO in an AIDS patient is strong evidence against *Pneumocystis carinii* pneumonia. An abnormal result indicates the need for further diagnostic evaluation. Routine measurement of D$_L$CO and other pulmonary function tests in AIDS patients with pulmonary disease is not advised, because of expense and lack of specificity.

Arterial blood gas analysis is fundamental to the modern practice of pulmonary medicine (see Chapter 20). An arterial blood gas profile (total charges range from $80.00 to $120.00) is indicated whenever a clinically important acid-base disturbance, hypoxemia, or hypercapnia is suspected. **Oximetry** provides an inexpensive, noninvasive alternative means of monitoring oxyhemoglobin saturation with oxygen. Pulse oximeters are accurate and portable and monitor heart rate as well as saturation. It is important to recognize that all oximeters monitor oxygen saturation and not oxygen tension. Table 9–3 displays the nor-

$$*\text{Corrected } D_L\text{CO} = \frac{\text{Measured } D_L\text{CO}}{0.0697 \times \text{Hb level (g/dL)}}$$

Table 9–3. Relationship of oxyhemoglobin saturation and partial pressure of oxygen in blood.[1,2]

Saturation (%)	Partial Pressure (mm Hg)[3]
50	27
55	29
60	31
65	34
70	37
75	40
80	45
85	50
90	58
91	60
92	63
93	66
94	69
95	74
96	81
97	92
98	111
99	159
99.9	500

[1]Modified and reproduced, with permission, from Severinghaus JW: Values for a standard blood oxygen dissociation curve. In: *Respiration and Circulation.* Altman PC, Dittmer DS (editors): Federation of American Societies for Experimental Biology, 1971.
[2]This relationship assumes a normal position of the oxyhemoglobin dissociation curve.
[3]Rounded to the nearest whole number.

mal relationship between oxyhemoglobin saturation and partial pressure of oxygen in blood. This relationship is not linear. Table 9–4 displays the effect of altitude on arterial PO_2.

American Thoracic Society: Lung function testing: Selection of reference values and interpretative strategies. Am Rev Respir Dis 1991;144:1202. (Expert consensus opinion.)
Zibrak JD, O'Donnell CR, Morton K: Indications for pulmonary function testing. Ann Intern Med 1990;112:763. (Review of original studies on the utility of preoperative pulmonary function tests in predicting postoperative outcomes.)

Table 9–4. The effect of altitude on PO_2 in normals.

Altitude (feet)	Barometric Pressure (mm Hg)	Atmospheric[1] PO_2 (mm Hg)	Tracheal[2] PO_2 (mm Hg)	Arterial[3] PO_2 (mm Hg)
Sea level	760	159	149	99
2,000	707	148	138	88
4,000	656	137	127	77
6,000	609	127	118	68
8,000	564	118	108	58
10,000	523	109	100	50
15,000	428	90	80	30

[1]Dry gas.
[2]Saturated with water vapor.
[3]Actual values at altitude will be higher, depending on the degree of adaptation (ventilatory response to hypoxia).

Pulmonary Exercise Stress Testing

Pulmonary exercise testing is usually performed to evaluate patients with unexplained exertional dyspnea. A bicycle ergometer or treadmill is used. Minute ventilation, expired oxygen and carbon dioxide tension, heart rate, blood pressure, and respiratory rate are monitored. The exercise protocol is determined by the indications for the test and the ability of the patient to exercise. Complications are rare. Total charges for a full exercise study (without arterial catheterization) approximate $400.00 to $500.00.

Eschenbacher WL, Mannina A: An algorithm for the interpretation of cardiopulmonary exercise tests. Chest 1990;97:263. (Standard parameters to simplify interpretation.)

Bronchoscopy

Flexible **fiberoptic bronchoscopy** is an essential tool in the diagnosis and management of many pulmonary diseases. Bronchoscopy is of value for evaluation of the airway, diagnosis and staging of bronchogenic carcinoma, evaluation of hemoptysis, biopsy of lung infiltrates, diagnosis of pulmonary infections, facilitation of bronchoalveolar lavage, and removal of retained secretions and foreign bodies from the airway. The procedure is contraindicated in patients with severe bronchospasm. A bleeding diathesis is a contraindication to biopsy and brushing. Complications include hemoptysis, fever, and a transient reduction in PO_2 (< k 10 mm Hg). The rate of major complications is less than 2%, and deaths are rare. Hospitalization for fiberoptic bronchoscopy is rarely necessary. The total cost of the procedure ranges from $600.00 to over $1500.00, depending on the need for fluoroscopy, processing of specimens in the laboratory, hospital outpatient stay charges, and other variables.

Rigid bronchoscopy is performed infrequently but is valuable in selected situations. These include massive bleeding, extraction of large obstructing objects (foreign bodies, blood clots, tumor masses, broncholiths), biopsy of tracheal or main stem bronchus tumors and bronchial carcinoids, facilitation of ventilation during bronchoscopy, and facilitation of laser therapy. Unlike fiberoptic bronchoscopy, rigid bronchoscopy usually requires general anesthesia.

DISORDERS OF THE AIRWAYS

Diseases of the airways have diverse causes but share certain pathophysiologic and clinical features. Limitation of airflow is characteristic and results from intraluminal airway obstruction, thickening of airway walls, or the loss of distending support by interstitial tissues necessary to maintain patency of the airways. Hypersecretion of mucus, airway irritability, and gas exchange abnormalities result in cough, sputum production, wheezing, and dyspnea.

ASTHMA

Essentials of Diagnosis

- Episodic or chronic wheezing, dyspnea, cough, and feeling of tightness in the chest.
- Prolonged expiration and diffuse wheezing on physical examination.
- Limitation of airflow on pulmonary function testing, or positive bronchoprovocation challenge test.
- Complete or partial reversibility of obstructive dysfunction after bronchodilator therapy.

General Considerations

Asthma is defined as a "disease characterized by an increased responsiveness of the trachea and bronchi to various stimuli, and manifested by widespread narrowing of the airways that changes in severity either spontaneously or as a result of treatment" (American Thoracic Society). Asthma is characterized by such pathologic changes as hypertrophy of bronchial smooth muscle, mucosal edema and hyperemia, thickening of epithelial basement membrane, hypertrophy of mucous glands, acute inflammation, and plugging of airways by thick, viscid mucus. These changes result in obstruction of airways of all calibers.

The pathogenesis of asthma is poorly understood. Asthma is now regarded primarily as subacute inflammatory disease of airways. The pivotal role of allergic mechanisms in the large majority of patients with asthma is gaining more attention. Multiple complex mechanisms probably are involved in reversible airflow obstruction. The sensitized tissue mast cell plays a pivotal role in asthma by degranulating and releasing mediators such as histamine, bradykinin, chemotactic factors, platelet-activating factor, and metabolites of arachidonic acid such as prostaglandins and leukotrienes. Neural factors may augment this response. These mediators act locally to effect bronchoconstriction, cellular infiltration, platelet activation, increased vascular permeability, edema, and increased secretion of mucus. Airway narrowing in asthma results from a combination of bronchoconstriction, airway edema and inflammation, and mucus plugging. Successful therapy depends upon reversing each of these factors.

Asthma is common in adults and even more common in children. Men and women are equally affected. About 4–5% of the population has asthma.

Exercise-induced asthma occurs 5–10 minutes after the patient starts to exercise and may be related to heat loss or water loss from the bronchial surface. **Triad asthma,** a combination of asthma, aspirin sensitivity, and nasal polyposis, occurs in fewer than 10% of asthma patients. Bronchoconstriction in this condition is due to the effects on arachidonic acid metabolism of aspirin and other nonsteroidal anti-inflammatory agents, tartrazine dyes, and other compounds. **Occupational asthma** may be triggered by various agents found in the workplace and occurs a few weeks to many years after initial exposure to an offending agent. Nocturnal cough may be the only symptom. **Cardiac asthma** represents bronchospasm precipitated by congestive heart failure. **Asthmatic bronchitis** denotes chronic bronchitis with features of bronchospasm that quickly responds to bronchodilator therapy. **Drug-induced asthma** is caused by many commonly used agents (Table 9–19).

Clinical Findings

A. Symptoms and Signs: Asthma is characterized by episodic wheezing, feelings of tightness in the chest, dyspnea, and cough. The frequency of asthma attacks is highly variable. Some patients may have very infrequent, brief attacks of asthma; others may suffer nearly continuous symptoms. Asthma is often worse at night. Nocturnal asthma is usually most severe around 4 AM, when circadian variations in bronchomotor tone and bronchial reactivity result in bronchoconstriction.

Asthma attacks occur spontaneously or result from various "trigger factors," including nonspecific irritants (dusts, odors, cold air, sulfur dioxide fumes), emotional stress, upper respiratory infections, exertion, exposure to aeroallergens, aspiration, and abrupt changes in weather. The antigens of the ubiquitous house dust mite represent an important aeroallergen for many patients with asthma. Inhalation of aeroallergens often initiates wheezing, chest tightness, dyspnea, and cough both immediately (immediate asthmatic response) and 4–6 hours later (late asthmatic response). Aspirin, other nonsteroidal anti-inflammatory drugs, sulfites added to foods and certain medications, beta-blockers, and other drugs (Table 9–19) can trigger attacks of asthma. Patients may present with chronic dry or nonproductive cough rather than with dyspnea and wheezing. In patients with this so-called "cough-variant asthma," baseline pulmonary function tests are normal but bronchial hyperreactivity can be demonstrated with bronchial provocation testing. Inhaled bronchodilators are often effective in controlling cough symptoms in these patients.

Physical findings vary with the severity of the attack. A mild attack may produce only slight tachycardia and tachypnea, with prolonged expiration and mild diffuse wheezing. More severe attacks are associated with use of accessory muscles of respiration, distant breath sounds, loud wheezing, hyperresonance, and intercostal retraction. Ominous signs in severe asthma include fatigue, pulsus paradoxus (> 20 mm Hg), diaphoresis, inaudible breath sounds with diminished wheezing, inability to maintain recumbency, and cyanosis.

B. Laboratory Findings: The total white blood cell count may be slightly increased during an acute attack, and eosinophilia is common. Expectorated sputum is viscid on gross examination; microscopic findings include mucus casts of small airways (Curschmann's spirals), eosinophils, and elongated rhomboid crystals derived from eosinophil cytoplasm (Charcot-Leyden crystals). Pulmonary function tests (Table 9–2) reveal abnormalities typical of obstructive dysfunction, and partial reversibility (improvement in FVC or FEV_1 of at least 15% or improvement in FEF_{25-75} of at least 25%) is often demonstrated after an inhaled bronchodilator is administered. It is important to emphasize that the absence of improvement in the pulmonary function test after bronchodilator does not constitute proof of irreversible airflow obstruction. Measuring the peak expiratory flow rate (PEFR) with a simple hand-held device can also indicate (inexpensively) the severity of airflow limitation. Predicted values vary with sex, age, and height. Values under 200 L/min indicate severe obstructive dysfunction.

Arterial blood gas measurements in asthma may be normal during a mild attack, but respiratory alkalosis and mild hypoxemia are usually observed. In more severe cases, hypoxemia worsens and respiratory alkalosis disappears when respiratory muscle fatigue prevents hyperventilation. Normalization of the PCO_2 or development of respiratory acidosis in this circumstance usually indicates the need for mechanical ventilation.

C. Imaging: Routine chest radiographs in adults and children with uncomplicated attacks reveal only hyperinflation; they are unnecessary in acute asthma unless pneumothorax, pneumonia, or another disorder mimicking asthma (see below) is suspected. Bronchial wall thickening and absence of vascular shadows in the periphery of the lung are sometimes observed.

D. Special Examinations: Skin testing for allergens that trigger attacks is most useful in young patients with extrinsic asthma. **Bronchial provocation testing** with methacholine or histamine is helpful in confirming asthma when the diagnosis is uncertain. This test is highly sensitive in the detection of bronchial hyperresponsiveness, the hallmark of asthma. It is not, however, entirely specific for asthma (including cough-variant asthma). Elevated serum levels of immunoglobulin E (IgE) are found in many patients with asthma but are not specific. Serum-specific IgE antibody against a specific allergen can be measured with the radioallergosorbent (RAST) test, but this test is expensive and less sensitive than intradermal skin testing.

Differential Diagnosis

Wheezing occurs not only in bronchial asthma but also in chronic obstructive pulmonary disease (COPD), left ventricular failure, pulmonary embolism, and bronchogenic carcinoma. Stridor in upper airway obstruction or in vocal cord dysfunction may simulate wheezing. Asthma must be distinguished from functional disorders of the larynx. Foreign body aspiration may also present with features suggesting bronchial asthma. Reversible bronchial obstruction with eosinophilia occurs in infestations with parasitic infection (particularly *Strongyloides*), bronchopulmonary aspergillosis, and Churg-Strauss syndrome.

Complications

Complications of asthma include exhaustion, dehydration, airway infection, cor pulmonale, and tussive syncope. Pneumothorax is a rare complication. Acute respiratory failure with hypoxemia and hypercapnia occurs in severe disease. In most western countries, there has been over the last decade a gradual increase in the asthma mortality rate, despite advances in understanding the pathogenesis of this disorder and the availability of new pharmacologic agents. The explanation for this increased death rate is not clear. The death rate from asthma in the United States is conservatively estimated to be approximately 0.4 cases per 100,000 population per year.

Prevention

Asthma is often preventable if environmental and occupational agents and other "trigger factors" known to provoke asthma attacks can be identified and eliminated. The importance of environmental control measures in both the home and the workplace cannot be overemphasized. For example, measures to control house dust mite antigen (pillow and mattress covers, removal of carpets, air filtering and conditioning, etc) and animal danders (washing the household dog weekly) should be employed. Early treatment of chest infections, recognition and effective management of nasal and paranasal disorders, discontinuance of cigarette smoking, and a sympathetic attitude on the part of the physician are essential aspects of preventive care. Patient compliance with prescribed medication is essential to prevent flare-ups of asthma. Many patients with asthma will benefit from recording PEFR at home and at work while correlating their symptoms with PEFR values.

Treatment

A. Ambulatory Patients With Asthma:

1. Mild asthma–Most patients require bronchodilator therapy to control symptoms. Patients with infrequent attacks may use, on an "as needed" basis, inhaled sympathomimetic bronchodilator drugs. Agents available in the United States include albuterol (salbutamol), metaproterenol, bitolterol, pirbuterol, terbutaline, isoetharine, isoproterenol, and epinephrine. All activate beta-agonist receptors on smooth muscle cells in the respiratory tract, thereby stimulating the intracellular enzyme adenylyl cyclase. This increases production of cAMP, resulting in relaxation of bronchial smooth muscle (bronchodilation). Inhaled sympathomimetics have replaced oral theophylline as the bronchodilator of choice for bronchial asthma. Metered-dose inhaler (MDI) devices are the most convenient and practical way of administering these drugs.

Oral sympathomimetics should, in general, be avoided because of cardiac and neuromuscular side effects, but they may be useful in patients unable to use inhalers. Continuous treatment with theophylline derivatives is not recommended for infrequent, mild attacks of asthma; however, a long-acting theophylline compound taken at bedtime may be helpful for patients with nocturnal asthma. An extended-release albuterol tablet may accomplish the same purpose. Exercise-induced asthma may be avoided by treatment with inhaled bronchodilators or cromolyn sodium before exercise.

2. Moderate to severe asthma–Patients who experience more frequent symptoms or more severe attacks of asthma require daily maintenance drug therapy. Anti-inflammatory agents are the treatment of choice in such patients because of their ability to prevent attacks of asthma. Regular use of inhaled corticosteroids is now advised for the majority of patients with moderate to severe asthma. Inhaled cromolyn is an alternative in selected patients. Most experts now advise that inhaled sympathomimetics be reserved for use as "rescue" drugs to treat attacks of asthma, not for maintenance therapy. Maintenance therapy with oral theophylline preparations in ambulatory patients with severe asthma is losing favor. Table 9–5 summarizes drugs used in the treatment of asthma and COPD.

a. Inhaled sympathomimetics–Albuterol, bitolterol, and terbutaline are relatively long-acting and may be administered every 4–6 hours for relief of symptoms. Metaproterenol, a shorter-acting agent, is given every 4 hours. One or two inhalations are usually sufficient. For severe asthma, up to four inhalations of any of these agents, administered as often as every 3 hours, may be required temporarily. Some patients may benefit from even more than four puffs. Sequential inhalations, separated by at least 1 minute, may enhance the bronchodilator effect. Excessive patient use of inhaled beta-sympathomimetic agents—arbitrarily defined as the use of more than three metered-dose inhalers monthly—should alert both the patient and the physician to the need for more careful evaluation and institution of alternative therapy, particularly anti-inflammatory agents. There is concern that regular excessive use of inhaled sympathomimetics increases the mortality rate in asthma.

The metered-dose inhaler (MDI) is the preferred means of delivery of sympathomimetic and cortico-steroid aerosol drugs. Unfortunately, a single inhaler may cost the patient as much as $20.00–30.00. Various extension devices ("spacers") may be attached to the inhaler to facilitate use and enhance aerosol deposition in the lung. Unfortunately, MDIs are used incorrectly by at least half of patients, and many physicians are uncertain about the proper technique. Optimal use of these devices requires one actuation (puff) just after beginning a slow, deep breath from functional residual capacity, followed by a 10-second breath-hold. Inspiration should take about 5 seconds. Maximal inspiration to total lung capacity is not required. The 10-second breath-hold is essential to allow deposition of the aerosol in the periphery of the lung. Careful patient instruction in MDI use and reinforcement of training on follow-up office visits are essential. Physically or mentally handicapped patients may be unable to use MDIs.

Hand-bulb nebulizers have no practical advantage. Compressed air or oxygen may be used to nebulize certain sympathomimetic drug solutions and cromolyn solution. Jet nebulizers are expensive and inconvenient and have not been demonstrated to be more effective than metered-dose inhalers. Their use should be reserved for patients who are unable to use the metered dose inhalers effectively. Liquid solutions of different medications (eg, a sympathomimetic drug and cromolyn) may be mixed together in the nebulizer unit.

b. Corticosteroids–Corticosteroids are effective in asthma because they suppress both acute and chronic airway inflammation. Their complex actions include attenuation of the release of and response to mediators of inflammation. These drugs may also potentiate the action of β_2-adrenergic agents.

Oral corticosteroid therapy is used only when other measures fail to relieve symptoms. Prednisone or prednisolone is preferred; the dosage is 40–60 mg/d orally to start, tapered in increments of 5–10 mg every 2–3 days over 1–3 weeks. Early treatment of severe asthma attacks with adequate doses of corticosteroids usually relieves symptoms and prevents hospitalization. Chronic maintenance therapy with systemic corticosteroids is unfortunately sometimes necessary and is associated with many adverse effects. Repeated efforts should be made to eliminate daily oral corticosteroids or reduce the dose to the minimal amount necessary to control symptoms. Treatment every other day is preferred to daily treatment for corticosteroid-dependent patients to reduce adverse effects, but control of asthma may be difficult. Some patients will experience repeated severe exacerbations of asthma if corticosteroids are tapered too quickly. Inhaled corticosteroids are helpful for many such patients and may eliminate the need for oral corticosteroids or permit a substantial reduction in their dosage.

Inhaled corticosteroids are now considered first-line maintenance therapy for the majority of patients

Table 9–5. Selected drugs for obstructive airway diseases.[1]

Drug	Important Formulations	Usual Adult Dosage (Stable Patient)	Comments
BRONCHODILATORS **Sympathomimetics** Albuterol (Proventil, Ventolin)[2]	Metered-dose inhaler (90 μg/puff; 200 puffs/inhaler)	1–4 puffs every 4–6 hours[3]	Preferred formulation in most cases. Clinically similar to metaproterenol but slightly longer duration of action.
	Nebulized solution (0.5%)	0.5 mL plus 2.5 mL normal saline every 4–6 hours[3]	Administer with powered nebulizer or, rarely, by IPPB.
	Tablets (2 mg, 4 mg)	2–4 mg orally every 6–8 hours	An extended-release 4 mg tablet is available for use every 12 hours (Proventil).
Metaproterenol (Alupent, Metaprel)	Metered-dose inhaler (0.65 mg/puff; 200 puffs/inhaler)	1–4 puffs every 3–4 hours (or more frequently)[3]	Preferred formulation in most cases.
	Nebulized solution (5%)	0.3 mL plus 2.5 mL normal saline every 3–4 hours[3]	Administer with powered nebulizer or, rarely, by IPPB. Also available as single-dose vial.
	Syrup (10 mg/5 mL)	2 tsp orally every 6–8 hours	
	Tablets (10 mg, 20 mg)	20 mg orally every 6–8 hours	
Bitolterol (Tornalate)[2]	Metered-dose inhaler (0.37 mg/puff; 300 puffs/inhaler)	2–3 puffs every 6–8 hours[3]	Longest duration of action.
Pirbuterol (Maxair)[2]	Metered-dose inhaler (200 μg/puff; 300 puffs/inhaler)	2 puffs every 4–6 hours[3]	
Terbutaline[2] (Brethaire, Brethine, Bricanyl)	Metered-dose inhaler (0.2 mg/puff; 300 puffs/inhaler) (Brethaire)	2–3 puffs every 4–6 hours[3]	
	Tablets (2.5 mg, 5 mg) (Brethine, Bricanyl)	2.5–5 mg orally 3 times daily	Tremor, nervousness, palpitations common. Oral formulation therefore not recommended.
	Subcutaneous injection (1 mg/mL) (Brethine, Bricanyl)	0.25 mg subcutaneously; may be repeated once in 30 minutes	Slow onset of action (30 minutes). Not limited to β2-adrenergic stimulation.
Isoetharine (Bronkometer, Bronkosol)	Metered-dose inhaler (340 μg/puff; 200 puffs/10 mL inhaler) (Bronkometer)	1–4 puffs every 3–4 hours[3]	
	Nebulized solution (1%) (Bronkosol)	0.5 mL of 1% solution plus 1.5 mL normal saline every 2–4 hours	Administer with powered nebulizer or, rarely, by IPPB.
Isoproterenol (Isuprel, others)	Metered-dose inhaler (131 μg/puff; 200 puffs/10 mL)	1–3 puffs every 2–4 hours	
	Nebulized solution (0.5%; 1% also available)	0.5 mL of 0.5% solution plus 1.5 mL normal saline every 2–4 hours	Administer with powered nebulizer or, rarely, by IPPB.
Epinephrine (many brands)	Metered-dose inhaler (0.2 mg/puff)	1 or 2 puffs every 2–4 hours	Available without prescription. β1 and α stimulation limit usefulness.
	Subcutaneous injection (0.1%; 1:1000)	0.3–0.5 mL subcutaneously; may be repeated once in 30 minutes	Use with caution in older patients or those with tachycardia, hypertension, or arrhythmia. No more effective than inhaled β2 agonist.
Anticholinergics Ipratropium bromide (Atrovent)	Metered-dose inhaler (18 μg/puff; 200 puffs/inhaler)	2–4 puffs every 6 hours	More potent than sympathomimetics in COPD. Minimal side effects.

(*continued*)

Table 9–5. Selected drugs for obstructive airway diseases.[1] (continued)

Drug	Important Formulations	Usual Adult Dosage (Stable Patient)	Comments
Anticholinergics (cont'd) Atropine sulfate	Nebulized solution (1 mg/mL)	0.025 mg/kg by inhalation every 6 hours; volume diluted to 2.5 mL with normal saline	Administer with powered nebulizer. Side effects common. Contraindicated in narrow-angle glaucoma or prostatic hypertrophy. Outpatient use is now practically obsolete because of availability of ipratropium bromide.
Theophyllines Theophylline, oral (many brands)	Sustained-release tablets and bead-filled capsules	200 mg orally every 12 hours initially; thereafter, 200–600 mg orally every 8–12 hours	Maintenance dose is guided by serum theophylline level. Therapeutic level is 10–20 µg/mL. Absorption varies with brand. Formulations are also available for administration every 24 hours.
Aminophylline	Intravenous	Loading dose is 5.6 mg/kg over 30 minutes for a person not using oral theophylline; maintenance dose is 0.7 mg/kg/h by constant infusion pump—lower if patient has liver disease or heart failure or is receiving erythromycin or cimetidine.	Seldom indicated. Calculate dose from lean body mass. Monitor serum theophylline level.
CORTICOSTEROIDS Beclomethasone dipropionate (Beclovent, Vanceril)	Metered-dose inhaler (42 µg/puff; 200 puffs/inhaler)	2–4 puffs every 6–12 hours	Rinse mouth with water after use to prevent oral candidiasis; use 30 seconds after inhaled sympathomimetic to control cough and airway irritation. Spacer devices also helpful to prevent oral candidiasis.
Triamcinolone acetonide (Azmacort)	Metered-dose inhaler with spacer (100 µg/puff; 240 puffs/inhaler)	2–4 puffs every 6–8 hours	Cough and wheezing after inhalation are reported to be less than after inhalation of beclomethasone.
Flunisolide (AeroBid)	Metered-dose inhaler (250 µg/puff; 100 puffs/inhaler)	2–4 puffs every 12 hours	Dosing frequency of twice daily offers an advantage.
Prednisone (several brands)	Tablets (2.5, 5, 10, 20, and 50 mg)	Acute bronchospasm: 40–60 mg (1 mg/kg) every 24 hours Chronic bronchospasm: 5–40 mg daily to every other day	
Methylprednisolone sodium succinate (several brands)	Intravenous injection (vials of 40, 125, 500, 1000, and 2000 mg)	0.5–1 mg/kg every 6 hours	Clinical response may be delayed for several hours.
Hydrocortisone sodium succinate (several brands)	Intravenous injection (100, 250, 500, and 1000 mg)	4 mg/kg every 6 hours	Clinical response may be delayed for several hours.
ANTIMEDIATORS Cromolyn sodium (Intal)	Metered-dose inhaler (800 µg/puff; 200 puffs/14.2 g canister) Nebulized solution (20 mg/3 mL ampule)	2 puffs 4 times daily 20 mg 4 times daily by powered nebulizer	Clinical response may require 2–4 weeks of treatment. Useful only for prophylaxis; younger patients with asthma are more likely to benefit. To prevent bronchospasm, cromolyn may be used 15–30 minutes before exercise or exposure to cold air or allergens.

[1]Only drugs available in the United States are listed.
[2]Preferential effect is on β_2-adrenergic receptors.
[3]More frequent dosing for acute or severe episodes of bronchoconstriction is acceptable.

with asthma. They are best started when patients are stable or adequately controlled with other antiasthma medications. Choices include beclomethasone, beginning with two inhalations (84 μg) two to four times daily and progressing, if necessary, to six inhalations four times daily; flunisolide, beginning with two inhalations (500 μg) every 12 hours and progressing to four inhalations every 12 hours; or triamcinolone, beginning with two inhalations (200 μg) four times daily and progressing to four inhalations four times daily. Corticosteroid aerosols may irritate the airway and stimulate transient cough and wheezing. Triamcinolone preparations may be better tolerated than beclomethasone preparations in this regard. Use of spacer devices for inhalation and mouth rinsing after dosing help prevent oral candidiasis. If inhalation provokes cough and wheezing, prescribe these drugs 20 minutes after inhalation of a sympathomimetic agent. Too rapid transfer from chronic systemic to inhaled corticosteroids may precipitate adrenal insufficiency.

c. Cromolyn sodium–Inhaled cromolyn sodium is an important, albeit expensive, maintenance drug for children and adults with chronic allergen- or exercise-induced asthma. Cromolyn is particularly useful in preventing exercise- or allergen-induced asthma but is ineffective in acute exacerbations of asthma. Cromolyn is sometimes effective in reducing the amount of corticosteroids needed by patients with severe asthma. The precise mechanism of action of cromolyn sodium is unknown. It probably stabilizes mast cell membranes, preventing mediator release, and inhibits reflux of calcium ions into mast cells, blocking bronchoconstriction. Cromolyn displays no anti-inflammatory or intrinsic bronchodilator activity. Patients should be advised that cromolyn may require several weeks until improvement occurs and that it is not a bronchodilator. Unlike sympathomimetics, cromolyn inhibits late asthmatic responses. Aerosol (two puffs, 1 mg each) and nebulizer solution (20 mg/2 mL) formulations are most convenient and should be used four times daily or 10–15 minutes before exercise. Toxicity is minimal. The powder formulation is now rarely used because of its inconvenience and tendency to promote cough and airway irritation.

d. Anticholinergics–Ipratropium bromide antagonizes acetylcholine and prevents increases in intracellular levels of cyclic guanosine monophosphate, a substance that promotes contraction of bronchial smooth muscle. Ipratropium may benefit selected ambulatory patients with asthma, such as older patients, those with nonallergic asthma, and those whose symptoms are poorly controlled by sympathomimetics alone. This drug is less effective than sympathomimetics in counteracting bronchospasm from specific stimuli. The dose of ipratropium is two to four inhalations by metered-dose inhaler every 6 hours. Systemic toxicity is minimal.

e. Oral theophylline–Oral theophyllines, once the cornerstone of maintenance therapy for asthma, are now considered third- or fourth-line agents for this purpose in both children and adults. In fact, some consider these drugs to be obsolete because of the shift to treatment with inhaled corticosteroids, sympathomimetics, and cromolyn. These authorities would limit their use to patients dependent on oral corticosteroids for a possible "steroid-sparing" effect. The mechanism of action of theophylline in producing bronchodilation is unknown. Airway smooth muscle cell adenosine receptor antagonism is the most popular of several proposed mechanisms. Phosphodiesterase inhibition is minimal at therapeutic dosage ranges. Long-acting oral theophylline preparations allow infrequent dosing. The usual starting dose for adults is 400–1000 mg/d in two divided doses. Serum theophylline levels should be measured 3–5 days after therapy is started and 4–5 hours after administration of a sustained-release formulation. Therapeutic levels of theophylline are 5–20 μg/mL; higher concentrations are associated with gastrointestinal, cardiac, and central nervous system side effects. Therapeutic benefits may be seen with levels between 5 and 10 μg/mL. Short-acting theophylline derivatives such as aminophylline and oxtriphylline require dosing every 6 hours and are rarely (if ever) indicated. Drug interactions with theophylline are common. Decreases in theophylline clearance accompany the use of cimetidine, erythromycin and other macrolide antibiotics, quinolone antibiotics, and oral contraceptives. Increases in theophylline clearance are caused by rifampin, phenytoin, and barbiturates.

f. Antimicrobial drugs–The routine use of antibiotic therapy for acute or chronic asthma is not warranted. In a few cases, bacterial tracheobronchitis may occur simultaneously with an attack of asthma or may follow an attack, indicating the need for sputum Gram stain and treatment with the appropriate antibiotic. Empirical antibiotic therapy, which saves the additional cost of sputum Gram stain, is a reasonable alternative approach. Amoxicillin (500 mg orally every 8 hours for 7–10 days), tetracycline (250–500 mg four times daily by mouth for 7–10 days), and trimethoprim-sulfamethoxazole (160/800 mg orally every 12 hours for 7–10 days) are reasonable alternative choices for empirical therapy.

g. Hyposensitization–Desensitization therapy is indicated for selected patients with asthma who fail to respond to environmental control measures and other forms of conventional therapy and who have documented specific reactivity to allergens that have consistently induced asthma attacks. Overall, only a few adult patients with bronchial asthma are likely to benefit from hyposensitization.

h. Immunosuppressive therapy–In corticosteroid-dependent adult patients with severe, chronic asthma, weekly intramuscular methotrexate (15 mg) has been tried as steroid-sparing adjunctive treatment. Contradictory reports on the efficacy of methotrexate therapy have emerged, and a large, well-designed, multicenter study has not been performed. The role of methotrexate in asthma management therefore remains unsettled.

i. Avoiding drugs that worsen symptoms– Beta-blocking drugs may worsen bronchospasm and should be avoided in patients with asthma. Even ophthalmic beta-blocker preparations can cause severe bronchospasm. Angiotensin converting enzyme inhibitors may aggravate cough in patients with bronchial hyperresponsiveness.

B. Patients With Acute, Severe Asthma: Patients with acute, severe asthma are often exhausted, irritable, and apprehensive. Dehydration and toxic effects resulting from overuse of medications are common. Objective measurement of airflow is important in patients with acute asthma because the intensity of wheezing on auscultation is an unreliable indicator of the extent of airflow limitation; however, in severe cases, patients may be unable to cooperate. The PEFR, the preferred index of airflow in an emergency setting, is measured initially to provide a baseline and at successive intervals during treatment. A PEFR under 100 L/min indicates very severe airway obstruction.

All patients with acute, severe asthma should receive supplemental oxygen, 1–3 L/min by nasal cannula. Monitoring with oximetry is desirable. An inhaled sympathomimetic drug such as metaproterenol (0.3 mL of 5% solution) or albuterol (0.5 mL of 0.5% solution) may be tried, diluted in 2.5 mL sterile normal saline, using a powered nebulizer. A metered-dose inhaler is satisfactory if the patient is able to inspire deeply. If the patient fails to respond within 30 minutes, the dose may be repeated. Inhaled sympathomimetic therapy is superior to intravenous aminophylline, which is now seldom used, in improving airflow. Subcutaneous epinephrine (0.3 mL of 1:1000 dilution) or terbutaline (0.25 mg) is an alternative form of sympathomimetic therapy, indicated only in young or middle-aged patients unable to use aerosolized drugs.

Corticosteroids are administered intravenously if the patient has very severe acute asthma or fails to respond to sympathomimetic therapy. Hydrocortisone (4 mg/kg) or methylprednisolone (1–2 mg/kg) is given initially and every 6 hours thereafter. A lag period of 4–6 hours before improvement occurs is common. Larger doses have no proved benefit. Although early emergency room treatment with intravenous corticosteroids has not demonstrated benefit in all asthma outcome studies, most physicians readily administer intravenous steroids to emergency room patients with acute, severe asthma. It is not yet clear whether oral therapy is an acceptable alternative to intravenous therapy. Inhaled corticosteroids have no proved role in acute, severe asthma and may worsen bronchospasm. Inhaled cromolyn is also not useful in severe acute asthma. The role of inhalation of ipratropium bromide aerosol in acute severe asthma is controversial. Further studies are needed before it can be concluded that this drug should be routinely added to sympathomimetic therapy.

Patients with severe, acute asthma who fail to respond to sympathomimetic and corticosteroid therapy are sometimes given intravenous aminophylline, though data supporting the efficacy of this approach are lacking. Simultaneous administration of intravenous aminophylline and sympathomimetic may increase toxicity. If aminophylline is used at all, treatment must be guided by serum theophylline levels.

The patient should be admitted to the hospital if any of the following are noted: failure to respond to the above regimen, a persistently low PEFR (< 30–40% of predicted value or < 200 L/min), respiratory acidosis, electrocardiographic abnormalities (supraventricular arrhythmias, including multifocal atrial tachycardia, conduction disturbances, ventricular ectopy), pneumothorax or pneumomediastinum, respiratory fatigue, suspected airway infection, and a history of status asthmaticus or previous intubation for acute respiratory failure.

Status asthmaticus is severe, prolonged asthma refractory to conventional modes of therapy. Management is similar to that for acute, severe asthma; it consists of controlled-flow oxygen therapy, intravenous corticosteroids, inhaled sympathomimetics, and antibiotics for presumed or proved airway infection. Intravenous aminophylline has no proved value when added to this regimen. Intravenous fluids are given as needed to maintain a state of normal hydration; overhydration has no benefit and may be deleterious. Treatment in an intensive care unit with careful monitoring of arterial blood gases and continuous oximetry is necessary. The role of ipratropium bromide has not been established.

Most patients with status asthmaticus improve with this regimen; however, some develop progressive respiratory acidemia and require tracheal intubation and mechanical ventilation. The decision to intubate is a complex one and is better based on the general appearance of the patient (fatigue, respiratory distress, apprehension) than on any single laboratory finding. Status asthmaticus not controlled after intubation and mechanical ventilation requires highly aggressive therapy, eg, sedation with a benzodiazepine, general anesthesia with a bronchodilating anesthetic agent, such as halothane, or segmental bronchial lavage to remove plugs of mucus. Fortunately, these extreme measures are rarely necessary.

Prognosis

The outlook for patients with bronchial asthma is excellent despite the small recent increase in the death rate. Attention to general health measures and use of pharmacologic agents permit control of symptoms in nearly all cases. The outlook is better for patients with extrinsic asthma who develop asthma early in life. Pneumococcal and yearly influenzal immunization should be part of every patient's regimen. A rigorous medical regimen may reduce hospitalization rates for patients with frequent exacerbations of asthma. Recently, the mortality rate from asthma has been increasing in the United States.

Drugs for ambulatory asthma. Med Lett Drugs Ther 1993;35:11.

McFadden ER Jr, Gilbert IA: Asthma. (Current Concepts.) N Engl J Med 1992;327:1928. (Pathogenesis and management.)

National Asthma Education Program, National Heart, Lung, and Blood Institute: Executive summary: Guidelines for the diagnosis and management of asthma. National Institutes of Health, Publication No. 91–3042A, June, 1991.

Spitzer WO et al: The use of β-agonists and the risk of death and near death from asthma. N Engl J Med 1992; 326:501. (Suggests that excessive use of inhalers should prompt reevaluation.)

CHRONIC OBSTRUCTIVE PULMONARY DISEASE (COPD)

Essentials of Diagnosis

- History of cigarette smoking (most cases).
- Chronic cough and sputum production (in chronic bronchitis) and dyspnea (in emphysema).
- Rhonchi, decreased intensity of breath sounds, and prolonged expiration on physical examination.
- Airflow limitation on pulmonary function testing.

General Considerations

The term chronic obstructive pulmonary disease (COPD) identifies patients with emphysema or chronic bronchitis. Although emphysema and chronic bronchitis must be diagnosed and treated as specific diseases, most patients with COPD have features of both conditions. About 10 million Americans are affected. As a group, the chronic obstructive lung diseases, including COPD and asthma, represent the fifth leading cause of death in the United States. The death rate from COPD is increasing, especially among elderly men.

Chronic bronchitis is characterized by excessive secretion of bronchial mucus and is manifested by productive cough for 3 months or more in at least 2 consecutive years in the absence of any other disease that might account for this symptom. **Emphysema** denotes abnormal, permanent enlargement of air spaces distal to the terminal bronchiole, with destruction of their walls and without obvious fibrosis (American Thoracic Society). Cigarette smoking is clearly the most important cause of COPD, even though only 10–15% of smokers develop COPD. Air pollution, airway infection, familial factors, and allergy have also been implicated in chronic bronchitis,

and hereditary factors (deficiency of α_1-antiprotease) have been implicated in emphysema. The pathogenesis of emphysema may be excessive lysis of elastin and other structural proteins in the lung matrix by elastase and other proteases derived from lung neutrophils, macrophages, and mononuclear cells. Atopy and the tendency for bronchoconstriction to develop in response to nonspecific airway stimuli may be important risks for COPD.

Clinical Findings

A. Symptoms and Signs: The clinical, roentgenographic, and laboratory findings in chronic bronchitis and emphysema are summarized in Table 9–6.

Patients with COPD characteristically present in the fifth or sixth decade of life complaining of excessive cough, sputum production, and shortness of breath that have often been present for 10 years or more. Productive cough usually occurs in the morning. Dyspnea is noted initially only on extreme exertion, but as the condition progresses, it becomes more severe and occurs with mild activity. In severe disease, dyspnea occurs at rest. Frequent exacerbations of illness are common and result in absence from work and eventual disability. Pneumonia, pulmonary hypertension, cor pulmonale, and chronic respiratory failure characterize the late stage of COPD. Death usually occurs during an exacerbation of illness in association with acute respiratory failure. Hemoptysis occurs occasionally, often following the use of aspirin, presumably because of its antiplatelet action.

Clinical findings may be completely absent early in the course of COPD. Diminished breath sounds and prolonged expiration may be detectable during exacerbations of the disease. The physical findings presented in Table 9–6 become apparent as the disease progresses.

B. Laboratory Findings: Secondary polycythemia may be found in advanced COPD as a result of hypoxemia. During exacerbations of illness, examination of the sputum may reveal *Streptococcus pneumoniae* or *Haemophilus influenzae,* though these may be present in the carrier state between episodes of deterioration. The ECG may show sinus tachycardia, and in advanced disease, chronic pulmonary hypertension may produce electrocardiographic abnormalities typical of cor pulmonale. Supraventricular arrhythmias (multifocal atrial tachycardia, atrial flutter, and atrial fibrillation) and ventricular irritability also occur.

Arterial blood gas measurements characteristically show no abnormalities early in COPD; indeed, they are unnecessary unless hypoxia or hypercapnia is suspected. Hypoxemia occurs in advanced disease, particularly when chronic bronchitis predominates. Compensated respiratory acidosis occurs in patients with chronic respiratory failure, particularly in chronic bronchitis, with worsening of acidemia during acute exacerbations. (See Chapter 18.)

Table 9–6. Emphysema versus chronic bronchitis: Clinical, roentgenographic, and laboratory findings.[1]

	Emphysema	Chronic Bronchitis
History		
Onset of symptoms	After age 50.	After age 35.
Dyspnea	Progressive, constant, severe.	Intermittent, mild to moderate.
Cough	Absent or mild.	Persistent, severe.
Sputum production	Absent or mild.	Copious.
Sputum appearance	Clear, mucoid.	Mucopurulent or purulent.
Other features	Weight loss.[2]	Airway infections, right heart failure, obesity.
Physical examination		
Body habitus	Thin, wasted.[2]	Stocky, obese.
Central cyanosis	Absent.	Present.[2]
Plethora	Absent.	Present.
Accessory respiratory muscles	Hypertrophied.	Unremarkable.
Anteroposterior chest diameter	Increased.	Normal.
Percussion note	Hyperresonant.	Normal.
Auscultation	Diminished breath sounds.	Wheezes, rhonchi.
Chest x-ray		
Bullae, blebs	Present.	Absent.
Overall appearance	Decreased markings in periphery.	Increased markings ("dirty lungs").
Hyperinflation	Present.	Absent.
Heart size	Normal or small, vertical.	Large, horizontal.
Hemidiaphragms	Low, flat.	Normal, rounded.
Laboratory studies		
Hematocrit	Normal.	Increased.
ECG	Normal.	Right axis deviation, right ventricular hypertrophy, "p" pulmonale.[2]
Hypoxemia	Absent, mild.	Moderate, severe.
Hypercapnia	Absent.	Moderate, severe.
Respiratory acidosis	Absent.	Present.
Total lung capacity	Increased.	Normal.
Static lung compliance	Increased.	Normal.
Diffusing capacity	Decreased.	Normal.

[1]As noted in the text, most patients with COPD have features of both emphysema and chronic bronchitis.
[2]In advanced disease.

Spirometry provides objective information about pulmonary function and assesses the results of therapy. Pulmonary function tests early in the course of COPD reveal only evidence of dysfunction in small airways (abnormal closing volume, reduced midexpiratory flow rate). Reduction in forced expiratory volume in 1 second (FEV_1) and in the ratio of forced expiratory volume to forced vital capacity (FEV_1:FVC) occurs later. In severe disease, the forced vital capacity is markedly reduced. Lung volume measurements reveal an increase in the total lung capacity (TLC), a marked increase in the residual volume (RV), and an elevation of the RV:TLC ratio, indicative of air trapping, particularly in emphysema.

C. Imaging: When emphysema is the main clinical feature, hyperinflation is apparent. Parenchymal bullae or subpleural blebs are pathognomonic of emphysema. Radiographs of patients with chronic bronchitis may show only nonspecific peribronchial and perivascular markings. Pulmonary hypertension becomes evident as enlargement of pulmonary arteries in advanced disease. Doppler echocardiography is an effective way to estimate pulmonary artery pressure if pulmonary hypertension is suspected. Thoracic CT scanning may detect emphysema not apparent on the chest x-ray, but it is very costly and therefore rarely indicated for this purpose.

Differential Diagnosis

Clinical, roentgenographic, and laboratory findings usually enable the clinician to distinguish COPD from other obstructive pulmonary disorders such as bronchial asthma, bronchiectasis, cystic fibrosis, bronchopulmonary aspergillosis, and central airway obstruction. Bronchiectasis is distinguished from COPD by features such as recurrent pneumonia and hemoptysis, digital clubbing, and radiographic abnormalities. Patients with severe α_1-antiprotease deficiency are recognized by the appearance of panacinar emphysema early in life, usually in the third or fourth decade. Hepatic cirrhosis and hepatoma may occur. Cystic fibrosis occurs in children and younger adults. Rarely, mechanical obstruction of the central airways simulates COPD. Flow-volume curves may help separate patients with central airway obstruction from those with diffuse intrathoracic airway obstruction characteristic of COPD.

Complications

Acute bronchitis, pneumonia, pulmonary embolization, and concomitant left ventricular failure may worsen otherwise stable COPD. Pulmonary hypertension, cor pulmonale, and chronic respiratory failure are common in advanced COPD. Spontaneous pneumothorax occurs in a small fraction of patients with emphysema. Hemoptysis may result from chronic bronchitis or may signal bronchogenic carcinoma.

Prevention

COPD is largely preventable. Many believe that early recognition of small airways dysfunction in patients who smoke, combined with appropriate treatment and cessation of smoking, may prevent relentless progression of the disease. Early treatment of airway infections and vaccination against influenza and pneumococcal disease may also be of benefit but have no effect on the progression of the disease.

Treatment

Management of COPD includes discontinuance of cigarette smoking, education of the patient about his or her disease, relief of bronchospasm, aerosol therapy, chest physiotherapy, treatment of complications such as airway infections and heart failure, use of supplemental oxygen, and other measures designed to promote rehabilitation. See Chapter 38 for a discussion of air travel in patients with lung disease.

A. Ambulatory Patients: The general health maintenance measures for patients with bronchial asthma are also important for patients with COPD. Goals in the treatment of COPD include control of symptoms, improvement in ability to carry out daily activities, reduction in the need for hospitalization, and rehabilitation. Controlling the frequency and severity of respiratory infections and acute exacerbations of COPD is also important.

A trial of bronchodilator drugs is warranted in all patients with symptomatic COPD. Inhaled ipratropium bromide or sympathomimetic drugs are the mainstay of this therapy. The response to bronchodilator therapy is assessed with spirometry. Patients with asthmatic bronchitis and those with partially reversible airflow obstruction, frequent acute exacerbations of disease, or wheezing may benefit the most from bronchodilator therapy. The routine use of maintenance bronchodilator drugs in all patients with COPD is controversial. These drugs probably have little value in patients with pure emphysema. If a clinical trial of bronchodilators over several months demonstrates no objective (spirometric) or symptomatic improvement, they may be discontinued; however, this is not often the case.

Ipratropium bromide is superior to sympathomimetic aerosols in achieving bronchodilation in patients with moderate to severe COPD. Ipratropium has a slower onset but a longer duration of action than sympathomimetic agents in stable COPD. In combination with other bronchodilators, it enhances and prolongs bronchodilation. Side effects are minimal, and effects on sputum production and viscosity are negligible. Two to four inhalations (18 μg each) every 6 hours is recommended.

Maintenance therapy with oral theophylline in ambulatory patients with COPD is controversial. Although theophylline has value as a bronchodilator in COPD patients with partial reversibility of airflow limitation, its principal value in COPD may relate to improving respiratory muscle performance. Improvements in dyspnea, exercise performance, and pulmonary function have been reported in some studies but not in others. A recent report noted improved oxygenation during non-REM sleep when oral theophylline was added to a beta-agonist in treating patients with moderate to severe COPD. Many pulmonary specialists now regard oral theophylline as a third-line agent in COPD—behind ipratropium and sympathomimetic agents—reserving its use for those patients who fail to respond to or cannot use inhaled bronchodilators or those with sleep-related respiratory disturbances. Theophylline use is the same as described for asthma (see above). Once-daily theophylline dosing, preferably at 8 PM, is advocated by some authorities.

Oral corticosteroids are prescribed in the same fashion as in asthma. Candidates for a trial of oral corticosteroid therapy include patients with asthmatic bronchitis and those with frequent exacerbations or disabling symptoms who fail to respond to conventional therapy with ipratropium bromide, sympathomimetics and theophylline; eosinophils in peripheral blood or sputum may also predict a response. Corticosteroids should be discontinued after 2–4 weeks if there is no objective (spirometric) improvement. Inhaled corticosteroids may be of value for corticosteroid-responsive patients, particularly those requiring less than 20 mg of prednisone (or equivalent) daily. Inhaled corticosteroids may permit discontinuance of systemic therapy. Cromolyn has no role in treatment of chronic bronchitis or emphysema; a trial in those with chronic asthmatic bronchitis may be warranted.

Bronchial hygiene decreases production of bronchopulmonary secretions and enhances their mobilization and clearance. Smoking cessation, avoiding airway irritants and allergens, controlling airway infection with broad-spectrum oral antimicrobials and preventing pulmonary aspiration may reduce the production of mucus. If airway infection is suspected, amoxicillin (500 mg every 8 hours), ampicillin or tetracycline (250–500 mg four times daily), or trimethoprim-sulfamethoxazole (160/800 mg every 12 hours) may be given orally for 7–10 days. Although routine antibiotic therapy for exacerbations of COPD is controversial, one recent study shows that COPD patients with increasing dyspnea and purulent sputum are particularly likely to benefit from antibiotics. Nicotine chewing gum (2 mg pieces chewed slowly over 30 minutes) and nicotine patches are effective aids to smoking cessation for patients highly motivated to stop smoking.

Increased mobilization of secretions may be accomplished through the use of adequate systemic hydration, effective cough training methods, and postural drainage, sometimes with chest percussion or vibration. One effective method of coughing up retained secretions is to have the patient lean forward and "huff" repeatedly, interspersed with relaxed breaths. Forceful paroxysms of cough should be discouraged. Inhalation of bland water aerosols is sometimes helpful. Postural drainage and chest percussion should be used only in selected patients with excessive amounts of retained secretions that cannot be cleared by coughing and other methods; these measures are of no benefit in pure emphysema. Expectorant-mucolytic therapy has generally been regarded as unhelpful in patients with chronic bronchitis, though a recent multicenter study suggested possible symptomatic benefit from iodinated glycerol (60 mg orally four times daily). Cough suppressants and sedatives should be avoided as routine measures.

Graded aerobic physical exercise programs (eg, walking 20 minutes three times weekly, or bicycling) are helpful to prevent deterioration of physical condition and to improve the patient's ability to carry out daily activities. Pursed-lip breathing to slow the rate of breathing and abdominal breathing exercises to relieve fatigue of accessory muscles of respiration may reduce dyspnea in some patients. Training of inspiratory muscles by inspiring against progressively larger resistive loads improves exercise tolerance in some but not all patients.

Severe dyspnea in spite of optimal medical management may respond to a trial of an opiate drug (eg, hydrocodone, 5 mg orally four times daily). Constipation is a common side effect. Sedative-hypnotic drugs (eg, diazepam, 5 mg three times daily) are controversial in intractable dyspnea but may benefit very anxious patients. Intermittent negative-pressure (cuirass) ventilation and transnasal positive-pressure ventilation at home to rest the respiratory muscles are promising new approaches to improve respiratory muscle function and reduce dyspnea in patients with severe COPD. The routine use of intermittent positive-pressure breathing (IPPB) for stable ambulatory COPD patients has been proved to confer no benefits and is very expensive.

Home oxygen therapy is prescribed for selected patients with COPD or other severe lung diseases who have significant hypoxemia. Requirements for Medicare coverage for a patient's home use of oxygen and oxygen equipment are listed in Table 9–7. Arterial blood gas analysis is preferable to ear or pulse oximetry to guide initial oxygen therapy. Oxygen may be prescribed for continuous use, only at night, or with exercise. Cardiovascular disorders such as angina pectoris, peripheral vascular disease, and terminal illnesses without hypoxemia are not indications for this expensive therapy. Hypoxemic patients with pulmonary hypertension, chronic cor pulmonale, erythrocytosis, impaired cognitive function, exercise intolerance, nocturnal restlessness, or morning headache are particularly likely to benefit from home oxygen therapy. Proved benefits of home oxygen

Table 9–7. Home oxygen therapy: Requirements for Medicare coverage.[1]

Group I (any of the following):

1. $PaO_2 \le 55$ mm Hg, or $SaO_2 \le 88\%$, taken at rest, breathing room air, while awake.

2. During sleep (prescription for nocturnal oxygen use only):

   a. $PaO_2 \le 55$ mm Hg, or $SaO_2 \le 88\%$, for a patient whose awake, resting, room air PaO_2 is $\ge 89\%$,

   or

   b. Decrease in $PaO_2 > 10$ mm Hg or decrease in $SaO_2 > 5\%$ associated with symptoms or signs reasonably attributed to hypoxemia (eg, impaired cognitive processes, nocturnal restlessness, insomnia).

3. During exercise (prescription for oxygen use only during exercise):

   a. $PaO_2 \le 55$ mm Hg, or $SaO_2 \le 88\%$ taken during exercise for a patient whose awake, resting, room air PaO_2 is ≥ 56 mm Hg or $SaO_2 \ge 89\%$.

   and

   b. There is evidence that the use of supplemental oxygen during exercise improves the hypoxemia that was demonstrated during exercise while breathing room air.

Group II:[2]

$PaO_2 = 56–59$ mm Hg or $SaO_2 = 89\%$ if there is evidence of any of the following:

1. Dependent edema suggesting congestive heart failure.

2. P pulmonale on ECG (P wave > 3 mm in standard leads II, III, or AVF).

3. Hematocrit > 56%.

[1]Health Care Financing Administration, 1989.
[2]Patients in this group must have a second oxygen test 3 months after the initial oxygen set-up.

therapy in advanced COPD include longer survival, reduced hospitalization needs, and better quality of life. Survival in hypoxemic patients with COPD treated with supplemental oxygen therapy is directly proportionate to the number of hours per day oxygen is administered. In such patients who are treated with continuous oxygen, the survival after 36 months is about 65%—significantly better than the survival rate of about 45% in those who are treated with only nocturnal oxygen.

Home oxygen may be supplied by liquid oxygen systems (LOX), compressed gas cylinders, or oxygen concentrators. Most patients benefit from having both stationary and portable systems. Oxygen by nasal prongs must be given at least 15 hours a day unless therapy is intended only for exercise or sleep. For most patients, a flow rate of 1–3 L/min achieves a PaO_2 greater than 55 mm Hg. The monthly cost of home oxygen therapy ranges from $300.00 to $500.00 or more, being higher for liquid oxygen systems. Medicare covers approximately 80% of home oxygen expenses. **Transtracheal oxygen** is an alternative method of delivery. Reservoir nasal cannulas or "pendants" and demand (pulse) oxygen delivery systems are also available to conserve oxygen.

Human α_1-proteinase inhibitor is available for replacement therapy of emphysema due to congenital deficiency of $\alpha_1$antiproteinase. The efficacy of this new agent is unknown, and it is very expensive.

Lung transplantation for end-stage COPD is currently being evaluated in several centers. Experience with both single and bilateral sequential lung transplantation for severe COPD is growing rapidly. Requirements for lung transplantation are severe lung disease, limited activities of daily living, exhaustion of medical therapy, ambulatory status, potential for pulmonary rehabilitation, limited life expectancy without transplantation, adequate function of other organ systems, and a good social support system. Average total charges for lung transplantation through the end of the first postoperative year approximate $300,000. Substantial improvements in pulmonary function and exercise performance have been noted after transplantation. The two-year survival rate after lung transplantation for COPD is 75%.

B. Hospitalized Patients: Hospitalization is indicated for acute worsening of COPD that fails to respond to measures for ambulatory patients. Patients with acute respiratory failure or complications such as cor pulmonale and pneumothorax should also be hospitalized.

Management of the hospitalized patient with an **acute exacerbation of COPD** uses a comprehensive approach similar to that for patients hospitalized with asthma. Therapeutic options include supplemental oxygen, ipratropium bromide, inhaled sympathomimetics, and intravenous aminophylline, as well as broad-spectrum antibiotics, corticosteroids, and, in selected cases, chest physiotherapy. Intravenous aminophylline has not been found to add significant benefit to inhaled bronchodilator therapy in patients with acute exacerbation of COPD. Its role remains controversial. Oxygen therapy should not be withheld for fear of worsening respiratory acidemia; hypoxemia is more detrimental than hypercapnia. Cor pulmonale usually responds to measures that reduce pulmonary artery pressure, such as supplemental oxygen and correction of acidemia; bed rest, salt restriction, and diuretics may add some benefit. Cardiac arrhythmias usually respond to aggressive treatment of COPD itself. Verapamil (240–480 mg/d in divided doses every 8 hours, or 0.075–0.15 mg/kg given intravenously at a rate of 1–2 mg/min) is sometimes effective in multifocal atrial tachycardia. If progressive respiratory failure ensues, tracheal intubation and mechanical ventilation are necessary. Inspiratory positive-pressure assistance with a face mask has recently been reported as a noninvasive alternative to conventional mechanical ventilation.

Prognosis

The outlook for patients with clinically significant COPD is poor. The median survival time of patients with severe COPD (FEV$_1$ ≤ 1 L) is about 4 years. The degree of pulmonary dysfunction (as measured by FEV$_1$) at the time the patient is first seen is probably the most important predictor of survival. Comprehensive care programs and cessation of smoking apparently reduce the rate of decline of pulmonary function, but therapy with bronchodilators and other approaches probably has little, if any, impact on the natural course of COPD. Survival time varies widely and cannot be easily predicted. The prognosis is better in the chronic asthmatic form of COPD (chronic asthmatic bronchitis) than in the emphysematous form.

American Thoracic Society: Guidelines for the approach to the patient with severe hereditary alpha-1-antitrypsin deficiency. Am Rev Respir Dis 1989;140:1494. (Practical guidelines for diagnosis and treatment.)

American Thoracic Society: Standards for the diagnosis and care of patients with chronic obstructive pulmonary disease (COPD) and asthma. Am Rev Respir Dis 1987; 136:225. (Official statement on definition and management.)

Derenne JP, Fleury B, Pariente R: Acute respiratory failure of chronic obstructive pulmonary disease. Am Rev Respir Dis 1989;138:1006. (Mechanisms, diagnosis, and therapy.)

Ferguson GT, Cherniack RM: Management of chronic obstructive pulmonary disease. N Engl J Med 1993; 328:1017.

CYSTIC FIBROSIS
(See also Chapter 22.)

Essentials of Diagnosis

- Chronic obstructive pulmonary disease in childhood and early adulthood.
- Chronic *Pseudomonas aeruginosa* or *Staphylococcus aureus* bronchitis and bronchiectasis with recurrent exacerbations.
- Positive family history of cystic fibrosis.
- Sweat chloride concentration above 80 meq/L in adults (> 60 meq/L under age 20) on two occasions.
- Idiopathic obstructive azoospermia in males.

General Considerations

Cystic fibrosis is a generalized autosomal recessive disorder of the exocrine glands. About one in 2500 Caucasians is affected, and one in 25 is a carrier of the cystic fibrosis gene (transmembrane conductance regulator). Deletion of a single phenylalanine residue from a 1480-amino-acid protein coded by the cystic fibrosis gene, resulting from a mutation of the long arm of chromosome 7 (band q31), accounts for the large majority of cases of cystic fibrosis. Almost all exocrine glands are affected by secretion of an abnormal mucus that obstructs glands and ducts in various organs. Obstruction results in dilation of the secretory glands and eventual damage to exocrine tissue. High concentrations of DNA in airway secretions render the sputum thick and viscous. Pulmonary manifestations, which occur in all patients who survive infancy, include acute and chronic bronchitis, bronchiectasis, pneumonia, atelectasis, and peribronchial and parenchymal scarring. Pneumothorax and mild hemoptysis are common. Cor pulmonale occurs in advanced cases and signifies a poor prognosis.

Cystic fibrosis is the most common fatal hereditary disorder of Caucasians in the USA and is the most common cause of chronic lung disease in children and young adults. About half of children with cystic fibrosis live beyond age 20. About one-third of the nearly 30,000 cystic fibrosis patients in the USA are adults. Clinicians should recognize that cystic fibrosis may be occult and may present with a variety of pulmonary and nonpulmonary manifestations in the adult.

Clinical Findings

A. Symptoms and Signs: The diagnosis should be suspected in a young adult presenting with a history of chronic lung disease (especially bronchiectasis), pancreatitis, or infertility. Cough, exercise intolerance, and recurrent pneumonia are typical. Steatorrhea is common. Digital clubbing, increased anteroposterior chest diameter, hyperresonance to percussion, and basilar crackles are noted on physical examination. Nasal polyps occur in as many as 15% of patients with cystic fibrosis. Biliary cirrhosis and gallstones may occur.

B. Laboratory Findings: Arterial blood gas studies reveal hypoxemia. Pulmonary function studies show reduction in forced vital capacity, airflow rates, and total lung capacity. Air trapping (high ratio of residual volume to total lung capacity) and reduction in pulmonary diffusing capacity are common. A mixed obstructive and restrictive pattern of dysfunction characterizes advanced disease.

C. Imaging: Hyperinflation is seen early in the disease process. Peribronchial cuffing, mucus plugging, bronchiectasis (ring shadows and cysts), increased interstitial markings, small rounded peripheral opacities, and focal atelectasis may be seen separately or in various combinations. Thin-section CT scanning may confirm the presence of bronchiectasis.

D. Special Examinations: The pilocarpine iontophoresis "sweat test" reveals elevated sodium and chloride levels (> 60 meq/L) in the sweat of patients with cystic fibrosis. Values higher than 80 meq/L are diagnostic. Two separate tests on consecutive days are required for accurate diagnosis.

Treatment

Early recognition and comprehensive, multidisciplinary therapy lengthen survival time and ameliorate symptoms. Referral to regional ambulatory care centers with diagnostic and therapeutic expertise in cystic fibrosis should be strongly considered. Treatment

of the psychosocial aspects is of paramount importance in young people; genetic and occupational counseling is also critical. Antibiotics are used to treat active airway infections based on results of culture and susceptibility testing of sputum. *S aureus* (including methicillin-resistant strains) and a mucoid variant of *P aeruginosa* are commonly present. *Haemophilus influenzae* and *Pseudomonas cepacia*—the latter a highly drug-resistant organism—are occasionally isolated. The use of aerosolized antibiotics (gentamicin and others) for prophylaxis or treatment of lower respiratory tract infections in patients with cystic fibrosis is sometimes helpful. Although some studies demonstrate reduced exacerbations in patients chronically infected with *P aeruginosa,* there is concern about the emergence of drug-resistant organisms, equipment contamination with *P cepacia,* and side effects such as bronchospasm.

Inhaled bland aerosols, chest physiotherapy, and inhaled bronchodilators are used to promote clearance of inspissated airway secretions. Cough suppressants should be avoided. Chronic use of mucolytic agents such as acetylcysteine is of no proved benefit and is potentially harmful. Yearly influenza vaccination is advised. Daily postural drainage and chest percussion are very helpful for patients with copious sputum production. Children with cystic fibrosis who were treated with alternate-day prednisone (2 mg/kg for 4 years) demonstrated improved height, weight, and pulmonary function and reduced hospitalization needs compared to controls in one study. The routine use of corticosteroids in adults with cystic fibrosis cannot be recommended in the absence of controlled clinical trials.

Screening of members of the family of a cystic fibrosis patient by DNA analysis may detect the cystic fibrosis gene in 70–75% of carriers. Screening raises many social and ethical issues, and population screening is not recommended.

Lung transplantation is currently the only definitive treatment for cystic fibrosis. Experience with double-lung and heart-lung transplantation is accumulating rapidly, and early results suggest a greatly improved quality of life in survivors.

Experimental approaches now under investigation include the use of aerosols of recombinant human deoxyribonuclease I to cleave DNA in airway secretions, gene therapy, and inhibitors of neutrophil elastase.

Prognosis

The longevity of patients with cystic fibrosis is increasing, and the median survival age is now 25 years. Few patients survive beyond 35 years. Death occurs from pulmonary complications, eg, pneumonia, pneumothorax, or hemoptysis, or as a result of terminal chronic respiratory failure and cor pulmonale.

Davis PB: Cystic fibrosis from bench to bedside. N Engl J Med 1991;325:575. (The potential impact of discovery of the basic genetic defect on airway inflammation and its management.)

Fick RB Jr, Stillwell PC: Controversies in the management of pulmonary disease due to cystic fibrosis. Chest 1989;95:1319. (Antibiotic therapy, corticosteroids, hospitalization, nutritional support, exercise conditioning, and other matters.)

UPPER AIRWAY OBSTRUCTION

Acute upper airway obstruction may cause life-threatening asphyxia and must be relieved promptly. Acute upper airway obstruction due to foreign body aspiration is discussed below. Other causes of acute upper airway obstruction include laryngospasm, trauma to the larynx and pharynx, laryngeal edema from airway burns, acute angioedema, and various inflammatory conditions (Ludwig's angina, peritonsillar and retropharyngeal abscess, acute epiglottitis, and acute allergic laryngitis).

Chronic obstruction of the upper airway may be caused by carcinoma of the pharynx or larynx, laryngeal or subglottic stenosis, laryngeal granulomas or webs, or bilateral vocal cord paralysis. Laryngeal or subglottic stenosis may become evident weeks or months following a period of translaryngeal endotracheal intubation. Inspiratory stridor, intercostal retractions on inspiration, and a palpable inspiratory thrill over the throat are characteristic findings. Flow-volume curves may reveal evidence of fixed airway obstruction or variable extrathoracic obstruction. Plain films (soft tissue views of the neck) may demonstrate supra- and infraglottic narrowing, and CT scanning and MRI may be useful to image lesions in the pharynx and larynx. Fiberoptic endoscopy is helpful in diagnosis of upper airway obstruction, but caution is necessary because this procedure may exacerbate upper airway edema, leading to critical airway narrowing.

Occasionally, a functional disorder of the larynx may mimic bronchial asthma. This condition, variously called "episodic laryngeal dyskinesia," "factitious asthma," and "emotional laryngeal wheezing," may be distinguished from true asthma by the finding of variable extrathoracic airway obstruction on the flow-volume loop, a normal alveolar-arterial oxygen tension gradient, laryngoscopic evidence of adduction of the vocal cords on both inspiration and expiration, and lack of response to bronchodilator therapy. Fluoroscopy may also be helpful in diagnosis. Pulmonary function testing is normal immediately after the attack resolves. Treatment consists of speech therapy and psychotherapy. Bronchodilator drugs are of no benefit.

LOWER AIRWAY OBSTRUCTION

Tracheal obstruction may be intrathoracic (below the suprasternal notch) or extrathoracic. Fixed tracheal obstruction may be caused by acquired or congenital tracheal stenosis, primary and secondary tracheal neoplasms, compression by extrinsic diseases (tumors of the lung, thymus, or thyroid; lymphadenopathy; congenital vascular rings; aneurysms, etc), foreign body aspiration, tracheal granulomas and papillomas, and tracheal trauma.

Acquired **tracheal stenosis** is usually secondary to tracheostomy or endotracheal intubation. Dyspnea, cough, and inability to clear pulmonary secretions occur weeks to months after tracheal decannulation or extubation. Physical findings may be absent until tracheal diameter is reduced 50% or more, when wheezing, a palpable tracheal thrill, and harsh breath sounds may be detected. Stridor implies severe stenosis. The diagnosis is usually confirmed by plain films, CT of the trachea when plain films are not adequate, and characteristic findings of the fixed airway obstruction on the flow-volume loop. Complications include recurring pulmonary infection and life-threatening respiratory failure. Management is directed toward ensuring adequate ventilation and oxygenation and avoiding manipulative procedures that may increase edema of the tracheal mucosa. Surgical reconstruction or laser photoresection is required in severe cases.

Bronchial obstruction is caused by retained pulmonary secretions, aspiration, primary lung cancer, compression by extrinsic masses, and (rarely) tumors metastatic to the airway. Clinical and radiographic findings vary depending on the location of the obstruction and the degree of airway narrowing. Symptoms include dyspnea, cough, wheezing, and if infection is present, fever and chills. A history of recurrent pneumonia in the same lobe or segment or slow resolution (> 3 months) of pneumonia on successive x-rays suggests the possibility of bronchial obstruction and the need for bronchoscopy. Complete obstruction of a main stem bronchus may be obvious on physical examination (asymmetric chest expansion, mediastinal shift, absence of breath sounds on the affected side, and dullness to percussion), but partial obstruction is often difficult or impossible to detect. Prolonged expiration and localized wheezing may be the only clues. Alterations of the flow-volume loop may be helpful in diagnosis. Segmental or subsegmental bronchial obstruction may produce no abnormalities on physical examination.

Roentgenographic findings range from **atelectasis** (lung collapse) to air trapping. The latter may be caused by unidirectional expiratory obstruction. Expiratory films may be particularly useful to show air trapping. CT scanning may demonstrate the nature and the exact location of obstruction of the central bronchi. MRI may be superior to CT for delineating the extent of the underlying disease in the hilum, but it is usually reserved for cases in which CT findings are equivocal. Bronchoscopy is the definitive diagnostic study, particularly if tumor or foreign body aspiration is suspected. The finding of tubular breath sounds on physical examination or an air bronchogram on chest x-ray in an area of atelectasis rules out complete airway obstruction. Bronchoscopy is unlikely to be of therapeutic benefit in this situation.

Right middle lobe syndrome is recurrent or persistent atelectasis of the right middle lobe, probably related to inadequate collateral ventilation. Fiberoptic bronchoscopy or CT scan is often necessary to rule out obstructing tumor or foreign body.

ALLERGIC BRONCHOPULMONARY ASPERGILLOSIS

Allergic bronchopulmonary aspergillosis is a pulmonary hypersensitivity disorder that is being recognized with increasing frequency in the USA. It is caused by allergy to antigens of *Aspergillus* species that colonize the tracheobronchial tree and usually occurs in atopic asthmatic individuals who are 20–40 years of age. Primary criteria for the diagnosis of allergic bronchopulmonary aspergillosis include a clinical history of asthma, peripheral eosinophilia, immediate skin reactivity to *Aspergillus* antigen, precipitating antibodies to *Aspergillus* antigen, elevated serum IgE levels, pulmonary infiltrates (transient or fixed), and central bronchiectasis. If the first six of these seven primary criteria are present, the diagnosis is almost certain. Secondary diagnostic criteria include identification of *Aspergillus* in sputum, a history of brown-flecked sputum, and late skin reactivity to *Aspergillus* antigen. Corticosteroids are the treatment of choice, and the response is usually excellent. Prednisone (0.5 mg/kg/d) is given as a single morning dose for several weeks before a transition is made to alternate-day dosing. Several months of prednisone therapy may be required. Inhaled corticosteroids and cromolyn sodium are not currently recommended. Bronchodilators (Table 9–5) are also helpful. Complications include hemoptysis, severe bronchiectasis, and pulmonary fibrosis.

BRONCHIECTASIS

Bronchiectasis is a congenital or acquired disorder of the large bronchi characterized by permanent, abnormal dilation and destruction of bronchial walls. It may be caused by recurrent inflammation or infection of the airways. Cystic fibrosis causes about half of all cases of bronchiectasis. Other causes include lung infection (tuberculosis, fungal infections, lung abscess, pneumonia), abnormal lung defense mechanisms (humoral immunodeficiency, α_1-antiprotease defi-

ciency with cigarette smoking, mucociliary clearance disorders, rheumatic diseases), and localized airway obstruction (foreign body, tumor, mucoid impaction). Immunodeficiency states that may lead to bronchiectasis include congenital or acquired panhypogammaglobulinemia; common variable immunodeficiency; selective IgA, IgM, and IgG subclass deficiencies; and acquired immunodeficiency from cytotoxic therapy, AIDS, lymphoma, multiple myeloma, leukemia, and chronic renal and hepatic diseases. However, most patients with bronchiectasis have panhypergammaglobulinemia, presumably reflecting an immune system response to chronic airway infection. Acquired primary bronchiectasis is now uncommon in the USA because of improved control of bronchopulmonary infections.

Symptoms of bronchiectasis include chronic cough, production of copious amounts of purulent sputum, hemoptysis, and recurrent pneumonia. Weight loss, anemia, and other systemic manifestations are common. Physical findings are nonspecific, but persistent crackles at the lung bases are common. Clubbing is infrequent. Copious, foul-smelling, purulent sputum that separates into three layers in a cup is characteristic. Obstructive pulmonary dysfunction with hypoxemia is seen in moderate or severe disease. Roentgenographic abnormalities include crowded bronchial markings related to peribronchial fibrosis and small cystic spaces at the base of the lungs. Thin-section (1.5 mm) CT scanning may detect moderate to severe cases. Bronchography is now performed infrequently.

Treatment consists of antibiotics (selected on the basis of sputum smears and cultures), daily chest physiotherapy with postural drainage and chest percussion, and inhaled bronchodilators. Empiric oral antibiotic therapy for 10–14 days with amoxicillin (500 mg every 8 hours), ampicillin or tetracycline (250–500 mg four times daily), or trimethoprim-sulfamethoxazole (160/800 mg every 12 hours) is reasonable therapy in an acute exacerbation if a specific bacterial pathogen cannot be isolated. Alternating cycles of two or three of these antibiotics, given orally for 2–4 weeks, is sometimes employed in stable bronchiectasis patients with copious, purulent sputum. The role of aerosolized antibiotics has not been established. Bronchoscopy is sometimes necessary to evaluate hemoptysis, remove retained secretions and rule out obstructing airway lesions. Surgical resection is reserved for a few patients with localized bronchiectasis and adequate pulmonary function who fail to respond to conservative management. Surgery is also indicated for massive hemoptysis. Complications of bronchiectasis include cor pulmonale, amyloidosis, and secondary visceral abscesses at distant sites, eg, brain.

Neeld DA et al: Computerized tomography in the evaluation of allergic bronchopulmonary aspergillosis. Am Rev

Respir Dis 1990;142:1200. (High-resolution CT scanning is emerging as the diagnostic test of choice in bronchiectasis.)

BRONCHIOLITIS OBLITERANS

Bronchiolitis is an acute, common, often severe respiratory illness of children under 2 years of age caused by respiratory syncytial virus, other viruses (occasionally), and *Mycoplasma pneumoniae.* An acute infectious bronchiolitis has not been recognized as a distinct entity in adults. However, bronchiolitis obliterans does occur. Once classified as a type of chronic interstitial pneumonia, bronchiolitis obliterans has been recently reclassified. Five clinical types have been described by Epler et al (1985): (1) toxic fume bronchiolitis obliterans, (2) postinfectious bronchiolitis obliterans, (3) bronchiolitis obliterans associated with connective tissue disease and organ transplantation, (4) bronchiolitis obliterans associated with localized lung lesions, and (5) idiopathic bronchiolitis obliterans with organizing pneumonia.

Bronchiolitis obliterans in adults is probably underrecognized. Cough, dyspnea, crackles on chest auscultation, and obstructive pulmonary dysfunction are characteristic.

Toxic fume bronchiolitis obliterans follows 1–3 weeks after exposure to oxides of nitrogen, phosgene, and other noxious gases. The chest x-ray shows diffuse nonspecific alveolar or "ground-glass" densities.

Postinfectious bronchiolitis obliterans is a late response to mycoplasmal or viral lung infection in adults and has a highly variable radiographic appearance.

Bronchiolitis obliterans may occur in association with rheumatoid arthritis, polymyositis, and dermatomyositis. Penicillamine therapy has been implicated as a possible cause of bronchiolitis obliterans in patients with rheumatoid arthritis. Bronchiolitis obliterans is a common complication of heart-lung transplantation and a rare complication of allogeneic bone marrow transplantation, the latter occurring in the setting of chronic graft-versus-host disease.

It is important to recognize **bronchiolitis obliterans with organizing pneumonia (BOOP).** This idiopathic disorder affects men and women equally. Most patients are between the ages of 50 and 70. Dry cough, dyspnea, and a flu-like illness, ranging in duration from a few days to several months, are typical. Fever and weight loss are common. Physical examination demonstrates crackles in most patients, and wheezing is present in about a third. Clubbing is uncommon. Pulmonary function studies demonstrate restrictive dysfunction and hypoxemia. The chest x-ray typically shows patchy, bilateral, ground glass or alveolar infiltrates. Solitary pneumonia-like infiltrates and a diffuse interstitial pattern have also recently been described.

BOOP is usually a difficult diagnosis to make on clinical grounds alone. The presence of fever and weight loss, abrupt onset of symptoms (often with an upper respiratory tract infection), a relatively short duration of symptoms, the absence of clubbing, and the presence of alveolar infiltrates help the clinician distinguish this entity from idiopathic pulmonary fibrosis. However, open lung biopsy may be necessary. Buds of loose connective tissue and inflammatory cells fill alveoli and distal bronchioles. Corticosteroid therapy is effective in two-thirds of cases, often abruptly. Relapses are common if corticosteroids are stopped prematurely, and most patients require at least 9–12 months of therapy. Prednisone is usually given initially in doses of 1 mg/kg/d for 2–3 months. The dose is then tapered slowly to 20–40 mg/d, depending on response, and eventually to an alternate-day regimen.

Respiratory bronchiolitis is a disorder of small airways in young cigarette smokers. Clinically and radiographically, this disorder resembles idiopathic pulmonary fibrosis. Cough, dyspnea, and crackles on chest auscultation are typical. However, the reduction in lung compliance seen in idiopathic pulmonary fibrosis is not found in this disorder. The condition may be recognized only on open lung biopsy, which demonstrates characteristic metaplasia of terminal and respiratory bronchioles and filling of respiratory and terminal bronchioles, alveolar ducts, and alveoli by pigmented alveolar macrophages.

Diffuse panbronchiolitis is an idiopathic disorder of respiratory bronchioles that is frequently diagnosed in Japan. The condition appears to be extremely rare in the United States. Men are affected about twice as often as women and are most often between ages 20 and 80. About two-thirds of patients are nonsmokers. The large majority have a history of chronic pansinusitis. Marked dyspnea, cough, and sputum production are cardinal features. Crackles and rhonchi are noted on physical examination. Pulmonary function tests reveal obstructive abnormalities. The chest x-ray shows a distinct pattern of diffuse small nodular shadows and hyperinflation. Open lung biopsy is necessary for diagnosis. This demonstrates thickening of the walls of respiratory bronchioles and extension of a chronic inflammatory cell infiltrate into peribronchiolar tissues. Airway infection, often by *P aeruginosa,* and features of bronchiectasis are common in advanced stages. Treatment is supportive, including smoking cessation, bronchodilators, and trials of antibiotics and corticosteroids. The prognosis is poor, and a rapidly progressive downhill course is typical.

Cordier JF, Loire R, Brune J: Idiopathic bronchiolitis obliterans organizing pneumonia: Definition of characteristic clinical profiles in a series of 16 patients. Chest 1989;96:999. (Three varieties may be distinguished clinically and radiographically.)

Kindt GC et al: Bronchiolitis in adults: A reversible cause of airway obstruction associated with airway neutrophils and neutrophil products. Am Rev Respir Dis 1989; 140:483.

PLEUROPULMONARY INFECTIONS

ACUTE TRACHEOBRONCHITIS

Acute tracheobronchitis is a poorly defined but common clinical condition caused by acute inflammation of the trachea and bronchi. This syndrome is usually attributed to infectious agents, though it may be difficult to distinguish from inflammation of the tracheobronchial tree by nonspecific irritants such as dust and smoke. Infectious agents causing acute tracheobronchitis in older children and adults include influenza A and B viruses, parainfluenza viruses, respiratory syncytial virus, adenovirus, rhinovirus, and others. Acute infectious tracheobronchitis often presents with cough (initially nonproductive but later productive of mucopurulent sputum) and substernal discomfort worsened by coughing. Symptoms of upper respiratory tract infection often precede and overlap the manifestations of tracheobronchitis.

Physical findings are minimal or absent. Rhonchi, which may disappear after productive cough, and wheezing may be evident. Signs of pulmonary consolidation are absent. The chest x-ray is normal.

Fever is usually minimal or absent except in cases of influenza. Chest x-ray examination should be reserved for those patients in whom influenza is suspected, those with underlying chronic obstructive pulmonary disease, and those with physical findings suggestive of pneumonia.

Treatment is symptomatic, aimed at controlling cough, chest discomfort, and fever. An inhaled bronchodilator, such as metaproterenol or albuterol, two puffs every 4 hours, may be tried if chest tightness or wheezing is present. Persistent dry cough after other symptoms of tracheobronchitis have cleared should alert the clinician to the possible diagnosis of cough-variant asthma. Sputum Gram stain or culture is generally not indicated. Empiric antibiotic therapy is generally not indicated except in patients with underlying chronic obstructive pulmonary disease or those with persistent cough productive of purulent sputum, which suggests possible secondary bacterial infection with S pneumoniae or H influenzae. In this situation, amoxicillin (500 mg every 8 hours); ampicillin, erythromycin, or tetracycline (each in a dose of 250–500 mg four times daily); or trimethoprim-sulfamethoxazole (160/800 mg every 12 hours) may be given orally for 7–10 days.

PNEUMONIA

Pneumonia continues to be a major health problem despite the availability of potent antimicrobial drugs. Microorganisms gain access to the lower respiratory tract by aspiration of oropharyngeal secretions and associated bacterial flora, inhalation of infected aerosols, and hematogenous dissemination. Characteristics of pneumonia caused by specific agents and appropriate antimicrobial therapy are presented in Table 9–8.

Approach to the Immunocompetent Patient With Possible Pneumonia

A chest radiograph is included in the initial evaluation of a patient with symptoms and signs suggestive of pneumonia. The pattern of the infiltrate is not pathognomonic of a specific cause of pneumonia.

The attempt to establish a specific causative diagnosis should always begin with a Gram-stained smear of expectorated sputum, which often reveals the predominant organism. An adequate sputum specimen demonstrates at least 25 polymorphonuclear leukocytes and fewer than ten squamous epithelial cells per low-power field.

Sputum induction should be performed if the patient cannot produce an adequate sputum specimen by spontaneous cough. Direct instruction by the physician is often all that is necessary. Merely leaving a sputum container at the patient's bedside is futile. The mouth should be rinsed with water initially. The patient is instructed to take several deep breaths and then inhale deeply before coughing vigorously. Simultaneous chest clapping over the lower lobes posteriorly may assist the cough. Complementary techniques include chest percussion or vibration, inhalation of bland aerosols of water from a face mask or ultrasonic nebulizer, inhalation of sympathomimetic bronchodilators, intermittent positive-pressure breathing (IPPB), and combinations of these approaches.

In examining expectorated sputum, one must discriminate between lower respiratory tract pathogens and organisms that colonize the pharynx. For example, the presence of gram-negative bacteria and fungi such as Candida albicans and Aspergillus species on a smear of expectorated sputum may represent pharyngeal colonization and not lower respiratory tract infection. The presence of bacteria within polymorphonuclear leukocytes is highly suggestive of infection by that organism.

The absence of a definitive bacterial organism on sputum Gram stain in a patient with pneumonia raises the possibility of lung infection by viruses, Mycoplasma pneumoniae, Chlamydia, Legionella, anaerobic organisms, and fungal or mycobacterial organisms. Cultures of sputum representative of lower respiratory tract secretions (ie, devoid of epithelial cells) should be obtained. Results of sputum cultures

Table 9–8. Characteristics and treatment of selected pneumonias.

Organism	Clinical Setting	Gram-Stained Smears of Sputum	Chest Radiograph[1]	Laboratory Studies	Complications	Antimicrobial Therapy[2]
Streptococcus pneumoniae (pneumococcus)	Chronic cardiopulmonary disease; follows upper respiratory tract infection.	Gram-positive diplococci.	Lobar consolidation.	Gram-stained smear of sputum; culture of blood, pleural fluid.	Bacteremia, meningitis, endocarditis, pericarditis, empyema.	Preferred: Penicillin G (or V, oral). Alternative: Erythromycin, cephalosporin.
Haemophilus influenzae	Chronic cardiopulmonary disease; follows upper respiratory tract infection.	Pleomorphic gram-negative coccobacilli.	Lobar consolidation.	Culture of sputum, blood, pleural fluid.	Empyema, endocarditis.	Preferred: Ampicillin (or amoxicillin). Cefotaxime or ceftriaxone for severe infections. Alternative: Cefuroxime, trimethoprim-sulfamethoxazole, amoxicillin-clavulanic acid, tetracycline.
Staphylococcus aureus	Influenza epidemics; nosocomial.	Plump gram-positive cocci in clumps.	Patchy infiltrates.	Culture of sputum, blood, pleural fluid.	Empyema, cavitation.	Preferred: Nafcillin.[3] Alternative: A cephalosporin, vancomycin, clindamycin, ciprofloxacin, amoxicillin-clavulanic acid, ticarcillin-clavulanic acid, ampicillin-sulbactam.
Klebsiella pneumoniae	Alcohol abuse, diabetes mellitus; nosocomial.	Plump gram-negative encapsulated rods.	Lobar consolidation.	Culture of sputum, blood, pleural fluid.	Cavitation, empyema.	Preferred: A cephalosporin; for severe infection, a cephalosporin plus gentamicin, tobramycin, or amikacin. Alternative: Mezlocillin or piperacillin, amoxicillin-clavulanic acid, ticarcillin-clavulanic acid, imipenem, aztreonam.
Escherichia coli	Nosocomial; rarely, community-acquired.	Gram-negative rods.	Patchy infiltrates, pleural effusion.	Culture of sputum, blood, pleural fluid.	Empyema.	Preferred: Aminoglycoside or a cephalosporin. Alternative: Ampicillin, carbenicillin, mezlocillin, ticarcillin, piperacillin, ciprofloxacin, ticarcillin-clavulanic acid, imipenem.
Pseudomonas aeruginosa	Nosocomial; cystic fibrosis.	Gram-negative rods.	Patchy infiltrates, cavitation.	Culture of sputum, blood.	Cavitation.	Preferred: Aminoglycoside plus anti-*Pseudomonas* penicillin, eg, ticarcillin, piperacillin. Alternative: Aminoglycoside plus ceftazidime, imipenem, or aztreonam; ciprofloxacin.

(*continued*)

Table 9–8. Characteristics and treatment of selected pneumonias. (continued)

Organism	Clinical Setting	Gram-Stained Smears of Sputum	Chest Radiograph[1]	Laboratory Studies	Complications	Antimicrobial Therapy[2]
Anaerobes	Aspiration, periodontitis.	Mixed flora.	Patchy infiltrates in dependent lung zones.	Culture of pleural fluid or of material obtained by transtracheal or transthoracic aspiration.	Necrotizing pneumonia, abscess, empyema.	Preferred: Penicillin G. Alternative: Clindamycin, chloramphenicol; metronidazole with penicillin.
Mycoplasma pneumoniae	Young adults; summer and fall.	PMNs and monocytes; no bacterial pathogens.	Extensive patchy infiltrates.	Complement fixation titer.[4] Cold agglutinin serum titers are not helpful as they lack sensitivity and specificity.	Skin rashes, bullous myringitis; hemolytic anemia.	Preferred: Erythromycin. Alternative: Tetracycline or doxycycline.
Legionella species	Summer and fall; exposure to contaminated construction site, water source, air conditioner; community-acquired or nosocomial.	Few PMNs; no bacteria.	Patchy or lobar consolidation.	Direct immunofluorescent examination of sputum or tissue; immunofluorescent antibody titer,[4] culture of sputum or tissue.[5]	Empyema, cavitation, endocarditis, pericarditis.	Preferred: Erythromycin, with or without rifampin. Alternative: Trimethoprim-sulfamethoxazole.
Chlamydia pneumoniae	Clinically similar to *M pneumoniae*, but prodromal symptoms last longer (up to 2 weeks). Sore throat with hoarseness common. Mild pneumonia in teenagers and young adults.	Nonspecific.	Subsegmental infiltrate, less prominent than in *M pneumoniae* pneumonia. Consolidation rare.	Isolation of the organism is very difficult. Serologic studies include microimmunofluorescence with TWAR antigen and a nonspecific complement fixation antibody test.	Reinfection in older adults with underlying COPD or heart failure may be severe or even fatal.	Preferred: Tetracycline. Alternative: Erythromycin, clarithromycin.
Moraxella catarrhalis	Preexisting lung disease; elderly; corticosteroid or immunosuppressive therapy.	Gram-negative diplococci.	Patchy infiltrates; occasional lobar consolidation.	Gram stain and culture of sputum or bronchial aspirate.	Rarely, pleural effusions and bacteremia.	Preferred: Trimethoprim-sulfamethoxazole. Alternative: Amoxicillin-clavulanic acid, an erythromycin, a tetracycline, cefuroxime.
Pneumocystis carinii	AIDS, immunosuppressive or cytotoxic drug therapy, cancer.	Not helpful in diagnosis.	Diffuse interstitial and alveolar infiltrates; apical or upper lobe infiltrates in patients on aerosolized pentamidine.	Cysts and trophozoites of *P carinii* on methenamine silver or Giemsa stains of sputum or bronchoalveolar lavage fluid.	Pneumothorax, respiratory failure, ARDS, death.	Preferred: Trimethoprim-sulfamethoxazole, pentamidine isethionate. Alternatives: Dapsone and trimethoprim; clindamycin and primaquine, trimetrexate; prednisone.

[1]X-ray findings lack specificity. See text.
[2]Antimicrobial sensitivities should guide therapy when available.
[3]Methicillin-resistant *S aureus* infections are treated with vancomycin.
[4]Fourfold rise in titer is diagnostic.
[5]Selective media are required.

may be misleading because of contamination with flora of the upper respiratory tract; cultures are most helpful when correlated with Gram-stained smears. It is important to emphasize that *the diagnosis of pneumonia cannot be based solely on the results of culture of expectorated sputum*. In patients appearing especially ill, blood cultures should also be obtained before antimicrobial therapy is started; if cultures are positive, the causative organism has been definitively identified.

Thoracentesis should be performed in most cases of suspected bacterial pneumonia if a significant pleural effusion is present. Gram-stained smears and cultures of pleural fluid may reveal the causative organism. Pleural fluid with characteristics diagnostic of empyema (see Table 9–23) represents an indication for tube thoracostomy in most cases.

Antimicrobial therapy should be started after initial diagnostic studies have been performed. Empiric antibiotic therapy is initiated in most cases, because the clinical presentation and initial sputum Gram stain do not commonly indicate infection caused by a specific infectious agent. If the physician judges that the specific infecting organism must be identified with precision before antibiotic therapy is started, an invasive procedure such as fiberoptic bronchoscopy with bronchoalveolar lavage or protected brushing (see below), or transthoracic needle aspiration must be performed. Such procedures are rarely necessary in patients with uncomplicated community-acquired pneumonia.

Empiric Treatment of Community-Acquired Pneumonia

Erythromycin is the drug of choice for *empiric* treatment of community-acquired atypical pneumonia in the young or middle-aged adult; the usual dose is 250–500 mg orally four times daily for 10–14 days. Azithromycin and clarithromycin are effective alternatives with less gastrointestinal toxicity than erythromycin, but these new agents are expensive. In contrast, if typical pneumonia is suspected in this setting and a Gram stain of sputum is consistent with pneumococcal infection, penicillin G or V is the drug of choice. The usual dose of penicillin G or V for pneumococcal pneumonia in an adult is 250 mg orally four times daily for 1 week. Cefuroxime is favored for empirical therapy of community-acquired typical pneumonia if the patient is elderly or has underlying COPD, chronic alcoholism, or a history of recent influenza. In such patients, hospitalization is usually necessary, and cefuroxime is given in doses of 0.75–1.5 g intravenously every 8 hours for 5–10 days, with adjustments as necessary for impaired renal function. If ambulatory treatment is considered acceptable, cefuroxime axetil is given in doses of 250–500 mg orally every 12 hours for 10–14 days. In patients with COPD, chronic heart disease, or alcoholism who are elderly or who have limited pulmonary reserve, em-

piric therapy for nonspecific community-acquired pneumonia often consists of both erythromycin and cefuroxime. Pneumonia caused by *Moraxella catarrhalis* is treated with trimethoprim-sulfamethoxazole (160 mg trimethoprim/800 mg sulfamethoxazole orally every 12 hours for 10–14 days) or amoxicillin-clavulanic acid (250–500 mg orally every 8 hours for 10–14 days).

Invasive procedures may be justified in immunodeficient patients or patients who fail to respond to conventional therapy. The benefits of invasive methods to pinpoint a specific organism causing pneumonia must be weighed against their risks and costs. Knowledge of indigenous hospital flora and their antimicrobial sensitivities is vital in selecting empiric therapy for nosocomial pneumonia; therapy is modified when antimicrobial sensitivities become known or if the patient fails to respond.

Prevention

Polyvalent pneumococcal vaccine (containing capsular polysaccharide antigens of 23 strains of *S pneumoniae*) has the potential to prevent or lessen the severity of 85–90% of pneumococcal infections in immunocompetent patients Indications for pneumococcal vaccination include any chronic cardiopulmonary disease (see Chapter 32).

Annual vaccination against influenza is recommended for those at risk. Guidelines are updated yearly by the Centers for Disease Control and Prevention (Influenza Branch, 7–112, Centers for Disease Control and Prevention, Atlanta, GA, 30333; [404] 639–3311).

Douglas RG., Jr: Prophylaxis and treatment of influenza. N Engl J Med 1990;322:443. (Vaccine and amantadine.)

Fang GD et al: New and emerging etiologies for community-acquired pneumonia with implications for therapy: A prospective multicenter study of 359 cases. Medicine 1990;68:307. (Five leading causes of community-acquired pneumonia in adults requiring hospitalization.)

Pachon J et al: Severe community-acquired pneumonia: Etiology, prognosis, and treatment. Am Rev Respir Dis 1990;142:369.

Shapiro ED et al: The protective efficacy of polyvalent pneumococcal polysaccharide vaccine. N Engl J Med 1991;325: 1453. (Vaccine should be used more widely.)

1. ACUTE BACTERIAL PNEUMONIA

Essentials of Diagnosis

- Fever, chills, pleuritic chest pain, cough, purulent sputum.
- Evidence of consolidation on examination of the chest.
- Leukocytosis with leftward shift; leukopenia in some.
- Patchy or lobar infiltrates on chest x-ray.

- Diagnostic sputum Gram stain or culture of blood or pleural fluid.

General Considerations

Information about the cause of acute bacterial pneumonia is often incomplete because of the difficulty encountered in isolating the responsible organisms. Sputum cultures may fail to reveal the bacterial pathogen while demonstrating other organisms that have merely colonized the upper respiratory tract. Blood cultures and cultures of pleural fluid are positive in a minority of patients. Most studies of community-acquired acute bacterial pneumonia identify *S pneumoniae* (pneumococcus) as the causative organism in about two-thirds of cases; *H influenzae, S aureus, Legionella pneumophila,* enteric gram-negative rods, and anaerobes account for most of the remainder.

The bacterial pathogens of nosocomial acute bacterial pneumonia differ from those of the community-acquired variety. Hospitalized patients commonly develop oropharyngeal colonization with enteric gram-negative rods, particularly *P aeruginosa,* and *S aureus,* which are usually responsible for lower respiratory tract infections in these patients. *S pneumoniae* is an infrequent cause of nosocomial pneumonia.

In HIV-infected patients, the frequency of pneumococcal pneumonia is much higher than in the general population. Multiple defects in the systemic immune system and abnormal pulmonary defense mechanisms are presumably responsible for this increased risk. Bacteremia and multilobar involvement are more commonly seen in HIV-infected patients with bacterial pneumonia than in immunologically normal patients.

Clinical Findings

A. Symptoms and Signs: Acute bacterial pneumonia is usually manifested by the abrupt onset of fever, chills, cough productive of purulent sputum, and pleuritic chest pain. Physical examination reveals a toxic-appearing, febrile patient with tachypnea and tachycardia. Evidence of consolidation may be present. In elderly patients, however, acute pneumonia may be heralded only by an alteration in mental status or an apparent worsening of underlying disease such as chronic obstructive pulmonary disease or congestive heart failure.

B. Laboratory Findings: An initial pair of blood cultures is necessary. Hematologic evaluation reveals leukocytosis with a shift to the left or sometimes leukopenia. Sputum is purulent or mucopurulent. Gram-stained smears of sputum reveal neutrophils and (usually) a single predominant organism. The finding of intracellular organisms helps to establish the specific bacterial etiology.

Bronchoscopy may be helpful in evaluating patients with suspected nosocomial pneumonia, particularly in critical care settings. Insertion of a protected brush catheter through the fiberoptic bronchoscope permits a highly accurate (> 90%) diagnosis of nosocomial pneumonia, using a cutoff level of 10^3 bacteria colony-forming units/mL. Such accuracy cannot be achieved with clinical and radiographic assessment alone. Bronchoalveolar lavage with microscopic identification of a high percentage of intracellular bacteria is another useful tool. However, the physician must decide in each case whether the risks and expense of bronchoscopy with brushing or lavage, accompanied by the delays in obtaining a final culture and sensitivity report, are acceptable when compared with the results of empiric antibiotic therapy.

C. Imaging: Chest radiography shows lobar or segmental ("patchy") infiltrates. Ipsilateral pleural effusion may be present, particularly in *S aureus* or *Streptococcus pyogenes* pneumonia. Cavitation also suggests *S aureus* or *S pyogenes* infection.

Treatment

The patient who is otherwise healthy and free of respiratory distress or complications of pneumonia may be managed as an outpatient with oral antibiotics (Table 9–8) and appropriate supportive care. Careful follow-up is important to ensure compliance with therapy and to examine for complications. However, many patients with acute bacterial pneumonia should be hospitalized (1–4 days is usually adequate).

Neutropenia, involvement of more than one lobe, and poor host resistance (eg, alcoholism, diabetes mellitus, malnutrition) suggest the possibility of a poor response to therapy and indicate the need for hospitalization. Bed rest, supplemental oxygen if hypoxemia is present, and antibiotics (Table 9–8) are the cornerstones of therapy. Respiratory and chest physical therapy are helpful in patients with specific problems such as bronchoconstriction and retained lung secretions but should not be routinely ordered.

The choice of antimicrobial drugs. Med Lett Drugs Ther 1990;32:41. (First-choice and alternative drugs for most important human pathogens.)

Meduri GU, Baselski V: The role of bronchoalveolar lavage in diagnosing nonopportunistic bacterial pneumonia. Chest 1991;100:179.

Meduri GU: Ventilator-associated pneumonia in patients with respiratory failure: A diagnostic approach. Chest 1990;97:1208. (Reliable diagnosis of pneumonia in mechanically ventilated patients may require the use of invasive diagnostic procedures such as protected specimen brush and bronchoalveolar lavage.)

Scheld WM, Mandell GL: Nosocomial pneumonia: Pathogenesis and recent advances in diagnosis and therapy. Rev Infect Dis 1991;13(Suppl 9):S743. (Including the role of gastric colonization in pathogenesis, the utility of bronchoscopic techniques in diagnosis, and the use of newer antibiotics.)

2. ATYPICAL PNEUMONIA

Essentials of Diagnosis

- Prominent constitutional symptoms, often including headache, myalgias, malaise, low-grade fever; cough, minimal chest pain; scanty sputum production.
- Minimal physical findings; absence of respiratory distress.
- Mucoid, rather purulent sputum that lacks a predominant bacterial organism on Gram stain.
- Normal or slightly elevated white blood cell count.
- Segmental, unilateral lower lung zone infiltrate on chest x-ray in most cases.

General Considerations

The most common cause of atypical pneumonia is *Mycoplasma pneumoniae*. Other less common causative agents include *Legionella* sp, *Chlamydia psittaci* (psittacosis), *Chlamydia pneumoniae* (TWAR strain), *Coxiella burnetii* (Q fever), *Pneumocystis carinii, Mycobacterium tuberculosis,* and, in endemic areas, *Coccidioides immitis* and *Histoplasma capsulatum.* Viral pneumonia produces a similar clinical picture; influenza (types A and B) and adenoviruses are the most common causes.

Clinical Findings

The clinical picture in atypical pneumonia is dominated by constitutional symptoms such as fever, malaise, and headache rather than by respiratory symptoms, though a nonproductive cough is usually present. Unfortunately, overlap of these symptoms with similar ones in bacterial processes precludes their use in establishing a diagnosis. Physical findings of consolidation are absent. Leukocytosis, if present, is mild. Gram-stained smears of sputum (if obtainable) reveal neutrophils or mononuclear cells but no predominant bacterial pathogens. Chest radiographs reveal patchy nonlobar infiltrates that are more extensive than might be predicted from the clinical presentation. Pleural effusions are uncommon.

Treatment

Antibiotic regimens are as follows: mycoplasmal pneumonia (erythromycin, 500 mg orally four times daily for 2 weeks); *Legionella* pneumonia (erythromycin, 1 g intravenously every 6 hours for 2 weeks); psittacosis or Q fever (tetracycline, 500 mg orally four times daily for 2–3 weeks); *C pneumoniae* pneumonia (tetracycline, 500 mg orally four times daily for 2 weeks).

Amantadine is 65–80% effective in prevention of symptomatic influenza A infection during outbreaks. If given during the first 1–2 days of illness, it also shortens the duration of symptoms of influenza A infection. Adults should receive 100 mg of amantadine twice daily for 10 days. The dose is reduced in those over age 65, in children, and in patients with a seizure disorder or renal impairment. Treatment guidelines are available from the Influenza Branch, 7–112, Centers for Disease Control, Atlanta, GA 30333.

Grayston JT et al: A new respiratory tract pathogen: *Chlamydia pneumoniae* strain TWAR. J Infect Dis 1990;161;618. (Microbiology, clinical features, and treatment.)

Mansel JK et al: *Mycoplasma pneumoniae* pneumonia. Chest 1989;95:639. (Clinical, radiographic, and laboratory features.)

Winterbauer RH (editor): Atypical pneumonia syndromes. Clin Chest Med 1991;12:203. (Clinical features of important types of atypical pneumonia.)

3. ANAEROBIC PNEUMONIA & LUNG ABSCESS

Essentials of Diagnosis

- Predisposition to aspiration.
- Poor dental hygiene.
- Fever, weight loss, malaise.
- Foul-smelling sputum (fewer than half of patients).
- Infiltrate in dependent lung zone, with single or multiple areas of cavitation or pleural effusion.

General Considerations

Aspiration of small amounts of oropharyngeal secretions occurs during sleep in normal individuals and rarely causes disease. Sequelae of aspiration of larger amounts of material include nocturnal asthma, bronchiectasis, chemical pneumonitis, mechanical obstruction of airways by particulate matter, and pleuropulmonary infection. Individuals predisposed to disease induced by aspiration include those with depressed levels of consciousness due to drug or alcohol use, seizures, general anesthesia, or central nervous system disease; those with impaired deglutition due to esophageal disease or neurologic disorders; and those with tracheal or nasogastric tubes, which disrupt the mechanical defenses of the airways.

Periodontal disease, which increases the number of anaerobic bacteria in aspirated material, is associated with a greater likelihood of anaerobic pleuropulmonary infection. Aspiration of infected oropharyngeal contents initially leads to pneumonia in dependent lung zones, such as the posterior segments of the upper lobes and superior and basilar segments of the lower lobes. Body position at the time of aspiration determines which lung zones are dependent. The onset of symptoms is insidious. By the time the patient seeks medical attention, necrotizing pneumonia, lung abscess, or empyema may be apparent.

About two-thirds of patients with necrotizing pneumonia, lung abscess, and empyema are found to be infected with multiple species of anaerobic bacteria only. Most of the remainder are infected with both anaerobic and aerobic bacteria. *Bacteroides mela-*

ninogenicus, anaerobic streptococci, and *Fusobacterium nucleatum* are commonly isolated anaerobic bacteria.

Clinical Findings

A. Symptoms and Signs: Patients with anaerobic pleuropulmonary infection usually present with constitutional symptoms such as fever, weight loss, and malaise. Cough with expectoration of foul-smelling purulent sputum suggests anaerobic infection, though the absence of productive cough does not rule out such an infection. Dental hygiene is poor, but patients are rarely edentulous; if the patient is edentulous, an obstructing bronchial lesion is commonly present.

B. Laboratory Findings: Expectorated sputum is inappropriate for culture of anaerobic organisms because of contaminating mouth flora. Representative material for culture can be obtained only by transtracheal or transthoracic aspiration, thoracentesis, or bronchoscopy with a protected brush. Transthoracic or transtracheal aspiration is rarely indicated, because anaerobic pleuropulmonary infections respond well to penicillin or clindamycin.

C. Imaging: The different types of anaerobic pleuropulmonary infection are distinguished on the basis of their radiographic appearance. **Lung abscess** appears as a thick-walled solitary cavity surrounded by consolidation. An air-fluid level is usually present. Other causes of cavitary lung disease (tuberculosis, mycosis, cancer, infarction, Wegener's granulomatosis) should be excluded. **Necrotizing pneumonia** is distinguished by multiple areas of cavitation within an area of consolidation. **Empyema** is characterized by the presence of pleural fluid (purulent on thoracentesis) and may accompany either of the other two radiographic findings. Ultrasonography is of value in locating fluid and may also reveal pleural loculations.

Treatment

Penicillin G (1–2 million units intravenously every 4 hours) is the usual treatment for anaerobic pleuropulmonary infections. Penicillin V (0.5–1 g orally every 6 hours) may be used after improvement with intravenous penicillin G has occurred. Clindamycin (600 mg intravenously every 8 hours until improvement, then 300 mg orally every 6 hours) is regarded by most authorities as an acceptable alternative to penicillin for treatment of anaerobic pleuropulmonary infections. However, two recent studies suggest that it is more effective than penicillin for treatment of community-acquired anaerobic lung infection. Antibiotic therapy should be continued until the chest x-ray stabilizes, a process that may take a month or more. The treatment of anaerobic pleuropulmonary disease requires adequate drainage. Tube thoracostomy is required for the treatment of empyema, but open pleural drainage is sometimes necessary because of the propensity of these infections to produce loculations in the pleural space.

Gudiol F et al: Clindamycin vs penicillin for anaerobic lung infections: High rate of penicillin failures associated with penicillin-resistant *Bacteroides melaninogenicus.* Arch Intern Med 1990;150:2525. (Clindamycin favored.)

Styrt B, Gorbach SL: Recent developments in the understanding of the pathogenesis and treatment of anaerobic infections. (Two parts.) N Engl J Med 1989;321:240, 298. (Pathogenetic mechanisms and clinical syndromes.)

PULMONARY INFILTRATES IN THE COMPROMISED HOST

Pneumonia in immunocompromised patients may be caused by bacterial, mycobacterial, fungal, protozoal, helminthic, or viral pathogens, but not all pulmonary infiltrates in compromised hosts are due to infection. Noninfectious processes such as pulmonary edema, drug reaction, pulmonary infarction, underlying malignant disease, and radiation pneumonitis may mimic infection. Although almost any pathogen can cause pneumonia in a compromised host, two clinical tools help the clinician narrow the differential diagnosis. The first of these is knowledge of the underlying immunologic defect: specific types of immunologic defects predispose to particular infections; eg, defects in humoral immunity predispose mainly to bacterial infections against which antibodies play an important role, whereas defects in cellular immunity predispose to infections with viruses, fungi, mycobacteria, and protozoa. Chest radiography is also helpful in clarifying the differential diagnosis. Diffuse infiltrates are usually seen with *Pneumocystis carinii* or viral pneumonias. Bacterial and fungal infections are typically associated with more localized infiltrates.

The time course of infection also provides clues to the etiology of pneumonia in immunocompromised patients. A fulminant pneumonia is probably caused by bacterial infection, whereas an insidious pneumonia is more apt to be caused by viral, fungal, protozoal, or mycobacterial infection. Pneumonia occurring within 2–4 weeks after organ transplantation is most likely to be bacterial, whereas several months or more after transplantation, infection caused by *P carinii,* viruses (CMV, others), and fungi (*Aspergillus,* others) is more likely.

Diagnostic procedures should include blood cultures and examination and culture of sputum and pleural fluid, if present. Examination of expectorated sputum for bacteria, fungi, mycobacteria, *Legionella,* and *P carinii* is important and may preclude the need for an expensive, invasive diagnostic procedure. An adequate sputum sample is frequently difficult to obtain. Sputum induction then becomes necessary. Repeated efforts to obtain sputum should be made.

Frequently, routine evaluation fails to identify the causative organism. The clinician must then either begin empirical antimicrobial therapy or proceed to invasive procedures such as bronchoscopy, transthoracic aspiration, or open lung biopsy. **Bronchoalveolar lavage** using the flexible fiberoptic bronchoscope is a safe and effective method for obtaining representative pulmonary secretions for microbiologic studies. It involves less risk of bleeding than transbronchial brushing and transbronchial biopsy. Lavage is especially suitable for the diagnosis of *P carinii* pneumonia in patients with AIDS (see Chapters 27 and 34), the yield being 90–97%. Examination of expectorated sputum for *P carinii* is a less expensive and noninvasive alternative to bronchoalveolar lavage. The sensitivity of induced sputum for detection of *P carinii* varies from 28% to 92% in large series and depends upon institutional expertise, number of specimens analyzed, and detection methods. Selection of the approach to management must be based on the severity of the pulmonary infection, the underlying disease, the risks of empiric therapy, and local expertise and experience with the diagnostic procedures. Open lung biopsy is considered the standard procedure for diagnosis of pulmonary infiltrates in the compromised host, but choice of this procedure should be tempered by the realization that the information obtained rarely affects the ultimate outcome. Moreover, a specific diagnosis is obtained in only about two-thirds of cases in which this test is performed. Therefore, empiric treatment is generally preferred, especially when the risk-benefit ratio of lung biopsy is high.

Drugs for AIDS and associated infections. Med Lett Drugs Ther 1991;33:95.

Dunn DL: Problems related to immunosuppression: Infection and malignancy occurring after solid organ transplantation. Crit Care Clin 1990;6:955. (Complications following solid organ transplantation, including bacterial pneumonia.)

Murray JF, Mills J: Pulmonary infectious complications of human immunodeficiency virus infection. (Two parts.) Am Rev Respir Dis 1990;141:1356, 1582. (Bacterial, fungal, mycobacterial, *Pneumocystis,* and parasitic lung infections in AIDS.)

PULMONARY TUBERCULOSIS

Essentials of Diagnosis

- Fatigue, weight loss, fever, night sweats.
- Productive cough. Pulmonary infiltrates on chest radiograph.
- Positive tuberculin skin test reaction (most cases).
- Acid-fast bacilli on smear of sputum.
- Sputum culture positive for *Mycobacterium tuberculosis.*

General Considerations

Infection with *M tuberculosis* begins when aerosolized droplets containing viable organisms are inhaled by a person susceptible to the disease. When they reach the lungs, the organisms are ingested by macrophages and either die or persist and multiply. Widespread lymphatic and hematogenous dissemination of organisms occurs before development of an effective immune response when mycobacteria throughout the body are walled off by granulomatous inflammation. This type of infection, called **primary tuberculosis,** is usually asymptomatic. Uncommonly, the immune response is inadequate, and progressive primary tuberculosis develops, accompanied by both pulmonary and constitutional symptoms. Hematogenous dissemination from the primary focus throughout the lungs ("miliary" tuberculosis), to the pleural space (tuberculous pleural effusion), or to extrapulmonary sites (meninges, bone) is a rare complication of primary tuberculosis. Dormant but viable organisms persist for years, and reactivation of disease in any of these sites ("pulmonary" focus, "Simon" focus) may occur if the host's defense mechanisms become impaired. Most cases of tuberculosis in adults are due to reactivation of disease (postprimary or reactivation tuberculosis) and not to recent infection. The percentage of patients with atypical presentations—particularly elderly patients, patients with late stage HIV infection, and those in nursing homes—has increased. Extrapulmonary tuberculosis is especially common in patients with HIV infection, who often display lymphadenitis or miliary disease.

Persons infected with the human immunodeficiency virus (HIV), with or without AIDS, are at increased risk of developing tuberculosis. HIV infection has emerged as the most important risk factor for the development of tuberculosis. The alarming increase in the incidence of tuberculosis in the United States since 1986 can in large part be attributed to the HIV epidemic. Poverty, immigration, homelessness, and poor health care may also be important in this increase. Tuberculosis is also common in the homeless and in refugees from Asia and Central America.

Clinical Findings

A. Symptoms and Signs: The patient with reactivated tuberculosis typically presents with constitutional symptoms of fatigue, weight loss, anorexia, low-grade fever, and night sweats. Pulmonary symptoms include cough, which is initially dry but later productive of purulent sputum and (sometimes) blood. Occasionally, there may be no symptoms. On physical examination, patients often appear chronically ill and exhibit evidence of weight loss. Examination of the chest may reveal findings such as posttussive apical rales or may be normal.

B. Laboratory Findings: A high index of suspicion is critical to the diagnosis of tuberculosis. Definitive diagnosis depends on recovery of *M tuberculosis* from cultures or identification of the organism by DNA probe. Diagnosis therefore starts with collection of an adequate sputum specimen for stain and culture. Induction of sputum may be helpful in patients who cannot voluntarily produce good specimens. Multiple sputum specimens are often required to identify acid-fast bacilli. The fluorochrome rhodamine-auramine stain of concentrated, digested sputum specimens is performed initially as a screening method, with confirmation by the Kinyoun or Ziehl-Neelsen stains. Demonstration of acid-fast bacilli on sputum smear does not confirm a diagnosis of tuberculosis, since saprophytic nontuberculous mycobacteria may colonize the airways or cause pulmonary disease. False-positive sputum cultures of *M tuberculosis* are, however, very rare.

In patients who are unable to produce sputum or in those who are still thought to have tuberculosis despite negative sputum smears, fiberoptic bronchoscopy is usually the next diagnostic step. Bronchial washings are particularly helpful. Postbronchoscopy expectorated sputum specimens may also be useful. Early morning aspiration of gastric contents after an overnight fast is an alternative to bronchoscopy. Gastric aspirates are suitable only for culture and not for stained smear, because nontuberculous mycobacteria may be present in the stomach in the absence of tuberculous infection.

Cultures on solid media to identify *M tuberculosis* require 6 to 8 weeks, imposing a long delay in definitive diagnosis. Current methods utilizes DNA probes to identify *M tuberculosis* complex and other mycobacterial complexes much more rapidly. A radiometric culture system (Bactec) may allow detection of mycobacterial growth in as little as several days. Once *M tuberculosis* is identified on culture, drug susceptibility testing is obtained whenever there is a suspicion of drug resistance. In state-run laboratories and many hospitals this practice is now routine because of the increase in drug-resistant tuberculosis in the United States.

Serologic diagnosis of tuberculosis using ELISA methodology to measure IgG antibody against mycobacterial antigens is a new and promising alternative to standard culture techniques. Experience with this approach is still limited. Polymerase chain reaction technology for immediate identification of mycobacteria is under investigation.

In patients with pleural effusions caused by *M tuberculosis*, needle biopsy of the pleura reveals granulomas in 50% to 80% of patients. Pleural fluid cultures for *M tuberculosis* are positive in less than 25% of cases.

C. Imaging: Because primary tuberculosis is usually asymptomatic, a chest x-ray is infrequently obtained. Radiographic abnormalities in primary tuberculosis are particularly likely to occur in children and include small homogeneous infiltrates (usually in the upper lobe), hilar and paratracheal lymph node enlargement, and segmental atelectasis. Pleural effusion may be present, especially in adults, sometimes as the sole radiographic abnormality. Ghon (calcified primary focus) and Ranke (calcified primary focus and calcified hilar lymph node) complexes are detected as residual evidence of healed primary tuberculosis in a minority of patients.

Postprimary or reactivation tuberculosis is associated with various radiographic manifestations, including fibrocavitary apical disease, nodules, and pneumonic infiltrates. The usual location is in the apical or posterior segments of the upper lobes or in the superior segments of the lower lobes; as many as 30% of patients may present with radiographic evidence of disease in other locations, however. This is especially true in elderly patients, in whom lower lobe infiltrates with or without pleural effusion are encountered with increasing frequency. Lower lung zone tuberculosis, which may occur with endobronchial tuberculosis, may masquerade as pneumonia or lung cancer. In HIV-infected patients who develop pulmonary tuberculosis, the radiographic features of tuberculosis may vary with the stage of HIV disease. In patients with "early" HIV infection, the radiographic features of tuberculosis resemble those in patients without HIV infection. In contrast, atypical radiographic features predominate in patients with "late" stage HIV infection (AIDS). These patients often display lower lung zone, diffuse, or miliary infiltrates, pleural effusions, and enlargement of hilar and mediastinal lymph nodes.

D. Special Examinations: The **tuberculin skin test** identifies individuals who have been infected at some time with *M tuberculosis* but does not distinguish between current disease and past infection. The standard Mantoux test is used for diagnosis of tuberculosis in individuals, while the multiple puncture test is used for population screening. In the Mantoux test, 0.1 mL of standard purified protein derivative (PPD-S), containing 5 TU, is injected intradermally on the volar surface of the forearm using a 27-gauge needle on a tuberculin syringe. The transverse width (in millimeters) of the induration at the skin test site should be recorded after 48–72 hours. The reaction should be measured and interpreted by individuals who are experienced with the test. Two important principles must be remembered: (1) a negative reaction does not rule out the diagnosis of tuberculosis; and (2) the larger the reaction, the greater the likelihood of infection due to *M tuberculosis*. Table 9–9 summarizes American Thoracic Society criteria for interpretation of the Mantoux tuberculin skin test.

HIV-seropositive patients should be monitored very closely with tuberculin skin tests. It is important to know that the criterion for a significant skin test reaction in patients with HIV infection or those with defects in cellular immunity is 5 mm or more of induration. In the early (asymptomatic) stage of HIV in-

Table 9–9. Classification of positive tuberculin skin tests reactions.[1,2]

Reaction Size	Group
≥ 5 mm	1. Persons with HIV infection or those at risk for HIV infection. 2. Close contacts of individuals with tuberculosis. 3. Persons with chest x-rays consistent with old healed tuberculosis.
≥ 10 mm	1. Persons from countries with a high incidence of tuberculosis in Asia, Africa, and Latin America. 2. Intravenous drug users. 3. Medically underserved, low-income populations, including blacks, Hispanics, and Native Americans. 4. Long-term residents of correctional institutions, nursing homes, and mental institutions. 5. Persons with the following medical conditions that increase the risk of tuberculosis: gastrectomy, being ≥ 10% below ideal body weight, jejunoileal bypass, diabetes mellitus, silicosis, chronic renal failure, corticosteroid or other immunosuppressive therapy, leukemia, lymphoma, and other malignancies.
≥ 15 mm	6. Other high-risk populations. All other persons.

[1]Recommendations of American Thoracic Society: Am Rev Respir Dis 1990;142:725.

[2]A Mantoux skin test reaction is considered **positive** if the transverse diameter of the indurated area reaches the size required for the specific group. All other reactions are considered **negative**.

fection, cutaneous reactivity to tuberculin is intact. Patients with AIDS are usually anergic.

Both false-positive and false-negative tuberculin reactions occur. False-positive reactions are due to infection with nontuberculous mycobacteria. False-negative reactions occur because of concurrent infection, malnutrition, old age, immunologic disorders, lymphoreticular malignancies, corticosteroid therapy, chronic renal failure, virus vaccinations, stress, fulminant tuberculosis, and improper testing technique.

"Boosting" of the skin test reaction by serial testing may cause a false impression of conversion, as dormant mycobacterial sensitivity is restored by the antigenic challenge of the initial skin test. This boosting phenomenon may increase the reaction size on a subsequent tuberculin test and is most commonly seen in those over age 55. A two-step testing procedure may identify a boosted tuberculin reaction. If the initial test is negative, it may be repeated a week later. If the second test result is negative, the person is uninfected or anergic. If it is positive, a boosted reaction is most likely. This effect may persist for at least 1 year.

Vaccination with BCG has a variable effect on the tuberculin skin test reaction. A history of BCG vaccination should not alter the interpretation of the tuberculin skin test. A significant skin test reaction in a person vaccinated with BCG should be regarded as evidence of infection with *M tuberculosis*.

An anergy skin test panel should be placed at the time of tuberculin testing if the patient is judged likely to be anergic for any reason.

Treatment

All possible or proved cases of tuberculosis should be reported to local and state public health departments. Treatment of patients with tuberculosis should be conducted by physicians who are skilled and highly experienced in the management of this condition. This is especially important in cases of drug-resistant tuberculosis.

A. Hospitalization: Hospitalization for initial therapy of tuberculosis is not necessary in most patients, though it should be considered if a patient is incapable of self-care or is likely to expose susceptible individuals to the risk of tuberculosis. Monthly follow-up of compliant outpatients is recommended, including sputum smear and culture until conversion occurs. A private room with appropriate ventilation and instruction in the importance of covering the mouth while coughing are sufficient infection control measures for hospitalized patients receiving effective chemotherapy.

B. Drug Therapy: (Table 9–10.) (See also Chapter 32.) Standard therapy for pulmonary infection due to fully susceptible *M tuberculosis* in compliant adults and children over the age of 12 consists of isoniazid, rifampin, and pyrazinamide daily for 2 months, followed by isoniazid and rifampin for 4 more months. If isoniazid resistance is suspected, ethambutol should be added for the first 2 months or until drug susceptibility studies are available. Twice-weekly administration of isoniazid and rifampin is acceptable for the last 4 months of the 6-month regimen, with dosage modification as in Table 9–10. A 9-month regimen of daily isoniazid and rifampin, supplemented as above with ethambutol when isoniazid resistance is suspected, is an alternative, but recent data suggest that the 6-month regimen is preferable. Treatment regimens of less than 6 months are unacceptable because of higher relapse rates. In patients with AIDS or HIV infection, drug-sensitive tuberculosis is treated with isoniazid, rifampin, and pyrazinamide for 2 months, followed by isoniazid and rifampin for at least 7 more months. The total duration of treatment is either 9 months or at least 6 months after sputum culture conversion to negative, whichever is longer. Patients who are expected to be noncompliant with treatment programs should have supervised administration of medications, including confinement if necessary. The importance of supervision of drug therapy cannot be overemphasized, because noncompliance is a major problem in control of tuberculosis in the United States.

A single recent study suggests that adult patients

Table 9–10. First-line antituberculous drugs.[1]

	Adult Dosages[2]		Most Common Side Effects	Tests for Side Effects	Drug Interactions	Remarks
	Daily	Twice Weekly				
Isoniazid (INH)	5 mg/kg orally or IM; maximum 300 mg	15 mg/kg; maximum 900 mg	Peripheral neuritis, hepatitis, hypersensitivity.	AST and ALT	Phenytoin (synergistic); disulfiram.	Bactericidal to both extracellular and intracellular organisms. Pyridoxine, 10 mg orally as prophylaxis for neuritis; 50–100 mg as treatment.
Rifampin	10 mg/kg orally; maximum 600 mg	10 mg/kg; maximum 600 mg	Hepatitis, febrile reaction, purpura (rare).	AST and ALT	Rifampin inhibits the effect of oral contraceptives, quinidine, corticosteroids, warfarin, methadone, digoxin, oral hypoglycemics; aminosalicylic acid may interfere with absorption of rifampin.	Bactericidal to all populations of organisms. Colors urine and other body secretions orange. Discoloring of contact lenses.
Pyrazinamide	15–30 mg/kg orally; maximum 2 g	50–70 mg/kg	Hyperuricemia, hepatotoxicity.	Uric acid, AST, ALT	. . .	Bactericidal to intracellular organisms. Combination with an aminoglycoside is bactericidal.
Ethambutol	15 mg/kg orally; maximum 2.5 g	50 mg/kg	Optic neuritis (reversible with discontinuance of drug; rare at 15 mg/kg); rash.	Red-green color discrimination and visual acuity (difficult to test in children under 3 years of age).	. . .	Bacteriostatic to both intracellular and extracellular organisms. Mainly used to inhibit development of resistant mutants. Use with caution in renal disease or when ophthalmologic testing is not feasible.
Streptomycin	15 mg/kg IM[3]; maximum 1 g[3]	25–30 mg/kg IM	Eighth nerve damage, nephrotoxicity.	Vestibular function (audiograms); BUN and creatinine.	Neuromuscular blocking agents may be potentiated and cause prolonged paralysis.	Bactericidal to extracellular organisms. Use with caution in older patients or those with renal disease.

[1]Modified and reproduced, with permission, from Bailey WC et al: Treatment of tuberculosis and other mycobacterial diseases. Am Rev Respir Dis 1983;127:790.
[2]Recommendations of American Thoracic Society: Am Rev Respir Dis 1986;134:355.
[3]In patients aged 60 years or older, the daily streptomycin dosage is 10 mg/kg; maximum 750 mg.

with smear-negative, culture-positive pulmonary tuberculosis can be effectively treated with a regimen of isoniazid, 300 mg, and rifampin, 600 mg, daily for 1 month, followed by isoniazid, 900 mg, and rifampin, 600 mg, twice weekly for 5 months. However, drug side effects are common with this regimen.

Strains of *M tuberculosis* resistant to one or more first-line antituberculous drugs are being encountered with an alarmingly increasing frequency, especially in large inner city populations. Risk factors for drug resistance include immigration from parts of the world with a high prevalence of tuberculosis and drug-resistant tuberculosis, HIV infection, cavitary disease, intravenous drug abuse, close and prolonged contact with individuals with drug-resistant tuberculosis, unsuccessful previous therapy, and patient noncompliance.

Until drug susceptibility tests are available, treatment must consist of at least two and preferably three drugs (bactericidal if possible) to which the patient

has not been exposed. If isoniazid resistance is confirmed, rifampin and ethambutol are given for 12 months. In the HIV-infected patient with isoniazid resistance (or intolerance), rifampin and ethambutol are given either for 18 months or for at least 12 months after sputum culture conversion to negative, whichever is longer. The possibility of drug resistance must also be considered when re-treatment of tuberculosis is necessary. Re-treatment requires at least two drugs (bactericidal if possible) to which the patient has not been exposed and against which microbial resistance has not been demonstrated.

Therapy of patients with multidrug-resistant tuberculosis requires the use of second-line antituberculous drugs that are often toxic. Treatment should be continued for at least 18–24 months after sputum cultures have converted to negative. Surgery also has a role in the management of these patients. Referral to an expert in tuberculosis is highly recommended.

The physician will occasionally encounter patients

with clinical and radiographic abnormalities consistent with tuberculosis, positive tuberculin reactions, and negative bacteriologic findings. In these patients, the bacillary population is presumed to be lower than in cases where sputum smears or cultures are positive. Evidence suggests the value of treatment of smear- and culture-negative pulmonary tuberculosis. A 4-month regimen of isoniazid and rifampin has been found to be effective.

Extrapulmonary tuberculosis due to fully susceptible *M tuberculosis* should be treated with a 9-month daily regimen of isoniazid (300 mg orally) and rifampin (600 mg orally). Twice weekly therapy with 900 mg of isoniazid and 600 mg of rifampin for the last 8 months of this regimen appears to be acceptable. One study suggests that a four-drug, largely twice-weekly, 6-month regimen for extrapulmonary tuberculosis is also effective. Treatment of skeletal tuberculosis is enhanced by early drainage and debridement of necrotic bone.

Consultation with experts in the treatment of tuberculosis is advised, since therapeutic errors by inexperienced physicians are commonly observed. The reader is referred to recent guidelines on the treatment of tuberculosis (American Thoracic Society).

Adults should have measurements of serum bilirubin, hepatic enzymes, urea nitrogen, and creatinine and a complete blood count, including platelets, before starting chemotherapy for tuberculosis. Visual acuity tests are recommended before initiation of ethambutol, and serum uric acid should be measured before starting pyrazinamide. The patient beginning therapy should be cautioned to watch for symptoms of drug toxicity (Table 9–10). Routine monitoring of laboratory tests for evidence of toxicity is not recommended, but monthly questioning for symptoms of drug toxicity is advised. Appropriate laboratory tests are mandatory if signs or symptoms of toxicity develop.

C. Chemoprophylaxis: Patients infected with *M tuberculosis* but without active disease harbor small numbers of organisms. Isoniazid prophylaxis (300 mg/d for adults and 10–14 mg/kg/d—up to 300 mg/d—for children) for 12 months in such patients may reduce the expected incidence of reactivated tuberculosis by 93%. Six months of isoniazid therapy may offer equal protection and improved patient compliance. Chemoprophylaxis of close contacts of patients with isoniazid-resistant tuberculosis could consist of (1) standard chemoprophylaxis with isoniazid, (2) treatment with standard doses of rifampin for 12 months, or (3) close observation only. The second approach is advised for those at greatest risk (children, immunocompromised hosts).

The following groups of individuals, regardless of age, should be offered isoniazid prophylaxis if they have significant tuberculin skin test results:

(1) Household members and other close contacts of individuals with potentially infectious tuberculosis. Children should be treated even if their initial skin test results are nonsignificant, and such tests should be repeated after 3 months of isoniazid therapy. If the skin test reaction becomes significant, isoniazid should be continued for a total of 12 months.

(2) Newly infected persons (conversion of skin test reaction from nonsignificant to significant within 2 years).

(3) Persons with a history of untreated or inadequately treated tuberculosis.

(4) Individuals with positive skin test reactions and chest x-ray abnormalities consistent with tuberculosis but without bacteriologic evidence of active disease. A course of 12 months of chemoprophylactic therapy is offered in this circumstance.

(5) Individuals with previous or current positive skin test reactions and underlying conditions that increase the risk of reactivated tuberculosis, including silicosis, diabetes mellitus, prolonged corticosteroid therapy, immunosuppressive therapy, end-stage renal disease, chronic malnutrition due to any cause, hematologic and reticuloendothelial cancers, and AIDS or positive tests for antibodies to HIV. In HIV-infected patients with positive tuberculin skin test reactions (and in intravenous drug users with positive tuberculin reactions and either confirmed *or* suspected HIV infection), isoniazid chemoprophylaxis is given for 12 months.

(6) Individuals with positive skin test reactions who are under 35 years of age and who have none of the risk factors discussed above. This particular indication for chemoprophylaxis has remained somewhat controversial.

The major risk of isoniazid prophylaxis is drug-induced hepatitis, the incidence of which increases with age. Isoniazid should be discontinued if a patient develops clinical evidence of hepatitis during therapy. Failure to discontinue the drug may result in progressive and possibly fatal hepatic necrosis. The routine monitoring of biochemical tests of liver function periodically during isoniazid prophylaxis is recommended for persons 35 and older. Elevations of transaminase up to three times normal without symptoms do not constitute an indication to stop therapy.

D. Vaccine: A number of live tuberculosis vaccines are available and are known collectively as BCG after the original strain of bacterium used in the vaccine (bacillus Calmette-Guérin). BCG vaccination should be considered only if isoniazid chemoprophylaxis cannot be used. Current recommendations are that BCG vaccination be considered for tuberculin-negative persons, especially children, who are repeatedly exposed to individuals with untreated or ineffectively treated tuberculosis. Vaccination should be considered for communities or groups in which a high rate of new infections occurs despite aggressive treatment and surveillance programs.

Prognosis

Almost all properly treated patients with tuberculosis are cured. Relapse rates are less than 5% with current regimens. The main cause of treatment failure is noncompliance.

American Thoracic Society: Diagnostic standards and classification of tuberculosis. Am Rev Respir Dis 1990; 142:725. (Official statement of the American Thoracic Society.)

Barnes PF et al: Tuberculosis in patients with human immunodeficiency virus infection. N Engl J Med 1991; 324:1644. (Epidemiology, clinical features, treatment, and prevention.)

Drugs for tuberculosis. Med Lett Drugs Ther 1992;34:10. (This statement summarizes modern treatment of tuberculosis.)

Frieden TR et al: The emergence of drug-resistant tuberculosis in New York City. N Engl J Med 1993;328:521.

DISEASE CAUSED BY NONTUBERCULOUS MYCOBACTERIA

Mycobacteria other than *M tuberculosis* ("atypical" mycobacteria) are ubiquitous in nature. Only *Mycobacterium kansasii* and *Mycobacterium avium-intracellulare* complex are important causes of pulmonary disease in humans, which is clinically indistinguishable from *M tuberculosis*. The diagnosis rests on recovery of the pathogen from cultures. Infections with *M avium-intracellulare* are being seen with increasing frequency in patients with AIDS, in whom the disease is likely to be disseminated.

Sputum cultures positive for atypical mycobacteria do not in themselves prove the presence of atypical tuberculosis, because atypical bacteria may exist as saprophytes in the airways or as environmental contaminants. Sputum cultures are meaningful if the following criteria are met: (1) The patient has clinical and radiographic evidence of disease compatible with a diagnosis of pulmonary tuberculosis and other causes of the lung disease have been excluded; and (2) two or more sputum specimens or bronchial washings are positive for acid-fast bacilli by smear or culture. A positive result on culture of material obtained from tissue biopsies or pleural fluid is also diagnostic. Drug susceptibility testing on cultures of nontuberculous mycobacteria is in general unhelpful clinically and not routinely indicated.

Disease caused by *M kansasii* responds well to drug therapy. Recent data suggest that a daily regimen of rifampin, isoniazid, and ethambutol for 18–24 months is sufficient.

In contrast, *M avium-intracellulare* is resistant in vitro to most antituberculosis drugs. Most nonimmunocompromised patients with lung infection caused by *M avium-intracellulare* are middle-aged or older men with underlying chronic lung disease. The treatment of *M avium-intracellulare* infection is controversial. Whether to use a standard or an individualized regimen, whether to use isoniazid, and whether to perform in vitro drug susceptibility testing are debated, largely because of insufficient data and experience.

Traditional chemotherapeutic regimens have taken an aggressive approach using five or six drugs, but these have been associated with drug-induced side effects and patient noncompliance. An alternative regimen uses isoniazid, ethambutol, and rifampin for 18–24 months, plus streptomycin during the first 2–3 months. The optimal duration of treatment is unknown, but therapy should be continued for 12 months after sputum conversion to negative. Second-line drugs include cycloserine, ethionamide, ciprofloxacin, and clofazimine. Medical treatment is initially successful in about two-thirds of cases, but relapses after treatment are common. Long-term benefit is demonstrated in about half of all patients treated medically. Those who do not respond favorably generally have active but stable disease. Surgical resection is an alternative for the patient with progressive disease that responds poorly to chemotherapy. The overall success with surgical therapy is favorable.

Dissemination of *M avium-intracellulare* infection is rare in immunocompetent patients. In contrast, in patients with AIDS, *M avium-intracellulare* infections are systemic and tend to occur late in the course. The prognosis is dismal in such cases (see Chapter 30). Treatment of *M avium-intracellulare* infections in patients with AIDS is controversial. The drug regimens used for immunocompetent patients are not applicable to those with AIDS. Multiple combinations of drugs such as isoniazid, ethambutol, rifampin, clofazimine, cycloserine, amikacin, ciprofloxacin, pyrazinamide, and ansamycin have been tried. No survival benefit has been demonstrated, but recent experience suggests that symptomatic benefit follows therapy with combinations of drugs such as ethambutol, rifampin, ciprofloxacin, clofazimine, and amikacin. Cycloserine and ethionamide should be avoided because of troublesome side effects. Clarithromycin is a promising new addition to the array of drugs for *M avium-intracellulare* infection in AIDS, but experience is limited. Rifabutin is now available for prevention of disseminated *M avium-intracellulare* infection in AIDS patients with low CD4 counts and for treatment of the disease.

American Thoracic Society: Diagnosis and treatment of disease caused by nontuberculous mycobacteria. Am Rev Respir Dis 1990;142:940. (Official statement of the American Thoracic Society.)

Heifets LB, Iseman MD: Individualized therapy versus standard regimens in the treatment of *Mycobacterium avium* infections. Am Rev Respir Dis 1991;144:1. (Questions the wisdom of the four-drug standard regimen recommended by the American Thoracic Society.)

Horsburgh CR Jr: *Mycobacterium avium* complex infection in the acquired immunodeficiency syndrome. (Current Concepts.) N Engl J Med 1991;324:1332. (Epidemiology, pathogenesis, clinical features, and treatment.)

NEOPLASTIC & RELATED DISEASES

BRONCHOGENIC CARCINOMA

Essentials of Diagnosis

- Cough, dyspnea, hemoptysis, anorexia, or weight loss in most patients.
- Variable findings on physical examination depending on stage of disease.
- Enlarging mass, infiltrate, atelectasis, cavitation, or pleural effusion on chest x-ray in most patients.
- Cytologic or histologic findings diagnostic of (primary) lung cancer in sputum, pleural fluid, or tissue.

General Considerations

About 170,000 new cases of lung cancer are expected in the USA in 1994. Lung cancer accounts for 34% of cancer deaths in men and 22% of cancer deaths in women, and its incidence in women is rising rapidly. Most cases present between the ages of 50 and 70. Fewer than 5% of lung cancer patients are under 40 years of age. Cigarette smoking is the most important cause of lung cancer in both men and women in the USA. Ionizing radiation (indoor radon gas, therapeutic radiation, atomic bomb blasts), asbestos, heavy metals (nickel, chromium), and industrial carcinogens (chloromethyl ether) are established but less potent pulmonary carcinogens. Lung scars, air pollution, and genetic factors are also implicated, but the data supporting these associations are not conclusive. Chronic obstructive pulmonary disease may represent a risk factor for lung cancer even after controlling for cigarette smoking. Primary lung cancer in nonsmokers is uncommon.

More than 20 benign and malignant primary neoplasms of the lung have been identified and classified histologically. Ninety percent of malignant cancers belong to one of the four major cell types of bronchogenic carcinoma, a term denoting primary malignant tumors of the airway epithelium. **Squamous cell carcinoma** and **adenocarcinoma** are the most common types of bronchogenic carcinoma and account for about 30–35% of primary tumors each. **Small cell carcinoma** and **large cell carcinoma** account for about 20–25% and 15%, respectively. Other malignant epithelial tumors of the lung include adenosquamous carcinoma, carcinoid tumor, bronchial gland carcinomas, and a few rare tumors.

Squamous cell carcinoma of the lung tends to originate in the central bronchi as an intraluminal growth and is thus more amenable to early detection through cytologic examination of sputum than are the other types of carcinoma. Squamous cell carcinoma tends to metastasize to regional lymph nodes. About 10% of squamous cell carcinomas cavitate. Small-cell carcinoma also occurs centrally and tends to narrow bronchi by extrinsic compression; widespread metastases are common. Adenocarcinoma and large-cell carcinoma resemble each other in their clinical behavior. These tumors usually appear in the periphery of the lung and therefore are not amenable to early detection through examination of sputum. They typically metastasize to distant organs. **Bronchioloalveolar cell carcinoma,** a subtype of adenocarcinoma, is a low-grade carcinoma that represents about 2% of cases of bronchogenic carcinoma and presents as single or multiple pulmonary nodules or an alveolar infiltrate.

Clinical Findings

The clinical features of lung cancer depend on the primary cancer itself, its metastases, systemic effects of the cancer, and any coexisting paraneoplastic syndromes.

A. Symptoms and Signs: Only 10–25% of patients are asymptomatic at the time of diagnosis of lung cancer. Symptomatic lung cancer is generally advanced and often not resectable. Initial symptoms include nonspecific complaints such as cough, weight loss, dyspnea, chest pain, and hemoptysis that are associated with other disorders. Any change in the pattern of cough, blood-streaked sputum, anorexia with weight loss, and hoarseness are symptoms that point to a diagnosis of bronchogenic carcinoma in the appropriate clinical setting.

Physical findings vary and may be totally absent. Central tumors that obstruct segmental, lobar, or main stem bronchi may cause atelectasis and postobstructive pneumonitis with typical physical findings. Peripheral tumors may cause no abnormalities on physical examination. Extension of the tumor to the pleural surface may cause pleural effusion. In one large series, lymphadenopathy, hepatomegaly, and clubbing were noted in about 20% of patients with lung cancer. Superior vena cava syndrome, **Horner's syndrome** (miosis, ptosis, enophthalmos, and loss of sweating on the affected side), **Pancoast's syndrome** (neurovascular complications of superior pulmonary sulcus tumor), recurrent laryngeal nerve palsy with hoarseness, phrenic nerve palsy with hemidiaphragm paralysis, and skin metastases are each seen in fewer than 5% of cases.

Paraneoplastic syndromes (extrapulmonary organ dysfunction not related to space-occupying metastases) occur in 15–20% of lung cancer patients (see Chapter 5). A number of tumor secretory products have been associated with lung cancer. The manifestations of paraneoplastic syndromes may precede, coincide with, or follow the diagnosis of lung cancer. Recognition of paraneoplastic syndromes in lung cancer is important, because treatment of the associated symptoms may improve the patient's well-being even though the primary tumor itself is not curable; occasionally, resection of the tumor is followed by immediate resolution of the paraneoplastic syndrome. Table 9–11 lists important paraneoplastic syndromes associated with lung cancer.

B. Laboratory Findings: All patients with suspected lung cancer should receive a complete blood count, liver function tests, and measurement of serum electrolytes and calcium in addition to a chest radiograph. Definitive diagnosis requires cytologic or histologic evidence of cancer.

Cytologic examination of sputum permits definitive diagnosis of lung cancer in 40–60% of cases, especially in centrally located tumors. This test is inexpensive and highly specific; unfortunately, the sensitivity averages only about 50% and is and influenced by a number of variables. However, a definitive diagnosis of lung cancer by sputum cytologic examination may spare the patient from having to submit to bronchoscopy or another invasive procedure. Examination of pleural fluid reveals cytologic findings positive for cancer in 40–50% of patients with malignant pleural effusion from lung cancer. Closed pleural biopsy (Cope or Abrams needle) yields a histologic diagnosis of cancer in about 55% of patients. Biopsy and cytologic study of pleural fluid combined establish a diagnosis of cancer in about 80% of patients with malignant pleural effusion.

Tissue for histologic confirmation of lung cancer may be obtained by various techniques, including bronchoscopy, percutaneous needle aspirate, mediastinoscopy, lymph node biopsy, or biopsy of other metastatic sites (eg, skin), and thoracotomy. Biopsy of mediastinal lymph nodes reveals cancer in about a third of lung cancer patients. Fine-needle aspiration of supraclavicular or cervical lymph nodes is useful if these nodes are enlarged on palpation. Thoracotomy is occasionally necessary to diagnose lung cancer when simpler cytologic and histologic evaluations are negative.

C. Imaging: Chest radiography demonstrates abnormal findings in nearly all patients with lung cancer. Comparison of old and current chest radiographs is especially important.

Radiographic abnormalities in primary lung cancer are not specific. Common abnormalities are hilar masses or enlargement, peripheral masses, atelectasis, infiltrates, cavitation, and pleural effusions. Multiple masses, consolidation, and chest wall involvement are unusual. Squamous cell and small-cell carcinomas commonly produce a hilar mass and mediastinal widening. Cavitation suggests squamous cell carcinoma and is exceedingly rare in small-cell carcinoma. Small peripheral masses usually are adenocarcinomas.

CT scanning, MRI, and ultrasound are useful imaging methods in selected patients with suspected or proved lung cancer. All depend upon initial detection of a suspicious lesion on the plain chest x-ray. CT scanning is particularly useful for evaluation of the lung parenchyma and pleura. MRI excels in evaluation of the hilum and mediastinum, but experience is less extensive than with CT scanning at this time.

D. Special Examinations: Early detection of lung cancer in an asymptomatic stage is feasible with cytologic examination of sputum and chest radiography. However, routine screening for lung cancer with chest radiography or cytologic studies of sputum is not recommended because the mortality rate from lung cancer is not appreciably reduced by early detection. Small-cell carcinoma is nearly always metastatic when first detected.

Staging of lung cancer utilizes the TNM international staging system for lung carcinoma, in which T describes the primary tumor, N the nodal involvement, and M any distant metastases. Small-cell carcinoma is staged as "limited" (tumor confined to one

Table 9–11. Paraneoplastic syndromes in lung cancer.

Classification	Syndrome	Common Histologic Type of Cancer
Endocrine and metabolic	Cushing's syndrome	Small cell
	Inappropriate secretion of antidiuretic hormone (SIADH)	Small cell
	Hypercalcemia	Squamous cell
	Gynecomastia	Large cell
Connective tissue and osseous	Clubbing and hypertrophic pulmonary osteoarthropathy	Squamous cell, adenocarcinoma, large cell
Neuromuscular	Peripheral neuropathy (sensory, sensorimotor)	Small cell
	Subacute cerebellar degeneration	Small cell
	Myasthenia (Eaton-Lambert syndrome)	Small cell
	Dermatomyositis	All
Cardiovascular	Thrombophlebitis	Adenocarcinoma
	Nonbacterial verrucous (marantic) endocarditis	
Hematologic	Anemia	All
	Disseminated intravascular coagulation	
	Eosinophilia	
	Thrombocytosis	
Cutaneous	Acanthosis nigricans	All
	Erythema gyratum repens	

hemithorax and hilar, mediastinal, and supraclavicular nodes) or "extensive" (spread to more distant sites). CT scan of the lungs, mediastinum, and upper abdomen (liver, adrenal glands, and periaortic lymph nodes) is usually helpful in staging lung cancer. In a patient with known lung cancer, the finding of mediastinal lymph nodes larger than 2 cm in diameter on CT scan is strong evidence of mediastinal spread of the tumor; however, occasional false-positive results occur with this technique. Nodes smaller than 1 cm have a low probability of tumor involvement. At least 85% of lung cancer patients with negative results on mediastinal CT scans have no evidence of mediastinal lymphadenopathy at the time of surgery.

History, physical examination, and simple laboratory studies (complete blood count, including differential white blood count, liver function tests, bone alkaline phosphatase, and serum calcium) are usually sufficient to detect metastases to distant sites such as liver, brain, bone, heart, abdomen, and skin. Routine radionuclide scans to detect occult distant metastases are not recommended. Radionuclide bone scanning for asymptomatic skeletal metastases is more sensitive than plain x-rays of the skeleton, but it lacks specificity. Patients with skeletal complaints should have bone x-rays. If these are negative, a radionuclide bone scan should be ordered. Those with abnormal central nervous system findings should have a CT scan or MRI of the brain. The latter is preferred for infratentorial lesions. Routine CT scanning of the brain in patients with adenocarcinoma of the lung who have no clinical features of brain metastases is not advised.

Surgical exploration of the mediastinum from the suprasternal or parasternal approach should be strongly considered before thoracotomy if radiographic studies suggest significant mediastinal lymphadenopathy or direct extension of the lung cancer into the mediastinum. This approach reduces the number of thoracotomies that do not permit curative lung resection.

Complications

A. Superior Vena Cava Syndrome: See Chapter 12.

B. Phrenic Nerve Palsy: Tumor destruction of the phrenic nerve, which courses through the mediastinum to innervate the hemidiaphragm, occurs in about 1% of patients with lung cancer and results in hemidiaphragmatic paralysis.

C. Recurrent Laryngeal Nerve Palsy: Recurrent laryngeal nerve palsy due to destruction of the recurrent laryngeal nerve by tumor causes paralysis of the muscles of the larynx, resulting in hoarseness. This palsy almost always occurs on the left side and is seen in fewer than 3% of patients with lung cancer.

Treatment

The main treatment options in lung cancer include surgery, chemotherapy, and radiation therapy. Laser photoresection is sometimes performed on obstructing central tumors to relieve dyspnea and control hemoptysis.

Surgery remains the treatment of choice for patients with non-small-cell carcinoma. Unfortunately, only about 25% of patients with lung cancer are appropriate candidates for surgery, and many of these are found to have unresectable disease at the time of thoracotomy. Contraindications to surgery include extrathoracic metastases; tumor involving the trachea, carina, or proximal main stem bronchi (< 2 cm from the carina); malignant pleural effusion; recurrent laryngeal nerve or phrenic nerve palsy; superior vena cava syndrome; tumor involving the esophagus or pericardium; spread to contralateral mediastinal lymph nodes; poor general health; and extensive involvement of the chest wall. Brain metastases of bronchogenic carcinoma have traditionally been considered unresectable and managed with radiation therapy and corticosteroids. However, a recent study indicates improved survival and quality of life when selected patients with *solitary* brain metastases are treated with surgical resection followed by radiation therapy compared to those given radiation therapy alone (Patchell et al, 1990). Patients with lung cancer often have severe obstructive pulmonary dysfunction. Those whose FEV_1 is less than 2 L, those whose FVC is less than 70% of predicted, and those whose maximum voluntary ventilation is less than 50% of predicted will tolerate pneumonectomy poorly. The preferred approach is to estimate the postresection FEV_1. A quantitative ventilation-perfusion lung scan is performed. The percentage of total ventilation or perfusion that will remain after resection is estimated and multiplied by the optimal preoperative FEV_1. Values greater than 800 mL or 40% of predicted FEV_1 suggest that the patient will have adequate postoperative ventilatory function. Elderly patients with severe COPD are especially likely to be functionally inoperable.

In patients with non-small-cell carcinoma, adjuvant therapy (chemotherapy, radiation therapy, or both given in the postoperative period) has in general yielded disappointing results. Single agent chemotherapy given postoperatively is of no value. In patients with stage II and stage III adenocarcinoma and large-cell carcinoma, chemotherapy with a combination of three drugs for completely resected tumors apparently increases disease-free survival. In patients with incompletely resected non-small-cell carcinoma, postoperative radiation therapy is frequently administered, and recent data suggest that the disease-free survival is further extended when postoperative radiation therapy is used with multidrug chemotherapy. Studies are currently under way to determine whether neoadjuvant therapy (combination chemotherapy given prior to surgical resection) improves resectability and survival in patients with non-small-cell carcinoma.

Combination chemotherapy (see Chapter 5) is the treatment of choice for small-cell carcinoma and results in considerable improvement in median survival. Single-agent chemotherapy has no proved value. Occasionally, posttreatment surgical debulking of primary lesions is carried out. Prophylactic cranial radiation is performed in patients with small-cell carcinoma who have responded to chemotherapy. Although tumor regression in non-small-cell carcinoma is possible with combination chemotherapy, median survival is improved only modestly, often at the expense of considerable drug toxicity.

Radiation therapy is often used to palliate symptoms of lung cancer such as cough, hemoptysis, pain due to bone metastases, and dyspnea from bronchial or tracheal obstruction. It is also employed to treat bronchial obstruction (atelectasis, pneumonia). Radiation therapy is only about 20% successful for treatment of bronchial obstruction by lung cancer; laser therapy is superior when the obstructing lesion is in a main stem bronchus. Radiation therapy is also useful to treat superior vena cava syndrome resulting from non-small-cell carcinoma. Superior vena cava syndrome from small cell carcinoma may be treated with chemotherapy or radiation therapy. Symptomatic brain metastases are treated with radiation therapy and corticosteroids. Selected patients with unresectable lung cancer also receive external beam radiation to the primary tumor site. In patients with limited-stage small-cell carcinoma, this improves complete response rates and survival when compared to chemotherapy alone. However, in non-small-cell lung cancer, survival is not improved. Intraluminal radiation ("brachytherapy") is a new approach to relief of symptoms of recurrent endobronchial lung cancer, but experience with this new modality is quite limited.

Prognosis

The overall 5-year survival rate for lung cancer is 10–15%. Determinants of survival include the stage of disease at the time of presentation, the patient's general health, age, histologic type of tumor, tumor growth rate, and type of therapy. Overall, the 5-year survival rate after "curative" resection of squamous cell carcinoma is 35–40%, compared with 25% for adenocarcinoma and large-cell carcinoma. Patients with small-cell carcinoma rarely live for 5 years after the diagnosis is made.

Batra P et al: Imaging techniques in the evaluation of pulmonary parenchymal neoplasms. Chest 1992;101:239. (The conventional chest x-ray is the imaging method of choice, with CT scanning reserved for staging and MRI for evaluating selected parenchymal neoplasms.)

Ginsberg RJ, Joss RA, Feld R (editors): Fifth World Conference on Lung Cancer. Chest 1989;96(Suppl):1S. (Epidemiology, biology, pathology, and therapy.)

Hazuka MB, Bunn PA Jr: Controversies in the nonsurgical treatment of stage III non-small cell lung cancer. Am Rev Respir Dis 1992;145:967. (Some improvement in survival when radiation therapy is combined with cisplatin.)

Ihde DC: Chemotherapy of lung cancer. N Engl J Med 1992;327:1434. (Current strategy in chemotherapy of various stages of non-small-cell and small-cell lung cancer.)

Little AG, Stitik FP: Clinical staging of patients with non-small cell lung cancer. Chest 1990;97:1431. (Summary of the TNM classification system and methods for staging.)

Murren JR, Buzaid AC, Hait WN: Critical analysis of neoadjuvant therapy for stage IIIa non-small cell lung cancer. Am Rev Respir Dis 1991;143:889. (Remission with preoperative chemotherapy, but the impact on survival is unknown.)

Patchell RA et al: A randomized trial of surgery in the treatment of single metastases to the brain. N Engl J Med 1990;322:494. (Benefits from surgical resection of a solitary brain metastasis combined with radiotherapy compared with radiotherapy alone.)

SOLITARY PULMONARY NODULE

A solitary pulmonary nodule is a round or oval, sharply circumscribed pulmonary lesion (up to 5 cm in diameter; larger lesions are termed "masses") surrounded by normal lung tissue. Central cavitation, calcification, or surrounding ("satellite") lesions may occur. Although mass population screening for lung cancer by chest x-ray is not advised, the finding of a solitary pulmonary nodule on chest x-ray in an individual patient is important. About 25% of cases of bronchogenic carcinoma present as solitary pulmonary nodule, and the 5-year survival rate for bronchogenic carcinoma that is detected in this form approaches 50%, which is considerably higher than the 10–15% 5-year survival rate of lung cancer overall.

In large surgical series, about 60% of solitary pulmonary nodules are benign lesions and 40% are malignant. Infectious granulomas account for most benign lesions, whereas primary lung cancer accounts for more than three-quarters of all malignant solitary pulmonary nodules. Solitary pulmonary nodules occasionally represent metastases from another primary tumor (see below). Determining whether the lesion is likely to be benign or malignant preoperatively is more important than establishing its precise cause.

A lesion is almost certainly benign if the volume doubling time is less than 30 days or more than 500 days or if the lesion is calcified (central, "clustered," or laminated calcium pattern). Factors favoring a benign diagnosis are young age, absence of symptoms, small size (< 2 cm in diameter), smooth margins on CT, and presence of satellite lesions, but none of these criteria are foolproof. Malignant solitary pulmonary nodules are occasionally symptomatic, tend to occur in patients over 45 years of age, are usually larger than 2 cm, often have indistinct margins, and are rarely calcified. Typical features of solitary pulmonary metastases include smooth or lobulated margins, peripheral location, location in the lower lobe, and absence of satellite lesions.

Skin tests and serologic studies for fungal infection are generally not helpful. Cytologic examination of sputum should be considered for evaluation of a large centrally located pulmonary nodule; a positive result might preclude the need for bronchoscopy or needle biopsy. However, sputum cytology is rarely diagnostic of malignancy in small or peripheral pulmonary nodules. Radiographic studies and *comparisons with old chest radiographs* are of utmost importance. CT scanning is particularly useful. Thin section (1.5–5 mm) CT scanning is the preferred method for detection of calcification within the nodule. Investigations for primary cancer elsewhere in the body are not indicated unless abnormal symptoms, signs, and results of simple laboratory studies (complete blood count and differential, urinalysis, stool sample for occult blood) suggest an extrapulmonary cancer. Routine percutaneous needle aspiration of all solitary pulmonary nodules is not advised; it seldom changes subsequent therapy, and false negatives are common.

Treatment

The important steps in the management of a patient with a solitary pulmonary nodule are as follows: (1) Review the chest x-ray in detail. (2) Obtain previous x-rays for comparison. (3) Take a complete medical history and perform a thorough physical examination. (4) Perform additional radiographic studies, such as CT scanning, if necessary. (5) Inform the patient about the findings, and—with the patient's participation—select the best of four approaches: "watchful waiting," fiberoptic bronchoscopy, percutaneous needle aspiration, or resection. As a general rule, all solitary pulmonary nodules in patients over age 35 should be considered potentially malignant and should be resected unless calcification typical of benign lesions or stability on radiography for 2 years is documented. Prospective evaluation ("watchful waiting") is generally not appropriate if calcification is not present or if stability cannot be documented.

Strong indications of a benign diagnosis or contraindications to surgery may justify a conservative approach. Otherwise, exploratory thoracotomy—or in some cases thoracoscopy— is advised as soon as possible after a solitary pulmonary nodule is detected. Decision analysis suggests that the average life expectancy of patients with solitary pulmonary nodules is similar, whether immediate surgery, biopsy, or observation is chosen as the initial approach. However, such an outcome has not been established by prospec-

tive clinical trials. Having the informed patient participate in the decision-making process is important.

Swensen SJ et al: An integrated approach to evaluation of the solitary pulmonary nodule. Mayo Clin Proc 1990; 65:173.
Viggiano RW et al: Evaluation and management of solitary and multiple pulmonary nodules. Clin Chest Med 1992; 13:83.

SECONDARY LUNG CANCER

Secondary lung cancers represent metastases from extrapulmonary malignant neoplasms that spread to the lungs through vascular or lymphatic channels or by direct extension. Almost any cancer can metastasize to the lung. Metastases to the lung usually occur via the pulmonary artery and typically present as multiple masses on chest radiography. Metastases to the lungs are found in 20–54% of patients dying of various malignancies.

Lymphangitic carcinoma denotes diffuse involvement of the pulmonary lymphatic network by secondary lung cancer, probably a result of extension of tumor from lung capillaries to the lymphatics. **Tumor embolization** from extrapulmonary cancer (renal cell carcinoma, hepatocellular carcinoma, choriocarcinoma) is an uncommon route tumor spread to the lungs. Endobronchial metastases occur in fewer than 5% of patients dying of nonpulmonary cancer; most metastases are intraparenchymal. Carcinoma of the kidney, breast, colon, and cervix and malignant melanoma are the tumors most likely to cause endobronchial metastases. Secondary lung cancer may also present as malignant pleural effusion.

Clinical Findings

A. Symptoms and Signs: Symptoms are uncommon but include cough, hemoptysis, and, in advanced cases, dyspnea. Symptoms are more often referable to the site of the primary tumor.

B. Laboratory Findings: The diagnosis of secondary lung cancer is usually established by identifying the primary tumor. Appropriate studies should be ordered if there is a suspicion of any primary cancer, such as breast, thyroid, testis, or prostate, for which specific treatment is available. If the history and physical examination fail to reveal the site of the primary tumor, attention is better focused on the lung, where tissue samples obtained by bronchoscopy, needle biopsy, or thoracotomy establish the histologic diagnosis and suggest the most likely primary. Occasionally, cytologic studies of pleural fluid or pleural biopsy reveal the diagnosis. Sputum cytology is not often helpful. If a solitary lung lesion is detected in a patient with known extrapulmonary cancer, primary lung cancer is still the most likely diagnosis. Sarcoma and melanoma are exceptions to this rule. Only about

3% of all resected solitary pulmonary nodules represent solitary metastases.

C. Imaging: Chest radiographs usually show multiple spherical densities with sharp margins. The size of metastatic lesions varies from a few millimeters (miliary densities) to large masses. Nearly all are less than 5 cm in diameter. The lesions are usually bilateral, pleural or subpleural in location, and more common in lower lung zones. Cavitation suggests primary squamous cell tumor; calcification suggests osteosarcoma. Conventional chest radiography is less sensitive than CT scan in detecting pulmonary metastases. Whole lung conventional tomography for determining the extent of pulmonary metastases has been rendered almost obsolete by CT scanning. The radiographic differential diagnosis of multiple pulmonary nodules includes pulmonary arteriovenous malformation, pulmonary abscesses, granulomatous infection, sarcoidosis, rheumatoid nodules, and Wegener's granulomatosis.

Diffuse lymphangitic spread and the solitary pulmonary nodule are less common radiographic presentations of secondary lung cancer.

Treatment

Surgical resection of a *solitary* pulmonary nodule is often prudent in the patient with known current or previous extrapulmonary cancer.

Once the diagnosis of secondary lung cancer has been established (usually by percutaneous needle biopsy or transbronchial biopsy), management consists of treatment of the primary neoplasm and any pulmonary complications. Local resection of one or more pulmonary metastases via thoracotomy or median sternotomy is feasible in a few carefully selected patients with various sarcomas and carcinomas (breast, testis, colon, kidney, and head and neck). Surgical resection should be considered only if the primary tumor is under control, if the patient is a good surgical risk, if all of the metastatic tumor can be resected, if nonsurgical approaches are not available, and if there are no metastases elsewhere in the body. Relative contraindications to resection of pulmonary metastases include (1) malignant melanoma, (2) requirement for pneumonectomy, (3) pleural involvement, and (4) simultaneous appearance of two or more metastases. The overall 5-year survival rate in secondary lung cancer treated surgically is 20–35%.

MESOTHELIOMA

Mesotheliomas are primary tumors arising from the surface lining of the pleura (80% of cases) or peritoneum (20% of cases). About three-fourths of pleural mesotheliomas are diffuse (usually malignant) tumors, and the remaining one-fourth are localized (usually benign). Men outnumber women by a 3:1 ratio. Numerous studies have confirmed the associa-

tion of **malignant pleural mesothelioma** with exposure to asbestos (particularly the crocidolite form). The lifetime risk to asbestos workers of developing malignant pleural mesothelioma is about 8%. The physician should inquire about asbestos exposure through mining, milling, manufacturing, shipyard work, insulation, brake linings, building construction and demolition, roofing materials, and a variety of asbestos products (pipe, textiles, paint, tile, gaskets, panels). Although cigarette smoking increases the risk of bronchogenic carcinoma in asbestos workers and aggravates asbestosis, there is no association between smoking and mesothelioma.

The mean age at onset of symptoms of malignant pleural mesothelioma is about 60 years. The latent period between exposure and onset of symptoms ranges from 20 to 40 years. Symptoms include the insidious onset of shortness of breath, nonpleuritic chest pain, and weight loss. Physical findings include dullness to percussion, diminished breath sounds, and, in some cases, finger clubbing. Radiographic abnormalities consist of nodular, irregular, unilateral pleural thickening and varying degrees of unilateral pleural effusion. CT scan helps demonstrate the extent of pleural involvement.

Pleural fluid is exudative and often hemorrhagic. Open pleural biopsy is usually necessary to obtain an adequate specimen for histologic diagnosis; even then, distinction from benign inflammatory conditions and from metastatic adenocarcinoma may be difficult.

Malignant pleural mesothelioma progresses rapidly as the tumor spreads quickly along the pleural surface to involve the pericardium, mediastinum, and contralateral pleura. The tumor may eventually extend beyond the thorax to involve abdominal lymph nodes and organs. Progressive pain and dyspnea are characteristic. Median survival time from onset of symptoms is 8–14 months, and about 75% of patients are dead within 1 year of diagnosis. Treatment with surgery, radiotherapy, chemotherapy, and a combination of methods has been attempted but is generally unsuccessful. Some surgeons claim that extrapleural pneumonectomy is the preferred surgical approach.

BENIGN TUMORS OF THE LUNG

Benign neoplasms of the lung typically present as asymptomatic solitary pulmonary nodules detected on routine chest radiography. They account for about 2% of all solitary pulmonary nodules.

Hamartoma is the most common benign lung tumor. Fibromas, lipomas, leiomyomas, hemangiomas, and papillomas account for most of the remainder. The clustered ("popcorn") pattern of calcification on chest x-ray or CT scans is a helpful diagnostic clue to hamartoma.

The medical history, physical examination, and radiographic studies do not permit reliable differentiation of malignant and benign lung tumors. Percutaneous needle biopsy, guided by fluoroscopy or CT scanning and using a needle large enough (18- to 20-gauge) to obtain a core of tissue, is occasionally successful in establishing a *specific* benign diagnosis. However, because of the suspicion of bronchogenic carcinoma, most patients will require thoracotomy for definitive diagnosis. Patients who are poor operative risks may be followed with serial chest films for progression. Even if cancer is present, short periods of observation do not appreciably affect the prognosis.

American Thoracic Society: Guidelines for percutaneous transthoracic needle biopsy. Am Rev Respir Dis 1989;140:255. (An accepted and safe technique, particularly for malignant and infectious conditions.)

BRONCHIAL CARCINOID TUMORS

Carcinoid and bronchial gland tumors are sometimes termed **bronchial adenomas,** but this classification is a misnomer, because it implies that the lesions are benign, when in fact carcinoid tumors and bronchial gland carcinomas are low-grade malignant neoplasms.

Carcinoid tumors are about six times more common than bronchial gland carcinomas, and most of them occur as pedunculated or sessile growths in central bronchi. Men and women are equally affected. Most patients are under 60 years of age. Common symptoms of bronchial carcinoid tumors are hemoptysis, cough, wheezing, and recurrent pneumonia. Peripherally located bronchial carcinoid tumors are rare and present as asymptomatic solitary pulmonary nodules. Carcinoid syndrome (flushing, diarrhea, wheezing, hypotension, etc) is rare. Fiberoptic bronchoscopy reveals a pink or purple tumor in a central airway, and biopsy may be complicated by significant bleeding, because these lesions have a well-vascularized stroma. CT scanning is helpful to localize the lesion and to follow its growth over time.

Bronchial carcinoid tumors grow slowly and rarely metastasize. Complications involve bleeding and airway obstruction rather than invasion by tumor and metastases. Surgical excision is necessary in some cases, and the prognosis is generally favorable. Most bronchial carcinoid tumors are resistant to radiation and chemotherapy.

MEDIASTINAL MASSES

Various developmental, neoplastic, infectious, traumatic, and cardiovascular disorders may cause masses that appear in the mediastinum on chest x-ray. A useful convention arbitrarily divides the mediastinum into three compartments—anterior, middle, and posterior—in order to classify mediastinal masses and assist in differential diagnosis. Specific mediastinal masses have a predilection for one or more of these compartments; most are located in the anterior or middle compartment. The differential diagnosis of an anterior mediastinal mass includes thymoma, teratoma, thyroid lesions, lymphoma, and mesenchymal tumors (lipoma, fibroma). The differential diagnosis of a middle mediastinal mass includes lymphadenopathy, pulmonary artery enlargement, aneurysm of the aorta or innominate artery, developmental cyst (bronchogenic, enteric, pleuropericardial), dilated azygous or hemiazygous vein, and foramen of Morgagni hernia. The differential diagnosis of a posterior mediastinal mass includes hiatus hernia, neurogenic tumor, meningocele, esophageal tumor, foramen of Bochdalek hernia, thoracic spine disease, and extramedullary hematopoiesis.

Symptoms and signs of mediastinal masses are nonspecific and are usually caused by the effects of the mass on surrounding structures. Insidious onset of retrosternal chest pain, dysphagia, or dyspnea is often an important clue to the presence of a mediastinal mass. In about half of cases, symptoms are absent, and the mass is detected on routine chest x-ray. Physical findings vary depending upon the nature and location of the mass.

CT scanning is helpful in management; additional radiographic studies of benefit include barium swallow if esophageal disease is suspected, Doppler sonography or venography of brachiocephalic veins and the superior vena cava, and arteriography. MRI is also useful; its advantages include distinction between vessels and masses, no need for contrast media, and better delineation of hilar structures. MRI also allows imaging in multiple planes, whereas CT permits only axial imaging. Tissue diagnosis is necessary if a neoplastic disorder is suspected. Treatment and prognosis depend on the underlying cause of the mediastinal mass.

Brown K et al: Current use of imaging in the evaluation of primary mediastinal masses. Chest 1990;98:466.
Gamsu G, Sostman D: Magnetic resonance imaging of the thorax. Am Rev Respir Dis 1989;139:254. (Advantages and limitations in comparison with CT.)

INTERSTITIAL LUNG DISEASES

Interstitial lung diseases comprise a heterogeneous group of disorders that have in common the features of inflammation and fibrosis of the interalveolar septum, which represent a nonspecific reaction of the lung to injury of diverse cause. About 180 disease entities share the manifestations of interstitial lung disease (Table 9–12). In the majority of patients, no specific cause can be identified. In the remainder, drugs and a variety of inorganic and organic dusts are the predominant causes.

The pathogenesis of interstitial lung disease of unknown etiology is believed to be lung injury that leads to inflammation of the interalveolar septum (alveolitis). Persistent alveolitis may lead to eventual irreversible interstitial fibrosis.

Interstitial lung diseases share common clinical, physiologic, and radiographic features. Exertional dyspnea and dry cough of insidious onset are the usual presenting symptoms. Chest examination is notable for fine inspiratory crackles at the bases of the lung. Digital clubbing is common. Pulmonary func-

tion testing reveals a restrictive ventilatory defect and a decreased diffusing capacity for carbon monoxide. Hypoxemia, especially with exercise, is common. Diffuse ground-glass, nodular, reticular, or reticulonodular infiltrates that may progress to "honeycomb lung" are noted on chest x-ray. Infrequently, the chest x-ray is normal when lung biopsy demonstrates interstitial lung disease. Conventional and high-resolution CT scanning of the chest has recently proved to be valuable in the assessment of patients with chronic diffuse infiltrative lung disease. Experienced radiologists are most accurate in diagnosing silicosis, interstitial pneumonia, lymphangitic carcinomatosis, and sarcoidosis by CT scanning.

The history, physical examination, chest x-ray, and laboratory studies may provide evidence of a specific cause of interstitial lung disease. Sputum is usually minimal or nonexistent. Induced sputum is likely to yield useful diagnostic information only if pulmonary infection or malignancy is suspected.

Techniques to evaluate the progression of alveolitis have been devised in an attempt to identify patients suitable for anti-inflammatory therapy. These techniques include lung biopsy, bronchoalveolar lavage, and gallium-67 lung scanning.

Transbronchial biopsy using a fiberoptic bronchoscope is easily performed and is associated with a low morbidity rate, but the tissue specimens obtained are small, and sampling errors are common. Open lung biopsy produces large specimens but has a higher rate of complications. Thoracoscopy is becoming a popular alternative to thoracotomy to obtain surgical lung biopsy specimens. Transbronchial biopsies and washings may be adequate to permit the diagnosis of diseases such as sarcoidosis, histiocytosis X, *Pneumocystis carinii* pneumonia, miliary tuberculosis, pulmonary alveolar proteinosis, and lymphangitic carcinomatosis. On the other hand, patients who are rapidly deteriorating may be best served by definitive surgical biopsy rather than potentially nondiagnostic transbronchial biopsy. The choice between transbronchial biopsy and surgical biopsy is often difficult. It is probably reasonable to begin with transbronchial biopsy in most patients because of the low rate of complications associated with this procedure. The risks of transbronchial biopsy include all the risks of routine bronchoscopy as well as of pneumothorax (about 5%) and bleeding (1–9%). If the results of bronchoalveolar lavage or transbronchial biopsy are nondiagnostic and it is felt that a specific diagnosis must be obtained, surgical lung biopsy by thoracoscopy or thoracotomy is necessary.

Bronchoalveolar lavage is useful in the diagnosis of *P carinii* pneumonia and in selected patients with lung infection from other organisms (mycobacteria, fungi, cytomegalovirus, and *Legionella* species). It is occasionally employed for specific diagnosis of lung cancer, pulmonary alveolar proteinosis, histiocytosis X, beryllium-induced lung disease, amiodarone-

Table 9–12. Selected interstitial lung diseases.[1]

Known Cause	Unknown Cause
Inorganic dusts	Cryptogenic fibrosing alveolitis
Silica	Sarcoidosis
Silicates (including asbestos)	Langerhans cell granulomatosis
Aluminum	Rheumatic disease-associated
Antimony	Goodpasture's syndrome
Carbon	Idiopathic pulmonary
Beryllium	hemosiderosis
Hard metal dusts	Wegener's granulomatosis
Organic dusts (hypersensitivity pneumonitis)	Lymphomatoid granulomatosis
Gases, fumes, vapors	Churg-Strauss syndrome
Chlorine	Angioimmunoblastic
Sulfur dioxide	lymphadenopathy
Mercury	Inherited diseases
Drugs	Tuberous sclerosis
Antineoplastic agents	Neurofibromatosis
Antibiotics	Pulmonary veno-occlusive disease
Sulfonamides	Ankylosing spondylitis
Penicillins	Amyloidosis
Nitrofurantoin	Chronic eosinophilic pneumonia
Drugs inducing lupus erythematosus	Pulmonary lymphangiomyomatosis
Sulfonylureas	Whipple's disease
Gold	Alveolar proteinosis
Phenytoin	Inflammatory bowel disease-associated
Penicillamine	
Amiodarone	
Poisons	
Paraquat	
Radiation	
Infections	
Disseminated mycobacterial or fungal infections	
Viral pneumonia	
Pneumocystis carinii pneumonia	
Residue of active infection of any type	
Pulmonary edema	
Lymphangitic carcinoma	

[1]Modified and reproduced, with permission, from Crystal RG et al: Interstitial lung disease: Current concepts of pathogenesis, staging, and therapy, Am J Med 1981;70:542.

induced pneumonitis, or pulmonary hemorrhage in thrombocytopenic patients. In ongoing studies, a very high percentage of T lymphocytes in bronchoalveolar lavage fluid suggests sarcoidosis or hypersensitivity pneumonitis; a predominance of neutrophils, eosinophils, and macrophages suggests idiopathic pulmonary fibrosis. Lung scanning with Ga 67 is nonspecific and has no proved value in diagnosis or management of patients with interstitial lung disease, though it may have some role in the management of outpatients with *Pneumocystis carinii* pneumonia.

Known causes of interstitial lung disease are dealt with in their specific sections. The important idiopathic forms are discussed below.

Muller NL, Miller RR: Computed tomography of chronic diffuse infiltrative lung disease. (2 parts.) Am Rev Respir Dis 1990;142:1206,1440.

Reynolds HY: Interstitial lung diseases. In: *Harrison's Principles of Internal Medicine,* 12th ed. Wilson JD et al (editors). McGraw-Hill, 1991.

CRYPTOGENIC FIBROSING ALVEOLITIS (Idiopathic Pulmonary Fibrosis)

Cryptogenic fibrosing alveolitis is the most common diagnosis among patients presenting with interstitial lung disease. Patients usually present in the sixth or seventh decade with the insidious onset of cough and dyspnea of months' to years' duration. Hamman-Rich syndrome is an uncommon rapidly progressive form of the illness. The disease is more common in men than in women. A familial form of the disease (autosomal dominant trait with variable penetrance) has been described. Symptoms, physical findings, and results on pulmonary function tests are typical of those of interstitial lung disease and are described above. Chest x-ray abnormalities are highly variable and correlate poorly with functional and clinical status. Lower lung zone interstitial infiltrates of a reticular pattern are typical when the patient is first seen. High-resolution CT scan best demonstrates the extent of lung parenchymal fibrosis. Patchy subpleural reticular infiltrates and cystic air spaces, most apparent in the lower lung zones, are typical.

Serologic tests for antinuclear antibody and rheumatoid factor are frequently positive (20–40% of cases). The diagnosis of cryptogenic fibrosing alveolitis is usually based on the clinical presentation and exclusion of other specific diagnoses, usually by means of bronchoalveolar lavage or lung biopsy. Histologic examination of lung tissue reveals a combination of cellular infiltration and fibrosis of the alveolar septum. Desquamated mononuclear cells, mainly macrophages, may be observed within alveoli. Open or thoracoscopic lung biopsy for the diagnosis of cryptogenic fibrosing alveolitis is helpful to exclude

other specific causes of interstitial lung disease. Its routine use for this purpose is controversial.

Treatment consists of supportive measures, supplemental oxygen, and corticosteroids. A clinical trial of corticosteroids is generally indicated in patients with progressive symptoms or deterioration in lung function. Daily prednisone—beginning at 1.5–2 mg/kg/d (up to 100 mg/d) for 6 weeks and tapering slowly over 3–6 months to a minimum maintenance dose of 0.25 mg/kg/d—is the mainstay of therapy. Cytotoxic drugs such as cyclophosphamide and azathioprine have also been used. The PaO_2 at rest and during pulmonary exercise stress testing is superior to traditional pulmonary function tests to monitor the physiologic response to therapy. Almost half of patients experience subjective improvement with corticosteroid therapy, but only about one-fourth demonstrate objective improvement. Younger patients, those with a shorter duration of illness, and those with a histopathologic pattern that is more cellular than fibrotic are more likely to have a favorable response. Relentless progression of the disease with eventual respiratory insufficiency is the rule, and the average survival time is about 4 years after the onset of symptoms. Heart-lung and single-lung transplantation for highly selected patients with end-stage pulmonary fibrosis is now available. It is important to distinguish cryptogenic fibrosing alveolitis from bronchiolitis obliterans organizing pneumonia (BOOP) by clinical and radiographic features and lung biopsy if necessary because of the excellent response of the latter disorder to corticosteroid therapy.

Cherniack RM, Crystal RG, Kalica AR: Current concepts in idiopathic pulmonary fibrosis: A road map for the future. Am Rev Respir Dis 1991;143:680. (Pathogenesis, clinical markers of disease activity, and implications for treatment.)

SARCOIDOSIS

Sarcoidosis is a systemic disease of unknown cause characterized by granulomatous inflammation of the lung in about 90% of patients. The incidence is highest in North American blacks and northern European whites; among blacks, women are more frequently affected than men. Onset of disease is usually in the third or fourth decade.

Patients may present with malaise, fever, and dyspnea of insidious onset. Alternatively, sarcoidosis may present with symptoms referable to the skin, eyes, peripheral nerves, liver, or heart. Some patients are asymptomatic and come to medical attention after abnormal findings (typically bilateral hilar and paratracheal lymphadenopathy) on routine chest radiographs. Physical findings in the chest are typical of those associated with interstitial lung involvement, if the parenchyma is involved. Other findings may include skin rashes, erythema nodosum, parotid gland enlargement, hepatosplenomegaly, and lymphadenopathy.

Laboratory tests may show leukopenia, eosinophilia, an elevated erythrocyte sedimentation rate, and hypercalcemia (about 10% of patients) or hypercalciuria (20%). Angiotensin-converting enzyme (ACE) levels are elevated in 40–80% of patients with active sarcoidosis. This finding is neither sensitive nor specific enough to have diagnostic significance. ACE is derived from the cell membrane of epithelioid cells of the sarcoid granuloma. Its synthesis is controlled by T lymphocytes. Physiologic testing may reveal evidence of airflow obstruction, but restrictive changes of decreased lung volumes and diffusing capacity are more common signs. Skin test anergy is present in 70%.

Radiographic findings are variable and include bilateral hilar adenopathy alone (stage I), hilar adenopathy and parenchymal involvement (stage II), or parenchymal involvement alone (stage III). Parenchymal involvement is usually manifested radiographically by diffuse reticular infiltrates, but focal infiltrates, acinar shadows, nodules, and, rarely, cavitation may be seen. Pleural effusion is noted in fewer than 10% of patients.

The diagnosis of sarcoidosis generally requires histologic demonstration of noncaseating granulomas in biopsies from a patient with other typical associated manifestations. Other granulomatous diseases (eg, berylliosis, tuberculosis) must be ruled out. If indicated, biopsy of easily accessible sites, eg, palpable lymph nodes, skin lesions, or salivary glands, is likely to provide positive findings. Transbronchial lung biopsy has a high yield of positive findings, especially in patients with radiographic evidence of parenchymal involvement. Most clinicians would agree that tissue biopsy is not necessary when stage I radiographic findings are detected in a clinical situation that strongly favors the diagnosis of sarcoidosis (eg, a young black female with erythema nodosum). Biopsy is essential whenever clinical and radiographic findings suggest the possibility of an alternative diagnosis such as lymphoma. Bronchoalveolar lavage is useful in following the activity of sarcoidosis in selected patients but does not provide a specific diagnosis.

Indications for treatment with corticosteroids include constitutional symptoms, hypercalcemia, iritis, arthritis, central nervous system involvement, granulomatous hepatitis, cutaneous lesions, and symptomatic pulmonary lesions. Long-term therapy is usually required over months to years. ACE serum levels usually fall with clinical improvement. About 20% of patients with lung involvement suffer irreversible lung impairment. The outlook is best for patients with hilar adenopathy alone; radiographic involvement of the lung parenchyma is associated with a worse prognosis. Death due to pulmonary insufficiency occurs in about 5% of patients.

INTERSTITIAL LUNG INVOLVEMENT IN OTHER DISEASES

Interstitial lung disease that clinically resembles cryptogenic fibrosing alveolitis has been described in a variety of rheumatic diseases. It also occurs with chronic active hepatitis, inflammatory bowel disease, biliary cirrhosis, autoimmune thrombocytopenia, and hemolytic anemia. Although other manifestations of these diseases usually dominate the clinical picture, interstitial lung disease may be symptomatic and progress to respiratory insufficiency, in which case treatment with anti-inflammatory drugs similar to those used in cryptogenic fibrosing alveolitis should be started. Nonspecific interstitial pneumonitis characterized by diffuse alveolar damage but lacking evidence of infection has been reported to account for one-third of all episodes of clinical pneumonitis in patients with AIDS.

Tazelaar HD et al: Interstitial lung disease in polymyositis and dermatomyositis: Clinical features and prognosis as correlated with histologic findings. Am Rev Respir Dis 1990;141:727. (Histologic classification may predict survival better than clinical and radiographic features.)
White DA, Matthay RA: Noninfectious pulmonary complications of infection with the human immunodeficiency virus. Am Rev Respir Dis 1989;140:1763. (Kaposi's sarcoma, non-Hodgkin's lymphoma, and interstitial pneumonitis associated with HIV infection.)

MISCELLANEOUS INFILTRATIVE LUNG DISEASES

PULMONARY ANGIITIS & GRANULOMATOSIS

Wegener's granulomatosis is an idiopathic disease manifested by a combination of glomerulonephritis, necrotizing granulomatous vasculitis of the upper and lower respiratory tracts, and varying degrees of small vessel vasculitis. Complaints of chronic sinusitis is a common presentation; pulmonary symptoms occur less often. Arthralgias, fever, skin rash, and weight loss are frequent symptoms. Multiple nodular infiltrates, often with cavitation, are present on chest radiography. Tracheal stenosis and endobronchial disease are sometimes seen. Antineutrophil cytoplasmic autoantibodies are helpful in diagnosis but are not entirely specific for this disorder. Normochromic, normocytic anemia, mild leukocytosis, and thrombocytosis are common, and virtually all patients have an elevated erythrocyte sedimentation rate. Serum anti-neutrophil cytoplasmic autoantibody (ANCA) levels are elevated in about 95% of patients with active disease and in half that many with disease in remission. This marker is 99% specific for the diagnosis. Establishing a specific diagnosis has traditionally required biopsy of lung, sinus tissue, or kidney with demonstration of necrotizing granulomatous vasculitis. As experience with measurement of serum ANCA levels increases, the role of tissue biopsy in patient management is evolving.

Lymphomatoid granulomatosis is a systemic disease manifested by granulomatous angiitis and a polymorphic cellular infiltrate consisting of atypical lymphocytoid and plasmacytoid cells. Any organs may be involved, but lung, brain, and skin are the most frequently affected. In contrast to Wegener's granulomatosis, the upper airway and kidneys are rarely involved clinically, though histologic evidence of cellular infiltration of the kidneys is frequently seen. The glomeruli are spared. Radiographic manifestations may include multiple nodular infiltrates or diffuse reticular infiltrates. The diagnosis is suggested by the characteristic pattern of lung, brain, and skin involvement and is confirmed by histologic findings. Lymphomatoid granulomatosis has a poor prognosis, since it evolves into malignant lymphoma in nearly half of patients.

Allergic angiitis and granulomatosis (Churg-Strauss syndrome) is an idiopathic multisystem vasculitis of small and medium-sized arteries that occurs in patients with asthma. Histologic features include fibrinoid necrotizing epithelioid and eosinophilic granulomas. The skin and lungs are most often involved, but other organs, including the heart, gastrointestinal tract, liver, and peripheral nerves, may also be affected. Marked peripheral eosinophilia is the rule. Abnormalities on chest radiographs range from transient infiltrates to multiple nodules. This illness may be part of a spectrum that includes polyarteritis nodosa.

Treatment of these disorders consists of combination therapy with corticosteroids and cyclophosphamide. Oral prednisone (1 mg/kg ideal body weight per day initially, tapering slowly to alternate-day therapy over 3–6 months) is the corticosteroid of choice; in Wegener's granulomatosis, some clinicians may omit the use of steroids. For fulminant vasculitis, therapy may be initiated with intravenous methylprednisolone for several days. Cyclophosphamide (2 mg/kg ideal body weight per day initially, with dosage adjustments to avoid neutropenia) is given daily by mouth for at least 1 year after complete remission is obtained. Five-year survival rates in patients with these vasculitis syndromes have been improved to about 90% by the combination therapy.

Complete remissions can be achieved in over 90% of patients with Wegener's granulomatosis. The addition of daily trimethoprim-sulfamethoxazole to standard therapy is currently being investigated.

Cordier JF et al: Pulmonary Wegener's granulomatosis: A clinical and imaging study of 77 cases. Chest 1990; 97:906. (Clinical and radiographic features.)
Hoffman GS et al: Wegener granulomatosis: An analysis of 158 patients. Ann Intern Med 1992;116:488. (Update on experience at NIH.)

ALVEOLAR HEMORRHAGE SYNDROMES

Diffuse alveolar hemorrhage may occur in a variety of immune and nonimmune disorders. Causes of **immune alveolar hemorrhage** have been classified as anti-basement membrane antibody disease (Goodpasture's syndrome), vasculitis and collagen vascular disease (systemic lupus erythematosus and others), idiopathic rapidly progressive glomerulonephritis, chemical or drug-related (penicillamine, trimellitic anhydride), and idiopathic. Hemoptysis, alveolar infiltrates on chest x-ray, anemia, dyspnea, and occasionally fever are characteristic. **Nonimmune disorders** causing diffuse hemorrhage include coagulopathy, mitral stenosis, and necrotizing pulmonary infection. Bronchoalveolar lavage is helpful to determine whether diffuse alveolar hemorrhage has an immune or an infectious basis.

Goodpasture's syndrome is idiopathic recurrent alveolar hemorrhage and rapidly progressive glomerulonephritis. The disease is mediated by anti-glomerular basement membrane antibodies detected as a linear fluorescent pattern on immunofluorescence studies of the lung and kidneys. Goodpasture's syndrome occurs mainly in men who are in their 30s and 40s. Hemoptysis is the usual presenting symptom, but pulmonary hemorrhage may be occult. Dyspnea, cough, hypoxemia, and diffuse bilateral alveolar infiltrates are typical features. Iron deficiency anemia and microscopic hematuria are usually present. The diagnosis is based on characteristic linear IgG deposits in glomeruli by immunofluorescence and on the presence of anti-glomerular basement membrane antibody in serum. The physician should attempt to distinguish Goodpasture's syndrome from other pulmonary-renal syndromes, which include systemic lupus erythematosus, idiopathic rapidly progressive glomerulonephritis, Wegener's granulomatosis, systemic necrotizing vasculitis, and drug-induced disease (penicillamine, trimellitic anhydride). Combinations of immunosuppressive drugs (methylprednisolone with cyclophosphamide) and plasmapheresis have yielded excellent results in recent years. Long-term remissions are occasionally observed.

Idiopathic pulmonary hemosiderosis is a disease

of children or young adults characterized by recurrent pulmonary hemorrhage; in contrast to Goodpasture's syndrome, renal involvement and anti-glomerular basement membrane antibodies are absent. Treatment of acute episodes of hemorrhage with corticosteroids may be useful. Recurrent episodes of pulmonary hemorrhage may result in interstitial fibrosis.

PULMONARY ALVEOLAR PROTEINOSIS

Pulmonary alveolar proteinosis is a disease in which a phospholipid material similar to surfactant accumulates within alveolar spaces. The condition may be primary (idiopathic) or secondary (occurring in immune deficiency; following lung infections, including tuberculosis and viral infections). Progressive dyspnea is the usual presenting symptom, and chest x-ray shows bilateral alveolar infiltrates suggestive of pulmonary edema. The diagnosis is based on demonstration of characteristic intra-alveolar phospholipid on open lung biopsy.

The course of the disease varies; some patients experience spontaneous remission, whereas in others, progressive respiratory insufficiency develops. Pulmonary infection with *Nocardia* or fungi may occur. Therapy for alveolar proteinosis consists of periodic whole lung lavage, which is effective in reducing exertional dyspnea.

EOSINOPHILIC PNEUMONIA

The term "eosinophilic pneumonia" denotes a syndrome characterized by peripheral lung infiltrates shown to be eosinophilic by bronchoalveolar lavage or lung biopsy. Blood eosinophilia is present in most cases. Symptoms may be mild and transient and can include fever, cough, and wheezing (Löffler's syndrome); or severe and progressive (chronic eosinophilic pneumonia). Fever, weight loss, and dyspnea may occur in chronic eosinophilic pneumonia. A severe acute form of eosinophilic pneumonia has recently been described, characterized by fever, respiratory failure, a high percentage of eosinophils in bronchoalveolar lavage fluid, rapid response to treatment with erythromycin and corticosteroids, and lack of recurrence.

Eosinophilic pneumonia may be associated with exposure to various drugs or infestation with roundworm parasites such as filariae, *Ascaris* (Löffler's syndrome), or *Strongyloides*. No precipitating cause may be apparent in as many as one-third of cases. If an extrinsic cause is identified, therapy consists of removal of the offending drug or treatment of the underlying parasitic infestation. Corticosteroid treatment should be instituted if no treatable extrinsic cause is discovered. The response to corticosteroids is usually dramatic. Recurrences are common.

Allen JN et al: Acute eosinophilic pneumonia as a reversible cause of noninfectious respiratory failure. N Engl J Med 1989;321:569. (A hypersensitivity basis is proposed.)

DISORDERS OF THE PULMONARY CIRCULATION

PULMONARY THROMBOEMBOLISM

Essentials of Diagnosis

- Predisposition to venous thrombosis, usually of the lower extremities.
- Abrupt onset of dyspnea, chest pain, apprehension, hemoptysis, or syncope.
- Acute respiratory alkalosis and hypoxemia in most patients.
- Characteristic defects on ventilation-perfusion lung scan.
- Diagnostic findings on pulmonary angiogram.

General Considerations

Pulmonary emboli arise from thrombi in the venous circulation or right side of the heart (thromboembolism), from tumors that have invaded the venous circulation (tumor emboli), or from other sources (amniotic fluid, air, fat, bone marrow, and foreign intravenous material).

Pulmonary thromboembolism is associated with as many as 200,000 deaths per year; about 10% of victims die within the first hour. Fewer than 10% of patients who die of pulmonary embolism have received treatment for the condition, a fact underscoring the difficulty encountered in diagnosis.

More than 90% of pulmonary emboli originate as clots in the deep veins of the lower extremities. Most deep venous thrombi originate in the calves, and some 80% of these spontaneously resolve without embolizing. The remainder may propagate into the iliofemoral veins. Fracture of the propagating thrombus in these proximal veins allows a clot to migrate into the inferior vena cava and ultimately to the lungs. One-third to one-half of patients with deep venous thrombosis of the iliofemoral system have clinically significant pulmonary embolism.

Physiologic risk factors for venous thrombosis include venous stasis, venous endothelial injury, and hypercoagulability (eg, oral contraceptives, cancer, protein C or S deficiency, and antithrombin III deficiency). Clinical risk factors include prolonged bed rest or inactivity, surgery, childbirth, advanced age, stroke, myocardial infarction, congestive heart failure, obesity, and fractures of the hip or femur. Occasionally, in situ thrombosis in the pulmonary arteries occurs without embolization; predisposing factors include sickle cell anemia, chest trauma, and certain congenital cardiac anomalies.

Discharge of thrombus into the pulmonary artery has both hemodynamic and pulmonary consequences. The hemodynamic consequences of pulmonary thromboembolism are related to mechanical obstruction of the pulmonary vascular bed and neurohumoral reflexes causing vasoconstriction. Both factors result in increased pulmonary vascular resistance and, in severe cases, pulmonary hypertension and right ventricular failure. The pulmonary consequences of thromboembolism result from reflex bronchoconstriction in the embolized lung zone, wasted ventilation (increased physiologic dead space), and loss of alveolar surfactant. Frank pulmonary infarction is uncommon.

Clinical Findings

A. Symptoms and Signs: The clinical findings in acute pulmonary thromboembolism (Table 9–13) depend on the size of the embolus and the patient's preexisting cardiopulmonary status. In pulmonary embolism that is less than massive, clot obstructs less than two-thirds of the pulmonary arterial tree. In *massive* pulmonary embolism, acute right ventricular failure and systemic hypotension result. Recognizing pulmonary thromboembolism is more difficult in patients with underlying cardiopulmonary disease. No single symptom or sign or combination of clinical

findings is pathognomonic of pulmonary thromboembolism.

Symptoms of pulmonary thromboembolism include chest pain, which is often pleuritic, dyspnea, apprehension, cough, hemoptysis, and diaphoresis. Pulmonary embolism occasionally presents as syncope, especially in patients with massive pulmonary embolism.

The signs of pulmonary thromboembolism include tachycardia, tachypnea, crackles, and accentuation of the pulmonary component of the second heart sound. Low-grade fever occurs in about 40% of cases. Thrombophlebitis, diaphoresis, and right-sided cardiac gallop each are noted in about a third of cases. Cyanosis, wheezing, and cardiac arrhythmias are noted in fewer than one-fourth of cases. Shock is unusual. Signs and symptoms do not generally differ between massive and less severe thromboembolism. Pulmonary embolism may mimic pneumonia, myocardial infarction, pneumothorax, and even rib fractures. The clinician should be alert to other conditions that mimic thrombophlebitis of the calf, including cellulitis, muscle strain or rupture, lymphangitis, and rupture of a Baker's cyst.

B. Laboratory Findings: The results of routine laboratory tests are not helpful in diagnosing pulmonary thromboembolism. Arterial blood gas measurements usually reveal acute respiratory alkalosis due to hyperventilation. About 90% of patients with proved pulmonary embolism have an arterial PO_2 under 80 mm Hg. Electrocardiographic findings are likewise not diagnostic. Nearly all patients with pulmonary thromboembolism have an abnormal ECG. Tachycardia and nonspecific ST–T wave changes are the most common abnormalities, being noted in about 44% and 35–49% of cases, respectively. A pattern of acute right heart strain (S_1Q_3, T wave inversion in leads V_{1-3}) is more characteristic but uncommon. Right axis deviation, right bundle branch block, clockwise rotation, and P pulmonale each are seen in less than 10% of cases of documented pulmonary thromboembolism. Standard pulmonary function tests are helpful only in consideration of alternative diagnoses. Specialized pulmonary function tests may reveal a nonspecific increase in wasted ventilation (increased physiologic dead space) and a failure of the ratio of tidal volume to dead space to fall with exercise, but such tests are not useful clinically.

C. Imaging and Special Examinations:

1. Chest radiography–The chest radiograph is usually abnormal in patients with pulmonary embolism, but the abnormalities are often related to chronic pulmonary or cardiac disease. No pathognomonic findings are present. Elevation of a hemidiaphragm and pulmonary infiltration are the most common abnormalities. Plate-like atelectasis, oligemia in the embolized lung zone (Westermark sign), and prominence of the pulmonary artery are sometimes seen. A small unilateral pleural effusion is oc-

Table 9–13. Incidence of symptoms and signs of angiographically proved pulmonary thromboembolism in 327 patients.[1]

	(%)
Symptoms	
Chest pain	88
Pleuritic	(74)
Nonpleuritic	(14)
Dyspnea	84
Apprehension	59
Cough	53
Hemoptysis	30
Sweats	27
Syncope	13
Signs	
Respiratory rate >16/min	92
Crackles	58
Accentuated S_2P	53
Pulse > 100/min	44
Temperature > 37.8°C	43
Phlebitis	32
Gallop	34
Diaphoresis	36
Edema	24
Murmur	23
Cyanosis	19

[1]Data from Bell WR, Simon TL, DeMets DL: The clinical features of submassive and massive pulmonary emboli. Am J Med 1977;62:355.

casionally present. A homogeneous, wedge-shaped density based on the pleura and pointing toward the hilum (Hampton's hump) is highly suggestive of pulmonary infarction but is uncommon.

2. Lung scanning–Most if not all patients with suspected pulmonary embolism should undergo a perfusion scan. Though perfusion lung scans may be abnormal in other diseases, including COPD, asthma, pneumonia, and heart failure, their results may be used to direct subsequent pulmonary arteriography and reduce the load of contrast media in these patients. A ventilation scan may be performed prior to the perfusion scan if concurrent disease of the airways or lung parenchyma is present.

A combined ventilation-perfusion lung scan is usually obtained. Results are interpreted as being normal, low probability, intermediate probability, or high probability for the presence of a pulmonary thromboembolism. Criteria for these interpretations are complex and are summarized by the PIOPED investigators (see JAMA 1990;263:2753).

Some important principles underlie lung scan interpretation. First, a normal perfusion scan rules out clinically significant pulmonary thromboembolism, and no further diagnostic studies are necessary. A perfusion scan is normal if no perfusion defects are present or if the perfusion pattern matches exactly the shape of the lungs as shown on the chest x-ray. A high-probability ventilation-perfusion lung scan is one in which two or more large (or four or more moderate) segmental perfusion defects are present without corresponding ventilation defects or abnormalities on the chest x-ray or are substantially larger than those abnormalities. Interpretation of low and intermediate probabilities requires more expertise. Consultation with a specialist in nuclear medicine is advised when interpreting lung scans.

It is important to recognize that a "low-probability" ventilation-perfusion scan *does not rule out pulmonary thromboembolism.* Between 14% and 31% of patients with such scans demonstrate pulmonary thromboemboli when pulmonary angiograms are performed. However, a high probability (85–90%) of pulmonary embolism exists when there is a lobar perfusion defect with ventilation mismatch. One-third of patients with an "intermediate probability" lung scan have positive pulmonary angiograms. Because of the high frequency of pulmonary embolism in patients with "low" or "intermediate" probability lung scan interpretations, some experts have advocated abandoning the current lung scan classification system and reporting scans as either normal, nondiagnostic, or of high probability. The diagnostic value of lung scanning is enhanced greatly when combined with the clinical estimate of the likelihood of pulmonary embolism or with the results of noninvasive studies for proximal deep vein thrombosis. For example, in patients with low-probability lung scans, pulmonary embolism is present in 40% of those with a high clinical suspicion of pulmonary thromboembolism but only 4% of those with a low clinical suspicion (PIOPED, 1990).

3. Venous thrombosis studies–Because the history and physical examination are neither sensitive nor specific in detecting thrombi in the deep veins of the lower extremities, specific tests such as contrast venography, impedance plethysmography, and duplex ultrasonography are necessary (see Chapter 12). None of these tests is ideal, and there is no consensus about which should be used. However, documentation of deep venous thrombosis in a patient with suspected pulmonary thromboembolism may preclude the need for pulmonary angiography.

Because of its high sensitivity and specificity, contrast venography remains the "gold standard" in testing for venous thrombosis. An intraluminal filling defect is pathognomonic of venous thrombosis. However, about 30% of patients with angiographically proved pulmonary embolism have negative contrast venograms. Disadvantages of contrast venography include discomfort, difficulty in interpretation, expense, difficult technical requirements, and complications such as phlebitis in 3–4% of patients. It is less accurate below the knee. Impedance plethysmography has both a sensitivity and a specificity of about 95% in the detection of thrombi in the popliteal, femoral, and iliac veins. Serial impedance plethysmography is a safe, effective, noninvasive, and inexpensive approach to detection of proximal thrombi in outpatients with suspected acute deep venous thrombosis. Duplex ultrasonography is an alternative approach with similar sensitivity and specificity. Impedance plethysmography and duplex ultrasonography may not detect proximal vein thrombi if obstruction is not complete, and neither method is sensitive in detection of thrombi in calf veins. However, either study may be used to follow the patient for propagation of a calf vein thrombus into the popliteal vein. ^{125}I fibrinogen leg scanning is very sensitive in detecting fresh thrombi in calf, popliteal, and lower thigh veins. It is not sensitive to thrombi above the mid thigh and requires 24 hours for interpretation. For these reasons it has become less popular than the impedance plethysmography and duplex ultrasonography. Bilateral radionuclide venography has a sensitivity similar to that of contrast venography but lacks its specificity. This procedure may be combined with perfusion lung scanning and does not cause phlebitis.

If the physician suspects deep venous thrombosis, intravenous heparin should be started and a noninvasive study ordered. Impedance plethysmography and duplex ultrasonography are currently the noninvasive methods of choice. If either is positive, continued treatment is advised. If the noninvasive study is negative, it should be repeated serially (every 2 days for 7–10 days) until a positive result is obtained; if the results are repeatedly negative, therapy may be terminated. Contrast venography is advised if the non-invasive study yields equivocal results.

The sensitivity and specificity of various studies for the detection of deep venous thrombosis depend upon the expertise of the team performing the studies. Thus, practitioners should be aware of which studies are most likely to be accurate in the setting of their own practice.

4. Pulmonary angiography–Pulmonary angiography—which can detect emboli as small as 3 mm in diameter—remains the definitive test for diagnosis of pulmonary embolism because of its high sensitivity and specificity. Emboli smaller than 3 mm in diameter are unlikely to be of clinical significance. The finding of an intraluminal defect or an arterial cutoff on the pulmonary angiogram is diagnostic. Oligemia and asymmetry of blood flow are suggestive but not specific. After 5 days, negative results on angiography do not rule out the possibility that an embolism has occurred.

Pulmonary angiography is expensive and invasive, occasionally difficult to interpret, and may be associated with complications; in experienced hands, however, the procedure is associated with a morbidity and mortality rate of less than 1%. The procedure is advised when the diagnosis of pulmonary embolism must be established with certainty, as in situations where anticoagulation is considered especially risky. Ventilation-perfusion lung scans of "intermediate" probability for pulmonary thromboembolism are frequently encountered. Moreover, lung scans of suboptimal quality because of patient performance and technical limitations are commonplace. In these situations, pulmonary angiography is often valuable. Pulmonary angiography is required if any type of surgical procedure for prevention of recurrent thromboemboli is planned, eg, interruption of the inferior vena cava. It is indicated in patients with suspected embolism whenever the diagnosis remains in doubt after preliminary studies (clinical evaluation, lung scans, tests for deep venous thrombosis) have been performed. Relative contraindications include severe pulmonary hypertension, ventricular arrhythmias, left bundle branch block, and renal failure. As in the use of radiocontrast materials for any purpose, precautions must be taken to prevent radiocontrast-induced acute renal failure and allergic reactions.

Prevention

Prevention of deep venous thrombosis and pulmonary thromboembolism may be accomplished by using physical measures, low-dose heparin, and antiplatelet drugs in patients at risk.

Intraoperative and postoperative intermittent external pneumatic compression of the legs is recommended for patients undergoing neurosurgery, urologic surgery, or major hip or knee surgery. Early ambulation after surgery, elevation of the legs for immobilized patients, and active and passive leg exer-cises are reasonable approaches to preventing deep venous thrombosis.

Low-dose heparin is of proved benefit in reducing the risk of deep vein thrombosis and fatal pulmonary embolism in general surgery patients; in patients undergoing surgery of the thorax, abdomen, or extremities; in patients who have suffered myocardial infarction, respiratory failure, and acute spinal cord injury; and in patients with stroke. If low-dose heparin is indicated, 5000 units subcutaneously is given every 8–12 hours, beginning 2 hours before surgery or upon admission to the hospital and continuing until the risk for deep vein thrombosis has lessened. Continuous monitoring of clotting studies is not necessary, though the partial thromboplastin time and platelet count should be checked occasionally, since some patients show increased sensitivity to heparin. Low-dose heparin is not effective in preventing pulmonary embolism in patients with major long bone fractures or those undergoing hip surgery or above-the-knee amputation. Intravenous dextran, adjusted-dose heparin, and moderate-dose warfarin are effective approaches to prophylaxis against postoperative venous thrombosis in these high-risk patients. The *adjusted-dose* heparin regimen is to administer just enough heparin subcutaneously every 8 hours to maintain the activated partial thromboplastin time, measured 6 hours after injection, at 31.5–36 seconds. The *moderate-dose* warfarin protocol raises the prothrombin time to an international normalized ratio (INR) of 2.0–3.0 (1.3–1.5 times control, using rabbit brain thromboplastin). Recent studies suggest that low-molecular-weight heparin slightly reduces the rate of deep venous thrombosis in patients undergoing elective hip surgery and may be superior to standard heparin in preventing thromboembolism after spinal cord injury. Furthermore, low-molecular-weight heparin is less hemorrhagic than standard heparin. Low-molecular-weight heparin is superior to standard heparin in reducing the risks of deep venous thrombosis and pulmonary thromboembolism in patients undergoing orthopedic surgery. However, further studies of this agent are needed before its routine use can be recommended for prevention of deep venous thrombosis. Antiplatelet drugs such as aspirin are not recommended for the prevention (or treatment) of venous thrombosis or pulmonary thromboembolism.

Treatment

A. Anticoagulation: Anticoagulation for established pulmonary embolism is preventive rather than definitive therapy. For acute pulmonary thromboembolism or proximal (thigh) deep venous thrombosis, heparin is the anticoagulant of choice. Distal (calf) deep venous thrombosis does not require systemic anticoagulation *if* coexisting proximal deep venous thrombosis has been excluded by noninvasive studies or contrast venography. In the absence of such evidence, anticoagulation for 3 months is advised for isolated calf vein thrombosis. Heparin inhibits thrombin and other clotting factors by potentiating antithrombin III; it does not dissolve established thrombi but does prevent their distal propagation. Heparin reduces the rate of recurrence of pulmonary embolism; it may reduce the incidence of death due to recurrence.

Heparin is given intravenously by continuous infusion. Intermittent subcutaneous heparin is clearly less effective in patients with acute proximal deep vein thrombosis. After a loading dose of 5000–10,000 units by bolus intravenous injection, the drug is given at a rate of 1000–1500 units/h. The activated partial thromboplastin time is determined 4–6 hours after therapy has been started and is maintained at 1.5–2.5 times the pretreatment control value until it has stabilized; the requirements for heparin are greater early in the clinical course. The platelet count is monitored every 2–3 days, because heparin may induce thrombocytopenia.

Oral anticoagulant therapy with warfarin may be started concurrently with heparin. A recent study suggests that institution of warfarin on the first day of anticoagulation with heparin is as effective as the old practice of instituting it several days later. Earlier hospital discharge and cost savings under should occur from this change in practice. Heparin is usually continued for at least 5 days in order to allow time for warfarin to exert its full anticoagulant effects. Warfarin alters the synthesis of vitamin K-dependent procoagulants (factors II, VII, IX, and X) and proteins C and S and requires 6–7 days to achieve full effectiveness. Begin treatment with 10 mg of warfarin daily (usually for 3–5 days) until the prothrombin time is 1.3–1.5 times control (using North American thromboplastin), which corresponds to an international normalized ratio (INR) of 2.0–3.0. Maintenance therapy with warfarin may require 2–15 mg daily, the required dose varying widely among patients. If warfarin is contraindicated or inconvenient, subcutaneous heparin may be substituted for warfarin, the dose being adjusted to maintain an activated partial thromboplastin time of 1.5 times the control value at the mid-dosing interval. Warfarin is contraindicated in pregnancy. Alterations in the prothrombin time in patients receiving warfarin may be caused by a number of drugs (Table 9–14). These effects require the physician to change the dose of warfarin and monitor the prothrombin time closely.

The duration of warfarin therapy after thromboembolic disease has been diagnosed depends on the individual patient's clinical situation, and insufficient data have accrued to define the optimal duration of therapy for each circumstance. If risk factors such as oral contraceptive use or immobility following a bone fracture have been eliminated, warfarin therapy for 1–3 months is reasonable. A minimum of 3 months of therapy is advised if risk factors cannot be quickly eliminated, as in patients with congestive

Table 9–14. Some important drugs that alter the prothrombin time in patients taking warfarin.

Prothrombin Time Increased By	Prothrombin Time Decreased By
Allopurinol	Aminoglutethimide
p-Aminosalicylic acid	Antihistamines
Amiodarone	Barbiturates
Androgens	Carbamazepine
Antibiotics	Contraceptives, oral
Tetracyclines	Diuretics
Some cephalosporins	Ethchlorvynol
(especially cefamandole,	Glutethimide
cefaperazone, moxalac-	Griseofulvin
tam)	Rifampin
Erythromycin	Vitamin K (in polyvitamin
Chloramphenicol	preparations and some
Metronidazole	diets)
Sulfonamides	
Chloral hydrate	
Cimetidine	
Clofibrate	
Disulfiram	
Glucagon	
Heparin (Quick test increased;	
no effect on prothrombin-	
proconvertin [P and P] test)	
Indomethacin	
Mefenamic acid	
Nalidixic acid	
Naproxen	
Phenylbutazone	
Phenytoin	
Propylthiouracil	
Quinidine	
Quinine	
Salicylates (> 3–5 g/d)	
Sufinpyrazone	
Thyroid hormones	

heart failure, prolonged immobility, or venous stasis. If the patient has continuing, unresolvable risk factors, such as cancer, antithrombin III deficiency, or protein C deficiency, or a second pulmonary embolism after discontinuance of warfarin, permanent anticoagulant therapy is recommended.

The major risk of anticoagulant therapy is bleeding. Independent risk factors for in-hospital bleeding in patients started on long-term anticoagulant therapy include comorbid disorders such as heart, liver, and kidney disease; the use of heparin in patients over age 60; unusually prolonged prothrombin or partial thromboplastin times; and worsening liver function. Major hemorrhage occurs in about 5% of patients receiving intravenous heparin, and the death rate is 0.6%. The risk of hemorrhage is increased in women over 60 years of age and in patients taking aspirin. The rate of major hemorrhage is similar for warfarin (2–10%), but serious hemorrhage is unusual in patients with adequately controlled prothrombin times (1.3–1.5 × control value, or INR 2.0–3.0). Longer prothrombin times invite more bleeding complications without enhancing efficacy. Subcutaneous heparin, administered in adjusted doses, may be as effective as warfarin in long-term treatment of deep venous thrombosis and is less likely to cause bleeding.

B. Thrombolytic Therapy: Lysis of pulmonary thromboemboli in situ represents the only available definitive medical treatment and is achieved by use of streptokinase, urokinase, and recombinant tissue plasminogen activator, which enhance endogenous fibrinolysis by activating plasminogen, thereby generating plasmin. Plasmin directly lyses thrombi both in the pulmonary artery and in the venous circulation and also has a secondary anticoagulant effect. Thrombolytic therapy, when compared to heparin alone, accelerates the resolution of pulmonary emboli, reduces pulmonary artery and right heart pressures, and improves right and left ventricular function in patients with established pulmonary embolism. Thrombolytic therapy may also preserve the anatomy and function of the valves in deep veins of the lower extremities. It has not been proved to affect the mortality rate from pulmonary thromboembolism, however. Critics of thrombolytic therapy point to its high cost compared to heparin therapy, lack of evidence of improved survival, and risks of bleeding.

The use of thrombolytic therapy in clinical practice is controversial. Most physicians reserve its use for patients with acute massive pulmonary embolism confirmed by pulmonary angiography and for selected patients with established deep venous thrombosis. Suitable candidates for thrombolytic therapy include patients with hemodynamic compromise due to pulmonary embolism, those with underlying severe cardiopulmonary disease, those with hemodynamic instability when surgical embolectomy is not available, and those who fail to show hemodynamic improvement after heparin therapy.

Care and expertise in monitoring therapy, managing bleeding, and controlling subsequent anticoagulation are essential. The duration of symptoms prior to starting thrombolytic therapy should be less than 7 days. Puncture of noncompressible arteries or veins, or intramuscular injections are not permitted during thrombolytic therapy. Anticoagulants and antiplatelet drugs should not be given concurrently. Absolute contraindications to thrombolytic therapy include active internal bleeding and recent (within 2 months) cerebrovascular accident. Other major contraindications include severe hypertension, recent trauma, gastrointestinal bleeding, and major surgical or obstetric procedures. Hemorrhage is the major complication of thrombolytic therapy and can usually be avoided by strict adherence to treatment guidelines. Intracranial bleeding has occurred in 0.3–0.7% of patients given thrombolytic therapy for myocardial infarction.

Urokinase or streptokinase is given as a continuous intravenous infusion by an infusion pump. Streptokinase is usually preferred because it is less expensive, but development of antibodies may prevent future use of the drug. Streptokinase, 250,000 units intravenously over 30 minutes as a loading dose, is followed by a maintenance dose of 100,000 units/h for 24–72 hours. Urokinase is given as a 2000 units/lb loading dose over 10 minutes, followed by continuous infusion of 2000 units/lb/h for 12–24 hours. A thrombin time or activated partial thromboplastin time is usually checked 2–4 hours after starting an infusion of streptokinase or urokinase to ensure that fibrinolysis has occurred, as indicated by prolongation of either test by 10 seconds or more. Administration of intravenous heparin is resumed upon completion of thrombolytic therapy. Recombinant tissue plasminogen activator is administered by peripheral vein in a dose of 100 mg over 2 hours. Bolus therapy with recombinant tissue plasminogen activator is now being investigated. No tests of coagulation are needed during infusion of recombinant tissue plasminogen activator.

C. Additional Measures: Surgical interruption of the inferior vena cava is indicated when recurrent pulmonary embolism would be life-threatening in a patient with major contraindications to anticoagulation or failure or complications of anticoagulant or thrombolytic therapy. Life-threatening paradoxic thromboembolism or septic thromboembolism may also justify surgical interruption, which may be achieved by ligation, plication, clipping, and insertion of intraluminal filters in the inferior vena cava just below the renal veins. Percutaneous transjugular placement of a filter has become the preferred mode of inferior vena cava interruption when the patient is at continued risk for recurrent pulmonary thromboembolism from pelvic or lower extremity thrombi. The risks of recurrent pulmonary thromboembolism and inferior vena cava occlusion after filter placement are low (2–3%). Infrequent complications have included inferior vena cava thrombosis or trapping of thrombi, hematoma at the insertion site, and, if improper technique has been used, filter migration and perforation of the vena cava wall.

Surgical removal of acute pulmonary embolism (pulmonary embolectomy) is now rarely performed. The mortality rate of this procedure approaches 50%.

Prognosis

Pulmonary embolism may cause sudden death, though the prognosis for survivors is generally favorable. The prognosis depends on the underlying disease and on proper diagnosis and treatment. The mortality rate in patients with undiagnosed pulmonary thromboembolism is about 30%. After diagnosis and treatment of pulmonary thromboembolism, death from a recurrence is unusual, occurring in less than 3% of cases. Perfusion defects resolve in most survivors. Pulmonary hypertension may be a complication of chronic recurrent pulmonary thromboembolism.

Carson JL et al: The clinical course of pulmonary embolism. N Engl J Med 1992;326:1240. (The recurrence rate within 1 year after treatment is 8.3% and the death rate from recurrences 2.5%, mostly within 2 weeks after the original diagnosis.)

Dalen JE, Hirsh J (editors): American College of Chest Physicians: Third ACCP Conference on Antithrombotic Therapy. Chest 1992;102(Suppl):S1. (Consensus conference on antithrombotic therapy, emphasizing cardiovascular disease.)

Goldhaber SZ: Evolving concepts in thrombolytic therapy for pulmonary embolism. Chest 1992;101(Suppl):183S.

Goldhaber SZ: Recent advances in the diagnosis and lytic therapy of pulmonary embolism. Chest 1991;99:173S. (Current thinking following the PIOPED study.)

Hirsh J: Heparin. N Engl J Med 1991;324:1565. (Pharmacology and clinical use.)

Hirsh J: Oral anticoagulant drugs. N Engl J Med 1991; 324:1865. (Pharmacology and clinical use of warfarin.)

Hyers TN et al: Antithrombotic therapy for venous thromboembolic disease. Chest 1992;102(4 Suppl):408S.

Levine MN et al: Hemorrhagic complications of anticoagulant therapy. Chest 1992;102(4 Suppl):352S. (Complications of heparin and oral anticoagulants with recommendations for prevention.)

Moser KM: Venous thromboembolism. Am Rev Respir Dis 1990;141:235. (Diagnosis, prevention, and treatment.)

Value of the ventilation/perfusion scan in acute pulmonary embolism: Results of the prospective investigation of pulmonary embolism diagnosis (PIOPED). JAMA 1990; 263:2753. (The high-probability scan is only 41% sensitive in detecting pulmonary thromboembolism.)

PULMONARY HYPERTENSION

Essentials of Diagnosis

- Dyspnea, fatigue, chest pain, and occasionally syncope on exertion.
- Narrow splitting of second heart sound with loud pulmonary component; findings of right ventricular hypertrophy and cardiac failure in advanced disease.
- Hypoxemia: wasted ventilation on pulmonary function tests in most cases.
- Electrocardiographic evidence of right ventricular strain or hypertrophy and right atrial enlargement.
- Enlarged central pulmonary arteries on chest x-ray.

General Considerations

The pulmonary circulation is unique because of its high blood flow, low pressure (normally 25/8 mm Hg, mean 12), and low resistance (normally 200–250 dynes/sec/cm^{-5}). It can accommodate large increases in blood flow during exercise with only modest increases in pressure because of its ability to recruit and distend blood vessels. The normal pulmonary circulation is also largely passive, since its pressures are determined mainly by the function of the right and left ventricles. Contraction of smooth muscle in the walls of pulmonary arteriolar resistance vessels becomes an important factor in numerous pathologic states.

Pulmonary hypertension is present when pulmonary artery pressure rises to a high level inappropriate for a given level of cardiac output. **Primary (idiopathic) pulmonary hypertension** (see Chapter 10) is a rare disorder of the pulmonary circulation occurring mostly in young and middle-aged women; it is characterized by progressive dyspnea, a rapid downhill course, and an invariably fatal outcome. This condition is also called plexogenic pulmonary arteriopathy, in reference to the characteristic histopathologic plexiform lesion found in muscular pulmonary arteries. Secondary pulmonary hypertension is more common.

Selected mechanisms responsible for pulmonary hypertension and examples of corresponding clinical conditions are set forth in Table 9–15. Pulmonary hypertension is usually caused by reduction of the cross-sectional area of the pulmonary vasculature at the arterial, capillary, or venous level. Hypoxia of any cause is the most important and potent stimulus of pulmonary arterial vasoconstriction. The mechanisms by which hypoxia causes pulmonary hypertension are poorly understood. Factors operating at the alveolar level and direct stimulation of arteriolar smooth muscle have been implicated. Recent interest has focused on the release of vasoactive substances from the endothelial cells of pulmonary arteries, such as endothelium-derived relaxing factor and endothelin-1, a potent vasoconstrictor peptide. Hypoxia

Table 9–15. Mechanisms of pulmonary hypertension and examples of corresponding clinical conditions.

Reduction in cross-sectional area of pulmonary arterial bed
Vasoconstriction
Hypoxia of any cause
Acidosis
Loss of vessels
Lung resection
Emphysema
Vasculitis
Pulmonary fibrosis
Connective tissue disease
Obstruction of vessels
Pulmonary embolism (thromboemboli, tumor emboli, foreign body emboli, etc)
In situ thrombosis
Schistosomiasis
Narrowing of vessels
Secondary structural changes due to pulmonary hypertension
Increased pulmonary venous pressure
Constrictive pericarditis
Left ventricular failure or reduced compliance
Mitral stenosis
Left atrial myxoma
Pulmonary veno-occlusive disease
Mediastinal diseases compressing pulmonary veins
Increased pulmonary blood flow
Congenital left-to-right intracardiac shunts
Increased blood viscosity
Polycythemia
Miscellaneous
Pulmonary hypertension occurring in association with hepatic cirrhosis and portal hypertension

is partially or fully responsible for the pulmonary hypertension observed in chronic bronchitis, infiltrative lung disease due to various causes, kyphoscoliosis, obesity-hypoventilation syndrome, chronic mountain sickness, obstructive sleep apnea, and neuromuscular disease. Acidosis is also a potent stimulus of pulmonary arterial vasoconstriction and exerts a synergistic vasoconstrictive effect with hypoxia.

Extensive obliteration and obstruction of the pulmonary arterial tree may cause pulmonary hypertension. Once present, pulmonary hypertension is self-perpetuating. It introduces secondary structural abnormalities in pulmonary vessels, including smooth muscle hypertrophy and intimal proliferation, and these may eventually stimulate atheromatous changes and in situ thrombosis, leading to further narrowing of the arterial bed.

Increased pulmonary venous pressure, when sustained, may cause "postcapillary" pulmonary hypertension; left ventricular failure is the most common cause.

Pulmonary veno-occlusive disease is a rare cause of postcapillary pulmonary hypertension occurring in children and young adults. The cause is unknown, but associations with various conditions such as viral infection, bone marrow transplantation, chemotherapy, and malignancy have been described. The disease is characterized by progressive fibrotic occlusion of pulmonary veins and venules, along with secondary hypertensive changes in the pulmonary arterioles and muscular pulmonary arteries. Nodular areas of pulmonary congestion, edema, hemorrhage, and hemosiderosis are found. Chest radiography reveals prominent, symmetric interstitial markings, Kerley B lines, pulmonary artery dilation, and normally sized left atrium and left ventricle. Premortem diagnosis is often difficult but is occasionally established by open lung biopsy. There is no effective therapy, and most patients die within 2 years as a result of progressive pulmonary hypertension.

Pulmonary hypertension is readily recognized when an obvious cause, such as severe COPD, is present. In adults, pulmonary hypertension in the absence of COPD is often caused by chronic pulmonary thromboembolism, interstitial fibrosis, sleep apnea, or obesity-hypoventilation syndrome. Other disorders listed in Table 9–15 should be excluded before the diagnosis of primary pulmonary hypertension is entertained.

Clinical Findings

A. Symptoms and Signs: Secondary pulmonary hypertension is difficult to recognize clinically in the early stages, when symptoms and signs are primarily those of the underlying disease. Pulmonary hypertension may cause or contribute to dyspnea, which is present initially on exertion and later at rest. Dull, retrosternal chest pain resembling angina pectoris may be present. Fatigue and syncope on exertion

also occur, presumably a result of reduced cardiac output related to elevated pulmonary artery pressures or bradycardia.

The signs of pulmonary hypertension include narrow splitting of the second heart sound, accentuation of the pulmonary component of the second heart sound, and a systolic ejection click. In advanced cases, tricuspid and pulmonary valve insufficiency and signs of right ventricular failure and cor pulmonale are found.

B. Laboratory Findings: Polycythemia is found in many cases of pulmonary hypertension that are associated with chronic hypoxemia. Electrocardiographic changes are those of right axis deviation, right ventricular hypertrophy, right ventricular strain, or right atrial enlargement.

C. Imaging and Special Examinations: Radiographic findings depend on the cause of pulmonary hypertension. In chronic disease, dilation of the right and left main and lobar pulmonary arteries and enlargement of the pulmonary outflow tract are seen; in advanced disease, right ventricular and right atrial enlargement are seen. Peripheral "pruning" of large pulmonary arteries is characteristic of pulmonary hypertension in severe emphysema.

Echocardiography is helpful in evaluating patients thought to have mitral stenosis, left atrial myxoma, and pulmonary valvular disease. Echocardiography may also reveal right ventricular enlargement and paradoxic motion of the interventricular septum. Doppler ultrasonography is a reliable noninvasive means of estimating systolic pulmonary artery pressure. However, other precise hemodynamic measurements can only be obtained with right heart catheterization, which is often helpful when postcapillary pulmonary hypertension, intracardiac shunting, or thromboembolic disease is considered as part of the differential diagnosis.

Routine pulmonary function tests reveal no findings diagnostic of pulmonary hypertension. Diminution of the pulmonary capillary bed may cause reduction in the single breath diffusing capacity.

Depending upon the suspected cause of pulmonary hypertension, ventilation-perfusion lung scanning, pulmonary angiography, and open lung biopsy are occasionally helpful. Ventilation-perfusion lung scanning is very helpful in identifying patients with pulmonary hypertension caused by recurrent pulmonary thromboemboli. Transbronchial biopsy carries an increased risk of bleeding.

Treatment

Treatment of primary pulmonary hypertension is discussed in Chapter 10. Treatment of secondary pulmonary hypertension consists mainly of treating the underlying disorder, such as COPD, sleep apnea, obesity-hypoventilation syndrome, and mitral stenosis. Early recognition of pulmonary hypertension is crucial to interrupt the self-perpetuating cycle responsible for the rapid progression of this disorder. By the time most patients present with signs and symptoms of pulmonary hypertension, however, the condition is far advanced. If hypoxemia or acidosis is detected, corrective measures should be started immediately. Supplemental oxygen administered for at least 15 hours per day has been demonstrated to be of benefit in patients with hypoxemic COPD.

Other disorders responsible for pulmonary hypertension should be treated appropriately. Patients with documented recurrent pulmonary thromboembolism should receive permanent anticoagulation therapy; some clinicians employ this therapy in pulmonary hypertension of unknown cause, since multiple, very small pulmonary emboli may produce this picture and be difficult to recognize clinically. Postcapillary pulmonary hypertension usually responds to treatment of the underlying cardiac disease.

Vasodilator therapy using various pharmacologic agents (eg, calcium antagonists, hydralazine, isoproterenol, diazoxide, nitroglycerin) has been tried in primary pulmonary hypertension and a few patients with secondary pulmonary hypertension with disappointing results. Short-term benefits have been demonstrated with some of these agents, but improved outcome has not been documented. Complications of pulmonary vasodilator therapy have occurred, including systemic hypotension, hypoxemia, and even death. Routine clinical use of these agents is not currently recommended. Continuous long-term infusion of prostacyclin (PGI_2), a potent pulmonary vasodilator, shows some promise in preliminary studies of patients with primary pulmonary hypertension, but recommendations for its use must await the completion of large clinical trials.

It is important to distinguish primary pulmonary hypertension with pulmonary vasoconstriction, a potentially reversible condition, from fixed obstruction of the pulmonary vascular bed. Patients most likely to benefit from long-term pulmonary vasodilator therapy are those who respond favorably to a vasodilator challenge at right heart catheterization. It is clear that long-term vasodilator therapy should be employed only if hemodynamic benefit is documented. Some experts advise a baseline hemodynamic assessment by right heart catheterization and a repeat study after oral therapy with a vasodilator agent such as a calcium channel blocker. Routine use of vasodilator therapy is not advised.

Patients with marked polycythemia (hematocrit > 60%) should undergo repeated phlebotomy in an attempt to reduce blood viscosity. Cor pulmonale complicating pulmonary hypertension is treated by managing the underlying pulmonary disease and by using diuretics, salt restriction, and, in appropriate patients, supplemental oxygen. The use of digitalis in cor pulmonale remains controversial. Pulmonary thromboendarterectomy may benefit selected patients with pulmonary hypertension secondary to chronic thrombotic obstructions of major pulmonary arteries.

Combined heart-lung transplantation (see Chapter 10) has been performed on patients with end-stage primary pulmonary hypertension as well as those with Eisenmenger's complex. The two-year survival rate in either condition after transplantation is 49%. Bronchiolitis obliterans is common in those who survive the operation.

Prognosis

The prognosis in secondary pulmonary hypertension depends on the course of the underlying disease. Patients with pulmonary hypertension due to fixed obliteration of the pulmonary vascular bed generally respond poorly to therapy; development of cor pulmonale in these cases implies a poor prognosis. The prognosis is favorable when pulmonary hypertension is detected early and the conditions leading to it are readily reversed.

Gilroy RJ Jr, Teague MW, Loyd JE: Pulmonary veno-occlusive disease: Fatal progression of pulmonary hypertension despite steroid-induced remission of interstitial pneumonitis. Am Rev Respir Dis 1991;143:1130. (Case report and literature review, emphasizing the interstitial component of this disorder.)

Rubin LJ et al: Treatment of primary pulmonary hypertension with continuous intravenous prostacyclin (epoprostenol): Results of a randomized trial. Ann Intern Med 1990;112:485. (Improvement in pulmonary vascular resistance and cardiac output with long-term infusion.)

DISORDERS DUE TO CHEMICAL & PHYSICAL AGENTS

INHALATION OF AIR POLLUTANTS

The respiratory tract is exposed to numerous potentially harmful substances in the environment, including air pollutants. Respiratory tract defense mechanisms protect the lung from noxious substances, but when these defenses are breached, serious respiratory tract injury may result.

Clinical Findings

Exposure to low levels of air pollutants is usually inconsequential; exposure to higher levels produces symptoms of upper and lower respiratory tract irritation, particularly in patients with asthma and COPD (Table 9–16).

Treatment

Healthy persons exposed to the usual ambient lev-

Table 9–16. Major air pollutants, their sources, and adverse effects.

Noxious Agent	Sources	Adverse Effects
Oxides of nitrogen	Automobile exhaust; gas stoves and heaters, wood-burning stoves, kerosene space heaters.	Respiratory tract irritation, bronchial hyperreactivity, impaired lung defenses, bronchiolitis obliterans.
Hydrocarbons	Automobile exhaust, cigarette smoke.	Lung cancer.
Ozone	Automobile exhaust, high-altitude aircraft cabins.	Cough, substernal discomfort, bronchoconstriction, decreased exercise performance, respiratory tract irritation.
Sulfur dioxide	Power plants, smelters, oil refineries, kerosene space heaters.	Exacerbation of asthma and COPD, respiratory tract irritation. Hospitalization may be necessary, and death may occur in severe exposure.

els of air pollutants need not observe special precautions. Patients with severe COPD or asthma should be advised to stay indoors and not engage in strenuous activity when high concentrations of air pollutants are present.

Prognosis

The outcome of lung injury from inhalation of air pollutants depends upon the severity and type of exposure and the patient's preexisting pulmonary status. After exposure to oxides of nitrogen, hydrocarbons, or ozone, healthy individuals usually recover fully. Occasionally, bronchiolitis obliterans results. Patients with underlying obstructive lung disease may experience severe exacerbations and even death after intense exposure to sulfur dioxide.

SMOKE INHALATION

The inhalation of products of combustion may cause serious respiratory complications. As many as one-third of patients admitted to burn treatment units have pulmonary injury from smoke inhalation. Morbidity and deaths due to smoke inhalation exceed those attributed to the burns themselves. The death rate of patients with both severe body burns and smoke inhalation exceeds 50%. All patients suspected to have had significant smoke inhalation should be admitted to the hospital for observation and treatment.

It is important to look for and recognize three consequences of smoke inhalation: impaired tissue oxygenation, thermal upper airway injury, and chemical injury to the lung. Impaired tissue oxygenation results from inhalation of carbon monoxide or cyanide and is an immediate threat to life. The management of patients with carbon monoxide poisoning and cyanide poisoning is discussed in Chapter 39. The clinician must recognize that patients with carbon monoxide poisoning display a normal partial pressure of oxygen in arterial blood (PaO_2) but have a low *measured* oxyhemoglobin saturation (SaO_2). Immediate treatment with 100% oxygen is essential and should be continued until the measured carboxyhemoglobin

level falls to less than 10% and concomitant metabolic acidosis has resolved.

Thermal injury to the mucosal surfaces of the upper airway occurs from inhalation of hot gases. Complications become evident by 18–24 hours. These include impaired ability to clear oral secretions and airway obstruction, producing inspiratory stridor. Respiratory failure with hypercapnia and hypoxemia occurs in severe cases. Early management (see also Chapter 38) includes the use of a high-humidity face mask with supplemental oxygen, gentle suctioning to evacuate oral secretions, elevation of the head 30 degrees to promote clearing of secretions, and topical epinephrine to reduce edema of the oropharyngeal mucous membrane. Helium-oxygen gas mixtures may reduce labored breathing. Close monitoring with arterial blood gases and later with oximetry is important. Examination of the upper airway with a fiberoptic laryngoscope or bronchoscope is superior to routine physical examination. Endotracheal intubation is often necessary to establish airway patency and is likely to be necessary in patients with deep facial burns, oropharyngeal or laryngeal edema, or respiratory failure. Tracheostomy should be avoided if possible because of an increased risk of pneumonia and death from sepsis.

Chemical injury to the lung results from inhalation of toxic gases and products of combustion, including aldehydes and organic acids. The site of lung injury depends upon the solubility of the gases inhaled, the duration of exposure, and the size of inhaled particles that transport noxious gases to distal lung units. Bronchorrhea and bronchospasm are seen early after exposure along with dyspnea, tachypnea, and tachycardia. Labored breathing and cyanosis may follow. Physical examination at this stage reveals diffuse wheezing and rhonchi. Bronchiolar edema and high-permeability pulmonary edema (ARDS) may develop within 1–2 days after exposure. Sloughing of the bronchiolar mucosa may occur within 2–3 days, leading to airway obstruction, atelectasis and worsening hypoxemia. Bacterial colonization and pneumonia are common by 5–7 days after the exposure.

Treatment of the pulmonary component of smoke inhalation consists of supplemental oxygen, bronchodilators, suctioning of mucosal debris and mucopurulent secretions via an indwelling endotracheal tube, chest physical therapy to aid clearance of secretions, and adequate humidification of inspired gases. Positive end-expiratory pressure (PEEP) has been advocated to treat bronchiolar edema. Judicious fluid management and close monitoring for secondary bacterial infection with daily sputum Gram stains round out the management protocol.

The routine use of corticosteroids for chemical lung injury from smoke inhalation has been shown to be ineffective and may even be harmful. Routine or prophylactic use of antibiotics is not recommended.

Those patients who survive should be watched for the development of late bronchiolitis obliterans.

Baud FJ et al: Elevated blood cyanide concentrations in victims of smoke inhalation. N Engl J Med 1991;325:1761. (Residential fires may result in cyanide poisoning as well as carbon monoxide poisoning.)
Haponik EF et al: Smoke inhalation. Am Rev Respir Dis 1988;138:1060. (Pathogenesis and management.)

PULMONARY ASPIRATION SYNDROMES

Aspiration of foreign material, such as liquids with pH > 2.5, into the tracheobronchial tree results from various disorders that impair normal deglutition, especially disturbances of consciousness and esophageal dysfunction.

Aspiration of Inert Material

Aspiration of inert material may cause asphyxia if the amount aspirated is massive and if cough is impaired, in which case immediate tracheobronchial suctioning is necessary. Most patients suffer no serious sequelae from aspiration of inert material.

Aspiration of Toxic Material

Aspiration of toxic material into the lung usually results in clinically evident pneumonia. **Hydrocarbon pneumonitis** is caused by ingestion of petroleum distillates, eg, gasoline, kerosene, furniture polish, and other household petroleum products. Lung injury results mainly from vomiting and secondary aspiration. Therapy is supportive. The lung should be protected from repeated aspiration with a cuffed endotracheal tube if necessary. **Lipid pneumonia** is a chronic syndrome related to the repeated aspiration of oily materials, eg, mineral oil, cod liver oil, and oily nose drops; it often occurs in elderly patients with impaired swallowing. Patchy infiltrates in dependent lung zones and lipid-laden macrophages in expectorated sputum are characteristic findings.

"Café Coronary"

Acute obstruction of the upper airway by food usually occurs in intoxicated individuals. Other predisposing factors include difficulty in swallowing, old age, poor dentition, dental problems that impair chewing, and use of sedative drugs. The Heimlich procedure may be lifesaving.

Retention of an Aspirated Foreign Body

Retention of an aspirated foreign body in the tracheobronchial tree may produce various acute and chronic conditions, including recurrent pneumonia, bronchiectasis, lung abscess, atelectasis, and postobstructive hyperinflation. Children are at greater risk than adults for foreign body aspiration. Occasionally, a misdiagnosis of asthma, COPD, or lung cancer is made in adult patients who have aspirated a foreign body. The plain chest x-ray usually suggests the site of the foreign body. In some cases, an expiratory film, demonstrating regional hyperinflation due to a check-valve effect, is helpful. Bronchoscopy is usually necessary to establish the diagnosis and attempt removal of the foreign body.

Chronic Aspiration of Gastric Contents

Chronic aspiration of gastric contents may result from primary disorders of the esophagus, eg, achalasia, esophageal stricture, scleroderma, esophageal carcinoma, esophagitis, and gastroesophageal reflux. In the last condition, relaxation of the tone of the lower esophageal sphincter allows reflux of gastric contents into the esophagus and predisposes to chronic pulmonary aspiration, especially at night. Cigarette smoking, consumption of alcohol, and use of theophylline are known to relax the lower esophageal sphincter. Pulmonary disorders linked to gastroesophageal reflux and chronic aspiration include bronchial asthma, idiopathic pulmonary fibrosis, and bronchiectasis. Even in the absence of aspiration, acid in the esophagus may trigger bronchospasm through reflex mechanisms.

The diagnosis of chronic aspiration is difficult. Barium swallow is usually necessary to rule out esophageal disease. Management consists of elevation of the head of the bed, cessation of smoking, weight reduction, and antacids or H_2 receptor antagonists (eg, cimetidine, 300–400 mg) at night. Metoclopramide (10–20 mg at bedtime) or bethanechol (10–25 mg at bedtime) is helpful in some patients with gastroesophageal reflux, as they elevate pressure in the lower esophageal sphincter.

Acute Aspiration of Gastric Contents (Mendelson's Syndrome)

Acute aspiration of gastric contents is often catastrophic. The pulmonary response depends on the characteristics and amount of the gastric contents aspirated. The more acidic the material, the greater the degree of chemical pneumonitis. Aspiration of pure gastric acid (pH < 2.5) causes extensive desquamation of the bronchial epithelium, bronchiolitis, hemorrhage, and pulmonary edema. Acute gastric aspiration is one of the commonest causes of adult respiratory distress syndrome. The clinical picture is one of abrupt onset of respiratory distress, with cough, wheezing, fever, and tachypnea. Crackles are audible at the bases of the lungs. Hypoxemia may be noted immediately after aspiration occurs. Radiographic abnormalities, consisting of patchy alveolar infiltrates in dependent lung zones, appear within a few hours. If particulate food matter has been aspirated along with gastric acid, radiographic features of bronchial obstruction may be observed. Even without superinfection, fever and leukocytosis occur.

Treatment of acute aspiration of gastric contents consists of supplemental oxygen, measures to maintain the airway, and the usual measures for treatment of acute respiratory failure. There is no evidence to support the routine use of corticosteroids or prophylactic antibiotics after gastric aspiration has occurred. Secondary pulmonary infection, which occurs in about one-fourth of patients, typically appears 2–3 days after aspiration. Management of this complication depends upon the observed flora of the tracheobronchial tree (Table 9–8). Hypotension secondary to alveolocapillary membrane injury and intravascular volume depletion is common and is managed with the judicious administration of intravenous fluids.

Finegold SM: Aspiration pneumonia. Rev Infect Dis 1991;13(Suppl 9):S737. (Key role of anaerobic organisms.)

Hoyt J: Aspiration pneumonitis: Patient risk factors, prevention, and management. J Intensive Care Med 1990;5(Suppl):S2. (Predisposing factors, prevention, and treatment.)

OCCUPATIONAL PULMONARY DISEASES

Many acute and chronic pulmonary diseases are directly related to inhalation of noxious substances encountered in the workplace; those disorders that are due to chemical agents may be classified as follows: (1) pneumoconioses, (2) hypersensitivity pneumonitis, (3) obstructive airway disorders, (4) toxic lung injury, (5) lung cancer, (6) pleural diseases, and (7) miscellaneous disorders.

Pneumoconioses

Pneumoconioses are chronic fibrotic lung diseases caused by the inhalation of coal dust and various inert, inorganic, or silicate dusts (Table 9–17). Pneumoconioses due to inhalation of inert dusts are usually asymptomatic disorders with diffuse nodular infiltrates on chest x-ray. Clinically important pneumoconioses include coal workers' pneumoconiosis,

Table 9–17. Selected pneumoconioses.

Disease	Agent	Occupational Sources
Metal dusts Siderosis	Metallic iron or iron oxide	Mining, welding, foundry work.
Stannosis	Tin, tin oxide	Mining, tinwork, smelting.
Baritosis	Barium salts	Glass and insecticide manufacturing.
Coal dust Coal worker's pneumoconiosis	Coal dust	Coal mining.
Inorganic dusts Silicosis	Free silica (silicon dioxide)	Rock mining, quarrying, stone cutting, tunneling, sandblasting, pottery, diatomaceous earth.
Silicate dusts Asbestosis	Asbestos	Mining, insulation, construction, shipbuilding.
Talcosis	Magnesium silicate	Mining, insulation, construction, shipbuilding.
Kaolin pneumoconiosis	Sand, mica, aluminum silicate	Mining of china clay; pottery and cement work.
Shaver's disease	Aluminum powder	Manufacture of corundum.

silicosis, and asbestosis. Treatment for each is supportive.

A. Coal Worker's Pneumoconiosis: In coal worker's pneumoconiosis, ingestion of inhaled coal dust by alveolar macrophages leads to the formation of coal macules, usually 2–5 mm in diameter, which appear on chest x-ray as diffuse small opacities but are especially prominent in the upper lung. Simple coal worker's pneumoconiosis is usually asymptomatic; pulmonary function abnormalities are unimpressive. Cigarette smoking does not increase the prevalence of coal worker's pneumoconiosis but may have an additive detrimental effect on ventilatory function. In complicated coal worker's pneumoconiosis ("progressive massive fibrosis"), conglomeration and contraction in the upper lung zones occur, with radiographic and clinical features resembling complicated silicosis. **Caplan's syndrome** is a rare condition characterized by the presence of necrobiotic rheumatoid nodules (1–5 cm in diameter) in the periphery of the lung in coal workers with rheumatoid arthritis.

B. Silicosis: In silicosis, extensive or prolonged inhalation of free silica (silicon dioxide) particles in the respirable range (0.3–5 μm) causes the formation of small rounded opacities (silicotic nodules) throughout the lung. Calcification of the periphery of hilar lymph nodes ("eggshell" calcification) is an unusual finding that strongly suggests silicosis. Simple silicosis is usually asymptomatic and has no effect on routine pulmonary function tests; in complicated silicosis, large conglomerate densities appear in the upper lung and are accompanied by dyspnea and obstructive and restrictive pulmonary dysfunction. A chronic lymphocytic alveolitis has been identified in silicosis, and one report suggests that this alveolitis may be responsive to corticosteroids. The incidence of tuberculosis is increased in patients with chronic silicosis. All patients with silicosis should have a tuberculin skin test. Chemoprophylaxis with isoniazid is recommended for silicotic patients who are tuberculin-reactive.

C. Asbestosis: Asbestosis, a nodular interstitial fibrosis occurring in asbestos workers and miners, is characterized by dyspnea, inspiratory crackles, and in some cases, clubbing and cyanosis. The radiographic features include interstitial fibrosis, thickened pleura, and calcified plaques (pleural) on the diaphragms or lateral chest wall. The lower lungs are more often involved than the upper. High-resolution CT scanning is the best imaging method in asbestosis because of its ability to detect parenchymal fibrosis and define the presence of coexisting pleural plaques. Cigarette smoking in asbestos workers increases the prevalence of radiographic pleural and parenchymal changes. It may also interfere with the clearance of short asbestos fibers from the lung. Pulmonary function studies show restrictive dysfunction and reduced diffusing capacity.

Hypersensitivity Pneumonitis

The term "hypersensitivity pneumonitis" (or "extrinsic allergic alveolitis") denotes nonatopic, nonasthmatic, allergic pulmonary disease. Hypersensitivity pneumonitis is manifested mainly as occupational disease (Table 9–18), in which exposure to inhaled organic agents leads to acute and eventually chronic pulmonary disease. Antibodies directed against the inhaled agent can be identified in serum. Acute illness is characterized by sudden onset of malaise, chills, fever, cough, dyspnea, and nausea 4–8 hours after exposure to the offending agent. This may occur after the patient has left work or even at night and thus may mimic paroxysmal nocturnal dyspnea. Bibasilar crackles, tachypnea, tachycardia, and (occasionally) cyanosis are noted. Small nodular densities sparing the apexes and bases of the lungs are noted on chest x-ray. Pulmonary function studies reveal restrictive dysfunction and reduced diffusing capacity. Laboratory studies reveal an increase in the white blood cell count with a shift to the left, hypoxemia, and the presence of precipitating antibodies to the offending agent in serum. Hypersensitivity pneumonitis antibody panels against common fungal antigens (cost approximately $95.00) are available.

A subacute hypersensitivity pneumonitis syndrome has been described that is characterized by the insidious onset of chronic cough and slowly progressive dyspnea, anorexia, and weight loss. Chronic re-

Table 9–18. Selected causes of hypersensitivity pneumonitis.

Disease	Antigen	Source
Farmer's lung	*Micropolyspora faeni, Thermoactinomyces vulgaris.*	Moldy hay.
"Humidifier lung"	Thermophilic actinomycetes.	Contaminated humidifiers, heating systems, or air conditioners.
Bird-fancier's lung ("pigeon-breeder's disease")	Avian proteins.	Bird serum and excreta.
Bagassosis	*Thermoactinomyces sacchari* and *T vulgaris.*	Moldy sugar cane fiber (bagasse).
Sequoiosis	*Graphium, Aureobasidium,* and other fungi.	Moldy redwood sawdust.
Maple bark stripper's disease	*Cryptostroma (Coniosporium) corticale.*	Rotting maple tree logs or bark.
Mushroom picker's disease	Same as farmer's lung.	Moldy compost.
Suberosis	*Penicillium frequentans.*	Moldy cork dust.
Detergent worker's lung	*Bacillus subtilis* enzyme.	Enzyme additives.

spiratory insufficiency and the appearance of pulmonary fibrosis on radiographs may or may not occur after repeated exposure to the offending agent. Lung biopsy by thoracotomy or thoracoscopy is occasionally necessary for diagnosis. Acute hypersensitivity pneumonitis is characterized by interstitial infiltrates of lymphocytes and plasma cells, with noncaseating granulomas in the interstitium and air spaces. Diffuse fibrosis is the hallmark of the subacute and chronic phases.

Treatment of hypersensitivity pneumonitis consists of identification of the offending agent, avoidance of further exposure, and, in severe acute or protracted cases, oral corticosteroids (prednisone, 0.5 mg/kg daily as a single morning dose, tapered to nil over 4–6 weeks). Change in occupation is advisable in some cases.

Obstructive Airway Disorders

Occupational pulmonary diseases manifested as obstructive airway disorders include occupational asthma, industrial bronchitis, and byssinosis.

A. Occupational Asthma: It has been estimated that from 2% to 5% of all cases of asthma are related to occupation. Offending agents in the workplace are numerous; they include grain dust, wood dust, tobacco, pollens, enzymes, gum arabic, synthetic dyes, isocyanates (particularly toluene diisocyanate), rosin (soldering flux), inorganic chemicals (salts of nickel, platinum, and chromium), trimellitic anhydride, phthalic anhydride, formaldehyde, and various pharmaceutical agents. Diagnosis of occupational asthma depends on a high index of suspicion, an appropriate history, spirometric studies before and after exposure to the offending substance, and peak flow rate measurements in the workplace. Bronchial provocation testing (a pulmonary function laboratory test demonstrating bronchial hyperreactivity to pharmacologic or antigenic agents) is helpful in some cases. Treatment consists of avoidance of further exposure to the offending agent and bronchodilators (Table 9–5), but symptoms may persist for years after workplace exposure has been terminated.

B. Industrial Bronchitis: Industrial bronchitis is chronic bronchitis found in coal miners and others exposed to cotton, flax, or hemp dust. Chronic disability does not often occur from industrial bronchitis.

C. Byssinosis: Byssinosis is an asthma-like disorder in textile workers caused by inhalation of cotton dust. The pathogenesis is obscure. Chest tightness, cough, and dyspnea are characteristically worse on Mondays or the first day back at work, with symptoms subsiding later in the week. Repeated exposure leads to chronic bronchitis.

Toxic Lung Injury

Toxic lung injury from inhalation of irritant gases is discussed in the section on smoke inhalation. **Silofiller's disease** is acute toxic noncardiogenic pulmonary edema caused by inhalation of nitrogen dioxide encountered in recently filled silos. Bronchiolitis obliterans is a common late complication, which perhaps can be prevented by early treatment of the acute reaction with corticosteroids. Extensive exposure to silage gas may cause sudden death.

Lung Cancer

Many industrial pulmonary carcinogens have been identified, including asbestos, radon gas, arsenic, iron, chromium, nickel, coal tar fumes, petroleum oil mists, isopropyl oil, mustard gas, and printing ink. Cigarette smoking acts as a cocarcinogen with asbestos and radon gas to cause bronchogenic carcinoma. Asbestos alone causes malignant mesothelioma. Almost all histologic types of lung cancer have been associated with these carcinogens. Chloromethylmethyl ether specifically causes small-cell carcinoma of the lung.

Pleural Diseases

Occupational diseases of the pleura may result from exposure to asbestos (see above) or talc. Inhalation of talc causes pleural plaques that are similar to those caused by asbestos. Benign asbestos pleural effusion occurs in some asbestos workers and may cause chronic blunting of the costophrenic angle on chest x-ray.

Other Occupational Pulmonary Diseases

Occupational agents are also responsible for other pulmonary disorders. These include **berylliosis,** an acute or chronic pulmonary disorder related to exposure to beryllium, which is absorbed through the lungs or skin and widely disseminated throughout the body. Acute berylliosis is a toxic, ulcerative tracheobronchitis and chemical pneumonitis following intense and severe exposure to beryllium. Chronic berylliosis, a systemic disease closely resembling sarcoidosis, is more common. Chronic pulmonary beryllium disease is thought to be an alveolitis mediated by the proliferation of beryllium-specific helper-inducer T cells in the lung. Exposure to beryllium now occurs in machining and handling of beryllium products and alloys. Beryllium miners are not at risk for berylliosis. Beryllium is no longer used in fluorescent lamp production, which was a source of exposure before 1950.

Cullen MR, Cherniack MG, Rosenstock L: Occupational medicine. (Two parts.) N Engl J Med 1990;322:594, 675. (Spectrum of occupational diseases, including lung diseases.)

Kokkarinen JI, Tukiainen HO, Terho EO: Effect of corticosteroid treatment on the recovery of pulmonary function in farmer's lung. Am Rev Respir Dis 1992;145:3. (Corticosteroids hasten the recovery of pulmonary function but do not influence long-term outcome.)

Merchant JA (editor): Environmental and occupational asthma. Chest 1990;98(Suppl):145S. (Epidemiologic and clinical aspects.)

Rom WN, Travis WD, Brody AR: Cellular and molecular basis of the asbestos-related diseases. Am Rev Respir Dis 1991;143:408. (Pathogenesis of asbestosis and pleural fibrosis.)

Sferlazza SJ, Beckett WS: The respiratory health of welders. Am Rev Respir Dis 1991;143:1134. (Adverse respiratory effects of welding.)

DRUG-INDUCED LUNG DISEASE

Typical patterns of pulmonary response to various drugs implicated in drug-induced respiratory disease are summarized in Table 9–19. Pulmonary injury due to drugs occurs as a result of allergic reactions, idiosyncratic reactions, overdose, or undesirable side effects. In most patients, the mechanism of pulmonary injury is unknown.

Precise diagnosis of drug-induced pulmonary disease is often difficult, because results of routine laboratory studies are not helpful and radiographic findings are not specific. A high index of suspicion and a thorough medical history of drug usage are critical to establishing the diagnosis of drug-induced lung dis-

Table 9–19. Pulmonary manifestations of selected drug toxicities.

Asthma	**Pulmonary edema**
Propranolol and other beta blockers	Noncardiogenic
Aspirin	Aspirin
Nonsteroidal anti-inflammatory drugs	Chlordiazepoxide
Histamine	Cocaine
Methacholine	Ethchlorvynol
Acetylcysteine	Heroin
Any nebulized medication	Cardiogenic
Cough	Propranolol
Captopril	**Pleural effusion**
Enalapril	Bromocriptine
Inhaled beclomethasone	Nitrofurantoin
Inhaled cromolyn	Any drug inducing systemic lupus erythematosus
Pulmonary infiltration	Methysergide
Without eosinophilia	Chemotherapeutic agents
Amitriptyline	**Mediastinal widening**
Azathioprine	Phenytoin
Amiodarone	Corticosteroids
With eosinophilia	Methotrexate
Sulfonamides	**Respiratory failure**
L-Tryptophan	Neuromuscular blockade
Nitrofurantoin	Aminoglycosides
Penicillin	Succinylcholine
Methotrexate	Gallamine
Crack cocaine	Dimethyltubocurarine (metocurine)
Drug-induced systemic lupus erythematosus	Central nervous system depression
Hydralazine	Sedatives
Procainamide	Hypnotics
Isoniazid	Narcotics
Chlorpromazine	Alcohol
Phenytoin	Tricyclic antidepressants
Interstitial fibrosis	Oxygen
Nitrofurantoin	
Bleomycin	
Busulfan	
Cyclophosphamide	
Methysergide	

ease. The clinical response to cessation of the suspected offending agent is also helpful. Acute episodes of drug-induced pulmonary disease usually disappear 24–48 hours after the drug has been discontinued, but chronic syndromes may take longer to resolve. Challenge tests to confirm the diagnosis are risky and rarely performed.

Treatment of drug-induced lung disease consists of discontinuing the offending agent immediately and managing the pulmonary symptoms appropriately.

Inhalation of freebase (crack) cocaine may cause a spectrum of acute pulmonary syndromes, including pulmonary infiltration with eosinophilia, pneumothorax and pneumomediastinum, bronchiolitis obliterans, and acute respiratory failure associated with diffuse alveolar damage and alveolar hemorrhage. Corticosteroids have been used successfully to treat the latter.

Cooper JAD (editor): Drug-induced pulmonary disease. Clin Chest Med 1990;11:1. (Comprehensive review of the topic.)

Drugs that cause pulmonary toxicity. Med Lett Drugs Ther 1990;32:88. (Commonly used systemic drugs with direct pulmonary toxicity.)

RADIATION LUNG INJURY

The lung is a radiosensitive organ that can be affected by external beam radiation therapy. The pulmonary response is determined by the volume of lung radiated, the dose and rate of therapy, and potentiating factors, eg, concurrent chemotherapy, previous radiation therapy in the same area, and simultaneous withdrawal of corticosteroid therapy. Symptomatic radiation lung injury occurs in about 10% of patients treated with megavoltage therapy for carcinoma of the breast, 5–15% of patients treated for carcinoma of the lung, and 5–35% of patients treated for lymphoma. Two phases of the pulmonary response to radiation are apparent: an acute phase (radiation pneumonitis) and a chronic phase (radiation fibrosis).

Radiation Pneumonitis

Radiation pneumonitis usually occurs 2–3 months (range 1–6 months) after completion of radiotherapy and is characterized by insidious onset of dyspnea, intractable dry cough, chest fullness or pain, weakness, and fever. The dominant histopathologic finding is that of a lymphocytic interstitial pneumonitis. Inspiratory crackles may be heard in the involved area. In severe disease, respiratory distress and cyanosis occur that are characteristic of adult respiratory distress syndrome (ARDS). An increased white blood cell count and elevated sedimentation rate are common. Pulmonary function studies reveal reduced lung volumes, reduced lung compliance, hypoxemia, reduced diffusing capacity, and reduced maximum voluntary ventilation. Chest x-ray, which correlates poorly with the presence of symptoms, usually demonstrates an alveolar or nodular infiltrate with a ground-glass opacification limited to the irradiated area. Air bronchograms are often observed. The sharp borders of the infiltrate help distinguish radiation pneumonitis from other conditions, eg, infectious pneumonia, lymphangitic spread of carcinoma, and recurrent tumor. Treatment consists of aspirin, cough suppressants, and bed rest. Acute respiratory failure, if present, is treated appropriately. Although there is no proof that corticosteroids are effective in radiation pneumonitis, prednisone (1 mg/kg/d orally) is usually given immediately for about 1 week. Thereafter, the dose is reduced and maintained at 20–40 mg/d for several weeks, then slowly tapered. Radiation pneumonitis usually resolves in 2–3 weeks. Death from ARDS is unusual.

Pulmonary Radiation Fibrosis

Pulmonary radiation fibrosis occurs in nearly all

patients who receive a full course of radiation therapy for cancer of the lung and breast. Patients who experience radiation pneumonitis develop pulmonary fibrosis after an intervening period (6–12 months) of well-being. Most patients are asymptomatic, though slowly progressive dyspnea occurs in some. Radiation fibrosis may occur with or without antecedent radiation pneumonitis. Cor pulmonale and chronic respiratory failure are rare. Radiographic findings include obliteration of normal lung markings, dense interstitial and pleural fibrosis, reduced lung volumes, tenting of the diaphragm, and sharp delineation of the irradiated area. No specific therapy is necessary, and corticosteroids have no value.

Other Complications of Radiation Therapy

Other complications of radiation therapy directed to the thorax include pericardial effusion, constrictive pericarditis, tracheoesophageal fistula, esophageal candidiasis, radiation dermatitis, and rib fractures. Small pleural effusions, radiation pneumonitis outside the irradiated area, spontaneous pneumothorax, and complete obstruction of central airways are unusual occurrences.

Roberts CM et al: Radiation pneumonitis: A possible lymphocyte-mediated hypersensitivity reaction. Ann Intern Med 1993;118:696. May be a generalized lymphocytic hypersensitivity alveolitis.)

DISORDERS OF VENTILATION

The principal influences on ventilatory control are arterial PCO_2, pH, and PO_2 and cerebrospinal fluid pH. These variables are monitored by **peripheral and central chemoreceptors.** Under normal conditions, the ventilatory control system maintains arterial pH and PCO_2 within narrow limits; arterial PO_2 is more loosely controlled.

PRIMARY ALVEOLAR HYPOVENTILATION

Primary alveolar hypoventilation ("Ondine's curse") is an uncommon syndrome of unknown cause characterized by inadequate alveolar ventilation despite normal neurologic function and normal airways, lungs, chest wall, and ventilatory muscles. Hypoventilation is even more marked during sleep. Individuals with this disorder are usually nonobese males in their third or fourth decades who present with lethargy, headache, and somnolence. Dyspnea is absent.

Physical examination may reveal cyanosis and evidence of pulmonary hypertension and cor pulmonale. Hypoxemia and hypercapnia are present and improve with voluntary hyperventilation. Erythrocytosis is common. Treatment with ventilatory stimulants is usually unrewarding. Augmentation of ventilation by mechanical methods (phrenic nerve stimulation, rocking bed, mechanical ventilators) has been helpful to some patients. Adequate oxygenation should be maintained with supplemental oxygen, but nocturnal oxygen therapy should be prescribed only if diagnostic nocturnal polysomnography has demonstrated its efficacy and safety. Primary alveolar hypoventilation resembles—but should be distinguished from—**central alveolar hypoventilation,** in which impaired ventilatory drive with chronic respiratory acidemia and hypoxemia follows an insult to the brain stem (eg, bulbar poliomyelitis, encephalitis, trauma).

OBESITY-HYPOVENTILATION SYNDROME (Pickwickian Syndrome)

A few obese individuals demonstrate hypoventilation during wakefulness indicative of the obesity-hypoventilation syndrome. This is distinguished from primary alveolar hypoventilation by the presence of extreme obesity. Symptoms, physical findings, and laboratory data are otherwise similar in the two syndromes. Hypercapnia, hypoxemia, and elevated hematocrit are characteristic features. Having the patient voluntarily hyperventilate for about 1 minute normalizes the PCO_2 and the PO_2, in contrast to lung diseases causing chronic respiratory failure such as COPD. In obesity-hypoventilation syndrome, hypoventilation appears to result from a synergistic combination of blunted ventilatory drives and the mechanical load imposed upon the ventilatory apparatus by obesity. Most patients with obesity-hypoventilation syndrome also suffer from obstructive sleep apnea (see below). Therapy of obesity-hypoventilation syndrome consists mainly of weight loss, which improves hypercapnia and hypoxemia as well as the ventilatory responses to hypoxia and hypercapnia; and medroxyprogesterone acetate, 10–20 mg every 8 hours orally. Marked improvement in hypoxemia, hypercapnia, erythrocytosis, and cor pulmonale may result. The obesity-hypoventilation syndrome should not be confused with **narcolepsy,** a disorder of excessive daytime sleepiness and irresistible sleep attacks (see Chapter 24).

SLEEP-RELATED BREATHING DISORDERS

Abnormal ventilation during sleep is manifested by apnea (breath cessation for at least 10 seconds) or hypopnea (decrement in airflow with drop in oxyhemoglobin saturation of at least 4%). Episodes of apnea are **central** if ventilatory effort is absent for the duration of the apneic episode, **obstructive** if ventilatory effort persists throughout the apneic episode but no airflow occurs because of transient obstruction of the upper airway, and **mixed** if absent ventilatory effort precedes upper airway obstruction during the apneic episode. Pure central sleep apnea is uncommon; it may occur in normals, in patients with primary alveolar hypoventilation, or in patients with lesions of the brain stem. Cheyne-Stokes respiration, an accentuated form of periodic breathing with apnea, is a type of central sleep apnea found in patients with congestive heart failure. Obstructive and mixed sleep apneas are more common and may be associated with life-threatening cardiac arrhythmias, severe hypoxemia during sleep, and daytime consequences of nocturnal hypoxemia, including congestive heart failure, pulmonary hypertension, cor pulmonale, and secondary erythrocytosis.

Definitive diagnostic evaluation should include otolaryngologic examination and polysomnography, the monitoring of multiple physiologic factors during sleep. Electroencephalography, electro-oculography, electromyography, electrocardiography, oximetry, and measurement of respiratory effort and airflow are performed in a complete evaluation. Screening may be performed using oximetry and electrocardiography only. Indications for polysomnography include a history of nocturnal breath cessation, restless sleep, and loud snoring from a bed partner, daytime hypersomnolence, unexplained erythrocytosis, pulmonary hypertension or cor pulmonale, and nocturnal cardiac arrhythmias (particularly bradycardia) noted on Holter monitoring.

Obstructive Sleep Apnea

Upper airway obstruction during sleep occurs when loss of normal pharyngeal muscle tone allows the pharynx to collapse passively during inspiration. Patients with anatomically narrowed upper airways (eg, micrognathia, macroglossia, obesity, tonsillar hypertrophy) are predisposed to the development of obstructive sleep apnea. Alcohol or sedatives before sleeping may precipitate or worsen the condition. Before making the diagnosis of obstructive sleep apnea, a drug history should be obtained and a seizure disorder, narcolepsy, or psychiatric depression excluded.

Most patients with obstructive or mixed sleep apnea are obese middle-aged men. Systemic hypertension is common. Patients complain of excessive daytime somnolence, morning sluggishness and headaches, daytime fatigue, cognitive impairment,

recent weight gain, and impotence. Bed partners usually report loud cyclical snoring, breath cessation, restlessness, and often thrashing movements of the extremities during sleep. Personality changes, poor judgment, work-related problems, and intellectual deterioration (memory impairment, inability to concentrate) may also be observed. Physical examination may be normal or may reveal systemic and pulmonary hypertension with cor pulmonale. The oronasopharynx is sometimes found to be narrowed by facial deformities, macroglossia, septal deviation, tumors, enlarged adenoids, or excessive pharyngeal soft tissue. Erythrocytosis is common. A hemoglobin level, and thyroid function tests should be obtained. Observation of the sleeping patient reveals loud snoring interrupted by episodes of increasingly strong ventilatory effort that fail to produce airflow. A loud snort accompanies the first breath following an apneic episode. Polysomnography reveals apneic episodes lasting as long as 1–2 minutes. Oxygen saturation falls, often to very low levels. Bradyarrhythmias such as sinus bradycardia, sinus arrest, or atrioventricular block may occur. Tachyarrhythmias, including paroxysmal supraventricular tachycardia, atrial fibrillation, and ventricular tachycardia, are common once airflow is reestablished.

Weight loss and strict avoidance of alcohol and hypnotic medications are the first steps in management and may be curative, but few patients lose weight successfully. Nasal continuous positive airway pressure (nasal CPAP) is very helpful in such circumstances. Polysomnography is necessary to determine what level of CPAP (usually 5 or 10 cm H_2O) is necessary to abolish obstructive apneas. Patients must use the nasal CPAP system nightly. Unfortunately, only about 75% of patients continue to use nasal CPAP after 1 year. Pharmacologic therapy for obstructive sleep apnea is disappointing. Protriptyline (10–20 mg orally at bedtime) is helpful in a small number of patients. Supplemental oxygen may lessen the severity of nocturnal desaturation but may also lengthen apneas. Polysomnography is necessary to assess the effects of oxygen therapy; it should not be routinely prescribed. Mechanical devices inserted into the mouth at bedtime to hold the jaw forward and prevent pharyngeal occlusion appear promising in preliminary studies.

Uvulopalatopharyngoplasty, a procedure consisting of resection of pharyngeal soft tissue and amputation of approximately 15 mm of the free edge of the soft palate and uvula, may be helpful in selected patients with retropalatal airway occlusion during sleep. Identifying patients who will benefit is difficult. Only about half of these operations are successful. **Nasal septoplasty** is performed if gross anatomic nasal septal deformity is present. **Tracheostomy** relieves upper airway obstruction and its physiologic consequences and represents the definitive treatment for obstructive sleep apnea. However, it has numerous adverse effects, including granuloma formation, difficulty with speech, and stoma and airway infection. Furthermore, the long-term care of the tracheostomy, especially in obese patients, can be difficult. Tracheostomy and other maxillofacial surgery approaches are reserved for patients with life-threatening arrhythmias or severe disability who have failed to respond to conservative therapy. In severe cases, it is prudent to combine tracheostomy with uvulopalatopharyngoplasty and attempt decannulation at a later time. This avoids the risk of acute airway obstruction due to postoperative edema.

American Thoracic Society: Indications and standards for cardiopulmonary sleep studies. Am Rev Respir Dis 1989;139:559. (The basic reference on modern standards for polysomnography.)
Hanly PJ: Mechanisms and management of central sleep apnea. Lung 1992;170:1. (Pathophysiology and management of central sleep apnea.)
Hudgel DW: Mechanisms of obstructive sleep apnea. Chest 1992;101:541. (Anatomic and functional variables.)
Hudgel DW et al: Uvulopalatopharyngoplasty in obstructive sleep apnea: Value of preoperative localization of site of upper airway narrowing during sleep. Am Rev Respir Dis 1991;143:942. (Airway obstruction may occur at the level of the palate or in the hypopharynx. Patients with obstruction benefit most.)
Kribbs NB et al: Objective measurement of patterns of nasal CPAP use by patients with obstructive sleep apnea. Am Rev Respir Dis 1993;147:887. (Patients are not very compliant with CPAP and overstate its actual use.)
Viner S, Szalai JP, Hoffstein V: Are history and physical examination a good screening test for sleep apnea? Ann Intern Med 1991;115:356. (Clinical judgment is not particularly accurate.)

HYPERVENTILATION SYNDROME

Hyperventilation is an increase in alveolar ventilation that leads to hypocapnia. It may be caused by a variety of conditions, such as hypoxemia, obstructive and infiltrative lung diseases, sepsis, hepatic dysfunction, fever, and pain. The term "central neurogenic hyperventilation" denotes a monotonous, sustained pattern of rapid and deep breathing seen in comatose patients with brain stem injury of multiple causes. Functional hyperventilation may be acute or chronic. Acute hyperventilation presents with hyperpnea, paresthesias, carpopedal spasm, tetany, and anxiety. Chronic hyperventilation may present with various nonspecific symptoms, including fatigue, dyspnea, anxiety, palpitations, and dizziness. The diagnosis of chronic hyperventilation syndrome is established if symptoms are reproduced during voluntary hyperventilation. Once organic causes of hyperventilation have been excluded, treatment of acute hyperventilation consists of rebreathing expired gas from a paper bag held over the face in order to decrease respiratory alkalemia and its associated symptoms. Anxiolytic drugs are also useful.

Tavel ME: Hyperventilation syndrome: Hiding behind pseudonyms? Chest 1990;97:1285. (Relationship to panic disorders. Treatment discussed.)

ACUTE RESPIRATORY FAILURE

Respiratory failure is defined as respiratory dysfunction resulting in abnormalities of oxygenation or CO_2 elimination severe enough to impair or threaten the function of vital organs. Arterial blood gas criteria for respiratory failure are not absolute but may be arbitrarily established as a PO_2 under 60 mm Hg and a PCO_2 over 50 mm Hg. Acute respiratory failure may occur in both pulmonary and nonpulmonary disorders (Table 9–20). Respiratory failure may be considered a failure of oxygenation, failure of ventilation, or both. A complete discussion of treatment of acute respiratory failure is beyond the scope of this chapter. Only general principles of management will be reviewed here.

Clinical Findings

Symptoms and signs of acute respiratory failure are those of the underlying disease combined with those of hypoxemia and hypercapnia. The chief symptom of hypoxemia is dyspnea, though profound hypoxemia may exist in the absence of complaints. Signs of hypoxemia include cyanosis, restlessness, confusion, anxiety, delirium, tachypnea, tachycardia,

Table 9–20. Selected causes of acute respiratory failure in adults.

Airway disorders
  Asthma
  Chronic bronchitis or emphysema in acute exacerbation
Parenchymal lung disorders
  Adult respiratory distress syndrome
  Congestive heart failure
  Pneumonia
  Hypersensitivity pneumonitis
Pulmonary vascular disorders
  Pulmonary thromboembolism
Chest wall and pleural disorders
  Flail chest
  Pneumothorax
Neuromuscular disorders
  Narcotic or sedative-hypnotic overdose
  Guillain-Barré syndrome
  Botulism
  Spinal cord injury
  Myasthenia gravis
  Poliomyelitis
  Stroke

hypertension, cardiac arrhythmias, and tremor. Dyspnea and headache are the cardinal symptoms of hypercapnia. Signs of hypercapnia include peripheral and conjunctival hyperemia, hypertension, tachycardia, tachypnea, impaired consciousness, papilledema, and asterixis. The symptoms and signs of acute respiratory failure are both insensitive and nonspecific; therefore, the physician must maintain a high index of suspicion and request an arterial blood gas analysis if respiratory failure is suspected.

Treatment

Treatment of the patient with acute respiratory failure consists of (1) specific therapy directed toward the underlying disease; (2) respiratory supportive care directed toward the maintenance of adequate gas exchange; and (3) general supportive care. Only the last two aspects are discussed below.

A. Respiratory Support: Respiratory support has both nonventilatory and ventilatory aspects.

1. Nonventilatory aspects–*The main therapeutic goal in acute hypoxemic respiratory failure is to ensure adequate oxygenation of vital organs.* Inspired oxygen concentration should be the lowest value that results in an oxygen saturation of $\geq 90\%$ (PaO_2 about 60 mm Hg). Higher arterial oxygen tensions are of no benefit and may cause hypoventilation in patients with chronic hypercapnia; however, *oxygen therapy should not be withheld for fear of causing progressive respiratory acidemia.* Hypoxemia in patients with obstructive airway disease is usually easily corrected by administering low-flow oxygen by nasal cannula (1–3 L/min) or Venturi mask (24–28%). Higher concentrations of oxygen are necessary to correct hypoxemia in patients with adult respiratory distress syndrome (ARDS), pneumonia, and other parenchymal lung diseases.

2. Ventilatory aspects–Ventilatory support consists of maintaining patency of the airway and ensuring adequate alveolar ventilation. Tracheal intubation and mechanical ventilation are often required.

a. Tracheal intubation–Indications for tracheal intubation are (1) hypoxemia which is not quickly reversed by supplemental oxygen, (2) upper airway obstruction, (3) impaired airway protection, (4) poor handling of secretions, and (5) need for positive-pressure mechanical ventilation. In general, orotracheal intubation is preferred to nasotracheal intubation in urgent or emergency situations because it is easier, faster, and less traumatic. Nasotracheal tubes are more comfortable and may be preferable if prolonged intubation is anticipated. The position of the tip of the endotracheal tube at the level of the aortic arch should be verified by chest x-ray immediately following intubation, and auscultation should be performed to verify that both lungs are being inflated. Only tracheal tubes with "floppy" (high-volume, low-pressure) air-filled or foam cuffs should be used.

b. Mechanical ventilation–Indications for mechanical ventilation include (1) apnea, (2) acute hypercapnia that is not quickly reversed by appropriate specific therapy, (3) severe hypoxemia, and (4) progressive patient fatigue despite appropriate treatment. In general, positive-pressure, volume-cycled ventilators should be used to provide mechanical ventilatory support.

Several modes of ventilation are available. Assisted mechanical ventilation (AMV), or assist/control (A/C), is a ventilatory mode in which the ventilatory frequency set on the ventilator serves as a backup rate, but the patient may trigger the ventilator to deliver additional positive-pressure breaths, each at the prescribed tidal volume. Continuous mechanical ventilation (CMV) provides ventilation at a specified rate for patients who are apneic. Intermittent mandatory ventilation (IMV) is a ventilatory technique in which the rate set on the ventilator serves as a backup rate, but the patient is able to augment the minute ventilation by taking spontaneous breaths through a one-way valve from a reservoir. Ventilator breaths are customarily delivered between spontaneous breaths (synchronized IMV, or SIMV). Intermittent mandatory ventilation may be of value for patients whose breathing cannot be synchronized with the ventilator; for tachypneic or agitated patients who develop respiratory alkalemia on assist/control ventilation; and for patients in whom strictly positive-pressure ventilation results in a reduction of cardiac output and in whom the negative-pressure breaths of intermittent mandatory ventilation produce an improvement in cardiac output. Numerous alternative modes of mechanical ventilation now exist.

Positive end-expiratory pressure (PEEP) is useful in improving oxygenation in patients with diffuse parenchymal lung disease such as ARDS. It should be used cautiously in patients with localized parenchymal disease, hyperinflation, or very high airway pressure requirements during mechanical ventilation.

c. Complications of mechanical ventilation–Potential complications of mechanical ventilation are numerous. Migration of the tip of the endotracheal tube into the right main bronchus can cause atelectasis of the left lung and overdistention of the right lung. **Barotrauma,** manifested by subcutaneous emphysema, pneumomediastinum, subpleural air cysts, pneumothorax, or systemic gas embolism, may occur in patients whose lungs are overdistended by excessive tidal volumes, especially those with hyperinflation caused by airflow obstruction or PEEP. Subtle parenchymal lung injury due to overdistention of alveoli is another potential hazard.

Acute respiratory alkalosis caused by overventilation is common. Hypotension induced by elevated intrathoracic pressure that results in decreased return of systemic venous blood to the heart may occur in patients treated with PEEP, those with severe airflow obstruction, and those with intravascular volume depletion.

B. General Supportive Care: Patients with acute respiratory failure are seriously ill, and careful attention must be paid to general supportive measures. Maintenance of adequate nutrition is vital; parenteral nutrition should be used only when conventional feeding methods are not possible. Overfeeding, especially with carbohydrate-rich formulas, should be avoided, because it increases CO_2 production and may potentially worsen or induce hypercapnia in patients with limited ventilatory reserve; however, failure to provide adequate nutrition is more common. Hypokalemia and hypophosphatemia may worsen hypoventilation due to muscle weakness. The hematocrit should be determined regularly and transfusions given if necessary. Sedative-hypnotics and narcotic analgesics are avoided if possible. If sedation is necessary, short-acting drugs such as triazolam, lorazepam, or oxazepam are preferred. Psychologic and emotional support, skin care to avoid decubitus ulcers, and meticulous avoidance of nosocomial infection and complications of tracheal tubes are vital aspects of comprehensive care for patients with acute respiratory failure.

Attention must also be paid to preventing complications associated with serious illness. Stress gastritis and ulcers may be avoided by administering sucralfate, antacids, or histamine H_2 receptor antagonists. There is some concern that the latter two agents, which raise the gastric pH, may permit increased growth of gram-negative bacteria in the stomach, predisposing to pharyngeal colonization and ultimately nosocomial pneumonia. The risk of deep venous thrombosis and pulmonary embolism may be reduced by subcutaneous administration of heparin (5000 units every 12 hours).

Course & Prognosis

The course and prognosis of acute respiratory failure vary and depend on the underlying disease. The prognosis of acute respiratory failure caused by uncomplicated sedative or narcotic drug overdose is excellent. Acute respiratory failure in patients with COPD who do not require intubation and mechanical ventilation has a good immediate prognosis. On the other hand, ARDS associated with sepsis has an extremely poor prognosis, with mortality rates of about 90%. Overall, adults requiring mechanical ventilation for all causes of acute respiratory failure have survival rates of 62% to weaning, 43% to hospital discharge, and 30% to 1 year after hospital discharge.

American Thoracic Society: Withholding and withdrawing life-sustaining therapy. Am Rev Respir Dis 1991; 144:726. (Ethical principles.)

Brochard L et al: Reversal of acute exacerbations of chronic obstructive lung disease by inspiratory assistance with a face mask. N Engl J Med 1990;323:1523. (May obviate the need for intubation and standard mechanical ventilation.)

Weinberger SE, Schwartzstein RM, Weiss JW: Hypercapnia. N Engl J Med 1989;321:1223. (Pathophysiology and differential diagnosis.)

Yang KL, Tobin MJ: A prospective study of indexes predicting the outcome of trials of weaning from mechanical ventilation. N Engl J Med 1991;324:1445. (Rapid shallow breathing was the most accurate predictor of weaning failure.)

ADULT RESPIRATORY DISTRESS SYNDROME (ARDS)

Essentials of Diagnosis

- History of systemic or pulmonary insult.
- Respiratory distress.
- Diffuse pulmonary infiltrates.
- Severe hypoxemia refractory to treatment with supplemental oxygen.
- Normal pulmonary capillary wedge pressure.

General Considerations

Adult respiratory distress syndrome denotes acute respiratory failure following a systemic or pulmonary insult; it is characterized by respiratory distress, diffuse infiltrates, hypoxemia, noncompliant lungs, and normal pulmonary capillary wedge pressure. ARDS may follow a wide variety of catastrophic clinical events (Table 9–21). Common risk factors for ARDS include sepsis, aspiration of gastric contents, shock, trauma, severe pneumonia, and multiple blood trans-

Table 9–21. Selected disorders associated with ARDS.

Systemic insults	Pulmonary insults
Trauma	Embolism of thrombus, fat, or amniotic fluid
Sepsis	
Pancreatitis	Miliary tuberculosis
Shock	Aspiration of gastric contents
Multiple transfusions	Diffuse pneumonia
Disseminated intravascular coagulation	Viral
	Mycoplasma
Burns	Legionnaire's
Drugs	(*Legionella*
Narcotics	*pneumophila*)
Aspirin	*Pneumocystis*
Chlordiazepoxide	Near-drowning
Phenylbutazone	Toxic gas inhalation
Colchicine	Nitrogen dioxide
Ethchlorvynol	Chlorine
Hydrochlorothiazide	Sulfur dioxide
Paraldehyde	Ammonia
Lidocaine	Smoke inhalation
Thrombotic thrombocytopenic purpura	Oxygen toxicity
	Lung contusions
Cardiopulmonary bypass	Radiation
Venous air embolism	High altitude
Head injury	Hanging
Paraquat	Reexpansion

fusions. About one-third of ARDS patients initially have sepsis syndrome. Pro-inflammatory cytokines (eg, tumor necrosis factor, interleukin-1) released from stimulated lymphocytes and macrophages appear to be pivotal in lung injury. Although the mechanism of lung injury varies with the cause, damage to capillary endothelial cells and alveolar epithelial cells (type I pneumocytes) is common to ARDS regardless of cause. Damage to these cells causes increased vascular permeability and inactivation of surfactant; both of these lead to interstitial and alveolar pulmonary edema and alveolar collapse.

Clinical Findings

ARDS is marked by the rapid onset of profound dyspnea that usually occurs 12–48 hours after the initiating event. Labored breathing, tachypnea, intercostal retractions, and crackles are noted on physical examination. Chest radiograph shows diffuse or patchy bilateral infiltrates that are initially interstitial but rapidly become alveolar; these characteristically spare the costophrenic angles. Air bronchograms occur in about 80% of cases. Upper lung zone venous engorgement (flow inversion) is distinctly uncommon. Heart size is normal, and pleural effusions are small or nonexistent. Marked hypoxemia occurs that is refractory to treatment with supplemental oxygen, indicating shunting. Most patients with ARDS demonstrate multiple organ failure, particularly involving the kidneys, liver, gut, central nervous system, and cardiovascular system.

Differential Diagnosis

Since ARDS is a physiologic and radiographic syndrome rather than a specific disease, the concept of differential diagnosis does not strictly apply. Normal-permeability ("cardiogenic") pulmonary edema must be ruled out, however, because specific therapy is available for that disorder. Measurement of pulmonary capillary wedge pressure by means of a flow-directed pulmonary artery catheter may be required, though routine use of the Swan-Ganz catheter in ARDS is discouraged.

Prevention

No measures that effectively prevent ARDS have been identified; specifically, prophylactic use of PEEP in patients at risk for ARDS has not been shown to be effective. Intravenous methylprednisolone does not prevent ARDS when given early to patients with sepsis syndrome or septic shock.

Treatment

Treatment of ARDS must include identification and specific treatment of the underlying condition (eg, sepsis). Aggressive supportive care must then be provided to compensate for the severe dysfunction of the respiratory system associated with ARDS. Supportive therapy almost always includes tracheal intubation and mechanical ventilation. The use of positive end expiratory pressure (PEEP) usually improves oxygenation in patients with ARDS but does not affect the natural history of this condition. PEEP should not be used routinely. The lowest level of PEEP that produces adequate oxygenation combined with an acceptable FIO_2 should be used. The lowest possible FIO_2 to keep the PaO_2 above 60 mm Hg or the SaO_2 above 90% should be used. High levels of PEEP may improve arterial PO_2 but may depress cardiac output and reduce oxygen delivery. Cardiac output must be monitored with a thermodilution pulmonary artery catheter whenever there is concern about adequacy of systemic oxygen transport (a product of cardiac output and arterial oxygen content) or the fluid balance of the patient. Cardiac output that falls when PEEP is used may be improved by reducing the level of PEEP or by administering inotropic drugs (eg, dopamine); administering fluids to increase intravascular volume should be done only with great caution, because doing so may worsen alveolar edema.

Elevated pulmonary capillary pressure worsens pulmonary edema in the presence of increased capillary permeability; therefore, the goal of fluid management is to maintain pulmonary capillary wedge pressure at the lowest possible level compatible with adequate cardiac output. Crystalloid solutions should be used when intravascular volume expansion is necessary. Diuretics should be used to reduce intravascular volume if pulmonary capillary wedge pressure is elevated. Packed red blood cell transfusions (see Chapter 13) are given to keep the hematocrit above 25%, a practice that maintains a reasonable arterial oxygen content.

Oxygenation in patients with ARDS may sometimes be improved by turning them from the supine to the prone position.

Extracorporeal membrane oxygenation, PEEP, corticosteroids, and prostaglandin E_1 have been shown not to improve survival. Corticosteroid therapy may benefit patients with ARDS due to radiation pneumonitis and possibly fat embolism syndrome. However, in patients with sepsis syndrome and ARDS, intravenous methylprednisolone has been shown to impede reversal of ARDS and increase its mortality rate.

Broad-spectrum antimicrobial treatment should be started promptly when infection is known or suspected.

New treatment approaches under investigation include surfactant supplementation, monoclonal antibodies to tumor necrosis factor, human recombinant interleukin-1 receptor antagonist, neutrophil inhibitors such as pentoxifylline, arachidonic acid metabolism inhibitors such as ibuprofen, new modes of mechanical ventilation, and extracorporeal CO_2 removal. Monoclonal antibodies (such as HA-1A against endotoxins have been used in patients with sepsis and gram-negative bacteremia, but recent results have been disappointing.

Course & Prognosis

The mortality rate associated with ARDS exceeds 50%. If ARDS is accompanied by sepsis, the mortality rate may reach 90%. The major cause of death in ARDS is nonpulmonary multiple organ system failure, often with sepsis. Median survival is about 2 weeks. Most survivors are asymptomatic within a few months, though abnormalities of oxygenation, diffusing capacity, and lung mechanics may persist in some.

Bone RC: A critical evaluation of new agents for the treatment of sepsis. JAMA 1991;266:1686. (Definition of sepsis and review of current therapy against endotoxin, tumor necrosis factor, and interleukin-1 receptors.)

Bone RC et al: Adult respiratory distress syndrome: Sequence and importance of development of multiple organ failure. Chest 1992;101:320. (ARDS is the pulmonary manifestation of a systemic disease characterized by increased endothelial permeability which causes multiple organ dysfunction or failure.)

Wiedemann HP, Matthay MA, Matthay RA (editors): Adult respiratory distress syndrome. Clin Chest Med 1990; 11:575. [Entire issue.] (Pathogenesis, pathophysiology, management, and outcome.)

Ziegler EJ et al: Treatment of gram-negative bacteremia and septic shock with HA-1A human monoclonal antibody against endotoxin: A randomized, double-blind, placebo-controlled trial. N Engl J Med 1991;324:429. (HA-1A human monoclonal antibody against endotoxin is reported to reduce mortality in patients with sepsis who have gram-negative bacteremia but not in others.)

PLEURAL DISEASES

PLEURITIS

Pain due to acute pleural inflammation is caused by irritation of the parietal pleura. Such pain is localized, sharp, and fleeting and is made worse by cough, sneezing, deep breathing, or movement. When the central portion of the diaphragmatic parietal pleura is irritated, pain may be referred to the shoulder. There are numerous causes of pleuritis. The setting in which pleuritic pain develops helps to narrow the differential diagnosis; eg, in young, otherwise healthy individuals, pleuritis is usually caused by viral respiratory infections or pneumonia. The presence of pleural effusion, pleural thickening, or air in the pleural space requires further diagnostic and therapeutic measures. It should also be recalled that simple rib fracture may cause severe pleurisy.

Treatment of pleuritis consists of treating the un-

derlying disease. Simple analgesics and anti-inflammatory drugs (eg, indomethacin, 25 mg orally two or three times daily) are often helpful for pain relief. Codeine (30–60 mg orally every 8 hours) may be used to control cough associated with pleuritic chest pain if retention of airway secretions is not a likely complication. Intercostal nerve blocks are sometimes helpful.

PLEURAL EFFUSION

Essentials of Diagnosis

- Asymptomatic in many cases; pleuritic chest pain if pleuritis is present; dyspnea if effusion is large.
- Decreased tactile fremitus; dullness to percussion; distant breath sounds; egophony if effusion is large.
- Radiographic evidence of pleural effusion.
- Diagnostic findings on thoracentesis.

General Considerations

Pleural fluid is formed in the normal individual mostly on the parietal pleural surface at the rate of about 0.1 mL/kg/h. Absorption of this fluid on the visceral pleural surface is thought to occur, keeping the pleural space nearly dry. However, the parietal pleura may also contribute to absorption. Up to 25 mL of pleural fluid is normally present in the pleural space, an amount not detectable on conventional chest radiographs. Movement of fluid into and out of the pleural space is dependent mostly on hydrostatic and osmotic forces in parietal and visceral pleural capillaries. **Pleural effusion** is an abnormal accumulation of fluid in the pleural space. The five major types of pleural effusion are transudates, exudates, empyema, hemorrhagic pleural effusion or hemothorax, and chylous or chyliform effusion.

Pleural effusions are classified as **transudates** or **exudates** to help in differential diagnosis. An exudate is a pleural fluid having *one or more* of the following features:

(1) Pleural fluid protein to serum protein ratio greater than 0.5.

(2) Pleural fluid LDH to serum LDH ratio greater than 0.6.

(3) Pleural fluid LDH greater than two-thirds the upper limit of normal serum LDH.

Transudates have none of these features.

Causes of transudates and exudates are listed in Table 9–22. Congestive heart failure accounts for most transudates and is the most common cause of pleural effusion. Mechanisms (and examples) leading to formation of transudates include increase in hydrostatic pressure (congestive heart failure), decreased oncotic pressure (hypoalbuminemia), and greater negative intrapleural pressure (acute atelectasis). Bacterial pneumonia and cancer are the commonest

Table 9–22. Causes of pleural fluid transudates and exudates.

Transudates	Exudates
Congestive heart failure	Parapneumonic effusion
Cirrhosis with ascites	Cancer
Nephrotic syndrome	Pulmonary embolism
Peritoneal dialysis	Empyema
Myxedema	Tuberculosis
Acute atelectasis	Connective tissue disease
Constrictive pericarditis	Viral infection
Superior vena cava obstruction	Fungal infection
Pulmonary embolism	Rickettsial infection
	Parasitic infection
	Asbestos pleural effusion
	Meigs' syndrome
	Pancreatic disease
	Uremia
	Chronic atelectasis
	Trapped lung
	Chylothorax
	Sarcoidosis
	Drug reaction
	Postmyocardial infarction syndrome

causes of exudative effusion. Exudates form as a result of disease of the pleura itself in association with increased capillary permeability (eg, pneumonia) or reduced lymphatic drainage (eg, carcinoma obstructing lymphatic drainage).

The gross appearance of pleural fluid helps to identify the other major types of pleural effusion. **Empyema** is an exudative pleural effusion caused by direct infection of the pleural space, causing the pleural fluid to appear purulent or turbid. **Hemothorax** is the presence of gross blood in the pleural space, usually a result of chest trauma. **Hemorrhagic pleural effusion** is a mixture of blood and pleural fluid. About 10,000 red blood cells per microliter are necessary to create blood-tinged pleural fluid; 100,000 red blood cells per microliter make pleural fluid appear grossly bloody. If the hematocrit of pleural fluid is more than 50% of the hematocrit of peripheral blood, hemothorax is present. In the absence of trauma, grossly bloody pleural fluid suggests cancer or, less commonly, pulmonary embolism.

Pleural fluid that is milky in appearance should be centrifuged. Clearing of the milky appearance from the supernatant suggests empyema, whereas persistent cloudy or turbid supernatant signifies **chylous** or **chyliform pleural effusion.** Chylous pleural effusion occurs acutely in chylothorax as a result of disruption of the thoracic duct. Chyliform pleural effusion occurs in pseudochylothorax as a result of accumulation of cholesterol complexes in a chronically thickened pleural space, a phenomenon sometimes seen in cases of trapped lung (entrapment of lung by a fibrous "peel" on the visceral pleura), tuberculous pleuritis (especially with previous therapeutic pneumothorax), or rheumatoid pleural effusion. Chylous pleural effusion may be distinguished from

chyliform pleural effusion on the basis of lipid analysis of the fluid, acute or subacute onset, and absence of pleural thickening on chest x-ray. A chylous pleural effusion has chylomicrons and a high triglyceride level, usually above 100 mg/dL.

Clinical Findings

A. Symptoms and Signs: Small pleural effusions are usually asymptomatic, whereas large pleural effusions may cause dyspnea, particularly in the presence of underlying cardiopulmonary disease. Pleuritic chest pain and dry cough may occur; any pleural fluid found in association with pleuritic chest pain is invariably an exudate. Physical findings are absent if less than 200–300 mL of pleural fluid is present. Findings consistent with the presence of a larger pleural effusion include decrease in tactile fremitus, dullness to percussion, and diminution of breath sounds over the effusion. In large effusions that compress the lung, accentuation of breath sounds and egophony may be noted just above the effusion. A pleural friction rub indicates pleuritis. A massive pleural effusion with high intrapleural pressure may cause contralateral shift of the trachea and bulging of the intercostal spaces.

B. Laboratory Findings: Diagnostic thoracentesis should be performed whenever a pleural effusion is detected and no cause for the effusion is clinically apparent. Not all pleural effusions require diagnostic thoracentesis. More than 1 cm of free pleural fluid should be evident on a lateral decubitus x-ray before diagnostic thoracentesis is attempted. Decubitus films are the preferred method to demonstrate free pleural fluid. Ultrasound examination is useful to find the site for thoracentesis of a loculated pleural effusion.

Transudates lack the distinguishing protein and LDH findings described above and often have other typical characteristics (white blood cell count < 1000/μL, predominance of mononuclear cells in the differential, glucose level in pleural fluid equal to that of serum, and normal pH). Laboratory findings in exudative pleural effusions are more variable and are summarized in Table 9–23. If an exudate is suspected, thoracentesis should be performed quickly. One should have a low threshold for performing pleural biopsy at this time. The presence of malignant cells or positive results on smear or culture are pathognomonic findings in pleural fluid; determination of other causes depends on a constellation of findings on gross examination and laboratory studies or on biopsy results. Routine laboratory tests of pleural fluid should include total and differential white blood cell count, protein, glucose, and LDH. Additional tests may be ordered as required after thoracentesis. Pleural fluid pH is helpful in narrowing the differential diagnosis of exudative effusions. A pH less than 7.30 indicates cancer, complicated parapneumonic effusion, lupus or rheumatoid effusion, tuberculosis, or

Table 9–23. Characteristics of important exudative pleural effusions.

Etiology or Type of Effusion	Gross Appearance	White Blood Cell Count (cells/μL)	Red Blood Cell Count (cells/μL)	Differential[1]	Glucose	Comments
Malignant effusion	Turbid to bloody; occasionally serous.	1000–<100,000	100 to several hundred thousand.	M	Equal to serum levels; <60 mg/dL in 15% of cases.	Eosinophilia uncommon; positive results on cytologic examination.
Uncomplicated parapneumonic effusion	Clear to turbid.	5000–25,000	<5000	P	Equal to serum levels.	Tube thoracostomy unnecessary.
Empyema	Turbid to purulent.	25,000–100,000	<5000	P	Less than serum levels; often very low.	Drainage necessary; putrid odor suggests anaerobic infection.
Tuberculosis	Serous to serosanguineous.	5000–10,000	<10,000	M	Equal to serum levels; occasionally <60 mg/dL.	Protein may exceed 5 g/dL; eosinophils (>10%) or mesothelial cells (>5%) make diagnosis unlikely.
Rheumatoid effusion	Turbid; greenish-yellow.	1000–20,000	<1000	M or P	<40 mg/dL.	Secondary empyema common; high LDH, low complement, high rheumatoid factor, cholesterol crystals are characteristic.
Pulmonary infarction	Serous to grossly bloody.	1000–50,000	100 to >100,000	M or P	Equal to serum levels.	Variable findings; no pathognomonic features.
Esophageal rupture	Turbid to purulent; red-brown	<5000–>50,000	…	P	Usually low.	High amylase level (salivary origin); pneumothorax in 25% of cases; effusion usually on left side; pH <6.0 strongly suggests diagnosis.
Pancreatitis	Turbid to serosanguineous.	1000–50,000	1000–10,000	P	Equal to serum levels.	Usually left-sided; high amylase level.

[1]M = mononuclear cell predominance; P = polymorphonuclear leukocyte predominance.

esophageal rupture. A high percentage of lymphocytes in pleural fluid suggests tuberculosis or cancer. Low levels of glucose in pleural fluid point toward cancer, empyema, tuberculosis, esophageal rupture, or connective tissue disease (rheumatoid pleuritis or systemic lupus erythematosus). Elevated levels of amylase in pleural fluid suggest one of four diagnoses: pancreatitis, pancreatic pseudocyst, pancreatic cancer, or esophageal rupture.

Closed pleural biopsy with a Cope or Abrams needle should be considered whenever malignancy or tuberculosis is considered in the differential diagnosis of a pleural effusion that is unexplained after routine studies and thoracentesis. Contraindications include bleeding diathesis, poor respiratory reserve, empyema, and absence of pleural fluid. The expected yield of the procedure approximates 55% in pleural malignancy, somewhat less than with cytologic examination of pleural fluid, and over 75% in pleural tuberculosis if the tissue fragments are submitted for culture as well as histology. Open pleural biopsy is sometimes required to establish the diagnosis of pleural malignancy and is especially indicated for the diagnosis of malignant pleural mesothelioma. Thoracoscopy with a flexible or rigid instrument is an alternative procedure with excellent diagnostic accuracy in experienced hands.

C. Imaging: About 250 mL of pleural fluid must be present before effusion can be detected on conventional erect posteroanterior chest x-ray. Lateral decubitus views can detect much smaller amounts of free (nonloculated) pleural fluid. Free pleural fluid collects in the subpulmonary area. Larger amounts of fluid spill over into the costophrenic sulcus to form a meniscus. Thickening of major and minor fissures is common. Atypical collections of pleural fluid are frequently seen. Lateral displacement of the apex of the diaphragm and abrupt obliteration of lung markings at the level of the diaphragm are features of subpulmonary effusion. Pleural fluid may become trapped ("loculated") by pleural adhesions, forming unusual collections along the chest wall or in the lung fissures. Shadows with a broad base on the chest wall that point inward toward the hilum are characteristic of loculated effusions. Round or oval collections of loculated fluid in fissures resemble tumors ("pseudotumors"). Ultrasound is useful to locate loculated or small effusions.

Massive pleural effusion (opacification of an entire hemithorax) is usually caused by cancer but has been observed in tuberculosis and other diseases. CT scanning is sensitive in the detection of small amounts of free or loculated pleural fluid, but this imaging method is costly.

Treatment

Treatment should address both the disease causing the pleural effusion and the effusion itself. Because a specific diagnosis can be established in most cases of pleural effusion, a diagnosis of "idiopathic" effusion may delay or even prevent successful therapy.

A. Transudative Pleural Effusion: Transudative pleural effusions generally respond to treatment of the underlying condition; therapeutic thoracentesis is indicated only if massive effusion causes dyspnea. Pleurodesis and tube thoracostomy are rarely if ever indicated. When bilateral pleural effusions are detected in a patient with congestive heart failure, neither diagnostic nor therapeutic thoracentesis is routinely indicated. Such effusions are likely to be transudates and will resolve with treatment of the underlying cardiac disease.

B. Malignant or Paramalignant Pleural Effusion: Pleural effusion in a patient with known cancer may be either malignant or paramalignant. In cancer patients with **paramalignant pleural effusion,** the pleural surface is directly invaded by malignant cells (pleural fluid cytology or pleural tissue biopsy reveals evidence of malignancy). In such cases the tumor causing the effusion is unresectable, and treatment with chemotherapy or radiotherapy is directed at the underlying cancer. The term "paramalignant pleural effusion" denotes a pleural effusion in a patient with cancer when the pleural space is not directly invaded by tumor and repeated thoracentesis and needle biopsy of the pleura give negative results. In this situation, the underlying tumor may or may not be resectable. Chemical **pleurodesis** (obliteration of the pleural space by producing fibrous adhesion between the visceral and the parietal pleura) is advised for selected patients with symptomatic malignant pleural effusion who fail to respond to chemotherapy or mediastinal radiation or who are not candidates for these forms of therapy (see Chapter 5). Repeated therapeutic thoracentesis, pleuroperitoneal shunting, and surgical pleurectomy are alternative approaches for certain patients with rapidly recurring malignant pleural effusion.

C. Parapneumonic Pleural Effusion: Pleural effusion in the setting of pneumonia ("parapneumonic effusion") usually responds to systemic antibiotic therapy. Management steps include sputum Gram stain and culture, blood cultures, diagnostic thoracentesis, antibiotic therapy, and a decision regarding closed chest drainage (tube thoracostomy). *Effective therapy requires early intervention* to avoid progression of the effusion from the exudative to subsequent (fibrinopurulent and organized) stages. Loculation of pleural fluid collections is likely once organization has occurred. Laboratory findings—especially the pH, glucose concentration, and the white cell count of pleural fluid—are important in guiding additional therapy. In "uncomplicated" parapneumonic effusion, no pleural infection is present, and the pleural fluid glucose and pH are normal. Such effusion is likely to resolve spontaneously, and chest tube drainage is not required. In "complicated" parapneumonic effusion, pleural fluid is either frank empyema or has the potential to organize into a fibrous "peel." A low pH (< 7.2), low glucose (< 50 mg/dL), and high LDH (> 1000 IU/L)—but not a high pleural fluid white blood cell count or protein concentration—help to separate complicated from uncomplicated parapneumonic effusions.

Tube thoracostomy is required for parapneumonic effusion if any of the following is present: (1) the fluid resembles frank pus, (2) pleural fluid glucose is < 40 mg/dL, or (3) pleural fluid pH is < 7.0. If the pleural fluid pH is between 7.0 and 7.2 or the LDH is > 1000 IU/L, the physician should strongly consider chest tube placement or should monitor the effusion carefully with serial thoracenteses. Serial thoracentesis is not an effective strategy for *treatment* of complicated parapneumonic effusions. The treatment of nonpurulent complicated parapneumonic effusions (Gram stain- or culture-positive and pH < 7.20) requires appropriate antibiotic therapy. However, the routine use of tube thoracostomy in such cases is controversial.

A parapneumonic effusion that does not respond to drainage within 24 hours may have become loculated. The clinician should be aware that localized pockets of empyema may be present in this circumstance, even though thoracentesis from another localized fluid collection did not reveal empyema. In such cases, ultrasound examination is required to guide placement of an additional chest tube in the proper location. Intrapleural injection of streptokinase via the chest tube (250,000 units in 100 mL normal saline daily for up to 10 days) may accelerate drainage. Open surgical drainage may be necessary if these measures are ineffective. A thick pleural "peel" developing after treatment of complicated parapneumonic effusion may resolve slowly over several months. Surgical decortication should be reserved for selected patients with established fibrothorax.

D. Hemothorax: Hemothorax is generally managed by the immediate insertion of one or more large chest tubes in order to control bleeding by causing apposition of pleural surfaces; chest tubes help the physician determine the amount of bleeding and decrease the risk of complications such as empyema and eventual fibrothorax. As much blood as possible should be drained before the chest tube is removed. Thoracotomy is occasionally required to control bleeding, remove large volumes of blood clots, and treat coexisting complications of trauma such as bronchopleural fistula. A very small hemothorax that is stable or improving on chest x-ray can be managed without tube drainage.

E. Other Types of Pleural Effusion: Management of patients with exudative pleural effusion due to other causes consists mainly of treating the underlying disease. Pleural fluid acidosis outside the setting of pneumonia is not an automatic indication for chest tube drainage. Patients with rheumatoid pleural

effusions should be watched closely for the development of secondary empyema.

Prognosis

The prognosis of patients with pleural effusion depends on the prognosis of the underlying disease. The prognosis of patients with documented malignant pleural effusion is poor, particularly if pleural fluid pH or glucose levels are low.

Aelony Y, King R, Boutin C: Thoracoscopic talc poudrage pleurodesis for chronic recurrent pleural effusions. Ann Intern Med 1991;115:778. (Effective and relatively painless.)

American Thoracic Society: Guidelines for thoracentesis and needle biopsy of the pleura. Am Rev Respir Dis 1989;140:257.

Berger HA, Morganroth ML: Immediate drainage is not required for all patients with complicated parapneumonic effusions. Chest 1990;97:731. (Challenges the practice of immediate tube thoracostomy.)

Menzies R, Charbonneau M: Thoracoscopy for the diagnosis of pleural disease. Ann Intern Med 1991;114:271. (Rigid thoracoscopy under local anesthesia is reported to have a diagnostic accuracy of 96%.)

Sahn SA: The pleura. Am Rev Respir Dis 1988;138:184.

SPONTANEOUS PNEUMOTHORAX

Essentials of Diagnosis

- Acute onset of ipsilateral chest pain and dyspnea, often of several days' duration.
- Minimal physical findings in mild cases; unilateral chest expansion, decreased tactile fremitus, hyperresonance, diminished breath sounds, mediastinal shift, cyanosis in tension pneumothorax.
- Presence of pleural air on chest x-ray.

General Considerations

Pneumothorax, or accumulation of air in the pleural space, is classified as spontaneous (primary or secondary) or traumatic. Primary pneumothorax occurs in the absence of an underlying cause, whereas secondary pneumothorax is a complication of preexisting pulmonary disease. Traumatic pneumothorax results from penetrating or nonpenetrating trauma and is often iatrogenic. Iatrogenic pneumothorax may follow procedures such as thoracentesis, pleural biopsy, subclavian line placement, percutaneous lung biopsy, bronchoscopy with transbronchial biopsy, and positive-pressure mechanical ventilation. In tension pneumothorax, the pressure of air in the pleural space exceeds ambient pressure throughout the respiratory cycle. A check-valve mechanism allows air to enter the pleural space on inspiration and prevents egress of air on expiration.

The incidence of primary pneumothorax is about nine per 100,000 per year; the disease affects mainly tall, thin men between the ages of 20 and 40 years.

Primary pneumothorax is thought to occur from rupture of subpleural apical blebs in response to high negative intrapleural pressures. Familial factors and cigarette smoking may also be important.

Secondary pneumothorax occurs as a complication of COPD, asthma, cystic fibrosis, tuberculosis, and a wide variety of infiltrative lung diseases, including *P carinii* pneumonia. Pneumothorax in association with menstruation (catamenial pneumothorax) is another well-established form of secondary pneumothorax. Because of underlying disease, secondary pneumothorax is usually a more serious condition than primary spontaneous pneumothorax.

Clinical Findings

A. Symptoms and Signs: Chest pain on the affected side and dyspnea occur in nearly all patients. Symptoms usually begin during rest or sleep. Many patients wait for several days before seeking medical attention. Alternatively, this may be present with life-threatening respiratory failure if underlying COPD or asthma is present; this is true irrespective of the size of the pneumothorax.

If pneumothorax is small, physical findings, other than mild tachycardia, are unimpressive. If pneumothorax is large, diminished breath sounds, decreased tactile fremitus, and hyperresonance are noted. Tension pneumothorax should be suspected in the presence of severe tachycardia, hypotension, and mediastinal or tracheal shift.

B. Laboratory Findings: Arterial blood gas analysis reveals hypoxemia in most patients but is often unnecessary. Left-sided primary pneumothorax may produce QRS axis and precordial T wave changes on the ECG that may be misinterpreted as acute myocardial infarction.

C. Imaging: Demonstration of a visceral pleural line is diagnostic and is best revealed on an expiratory film. A few patients have secondary pleural effusion that demonstrates a characteristic air-fluid level on chest radiography. In supine patients, pneumothorax on a conventional chest x-ray may appear as an abnormally radiolucent costophrenic sulcus (the "deep sulcus" sign). In patients with tension pneumothorax, chest x-rays show a large amount of air in the affected hemithorax and contralateral shift of mediastinal structures. Tension pneumothorax usually occurs in the setting of penetrating trauma, lung infection, cardiopulmonary resuscitation, or positive-pressure mechanical ventilation.

Differential Diagnosis

If the patient is a young, tall, thin, cigarette-smoking man, the diagnosis of primary spontaneous pneumothorax is usually obvious and can be confirmed by chest x-ray. In secondary pneumothorax, it is sometimes difficult to distinguish loculated pneumothorax from an emphysematous bleb. Occasionally, pneu-

mothorax may mimic myocardial infarction, pulmonary embolization, or pneumonia.

Complications

Tension pneumothorax may result in acute respiratory failure. Cardiopulmonary arrest and death are extremely rare. Pneumomediastinum may occur as a complication of spontaneous pneumothorax. If this is detected, rupture of the esophagus or a bronchus should be considered.

Treatment

Treatment depends upon the severity of pneumothorax. The patient with a new small (< 15%) pneumothorax should be hospitalized and placed at bed rest, treated symptomatically for cough and chest pain, and followed with serial chest x-rays every 12–24 hours. Observation in the hospital for 2 days is adequate in most cases. A patient with a small pneumothorax that has been observed to be stable in size for several days to a week can be followed closely with serial chest x-rays without hospitalization. Many small pneumothoraces resolve spontaneously as air is absorbed from the pleural space; however, pneumothorax may unpredictably progress to tension pneumothorax. Progression to tension pneumothorax is accelerated during positive-pressure mechanical ventilation. In this situation, or in patients who are severely symptomatic or who have a larger pneumothorax (> 15%), chest tube placement (tube thoracostomy) is performed. The chest tube is placed under water-seal drainage, and suction is applied until the lung expands. Intravenous catheters and emergency pneumothorax treatment tubes should not be used in the hospital setting because of a high rate of technical failures. Air leaks persisting after 3 days are unusual. Tube thoracostomy alone does not cause enough pleural scarification to prevent recurrence of spontaneous pneumothorax. Pulmonary edema on the affected side may follow abrupt evacuation of pneumothorax. If tension pneumothorax is suspected, a large-bore needle should be inserted immediately in the affected side; tube thoracostomy may be performed thereafter.

Chemical pleurodesis (see Chapter 5) has been recommended by some authorities for management of a first episode of spontaneous pneumothorax, but this procedure causes considerable pain, requiring premedication with adequate doses of parenteral meperidine or morphine. Intrapleural lidocaine is ineffective for prevention or relief of this intense pain. Powdered talc is an older agent that has been used successfully for chemical pleurodesis to prevent recurrent pneumothorax.

All patients should be advised to discontinue smoking and warned that the risk of recurrence is 50%. Exposure to high altitudes, flying in unpressurized aircraft, and scuba diving should be avoided. If spontaneous pneumothorax recurs, the second episode should be managed in a manner similar to that of the first episode. Some experts advocate surgery for any recurrence.

Indications for thoracoscopy or open thoracotomy include recurrences of spontaneous pneumothorax (the minimum number of episodes being controversial), any occurrence of bilateral pneumothorax, and failure of tube thoracostomy for the first episode (failure of lung to reexpand or persistent air leak). Surgery permits oversewing of the ruptured blebs responsible for the pneumothorax and greatly reduces the risk of recurrence. Pleural symphysis may be obtained by scarification from abrasion of the pleural surface. Pleurectomy is of no particular value.

Prognosis

About half of patients with spontaneous pneumothorax experience recurrence of the disorder after either observation or tube thoracostomy for the first episode. Recurrence after surgery is rare. Following successful therapy, there are no long-term complications.

Almind M, Lange P, Viskum KAJ: Spontaneous pneumothorax: Comparison of simple drainage, talc pleurodesis, and tetracycline pleurodesis. Thorax 1989;44:627. (Talc compares favorably.)

Baumann MH, Sahn SA: Medical management and therapy of bronchopleural fistulas in the mechanically ventilated patient. Chest 1990;97:721. (Proper use of chest tubes and ventilation management.)

Carter EJ, Ettensohn DB: Catamenial pneumothorax. Chest 1990;98:713. (Importance of the menstrual history.)

Powner DJ, Bierman MI: Thoracic and extrathoracic bronchial fistulas. Chest 1991;100:480. (Practical uses of bronchoscopy and thoracoscopy.)

REFERENCES

Baum GL, Wolinsky E (editors): *Textbook of Pulmonary Diseases,* 4th ed. Little, Brown, 1989.

Bone RC et al: *Pulmonary and Critical Care Medicine.* Mosby-Year Book, 1993.

Chang HK, Paiva M (editors): *Respiratory Physiology: Lung Biology in Health and Disease,* Vol 40. Marcel Dekker, 1989.

Crystal RG, West JB (editors): *The Lung: Scientific Foundations.* Raven Press, 1990.

Fishman AP (editor): *Pulmonary Diseases and Disorders,* 2nd ed. McGraw-Hill, 1991.

Fraser RG et al: *Diagnosis of Diseases of the Chest,* 3rd ed. Saunders, 1988.

George RB et al: Chest Medicine. *Essentials of Pulmonary and Critical Care Medicine,* 2nd ed. Williams & Wilkins, 1990.

Hall JB, Schmidt GA, Wood LDH (editors): *Principles of Critical Care.* McGraw-Hill, 1992.

Kryger MH, Roth T, Dement WC (editors): *Principles and Practice of Sleep Medicine.* Saunders, 1989.

Kryger MH (editor): *Introduction to Respiratory Medicine,* 2nd ed. Churchill Livingstone, 1990.

Light RW: *Pleural Diseases,* 2nd ed. Lea & Febiger, 1990.

Mahler DA (editor): *Dyspnea.* Futura, 1990.

Martin RJ (editor): *Cardiorespiratory Disorders During Sleep,* 2nd ed. Futura, 1990.

Murray JF, Nadel JA: *Textbook of Respiratory Medicine,* Saunders, 1988.

Naidich DP, Zerhouni EA, Siegelman SS: *Computed Tomography and Magnetic Resonance of the Thorax,* 2nd ed. Raven Press, 1991.

Parrillo JE (editor): *Current Therapy in Critical Care Medicine,* 2nd ed. BC Decker, 1991.

Phelan PD, Landau LI, Olinsky A: *Respiratory Illness in Children,* 3rd ed. Blackwell, 1989.

Pickard LR: *Decision Making in Surgery of the Chest.* Saunders, 1989.

Pierson DJ, Kacmarek RM: *Foundations of Respiratory Care.* Churchill Livingstone, 1992.

Rippe JM et al (editors): *Intensive Care Medicine,* 3rd ed. Little, Brown, 1991.

Schwarz MI, King TE Jr (editors): *Interstitial Lung Disease,* 2nd ed. CRC Press, 1993.

Shoemaker WC, et al: *The Society of Critical Care Medicine: Textbook of Critical Care,* 2nd ed. Saunders, 1988.

Thurlbeck WM (editor): *Pathology of the Lung.* Thieme Medical Publishers, 1988.

Tobin MJ: *Essentials of Critical Care Medicine.* Churchill Livingstone, 1989.

West JB: *Pulmonary Pathophysiology: The Essentials,* 3rd ed. Williams & Wilkins, 1987.

West JB: *Respiratory Physiology: The Essentials,* 4th ed. Williams & Wilkins, 1990.

Weir EK, Reeves JT (editors): *Pulmonary Vascular Physiology and Pathophysiology. (Lung Biology in Health and Disease,* vol 38.) Marcel Dekker, 1989.

Zagelbaum GL, Welch MA Jr, Doyle PR: *Basic Arterial Blood Gas Interpretation.* Little, Brown, 1988.

10   Cardiovascular Disease

Barry M. Massie, MD

SYMPTOMS & SIGNS; DIAGNOSTIC PROCEDURES

COMMON SYMPTOMS

The most common symptoms of heart disease are dyspnea, chest pain, palpitations, presyncope or syncope, and fatigue. None are specific, and interpretation depends on the entire clinical picture and, in many cases, diagnostic testing.

Many of the textbooks listed at the end of this chapter have excellent discussions of signs and symptoms of heart disease, including pathophysiology and differential diagnosis; see especially Fowler, Gazes.

Dyspnea

Dyspnea due to heart disease is precipitated or exacerbated by exertion and results from elevated left atrial and pulmonary venous pressures or hypoxia. The former are most commonly caused by left ventricular systolic dysfunction, left ventricular diastolic dysfunction (due to hypertrophy, fibrosis, or pericardial disease), or valvular obstruction. The acute onset or worsening of left atrial hypertension may result in **pulmonary edema.** Hypoxia may be due to pulmonary edema or intracardiac shunting. Dyspnea should be quantified by the amount of activity that precipitates it. Dyspnea is also a common symptom of pulmonary disease, and the etiologic distinction may be very difficult. Shortness of breath is also found in deconditioned or obese individuals, anxiety states, anemia, and many other illnesses.

Orthopnea is dyspnea that occurs in recumbency and results from an increase in central blood volume. Orthopnea may also result from pulmonary disease and obesity. **Paroxysmal nocturnal dyspnea** is relieved by sitting up or standing; this symptom is more specific for cardiac disease.

Tobin MJ: Dyspnea: Pathophysiologic basis, clinical presentation, and management. Arch Intern Med 1990; 150:1604. (Review of physiology, especially of noncardiac dyspnea.)

Wasserman K: Dyspnea on exertion: Is it the heart or the lungs? JAMA 1982;248:2039. (Although 12 years old, still a useful discussion of this difficult problem.)

Chest Pain

Chest pain is a common symptom that can occur as a result of pulmonary or musculoskeletal disease, esophageal or other gastrointestinal disorders, cervicothoracic nerve root irritation, or anxiety states, as well as many cardiovascular diseases. The commonest cause of cardiac chest pain is myocardial ischemia. This is usually described as dull, aching, or as a sensation of "pressure," "tightness," "squeezing," or "gas," rather than as sharp or spasmodic; and it is often perceived as an uncomfortable sensation rather than "pain." **Ischemic pain** usually subsides within 30 minutes but may last longer. Protracted episodes often represent **myocardial infarction.** The pain is commonly accompanied by a sense of anxiety or uneasiness. The location is usually retrosternal or left precordial. Though the pain may radiate to or be localized in the throat, lower jaw, shoulders, inner arms, upper abdomen, or back, it nearly always also involves the sternal region. Ischemic pain is often precipitated by exertion, cold temperature, meals, stress, or combinations of these factors and is usually relieved by rest. It is not related to position or respiration and is usually not elicited by chest palpation.

Hypertrophy of either ventricle and aortic valvular disease may also give rise to ischemic pain or pain with less typical features. Myocarditis, cardiomyopathy, and mitral valve prolapse are associated with chest pain of a more atypical nature. Pericarditis may produce pain that changes with position or respiration. Aortic dissection produces an instantaneous tearing pain of great intensity that often radiates to the back.

Richter JE et al(editors): Unexplained chest pain. Med Clin North Am 1991;75:No 5. (Differential diagnosis and management.)

Palpitations, Dizziness, Syncope

Awareness of the heartbeat may be a normal phenomenon or may reflect increased cardiac or stroke output in patients with many noncardiac conditions (eg, exercise, thyrotoxicosis, anemia, anxiety). It may also be due to cardiac abnormalities that increase stroke volume (regurgitant valvular disease, bradycardia) or may be a manifestation of cardiac arrhythmias. Ventricular premature beats may be sensed as extra or "skipped" beats. Supraventricular or ventricular tachycardia may be felt as rapid, regular or irregular palpitations or "fluttering"; many patients are asymptomatic, however.

If the abnormal rhythm is associated with a sufficient decline in arterial pressure or cardiac output, it may—especially in the upright position—impair cerebral blood flow, causing dizziness, blurring of vision, loss of consciousness (syncope), or other symptoms.

Cardiogenic syncope most commonly results from sinus node arrest or exit block, atrioventricular conduction block, or ventricular tachycardia or fibrillation. It is associated with few prodromal symptoms and may thus be an occasion for injuries. The absence of premonitory symptoms helps distinguish cardiogenic syncope (often called Stokes-Adams attacks) from vasovagal faint, postural hypotension, or seizure. Although recovery is often immediate, some patients may exhibit seizure-like movements. Aortic valve disease and hypertrophic obstructive cardiomyopathy may also cause syncope, which is usually exertional or postexertional.

Olsky M, Murray J: Dizziness and fainting in the elderly. Emerg Med Clin North Am 1990;8:295.

Kapoor WN: Diagnostic evaluation of syncope. Am J Med 1991;90:91. (Concentrating on recurrent cases.)

Edema

Subcutaneous fluid collections appear first in the lower extremities in ambulatory patients or in the sacral region of bedridden individuals. In heart disease, edema results from elevated right atrial pressures. Right heart failure most commonly results from left heart failure, although the right-sided signs may predominate. Other cardiogenic causes of edema include pericardial disease, right-sided valve lesions, and cor pulmonale. Edema may also be due to peripheral venous insufficiency, venous obstruction, nephrotic syndrome, cirrhosis, or premenstrual fluid retention, or it may be idiopathic. Advanced right heart failure can produce ascites, almost always in conjunction with edema.

FUNCTIONAL CLASSIFICATION OF HEART DISEASE

As a means of quantifying the limitation on activity of cardiac patients imposed by their symptoms, the classification system of the New York Heart Association is commonly employed. In following individual patients, it is important to document specific activities that produce symptoms.

Class I: No limitation of physical activity. Ordinary physical activity does not cause undue fatigue, dyspnea, or anginal pain.

Class II: Slight limitation of physical activity. Ordinary physical activity results in symptoms.

Class III: Marked limitation of physical activity. Comfortable at rest, but less than ordinary activity causes symptoms.

Class IV: Unable to engage in any physical activity without discomfort. Symptoms may be present even at rest.

SIGNS OF HEART DISEASE

Although the cardiovascular examination centers on the heart, peripheral signs are often invaluable.

Appearance

While cardiac patients may appear healthy and comfortable at rest, many with acute myocardial infarction appear anxious and restless. **Diaphoresis** suggests hypertension or a hyperadrenergic state, such as during pericardial tamponade, tachyarrhythmias, or myocardial infarction. Patients with severe congestive heart failure or other chronic low cardiac output states may appear **cachectic.**

Cyanosis may be central, due to arterial desaturation, or peripheral, reflecting impaired tissue delivery of adequately saturated blood in low-output states, polycythemia, or peripheral vasoconstriction. Central cyanosis may be caused by pulmonary disease, left heart failure, or right-to-left shunting; the latter will not be improved by increasing the inspired oxygen concentration. **Pallor** usually indicates anemia but may be a sign of low cardiac output.

Vital Signs

Although the normal **heart rate** ranges from 50 to 100 beats/min, both slower and more rapid rates may occur in normal individuals or may reflect noncardiac conditions such as anxiety or pain, medication effect, thyroid disease, pulmonary disease, anemia, or hypovolemia. If symptoms or clinical suspicion warrants, an electrocardiogram (ECG) should be performed to diagnose arrhythmia, conduction disturbance, or other abnormality. The range of normal **blood pressure** is wide, but even in asymptomatic individuals systolic pressures below 90 mm Hg or above 140 mm Hg and diastolic pressures above 90 mm Hg warrant further clinical evaluation and follow-up. Initially elevated pressures may decline if the patient is allowed to relax and rest comfortably. **Tachypnea** is also nonspecific, but pulmonary disease and heart failure should be considered when respiratory rates exceed 16/min under basal conditions. **Periodic breathing** (Cheyne-Stokes respiration) is not uncommon in severe heart failure.

Peripheral Pulses & Venous Pulsations

Diminished peripheral pulses most commonly result from arteriosclerotic peripheral vascular disease and may be accompanied by localized **bruits.** Asymmetry of pulses should also arouse suspicion of coarctation of the aorta or aortic dissection; previous cardiac catheterization may also be responsible. **Exaggerated pulses** may indicate aortic regurgitation, coarctation, patent ductus arteriosus, or other conditions that increase stroke volume. The carotid pulse is a valuable aid to assessment of left ventricular ejection. It has a **delayed upstroke** in aortic stenosis and a **bisferiens** quality (two palpable peaks) in mixed aortic stenosis and regurgitation or hypertrophic obstructive cardiomyopathy. **Pulsus paradoxus** (a decrease in systolic blood pressure during inspiration greater than the normal 10 mm Hg) is a valuable sign of pericardial tamponade, though it also occurs in asthma and chronic obstructive pulmonary disease.

Jugular venous pulsations provide insight into right atrial pressure. They indicate (1) **elevated central venous pressure** if they are more than 3 vertical centimeters above the angle of Louis, (2) increased central blood volume if they rise more than 1 cm with sustained (30 seconds) right upper quadrant abdominal pressure **(hepatojugular reflux),** (3) tricuspid obstruction or pulmonary hypertension if the *a* wave is exaggerated, and (4) tricuspid regurgitation if **large *cv* waves** are seen. The latter may be associated with hepatic pulsations. Atrioventricular dissociation due to conduction block or ventricular arrhythmia can be recognized by intermittent **cannon *a*** waves.

Pulmonary Examination

Rales heard at the lung bases are a sign of congestive heart failure but may be caused by similarly localized pulmonary disease. **Wheezing** and **rhonchi** suggest obstructive pulmonary disease but may occur in left heart failure. **Pleural effusions** with bibasilar percussion dullness and reduced breath sounds are common in congestive heart failure.

Precordial Pulsations

A **parasternal lift** usually indicates right ventricular hypertrophy, pulmonary hypertension (systolic pressure > 50 mm Hg), or left atrial enlargement; pulmonary artery pulsations may also be visible. The left ventricular **apical impulse,** if sustained and enlarged, suggests myocardial hypertrophy or dysfunction. If forceful but not sustained, the apical impulse may indicate volume overload or high-output states. Additional precordial pulsations may reflect regional abnormalities of left ventricular contraction.

Heart Sounds & Murmurs

Auscultation is diagnostic of—or helpful in diagnosis of—many heart diseases, including cardiac failure. Specific findings are discussed under diagnostic headings.

The **first heart sound (S_1)** may be diminished with severe left ventricular dysfunction or accentuated with mitral stenosis or short PR intervals. S_2 is usually split, with the two components (aortic preceding pulmonary) being separated more during inspiration; **splitting** is *fixed* in atrial septal defect, *wide* with right bundle branch block, and *absent* or *reversed* **(paradoxic splitting)** with aortic stenosis, left ventricular failure, or left bundle branch block. With normal splitting, an accentuated P_2 is an important sign of pulmonary hypertension. **Third and fourth heart sounds** (ventricular and atrial gallops, respectively) indicate ventricular volume overload or impaired compliance and may be heard over either ventricle. An apical S_3 is a normal finding in younger individuals and in pregnancy. Additional auscultatory findings include sharp, high-pitched sounds classified as **"clicks."** These may be early systolic and represent **ejection sounds** (as with a bicuspid aortic valve or pulmonary stenosis) or may occur in mid or late systole, indicating myxomatous changes in the mitral valve.

While many **murmurs** indicate valvular disease, a soft, short systolic murmur, usually localized along the left sternal border or toward the apex, may be innocent, reflecting pulmonary flow. **Innocent murmurs** often vary with inspiration, diminish in the upright position, and are most frequently heard in thin individuals. **Systolic murmurs** are **pansystolic (holosystolic)** when they merge with the first sound and persist through all of systole or **"ejection" murmurs** when they begin after the first sound and end before the second sound, with a peak in early or mid systole. The former represent mitral regurgitation if maximal at the apex or in the axilla and tricuspid regurgitation or ventricular septal defect if best heard at the sternal border. Short aortic ejection murmurs with a preserved A_2 are common in older individuals, especially when hypertension has been present, and even if they are moderately loud they usually reflect thickening (sclerosis) of the valve rather than stenosis. Association of murmurs with palpable vibrations **("thrills")** is always clinically significant, as are **diastolic murmurs.**

Constant J: *Bedside Cardiology,* 4th ed. Little, Brown, 1993. (The disappearing art of clinical assessment.)
Marriott HJ: *Bedside Cardiac Diagnosis.* Lippincott, 1993. (Clinical wisdom from an accomplished teacher.)
Perloff JK: *Physician Examination of the Heart and Circulation,* 2nd ed. Saunders, 1990. (Directed at the level of physicians in training.)

Edema

Peripheral edema, especially if it is bilateral and associated with other symptoms and signs, may indicate heart failure. Other causes of edema include peripheral venous abnormalities; hepatic, renal, and thyroid disease; and fluid retention due to medications (especially calcium blockers or nonsteroidal agents) or estrogen effect.

DIAGNOSTIC TESTING

The **chest radiograph** will provide information about heart size, the pulmonary circulation (with characteristic signs suggesting both pulmonary artery or pulmonary venous hypertension), primary pulmonary disease, and aortic abnormalities. The **echocardiogram** provides much more reliable information about chamber size, hypertrophy, pericardial effusions, valvular abnormalities, and congenital abnormalities, and where readily available this procedure has replaced x ray for evaluation of cardiac disease. The **ECG** indicates cardiac rhythm, reveals conduction abnormalities, and provides evidence of ventricular hypertrophy, myocardial infarction, or ischemia. Nonspecific ST segment and T wave changes may reflect these processes but are also noted with electrolyte imbalance, drug effects, and many other conditions. Routine x-rays and ECGs are not recommended to screen for heart disease and have a limited role in the follow-up of patients with known heart disease. However, a baseline ECG is helpful in older patients.

Goldschlager N, Goldman MJ: *Principles of Clinical Electrocardiography,* 13th ed. Lange, 1989.
Marriott HJ: *Practical Electrocardiography,* 8th ed. Williams & Wilkins, 1988.
Schlant R et al: Guidelines for electrocardiography. A report of the American College of Cardiology/AHA Task Force of Assessment of Diagnostic and Therapeutic Cardiovascular Procedure. J Am Coll Cardiol 1992; 19;473.
Sox HC: The baseline electrocardiogram. Am J Med 1991; 91:573.

SPECIAL DIAGNOSTIC PROCEDURES

Noninvasive diagnostic procedures are growing in number and application. However, they are frequently overutilized. The clinician should carefully consider what question is being asked and how the results will alter patient management before ordering these tests. They have limited applicability in screening for asymptomatic disease and should not be substituted for a careful clinical evaluation.

Exercise Electrocardiography

The resting ECG is often insensitive to ischemia, but horizontal or downsloping exercise-induced ST segment depression, particularly when it exceeds 0.15 mV (1.5 mm with usual standardization), is strongly suggestive. Exercise-induced chest pain and

hypotension also suggest coronary disease. Exercise testing has a sensitivity of 60–80% and a specificity of 70–80%, and these figures may increase with concomitant scintigraphy. This procedure helps to diagnose or exclude disease, to estimate its severity, and to provide guidelines for activity in patients with known ischemic heart disease. However, it has not proved very useful in screening asymptomatic individuals, since false-positive results are common and the sensitivity for predicting future events is low.

Coplan NL, Fuster V: Limitations of the exercise test as a screen for acute cardiac events in asymptomatic patients. Am Heart J 1990;119:987.
Fletcher GF et al: Exercise standards: A statement for health professionals from the American Heart Association. Circulation 1990;82:2286. (Consensus on procedures, interpretation, and indications for exercise testing. Also discusses risks and procedures for exercise training.)
Sisconick DS et al: Sensitivity of exercise electrocardiography for acute cardiac events during moderate and strenuous physical activity. Arch Intern Med 1991;151:325. (Most events are not predicted even in a high-risk population undergoing serial testing.)
Sox HC et al: The role of exercise testing in screening for coronary artery disease. Ann Intern Med 1989;110:456. (Not currently indicated.)

Echocardiography

M-mode and **two-dimensional echocardiograms** yield semiquantitative measurements of left ventricular size, function, and thickness and qualitative information about aortic and mitral stenosis. Left ventricular segmental wall motion can be assessed, and the size of all four cardiac chambers can be determined. Hypertrophic cardiomyopathy, pericardial effusion, mitral valve prolapse, valvular vegetations, and cardiac tumors may all be diagnosed. **Two-dimensional echocardiograms** visualize more of the heart. **Doppler ultrasound** now permits the quantitative estimation of transvalvular gradients and pulmonary artery pressure and qualitative evaluation of valvular regurgitation and intraventricular shunts. **Color Doppler** visually demonstrates patterns and directionality of flow; it has been particularly useful in evaluating congenital heart disease. Doppler studies frequently detect *clinically insignificant* valvular regurgitation; care should be taken not to overinterpret those findings.

Transesophageal echocardiography is used in an increasing number of centers to improve the quality of echocardiograms, to derive information about posterior structures and prosthetic valves, and to monitor patients during surgery. It is superior to surface echocardiography in diagnosing dissection of the aorta and left atrial thrombi. It is also quite sensitive in detecting dissection of the ascending aorta.

Stress echocardiography is being used increasingly to enhance the information available from ECGs and as an alternative to nuclear medicine procedures. Echocardiograms may be performed during or immediately following exercise. Changes in segmental wall motion suggest myocardial ischemia. Dobutamine infusions can also be utilized as a form of stress testing in patients unable to exercise.

ACC/AHC guidelines for the clinical application of echocardiography. Circulation 1990;82:2323.

Feigenbaum H: *Echocardiography*, 5th ed. Lea & Febiger, 1993. (New edition of a practical textbook.)

Fisher EA et al: Transesophageal echocardiography: Procedures and clinical application. J Am Coll Cardiol 1991;18:1333.

Marwick TH et al: Accuracy and limitations of exercise echocardiography in a routine clinical setting. J Am Coll Cardiol 1992;19:74. (Series of 150 patients showing improvement over exercise ECG alone.)

Popp RL: Echocardiography. (Two parts.) N Engl J Med 1990;323:101, 165. (Concise review of applications and advances.)

Ambulatory Electrocardiographic Monitoring

Ambulatory electrocardiographic (Holter) monitoring is most useful for determining the need for therapy in patients with symptoms consistent with arrhythmia. Since these symptoms are often nonspecific, their temporal association with a conduction or rhythm disturbance provides a definitive indication for treatment. Documentation of asymptomatic "premonitory" abnormalities such as second-degree atrioventricular block, transient sinus node arrest, or nonsustained ventricular tachycardia may by association suggest the basis for previous symptomatic episodes. Although ambulatory electrocardiographic monitoring is frequently performed in patients with heart disease without symptoms consistent with arrhythmia— and although the detection of frequent or repetitive ventricular ectopy is sometimes associated with a poor prognosis—there are no studies which indicate that interventions alter prognosis. Thus, ambulatory monitoring is rarely indicated except for symptom evaluation.

A number of studies have employed ambulatory monitoring to detect and quantify silent ischemia, which is diagnosed by ST segment shifts. However, the routine clinical use of this approach is not justified by current data, since most patients with silent ischemic episodes also have symptomatic episodes, and the value of treating silent ischemia has not been proved.

DiMarco JP, Philbrick JT: Use of ambulatory electrocardiographic (Holter) monitoring. Ann Intern Med 1990; 113:53. (Diagnosis of arrhythmia, monitoring of therapy, and detection of ischemia. Followed by American College of Physicians position paper on this test.)

Knoebel SB et al: Guidelines for ambulatory electrocardiography: A report of the American College of Cardiology–American Heart Association joint task force on assessment of diagnostic and therapeutic cardiovascular procedures. Circulation 1989;79:206. (Position paper on role of ambulatory monitoring.)

Radionuclide Techniques

Several nuclear medicine studies are useful in the assessment of heart disease.

Scintigraphy with **thallium-201** or the newer technetium-complexed agents demonstrates relative myocardial perfusion. It is most commonly employed in conjunction with exercise testing to detect ischemia, which appears as a perfusion defect. After 3–24 hours, the defect will usually fill in or "redistribute" with reversible ischemia but will remain fixed in regions of infarction. A second injection after 3 hours or on another occasion at rest is often required to differentiate viable ischemic myocardium from scar with certainty. Scintigraphy following **dipyridamole-** or **adenosine-induced vasodilation** provides similar information in patients unable to exercise. The sensitivity of exercise scintigraphy is in the 80–90% range, which is somewhat superior to the exercise ECG, but its expense should limit its use to situations in which ordinary exercise testing needs corroboration or is not accurate (eg, bundle branch block, digitalis effect, left ventricular hypertrophy with "strain" pattern, or other baseline repolarization changes) or when regional localization is required. Both exercise and dipyridamole scintigraphy also provide useful prognostic information in patients with prior myocardial infarction and angina pectoris.

The newer technetium-based perfusion agents may provide better image resolution, but no superiority has been demonstrated by clinical criteria. They differ from thallium-201 physiologically (with Tc-99m sestamibi remaining "fixed" in the myocardium and Tc-99m teboroxime washing out very rapidly). Since these agents are more expensive and not clearly more useful for most applications, their appropriate role is not clear.

Radionuclide angiography provides accurate measurements of left and, in some laboratories, right ventricular ejection fractions. Segmental wall motion may be examined, and semiquantitative estimates of valvular regurgitation are possible. Radionuclide angiography may be performed during **exercise,** so that changes in global or segmental left ventricular function can be employed to diagnose ischemia or impaired functional reserve. Thallium scintigraphy is a more accurate test for evaluating ischemic heart disease, but the exercise ejection fraction response provides useful prognostic information, especially postmyocardial infarction. Radionuclide angiography can also be used to quantify the pulmonary-to-systemic flow ratio in **left-to-right shunts.** Ratios above 1.3–1.5 can be accurately detected.

Technetium-99m pyrophosphate scintigraphy detects radiotracer uptake in areas of recent infarction. Its usefulness is limited by an 18- to 24-hour lag time after acute infarction before the test becomes positive and a limited sensitivity for small, especially nontransmural infarctions. This technique is most useful when the ECG and cardiac enzymes are non-diagnostic, such as after cardiac surgery or when chest pain has occurred more than 48 hours prior to assessment.

Cardiovascular Nuclear Medicine: An update. Semin Nucl Med 1991;21:169. (Eight articles covering new imaging agents and new stress procedures.)

Kotler TS, Diamond GA: Exercise thallium-201 scintigraphy in the diagnosis and prognosis of coronary artery disease. Ann Intern Med 1990;113:684. (Accuracy and prognostic value. Followed by American College of Physicians position paper on use of this test.)

Zaret BL, Beller GA (editors): *Nuclear Cardiology: State of the Art and Future Directions.* Mosby, 1993. (Update on new radiopharmaceuticals, PET scanning, and clinical results.)

Newer Imaging Modalities

Many new imaging techniques have been developed, but their application in cardiovascular disease remains to be determined. **Computed tomography (CT scan)** can image the heart and, with contrast medium, the vascular system, but the relatively slow speed of most instruments limits its utility. The main application of CT is the evaluation of pericardial disease. **Ultrafast** or **cine CT** involves a specially designed instrument with high temporal resolution. Its availability is limited, but it provides excellent assessments of cardiac structure and function. Detection of coronary artery calcifications with this extremely sensitive test has been advocated as a screening procedure, but it is unclear how this information should be used in clinical practice.

Cardiac magnetic resonance imaging (MRI) is an evolving modality that provides high-resolution images of the heart and great vessels without radiation exposure or use of iodinated contrast media. It provides excellent anatomic definition, permitting assessment of pericardial disease, neoplastic disease of the heart, myocardial thickness, chamber size, and many congenital heart defects. It is the best noninvasive test for evaluating dissection of the aorta. Rapid acquisition sequences can produce excellent cine-mode images demonstrating left ventricular function and wall motion, and it is thus a useful alternative when the echocardiogram is suboptimal.

Positron emission tomography (PET) can provide both qualitative and quantitative information concerning myocardial metabolism and blood flow, but its availability is limited, and a nearby cyclotron is required for many applications. PET can accurately distinguish between myocardium which is transiently dysfunctional ("stunned") due to ischemia and infarcted myocardium—a distinction that is important in considering revascularization. However, it is unclear whether this technique provides adequate incre-

mental information over stress and rest perfusion scintigraphy to justify its use.

Marcus ML et al (editors): *Cardiac Imaging: A Companion to Braunwald's Heart Disease.* Saunders, 1991. (By experts in fields of noninvasive and invasive techniques.)

Rehr RB: Cardiovascular nuclear magnetic resonance imaging and spectroscopy. Curr Probl Cardiol 1991; 16(3):127. (Current and potential future applications.)

Ritman EL: Fast computed tomography for quantitative cardiac analysis: State of the art and future perspectives. Mayo Clin Proc 1990;65:1336.

Schwaiger M, Hutchins GD: Evaluation of coronary artery disease with positron emission tomography. Semin Nucl Med 1992;22:210.

Cardiac Catheterization

Right heart catheterization is convenient to perform and allows measurement of right atrial, right ventricular, pulmonary artery and pulmonary capillary wedge pressures (the latter an indicator of left atrial pressure), oxygen saturation, and cardiac output. These data may diagnose intracardiac shunts, physiologically significant pericardial disease, and right-sided valve lesions and can distinguish between cardiac and pulmonary disease. Balloon flotation catheters permit hemodynamic measurements and continuous monitoring at the bedside. These data can be critical in the evaluation and treatment of shock, heart failure, myocardial infarction, respiratory failure, postoperative state, and many other situations. Bedside echocardiography can also be used in the evaluation and treatment of these entities when continuous monitoring is not required, and it is less invasive. Complications of right heart catheterization include bleeding, pneumothorax, arrhythmias, pulmonary emboli, pulmonary artery rupture, and sepsis.

Left heart catheterization permits quantitative assessment of mitral and aortic stenosis. With contrast angiography, valvular regurgitation and global and regional left ventricular function can be examined. Its main application is to produce selective coronary arteriograms. Since much of this information is available noninvasively, its main role is to confirm assessments of valvular abnormalities preoperatively and to obtain selective coronary arteriograms. Increasingly, the catheterization laboratory is being used for interventional procedures.

ACC/AHA guidelines for cardiac catheterization and cardiac catheterization laboratories. J Am Coll Cardiol 1991;18:1149.

Grossman W, Baim DS (editors): *Cardiac Catheterization, Angiography and Intervention,* 4th ed. Lea & Febiger, 1991.

Matthay MA, Chatterjee K: Bedside catheterization of the pulmonary artery: Risks compared with benefits. Ann Intern Med 1988;109:826. (A sobering perspective on the role of hemodynamic monitoring.)

Swan HJC: The pulmonary artery catheter. Dis Mon (Aug)

1991;37:475. (In-depth review of methodology and applications.)

Electrophysiologic Testing

Intracardiac electrocardiographic recording and stimulation studies have revolutionized the diagnosis and treatment of severe arrhythmias. Electrophysiologic testing is important for evaluating unexplained syncope. The location and severity of atrioventricular conduction disturbances and sinus node dysfunction can be assessed in symptomatic patients in whom diagnostic information cannot be obtained by ambulatory monitoring. The mechanism and optimal therapy of complex supraventricular arrhythmias—particularly those associated with accessory conduction pathways—can be elucidated and the approach to ventricular arrhythmias similarly refined. Catheter ablation procedures can definitively treat many supraventricular arrhythmias and some cases of ventricular tachycardia.

ACC/AHA Task Force Report: Guidelines for clinical intracardiac electrophysiologic studies. J Am Coll Cardiol 1989;14:1827.

CONGENITAL HEART DISEASES

Congenital lesions account for only about 2% of heart disease in adults. Only the most common acyanotic lesions are discussed here. The reader is referred to the following references for full discussions:

Beekman RH, Rocchini AP: Transcatheter treatment of congenital heart disease. Prog Cardiovasc Dis 1989;32:1. (Valve stenosis, coarctation, ASD, and VSD.)
Higgins CB (editor): Congenital Heart Disease: Echocardiography and Magnetic Resonance Imaging. Raven Press, 1990.
Hess J, Sutherland GR (editors): Congenital Heart Disease in Adolescents and Adults. Kluger, 1992.
McNamara DG: The adult with congenital heart disease. Curr Probl Cardiol 1989;14(2):57. (Concise review of main lesions.)
Perloff JK, Child JS: Congenital Heart Disease in Adults. Saunders, 1991.

PULMONARY STENOSIS

Essentials of Diagnosis

- No symptoms in patients with mild or moderately severe lesions.
- Severe cases may present with right-sided heart failure and cause sudden death.
- High-pitched systolic ejection murmur maximal in the second left interspace. S_2 delayed and soft or absent. Ejection click often present. Increased right ventricular impulse.
- Right ventricular hypertrophy on ECG; pulmonary artery dilation on x-ray. Echo-Doppler diagnostic.

General Considerations

Stenosis of the pulmonary valve or infundibulum increases the resistance to outflow, raises the right ventricular pressure, and limits pulmonary blood flow. In the absence of associated shunts, arterial saturation is normal, but severe stenosis causes peripheral cyanosis by reducing cardiac output. Clubbing and polycythemia do not develop unless a patent foramen ovale or atrial septal defect is present, permitting right-to-left shunting.

Clinical Findings

A. Symptoms and Signs: Mild cases (right ventricular-pulmonary artery gradient < 30 mm Hg) are asymptomatic. Moderate to severe stenosis (gradients 50 to > 80 mm Hg) may cause dyspnea on exertion, syncope, chest pain, and eventually right ventricular failure.

There is a palpable parasternal lift. A loud, harsh systolic murmur and a prominent thrill are present in the left second and third interspaces parasternally; the murmur is in the third and fourth interspaces in infundibular stenosis. The second sound is obscured by the murmur in severe cases; the pulmonary component is diminished, delayed, or absent. Both components are audible in mild cases. A right-sided S_4 and a prominent *a* wave in the venous pulse are present in severe cases.

B. Electrocardiography and Chest X-Ray: Right axis deviation or right ventricular hypertrophy is noted; peaked P waves provide evidence of right atrial overload. Heart size may be normal on radiographs, or there may be a prominent right ventricle and atrium or gross cardiac enlargement, depending upon the severity. There is often poststenotic dilation of the main and left pulmonary arteries. Pulmonary vascularity is normal or diminished.

C. Diagnostic Studies: Echocardiography usually demonstrates the anatomic abnormality and assesses right ventricular size and function. Doppler ultrasound can estimate the gradient accurately; its findings are usually confirmed by cardiac catheterization.

Prognosis & Treatment

Patients with mild pulmonary stenosis may have a normal life expectancy. Severe stenosis is associated with sudden death and can cause heart failure in the 20s and 30s. Moderate stenosis may be asymptomatic in childhood and adolescence, but symptoms increase as patients grow older.

Symptomatic patients or those with evidence of right ventricular hypertrophy and resting gradients over 75–80 mm Hg require correction in most cases. Percutaneous balloon valvuloplasty has proved successful and is usually the treatment of choice. Surgery can be performed with an operative mortality rate of 2–4% and an excellent long-term result in most cases.

Kopecky SL et al: Long-term outcome of patients undergoing surgical repair of isolated pulmonary valve stenosis. Follow-up at 20–30 years. Circulation 1988;78:1150. (Good results.)

Stanger P et al: Balloon pulmonary valvuloplasty: Results of the Valvuloplasty and Angioplasty of Congenital Anomalies Registry. Am J Cardiol 1990;65:775. (Extremely effective.)

COARCTATION OF THE AORTA

Essentials of Diagnosis
- Infants may have severe heart failure; children and adults are usually asymptomatic, presenting with hypertension.
- Absent or weak femoral pulses.
- Systolic pressure higher in upper extremities than in lower extremities; diastolic pressures are similar.
- Harsh systolic murmur heard in the back.
- ECG shows left ventricular hypertrophy; chest x-ray shows rib notching. Echo-Doppler is diagnostic.

General Considerations
Coarctation of the aorta consists of localized narrowing of the aortic arch just distal to the origin of the left subclavian artery. A bicuspid aortic valve is present in 25% of cases. Blood pressure is elevated in the aorta and its branches proximal to the coarctation and decreased distally. Collateral circulation develops through the intercostal arteries and branches of the subclavian arteries.

Clinical Findings
A. Symptoms and Signs: If cardiac failure does not occur in infancy, there are usually no symptoms until the hypertension produces left ventricular failure or cerebral hemorrhage; the latter may also occur from associated cerebral aneurysms. Strong arterial pulsations are seen in the neck and suprasternal notch. Hypertension is present in the arms, but the pressure is normal or low in the legs. This difference is exaggerated by exercise. Femoral pulsations are weak and are delayed in comparison with the brachial pulse. Patients with large collaterals may have relatively small gradients but still have severe coarctation. Late systolic ejection murmurs at the base are often heard better posteriorly, especially over the spinous processes. There may be an associated aortic insufficiency murmur due to a bicuspid aortic valve.

B. Electrocardiography and Chest X-Ray: The ECG usually shows left ventricular hypertrophy. Radiography shows scalloping of the ribs due to enlarged collateral intercostal arteries, dilation of the left subclavian artery and poststenotic aortic dilation, and left ventricular enlargement.

C. Diagnostic Studies: Measurement of the gradient across the lesion by catheterization and aortography remain the primary methods of diagnosis. MRI is a useful imaging adjunct, and Doppler ultrasound can also estimate the severity of obstruction.

Prognosis & Treatment
Cardiac failure is common in infancy and in older untreated patients; it is uncommon in late childhood and young adulthood. Most untreated patients with the adult form of coarctation die before age 40 from the complications of hypertension, rupture of the aorta, infective endarteritis, or cerebral hemorrhage (associated in some cases with congenital cerebral aneurysms). Aortic dissection also occurs with increased frequency in coarctation.

Resection of the coarcted site has a surgical mortality rate of 1–4%. The risks of the disease are such, however, that all coarctations in patients up to age 20 years should be resected. In patients under 40 years of age, surgery is advisable if the patient has refractory hypertension or significant left ventricular hypertrophy. The surgical mortality rate rises considerably in patients over age 50 and is of doubtful value. Balloon angioplasty of the stenosis has been accomplished successfully and may become the procedure of choice, but aortic tears have been described. About one-fourth of corrected patients continue to be hypertensive years after surgery and they have all the complications associated with hypertension.

Bobby JJ et al: Operative survival and 40 year follow-up of surgical repair of aortic coarctation. Br Heart J 1991;65;271. (Generally good results.)

Stern HC et al: Noninvasive assessment of coarctation of the aorta. Pediatr Cardiol 1991;12:1. (Role of Doppler and MRI.)

Tynan M et al: Balloon angioplasty for the treatment of native coarctation: Results of Valvuloplasty and Angioplasty of Congenital Anomalies Registry. Am J Cardiol 1990;65:790. (Procedure generally effective.)

ATRIAL SEPTAL DEFECT

Essentials of Diagnosis
- Usually asymptomatic until middle age.
- Right ventricular lift; S_2 widely split and fixed.
- Grade I–III/VI systolic ejection murmur at pulmonary area.
- ECG shows right ventricular conduction delay; x-ray shows dilated pulmonary arteries and in-

creased vascularity. Echo-Doppler usually diagnostic.

General Considerations

The most common form of atrial septal defect (80% of cases) is persistence of the ostium secundum in the mid septum; less commonly, the ostium primum (which is low in the septum) persists, in which case mitral or tricuspid abnormalities may also be present. A third form is the sinus venosus defect of the upper part of the septum. This is often associated with partial anomalous drainage of the pulmonary veins into the superior vena cava. In all cases, normally oxygenated blood from the left atrium passes into the right atrium, increasing right ventricular output and pulmonary blood flow.

Clinical Findings

A. Symptoms and Signs: Most patients with small or moderate defects are asymptomatic. With large shunts, exertional dyspnea or cardiac failure may develop, most commonly in the fourth decade or later. Prominent right ventricular and pulmonary artery pulsations are readily visible and palpable. A moderately loud systolic ejection murmur can be heard in the second and third interspaces parasternally as a result of increased pulmonary artery flow. S_2 is widely split and does not vary with breathing.

B. Electrocardiography and Chest X-Ray: Right axis deviation or right ventricular hypertrophy may be present in ostium secundum defects. Incomplete or complete right bundle branch block is present in nearly all cases of atrial septal defect, and superior axis deviation is noted in ostium primum defect. With sinus venosus defects, the P axis is leftward of +15 degrees. The chest radiograph shows large pulmonary arteries, increased pulmonary vascularity, an enlarged right atrium and ventricle, and a small aortic knob.

C. Diagnostic Studies: Echocardiography can demonstrate right ventricular volume overload with a large right ventricle and atrium, and sometimes the defect itself. Echocardiography with saline bubble contrast and Doppler flow studies can demonstrate shunting and increased pulmonary flow. Radionuclide flow studies quantify left-to-right shunting, and MRI can also elucidate the anatomy. Cardiac catheterization remains the definitive diagnostic procedure, since it can demonstrate an increase in oxygen saturation between the venae cavae and right ventricle due to the admixture of oxygenated blood from the left atrium, quantify the shunt, and measure pulmonary vascular resistance. Right and left ventricular contrast angiography may demonstrate associated valvular abnormalities or anomalous pulmonary venous drainage.

Prognosis & Treatment

Patients with small shunts may live a normal life span. Large shunts cause disability by age 40. Raised pulmonary vascular resistance secondary to pulmonary hypertension rarely occurs in childhood or young adult life in secundum defects but is more common in primum defects; after age 40, pulmonary hypertension, cardiac arrhythmias (especially atrial fibrillation), and heart failure may occur in secundum defects. Paradoxic systemic arterial embolization is a concern, especially in patients with pulmonary hypertension or venous thrombosis. Infective endocarditis does not occur with increased frequency.

Small atrial septal defects do not require surgery. The risks are now sufficiently low so that patients with left-to-right shunts and pulmonary-to-systemic flow ratios between 1.5 and 2.0 may be operated on if the total clinical picture warrants. Ratios exceeding 2.0 are an indication for surgical closure of the defect.

Surgery should be withheld from patients with pulmonary hypertension with reversed (right-to-left) shunting because of the risk of acute right heart failure. Relocation of pulmonary veins is required in patients with partial anomalous venous drainage. In ostium primum defects, in addition to closure of the defect, suture of the valve clefts—especially those of the mitral valve—is advisable if mitral regurgitation of any significant degree is present. The surgical mortality rate is low (< 1%) in patients under age 45 who are not in cardiac failure and those who have systolic pulmonary artery pressures less than 60 mm Hg. It increases to 5–10% in patients over age 40 with cardiac failure or with systolic pulmonary artery pressures greater than 60 mm Hg.

Borow KM, Karp R: Atrial septal defect: Lessons from the past, directions for the future. (Editorial.) N Engl J Med 1990;323:1698.

Konstantinides S et al: The natural course of atrial septal defect in adults: A still unsettled issue. Klin Wochenschr 1991;69:506.

Lin SL et al: Transesophageal echocardiographic detection of atrial septal defect in adults. Am J Cardiol 1992;69:280.

PATENT DUCTUS ARTERIOSUS

Essentials of Diagnosis

- Adults with small or moderately large patent ductus are usually asymptomatic at least until middle age.
- Widened pulse pressure; loud S_2.
- Continuous murmur over pulmonary area; thrill common.
- Echo-Doppler is helpful, but the lesion is best visualized by aortography.

General Considerations

The embryonic ductus arteriosus fails to close normally and persists as a shunt connecting the left pulmonary artery and aorta, usually near the origin of the left subclavian artery. Prior to birth, the ductus is kept patent by the effect of circulating prostaglandins; in early infancy, a patent ductus can often be closed by administration of intravenous indomethacin (0.2 mg/kg intravenously). If the defect is not closed, blood flows continuously from the aorta through the ductus into the pulmonary artery in both systole and diastole; the defect is a form of arteriovenous fistula, increasing the work of the left ventricle. If it remains open, obliterative changes in the pulmonary arterioles can cause pulmonary hypertension. Then the shunt is bidirectional or right-to-left (Eisenmenger's syndrome). This complication does not correlate with shunt size.

Clinical Findings

A. Symptoms and Signs: There are no symptoms unless left ventricular failure or pulmonary hypertension develops. The heart is of normal size or slightly enlarged, with a hyperdynamic apical impulse. The pulse pressure is wide, and diastolic pressure is low. A continuous rough "machinery" murmur, accentuated in late systole at the time of S_2, is heard best in the left first and second interspaces at the left sternal border. Thrills are common.

B. Electrocardiography and Chest X-Ray: A normal tracing or left ventricular hypertrophy is found, depending upon the magnitude of shunting. On chest radiographs, the heart is normal in size and contour, or there may be left ventricular and left atrial enlargement. The pulmonary artery, aorta, and left atrium are prominent.

C. Diagnostic Studies: Echocardiography quantifies left ventricular and atrial size. The magnitude of the shunt can also be determined by radionuclide flow studies. Cardiac catheterization establishes the presence and severity of a left-to-right shunt and whether pulmonary hypertension is present; angiography can define its anatomy.

Prognosis & Treatment

Large shunts cause a high mortality rate from cardiac failure early in life. Smaller shunts are compatible with long survival, congestive heart failure being the most common complication. Infective endarteritis or endarteritis may also occur, and antibiotic prophylaxis is required. A small percentage of patients develop pulmonary hypertension and reversal of shunt (right-to-left shunting), such that the lower legs, especially the toes, appear cyanotic and clubbed in contrast to normally pink fingers. At this stage, the patient is inoperable.

Surgical ligation of the patent ductus can be accomplished with excellent results in uncomplicated patients. Recent experience with catheter closure using an "umbrella" device has also been favorable, indicating that where available, this newer option is the procedure of choice for most patients. Closure is recommended for children or adults with symptoms or large shunts. Asymptomatic adults with no left ventricular hypertrophy and small left-to-right shunts are at low risk of developing pulmonary hypertension or congestive heart failure. The indications for closure of a patent ductus arteriosus in the presence of pulmonary hypertension are controversial. Opinion favors closure whenever the pulmonary vascular resistance is low and the flow through the ductus is from left to right.

Transcatheter occlusion of persistent arterial duct. Report of the European Registry. Lancet 1992;340:1062.(Greater than 90% success at 30 months.)

Yilmaz AJ et al: Ligation in adult persistent ductus arteriosus. J Cardiovasc Surg 1991;32:575. (Recent series with excellent results.)

VENTRICULAR SEPTAL DEFECT

Essentials of Diagnosis

- Adults asymptomatic if defect is small to moderate.
- Grade II–VI/VI pansystolic murmur maximal at the left sternal border; associated thrill common.
- ECG may show left or right ventricular hypertrophy if shunt is reversed; x-ray shows increased pulmonary vascularity. Echo-Doppler is diagnostic.

General Considerations

In this lesion, a persistent opening in the upper interventricular septum resulting from failure of fusion with the aortic septum permits blood to pass from the high-pressure left ventricle into the low-pressure right ventricle. The subsequent natural history and pathophysiology depend on the size of the defect and the magnitude of left-to-right shunting. Large defects are associated with early left ventricular failure. Chronic but more moderate left-to-right shunts may lead to pulmonary vascular disease and right-sided failure. Many ventricular defects close spontaneously in early childhood.

Clinical Findings

A. Symptoms and Signs: The clinical features are dependent upon the size of the defect and the presence or absence of a raised pulmonary vascular resistance. Large shunts are associated with loud, harsh holosystolic murmurs in the left third and fourth interspaces along the sternum and, in some cases, middiastolic flow murmurs and an S_3 at the apex. Smaller shunts may produce only an early systolic murmur or a diamond-shaped murmur. A systolic thrill is common. Clinical evidence of pulmonary hypertension is often more informative than the murmur itself. High defects may be associated with aortic regurgitation owing to prolapse of a valve leaflet.

B. Electrocardiography and Chest X-Ray:
The ECG may be normal or may show right, left, or biventricular hypertrophy, depending on the size of the defect and the pulmonary vascular resistance. With large shunts, the right or left ventricle (or both), the left atrium, and the pulmonary arteries are enlarged, and pulmonary vascularity is increased on chest radiographs. If pulmonary vascular disease evolves, an enlarged pulmonary artery with diminished distal vascularity is seen.

C. Diagnostic Studies: Echocardiography can demonstrate chamber size and may demonstrate the defect. Doppler ultrasound can qualitatively assess the magnitude of shunting and the pulmonary artery pressure. Magnetic resonance imaging can often visualize the defect, while radionuclide flow studies quantify pulmonary-to-systemic flow ratios. Cardiac catheterization permits definitive diagnosis in all but the most trivial defects; it is the only technique that can measure pulmonary vascular resistance.

Prognosis & Treatment

Patients with the typical murmur as the only abnormality have a normal life expectancy except for the threat of infective endocarditis. The latter is more typical of smaller shunts. Antibiotic prophylaxis is mandatory. With large shunts, congestive heart failure may develop early in life, and survival beyond age 40 is unusual. Shunt reversal occurs in an estimated 25%, producing Eisenmenger's syndrome.

Small shunts (pulmonary-to-systemic flow ratio < 1.5) in asymptomatic patients do not require surgery. Defects causing large shunts should be repaired to prevent irreversible pulmonary vascular disease or late heart failure. When severe pulmonary hypertension is present (systolic pulmonary arterial pressures > 85 mm Hg) and the left-to-right shunt is small, the surgical mortality risk is at least 50%. If the shunt is reversed, surgery is contraindicated. If surgery is required because of unrelenting cardiac failure in infancy due to a large left-to-right shunt, early closure of the defect is now the preferred procedure. The surgical mortality rate is 2–3% for primary repair. Some defects (perhaps as many as 40%) close spontaneously. Therefore, surgery should be deferred until late childhood unless the disability is severe or unless pulmonary hypertension is observed to develop or progress. It is now possible to close ventricular septal defects percutaneously in some cases.

Ellis JH et al: Ventricular septal defect in the adult: Natural and unnatural history. Am Heart J 1987;114(1 Part 1):115. (Useful management recommendations.)

Frontera-Izquierdo P, Cabezudo-Huerta G: Natural and modified history of isolated ventricular septal defect: A 17-year study. Pediatr Cardiol 1992;13:193. (Follow-up in 882 cases.)

O'Laughlin MP, Mullins CE: Transcatheter occlusion of ventricular septal defect. Cathet Cardiovasc Diagn 1989;17:175.

VALVULAR HEART DISEASE

While most cases of valvular disease were at one time due to rheumatic heart disease (still true in developing countries), other causes are now more common. The typical findings of each lesion are described in Figure 10–1 and Table 10–1. Table 10–2 shows how to use bedside maneuvers to distinguish murmurs. The references below deal with valve disease in general. Specific lesions are discussed and referenced subsequently.

Bansal RC, Shah PM: Usefulness of echo-Doppler in management of patients with valvular heart disease. Curr Probl Cardiol 1989;14(6):281.

Bashore TM, Davidson CJ (editors): *Percutaneous Balloon Valvuloplasty and Related Techniques.* Williams & Wilkins, 1991.

Carabello BA (editor): Valvular heart disease. Saunders Cardiology Clinics 1991;9(2):1. (All lesions, diagnostic techniques, and treatment.)

Frankl WS, Brest AN (editors): *Valvular Heart Disease: Evaluation and Treatment,* 2nd ed. Davis, 1993. (Chapters on natural history, diagnostic procedures, surgery and other treatments.)

MITRAL STENOSIS

Essentials of Diagnosis

- Dyspnea, orthopnea, and paroxysmal nocturnal dyspnea.
- Symptoms often precipitated by onset of atrial fibrillation or pregnancy.
- Prominent mitral first sound, opening snap (usually), and apical crescendo rumble.
- ECG shows left atrial abnormality and, commonly, atrial fibrillation. Echo-Doppler confirms diagnosis and quantitates severity.

General Considerations

Nearly all patients with mitral stenosis have underlying rheumatic heart disease, though a history of rheumatic fever is often absent.

Clinical Findings

A. Symptoms and Signs: A characteristic finding of mitral stenosis is a localized middiastolic murmur low in pitch whose duration varies with the severity of the stenosis and the heart rate (Table 10–1). Because it is thickened, the valve opens in early diastole with an opening snap. The sound is sharp, is widely distributed over the chest, and occurs early after A_2 in severe and later in milder varieties of mitral stenosis. In severe mitral stenosis with low flow across the mitral valve, the murmur may be soft

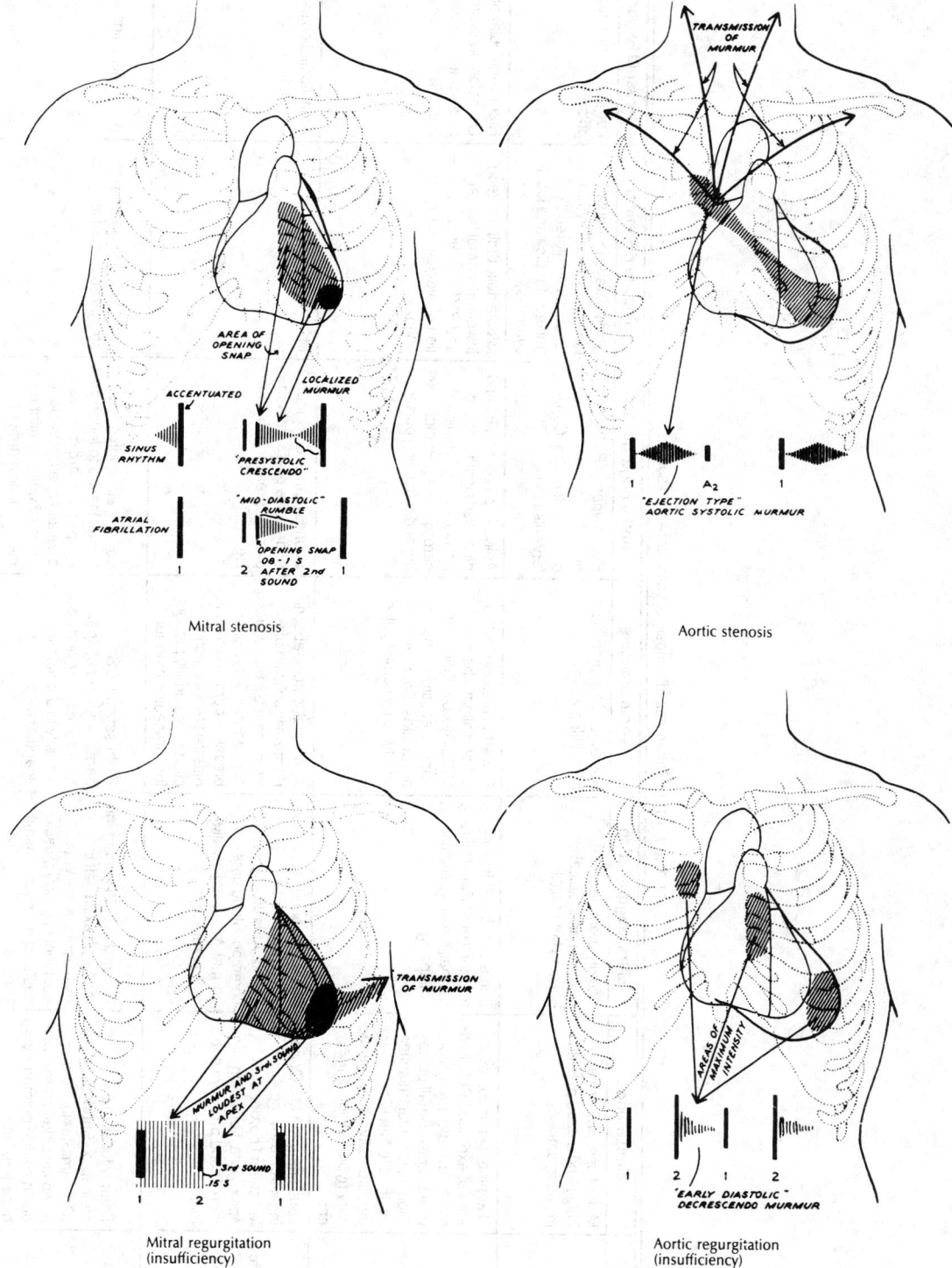

Figure 10–1. Murmurs and cardiac enlargement in common valve lesions.

Table 10–1. Differential diagnosis of valvular heart disease.

	Mitral Stenosis	Mitral Regurgitation	Aortic Stenosis	Aortic Regurgitation	Tricuspid Stenosis	Tricuspid Regurgitation
Inspection	Malar flush, precordial bulge and diffuse pulsation in young patients.	Usually prominent and hyperdynamic apical impulse to left of MCL.	Sustained PMI, prominent atrial filling wave.	Hyperdynamic PMI to left of MCL and down. Visible carotid pulsations. Capillary pulsations.	Giant *a* wave in jugular pulse with sinus rhythm. Often olive-colored skin (mixed jaundice and local cyanosis).	Large *v* wave in jugular pulse.
Palpation	"Tapping" sensation over area of expected PMI. Middiastolic and/or presystolic thrill at apex. Small pulse. Right ventricular pulsation left third to fifth ICS parasternally when pulmonary hypertension is present.	Forceful, brisk PMI; systolic thrill over PMI. Pulse normal, small, or slightly collapsing.	Powerful, heaving PMI to left and slightly below MCL. Systolic thrill over aortic area, sternal notch, or carotids. Small and slowly rising carotid pulse.	Apical impulse forceful and displaced significantly to left and down. Prominent carotid pulses. Rapidly rising and collapsing pulses.	Middiastolic thrill between lower left sternal border and PMI. Presystolic pulsation of liver (sinus rhythm only).	Right ventricular pulsation. Occasionally systolic thrill at lower left sternal edge. Systolic pulsation of liver.
Heart sounds, rhythm, and blood pressure	Loud snapping M_1. Opening snap following A_2 along left sternal border or at apex. Atrial fibrillation common. Blood pressure normal.	M_1 normal or buried in murmur. Prominent third heart sound. Atrial fibrillation common. Blood pressure normal. Midsystolic clicks may be present.	A_2 normal, soft, or absent. Paradoxic splitting of S_2. Prominent S_4. Blood pressure normal or systolic pressure normal with high diastolic level. Ejection click occasionally present just preceding murmur.	Sounds normal or A_2 loud. Wide pulse pressure with diastolic pressure <60 mm Hg.	M_1 often loud.	Atrial fibrillation usually present.
Murmurs: Location and transmission	Sharply localized at or near apex. Short diastolic (Graham Steell) murmur along lower left sternal border in severe pulmonary hypertension.	Loudest over PMI; transmitted to left axilla, left infrascapular area. With posterior papillary muscle dysfunction, may transmit to base.	Right second ICS parasternally or at apex; heard in carotids and occasionally in upper interscapular area.	Loudest along left sternal border in third to fourth interspace. Heard over aortic area and apex. May be associated with low-pitched mid-diastolic murmur at apex (Austin Flint).	Third to fifth ICS along left sternal border out to apex.	As for tricuspids stenosis.

Murmurs (cont'd): Timing	Onset at opening snap ("middiastolic") with presystolic accentuation if in sinus rhythm. Graham Steell begins with P_2 (immediate diastolic).	Pansystolic: begins with M_1 and ends at or after A_2. May be late systolic in prolapse.	Midsystolic: begins after M_1, ends before A_2; reaches maximum intensity in mid systole.	Begins immediately after aortic second sound and ends before first sound.	As for mitral stenosis.	As for mitral regurgitation.
Character	Low-pitched, rumbling; presystolic murmur merges with loud M_1 in a "crescendo." Graham Steell high-pitched, blowing.	Blowing, high-pitched; occasionally harsh or musical.	Harsh, rough.	Blowing, often faint.	As for mitral stenosis.	Blowing, coarse, or musical.
Optimum auscultatory conditions	After exercise, left lateral recumbency. Bell chest piece lightly applied.	After exercise; diaphragm chest piece. In prolapse, findings most prominent while standing.	Patient resting, leaning forward, breath held in full expiration. Bell chest piece lightly applied.	Patient resting, leaning forward, breath held in expiration. Diaphragm chest piece.	Murmur usually louder during and at peak of inspiration. Patient recumbent. Bell chest piece.	Murmur usually becomes louder during inspiration.
X-ray	Straight left heart border. Large left atrium sharply indenting esophagus. Elevation of left bronchus. Large right ventricle and pulmonary artery if pulmonary hypertension is present. Calcification occasionally seen in mitral valve.	Enlarged left ventricle and left atrium.	Concentric left ventricular hypertrophy. Prominent ascending aorta, small knob. Calcified valve common.	Moderate to severe left ventricular enlargement. Prominent aortic knob.	Enlarged right atrium only.	Enlarged right atrium and ventricle.

(continued)

Table 10–1. Differential diagnosis of valvular heart disease. (continued)

	Mitral Stenosis	Mitral Regurgitation	Aortic Stenosis	Aortic Regurgitation	Tricuspid Stenosis	Tricuspid Regurgitation
ECG	Broad P waves in standard leads; broad negative phase of diphasic P in V_1. If pulmonary hypertension is present, tall peaked P waves, right axis deviation, or right ventricular hypertrophy appears.	Left axis deviation or frank left ventricular hypertrophy. P waves broad, tall, or notched in standard leads; broad negative phase of diphasic P in V_1.	Left ventricular hypertrophy.	Left ventricular hypertrophy.	Tall, peaked P waves. Normal axis.	Right axis usual.
Echocardiography M mode	Thickened, immobile mitral valve with anterior and posterior leaflets moving together. Slow early diastolic filling slope, left atrial enlargement, normal to small left ventricle.	Thickened mitral valve in rheumatic disease; mitral valve prolapse; flail leaflet or vegetations may be seen. Enlarged left ventricle with above-normal, normal, or decreased function.	Dense persistent echoes from the aortic valve with poor leaflet excursion, left ventricular hypertrophy with preserved contractile function.	Diastolic vibrations of the anterior leaflet of the mitral valve and septum, early closure of the mitral valve when severe, dilated left ventricle with normal or decreased contractility.	Tricuspid valve thickening, decreased early diastolic filling slope of the tricuspid valve. Mitral valve also usually abnormal.	Enlarged right ventricule, prolapsing valve, mitral valve often abnormal.
Two-dimensional	Maximum diastolic orifice size reduced, subvalvular apparatus foreshortened, variable thickening of other valves.	Same as M-mode but more reliable.	Above plus poststenotic dilatation of the aorta, restricted opening of the aortic leaflets, bicuspid aortic valve in about 30%.	Above plus may show vegetations in endocarditis, bicuspid valve, root dilatation.	Above plus enlargement of the right atrium.	Same as above.
Doppler	Prolonged pressure half-time across mitral valve; indirect evidence of pulmonary hypertension.	Regurgitant flow mapped into left atrium; indirect evidence of pulmonary hypertension.	Increased transvalvular flow velocity, yielding calculated gradient. Valve area estimate using continuity equation.	Demonstrates regurgitation and qualitatively estimates severity.	Prolonged pressure half-time across tricuspid valve.	Regurgitant flow mapped into right atrium and venae cavae; right ventricular systolic pressure estimated.

A_2 = Aortic second sound MCL = Midclavicular line
ICS = Intercostal space P_2 = Pulmonary second sounds
M_1 = Mitral first sound PMI = Point of maximal impulse

Table 10–2. Effect of various interventions on systolic murmurs.[1]

Intervention	Hypertrophic Obstructive Cardiomyopathy	Aortic Stenosis	Mitral Regurgitation	Mitral Prolapse
Valsalva	↑	↓	↓ or ↔	↑ or ↓
Standing	↑	↑ or ↔	↓ or ↔	↑
Handgrip or squatting	↓	↓ or ↔	↑	↓
Supine position with legs elevated	↓	↑ or ↔	↔	↓
Exercise	↑	↑ or ↔	↑	↑
Amyl nitrite	↑↑	↑	↓	↑
Isoproterenol	↑↑	↑	↓	↑

Key: ↑ = increased; ↑↑ = markedly increased; ↓ = decreased; ↔ = unchanged

[1] Modified from Paraskos JA: Combined valvular disease. In: *Valvular Heart Disease.* Dalen JE, Alpert JS (editors). Little, Brown, 1987.

and difficult to find, but the opening snap can usually be heard. If the patient has both mitral stenosis and mitral regurgitation, the dominant features may be the systolic murmur of mitral regurgitation with or without a short diastolic murmur and a delayed opening snap.

When the valve has narrowed to less than 1.5 cm² (normal, 4–6 cm²), the left atrial pressure must rise to maintain normal flow across the valve and a normal cardiac output. This results in a pressure difference between the left atrium and left ventricle during diastole. The pressure gradient and the length of the diastolic murmur reflect the severity of mitral stenosis; they persist throughout the diastole when the lesion is severe or when the ventricular rate is rapid.

In mild cases, left atrial pressure and cardiac output may be essentially normal and the patient asymptomatic, but in moderate stenosis (valve area < 1.5 cm²)—especially with tachycardia, which shortens diastole and increases mitral flow rate—dyspnea and fatigue appear as the left atrial pressure rises. With severe stenosis, the left atrial pressure is high enough to produce pulmonary venous congestion at rest and reduce cardiac output, with resulting dyspnea, fatigue, and right heart failure. Recumbency at night further increases the pulmonary blood volume, causing orthopnea and paroxysmal nocturnal dyspnea. Severe pulmonary congestion may also be initiated by any acute respiratory infection, excessive salt and fluid intake, endocarditis, or recurrence of rheumatic carditis. As a result of long-standing pulmonary venous hypertension, anastomoses develop between the pulmonary and bronchial veins in the form of bronchial submucosal varices. These often rupture, producing mild or severe hemoptysis. In a few patients, the pulmonary arterioles become narrowed; this greatly increases the pulmonary artery pressure and accelerates the development of right ventricular hypertrophy and failure. These patients have relatively little dyspnea but experience fatigue on exertion.

Fifty to 80 percent of patients develop paroxysmal or chronic atrial fibrillation that, until the ventricular rate is controlled, may precipitate dyspnea or pulmonary edema.

B. Diagnostic Studies: Echocardiography is the most valuable technique for assessing mitral stenosis. The valve is thickened, opens poorly, and closes slowly. The anterior and posterior leaflets are fixed and move together, rather than in opposite directions. Left atrial size can be determined by echocardiography: increased size denotes an increased likelihood of atrial fibrillation or systemic emboli. The mitral valve area can be measured, and the gradient and pulmonary artery pressure can be estimated by Doppler techniques. Echocardiography also detects atrial myxoma, which sometimes presents clinically in a fashion resembling mitral stenosis.

Because echocardiography provides most of the needed information, cardiac catheterization is employed primarily to detect associated valve, coronary, or myocardial disease—usually preoperatively.

Treatment & Prognosis

Mitral stenosis may be present for a lifetime with few or no symptoms, or it may become severe in a few years. In most cases, there is a long asymptomatic phase, followed by subtle limitation of activity. The onset of atrial fibrillation often precipitates more severe symptoms, although with return to sinus rhythm (using digoxin and, often, class I or III antiarrhythmic agents) or ventricular rate control, the patient may improve. Conversion to and subsequent maintenance of sinus rhythm is most commonly successful when the duration of atrial fibrillation is brief (< 6–12 months) and the left atrium is not severely dilated (diameter < 4.5 cm). Once atrial fibrillation occurs, the patient should receive warfarin anticoagulation therapy even if sinus rhythm is restored, since 20–30% of these patients will have systemic embolization if untreated. Systemic embolization in the presence of only mild to moderate disease is not an indication for surgery but should be treated with warfarin anticoagulation.

Indications for relieving the stenosis include the following: (1) uncontrollable pulmonary edema; (2) limiting dyspnea and intermittent pulmonary edema; (3) evidence of pulmonary hypertension with right ventricular hypertrophy or hemoptysis; (4) limitation of activity despite ventricular rate control and medical therapy; and (5) recurrent systemic emboli despite anticoagulation with moderate or severe stenosis.

Open mitral commissurotomy may be effective in patients without substantial mitral regurgitation. Replacement of the valve is indicated when combined stenosis and insufficiency are present or when the mitral valve is so distorted and calcified that a satisfactory valvulotomy is not possible. Operative mortality rates are low: 1–5% in most institutions. Balloon valvuloplasty is becoming increasingly popular. Initial success rates are high, especially if valve calcification is not excessive. The rate of restenosis is not yet known but appears to be lower than that with aortic stenosis. As a result, this option appears to be a suitable alternative to surgery for many patients in experienced centers.

Problems associated with prosthetic valves are thrombosis (especially at the mitral position), paravalvular leak, endocarditis, and degenerative changes in tissue valves. Warfarin anticoagulant therapy is mandatory with mechanical prostheses and is usually employed for at least the initial 3 months with bioprostheses, especially if the patient has significant left atrial enlargement and remains in atrial fibrillation.

Keren G et al: Atrial fibrillation and atrial enlargement in patients with mitral stenosis. Am Heart J 1987;114:1146.

Kulick DL et al: Catheter balloon commissurotomy in adults. Part II: Mitral and other stenoses. Curr Probl Cardiol 1990;15(8):397. (Techniques and results.)

NHLBI Balloon Valvuloplasty Registry: Multicenter experience with balloon mitral commissurotomy. Circulation 1992;85:448. (Improving results make this an effective treatment option.)

MITRAL REGURGITATION
(Mitral Insufficiency)

Essentials of Diagnosis

- Variable causes determine clinical presentation.
- May be asymptomatic for many years (or for life) or may cause left-sided heart failure.
- Pansystolic murmur at the apex, radiating into the axilla; associated with S_3.
- ECG shows left atrial abnormality or atrial fibrillation and left ventricular hypertrophy; x-ray shows left atrial and ventricular enlargement. Echo-Doppler confirms diagnosis and estimates severity.

General Considerations

Mitral regurgitation may result from many processes. Rheumatic disease is associated with a thickened valve with reduced mobility and often a mixed picture of stenosis and regurgitation. Rheumatic disease has been replaced as the commonest cause of mitral regurgitation in most developed countries by other processes, which include myxomatous degeneration (eg, **mitral valve prolapse** with or without connective tissue diseases such as Marfan's syndrome), infective endocarditis, and subvalvular dysfunction (due to papillary muscle dysfunction or ruptured chordae tendineae). Cardiac tumors, chiefly left atrial myxoma, are a rare cause of mitral regurgitation.

Clinical Findings

A. Symptoms and Signs: During left ventricular systole, the mitral leaflets do not close normally, and blood is ejected into the left atrium as well as through the aortic valve. The net effect is an increased volume load on the left ventricle, and the presentation depends on the rapidity with which the lesion develops. In acute regurgitation, left atrial pressure rises abruptly, leading to pulmonary edema if severe. When it is chronic, the left atrium enlarges progressively, but the pressure in pulmonary veins and capillaries rises only transiently during exertion. Exertional dyspnea and fatigue progress gradually over many years.

Mitral regurgitation, like mitral stenosis, predisposes to atrial fibrillation; but this arrhythmia is less likely to provoke acute pulmonary congestion, and fewer than 5% of patients have peripheral arterial emboli. Mitral regurgitation more often predisposes to infective endocarditis.

Clinically, mitral regurgitation is characterized by a pansystolic murmur maximal at the apex, radiating to the axilla and occasionally to the base; a hyperdynamic left ventricular impulse and a brisk carotid upstroke; and a prominent third heart sound. Left atrial enlargement is usually considerable in chronic mitral regurgitation; the degree of left ventricular enlargement usually reflects the severity of regurgitation. Calcification of the mitral valve is less common than in pure mitral stenosis. The same is true of enlargement of the main pulmonary artery on radiographs. Hemodynamically, left ventricular volume overload may ultimately lead to left ventricular failure and reduced cardiac output, but for many years the left ventricular end-diastolic pressure and the cardiac output may be normal at rest, even with considerable increase in left ventricular volume.

Nonrheumatic mitral regurgitation may develop abruptly, such as with papillary muscle dysfunction following myocardial infarction, valve perforation in infective endocarditis, or ruptured chordae tendineae in mitral valve prolapse. In acute mitral regurgitation, patients are in sinus rhythm rather than atrial fibrillation, have little or no enlargement of the left atrium, no calcification of the mitral valve, no associated mitral stenosis, and in many cases little left ventricular dilation.

Myxomatous mitral valve ("floppy" or "billowing" mitral valve, or mitral valve prolapse) is usually asymptomatic but may be associated with nonspecific chest pain, dyspnea, fatigue, or palpitations. Most patients are female, many are thin, and some have minor chest wall deformities. There are characteristic midsystolic clicks, which may be multiple, often but not always followed by a late systolic murmur. These findings are accentuated in the standing position. The diagnosis is primarily clinical but can be confirmed echocardiographically. Its significance is in dispute because of the frequency (up to 10%) with which it is diagnosed in healthy young women and men, but in occasional patients this lesion is not benign. Patients who have only a midsystolic click usually have no sequelae, but patients with a late or pansystolic murmur may develop significant mitral regurgitation, often due to rupture of chordae tendineae. The need for valve replacement is commonest in men and increases with aging, so that approximately 2% of patients with clinically significant regurgitation over age 60 will require surgery. Infective endocarditis may occur, chiefly in patients with murmurs; such patients should have antibiotic prophylaxis prior to dental work and surgical procedures. Sudden death is rare and is probably related to ventricular tachycardias; β-adrenergic blocking agents are often effective for supraventricular arrhythmias. If symptomatic ventricular tachycardia or fibrillation is present, antiarrhythmic therapy and, in many cases, electrophysiologic studies are indicated. An association between mitral prolapse and embolic cerebrovascular events has also been reported.

Papillary muscle dysfunction or infarction following acute myocardial infarction is less common. When mitral regurgitation is due to papillary dysfunction, it may subside as the infarction heals or left ventricular dilation diminishes. If severe regurgitation persists, these patients have a poor prognosis with or without surgery and a natural history that reflects their underlying heart disease. Transient—but sometimes severe—mitral regurgitation may occur during episodes of myocardial ischemia. Patients with dilated cardiomyopathies of any origin may have **secondary mitral regurgitation** due to papillary muscle dysfunction or dilation of the mitral annulus. In these, mitral valve surgery is not helpful.

B. Diagnostic Studies: Echocardiography is useful in demonstrating the underlying pathologic process (rheumatic, prolapse, flail leaflet) but provides only estimates of its severity, even by Doppler techniques. The accompanying information concerning left ventricular size and function, left atrial size,

pulmonary artery pressure, and right ventricular function can be invaluable in planning treatment as well as in recognizing associated lesions. Nuclear medicine techniques as well as MRI permit measurement of left ventricular function and estimation of the severity of regurgitation.

Cardiac catheterization provides the best assessment of regurgitation and, additionally, of left ventricular function and pulmonary artery pressure. Coronary arteriography is often indicated to determine the cause of the lesion and for preoperative evaluation.

Treatment & Prognosis

Acute mitral regurgitation due to endocarditis, myocardial infarction, and ruptured chordae tendineae often requires emergency surgery. Some patients can be stabilized with vasodilators or intra-aortic balloon counterpulsation, which reduce the amount of regurgitant flow by lowering systemic vascular resistance. Patients with chronic lesions may remain asymptomatic for many years. Operation is necessary when activity becomes limited or if left ventricular function deteriorates progressively. When left ventricular function is poor (ejection fraction < 40%), due either to chronic volume overload or to another process, the surgical risk is high and the subsequent outcome poor. There has been growing success with valve repair in nonrheumatic lesions, which avoids the complications of prosthetic valves described earlier. In addition, left ventricular function appears to be better preserved when the subvalvular structures can be maintained intact by valve repair.

Crawford MH et al: Determinants of survival and left ventricular performance after mitral valve replacement. Circulation 1990;81:1173. (Results better if surgery is performed before advanced left ventricular dysfunction and dilation are present.)

Fontana ME et al: Mitral valve prolapse and the mitral valve prolapse syndrome. Curr Probl Cardiol 1991;16(5):311.

Galloway AC et al: Current concepts of mitral valve reconstruction for mitral insufficiency. Circulation 1988;78(5 Part 1):1087. (The preferred approach where feasible.)

Rankin JS et al: Ischemic mitral regurgitation. Circulation 1989;79(6 Part 2):116. (High risk for surgery.)

Wooley CF et al: The floppy, myxomatous mitral valve, mitral valve prolapse, and mitral regurgitation. Prog Cardiovasc Dis 1991;33:397. (A somewhat different perspective.)

AORTIC STENOSIS

Essentials of Diagnosis

- In adults, usually asymptomatic until middle or old age.
- Delayed and diminished carotid pulses.
- Soft, absent, or paradoxically split S_2.
- Harsh systolic murmur, sometimes with thrill

along left sternal border, often radiating to the neck; may be louder at apex in older patients.

- ECG usually shows left ventricular hypertrophy; calcified valve on x-ray or fluoroscopy. Echo-Doppler is diagnostic in most cases.

General Considerations

Aortic valvular stenosis may follow rheumatic fever but is more commonly caused by progressive valvular calcification superimposed upon a congenitally bicuspid valve, or in the elderly, a previously normal valve. Aortic stenosis has become the commonest surgical valvular lesion in developed countries. Over 80% of patients are men. Valvular stenosis must be distinguished from supravalvular obstruction and from outflow obstruction of the left ventricular infundibulum, both relatively rare.

Clinical Findings

A. Symptoms and Signs: Slightly narrowed, thickened, or roughened valves (aortic sclerosis) or aortic dilation may produce the typical murmur and thrill without causing significant hemodynamic effects. In mild or moderate cases, the characteristic signs are a systolic ejection murmur at the aortic area transmitted to the neck and apex; in severe cases, a palpable left ventricular heave or thrill, a weak to absent aortic second sound, or reversed splitting of the second sound are present (see Table 10–1). When the valve area is less than $0.8–1$ cm^2 (normal, $3–4$ cm^2), ventricular systole becomes prolonged and the typical carotid pulse pattern of delayed upstroke and low amplitude is present, but this may be an unreliable finding in older patients with extensive arteriosclerotic vascular disease. Left ventricular hypertrophy increases progressively, with resulting elevations in diastolic pressure. Cardiac output is maintained until the stenosis is severe (with a valve area < 0.8 cm^2). Patients may present with left ventricular failure, angina pectoris, or syncope.

Symptoms of failure may be sudden in onset or may progress gradually. Angina pectoris frequently occurs in aortic stenosis. One-half of patients with calcific aortic stenosis and angina have significant associated coronary artery disease, whereas coronary disease is noted at only half this rate in the absence of angina. Syncope is typically exertional and may be due to arrhythmias (usually ventricular tachycardia but sometimes sinus bradycardia), hypotension, or decreased cerebral perfusion resulting from increased blood flow to exercising muscle without compensatory increase in cardiac output. Sudden death may occur even in previously asymptomatic individuals.

B. Diagnostic Studies: The clinical assessment of aortic stenosis may be difficult, especially in older patients. The ECG reveals left ventricular hypertrophy or suggestive repolarization changes in most patients but may be normal in up to 10%. The chest radiograph may show a normal or enlarged cardiac silhouette, calcification of the aortic valve, and dilation and calcification of the ascending aorta. The echocardiogram provides useful data about aortic valve calcification and opening and left ventricular thickness and function, while Doppler can estimate the aortic valve gradient. These data can reliably exclude or diagnose severe stenosis. In patients with moderate obstruction, especially with low cardiac output or concomitant regurgitation, these evaluations may be inaccurate.

Cardiac catheterization is the definitive diagnostic procedure. The valve gradient is measured and the valve area calculated; a valve area below 0.8 cm^2 indicates severe stenosis. Aortic regurgitation can be quantified by aortic root angiography. Coronary arteriography should be performed in most adults with aortic stenosis.

Prognosis & Treatment

Following the onset of heart failure, angina, or syncope, the prognosis without surgery is poor (50% 3-year mortality rate). Medical treatment may stabilize patients in heart failure, but surgery is indicated for all symptomatic patients, including those with left ventricular dysfunction, which often improves postoperatively. Asymptomatic patients are at risk for sudden death, though this is usually preceded by symptoms; valve replacement should be considered in such cases only when the gradient is severe (> 60–80 mm Hg) or left ventricular hypertrophy is advanced.

The surgical mortality rate for valve replacement is 2–5%, but it rises to 10% above the age of 70. Severe coronary lesions are usually bypassed at the same time. Anticoagulation with warfarin is required for mechanical prostheses but is not essential with bioprostheses. The latter undergo degenerative changes and often require reoperation in 7–10 years. Many patients continue to exhibit conduction system disease or ventricular arrhythmias postoperatively.

Recently, many centers have begun performing balloon valvuloplasty for aortic stenosis. The stenosis can be relieved in the majority of subjects, but the mortality rate of the procedure approaches that of surgery—except in very high risk individuals—and restenosis occurs in up to 50% of cases within the first 6–12 months. This approach should be considered an alternative limited to individuals who are poor candidates for surgery or as an intermediate procedure to stabilize high-risk patients prior to surgery.

Bernard Y et al: Long term results of percutaneous aortic valvuloplasty compared with aortic valve replacement in patients more than 75 years old. J Am Coll Cardiol 1992;20:796. (Results better with surgery.)

Kennedy KD et al: Natural history of moderate aortic stenosis. J Am Coll Cardiol 1991;17:313. (Once symptoms occur, complications are common even when stenosis is not critical.)

Lombard JT, Selzer A: Valvular aortic stenosis: A clinical and hemodynamic profile of patients. Ann Intern Med 1987;106:292. (Review of changing presentations.)

NHLBI Balloon Valvuloplasty Registry: Percutaneous balloon aortic valvuloplasty: Acute and 30 day follow-up results in 674 patients. Circulation 1991;84:2388. (Results are improving, but the 30-day mortality rate is 14% in the high-risk group undergoing the procedure; surgery remains preferable when feasible.)

Pellikka PA et al: Natural history of adults with asymptomatic hemodynamically significant aortic stenosis. J Am Coll Cardiol 1990;15:1012. (While many become symptomatic, sudden death is rare.)

AORTIC REGURGITATION
(Aortic Insufficiency)

Essentials of Diagnosis
(Chronic Regurgitation)

- Usually asymptomatic until middle age; presents with left-sided failure or chest pain.
- Wide pulse pressure with associated peripheral signs.
- Hyperactive, enlarged left ventricle.
- Diastolic murmur along left sternal border.
- ECG shows left ventricular hypertrophy; x-ray shows left ventricular dilation. Echo-Doppler confirms diagnosis and estimates severity.

General Considerations

Rheumatic aortic regurgitation has become less common than in the preantibiotic era, but nonrheumatic causes are frequent and are the major cause of isolated aortic regurgitation. These include congenitally bicuspid valves, infective endocarditis, and hypertension. Many patients have aortic regurgitation secondary to aortic root diseases such as cystic medial necrosis (especially Marfan's syndrome), aortic dissection, ankylosing spondylitis, Reiter's syndrome, and syphilis.

Clinical Findings

A. Symptoms and Signs: The clinical presentation is determined by the rapidity with which regurgitation develops. In chronic regurgitation, the only sign for many years may be a soft aortic diastolic murmur. As the valve deformity increases, larger amounts regurgitate, diastolic blood pressure falls, and the left ventricle progressively enlarges. Most patients remain asymptomatic even at this point, and an often prolonged plateau phase, characterized by stable left ventricular dilation, occurs. Left ventricular failure is a late event and may be sudden in onset. Exertional dyspnea and fatigue are the most frequent symptoms, but paroxysmal nocturnal dyspnea and pulmonary edema may also occur. Angina pectoris or atypical chest pain may be present. Associated coronary artery disease and syncope are less common than in aortic stenosis.

Hemodynamically, because of compensatory left ventricular dilation, patients eject a large stroke volume which is adequate to maintain forward cardiac output until late in the course of the disease. Left ventricular diastolic pressure remains normal also but may abruptly rise when heart failure occurs. Abnormal left ventricular systolic function, as manifested by reduced ejection fraction and increasing end-systolic left ventricular volume, is a late sign.

The major physical findings relate to the wide arterial pulse pressure. The pulse has a rapid rise and fall (Corrigan's pulse), with an elevated systolic and low diastolic pressure, owing to the large stroke volume and rapid diastolic runoff back into the left ventricle, respectively. The large stroke volume is also responsible for characteristic findings such as Quincke's pulses (subungual capillary pulsations) and Duroziez's sign (diastolic murmur over a partially compressed peripheral artery, commonly the femoral). The apical impulse is prominent, laterally displaced, and usually hyperdynamic and may be sustained. The murmur itself may be quite soft and localized; the aortic diastolic murmur is high-pitched and decrescendo. A mid or late diastolic low-pitched mitral murmur (Austin Flint murmur) may be heard in advanced aortic insufficiency, owing to obstruction of mitral flow produced by partial closure of the mitral valve by the regurgitant jet.

When aortic insufficiency develops acutely (as in aortic dissection or infective endocarditis), left ventricular failure, manifested primarily as pulmonary edema, may develop rapidly, and surgery is urgently required. Patients with acute aortic insufficiency do not have the dilated left ventricle of chronic aortic insufficiency. In the same way, the diastolic murmur is shorter and may be minimal in intensity, and the pulse pressure may not be widened, making clinical diagnosis difficult.

B. Diagnostic Studies: The ECG usually shows moderate to severe left ventricular hypertrophy. Radiographs show cardiomegaly with left ventricular prominence.

Echocardiography can demonstrate diastolic fluttering of the anterior mitral leaflet or septum produced by the regurgitant jet. Serial assessments of left ventricular size and function are critical in determining the timing for valve replacement. Doppler techniques can qualitatively estimate the severity of regurgitation, though it should be noted that "mild" regurgitation is not uncommon and should not be overinterpreted. Scintigraphic studies can quantify left ventricular function and functional reserve during exercise—a useful predictor of prognosis.

Cardiac catheterization can help quantify severity and is used to evaluate the coronary and aortic root anatomy preoperatively.

Treatment & Prognosis

Aortic regurgitation that appears or worsens during

or after an episode of infective endocarditis or aortic dissection may lead to acute severe left ventricular failure or subacute progression over weeks or months. The former usually presents as pulmonary edema; surgical replacement of the valve is indicated even during active infection. These patients may be transiently improved or stabilized by vasodilators.

Chronic regurgitation has a long natural history, but the prognosis without surgery becomes poor when significant symptoms occur. Vasodilators, such as hydralazine and angiotensin-converting enzyme inhibitors, can reduce the severity of regurgitation, and prophylactic treatment may postpone or avoid surgery in asymptomatic patients with severe regurgitation and dilated left ventricles. In symptomatic patients, medical therapy with diuretics, vasodilators, and digoxin can stabilize or improve symptoms but should usually be employed only as a preliminary to surgical correction. Surgery is also indicated for those with few or no symptoms who present with significant left ventricular dysfunction (ejection fraction < 45–50%) or who exhibit progressive deterioration of left ventricular function, irrespective of symptoms.

The operative mortality rate is usually in the 3–5% range. Surgeons are attempting valve repair more frequently in patients with leaflet prolapse (most frequently in individuals with bicuspid valves). Aortic regurgitation due to aortic root disease requires repair or replacement of the root, a more difficult operation. Following surgery, left ventricular size usually decreases and left ventricular function improves, except where dysfunction has been present chronically.

Cosgrove DM et al: Valvuloplasty for aortic insufficiency. J Thorac Cardiovasc Surg 1991;102:571.

Greenberg B et al: Long-term vasodilator therapy of chronic aortic insufficiency: A randomized double-blinded, placebo-controlled clinical trial. Circulation 1988;78:92. (Large trial indicating value of prophylactic therapy.)

Michel PL et al: Degenerative aortic regurgitation. Eur Heart J 1991;12:875. (In one-third of patients undergoing valve replacement for isolated chronic aortic insufficiency, aortic root disease is the cause.)

Siemienczuk D et al: Chronic aortic insufficiency: Factors associated with progression to aortic valve replacement. Ann Intern Med 1989;110:587. (Left ventricular size and function determine outcome.)

TRICUSPID STENOSIS

Tricuspid stenosis is usually rheumatic in origin. It should be suspected when "right heart failure" appears in the course of mitral valve disease, marked by hepatomegaly, ascites, and dependent edema. The typical diastolic rumble along the lower left sternal border mimics mitral stenosis. In sinus rhythm, a presystolic liver pulsation may be found.

Hemodynamically, a diastolic pressure gradient of 5–15 mm Hg is found across the tricuspid valve in conjunction with raised pressure in the right atrium and jugular veins, with prominent *a* waves and with a slow *y* descent because of slow right ventricular filling.

Echocardiography usually demonstrates the lesion, and Doppler flow studies can measure the gradient; accompanying valve lesions can also be detected. Right heart catheterization is diagnostic.

Acquired tricuspid stenosis may be amenable to valvotomy under direct vision, but it usually requires a prosthetic valve replacement. Although experience is limited, balloon valvuloplasty may be the initial procedure of choice in many patients.

TRICUSPID REGURGITATION

Tricuspid regurgitation may occur in a variety of situations other than disease of the tricuspid valve itself. The most common is right ventricular overload resulting from left ventricular failure due to any cause. Tricuspid insufficiency occurs in association with right ventricular and inferior myocardial infarction. Tricuspid valve endocarditis and resulting regurgitation are common in intravenous drug users. Other causes include the carcinoid syndrome, lupus erythematosus, and myxomatous degeneration of the valve (associated with mitral valve prolapse). The symptoms and signs are identical to those resulting from right ventricular failure due to any cause. In the presence of mitral valve disease, the tricuspid valvular lesion can be suspected on the basis of early onset of right heart failure and a harsh systolic murmur along the lower left sternal border which is separate from the mitral murmur and which often increases in intensity during and just after inspiration.

Hemodynamically, tricuspid insufficiency is characterized by a prominent regurgitant systolic (*v*) wave in the right atrium and jugular venous pulse, with a rapid *y* descent and a small or absent *x* descent. The regurgitant wave, like the systolic murmur, is increased with inspiration, and its size depends upon the size of the right atrium. In tricuspid regurgitation, especially with right ventricular failure, an inspiratory S_3 may be present.

Tricuspid insufficiency secondary to severe mitral valve disease or other left-sided lesions may regress when the underlying disease is corrected. When surgery is required, valve repair or valvuloplasty of the tricuspid ring is often preferable to valve replacement. Replacement of the tricuspid valve is infrequently done now.

Choice & Management of Prosthetic Valves

Valve repair for tricuspid and mitral regurgitation—and, to a lesser extent, aortic regurgitation and percutaneous or open valvulotomy—may be optimal for many patients with mitral, pulmonary, and tricuspid stenosis. Nonetheless, the number of valve replacement procedures continues to increase as a result of the aging of the population. The choice of a mechanical device versus a bioprosthesis is often a difficult one, balancing the risk of chronic anticoagulation and thromboembolism versus the need for eventual reoperation. In general, otherwise healthy patients below age 65 should receive mechanical valves unless anticoagulation is contraindicated because their life expectancy is greater than the durability of tissue prostheses. Deterioration of bioprostheses is accelerated in younger patients, in particular. In patients with a small left ventricular cavity or aortic annulus, several mechanical disk valves have significant hemodynamic advantages. Finally, patients who will require anticoagulation in any case, such as those in atrial fibrillation, should receive mechanical valves. Bioprostheses are preferable in older patients and those with life expectancies less than 10 years and when anticoagulation is contraindicated. However, hemodialysis patients should not receive tissue valves because they have a high failure rate.

The identification of valve dysfunction may be difficult, but Doppler echocardiography, especially via the transesophageal approach, can identify regurgitation and stenosis in most cases. In patients with mechanical valves, careful anticoagulation is required with a target prothrombin time of 1.5–2 times control (INR 3-D4). Anticoagulation should rarely be discontinued. For elective surgery, oral warfarin can be stopped 2–3 days preoperatively with heparin coverage until effective anticoagulation is resumed. In pregnant women, warfarin should be continued until 2 weeks before expected delivery, when heparin can be substituted, though the risk of fetal hemorrhage is increased somewhat.

Bloomfield P et al: Twelve year comparison of a Bjork-Shiley mechanical heart valve with porcine bioprostheses. N Engl J Med 1991;324:573. (By 12 years, survival without reoperation is better with mechanical valve.)

Cobanoglu A, Ott GY: Tricuspid valve surgery: Indications, methods, and results. Cardiovasc Clinics 1993;23:265.

Grunkemeir GL et al: Prosthetic heart valve performance: LongDterm followDup. Curr Probl Cardiol 1992;17:329. (Extensive review of data.)

Jamieson WR: Modern cardiac valve devices—bioprostheses and mechanical prostheses: State of the art. J Cardiac Surg 1993;8:89. (Recommendations for choice of prosthetic valve.)

Stein PD et al: Antithrombotic therapy in patients with mechanical and biological prosthetic heart valves. Chest 1992;102(Suppl 4):445S. (Consensus statement.)

INFECTIVE ENDOCARDITIS

Essentials of Diagnosis
- Preexisting organic heart lesion (not necessary in intravenous drug users).
- Persistent fever, nonspecific systemic symptoms.
- New or changing heart murmur.
- Evidence of systemic emboli.
- Leukocytosis, elevated erythrocyte sedimentation rate, positive blood culture.

General Considerations
Endocarditis has traditionally been classified as acute or subacute based upon the pathogenic organism and the clinical presentation, but this distinction has become less clear and the less specific term "infective endocarditis" is now more commonly used. Important factors that determine the clinical presentation are (1) the nature of the infecting organism; (2) whether the infection is superimposed upon preexisting abnormal cardiac structures; and (3) the source of infection, since endocarditis in intravenous drug abusers and infections acquired during open heart surgery have special features.

More virulent organisms—*Staphylococcus aureus* in particular—tend to produce a more rapidly progressive and destructive infection. Patients are more likely to present with acute febrile illnesses, early embolization, and acute valvular regurgitation and myocardial abscess formation. Still, these organisms can produce a more gradual illness, and more indolent organisms can occasionally cause the acute presentation. *Streptococcus viridans,* enterococci, and a variety of other gram-positive and gram-negative bacilli, yeasts, and fungi tend to cause a more subacute picture. Streptococcal infection tends to be more chronic, though the average incubation period is 1–2 weeks. Systemic and peripheral manifestations may predominate, but acute deterioration due to valve perforations or large emboli may supervene at any time.

Most patients who develop infective endocarditis have underlying cardiac disease, although this is frequently not the case with intravenous drug users and hospital-acquired infections. Abnormal valves or endocardial changes due to jet flow effects in congenital lesions (most commonly ventricular septal defect, tetralogy of Fallot, coarctation of the aorta, or patent ductus arteriosus) provide a nidus for infection during bacteremic episodes. Predisposing valvular abnormalities include rheumatic involvement of any valve, bicuspid aortic valves, calcific or sclerotic aortic valves (which are very common in elderly hypertensives), hypertrophic subaortic stenosis, and mitral valve prolapse. Because of its high prevalence, the latter condition is the most controversial. Most experts use antibiotic prophylaxis only in patients with mitral valve prolapse who have a mitral insufficiency murmur. Although unproved, it may be prudent to employ prophylaxis in older patients with aortic ejection murmurs in the absence of aortic stenosis. In the past, rheumatic disease was the commonest predisposing condition, this is no longer the case in developed countries.

The initiating event in infective endocarditis is intravascular contamination by pathogenic organisms. Contamination may occur directly or may result from transient or persistent bacteremia. Transient bacteremia is common during dental, upper respiratory, urologic, and lower gastrointestinal diagnostic and surgical procedures. It is less common during upper gastrointestinal and gynecologic procedures, though a high incidence has been reported during suction abortion. Intravenous drug abuse is a major cause of endocarditis and is the commonest source of right-sided (especially tricuspid) lesions. Although staphylococcal infections are most frequent, these patients may be infected by unusual organisms such as gram-negative bacilli, yeasts, and fungi, and multiple pathogens are not infrequently involved. Intravenous drug use with fever of obscure origin should be investigated by blood culture and treated for presumed endocarditis. Hospital-acquired endocarditis may be related to infected intravascular or urinary catheters. Endocarditis may complicate prosthetic valve replacement—either early, as a result of surgical contamination, or late, as a result of bacteremia from other sources. Although many different pathogens have caused endocarditis in the first 2 months after valve replacement surgery, late prosthetic valve endocarditis is most commonly caused by *S viridans* or staphylococcal species.

Clinical Findings

A. Symptoms and Signs: Most patients present with a febrile illness that has lasted several days to 2 weeks. Nonspecific symptoms are common. Cough, dyspnea, arthralgias or arthritis, diarrhea, and abdominal or flank pain may occur as a result of embolization or immunologically mediated phenomena. The initial symptoms or signs of endocarditis may be caused by arterial emboli or cardiac damage, described below under complications.

Most patients have readily documented fever, though fever may be absent in older individuals. Ninety percent have heart murmurs, but murmurs may be absent in patients with right-sided infections. A changing murmur is common only in acute endocarditis. The characteristic peripheral lesions—petechiae (on the palate or conjunctiva or beneath the fingernails); subungual ("splinter") hemorrhages; Osler nodes (painful, violaceous raised lesions of the fingers, toes, or feet); Janeway lesions (painless erythematous lesions of the palms or soles); and Roth spots (exudative lesions in the retina)—occur in a substantial minority of patients. Pallor and splenomegaly are other helpful signs.

In acute endocarditis, leukocytosis is common; in subacute cases, anemia of chronic disease and a normal white count are the rule. Hematuria and proteinuria as well as renal dysfunction may result from emboli or immunologically mediated glomerulonephritis.

B. Diagnostic Studies: Blood cultures are the definitive diagnostic procedure and are essential to guide antibiotic therapy. At least six cultures should be obtained to increase the probability of establishing the diagnosis. The optimal time to obtain cultures is just before a temperature rise. Cultures should be obtained in duplicate to permit recognition of contaminants, and blood should be cultured anaerobically and aerobically. Special procedures and media may be required to detect unusual organisms, such as *Coxiella, Chlamydia,* and certain fungi. Extended growth periods are required for *Brucella* and *Aspergillus,* among other organisms.

Positive cultures are usually readily obtainable in acute endocarditis and infections caused by gram-positive cocci, but cultures may fail to grow organisms in certain gram-negative or anaerobic bacterial infections and in fungal infections. Prior antibiotic therapy may temporarily sterilize the blood for up to a week. If initial cultures are negative and antibiotics have been given, cultures should be obtained every 24–48 hours for 7–10 days in suspected cases. Negative blood cultures have been reported in up to 30% of proved infective endocarditis cases, but with adequate numbers of cultures and optimal techniques, this number should be below 10%.

The chest x-ray may show evidence for the underlying cardiac abnormality and, in right-sided endocarditis, scattered lung infiltrates and multiple abscesses. The ECG is nondiagnostic. Changing conduction abnormalities suggest myocardial abscess formation. Patients with proved endocarditis or in whom the level of suspicion is high should be investigated by echocardiography. The echocardiogram is useful in demonstrating underlying valvular lesions and in quantifying their severity (see sections on congenital and valvular disease). The echocardiogram is less accurate in diagnosing endocarditis. Characteristic vegetations are strongly suggestive of the diagnosis, but they are present only in a minority of cases. Echocardiograms are also helpful in demonstrating myocardial and aortic root involvement, which often indicates the need for early surgery. Transesophageal echocardiography increases the sensitivity of this technique for mitral valve lesions and vegetations. Unfortunately, the demonstration of vegetations—even when they are large—has not been either sensitive or specific in predicting future embolization in left-sided endocarditis.

Birmingham GD et al: Improved detection of infective endocarditis with transesophageal echocardiography. Am Heart J 1992;123:724. (Especially with the mitral valve, more frequent and better visualization of vegetations is provided.)

Heimberger TS, Dira RJ: Infections of prosthetic heart valves and cardiac pacemakers. Infect Dis Clin North Am 1989;3:221.

Molavi A: Endocarditis: Recognition, management and prophylaxis. Cardiovasc Clin 1993;23:139.

Roberts R, Slows CM: Endocarditis in intravenous drug abusers. Emerg Med Clin North Am 1990;8:655.

Complications

The clinical course of infective endocarditis is determined by the degree of damage to the heart, by the site of infection (right- versus left-sided, aortic versus mitral valve), by whether embolization from the site of infection occurs, and by immunologically mediated processes. Destruction of infected heart valves is especially common and precipitous with *S aureus* and often enterococci but can occur with any organism. The resulting regurgitation can be mild or severe and can progress even after bacteriologic cure. The infection can also extend into the myocardium, resulting in abscesses leading to conduction disturbances, and can also involve the wall of the aorta, creating sinus of Valsalva aneurysms. Rarely, a picture resembling acute myocarditis dominates.

Peripheral embolization can occur with any organism. The most catastrophic are cerebral and myocardial embolizations, with resulting infarctions. The spleen and kidneys are also common sites. Peripheral emboli may initiate metastatic infections or may become established in vessel walls, leading to mycotic aneurysms. Right-sided endocarditis, which usually involves the tricuspid valve, often leads to septic pulmonary emboli, causing infarction and lung abscesses.

Jaffe WM et al: Infective endocarditis, 1983–1988: Echocardiographic findings and factors influencing morbidity and mortality. J Am Coll Cardiol 1990;15:1227. (Series of 70 patients with emphasis on prognostic value of echocardiography.)

Steckelberg JM et al: Emboli in infectious endocarditis: The prognostic value of echocardiography. Ann Intern Med 1991;114:635. (Vegetations do not predict emboli.)

Prevention

Some cases of endocarditis occur after dental procedures or operations involving the upper respiratory, genitourinary, or intestinal tract. Prophylactic antibiotics should be given to patients with predisposing congenital or valvular anomalies who are to have any of these procedures (Tables 10–3 and 10–4). Current recommendations are given in Table 37–9.

Dajani AS et al: Prevention of bacterial endocarditis: Recommendations by the American Heart Association. JAMA 1990;264:2919.

van der Meer JJ et al: Efficacy of antibiotic prophylaxis for prevention of native valve endocarditis. Lancet 1992; 339:135. (Controversial case controlled study suggesting that only 50% of cases are prevented.)

Treatment

Antimicrobial treatment of endocarditis is outlined in Chapter 32.

While most cases can be successfully treated medically, operative management is sometimes required. Valvular regurgitation resulting in acute heart failure that does not resolve promptly after institution of medical therapy is an indication for valve replacement even if active infection is present, especially if the aortic valve is involved. Infections that do not respond to appropriate antimicrobial therapy after 7–10 days are more likely to be eradicated if the valve is replaced. Surgery is nearly always required for fungal

---

Table 10–3. Cardiac lesions for which bacterial endocarditis prophylaxis is or is not recommended.[1,2]

Endocarditis prophylaxis recommended
  Prosthetic cardiac valves, including bioprosthetic and homograft valves
  Previous bacterial endocarditis, even in the absence of heart disease
  Most congenital cardiac malformations
  Rheumatic and other acquired valvular dysfunction, even after valvular surgery
  Hypertrophic cardiomyopathy
  Mitral valve prolapse with valvular regurgitation and murmur
  Sclerotic aortic valve

Endocarditis prophylaxis not recommended
  Isolated secundum septal defect
  Surgical repair without residua beyond 6 months of secundum atrial septal defect, or patent ductus arteriosus
  Previous coronary artery bypass graft surgery
  Mitral valve prolapse without valvular regurgitation[3] or no murmur
  Physiologic, functional, or innocent heart murmurs
  Previous Kawasaki disease without valvular dysfunction
  Cardiac pacemakers and implanted defibrillators

[1]Modified and reproduced, with permission, from Dajani AS et al: Prevention of bacterial endocarditis. JAMA 1990;264;2929. Copyright © 1990 by American Medical Association.
[2]This table lists selected conditions and is not meant to be all-inclusive.
[3]Individuals who have a mitral valve prolapse associated with thickening or redundancy of the valve leaflets may be at increased risk for bacterial endocarditis, particularly men who are 45 years of age or older.

Table 10–4. Procedures for which bacterial endocarditis prophylaxis is or is not recommended.[1,2]

Endocarditis prophylaxis recommended
    Dental procedures known to induce gingival or mucosal bleeding, including professional cleaning
    Tonsillectomy or adenoidectomy
    Surgical operations that involve intestinal or respiratory mucosa
    Bronchoscopy with a rigid bronchoscope
    Sclerotherapy for esophageal varices
    Esophageal dilation
    Gallbladder surgery
    Cystoscopy
    Urethral dilation
    Urethral catheterization if urinary tract infection is present[3]
    Urinary tract surgery if urinary tract infection is present
    Prostatic surgery
    Incision and drainage of infected tissue
    Vaginal hysterectomy
    Vaginal delivery in the presence of infection[3]

Endocarditis prophylaxis not recommended[4]
    Dental procedures not likely to induce gingival bleeding, such as simple adjustment of orthodontic appliances or fillings above
        the gum line
    Injection of local intraoral anesthetic (except intraligamentary injections)
    Shedding of primary teeth
    Tympanostomy tube insertion
    Endotracheal intubation
    Bronchoscopy with a flexible bronchoscope, with or without biopsy
    Cardiac catheterization
    Endoscopy with or without gastrointestinal biopsy
    Cesarean section
    In the absence of infection; urethral catheterization, dilation and curettage, uncomplicated vaginal delivery, therapeutic
        abortion, sterilization procedures, or insertion or removal of intrauterine devices.

[1]Modified and reproduced, with permission, from Dajani AS et al: Prevention of bacterial endocarditis. JAMA 1990;264;2919. Copyright © 1990 by American Medical Association.
[2]This table lists selected conditions and is not meant to be all-inclusive.
[3]In addition to prophylactic regimen for genitourinary procedures, antibiotic therapy should be directed against the most likely bacterial pathogen.
[4]In patients who have prosthetic heart valves, a history of endocarditis, or surgically constructed systemic-pulmonary shunts or conduits, physicians may choose to administer prophylactic antibiotics even for low-risk procedures that involve the lower respiratory, genitourinary, or gastrointestinal tracts.

endocarditis and is more often necessary with gram-negative bacilli. Surgery is also indicated when the infection involves the sinus of Valsalva or produces septal abscesses. Recurrent infection with the same organism often indicates that surgery is necessary, especially with infected prosthetic valves. Continuing embolization presents a difficult problem when the infection is otherwise responding but may be an indication for surgery when large vegetations are detected by echocardiography after more than 3–5 days of treatment. Embolization after bacteriologic cure, however, does not necessarily imply recurrence of endocarditis. Some authors suggest that anticoagulation may be helpful to prevent emboli, but there is no good evidence to support its use, and it increases the risk of catastrophic intracerebral hemorrhage.

Kahn SS, Gray RJ: Valvular emergencies. Cardiol Clin 1991;9:689. (When valve replacement is required in the setting of endocarditis.)
Middlemost S et al: A case for early surgery in native left-sided endocarditis complicated by heart failure: Results in 203 patients. J Am Coll Cardiol 1991;18:663. (Once failure occurs, early intervention is required.)

CORONARY HEART DISEASE (Arteriosclerotic Coronary Artery Disease; Ischemic Heart Disease)

Coronary atherosclerotic heart disease is the commonest cause of cardiovascular disability and death in the USA. Men are more often affected than women by an overall ratio of 4:1, but before age 40 the ratio is 8:1, and beyond age 70 it is 1:1. In men, the peak incidence of clinical manifestations is at age 50–60; in women, at age 60–70.

Risk factors for the development of ischemic heart disease include age, male gender, genetic predisposition, blood lipid abnormalities, arterial hypertension, cigarette smoking, and diabetes mellitus. Other factors of less certain importance include obesity, physical inactivity, and personality type. Patients with clinical manifestations of coronary disease before age 50 tend to have predisposing risk factors, but this is often not the case in older individuals.

Pathophysiology

Knowledge concerning the pathophysiology of atherosclerosis and the clinical presentations of coronary artery disease is accumulating rapidly and is discussed in greater detail in Chapter 27. Abnormal lipid metabolism or excessive intake of cholesterol and saturated fats—especially when superimposed on a genetic predisposition—initiates the atherosclerotic process. The initial step is the "fatty streak," or subendothelial accumulation of lipids and lipid-laden monocytes (macrophages). Low-density lipoproteins (LDLs) are the major atherogenic lipid. High-density lipoproteins (HDLs), in contrast, are protective and probably assist in the mobilization of LDLs. The pathogenetic role of other lipids, including triglycerides, is less clear. LDLs undergo in situ oxidation, which makes them more difficult to mobilize as well as locally cytotoxic. Subsequent steps include altered endothelial function (inhibition of endothelium-derived relaxing factor [EDRF] production), disruption of the endothelium, adherence of platelets and release of platelet-derived growth factor (PDGF) and other growth factors, cell proliferation, and formation of the "mature" fibrous plaque.

These processes are slowly progressive over decades in most cases. In contrast, the natural history of the mature plaque is less predictable. Plaque ulceration, fracture, or hemorrhage can initiate a cascade of further injury, platelet adherence, and thrombus formation that can either heal, often with more severe luminal obstruction, or cause the various ischemic syndromes described below.

Fuster V et al: The pathogenesis of coronary artery disease and the acute coronary syndromes. (Two parts.) N Engl J Med 1992;326:242, 310.
Steinberg D, Witzum JL: Lipoproteins and atherogenesis: Current concepts. JAMA 1990;264:3047.

Prevention of Ischemic Heart Disease

It is now clear that reducing certain risk factors, such as smoking and hyperlipidemia, can both prevent coronary disease and delay its progression and complications after it has become manifest. Treatment of lipid abnormalities (Chapter 27) has now been shown to delay the progression of atherosclerosis and in some cases to produce regression.

Another preventive measure is aspirin prophylaxis. Aspirin (325 mg every other day) in males over the age of 50 reduces the incidence of myocardial infarction. Whether this approach should be employed in the general population or only in those at higher risk is unclear, and the optimal dosage is not known. A prudent approach would be to administer 325 mg daily to men with at least one risk factor if no contraindication is present. The same approach is probably warranted for women, commencing 5–10 years later. The value of other platelet-inhibiting agents or dietary supplements, such as fish oil or omega-3 fats, is unknown.

Control of blood pressure has now been shown to prevent infarctions in older patients. Although unproved, it seems likely that control of blood pressure in younger individuals also prevents subsequent coronary events. The role of exercise remains controversial. The decrease in number of coronary deaths over the last 2 decades may be due to a decrease in the prevalence of risk factors but probably reflects also the role of coronary care units, better treatment of angina, arrhythmias, and heart failure, and improved survival after coronary revascularization in some patient subsets.

Brown G et al: Regression of coronary artery disease as a result of intensive lipid-lowering therapy in men with high levels of apolipoprotein B. N Engl J Med 1990; 323:1289. (Most dramatic demonstration of regression of coronary artherosclerosis.)
Chandrasheckhar Y, Anand IS: Exercise as a coronary protective factor. Am Heart J 1991;122:1723. (Exercise is probably protective.)
McIntosh HD: Risk factors for cardiovascular disease and death: A clinical perspective. J Am Coll Cardiol 1989; 14:24. (Exercise, smoking, and hyperlipidemia.)
Muldoon MF et al: Lowering cholesterol concentrations and mortality: A quantitative review of primary prevention trials. Brit Med J 1990;301:309. (Meta-analysis makes the often overlooked point that the total mortality rate has not been reduced by lowering cholesterol because of the increase in the noncardiac death rate.)
Willard JE et al: The use of aspirin in ischemic heart disease. N Engl J Med 1992;327:175.

Pathophysiology of Symptomatic & Silent Ischemia & Coronary Syndromes

Advanced coronary atherosclerosis and even complete occlusion may remain clinically silent. There is only a modest correlation between the clinical symptoms and the anatomic extent of disease. At present, the only means of determining the location and extent of narrowing is coronary arteriography, although ischemia can be recognized by other less invasive studies. Myocardial ischemia may be provoked by either increased myocardial oxygen requirements (exercise, mental stress, or spontaneous fluctuations in heart rate and blood pressure) or by decreased oxygen supply (caused by coronary vasospasm, platelet plugging, or partial thrombosis). Abnormal endothelial function appears to play a role in the fluctuating threshold for ischemia; impaired release of endothelium-derived relaxing factor may permit unopposed vasoconstriction and facilitate platelet adhesion.

Most studies indicate that in angina pectoris, increased oxygen demand is the most frequent mechanism. In contrast, the acute coronary syndromes of unstable angina and myocardial infarction are caused by plaque disruption, platelet plugging, and coronary thrombosis. Of interest is the predilection for these episodes to occur in the early morning or shortly after arising. Whether the vessel becomes occluded or whether thrombolysis occurs and the plaque is stabilized determine the outcome. Thus, therapy is primarily directed toward inhibition of platelet activity (aspirin) and thrombolysis in acute syndromes and toward minimizing myocardial oxygen requirements—as well as preventive measures—in chronic angina.

Some episodes of myocardial ischemia are painful, causing angina pectoris; others are completely silent. Many silent episodes are brought on by emotional and mental stress. In patients with diagnosed coronary disease, as evidenced by prior myocardial infarction or angina, silent ischemic episodes have the same prognostic import as painful ones. The prognosis for patients with only silent ischemia is not well established, nor is the potential benefit of preventing silent ischemia.

Cohn PF: Should silent ischemia be treated in asymptomatic individuals? Circulation 1990;82(Suppl II):149. (Important question, but answer unclear.)

Muller JE et al: Circadian variation and triggers of onset of acute cardiovascular disease. Circulation 1989;79:733. (More common in early morning.)

Selwyn AP et al: Pathophysiology of ischemia in patients with coronary artery disease. Prog Cardiovasc Dis 1992;35:27.

Yeung A et al: The effect of atherosclerosis on the vascular response of coronary arteries to mental stress. N Engl J Med 1991;325:1551. (Impaired endothelial function may be the mechanism.)

SUDDEN DEATH

Sudden death may be the first clinical manifestation of coronary disease in as many as one-fourth of patients but is more likely to occur in patients with prior infarction and moderate to severe left ventricular dysfunction. In addition, 20% of patients with acute myocardial infarction will die before reaching a hospital. Most of these deaths are caused by ventricular fibrillation. It is noteworthy that transient ischemia (as opposed to infarction or coronary occlusion) is rarely the cause of sudden death. See section on ventricular arrhythmias and evaluation of survivors of sudden death for management of patients at risk for sudden death and of survivors.

Akhtar M, Myerburg RJ: Current perspectives on the problem of sudden cardiac death. Circulation 1992;85(Suppl I):I–1. (Entire issue. Cupples articles show that underlying coronary artery disease is the main risk factor. Davies article shows that 73% of victims have recent coronary thrombotic lesions.)

Josephson ED (editor): *Sudden Cardiac Death.* Blackwell, 1993.

ANGINA PECTORIS

Essentials of Diagnosis

- Precordial chest pain, usually precipitated by stress or exertion, relieved rapidly by rest or nitrates.
- Electrocardiographic or scintigraphic evidence of ischemia during pain or stress testing.
- Angiographic demonstration of significant obstruction of major coronary vessels.

General Considerations

Angina pectoris is usually due to atherosclerotic heart disease. Coronary vasospasm may occur at the site of a lesion or, less frequently, in apparently normal vessels. Other unusual causes of coronary artery obstruction such as congenital anomalies, emboli, arteritis, or dissection may cause ischemia or infarction. Angina may also occur in the absence of coronary artery obstruction as a result of severe myocardial hypertrophy, severe aortic stenosis or insufficiency, or in response to increased metabolic demands, as in hyperthyroidism, marked anemia, or paroxysmal tachycardias with rapid ventricular rates.

Clinical Findings

A. History: The diagnosis of angina pectoris depends principally upon the history, which should specifically include the following information.

1. Circumstances that precipitate and relieve angina–Angina occurs most commonly during activity and is relieved by resting. Exertion that involves straining the thoracic or upper extremity muscles (eg, lifting) or walking rapidly uphill precipitates attacks most consistently. Patients prefer to remain upright rather than lie down. The amount of activity required to produce angina may be relatively consistent under comparable physical and emotional circumstances or may vary from day to day. It is usually less after meals, during excitement, or on exposure to cold. The threshold for angina is often lower in the morning or after strong emotion; the latter can provoke attacks in the absence of exertion. In addition, discomfort may occur during sexual activity, at rest, or at night as a result of coronary spasm.

2. Characteristics of the discomfort–Patients often do not refer to angina as "pain" but as a sensation of tightness, squeezing, burning, pressing, choking, aching, bursting, "gas," indigestion, or an ill-characterized discomfort. It is often characterized by clenching a fist over the mid chest. The distress of angina is never sharply localized and is not spasmodic.

3. Location and radiation–The distribution of the distress may vary widely in different patients but is usually the same for each patient unless unstable angina or myocardial infarction supervenes. In 80–90% of cases, the discomfort is felt behind or slightly to the left of the mid sternum. When it begins farther to the left or, uncommonly, on the right, it characteristically moves centrally to include the sternum. Although angina may radiate to any dermatome from C8 to T4, it radiates most often to the left shoulder and upper arm, frequently moving down the inner volar aspect of the arm to the elbow, forearm, wrist, or fourth and fifth fingers. Radiation to the right shoulder and distally is less common, but the characteristics are the same. Occasionally, angina may be felt initially in the lower jaw, the back of the neck, the interscapular area, high in the left back, or in the volar aspect of the wrist. If the patient identifies the site of pain by pointing to the area of the apical impulse with one finger, angina is unlikely.

4. Duration of attacks–Angina is of short duration and subsides completely without residual discomfort. If the attack is precipitated by exertion and the patient promptly stops to rest, it usually lasts less than 3 minutes. Attacks following a heavy meal or brought on by anger often last 15–20 minutes. Attacks lasting more than 30 minutes are unusual and suggest the development of unstable angina, myocardial infarction, or an alternative diagnosis.

5. Effect of nitroglycerin–The diagnosis of angina pectoris is strongly supported if sublingual nitroglycerin invariably shortens an attack and if prophylactic nitrates permit greater exertion or prevent angina entirely.

6. Risk factors–The presence of risk factors described previously makes the diagnosis of angina more likely, but their absence does not exclude angina since most patients do not have a risk profile markedly different from that of the general population.

B. Signs: Examination during a spontaneous or induced attack frequently reveals a significant elevation in systolic and diastolic blood pressure, although hypotension may also occur; occasionally, a gallop rhythm and an apical systolic murmur due to transient mitral regurgitation from papillary muscle dysfunction are present during pain only. Supraventricular or ventricular arrhythmias may be present, either as the precipitating factor or as a result of ischemia.

It is important to detect signs of diseases that may contribute to or accompany atherosclerotic heart disease, eg, diabetes mellitus (retinopathy or neuropathy), xanthelasma, tendinous xanthomas, hypertension, thyrotoxicosis, myxedema, or peripheral vascular disease. Aortic stenosis or regurgitation, hypertrophic cardiomyopathy, and mitral valve prolapse should be sought, since they may produce angina or other forms of chest pain.

C. Laboratory Findings: It is important to evaluate risk factors associated with the development of atherosclerosis, particularly serum lipids. Contributing factors such as diabetes, anemia, renal disease, thyrotoxicosis, or myxedema should be sought if suggested by the history and physical examination.

D. Electrocardiography: The resting ECG is normal in about a quarter of patients with angina. In the remainder, abnormalities include old myocardial infarction, nonspecific ST–T changes, atrioventricular or intraventricular conduction defects, and changes of left ventricular hypertrophy. During anginal episodes, the characteristic electrocardiographic change is horizontal or downsloping ST segment depression that reverses after the ischemia disappears. T wave flattening or inversion may also occur. Less frequently, ST segment elevation is observed; this finding suggests severe (transmural) ischemia and often occurs with coronary spasm.

E. Exercise Electrocardiography: Exercise testing is the most useful noninvasive procedure for evaluating the patient with angina. Ischemia that is not present at rest is detected by precipitation of typical chest pain or ST segment depression (or, rarely, elevation). Exercise testing is often combined with scintigraphic studies or echocardiography (see below), but in patients without baseline ST segment abnormalities or in whom anatomic localization is not necessary, the exercise ECG should be the initial procedure because of considerations of cost and convenience.

Exercise testing can be done on a motorized treadmill or with a bicycle ergometer. A variety of exercise protocols are utilized, the most common being the Bruce protocol, which increases the treadmill speed and elevation every 3 minutes until limited by symptoms. At least two electrocardiographic leads should be monitored continuously.

1. Precautions and risks–The usually quoted risk of exercise testing is one infarction or death per 1000 tests, but individuals with unstable angina or pain at rest or minimal activity are at higher risk and should not be tested. Many of the traditional exclusions, such as recent myocardial infarction or congestive heart failure, are no longer employed *if the patient is stable and ambulatory,* but aortic stenosis remains a contraindication. A physician should monitor the test, and full resuscitation equipment should be available. While most tests are carried to a symptom-limited end point (except submaximal testing early postinfarction), the test should be terminated when hypotension, significant ventricular or supraventricular arrhythmias, more than mild to moderate angina, or more than 3- to 4-mm ST segment depression occurs.

2. Indications–Exercise testing is employed (1) to confirm the diagnosis of angina; (2) to determine the severity of limitation of activity due to angina; (3) to assess prognosis in patients with known coronary disease, including those recovering from myocardial infarction, by detecting groups at high or low risk; (4) to evaluate responses to therapy; and (5) less successfully, to screen asymptomatic populations for silent coronary disease. The latter application is controversial. Because false-positive tests often exceed true positives, leading to much patient anxiety and self-imposed or mandated disability, exercise testing of asymptomatic individuals should be done only for those at high risk (usually a strong family history of premature coronary disease or hyperlipidemia), those whose occupations place them or others at special risk (eg, airline pilots), and older individuals commencing strenuous activity.

3. Interpretation–The usual electrocardiographic criterion for a positive test is 1 mm (0.1 mV) horizontal or downsloping ST segment depression (beyond baseline) measured 80 ms after the J point. By this criterion, 60–80% of patients with anatomically significant coronary disease will have a positive test, but 10–20% of those without significant disease will also be positive. False-positives are uncommon when a 2-mm depression is present. Additional information is inferred from the time of onset and duration of the electrocardiographic changes, their magnitude and configuration, blood pressure and heart rate changes, the duration of exercise, and the presence of associated symptoms. In general, patients exhibiting more severe ST segment depression (> 2 mm) at low workloads (< 6 minutes on the Bruce protocol) or heart rates (< 70% of age-predicted maximum)—especially when the duration of exercise and rise in blood pressure are limited or when hypotension occurs during the test—have more severe disease and a poorer prognosis. Depending on symptom status, age, and other factors, such patients should be referred for coronary arteriography and possible revascularization. On the other hand, less impressive positive tests in asymptomatic patients are often "false-positives." Therefore, exercise testing results that do not conform to the clinical picture should be confirmed by scintigraphic study (see below).

F. Scintigraphic Assessment of Ischemia: Two nuclear medicine studies provide additional information about the presence, location, and extent of coronary disease.

1. Myocardial perfusion scintigraphy–This test provides images in which radionuclide uptake is proportionate to blood flow at the time of injection. Thallium-201 or one of the newer technetium-based imaging agents is used. Areas of diminished uptake reflect relative hypoperfusion (compared to other myocardial regions). If the radiotracer is injected during exercise or dipyridamole- or adenosine-induced coronary vasodilation, scintigraphic defects indicate a zone of ischemia or hypoperfusion. Over time, as relative blood flow equalizes, these defects tend to "fill in" if the abnormality is transient, indicating reversible ischemia. Defects observed when the radiotracer is injected at rest or still present 3–4 hours after an injection during exercise or dipyridamole vasodilation usually indicate myocardial infarction (old or recent) but may be present with severe ischemia. Occasionally, other conditions, including infiltrative diseases (sarcoidosis, amyloidosis), left bundle branch block, and dilated cardiomyopathy, may produce resting or persistent perfusion defects.

In experienced laboratories, thallium-201 scintigraphy is positive in 75–90% of patients with anatomically significant coronary disease and in only about 20% of those without it. False-positive tests in women may be due to attenuation through breast tissue.

Myocardial scintigraphy is indicated (1) when the resting ECG makes an exercise ECG difficult to interpret (LBBB, baseline ST-T changes, low voltage, etc); (2) for confirmation of the results of the exercise ECG when they are contrary to the clinical impression (eg, a positive test in an asymptomatic patient); (3) to localize the region of ischemia; (4) to distinguish ischemic from infarcted myocardium; (5) to assess the completeness of vascularization following bypass surgery or coronary angioplasty; or (6) as a prognostic indicator in patients with known coronary disease.

2. Radionuclide angiography–This procedure images the left ventricle and measures its ejection fraction and wall motion. In coronary disease, resting abnormalities usually represent infarction, and those that occur with exercise usually indicate stress-induced ischemia. Normal subjects usually exhibit an increase in ejection fraction with exercise or no change; patients with coronary disease may exhibit a decrease. Exercise radionuclide angiography has approximately the same sensitivity as thallium-201 scintigraphy, but it is less specific in older individuals and those with other forms of heart disease. The indications are similar to those for thallium-201 scintigraphy.

G. Echocardiography: Echocardiography can image the left ventricle and reveal segmental wall motion abnormalities, which may indicate ischemia or prior infarction. It is a convenient technique for assessing left ventricular function, which is an important indicator of prognosis and determinant of therapy. An increasing number of laboratories are performing echocardiograms during supine exercise or immediately following upright exercise; exercise-induced segmental wall motion abnormalities are used as an additional indicator of ischemia. This technique requires considerable expertise; however, in experienced laboratories, the increment in test accuracy is comparable to that obtained with scintigraphy—though a higher proportion of tests are technically inadequate. Pharmacologic stress with high-dose (20–40 µg/kg/min) dobutamine can be used as an alternative to exercise.

H. Ambulatory Electrocardiographic Monitoring: With current ambulatory electrocardiographic recorders and with trained technicians, episodes of ischemic ST segment depression can be monitored. In patients with coronary artery disease, these episodes usually signify ischemia, even when asymptomatic ("silent"). In many, silent episodes are more frequent than symptomatic ones. In most cases, they occur in patients with other evidence of ischemia, and they respond to the same treatments, so that the role of ambulatory monitoring is unclear, as is the benefit of abolishing all such episodes in patients who are otherwise being managed properly.

I. Coronary Angiography: Selective coronary arteriography is the definitive diagnostic procedure for coronary artery disease. It can be performed with low mortality (about 0.1%) and morbidity (1–5%), but the cost is high, and with currently available noninvasive techniques it is usually not indicated solely for diagnosis.

Coronary arteriography should be performed in the following groups:

(1) Patients being considered for coronary artery revascularization because of limiting stable angina who have failed to improve on an adequate medical regimen.

(2) Patients in whom coronary revascularization is being considered because the clinical presentation (unstable angina, postinfarction angina, etc) or noninvasive testing suggests high-risk disease (see Indications for Revascularization).

(3) Patients with aortic valve disease who also have angina pectoris, in order to determine whether the angina is due to accompanying coronary disease. Coronary angiography is also performed in asymptomatic older patients undergoing valve surgery so that concomitant bypass may be done if the anatomy is propitious.

(4) Patients who have had coronary revascularization with subsequent recurrence of symptoms, to determine whether bypass grafts or native vessels are occluded.

(5) Patients with cardiac failure in whom a surgically correctable lesion, such as left ventricular aneurysm, mitral regurgitation, or reversible ischemic dysfunction, is suspected.

(6) Patients surviving sudden death or with symptomatic or life-threatening arrhythmias in whom coronary artery disease may be a correctable cause.

(7) Patients with chest pain of uncertain cause or cardiomyopathy of unknown cause.

Coronary arteriography visualizes the location and severity of stenoses. Narrowing greater than 50% of the luminal diameter is considered clinically significant, although most lesions producing ischemia are associated with narrowing in excess of 70%. This information has important prognostic value, since mortality rates are progressively higher in patients with one-, two-, and three-vessel disease and those with left main coronary artery obstruction (ranging from 1% per year to 25% per year). Among stable patients, 20%, 30%, and 50% have one-, two-, and three-vessel involvement, respectively, while left main disease is present in 10%. In those with strongly positive exercise ECGs or scintigraphic studies, three-vessel or left main disease may be present in 75–95% depending upon the criteria employed. Coronary arteriography also shows whether the obstructions are amena-

ble to bypass surgery or percutaneous transluminal coronary angioplasty (PTCA).

J. Left Ventricular Angiography: Left ventricular angiography is usually performed at the same time as coronary arteriography. Global and regional left ventricular function are visualized, as well as mitral regurgitation if present. Left ventricular function is the major determinant of prognosis in stable coronary disease and of the risk of bypass surgery.

Abrams J (editor): Angina pectoris: Mechanisms, diagnosis, and therapy. Cardiol Clin 1991;9(1):1. (Entire monograph.)

Cheitlin MD: Finding the high-risk patient with coronary artery disease. JAMA 1988;259:2271.

Gibbons RJ: The use of radionuclide techniques for identification of severe coronary disease. Curr Probl Cardiol 1990;15(6):301. (Results in relation to coronary anatomy and prognosis.)

Pollack SG et al: Independent and incremental prognostic value of tests performed in hierarchical order to evaluate patients with suspected coronary artery disease. Circulation 1992;85:237. (Scintigraphy adds to prognostic information obtained by clinical evaluation and exercise ECG as well as to information about coronary artery anatomy.)

Shub C: Stable angina pectoris: 1. Clinical patterns. 2. Cardiac evaluation and diagnostic testing. Mayo Clin Proc 1990;65:233, 243.

Coronary Vasospasm & Angina With Normal Coronary Arteriograms

Although most symptoms of myocardial ischemia result from fixed stenosis of the coronary arteries or thrombosis or hemorrhage at the site of lesions, some ischemic events may be precipitated by coronary vasoconstriction.

Spasm of the large coronary arteries with resulting decreased coronary blood flow may occur spontaneously or may be induced by exposure to cold, emotional stress, or vasoconstricting medications, such as ergot derivative drugs. Spasm may occur both in normal and in stenosed coronary arteries and may be silent or result in angina pectoris. Even myocardial infarction may occur as a result of spasm in the absence of visible obstructive coronary heart disease, although most instances of coronary spasm occur in the presence of coronary stenosis.

Cocaine-induced myocardial ischemia is a growing problem. While coronary artery vasoconstriction plays a role in many patients, coronary thrombosis and increased myocardial energy requirements may also be important factors.

Prinzmetal's (variant) angina is a clinical syndrome in which chest pain occurs without the usual precipitating factors and is associated with ST segment elevation rather than depression. It often affects women under 50 years of age. It characteristically occurs in the early morning, awakening patients from sleep, tends to involve the right coronary artery, and is apt to be associated with arrhythmias or conduction defects. There may be no fixed stenoses.

Patients with this pattern of pain or any chest pain syndrome associated with ST segment elevation should undergo coronary arteriography to determine whether fixed stenotic lesions are present. If they are, aggressive medical therapy or revascularization is indicated, since this may represent an unstable phase of the disease. If significant lesions are not seen and spasm is suspected, ergonovine may be administered intravenously to precipitate vasospasm. This must be done cautiously and with nitroglycerin prepared for intracoronary administration, since irreversible spasm may lead to infarction. Episodes respond well to nitrates or calcium channel blockers, and both drugs are effective prophylactically. Beta-blockers have exacerbated coronary vasospasm, but they may have a role in management of patients in whom spasm is associated with fixed stenoses.

There is a growing consensus that myocardial ischemia may also occur in patients with normal coronary arteries as a result of disease of the coronary microcirculation. This has been termed syndrome X.

Gitter MJ et al: Cocaine and chest pain: Clinical features and outcome of patients hospitalized to rule out myocardial infarction. Ann Intern Med 1991;115:277. (Symptoms and electrocardiographic changes may mimic ischemia or infarction.)

Cannon RD: Microvascular angina: Cardiovascular investigations regarding pathophysiology and management. Med Clin North Am 1991;75:1097. (Comprehensive and provocative.)

Maseri A et al: Mechanisms and significance of cardiac ischemic pain. Prog Cardiovasc Dis 1992;35:1. (Role of coronary spasm and microvascular disease.)

Rezkalla SH et al: Cocaine-induced heart disease. Am Heart J 1990;120:1403. (Coronary and noncoronary pathology.)

Differential Diagnosis

With an appropriate history, the diagnosis of angina pectoris is more than 90% certain. When atypical features are present—such as prolonged duration (hours or days); or darting, knifelike pains at the apex or over the precordium—ischemia is less likely.

"Anterior chest wall syndrome" is characterized by sharply localized tenderness of intercostal muscles. Sprain or inflammation of the chondrocostal junctions, which may be warm, swollen, and red, may result in diffuse chest pain that is also reproduced by local pressure (Tietze's syndrome). Intercostal neuritis (herpes zoster, diabetes mellitus, etc) also mimics angina.

Cervical or thoracic spine disease involving the dorsal roots produces sudden sharp, severe chest pain suggesting angina in location and "radiation" but related to specific movements of the neck or spine, recumbency, and straining or lifting. Pain due to cervical or thoracic disk disease involves the outer or dorsal aspect of the arm and the thumb and index fingers rather than the ring and little fingers.

Peptic ulcer, chronic cholecystitis, esophageal spasm, and functional gastrointestinal disease may produce pain suggestive of angina pectoris. Reflux esophagitis is characterized by lower chest and upper abdominal pain after heavy meals, occurring in recumbency or upon bending over. The pain is relieved by antacids, carafate, or H_2 receptor antagonists. The picture may be especially confusing because ischemic pain may also be associated with upper gastrointestinal symptoms, and esophageal motility disorders may be improved by nitrates and calcium channel blockers. Detailed assessment of esophageal motility may be necessary.

Degenerative and inflammatory lesions of the left shoulder and thoracic outlet syndromes may cause chest pain due to nerve irritation or muscular compression; the symptoms are usually precipitated by movement of the arm and shoulder and are associated with paresthesias.

Spontaneous pneumothorax may cause chest pain as well as dyspnea and may create confusion with angina as well as myocardial infarction. Even the ECG may resemble infarction because of changes in voltage from the pneumothorax. The same is true of pneumonia and pulmonary embolization. Dissection of the thoracic aorta can cause severe "tearing" chest pain that is commonly felt in the back; it is sudden in onset, reaches maximum intensity immediately, and may be associated with changes in pulses. Other cardiac disorders such as mitral valve prolapse, hypertrophic cardiomyopathy, myocarditis, pericarditis, aortic valve disease, or right ventricular hypertrophy may cause atypical chest pain or even myocardial ischemia. Noninvasive testing and, in many cases, cardiac catheterization may be required to establish the diagnosis.

Richter JE et al(editors): Unexplained chest pain. Med Clin North Am 1991;75:1045. (Differential diagnosis and management of chest pain.)

Treatment

A. Treatment of Acute Attack: Sublingual nitroglycerin is the drug of choice; it acts in about 1–2 minutes. Nitrates decrease arteriolar and venous tone, reduce preload and afterload, and lower the oxygen demand of the heart. Nitrates may also improve myocardial blood flow by dilating collateral channels and, in the presence of increased vasomotor tone, coronary stenoses. As soon as the attack begins, one fresh tablet is placed under the tongue. This may be repeated at 3- to 5-minute intervals. The dosage (0.3, 0.4, or 0.6 mg) and the number of tablets to be used before seeking further medical attention must be individualized. Nitroglycerin buccal spray is also available as a metered (0.4 mg) delivery system. It has the advantage of being more convenient for patients who have difficulty handling the pills and of being more stable. Nitroglycerin should also be used prophylactically before activities likely to precipitate angina. Pain not responding to three tablets or lasting more than 20 minutes may represent evolving infarction, and the patient should be instructed to seek immediate medical attention.

B. Prevention of Further Attacks:

1. Aggravating factors–Angina may be aggravated by hypertension, left ventricular failure, arrhythmia (usually tachycardias), strenuous activity, cold temperatures, and emotional states. These factors should be identified and treated or avoided where possible.

2. Nitroglycerin–Nitroglycerin, 0.3–0.6 mg sublingually or by spray, should be taken 5 minutes before any activity likely to precipitate angina. Sublingual isosorbide dinitrate (2.5–10 mg) is only slightly longer-acting than sublingual nitroglycerin.

3. Long-acting nitrates–A number of longer-acting nitrate preparations are available. These include isosorbide dinitrate, 10–40 mg orally three times daily; isosorbide mononitrate, 10–20 mg orally twice daily; oral sustained-release nitroglycerin preparations, 6.25–12.5 mg two to four times daily; nitroglycerin ointment, 6.25–25 mg applied two to four times daily; and transdermal nitroglycerin patches that deliver nitroglycerin at a predetermined rate (usually 5–20 mg/24 h). The main limitation to chronic nitrate therapy is tolerance, which occurs to some degree in most patients. The degree of tolerance can be limited by utilizing a regimen which includes a minimum 8- to 10-hour period without nitrates. Isosorbide dinitrate given three times daily, with the last dose after dinner, is the most commonly used approach in the United States. Isosorbide mononitrate is popular in Europe. Because it is the active metabolite of the dinitrate, it has more consistent bioavailability. Transdermal preparations should be removed overnight in most patients.

Nitrate therapy is often limited by headache. Other side effects include nausea, dizziness, and hypotension.

4. Beta-blockers–The beta-blockers prevent angina by reducing myocardial oxygen requirements during exertion and stress. This is accomplished by reducing the heart rate, myocardial contractility, and, to a lesser extent, blood pressure. The beta-blockers are the only antianginal agents that have been demonstrated to prolong life in patients with coronary disease (post-myocardial infarction). They are at least as effective as alternative agents in studies employing exercise testing, ambulatory monitoring, and symptom assessment. As a result, they should be considered for first-line therapy in most patients with chronic angina.

In the United States, only propranolol, metoprolol, nadolol, and atenolol are approved for angina. Nonetheless, all available beta-blockers appear to be effective for angina, though those with intrinsic sympathomimetic activity, such as pindolol, are less desirable because they may exacerbate angina in some individuals and have not been effective in secondary prevention trials. The pharmacology and side effects of the beta-blockers are discussed in Chapter 11 (Table 11–2). The dosages of all these drugs when given for angina are similar. The major contraindications are bronchospastic disease, bradyarrhythmias, and overt heart failure.

5. Calcium entry-blocking agents–Verapamil, diltiazem, nifedipine, nicardipine, and amlodipine are chemically and pharmacologically heterogeneous agents that prevent angina by reducing myocardial oxygen requirements and by inducing coronary artery vasodilation. Isradipine and felodipine are not approved in the USA for angina but probably are about as effective as nifedipine and other dihydropyridine agents. Myocardial oxygen demand is lessened by reducing blood pressure, left ventricular wall stress, and, in the case of verapamil and diltiazem, resting or exercise heart rate. Though these agents are all potent coronary vasodilators, it is unclear whether they improve myocardial blood flow in most patients with stable exertional angina. In those with coronary vasospasm, the calcium entry blockers may be the agent of choice.

Most calcium channel blockers have negative inotropic, chronotropic, and dromotropic properties in vitro, but the reflex sympathetic response may obscure these effects in vivo (except in the presence of beta blockade or severely depressed left ventricular function). Several newer calcium channel blockers of the dihydropyridine class, including felodipine and amlodipine, have less negative inotropic action, but their safety in patients with heart failure remains to be demonstrated. Unlike the beta-blockers, calcium channel blockers have not reduced mortality postinfarction and in some cases have increased ischemia and mortality rates. This appears to be the case with some dihydropyridines and with diltiazem and verapamil in patients with clinical heart failure or moderate to severe left ventricular dysfunction. Thus, calcium blockers should not be the initial antianginal medication in most patients.

The pharmacologic effects and side effects of the calcium channel blockers are discussed in Chapter 11 and summarized in Table 11–4. Although all have been shown to be efficacious for angina, not all preparations and agents are approved for this indication. By and large, diltiazem and verapamil are preferable as first-line agents because they produce less reflex tachycardia and because the former, at least, may cause fewer side effects. Nifedipine, nicardipine, and amlodipine are also approved agents for angina. Bepridil is a unique calcium channel blocker similar to verapamil in its effects on automatic tissues but with additional properties similar to those of quinidine (prolonging ventricular refractoriness and the

QT interval). It is not approved for hypertension and should be used only for refractory angina because of its potential to induce ventricular arrhythmias.

6. Combination therapy–Patients remaining symptomatic when given one class of preventive agent should be treated with combinations. A beta-blocker and a long-acting nitrate or a beta-blocker and a calcium channel blocker (other than verapamil, where the risk of atrioventricular block or heart failure is higher) are the most appropriate combinations. A few patients will have a further response to a regimen including all three agents.

7. Platelet-inhibiting agents–Coronary thrombosis is responsible for most episodes of myocardial infarction and many unstable ischemic syndromes. Several studies have demonstrated the benefit of antiplatelet drugs following unstable angina and infarction. Therefore, unless contraindicated, small doses of aspirin (162–325 mg daily or 325 mg every other day) should be prescribed for patients with angina.

8. Revascularization–The indications for coronary artery revascularization and the choice of procedure are discussed below.

Prognosis

The prognosis of angina pectoris has improved with advances in the understanding of its pathophysiology and in pharmacologic therapy. Mortality rates range from 1% to 25% per year depending on the number of vessels diseased, the severity of obstruction, the status of left ventricular function, and the presence of complex arrhythmias. In patients with stable symptoms and normal ejection fractions (> 55%, depending on the laboratory), the mortality rate is less than 4% per year. However, the outlook in individual patients is unpredictable, and nearly half of the deaths are sudden. Therefore, risk stratification is often attempted. Patients with accelerating symptoms have a poorer outlook. Among stable patients, those whose exercise tolerance is severely limited by ischemia (less than 6 minutes on the Bruce treadmill protocol) and those with extensive ischemia by exercise electrocardiography or scintigraphy have more severe anatomic disease and a poorer prognosis.

Elkayam U: Tolerance to organic nitrates: Evidence, mechanisms, clinical relevance, and strategies for prevention. Ann Intern Med 1991;114:667. (Emphasizes need for intermittent therapy.)

Maseri A: Medical therapy of chronic stable angina pectoris. Circulation 1990;82:2258.

Packer M: Combined beta-adrenergic and calcium entry blockade in angina pectoris. N Engl J Med 1989; 320:709. (Two drugs not always better than one.)

Ridker PM et al: Low dose aspirin therapy for chronic stable angina. Ann Intern Med 1991;114:835. (First myocardial infarction prevented.)

Shub C: Stable angina pectoris: 3. Medical treatment. Mayo Clin Proc 1990;65:256.

REVASCULARIZATION PROCEDURES FOR PATIENTS WITH ANGINA PECTORIS

Indications

The indications for coronary artery revascularization in patients with stable angina pectoris are often debated. There is general agreement that otherwise healthy patients in the following groups should undergo revascularization. (1) Patients with unacceptable symptoms despite medical therapy to its tolerable limits. (2) Patients with left main coronary artery stenosis greater than 50% with or without symptoms. (3) Patients with three-vessel disease with left ventricular dysfunction (ejection fraction < 50% or previous transmural infarction). (4) Patients with unstable angina who after symptom control by medical therapy continue to exhibit ischemia on exercise testing or monitoring. (5) Post-myocardial infarction patients with continuing angina or ischemia on noninvasive testing, particularly if they have received thrombolytic treatment (see sections on Unstable Angina and Myocardial Infarction).

In addition, many cardiologists feel that patients with less severe symptoms should be revascularized if they have anatomically critical lesions (> 90% proximal stenoses, especially of the proximal left anterior descending artery) or physiologic evidence of severe ischemia (early positive exercise tests, large exercise-induced thallium scintigraphic defects, or frequent episodes of ischemia on ambulatory monitoring). This trend toward aggressive intervention has accelerated as a result of the growing availability of coronary angioplasty. While such patients are at increased risk, it has not been proved that their prognosis is better after coronary revascularization by either surgery or angioplasty. In most, a trial of medical therapy is warranted to determine whether symptoms and other evidence of ischemia improve.

Type of Procedure

A. Coronary Artery Bypass Grafting (CABG): CABG can be accomplished with a very low mortality rate (1–3%) in otherwise healthy patients with preserved cardiac function. However, the mortality rate of this procedure has increased to 4–8% or higher in recent years because the surgical population includes a greater proportion of high-risk and older patients. Increasingly, younger individuals with focal lesions of one or several vessels are undergoing coronary angioplasty as the initial revascularization procedure.

Grafts employing one or both internal mammary arteries (usually to the left anterior descending artery or its branches) provide the best long-term results in terms of patency and flow. Segments of the saphenous vein (or, less optimally, other veins) interposed between the aorta and the coronary arteries distal to the obstructions are also utilized. One to five distal anastomoses are commonly performed. After successful surgery, symptoms generally abate. The need for antianginal medications diminishes, and left ventricular function may improve.

The operative mortality rate is increased in patients with poor left ventricular function (left ventricular ejection fraction < 35%) or those requiring additional procedures (valve replacement or ventricular aneurysmectomy). Patients over 70 years of age, patients undergoing repeat procedures, or those with important noncardiac disease (especially renal insufficiency, diabetes, or poor general health) also have higher operative mortality and morbidity rates, and full recovery is slow. Thus, CABG should be reserved for more severely symptomatic patients in this group. Early (1–6 months) graft patency rates average 85–90% (higher for internal mammary grafts), and subsequent graft closure rates are about 4% annually. Early graft failure is common in vessels with poor distal flow, while late closure is more frequent in patients who continue smoking and those with untreated hyperlipidemia. Antiplatelet therapy with aspirin alone or combined with dipyridamole improves graft patency rates. Vigorous treatment of blood lipid abnormalities is warranted, with a goal for LDL cholesterol of < 130 mg/dL and of HDL cholesterol > 45 mg/dL. Long-term dipyridamole therapy is expensive, inconvenient, and of limited value. Repeat CABG or angioplasty (see below) is often necessitated by progressive native vessel disease and graft occlusions. Reoperation is technically demanding and less often fully successful than the initial operation.

B. Percutaneous Transluminal Coronary Angioplasty (PTCA): Coronary artery stenoses can be effectively dilated by inflation of a balloon under high pressure. This procedure is performed in the cardiac catheterization laboratory under local anesthesia either at the same time as diagnostic coronary arteriography or at a later time. The mechanism of dilation is rupture of the atheromatous plaque, with subsequent resorption of intraluminal debris.

This procedure was at one time reserved for proximal single-vessel disease, but now it is widely employed in multivessel disease with multiple lesions, though only rarely in left main disease. PTCA is also effective in CABG stenoses. Optimal lesions for PTCA are relatively proximal, noneccentric, free of plaque dissection, and removed from the origin of large branches. In the USA, the number of PTCA procedures now exceeds that of CABG operations. With improved catheter systems, experienced operators are able to manipulate the balloon catheter across approximately 90% of approachable lesions and successfully dilate 90% of those. The major early complication is intimal dissection with vessel occlusion. This can sometimes be treated by repeat PTCA, but urgent CABG is required in 3–5% of cases, and morbidity and mortality rates are high. Therefore, these procedures must be done in a laboratory where surgery is available on short notice.

In the United States, the number of PTCA procedures now exceeds that of CABG operations, but the justification for many of these is weak. One controlled study showed PTCA to be superior to medical therapy for symptom relief but not in preventing infarction or death. Controlled studies of PTCA versus either medical treatment or CABG in multivessel disease are not yet available.

The major limitation with PTCA has been restenosis, which occurs in the first 6 months in 25–35% of vessels dilated. The mechanism of restenosis is unclear, and it can often be treated successfully by repeat PTCA.

C. Investigational Revascularization Procedures: There is considerable interest in the use of laser catheters and catheter devices to remove atheromatous material ("atherectomy"). These approaches are now available on an investigational basis. Current data do not indicate a significant improvement in either initial success or restenosis rates with these experimental techniques, but the technologies are evolving. Intracoronary stents have been used to maintain vessel patency in patients with acute closure during PTCA or with restenosis. Long-term results have not been impressive.

Results

The mortality rates of PTCA and CABG are comparable in stable angina. Recovery after PTCA is obviously faster, but the early success rate of CABG is probably higher. The increasing popularity of PTCA primarily reflects its lower cost, shorter hospitalization, the perception that CABG is best done only once and can be reserved for later, and the preference of patients for less invasive treatment. However, preliminary results from a number of trials suggest that the high rate of repeat procedures and eventual CABG in patients undergoing PTCA may outweigh these advantages. It should also be noted that the excellent outcome of patients treated medically has made it difficult to show an advantage with either revascularization approach except in patients who remain symptom-limited or have left main lesions or three-vessel disease and left ventricular dysfunction.

Alderman EL et al: Ten-year follow-up of survival and myocardial infarction in the randomized Coronary Artery Surgery Study. Circulation 1990;82:1629. (Patients with initial left ventricular dysfunction do better with surgery; others do not.)

Guidelines and indications for coronary artery bypass graft surgery. ACC/AHA Task Force Report: J Am Coll Cardiol 1991;17:543.

Hoffman JL: Myocardial revascularization: Coronary angioplasty and bypass indications. Med Clin North Am 1992;76:1083. (Balanced discussion of pros and cons.)

Topol EJ: Promises and pitfalls of new devices for coronary

artery disease. Circulation 1991;83:689. (Great enthusiasm and promise, few positive results.)

Weintraub WS et al: Influence of age on the results of coronary artery surgery. Circulation 1991;84:(Suppl III):III–226. (Mortality rate increased from 2% in patients under 70 to 8% in those over 80. Neurologic events and wound infections were also more frequent.)

UNSTABLE ANGINA

Most clinicians use the term "unstable angina" to denote an accelerating or "crescendo" pattern of pain in cases where previously stable angina occurs with less exertion or at rest, lasts longer, and is less responsive to medication. Coronary angioscopy has shown that a high proportion of patients with this pattern of symptoms have "complex" coronary stenosis characterized by plaque ulceration, hemorrhage, or thrombosis. This inherently unstable situation may progress to complete occlusion and infarction or may heal, with reendothelialization and a return to a stable though possibly more severe pattern of ischemia. New-onset angina is sometimes considered unstable, but if it is exertional and responsive to rest and medication, it does not carry the same poor prognosis.

Diagnosis

Most patients with unstable angina will exhibit electrocardiographic changes during pain—commonly ST segment depression or T wave flattening or inversion but sometimes, and more ominously, ST segment elevation. They may exhibit signs of left ventricular dysfunction during pain and for a time thereafter.

Treatment

A. General Measures: Treatment of unstable angina should be multifaceted and vigorous. Patients should be hospitalized, maintained at bed rest or at very limited activity, monitored, and given supplemental oxygen. Sedation with a benzodiazepine agent is usually indicated. The systolic blood pressure is usually maintained at 100–120 mm Hg, except in previously severe hypertensives. Patients with heart rates above 70–80/min should be given beta-blockers unless heart failure or other medical contraindications are present.

B. Nitroglycerin: The nitrates are first-line therapy for unstable angina. Nonparenteral therapy with sublingual or oral agents or nitroglycerin ointment is usually sufficient. If pain persists despite the addition of other agents, intravenous nitroglycerin should be started. The usual initial dosage is 10 µg/min. The dosage should be titrated to 1–2 µg/kg/min over 30–60 minutes and further increased as tolerated if pain recurs. Dosages up to 10 µg/kg/min or higher may be used. Tolerance to continuous nitrate infusion is common. Careful—usually continuous—blood pressure

monitoring is required when intravenous nitroglycerin is used.

C. Beta-Blockers: These agents are effective in unstable angina, particularly when tachycardia is present or precipitated by other medications. If the patient has no history or physical findings of heart failure, these agents can usually be started without measurements of left ventricular function. Patients with evidence of large or multiple old infarctions are an exception. The pharmacology of these agents is discussed in Chapter 11 and summarized in Table 11–2. Use of agents with intrinsic sympathomimetic activity should be avoided in this setting. The goal of acute treatment is to reduce the heart rate below 60–70/min. Intravenous treatment with esmolol (500 µg/kg followed by 50–200 µg/kg/min) or longer-acting agents may be preferable in very unstable patients. Oral therapy should be aggressively titrated as blood pressure permits.

D. Calcium Entry Blockers: Although the data on efficacy of calcium channel blockers are less extensive than with beta-blockers—since alterations in coronary vasomotor tone may play a role in unstable ischemic syndromes, these agents are commonly employed. In the presence of nitrates and without accompanying beta-blockers, diltiazem or verapamil is preferred, since nifedipine and the other dihydropyridines are more likely to cause reflex tachycardia or hypotension. The initial dosage should be low, but upward titration should proceed rapidly. (See Table 11–4.)

E. Anticoagulation, Antiplatelet, and Thrombolytic Therapy: As noted above, intravascular thrombosis plays a prominent role in the pathophysiology of unstable angina and its progression to myocardial infarction. Therefore, antithrombotic therapy is an important part of treatment for unstable angina. Heparin may be more effective than aspirin, but it is likely that the two are additive. Aspirin, 325 mg daily (lower doses may be adequate), should be commenced on admission, and intravenous heparin should be started if symptoms persist. Studies employing thrombolytic agents have yielded mixed results, and their use should be limited to patients with marked electrocardiographic changes who are refractory to other approaches.

F. Intra-aortic Balloon Counterpulsation (IABC): If pain persists with accompanying electrocardiographic changes despite the above measures, IABC should be considered both to reduce myocardial energy requirements (systolic unloading) and to improve diastolic blood flow. While this approach is often effective, many experts will proceed directly to coronary arteriography and revascularization. Intra-aortic balloon counterpulsation is best applied only if CABG or PTCA is planned. Aortic insufficiency is a contraindication, and IABC must be used cautiously in patients with peripheral vascular disease.

Prognosis & Indications
for Revascularization

Over 90% of patients can be rendered pain-free with these measures. Patients who do not become ischemia-free on medical therapy should have early coronary arteriography and revascularization. Controlled trials have not shown any advantage in increased survival or lower infarction rates with CABG compared to medical therapy, although many patients treated medically will need revascularization later for recurrent symptoms. Depending on the stringency of the definition of unstable angina, 10–30% of patients will have an early infarction, and the 1-year mortality rate is 10–20%. Recent data from ambulatory monitoring indicate that many patients without pain continue to have "silent" episodes of ST segment depression or, less commonly, elevation. These individuals have a poorer prognosis.

Because recurrent episodes, infarction, and sudden death may occur following relief of unstable angina, additional evaluations should be performed in patients who have been stabilized, consisting of either (1) early exercise or dipyridamole stress testing to identify high-risk subsets for further invasive evaluation, or (2) coronary arteriography. The choice of approach should be individualized based on the patient's age and general health as well as the severity of symptoms and signs of ischemia. The artery responsible for the ischemia can usually be determined from electrocardiographic or scintigraphic changes during pain, and the lesion is often amenable to PTCA. If revascularization is not performed, long-term management is the same as that outlined for stable angina pectoris.

Freeman MR et al: Thrombolysis in unstable angina. Randomized double-blind trial of t-PA and placebo. Circulation 1992;85:150. (No improvement in outcome observed.)

Lubsen J: Medical management of unstable angina: What have we learned from the randomized trials? Circulation 1990;82(3 Suppl):1182. (Best evidence for efficacy is with beta-blockers and aspirin. Heparin and calcium blockers may be useful. Nitrates are less well studied.)

Munger T, Jae KO: Unstable angina. Mayo Clin Proc 1990;65:384. (Comprehensive review.)

Rutherford JD (editor): *Unstable Angina.* Marcel Dekker, 1992.

Theroux P et al: Aspirin, heparin, or both to treat acute unstable angina. N Engl J Med 1988;319:1105. (Study showing benefit of heparin with or without aspirin.)

ACUTE MYOCARDIAL INFARCTION

Essentials of Diagnosis

- Sudden but not instantaneous development of prolonged (> 30 minutes) anterior chest discomfort (sometimes felt as "gas") that may produce arrhythmias, hypotension, shock, or cardiac failure.
- Rarely painless, masquerading as acute congestive heart failure, syncope, cerebral vascular accident, or "unexplained" shock.
- Electrocardiography: ST segment elevation or depression, evolving Q waves, symmetric inversion of T waves.
- Elevation of cardiac enzymes (CK-MB, LDH fraction 1).
- Appearance of segmental wall motion abnormality.

General Considerations

Myocardial infarction results from prolonged myocardial ischemia, precipitated in most cases by an occlusive coronary thrombus at the site of a preexisting (though not necessarily severe) atherosclerotic stenosis. More rarely, infarction may result from prolonged vasospasm, inadequate myocardial blood flow (eg, hypotension), or excessive metabolic demand. These processes also occur most commonly in patients with atherosclerotic disease. Very rarely, myocardial infarction may be caused by embolic occlusion, vasculitis, aortic root or coronary artery dissection, or aortitis. Cocaine is a rare cause of infarction but should be considered in young individuals without risk factors.

The location and extent of infarction depend upon the anatomic distribution of the occluded vessel, the presence of additional stenotic lesions, and the adequacy of collateral circulation. Thrombosis in the anterior descending branch of the left coronary artery results in infarction of the anterior left ventricle and interventricular septum. Occlusion of the left circumflex artery produces anterolateral or posterolateral infarction. Right coronary thrombosis leads to infarction of the posteroinferior portion of the left ventricle and may involve the right ventricular myocardium and interventricular septum. The arteries supplying the atrioventricular node and the sinus node more commonly arise from the right coronary; thus, atrioventricular block at the nodal level and sinus node dysfunction occur more frequently during inferior infarctions. However, because there are great individual variations in coronary anatomy and because associated lesions and collaterals may confuse the picture, prediction of coronary anatomy from the infarct location may be inaccurate.

Infarctions are often classified as transmural, if the classic electrocardiographic evolution of ST segment elevation to Q waves is observed; or nontransmural or subendocardial, if pain, enzyme elevations, and ST–T wave changes occur in the absence of new Q waves. However, on pathologic examination, most infarctions involve the subendocardium predominantly, and some transmural extension is common even in the absence of Q waves. Thus, the better classification is Q wave versus non-Q wave infarction. The latter may result from spontaneous lysis of the thrombus and often signifies the presence of additional jeopardized myocardium; it is associated with a higher incidence of reinfarction and recurrent ischemia.

The size and anatomic location of the infarction determines the acute clinical picture, the early complications, and the long-term prognosis. The hemodynamic findings are related directly to the extent of necrosis (together with the amount of damage from previous infarctions). In small infarctions, cardiac function is normal, whereas with more extensive damage, early heart failure and hypotension (cardiogenic shock) may appear. Additional myocardium beyond that initially infarcted is often threatened, being maintained by collateral circulation or by blood flow through a partially recanalized vessel. Thus, preventing extension of the infarct is one of the major goals of early management. The complications of acute infarction are discussed below.

ACC/AHA guidelines for the early management of patients with acute myocardial infarction. Circulation 1990; 82:664. (Covers everything from transportation to predischarge evaluation. Many references.)

Alpert JS, Francis GS: Handbook of Coronary Care, 5th ed. Little, Brown, 1993. (Very well done pocket "cookbook.")

Anderson JL (editor): Modern Management of Acute Myocardial Infarction in the Community Hospital. Marcel Dekker, 1991 (Pragmatic but aggressive.)

Gersh BJ, Rahimtoola SH (editors): Acute Myocardial Infarction. Elsevier, 1991. (Pathophysiology, diagnosis, and short- and long-term management.)

Clinical Findings

A. Symptoms:

1. Premonitory pain–One-third of patients give a history of alteration in the pattern of angina, recent onset of typical or atypical angina, or unusual "indigestion" felt in the chest.

2. Pain of infarction–Most infarctions occur at rest unlike anginal episodes, and more commonly in the early morning. The pain is similar to angina in location and radiation but is more severe, and it builds up rapidly or in waves to maximum intensity over a few minutes or longer. Nitroglycerin has little effect; even narcotics may not relieve the pain.

3. Associated symptoms–Patients may break out in a cold sweat, feel weak and apprehensive, and move about, seeking a position of comfort. They prefer not to lie quietly. Light-headedness, syncope, dyspnea, orthopnea, cough, wheezing, nausea and vomiting, or abdominal bloating may be present singly or in any combination.

4. Painless infarction–In a minority of cases, pain is absent or minor and is overshadowed by the immediate complications. As many as 25% of infarctions are detected on routine ECG without there having been any recallable acute episode.

5. Sudden death and early arrhythmias–Approximately 20% of patients with acute infarction will die before reaching the hospital; these deaths are usually in the first hour and are chiefly due to ventricular fibrillation.

B. Signs:

1. General–Patients usually appear anxious and are often sweating profusely. The heart rate may range from marked bradycardia (most commonly in inferior infarction) to tachycardia resulting from increased sympathetic nervous system activity, low cardiac output, or arrhythmia. The blood pressure may be high, especially in former hypertensives, or low in patients with shock. Respiratory distress usually indicates heart failure. Fever, usually low-grade, may appear after 12 hours and persist for several days.

2. Chest–Clear lung fields are a good prognostic sign, but basilar rales are common and do not necessarily indicate heart failure. More extensive rales or diffuse wheezing may indicate pulmonary edema.

3. Heart–The cardiac examination may be unimpressive or very abnormal. An abnormally located ventricular impulse often represents the dyskinetic infarcted region. Soft heart sounds may indicate left ventricular dysfunction. Atrial gallops (S_4) are the rule, whereas ventricular gallops (S_3) are less common and indicate significant left ventricular dysfunction. Mitral regurgitation murmurs are not uncommon and usually indicate papillary muscle dysfunction or, rarely, rupture. Pericardial friction rubs are uncommon in the first 24 hours but may appear later.

4. Extremities–Edema is usually not present. Cyanosis and cold temperature indicate low output. The peripheral pulses should be noted, since later shock or emboli may alter the examination.

C. Laboratory Findings: Leukocytosis of $10,000–20,000/\mu L$ often develops on the second day and disappears within a week. The most valuable diagnostic test is serial measurement of cardiac enzymes, of which creatine kinase (CK or CPK) rises the earliest and is the most specific for infarction. In the coronary care unit, CK has a sensitivity of 97% and a specificity of 67% for the diagnosis of acute myocardial infarction. False positives are usually from skeletal muscle. The CK-MB isoenzyme is very specific for the heart and remains sensitive. It appears in serum 4–6 hours post-myocardial infarction, peaks at 12–24 hours (earlier following thrombolysis), and declines over 48–72 hours. The peak CK value correlates with the size of the infarction. Serum lactic acid dehydrogenase may remain elevated for 5–7 days, and fraction 1 is relatively specific for myocardial damage. Serial determinations may be helpful in equivocal instances.

D. Electrocardiography: Most patients with acute infarction have ECG changes, and a normal tracing is rare. The extent of the electrocardiographic abnormalities provides only a crude estimate of the magnitude of infarction. The classic evolution of changes is from peaked ("hyperacute") T waves, to

ST segment elevation, to Q wave development, to T wave inversion. This may occur over a few hours to several days. The evolution of new Q waves (> 30 ms in duration and 25% of the R wave amplitude) is diagnostic, but Q waves do not occur in 30–50% of acute infarctions (subendocardial or non-Q wave infarctions). If these patients have an appropriate clinical presentation, characteristic cardiac enzymes, and ST segment changes (usually depression) or T wave inversion lasting at least 48 hours, they are classified as having non-Q wave infarctions.

E. Chest X-Ray: The chest x-ray may demonstrate signs of congestive heart failure, but these changes often lag behind the clinical findings. Signs of aortic dissection should be sought as a possible alternative diagnosis.

F. Echocardiography: Echocardiography provides convenient bedside assessment of left ventricular global and regional function. This can help with the diagnosis and management of infarction; echocardiography has been used successfully to make judgments about admission and management of patients with suspected infarction, since normal wall motion makes an infarction unlikely. Doppler echocardiography is probably the most convenient procedure for diagnosing postinfarction mitral regurgitation or ventricular septal defect.

G. Scintigraphic Studies: Technetium-99m pyrophosphate scintigraphy can be used to diagnose acute myocardial infarction. When injected at least 18 hours postinfarction, the radiotracer complexes with calcium in necrotic myocardium to provide a "hot spot" image of the infarction. This test is insensitive to small infarctions, and false-positive studies occur, so its use is limited to patients in whom the diagnosis by electrocardiography and enzymes is not possible—principally those who present several days after the event or have intraoperative infarctions.

Radionuclide angiography demonstrates akinesis or dyskinesis in areas of infarction and also measures ejection fraction, which can be valuable. Right ventricular dysfunction may indicate infarction of this chamber.

H. Hemodynamic Measurements: These can be invaluable in managing the complicated patient. Their use is described below and in Table 10–4.

Schweitzer P: The electrocardiographic diagnosis of acute myocardial infarction in the thrombolytic era. Am Heart J 1990;119:642. (Review emphasizing limitations.)

Treatment

A. Thrombolytic Therapy: Thrombolytic ther-

apy reduces the mortality rate and limits infarct size in many patients when started within 3–6 hours after the onset of infarction. Some investigators have suggested that it may have a lesser effect for up to 24 hours in some patients (probably those with extensive collateral circulation), but this is controversial. The benefit is greatest in patients with potentially large infarcts, ie, those with anterior or multifocal electrocardiographic changes, but also occurs with inferior infarctions, who have a relatively good prognosis in any case. Patients with non-Q wave infarctions generally have incomplete or partially recanalized occlusions and have not benefited as consistently from thrombolysis. Serious bleeding complications occur in 0.5–5% of patients. Contraindications include known bleeding diatheses, a history of any cerebrovascular disease, uncontrolled hypertension (> 190/110 mm Hg), pregnancy, and recent trauma or surgery of the head or spine. Relative contraindications include recent major thoracoabdominal surgery or biopsies, gastrointestinal or genitourinary bleeding, diabetic retinopathy, current oral anticoagulant therapy, prolonged cardiopulmonary resuscitation, and noncompressible puncture sites. Older patients have a higher complication rate but may benefit, especially if the potential infarction is large.

Therefore, the current recommendation is to administer thrombolytic therapy to patients up to age 80—or even older if the benefit-to-risk ratio seems favorable—with ST elevation or Q waves who present within 6 hours after onset of pain unless otherwise contraindicated. Adjunctive aspirin causes a significant further reduction in mortality rate and should therefore be administered acutely. Therapy can be initiated in the emergency room or ambulance if personnel are appropriately trained and equipped.

Prior to initiating thrombolytic therapy, a large-bore peripheral intravenous line should be established and not removed until 6 hours after the thrombolytic agent is discontinued. Arterial punctures and other invasive procedures should be avoided if possible. Samples should be drawn for baseline coagulation tests (prothrombin time, partial thromboplastin time, fibrinogen level, and platelet count), blood typing, and other blood tests. Automated blood pressure monitoring (preferably noninvasive) should be instituted.

Three thrombolytic agents have been evaluated extensively in acute infarction and are characterized in Table 10–5. All are associated with higher reperfusion rates when administered within 3 hours after onset of infarction. Two large international studies have compared the results with different thrombolytic therapies. The recently reported ISIS-3 trial compared three agents (tissue plasminogen activator [t-PA], streptokinase, and anistreplase) in over 40,000 patients. No difference in mortality rate was observed between treatments, though cerebral hemorrhage was more common with t-PA. GISSI-2 com-

Table 10–5. Thrombolytic therapy for acute myocardial infarction.

	Streptokinase	Tissue Plasminogen Activator (t-PA)	Anistreplase (APSAC)
Source	Group C *Streptococcus*	Recombinant DNA	Group C *Streptococcus*
$T_{1/2}$	10–12 minutes	5 minutes	90 minutes
Usual dose	1.5 million units	100 mg	30 units
Administration	750,000 units over 20 minutes followed by 750,000 units over 40 minutes	Infuse 10 mg initially, then 50 mg over first hour, followed by 10 mg/h for 4 hours[1]	Infuse over 2–5 minutes
Anticoagulation after infusion	Aspirin, 325 mg daily. Heparin, 1000 units/h adjusted to keep PTT 1½ times control. (Need for heparin uncertain.)	Aspirin, 325 mg daily. Heparin, 5000 units as bolus, followed by same procedure as for streptokinase.	Same as streptokinase
Clot selectivity	Low	High	Moderate
Fibrinogenolysis	+++	+	+
Bleeding	+	+[2]	+
Hypotension	+++	+	+
Allergic reactions	++	0	+
Reperfusion[3]	55–60%	70%	60%
Reocclusion	5–20%	10–30%	5–20%
Approximate cost	$125	$2800	$1800

[1]Recent studies employing "front-loaded" t-PA (such as the administration of an initial bolus of 15 mg, 50 mg over the next 30 minutes, and 35 mg over the next 60 minutes) have shown higher early patency rates, but that approach has not received regulatory approval or extensive validation.
[2]t-PA causes a higher incidence of cerebral hemorrhage than other agents, especially when utilized with heparin. This incremental risk is substantial in patients over age 70 years or those with systolic blood pressure >160 mm Hg, in whom t-PA should be avoided.
[3]Estimated reperfusion rates when administered in the first 3 hours. After 3 hours, t-PA reperfusion rate is higher than that of streptokinase.

pared the first two of these agents and also failed to show a significant difference.

Tissue plasminogen activator (t-PA) is a naturally occurring thrombolytic factor that is theoretically the most thrombus-specific, but bleeding complications have not been less frequent with t-PA, even though fibrinogen levels are better maintained, and hemorrhagic strokes appear to be more frequent. In patients over age 70 or with elevated blood pressure, the rate of intracranial hemorrhage rises substantially, and t-PA should be avoided in these. Incomplete data suggest that t-PA produces higher reperfusion rates, especially if given more than 3 hours after the onset of pain. Reocclusion rates are higher with t-PA because of its shorter half-life, so intravenous heparin is recommended for at least 24 hours. Since t-PA is significantly more expensive than alternative agents and has not been demonstrated to reduce mortality more strikingly or to preserve left ventricular function better than other agents, it should be reserved for patients in whom streptokinase is relatively contraindicated (by previous exposure, hypotension, or potential need for early surgery).

Streptokinase is more likely to produce allergic reactions, including fever, chills, rashes, and anaphylaxis. This agent should be avoided if the patient has received it previously. Streptokinase also has a tendency to produce severe hypotension and therefore must be administered slowly. Hypotension should be treated by slowing or interrupting the infusion, placing the patient in the Trendelenburg position, and administering fluids.

Anisoylated plasminogen streptokinase activator complex (anistreplase; APSAC) is a conjugate of streptokinase that is inactive until the anisoyl group is hydrolyzed, which occurs gradually after injection (half-time, 90 minutes). The drug is concentrated at the site of the thrombus and is activated locally. Thus, it can be injected as a bolus but will provide continuing thrombolytic activity. This makes APSAC a convenient agent to administer out of the hospital or in a busy emergency room. Otherwise, it has many of the same features of streptokinase, including the potential to produce allergic reactions and hypotension, but it is far more expensive.

Urokinase has not been specifically approved for acute myocardial infarction, but small studies have demonstrated that it induces coronary thrombolysis.

After completion of the thrombolytic infusion, aspirin should be continued. Anticoagulation with intravenous heparin is advocated by many authorities especially if t-PA has been employed, but its risk/benefit ratio has been questioned. Prophylactic treatment with antacids and an H_2 blocker is indicated.

Reperfusion rates of 40–80% can be expected, determined primarily by the interval between onset of the infarction and treatment. Reperfusion is recognized clinically by the abrupt cessation of pain, ventricular arrhythmias (most characteristically accelerated idioventricular rhythm), rapid evolution of the ECG to Q waves, and an early peak of CK (by 12 hours); however, all of these signs may be misleading. Even with anticoagulation, 10–20% of reperfused vessels will reocclude during hospitalization. This is usually recognized by the recurrence of pain and ST segment elevation and is treated by readministration of a thrombolytic agent or immediate angiography and PTCA.

The optimal management of myocardial infarction after thrombolysis is controversial but has been clarified considerably by the TIMI 2 trial. Patients with recurrent ischemic pain prior to discharge should undergo catheterization and, if indicated, revascularization. Asymptomatic, clinically stable patients should undergo predischarge evaluation to determine whether residual jeopardized myocardium is present. This can be accomplished by exercise or dipyridamole scintigraphy. Those with significantly positive tests or a low threshold for symptomatic ischemia should undergo angiography and revascularization where feasible. Patients with negative tests have an excellent prognosis without intervention, though they may require revascularization for symptoms at a later time.

B. Acute PTCA: A number of centers are now performing immediate coronary arteriography in patients presenting within 3 hours after infarction. The results of this approach in specialized centers are not excellent, but this experience may not be generalizable, so acute thrombolytic therapy is followed by elective catheterization and PTCA 5–10 days later in selected patients. Patients with acute pump failure may be an exception.

C. General Measures: CCU monitoring should be instituted as soon as possible. Uncomplicated patients can be transferred to less intensively monitored settings after 24–48 hours. Activity should initially be limited to bed rest, with the availability of a nearby toilet or commode in more stable patients. Progressive ambulation should be started after 48–72 hours if tolerated. Low-flow oxygen therapy (2–4 L/min) is usually given. A liquid diet is recommended during the initial 24 hours.

D. Analgesia: An initial attempt should be made to relieve pain with sublingual nitroglycerin. However, if no response occurs after two or three tablets, intravenous opiates provide the most rapid and effective analgesia. Morphine sulfate, 4–8 mg, or meperidine, 50–75 mg, should be given. Subsequent small doses can be given every 15 minutes until pain abates.

E. Antiarrhythmic Prophylaxis: The incidence of ventricular fibrillation in hospitalized patients is approximately 5%, with 80% of episodes occurring in the first 12–24 hours. Prophylactic lidocaine infusions (1–2 mg/min) prevent most episodes, but this therapy has not reduced the mortality rate and it increases the risk of asystole, so this approach is no longer recommended except in patients with very frequent ectopic beats or nonsustained ventricular tachycardia. Intravenous magnesium sulfate has been effective in one study, but confirmation is required before it can be recommended routinely.

F. Beta-Adrenergic Blocking Agents: Several studies have shown modestly improved short-term survival when intravenous beta-blockers are given immediately after acute myocardial infarction. These agents reduce the duration of ischemic pain and the incidence of ventricular fibrillation. A favorable effect appears to persist even after thrombolytic therapy. However, the survival benefit is small, so beta-blockers should not be given to patients with relative contraindications. Long-term beta-blocker therapy is discussed below.

G. Nitrates and Calcium Channel-Blocking Agents: While both of these groups of medications effectively treat ischemia, they have not been shown to improve outcome in acute infarction. Indeed, they may provoke reflex tachycardia or excessive hypotension with deleterious consequences, as has occurred in several studies with nifedipine. They should be reserved for patients with recurrent ischemia unresponsive to beta-blockers or for the treatment of hypertension. Diltiazem and verapamil appear to prevent reinfarction and ischemia in the subset of patients with non-Q wave disease. The former agent is preferable because it causes less myocardial depression. The dosage is 240–360 mg daily.

H. Anticoagulation: With the exception of patients undergoing thrombolysis and subsequent heparin therapy, the use of full anticoagulation remains controversial. Patients who will be at bed rest or on limited activity status for some time should be given 5000 units of heparin subcutaneously every 8–12 hours unless contraindicated. Aspirin, 325 mg daily, should be given unless contraindicated.

Granger CB et al: Thrombolytic therapy for acute myocardial infarction: A review. Drugs 1992;44:293.

Grines CL et al: A comparison of immediate angioplasty with thrombolytic therapy for acute myocardial infarction. N Engl J Med 1993;328:673. (Results suggest potential benefit of acute PTCA. See also editorial comment on page 726 suggesting caution in applying these results.)

Muller DWM, Topol EJ: Selection of patients with acute myocardial infarction for thrombolytic therapy. Ann Intern Med 1990;118:949. (Review emphasizing failure to treat most eligible patients.)

Popma JJ, Topol EJ: Adjuncts to thrombolysis for myocardial reperfusion. Ann Intern Med 1991;115:34. (Aspirin is beneficial; intravenous beta-blockers should be considered; heparin remains controversial.)

TIMI Study Group: Comparison of invasive and conservative strategies after treatment with intravenous tissue plasminogen activator in acute myocardial infarction: Results of the thrombolysis in myocardial infarction. N Engl J Med 1989;320:618. (Definitive trial demonstrating that PTCA can be reserved for those with predischarge evidence of ischemia.)

Woods KL et al: Intravenous magnesium sulfate in suspected acute myocardial infarction: Results of the second Leicester Intravenous Magnesium Intervention Trial (LIMIT-2). Lancet 1992;339:1553.

Yusuf S et al: Routine medical management of acute myocardial infarction: Lessons from overviews of recent randomized controlled trials. Circulation 1990;82(2 Suppl):II–117. (Comprehensive review, concluding that aspirin and beta-blockers are the only proved agents.)

Complications

Most patients have one or more complications of myocardial infarction, though the response to treatment is usually prompt.

A. Infarct Extension and Postinfarction Ischemia: Recurrent infarction in the region of infarction (infarct extension) in the first 10–14 days occurs in approximately 10% of patients. It may be associated with prolonged or intermittent episodes of chest pain. In many cases, the process is relatively silent, being detected on routine ECG, by laboratory testing, or by onset or worsening of heart failure. Infarct extension is at least twice as common in non-Q wave infarcts and is more likely to occur after successful thrombolytic therapy owing to residual jeopardized myocardium. Diltiazem, 60–90 mg four times daily, has been shown to reduce the rate of extension following non-Q wave infarction.

Approximately 30% of patients will have anginal episodes postinfarction. These are more common in patients with angina prior to infarction and in non-Q wave infarction. Postinfarction angina is associated with increased short- and long-term mortality rates. The underlying mechanism is usually inadequate blood flow through a recanalized vessel or reocclusion. Vigorous medical therapy should be instituted, including nitrates, calcium channel blockers, and beta-blockers, as well as aspirin and heparin. Thrombolytic therapy may also be helpful. Most patients with postinfarction angina—and all who are refractory to medical therapy—should undergo early catheterization and revascularization by PTCA or CABG.

B. Arrhythmias: Abnormalities of rhythm and conduction are common.

1. Sinus bradycardia–This is most common in inferior infarctions or may be precipitated by medications. Observation or withdrawal of the offending agent is usually sufficient. If accompanied by signs of low cardiac output, atropine, 0.5–1 mg intravenously, is usually effective. Temporary pacing is rarely required.

2. Supraventricular tachyarrhythmias–Sinus tachycardia is common and may reflect either increased adrenergic stimulation or hemodynamic compromise due to hypovolemia or pump failure. If the latter, beta blockade is contraindicated. Supraventricular premature beats are common and may be premonitory for atrial fibrillation. Electrolyte abnormalities and hypoxia should be corrected and causative agents (especially aminophylline) stopped. Atrial fibrillation should be rapidly controlled or converted to sinus rhythm. Intravenous verapamil (given cautiously in 2- to 5-mg increments up to 20 mg) or the short-acting beta-blocker esmolol (500 μg/kg, followed by 50–200 μg/kg/min) are the agents of choice if cardiac function is adequate. Digoxin (0.5 mg as initial dose, then 0.25 mg every 90–120 minutes [up to 1–1.25 mg] for a loading dose, followed by 0.25 mg daily if renal function is normal) is preferable if heart failure is present with atrial fibrillation, but it takes longer. Electrical cardioversion (commencing with 100 J) may be necessary if atrial fibrillation is complicated by hypotension, heart failure, or ischemia, but the arrhythmia often recurs. A class Ia agent such as procainamide or quinidine may be required in addition to verapamil, a beta-blocker, or digoxin to maintain sinus rhythm.

3. Ventricular arrhythmias–Ventricular arrhythmias are most common in the first few hours after infarction. Ventricular premature beats (VPBs) may be premonitory for ventricular tachycardia or fibrillation. Prophylactic lidocaine should be started (1 mg/kg bolus followed by an infusion of 2 mg/min) if more than 6 VPB/min, early (R on T wave) VPB, couplets or nonsustained ventricular tachycardia are observed. Additional boluses of 0.5 mg/kg followed by an increased infusion rate (up to 4 mg/min) may be necessary, but toxicity (tremor, anxiety, confusion, seizures) is common, especially in older patients and those with hypotension, heart failure, or liver disease. The infusion rate should be reduced after 3–4 hours, since blood levels tend to rise, but generally, once initiated, lidocaine should be continued for at least 24 hours.

Ventricular tachycardia should be treated with a 1 mg/kg bolus of lidocaine if the patient is stable or by electrical cardioversion (100–200 J) if not. If the arrhythmia cannot be suppressed with lidocaine, procainamide should be initiated (100 mg boluses over 1–2 minutes every 5 minutes to a cumulative dose of 750–1000 mg, followed by an infusion of 20–80 μg/kg/min). Hypotension may occur acutely, and depression of myocardial function or conduction may complicate maintenance therapy. Refractory ventricular arrhythmias may rarely respond to beta blockade (esmolol [500 μg/kg intravenously, followed by 50–200 μg/kg/min] is recommended because of its rapid onset and short duration of action), phenytoin (loading dose: boluses of 100 mg over 5 minutes every 5–10 minutes to a total of 1000 mg; maintenance 300–500 mg/d in divided doses), or bretylium tosylate (5 mg/kg intravenously over 3–5 minutes, repeated after 20 minutes if necessary, followed by an infusion of

1–2 mg/min). Intravenous amiodarone can be very effective, but in the USA it is available only in a few centers. Ventricular fibrillation is treated electrically (300–400 J). Unresponsive ventricular fibrillation should be treated by bretylium and repeat cardioversion while CPR is administered. Accelerated idioventricular rhythm is a regular, wide complex rhythm at a rate of 70–100/min. It often follows reperfusion after thrombolytic therapy. The need for treating it in the absence of other ventricular arrhythmias is controversial.

4. Conduction disturbances–All degrees of atrioventricular block may occur in the course of acute myocardial infarction. Block at the level of the atrioventricular node is more common than infranodal block and occurs in approximately 20% of inferior myocardial infarctions. First-degree block is the most usual and requires no treatment. Seconddegree block is usually of the Mobitz type I form (Wenckebach), is often transient, and requires treatment only if associated with a heart rate slow enough to cause symptoms. Complete atrioventricular block occurs in up to 5% of acute inferior infarctions, usually is preceded by second-degree block, and usually resolves spontaneously, though it may persist for hours to several weeks. The escape rhythm originates in the distal atrioventricular node or atrioventricular junction and hence has a narrow QRS complex and is reliable, albeit often slow (30–50 beats/min). Treatment is often necessary because of resulting hypotension and low cardiac output. Intravenous atropine (1 mg) usually restores atrioventricular conduction temporarily, but if the escape complex is wide or if repeated atropine treatments are needed, temporary ventricular pacing is indicated. The prognosis for these patients is only slightly worse than that of patients who do not develop atrioventricular block.

In anterior infarctions, the site of block is distal, below the atrioventricular node, and usually a result of extensive damage of the His-Purkinje system and bundle branches. New first-degree block (prolongation of the PR interval) is unusual in anterior infarction; Mobitz type II atrioventricular block or complete heart block may be preceded by intraventricular conduction defects or may occur abruptly. The escape rhythm, if present at all, is an unreliable widecomplex idioventricular rhythm. Urgent ventricular pacing is mandatory, but even with successful pacing, mortality rates following the onset of complete heart block approach 80% because of the associated extensive myocardial change. New conduction abnormalities such as right or left bundle branch block or posterior or anterior fascicular blocks may presage progression, often sudden, to second- or third-degree atrioventricular block. Prophylactic temporary ventricular pacing is recommended for new-onset alternating bilateral bundle branch block, bifascicular block, or bundle branch block with worsening firstdegree atrioventricular block. Patients with anterior infarction who progress to second- or third-degree block even transiently should be considered for insertion of a prophylactic permanent ventricular pacemaker before discharge.

C. Myocardial Dysfunction: The severity of cardiac dysfunction is proportionate to the extent of myocardial necrosis but is exacerbated by preexisting dysfunction and ongoing ischemia. Patients who have no signs of heart failure, normal blood pressure, and normal urine output have a good prognosis. Patients with hypotension or evidence of more than mild heart failure should have bedside right heart catheterization and continuous measurements of arterial pressure. These measurements permit the accurate assessment of cardiac function, facilitate the correct choice of therapy, and provide important prognostic information. Table 10–4 categorizes patients based upon these hemodynamic findings.

1. Acute left ventricular failure–Basilar rales are common in acute myocardial infarction, but dyspnea, more diffuse rales, and arterial hypoxemia usually indicate left ventricular failure. Since both the physical examination and chest x-ray correlate poorly with hemodynamic measurements and since the central venous pressure does not correlate with the pulmonary capillary wedge pressure (PCWP), right heart catheterization may be essential in monitoring therapy. General measures include supplemental oxygen to increase arterial saturation to above 95% and elevation of the trunk. Diuretics are usually the initial therapy unless right ventricular infarction is present. Intravenous furosemide (10–40 mg) or bumetanide (0.5–1 mg) is preferred because of the reliably rapid onset and short duration of action of these drugs. Higher dosages can be given if an inadequate response occurs. Morphine sulfate (4 mg intravenously followed by increments of 2 mg) is valuable in acute pulmonary edema.

Diuretics are usually effective; however, since most patients with acute infarction are not volume overloaded, the hemodynamic response may be limited and may be associated with hypotension. Vasodilators will reduce PCWP and improve cardiac output by a combination of venodilation (increasing venous capacitance) and arteriolar dilation (reducing afterload and left ventricular wall stress). In mild heart failure, sublingual isosorbide dinitrate (2.5–10 mg every 2 hours) or topical nitroglycerin ointment (6.25–25 mg every 4 hours) may be adequate to lower PCWP. In more severe failure, especially if cardiac output is reduced, sodium nitroprusside is the preferred agent. It should be initiated only with hemodynamic monitoring; the initial dosage should be low (0.25 μg/kg/min) to avoid excessive hypotension, but the dosage can be increased by increments of 0.5 μg/kg/min every 5–10 minutes up to 5–10 μg/kg/min until the desired hemodynamic response (PCWP < 18 mm Hg, CI > 2.5) is obtained. Excessive hypotension (mean blood pressure < 65–75 mm Hg) or tachycardia (> 10/min increase) should be avoided. Combination of nitroprusside with inotropic agents may be necessary to preserve blood pressure or maximize benefit.

Intravenous nitroglycerin (starting at 10 mg/min and titrating up to 10 μg/kg/min) is usually less effective but may lower PCWP with less hypotension. Oral or transdermal vasodilator therapy with nitrates or angiotensin-converting enzyme inhibitors is often necessary after the initial 24–48 hours (see below).

Inotropic agents should be avoided if possible, because they often increase heart rate and myocardial oxygen requirements. Dobutamine has the best hemodynamic profile, increasing cardiac output and modestly lowering PCWP, usually without excessive tachycardia, hypotension, or arrhythmias. The initial dosage is 2.5 μg/kg/min, and it may be increased by similar increments up to 15–20 μg/kg/min at intervals of 5–10 minutes. Dopamine is more useful in the presence of hypotension (see below), since it produces peripheral vasoconstriction, but it has a less beneficial effect on PCWP. Amrinone is a positive inotrope and vasodilator that produces hemodynamic effects similar to those of dobutamine but with a greater decrease in PCWP. However, its longer duration of action makes it less useful in unstable situations. Milrinone is a more potent and newer congener of amrinone with fewer side effects. It should be commenced in a loading dose of 50 μg/kg over 10 minutes, followed by an infusion of 0.375–0.75 μg/kg/min. Digoxin has not been helpful in acute infarction except to control the ventricular response in atrial fibrillation, but it may be beneficial if chronic heart failure persists.

2. Hypotension and shock–Patients with hypotension (systolic blood pressure < 100 mm Hg, individualized depending on prior blood pressure) and signs of diminished perfusion (low urine output, confusion, cold extremities) should be hemodynamically monitored. Up to 20% will have findings indicative of intravascular hypovolemia (due to diaphoresis, vomiting, decreased venous tone, medications—such as diuretics, nitrates, morphine, beta-blockers, calcium channel blockers, and thrombolytic agents— and lack of oral intake). These should be treated with successive boluses of 100 mL of normal saline until PCWP reaches 15–18 mm Hg to determine whether cardiac output and blood pressure respond. Pericardial tamponade due to hemorrhagic pericarditis (especially after thrombolytic therapy or cardiopulmonary resuscitation) or ventricular rupture should be considered and excluded by echocardiography if clinically indicated. Right ventricular infarction, characterized by a normal PCWP but elevated right atrial pressure, can produce hypotension. This is discussed below.

Most hypotensive patients will have moderate to severe left ventricular dysfunction; pathologic studies indicate that more than 20% of the left ventricle is infarcted (> 40% in cardiogenic shock). If hypotension is only modest (systolic pressure > 90 mm Hg) and the PCWP is elevated, diuretics and an initial trial of nitroprusside (see above for dosing) are indicated. If the blood pressure falls, inotropic support will need to be added or substituted. Such patients may also be treated with intra-aortic balloon counterpulsation. This device unloads the left ventricle during systole and increases diastolic coronary artery filling pressure. It often facilitates the use of vasodilators in patients who previously did not tolerate them.

Dopamine is the most appropriate pressor for cardiogenic hypotension. It should be initiated at a rate of 2 μg/kg/min and increased at 5-minute intervals to the appropriate hemodynamic end point. At low dosages (< 5 μg/kg/min), it improves renal blood flow; at intermediate dosages (2.5–10 μg/kg/min), it stimulates myocardial contractility; at higher dosages (> 8 μg/kg/min), it is a potent α_1-adrenergic agonist. In general, blood pressure and cardiac index rise, but PCWP does not fall. Dopamine may be combined with nitroprusside or dobutamine (see above for dosing), or the latter may be used in its place if hypotension is not severe. Amrinone has hemodynamic effects similar to those of dobutamine, but its longer duration of action precludes rapid dosage adjustment. Norepinephrine (0.1–0.5 μg/kg/min) is the usual pressor of last resort, since isoproterenol and epinephrine produce less vasoconstriction, do not increase coronary perfusion pressure (aortic diastolic pressure), and tend to worsen the balance between myocardial oxygen delivery and utilization.

Patients with cardiogenic shock have a poor prognosis. If they do not respond rapidly, the previously described measure—intra-aortic balloon counterpulsation—should be instituted. Early PTCA may preserve enough viable myocardium to reverse the hypotension and should be attempted whenever feasible. Operation to repair mechanical defects (see below), revascularize ischemic myocardium, and resect aneurysms should be considered. Left ventricular assist devices as a bridge to early transplantation can be used in refractory patients under age 60 without other systemic illnesses.

D. Right Ventricular Infarction: Right ventricular infarction is present in one-third of patients with inferior wall infarction but is clinically significant in less than 50% of these. It presents as hypotension with relatively preserved left ventricular function and should be considered whenever patients with inferior infarction exhibit signs of low cardiac output and raised venous pressure. Hypotension is often exacerbated by medications that decrease intravascular volume or produce venodilation, such as diuretics, nitrates, and narcotics. Right atrial pressure and jugular venous pulsations are high, while PCWP is normal or low and the lungs are clear. The diagnosis is suggested by right precordial ST segment elevation using V_1 and leads to the right of the sternum corresponding to the location of V_3 and V_4. The diagnosis can be confirmed by echocardiography or hemodynamic measurements. When hypotension is present, hemodynamic measurements are necessary to monitor therapy. Treatment consists of fluid loading to improve left ventricular filling; inotropic agents may also be useful.

E. Mechanical Defects: Partial or complete rupture of a papillary muscle or of the interventricular septum occurs in less than 1% of acute myocardial infarctions and carries a poor prognosis. These complications occur in both anterior and inferior infarctions, usually 3–7 days after the acute event. They are detected by the appearance of a new systolic murmur and clinical deterioration, often with pulmonary edema. The two lesions are distinguished by the location of the murmur (apical versus parasternal) and by Doppler echocardiography. Hemodynamic monitoring is essential for appropriate management and demonstrates an increase in oxygen saturation between the right atrium and pulmonary artery in ventricular septal defect and, often, a large v wave with mitral regurgitation. Treatment by nitroprusside and, preferably, intra-aortic balloon counterpulsation reduces the regurgitation or shunt, but surgical correction is mandatory. In patients remaining hemodynamically unstable or requiring continuous parenteral pharmacologic treatment or counterpulsation, early surgery is recommended, though mortality rates are high (15% to nearly 100%, depending on residual ventricular function and clinical status). Patients who are stabilized medically can have delayed surgery with lower risks (10–25%).

F. Myocardial Rupture: Complete rupture of the left ventricular free wall occurs in less than 1% of patients and usually results in immediate death. It occurs 2–7 days postinfarction, usually involves the anterior wall, and is more frequent in older women. Incomplete or gradual rupture may be sealed off by the pericardium, creating a **pseudoaneurysm.** This may be recognized by echocardiography, radionuclide angiography, or left ventricular angiography, often as an incidental finding. It demonstrates a narrow-neck connection to the left ventricle. Early surgical repair is indicated, since delayed rupture is common.

G. Left Ventricular Aneurysm: Ten to 20 percent of patients surviving an acute infarction develop a left ventricular aneurysm, a sharply delineated area of scar that bulges paradoxically during systole. This usually follows anterior Q wave infarctions. Aneurysms are recognized by persistent ST segment elevation (beyond 4–8 weeks), and a wide neck from the left ventricle can be demonstrated by echocardiography, scintigraphy, or contrast angiography. They rarely rupture but may be associated with arterial emboli, ventricular arrhythmias, and congestive heart failure. Surgical resection may be performed for

these indications if other measures fail. The best results (mortality rates of 10–20%) are obtained when the residual myocardium contracts well and when significant coronary lesions supplying adjacent regions are bypassed.

H. Pericarditis: The pericardium is involved in approximately 50% of infarctions, but pericarditis is often not clinically significant. Twenty percent of patients with Q wave infarctions will have an audible friction rub if examined repetitively. Pericardial pain occurs in approximately the same proportion after 2–7 days and is recognized by its variation with respiration and position (improved by sitting). Often, no treatment is required, but aspirin (650 mg every 4–6 hours) or indomethacin (25 mg three or four times daily) will usually relieve the pain. Anticoagulation should be avoided, since hemorrhagic pericarditis may result.

From 1 to 12 weeks after infarction, Dressler's syndrome (post-myocardial infarction syndrome) occurs in less than 5% of patients. This is an autoimmune phenomenon and presents as pericarditis with associated fever, leukocytosis, and, occasionally, pericardial or pleural effusion. It may recur over months. Treatment is the same as for other forms of pericarditis. A short course of corticosteroids may help if nonsteroidal agents do not relieve symptoms.

I. Mural Thrombus: Mural thrombi are common in large anterior infarctions but not in infarctions at other locations. Arterial emboli occur in approximately 2% of patients with known infarction, usually within 6 weeks. Anticoagulation with heparin followed by short-term (3-month) warfarin therapy prevents most emboli and should be considered in all patients with large anterior infarctions. Mural thrombi can be detected by echocardiography or CT scan (MRI has yielded frequent false-positive results) but with only moderate reliability, and only a small percentage (0–25%) embolize, so these procedures should not be relied upon for determining the need for anticoagulation.

Bolooki H: Surgical treatment of complications of acute myocardial infarction. JAMA 1990;263:1237. (When and how.)

Bosch X et al: Clinical and angiographic features and prognostic significance of early postinfarction angina. Am J Med 1991;91:493. (Large series showing that when electrocardiographic changes accompany pain, the event rate is high.)

Brugada P, Andries EW: Early postDmyocardial infarction ventricular arrhythmias. Cardiovasc Clin 1992;22:165.

Chatterjee K: Complications of acute myocardial infarction. Curr Probl Cardiol 1993;18:1.

Fitzpatrick A, Sutton R: A guide to temporary pacing. Br Med J 1992;304:365. (When to pace.)

Gacioch GM et al: Cardiogenic shock complicating acute myocardial infarction: The use of coronary angioplasty and the integration of the new support devices in patient management. J Am Coll Cardiol 1992;19:647. (PTCA may be helpful, but the role of other "high-tech" approaches is unclear.)

Left ventricular thrombosis and stroke following myocardial infarction. (Editorial.) Lancet 1990;335:759.

Setaro JF, Cabin HS: Right ventricular infarction. Cardiol Clin 1992;10:69.

Topaz O et al: Acute ventricular septal rupture. Am Heart J 1990;120:412. (Early surgery indicated.)

Postinfarction Management

Twenty percent of patients with acute myocardial infarction die before they reach the hospital. Mortality rates in hospitalized patients range from 5% to 15% and are determined chiefly by the size of the infarction and the age and general condition of the patient. Patients developing heart failure or hypotension have high early mortality rates. Several classification criteria have been developed to estimate early prognosis for survival. The most accurate is hemodynamic subsetting (Table 10–6). The prognosis after discharge is determined by three major factors: the degree of left ventricular dysfunction, the extent of residual ischemic myocardium, and the presence of ventricular arrhythmias. The mortality rate in the first year after discharge is approximately 6–8%, with over half of deaths occurring in the first 3 months, chiefly in patients with postinfarction heart failure. Subsequently, the mortality rate averages 4% per year.

A. Risk Stratification: A number of findings indicate increased risk after infarction. These include: (1) postinfarction angina; (2) non-Q wave infarction; (3) heart failure; (4) left ventricular ejection fraction less than 40%; (5) exercise-induced ischemia, diagnosed by electrocardiography or scintigraphy; and (6) ventricular ectopy (> 10 VPBs/h).

Patients with postinfarction angina should undergo coronary arteriography. Authorities differ about which tests should be performed routinely in other patients. Significant left ventricular dysfunction is most likely with anterior infarction or multiple infarctions. In these, noninvasive assessment of left ventricular function by echocardiography or scintigraphy will help assess prognosis and facilitate medical management. Submaximal exercise testing before discharge or a maximal test after 3–6 weeks (the latter being more sensitive for ischemia) helps patients and physicians plan the return to normal activity. Scintigraphy in conjunction with stress testing adds additional sensitivity for ischemia and provides localizing information. Both exercise and pharmacologic stress scintigraphy have successfully predicted subsequent outcome. One of these tests should usually be employed prior to discharge in patients who have received thrombolytic therapy as a means of selecting appropriate candidates for coronary angiography.

Ambulatory electrocardiographic monitoring for arrhythmias is of less clear value; though it has some prognostic value beyond measurements of left ventricular function, no benefit from antiarrhythmic therapy for asymptomatic patients has been demonstrated. Ischemia detected during ambulatory monitoring is an indicator of poor prognosis, but it is unclear how much additional information is obtained in patients who have also undergone exercise testing or scintigraphic studies.

A conservative approach to postinfarction evaluation would include measurement of left ventricular function in patients with signs of heart failure or large infarctions and a test for ischemia in patients without recurrent chest pain. The latter should occur before discharge if the patient has undergone thrombolytic therapy but may be delayed for 3–6 weeks in most other patients.

B. Prophylactic Therapy: Postinfarction management should begin with identification and modification of risk factors. Treatment of hyperlipidemia and smoking cessation both prevent recurrent infarctions. Blood pressure control, weight loss, and exer-

Table 10–6. Hemodynamic subsets in acute myocardial infarction.

Category	CI or SWI	PCWP	Treatment	Comment
Normal	>2.2, >30	<15	None	Mortality rate <5%.
Hyperdynamic	>3.0, >40	<15	Beta-blockers	Characterized by tachycardia; mortality rate <5%.
Hypovolemic	<2.5, <30	<10	Volume expansion	Hypotension, tachycardia, but preserved left ventricular function by echocardiography; mortality rate 4–8%.
Left ventricular failure	<2.2, <30	>15	Diuretics	Mild dyspnea, rales, normal blood pressure; mortality rate 10–20%.
Severe failure	<2.0, <20	>20	Diuretics, vasodilators	Pulmonary edema, mild hypotension; inotropic agents, IABC may be required; mortality rate 20–40%.
Shock	<1.8, <30	>18	Inotropic agents, IABC	IABC early unless rapid reversal; mortality rate >60%.

CI = cardiac index (L/min/m^2); SWI = stroke work index (g-m/m^2, calculated as [mean arterial pressure – PCWP] × stroke volume index × 0.0136); PCWP = pulmonary capillary wedge pressure (in mm Hg; pulmonary artery diastolic pressure may be used instead); IABC = intra-aortic balloon counterpulsation.

cise are recommended, though definite benefit on postinfarction prognosis has not been demonstrated.

Many drugs have been studied, and some have been shown to be beneficial in preventing death or reinfarction. However, their usefulness in the era of thrombolysis and revascularization is unclear. Beta-blockers improve survival rates, primarily by reducing the incidence of sudden death in high-risk subsets of patients. Beta-blockers should be given to such individuals, except those with overt heart failure, but are of limited value in uncomplicated patients with small infarctions and normal exercise tests. No advantage of one preparation over another has been demonstrated except that those with intrinsic sympathomimetic activity have not proved beneficial in postinfarction patients.

Calcium channel blockers have not been shown to improve prognosis overall, but both diltiazem and verapamil appear to reduce mortality rates in patients with preserved left ventricular function. Diltiazem may help to prevent reinfarction after non-Q wave infarction.

Antiplatelet agents are beneficial; low-dose aspirin (325 mg daily) is recommended. Warfarin anticoagulation for 3–6 months reduces the incidence of arterial emboli after large anterior infarctions, and according to the results of at least one study it improves long-term prognosis, but an additive benefit to aspirin after 6 months has not been confirmed.

Antiarrhythmic therapy other than with beta-blockers has not been shown to be effective except in patients with symptomatic arrhythmias and, in fact, class Ic agents increase the mortality rate in postinfarction patients. However, a recent relatively small study indicated that low-dose amiodarone may be beneficial.

Cardiac rehabilitation programs and exercise training can be of considerable psychologic benefit, but it is not known whether they alter prognosis.

C. ACE Inhibitors in Patients With Left Ventricular Dysfunction: Patients who sustain substantial myocardial damage often experience subsequent progressive left ventricular dilation and dysfunction, leading to clinical heart failure and reduced long-term survival. A recent trial demonstrated that in patients with ejection fractions less than 40%, captopril (25–50 mg three times daily commencing 3–16 days postinfarction) prevents left ventricular dilation and the onset of heart failure and also reduces the mortality rate.

D. Revascularization: Because of the increasing use of thrombolytic therapy and accumulating experience with PTCA, the indications for revascularization are rapidly evolving. Postinfarction patients who appear likely to benefit from early revascularization if the anatomy is appropriate are (1) those who have undergone thrombolytic therapy and have residual symptoms or laboratory evidence of ischemia; (2) patients with left ventricular dysfunc-

tion (ejection fraction < 30–40%) and evidence of ischemia; (3) patients with non-Q wave infarction and evidence of more than mild ischemia; and (4) patients with markedly positive exercise tests and multivessel disease. The value of revascularization in the following groups is less clear: (1) patients treated with thrombolytic agents, with little evidence of reperfusion or residual ischemia; (2) patients with left ventricular dysfunction but no detectable ischemia; and (3) patients with preserved left ventricular function who have mild ischemia and are not symptom-limited. Patients who survive infarctions without complications, have preserved left ventricular function (ejection fraction > 50%), and have no exercise-induced ischemia have an excellent prognosis and do not require invasive evaluation.

American College of Physicians Position Paper: Evaluation of patients after recent acute myocardial infarction. Ann Intern Med 1989;110:485.

Case RB et al: Living alone after myocardial infarction: Impact on prognosis. JAMA 1992;267:515. (Social factors are cultural determinants of outcome.)

Gheorghiade M, Goldstein S: Calcium channel blockers in post-myocardial infarction patients. Prog Cardiovasc Dis 1991;34:37. (To be avoided if heart failure or significant left ventricular dysfunction is present.)

Jafri SM et al: Medical therapy after acute myocardial infarction. Curr Probl Cardiol 1991;16(9):585. (Comprehensive review, including beta-blockers, anticoagulation, and other potential treatments.)

Krone RJ: The role of risk stratification in the early management of a myocardial infarction. Ann Intern Med 1992;116:223.

Moss AJ, Benhorn J: Prognosis and management after a first myocardial infarction. N Engl J Med 1990;322:743.

Pfeffer M et al: Effect of captopril on mortality and morbidity in patients with left ventricular dysfunction after myocardial infarction: Results of the Survival and Ventricular Enlargement Trial. N Engl J Med 1992;327:669.

Siegel D et al: Risk factor modification after myocardial infarction. Ann Intern Med 1988;109:213. (Often forgotten in the high-tech world.)

Smith P et al: The effect of warfarin on mortality and reinfarction after myocardial infarction. N Engl J Med 1990;323:147. (Anticoagulation appears to be beneficial.)

Yusuf S, Wittes J, Friedman L: Overview of results of randomized clinical trials in heart disease: 1. Treatments following myocardial infarction. JAMA 1988;260:2088. (Includes thrombolysis, beta-blockers, nitrates, calcium channel blockers, antiarrhythmics, anticoagulants, and antiplatelet drugs.)

DISTURBANCES OF RATE & RHYTHM

Abnormalities of cardiac rhythm and conduction can be lethal (sudden cardiac death), symptomatic (syncope, near syncope, dizziness, or palpitations), or asymptomatic. They are dangerous to the extent that they reduce cardiac output, so that perfusion of the brain or myocardium is impaired, or tend to deteriorate into more serious arrhythmias with the same consequences. Stable supraventricular tachycardia is generally well tolerated in patients without underlying heart disease but may lead to myocardial ischemia or congestive heart failure in patients with coronary disease, valvular abnormalities, and systolic or diastolic myocardial dysfunction. Ventricular tachycardia is prolonged (lasting more than 10–30 seconds), is less well tolerated, and is more likely to deteriorate into ventricular fibrillation.

Whether slow heart rates produce symptoms at rest or on exertion depends upon the underlying state of the cardiac muscle and its ability to increase its stroke output. If the heart rate abruptly slows, as with the onset of complete heart block or transient standstill, syncope or convulsions may result.

Arrhythmias are detected either because they present with symptoms or because they are detected during the course of monitoring. Symptomatic arrhythmias (especially sudden death, syncope, or near syncope) require further evaluation and treatment unless they are related to conditions that are unlikely to occur (eg, electrolyte abnormalities or acute myocardial infarction). In contrast, there is controversy over when and how to evaluate and treat rhythm disturbances that are not symptomatic but are possible markers for more serious abnormalities (eg, nonsustained ventricular tachycardia). This uncertainty reflects two issues: (1) the difficulty in reliably stratifying patients into high-risk and low-risk groups; and (2) the lack of treatments which are both effective and safe. Thus, screening patients for these so-called "premonitory" abnormalities is often not productive.

A number of procedures are employed to evaluate patients with symptoms who are felt to be at risk for life-threatening arrhythmias, including in-hospital and ambulatory electrocardiographic monitoring, event recorders (instruments that can be worn for prolonged periods in order to record or transmit rhythm tracings when infrequent episodes occur), exercise testing, intracardiac electrophysiologic studies (to assess sinus node function, atrioventricular conduction, and inducibility of arrhythmias), signal-average ECGs, and tests of autonomic nervous system function (especially tilt-table testing). These are discussed below and in the subsequent sections on individual rhythm disturbance and symptomatic presentation. In general, these techniques are more successful in diagnosing symptomatic arrhythmias than in predicting the outcome of asymptomatic ones.

Josephson ME: *Clinical Cardiac Electrophysiology: Techniques and Interpretations,* 2nd ed. Lea & Febiger, 1993.
Kastor JA: *Arrhythmias.* Saunders, 1993. (Very practical text, appropriate for primary care physicians.)

MECHANISMS OF ARRHYTHMIAS

Electrophysiologic studies have greatly increased our understanding of the mechanisms underlying most arrhythmias. These include (1) disorders of impulse formation or automaticity, (2) abnormalities of impulse conduction, (3) reentry, and (4) triggered activity.

Altered automaticity is the mechanism for sinus node arrest, many premature beats, and automatic rhythms as well as an initiating factor in reentry arrhythmias.

Abnormalities of impulse conduction can occur at the sinus or atrioventricular node, in the intraventricular conduction system, and within the atria or ventricles. These are responsible for sinoatrial exit block, for atrioventricular block at the node or below, and for establishing reentry circuits.

Reentry is the underlying mechanism for many arrhythmias, including premature beats, most paroxysmal supraventricular tachycardias, and atrial flutter. For reentry to occur, there must be an area of unidirectional block with an appropriate delay to allow repeat depolarization at the site of origin. Reentry is confirmed if the arrhythmia can be terminated by interruption of the circuit by a spontaneous or induced premature beat.

Triggered activity occurs when afterdepolarizations (abnormal electrical activity persisting after repolarization) reach the threshold level required to trigger a new depolarization. This may be the mechanism of ventricular tachycardia in the prolonged QT syndrome and in some cases of digitalis toxicity.

Binah O, Rosen MR: Mechanisms of ventricular arrhythmias. Circulation 1992;85(Suppl I):I–25.

TECHNIQUES FOR EVALUATING RHYTHM DISTURBANCES

Electrocardiographic Monitoring

The ideal way of establishing a causal relationship between a symptom and a rhythm disturbance is to demonstrate the presence of the rhythm during the symptom. Unfortunately, this is not always easy because symptoms are usually episodic.

Patients with aborted sudden death and recent or recurrent syncope are often monitored in the hospital. Those with less potentially life-threatening symptoms may be monitored as outpatients. When episodes are infrequent, use of an event recorder is preferable. Exercise testing may be helpful when the symptoms are associated with exertion or stress. If symptomatic bradyarrhythmias or supraventricular tachyarrhythmias are detected, therapy can usually be initiated without additional diagnostic studies. Further electrophysiologic studies may be useful in evaluating ventricular tachyarrhythmias.

Extreme caution is required before attributing a patient's symptom to rhythm or conduction abnormalities observed during monitoring without concomitant symptoms. In many cases, the symptoms are due to a different arrhythmia or to noncardiac causes. For instance, in evaluating dizziness or syncope in older patients, bradycardia, sinus node abnormalities, and ventricular ectopy are all commonly found but may have nothing to do with the symptoms. Ambulatory monitoring is frequently used to quantify ventricular ectopy and detect asymptomatic ventricular tachycardia in post-myocardial infarction or heart failure patients. Unfortunately, while asymptomatic ventricular arrhythmias have negative prognostic implications, there are no data to support specific therapeutic intervention. Thus, monitoring in asymptomatic individuals is not usually indicated.

Electrophysiologic Testing

Electrophysiologic testing employing intracardiac electrocardiographic recordings and programmed atrial or ventricular (or both) stimulation has become increasingly important in the diagnosis and management of complex arrhythmias. The primary indications for electrophysiologic testing are (1) evaluation of recurrent syncope of possible cardiac origin, when the ambulatory ECG has not provided the diagnosis; (2) evaluation of the efficacy of pharmacotherapy in survivors of aborted sudden death or other patients with symptomatic or life-threatening ventricular tachycardia; (3) differentiation of supraventricular from ventricular arrhythmias; (4) evaluation of therapy in patients with accessory atrioventricular pathways; and (5) evaluation of patients for antitachycardia pacing devices and surgical or catheter ablation procedures.

Signal-Averaged ECG

A newer approach to arrhythmia evaluation and prediction is the signal-averaged ECG (SAECG). This procedure sums 100 or more cardiac cycles to provide a highly resolved electrocardiographic tracing which is then filtered to maximize detection of high-frequency potentials. The finding of late potentials following the QRS complex indicates a possible substrate for ventricular arrhythmias. They are most common and of greater prognostic value in patients who have sustained a myocardial infarction. In this latter group, absence of late potentials indicates a low risk for serious ventricular arrhythmias and sudden death. While the predictive accuracy of a positive SAECG is relatively low, it has been advocated as a screening test for patients who should undergo electrophysiologic testing. At present, however, data are not adequate to support this approach in asymptomatic postinfarction patients even when they exhibit nonsustained ventricular arrhythmias. Conversely, those with symptoms consistent with arrhythmia require further evaluation and treatment regardless of the SAECG results. The value of the SAECG in patients without ischemic heart disease is unclear.

ACC Policy Statement: Standard for analyses of ventricular late potentials using high-resolution or signal-averaged electrocardiography. J Am Coll Cardiol 1991;17:999. (Consensus statement.)

Podrid PJ, Bumio F, Fogel RI: Evaluating patients with ventricular arrhythmia: Role of the signalDaveraged electrocardiogram, exercise test, ambulatory electrocardiogram and electrophysiologic studies. Cardiol Clin 1992; 10:371.

Steinberg JS et al: Predicting arrhythmic events after acute myocardial infarction using the signal-averaged electrocardiogram. Am J Cardiol 1992;69:13.

Autonomic Testing

In many patients with recurrent syncope or near syncope, arrhythmias are not the cause. This is particularly true when the patient has no evidence of associated heart disease by history, examination, standard ECG, or noninvasive testing. Syncope may be neurocardiogenic in origin, mediated by excessive vagal stimulation or an imbalance between sympathetic and parasympathetic autonomic activity. With assumption of upright posture, there is venous pooling in the lower limbs. However, instead of the normal response, which consists of an increase in heart rate and vasoconstriction, a sympathetically mediated increase in myocardial contractility activates mechanoreceptors that trigger reflex *bradycardia* and *vasodilation*. Autonomic testing is an important component of the evaluation in these individuals and should usually precede invasive electrophysiologic procedures. Carotid sinus massage in patients who do not have carotid bruits or a history of cerebral vascular disease can precipitate sinus node arrest or atrioventricular block in patients with carotid sinus hypersensitivity. Head-up tilt-table testing can identify patients whose syncope may be on a vasovagal basis. Although different testing protocols are employed, passive tilting to at least 70 degrees for 10–40 minutes—in conjunction with isoproterenol infusion, if necessary—is typical. Syncope due to bradycardia, hypotension, or both will occur in approximately one-third of patients with recurrent syncope. Some recent studies have suggested that, at least with some of the more extreme protocols, false-positive responses may occur.

Fitzpatrick AP et al: Methodology of headDup tilt testing in patients with unexplained syncope. J Am Coll Cardiol 1991;17:125. (Discusses the variety of testing approaches.)

Kapoor WN, Brant NL: Evaluation of syncope by upright tiltDtesting with isoproterenol: A nonspecific test. Ann Intern Med 1992;116:358.

Antiarrhythmic Drugs
(Table 10–7)

Antiarrhythmic drugs have limited efficacy and produce frequent side effects. They are often divided into four classes based upon their electropharmacologic actions.

Class I agents block membrane sodium channels. Three subclasses are further defined by the effect of agents on the Purkinje fiber action potential. Class Ia drugs slow the rate of rise of the action potential (V_{max}) and prolong its duration, thus slowing conduction and increasing refractoriness. Class Ib agents shorten action potential duration; they do not affect conduction or refractoriness. Class Ic agents prolong V_{max} and slow repolarization, thus slowing conduction and prolonging refractoriness, but more so than class Ia drugs.

Class II agents are the beta-blockers, which decrease automaticity, prolong atrioventricular conduction, and prolong refractoriness.

Class III agents block potassium channels and prolong repolarization, widening the QRS and prolonging the QT interval. They decrease automaticity and conduction and prolong refractoriness.

Class IV agents are the slow calcium channel blockers, which decrease automaticity and atrioventricular conduction.

Although the in vitro electrophysiologic effects of most of these agents have been defined, their use remains largely empirical. All can exacerbate arrhythmias (proarrhythmic effect), and most depress left ventricular function.

The risk of antiarrhythmic agents has recently been highlighted by the Coronary Arrhythmia Suppression Trial (CAST), in which two class Ic agents (flecainide, encainide) and a class Ia agent (moricizine) increased mortality rates in patients with asymptomatic ventricular ectopy after myocardial infarction. Therefore, class Ic agents and perhaps any antiarrhythmic drug should not be used except for life-threatening arrhythmias and symptomatic supraventricular tachyarrhythmias. The decision to treat asymptomatic ventricular ectopy with any antiarrhythmic agent should be carefully considered.

The use of antiarrhythmic agents for specific arrhythmias is discussed below.

Gill J et al: Amiodarone: An overview of its pharmacologic properties and review of its therapeutic use in cardiac arrhythmias. Drugs 1992;43:69. (A drug that is becoming more widely used.)

Harrison DC, Bottorff MB: Advances in antiarrhythmic drug therapy. Adv Pharmacol 1992;23:179.

Morganroth J: Proarrhythmic effects of antiarrhythmic drugs: Evolving concepts. Am Heart J 1992;123:1137. (Treatment is always a twoDedged sword.)

Singh BW et al: Sotalol: A betaDblocker with unique antiarrhythmic properties. Am Heart J 1987;114:121. (A useful agent now available in the USA.)

Woosley RL: Antiarrhythmic drugs. Annu Rev Pharmacol Toxicol 1991;31:427. (Updated classification.)

SUPRAVENTRICULAR ARRHYTHMIAS

1. SINUS ARRHYTHMIA, BRADYCARDIA, & TACHYCARDIA

Sinus arrhythmia is a cyclic increase in normal heart rate with inspiration and decrease with expiration. It results from reflex changes in vagal influence on the normal pacemaker and disappears with breath holding or increase of heart rate due to any cause. It has no clinical significance. It is common in both the young and the elderly.

Sinus bradycardia is a heart rate slower than 50/min due to increased vagal influence on the normal pacemaker or organic disease of the sinus node. The rate usually increases during exercise or administration of atropine. In healthy individuals, and especially in patients who are in excellent physical condition, sinus bradycardia is a normal finding. However, severe sinus bradycardia may be an indication of sinus node pathology (see below), especially in elderly patients and individuals with heart disease. It may cause weakness, confusion, or syncope if cerebral perfusion is impaired. Atrial and ventricular ectopic rhythms are more apt to occur with slow sinus rates. Rarely, pacing is required if symptoms correlate with the bradycardia.

Sinus tachycardia is defined as a heart rate faster than 100 beats/min that is caused by rapid impulse formation from the normal pacemaker; it occurs with fever, exercise, emotion, pain, anemia, heart failure, shock, thyrotoxicosis, or drug effect. Alcohol and alcohol withdrawal are common causes of sinus tachycardia and other supraventricular arrhythmias. The onset and termination are usually gradual, in contrast to paroxysmal supraventricular tachycardia due to reentry. The rate infrequently exceeds 160/min but may reach 180/min in young persons. The rhythm is basically regular, but serial 1-minute counts of the heart rate indicate that it varies five or more beats per minute with changes in position, with breath holding or sedation.

Table 10–7. Antiarrhythmic drugs.

Agent	Intravenous Dosage	Oral Dosage	Therapeutic Plasma Level	Route of Elimination	Side Effects
Class Ia:	**Action:** Sodium channel blockers: Depress phase 0 depolarization; slow conduction; prolong repolarization. **Indications:** Supraventricular tachycardia, ventricular tachycardia, prevention of ventricular fibrillation, symptomatic ventricular premature beats.				
Quinidine	6–10 mg/kg (IM or IV) over 20 min (rarely used parenterally)	200–400 mg every 4–6 h (or every 8 h long-acting)	2–5 µg/mL	Hepatic	GI, ↓ LVF, ↑ Dig
Procainamide	100 mg/1–3 min to 500–1000 mg; maintain at 2–6 mg/min	50 mg/kg/d in divided doses every 3–4 h or every 6 h (long-acting)	4–10 µg/mL; NAPA (active metabolite), 10–20 µg/mL	Renal	SLE, hypersensitivity, ↓ LVF
Disopyramide		100–200 mg every 6–8 h	2–8 µg/mL	Renal	Urinary retention, dry mouth, markedly ↓ LVF
Moricizine		200–300 mg every 8 h	*Note:* Active metabolites	Hepatic	Dizziness, nausea, headache, ↓ theophylline level, ↓ LVF
Class Ib:	**Action:** Short repolarization. **Indications:** Ventricular tachycardia, prevention of ventricular fibrillation, symptomatic ventricular beats.				
Lidocaine	1–2 mg/kg at 50 mg/min; maintain at 1–4 mg/min		1–5 µg/mL	Hepatic	CNS, GI
Tocainide		200–400 mg every 6–8 h	3–10 µg/mL	Hepatic	CNS, GI, leukopenia
Mexiletine		100–300 mg every 6–12 h. Maximum: 1200 mg/d	0.5–2 µg/mL	Hepatic	CNS, GI, leukopenia
Phenytoin	50 mg/5 min to 1000 mg (12 mg/kg); maintain at 200–400 mg/d	200–400 mg every 12–24 h	5–20 µg/mL	Hepatic	CNS, GI
Class Ic:	**Action:** Depress phase 0 repolarization; slow conduction. *Propafenone* is a weak calcium channel- and beta-blocker and prolongs action potential and refractoriness. **Indications:** Life-threatening ventricular tachycardia or fibrillation; refractory supraventricular tachycardia.				
Flecainide		100–200 mg twice daily	0.2–1 µg/mL	Hepatic	CNS, GI, ↓↓ LVF, incessant VT, sudden death
Propafenone		150–300 mg every 8–12 h	*Note:* Active metabolites	Hepatic	CNS, GI, ↓↓ LVF, ↑ Dig
Class II:	**Action:** Beta-blocker, slows AV conduction. *Note:* Other beta-blockers may also have antiarrhythmic effects but are not yet approved for this indication in the USA. **Indications:** Supraventricular tachycardia, may prevent ventricular fibrillation.				
Esmolol	500 µg/kg over 1–2 min; maintain at 25–200 µg/kg/min	Other beta-blockers may be used	0.15–2 µg/mL	Hepatic	↓ LVF, bronchospasm
Propranolol	1–5 mg at 1 mg/min	40–320 mg in 1–4 doses (depending on preparation)	Not established	Hepatic	↓ LVF, bradycardia, AV block, bronchospasm
Acebutolol		200–600 mg twice daily	Not established	Hepatic	↓ LVF, bradycardia, positive ANA, lupus-like syndrome

(continued)

Table 10–7. Antiarrhythmic drugs. (continued)

Agent	Intravenous Dosage	Oral Dosage	Therapeutic Plasma Level	Route of Elimination	Side Effects
Class III:	**Action:** Prolong action potential. **Indications:** *Amiodarone:* refractory ventricular tachycardia, supraventricular tachycardia, prevention of ventricular tachycardia, ventricular fibrillation; *sotalol:* ventricular tachycardia; *bretylium:* ventricular fibrillation, ventricular tachycardia.				
Amiodarone	Same as oral	800–1600 mg/d for 7–21 days; maintain at 100–400 mg/d (higher doses may be needed)	1–5 µg/mL	Hepatic	Pulmonary fibrosis, hypothyroidism, hyperthyroidism, corneal and skin deposits, hepatitis, ↑ Dig, neurotoxicity, GI
Sotalol		80–160 mg every 12 h (higher doses may be used for life-threatening arrhythmias)		Renal (dosing interval should be extended if creatinine clearance is <60 mL/min)	↓ LVF, bradycardia, fatigue (and other side effects associated with beta-blockers)
Bretylium	5–10 mg/kg over 5–10 min; maintain at 0.5–2 mg/min. Maximum: 30 mg/kg		0.5–1.5 µg/mL	Renal	Hypotension, nausea
Class IV:	**Action:** Slow calcium channel blockers. **Indications:** Supraventricular tachycardia.				
Verapamil	10–20 mg over 2–20 min; maintain at 5 µg/kg/min	80–120 mg every 6–8 h; 240–360 mg once daily with sustained-release preparation (not approved for arrhythmia)	0.1–0.15 µg/mL	Hepatic	↓ LVF, constipation, ↑ Dig
Diltiazem	0.25 mg/kg over 2 min; second 0.35 mg/kg bolus after 15 min if response is inadequate; infusion rate, 5–15 mg/h	180–360 mg daily in 1–3 doses depending on preparation (oral forms not approved for arrhythmias)		Hepatic metabolism, renal excretion	Hypotension, ↓ LVF
Class V:	**Indications:** Supraventricular tachycardia.				
Adenosine	6 mg rapidly followed by 12 mg after 1–2 min if needed			Adenosine receptor stimulation, metabolized in blood	Transient flushing, dyspnea, chest pain, AV block, sinus bradycardia; effect ↓ by theophylline, ↑ by dipyridamole
Digoxin	0.5 mg over 20 min followed by increment of 0.25 or 0.125 mg to 1–1.5 mg over 24 hours	1–1.5 mg over 24–36 hours in 3 or 4 doses; maintenance, 0.125–0.5 mg/d	0.7–2 mg/mL	Renal	AV block, arrhythmias, GI, visual changes

Key: AV = atrioventricular; CNS = central nervous system; ↑ Dig = elevation of serum digoxin level; GI = gastrointestinal (nausea, vomiting, diarrhea); ↓ LVF = reduced left ventricular function; SLE = systemic lupus erythematosus; VT = ventricular tachycardia

2. ATRIAL PREMATURE BEATS (Atrial Extrasystoles)

Atrial premature beats occur when an ectopic focus in the atria fires before the next sinus node impulse or a reentry circuit is established. The contour of the P wave usually differs from the patient's normal complex. Ventricular systole occurs prematurely, and the compensatory pause following this is only slightly longer than the normal interval between beats. Such premature beats occur frequently in normal hearts and are never a sufficient basis for a diagnosis of heart disease. Speeding of the heart rate by any means usually abolishes most premature beats. Early atrial premature beats may cause aberrant QRS complexes (wide and bizarre) or may be nonconducted to the ventricles because the latter are still refractory.

3. DIFFERENTIATION OF ABERRANTLY CONDUCTED SUPRAVENTRICULAR BEATS FROM VENTRICULAR BEATS

This distinction can be very difficult in patients with a wide QRS complex; it is important because of the differing prognostic and therapeutic implications of each type. Findings favoring a ventricular origin include (1) atrioventricular dissociation; (2) a QRS duration exceeding 0.14 s; (3) capture or fusion beats (infrequent); (4) left axis deviation with right bundle branch block morphology; (5) monophasic (R) or biphasic (qR, QR, or RS) complexes in V_1; and (6) a qR or QS complex in V_6. Supraventricular origin is favored by (1) a triphasic QRS complex, especially if there was initial negativity in leads I and V_6; (2) ventricular rates exceeding 170/min; (3) QRS duration longer than 0.12 s but not longer than 0.14 s; and (4) the presence of preexcitation syndrome.

The relationship of the P waves to the tachycardia complex is helpful. A 1:1 relationship usually means a supraventricular origin, except in the case of ventricular tachycardia with retrograde P waves. If the P waves are not clearly seen, Lewis leads (in which the right arm electrode is placed in the V_1 position two interspaces higher than usual and the left arm electrode is placed in the usual V_1 position) may be employed. This accentuates the size of the P waves. Esophageal leads, in which the electrode is placed directly posterior to the left atrium, achieve the same effect even more clearly. Right atrial electrograms may also help to clarify the diagnosis by accentuating the P waves.

Akhtar M et al: Wide QRS complex tachycardia: Reappraisal of a common clinical problem. Ann Intern Med 1988;109:905. (Most wide-complex arrhythmias are ventricular tachycardia.)

4. PAROXYSMAL SUPRAVENTRICULAR TACHYCARDIA (Atrial or Junctional Tachycardia)

This is the commonest paroxysmal tachycardia. It occurs more often in young patients with normal hearts. Attacks begin and end abruptly and may last several hours or longer. The heart rate may be 140–240/min (usually 160–220/min) and is perfectly regular (despite exercise or change in position). The P wave usually differs in contour from sinus beats. Patients may be asymptomatic except for awareness of rapid heart action, but some experience mild chest pain or shortness of breath, especially when episodes are prolonged, even in the absence of associated car-

diac abnormalities. Paroxysmal supraventricular tachycardia may result from digitalis toxicity and then is commonly associated with atrioventricular block.

The most common mechanism for paroxysmal supraventricular tachycardia is reentry, which may be initiated or terminated by a fortuitously timed atrial or ventricular premature beat. The reentry circuit may involve the sinus node, the atrioventricular node, or an accessory pathway. Recent evidence indicates that about one-third of patients have aberrant pathways to the ventricles. The pathophysiology and management of arrhythmias due to accessory pathways differs in important ways and is discussed separately below.

Treatment of the Acute Attack

In the absence of heart disease, serious effects are rare. Most attacks break spontaneously, and the physician should not use remedies that are more dangerous than the disease. Particular effort should be made to terminate the attack quickly if cardiac failure, syncope, or anginal pain develops or if there is underlying cardiac or (particularly) coronary disease. Because reentry is the most common mechanism for paroxysmal atrial tachycardia, effective therapy requires that conduction be interrupted at some point in the reentry circuit.

A. Mechanical Measures: A variety of methods have been used to interrupt attacks, and patients may learn to perform these themselves. These include Valsalva's maneuver, stretching the arms and body, lowering the head between the knees, coughing, and breath holding. These maneuvers, as is true also of carotid sinus pressure (see below), stimulate the vagus, delay atrioventricular conduction, and block the reentry mechanism, terminating the arrhythmias.

B. Vagal Stimulation With Carotid Sinus Pressure: *Caution: This procedure should not be performed if the patient has carotid bruits or a history of transient cerebral ischemic attacks.* With the patient relaxed in the semirecumbent position, firm but gentle pressure and massage are applied first over one carotid sinus for 10–20 seconds and then over the other. *Pressure should not be exerted on both carotid sinuses at the same time.* Continuous electrocardiographic or auscultatory monitoring of the heart rate is required so that carotid sinus pressure can be relieved as soon as the attack ceases or if excessive slowing occurs. Carotid sinus pressure will interrupt up to half the attacks, especially if the patient has been digitalized or sedated. Eyeball pressure has been recommended by some, but it should be avoided because of the danger of retinal detachment.

C. Drug Therapy: If mechanical measures fail, two rapidly acting intravenous agents will terminate more than 90% of episodes. Intravenous adenosine has become the treatment of choice in most patients because of its very brief duration of action and minimal negative inotropic activity. A 6-mg bolus is administered. If no response is observed after 1–2 minutes, a second and third 12-mg bolus should be given. Since the half-life of adenosine is less than 10 seconds, the drug must be given rapidly (in 1–2 seconds from a proximal intravenous port). Adenosine is very well tolerated, but nearly 20% of patients will experience transient flushing, and some patients experience severe chest discomfort.

Intravenous verapamil may be given as a 2.5 mg-bolus, followed by additional doses of 2.5 mg to 5 mg every 1–3 minutes up to a total of 20 mg if blood pressure and rhythm are stable. If the rhythm recurs, further doses can be given. Oral verapamil, 80–120 mg every 4–6 hours, can be used as well in stable patients who are tolerating the rhythm without difficulty.

Esmolol, a short-acting beta-blocker, is also highly effective; the initial dose is 500 μg/kg intravenously over 1 minute followed by an infusion of 25–200 μg/min. Parasympathetic stimulating drugs such as edrophonium, 5–10 mg intravenously, which delay atrioventricular conduction, may break the reentry mechanism. Because it frequently causes nausea and vomiting, it should be used only if the previously discussed agents fail. Metaraminol or phenylephrine, alpha-adrenergic stimulants that activate the baroreceptors by raising the blood pressure and causing vagal stimulation, can break attacks but should be used cautiously because they may provoke excessive hypertension. Digoxin is effective, but it often requires several hours to safely administer an adequate dose. An initial dose of 0.5–0.75 mg intravenously, followed by 0.25-mg or 0.125-mg increments every 2–4 hours up to a total of 1–1.25 mg, is used. Outpatients who are tolerating the rhythm can be treated with oral digitalis. Intravenous procainamide may terminate supraventricular tachycardia; however, since it facilitates atrioventricular conduction and an initial increase in rate may occur, it is usually not given until after digoxin, verapamil, or a beta-blocker has been administered. In patients with Wolff-Parkinson-White syndrome, in which an accessory pathway is involved, these agents may be contraindicated (see below).

D. Cardioversion: If the clinical situation is severe enough to warrant immediate termination and adenosine and verapamil are contraindicated or ineffective, synchronized electrical cardioversion (beginning at 50–100 J) is almost universally successful. If digitalis toxicity is present or strongly suspected, as in the case of paroxysmal tachycardia with block, electrical cardioversion should be avoided.

Prevention of Attacks

A. Drugs: Digoxin orally is the usual drug of first choice because of its convenience and efficacy. Verapamil, alone or in combination with digitalis, is a second choice, though oral therapy is not as effective as intravenous therapy. (*Note:* Verapamil in-

creases digoxin serum levels.) Beta-blockers are also effective. Patients who do not respond to these agents should be treated with a class Ia agent such as quinidine, perhaps in combination with digoxin or another agent that inhibits atrioventricular conduction. In patients taking quinidine, digoxin levels also increase by about 30%.

Procainamide and disopyramide are also effective. The newer class Ic agents, flecainide and propafenone, are especially successful in patients with bypass tracts. Amiodarone is highly effective, but because of its toxicity it should be employed only in refractory and symptomatic patients.

B. Atrioventricular Node Modification and His Bundle Ablation: In patients with repeated or near-incessant symptomatic attacks that are difficult to control, delivery of radiofrequency energy to the atrioventricular node via a properly positioned catheter may modify conduction to eliminate the reentry circuit. Failing this, the bundle of His can be interrupted by catheter techniques. In this case, a ventricular pacemaker is necessary, because complete atrioventricular block is often produced. There is growing experience with ablation, and that procedure has become the treatment of choice in many patients.

C. Antitachycardia Pacemakers: Specially programmed permanent pacemakers have been employed to sense the appearance of supraventricular tachycardia and pace to interrupt the reentry circuit and stop the arrhythmia. This approach requires the involvement of highly specialized electrophysiologists.

AHA Medical/Scientific Statement: Current role of catheter ablative procedures in patients with cardiac arrhythmias. Circulation 1991;83:2146. (Consensus statement covering supraventricular and ventricular arrhythmias.)

Camm AJ, Garra CJ: Adenosine and supraventricular tachycardia. N Engl J Med 1991;325;1621.

Haines DE, DiMarco JP: Current therapy for supraventricular tachycardia. Curr Probl Cardiol 1992;17(7):411. (Extensive review of all supraventricular arrhythmias, emphasizing ablation.)

Scheinman MM (editor): Supraventricular tachycardia. Cardiol Clin 1990;8(3):1. (Mechanisms, diagnosis, and treatment, including ablation techniques.)

Scheinman MM: Catheter ablation. Circulation 1991; 83:1489. (The procedure of choice for many patients.)

5. ATRIAL FIBRILLATION

Atrial fibrillation is the commonest chronic arrhythmia. It occurs in rheumatic heart disease, dilated cardiomyopathy, atrial septal defect, hypertension, mitral valve prolapse, and hypertrophic cardiomyopathy as well as in patients with no apparent cardiac disease. Atrial fibrillation may be the initial presenting sign in thyrotoxicosis, which should always be excluded. Atrial fibrillation often appears paroxysmally before becoming the established rhythm. Pericarditis, chest trauma or surgery, or pulmonary disease (as well as medications such as theophylline and betaDadrenergic agonists) may cause attacks in patients with normal hearts. Alcohol intoxication and alcohol withdrawal—and, in predisposed individuals, even consumption of small amounts of alcohol—may precipitate atrial fibrillation. This syndrome, which is often termed "holiday heart," is usually transient and self-limited. Short-term rate control with digoxin usually suffices as treatment.

Atrial fibrillation is the only common arrhythmia in which the ventricular rate is rapid and the rhythm very irregular. The atrial rate is 400–600/min, but most impulses are blocked at the atrioventricular node. The ventricular response is completely irregular, ranging from 80 to 180/min in the untreated state. Because of the varying stroke volumes resulting from varying periods of diastolic filling, not all ventricular beats produce a palpable peripheral pulse. The difference between the apical rate and the pulse rate is the "pulse deficit"; this deficit is greater when the ventricular rate is high.

The major morbidity from atrial fibrillation (other than precipitation of cardiac failure or ischemia) is arterial emboli from the poorly contracting and often enlarged left atrium. Because atrial fibrillation is associated with a significantly increased risk of stroke and other embolic complications, conversion to normal sinus rhythm is preferred. If conversion is not possible, anticoagulation should be initiated in patients with atrial fibrillation and mitral valve disease. Atrial fibrillation due to other causes is also associated with a higher risk of arterial emboli. The risk is highest in those with prior emboli, congestive heart failure, and hypertension. Anticoagulation with warfarin reduces thromboembolic complications in patients under 75 years of age. Aspirin is also beneficial in patients under 75 years of age, though the results with aspirin in different trials have been mixed. The recently presented preliminary results of the Second Stroke Prevention in Atrial Fibrillation Trial (SPAFD2) suggest that in the absence of valvular disease, heart failure, or systolic blood pressure over 160 mm Hg, aspirin is as effective as warfarin except in women over 75 years of age, where additional data are required. In "lone" atrial fibrillation (when significant heart disease and hypertension are excluded), the incidence of emboli in patients under age 60 is sufficiently low as not to require anticoagulation. In older patients with "lone" atrial fibrillation, anticoagulation is warranted.

Acute Ventricular Rate Control

The initial goal of therapy is to control the ventricular response. This should be accomplished rapidly if the patient manifests ischemia, hypotension, or heart failure but can be accomplished more gradually and on an outpatient basis in those who are tolerating the

rhythm. For inpatients, intravenous verapamil is the agent of choice and will control the ventricular response in 90% of patients. It selectively increases atrioventricular block and slows the ventricular rate. Intravenous diltiazem (0.25 mg/kg over 2 minutes, followed by a second injection of 0.35 mg/kg if needed) has recently become available and is preferable in patients with left ventricular dysfunction. The short-acting beta-blocker esmolol (500 µg/kg intravenously over 1 minute followed by an infusion of 25–200 µg/min) is an alternative approach. Digoxin remains highly effective, though control takes longer to accomplish. For outpatients, digoxin is the usual drug of choice. An initial dose of 0.5 mg can be followed by two or three additional doses of 0.25 mg every 6 hours to a total dose of 1–1.5 mg; a maintenance dose of 0.125–0.5 mg daily can then be started. None of these agents should be given to patients with Wolff-Parkinson-White syndrome conducting antegrade through the accessory pathway (wide ventricular complexes), since conduction may accelerate and the rhythm degenerate into ventricular fibrillation (see below).

Cardioversion

Immediate electrical cardioversion is required for patients with hypotension, heart failure, or angina. Other patients should be controlled medically; however, even when the ventricular rate is controlled medically, a decision must be made about whether to attempt conversion to sinus rhythm. In general, if atrial fibrillation is of recent onset (< 12 months) and left atrial dilation is not severe (left atrial dimension > 45–50 mm by echocardiography), conversion is recommended. Except in young patients without underlying heart disease, there is a risk of embolization following the return of sinus rhythm that persists for 2–3 weeks after cardioversion. Therefore, except in emergent situations, anticoagulation with warfarin should be maintained for 3–4 weeks prior to elective cardioversion. Electrical conversion can also be performed on an ambulatory or in-patient basis. Quinidine, 300 mg every 6 hours, is often given for 24 hours before the procedure to prevent early recurrence. In some patients, conversion will occur. If it does not, synchronized DC shock should be employed, with the initial dosage being 100 J, though more current may be needed. Cardioversion can also be attempted by pharmacologic means. Quinidine is the usual agent. It is started at 200–300 mg every 6 hours and may be increased to 400 mg every 6 hours. Electrocardiographic monitoring is required in patients with heart disease, since ventricular arrhythmias may occur. Care should be taken to avoid digoxin toxicity, since quinidine increases digoxin levels. Atrial fibrillation will recur in 50–70% of patients unless the precipitating cause is removed (eg, thyrotoxicosis, alcoholic excess, or mitral stenosis). Therapy with digoxin may prevent recurrence, but the addition of quinidine or other class Ia agents will more effectively maintain sinus rhythm. However, these drugs may have an adverse effect on patient survival. Flecainide, propafenone, sotalol, and amiodarone are all probably more effective but potentially more toxic.

Treatment of Chronic Atrial Fibrillation

Digoxin is the preferred drug for chronic ventricular rate control in the absence of preexcitation. Higher than normal dosages and serum levels are often required to maintain the resulting ventricular response in the 60–80/min range and to prevent excessive rise with modest exertion. Often a second agent, such as verapamil or a beta-blocker, facilitates ventricular rate control, especially with activity. Sotalol offers another option.

Albers AW et al: Stroke prevention in non-valvular atrial fibrillation. Ann Intern Med 1991;115:727. (Round table discussion reviewing most recent data and recommendations.)

Falk RH: Proarrhythmia in patients treated with atrial fibrillation. Ann Intern Med 1992;117:141. (Decision to use antiarrhythmic drugs must be considered carefully, since mortality rate appears to be increased.)

Gosselink AT et al: LowDdose amiodarone for maintenance of sinus rhythm after cardioversion of atrial fibrillation or flutter. JAMA 1992;267:3289. (Very effective and perhaps the safest antiarrhythmic agent.)

Pritchett EL: Management of atrial fibrillation. N Engl J Med 1992;326:1264. (Covers all the issues.)

The Stroke Prevention on Atrial Fibrillation Investigators: Predictors of thromboembolism in atrial fibrillation. (Two parts.) Ann Intern Med 1992;116:1, 6. (Prior embolism, heart failure, hypertension, left ventricular dysfunction on echo, and left atrial size on echo were predictors of stroke. High and low risk patients could be identified.)

6. ATRIAL FLUTTER

Atrial flutter is less common than fibrillation and usually occurs in patients with COPD, rheumatic or coronary heart disease, congestive heart failure, or atrial septal defect. Ectopic impulse formation occurs at atrial rates of 250–350/min, with transmission of every second, third, or fourth impulse through the atrioventricular node to the ventricles. Atrial flutter is often an unstable rhythm, frequently exhibiting a variable degree of atrioventricular block leading to highly variable ventricular rates. Spontaneous conversion to atrial fibrillation is common. In the acute situation, rate control may be attempted if the patient is stable, but cardioversion is often required. Chronic atrial flutter presents a difficult management problem, and conversion to sinus rhythm is preferable.

Atrial flutter is often not responsive to pharmacologic therapy. Unlike paroxysmal supraventricular tachycardia, atrial flutter does not respond to adenosine, but verapamil may transiently slow the ventricular rate by increasing atrioventricular block, and a combination of digoxin and quinidine may cause the rhythm to revert to sinus rhythm. In contrast, the rhythm is exquisitely sensitive to electrical cardioversion, which can often be accomplished with less than 50 J and is therefore the treatment of choice for acute episodes. Class Ia or Ic agents should be avoided unless an agent that delays atrioventricular conduction (eg, digoxin, verapamil, or a beta-blocker) has been administered, because they can lead to increased atrioventricular conduction. The same approaches discussed under atrial fibrillation are used to prevent further episodes. Because the risk of embolization is lower with atrial flutter than fibrillation, anticoagulation should be reserved for patients with mitral valve disease.

Olshansky B et al: Atrial flutter: Update on the mechanism and treatment. PACE 1992;15:2308.

7. MULTIFOCAL (CHAOTIC) ATRIAL TACHYCARDIA

This is a rhythm characterized by varying P-wave morphology and markedly irregular PP intervals. The rate is usually between 100 and 140/min, and atrioventricular block is unusual. Most patients have severe associated illnesses, especially COPD. Treatment of the underlying condition is the most effective approach; verapamil, 240–480 mg daily in divided doses, is also of value in some patients.

Kastor JA: Multifocal atrial tachycardia. N Engl J Med 1990;322:1713.

8. ATRIOVENTRICULAR JUNCTIONAL RHYTHM

The atrial-nodal junction or the nodal-His bundle junctions may assume pacemaker activity for the heart, usually at a rate of 40–60/min. This may occur in patients with myocarditis, coronary artery disease, and digitalis toxicity as well as in individuals with normal hearts. The rate responds normally to exercise, and the diagnosis is often an incidental finding on electrocardiographic monitoring, but it can be suspected if the jugular venous pulse shows cannon *a* waves. Junctional rhythm is often an escape rhythm because of depressed sinus node function with sinoatrial block or delayed conduction in the atrioventricular node. **Nonparoxysmal junctional tachycardia** results from increased automaticity of the junctional tissues in digitalis toxicity or ischemia and is associated with a narrow QRS complex and a rate usually less than 120–130/min. It is usually considered benign when it occurs in acute myocardial infarction, but the ischemia that induces it may also induce ventricular tachycardia and ventricular fibrillation.

9. SUPRAVENTRICULAR TACHYCARDIAS DUE TO ACCESSORY ATRIOVENTRICULAR PATHWAYS
(Preexcitation Syndromes)

Pathophysiology & Clinical Findings

Accessory pathways between the atria and the ventricle which avoid the conduction delay of the atrioventricular node predispose to reentry tachycardias, such as paroxysmal supraventricular tachycardia and atrial flutter, and to atrial fibrillation. These may be wholly or partly within the node (Mahaim fibers), yielding a short PR interval and normal QRS morphology (**Lown-Ganong-Levine syndrome**). More commonly, they make direct connections between the atria and ventricle through Kent bundles (**Wolff-Parkinson-White syndrome**). This produces a short PR interval but an early delta wave at the onset of the wide, slurred QRS complex owing to early ventricular depolarization of the region adjacent to the pathway. While the morphology and polarity of the delta wave can suggest the location of the bypass tract, mapping by intracardiac recordings is required for precise anatomic localization.

Accessory pathways occur in 0.1–0.3% of the population and facilitate reentry arrhythmias owing to the disparity in refractory periods of the atrioventricular node and accessory pathway. Whether the tachycardia is associated with a narrow or wide QRS complex is determined by whether antegrade conduction is through the node (narrow) or the bypass tract (wide). Many patients with Wolff-Parkinson-White syndrome never conduct antegrade through the bypass tract which is therefore "concealed." Although reentry supraventricular tachycardias involving the AV node are commonest, 20–30% of patients with tachyarrhythmias have atrial fibrillation or flutter. Many have no arrhythmia. A minority of patients conduct antegrade through the accessory pathway, but these individuals may develop very fast rates, especially during atrial fibrillation. Patients with RR intervals less than 220 ms are at highest risk. Digoxin and, to a lesser extent, verapamil and beta-blockers may decrease accessory pathway refractoriness and increase ventricular response and should be avoided in atrial fibrillation with accessory pathways.

Pharmacologic Therapy

Narrow complex reentry rhythms can be managed as discussed for paroxysmal supraventricular tachycardias other than atrial fibrillation or flutter. Adenosine has proved to be very effective; digoxin is best avoided in patients with known Wolff-Parkinson-White syndrome. The class Ia antiarrhythmics, as well as the newer class Ic and class III agents, will increase the refractoriness of the bypass tract and are the drugs of choice for wide-complex tachycardias. If hemodynamic compromise is present, electrical cardioversion is warranted.

Long-term therapy often involves a combination of agents that increase refractoriness in the bypass tract (class Ia or Ic agents) and in the atrioventricular node (verapamil, digoxin, and beta-blockers), provided that atrial fibrillation or flutter with short RR cycle lengths is not present (see above). Amiodarone is effective in refractory cases. Patients who are difficult to manage should undergo electrophysiologic evaluation.

Electrophysiologic Evaluation & Specialized Treatment

Patients with preexcitation syndromes who have episodes of atrial fibrillation or flutter should be tested by induction of atrial fibrillation in the electrophysiologic laboratory, noting duration of the RR cycle; if it is less than 220 ms, a short refractory period is present, and these individuals are at highest risk for sudden death. Patients with frequent tachycardia, especially if refractory to therapy, and those who conduct antegrade through the accessory pathway should be evaluated by electrophysiologic studies. These can determine the location of the accessory pathway and the feasibility of catheter ablation, assess the risk of excessively rapid conduction, and facilitate appropriate drug selection. Success rates for ablation of accessory pathways with radiofrequency catheters exceed 90% in appropriate patients, so this procedure has become the treatment of choice in patients with recurrent arrhythmias or rapid antegrade conduction. Surgical interruption of the pathway is another alternative if catheter ablation fails. Some patients can be managed with antitachycardia pacemakers that deliver properly timed impulses to interrupt the reentry cycle.

Arai A, Kron J: Current management of the Wolff-Parkinson-White syndrome. West J Med 1990;152:383. (Review of diagnosis, pharmacologic management, and interventional procedures.)

Cain ME et al: Diagnosis and localization of accessory pathways. PACE 1992;15:801.

Prystowsky EN et al: Non-pharmacologic treatment of the Wolff-Parkinson-White syndrome and other supraventricular tachycardias. Annu Rev Med 1990;41:239.

Scheinman MM: Catheter ablation. Circulation 1991;83:1489. (The procedure of choice for many patients.)

VENTRICULAR ARRHYTHMIAS

1. VENTRICULAR PREMATURE BEATS (Ventricular Extrasystoles)

Ventricular premature beats are similar to atrial premature beats in mechanism and manifestations but are more common. They are characterized by wide QRS complexes that differ in morphology from the patient's normal beats. They are usually not preceded by a P wave, although retrograde ventriculoatrial conduction may occur. Unless the latter is present, there is a fully compensatory pause. Bigeminy and trigeminy are arrhythmias in which every second or third beat is premature. Exercise generally abolishes premature beats in normal hearts, and the rhythm becomes regular. The patient may or may not sense the irregular beat, usually as a skipped beat.

Ambulatory electrocardiographic monitoring or monitoring during graded exercise reveals more frequent and complex ventricular premature beats than occur in a single routine ECG. Premature beats induced by a low level of exercise may have a worse prognosis than those which occur spontaneously.

Premature beats have questionable significance in the absence of heart disease. Sudden death occurs more frequently (presumably as a result of ventricular fibrillation) when ventricular premature beats occur in the presence of organic heart disease but not in individuals with no known cardiac disease.

If no associated cardiac disease is present and if the ectopic beats are asymptomatic (especially hypo- or hyperkalemia and hypomagnesemia), no specific therapy is indicated. If they are frequent, electrolyte abnormalities, hyperthyroidism, and occult heart disease should be excluded. Pharmacologic treatment is probably indicated only for patients who are symptomatic. The value of ventricular premature beat suppression in asymptomatic patients is unproved even when they occur as couplets or brief runs. Recent data from the Coronary Arrhythmia Suppression Trial (CAST) suggest that at least in the setting of coronary artery disease and with class Ic agents, the risk-benefit ratio of such prophylactic therapy is unfavorable. If the underlying condition is mitral prolapse, hypertrophic cardiomyopathy, left ventricular hypertrophy, or coronary disease—or if the QT interval is prolonged—a trial of a beta-blocker may be worthwhile even though these agents are often unsuccessful. The class Ia and Ib agents (see Table 10–5) are all effective in reducing ventricular premature beats but often cause side effects and may exacerbate arrhythmias in 5–20% of patients. Class Ic agents, though highly effective, should not be used because of their potential for increased mortality rates. The class III agent sotalol may be the safest approach, but side effects are more frequent than with other beta-blockers.

Echt DS et al: Mortality and morbidity in patients receiving encainide, flecainide or placebo: The Cardiac Arrhythmia Suppression Trial. N Engl J Med 1991;324:781. (These agents increased the mortality rate compared to placebo.)

Kennedy HL et al: Long-term follow-up of asymptomatic healthy subjects with frequent and complex ventricular ectopy. N Engl J Med 1985;312:193. (Most do well.)

2. VENTRICULAR TACHYCARDIA

Ventricular tachycardia is defined as three or more consecutive ventricular premature beats. The usual rate is 160–240/min and is moderately regular but less so than atrial tachycardia. Carotid sinus pressure has no effect. The distinction from aberrant conduction of supraventricular tachycardia may be difficult and is discussed above. The usual mechanism is reentry, but abnormally triggered rhythms occur. Ventricular tachycardia is either *nonsustained* (lasting less than 30 seconds) or *sustained.* It may be asymptomatic or associated with syncope or milder symptoms of impaired cerebral perfusion.

Ventricular tachycardia is a frequent complication of acute myocardial infarction and dilated cardiomyopathy but may occur in hypertrophic cardiomyopathy, mitral valve prolapse, myocarditis, and in most other forms of myocardial disease. **Torsade de pointes,** a form of ventricular tachycardia in which QRS morphology varies, may occur spontaneously or after quinidine or any drug that prolongs the QT interval; it has a particularly poor prognosis. In nonacute settings, most patients with ventricular tachycardia have known or easily detectable cardiac disease, and the finding of ventricular tachycardia is an unfavorable prognostic sign.

Treatment

A. Acute Ventricular Tachycardia: The treatment of acute ventricular tachycardia is determined by the degree of hemodynamic compromise and the duration of the arrhythmia. The management of ventricular tachycardia in acute infarction has been discussed. In other patients, if severe hypotension, heart failure, or angina is present, synchronized DC cardioversion with 100–400 J should be performed immediately. If the patient is tolerating the rhythm, lidocaine, 1 mg/kg as an intravenous bolus injection, may terminate it. If the patient is stable and lidocaine is not effective, a trial of intravenous procainamide, 100 mg intravenously slowly every 5 minutes (up to 1000 mg), followed by an infusion of 20–80 μg/kg/min, or bretylium, 5 mg/kg intravenously over 3–5 minutes, repeated after 20 minutes if necessary, followed by an infusion of 1–2 mg/min, may be successful. Ventricular tachycardia can be terminated by ventricular overdrive pacing, and this approach is useful when the rhythm is recurrent.

Amiodarone takes time to achieve a therapeutic level, but intravenous or oral loading with 1000–2000 mg/d may deliver a therapeutic response in 24–72 hours or even earlier in refractory patients.

B. Chronic Recurrent Ventricular Tachycardia: The treatment of recurrent, **nonsustained ventricular tachycardia** (runs of three or more beats lasting less than 30 seconds) not associated with symptoms is controversial. In subjects without heart disease, this rhythm is not clearly associated with a poor prognosis, whereas in patients with organic heart disease, it is a marker for increased mortality rates from the underlying disease and, in some studies, from arrhythmias. Whether antiarrhythmic therapy is beneficial in these patients with nonsustained ventricular tachycardia is unclear, but it is often initiated. In the patient with coronary artery disease post myocardial infarction, the risk for developing symptomatic ventricular tachycardia or sudden death can be stratified with moderate success. The lack of occurrence of late potentials on the noninvasively recorded signal-averaged ECG and the presence of a normal left ventricular ejection fraction usually imply a good prognosis; however, many patients with late potentials and left ventricular dysfunction also will not become symptomatic, and late potentials are of little prognostic value in patients without coronary artery disease. One strategy is to perform ventricular stimulation in the latter group. Patients with inducible sustained ventricular tachycardia should be treated. Given current data, treatment of patients with nonsustained ventricular arrhythmias should be limited to patients who are either symptomatic or have inducible sustained arrhythmias. In these, class Ia agents have traditionally been the initial approach; class Ib agents are less successful, and class Ic agents have a greater risk of inducing proarrhythmias (Table 10–5). Beta-blockers are occasionally effective. More recent data favor the class III agents, sotalol or amiodarone, because proarrhythmia may be less frequent and because the latter agent has improved outcomes in some studies. The efficacy of treatment is assessed by ambulatory electrocardiographic monitoring or repeat stimulation studies. The signal-averaged ECG has not proved useful for monitoring therapy.

Patients with symptomatic or asymptomatic **sustained ventricular tachycardia** require effective suppressive therapy. To develop a therapeutic regimen, the rhythm either must be present spontaneously or be induced by programmed stimulation in the electrophysiology laboratory. The recent ESVEM (Electrophysiology Study Versus Electrocardiography Monitoring) study suggests that either approach is appropriate, but neither is optimal. Various antiarrhythmic drugs can then be given in sequence to determine which agents prevent ventricular tachycardia. Drugs that prevent the electrical induction of ventricular tachycardia in the laboratory or suppress its occurrence during monitoring are more likely to be effective in vivo for long-term therapy; some agents, such as sotalol and amiodarone, may still be effective even if the arrhythmia is not fully prevented in the laboratory. This is the case especially with amiodarone, which has emerged as a very effective though toxic agent for this select group of patients. The potential of all antiarrhythmia drugs to exacerbate ventricular arrhythmias in some patients should be kept in mind in initiating and monitoring therapy.

Patients with sustained ventricular tachycardia who do not respond to or tolerate antiarrhythmic medications are candidates for an automatic implantable cardiac defibrillator (AICD), which can be programmed to sense tachycardias above a predetermined rate and deliver a shock after a predetermined latent period (sufficient to allow charging and for many patients to lose consciousness). Because of the risks and poor tolerability of antiarrhythmic therapy, many experts are using these devices earlier in patients with symptomatic ventricular tachycardia, but the substantial morbidity and mortality rates (about 5%), their high cost (over $20,000), and the associated psychologic disability in many patients should be kept in mind. Another approach in specialized centers is to determine the site of origin of the ventricular tachycardia by mapping studies in the electrophysiology laboratory. Some foci (especially in the right ventricle) are amenable to radiofrequency catheter ablation. Other foci can be surgically resected or isolated.

Burkart F et al: Effect of antiarrhythmia therapy on mortality in survivors of myocardial infarction with asymptomatic complex ventricular arrhythmias. J Am Coll Cardiol 1990;16:1711. (Amiodarone reduced mortality and arrhythmia events—the first study showing a beneficial effect of antiarrhythmia therapy postinfarction.)

Greenspan AJ, Waxman HL: Contemporary management of ventricular arrhythmias. Cardiovasc Clin 1992;22:1. (Entire volume deals with this issue.)

Josephson ME (editor): *Sudden Cardiac Death.* Blackwell, 1993.

Weiss JN et al: Ventricular arrhythmias in ischemic heart disease. Ann Intern Med 1991;114:784.

Wellens HJ: The approach to nonsustained ventricular tachycardia after a myocardial infarction. Circulation 1990;82:633. (Common-sense approach.)

3. VENTRICULAR FIBRILLATION

The acute treatment of ventricular fibrillation is discussed under complications of myocardial infarction, and the chronic management of survivors is discussed under survivors of sudden death.

4. ACCELERATED IDIOVENTRICULAR RHYTHM

Accelerated idioventricular rhythm is a relatively regular wide complex rhythm with a rate of 60–120/min, usually with a gradual onset. Because the rate is often similar to the sinus rate, fusion beats and alternating rhythms are common. Two mechanisms have been invoked: (1) an escape rhythm due to suppression of higher pacemakers resulting from sinoatrial and atrioventricular block or from depressed sinus node function; and (2) slow ventricular tachycardia due to increased automaticity or, less frequently, reentry. It occurs commonly in acute infarction and following reperfusion after thrombolytic drugs. The incidence of associated ventricular fibrillation is much less than that of ventricular tachycardia with a rapid rate, and treatment is not indicated unless there is hemodynamic compromise or more serious arrhythmias. This rhythm also is common in digitalis toxicity.

Accelerated idioventricular rhythm must be distinguished from the idioventricular or junctional rhythm with rates less than 40–45/min that occurs in the presence of complete atrioventricular block. Atrioventricular dissociation—where ventricular rate exceeds sinus—but not atrioventricular block occurs in most cases of accelerated idioventricular rhythm.

5. LONG QT SYNDROME

Idiopathic long QT syndrome is an uncommon disease that was first described in deaf siblings. It is characterized by recurrent syncope, a long QT interval (usually 0.5–0.7 s), documented ventricular arrhythmias, and sudden death. The sympathetic nervous system (especially the left stellate ganglion) may be important in pathogenesis.

Beta-blockers are the most effective therapy for "congenital" long QT syndrome, though phenytoin and the class Ib agents have also been beneficial. Agents that prolong the QT (classes Ia, Ic, and III) are contraindicated. Refractory acute arrhythmic episodes may be treated by local anesthetic block of the left stellate ganglion, and recurrent episodes can be treated by resection of this ganglion as well as of the first three to five thoracic ganglia.

Acquired long QT interval secondary to use of antiarrhythmic agents or antidepressant drugs, electrolyte abnormalities, myocardial ischemia, or significant bradycardia may result in ventricular tachycardia (torsade de pointes, ie, twisting about the baseline into varying QRS morphology). The role of a prolonged QT interval is difficult to evaluate because classes Ia, Ic, and III antiarrhythmic agents increase the QT interval and yet are effective in treating the ventricular tachyarrhythmias; it may be the reason that these drugs paradoxically cause ventricular tachycardia in some patients. Acquired QT interval prolongation requires further study, but prudence speaks against continuing therapy that prolongs the QT interval beyond 500 ms.

The management of **torsade de pointes** differs from that of other forms of ventricular tachycardia. Class I, Ic, or III antiarrhythmics, which prolong the QT interval, should be avoided—or withdrawn immediately if being used. Intravenous beta-blockers may be effective, especially in the congenital form; intravenous magnesium has also worked. An effective approach is temporary ventricular or atrial pacing, which can both break and prevent the rhythm.

Jackman WM et al: The long QT syndromes: A critical review, new clinical observations, and a unifying hypothesis. Prog Cardiovasc Dis 1988;31:115.
Stratmann HG, Kennedy HL: Torsades de pointes associated with drugs and toxins: Recognition and management. Am Heart J 1987;113:1470.

CONDUCTION DISTURBANCES

Abnormalities of conduction can occur between the sinus node and atrium, within the atrioventricular node, and in the intraventricular conduction pathways.

SINOATRIAL EXIT BLOCK

Sinoatrial exit block produces a pause of duration equal to a multiple of the underlying PP interval. Often there is progressive shortening of the PP interval prior to the pause (sinoatrial Wenckebach). This disturbance may be due to excessive vagal tone, ischemia, fibrosis or calcification of the conduction fibers, or drug effect (especially digitalis, calcium channel blockers, antiarrhythmic agents, and sympatholytic medications). Sinoatrial exit block is usually asymptomatic, though prolonged pauses equivalent to sinus arrest rarely occur as part of the sick sinus syndrome and are treated as outlined below.

SICK SINUS SYNDROME

This imprecise diagnosis is applied to patients with sinus arrest, sinoatrial exit block, or persistent sinus bradycardia. These rhythms are often caused or exacerbated by drug therapy (digitalis, calcium channel blockers, beta-blockers, sympatholytic agents, antiarrhythmics), and agents that may be responsible should be withdrawn prior to making the diagnosis.

Another presentation is of recurrent supraventricular tachycardias (paroxysmal reentry tachycardias, atrial flutter, and atrial fibrillation), associated with bradyarrhythmias ("tachy-brady syndrome"). The long pauses that often follow the termination of tachycardia cause the associated symptoms.

The electrocardiographic features of sick sinus syndrome are noted mostly in elderly patients. The pathologic changes are usually nonspecific, characterized by patchy fibrosis of the sinus node and cardiac conduction system. Cardiac amyloidosis also preferentially affects these structures. Sick sinus syndrome may also be caused by other conditions, including sarcoidosis, amyloidosis, Chagas' disease, and various cardiomyopathies. Coronary disease is an uncommon cause.

Most patients with electrocardiographic evidence of sick sinus syndrome are asymptomatic, but rare individuals may experience syncope, dizziness, confusion, palpitations, heart failure, or angina. Because—particularly in older patients—these symptoms are either nonspecific or are due to other causes, it is essential that they be demonstrated to coincide with arrhythmias. This may require prolonged ambulatory monitoring or the use of an event recorder. Pharmacologic therapy for sick sinus syndrome has been difficult, but recent studies have indicated that oral theophylline may be effective, especially when sinus bradycardia is the major manifestation. Most symptomatic patients will require permanent pacing. Since atrioventricular node disease is often also present, ventricular or dual chamber pacing is preferred unless electrophysiologic studies indicate normal atrioventricular conduction. Treatment of associated tachyarrhythmias is often difficult without first instituting pacing, since digoxin and other antiarrhythmic agents may exacerbate the bradycardia. Unfortunately, symptomatic relief following pacing has not been consistent, largely because of inadequate documentation of the etiologic role of bradyarrhythmias in producing the symptom. Furthermore, many of these patients may have associated ventricular arrhythmias that may require treatment; however, carefully selected patients may become asymptomatic with permanent pacing alone.

Alboni P et al: Clinical effects of oral theophylline in sick sinus syndrome. Am Heart J 1991;122:1361. (Favorable report.)

Rodriguez RD, Schocken DD: Update on sick sinus syndrome, a cardiac disorder of aging. Geriatrics 1990; 45:26.

Sneddon JF, Camm AJ: Sinus node disease: Current concepts in diagnosis and therapy. Drugs 1992;44:728.

ATRIOVENTRICULAR BLOCK

Atrioventricular block is categorized as first-degree (PR interval > 0.21 s with all atrial impulses conducted), second-degree (intermittent blocked beats), or third-degree (complete heart block, in which no supraventricular impulses are conducted to the ventricles).

Second-degree block is subclassified. In **Mobitz type I (Wenckebach)** atrioventricular block, the atrioventricular conduction time (PR interval) progressively lengthens, with the RR interval shortening, before the blocked beat; this phenomenon is almost always due to abnormal conduction within the atrioventricular node. **Mobitz type II** atrioventricular block is abrupt and is not preceded by a lengthening atrioventricular conduction time; it is usually due to block within the His bundle system. The classification as Mobitz type I or Mobitz type II is only partially reliable, because patients may appear to have both types on the surface ECG, and one cannot predict the site of origin of the 2:1 atrioventricular block from the ECG. The width of the QRS complexes assists in determining whether the block is nodal or infranodal. When they are narrow, the block is usually nodal; when they are wide, the block is usually infranodal. His bundle readings may be necessary for accurate localization. Management of atrioventricular block in acute myocardial infarction has already been discussed. This section deals with patients in the nonacute setting.

First-degree and **Mobitz type I block** may occur in normal individuals with heightened vagal tone. They may also occur as a drug effect (especially digitalis, calcium channel blockers, beta-blockers, or other sympatholytic agents), often superimposed on organic disease. These disturbances also occur transiently or chronically due to ischemia, infarction, inflammatory processes, fibrosis, calcification, or infiltration. The prognosis is usually good, since reliable alternative pacemakers arise from the atrioventricular junction below the level of block if higher degrees of block occur.

Mobitz type II block is almost always due to organic disease involving the infranodal conduction system. In the event of progression to complete heart block, alternative pacemakers are not reliable. Thus, prophylactic ventricular pacing is required.

Complete (third-degree) heart block is a more advanced form of block often due to a lesion distal to the His bundle and associated with bilateral bundle branch block. The QRS is wide and the ventricular rate is slower, usually less than 50/min. Transmission of atrial impulses through the atrioventricular node is completely blocked, and a ventricular pacemaker maintains a slow, regular ventricular rate, usually less than 45/min. Exercise does not increase the rate. The first heart sound varies in intensity; wide pulse pressure, a changing systolic blood pressure level, and cannon venous pulsations in the neck are also present. Patients may be asymptomatic or may complain of weakness or dyspnea if the rate is less than 35/min; symptoms may occur at higher rates if the left ventricle cannot increase its stroke output. During periods of transition from partial to complete heart block, some patients have ventricular asystole that lasts several seconds to minutes. Syncope occurs abruptly.

Patients with episodic or chronic infranodal complete heart block require permanent pacing, and temporary pacing is indicated if implantation is delayed.

Shen WK, Wharton JM, Strauss HC: Mechanisms of bradyarrhythmias and blocks. Hosp Pract (July 15) 1988;23:93. (Practical review including sinus node diseases.)

ATRIOVENTRICULAR DISSOCIATION

When a ventricular pacemaker is firing at a rate faster than or close to the sinus rate (accelerated idioventricular rhythm, ventricular premature beats, or ventricular tachycardia), atrial impulses arriving at the atrioventricular node when it is refractory may not be conducted. This phenomenon is atrioventricular dissociation but does not necessarily indicate atrioventricular block. No treatment is required aside from management of the causative arrhythmia.

INTRAVENTRICULAR CONDUCTION DEFECTS

Intraventricular conduction defects, including bundle branch block, are common in individuals with otherwise normal hearts and in many disease processes, including ischemic heart disease, inflammatory disease, infiltrative disease, cardiomyopathy, and postcardiotomy. Below the atrioventricular node and bundle of His, the conduction system trifurcates into a right bundle and anterior and posterior fascicles of the left bundle. Conduction block in each of these fascicles can be recognized on the surface ECG. Although such conduction abnormalities are often seen in normal hearts, they are more commonly due to organic heart disease—either an isolated process of fibrosis and calcification (Lev's or Lenegre's disease) or more generalized myocardial disease. Bifascicular block is present when two of these— right bundle, left anterior and posterior hemibundle—are involved. Trifascicular block is defined as right bundle branch block with alternating left hemiblock, alternating right and left bundle branch block, or bifascicular block with documented prolonged infranodal conduction (long HV interval).

The prognosis of intraventricular block is generally that of the underlying myocardial process. Even in bifascicular block, the incidence of occult complete heart block or progression to it is low, and pacing is not usually warranted. In patients with symptoms (eg, syncope) consistent with heart block and intraventricular block, pacing should be reserved for those with documented concomitant complete heart block on monitoring or those with a very prolonged HV interval (> 90 ms) with no other cause for symptoms. Even in the latter group, prophylactic pacing has not improved the prognosis significantly, probably because of the high incidence of ventricular arrhythmias in the same population.

Kreger BE et al: Prevalence of intra-ventricular block in the general population: The Framingham Study. Am Heart J 1989;117:903. (Common in older patients. Prognosis depends chiefly on that of associated disease.)

Scheinman MM et al: Electrophysiologic studies in patients with bundle branch block. PACE 1983;6:1157. (Follow-up study with suggested guidelines on when to measure HV and when to pace.)

PERMANENT PACING

The indications for permanent pacing have been discussed: symptomatic bradyarrhythmias, asymptomatic Mobitz II AV block, or complete heart block. The versatility of pacemaker generator units has increased markedly, and dual-chamber multiple programmable units being implanted with increasing frequency. A standardized nomenclature for pacemaker generators is employed, usually consisting of four letters. The first letter refers to the chamber which is simulated (A = atrium, V = ventricle, D = dual for both). The second letter refers to the chamber where sensing occurs (also A, V or D). The third position refers to the sensory mode (I = inhibition by a sensed impulse, T = triggering by a sensed impulse, D = dual modes of response). The fourth letter refers to the programmability or rate modulation capacity (usually P for programming for two functions, M for programming more than two, and R for rate modulation).

Conceptually, a pacemaker that senses and paces in both chambers is the most physiologic approach to pacing patients who remain in sinus rhythm. However, because of the substantially increased cost and complexity of dual-chamber pacing and rate-modulability and the shorter projected battery life, their use should be limited to patients in whom atrial contraction produces a substantial increment in stroke volume and to those in whom sensing the atrial rate to provide rate-responsive ventricular pacing is useful. Dual-chamber pacing is most useful for individuals with left ventricular systolic or—perhaps more importantly—diastolic dysfunction and for physically active individuals. In patients with single-chamber pacemakers, the lack of an atrial kick may lead to the so-called pacemaker syndrome, in which the patient experiences signs of low cardiac output while upright. Pacers are also available that can increase their rate in response to motion or respiratory rate when the atrial rate is not an indication of optimal heart rate. However, patients with intermittent or potential bradyarrhythmias or conduction disturbances in whom pacing is primarily prophylactic should undergo ventricular pacing. Follow-up after pacemaker implantation, usually by telephonic monitoring, is essential. All pulse generators and lead systems have an early failure rate that is now below 5% as well as a finite life expectancy varying from 4 to 10 years.

ACC/AHA Task Force Report: Guidelines for implantation of cardiac pacemakers and antiarrhythmia devices. J Am Coll Cardiol 1991;18:1. (Consensus statement on indications.)

Baig MW, Perrins EJ: The hemodynamics of cardiac pacing: Clinical and physiological aspects. Prog Cardiovasc Dis 1991;33:283. (When and how atrial contraction is important.)

Furman S: Rate-modulated pacing. Circulation 1990; 82:1081. (State of the art technology, but do many patients really need it?)

Furman S, Gross J: Dual-chamber pacing and pacemakers. Curr Probl Cardiol 1990;15(3):119. (Indications and technology.)

Griffin JC (editor): Cardiac pacing. Cardiol Clin 1992; 10(4):S61.

EVALUATION OF SYNCOPE & SURVIVORS OF SUDDEN DEATH

SYNCOPE

Syncope—transient loss of consciousness due to inadequate cerebral blood flow—is a common clinical problem, especially in the elderly. More common still are episodes of dizziness, feeling "faint" (ie, a perception that loss of consciousness is imminent), seizures, and transient neurologic deficits associated with impaired consciousness. Thus, before a diagnosis of syncope can be established, epileptic seizures, transient ischemic attacks, and episodes of vertigo, hypoglycemia, and anxiety attacks (often accompanied by hyperventilation) must be excluded. Syncope can be psychogenic in origin, so a psychologic evaluation is an important part of the assessment of recurrent syncope.

Syncope usually *does not have* the following features: premonitory aura, preceding autonomic signs and symptoms characteristic of hypoglycemia, vertigo, hyperventilation, gradual onset, convulsive movements and incontinence (though these may occur inconsistently), confusion postrecovery, and residual neurologic deficits.

Syncope is more likely to occur in patients with known heart disease, older men, and young women (who are prone to vasovagal episodes). Syncopal episodes are characteristically abrupt in onset (so much so that they frequently cause traumatic injuries), transient (lasting for seconds to a few minutes), and followed by prompt recovery of full consciousness.

Vasomotor syncope may be due to excessive vagal tone or impaired reflex control of the peripheral circulation. The most frequent type of vasodepressor syncope is vasovagal hypotension or the "common faint," which is often initiated by stressful, painful, or claustrophobic experience, especially in young women. Premonitory symptoms, such as nausea, diaphoresis, tachycardia, and loss of color, are usual. Episodes can be aborted by lying down or removing the inciting stimulus. Enhanced vagal tone with resulting hypotension is the cause of syncope in carotid sinus hypersensitivity and postmicturition syncope; vagal-induced sinus bradycardia, sinus arrest, and atrioventricular block are common accompaniments and may themselves be the cause of syncope. Carotid sinus massage under carefully monitored conditions or tilt-table testing may be diagnostic (see above under Autonomic Testing). Treatment consists largely of counseling patients to avoid predisposing situations. Paradoxically, beta-blockers may be helpful in patients with altered autonomic function uncovered by head-up tilt testing. Permanent pacing may benefit patients with documented bradycardiac responses.

Orthostatic (postural) hypotension is another common cause of vasomotor syncope, especially in the elderly, in diabetics or other patients with autonomic neuropathy, in patients with blood loss or hypovolemia, and in patients taking vasodilators, diuretics, and adrenergic blocking drugs. In addition, a syndrome of chronic idiopathic orthostatic hypotension exists primarily in older men. In most of these conditions, the normal vasoconstrictive response to assuming upright posture, which compensates for the abrupt decrease in venous return, is impaired. A greater than normal decline (20 mm Hg) in blood pressure immediately upon arising from the supine to the standing position is observed, with or without tachycardia depending on the status of autonomic (baroreceptor) function. Studying patients with a tilt table can establish the diagnosis with more certainty. Autonomic function can be assessed by observing blood pressure and heart rate responses to Valsalva's maneuver and by tilt testing. In older patients, vasoconstrictor abnormalities and autonomic insufficiency are perhaps the most common causes of syncope. Thus, tilt testing should be employed before proceeding to invasive studies unless clinical and ambulatory electrocardiographic evaluation suggests a cardiac abnormality.

Cardiogenic syncope can occur on a mechanical or arrhythmic basis. Mechanical problems that can cause syncope include aortic stenosis (where syncope may occur from autonomic reflex abnormalities or ventricular tachycardia), pulmonary stenosis, hypertrophic obstructive cardiomyopathy, congenital lesions associated with pulmonary hypertension or right-to-left shunting, and left atrial myxoma obstructing the mitral valve. Episodes are commonly exertional or postexertional. More commonly, cardiac syncope is due to disorders of automaticity (sick sinus syndrome), conduction disorders (atrioventricular block), or tachyarrhythmias (especially ventricular tachycardia and supraventricular tachycardia with rapid ventricular rate).

The evaluation for syncope depends heavily on a careful history and physical examination (especially orthostatic blood pressure evaluation, examination of carotid and other arteries, cardiac examination, and, if appropriate, carotid sinus massage). The resting ECG may reveal arrhythmias, evidence of accessory pathways, prolonged QT interval, and other signs of heart disease (such as infarction or hypertrophy). If the history is consistent with syncope, ambulatory electrocardiographic monitoring is essential. This may need to be repeated several times, since yields increase with longer periods of monitoring, at least up to 3 days. Event recorder and transtelephone electrocardiographic monitoring may be helpful in patients with intermittent presyncopal episodes. Electrophysiologic studies to assess sinus node function and atrioventricular conduction and to induce supraventricular or ventricular tachycardia are indicated in patients with recurrent episodes and nondiagnostic ambulatory ECGs. They reveal an arrhythmic cause in 20–50% of patients, depending on the study criteria, and are most often diagnostic when the patient has had multiple episodes and has identifiable cardiac abnormalities.

Kapoor WN: Evaluation and management of the patient with syncope. JAMA 1992;268:2553.

Linzer M et al: Psychiatric syncope: A new look at an old disease. Psychosomatics 1990;31:181. (An important cause of recurrent syncope.)

Mader SL: Orthostatic hypotension. Med Clin North Am 1989;73:1337. (A common cause of syncope in the elderly, often exacerbated by medications.)

Schaal ST et al: Syncope. Curr Probl Cardiol 1992; 17(4):205.

Strasberg B: Carotid sinus hypersensitivity and the carotid sinus syndrome. Prog Cardiovasc Dis 1989;31:379.

SURVIVORS OF SUDDEN DEATH

Sudden cardiac death is defined as unexpected nontraumatic death in clinically well or stable patients who die within 1 hour after onset of symptoms. The causative rhythm in most cases is ventricular fibrillation, which is usually preceded by ventricular tachycardia; complete heart block and sinus node arrest may also cause sudden death. A disproportionate number of sudden deaths occur in the early morning hours. Over 75% of victims of sudden cardiac death have had severe coronary artery disease. Many have old infarctions. Sudden death may be the initial manifestation of coronary disease in up to 20% of patients and accounts for approximately 50% of deaths from coronary disease. When ventricular fibrillation occurs in the initial 24 hours after infarction, long-term management is no different from that of other patients with acute infarction. Other conditions that predispose to sudden death include severe left ventricular hypertrophy, hypertrophic cardiomyopathy, congestive cardiomyopathy, aortic stenosis, pulmonary stenosis, primary pulmonary hypertension, cyanotic congenital heart disease, atrial myxoma, mitral valve prolapse, hypoxia, electrolyte abnormalities, prolonged QT interval syndrome, and conduction system disease. Recent studies suggest that detection of late potentials (after the QRS complex) on a signal-averaged surface ECG in patients with prior myocardial infarction may identify a group of patients at risk of ventricular arrhythmias and sudden death.

Unless ventricular fibrillation occurred early postmyocardial infarction or an unusual correctable process was present (such as an electrolyte abnormality, drug toxicity, or aortic stenosis), these patients should undergo intensive investigation. Exercise testing or coronary arteriography should be performed to exclude coronary disease as the underlying cause. Conduction disturbances should be managed as described above. If serious prodromal ventricular arrhythmias such as sustained or nonsustained ventricular tachycardia or frequent ventricular premature beats are found by ambulatory electrocardiographic monitoring, their elimination by therapy may prevent further episodes. Ventricular stimulation studies are also indicated, especially if monitoring does not reveal significant arrhythmias. If inducibility cannot be prevented by the usual agents or if monitored arrhythmias are not obliterated, amiodarone and beta-blockers may still be effective. The automatic implantable difibrillator is an alternative approach, particularly in patients in whom a sustained arrhythmia cannot be induced or suppressed.

Patients who have recurrent sudden death, syncope due to ventricular arrhythmias, or documented sustained ventricular tachycardia despite these measures should be referred for ablation of foci or implantation of an automatic defibrillator.

Recommendations for Resumption of Driving

An important management problem in patients who have experienced syncope, symptomatic ventricular tachycardia, or aborted sudden death is to provide recommendations concerning automobile driving. According to a survey published in 1991, only eight states had specific laws dealing with this issue, whereas 42 had laws restricting driving in patients with seizure disorders. There are not adequate data to support driving restrictions in patients who have not experienced symptomatic arrhythmias, though patients with frequent nonsustained ventricular tachycardia, associated heart disease, and significant left ventricular dysfunction are at high enough risk to warrant cautioning. Patients with syncope or aborted sudden death thought to have been due to temporary factors (acute myocardial infarction, bradyarrhythmias subsequently treated with permanent pacing, drug effect, electrolyte imbalance) should be permitted to resume driving after recovery and an appropriate period of observation (usually 1 month). Other patients with symptomatic ventricular tachycardia or aborted sudden death, whether treated pharmacologically, with antitachycardia devices, or with ablation therapy, should not drive for a least 6 months. Longer restrictions are warranted in many such patients if spontaneous arrhythmias persist. The physician should comply with local regulations and consult local authorities concerning individual cases.

Akhtar M et al: Sudden cardiac death: Management of high-risk patients. Ann Intern Med 1991;114:499.
Akhtar M, Myenburg RJ: Current perspectives on the problem of sudden cardiac death. Circulation 1992;85(Suppl I):1. (Entire volume covering mechanisms, epidemiology, specific populations such as athletes and children, and treatment.)
Amsterdam EH: Sudden death during exercise. Cardiology 1990;77:411. (Sudden death in young people, athletes, and older patients.)
Greenspan AJ, Waxman HL (editors): Contemporary management of ventricular arrhythmias. Cardiovasc Clin 1992;22(1). (Several articles deal with management and prevention of lethal ventricular arrhythmias.)
Strizkberger SA et al: When should patients with lethal ventricular arrhythmias resume driving? Ann Intern Med 1991;115:560.

CARDIAC FAILURE

Essentials of Diagnosis

- Left ventricular failure: Exertional dyspnea, cough, fatigue, orthopnea, paroxysmal nocturnal dyspnea, cardiac enlargement, rales, gallop rhythm, and pulmonary venous congestion.
- Right ventricular failure: Elevated venous pressure, hepatomegaly, dependent edema.
- Both: Combination of above.
- Diagnosis should be confirmed by noninvasive or hemodynamic measurements.

General Considerations

Systolic function of the heart is governed by four major determinants: the contractile state of the myocardium, the preload of the ventricle (the end-diastolic volume and the resultant fiber length of the ventricles prior to onset of the contraction), the afterload applied to the ventricles (the impedance to left ventricular ejection), and the heart rate.

Cardiac function may be inadequate as a result of alterations in any of these determinants. In most instances, the primary derangement is depression of myocardial contractility caused either by loss of functional muscle (due to myocardial infarction, etc) or by processes diffusely affecting the myocardium. However, the heart may fail as a pump because preload is excessively elevated, such as in valvular regurgitation, or when afterload is excessive, such as in aortic stenosis or in severe hypertension. Pump function may also be inadequate when the heart rate is too slow or too rapid. While the normal heart can tolerate wide variations in preload, afterload, and heart rate, the diseased heart often has limited reserve for such alterations. Finally, cardiac pump function may be supranormal but nonetheless inadequate when metabolic demands or requirements for blood flow are excessive. This situation is termed **high-output heart failure** and, though uncommon, tends to be specifically treatable. Causes of high output include thyrotoxicosis, beriberi, severe anemia, arteriovenous shunting, and Paget's disease of bone.

Manifestations of cardiac failure can also occur as a result of isolated or predominant **diastolic dysfunction** of the heart. In these cases, filling of the left or right ventricle is impaired because the chamber is noncompliant ("stiff") due to excessive hypertrophy or changes in composition of the myocardium. Even though contractility may be preserved, diastolic pressures are elevated and cardiac output may be reduced.

Pathophysiology

When the heart fails, a number of adaptations occur both in the heart and systemically. If the stroke volume of either ventricle is reduced by depressed contractility or excessive afterload, end-diastolic volume and pressure in that chamber will rise. This increases end-diastolic myocardial fiber length, resulting in a greater systolic shortening (Starling's law of the heart). If the condition is chronic, ventricular dilation will occur. While this may restore resting cardiac output, the resulting chronic elevation of diastolic pressures will be transmitted to the atria and to the pulmonary and systemic venous circulation. Ultimately, increased capillary pressure may lead to transudation of fluid with resulting pulmonary or systemic edema. Reduced cardiac output, particularly if associated with reduced arterial pressure or perfusion of the kidneys, will also activate several neural and humoral systems. Increased activity of the sympathetic nervous system will stimulate myocardial contractility, heart rate, and venous tone; the latter change results in a rise in the effective central blood volume, which serves to further elevate preload. Though these adaptations are designed to increase cardiac output, they may themselves be deleterious. Thus, tachycardia and increased contractility may precipitate ischemia in patients with underlying coronary artery disease, and the rise in preload may worsen pulmonary congestion. Sympathetic nervous system activation also increases peripheral vascular resistance; this adaptation is designed to maintain perfusion to vital organs, but when it is excessive it may itself reduce renal and other tissue blood flow. Peripheral vascular resistance is also a major determinant of left ventricular afterload, so that excessive sympathetic activity may further depress cardiac function.

One of the more important effects of lower cardiac output is reduction of renal blood flow and glomerular filtration rate, which leads to sodium and fluid retention. The renin-angiotensin-aldosterone system is also activated, leading to further increases in peripheral vascular resistance and left ventricular afterload as well as sodium and fluid retention. Heart failure is associated with increased circulating levels of arginine vasopressin, which also serves as a vasoconstrictor and inhibitor of water excretion. While release of atrial natriuretic peptide is increased in heart failure owing to the elevated atrial pressures, there is evidence of resistance to its natriuretic and vasodilating effects.

Hemodynamic Alterations

Myocardial failure is characterized by two hemodynamic derangements, and the clinical presentation is determined by their severity. The first is reduction in cardiac output, ie, the ability to increase cardiac output in response to increased demands imposed by exercise or even ordinary activity (cardiac reserve). The second abnormality, elevation of ventricular diastolic pressures, is primarily a result of the compensatory processes.

Heart failure may be right-sided or left-sided. Patients with the picture of **left heart failure** have symptoms of low cardiac output and elevated pulmonary venous pressure; dyspnea is the predominant feature. Signs of fluid retention predominate in **right heart failure,** with the patient exhibiting edema, hepatic congestion, and, on occasion, ascites. Most patients exhibit signs or symptoms of both right- and left-sided failure, and left ventricular dysfunction is the primary cause of right ventricular failure. Surprisingly, some individuals with severe left ventricular dysfunction will display few signs of left heart failure and appear to have isolated right heart failure. Indeed, they may be clinically indistinguishable from patients with cor pulmonale, who have right heart failure secondary to pulmonary disease.

Although this section concerns cardiac failure due to systolic left ventricular dysfunction, patients with diastolic dysfunction experience many of the same symptoms and may be difficult to distinguish clinically. Diastolic pressures are elevated even though diastolic volumes are normal or small. These pressures are transmitted to the pulmonary and systemic venous systems, resulting in dyspnea and edema. The most frequent cause of diastolic cardiac dysfunction is left ventricular hypertrophy, commonly resulting from hypertension, but conditions such as hypertrophic or restrictive cardiomyopathy, diabetes, and pericardial disease can produce the same clinical picture. While diuretics are often useful in these patients, the other therapies discussed in this section (digitalis, vasodilators, inotropic agents) may be inappropriate.

Causes of Cardiac Failure

The syndrome of cardiac failure can be produced by many diseases. In developed countries, coronary artery disease with resulting myocardial infarction and loss of functioning myocardium (ischemic cardiomyopathy) is the commonest cause. A number of processes may present with dilated or congestive cardiomyopathy, which is characterized by left ventricular or biventricular dilation and generalized systolic dysfunction. These are discussed elsewhere in this chapter, but the most common are alcoholic cardiomyopathy, viral myocarditis (including infections by HIV), and dilated cardiomyopathies with no obvious underlying cause (idiopathic cardiomyopathy). Rare causes of dilated cardiomyopathy include infiltrative diseases (hemochromatosis, sarcoidosis, amyloidosis, etc), other infectious agents, metabolic disorders, cardiotoxins, and drug toxicity.

Systemic hypertension remains an important cause of congestive heart failure and, even more commonly in the USA, an exacerbating factor in patients with cardiac dysfunction due to other causes. Valvular heart disease has become a less frequent cause of heart failure with the declining incidence and severity of rheumatic fever. However, aortic stenosis remains a common and reversible cause. Patients with chronic volume overload of the left ventricle, such as mitral or aortic regurgitation, may develop progressive myocardial dysfunction and have a picture of cardiomyopathy even after the underlying condition is corrected. This form of congestive heart failure is preventable by early diagnosis and treatment of the valvular lesion.

Hosenpud JD, Greenberg BH (editors): *Congestive Heart Failure: Pathophysiology of Differential Diagnosis and Comprehensive Approach to Therapy.* Springer-Verlag, 1993.

Packer M: Role of the sympathetic nervous system in heart failure: Basic mechanisms and clinical directions. Circulation 1990;82(2 Suppl I):I–1.

Shah PM, Pai RG: Diastolic heart failure. Curr Probl Cardiol 1992;17(12):781.

Weber KT (editor): Heart failure: Current concepts and management. Cardiol Clin 1989;7(1):1.

Woeber KA: Thyrotoxicosis and the heart. N Engl J Med 1992;327:94. (Thyroid disease should be excluded as a reversible cause of heart failure.)

Clinical Findings

A. Symptoms: The symptoms of cardiac failure have been discussed in part in earlier sections. The most common complaint is shortness of breath often chiefly exertional dyspnea at first and progressing to orthopnea, paroxysmal nocturnal dyspnea, and rest dyspnea. A more subtle and often overlooked symptom of heart failure is a chronic nonproductive cough, which is often worse in the recumbent position. Nocturia due to excretion of fluid retained during the day and increased renal perfusion in the recumbent position is a common nonspecific symptom of heart failure. Patients with heart failure also complain of fatigue and exercise intolerance. These symptoms correlate poorly with the degree of cardiac dysfunction and result in part from changes in peripheral blood flow and blood flow to skeletal muscle which are part of the syndrome of heart failure. Patients with right heart failure may experience right upper quadrant pain due to passive congestion of the liver, loss of appetite and nausea due to edema of the gut or impaired gastrointestinal perfusion, and peripheral edema.

Cardiac failure may present acutely in a previously asymptomatic patient. Causes include myocardial infarction, myocarditis, and acute valvular regurgitation due to endocarditis or other conditions. These patients usually present with pulmonary edema. The management of acute heart failure has been discussed under myocardial infarction and centers around initial stabilization with diuretics and parenteral vasodilators or inotropic agents.

Patients may also present with acute exacerbations of chronic, stable heart failure. Exacerbations are usually caused by alterations in therapy (or patient noncompliance), excessive salt and fluid intake, arrhythmias, excessive activity, pulmonary emboli, intercurrent infection, or progression of the underlying disease.

B. Signs: Many patients with heart failure, including some with severe symptoms, appear comfortable at rest. Others will be dyspneic during conversation or minor activity, and those with longstanding severe heart failure may appear cachectic or cyanotic. The vital signs may be normal, but tachycardia, hypotension, and reduced pulse pressure may be present. Patients often show signs of increased sympathetic nervous system activity, including cold extremities and diaphoresis. Important peripheral signs of heart failure can be detected by examination of the neck, the lungs, the abdomen, and the extremities. Right atrial pressure may be estimated through the height of the pulsations in the jugular venous system. In addition to the height of the venous pressure, abnormal pulsations such as regurgitant *v* waves

should be sought. Examination of the carotid pulse allows estimation of pulse pressure as well as detection of aortic stenosis. The thyroid examination is important, since occult hyperthyroidism and hypothyroidism are readily treatable causes of heart failure. In the lungs, crackles at the bases reflect transudation of fluid into the alveoli. Pleural effusions may cause bibasilar dullness to percussion. Expiratory wheezing and rhonchi may be signs of heart failure. Patients with severe right heart failure may have hepatic enlargement—tender or nontender—due to passive congestion. Systolic pulsations may be felt in tricuspid regurgitation. Sustained moderate pressure on the liver may increase jugular venous pressure (a positive hepatojugular reflux is an increase of > 1 cm). Ascites may also be present. Peripheral pitting edema is a common sign in patients with right heart failure and may extend into the thighs and abdominal wall.

The cardiac examination has been discussed. Cardinal signs in heart failure are a parasternal lift, indicating pulmonary hypertension; an enlarged and sustained left ventricular impulse, indicating left ventricular dilation and hypertrophy; a diminished first heart sound, suggesting impaired contractility; and S_3 gallops originating in the left and sometimes the right ventricle. Murmurs should be sought to exclude primary valvular disease; secondary mitral regurgitation and tricuspid regurgitation murmurs are common in patients with dilated ventricles.

C. Laboratory Findings: A blood count may reveal anemia, a cause of high-output failure and an exacerbating factor in other forms of cardiac dysfunction, or polycythemia. Biochemical studies may show renal insufficiency as a possible compounding factor. Renal function tests also determine whether cardiac failure is associated with prerenal azotemia, with serum urea nitrogen elevated disproportionately to serum creatinine. Electrolytes may disclose heightened neuroendocrine activity with resultant hyponatremia. Particularly in older patients and those with atrial fibrillation or accompanying pericardial effusion, thyroid function should be assessed to detect occult thyrotoxicosis or myxedema. Rectal, gingival, or skin biopsies may be performed to exclude amyloidosis. The additional diagnostic assessment of patients with dilated cardiomyopathy may include iron studies to exclude hemochromatosis. Other studies, including myocardial biopsy, may be appropriate to exclude specific causes of dilated cardiomyopathy.

D. Electrocardiography and Chest X-Ray: Electrocardiography may indicate an underlying or secondary arrhythmia, myocardial infarction, or nonspecific changes that often include low voltage, intraventricular conduction defects, left ventricular hypertrophy, and nonspecific repolarization changes. Chest radiographs provide information about the size and shape of the cardiac silhouette. Cardiomegaly is an important finding. Evidence of pulmonary venous hypertension includes relative dilation of the upper lobe veins, perivascular edema (haziness of vessel outlines), interstitial edema, and alveolar fluid. In acute heart failure, these findings correlate moderately well with pulmonary venous pressure, and when present in chronic failure they indicate elevated pressures. However, patients with chronic heart failure may show relatively normal pulmonary vasculature and have markedly elevated pressures. Pleural effusions are common and tend to be bilateral or right-sided.

E. Diagnostic Studies: Most patients with heart failure should undergo noninvasive cardiac testing because many of the symptoms are nonspecific and many studies have indicated that the clinical diagnosis of systolic myocardial dysfunction is often inaccurate. The primary confounding conditions are diastolic dysfunction of the heart with decreased relaxation and filling of the left ventricle (particularly in hypertension and in hypertrophic states) and pulmonary disease.

The most useful test is the echocardiogram. This will reveal the size and function of both ventricles and of the atria. It will also allow detection of pericardial effusion, valvular abnormalities, intracardiac shunts, and segmental wall motion abnormalities suggestive of old myocardial infarction as opposed to more generalized forms of dilated cardiomyopathy.

Radionuclide angiography measures left ventricular ejection fraction and permits analysis of regional wall motion. This test is especially useful when echocardiography is technically suboptimal, such as in patients with severe pulmonary disease.

F. Cardiac Catheterization: Cardiac catheterization is not necessary in most patients with heart failure. Clinical examination and noninvasive tests can determine left ventricular size and function well enough to confirm the diagnosis. Left heart catheterization is necessary when valvular disease must be excluded and when the presence and extent of coronary artery disease must be determined. The latter is particularly important when surgery to excise a left ventricular aneurysm is contemplated or when it is believed that left ventricular dysfunction may be partially reversible by revascularization. Right heart catheterization may be useful to select and monitor therapy in patients refractory to standard therapy.

Chakko S et al: Clinical, radiographic and hemodynamic correlations in chronic congestive heart failure: Conflicting results may lead to inappropriate care. Am J Med 1991;90:353. (X-ray and physical examination may underestimate the severity of cardiac dysfunction.)
Meyers J, Froelicher VF: Hemodynamic determinants of exercise capacity in chronic heart failure. Ann Intern Med 1991;115:377. (Exercise capacity and systolic dysfunction correlate poorly—discusses other mechanisms responsible for symptoms.)
Minotti JR et al: Skeletal muscle function, morphology, and metabolism in patients with congestive heart failure. Chest 1992;101(Suppl 5):333S. (Mechanism of exercise intolerance.)

Treatment

A. Correction of Reversible Causes: The major reversible causes have been discussed earlier and include thyrotoxicosis, myxedema, valvular lesions, intracardiac shunts, high-output states, arrhythmias, and alcohol- or drug-induced myocardial depression. Calcium channel blockers and antiarrhythmic agents are important causes of worsening heart failure in patients with left ventricular dysfunction. Some metabolic and infiltrative cardiomyopathies may be partially reversible, or their progression may be slowed; these include hypercalcemia, hemochromatosis, sarcoidosis, and primary amyloidosis. Acute myocarditis may respond to immunosuppressive therapy and corticosteroids. Reversible causes of diastolic dysfunction include pericardial disease and left ventricular hypertrophy due to hypertension. Once it is established that there is no reversible component to the heart failure and that the underlying pathophysiologic process is impaired contractility of the left ventricle, the measures outlined below are appropriate.

B. Diet and Activity: Patients should routinely be under moderate sodium (1.5–2 g) restriction. More severe sodium restriction is usually difficult to achieve and unnecessary because of the availability of potent diuretic agents. Alterations in life-style reduce symptoms and the need for additional medications. In severe heart failure, restriction of activity, including bed rest if necessary, often facilitates temporary recompensation. With such limitations, these patients may exhibit profound diuresis even though fluid retention was previously refractory. There is no convincing evidence that prolonged bed rest alters the natural history of congestive heart failure.

C. Diuretic Therapy: Diuretics are the most effective means of providing symptomatic relief to patients with moderate to severe congestive heart failure. Few patients with signs or symptoms of fluid retention can be optimally managed without a diuretic. However, excessive diuresis can lead to electrolyte imbalance and neurohormonal activation. In view of the beneficial effects of ACE inhibitors, a combination of a diuretic and an ACE inhibitor should be the initial treatment in most symptomatic patients. When fluid retention is mild, thiazide diuretics or a similar type of agent (hydrochlorothiazide, 25–100 mg; metolazone, 2.5–10 mg; chlorthalidone, 25–100 mg; etc) may be sufficient. These agents block sodium reabsorption in the cortical diluting segment at the terminal portion of the loop of Henle and in the proximal portion of the distal convoluted tubule. The result is natriuresis and kaliuresis. These agents also have weak carbonic anhydrase inhibitor activity, which results in proximal tubule inhibition of sodium reabsorption.

The thiazides are generally ineffective when the glomerular filtration rate falls below 30 mL/min, a not infrequent occurrence in patients with severe heart failure. Metolazone maintains its efficacy down to a glomerular filtration rate of approximately 10 mL/min. Adverse reactions to the thiazide diuretics include hypokalemia and intravascular volume depletion with resulting prerenal azotemia, skin rashes, neutropenia and thrombocytopenia, hyperglycemia, hyperuricemia, and hepatic dysfunction.

Patients with more severe heart failure should be treated with one of the "loop diuretics." These include furosemide (20–320 mg daily in single or divided doses), bumetanide (1–8 mg daily in single or divided doses), and ethacrynic acid (25–200 mg daily in single or divided doses). These agents have a rapid onset and short duration of action. In acute situations or when gastrointestinal absorption is in doubt, they should be given intravenously. The loop diuretics inhibit chloride reabsorption in the ascending limb of the loop of Henle, which results in natriuresis, kaliuresis, and metabolic alkalosis. They are active even in severe renal insufficiency, though very large doses (up to 500 mg of furosemide or equivalent) may be required. The major adverse reactions to loop diuretics relate to their potency; patients often develop excessive diuresis with resultant intravascular volume depletion, prerenal azotemia, and hypotension. Hypokalemia, particularly with accompanying digitalis therapy, is a major problem. Less common side effects include skin rashes, gastrointestinal distress, and ototoxicity (the latter more common with ethacrynic acid and possibly less common with bumetanide).

The potassium-sparing agents spironolactone, triamterene, and amiloride are often useful in combination with the loop diuretics and thiazides. Triamterene and amiloride act on the distal tubule to reduce potassium secretion. Their diuretic potency is only mild and not adequate for most patients with heart failure, but they may minimize the hypokalemia induced by more potent agents. Side effects include hyperkalemia, gastrointestinal symptoms, and renal dysfunction. Spironolactone is a specific inhibitor of aldosterone, which is often increased in congestive heart failure. Its onset of action is slower than the other potassium-sparing agents, and its side effects include gynecomastia. Combinations of potassium supplements or angiotensin converting enzyme inhibitors and potassium-sparing drugs can produce hyperkalemia.

Patients with refractory edema may respond to combinations of a loop diuretic and thiazide-like agents. Metolazone, because of its maintained activity with renal insufficiency, is the most useful agent for such a combination. Extreme caution must be observed with this approach, since massive diuresis and electrolyte imbalances often occur; 2.5 mg of metolazone should be added to the previous dosage of loop diuretic. In many cases this is necessary only once or twice a week, but dosages up to 10 mg daily have been used in some patients.

D. Digitalis Glycosides: Although digitalis was once the mainstay of treatment in congestive heart failure, it is now used somewhat more judiciously. Nonetheless, the efficacy of digitalis has recently been reconfirmed in several large studies.

1. Mechanism of action–Digitalis has a number of effects on the heart. Its positive inotropic effect is accomplished by increasing intracellular calcium and enhancing actin-myosin cross-bridge formation. Digitalis binds to the sodium-potassium ATPase on the cell membrane and inhibits the sodium pump. The resulting increase in intracellular sodium facilitates sodium-calcium exchange, resulting in increasing intracellular calcium concentrations.

The digitalis glycosides have electrophysiologic effects that may be beneficial or deleterious in individual patients. These effects are primarily the result of enhancement of the cardiac effects of the parasympathetic nervous system. Its primary therapeutic effect is inhibition of atrioventricular conduction. This decreases the ventricular response to supraventricular arrhythmias, such as atrial fibrillation or flutter. In addition, digitalis decreases sinus node automaticity. The increase in intracellular calcium and sodium may enhance automaticity of latent pacemakers. This increased excitability of ventricular myocardium underlies many of the arrhythmias associated with digitalis toxicity. Digitalis effect and toxicity are increased by reduced intracellular potassium concentrations and increased extracellular calcium concentrations.

2. Pharmacokinetics–Digitalis glycosides are available in a variety of preparations, but of these only digoxin (intravenously and orally) and digitoxin (primarily orally) are usually employed. The intravenous route is preferable if a rapid effect is desired; this is necessary chiefly when early control of rapid supraventricular arrhythmias is sought. Intravenous digoxin begins to have an effect after 15–30 minutes, and the peak effect is seen after 1½–3 hours. The usual initial dose is 0.5 mg given slowly over 10–20 minutes to avoid an immediate hypertensive response. Additional 0.25 or 0.125 mg doses may be administered after 3 hours. A total dosage of 1–1.25 mg is usually required to achieve full digitalis effect, but smaller dosages are sometimes adequate in older patients and in individuals with small lean body masses.

Therapeutic concentrations may also be achieved by the oral route. If a full effect is desired fairly rapidly, 1–1.25 mg are administered in divided dosages over the initial 24 hours. An additional 0.5 mg is added during the second 24 hours. In most instances, maximum effect is accomplished more gradually by administering 0.5 mg daily for 3 days, followed by the usual maintenance dosage. Digoxin is excreted principally by the kidneys and has a half-life ranging from 36 to 48 hours. The oral maintenance dose may range from 0.125 to 0.5 mg daily, depending on renal function, body size, age, thyroid function, and gastrointestinal absorption (ordinarily, approximately 60–70% of the oral dose is absorbed). Smaller doses are necessary in the presence of renal insufficiency. Unless the end point of therapy is control of the ventricular response in atrial fibrillation, it is worthwhile to measure serum digoxin levels after approximately 1 week of maintenance therapy; individual absorption rates and excretion rates may vary considerably. Digitoxin is less frequently used because of its long half-life (4–6 days), which will prolong the duration of toxicity if it occurs. Digitoxin is excreted by the liver, so blood levels may fluctuate less in patients with varying degrees of renal insufficiency.

A number of drugs have been found to affect digoxin pharmacology. Cholestyramine, some broad-spectrum oral antibiotics, antacids, and kaolin-pectin mixtures (eg, Kaopectate) may decrease absorption of digoxin. Quinidine, verapamil, amiodarone, and propafenone increase plasma levels of digoxin by reducing both the volume of distribution and the renal excretion of the agent. As noted previously, hypokalemia, hypercalcemia, and hypomagnesemia enhance the digitalis effect and potentiate its toxicity.

3. Digitalis toxicity–The therapeutic-to-toxic ratio of digitalis is quite narrow, and digitalis toxicity remains a potential problem. Its frequency has diminished as a result of improved understanding of its pharmacology, a trend toward employing lower dosages, and the availability of measurements of digoxin levels. Digoxin toxicity is uncommon with serum levels below 1.4 ng/mL and is present in approximately 50% of patients with levels above 3 ng/mL. Symptoms of digitalis toxicity include anorexia, nausea and vomiting, headache, visual symptoms (changes in color perception, halos, and scotomas), and disorientation. These symptoms may precede cardiotoxic effects.

Cardiac toxicity may take many forms, the most common being atrioventricular conduction disturbances, arrhythmias reflecting increased automaticity, and reentry arrhythmias. However, atrial flutter is rarely, if ever, secondary to digitalis toxicity. Arrhythmias due to digitalis toxicity include sinus node arrest, Mobitz type I second-degree atrioventricular block, ventricular premature beats or bigeminy, atrioventricular junctional tachycardia, paroxysmal supraventricular tachycardia with associated atrioventricular block, and ventricular tachycardia or fibrillation. When these arrhythmias are seen, digitalis toxicity should be suspected and the medication withheld. This, together with electrocardiographic monitoring, is adequate for many arrhythmias. Hypokalemia, if present, should be corrected, and any associated

tachyarrhythmias may resolve after blood potassium levels increase to the high-normal range. Potassium administration may exacerbate atrioventricular block, however. Ventricular tachycardia and very frequent ventricular premature beats should be treated with lidocaine or phenytoin. Class Ia and Ib agents are often less effective, and quinidine may exacerbate toxicity. Second-degree atrioventricular block usually does not require treatment, but complete heart block should be managed with atropine followed by temporary transvenous pacing. Electrical cardioversion for tachyarrhythmias should be avoided if possible, since digitalis toxicity may predispose to intractable ventricular fibrillation or cardiac standstill. If it cannot be avoided, patients should be pretreated with lidocaine (1 mg/kg) and low energy levels (10 J) should be employed initially.

Life-threatening episodes of digitalis toxicity or massive overdosages are characterized by severe hyperkalemia. They can be treated with digoxin-specific Fab antibody fragments. These are now commercially available and will rapidly reverse all manifestations of digitalis toxicity.

E. Vasodilators: Agents that dilate arteriolar smooth muscle and lower peripheral vascular resistance reduce left ventricular afterload. Medications that diminish venous tone and increase venous capacitance reduce the preload of both ventricles as their principal effect. Since, as noted earlier, most patients with moderate to severe heart failure have both elevated preload and reduced cardiac output, the maximum benefit of vasodilator therapy can be achieved by an agent or combination of agents with both actions. Many patients with heart failure have mitral or tricuspid regurgitation; agents that reduce resistance to left or right ventricular outflow tend to redirect regurgitant flow in a forward direction.

Several trials have indicated that vasodilator therapy with ACE inhibitors prolongs life in patients with moderate to severe heart failure. This evidence, plus many studies that show improvement in symptoms, has led to a wider use of these drugs. The combination of hydralazine and isosorbide dinitrate has also improved survival, but to a lesser extent than ACE inhibitors.

The intravenous vasodilating drugs and their dosages have been discussed in the section on complications in acute myocardial infarction.

1. Angiotensin-converting enzyme (ACE) inhibitors–The ACE inhibitors have become standard therapy for heart failure. Their beneficial effects include both vasodilation and inhibition of increased neurohormonal activity. These agents block the renin-angiotensin-aldosterone system, producing vasodilation by blocking angiotensin II-induced vasoconstriction and decreasing sodium retention by reducing aldosterone secretion. They also inhibit the degradation of bradykinin, increase the production of vasodilating prostaglandins, and indirectly inhibit the adrenergic nervous system. Although the other vasodilators tend to stimulate the renin-angiotensin system and often lose part of their effect due to the resulting fluid retention, tolerance to the ACE inhibitors is uncommon.

A growing number of ACE inhibitors are becoming available (see Table 10–3). Only captopril and enalapril have been approved for treatment of heart failure in the United States, but two others, lisinopril and quinipril, have been recommended for approval, and it is likely that all agents of this class are effective.

Acute hemodynamic studies show that the ACE inhibitors reduce left ventricular filling pressure and right atrial pressure and moderately increase cardiac output. During long-term follow-up, these hemodynamic benefits are maintained or increased. ACE inhibitors lessen symptoms and increase exercise tolerance. They also correct the electrolyte abnormalities that characterize severe heart failure, such as hyponatremia and diuretic-induced hypokalemia, which may reduce the propensity to arrhythmias. Survival rates are improved by ACE inhibitor therapy in patients with mild, moderate, and severe heart failure. In addition, recent data from two trials, SOLVD (Studies on Left Ventricular Dysfunction) and SAVE (Survival and Ventricular Enlargement), show that they can delay the onset and progression of heart failure in patients with asymptomatic left ventricular dysfunction.

Because the ACE inhibitors may produce significant hypotension in some patients with congestive heart failure, particularly after the initial doses, they must be started with caution. Hypotension is most prominent in patients with hypovolemia, prerenal azotemia (especially if it is diuretic-induced), and hyponatremia (an indicator of activation of the renin-angiotensin system). Before therapy with the ACE inhibitors is started, other vasodilators should be discontinued and the dosages of diuretics should be reduced or the drugs withheld for 24 hours. Captopril is the preferred agent for beginning ACE inhibitor therapy, especially in patients at risk for hypotension, because of its predictable onset and short duration of action (peak effect in 30–90 minutes). Treatment should be started with a low dose: either 12.5 mg or, in patients with hyponatremia or preexisting low blood pressure, 6.25 mg. The blood pressure should be monitored for the first 2 hours after dosing; if symptomatic or clinically significant hypotension does not occur, the patient may be sent home on a dosage of 12.5 mg three times daily. Patients should be questioned about symptoms of hypotension, and renal function should be checked during the first week. The chronically effective dose of captopril appears to be 25–100 mg three times daily, although some patients will not tolerate this high a dose because of hypotension.

Because enalapril must be deesterified in the liver,

which may be affected by passive congestion, its pharmacokinetics are less predictable in heart failure. However, maintenance therapy with enalapril is generally well tolerated, and this agent has been employed in most of the large survival studies. It is important to note that most of the trials which have led to the widespread use of ACE inhibitors have employed much higher doses (typically 15–20 mg daily of enalapril and 150 mg of captopril) than are used by many practitioners. Treatment should be titrated to these dosages unless limited by side effects, hypotension, or renal dysfunction. The doses of the newer agents should be comparable (see Table 10–3).

The major limitation to ACE inhibitor therapy in heart failure is hypotension and renal insufficiency due to inadequate renal perfusion pressures. Other side effects such as skin rashes, taste alterations, cough, neutropenia, and proteinuria are less serious or very uncommon. The ACE inhibitors tend to increase serum potassium concentrations. Potassium-sparing agents should be withdrawn before ACE inhibitor therapy is started; and although potassium supplements may be required in individuals receiving diuretics and digitalis, their dosage should be decreased and subsequently adjusted as needed.

2. Nitrates–Sodium nitroprusside is a potent dilator of both the arteriolar resistance and venous capacitance vessels, and it consistently increases cardiac output and reduces ventricular filling pressures. It is only occasionally employed in the management of chronic heart failure, usually during episodes of acute decompensation. In such cases it may produce excessive hypotension, and it has been combined with dopamine or dobutamine to produce optimal hemodynamic improvement. Intravenous nitroglycerin is less useful in chronic heart failure, since it produces only a limited increase in cardiac output.

Isosorbide dinitrate, 20–80 mg orally every 6–8 hours, has proved effective in several small studies. Nitroglycerin ointment, 12.5–50 mg (1–4 in) every 6 hours, appears to be equally effective although somewhat inconvenient for long-term therapy. The nitrates are moderately effective in relieving shortness of breath, especially in patients with mild to moderate symptoms, but less successful—probably because they have little effect on cardiac output—in advanced heart failure. Nitrate therapy is generally well tolerated, but headaches and hypotension may limit the dose of all agents. The development of tolerance to chronic nitrate therapy is now generally acknowledged. This is minimized by intermittent therapy, especially if a daily 8- to 12-hour nitrate-free interval is employed, but probably develops to some extent in most patients receiving these agents. Transdermal nitroglycerin patches have no sustained effect in patients with heart failure and should not be employed for this indication.

3. Hydralazine–Oral hydralazine is a potent arteriolar dilator and markedly increases cardiac output in patients with congestive heart failure. However, as a single agent, it has not been shown to improve symptoms or exercise tolerance during chronic treatment. The combination of nitrates and oral hydralazine produces greater hemodynamic and clinical effects.

Hydralazine therapy is frequently limited by side affects. Approximately 30% of patients are unable to tolerate the relatively high doses required to produce hemodynamic improvement in heart failure (200–400 mg daily in divided doses). The major side effect is gastrointestinal distress, but headaches, tachycardia, hypotension, and the drug-induced lupus syndrome are also relatively common.

4. Alpha-adrenergic blockers–These agents produce vasodilation by blocking postsynaptic alpha receptors. Although they cause short-term hemodynamic improvement, their efficacy is limited by the rapid development of tolerance. However, a recent study did indicate some benefit during chronic doxazosin treatment.

F. Newer Positive Inotropic Agents: The digitalis derivatives are the only available oral inotropic agents at this time in the USA. However, a number of drugs that increase myocardial contractility in experimental preparations have been or are being investigated. These include beta-adrenergic agonists, dopaminergic agents, and a group of nondigitalis, noncatecholamine agents that increase myocardial contractility by inhibiting myocardial phosphodiesterase. Two of the latter class, milrinone and amrinone, have been approved for intravenous use. However, several trials with newer inotropic agents (including milrinone and the beta-adrenergic agonist xamoterol) have demonstrated that they often *reduce* survival. Approval for any new oral positive inotropic agent is not anticipated for several years.

G. Calcium Channel Blockers: Data with the first generation of Ca^{2+} blockers have shown that these agents produce little benefit and may accelerate the progression of congestive heart failure. Whether this will be the case with newer agents is uncertain.

H. Beta-Blocker Therapy: A number of investigators have suggested that beta-blockers may produce symptomatic improvement in patients with chronic congestive heart failure. This approach runs counter to the usual practice of avoiding beta-blockers in heart failure but has been justified by the potentially harmful effects of circulating catecholamines and because it offers a means of reversing the "downregulation" of myocardial beta receptors. Metoprolol has been the most studied, but agents with adjunctive vasodilator effects (bucindolol or carvedilol, neither of which is currently available in the United States) may be equally or more effective. Obviously, this approach carries the risk of worsening heart failure, and these agents must be initiated at *very* low dosages (5 mg or less of metoprolol twice daily) and in-

creased very gradually. No multicenter controlled trial with beta-blockers has been reported, so their true role remains unclear.

I. Anticoagulation: Patients with severe left ventricular failure are prone to development of systemic arterial emboli, particularly when they are in atrial fibrillation. While these may be catastrophic, the routine use of anticoagulants is controversial, since these patients have short life expectancies and are taking multiple medications that may interfere with optimal regulation of anticoagulation. Most experts prescribe anticoagulants only to appropriate patients who have had embolic episodes or those with atrial fibrillation. Some also anticoagulate patients with severe dilated cardiomyopathy (ejection fraction < 20%) in normal sinus rhythm.

J. Antiarrhythmic Therapy: Patients with moderate to severe heart failure have a high incidence of both symptomatic and asymptomatic arrhythmias. Although fewer than 10% of patients have syncope or presyncope resulting from ventricular tachycardia, ambulatory monitoring reveals that up to 70% of patients have asymptomatic episodes of nonsustained ventricular tachycardia. These arrhythmias indicate a poor prognosis independent of the severity of left ventricular dysfunction, but many of the deaths are probably not arrhythmia-related, and there is no evidence that antiarrhythmic therapy improves prognosis in asymptomatic patients.

Patients with symptomatic ventricular arrhythmias should be treated vigorously as outlined elsewhere in this chapter. Whether patients with asymptomatic nonsustained ventricular tachycardia warrant therapy remains controversial, largely because such treatment is not without risk. Most effective antiarrhythmic agents may depress left ventricular function or may themselves worsen the arrhythmia. While most experts do not initiate treatment for frequent ventricular premature beats, they may attempt to suppress frequent episodes of nonsustained ventricular tachycardia. As more evidence accrues that type I antiarrhythmic drugs all may worsen the arrhythmia and exacerbate heart failure, amiodarone has become the agent of choice.

Prognosis

Despite advances in treatment of patients with congestive heart failure, their prognosis remains poor, with annual mortality rates ranging from 10% in stable patients with mild symptoms to over 50% in patients with advanced, progressive symptoms. Poorer prognosis is associated with severe left ventricular dysfunction (ejection fractions < 20%), severe symptoms and limitation of exercise capacity (maximal oxygen consumption < 10 mL/kg/min), secondary renal insufficiency, hyponatremia, and elevated plasma catecholamine levels. About 40–50% of patients with heart failure die suddenly, presumably due to ventricular arrhythmias. Nonsustained ventricular tachycardia is a poor prognostic sign, but its prevalence is so high that it cannot be used to predict which individuals are at risk of sudden death.

Cardiac Transplantation

Because of the poor prognosis in patients with advanced heart failure, cardiac transplantation is now performed in many centers throughout the world. Since the advent of cyclosporine immunosuppressive therapy and more careful screening of donor hearts, the survival of patients after cardiac transplantation has increased considerably. Many centers now have 1-year survival rates exceeding 80–90%, and 5-year survival rates are above 70% in the future. Infections, hypertension and renal dysfunction caused by cyclosporine, rapidly progressive coronary atherosclerosis, and immunosuppressant-related cancers have been the major complications. Clearly, cardiac transplantation is effective in selected individuals, but the high cost and limited number of donor organs require careful patient selection. Patients who are candidates for transplantation should be assessed early in their course, since the incidence of sudden death is high once they exhibit advanced symptoms.

Bousquet GL: Congestive heart failure: A review of non-pharmacologic therapies. J Cardiovasc Nursing 1990; 4:35. (Key management approaches.)

Cody RJ: Management of refractory congestive heart failure. Am J Cardiol 1992;69:141G. (What to do when usual approaches don't work.)

Cohn JN et al: A comparison of enalapril with hydralazine-isosorbide dinitrate in the treatment of chronic congestive heart failure. N Engl J Med 1991;325:303. (Survival better with enalapril, but exercise tolerance greater on hydralazine-isosorbide dinitrate.)

Feldman AM: Can we alter survival in patients with congestive heart failure? JAMA 1992;267:1956. (Review of data and implications for treatment.)

Goldstein RE et al: Diltiazem increases late-onset congestive heart failure in post-infarction patients with early reduction in ejection fraction. Circulation 1991;83:52. (Calcium channel blockers should be avoided in symptomatic heart failure, but studies show over 30% of these patients are receiving them.)

Minotti JR, Massie BM: Exercise training in heart failure patients. Does reversing the peripheral abnormalities protect the heart? Circulation 1992;85:2323. (Activity should be encouraged in patients with stable congestive heart failure.)

Mujais SK et al: Principles and clinical uses of diuretic therapy. Prog Cardiovasc Dis 1992;35:221.

O'Connell JB et al: Cardiac transplantation: recipient selection, donor procurement, and medical follow-up. Circulation 1992;86:1061. (Consensus statement with focus on patient selection.)

Om A, Hess MC: Inotropic therapy of the failing myocardium. Clin Cardiol 1993;16:5. (Updated review of old and new drugs.)

Parmley WW et al: Congestive heart failure: New frontiers. West J Med 1991;154:427. (Mechanisms and treatment.)

Podrid PJ, Wilson JS: Should asymptomatic ventricular arrhythmia in patients with congestive heart failure be treated? Am J Cardiol 1990;66:451. (The author argues no.)

SOLVD Investigators: Effect of enalapril on mortality and development of heart failure in asymptomatic patients with reduced left ventricular ejection fractions. N Engl J Med 1992;327:685. (ACE inhibitor therapy prevents or delays clinical CHF in these patients.)

SOLVD Investigators: Effect of enalapril on survival in patients with reduced left ventricular ejection fractions and congestive heart failure. N Engl J Med 1991; 325:293. (Major trial showing that enalapril prolongs survival and prevents hospitalization.)

Stambler BS et al: Sudden death in patients with congestive heart failure: Future directions. PACE 1992;15:451. (Pros and cons of antiarrhythmic drugs and devices.)

Stevenson LW, Fonarow G: Vasodilators: A reevaluation of their role in heart failure. Drugs 1992;43:15.

Stevenson LW, Perloff JK: The limited reliability of physical signs for estimating hemodynamics in chronic heart failure. JAMA 1989;261:884. (Left ventricular filling pressure cannot be estimated by examination.)

ACUTE PULMONARY EDEMA

Essentials of Diagnosis

- Acute onset or worsening of dyspnea at rest.
- Tachycardia, diaphoresis, cyanosis.
- Pulmonary rales, rhonchi; expiratory wheezing.
- X-ray shows interstitial and alveolar edema with or without cardiomegaly.
- Arterial hypoxemia.

General Considerations

The most common causes of cardiogenic pulmonary edema are acute myocardial infarction, acute volume overload of the left ventricle (valvular regurgitation or ventricular septal defect), and mitral stenosis.

Clinical Findings

Acute pulmonary edema presents with a characteristic clinical picture of severe dyspnea, the production of pink, frothy sputum, and diaphoresis and cyanosis. Examination of the lungs reveals rales in all lung fields or generalized wheezing and rhonchi. Pulmonary edema may appear suddenly in the setting of chronic heart failure or may be the first manifestation of cardiac disease, usually acute myocardial infarction, which may be painful or silent.

While most cases of pulmonary edema are due to left ventricular failure or mitral valve disease, a number of noncardiac conditions can also produce pulmonary edema. This occurs either because of imbalance in the Starling forces (such as can occur from a decrease in plasma proteins or an increase in pulmonary venous pressure) or a functional or anatomic abnormality of the alveolar-capillary membrane. Causes of noncardiogenic pulmonary edema include intravenous narcotics, increased intracerebral pressure, high altitude, sepsis, several medications, inhaled toxins, transfusion reactions, shock, and disseminated intravascular coagulation. These are usually distinguished from cardiogenic pulmonary edema by the clinical setting, the history, and the physical examination. Conversely, in most patients with cardiogenic pulmonary edema, an underlying cardiac abnormality can usually be detected clinically or by the ECG, chest x-ray, or echocardiogram.

The chest radiograph reveals signs of pulmonary vascular redistribution, blurriness of vascular outlines, increased interstitial markings, and, characteristically, the butterfly pattern of alveolar edema. The heart may be enlarged or normal in size depending on whether heart failure was previously present. An acute assessment of cardiac function by echocardiography or right heart catheterization is helpful in determining the cause. In cardiogenic pulmonary edema, the pulmonary capillary wedge pressure is universally elevated, usually over 25 mm Hg. Cardiac output may be normal or depressed. In noncardiogenic pulmonary edema, as in the acute respiratory distress syndrome, or severe pulmonary disease masquerading as pulmonary edema. the wedge pressure may be normal or even low.

Treatment

The patient should be placed in a sitting position with legs dangling over the side of the bed; this facilitates respiration and reduces venous return. Oxygen should be delivered by mask to obtain an arterial PO_2 greater than 60 mm Hg. If respiratory distress is severe, endotracheal intubation and mechanical ventilation may be necessary.

Morphine sulfate is highly effective in pulmonary edema. The initial dosage should be 4–8 mg intravenously (subcutaneous administration is effective in milder cases), and this may be repeated after 2–4 hours. Morphine increases venous capacitance, lowering left atrial pressure, and relieves anxiety, which can reduce the efficiency of ventilation. However, morphine may lead to CO_2 retention and reduce the ventilatory drive. Morphine should be avoided in patients with narcotic-induced pulmonary edema, who may improve with narcotic antagonists, and in those with neurogenic pulmonary edema.

Intravenous diuretic therapy (furosemide, 40 mg, or bumetanide, 1 mg—or higher doses if the patient has been receiving chronic diuretic therapy) is usually indicated even if the patient has not exhibited prior fluid retention. These agents produce immediate venodilation even prior to the onset of diuresis. Other approaches to therapy include further measures to reduce left ventricular preload. This may be accomplished by the administration of sublingual or intravenous nitrates and, in otherwise refractory cases, phlebotomy of approximately 500 mL of blood or plasmapheresis. Bronchospasm may occur in response to pulmonary edema and may itself exacerbate hypoxemia and dyspnea. Treatment with inhaled beta-adrenergic agonists or intravenous aminophylline may be helpful, but both may also provoke tachycardia and supraventricular arrhythmias. Particularly in patients with elevated arterial pressures, vasodilators such as intravenous nitroprusside may be worthwhile. In patients with low-output states, particularly when hypotension is present, positive inotropic agents are indicated. These approaches to treatment have been discussed previously.

Allison RC: Initial treatment of pulmonary edema: A physiologic approach. Am J Med Sci 1991;302:385.
Massie BM, Braun S: Pulmonary edema. In: *Current Therapy in Emergency Medicine,* 2nd ed. Callaham ML (editor). BC Decker, 1991.

MYOCARDITIS & THE CARDIOMYOPATHIES

ACUTE MYOCARDITIS

Acute myocarditis is focal or diffuse inflammation of the myocardium. Most cases are infectious, caused by viral, bacterial, rickettsial, spirochetal, fungal, or parasitic agents; but toxins, drugs, and immunologic reaction can also cause myocarditis.

1. INFECTIOUS MYOCARDITIS

Essentials of Diagnosis
- Often follows respiratory infection.
- May present with chest pain (pleuritic or nonspecific), signs of heart failure, or arrhythmias.
- ECG may show sinus tachycardia, nonspecific repolarization changes, intraventricular conduction abnormalities.
- Echocardiogram documents cardiomegaly and contractile dysfunction.
- Myocardial biopsy may reveal a characteristic inflammatory pattern.

General Considerations
Viral myocarditis is the most common form and is usually caused by coxsackieviruses, but a host of other agents have also been responsible. Rickettsial myocarditis occurs with scrub typhus, Rocky Mountain spotted fever, and Q fever. Diphtheritic myocarditis is caused by the toxin and often is manifested by conduction abnormalities as well as heart failure.

Chagas' disease, caused by the insect-borne protozoan *Trypanosoma cruzi,* is a common form of myocarditis in Central and South America. An acute inflammatory process may occur, but the major clinical manifestations appear after a latent period of more than a decade. At this stage, patients present with cardiomyopathy, congestive heart failure, conduction disturbances, and sudden death. Associated gastrointestinal involvement (megaesophagus and megacolon) is the rule. Toxoplasmosis causes myocarditis that is usually asymptomatic but can lead to heart failure. Among parasitic infections, trichinosis is the most common cause of cardiac involvement. The potential for the HIV virus to cause myocarditis is now well recognized, though the prevalence of this complication is not known, and it is an uncommon cause of morbidity and mortality in AIDS. In addition, other infectious myocarditides are more common in patients with AIDS.

Clinical Findings

A. Symptoms and Signs: Patients may present several days to a few weeks after the onset of acute febrile illness or a respiratory infection or with heart failure without antecedent symptoms. Pleural-pericardial chest pain is common. Nonspecific systemic symptoms are often present. Examination often reveals tachycardia, gallop rhythm, and other evidence of heart failure or conduction defect.

B. Electrocardiography and Chest X-Ray: Nonspecific ST–T changes and conduction disturbances are common. Ventricular ectopy may be the initial and only clinical finding. Chest x-ray is nonspecific.

C. Diagnostic Studies: Echocardiography provides the most convenient way of evaluating cardiac function and can exclude many other processes. Gallium-67 scintigraphy has been reported to yield cardiac uptake in acute or subacute myocarditis. Paired serum viral titers and serologic tests for other agents may indicate the cause.

D. Endomyocardial Biopsy: Pathologic examinations may reveal a round cell inflammatory reaction and patchy necrosis. This picture defines an "active" inflammatory stage and may persist for many months.

Treatment & Prognosis

Specific antimicrobial therapy is indicated if an infecting agent can be identified. Observational studies have suggested that immunosuppressive therapy with corticosteroids and other agents may improve the outcome when the process is acute (< 6 months) and the biopsy suggests ongoing inflammation. However, controlled trials have not been positive, so the value of routine myocardial biopsies in patients presenting with an acute myocarditic picture is uncertain. Empiric immunosuppressive therapy without histologic confirmation is unwarranted. Otherwise, treatment is directed toward the manifestations of heart failure and arrhythmias.

Many cases resolve spontaneously, but in others cardiac function deteriorates progressively and may evolve into dilated cardiomyopathy. Recent data using molecular biology techniques suggest that many cases of idiopathic dilated cardiomyopathy may represent the end stage of viral myocarditis.

Francis CK: Cardiac involvement in AIDS. Curr Probl Cardiol 1990;15(10):569. (Myocarditis, pericarditis, and other problems.)

Parrillo JE et al: A prospective, randomized controlled trial of prednisone for dilated cardiomyopathy. N Engl J Med 1989;321:1061. (No benefit.)

Mengel JO, Rossi MA: Chronic chagasic myocarditis pathogenesis. Am Heart J 1992;124:1052. (One of the world's commonest infectious cardiomyopathies.)

Rose NR et al: Coxsackie virus myocarditis. Adv Intern Med 1992;37:411. (Most common form.)

See DM, Tilles JG: Viral myocarditis. Rev Infect Dis 1991;13:951. (Causes and presentation.)

2. DRUG-INDUCED & TOXIC MYOCARDITIS

A variety of medications, illicit drugs, and toxic substances can produce acute inflammatory myocardial reactions or more chronic damage. The clinical presentation may vary widely, so this brief section will serve only to alert the physician to potential causative agents. Doxorubicin and other cytotoxic agents used for treatment of neoplasm, emetine (an antiparasitic agent for amebiasis), and catecholamines (especially with pheochromocytoma) can produce a pathologic picture of inflammation and necrosis together with clinical heart failure and arrhythmias; toxicity of the first two is dose-related. The phenothiazines, lithium, chloroquine, disopyramide, antimony-containing compounds, and arsenicals can also cause electrocardiographic changes, arrhythmias, or heart failure. Hypersensitivity reactions to sulfonamides, penicillins, and aminosalicylic acid as well as other drugs can result in cardiac dysfunction. Radiation can cause an acute inflammatory reaction as well as a chronic fibrosis, usually in conjunction with pericarditis.

The incidence of cocaine cardiotoxicity has increased markedly. Cocaine can cause coronary artery spasm, myocardial infarction, arrhythmias, and myocarditis. Because many of these processes are believed to be mediated by cocaine's inhibitory effect on norepinephrine reuptake by sympathetic nerves, beta-blockers have been used therapeutically. In coronary spasm, calcium channel blockers are more appropriate.

Kloner RA et al: The effects of acute and chronic cocaine use on the heart. Circulation 1992;85:407. (Mechanisms and clinical presentations.)

Lipshultz SE et al: Late cardiac effects of doxorubicin therapy for acute lymphoblastic leukemia in childhood.

N Engl J Med 1991;324:808. (Evidence of elevated wall stress and reduced contractility.)

THE CARDIOMYOPATHIES

The cardiomyopathies are a heterogeneous group of entities affecting the myocardium primarily and not associated with the major causes of cardiac disease, ie, ischemic heart disease, hypertension, valvular disease, or congenital defects. While some have specific causes, many cases are idiopathic. There is now general agreement on a classification of the cardiomyopathies into three categories based upon general features of their presentation and pathophysiology. Table 10–8 outlines this classification. Some patients have overlapping features, but this classification is of use in planning diagnostic evaluation and therapy.

Perloff JK et al: The cardiomyopathies. Cardiol Clin 1988;6(2):185. (Chapters on dilated, hypertrophic, and restrictive cardiomyopathy.)
Shaver JA (editor): Cardiomyopathies: Clinical presentation, differential diagnosis, and management. Cardiovasc Clin 1988;19(1):1.

Role of Myocardial Biopsy

The use of myocardial biopsy to make specific diagnoses in patients with cardiomyopathies is increasing. The indications for the procedure remain controversial, but it is essential for the early detection of transplant rejection. Biopsies have also been helpful in distinguishing restrictive cardiomyopathy from pericardial constriction, an often difficult problem. Occasionally, a specific diagnosis of amyloidosis, sarcoidosis, hemochromatosis, or an unusual infection can be made, but in most cases these conditions are suggested by other cardiac or systemic findings. Biopsies can reveal evidence of acute myocarditis and, if immunosuppressive therapy is contemplated, should be performed in appropriate patients.

Chow LC, Dittrich HC, Shabetai R: Endomyocardial biopsy in patients with unexplained congestive heart failure. Ann Intern Med 1988;109:535. (Low incidence of myocarditis and other diagnostic findings in a large series.)
Mason JW, O'Connell JB: Clinical merit of endomyocardial biopsy. Circulation 1989;79:971.

1. DILATED CARDIOMYOPATHY

Essentials of Diagnosis

- Symptoms and signs of heart failure.
- ECG may show low QRS voltage, nonspecific repolarization abnormalities, intraventricular conduction abnormalities.
- X-ray shows cardiomegaly.
- Echocardiogram confirms left ventricular dilation, thinning, and global dysfunction.

General Considerations

Dilated cardiomyopathies usually present with symptoms and signs of congestive heart failure (most commonly dyspnea). Occasionally, symptomatic ventricular arrhythmias are the presenting event. Left ventricular dilation and systolic dysfunction are essential for diagnosis. Often no cause can be identified, but chronic alcohol abuse and myocarditis are probably frequent causes. Indeed, many believe that idiopathic dilated cardiomyopathy often represents

Table 10–8. Classification of the cardiomyopathies.

	Dilated	Hypertrophic	Restrictive
Frequent causes	Idiopathic, alcoholic, myocarditis, postpartum, doxorubicin, endocrinopathies, genetic diseases	Hereditary syndrome, possibly chronic hypertension	Amyloidosis, postradiation, post-open heart surgery, diabetes, endomyocardial fibrosis
Symptoms	Left or biventricular CHF	Dyspnea, chest pain, syncope	Dyspnea, fatigue, right-sided CHF
Physical examination	Cardiomegaly, S₃, elevated JVP, rales	Sustained PMI, S₄, variable systolic murmur, bisferiens carotid pulse	Elevated JVP, Kussmaul's sign
ECG	ST–T changes, conduction abnormalities, ventricular ectopy	LVH, exaggerated septal Q waves	ST–T changes, conduction abnormalities, low voltage
Chest x-ray	Enlarged heart, pulmonary congestion	Mild cardiomegaly	Mild to moderate cardiomegaly
Echocardiogram, nuclear studies	LV dilation and dysfunction	LVH, asymmetric septal hypertrophy, small LV size, normal or supranormal function, systolic anterior mitral motion, diastolic dysfunction	Small or normal LV size, normal or mildly reduced LV function
Cardiac catheterization	LV dilation and dysfunction, high diastolic pressures, low cardiac output	Small, hypercontractile LV, dynamic outflow gradient, diastolic dysfunction	High diastolic pressures, "square root" sign, normal or mildly reduced LV function

the end stage of myocarditis. Histologically, the picture is one of extensive fibrosis.

Clinical Findings

A. Symptoms and Signs: In most patients, symptoms of heart failure develop gradually. They may be recognized because of asymptomatic cardiomegaly, electrocardiographic abnormalities, or ventricular ectopy. The initial presentation may be severe biventricular failure. The physical examination reveals cardiomegaly, S_3 gallop rhythm, and often a murmur of functional mitral regurgitation. Signs of left- and right-sided failure may be present on initial examination.

B. Electrocardiography and Chest X-Ray: The major findings are included in Table 10–6.

C. Diagnostic Studies: Laboratory tests should be performed to exclude treatable causes of cardiomyopathy. The role of myocardial biopsy has been discussed. An echocardiogram is indicated to exclude unsuspected valvular or other lesions and confirm the presence of dilated cardiomyopathy. Exercise thallium-201 scintigraphy may suggest the possibility of underlying coronary disease if a large reversible defect is found, but false-positives occur in cardiomyopathy. Cardiac catheterization is seldom of specific value unless myocardial ischemia or left ventricular aneurysm is suspected.

Treatment

Few cases of cardiomyopathy are amenable to specific therapy. Alcohol use should be discontinued. There is often marked recovery of cardiac function following a period of abstinence in alcoholic cardiomyopathy. Endocrine causes (thyroid dysfunction, acromegaly, pheochromocytoma) should be treated. Immunosuppressive therapy is not indicated in chronic dilated cardiomyopathy. The management of congestive heart failure is outlined in the section on heart failure.

Prognosis

The prognosis of dilated cardiomyopathy without clinical heart failure is variable, with some patients remaining stable, some deteriorating gradually, and others declining rapidly. Once heart failure is manifest, the natural history is similar to that of other causes of heart failure. Arterial and pulmonary emboli are more common in dilated cardiomyopathy than in ischemic cardiomyopathy; suitable candidates may benefit from chronic anticoagulation.

Abelmann WH, Lorell BH: The challenge of cardiomyopathy. J Am Coll Cardiol 1989;13:1219.

Davidson DM: Cardiovascular effects of alcohol. West J Med 1989;151:430.

Moushmoush B, Abi-Mansour P: Alcohol and the heart. Arch Intern Med 1991;151:36.

Zarich SW, Nesto RW: Diabetic cardiomyopathy. Am Heart J 1989;118:1000.

2. HYPERTROPHIC CARDIOMYOPATHY

Essentials of Diagnosis

- May present with dyspnea, chest pain, syncope.
- Examination shows sustained apical impulse, S_4, systolic ejection murmur.
- ECG shows left ventricular hypertrophy.
- Echocardiogram shows hypertrophy, which may be asymmetric; usually shows normal or enhanced contractility and signs of dynamic obstruction.

General Considerations

In hypertrophic cardiomyopathy, there is inappropriate—ie, unrelated to any pressure or volume overload—myocardial hypertrophy that tends to impinge upon the left ventricular cavity. Characteristically, the interventricular septum is disproportionately involved (asymmetric septal hypertrophy), but in some cases the hypertrophy is localized to the apex. The left ventricular outflow tract is often narrowed during systole between the bulging septum and an anteriorly displaced anterior mitral valve leaflet, causing a dynamic obstruction (hence the name idiopathic hypertrophic subaortic stenosis; IHSS). The obstruction is worsened by factors that increase myocardial contractility (sympathetic stimulation, digoxin, postextrasystolic beat) or that decrease left ventricular filling (Valsalva's maneuver, peripheral vasodilators).

Hypertrophic cardiomyopathy is in some cases inherited as an autosomal dominant trait with variable penetrance. These patients usually present in early adulthood. Others are elderly, and many of those patients have a long history of hypertension. Some cases occur sporadically.

Except in late stages, hypertrophic cardiomyopathy is characterized by a small, hypercontractile left ventricle. Although dyspnea is a common symptom, it results primarily from markedly impaired diastolic compliance rather than systolic dysfunction or outflow obstruction.

Clinical Findings

A. Symptoms and Signs: The most frequent symptoms are dyspnea and chest pain. Syncope is also common and is typically postexertional, when diastolic filling diminishes while outflow obstruction remains increased. Arrhythmias are an important problem. Atrial fibrillation is a long-term consequence of chronically elevated left atrial pressures and is a poor prognostic sign. Ventricular arrhythmias are also common, and sudden death may occur, often in athletes after extraordinary exertion.

Features on physical examination are a bisferiens carotid pulse, triple apical impulse (due to the prominent atrial filling wave and early and late systolic impulses), and a loud S_4. In cases with outflow obstruction, a loud systolic murmur is present that increases with upright posture or Valsalva's maneuver and decreases with squatting.

B. Electrocardiography and Chest X-Ray: Left ventricular hypertrophy is nearly universal. Exaggerated septal Q waves inferolaterally may suggest myocardial infarction. The chest x-ray is often unimpressive.

C. Diagnostic Studies: The echocardiogram is diagnostic, revealing asymmetric left ventricular hypertrophy, systolic anterior motion of the mitral valve, early closing followed by reopening of the aortic valve, a small and hypercontractile left ventricle, and delayed relaxation and filling of the left ventricle during diastole. Doppler ultrasound reveals turbulent flow and a dynamic gradient across the aortic valve and, commonly, mitral regurgitation. Cardiac catheterization may confirm the gradient but adds little to echocardiographic studies.

Treatment

Beta-blockers should be the initial drug in symptomatic individuals, especially when dynamic outflow obstruction is noted on the echocardiogram. Dyspnea, angina, and arrhythmias respond in about 50% of patients. Calcium channel blockers, especially verapamil, have also been effective in symptomatic patients. Their effect may be due primarily to improved diastolic function, but their vasodilating actions may also increase outflow obstruction. Excision of part of the myocardial septum has been successful in patients with severe symptoms when performed by surgeons experienced with the procedure. Recent studies have indicated that dual-chamber pacing may prevent the progression of hypertrophy and obstruction. Antiarrhythmic agents may be valuable because of the frequency of ventricular arrhythmias and their possible relation to sudden death.

Prognosis

The natural history of hypertrophic cardiomyopathy is highly variable. Some patients remain asymptomatic for many years or for life. Sudden death, especially during exercise, may be the initial event. Indeed, hypertrophic cardiomyopathy is the pathologic feature most frequently associated with sudden death in athletes. Other patients have a history of gradually progressive symptoms. A final stage may be a transition into dilated cardiomyopathy. Amiodarone, in particular, has been advocated in these patients.

Jeanrenaud X et al: Effects of dualDchamber pacing in hypertrophic obstructive cardiomyopathy. Lancet 1992; 339:1318. (Promising approach.)

Lewis JF, Maron BJ: Elderly patients with hypertrophic cardiomyopathy: A subset with distinctive left ventricular morphology and progressive clinical course late in life. J Am Coll Cardiol 1989;13:36.

Maron BJ, Fananapazir L: Sudden cardiac death in hypertrophic cardiomyopathy. Circulation 1992;85(Suppl I):I–57.

Maron BJ et al: Hypertrophic cardiomyopathy: Interrelations of clinical manifestations, pathophysiology, and therapy. (Two parts.) N Engl J Med 1987;316:780, 844.

3. RESTRICTIVE CARDIOMYOPATHY

Restrictive cardiomyopathy is characterized by impaired diastolic filling with preserved contractile function. This condition is relatively uncommon, with the most frequent causes being amyloidosis, radiation, and myocardial fibrosis after open heart surgery. In Africa, endomyocardial fibrosis, a specific entity in which there is severe fibrosis of the endocardium, often with eosinophilia (Löffler's syndrome) is common. Other causes of a restrictive picture are infiltrative cardiomyopathies (eg, sarcoidosis, hemo–chromatosis, carcinoid syndrome) and connective tissue diseases (eg, scleroderma).

Amyloidosis can affect the heart in several ways. Although it is a frequent cause of restrictive cardiomyopathy, it more frequently produces dilated cardiomyopathy with congestive heart failure. Almost invariably, conduction disturbances are present. Rectal, abdominal fat, or gingival biopsies—as well as myocardial biopsy—can be diagnostic.

The primary diagnostic problem with restrictive cardiomyopathy is differentiation from constrictive pericarditis. The clinical picture often strongly suggests the diagnosis, but the status of left ventricular function (usually normal with pericarditis, slightly depressed with restrictive cardiomyopathy) can be helpful, as can be evidence of a thickened pericardium. Myocardial biopsies are usually negative with pericarditis but not in restrictive cardiomyopathy. In some cases, only surgical exploration can make the diagnosis.

Unfortunately, little useful therapy is available for either the causative conditions or restrictive cardiomyopathy itself. Diuretics can help, but excessive diuresis can produce worsening symptoms.

Gertz MA, Kyle RA: Primary systemic amyloidosis: A diagnostic primer. Mayo Clin Proc 1991;64:1505. (Major cause of restrictive cardiomyopathy.)

Katritsis D et al: Primary restrictive cardiomyopathy: Clinical and pathologic characteristics. J Am Coll Cardiol 1991;18:1230.

Vaitkus PJ, Kussmaul WG: Constrictive pericarditis versus restrictive cardiomyopathy: A reappraisal and update of diagnostic criteria. Am Heart J 1991;122:1431. (Difficult distinction.)

ACUTE RHEUMATIC FEVER & RHEUMATIC HEART DISEASE

Essentials of Diagnosis

- Peak incidence ages 5–15 years.
- Diagnosis based on Jones criteria (see text) and confirmation of streptococcal infection.
- May involve mitral and other valves acutely, rarely leading to heart failure.
- Long-term damage to heart valves (especially mitral in women, aortic in men).

General Considerations

Rheumatic fever is a systemic immune process which is a sequela to hemolytic streptococcal infection of the pharynx. Recent studies have indicated that pyodermic infections are not associated with rheumatic fever. Signs of rheumatic fever usually commence 2–3 weeks after infection but may appear as early as 1 week or as late as 5 weeks. It had become uncommon in the USA, except in recent immigrants. However, there have been recent reports of new outbreaks in several regions of the USA. The peak incidence is between ages 5 and 15; rheumatic fever is rare before age 4 and after age 40. Rheumatic carditis and valvulitis may be selfDlimited or may lead to slowly progressive valvular deformity. The characteristic lesion is a perivascular granulomatous reaction with vasculitis. The mitral valve is attacked in 75–80% of cases, the aortic valve in 30%, and the tricuspid and pulmonary valves in under 5%.

Clinical Findings

Diagnostic criteria first described by Jones are still employed. The presence of two major criteria—or one major and one minor criterion—establishes the diagnosis.

A. Major Criteria:

1. Carditis–Carditis is most likely to be evident in children and adolescents. Any of the following signs establishes the presence of carditis. (1) Pericarditis, which is uncommon in adults and diagnosed by detection of a friction rub or evidence of effusion by echocardiogram. (2) Cardiomegaly, detected by physical signs, radiography, or echocardiography. (3) Congestive failure, right- or left-sided—the former perhaps more prominent in children, with painful liver engorgement due to tricuspid regurgitation. (4) Mitral or aortic regurgitation murmurs, indicative of dilation of a valve ring with or without associated valvulitis. The Carey-Coombs short middiastolic mitral murmur may be present.

In the absence of any of the above definitive signs, the diagnosis of carditis depends upon the following less specific abnormalities. (1) Electrocardiographic changes: The most significant abnormality is PR prolongation greater than 0.04 s above the patient's normal. Changing contour of P waves or inversion of T waves is less useful. (2) Changing quality of heart sounds. (3) Sinus tachycardia persisting during sleep and markedly increased by slight activity. (4) Arrhythmias, shifting pacemaker, ectopic beats.

2. Erythema marginatum and subcutaneous nodules–The former begin as rapidly enlarging macules that assume the shape of rings or crescents with clear centers. They may be raised, confluent, and either transient or persistent.

Subcutaneous nodules are uncommon except in children. They are small (≤ 2 cm in diameter), firm, and nontender and are attached to fascia or tendon sheaths over bony prominences. They persist for days or weeks, are recurrent, and are indistinguishable from rheumatoid nodules.

3. Sydenham's chorea–Sydenham's chorea—involuntary choreoathetoid movements primarily of the face, tongue, and upper extremities—may be the sole manifestation; half of cases have other overt signs of rheumatic fever. Girls are more frequently affected, and occurrence in adults is rare. This is the least common (3% of cases) but most diagnostic of the manifestations of rheumatic fever.

4. Arthritis–This is a migratory polyarthritis that involves the large joints sequentially. In adults, only a single joint may be affected. The arthritis lasts 1–5 weeks and subsides without residual deformity. Prompt response of arthritis to therapeutic doses of salicylates or nonsteroidal agents is characteristic.

B. Minor Criteria: These include fever, polyarthralgias, reversible prolongation of the PR interval, rapid erythrocyte sedimentation rate, evidence of an antecedent β-hemolytic streptococcal infection, or a history of rheumatic fever.

C. Laboratory Findings: There is nonspecific evidence of inflammatory disease, as shown by a rapid sedimentation rate. High or increasing titers of antistreptococcal antibodies (antistreptolysin O and anti-DNAse B) are used to confirm recent infection; 10% of cases lack this serologic evidence.

Differential Diagnosis

Rheumatic fever may be confused with the following: rheumatoid arthritis, osteomyelitis, endocarditis, chronic meningococcemia, systemic lupus erythematosus, Lyme disease, sickle cell anemia, "surgical abdomen," and many other diseases.

Complications

Congestive heart failure occurs in severe cases. In the longer term, the development of rheumatic heart disease is the major problem. Other complications include arrhythmias, pericarditis with effusion, and rheumatic pneumonitis.

Treatment

A. General Measures: Bed rest should be enforced until: return of temperature to normal without medications; normal sedimentation rate; normal resting pulse rate (< 100/min in adults); and return of ECG to baseline.

B. Medical Measures:

1. Salicylates–The salicylates markedly reduce fever and relieve joint pain and swelling. They have no effect on the natural course of the disease. Adults may require aspirin, 0.6–0.9 g every 4 hours; children are treated with lower doses. Toxicity includes tinnitus, vomiting, and gastrointestinal bleeding.

2. Penicillin–Penicillin (benzathine penicillin, 1.2 million units intramuscularly once, or procaine penicillin, 600,000 units intramuscularly daily for 10 days) is employed to eradicate streptococcal infection if present. Erythromycin (dosage as above) may be substituted.

3. Corticosteroids–There is no proof that cardiac damage is prevented or minimized by corticosteroids. A short course of corticosteroids (prednisone, 40–60 mg orally daily, with tapering over 2 weeks) usually causes rapid improvement and is indicated when response to salicylates has been inadequate.

Prevention of Recurrent Rheumatic Fever

The initial episode of rheumatic fever can usually be prevented by early treatment of streptococcal pharyngitis. (See Chapter 32.) Prevention of recurrent episodes is critical. Recurrences of rheumatic fever are most common in patients who have had carditis during their initial episode and in children, 20% of whom will have a second episode within 5 years. Recurrences are uncommon after 5 years and infrequent in patients over 25 years of age. Prophylaxis is usually discontinued after these times except in groups with a high risk of streptococcal infection—parents of young children, nurses, military recruits, etc.

A. Penicillin: The preferred method of prophylaxis is with benzathine penicillin G, 1.2 million units intramuscularly every 4 weeks. Oral penicillin (200,000–250,000 units twice daily) is less reliable.

B. Sulfonamides or Erythromycin: If the patient is allergic to penicillin, sulfadiazine (or sulfisoxazole), 1 g daily throughout the year, may be substituted, as may erythromycin, 250 mg orally twice daily.

Prognosis

Initial episodes of rheumatic fever may last months in children and weeks in adults. The immediate mortality rate is 1–2%. Persistent rheumatic carditis with cardiomegaly, heart failure, and pericarditis imply a poor prognosis; 30% of children thus affected die within 10 years after the initial attack. Eighty percent of affected children attain adult life, and half of these have little if any limitation of activity. After 10 years, two-thirds of surviving patients will have detectable valvular disease. In adults, residual heart damage occurs in less than 20%, with mitral regurgitation the commonest; aortic insufficiency is more common than in children. In developing countries, acute rheumatic fever appears earlier in life, and the evolution to chronic valvular disease is accelerated.

Bisno AL: Group A streptococcal infections and acute rheumatic fever. N Engl J Med 1991;325:783. (Pathophysiology and epidemiology.)

Dajani AS et al: Prevention of rheumatic fever. Circulation 1988;78:1082. (American Heart Association consensus statement on who needs prophylaxis and what to give.)

Guidelines for the diagnosis of rheumatic fever. Jones Criteria, 1992 update. JAMA 1992;268:2069.

RHEUMATIC HEART DISEASE

Chronic rheumatic heart disease results from single or repeated attacks of rheumatic fever that produce rigidity and deformity of valve cusps, fusion of the commissures, or shortening and fusion of the chordae tendineae. Stenosis or insufficiency results, and the two often coexist. The mitral valve alone is affected in 50–60% of cases; combined lesions of the aortic and mitral valves occur in 20%; pure aortic lesions are seen in only 10%. Tricuspid involvement occurs only in association with mitral or aortic disease in about 10% of cases. The pulmonary valve is rarely affected. A history of rheumatic fever is obtainable in only 60% of patients with rheumatic heart disease.

The first clue to organic valvular disease is a murmur. Physical examination permits accurate diagnosis of most valve lesions. Echocardiography will reveal valve cusp thickening with decreased opening in stenosis, estimate the magnitude of regurgitation, and demonstrate the earliest stages of specific chamber enlargement.

Recurrences of acute rheumatic fever can be prevented (see above). The patient should also receive prophylactic antibiotics preceding dental extraction, urologic and surgical procedures, etc, to prevent endocarditis (Table 37–9). With mitral valve disease, it is important to identify the onset of atrial fibrillation in order to institute anticoagulation. The important findings in each of the major valve lesions are summarized in Table 10–1. The hemodynamic changes, symptoms, associated findings, and course have been discussed previously.

DISEASES OF THE PERICARDIUM

ACUTE PERICARDITIS

The pericardium consists of two layers: the inner visceral layer, which is attached to the epicardium; and an outer parietal layer. The pericardium stabilizes the heart in anatomic position and reduces contact between the heart and surrounding structures. It is composed of fibrous tissue, and while it is loose enough to permit moderate changes in cardiac size, it cannot stretch rapidly enough to accommodate rapid dilation of the heart or accumulation of fluid without increasing intrapericardial (and, therefore, intracardiac) pressure.

The pericardium is often involved by processes that affect the heart, but it may also be affected by diseases of adjacent tissues and may itself be a primary site of disease.

INFLAMMATORY PERICARDITIS

Acute inflammation of the pericardium may be infectious in origin or may be due to systemic diseases (autoimmune syndromes, uremia), neoplastic invasion, radiation effects, drug toxicity, leakage of blood into the pericardial space, or extension of inflammatory processes from the myocardium or lung. In many of these conditions, the pathologic process involves both the pericardium and the myocardium, and they often are associated with varying degrees of cardiac dysfunction.

The presentation and course of inflammatory pericarditis depend on its cause, but all syndromes are often (not always) associated with chest pain, which is usually pleuritic and postural (relieved by sitting). The pain is substernal but may radiate to the neck, shoulders, back, or epigastrium. Dyspnea may also be present. A pericardial friction rub is characteristic, with or without evidence of fluid accumulation or constriction (see below). Fever and leukocytosis are often present. The ECG usually shows generalized ST and T wave changes and may manifest a characteristic progression beginning with generalized ST elevation, followed by a return to baseline and then to T wave inversion. The chest x-ray may show cardiac enlargement if fluid has collected, as well as signs of related pulmonary disease. The echocardiogram may disclose pericardial effusions and indicate their hemodynamic significance, but it is often normal in inflammatory pericarditis.

Several of the specific pericarditis syndromes are discussed below.

Viral Pericarditis

Viral infections (especially infections with coxsackieviruses and echoviruses but also influenza, Epstein-Barr, varicella, hepatitis, mumps, and HIV viruses) are the commonest cause of acute pericarditis and probably are responsible for many cases classified as idiopathic. Males—usually under age 50—are most commonly affected. Pericardial involvement often follows upper respiratory infection. The diagnosis is usually clinical, but rising viral titers in paired sera may be obtained for confirmation. Cardiac enzymes may be slightly elevated, reflecting a myocarditic component. The differential diagnosis is primarily with myocardial infarction.

Treatment is generally symptomatic. Aspirin (650 mg every 3–4 hours) or other nonsteroidal agents (eg, indomethacin, 100–150 mg daily in divided doses) are usually effective. Corticosteroids may be beneficial in unresponsive cases. In general, symptoms subside in several days to weeks. The major early complication is tamponade, which occurs in fewer than 5% of patients. There may be recurrences in the first few weeks or months. Rare patients will continue to experience recurrences chronically, sometimes leading to constrictive pericarditis. Pericardial resection may be required.

Tuberculous Pericarditis

Tuberculous pericarditis has become rare in developed countries but remains common in other areas. It results from direct lymphatic or hematogenous spread; clinical pulmonary involvement may be absent or minor, although associated pleural effusions are common. The presentation tends to be subacute, but nonspecific symptoms (fever, night sweats, fatigue) may be present for days to months. Pericardial effusions are usually small or moderate but may be large. The diagnosis can be inferred if evidence of acid-fast bacilli are found elsewhere. The yield of organisms by pericardiocentesis is low; pericardial biopsy has a higher yield but may also be negative, and pericardiectomy may be required. Standard antituberculous drug therapy is usually successful (Table 9–8), but constrictive pericarditis can occur.

Other Infectious Pericarditides

Bacterial pericarditis has become rare and usually results from direct extension from pulmonary infections. Signs and symptoms are similar to those of other types of inflammatory pericarditides, but patients appear toxic—often critically ill. *Borrelia burgdorferi,* the organism responsible for Lyme disease, can also cause myopericarditis.

Uremic Pericarditis

This syndrome is a common complication of renal failure whose pathogenesis is uncertain; it occurs both with untreated uremia and in otherwise stable dialysis patients. The pericardium is characteristically "shaggy," and the effusion is hemorrhagic and exudative. Uremic pericarditis can present with or without symptoms; fever is absent. The pericarditis usually resolves with the institution of—or with more aggressive—dialysis. Tamponade is fairly common, and partial pericardiectomy (pericardial window) may be necessary. While anti-inflammatory agents may relieve the pain and fever associated with uremic pericarditis, a recent prospective double-blind randomized trial showed that indomethacin and systemic glucocorticoids did not affect the natural history of uremic pericarditis.

Neoplastic Pericarditis

Spread of adjacent lung cancer as well as invasion by breast cancer, renal cell carcinoma, Hodgkin's disease, and lymphomas are the commonest neoplastic processes involving the pericardium and have become the most frequent cause of pericardial tamponade in many countries. Often the process is painless, and the presenting symptoms relate to hemodynamic compromise or the primary disease. The diagnosis can usually be made by cytologic examination of the effusion or by biopsy, but it may be difficult to establish clinically if the patient has received mediastinal radiation within the previous year. MRI and CT scan can visualize neighboring tumor when present. The prognosis with neoplastic effusion is dismal, with only a small minority surviving 1 year. If it is compromising the patient, the effusion is initially drained. Instillation of chemotherapeutic agents or tetracycline may also prevent recurrence. Pericardial windows are rarely effective, but partial pericardiectomy from a subxiphoid incision may be successful; patients may be too ill to tolerate this.

Postmyocardial Infarction or Postcardiotomy Pericarditis (Dressler's Syndrome)

Pericarditis may occur 2–5 days after infarction due to an inflammatory reaction to myocardial necrosis. It usually presents as a recurrence of pain with pleural-pericardial features. A rub is often audible, and repolarization changes may be confused with ischemia. Large effusions are uncommon, and spontaneous resolution usually occurs in a few days. Aspirin or nonsteroidal agents in the dosages given in the section on viral pericarditis provide symptomatic relief.

Dressler's syndrome occurs weeks to several months after myocardial infarction or open heart surgery, may be recurrent, and probably represents an autoimmune syndrome. Patients present with typical pain, fever, malaise, and leukocytosis. The sedimentation rate is usually high. Large pericardial effusions and accompanying pleural effusions are frequent. Tamponade is rare with Dressler's syndrome after infarction but not when it occurs postoperatively. Nonsteroidal agents are given, but recurrences are common; corticosteroids are effective but may be difficult to withdraw without relapse.

Radiation Pericarditis

Radiation can initiate a fibrinous and fibrotic process in the pericardium, presenting as subacute pericarditis or constriction. The clinical onset is usually within the first year but may be delayed for many years. Radiation pericarditis usually follows treatments of more than 4000 cGy delivered to ports including more than 30% of the heart. Symptomatic therapy is the initial approach, but recurrent effusions and constriction often require surgery.

Other Causes of Pericarditis

These include connective tissue diseases, such as lupus erythematosus, rheumatoid arthritis, and drug-induced pericarditis (minoxidil, penicillins), and myxedema.

Arsenian MA: Cardiovascular sequelae of therapeutic thoracic radiation. Prog Cardiovasc Dis 1991;33:299. (A growing problem, particularly involving the pericardium.)

Fowler NO: Tuberculous pericarditis. JAMA 1991;266:99.

Park S, Bayer AS: Purulent pericarditis. Curr Clin Top Infect Dis 1992;12:56.

Shabetai R (editor): Disease of the pericardium. Cardiol Clin 1990;8(4):579. (Entire volume devoted to pericardial disease—pathophysiology, diagnosis, and treatment.)

PERICARDIAL EFFUSION

Pericardial effusion can develop during any of the processes discussed in the preceding paragraphs. The speed of accumulation determines the physiologic importance of the effusion. Because the pericardium stretches, large effusions (> 1000 mL) that develop slowly may produce no hemodynamic effects. Smaller effusions that appear rapidly can cause tamponade. Tamponade is characterized by elevated intrapericardial pressure (> 15 mm Hg), which restricts venous return and ventricular filling. As a result, the stroke volume and pulse pressure fall, and the heart rate and venous pressure rise. Shock and death may result.

Clinical Findings

A. Symptoms and Signs: Pericardial effusions may be associated with pain if they occur as part of an acute inflammatory process or may be painless, as is often the case with neoplastic or uremic effusion. Dyspnea and cough are common, especially with tamponade. Other symptoms may result from the primary disease.

A pericardial friction rub may be present even with large effusions. In cardiac tamponade, tachycardia, tachypnea, a narrow pulse pressure, and a relatively preserved systolic pressure are characteristic. Pulsus paradoxus—a greater than 10 mm Hg decline in systolic pressure during inspiration due to further impairment of left ventricular filling—is the classic finding, but it may also occur with obstructive lung disease. Central venous pressure is elevated, and edema or ascites may be present; these signs favor a more chronic process.

B. Laboratory Findings: Laboratory tests tend to reflect the underlying processes.

C. Diagnostic Studies: Chest x-ray can suggest effusion by an enlarged cardiac silhouette with a "water-bottle" configuration. The ECG often reveals nonspecific T wave changes and low QRS voltage. Electrical alternans may be present. Echocardiography, however, is the primary method for demonstrating pericardial effusion. Tamponade presents a characteristic picture of inadequate ventricular filling (diastolic collapse of the right ventricle or right atrium). The echocardiogram readily discriminates pericardial effusion from congestive heart failure. MRI also demonstrates pericardial fluid and lesions. Diagnostic pericardiocentesis or biopsy is often indicated for microbiologic and cytologic studies; a pericardial biopsy may be performed relatively simply through a small subxiphoid incision.

Treatment

Small effusions can be followed clinically and with the aid of echocardiograms. When tamponade is present, urgent pericardiocentesis is required. Removal of a small amount of fluid often produces immediate hemodynamic benefit, but complete drainage with a catheter is preferable. Continued drainage may be indicated.

Additional therapy is determined by the nature of the primary process. Recurrent effusion in neoplastic disease and uremia, in particular, may require partial pericardiectomy.

Ameli S, Shah PK: Cardiac tamponade: Pathophysiology, diagnosis, and management. Cardiol Clin 1991;9:665.
Hancock EW: Neoplastic pericardial disease. Cardiol Clin 1990;8:673.
Press OW, Livingston R: Management of malignant pericardial effusion and tamponade. JAMA 1987;257:1088.

CHRONIC CONSTRICTIVE PERICARDITIS

Chronic inflammation can lead to a thickened, fibrotic, adherent pericardium that restricts diastolic filling and produces chronically elevated venous pressures. In the past, tuberculosis was the most common cause of constrictive pericarditis, but the process now more often occurs after radiation therapy, cardiac surgery, or viral pericarditis.

The principal symptoms are slowly progressive

dyspnea, fatigue, and weakness. Chronic edema, hepatic congestion, and ascites are usually present. The examination reveals these signs and a characteristically elevated jugular venous pressure with a rapid y descent. Kussmaul's sign—an increase in jugular venous pressure during inspiration—occurs in constrictive pericarditis and restrictive cardiomyopathy. Pulsus paradoxus is unusual. Atrial fibrillation is common.

The chest x-ray may show normal heart size or cardiomegaly. Pericardial calcification is best seen on the lateral view and is common. Echocardiography can demonstrate a thick pericardium and small chambers. CT scans and MRI are helpful in revealing pericardial thickening and may be more sensitive than echocardiography.

The primary differential diagnoses are restrictive cardiomyopathy and tamponade. The former distinction can be difficult and is best made by evaluating left ventricular function (more consistently depressed in cardiomyopathy), measuring hemodynamics (which show more complete equalization of diastolic pressures in all four chambers in constrictive pericarditis), and demonstrating pericardial thickening and calcification.

Acute treatment consists of gentle diuresis. Surgical removal of the pericardium, which should be complete, is usually required in symptomatic patients but is associated with a relatively high mortality rate.

Brockington GM et al: Constrictive pericarditis. Cardiol Clin 1990;8:645.
Killian DM et al: Constrictive pericarditis after cardiac surgery. Am Heart J 1989;118:563. (Not a rare problem.)
Vaitkus PT, Kussmaul WG: Constrictive pericarditis versus restrictive cardiomyopathy: A reappraisal and update of diagnostic criteria. Am Heart J 1991;122:1431. (A very difficult problem.)

PULMONARY HYPERTENSION & HEART DISEASE

PRIMARY PULMONARY HYPERTENSION

Primary pulmonary hypertension is defined as pulmonary hypertension and elevated pulmonary vascular resistance in the absence of other disease of the lungs or heart. Pathologically, it is characterized by diffuse narrowing of the pulmonary arterioles. Circumstantial evidence suggests that unrecognized recurrent pulmonary emboli or in situ thrombosis may play a role in some cases. The latter may well be an exacerbating factor (precipitated by local endothelial injury) rather than a cause of the syndrome. Primary pulmonary hypertension must be distinguished from chronic pulmonary heart disease (cor pulmonale), recurrent pulmonary emboli, mitral stenosis, congenital heart disease, and occult mitral stenosis. Exclusion of secondary causes by echocardiography and lung scanning—and, if necessary, pulmonary angiography—is essential.

The clinical picture is similar to that of pulmonary hypertension from other causes. Patients—characteristically young women—present with evidence of right heart failure that is usually progressive, leading to death in 2–8 years. Patients have manifestations of low cardiac output, with weakness and fatigue, as well as edema and ascites as right heart failure advances. Peripheral cyanosis is present, and syncope on effort may occur.

The chest x-ray shows enlarged main pulmonary arteries with reduced peripheral branches. The right ventricle is enlarged. The ECG shows right ventricular and atrial hypertrophy.

Some authorities advocate chronic oral anticoagulation. The efficacy of vasodilator drugs is controversial, in part because the responses are variable. The calcium channel blockers nifedipine and diltiazem appear to be the preferred agents. The best response may be in patients in the earlier stages of the disease, when a more reversible vasoconstrictive component is present. A recent trial with chronic home infusions of prostacyclin showed both hemodynamic and clinical benefit in patients with advanced disease.

The prognosis in primary pulmonary hypertension is poor. Although most patients have a downhill course within a few years, some patients survive for 5–6 years. Heart-lung transplantation is being employed more frequently now with encouraging successes, resulting primarily from the availability of cyclosporine to decrease rejection.

D'Alonzo GE et al: Survival in patients with primary pulmonary hypertension. Ann Intern Med 1991;115:343. (Median survival 2–8 years, with early death predicted by poor hemodynamics.)

Palevsky HI, Fishman AP: The management of primary pulmonary hypertension. JAMA 1991;265:1014.

Rubin LJ: Primary pulmonary hypertension: Practical therapeutic recommendations. Drugs 1992;43:37. (Review of new approaches.)

PULMONARY HEART DISEASE (Cor Pulmonale)

Essentials of Diagnosis

- Symptoms and signs of chronic bronchitis and pulmonary emphysema.
- Elevated jugular venous pressure, parasternal lift, edema, hepatomegaly, ascites.
- ECG shows tall, peaked P waves (P pulmonale),

right axis deviation, and right ventricular hypertrophy.

- Chest x-ray: Enlarged right ventricle and pulmonary artery.
- Echocardiogram or radionuclide angiography excludes primary left ventricular dysfunction.

General Considerations

The term "cor pulmonale" denotes right ventricular hypertrophy and eventual failure resulting from pulmonary disease. Its clinical features depend upon both the primary disease and its effects on the heart.

Cor pulmonale is most commonly caused by chronic obstructive pulmonary disease. Rare causes include pneumoconiosis, pulmonary fibrosis, kyphoscoliosis, primary pulmonary hypertension, repeated episodes of subclinical or clinical pulmonary embolization, Pickwickian syndrome, schistosomiasis, and obliterative pulmonary capillary or lymphangitic infiltration from metastatic carcinoma. Hypoxia is the common denominator of these conditions which ultimately lead to cor pulmonale.

Clinical Findings

A. Symptoms and Signs: The predominant symptoms of compensated cor pulmonale are related to the pulmonary disorder and include chronic productive cough, exertional dyspnea, wheezing respirations, easy fatigability, and weakness. When the pulmonary disease causes right ventricular failure, these symptoms may be intensified. Dependent edema and right upper quadrant pain may also appear. The signs of cor pulmonale include cyanosis, clubbing, distended neck veins, right ventricular heave or gallop (or both), prominent lower sternal or epigastric pulsations, an enlarged and tender liver, and dependent edema.

B. Laboratory Findings: Polycythemia is often present in cor pulmonale secondary to COPD. The arterial oxygen saturation is below 85%; PCO_2 may or may not be elevated.

C. Electrocardiography and Chest X-Ray: The ECG may show right axis deviation and peaked P waves. Deep S waves are present in lead V_6. Right axis deviation and low voltage may be noted in patients with pulmonary emphysema. Frank right ventricular hypertrophy is uncommon except in "primary pulmonary hypertension." The ECG often mimics myocardial infarction; Q waves may be present in leads II, III, and aVF because of the vertically placed heart, but they are rarely deep or wide, as in inferior myocardial infarction. Supraventricular arrhythmias are frequent and nonspecific.

The chest radiograph discloses the presence or absence of parenchymal disease and a prominent or enlarged right ventricle and pulmonary artery.

D. Diagnostic Studies: Pulmonary function tests usually confirm the underlying lung disease. The echocardiogram should show normal left ventricular size and function but right ventricular dilation. Perfusion lung scans are rarely of value, but, if negative, they help to exclude pulmonary emboli, an occasional cause of cor pulmonale. Pulmonary angiography is the most specific method of diagnosis for the pulmonary emboli, but it carries increased risk when performed in patients with pulmonary hypertension.

Differential Diagnosis

In its early stages, cor pulmonale can be diagnosed on the basis of radiologic, echocardiographic, or electrocardiographic evidence. Catheterization of the right heart will establish a definitive diagnosis but is usually performed to exclude left-sided heart failure, which may in some patients be an inapparent cause of right-sided failure. Differential diagnostic considerations relate chiefly to the specific pulmonary disease that has produced right ventricular failure (see above).

Treatment

The details of the treatment of chronic pulmonary disease (chronic respiratory failure) are discussed in Chapter 7. Otherwise, therapy is directed at the pulmonary process responsible for right heart failure. Oxygen, salt and fluid restriction, and diuretics are mainstays; digitalis has no place in right heart failure unless atrial fibrillation is present.

Prognosis

Compensated cor pulmonale has the same outlook as the underlying pulmonary disease. Once congestive signs appear, the average life expectancy is 2–5 years, but survival is significantly longer when uncomplicated emphysema is the cause.

Dell'Italia LJ: The right ventricle: Anatomy, physiology, and clinical importance. Curr Probl Cardiol 1991;16 (10):653. (Comprehensive review that includes cor pulmonale, pulmonary hypertension, and other topics.)
Klinger JR, Hill NS: Right ventricular dysfunction in chronic obstructive pulmonary disease. Evaluation and management. Chest 1991;99:715.
Sherman S: Cor pulmonale: Treatment implications of right versus left ventricular impairment. Postgraduate Med 1992;91:227.

where are more frequent. Tumors involving the heart are bronchogenic carcinoma, carcinoma of the breast, malignant melanoma, the lymphomas, renal cell carcinoma, and, in patients with AIDS, Kaposi's sarcoma. These are often "silent" but may lead to pericardial tamponade, arrhythmias and conduction disturbances, heart failure, and peripheral emboli. The diagnosis is often made by echocardiography, but MRI and CT scanning are also helpful. The prognosis is dismal; effective treatment is not available.

The commonest primary tumors of the heart are atrial myxomas. These tend to occur in middle age, more often in women than in men. They usually originate in the intraventricular septum, with over 80% growing into the left atrium. Myxomas are benign tumors, but they can metastasize by embolization.

Patients with myxoma can present with a picture of a systemic illness, obstruction of blood flow through the heart, or signs of peripheral embolization. The characteristic picture includes fever, malaise, weight loss, leukocytosis, elevated sedimentation rate, and emboli (peripheral or pulmonary, depending on the location of the tumor). This picture is often confused with infective endocarditis, lymphoma, other cancers, or autoimmune diseases. In other cases, the tumor may grow to considerable size and produce symptoms by obstructing mitral flow. Episodic pulmonary edema (classically occurring when an upright posture is assumed) and signs of low output may result. Physical examination may reveal a diastolic sound related to motion of the tumor ("tumor plop") or a diastolic murmur similar to that of mitral stenosis. Right-sided myxomas may cause symptoms of right-sided failure. The diagnosis is established by echocardiography or by pathologic study of embolic material. MRI is also useful. Contrast angiography is usually not necessary. Surgical excision is usually curative.

Other primary cardiac tumors include rhabdomyomas, fibrous histiocytomas, hemangiomas, and a variety of unusual sarcomas. The diagnosis may be supported by an abnormal cardiac contour on x-ray. Echocardiography is usually helpful but may miss tumors infiltrating the ventricular wall. It is likely that MRI will be useful as well.

Salcedo EE et al: Cardiac tumors: Diagnosis and management. Curr Probl Cardiol 1992;17(2):75.

NEOPLASTIC DISEASES OF THE HEART

THE CARDIAC PATIENT & SURGERY

Primary cardiac tumors are rare and constitute only a small fraction of all tumors that involve the heart or pericardium. Metastases from malignant tumors else-

Patients with known or suspected cardiac disease undergoing general surgery present a common management problem. Anesthesia and surgery are often associated with marked fluctuations of heart rate and blood pressure, changes in intravascular volume, myocardial ischemia or depression, arrhythmias, decreased oxygenation, increased sympathetic nervous system activity, and alterations in medical regimens and pharmacokinetics. Even with careful monitoring and management, the perioperative period can be very stressful to cardiac patients.

The risk of surgery in patients with heart disease depends primarily on three factors: the type of operation, the nature of the heart disease, and the degree of preoperative stability. The type of anesthesia is less important, though halothane, enflurane, and barbiturates are more severe myocardial depressants, while narcotics have little depressive effect. Spinal and epidural anesthesia were previously thought to be preferable in patients with heart disease, but this has not proved to be the case.

The highest-risk procedures are surgery of the aorta and vascular procedures, in part because these patients often have associated severe coronary disease but also because marked blood pressure and volume changes are common. Major abdominal and thoracic surgery are also associated with substantial cardiovascular risk, especially in older patients with associated cardiovascular disease.

Numerous studies have evaluated the excess risk of surgery in patients with various cardiac diseases. Recent (within 3 months) myocardial infarction, unstable angina, congestive heart failure, significant aortic stenosis, uncontrolled hypertension (> 180/110 mm Hg), and complex ventricular arrhythmias all are associated with substantial increases in operative morbidity and mortality rates. Any degree of instability in these conditions magnifies the potential risk. Although less common, cyanotic congenital heart disease and severe primary or secondary pulmonary hypertension pose great risks during major surgery. In patients with any of these problems, the risk-to-benefit ratio of the planned surgery should be carefully examined. If the procedure is necessary but elective, consideration should be given to delaying it until full recovery postinfarction and correction or optimal stabilization of the other conditions are achieved. Hypertension should be at least moderately controlled. Patients with severe angina should have increased medical therapy or be considered for revascularization before noncardiac surgery. Symptomatic arrhythmias, nonsustained ventricular tachycardia, or high-grade atrioventricular block and cardiac failure should be treated optimally.

Clinical assessment provides the most useful guidance in determining the risk of noncardiac surgery. The use of multifactorial indices is discussed in the articles by Abraham and Wong cited below. Important indicators of high risk have been discussed above. Patients with known but clinically stable heart disease, such as angina pectoris or prior myocardial infarction, are at intermediate risk, particularly for major operations such as vascular surgery. If a history or symptoms of heart failure are present, assessment of left ventricular function can be very helpful in perioperative management. Although frequently advocated, further noninvasive testing for myocardial ischemia for the purpose of risk stratification is probably overutilized. Tests such as stress myocardial perfusion scintigraphy or dobutamine echocardiography should be reserved for situations in which the results may alter patient management. There is no evidence that prophylactic revascularization by either PTCA or coronary artery bypass surgery alters long-Dterm outcome in patients (eg, the combined morbidity and mortality of the two surgical procedures) without the usual indications for these procedures. Only in the case of major vascular operations is perioperative mortality and morbidity high enough that this may be the case in selected individuals.

Once the decision to operate is made, careful management is essential. Most cardiac medications should be continued preoperatively and postoperatively. Monitoring is the best prophylactic measure; hemodynamic monitoring is critical for patients with heart failure, severe valve disease, or easily induced myocardial ischemia. Excessive hypertension, hypotension, and myocardial ischemia should be searched for and appropriately treated using rapidly acting agents. Transesophageal echocardiography provides another useful technique for continuous monitoring of cardiac function and detection of ischemic episodes. Ischemic events, whether symptomatic or silent, should be vigorously treated.

Abraham SA et al: Coronary risk of non-cardiac surgery. Prog Cardiovasc Dis 1991;34:205. (Comprehensive review, with emphasis on risk stratification by dipyridamole thallium scintigraphy.)

Massie BM, Mangano DT: Assessment of perioperative risk: Have we put the cart before the horse? J Am Coll Cardiol 1993;21:1356. (Editorial suggesting that risk stratification with expensive diagnostic tests is often not justified.)

Massie BM: Cardiac disease and the surgical patient. In: *Current Surgical Diagnosis & Treatment,* 10th ed. Way LW (editor). Appleton & Lange, 1993.

Salem DN et al: Assessment and management of cardiac disease in the surgical patient. Curr Probl Cardiol 1989;14(4):171.

Wong T, Detsky AS: Preoperative cardiac risk assessment for patients having peripheral vascular surgery. Ann Intern Med 1992;116:743. (Role of noninvasive cardiac tests.)

THE CARDIAC PATIENT & PREGNANCY

The management of cardiac disease in pregnancy is discussed in detail in the references listed below. Only a few major points can be covered in this brief section.

CARDIOVASCULAR CHANGES DURING PREGNANCY

Normal physiologic changes during pregnancy can exacerbate symptoms of underlying cardiac disease even in previously asymptomatic individuals. Maternal blood volume rises progressively until the end of the sixth or seventh month. Stroke volume increases over the same time course as a result of the volume change and an increase in ejection fraction. The latter reflects predominantly a decline in peripheral resistance due to vasodilation and the low-resistance shunting through the placenta. The heart rate tends to rise in the third trimester. Overall, cardiac output increases by 30–50%; systolic blood pressure tends to decline slightly or remain unchanged, but diastolic pressure falls significantly.

High cardiac output causes alterations in the cardiac examination. A third heart sound is prominent and normal, and a pulmonary flow murmur is common. Electrocardiographic changes include rate-related decreases in PR and QT intervals, a leftward axis shift, inferior Q waves due to the more horizontal position of the heart, and nonspecific ST–T wave changes.

MANAGEMENT OF PREEXISTING CONDITIONS

The physiologic changes imposed by pregnancy can cause cardiac decompensation in patients with any significant cardiac abnormality, but the most severe problems are encountered in patients with valvular stenosis (especially mitral and aortic stenosis), congenital or acquired abnormalities associated with pulmonary hypertension or right-to-left shunting, congestive heart failure due to any cause, coronary heart disease, and hypertension. Valvular insufficiency or left-to-right shunting often diminishes because of the fall in peripheral resistance and is better tolerated.

Mitral stenosis becomes more hemodynamically severe owing to the increase in diastolic flow and the rate-related shortening of diastole. Left atrial pressures rise, and dyspnea or pulmonary edema can

occur in previously asymptomatic individuals. The onset of atrial fibrillation often leads to acute decompensation. Patients with moderate to severe stenosis should have the condition corrected prior to becoming pregnant if possible. Patients who become symptomatic can undergo successful surgery, preferably in the third trimester. Balloon valvuloplasty is an attractive alternative, though radiation exposure to the fetus is unavoidable. Coarctation is usually well tolerated, but patients with symptoms should have corrective surgery before pregnancy. Patients with severe pulmonary hypertension and cyanotic congenital heart disease and those with severe aortic stenosis are at extremely high risk and should not become pregnant unless surgical correction is undertaken.

Asymptomatic arrhythmias should be closely observed unless underlying heart disease is present, in which case they should be treated with drugs. Paroxysmal supraventricular arrhythmias are quite common. Patients with Wolff-Parkinson-White syndrome often have more problems during pregnancy. Therapy is similar to that required for nonpregnant women.

Preexisting systemic hypertension is usually well tolerated and controllable, though the fetal morbidity rate is slightly increased. The incidence of preeclampsia and eclampsia (see Chapter 15) is increased.

Most experts discourage treatment with diuretics because hypovolemia may reduce uterine blood flow. Hydralazine and methyldopa have been well tolerated. Beta-blockers may retard fetal growth, but experience with them has been generally favorable. A recent advisory has noted injury to the fetus with ACE inhibitors. Little is known about the safety of most other antihypertensive agents.

CARDIOVASCULAR COMPLICATIONS OF PREGNANCY

Pregnancy-related hypertension (eclampsia and preeclampsia) is discussed in Chapter 15.

Cardiomyopathy of Pregnancy (Peripartum Cardiomyopathy)

In approximately one out of 4000–15,000 patients, dilated cardiomyopathy develops in the final month of pregnancy or within 6 months after delivery. The cause is unclear, but immune and viral causes have been postulated. The course of the disease is variable; many cases improve or resolve completely over several months, but others progress to refractory heart failure. Immunosuppressive therapy has been advocated, but few supportive data are available. Recently, beta-blockers have been administered judiciously to these patients, with at least anecdotal success. Recurrence in subsequent pregnancies has been reported.

Aortic Dissection

Pregnancy predisposes to aortic dissection, perhaps because of the accompanying connective tissue changes. Dissection usually occurs near term or shortly postpartum and is managed as it is in other patients; it may occur in the arteries in addition to the aorta, including the coronary arteries.

SPECIAL PROBLEMS

Prophylaxis for Infective Endocarditis

Although there is not universal agreement, many authorities recommend antibiotic prophylaxis during labor for patients at risk for endocarditis, especially if forceps or an episiotomy is employed. Ampicillin (2 g intravenously or intramuscularly) plus gentamicin (1.5 mg/kg intravenously or intramuscularly [up to 80 mg]) followed by amoxicillin, 1.5 g orally every 6 hours, is the recommended regimen.

Management of Labor

While vaginal delivery is usually well tolerated, unstable patients (including patients with severe hypertension and worsening heart failure) should have cesarean section. An increased risk of aortic rupture has been noted during delivery in patients with coarctation of the aorta and severe aortic root dilation with Marfan's syndrome, and vaginal delivery should be avoided in these conditions.

Cardiovascular Drugs During Pregnancy

Experience during pregnancy with many drugs is limited, and the effect on the fetus is often not well defined. Drugs with known potential for teratogenicity or fetal injury include phenytoin and the ACE inhibitors. Warfarin also presents a risk, but—at least in patients with prosthetic heart valves—many recommend that it be continued until the final 2 weeks. Self-injected heparin offers an alternative. Drugs that appear to be safe are hydralazine, methyldopa, digitalis, quinidine, procainamide, lidocaine, and short-term verapamil. Diuretics and beta-blockers are relatively safe but may have undesirable physiologic effects.

Burlew BS: Managing the pregnant patient with heart disease. Clin Cardiol 1990;13:757.

Douglas PS: *Heart Disease in Women.* Davis, 1989. (Six chapters deal with problems related to pregnancy.)

Elkayam U, Gleicher N (editors): *Cardiac Problems in Pregnancy: Diagnosis and Management of Maternal and Fetal Diseases,* 2nd ed. Alan R. Liss, 1989.

Midei MG et al: Peripartum myocarditis and cardiomyopathy. Circulation 1990;81:922. (Myocarditis may be the cause of peripartum myopathy, and immunosuppression may be effective.)

UCLA Conference: Pregnancy and congenital heart disease. Ann Intern Med 1990;112:445.

REFERENCES

Braunwald E (editor): *Heart Disease: A Textbook of Cardiovascular Medicine,* 4th ed. Saunders, 1992. (References up to 1990–1991 in many chapters.)

Chatterjee F et al (editors): *Cardiology: An Illustrated Text/Reference,* 2 vols. Lippincott, 1991. (Looseleaf text with beautiful illustrations.)

Fowler NO: *Diagnosis of Heart Disease.* Springer-Verlag, 1991.

Fozzard HA et al (editors): *The Heart and Cardiovascular System: Scientific Foundations,* 2 vols. Raven Press, 1991. (Outstanding reference book blending science and clinical medicine.)

Froelicher VF et al (editors): *Exercise and the Heart,* 3rd ed. Mosby, 1993.

Gazes PC: *Clinical Cardiology,* 3rd ed. Lea & Febiger, 1990. (For students and practitioners with an interest in cardiology.)

Hillis LD: *Manual of Clinical Problems in Cardiology: With Annotated Key References,* 4th ed. Little, Brown, 1992.

Katz AM: *Physiology of the Heart,* 2nd ed. Raven Press, 1992.

Kirklin JW, BarrattDBoyes B (editors): *Cardiac Surgery,* 2nd ed. Churchill Livingstone, 1993.

Marcus ML et al (editors): *Cardiac Imaging: A Companion to Braunwald's Heart Disease.* Saunders, 1991. (By experts in fields of noninvasive and invasive techniques.)

Opie LH (editor): *Drugs For The Heart,* 3rd ed. Saunders, 1991. (Multi-authored comprehensive monograph.)

Perloff JF: *Physical Examination of the Heart and Circulation,* 2nd ed. Saunders, 1990. (For readers at all levels of experience.)

Schlant RC et al (editors): *Hurst's The Heart,* 8th ed. McGraw-Hill, 1993.

Sokolow M, McIlroy MB, Cheitlin MD: *Clinical Cardiology,* 6th ed. Appleton & Lange, 1992. (More compact and practical book for the student, resident, and primary care physician.)

Willerson JT (editor): *Treatment of Heart Disease.* Gower, 1992. (Clinically oriented, beautifully illustrated.)

Systemic Hypertension

11

Barry M. Massie, MD

Hypertension is an important preventable cause of cardiovascular disease; untreated, it increases the incidence of stroke, coronary events, heart failure, and renal failure and shortens life expectancy. Hypertension alone increases the risk of each of these outcomes, but it also is synergistic with other risk factors such as hyperlipidemia, smoking, and diabetes. Although awareness of hypertension has increased, only about 20% of hypertensive patients have satisfactory blood pressure control. Although hypertension alone increases the risk of each of these outcomes, it is synergistic with other risk factors such as hyperlipidemia, smoking, and diabetes. Only about half of the hypertensive population are aware they have the condition, and only half of those who are aware of it have their pressure normalized by treatment.

Until recently, hypertension was diagnosed and categorized primarily based upon diastolic blood pressure readings. However, it has long been recognized that morbidity and mortality increase as both systolic and diastolic blood pressures rise, and that in individuals over age 50 the systolic blood pressure is a better predictor of complications. Recent trials have demonstrated the importance of treating patients with isolated or predominantly systolic hypertension. The importance of systolic hypertension has been recognized in the recently released Fifth Report of the Joint National Committee on Detection, Evaluation, and Treatment of High Blood Pressure (JNCDV). As shown in Table 11–1, hypertension is now diagnosed based upon elevations of either the systolic or diastolic blood pressure, and the objective of management is to achieve reductions in both.

Blood pressure should be measured with a well-calibrated sphygmomanometer using standard procedural guidelines. Because blood pressure readings in many individuals are highly variable—especially in the office setting—the diagnosis of hypertension should be made only after elevation is noted on three readings on different occasions, usually over a period of several months unless the elevations are severe or associated with symptoms (see Table 11–1). Transient elevation of blood pressure caused by excitement or apprehension does not constitute hypertensive disease but may indicate a propensity toward its evolution. Ambulatory 24-hour blood pressure monitoring may be helpful in evaluating patients with borderline or variable office blood pressure, as well as in assessing resistant hypertension and possible treatment-related hypotensive symptoms. This technique has become convenient and increasingly available, but it should be employed only to address specific management problems because of its high cost (approximately $300.00).

Continued hypertension does not necessarily indicate the need for pharmacologic treatment. Nonpharmacologic approaches and individualized assessment of the benefit-to-risk ratio of drug therapy should precede pharmacologic management in patients with mild hypertension (diastolic pressure < 100 mm Hg; systolic < 160 mm Hg).

The Fifth Report of the Joint National Committee on Detection, Education, and Treatment of High Blood Pressure (JNC V). Arch Intern Med 1993;153:154. (Newly revised guidelines for evaluation and treatment of hypertension.)

Littenberg B et al: Screening for hypertension. Ann Intern Med 1990;112:192. (Valuable and cost-effective.)

National High Blood Pressure Education Program Working Group report on ambulatory blood pressure monitoring. Arch Intern Med 1990;150:2270. (Standards, results, and applications.)

Recommendations for routine blood pressure measurement by indirect cuff sphygmomanometry. Am J Hypertens 1992;5:207. (Pitfalls and guidelines from the American Society of Hypertension.)

MANAGEMENT OF HYPERTENSION

Etiology & Classification

A. Primary (Essential) Hypertension: In about 95% of cases, no cause can be established. The condition occurs in 10–15% of white adults and 20–30% of black adults in the USA. The onset of essential hypertension is usually between ages 25 and 55. Hypertension is uncommon before age 20. In young people it is commonly caused by renal insufficiency, renal artery stenosis, or coarctation of the aorta.

Elevations in pressure are transient early in the course of the disease but eventually become permanent. Even in established cases, the blood pressure fluctuates widely in response to emotional stress and physical activity. Blood pressures taken by the pa-

Table 11–1. Classification and follow-up of blood pressure measurements.[1]

Category[2]	Systolic Blood Pressure (mm Hg)	Diastolic Blood Pressure (mm Hg)	Follow-Up Recommended
Normal	<130	<85	Recheck in 2 years.
High Normal	130–139	85–89	Recheck in 1 year.[3]
Hypertension[4]			
Stage 1 (mild)	140–159	90–99	Confirm within 2 months.
Stage 2 (moderate)	160–179	100–109	Evaluate or refer within 1 month.
Stage 3 (severe)	180–209	110–119	Evaluate or refer within 1 week.
Stage 4 (very severe)	≥210	≥120	Evaluate or refer immediately.

[1]The Fifth Report of the Joint National Committee on Detection, Education, and Treatment of High Blood Pressure (JNC-V). Arch Intern Med 1993;153:154.

[2]When systolic and diastolic pressures fall into different categories, the higher category should be selected to classify the individual's blood pressure. Isolated systolic hypertension is defined as a systolic blood pressure of 140 mm Hg or more and a diastolic blood pressure of less than 90 mm Hg.

[3]Consider offering counseling about life-style modifications.

[4]In individuals aged 18 years or older not taking antihypertensive drugs and not acutely ill. Based on the average of two or more readings on two or more occasions after initial screening.

tient at home or during daily activities using a portable apparatus are often lower than those recorded in the office, clinic, or hospital and may be more reliable in estimating prognosis.

The pathogenesis of essential hypertension is multifactorial. Genetic factors play an important role. Children with one—and even more so with two—hypertensive parents tend to have higher blood pressures. Abnormal cation exchange in red blood cells has been suggested to be a potential marker of a genetic defect.

Environmental factors also appear to play an important role. Increased salt intake has long been incriminated as a pathogenic factor in essential hypertension. Increased salt intake alone is probably not sufficient to elevate blood pressure to abnormal levels; a combination of too much salt plus a genetic predisposition is required. Cl^- may be as important as Na^+ in the pathogenesis of hypertension. Other factors that may be involved in the pathogenesis of essential hypertension are the following:

1. Sympathetic nervous system hyperactivity–Sympathetic nervous system hyperactivity is most apparent in younger hypertensives, who may exhibit tachycardia and an elevated cardiac output. However, this is usually transient, and correlations between plasma catecholamines and blood pressure have generally been poor. Insensitivity of the baroreflexes may play a role in the genesis of adrenergic hyperactivity. Sympathetic activation may also play a role in "labile" hypertension, characterized by marked blood pressure fluctuations under differing, or even similar, circumstances.

2. Renin-angiotensin system–Renin, a proteolytic enzyme, is secreted by the juxtaglomerular cells surrounding afferent arterioles in response to a number of stimuli, including reduced renal perfusion pressure, diminished intravascular volume, circulating catecholamines, increased sympathetic nervous system activity, increased arteriolar stretch, and hypokalemia. Renin acts on angiotensinogen or renin substrate to cleave off the ten-amino-acid peptide angiotensin I. This peptide is then acted upon by angiotensin-converting enzyme to create the eight-amino-acid peptide angiotensin II, a potent vasoconstrictor and a major stimulant of aldosterone release from the adrenal glands. Despite the important role of this system in the regulation of blood pressure, it probably does not play a primary role in the pathogenesis of essential hypertension in most individuals. Black hypertensives and older patients tend to have lower plasma renin activity. Patients with low plasma renin activity may have higher intravascular volumes. Plasma renin activity levels can be best classified in relation to dietary sodium intake or urinary sodium excretion. Approximately 10% of essential hypertension patients have relatively high levels, 60% have essentially normal levels, and 30% have relatively low levels. Although such measurements have contributed to our understanding of the pathophysiology of hypertension, there is little clinical utility to measuring plasma renin activity.

3. Defect in natriuresis–Normal individuals increase their renal sodium excretion in response to elevations in arterial pressure and to a sodium or volume load. Hypertensive patients, particularly when their blood pressure is normal, exhibit a diminished ability to excrete a sodium load. This defect may result in increased plasma volume and hypertension. However, during chronic hypertension, a sodium load is usually handled normally.

4. Intracellular sodium and calcium–There is growing evidence that intracellular Na^+ is elevated in blood cells and other tissues in essential hypertension. This may result from abnormalities in Na^+-K^+ exchange and other Na^+ transport mechanisms. Circulating "digitalis-like" substances may be responsible. An increase in intracellular Na^+ may lead to increased intracellular Ca^{2+} concentrations as a result of facilitated exchange. This could explain the increase in vascular smooth muscle tone that is characteristic of established hypertension.

5. Exacerbating factors–A number of conditions exacerbate or precipitate hypertension in predisposed individuals. The best-documented of these is **obesity,** which is associated with an increase in intravascular volume and an appropriately high output.

Weight reduction in the obese lowers blood pressure slightly. Excessive use of **alcohol** also raises blood pressure, perhaps by increasing plasma catecholamines. Hypertension can be difficult to control in patients who consume more than 40 g of ethanol (two drinks) daily or drink in "binges." **Cigarette smoking** acutely raises blood pressure, again by increasing plasma norepinephrine, but the long-term effect of smoking in essential hypertension is less clear. Blood pressure should not be measured within 1 hour after smoking or 12 hours after alcohol consumption. The relationship of **exercise** to hypertension is also uncertain, although exercise training can lower blood pressure modestly. Despite popular preconceptions, the relationship between stress and hypertension is not as close. **Polycythemia** increases the viscosity, whether it be primary or due to diminished plasma volume. This may raise blood pressure.

B. Secondary Hypertension: With complete evaluation, approximately 5% of patients with hypertension can be found to have specific causes. These are labeled secondary hypertension.

1. Estrogen use–The most common definable cause is the chronic use of oral contraceptive pills. A small increase in blood pressure occurs in most women taking oral contraceptives, but considerable rises may occur. This is caused by volume expansion due to increased activity of the renin-angiotensin-aldosterone system. The primary abnormality is an increase in the hepatic synthesis of renin substrate. Approximately 5% of women taking oral contraceptives chronically will exhibit a rise in blood pressure above 140/90 mm Hg; this represents twice the expected prevalence. Contraceptive-related hypertension is more common in women over 35 years of age, in those who have taken contraceptives for more than 5 years, and in obese individuals. It is less common in those taking low-dose estrogen tablets. In most cases, hypertension is reversible by discontinuing the contraceptive, but it may take several weeks. There is no evidence that postmenopausal estrogen use causes hypertension.

2. Renal disease–Virtually any disease of the renal parenchyma can produce secondary hypertension. The mechanism of renal hypertension is multifaceted, but most instances are related to increased intravascular volume or increased activity of the renin-angiotensin-aldosterone system. Hypertension exaggerates progression of renal insufficiency, so its early recognition and vigorous treatment is important. Hypertension may be reversed if plasma volume is controlled by drugs or dialysis or after bilateral nephrectomy (rarely necessary) and is often improved by renal transplantation. However, posttransplantation hypertension is also a problem; this is now recognized to be in part precipitated by immunosuppressive therapy with cyclosporine.

3. Renal vascular hypertension–Renal artery stenosis is a common cause of secondary hypertension and is present in 1–2% of hypertensive patients. The cause in younger individuals is most commonly fibromuscular hyperplasia. This accounts for approximately 30% of renal vascular disease, though it is more common in women under 50. The remainder of renal vascular disease is due to atherosclerotic stenoses of the proximal renal arteries. The mechanism of renal vascular hypertension is excessive renin release due to reduction in renal blood flow and perfusion pressure. Renal vascular hypertension may occur when a single branch of the renal artery is obstructed, but in as many as 25% of patients both arteries are obstructed.

Renal vascular hypertension may present in the same manner as essential hypertension but should be suspected in the following circumstances: (1) if the onset is below age 20 or after age 50, (2) if there are epigastric or renal artery bruits, (3) if there is atherosclerosis elsewhere, or (4) if there is abrupt deterioration in renal function after administration of angiotensin-converting enzyme inhibitors. Renal angiograms may be indicated if anatomic stenosis is strongly suggested by the history and signs and if the hypertensive disease is difficult to control medically.

There is no ideal "screening" test for renal vascular hypertension. All tests are sufficiently nonspecific so that in populations with a low incidence of the disease, false-positive results will exceed true-positives. In addition, none of these tests have more than 80% sensitivity. Additional diagnostic testing is appropriate only in the high-risk populations described in the previous paragraph. If the suspicion of renal vascular hypertension is sufficiently high, renal arteriography, the definitive diagnostic test, is the best approach. Where suspicion is moderate to low, radioisotope renography performed before and after administration of an angiotensin-converting enzyme inhibitor is probably the best noninvasive diagnostic test. The baseline study may show a smaller kidney with diminished function on the side of the stenosis. Postdrug (captopril, 100 mg orally, or enalaprilat, 2.5 mg intravenously) uptake and clearance of the radiotracer are delayed. However, bilateral disease may be difficult to detect if both kidneys are equally affected. The physiologic significance of the stenosis can be assessed by measuring differences in renin activity in the two renal veins.

The treatment of patients with recognized renal vascular hypertension is controversial. Young individuals and good-risk patients of any age who have not responded to medical therapy should have the lesion corrected. Although the surgical results from renal artery reconstruction are generally good, percutaneous transluminal angioplasty is now the preferred approach for fibromuscular hyperplasia and for discrete stenotic arteriosclerotic lesions that do not involve the renal artery ostium. Older individuals, particularly if they have bilateral disease or other risk factors, may be managed medically if renal function does not deteriorate. The use of converting enzyme inhibitors has improved the success rate of medical therapy, but these have been associated with marked hypotension and deterioration of renal function in individuals with bilateral renal artery stenosis.

4. Primary hyperaldosteronism and Cushing's syndrome–Most patients with adrenal hypertension have excess aldosterone secretion as the underlying pathophysiologic process. They make up less than 0.5% of all cases of hypertension. The usual lesion is an adrenal adenoma, although a minority of patients have bilateral adrenal hyperplasia. The diagnosis should be suspected when patients present with hypokalemia prior to diuretic therapy and when this is associated with excessive urinary potassium excretion and suppressed levels of plasma renin activity. Aldosterone concentrations in urine and blood are elevated. The lesion can be demonstrated by CT scanning as well as by MRI and abdominal ultrasound. Even less commonly, patients with Cushing's syndrome (glucocorticoid excess) may manifest hypertension as a first sign (see Chapter 25).

5. Pheochromocytoma–Although hypertension due to pheochromocytoma is often thought to be episodic, most patients have chronic blood pressure elevations. The majority of patients have exaggerated orthostatic blood pressure changes, and many develop glucose intolerance. The diagnosis and treatment of this entity are discuss in Chapter 25.

6. Coarctation of the aorta–This uncommon cause of hypertension is discussed in Chapter 10.

7. Hypertension associated with pregnancy–Hypertension occurring de novo or worsening during pregnancy is one of the commonest causes of maternal and fetal morbidity and mortality (see Chapter 17).

8. Other causes of secondary hypertension–Hypertension has also been associated with hyperparathyroidism, hypercalcemia due to any cause, acromegaly, hyperthyroidism, hypothyroidism, and a variety of neurologic disorders causing increased intracranial pressure.

Alcohol and hypertension—implications for management. A consensus statement by the World Hypertension League. J Hum Hypertens 1991;5:227. (Review of data and recommendations.)

Cunningham FG, Lindheimer MD: Hypertension in pregnancy. N Engl J Med 1992;326:927.

Hall JE et al: Abnormal pressure natriuresis. A cause or consequence of hypertension. Hypertension 1990; 15:547. (Good discussion of possible mechanism of essential hypertension.)

Mann SJ, Pickering TG: Detection of renovascular hypertension. State of the art: 1992. Ann Intern Med 1992; 117:845. (Several noninvasive tests are sensitive enough to screen high-risk patients.)

National High Blood Pressure Education Program Working Group report on primary prevention of hypertension. Arch Intern Med 1993;153:186. (Extensively documented report which discusses population and individual approaches to the prevention and non-drug treatment of hypertension.)

Pickering TG: Diagnosis and evaluation of renovascular hypertension: Indications for therapy. Circulation 1991; 83(Suppl I):I–147. (How and whom to evaluate. This supplement also includes articles on renal artery angioplasty and surgery.)

Ram CVS (editor): Secondary hypertension. Cardiol Clin 1988;6(4):465. (Good chapters on when to perform evaluation for secondary hypertension and on each of the potential causes.)

Stadel BV: Oral contraceptives and cardiovascular disease. N Engl J Med 1981;305:672. (Still useful review of contraceptive-related hypertension and other problems.)

van Hooft IMS et al: Renal hemodynamics and the renin-angiotensin-aldosterone system in normotensive subjects with hypertensive and normotensive parents. N Engl J Med 1991;324:1305. (Renal hemodynamics abnormal at an early age, prior to systemic hypertension.)

Young WF et al: Primary aldosteronism: Diagnosis and treatment. Mayo Clin Proc 1990;65:960.

Complications of Untreated Hypertension

Complications of hypertension are related either to sustained elevations of blood pressure, with consequent changes in the vasculature and heart, or to atherosclerosis that accompanies and is accelerated by long-standing hypertension. The excess morbidity and mortality related to hypertension are progressive over the whole range of systolic and diastolic blood pressures. However, target-organ damage varies markedly between individuals with similar levels of office hypertension. Ambulatory pressures are more closely related to end-organ damage. In general, blacks of both sexes and white males have a higher incidence of complications from hypertension. Specific complications include the following:

A. Hypertensive Cardiovascular Disease: Cardiac complications are the major causes of morbidity and mortality in essential hypertension, and preventing them is a major goal of therapy. Left ventricular hypertrophy is found in 10–30% of chronic hypertensives, depending on the level of blood pressure, the duration of hypertension, the technique of diagnosis (echocardiography is more sensitive than electrocardiography), and additional factors that remain poorly understood. Once established, left ventricular hypertrophy is an indication of increased risk for morbidity and mortality; for any level of blood pressure, its presence is associated with a several-fold increase in risk. A number of epidemiologic studies have shown that echocardiographic left ventricular hypertrophy is the best predictor of prognosis. Left ventricular hypertrophy may cause or facilitate many cardiac complications of hypertension, including congestive heart failure, ventricular arrhythmias, myocardial ischemia, and sudden death.

Left ventricular diastolic dysfunction, which may present with many of the signs and symptoms of congestive heart failure, is common in patients with long-standing hypertension. Hypertensive left ventricular hypertrophy regresses with therapy; it is uncertain whether this is a nonspecific response to blood pressure reduction or whether it is facilitated by treatment with certain classes of drugs such as the sympatholytic agents, calcium channel blockers, and angiotensin-converting enzyme inhibitors.

While hypertension alone can lead to many of these cardiac complications, the combination of hypertension with coronary artery disease or alcohol abuse is synergistic in producing these complications.

B. Hypertensive Cerebrovascular Disease: Hypertension is the major predisposing cause of stroke, especially intracerebral hemorrhage but also cerebral infarction. Cerebrovascular complications are more closely correlated with the systolic than the diastolic blood pressure. The incidence of these complications is markedly reduced by antihypertensive therapy.

C. Hypertensive Renal Disease: Chronic hypertension leads to nephrosclerosis, a common cause of renal insufficiency. Hypertensive renal damage is limited by successful therapy. Secondary renal disease is more common in blacks than whites.

D. Aortic Dissection: Hypertension is a major cause and exacerbating factor in many patients with dissection of the aorta. The diagnosis and treatment of aortic dissection are discussed in Chapter 12.

E. Atherosclerotic Complications: Most patients with hypertension in the USA die of complications of atherosclerosis, but the linkage between hypertension and atherosclerotic cardiovascular disease is much less close than that with the previously discussed complications. This reflects the multifactorial origin of atherosclerosis. Effective antihypertensive therapy is thus less successful in preventing complications of coronary heart disease, but recent trials have convincingly demonstrated that coronary events can be reduced in high-risk patients.

F. Malignant and Accelerated Hypertension: Any form of sustained hypertension, primary or secondary, may abruptly become accelerated, with resulting encephalopathy, nephropathy, retinopathy, heart failure, or myocardial ischemia. These complications are discussed below in the section on Hypertensive Urgencies and Emergencies.

Frohlich ED et al: The heart in hypertension. N Engl J Med 1992;327:998. (Pathophysiology and clinical impact.)

National High Blood Pressure Education Program Working Group Report on Hypertension and Chronic Renal Failure: Arch Intern Med 1991;151:1280. (Progressive renal failure during treatment remains a problem; more vigorous treatment is advocated.)

National Education Programs Working Group Report on the Management of Patients With Hypertension and High Blood Cholesterol: Ann Intern Med 1991;114:224. (Attention must be paid to associated hyperlipidemia if maximal benefit is to be obtained from antihypertensive therapy. Provides rationale and guidelines.)

O'Kelly BF et al: Coronary morbidity and mortality, preexisting silent coronary artery disease and mild hypertension. Ann Intern Med 1989;110:1017. (Therapy should focus on reducing coronary complications.)

Phillips SJ: Pathogenesis, diagnosis, and treatment of hypertension-associated stroke. Am J Hypertens 1989; 2:493.

Clinical Findings

The clinical and laboratory findings are mainly referable to involvement of the "target organs": heart, brain, kidneys, eyes, and peripheral arteries.

A. Symptoms: Mild to moderate essential hypertension is usually associated with normal health and well-being for many years. Vague symptoms often appear after patients learn they have "high blood pressure." Suboccipital pulsating headaches, characteristically occurring early in the morning and subsiding during the day, are common, but any type of headache may occur. Accelerated hypertension may be associated with somnolence, headache, confusion, visual disturbances, and nausea and vomiting (hypertensive encephalopathy).

Patients with pheochromocytomas that secrete predominantly norepinephrine usually have sustained hypertension but may have intermittent hypertension. Attacks (lasting minutes to hours) of anxiety, palpitation, profuse perspiration, pallor, tremor, and nausea and vomiting occur; blood pressure is markedly elevated, and angina or acute pulmonary edema may occur. In primary aldosteronism, patients may have recurrent episodes of generalized muscular weakness or paralysis as well as paresthesias, polyuria, and nocturia due to associated hypokalemia; malignant hypertension, however, is rare.

Chronic hypertension often leads to left ventricular hypertrophy, which may be associated with diastolic or, in late stages, systolic dysfunction. Exertional and paroxysmal nocturnal dyspnea may result. Severe left ventricular hypertrophy predisposes to myocardial ischemia (especially when concomitant coronary artery disease is present), ventricular arrhythmias, and sudden death.

Renal involvement may not produce symptoms, but hematuria is frequent in the malignant phase.

Cerebral involvement causes (1) stroke due to thrombosis or (2) small or large hemorrhage from microaneurysms of small penetrating intracranial arteries. Hypertensive encephalopathy is probably caused by acute capillary congestion and exudation with cerebral edema. The findings are usually reversible if adequate treatment is given promptly. Although there is no strict correlation of diastolic blood pressure with hypertensive encephalopathy, it usually exceeds 130 mm Hg.

B. Signs: Physical findings depend upon the

cause of hypertension, its duration and severity, and the degree of effect on target organs.

1. Blood pressure–Blood pressure should be measured after the patient has rested 10 or more minutes in familiar, quiet, warm surroundings. On the initial observation, pressure should be examined in both arms and, if lower extremity pulses are diminished, in the legs to exclude coarctation of the aorta. Supine and standing measurements should be made to detect postural changes, which are usually present in pheochromocytoma. Elderly patients may have falsely elevated readings by sphygmomanometry because of noncompressible vessels. This may be suspected in the presence of Osler's sign—a palpable brachial or radial artery when the cuff is inflated above systolic pressure. Occasionally, it may be necessary to maker direct measurements of intra-arterial pressure, especially in patients with apparent severe hypertension who do not tolerate therapy.

2. Retinas–The Keith-Wagener (KW) classification of retinal changes in hypertension, in spite of deficiencies, presage a worse prognosis when stage II or higher changes are present (see Table 7–2).

3. Heart and arteries–A loud aortic second sound and an early systolic ejection click may occur. Left ventricular enlargement with a left ventricular heave indicates well-established disease. Older patients frequently have systolic ejection murmurs resulting from aortic sclerosis, and these may evolve to significant aortic stenosis in some individuals. Aortic insufficiency may be auscultated in up to 5% of patients, and hemodynamically insignificant aortic insufficiency can be detected by Doppler echocardiography in 10–20%. A presystolic (S_4) gallop due to decreased compliance of the left ventricle is quite common.

4. Pulses–The timing of upper and lower extremity pulses should be compared to exclude coarctation of the aorta. All major peripheral pulses should be evaluated to exclude aortic dissection and peripheral atherosclerosis, which may be associated with renal artery involvement.

C. Laboratory Findings: Most laboratory examinations are normal in uncomplicated essential hypertension. Testing is recommended to detect secondary hypertension and important associated conditions. Thus, standard testing should include measurements of hemoglobin (to detect anemia or polycythemia), complete urinalysis (to detect hematuria, proteinuria, and casts, which may signify primary renal disease or nephrosclerosis), renal function testing (for the same reasons), measurement of serum K^+ (to detect hyperaldosteronism), measurement of fasting blood sugar (to detect diabetes and as evidence for pheochromocytoma), and measurement of plasma lipids (as an indicator of atherosclerosis risk).

D. Electrocardiography and Chest X-Ray: Electrocardiographic criteria are highly specific but not very sensitive for left ventricular hypertrophy.

The "strain" pattern of ST–T wave changes is a sign of more advanced disease and associated with a poor prognosis. A chest x-ray is not recommended in the routine evaluation of uncomplicated hypertension, since it usually does not yield additional information.

E. Echocardiography: The echocardiogram is much more sensitive than the ECG in detecting left ventricular hypertrophy, and measurements of left ventricular mass predict prognosis in populations. However, until it is found that these measurements are useful in determining the need for therapy or in selecting therapy, this test should not be employed in uncomplicated patients.

F. Diagnostic Studies: Only if the clinical presentation or routine tests suggest secondary or complicated hypertension are additional diagnostic studies indicated. These may include blood and urinary tests for endocrine causes of hypertension, intravenous urograms, or renal ultrasound to diagnose primary renal disease (polycystic kidneys, obstructive uropathy) or renovascular abnormalities, and isotope renograms for the latter diagnosis. Further evaluation may include abdominal imaging studies (CT scan, or MRI) or renal arteriography.

G. Summary: Since most hypertension is "primary," an extensive diagnostic evaluation is not indicated before starting therapy. Most clinicians obtain only a blood count, renal function test, electrolyte panel and urinalysis, and ECG after establishing the diagnosis. If conventional therapy is unsuccessful or if symptoms suggest a secondary cause, further studies are indicated.

Gifford RW et al: Office evaluation of hypertension. Circulation 1989;79:721. (How to approach the initial evaluation.)

Nonpharmacologic Therapy

All patients with high normal or elevated blood pressures (as defined in Table 11–1), those who have a family history of cardiovascular complications of hypertension, and those who have multiple coronary risk factors should be counseled about nonpharmacologic approaches to lowering blood pressure. Approaches of proved but modest value include weight reduction, reduced alcohol consumption, and in some patients reduced salt intake. Increased activity levels in previously sedentary patients may lower blood pressure, but strenuous exercise training programs in already active individuals may have less benefit. Stress reduction is of unclear value. Calcium and potassium supplements have been advocated, but their ability to lower blood pressure is limited and probably not applicable to most patients.

Beilin LJ, Puddey IB: Alcohol and hypertension. Clin Exp Hypertens 1992;14:119.
Cutler JA et al: An overview of randomized trials of sodium reduction and blood pressure. Hypertension 1991;

17(Suppl I):I–27. (Sodium restriction effective in some patients.)

The effects of nonpharmacologic events on blood pressure of persons with high normal levels. Trials of Hypertension Prevention Collaborative Research Group. JAMA 1992;267:1213. (Weight reduction and salt restriction were helpful, but dietary supplementation and stress reduction techniques were not.)

Nonpharmacologic approaches to the control of high blood pressure. Hypertension 1986;8:444. (Consensus statement by Joint National Committee.)

Who Should Be Treated With Medications?

Recommendations concerning which patients should be treated with medications after implementation of nonpharmacologic treatment remain controversial. Factors that unfavorably influence the prognosis in chronic arterial hypertension and so determine the threshold for drug therapy include the following: (1) the level of diastolic and systolic blood pressures; (2) a family history of hypertension-related complications; (3) male gender; (4) early age at onset; (5) black race; (6) the presence of additional risk factors for coronary artery disease; (7) accompanying cardiac disease, cerebral vascular disease, or diabetes; (8) left ventricular hypertrophy on ECG or echocardiogram; and (9) renal dysfunction.

Drug treatment of severe (systolic blood pressure ≥ 180 mm Hg or diastolic blood pressure ≥ 110 mm Hg) and moderate (systolic blood pressure 160-D179 mm Hg or diastolic blood pressure 100-109 mm Hg) chronic hypertension results in lower morbidity and mortality rates from cardiovascular disease (stroke and heart failure) than occur in untreated control patients. Recent trials have also demonstrated that coronary events, including nonfatal myocardial infarctions, can be prevented in severely hypertensive patients, including those with isolated systolic hypertension. In patients with diastolic pressures less than 100 mm Hg without accompanying moderate or severe systolic hypertension, the data are less clear, largely because complications are less frequent. Since insurance data have shown that even slight increases in blood pressure reduce longevity, most patients with diastolic blood pressures over 95 mm Hg should be treated, as should individuals with diastolic pressures of 90 mm Hg or more if there is evidence of target organ damage or associated systolic hypertension or if any of the risk factors listed above are present.

Collins R et al: Blood pressure, stroke, and coronary heart disease. 2. Short term reduction in blood pressure: Overview of randomized trials in their epidemiological context. Lancet 1990;335:827. (Stroke reduced by 42%, coronary events by 14%.)

Dahlof B et al: Morbidity and mortality in the Swedish Trial in Old Patients with Hypertension (STOP–Hyperten-

sion). Lancet 1991;338:1281. (Stroke and cardiovascular mortality reduced with diuretic or beta-blocker therapy.)

Medical Research Council Trial of Treatment of Hypertension in Older Adults: Principal results. MRC Working Party. Br Med J 1992;304:405. (Stroke and coronary events prevented, more so by diuretic than beta-blocker. Diuretic also reduced coronary events.)

SHEP Cooperative Research Group: Prevention of stroke by antihypertensive drug treatment in older persons with isolated systolic hypertension. JAMA 1991;265:3255. (Seminal study indicating the need to treat isolated systolic hypertension and the efficacy of diuretics in doing so.)

Antihypertensive Drug Therapy

An ideal antihypertensive drug would be effective as a single agent or in combination with other agents in all classes of patients; would lower blood pressure by a physiologic mechanism; would reduce morbidity and mortality rates; would have no long-term toxicity or unpleasant side effects that affect life-styles; could be taken once a day; would not require multiple-dose titration steps; and would be of moderate cost. No such agent currently exists, but the growing number of available drugs has allowed the physician to tailor treatment to the needs of individual patients. These agents are listed in Tables 11–2 to 11–5.

A. The Stepped Care Approach: Over the past 2 decades, the "stepped care" approach to treatment of hypertension has been advocated. Patients were initially started on a diuretic agent, or beta-blocker, and other drugs were added later if required. This approach was highly effective, with approximately 80% of compliant patients exhibiting adequate blood pressure control. It was also relatively inexpensive and straightforward.

In recent years, a number of considerations have led many experts to question this as a universal treatment plan. These include recognition of adverse effects of diuretics and beta-blockers, concern over the long-term implications of the metabolic changes (especially unfavorable changes in plasma lipids and insulin sensitivity) induced by these agents, realization that patients not controlled by one agent may be controlled by another without moving directly to combined therapy, and the more recent availability of other effective and well-tolerated agents with different mechanisms of action. However, recent positive trials have shown that the low-dose diuretic-based treatment can reduce the incidence of coronary events as well as stroke. Similar benefits have not been shown with the newer agents such as the calcium channel blockers and ACE inhibitors, so the pendulum has begun to swing back.

B. Potential Initial Medications: The recent recommendations of JNC-V are that diuretics and beta-blockers should be considered first-line therapy in most patients, but considerable latitude is permitted for individualized treatment. Additional choices include ACE inhibitors, calcium channel blockers,

Table 11–2. Antihypertensive drugs: Diuretics, alpha-adrenergic blocking agents, sympatholytics, and vasodilators.

Drug	Proprietary Name	Initial Dosage	Dosage Range	Cost for 30 Days (Average Dosage)	Adverse Effects	Comments
Thiazides and related diuretics						
Hydrochlorothiazide	Esidrix,* Hydro-Diuril*	12.5 or 25 mg once daily	12.5–50 mg once daily	$12.94 (60 cents generic) (25 mg once daily)	↓K⁺, ↓Mg²⁺, ↑Ca²⁺, ↓Na⁺, ↑uric acid, ↑glucose, ↑LDL cholesterol, ↑triglycerides, rash, impotence	Low dosages effective in many patients without associated metabolic abnormalities; metolazone more effective with concurrent renal insufficiency; indapamide may have additional vasodilator action.
Chlorthalidone	Hygroton*	12.5 or 25 mg once daily	12.5–50 mg once daily	$15.00 (1.45 cents generic) (25 mg once daily)		
Metolazone	Diulo, Zaroxolyn	1.25 or 2.5 mg once daily	1.25–5 mg once daily	$11.16 (2.5 mg once daily)		
	Mykrox	0.5 mg once daily	0.5–1 mg once daily	$18.40 (0.5 mg once daily)		
Indapamide	Lozol	2.5 mg once daily	2.5–5 mg once daily	$19.77 (2.5 mg once daily)		
Loop diuretics						
Furosemide	Lasix*	20 mg bid	40–320 mg in 2 or 3 doses	$7.78 ($2.34 generic) (20 mg bid)	Same as thiazides, but higher risk of excessive diuresis and electrolyte imbalance.	Short duration of action a disadvantage; should be reserved for patients with renal insufficiency or fluid retention.
Bumetanide	Bumex	0.25 mg bid	0.5–10 mg in 2 or 3 doses	$13.98 (0.5 mg bid)		
Combination products						
Hydrochlorothiazide/triamterene	Dyazide* (25/50 mg)	1 tab once daily	1 or 2 tabs once daily	$8.74 ($1.05 generic) (1 tab once daily)	Same as thiazides plus GI disturbances, hyperkalemia rather than hypokalemia, headache; triamterene can cause kidney stones and renal dysfunction; spironolactone causes gynecomastia and agranulocytosis.	Use should be limited to patients with demonstrable need for a potassium-sparing agent.
Hydrochlorothiazide/amiloride	Moduretic* (50/5 mg)	½ tab once daily	1–2 tabs once daily	$11.05 ($5.08 generic) (1 tab once daily)		
Hydrochlorothiazide/spironolactone	Aldactazide (25/25 mg)	1 tab once daily	1–2 tabs once daily	$10.35 ($1.15 generic) (1 tab once daily)		
Alpha-adrenergic blockers						
Prazosin	Minipress*	1 mg hs	2–20 mg in 2 or 3 doses	$48.58 ($31.17 generic) (5 mg bid)	Syncope with first dose; postural hypotension, dizziness, palpitations, headache, weakness, drowsiness, sexual dysfunction, anticholinergic effects, urinary incontinence; first-dose effects may be less with doxazosin.	May ↑HDL and ↓LDL cholesterol.
Terazosin	Hytrin	1 mg hs	1–20 mg in 1 or 2 doses	$24.53 (5 mg once daily)		May provide short-term relief of obstructive prostatic symptoms. Tachyphylaxis may occur.
Doxazosin	Cardura	1 mg hs	1–16 mg once daily	$20.90 (4 mg once daily)		

(continued)

Table 11–2. Antihypertensive drugs: Diuretics, alpha-adrenergic blocking agents, sympatholytics, and vasodilators. (continued)

Drug	Proprietary Name	Initial Dosage	Dosage Range	Cost for 30 Days (Average Dosage)	Adverse Effects	Comments
Central sympatholytics						
Clonidine	Catapres*	0.1 mg bid	0.2–0.6 mg in 2 doses	$27.86 ($3.68 generic)	Sedation, dry mouth, sexual dysfunction, headache, bradyarrhythmias; side effects may be less with guanfacine. Contact dermatitis with clonidine patch. Methyldopa also causes hepatitis, hemolytic anemia, fever.	"Rebound" hypertension may occur even after gradual withdrawal. Methyldopa should be avoided in favor of safer agents.
	Catapress TTS	0.1 mg/d patch weekly	0.1–0.3 mg/d patch weekly	$10.67 (0.2 mg weekly)		
Guanabenz	Wytensin	4 mg bid	8–64 mg in 2 doses	$25.46 (4 mg bid)		
Guanfacine	Tenex	1 mg once daily	1–3 mg once daily	$14.92 (1 mg once daily)		
Methyldopa	Aldomet*	250 mg bid	500–2000 mg in 2 doses	$26.68 ($22.39 generic) (500 mg bid)		
Peripheral neuronal antagonists						
Guanethidine	Ismelin	10 mg once daily	10–100 mg once daily	$21.44 (25 mg once daily)	Orthostatic hypotension, diarrhea, exercise hypotension, sexual dysfunction, salt and water retention. Depression, night terrors, nasal stuffiness, drowsiness, peptic disease, GI disturbances, bradycardia.	
Guanadrel	Hylorel	5 mg bid	10–70 mg in 2 doses	$36.40 (10 mg bid)		
Reserpine	Serpasil*	0.05 mg once daily	0.05–0.25 mg once daily	$1.46 ($1.08 generic) (0.1 mg once daily)		
Direct vasodilators						
Hydralazine	Apresoline*	25 mg bid	50–300 mg in 2–4 doses	$15.55 ($1.89 generic) (25 mg bid)	GI disturbances, tachycardia, headache, nasal congestion, rash, LE-like syndrome.	May worsen or precipitate angina.
Minoxidil	Loniten*	5 mg once daily	5–40 mg once daily	$14.17 ($1.50 generic) (10 mg once daily)	Tachycardia, fluid retention, headache, hirsutism, pericardial effusion, thrombocytopenia.	Should be used in combination with beta-blocker and diuretic.

*Generic preparation available.

alpha-blockers, and combined alpha- and beta-blockers. These medications are all effective and generally well tolerated (the alpha-blockers less so), but responses vary among demographic groups. Selection is based upon individual factors, which include age, race, life-style, cost, the experience of the physician, and the side effects of the agent. Accompanying illnesses are often the major factor in selection of medications, since these may exclude some medications or favor the use of others.

A recent Veterans Affairs Cooperative Study compared representatives of six classes of antihypertensive medications in a placebo-controlled trial. Over-all, the calcium channel blocker was the most broadly effective and well-tolerated agent, but responses varied among demographic subgroups (Figure 11–1). In older whites, the beta-blocker and calcium channel blocker produced the best responses, but the diuretic was the best agent in lowering systolic pressure. In younger whites, the beta-blocker and ACE inhibitor were most effective, and diuretic was quite ineffective. The calcium channel blocker was the most potent agent in blacks, although diuretic was also effective in older blacks. The ACE inhibitor had little effect as a single agent in blacks. It is unclear whether similar results occur in women, who were not in-

Table 11–3. Antihypertensive drugs: Beta-adrenergic blocking agents.

Drug	Proprietary Name	Initial Dosage	Dosage Range	Cost for 30 Days (Avg Dosage)	β_1 Selectivity	ISA	MSA	Lipid Solubility	Renal vs Hepatic Elimination	Comments
Acebutolol	Sectral	200 mg once daily	200–1200 mg in 1 or 2 doses	$23.22 (400 mg once daily)	+	+	+	+	H > R	Positive ANA; rare LE syndrome; also indicated for arrhythmias.
Atenolol	Tenormin*	25 mg once daily	25–200 mg once daily	$23.31 ($12.58 generic) (50 mg once daily)	+	0	0	0	R	Also indicated for angina pectoris and post-MI.
Betaxolol	Kerlone	10 mg once daily	10–40 mg once daily	$26.86 (20 mg once daily)	+	0	0	+	H > R	
Carteolol	Cartrol	2.5 mg once daily	2.5–10 mg once daily	$19.07 (5 mg once daily)	0	+	0	+	R > H	
Labetalol	Normodyne, Trandate	100 mg bid	200–1200 mg in 2 doses	$33.45 (200 mg bid)	0	0/+	0	+	H	α:β blocking activity 1:3; more orthostatic hypotension, fever, hepatotoxicity.
Metoprolol	Lopressor	50 mg in 1 or 2 doses	50–200 mg in 1 or 2 doses	$27.64 (50 mg bid)	+	0	+	+++	H	Also indicated for angina pectoris and post-MI.
	Toprol XL (SR preparation)	50 mg once daily	50–200 mg once daily	$14.20 (100 mg once daily)						
Nadolol	Corgard	20 mg once daily	20–160 mg once daily	$22.23 (40 mg once daily)	0	0	0	0	R	
Penbutolol	Levatol	20 mg once daily	20–80 mg once daily	$22.32 (20 mg once daily)	0	+	0	+	R > H	
Pindolol	Visken	5 mg bid	10–60 mg in 2 doses	$38.12 (5 mg bid)	0	+	+	+	H > R	
Propranolol	Inderal*	20 mg bid	40–320 mg in 2 doses	$21.47 ($4.71 generic) (40 mg bid)	0	0	+	+++	H	Once-daily SR preparation also available. Also indicated for angina pectoris and post-MI.
Timolol	Blocadren*	5 mg bid	10–40 mg in 2 doses	$19.08 ($13.72 generic) (10 mg bid)	0	0	0	+	H > R	Also indicated post-MI.

*Generic preparation available.
ISA = intrinsic sympathomimetic activity; MSA = membrane-stabilizing activity; 0 = no effect; +, ++, +++ = some, moderate, most effect.

Notes:
1. Adverse effects of all beta-blockers: bronchospasm, fatigue, sleep disturbance and nightmares, bradycardia and AV block, worsening of congestive heart failure, cold extremities, GI disturbances, impotence, ↑triglycerides, ↓HDL cholesterol, rare blood dyscrasias.
2. Agents with β_1 selectivity are less likely to precipitate bronchospasm and decreased peripheral blood flow *in low doses,* but selectivity is only relative.
3. Agents with ISA cause less resting bradycardia and lipid changes.

Table 11–4. Antihypertensive drugs: ACE inhibitors.

Drug	Proprietary Name	Initial Dosage	Dosage Range	Cost of 30 Days (Avg Dosage)	Adverse Effects	Comments
Benazepril	Lotensin	10 mg once daily	5–40 mg in 1 or 2 doses	$19.09 (20 mg once daily)	Cough, hypotension, dizziness, renal dysfunction, hyperkalemia, angioedema; taste alteration and rash (may be more frequent with captopril); proteinuria, blood dyscrasia.	**Benazepril** and **fosinopril** are excreted by the liver in patients with renal dysfunction (dose reduction may not be necessary). **Captopril** is active without metabolism; approved for congestive heart failure. **Enalapril** is approved for congestive heart failure. **Lisinopril** is active without metabolism.
Captopril	Capoten	25 mg bid	50–300 mg in 2 or 3 doses	$30.22 (25 mg bid)		
Enalapril	Vasotec	5 mg once daily	5–40 mg in 1 or 2 doses	$20.89 (10 mg once daily)		
Fosinopril	Monopril	10 mg once daily	10–80 mg in 1 or 2 doses	$22.75 (20 mg once daily)		
Lisinopril	Prinivil, Zestril	5–10 mg once daily	5–40 mg once daily	$19.66 (20 mg once daily)		
Quinapril	Accupril	10 mg once daily	10–80 mg in 1 or 2 doses	$17.67 (20 mg once daily)		
Ramipril	Altace	2.5 mg once daily	2.5–20 mg in 1 or 2 doses	$19.14 (5 mg once daily)		

cluded in this trial, but previous studies have not shown significant differences in blood pressure responses by gender.

C. Current Antihypertensive Agents: (See Tables 11–2 to 11–6 for dosages.)

1. Diuretics–(Table 11–2.) The diuretics remain the most widely used hypertensive medications and are the only agents shown to reduce mortality and morbidity related to coronary artery disease in major trials. Relative to the beta-blockers and the ACE inhibitors, they are more potent in blacks, older individuals, the obese, and other sub-groups with increased plasma volume or low plasma renin activity. Interestingly, they are relatively more effective in smokers than in nonsmokers. Overall, the diuretics administered alone, control blood pressure in 50% of patients and can be used effectively with all other agents. They are perhaps the most effective agents for lowering predominantly systolic hypertension.

Diuretics lower blood pressure initially by decreasing plasma volume (by suppressing tubular reabsorption of sodium, thus increasing the excretion of sodium and water) and cardiac output, but during chronic therapy their major hemodynamic effect is reduction of peripheral vascular resistance by an as yet unknown mechanism. It is now generally appreciated that most of the antihypertensive effect of these agents is achieved at lower dosages than used previously but that their biochemical effects are dose-related. The thiazide diuretics are the most widely used. The loop diuretics (such as furosemide) may lead to electrolyte and volume depletion more readily than the thiazides and have short durations of action; therefore, they are not ordinarily used in hypertension

except in the presence of renal dysfunction (serum creatinine above 2.5 mg/dL).

The adverse effects of diuretics relate chiefly to the metabolic changes listed in Table 11–2. Impotence, skin rashes, and photosensitivity are also less frequent side effects. Hypokalemia may lead to decreased renal blood flow with a potential rise in serum creatinine, especially in older patients. Hypokalemia can be minimized by employing very low doses (hydrochlorothiazide, 12.5–25 mg daily), eating a high-potassium diet (see Table 20–6 for the potassium content of foods), and limiting salt intake. With the lower doses of diuretics now commonly used, potassium replacement is usually not required and should be limited to individuals demonstrating hypokalemia (serum $K^+ < 3.5$ mmol/L) or a reduction greater than 0.6 mmol/L from baseline—or to patients at special risk from intracellular potassium depletion (patients taking digoxin or having ventricular arrhythmias and diabetics in whom insulin release and insulin sensitivity are reduced by hypokalemia). Combinations of thiazide diuretics and potassium-sparing agents (spironolactone, triamterene, amiloride) are often employed, but these medications are considerably more expensive, have additional side effects, impose a risk of hyperkalemia if potassium supplements are given, are often unnecessary in patients receiving low diuretic dosages, and are dangerous in the presence of oliguria. Diuretics also increase serum uric acid and may precipitate acute gout. Increases in blood glucose, triglycerides, low-density lipoprotein cholesterol, and plasma insulin are common also and may be deleterious in the long term. These changes may be blunted by time and by a

Table 11–5. Antihypertensive drugs: Calcium channel-blocking agents.

Drug	Proprietary Name	Initial Dosage	Dosage Range	Cost for 30 Days (Avg Dosage)	Special Properties			Adverse Effects	Comments
					Peripheral Vaso-dilation	Cardiac Automaticity and Conduction	Contrac-tility		
Nondihydropyridine agents									
Diltiazem	Cardizem	60 mg tid	180–360 mg in 3 doses	$93.94 ($23.07 generic) (120 mg tid)	++	↓↓	↓↓	Edema, headache, bradycardia, GI disturbances, dizziness, AV block, congestive heart failure, urinary frequency.	Also approved for angina
	Cardizem SR	90 mg bid	180–360 mg in 2 doses	$59.14 (240 mg once daily)					
	Cardizem CD	180 mg once daily	180–360 mg once daily	$48.31					
	Dilacor XR	180 or 240 mg once daily	180–480 mg daily	$28.26					
Verapamil	Calan, Isoptin*	80 mg tid	240–480 mg in 3 doses	$48.13 ($25.88 generic) (120 mg tid)	++	↓↓↓	↓↓↓	Same as diltiazem but more likely to cause constipation and congestive heart failure.	Also approved for angina and arrhythmias
	Calan SR, Isoptin SR, Verelan	240 mg SR once daily	240–480 in 1 or 2 doses	$32.41 (240 mg once daily)					
Dihydropyridines									
Amlodipine	Norvasc	5 mg once daily	5–10 mg once daily	$36.50 (5 mg once daily)	+++	↓/0	↓/0	Edema, dizziness, palpitations, flushing, headache, hypotension, tachycardia, GI disturbances, urinary frequency, worsening of congestive heart failure (may be less common with felodipine, amlodipine).	Nicardipine, nifedipine, and amlodipine also approved for angina
Felodipine	Plendil	5 mg once daily	5–20 mg once daily	$35.86 (10 mg once daily)	+++	↓/0	↓/0		
Isradipine	DynaCirc	2.5 mg bid	5–10 mg in 2 doses	$33.00 (5 mg bid)	+++	↓/0	↓		
Nicardipine	Cardene	20 mg tid	60–120 mg in 3 doses	$50.81 (30 mg tid)	+++	↓/0	↓		
Nifedipine	Adalat, Procardia	10 mg tid	30–120 mg in 3 doses	$83.88 ($72.00 generic) (20 mg tid)	+++	↓	↓↓		
	Procardia XL	30 mg once daily	30–120 mg once daily	$47.88 (60 mg once daily)	+++	↓	↓↓		

*Generic preparation available.

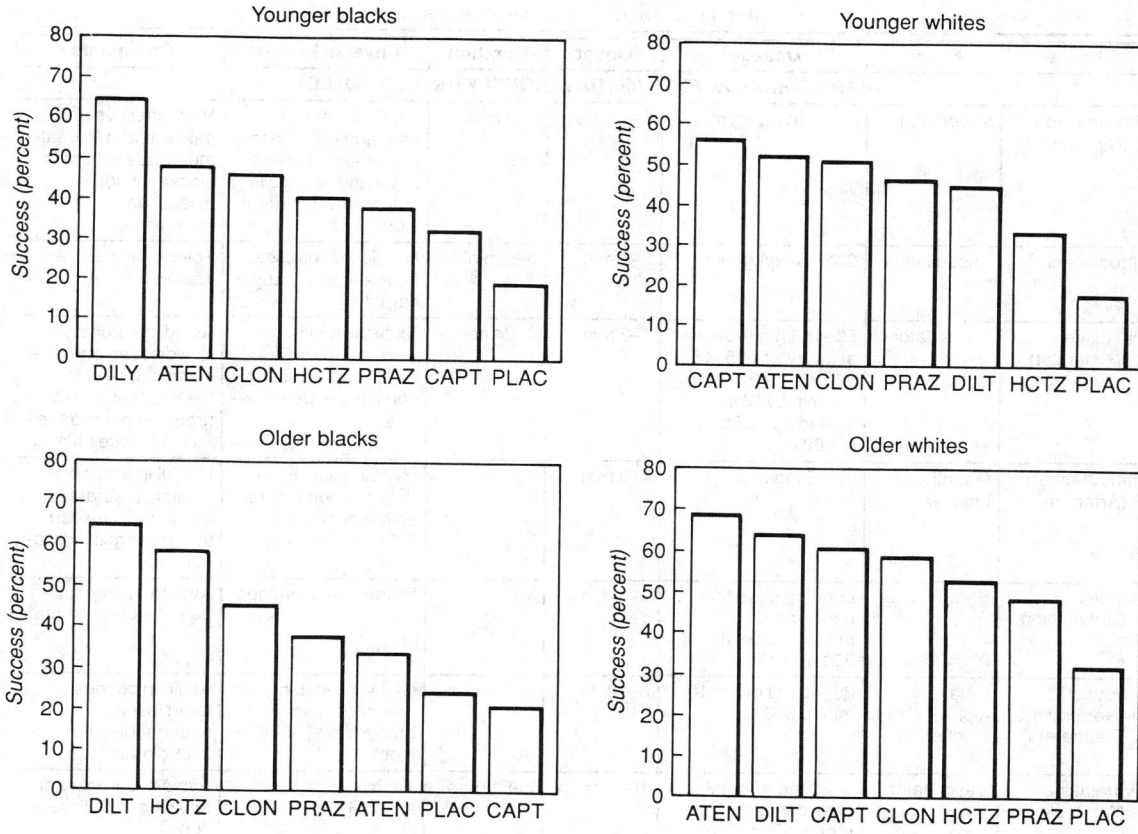

Figure 11–1. Single-drug therapy for hypertension in men. A comparison of six antihypertensive agents with placebo. The Department of Veterans Affairs Cooperative Study Group on Antihypertensive Agents.

shift to a low-cholesterol, low-saturated fat diet, but their long-term consequences are unknown. Some experts feel that these lipid changes may limit the beneficial effect of blood pressure reduction on the progression of atherosclerosis.

2. Beta-adrenergic blocking agents–(Table 11–3.) These drugs are effective in hypertension because they decrease the heart rate and cardiac output. Even after continued use of beta-blockers for a number of years, cardiac output remains decreased and systemic vascular resistance increased with agents that do not have intrinsic sympathomimetic or alpha-blocking activity. The beta-blockers also decrease renin release and are in general more efficacious in populations likely to have elevated plasma renin activity, such as younger white patients. They neutralize the reflex tachycardia caused by vasodilators such as hydralazine and alpha-adrenergic blockers in the treatment of hypertension. The beta-blockers are especially useful in patients with associated conditions that benefit from this mode of therapy. These include patients with angina pectoris, patients with previous myocardial infarction, and individuals with migraine headaches and somatic manifestations of anxiety.

Although all beta-blockers appear to be approximately equivalent in antihypertensive potency, controlling 50–60% of patients, they differ in a number of pharmacologic properties (these differences are summarized in Table 11–3). They differ with respect to whether their effect is relatively specific to the cardiac β_1 receptors (cardioselectivity) or whether they also block the β_2 receptors in the bronchi and vasculature; at higher dosages, however, all agents are nonselective. The beta-blockers also differ in their pharmacokinetics and lipid solubility—which determines whether they enter the brain and cause cerebral symptoms—and mechanisms of elimination. The effect on the pulse rate varies; agents with intrinsic sympathetic activity may be preferable in patients who develop more pronounced bradycardia (< 45/min) when given other beta-blockers. Labetalol is a combined alpha- and beta-blocker and, unlike most beta-blockers, decreases peripheral resistance more than the other agents.

Table 11–6. Drugs for hypertensive crises.

Agent	Action	Dosage	Onset	Duration	Adverse Effects	Comments
PARENTERAL AGENTS (INTRAVENOUSLY UNLESS NOTED)						
Nitroprusside (Nipride)	Vasodilator	0.25–10 µg/kg/min	Seconds	3–5 min	GI, CNS; thiocyanate and cyanide toxicity, especially with renal and hepatic insufficiency; hypotension.	Most effective and easily titratable treatment. Use with betablocker in aortic dissection.
Nitroglycerin	Vasodilator	0.25–5 µg/kg/min	2–5 min	3–5 min	Headache, nausea, hypotension, bradycardia.	Tolerance may develop.
Diazoxide (Hyperstat)	Vasodilator	50–150 mg repeated at intervals of 5–15 min, or 15–30 mg/min by IV infusion to a maximum of 600 mg	1–2 min	4–24 hours	Excessive hypotension, tachycardia, headache, nausea, vomiting, hyperglycemia.	Avoid in coronary artery disease and dissection. Use with betablocker and diuretic. Avoid extravasation (tissue irritant).
Trimethaphan (Arfonad)	Ganglionic blocker	0.5–5 mg/min	1–3 min	10 min	Hypotension, ileus, urinary retention, respiratory arrest.	Useful in aortic dissection. Liberates histamine; use caution in allergic individuals.
Esmolol (Breviblock)	Beta-blocker	Loading dose 500 µg/kg over 1 min; maintenance, 25–200 µg/kg/min	1–2 min	10–30 min	Bradycardia, nausea.	Avoid in congestive heart failure, asthma.
Labetalol (Normodyne, Trandate)	Beta- and alpha-blocker	20–40 mg every 10 min to 300 mg	5–10 min	3–6 hours	GI, hypotension, bronchospasm, bradycardia, heart block.	Avoid in congestive heart failure, asthma. May be continued orally.
Hydralazine (Apresoline)	Vasodilator	5–20 mg IV or IM (less desirable); may repeat after 20 min	10–30 min	2–6 hours	Tachycardia, headache, GI.	Avoid in coronary artery disease, dissection.
Enalaprilat (Vasotec)	ACE inhibitor	1.25 mg every 6 hours	15 min	6 hours or more	Excessive hypotension.	Additive with diuretics; may be continued orally.
Furosemide (Lasix)	Diuretic	10–80 mg	15 min	4 hours	Hypokalemia, hypotension.	Adjunct to vasodilator.
Nicardipine (Cardene)	Calcium channel blocker	5 mg/h; may increase by 1–2.5 mg/h every 15 min to 15 mg/h	1–5 min	3–6 hours	Hypotension, tachycardia, headache.	May precipitate myocardial ischemia.
ORAL AGENTS						
Nifedipine (Adalat, Procardia)	Calcium channel blocker	10 mg initially; may be repeated after 30 minutes	15 min	2–6 hours	Excessive hypotension, tachycardia, headache.	Response variable. May precipitate angina. Can be given by sublingual or buccal route.
Clonidine (Catapres)	Central sympatholytic	0.1–0.2 mg initially; then 0.1 mg every hour to 0.8 mg	30–60 min	6–8 hours	Sedation	Rebound may occur.
Captopril (Capoten)	ACE inhibitor	25 mg	15–30 min	4–6 hours	Excessive hypotension.	

The side effects of all beta-blockers include development of bronchial asthma in predisposed patients; bradycardia; atrioventricular conduction defects; left ventricular failure, because of the negative inotropic action of the sympatholytic action of the drugs; nasal congestion; Raynaud's phenomenon, especially in women; and central nervous system symptoms with nightmares, excitement, and confusion. Fatigue, lethargy, and impotence may occur. All beta-blockers tend to increase plasma triglycerides. The nonselective and, to a lesser extent, the cardioselective beta-blockers tend to depress the protective HDL fraction of plasma cholesterol. This is not seen in agents with intrinsic sympathomimetic activity, and as with diuretics, the changes are blunted with time and dietary changes. Some experts believe that these lipid changes may have an adverse effect on coronary artery disease.

These agents are contraindicated in patients with congestive heart failure or symptomatic bronchospasm. Beta-blockers are relatively contraindicated in insulin-dependent diabetes, since they inhibit gluconeogenesis and may prolong hypoglycemic episodes. However, recent studies have not confirmed earlier suggestions that they may worsen symptoms of peripheral vascular disease.

3. Angiotensin-converting enzyme (ACE) inhibitors–(Table 11–4.) These drugs are being increasingly used as the initial medication in mild to moderate hypertension. Their primary mode of action is inhibition of the renin-angiotensin-aldosterone system, but they also inhibit bradykinin degradation, stimulate vasodilating prostaglandin synthesis, and, sometimes, reduce sympathetic nervous system activity. These latter actions may explain why they exhibit some effect even in patients with low plasma renin activity. The ACE inhibitors appear to be most effective in younger whites. They are relatively less effective in blacks and in the elderly and in predominantly systolic hypertension. While as single therapy they achieve adequate antihypertensive control in only about 40–50% of patients, the combination of an ACE inhibitor and a diuretic or calcium channel blocker is potent.

An advantage of the ACE inhibitors is their relative freedom from troublesome side effects. Severe hypotension can occur in patients with bilateral renal artery stenosis; acute renal failure may ensue. Hyperkalemia may develop in patients with intrinsic renal disease and type IV renal tubular acidosis (commonly seen in diabetics) and in the elderly. A chronic dry cough due to bronchial or laryngeal irritation is seen in 5–15% of patients and may require stopping the drug. Skin rashes and taste alterations are seen more often with captopril than with the non-sulfhydryl-containing agents (enalapril and lisinopril) but often disappear with continued therapy. Angioneurotic edema is an uncommon but potentially dangerous side effect of all agents of this class. Pro-

teinuria and neutropenia are very uncommon at the lower dosages now employed except in individuals with preexisting renal insufficiency or autoimmune disease. Indeed, in the diabetic patient with microalbuminuria who is at risk for renal insufficiency, ACE inhibitors may delay the progression of renal disease, but this suggestion awaits confirmation by clinical trials. ACE inhibitors do not produce impotence or fatigue and therefore, unlike some other medications, do not impair quality of life.

4. Calcium channel blockers–(Table 11–5.) All the agents of this class reduce blood pressure, and a number of new agents with a longer duration of action and perhaps less negative inotropic activity are available. They act by causing peripheral vasodilation, which is associated with less reflex tachycardia and fluid retention than other vasodilators. These agents are effective as single-drug therapy in approximately 60% of patients and appear to be beneficial in all demographic groups and all grades of hypertension. As a result, they may be preferable to beta-blockers and ACE inhibitors in blacks and older subjects. Calcium channel blockers and diuretics are less additive when given together than when either is combined with beta-blockers or ACE inhibitors. However, verapamil and diltiazem should be combined cautiously with beta-blockers because of their potential for depressing atrioventricular conduction and sinus node automaticity.

The most common side effects of calcium channel blockers are headache, peripheral edema, bradycardia, and constipation (especially with verapamil in the elderly). The dihydropyridine agents—nifedipine, nicardipine, isradipine, felodipine, and amlodipine—are more likely to produce symptoms of vasodilation, such as headache, flushing, palpitations, and peripheral edema. Calcium channel blockers have negative inotropic effects and may cause or exacerbate heart failure in patients with cardiac dysfunction. This tendency may be less with the newer dihydropyridines—felodipine and amlodipine—but further studies are needed. Most of these agents are now available in preparations that can be administered once or twice daily.

5. Drugs with central sympatholytic action–(Table 11–2.) Methyldopa, clonidine, guanabenz, and guanfacine lower blood pressure by stimulating alpha-adrenergic receptors in the central nervous system, thus reducing efferent peripheral sympathetic outflow. These agents are effective as single therapy in some patients, but they are usually employed as second- or third-line agents because of the high frequency of drug intolerance, including sedation, fatigue, dry mouth, postural hypotension, and impotence. An important concern is rebound hypertension following withdrawal. Methyldopa also causes hepatitis and hemolytic anemia and should be avoided except in individuals who have already tolerated chronic therapy.

6. Alpha-receptor antagonists–(Table 11–2.) Prazosin, terazosin, and doxazosin block postsynaptic alpha receptors, relax smooth muscle, and reduce blood pressure by lowering peripheral vascular resistance. These agents are effective as single-drug therapy in some individuals, but tachyphylaxis may appear during long-term therapy and side effects are relatively common. The major side effects are marked hypotension and syncope after the first dose, which, therefore, should be small and be given at bedtime. Postdosing palpitations, headache, and nervousness may continue to occur during chronic therapy. These side effects may be less frequent or severe with doxazosin because of its more gradual onset of action. Unlike the beta-blockers and diuretics, the alpha-blockers have no adverse effect on serum lipid levels—in fact, they increase high-density lipoprotein cholesterol while reducing total cholesterol. Whether this is beneficial in the long term has not been established. These drugs are most useful in combination with other agents in less responsive patients. One interesting attribute is a reduction in symptoms of prostatism in some men.

7. Arteriolar dilators–(Table 11–2.) Hydralazine and minoxidil relax vascular smooth muscle and produce peripheral vasodilation. When given alone, they stimulate reflex tachycardia, increase myocardial contractility, and cause headache, palpitations, and fluid retention. They are usually given in combination with diuretics and beta-blockers in resistant patients. Hydralazine produces frequent gastrointestinal disturbances and may induce a lupus-like syndrome. Minoxidil causes hirsutism and marked fluid retention; this agent is reserved for the most refractory of patients.

8. Peripheral sympathetic inhibitors–(Table 11–2.) These agents are now used infrequently. Reserpine remains a cost-effective antihypertensive agent. Its reputation for inducing mental depression and its other side effects—sedation, nasal stuffiness, sleep disturbances, and peptic ulcers—have made it unpopular, though these problems are uncommon at low dosages. Guanethidine and guanadrel inhibit catecholamine release from peripheral neurons but frequently cause orthostatic hypotension (especially in the morning or after exercise), diarrhea, and fluid retention. These agents are used chiefly in refractory hypertension.

9. Combination therapy–Most patients with hypertension can be controlled with one agent or with two-drug combinations such as (1) a diuretic plus a beta-blocker, (2) a diuretic plus an ACE inhibitor, (3) a diuretic plus a calcium channel blocker, or (4) a calcium channel blocker plus an ACE inhibitor. A minority may require triple-drug therapy. Particularly useful multidrug regimens are (1) a diuretic plus a beta-blocker plus a vasodilator or a calcium channel blocker; (2) a diuretic plus an ACE inhibitor plus either a calcium channel blocker or a sympatholytic (or both); and (3) a calcium channel blocker plus an ACE inhibitor plus either a sympatholytic or a beta-blocker (or both). Patients who are compliant with their medications and who do not respond to these combinations should usually be evaluated for secondary hypertension before proceeding to more complex regimens.

Alderman MH: Which antihypertensive drugs first—And why! JAMA 1992;267:2786. (Cogent argument for use of diuretics and beta-blockers.)

Applegate WB et al: A randomized controlled trial of the effects of three antihypertensive agents on blood pressure control and quality of life in older women. Arch Intern Med 1991;151:1817. (As in older men, calcium channel blockers are somewhat better than beta-blockers and ACE inhibitors.)

Drugs for hypertension: Med Lett Drugs Ther 1991;33:33.

Epstein M, Sowers JR: Diabetes mellitus and hypertension. Hypertension 1992;19:403. (Mechanisms and clinical considerations.)

The Fifth Report of the Joint National Committee on Detection, Education, and Treatment of High Blood Pressure (JNC V). Arch Intern Med 1993;153:154. (Extensive discussion and tabular presentation of antihypertensive drugs and their use in different patient groups.)

Saunders E et al: A comparison of the efficacy and safety of a beta-blocker, a calcium channel blocker, and a converting enzyme inhibitor in hypertensive blacks. Arch Intern Med 1990;150:1707. (Calcium blocker most effective, ACE inhibitor least.)

Setaro JF, Black HR: Refractory hypertension. N Engl J Med 1992;327:543. (Most patients can be managed with combinations that include diuretics and newer agents.)

See also general references at the end of this chapter.

Goals of Treatment

The goal of treatment should be to reduce blood pressure to normal levels (ie, < 140/90 mm Hg) with minimal side effects. Since there may be additional benefits from further lowering of blood pressure, most authorities also seek to achieve a minimum of 10 mm Hg reduction in diastolic pressure in patients with mild hypertension (90–99 mm Hg). In older patients with predominantly systolic hypertension, a systolic pressure of less than 160 mm Hg may be an acceptable end point if further reduction cannot be obtained without unacceptable side effects. is a satisfactory end point. However, a significant decrease in hypertension-related morbidity from blood pressure reduction is possible even if these therapeutic goals are not achieved. Thus, a compromise between goal blood pressure and an adequately tolerated therapeutic regimen may be necessary in some individuals. Some data indicate that the risk of myocardial infarction and sudden death may rise when the diastolic blood pressure is lowered below 80–85 mm Hg (a phenomenon referred to as the "J" curve of morbidity versus blood pressure reduction), but this concept has not been supported by recent trials.

Fletcher AE, Bulpitt CS: How far should blood pressure be lowered? N Engl J Med 1992;326:251. (Discussion of the controversial questions: Is too low dangerous? How much is enough?)

Kaplan NM: The appropriate goals of antihypertensive therapy: Neither too much nor too little. Ann Intern Med 1992;116:686. (Benefits and risks must be balanced.)

HYPERTENSIVE URGENCIES & EMERGENCIES

Hypertensive emergencies have become less frequent in recent years but still require prompt recognition and aggressive but careful management. A spectrum of acute presentations exists, and the appropriate therapeutic approach varies.

Hypertensive urgencies are situations in which blood pressure must be reduced within a few hours. Examples are asymptomatic severe hypertension (systolic pressure > 240 mm Hg, diastolic pressure > 130 mm Hg) and symptomatic moderately severe hypertension (systolic pressure > 200 mg Hg, diastolic pressure > 120 mm Hg, or even lower levels) associated with headache, heart failure, or angina or occurring in the perioperative period. Parenteral therapy is rarely required, and partial reduction of blood pressure with relief of symptoms is the goal.

Hypertensive emergencies require substantial reduction of blood pressure within 1 hour to avoid serious morbidity or death. Although blood pressure is usually strikingly elevated (diastolic pressure > 130 mm Hg), the correlation between pressure and end-organ damage is often poor. It is the latter that determines the seriousness of the emergency and the approach to treatment. Emergencies include hypertensive encephalopathy (which presents with headache, irritability, confusion, and altered mental status due to cerebrovascular spasm), hypertensive nephropathy (which presents with hematuria, proteinuria, and progressive renal dysfunction due to arteriolar necrosis and intimal hyperplasia of the interlobular arteries), intracranial hemorrhage, dissecting aneurysm, preeclampsia-eclampsia, pulmonary edema, unstable angina, or myocardial infarction.

Malignant hypertension is a specific emergent syndrome characterized by encephalopathy or nephropathy with accompanying papilledema. Progressive renal failure usually ensues without therapy.

Parenteral therapy is indicated in most hypertensive emergencies, especially if encephalopathy is present. The initial goal of treatment should be rapid reduction of systolic and diastolic pressure by at least 20–40 mm Hg and 10–20 mm Hg, respectively, to levels below 180–200/110–120 mm Hg. A subsequent more gradual reduction to near-normal levels is appropriate.

Pharmacologic Management

A. Parenteral Agents: A growing number of agents are available for management of acute hypertensive problems. (Table 11–6 lists drugs, dosages, adverse effects.) Sodium nitroprusside is the agent of choice for the most serious emergencies because of its rapid and easily controllable action, but continuous monitoring is essential when this agent is used. In the presence of myocardial ischemia, intravenous nitroglycerin or an intravenous beta-blocker, such as labetalol or esmolol, is preferable.

1. Nitroprusside sodium–This agent is given by controlled intravenous infusion gradually titrated to the desired effect. It lowers the blood pressure within seconds by direct arteriolar and venous dilatation. Monitoring with an intra-arterial line is essential to avoid hypotension. Nitroprusside—in combination with a beta-blocker—is especially useful in patients with aortic dissection.

2. Nitroglycerin, intravenous–This agent is a less potent antihypertensive than nitroprusside and should be reserved for patients with accompanying acute ischemic syndromes.

3. Trimethaphan–The ganglionic blocking agent trimethaphan is titrated with the patient sitting; its activity depends upon this. The patient can be placed supine if the hypotensive effect is excessive. The effect occurs within a few minutes and persists for the duration of the infusion.

4. Diazoxide–Diazoxide acts promptly as a vasodilator without decreasing renal blood flow. It has been used often in preeclampsia-eclampsia. Side effects include hypotension, which may be severe; this necessitates starting with a smaller dose in elderly patients or administering by slow infusion over 30 minutes, which is usually just as effective and better tolerated. Hyperglycemia and sodium and water retention may occur. The drug should be used only for short periods and is best combined with a powerful diuretic such as furosemide.

5. Esmolol–This rapidly acting beta-blocker is approved by the FDA only for treatment of supraventricular tachycardia, but it is useful in acutely lowering blood pressure, especially when combined with a vasodilator such as nitroprusside, nitroglycerin, or hydralazine. Esmolol is especially useful during myocardial ischemia or dissecting aneurysm.

6. Labetalol–This combined beta- and alpha-adrenergic blocking agent is the only other beta-blocker that can lower blood pressure rapidly enough for emergency treatment.

7. Hydralazine–Hydralazine can be given intravenously or intramuscularly, but its effect is less predictable than that of other drugs in this group. It produces reflex tachycardia and should not be given without beta-blockers in patients with possible coronary disease or aortic dissection. Hydralazine is valuable in children and pregnant women.

8. Enalaprilat–This is the active form of the oral

ACE inhibitor enalapril. The onset of action is usually within 15 minutes, but the peak effect may be delayed for up to 6 hours. Therefore, enalaprilat is useful primarily as an adjunctive agent.

9. Diuretics—Intravenous loop diuretics can be very helpful when the patient has signs of heart failure or fluid retention. Low dosages should be used initially (furosemide, 20 mg; or bumetanide, 0.5 mg). They facilitate the response to vasodilators, which often stimulate fluid retention.

B. Oral Agents: Patients with less severe acute hypertensive syndromes can often be treated with oral therapy. They should be closely monitored until a therapeutic end point is achieved.

1. Clonidine—Clonidine, 0.2 mg orally initially, followed by 0.1 mg every hour to a total of 0.8 mg, will usually lower blood pressure over a period of several hours. Sedation is frequent, and rebound hypertension may occur if the drug is stopped.

2. Nifedipine—Nifedipine, 10–20 mg orally or sublingually, will reduce blood pressure within 5–20 minutes in most patients. An additional 10 mg dose may be needed. Excessive hypotensive responses may occur, and reflex tachycardia may induce angina.

3. Captopril—Captopril, 12.5–25 mg orally, will also lower blood pressure in 15–30 minutes. The response is variable and may be excessive.

C. Subsequent Therapy: When the blood pressure has been brought under control, combinations of oral antihypertensive agents can be added as parenteral drugs are tapered off over a period of 2–3 days. Most subsequent regimens should include a diuretic.

Calhoun DA, Oparil S: Treatment of hypertensive crisis. N Engl J Med 1990;323:1177. (Brief clinical review.)
Gifford RW Jr: Management of hypertensive crises. JAMA 1991;266:829.

HYPERTENSION IN THE PRESENCE OF RENAL FAILURE

In the presence of renal failure, hypertension is highly dependent on blood volume. If the blood pressure is not reduced by vigorous use of antihypertensive drugs—including furosemide, beta-blocking drugs, minoxidil, or diazoxide—dialysis should be employed; in most instances, the blood pressure will be reduced as the patient achieves a dry weight state. The presence of renal failure is an adverse prognostic sign, but vigorous therapy often can prolong life.

REFERENCES

Anastos K et al: Hypertension in women: What is really known? Ann Intern Med 1991;115:287. (The answer is very little.)
Cooke JP, Frohlich ED (editors): *Current Management of Hypertension and Vascular Diseases.* BC Decker, 1992.
Kaplan NM: *Clinical Hypertension,* 5th ed. Williams & Wilkins, 1990.
Laragh JH, Brenner BM (editors): *Hypertension: Pathophysiology, Diagnosis and Management.* 2 vols. Raven Press, 1990.

Blood Vessels & Lymphatics

12

Lawrence M. Tierney, Jr., MD

Atherosclerosis causes most degenerative arterial disease. Its incidence increases with age; although manifestations of the disease may appear in the fourth decade, people over 40 (particularly men) are most commonly affected. Risk factors include hypercholesterolemia, diabetes mellitus, smoking, and hypertension. Atherosclerosis tends to be a generalized disease, with some degree of involvement of all major arteries, but it produces its clinical manifestations by critical involvement of a limited number of arteries. Narrowing and occlusion of the artery are the most common manifestations of the disease, but weakening of the arterial wall from a loss of elastin and collagen, resulting in aneurysmal dilation, also occurs, and both processes may be present in the same individual. Less common arterial diseases include vasculitis (of both large and small arteries), thromboangiitis obliterans (Buerger's disease), fibrodysplasia of visceral arteries, syphilitic aortitis, and radiation arteritis.

DISEASES OF THE AORTA

ANEURYSMS OF THE ABDOMINAL AORTA

Essentials of Diagnosis

- Most aneurysms are asymptomatic, detected at incidental physical examination or sonography.
- Back or abdominal pain often precedes rupture.
- Atherosclerotic occlusive disease not usually associated.

General Considerations

More than 90% of abdominal atherosclerotic aneurysms originate below the renal arteries, and many involve the bifurcation of the aorta. Aneurysms of the upper aorta are much less common. The infrarenal aorta is normally 2 cm in diameter; an aneurysm is considered present when the diameter exceeds 4 cm.

Clinical Findings

A. Symptoms and Signs:

1. Asymptomatic–A pulsating mid and upper abdominal mass may be discovered on a routine physical examination, most frequently in men over 50. Also, sonography done for other purposes often detects asymptomatic aneurysms. It is also the most cost-effective test for confirming a suspicion of aneurysm raised by physical examination. Peripheral pulses are often strikingly prominent as a result of generalized arteriomegaly in these patients. Aneurysms of the popliteal artery often coexist.

2. Symptomatic–Pain is present in some form in one-fourth to one-third of cases and varies from mild to severe midabdominal or lower back discomfort. The pain may be constant or intermittent. Peripheral emboli may occur, even from small aneurysms, and symptomatic arterial insufficiency in the legs may result.

3. Rupture–Aortic aneurysm rupture results in death before hospitalization in 25–50% of patients, and others die before they reach the operating room. Those with bleeding confined to the retroperitoneal area may have severe pain in the abdomen, flank, or back and a pulsating abdominal mass without clinical evidence of rapid blood loss, and these are the patients that require emergency aneurysm resection, which has an operative mortality rate of 50% or more. Altogether, only 10–20% survive the acute rupture of an abdominal aortic aneurysm.

B. Laboratory Findings: Electrocardiography and renal function studies should be obtained to assess potential concomitant dysfunction in those systems.

C. Imaging: Abdominal ultrasonography is the diagnostic study of choice and is also valuable for following aneurysm size in patients not immediately treated surgically. Curvilinear calcifications outlining portions of the aneurysm wall may be visible on plain films of the aortic area in approximately three-fourths of those with an aneurysm, but this study is less sensitive than ultrasonography. Contrast-enhanced CT scanning may define the extent of the aneurysm, though some surgeons prefer preoperative aortography. This study may underemphasize the aneurysm's size if thrombus is present, as is often the case. MRI is probably as sensitive and specific as CT, and its use for this purpose is increasing. It has the advantage of sparing the patient exposure to nephrotoxic contrast.

Treatment

Surgical excision and grafting is the treatment of choice for most aneurysms of the distal abdominal aorta. Aneurysms usually progressively enlarge and ultimately rupture if left untreated. The size of the aneurysm correlates best with the risk of rupture: In asymptomatic patients, surgery is advised when the aneurysm is 5 or 6 cm in diameter; in symptomatic patients, repair is indicated irrespective of size. The risk of rupture cannot be safely predicted for individuals, but it obviously increases—as does intramural aortic wall tension—as a function of its radius. Opinion differs about whether asymptomatic aneurysms in poor-risk patients should be removed or followed closely by means of ultrasound measurements to detect signs of expansion. Long-term beta-blockade appears to be associated with a decreased rate of growth of aneurysms that are being followed. Patients with significant symptomatic coronary or carotid disease may be more likely to suffer myocardial infarction or stroke during and following aneurysm resection; coronary artery bypass grafting or coronary angioplasty to lessen this risk prior to elective aneurysm repair is advocated by some. Other experienced vascular surgeons, however, believe the aneurysms should be treated first or there may be a higher rate of rupture in patients postoperative for major surgery such as coronary artery bypass grafting. Likewise, prophylactic carotid endarterectomy has not been established as being useful in this setting. Finally, individuals over age 80 with good preoperative risk factors can undergo elective surgery with an acceptable mortality rate; those with significant associated disease generally should not undergo operation without compelling indications.

Complications

Irreversible renal injury can occur if hemodynamic instability is allowed to persist through surgery. Ischemia of the distal colon and of one or both legs occasionally occurs following this surgery; in most cases, it can be prevented by meticulous attention to detail before and during surgery. As noted above, these patients are susceptible to intra- and postoperative stroke and myocardial infarction. Gastrointestinal hemorrhage, even years after aortic surgery, should suggest the possibility of graft-enteric fistula; the incidence of this complication is higher when the initial surgery was performed on an emergent basis.

Prognosis

The mortality rate following elective surgical resection is 3–8%, though in certain clinics it has recently approached 1%; clinicians must be aware of surgical success rates in their own institutions before making the often difficult decision to operate, especially in high-risk patients. Of those who survive surgery, approximately 60% are alive 5 years later, and in those who die, myocardial infarction is the leading cause of death. Among unoperated patients, old studies indicate that less than 20% survive 5 years, and aneurysm rupture is the cause of 60% of the deaths; more recently, a less rapid rate of expansion has been reported, but some surgeons dispute this. In general, a patient with an aortic aneurysm has a three-fold greater chance of dying as a consequence of rupture of the aneurysm than of dying from surgical resection. If coronary or carotid artery surgery is done preoperatively, the added morbidity and mortality of these procedures must be considered in the overall approach to the patient.

Crawford ES, Hess KR: Abdominal aortic aneurysm. N Engl J Med 1989;321:1040. (Natural history.)

Fortner G, Johansen K: Abdominal aortic aneurysm. Surg Clin North Am 1989;69:4.

Katz DA, Littenberg B, Cronenwett JL: Management of small abdominal aortic aneurysms: Early surgery vs watchful waiting. JAMA 1992;268:2678. (A decision analysis tending to favor early surgery.)

ANEURYSMS OF THE THORACIC AORTA

Thoracic aortic aneurysms are most commonly due to atherosclerosis; syphilis is now a rare cause. Vasculitis and annuloaortic ectasia (with or without Marfan's syndrome) may also result in thoracic aneurysm. Traumatic aneurysms may occur just beyond the origin of the left subclavian artery when the wall of the aorta is incompletely torn as a result of a rapid deceleration accident. Less than 10% of aortic aneurysms are thoracic.

Clinical Findings

Manifestations depend largely on the size and position of the aneurysm and its rate of growth.

A. Symptoms and Signs: There may be no symptoms or signs if the aneurysm has been diagnosed by chest x-ray done for other reasons. Substernal, back, or neck pain may occur, as well as symptoms and signs due to pressure on (1) the trachea (dyspnea, stridor, a brassy cough), (2) the esophagus (dysphagia), (3) the left recurrent laryngeal nerve (hoarseness), or (4) the superior vena cava (edema in the neck and arms, distended neck veins). Aortic insufficiency may be present.

B. Imaging: In addition to chest x-rays, aortography may be necessary to substantiate the diagnosis and to delineate the precise location and extent of the aneurysm and its relation to the vessels arising from the arch. CT scan is of more use than ultrasound in scanning thoracic aneurysms and may be as sensitive and specific as aortography, as may MRI as well. The coronary vessels and the aortic valve should also be studied if the ascending aorta is involved; echocardiography provides adequate visualization of the valve.

Differential Diagnosis

It may be difficult to determine whether a mass in the mediastinum is an aneurysm, a neoplasm, or a cyst. The x-ray studies mentioned above will distinguish an aneurysm. Radioactive isotope studies (^{125}I) may be helpful in diagnosing a substernal goiter.

Treatment

Aneurysms of the thoracic aorta often progress, with increasing symptoms, and finally rupture. Resection of aneurysms is now considered the treatment of choice if a skilled surgical team is available and if the patient's general condition is such that the major surgical procedure usually required can be done with an acceptable risk. Small asymptomatic aneurysms, especially in poor-risk patients, are perhaps better treated only if progressive enlargement occurs. Control of hypertension may slow progression. The overall mortality rate of thoracic aneurysmectomy, however, is considerably higher than the 3–5% rate for abdominal aneurysms given the complicated nature of the surgery, but no studies allow precise risk assessment.

If the aortic valve is involved, an aortic valve replacement may be necessary, and reattachment of the coronary arteries or aortocoronary bypass grafts may also be indicated. Paraplegia due to anterior spinal artery compromise is a complication of excision and graft replacement in 3% of aneurysms involving the descending thoracic aorta.

Prognosis

Small aneurysms may change very little over a period of years, and death may result from causes other than rupture. If the aneurysm is large, symptomatic, and associated with hypertension or arteriosclerotic cardiovascular disease, the prognosis is poor. Saccular aneurysms, those distal to the left subclavian artery, and those limited to the ascending aorta may be approached surgically in good-risk candidates, with the caveats cited above. Resection of aneurysms of the transverse aortic arch involves major technical problems that can be dealt with only by skilled surgical teams using hypothermia to protect the nervous system.

Crawford ES et al: Thoracoabdominal aortic aneurysms: Preoperative and intraoperative factors determining immediate and long term results of operations in 605 patients. J Vasc Surg 1986;3:389. (Largest series by far, from a group with particular technical expertise.)

PERIPHERAL ARTERY ANEURYSMS (Popliteal & Femoral)

Popliteal artery aneurysms rank third in frequency among aneurysmal lesions; most of the other peripheral aneurysms are femoral. Almost all are atherosclerotic and occur in men; bilaterality is frequent.

Popliteal Aneurysms

Almost half are asymptomatic when diagnosed, and they are generally discovered in the popliteal fossa as a pulsating mass 2 cm or more in diameter. When a popliteal aneurysm is diagnosed, abdominal aneurysm may be present and should be excluded by ultrasonography. Most aneurysms present with symptoms generally related to varying degrees of reduced blood flow to the lower leg and foot, ie, intermittent claudication if it develops slowly, or severe ischemic manifestations of rest pain, pregangrene, or gangrene when sudden thrombosis of the aneurysm occurs or when distal embolization takes place. Large aneurysms may be associated with a degree of venous obstructive manifestations or pain from pressure on the nerves; thrombophlebitis is infrequent, and rupture is rare.

Angiography is of value in defining the distal arterial tree and the collateral vessels. The actual size of the aneurysm is more clearly determined by ultrasound examination.

Popliteal aneurysms rank second to abdominal aortic aneurysms in the incidence of potentially serious complications. Even small aneurysms (2 cm in size) can become thrombosed or give rise to emboli, particularly if laminated clot exists within the lumen of the aneurysm. When thrombosis occurs, amputation may be required. Thus, prophylactic surgery is advisable upon diagnosis, and a reversed saphenous vein bypass graft with proximal and distal ligation of the aneurysm is generally employed. In large aneurysms with manifestations of vein or nerve compression, resection of the aneurysm with grafting of the arterial defect may be necessary.

Femoral Aneurysms

Femoral aneurysms, as manifested by a pulsatile mass in the femoral area on one or both sides, have the potential for the same complications as popliteal aneurysms, although rupture is a more frequent complication and limb-threatening episodes are less frequent in femoral aneurysms. Because the incidence of serious complications in the asymptomatic group seems to be considerably less than for popliteal aneurysms, there is more reason to follow rather than operate on smaller, asymptomatic femoral aneurysms and to deal first with aortoiliac and then popliteal aneurysms in preference to femoral aneurysms when aneurysmal disease exists in all of these areas.

Anton GE et al: Surgical management of popliteal aneurysms: Trends in presentation, treatment and results from 1952 to 1984. J Vasc Surg 1986;3:1986.

AORTIC DISSECTION

Essentials of Diagnosis

- A history of hypertension or Marfan's syndrome is often present. Aortic insufficiency may be present.
- Sudden severe chest pain with radiation to the back, occasionally migrating to the abdomen and hips.
- Patient appears to be in shock, but blood pressure is normal or elevated; pulse discrepancy, aortic insufficiency found in many patients.

General Considerations

Extravasation of blood into and along the wall of the aorta may occur, resulting in aortic dissection. Dissection generally begins either in the proximal aorta just above the aortic valve or at a site just beyond the origin of the left subclavian artery. If the ascending aorta is involved, it is referred to as type A; all others are type B. The initial intimal tear probably results from the constant movement of the ascending and proximal descending aorta that occurs at these two points associated with the pulsatile blood flow from the heart. Dissection occurs on rare occasions in an aorta even without an intimal tear; these aortas invariably show histologic abnormalities of the media. Proximal dissections are more often in aortas involved with abnormalities of the smooth muscle, elastic tissue, or collagen; distal dissections occur in older patients with long-standing hypertension and is a relatively rare complication of long-standing hypertension. Pregnancy (types A and B), bicuspid aortic valves and coarctation (types A and B), and Marfan's syndrome (type A) are associated with dissection in younger individuals. Both hypertension and a forceful pulse are important in progression of dissection, which may extend from the ascending aorta distally to the abdominal aorta or beyond. Alternatively, dissection may remain limited to the ascending aorta and the aortic valve area, especially if hypertension is not present or is controlled early; furthermore, distal dissection may progress not only distally but also proximally. Death may occur after hours, days, or weeks and is usually due to rupture of the aorta into the pericardial sac (with cardiac tamponade), into the left pleural cavity, or into the retroperitoneal area. Dissection may rupture back into the true lumen of the aorta (recanalization) with blood flow through both the true and false lumens; long-term survival can thus occur.

Clinical Findings

A. Symptoms and Signs: Severe, persistent chest pain of sudden onset, nearly always anterior but often also posterior, which may later progress to the abdominal and hip areas, is characteristic. Radiation down the arms or into the neck may or may not occur. Usually there is only a mild decrease in the prerupture level of blood pressure. Partial or complete occlusion of the arteries arising from the aortic arch or of the intercostal and lumbar arteries may lead to such central nervous system findings as syncope, hemiplegia, or paralysis of the lower extremities. Peripheral pulses and blood pressures may be diminished or unequal. An aortic diastolic murmur may develop as a result of dissection close to the aortic valve, resulting in secondary valvular insufficiency, heart failure, and cardiac tamponade.

B. Laboratory Findings: Electrocardiographic changes indicating left ventricular hypertrophy from long-standing hypertension are often present; acute changes may not develop unless the dissection involves the coronary ostium. In that case, inferior wall abnormalities predominate, since dissection leads to compromise of the right rather than the left coronary artery. In some, the ECG may be perfectly normal.

C. Imaging: Chest radiographs often reveal an abnormal aortic contour or a wide superior mediastinum, with changes in the configuration and thickness of the aortic wall in successive films. There may be findings of pleural or pericardial effusion. CT scan with contrast enhancement and magnetic resonance imaging (MRI) are both sensitive studies but are too time-consuming if dissection is clinically likely. Such patients should have immediate angiography, because emergency surgery may be lifesaving in type A dissection and because most surgeons require angiographic confirmation preoperatively. Recently, transesophageal echo of the aorta has shown particular promise in the diagnosis of dissection. MRI or CT scanning is best employed when dissection is considered possible but unlikely; a normal image by either technique is strong evidence against dissection, since both studies are more than 90% sensitive.

Differential Diagnosis

Aortic dissection is most commonly confused with myocardial infarction (see Chapter 10) as well as other causes of chest pain, such as pulmonary embolization. However, it may simulate numerous neurologic lesions and even various abdominal conditions related to renal-visceral ischemia.

Treatment

A. Medical Measures: If hypertension is present, aggressive measures to lower the pressure should probably be initiated even before diagnostic studies have been completed, and while the need for surgery is being contemplated. Treatment generally includes the simultaneous reduction of the systolic blood pressure to 100 mm Hg and reduction of the pulsatile aortic flow by means of the following:

(1) A rapid-acting antihypertensive agent as an intravenous infusion at a flow rate regulated by very frequent blood pressure determinations. Nitroprusside or trimethaphan may be given as follows: (a) Nitroprusside (50 mg in 1000 mL of 5% dextrose in water) is started at a rate of 0.5 mL/min and the infusion rate increased by 0.5 mL every 5 minutes until adequate control of the pressure has been achieved. Thiocyanate levels should be obtained if treatment is continued for 48 hours, and the infusion should be stopped if the drug level reaches 10 mg/dL; (b) Trimethaphan (1 or 2 mg/mL) may be infused with the patient in the semi-Fowler position.

(2) Intravenous propranolol, 0.15 mg/kg given over a 5-minute period and repeated as necessary to maintain the pulse rate at 60/min. The rapid-acting beta-blocker esmolol may be tried first in patients in whom adverse effects are considered more likely to occur, although propranolol is preferred by many for ongoing therapy. Intravenous reserpine (0.1–0.2 mg) may be used if beta-blockers are contraindicated.

Failure of this pharmacologic approach and the need for urgent surgery is suggested if chest pain is not relieved or if it reappears; if significant compromise or occlusion of a major branch of the aorta develops; or if progressive aortic enlargement, suggesting impending rupture, occurs.

B. Surgical Measures: The emphasis in treatment has shifted toward surgery, as a result of increased proficiency in handling these very difficult technical problems. If a skilled cardiovascular team is available, all acute dissections involving the ascending aorta (type A) should be treated promptly with surgery to relieve or to prevent aortic valve insufficiency and to prevent rupture. The ascending aorta and, if necessary, the aortic valve and arch may be replaced with reattachment of the coronaries and brachiocephalic vessels. The mortality rate for such operations approaches 20% or more, but this is still less than the rate for untreated type A dissection.

Surgical treatment is increasingly popular for dissections arising in the descending thoracic aorta (type B); it may be delayed until the hypertension and dissection have been stabilized by medical means and oral antihypertensives instituted. The origin of the dissection is then removed; the false lumen is closed; and a graft is inserted to deliver all blood flow through the normal lumen, thus relieving the occlusive pressure on the aortic branches.

Since patients with type B dissections tend to be poor surgical risks, permanent medical therapy may be offered. Indeed, the surgical mortality rate is higher for this operation than for operation on the more technically challenging type A patient. Regimens should include beta-blockers and antihypertensive drugs; vasodilators are contraindicated unless used with beta-blockers.

Prognosis

Without treatment, the mortality rate at 3 months is over 90%. Twenty percent are dead in 24 hours and 60% in 2 weeks. These figures may be somewhat worse for type A dissections. Although the surgical mortality rate is high in both groups, is appreciably more so in type B patients because of co-morbid illnesses. Medical therapy of type A dissection is associated with a prohibitively high mortality rate (at least 30% in 24 hours, and up to 75% in 1 week). Survival without treatment, usually due to recanalization, does occasionally occur. Intensive pharmacologic methods to lower the pulse wave and blood pressure have led to healing of the dissected aorta in patients with acute dissection and will convert others to a subacute or chronic form, which may then be treated by surgery.

Crawford ES: The diagnosis and management of aortic dissection. JAMA 1990;264:2537. (Most recent review from a center with vast experience.)

Nienaber CA et al: Diagnosis of thoracic aortic dissection: Magnetic resonance imaging versus transesophageal echocardiography. Circulation 1992;85:434. (Both very sensitive, but transesophageal echo is less specific than in earlier studies.)

ATHEROSCLEROTIC OCCLUSIVE DISEASE

Occlusive disease of the aorta and its branches is a common cause of disability. It is also a predictor of morbidity for patients with cardiac disease and those undergoing general surgery. It is essential for the primary physician to emphasize its prevention, particularly in light of what is known about etiologic factors. Smoking must be interdicted in all individuals, and serum cholesterol should be determined in all adults under the care of physicians. Discontinuance of smoking and dietary or pharmacologic management when the serum cholesterol exceeds 200 mg/dL are prudent measures likely to reduce morbidity from atherosclerosis (see Chapters 1 and 27).

OCCLUSIVE DISEASE OF THE AORTA & ILIAC ARTERIES

Occlusive disease of the aorta and the iliac arteries begins most frequently just proximal to the bifurcation of the common iliac arteries and at or just distal to the bifurcation of the aorta. Atherosclerotic changes occur in the intima and media, often with associated perivascular inflammation and calcified plaques in the media. Progression involves the complete occlusion of one or both common iliac arteries and then the abdominal aorta up to the segment just below the renal vessels. Although atherosclerosis is a generalized disease, occlusion tends to be segmental in distribution, and when the involvement is in the aortoiliac vessels there may be minimal atherosclerosis in the more distal external iliac and femoral arteries. Patients with localized occlusions less than 10 cm in length at or just beyond the aortic bifurcation with relatively normal vessels proximally and distally are good candidates for angioplasty, atherectomy, and perhaps stenting. Conversely, patients with multisegmented arterial disease usually have more symptoms, are more apt to require surgical treatment and are at greater risk of losing a limb. Abrupt worsening of limb ischemia symptoms may be associated with plaque rupture (crescendo claudication), as may myocardial ischemia.

Clinical Findings

Intermittent claudication is almost always present in the calf muscles and is usually present in the thighs and buttocks. It is most often bilateral and progressive. Some complain only of weakness in the legs when walking or a feeling of "tiredness" in the buttocks. Impotence is a common complaint in men. Rest pain is infrequent.

Femoral pulses are absent or very weak, and distal pulses are absent. A bruit may be heard over the aorta or over the iliac or femoral arteries. Systolic blood pressure, normally higher in the leg, is greater in the brachial artery than at the ankle; the difference is exaggerated by exercise. Atrophic changes of the skin, subcutaneous tissues, and muscles of the distal leg are usually minimal, as are dependent rubor and coolness of the skin, unless distal arterial disease is also present. Aortography, including oblique views of the thigh and leg arteries, demonstrates the level and extent of the occlusion and the condition of the vessels distal to the block, but it is not indicated unless invasive restoration of flow is contemplated. It may be replaced by magnetic resonance angiography, which does not require contrast. Doppler ultrasonography and transcutaneous oximetry offer noninvasive evaluation of pressure and oxygenation; though not necessary for screening, they can be useful in following progression of disease.

Treatment

Surgical or angioplastic treatment is indicated if claudication interferes appreciably with the patient's essential activities or work. Discontinuation of smoking is essential; some surgeons insist on it as a prerequisite for operation.

Because many of these patients have coexisting ischemic heart disease, their medical management should be maximized preoperatively. The roles of exercise testing and coronary angiography are dis-

cussed in Chapter 10 (in the section on the Cardiac Patient and Surgery). Some clinicians obtain these studies with an eye toward prophylactic bypass grafting or coronary angioplasty; this has not been conclusively shown to be of benefit in this situation if patients are minimally symptomatic.

A. Conservative Care: A program of daily walking for fixed periods, stopping for claudication, may improve collateralization and function. Although its use is debated, pentoxifylline, 400 mg three times daily, may help some patients with symptomatic claudication of long duration. It appears to reduce the incidence of invasive therapeutic procedures such as surgery, though the overall cost of care is not affected. Many patients with claudication are receiving beta-blockers for angina or hypertension. Though in theory this may worsen symptoms by allowing unopposed alpha agonism, consensus holds that this is not a clinical problem.

The following therapies are best advanced for disabling symptoms, such as extremity pain at rest and skin ulceration.

B. Arterial Graft (Prosthesis): An arterial prosthesis bypassing the occluded segment or segments is effective treatment for complex aortoiliac occlusive disease. In general, the bifurcation graft extends from the infrarenal abdominal aorta, usually by means of an end-to-end anastomosis, to the distal external iliac or common femoral arteries as end-to-side anastomoses. A patient may also be treated surgically with less risk but also less favorable results by means of a graft from the axillary artery to one or both femoral arteries or, in the case of iliac unilateral disease, from the femoral artery with normal blood flow to the contralateral femoral artery distal to the stenotic iliac vessel.

C. Thromboendarterectomy: This procedure, which avoids the use of a prosthesis, is generally used when the occlusion is limited to the common iliac arteries and when the external iliac and common femoral arteries are free of significant occlusive disease.

D. Endovascular Surgical Techniques: Occlusive lesions that were formerly dealt with entirely by methods as described in paragraphs B and C, above, are now being treated by percutaneous transluminal angioplasty, atherectomy, and laser with increasing frequency. (See below for further details.)

Prognosis

The operative mortality rate is 2–6%—a great deal less for the angioplastic procedure. The immediate and long-term benefits are often impressive. In patients with no distal occlusive disease, improvement is both subjective and objective, with relief of all or most of the claudication and, usually, return of all the pulses in the extremities. Late occlusions in this group of patients are infrequent, and if proper judgment is used in patient selection, results are comparable for angioplasty, endarterectomy, and arterial grafting techniques.

Coffman JD: Intermittent claudication: Be conservative. N Engl J Med 1991;325:577. (Articulates a cautious approach based on attention to natural history.)

Wilt TJ: Current strategies in the diagnosis and management of lower extremity peripheral vascular disease. J Gen Intern Med 1992;7:87. (A balanced review.)

OCCLUSIVE DISEASE OF THE FEMORAL & POPLITEAL ARTERIES

In the region of the thigh and knee, the vessels most frequently blocked by occlusive disease are the superficial femoral artery and the popliteal artery. Atherosclerotic changes usually appear first at the most distal point of the superficial femoral artery, where it passes through the adductor magnus tendon into the popliteal space. In time, the whole superficial femoral artery may become occluded; the disease progresses into the popliteal artery less frequently. The common femoral and deep femoral arteries are usually patent and relatively free of disease, although the origin of the profunda femoris is sometimes narrowed. The distal popliteal and its three terminal branches may also be relatively free of occlusive disease.

Clinical Findings

A. Symptoms and Signs: Intermittent claudication is confined to the calf and foot. Atrophic changes in the lower leg and foot are distinct, with loss of hair, thinning of the skin and subcutaneous tissues, and diminution in the size of the muscles. Dependent rubor and blanching on elevation of the foot are usually present. When the leg is lowered after elevation, venous filling on the dorsal aspect of the foot may be slowed to 15–20 seconds or more. The foot is usually cool. The common femoral pulsations are usually of fair or good quality, although a bruit may be heard. No popliteal or pedal pulses can be felt. Pressure measurements in the distal leg, using ultrasound, will supply an objective functional assessment of the circulation and will aid in the decision to go on to x-ray studies and possibly surgery. In general, the greater the differentiation in pressure between proximal and distal extremity pressures, the worse the prognosis for limb preservation without revascularization.

B. Imaging: If surgery is being considered, a femoral arteriogram will show the location and extent of the block as well as the status of the distal vessels, and lateral or oblique views will reveal whether the origin of the profunda femoris is narrow. It is important to know the condition of the aortoiliac vessels also, since a relatively normal inflow as well as an adequate distal "run-off" is important in determining the likelihood of success of an arterial procedure. Magnetic resonance angiography holds promise for a less invasive way to acquire the same information.

Treatment

Walking is the most effective way to develop collateral circulation, and walking up to the point of claudication, followed by a 3-minute rest, should be done at least eight times a day. Smoking must be discontinued.

Surgery is indicated (1) if intermittent claudication is progressive or incapacitating, interfering significantly with the patient's essential physical activities such as ability to work; or (2) if there is rest pain or pregangrenous or gangrenous lesions on the foot.

A. Arterial Graft: An autogenous vein graft using a reversed segment of the great saphenous vein can be placed, bypassing the occluded segment. The distal anastomosis is usually to the popliteal artery, below the site of major occlusive disease. Another approach is to destroy the valves in the in situ saphenous vein before making the bypass anastomosis. When the entire popliteal artery is occluded and gangrene or advanced ischemic changes are present in the foot, it is generally better to perform an amputation below the knee rather than an anastomosis to one of the leg arteries, though bypass anastomosis to a tibial or peroneal artery is being done by skilled vascular surgeons with increasing success. Synthetic arterial prostheses, with the possible exception of the PTFE (polytetrafluoroethylene) grafts, have not proved to be very successful in this area because of the relatively high incidence of early or late thrombosis.

B. Thromboendarterectomy: Thromboendarterectomy with removal of the central occluding core may be successful if the occluded and stenotic segment is very short.

When significant aortoiliac or common femoral occlusive disease exists as well as superficial femoral and popliteal occlusions, it is usually better to relieve the obstructions in the larger, proximal arteries and deliver more blood flow to the profunda femoris than to operate on the smaller distal vessels, where the chances of success are less. If the origin of the profunda femoris is narrowed, a limited procedure at that site—a profundoplasty—may be successful in improving blood flow to the leg and foot and may be used, especially in poor-risk patients with rest pain.

C. Endovascular Surgery: As for aortoiliac disease, more distal lesions may be treated using one or more nonsurgical approaches, which include (1) balloon angioplasty, using balloon-tipped catheters capable of forcefully dilating narrow or occluded areas; (2) mechanical atherectomy devices to remove the occluding atheroma from the lumen of the artery; and (3) laser or thermal angioplasty equipment that can vaporize the occlusive material.

These techniques require arteriography. Anticoagulants, thrombolytics, antiplatelet drugs, and agents to counteract arterial spasm are frequently employed along with the procedure. Recurrent stenosis can often be re-treated by these techniques, or bypass surgery may be elected.

The most favorable lesions again include single, short discrete stenoses. Less favorable lesions are multiple stenoses in series, those longer than 5 cm, complete occlusions less than 5 cm long, lesions in the smaller arteries, and stenotic arterial anastomoses or grafts, particularly if the patient has diabetes or is a smoker.

After any of these procedures, the patient is generally maintained on permanent antiplatelet medication; one aspirin tablet daily is sufficient.

Prognosis

Thrombosis of the bypass graft or of the endarterectomized vessel either in the immediate postoperative period or months or years later is relatively frequent in the superficial femoral-popliteal area. This is particularly true if iliac arterial stenosis exists or if one or more of the three terminal branches of the distal popliteal artery are badly diseased. It is also observed after endarterectomy, when a synthetic prosthesis is used, or after an angioplastic procedure. For this reason, operation is usually not recommended for mild or moderate claudication, and approximately 80% of these patients will have relatively stable symptoms and will go for years without much progression. Some may improve as collateral circulation develops. The chances of improvement after surgery are less in patients with ischemia or early gangrene, but surgery or angioplasty is often justified because some limbs can be saved from amputation. The 5-year overall patency rate for the saphenous vein bypass grafts is in the range of 60–80%, or less if the bypass is to a tibial artery. The 2-year patency rate after transluminal angioplasty is over 80% and thus compares favorably with the venous bypass results over that period, although the long-term results may not be as good. Only about 50% of these patients survive 5 years; most deaths are due to complications of atherosclerosis, especially myocardial infarction. After 5 years, the yearly mortality rate exceeds the rate of loss of patency of the graft.

Higgins CB: The potential role of magnetic resonance imaging in ischemic vascular disease. (Editorial.) N Engl J Med 1992;326:1624.
Moore WS et al: Endovascular Surgery. Saunders, 1989. (State of the art in a rapidly developing field.)

OCCLUSIVE DISEASE OF THE ARTERIES IN THE LOWER LEG & FOOT

Occlusive processes in the lower leg and foot may involve, in order of incidence, the tibial and common peroneal arteries, the pedal vessels, and occasionally the small digital vessels. Symptoms depend upon the vessels that are narrowed or thrombosed, the suddenness and extent of the occlusion, and the status of the proximal and collateral vessels. The clinical picture may be a rather stable or a slowly progressive form of vascular insufficiency that over months or years may ultimately result in atrophy, ischemic pain, and, occasionally, gangrene.

Clinical Findings

Although all of the possible manifestations of vascular disease in the lower leg and foot cannot be described here, there are certain significant clinical aspects that enter into the evaluation of these patients.

A. Symptoms and Signs: Intermittent claudication is the commonest presenting symptom. Aching fatigue during exertion usually appears first in the calf muscles; in more severe cases, a constant or cramping pain may be brought on by walking only a short distance. Less commonly, the feet are the site of most of the pain. The distance the patient can walk before onset of pain is indicative of the degree of circulatory inadequacy: two blocks (360–460 meters) or more is mild, one block is moderate, and one-half block or less is severe. Rest pain may occur at night and is a dull, persistent ache. As in the case of femoral and popliteal disease, rest pain implies severe involvement. A degree of relief can often be obtained by uncovering the foot and letting it hang over the side of the bed.

On examination, although the popliteal pulse may be present, both pedal pulses are usually absent. Exercise may make pedal pulses disappear in some patients. Dependent rubor is prominent. The skin is cool, atrophic, and hairless. Again, these findings may be indistinguishable from those of occlusive disease higher in the leg. The presence of a popliteal pulse points to more distal occlusion when these symptoms and signs are present.

B. Imaging: Films of the lower leg and foot may show calcification of the vessels. If there is a draining sinus or an ulcer close to a bone or joint, osteomyelitis may be apparent on the film. If fairly strong popliteal pulses can be felt, arteriography is of little value. Doppler ultrasonography provides an accurate blood pressure assessment in the pedal pulses.

Treatment

A. Medical Measures: Low-dose aspirin (80–325 mg daily) has theoretical value and is innocuous as an antiplatelet agent; it should be given to all patients with severe peripheral vascular disease. Pentoxifylline (400 mg three times daily) may have some usefulness in patients with chronic symptomatology.

B. Circulatory Insufficiency in the Foot and Toes: Lumbar sympathectomy may be indicated when ischemic or pregangrenous changes are present in the distal foot or when small ulcers are present in a foot with diminished circulation. There is no change in the circulation to the muscles and thus no relief from claudication. Patients who cannot tolerate the surgical procedure may be considered for chemical sympathectomy with 6% phenol. Vasodilator drugs are of little or no value. The general care of the feet is most important (see Chapter 26.)

ARTERIAL DISEASE IN DIABETIC PATIENTS

Atherosclerosis develops more often and earlier in patients with diabetes mellitus, especially if the patient smokes. Either the large or small vessels may be involved, but occlusion of the smaller vessels is more frequent than in the nondiabetic, and diabetics thus more often have the form of the disease that may not be suitable for arterial surgery. Cigarette smoking is particularly harmful and must be strongly interdicted. Ulcers, when present, are more likely to be moist and infected; healing, if it occurs at all, may be very slow, and healed areas may break down easily.

Diabetic neuropathy with diminished or absent sensation of the toes or feet may occur, predisposing to injury or pressure ulcerations that may be neglected because of the absence of pain. These patients may not necessarily have diminished circulation to the feet.

Poor vision due to diabetic retinopathy makes the care of the feet more difficult and injury more likely. The best approach to diabetic lower limb loss is prevention, and the incidence can be reduced by up to 50% in communities with diabetic foot clinics. See Chapter 26 for instructions on care of the feet.

Moss SE, Klein R, Klein BEK: The prevalence and incidence of lower extremity amputation in a diabetic population. Arch Intern Med 1992;152:610.

OCCLUSIVE CEREBROVASCULAR DISEASE

Although episodes of weakness or dizziness, blurred vision, or sudden complete hemiplegia may be due to a variety of causes, atherosclerotic occlusive or ulcerative disease accounts for many of these problems (see Chapter 23). Single or multiple segmental lesions are often located in the extracranial arteries and account for ischemic stroke syndromes in over half of cases. The extracranial areas most often involved are (1) the common carotid bifurcation, including the origins of the internal and external carotid arteries (approximately 90%); (2) the origin of the vertebral artery; and (3) the intrathoracic segments of the aortic arch branches.

Clinical Findings

A. Symptoms: Transient ischemic attacks (TIAs) may be the earliest manifestation of carotid arterial stenosis or ulceration. Episodes usually last for only a few minutes but may continue for up to 24 hours. Significant carotid artery stenosis with temporary diminished blood flow to the brain or ulcerations with microemboli from the carotid ulcer to the brain or the ipsilateral retinal artery are responsible for many TIAs and may precede a complete stroke in half of these patients. The classic manifestations include contralateral weakness or sensory changes, speech alterations, and visual disturbance (usual temporary partial or complete loss of vision in the ipsilateral eye). Vertebrobasilar TIAs are characterized by brain stem and cerebellar symptoms, including dysarthria, diplopia, vertigo, ataxia, and alternating hemiparesis or quadriparesis.

Dizziness and unsteadiness, particularly when associated with a quick change in position, are nonspecific symptoms and more often the result of postural hypotension than of vertebrobasilar problems. Atypical neurologic symptoms or personality changes are seldom symptoms of cerebral ischemia.

B. Signs: Bruits in the lower neck, diminished or absent pulsations in the neck or arms, and a blood pressure difference in the two arms of more than 10 mm Hg may be indications of occlusive disease in the brachiocephalic arteries. More significant than a brachiocephalic bruit is one sharply localized high in the lateral neck close to the angle of the jaw (overlying the common carotid bifurcation), but a major stenosis of 75% or more and thus sufficient to reduce the blood flow through the vessel is present in a minority of patients with these bruits. The murmur of aortic stenosis may be heard as a bruit over the subclavian and carotid arteries; when there is no such heart murmur, the bruit generally denotes disease in these arteries. Bruits are often present without symptoms, and the absence of a bruit does not exclude the possibility of carotid artery stenosis. Thus, bruits heard over the carotid arteries are neither sensitive nor specific enough to alter the diagnostic approach in this patient group. Microemboli can arise from ulcerations of arteries to the brain without stenosis or bruit, particularly if the ulcer is large. Only the common carotid and superficial temporal pulses can be felt with accuracy; the internal carotid pulses cannot usually be palpated.

Additional Studies

Diagnostic studies of the cerebral circulation are both noninvasive and invasive. Of the former, duplex ultrasonography, when available, is now the investigation of choice. In duplex ultrasound, two ultrasonic techniques are used in concert, and the clinician is provided with both physiologic and anatomic information; indeed, ulcerating plaques, hemorrhage into an atherosclerotic lesion, and other abnormalities may be observed in images comparable to those obtained by angiography. Results in combined studies show high specificity and sensitivity for this test—in excess of any other current noninvasive technique. In addition, the hemodynamic degree of stenosis may be accurately determined. When duplex ultrasonography is unavailable, Doppler ultrasound provides an excellent alternative, though the information gleaned concerns mainly changes in blood flow caused by stenosis. Doppler ultrasound is not as sensitive as duplex ultrasonography; it has comparable specificity. When combined with the indirect information obtained by periorbital Doppler ultrasound—which detects collaterals in the periorbital circulation—its sensitivity may be increased. Doppler ultrasound does not identify anatomic abnormalities, however, as reliably as duplex ultrasound.

Arteriographic visualization of the cerebral vessels confirms the location and degree of stenoses and plaques, the presence of arterial occlusions, and the nature of collateral flow.

Treatment

A. Medical Measures: Acute strokes, most progressive or evolving strokes, and those with major neurologic deficits are treated by medical means as discussed in the section on cerebrovascular accidents in Chapter 23. Patients with transient ischemic attacks may be treated with antiplatelet drugs (aspirin, 100–325 mg/d) or with oral anticoagulants, though there is now some evidence that the former is safer and more effective than the latter, particularly in men.

B. Surgical Measures: Carotid endarterectomy, when expertly performed, may be offered for properly evaluated transient ischemic attacks. It is most effective when symptoms are specific for cerebral ischemia of recent origin involving the anterior circulation, and it is essential that the vascular surgeon be one who performs carotid endarterectomies regularly with a mortality-complication rate of less than 3%. Primary care physicians are obliged to know this information prior to referral, since even a slightly increased risk may outweigh the anticipated benefit.

Considerable controversy exists as to whether surgery should be offered to patients with asymptomatic carotid bruits. Many surgeons believe that with increasing ability to evaluate stenosis noninvasively, it is possible to easily identify patients with high-grade stenosis who might theoretically be helped by prophylactic carotid endarterectomy. The best data available, however, indicate that with few exceptions, the risk of stroke in untreated patients with asymptomatic carotid bruits is less than the combined risk of carotid angiography and surgery if preventing stroke is the aim. About 2% of patients per year with such a bruit suffer a stroke; this approximates 3% if the stenosis exceeds 75%. Thus, the risk of causing stroke from angiography and surgery should be less

than 3% if surgery is to be offered at all. The widespread variability in the skill of surgical teams has perhaps contributed to the nature of the controversy. It should also be noted that prophylactic carotid endarterectomy does not appear to alter the incidence of stroke complicating coronary artery bypass grafting. Stroke in this clinical setting may result from cardiac embolization and not from carotid disease.

Endarterectomy may be indicated as an emergency procedure in patients with very early and fluctuating neurologic deficits with significant carotid stenosis. It is not useful in acute stroke or progressing stroke or when there is also severe intracranial disease.

Prognosis

The prognosis and results of therapy are related to the number of vessels involved, the degree of stenosis in each, and the collateral flow in the circle of Willis. Expertly performed surgery may have a mortality rate of 1–2% and with 1–4% permanent major or minor neurologic complications; there is wide institutional variation in these figures. Transient ischemic attacks known to be secondary to significant carotid artery stenosis or ulceration can often be eliminated by surgery, and although future strokes can occur in such patients, other arterial lesions, such as a contralateral carotid stenosis or intracranial arterial lesions, are often responsible. Concomitant coronary artery disease results in an overall mortality rate that is similar in operated and unoperated groups. In the best hands, the operative procedure in patients with transient ischemic attacks may reduce the chance of developing a permanent neurologic deficit within 5 years from 34–35% to 10%. The incidence of later stroke after uncomplicated endarterectomy is around 5–15%, and although restenosis may occur in the operated artery, it may not be clinically symptomatic. Significant carotid artery stenosis without symptoms entails no more than a 5–20% stroke risk over 3–5 years.

Feussner JR, Matchar DB: When and how to study the carotid arteries. Ann Intern Med 1988;109:805. (Superb overall review of the subject, recommending a conservative approach.)

Mayberg MR et al: Carotid endarterectomy and prevention of cerebral ischemia in symptomatic carotid stenosis. JAMA 1991;266:3289. (Indicates benefit when stenosis is between 70% and 99%.)

North American Symptomatic Carotid Endarterectomy Trial Collaborators: Beneficial effects of carotid endarterectomy in symptomatic patients with high-grade carotid stenosis. N Engl J Med 1991;325:445. (Current status of indications for this procedure.)

VISCERAL ARTERY INSUFFICIENCY

Chronic intestinal ischemia generally results from atherosclerotic occlusive lesions at or close to the origins of the superior mesenteric, celiac, and inferior mesenteric arteries, leading to a significant reduction of blood flow to the intestines. Symptoms consist of epigastric or periumbilical postprandial pains that last for 1–3 hours. To avoid pain, the patient limits oral intake, and weight loss results; at this stage of the illness, pain may be absent. Diarrhea may be present. Such a history in a person over 45 years of age who appears chronically ill and who has peripheral arterial disease is probably an indication for arteriography if the patient is felt to be a candidate for surgery.

Acute intestinal ischemia results from (1) embolic occlusions of the visceral branches of the abdominal aorta, generally in patients with valvular heart disease or atrial fibrillation, or left ventricular mural thrombus; (2) thrombosis of one or more of the visceral vessels involved with arteriosclerotic occlusive changes, sometimes in patients with a history of chronic intestinal ischemia as described above; or (3) nonocclusive mesenteric vascular insufficiency, generally in patients with congestive heart failure receiving recently instituted digitalis or in those who are in shock. The acute onset of crampy or steady epigastric and periumbilical abdominal pain combined with minimal or no findings on abdominal examination and often a high leukocyte count should suggest one of these three events in the superior mesenteric system. Lactic acidosis, hypotension, and abdominal distention suggests bowel infarction rather than ischemia. Angiography of the superior mesenteric artery is essential for early diagnosis and should be performed promptly if surgery is contemplated. Mesenteric duplex scanning is a noninvasive technique for the anatomic and physiologic assessment of the visceral vessels and may be helpful in selecting patients for arteriography. If occlusion is present, antibiotics specific for intestinal flora should be instituted (eg, ampicillin and aminoglycoside plus clindamycin or metronidazole) and laparotomy should be performed to reestablish blood flow to the intestine if possible and remove necrotic bowel if at least some viable bowel exists. The clinical picture of **acute mesenteric vein occlusion** is similar to that of arterial syndromes, and therapy is identical. Patients at risk include those with systemic hypercoagulability, such as is observed with paroxysmal nocturnal hemoglobinuria or protein C, protein S, or antithrombin III deficiency.

Through early diagnosis and aggressive treatment, the very poor prognosis of the past should yield somewhat lower morbidity and mortality rates.

Ischemic colitis develops when the diminished circulation is most prominent in the distribution of the inferior mesenteric artery. Because of the nature of the collaterals, infarction is uncommon in this instance. However, the patient may have episodic bouts of crampy lower abdominal pain associated with mild diarrhea, often bloody. This picture may be indistinguishable from inflammatory bowel disease. Colonoscopy may reveal segmental inflammatory changes, most often in the rectosigmoid and the splenic flexure where the collateral circulation is most active. Because adequate collateral circulation usually develops, the prognosis is better than when the vascular insufficiency involves the superior mesenteric circulation, and maintenance of hydration may be all that is necessary.

Rapp JH et al: Durability of endarterectomy and antegrade grafts in the treatment of chronic visceral ischemia. J Vasc Surg 1986;3:799. (Shows that a surgical approach may provide appreciable benefit.)

ACUTE ARTERIAL OCCLUSION

Essentials of Diagnosis

- Symptoms and signs depend on the artery occluded, the organ or region supplied by the artery, and the adequacy of the collateral circulation to the area primarily involved.
- Occlusion in an extremity usually results in pain, numbness, tingling, weakness, and coldness.
- There is pallor or mottling; motor, reflex, and sensory alteration; and collapsed superficial veins.
- Pulsations are absent in arteries distal to the occlusion. Occlusions in other areas result in such conditions as cerebrovascular accidents, intestinal ischemia and gangrene, and renal or splenic infarcts.

Differential Diagnosis

The primary differentiation is between arterial embolism and thrombosis. In an older individual with both arteriosclerotic vascular disease and cardiac disease, the differentiation may be very difficult, and in 10–20% a definite diagnosis either cannot be made or turns out to be incorrect. Arterial trauma may result in either occlusion or spasm.

1. ARTERIAL EMBOLISM

Arterial embolism is generally a complication of heart disease; a minority of those with embolism have rheumatic heart disease, but most have ischemic heart disease, with or without myocardial infarction. Atrial fibrillation is often present. Other forms of heart disease and miscellaneous causes account for the rest. In 10%, there is more than one embolism, and recurrent emboli after initial successful treatment may occur.

Emboli tend to lodge at the bifurcation of major arteries, with over half going to the aortic bifurcation or the vessels in the lower extremities; the carotid system is involved in 20%, and the upper extremity and the mesenteric arteries in the remainder. Emboli from arterial ulcerations are usually small, giving rise to transient symptoms in the toes or brain.

Clinical Findings

In an extremity, the initial symptoms are usually pain (sudden or gradual in onset), numbness, coldness, and tingling. Signs include absence of pulsations in the arteries distal to the block, coldness, pallor or mottling, hypesthesia or anesthesia, and weakness, muscle spasm, or paralysis. The superficial veins are collapsed. Later, blebs and skin necrosis may appear, and gangrene may occur.

Treatment

Immediate embolectomy is the treatment of choice in almost all early cases of emboli in extremities. It is best done within 4–6 hours after the embolic episode; it is occasionally successful after longer delays if the supplied tissue remains viable.

A. Emergency Preoperative Care:

1. Heparin–Heparin sodium, 5000 units intravenously, should be given as soon as the diagnosis is made or suspected in an effort to prevent distal thrombosis and continued until the time of surgery, maintaining the partial thromboplastin time (PTT) at twice the normal level. It may also help relieve associated spasm.

2. Protect the part–The extremity is kept at or below the horizontal plane, and neither heat nor cold is applied. The limb must be protected from hard surfaces and overlying bedclothes.

3. Imaging–Arteriography is often of value either before or during surgery; contrast studies, though still the standard of care, may be supplanted by magnetic resonance angiography. There may be more than one embolus in an extremity. Echocardiography may confirm the source; the transesophageal approach increases the test's sensitivity.

B. Surgical Measures: Local anesthesia is generally used if the occlusion is in an artery to an extremity. After the embolus is removed through the arteriotomy, the proximal and distal artery should be explored for additional emboli or secondary thrombi by means of a specially designed catheter with a small inflatable balloon at the tip (Fogarty catheter). An embolus at the aortic bifurcation or in the iliac artery can often be removed under local anesthesia through common femoral arteriotomies with the use of these same catheters. Laparotomy is necessary for emboli to the mesenteric circulation. Heparinization for a week or more postoperatively is indicated, and prolonged anticoagulation with warfarin is usually desirable after that to prevent recurrence.

Delayed embolectomy carried out more than 12 hours following the embolism or when there is ischemia or necrosis—as evidenced by mottled cyanosis, muscle rigidity, anesthesia, or markedly elevated serum CK—involves a high risk of acute respiratory distress syndrome or acute renal failure (or both). Anticoagulation rather than surgery or catheter embolectomy is the proper initial therapy under such circumstances, accepting urgent or elective amputation as the necessary lifesaving procedure in most instances.

Prognosis

Arterial embolism is a threat not only to the limb (5–25% amputation rate) but also to the life of the patient (25–30% hospital mortality rate, with the underlying heart disease responsible for over half of these deaths).

Emboli in the aortoiliac area are more dangerous than more peripheral emboli, and the mortality rate rises if there are multiple peripheral emboli or carotid or visceral emboli, approaching 100% if all three areas are involved. Emboli associated with hypertensive or arteriosclerotic heart disease have a poorer prognosis than those arising from rheumatic valvular disease.

In patients with atrial fibrillation, an attempt may be made to restore normal rhythm pharmacologically or by cardioversion after the patient has been anticoagulated; restoration of normal rhythm tends to be permanent only in patients with recent onset or transitory fibrillation. Long-term anticoagulant therapy diminishes the danger of further emboli and in the majority of patients is the only long-term prophylactic measure that can be instituted.

If no heart disease exists, arteriography may reveal an atherosclerotic ulcer or small aneurysm to be the origin of the embolus; depending upon location, these may be treated surgically. Three-fourths of the patients that do survive the embolic episode and the associated hospital stay may then have a good quality of life.

2. ACUTE ARTERIAL THROMBOSIS

Acute arterial thrombosis generally occurs in an artery in which the lumen has become narrow as a result of arteriosclerotic changes in the wall of the artery. Blood flowing through such a narrow, irregular, or ulcerated lumen may clot, leading to a sudden, complete occlusion of the narrow segment. The thrombosis may then propagate either up or down the artery to a point where the blood is flowing rapidly through a somewhat less diseased artery (usually to a significant arterial branch proximally or one or more functioning collateral vessels distally). Occasionally, the thrombosis is precipitated when the bloodstream dissects and displaces an arteriosclerotic plaque, blocking the lumen; trauma to the artery may precipitate a similar event. Inflammatory involvement of the arterial wall will also lead to acute thrombosis. Chronic mechanical irritation of the subclavian artery compressed by a cervical rib may also lead to a complete occlusion. Thrombosis in a diseased artery may be secondary to an episode of hypotension or cardiac failure. Polycythemia and dehydration also increase the chance of thrombosis, as do repeated arterial punctures.

Chronic, incomplete arterial obstruction usually results in the establishment of some collateral flow, and further flow will develop relatively rapidly through the collaterals once complete occlusion has developed. The extremity may be threatened for hours or days, however, while the additional collateral circulation develops around the block.

Clinical Findings

The local findings in the extremity are usually very similar to those described in the section on arterial embolism. The following differential points should be checked: (1) Are there manifestations of advanced occlusive arterial disease in other areas, especially the opposite extremity (bruit, absent pulses, secondary changes)? Is there a history of intermittent claudication? These clinical manifestations are suggestive but not diagnostic of thrombosis. (2) Is there a history or are there findings of rheumatic heart disease or of a recent episode of atrial fibrillation or myocardial infarction? If so, an embolism is more likely than a thrombosis. (3) Electrocardiography, echocardiography, and serum enzyme studies may give added information regarding the presence of a silent myocardial infarction and its likelihood as a source of an embolus. Ultimately, arteriography is necessary for accurate differential diagnosis and for planning therapy.

Treatment

Whereas emergency embolectomy is the usual approach in the case of an early occlusion from an embolus, a nonoperative approach is generally used in the case of thrombosis for two reasons: (1) The segment of thrombosed artery may be quite long, requiring rather extensive and difficult surgery (thromboendarterectomy or artery graft). The removal of a single embolus in a normal or nearly normal artery is, by comparison, relatively easy and quick. (2) The extremity is more likely to survive without development of gangrene because some collateral circulation has usually formed during the slowly progressive stenosing phase before acute thrombosis. With an embolism, this is not usually the case; the block is most often at a major arterial bifurcation, occluding both branches, and the associated arterial spasm is usually more acute. Treatment—particularly if tissue necrosis is present—is as described for emergency preoperative care for arterial embolism. Thrombolytic therapy using streptokinase or the more expensive urokinase or tissue plasminogen activator (t-PA) may be tried in acute thrombosis if no tissue necrosis exists; lysis may be achieved in 50–80% of cases, and direct arterial infusion into the thrombus has fewer bleeding complications than systemic therapy with these drugs since the dose given locally is much smaller. A complication and amputation rate of al-

most 20% and a mortality rate of 2% dictates caution in the use of this form of therapy. If successful thrombolysis occurs, rethrombosis may be prevented by angioplasty. Otherwise, treatment is as outlined under emergency preoperative care for arterial embolism.

Prognosis

Limb survival usually occurs with acute thrombosis of the iliac or superficial femoral arteries; gangrene is more likely if the popliteal is suddenly occluded, especially if the period between occlusion and treatment is long or if there is considerable arterial spasm or proximal arterial occlusive disease. If the limb does survive the acute occlusion, significant functional recovery may occur gradually over a number of weeks. The later treatment and prognosis are outlined above in the section on occlusive disease of the iliac, femoral, and popliteal arteries.

Dacey LJ et al: Cost-effectiveness of intra-arterial thrombolytic therapy. Arch Surg 1988;123:1218. (May diminish morbidity and hospitalization time, thus reducing cost.)

THROMBOANGIITIS OBLITERANS (Buerger's Disease)

Essentials of Diagnosis

- Almost always in young men who smoke.
- Extremities involved with inflammatory occlusions of the more distal arteries, resulting in circulatory insufficiency of the toes or fingers.
- Thromboses of superficial veins may also occur.
- Course is intermittent and amputation may be necessary, especially if smoking is not stopped.

General Considerations

Buerger's disease is an episodic and segmental inflammatory and thrombotic process of the arteries and veins, principally in the limbs. The cause is not known. It is seen most commonly in men under 40 who smoke. The effects of the disease are almost solely due to occlusion of the arteries. The symptoms are primarily due to ischemia, complicated in the later stages by infection and tissue necrosis. The inflammatory process is intermittent, with quiescent periods lasting weeks, months, or years.

The arteries most commonly affected are the plantar and digital vessels in the foot and those in the lower leg. The arteries in the hands and wrists may also become involved. Different arterial segments may become occluded in successive episodes; a certain amount of recanalization occurs during quiescent periods. Superficial migratory thrombophlebitis is a common early indication of the disease.

Clinical Findings

The signs and symptoms are primarily those of arterial insufficiency, and the differentiation from arteriosclerotic peripheral vascular disease may be difficult; however, the following findings suggest Buerger's disease:

(1) The patient is a man under 40 who smokes.

(2) There is a history or finding of small, red, tender cords resulting from migratory superficial segmental thrombophlebitis, usually in the saphenous tributaries rather than the main vessel. A biopsy of such a vein often gives microscopic proof of Buerger's disease.

(3) Intermittent claudication is common and is frequently noted in the palm of the hand or arch of the foot. Rest pain is frequent and persistent. It tends to be more pronounced than in the patient with atherosclerosis. Numbness, diminished sensation, and pricking and burning pains may be present as a result of ischemic neuropathy.

(4) The digit or the entire distal portion of the foot may be pale and cold, or there may be rubor that may remain relatively unchanged by posture; the skin may not blanch on elevation, and on dependency the intensity of the rubor is often more pronounced than that seen in the atherosclerotic group. The distal vascular changes are often asymmetric, so that not all of the toes are affected to the same degree. Absence or impairment of pulsations in the dorsalis pedis, posterior tibial, ulnar, or radial artery is frequent.

(5) Trophic changes may be present, often with painful indolent ulcerations along the nail margins.

(6) There is usually evidence of disease in both legs and possibly also in the hands and lower arms. There may be a history or findings of Raynaud's phenomenon in the finger or distal foot.

(7) The course is usually intermittent, with acute and often dramatic episodes followed by rather definite remissions. When the collateral vessels as well as the main channels have become occluded, an exacerbation is more likely to lead to gangrene and amputation. The course in the patient with atherosclerosis tends to be less dramatic and more persistent.

Differential Diagnosis

Differences between thromboangiitis obliterans and atherosclerosis obliterans are discussed above.

Raynaud's disease causes symmetric bilateral color changes, primarily in young women. There is no impairment of arterial pulsations. Livedo reticularis and acrocyanosis are vasospastic diseases that do not affect peripheral pulsations; they do not show the early blanching of the digits seen in Raynaud's disease.

Treatment

The principles of therapy are the same as those outlined for atherosclerotic peripheral vascular disease, but the long-range outlook is better in patients with Buerger's disease, so that when possible the approach should be more conservative and tissue loss kept to a minimum.

A. General Measures: Smoking must be stopped; the physician must insist on it. The disease will progress if this advice is not followed.

B. Surgical Measures:

1. Sympathectomy–Sympathectomy may be useful in eliminating the vasospastic manifestations of the disease and aiding in the establishment of collateral circulation to the skin. It may also relieve the mild or moderate forms of rest pain. If amputation of a digit is necessary, sympathectomy may aid in healing of the surgical wound.

2. Amputation–The indications for amputation are similar in many respects to those outlined for the atherosclerotic group, although the approach should be more conservative from the point of view of preservation of tissue. Most patients with Buerger's disease who are managed carefully and who stop smoking do not require amputation of the fingers or toes. It is almost never necessary to amputate the entire hand, but amputation below the knee is occasionally necessary because of gangrene or severe pain in the foot.

Prognosis

Except in the case of the rapidly progressive form of the disease—and provided the patient stops smoking and takes good care of the feet—the prognosis for survival of the extremities is good.

IDIOPATHIC ARTERITIS OF TAKAYASU ("Pulseless Disease")

Pulseless disease, most frequent in young women, is an occlusive polyarteritis of unknown cause with a special predilection for the branches of the aortic arch. It occurs most commonly in Asians. Manifestations, depending upon the vessel or vessels involved, may include evidence of cerebrovascular insufficiency, with transient ischemic attacks and visual disturbances; and absent pulses in the arms, with a rich collateral flow in the shoulder, chest, and neck areas. The extent of the vascular involvement may be defined by angiography.

Pulseless disease must be differentiated from vascular lesions of the aortic arch due to atherosclerosis, though in the latter instance concomitant lower extremity disease is invariably present. Histologically, the arterial lesions are indistinguishable from those of giant cell arteritis. In the early stage of the disease, the progression of the vascular stenosis may be reversed by steroids; in the more advanced forms, bypass arterial grafts are necessary.

GIANT CELL ARTERITIS

This disorder is discussed in Chapter 19.

CHOLESTEROL ATHEROEMBOLIC DISEASE

In some patients with severe atherosclerosis involving the aorta and its branches, a distinct syndrome resulting from repeated microembolization from atherosclerotic plaques has been observed. This syndrome occurs spontaneously or following transfemoral aortographic procedures. Patients complain of pain in the abdomen and legs and of mottled lower extremities. Physical examination reveals cholesterol plaques in the optic fundi, livedo reticularis, and reduced arterial pulses (with or without bruits). Laboratory investigations disclose microhematuria, renal insufficiency, eosinophilia, and an accelerated sedimentation rate. Biopsies of the kidney and other tissues show cholesterol clefts in the small vessels.

Although no specific therapy exists, it is important to recognize this disease, since misdiagnosis of systemic vasculitis may result in inappropriate use of immunomodulating drugs.

O'Keeffe ST et al: Blue toe syndrome: Causes and management. Arch Intern Med 1992;152:2197.

VASOMOTOR DISORDERS

RAYNAUD'S DISEASE & RAYNAUD'S PHENOMENON

Essentials of Diagnosis

- Paroxysmal bilateral symmetric pallor and cyanosis followed by rubor of the skin of the digits.
- Precipitated by cold or emotional upset; relieved by warmth.
- Primarily a disorder of young women.

General Considerations

Raynaud's disease is the primary, or idiopathic, form of paroxysmal digital cyanosis. Raynaud's phenomenon, which is more common than Raynaud's disease, may be due to a number of regional or systemic disorders. In Raynaud's disease the digital arteries respond excessively to vasospastic stimuli. The cause is not known, but some abnormality of the sympathetic nervous system seems to be active in this entity.

Clinical Findings

Raynaud's disease and Raynaud's phenomenon are characterized by intermittent attacks of pallor or cyanosis—or pallor followed by cyanosis—in the fingers (and rarely the toes), precipitated by cold or occasionally by emotional upsets. In early attacks of Raynaud's phenomenon, only 1–2 fingertips may be affected; as it progresses, all the fingers down to the distal palm may be involved. The thumbs are rarely affected. During recovery there may be intense rubor, throbbing, paresthesia, and slight swelling. Attacks usually terminate spontaneously or upon returning to a warm room or putting the extremity in warm water. Between attacks there are no abnormal findings. Sensory changes that often accompany vasomotor manifestations include numbness, stiffness, diminished sensation, and aching pain. The condition may progress to atrophy of the terminal fat pads and the digital skin, and gangrenous ulcers may appear near the fingertips; they may heal during warm weather.

Raynaud's disease appears first between ages 15 and 45, almost always in women. It tends to be progressive, and, unlike Raynaud's phenomenon (which may be unilateral and may involve only 1–2 fingers), symmetric involvement of the fingers of both hands is the rule. Spasm becomes more frequent and prolonged.

Raynaud's disease may be diagnosed if the phenomenon persists for greater than 3 years without evidence of an associated disease (see below). There are no specific laboratory abnormalities; the diagnosis is a clinical one, though studies to exclude the conditions associated with Raynaud's disease are warranted.

Differential Diagnosis

Raynaud's disease must be differentiated from the numerous disorders that may be associated with Raynaud's phenomenon. The history and examination lead to the diagnosis of rheumatoid arthritis, systemic sclerosis (including its more localized CREST variant), systemic lupus erythematosus, and mixed connective tissue disease, with which Raynaud's phenomenon is commonly associated. Raynaud's phenomenon is occasionally the first manifestation of these disorders.

The differentiation from thromboangiitis obliterans is usually not difficult, since thromboangiitis obliterans is generally a disease of men; peripheral pulses are often diminished or absent; and, when Raynaud's phenomenon occurs in association with thromboangiitis obliterans, it is usually in only one or two digits.

Raynaud's phenomenon may occur in patients with the thoracic outlet syndromes. In these disorders, involvement is generally unilateral, and symptoms referable to brachial plexus compression tend to dominate the clinical picture. Carpal tunnel syndrome should also be considered, and nerve conduction tests are appropriate in selected cases.

In acrocyanosis, cyanosis of the hands is permanent and diffuse. Frostbite may lead to chronic Raynaud's phenomenon. Ergot poisoning, particularly due to prolonged or excessive use of ergotamine, must also be considered.

A particularly severe form of Raynaud's phenomenon occurs in up to one-third of patients receiving bleomycin and vincristine in combination, often for testicular cancer. Treatment is unsuccessful, and the problem persists even with discontinuance of the drugs.

Finally, Raynaud's phenomenon may be mimicked by cryoglobulinemia, in which serum proteins aggregate in the cooler distal circulation. Cryoglobulinemia may be idiopathic or associated with multiple myeloma and other hyperglobulinemic states.

Treatment

A. General Measures: The body should be kept warm, and the hands especially should be protected from exposure to cold; gloves should be worn when out in the cold. The hands should be protected from injury at all times; wounds heal slowly, and infections are consequently hard to control. Softening and lubricating lotion to control the fissured dry skin should be applied to the hands frequently. Smoking should be stopped.

B. Vasodilators: Vasodilators drugs are of limited value but may be of some benefit in those patients who are not adequately controlled by general measures and when there is peripheral vasoconstriction without significant organic vascular disease. Shortening of temperature recovery time may occur with the use of transdermal nitroglycerin or a longer-acting oral nitrate. Low doses of nifedipine (10 mg three times daily) have been employed with good effect in the treatment of Raynaud's phenomenon and disease.

C. Surgical Measures: Sympathectomy may be indicated when attacks have become frequent and severe, interfering with work and well-being—and particularly if trophic changes have developed and medical measures have failed. In the lower extremities, complete and permanent relief may result, whereas dorsal sympathectomies generally result in only temporary improvement in most patients treated with operation. Although vascular tone of the vessels in the hands usually ultimately reappears, the symptoms in the fingers that may thus recur in 1–5 years are usually milder and less frequent. Sympathectomies are of very limited value in far-advanced cases, particularly if significant digital artery obstructive disease with scleroderma is present.

Prognosis

Raynaud's disease is usually benign, causing mild discomfort on exposure to cold and progressing very slightly over the years. In a few cases rapid progression does occur, so that the slightest change in temperature may precipitate color changes. It is in this situation that sclerodactyly and small areas of gangrene may be noted, and such patients may become quite disabled by severe pain, limitation of motion, and secondary fixation of distal joints. The prognosis of Raynaud's phenomenon is that of the associated disease.

LIVEDO RETICULARIS

Livedo reticularis is an uncommon vasospastic disorder of unknown cause that results in constant mottled discoloration on large areas of the extremities, generally in a fishnet pattern with reticulated cyanotic areas surrounding a paler central core. It occurs primarily in young women. It may be associated with an occult malignant neoplasm, polyarteritis nodosa, or atherosclerotic microemboli to the skin.

Livedo reticularis is most apparent on the thighs and forearms and occasionally on the lower abdomen and is most pronounced in cold weather. The color may change to a reddish hue in warm weather but does not entirely disappear. A few patients complain of paresthesias, coldness, or numbness in the involved areas. Recurrent ulcers in the lower extremities may occur in severe cases.

Bluish mottling of the extremities is diagnostic. The peripheral pulses are normal. The extremity may be cold, with increased perspiration.

Treatment consists of protection from exposure to cold; use of vasodilators is seldom indicated. In most instances, livedo reticularis is entirely benign. In the rare patient who develops ulcerations or gangrene, underlying systemic disease should be considered.

ACROCYANOSIS

Acrocyanosis is an uncommon symmetric condition that involves the skin of the hands and feet and, to a lesser degree, the forearms and legs. It is associated with arteriolar vasoconstriction combined with dilation of the subpapillary venous plexus of the skin, through which deoxygenated blood slowly circulates. It is worse in cold weather but does not completely disappear during the warm season. It occurs in either sex, is most common in the teens and 20s, and usually improves with advancing age or during pregnancy. It is characterized by coldness, sweating, slight edema, and cyanotic discoloration of the involved areas. Pain, trophic lesions, and disability do not occur, and the peripheral pulses are present. The individual may thus be reassured and encouraged to dress warmly in cold weather.

ERYTHROMELALGIA

Erythromelalgia is a paroxysmal bilateral vasodilatory disorder of unknown cause. Idiopathic (primary) erythromelalgia occurs in otherwise healthy persons, rarely in children, and affects men and women equally. A secondary type is occasionally seen in patients with polycythemia vera, hypertension, gout, and organic neurologic diseases.

The chief symptom is bilateral burning distress that lasts minutes to hours, involving circumscribed areas on the soles or palms first and, as the disease progresses, the entire extremity. The attack occurs in response to stimuli producing vasodilation (eg, exercise, warm environment), especially at night when the extremities are warmed under bedclothes. Reddening or cyanosis as well as heat may be noted. Relief may be obtained by cooling the affected part and by elevation.

No findings are generally present between attacks. With onset of an attack, heat and redness are noted in association with the typical pain. Skin temperature and arterial pulsations are increased, and the involved areas may sweat profusely.

In primary erythromelalgia, aspirin may give excellent relief. The patient should avoid warm environments. In severe cases, if medical measures fail, section or crushing of peripheral nerves may be necessary to relieve pain.

Primary idiopathic erythromelalgia is uniformly benign.

REFLEX SYMPATHETIC DYSTROPHY

Essentials of Diagnosis

- Burning or aching pain following trauma to an extremity of a severity greater than that expected from the initiating injury.
- Manifestations of vasomotor instability are generally present and include temperature, color, and texture alterations of the skin of the involved extremity.

General Considerations

Pain—usually burning or aching—in an injured extremity is the single most common finding, and the disparity between the severity of the inciting injury and the degree of pain experienced is the most characteristic feature. Crushing injuries with lacerations and soft tissue destruction are the most common causes, but closed fractures, simple lacerations, burns (especially electric), and elective operative procedures are also responsible for this syndrome. It may also involve the left upper extremity after intrathoracic diseases such as myocardial infarction. It is rare in children. The manifestations of pain and the associated objective changes may be relatively mild or quite severe, and the initial manifestations often change if the condition proceeds to a chronic stage.

Clinical Findings

In the early stages, the pain, tenderness, and hyperesthesia may be strictly localized to the injured area, and the extremity may be warm, dry, swollen, and red

or slightly cyanotic. The involved extremity is held in a splinted position by the muscles, and the nails may become ridged and the hair long. In advanced stages, the pain is more diffuse and worse at night; the extremity becomes cool and clammy and intolerant of temperature changes (particularly cold); and the skin becomes glossy and atrophic. The joints become stiff, generally in a position that makes the extremity useless. Radiographs of the involved extremity reveal severe osteopenia in excess of that anticipated due to disuse. The dominant concern of the patient may be to avoid the slightest stimuli to the extremity and especially to the trigger points that may develop.

Prevention

During operations on an extremity, peripheral nerves should be handled only when absolutely necessary and then with utmost gentleness. Splinting of an injured extremity for an adequate period during the early, painful phase of recovery, together with adequate analgesics, may help prevent this condition.

Treatment & Prognosis

A. Conservative Measures: It is most important that the condition be recognized and treated in the early stages, when the manifestations are most easily reversed and major secondary changes have not yet developed. In mild, early cases with minimal skin and joint changes, physical therapy involving active and passive exercises combined with diazepam, 2 mg twice daily, or alprazolam, 0.125–0.25 mg every 12 hours, may relieve symptoms. Protecting the extremity from irritating stimuli is important, and the use of nonaddicting analgesics may be necessary.

B. Surgical Measures: If the condition fails to respond to conservative treatment or if there are more severe or advanced objective findings, sympathetic blocks (stellate ganglion or lumbar) may be helpful. Intensive physical therapy may be used during the pain-free periods following effective blocks. Patients who achieve significant temporary relief of symptoms after sympathetic blocks but fail to obtain permanent relief by the blocks may be cured by sympathectomy. In the advanced forms—particularly in association with major local changes and emotional reactions—the prognosis for a useful life is poor. The newer neurosurgical approaches using implantable electronic biostimulator devices to block pain impulses in the cervical spinal cord have met with some success.

Garrett WV et al: Posttraumatic pain syndromes: Causalgia and mimocausalgia. In: *Vascular Surgery: Principles and Practice.* Wilson SE, Williams RA (editors). McGraw-Hill, 1987. (Reasonable summary of a difficult clinical problem.)

VENOUS DISEASES

VARICOSE VEINS

Essentials of Diagnosis

- Dilated, tortuous superficial veins in the lower extremities.
- May be asymptomatic or may be associated with fatigue, aching discomfort, or pain.
- Edema, pigmentation, and ulceration of the skin of the distal leg may develop.
- Increased frequency after pregnancy.

General Considerations

Varicose veins develop predominantly in the lower extremities. They consist of abnormally dilated, elongated, and tortuous alterations in the saphenous veins and their tributaries. These vessels lie immediately beneath the skin and superficial to the deep fascia; they therefore do not have as adequate support as the veins deep in the leg, which are surrounded by muscles. An inherited defect seems to play a major role in the development of varicosities in many instances, but it is not known whether the basic valvular incompetence that exists is secondary to defective valves in the saphenofemoral veins or to a fundamental weakness of the walls of the vein, resulting in dilation of the vessel. Periods of high venous pressure related to prolonged standing or heavy lifting are contributing factors, and the highest incidence is in women who have been pregnant. Fifteen percent of adults develop varicosities.

Secondary varicosities can develop as a result of obstructive changes and valve damage in the deep venous system following thrombophlebitis, or occasionally as a result of proximal venous occlusion due to neoplasm. Congenital or acquired arteriovenous fistulas are also associated with varicosities.

The long saphenous vein and its tributaries are most commonly involved, but the short saphenous vein may also be affected. There may be one or many incompetent perforating veins in the thigh and lower leg, so that blood can reflux into the varicosities not only from above, by way of the saphenofemoral junction, but also from the deep system of veins through the incompetent perforators in the mid thigh or lower leg. Largely because of these valvular defects in the most proximal valve of the long saphenous vein or in the distal communicating veins, venous pressure in the superficial veins does not fall appreciably on walking; over the years, the veins progressively enlarge, and the surrounding tissue and skin develop secondary changes such as fibrosis, chronic edema, and skin pigmentation and atrophy.

Clinical Findings

A. Symptoms: The severity of the symptoms caused by varicose veins is not necessarily correlated with the number and size of the varicosities; extensive varicose veins may produce no subjective symptoms, whereas minimal varicosities may produce many symptoms, especially in women. Dull, aching heaviness or a feeling of fatigue brought on by periods of standing is the most common complaint. Cramps may occur, often at night, and elevation of the legs typically relieves symptoms. One must be careful to distinguish between the symptoms of arteriosclerotic peripheral vascular disease, such as intermittent claudication and coldness of the feet, and symptoms of venous disease, since occlusive arterial disease usually contraindicates the operative treatment of varicosities distal to the knee. Indeed, reduced blood flow due to atherosclerosis may improve varicosities by reducing blood flow through the veins. Itching from an associated eczematoid dermatitis may occur above the ankle.

B. Signs: Dilated, tortuous, elongated veins beneath the skin in the thigh and leg are generally readily visible in the standing individual, although in very obese patients palpation may be necessary to detect their presence and location. Secondary tissue changes may be absent even in extensive varicosities; but if the varicosities are of long duration, brownish pigmentation and thinning of the skin above the ankle are often present. Swelling may occur, but signs of severe chronic venous stasis such as extensive swelling, fibrosis, pigmentation, and ulceration of the distal lower leg usually denote the postphlebitic state. Doppler ultrasonography or the duplex scanner is useful diagnostically in detecting the precise location of incompetent valves, allowing reflux of blood from the femoral, popliteal, or more peripheral deep veins into the superficial veins; such knowledge allows more precise corrective surgery with better results.

Differential Diagnosis

Primary varicose veins should be differentiated from those secondary to (1) chronic venous insufficiency of the deep system of veins (the postphlebitic syndrome); (2) retroperitoneal vein obstruction from extrinsic pressure or fibrosis; (3) arteriovenous fistula (congenital or acquired)—a bruit is present and a thrill is often palpable; and (4) congenital venous malformation. Pain or discomfort secondary to arthritis, radiculopathy, or arterial insufficiency should be distinguished from symptoms associated with coexistent varicose veins.

Complications

If thin, atrophic, pigmented skin has developed at or above the ankle, secondary ulcerations may occur—often as a result of little or no trauma. An ulcer will occasionally extend into the varix, and the resulting fistula will be associated with profuse hemorrhage unless the leg is elevated and local pressure is applied to the bleeding point.

Chronic stasis dermatitis with fungal and bacterial infection may be a problem.

Thrombophlebitis may develop in the varicosities, particularly in postoperative patients, pregnant or postpartum women, or those taking oral contraceptives. Local trauma or prolonged periods of sitting may also lead to superficial venous thrombosis. Extension of the thrombosis into the deep venous system by way of the perforating veins or through the saphenofemoral junction may occur, resulting in deep thrombophlebitis and the risk of pulmonary embolism.

Treatment

A. Nonsurgical Measures: The use of elastic stockings (medium or heavy weight) to give external support to the veins of the proximal foot and leg up to but not including the knee is the best nonoperative approach to the management of varicose veins. These may be useful in early varicosities as well, in preventing progression of disease. When elastic stockings are worn during the hours that involve much standing and when this is combined with the habit of elevation of the legs when possible, reasonably good control can be maintained and progression of the condition and the development of complications can often be avoided. This approach may be used in elderly patients, in those who refuse or wish to defer surgery, sometimes in women with mild or moderate varicosities who plan to have more children, and in those with mild asymptomatic varicosities.

B. Surgical Measures: The surgical treatment of varicose veins consists of interruption or removal of the varicosities and the incompetent perforating veins. Accurate delineation and division of the latter are required to prevent formation of recurrent varicosities in previously uninvolved veins. Venous segments that are not demonstrated to be incompetent and varicosed should not be ligated or removed; they may be needed as artery grafts later in the patient's life.

Varicose ulcers that are small generally heal with local care, frequent periods of elevation of the extremity, and compression bandages or some form of compression boot dressing for the ambulatory patient. It is best to defer a stripping procedure until healing has been achieved and stasis dermatitis has been controlled. Some ulcers require skin grafting.

C. Compression Sclerotherapy: Sclerotherapy to obliterate and produce permanent fibrosis of the involved veins is generally reserved for the treatment of residual small varicosities following definitive varicose vein surgery. The injection of the sclerosing solution into the varicosed vein is followed by a period of compression of the segment, resulting in obliteration of the vein. Complications such as phlebitis, tissue necrosis, or infection may

occur, and vary in incidence with the skill of the operator.

Prognosis

Patients should be informed that even extensive and carefully performed surgery may not prevent the development of additional varicosities and that further (though usually more limited) surgery or sclerotherapy may become necessary. Good results with relief of symptoms are usually obtained in most patients. If extensive varicosities reappear after surgery, the completeness of the high ligation should be questioned, and reexploration of the saphenofemoral area may be necessary. Even after adequate treatment, secondary tissue changes may not regress.

THROMBOPHLEBITIS

Thrombophlebitis is partial or complete occlusion of a vein by a thrombus with secondary inflammatory reaction in the wall of the vein. Trauma to the endothelium of the vein wall resulting in exposure of subendothelial tissues to platelets in the venous blood may initiate thrombosis, especially if a degree of venous stasis also exists. Platelet aggregates form on the vein wall followed by the deposition of fibrin, leukocytes, and finally erythrocytes; a thrombus results that can then propagate along the veins as a free-floating clot. Within 7–10 days, this thrombus becomes adherent to the vein wall, and secondary inflammatory changes develop, although a free-floating tail may persist. The thrombus is ultimately invaded by fibroblasts, resulting in scarring of the vein wall and destruction of the valves. Central recanalization may occur later, with restoration of flow through the vein; however, because the valves do not recover function, directional flow is not reestablished, leading in turn to secondary functional and anatomic problems.

1. THROMBOPHLEBITIS OF THE DEEP VEINS

Essentials of Diagnosis

- Pain in the calf or thigh, occasionally associated with swelling; alternatively, there may be no symptoms.
- History of congestive heart failure, recent surgery, neoplasia, oral contraceptive use, or varicose veins; prolonged inactivity also predisposes.
- Physical signs unreliable.
- Ultrasound and plethysmography are abnormal; venography is diagnostic.

General Considerations

The deep veins of the lower extremities and pelvis are most frequently involved. The process begins approximately 80% of the time in the deep veins of the calf, although it can arise in the femoral or iliac veins. When the process begins in the calf, propagation into the popliteal and femoral veins takes place in approximately 10% of these cases. About 3% of patients undergoing major general surgical procedures will develop clinical manifestations of thrombophlebitis, which may develop up to 2 weeks postoperatively; many others with the process will have no detectable findings. Certain operations, such as total hip replacement, are associated with appreciably higher incidences of thromboembolic complications. Illnesses that involve periods of bed rest, such as cardiac failure or stroke, are associated with a high incidence of thrombophlebitis. Use of oral contraceptive drugs, especially by women over 30 and by those who smoke, may be associated with hypercoagulability, resulting in thrombophlebitis in some women. These drugs should not be prescribed for women with a history of phlebitis. Hypercoagulability is also observed in cancer, particularly adenocarcinoma.

Clinical Findings

Approximately half of patients with thrombophlebitis have no symptoms or signs in the extremity in the early stages. The patient may suffer a pulmonary embolism, presumably from the leg veins, without symptoms or demonstrable abnormalities in the extremities.

A. Symptoms: The patient may complain of a dull ache, a tight feeling, or frank pain in the calf or, in more extensive cases, the whole leg, especially when walking.

B. Signs: Typical findings, though variable and unreliable and in about half of cases absent, are as follows: slight swelling in the involved calf, distention of the superficial venous collaterals; and slight fever and tachycardia. Any of these signs may occur without deep vein thrombosis. When the femoral and iliac veins are also involved, there may be tenderness over these veins, and the swelling in the extremity may be marked. The skin may be cyanotic if venous obstruction is severe, or pale and cool if a reflex arterial spasm is superimposed.

C. Diagnostic Techniques: Because of the difficulty in making a precise diagnosis by history and examination and because of the morbidity associated with treatment, diagnostic studies are essential. (See Chapter 9, Disorders of the Pulmonary Circulation.)

1. Ascending contrast venography, the most accurate method of diagnosis, will define the location, extent, and degree of attachment of the thrombosis (thrombi in the profunda femoris and internal iliac veins will not be demonstrated). Because of the time, expense, and discomfort involved, this test is not used as a screening study and is unsuitable for repeated monitoring. It is particularly useful when the clinical picture strongly suggests calf vein thromboses but noninvasive tests are equivocal. It may on oc-

casion produce or exacerbate a thrombotic process, but this occurs in less than 5% of patients. It is the most accurate study for detection of calf vein or intra-abdominal venous thrombosis.

2. The Doppler ultrasound blood flow detector allows the major veins in an extremity to be examined for thrombosis. This test is of value as a rapid screening procedure for the detection of thrombosis in large veins, and it may be particularly helpful in detecting an extension of small thrombi in the calf veins into the popliteal and femoral veins. This test is inexpensive but operator-dependent; it relies on sonic differences in flow rates that occur with inspiration in normal veins. Incompetent venous valves in the legs may also be inferred from this investigation. Impedance plethysmography may similarly be used to detect the alteration of venous flow by obstruction of thrombi. High-resolution real time B-mode ultrasonography for detection of thrombosis may be used rather than phlebography to confirm positive or equivocal findings of plethysmography. These examinations may miss small thrombi in the calf veins when collateral channels are present. A multiple-center trial with either color Doppler or plethysmography has shown low sensitivity for proximal thrombosis in high-risk but asymptomatic patients. Positive studies in high-risk asymptomatic patients, however, allow initiation of therapy. Similarly, the tests appear to be far more sensitive in symptomatic deep venous thrombosis, though venography remains the most sensitive study.

Differential Diagnosis

Calf muscle strain or contusion may be difficult to differentiate from thrombophlebitis; phlebography may be required to determine the correct diagnosis.

Cellulitis may be confused with thrombophlebitis; with infection, there is usually an associated wound, and inflammation of the skin is more marked.

Obstruction of the lymphatics or the iliac vein in the retroperitoneal area from tumor or irradiation may lead to unilateral swelling, but it is usually more chronic and painless. An acute arterial occlusion is more painful, the distal pulses are absent, there is usually no swelling, and the superficial veins in the foot fill slowly when emptied.

Bilateral leg edema is more likely to be due to heart, kidney, or liver disease.

Occasionally, a ruptured Baker cyst may produce unilateral pain and swelling in the calf. A history of arthritis in the knee of the same leg is a clue to diagnosis, and the patient may report disappearance of the popliteal cyst at the time symptoms develop.

Complications

A. Pulmonary Thromboembolism: See Chapter 9.

B. Chronic Venous Insufficiency: Chronic venous insufficiency with or without secondary varicosities is a late complication of deep thrombophlebitis. (See Chronic Venous Insufficiency.)

Prevention

Prophylactic measures may diminish the incidence of venous thrombosis in hospitalized patients.

A. Nonpharmacologic Means: Venous stasis may be avoided by the following measures:

1. Elevation of the foot of the bed 15–20 degrees will encourage venous flow from the legs, particularly if the head of the bed is kept low or horizontal. Slight flexion of the knees is desirable. This position is also maintained on the operating table and in the recovery room. Sitting in a chair in the early postoperative period should be avoided.

2. Leg exercises, carried out by the surgical team immediately following major surgery and during the early postoperative period and practiced by the patient when in bed, are important. Intermittent pneumatic compression of the legs may be used prophylactically and may be the preventive measure of choice in patients in whom all anticoagulants are contraindicated, such as in patients undergoing neurosurgery.

3. Elastic antiphlebitic stockings may be employed, particularly in patients with varicose veins or a history of phlebitis who will require bed rest for a number of days. Walking for brief but regular periods postoperatively and during long airplane and automobile trips should be encouraged.

B. Anticoagulation: Anticoagulants may be used in patients considered at high risk for venous thrombosis.

1. Low-dose heparin, 5000 units every 8–12 hours subcutaneously 2 hours preoperatively and during the postoperative period of bed rest and limited ambulation, appears to be effective in reducing the incidence of thromboembolic complications in moderate-risk patients, although its effectiveness in major pelvic and hip procedures has been disappointing for these high-risk patients. Adjusted-dose heparin to a PTT in the upper half of the normal range—or warfarin to a PT 1.3–1.5 times control—is recommended. External pneumatic compression is significantly less effective than warfarin in this setting.

2. Aspirin, 80—325 mg daily, may have a prophylactic value when used both pre- and postoperatively in surgical patients.

Treatment

A. Local Measures: As for prophylaxis, the legs should be elevated 15–20 degrees, the trunk should be kept horizontal, and the head and shoulders may be supported with pillows. The legs should be slightly flexed at the knees. Bed rest should be maintained until local tenderness and swelling have disappeared, by which time the thrombus has generally become adherent to the vein wall; a week may be adequate for calf thrombosis and 10–14 days for thigh

or pelvic thrombosis. Walking but not standing or sitting is then permitted; the time out of bed and walking is increased each day.

B. Medical Measures (Anticoagulants): Therapy with anticoagulants is considered to be the preferred treatment in most cases of deep thrombophlebitis with or without pulmonary embolism. There is evidence that the incidence of fatal pulmonary embolism secondary to venous thrombosis is reduced by adequate anticoagulant therapy, and the incidence of death from additional emboli following an initial embolism is reduced. Progressive thrombosis with its associated morbidity is also reduced considerably, and the chronic secondary changes in the involved leg are probably also less severe. Heparin acts rapidly and must be considered the anticoagulant of choice for short-term therapy; hospitalization is generally necessary. Subcutaneous heparin may be as effective as continuous infusion, and there may be a marginal preference for low-molecular-weight heparin over the standard drug. LMW heparin is given subcutaneously and does not require PTT monitoring, but it is considerably more expensive than the standard heparin. Thus, its use is likely to remain sporadic. After the initial phase of therapy with heparin—and if a prolonged period of anticoagulation is advisable—warfarin can be used.

Treatment with heparin does not affect thrombi that have already developed but stops propagation and allows fibrinolysis to occur. The duration of therapy is purely an empirical decision—most clinicians administer heparin for 7–10 days and oral anticoagulants for at least 12 weeks, but data to support these regimens are sparse. Permanent anticoagulation may be considered if the stimulus to thrombosis is chronic—eg, congestive heart failure, postphlebitic syndrome—or if previous episodes have occurred. As experience with thrombolysis develops, it may replace heparin as the treatment of first choice; there is evidence that it reduces the incidence of postphlebitic syndrome.

Details on the use of heparin, oral anticoagulants, and thrombolytics may be found in Chapter 9.

Prognosis

With adequate treatment the patient usually returns to normal health and activity within 3–6 weeks. The prognosis in most cases is good once the period of danger of pulmonary embolism has passed. Occasionally, recurrent episodes of phlebitis will occur in spite of good local and anticoagulant management. Such cases may even have recurrent pulmonary emboli as well. Chronic venous insufficiency may result, with its associated complications; this is less likely when thrombolytics are used to treat acute phlebitis.

Davidson BL, Elliott CG, Lensing AWA: Low accuracy of
    color Doppler ultrasound in the detection of proximal leg

vein thrombosis in asymptomatic high-risk patients. Ann Intern Med 1992;117:735.

Hirsh J: Heparin. N Engl J Med 1991;324:1565. (Pharmacology and clinical use.)

Hirsh J: Oral anticoagulant drugs. N Engl J Med 1991; 324:1865.

Hyers JM, Hull RD, Weg JG: Antithrombotic therapy for venous thromboembolic disease. Chest 1989;95 (Suppl):37S. (Consensus conference of experts in the field.)

2. THROMBOPHLEBITIS OF THE SUPERFICIAL VEINS

Essentials of Diagnosis

- Induration, redness, and tenderness along a superficial vein.
- Often a history of recent intravenous line or trauma. No significant swelling of the extremity.

General Considerations

Superficial thrombophlebitis may occur spontaneously, as in pregnant or postpartum women or in individuals with varicose veins or thromboangiitis obliterans; or it may be associated with trauma, as in the case of a blow to the leg or following intravenous therapy with irritating solutions. It may also be a manifestation of abdominal cancer such as carcinoma of the pancreas and may be the earliest sign. The long saphenous vein is most often involved. Superficial thrombophlebitis may be associated with occult deep vein thrombosis in about 20% of cases. Pulmonary emboli are rare.

Short-term plastic venous catheterization of superficial arm veins is now in routine use. The catheter should be observed daily for signs of local inflammation. It should be removed if a local reaction develops in the veins. Serious thrombotic or septic complications can occur if this policy is not followed. The steel intravenous needle with the anchoring flange (butterfly needle) is less likely to be associated with phlebitis and infection than the plastic catheter, but this may be due to its remaining in place for shorter periods.

Clinical Findings

The patient usually experiences a dull pain in the region of the involved vein. Local findings consist of induration, redness, and tenderness along the course of a vein. The process may be localized, or it may involve most of the long saphenous vein and its tributaries. The inflammatory reaction generally subsides in 1–2 weeks; a firm cord may remain for a much longer period. Edema of the extremity and deep calf tenderness are absent unless deep thrombophlebitis has also developed. Chills and high fever suggest septic phlebitis and are often encountered when the phlebitis is secondary to an indwelling intravenous catheter.

Differential Diagnosis

The linear rather than circular nature of the lesion and the distribution along the course of a superficial vein serve to differentiate superficial phlebitis from cellulitis, erythema nodosum, erythema induratum, panniculitis, and fibrositis. Lymphangitis and deep thrombophlebitis must also be considered.

Treatment

If the process is well localized and not near the saphenofemoral junction, local heat and bed rest with the leg elevated are usually effective in limiting the thrombosis. Nonsteroidal anti-inflammatory drugs relieve symptoms.

If the process is very extensive or is progressing upward toward the saphenofemoral junction, or if it is in the proximity of the saphenofemoral junction initially, ligation and division of the saphenous vein at the saphenofemoral junction are indicated. The inflammatory process usually regresses following this procedure, though removal of the involved segment of vein (stripping) may result in a more rapid recovery.

Anticoagulation therapy is usually not indicated unless the disease is rapidly progressing. It is indicated if there is extension into the deep system.

Septic thrombophlebitis requires excision of the involved vein up to its junction with an uninvolved vein in order to control bacteremia. *Staphylococcus* is the commonest cause, and antibiotics with antistaphylococcal activity should be instituted pending results of blood cultures. If cultures are positive, therapy should be continued for 7–10 days—or for 4–6 weeks if complicating endocarditis cannot be excluded.

Prognosis

The course is generally benign and brief, and the prognosis depends on the underlying pathologic process. Phlebitis of a saphenous vein occasionally extends to the deep veins, in which case pulmonary embolism may occur.

CHRONIC VENOUS INSUFFICIENCY

Essentials of Diagnosis

- History of phlebitis or leg injury.
- Ankle edema is the earliest sign.
- Stasis pigmentation, dermatitis, subcutaneous induration, and often varicosities occur later.
- Ulceration at or above the ankle is common (stasis ulcer).

General Considerations

Chronic venous insufficiency generally results

from changes secondary to deep thrombophlebitis, although a definite history of phlebitis is not obtainable in about 25% of these patients. There is often a history of leg trauma. It can also occur in association with varicose veins and as a result of neoplastic obstruction of the pelvic veins or congenital or acquired arteriovenous fistula.

When insufficiency is secondary to deep thrombophlebitis (the postphlebitic syndrome), the valves in the deep venous channels of the lower leg have been damaged or destroyed by the thrombotic process. The recanalized, nonelastic deep veins are functionally inadequate because of the damaged valves in the deep and perforating veins. The antegrade venous flow ensured by the valves and the calf muscle pump is lost, resulting in bidirectional flow and abnormally high ambulatory venous pressures in the calf veins in particular. The high ambulatory venous pressure transmitted through the communicating veins to the subcutaneous veins and tissues of the calf and ankle areas results in a series of deleterious secondary changes, including edema, fibrosis of subcutaneous tissue and skin, pigmentation of skin, and, later, dermatitis, cellulitis, and ulceration. Dilation of the superficial veins may occur, leading to varicosities. Whereas primary varicose veins with no abnormality of the deep venous system may be associated with some similar changes, the edema is more pronounced in the postphlebitic extremities, and the secondary changes are more extensive and encircling.

Clinical Findings

Chronic venous insufficiency is characterized first by progressive edema of the leg (particularly the lower leg) and later also by secondary changes in the skin and subcutaneous tissues. The usual symptoms are itching, a dull discomfort made worse by periods of standing, and pain if an ulceration is present. The skin is usually thin, shiny, atrophic, and cyanotic; and a brownish pigmentation often develops. Eczema may be present, with superficial weeping dermatitis. The subcutaneous tissues become thick and fibrous. Recurrent ulcerations may occur, usually just above the ankle, on the medial or anterior aspect of the leg; healing results in a thin scar on a fibrotic base that often breaks down with minor trauma. Varicosities frequently appear that are associated with incompetent perforating veins.

Differential Diagnosis

Congestive heart failure and chronic renal disease may result in bilateral edema of the lower extremities, but generally there are other clinical or laboratory findings of heart or kidney disease.

Lymphedema is associated with a brawny thickening in the subcutaneous tissue that does not respond readily to elevation; varicosities are absent, and there is often a history of recurrent cellulitis.

Primary varicose veins may be difficult to differen-

tiate from the secondary varicosities that often develop in this condition, as discussed above. It may be impossible to exclude superimposed acute phlebitis from chronic venous insufficiency without diagnostic tests.

Other conditions associated with chronic ulcers of the leg include autoimmune diseases (eg, Felty's syndrome), arterial insufficiency (often very painful), sickle cell anemia, erythema induratum (bilateral and usually on the posterior aspect of the lower part of the leg), and fungal infections (cultures specific; no chronic swelling or varicosities).

Prevention

Irreversible tissue changes and associated complications in the lower legs can be minimized through early and energetic treatment of acute thrombophlebitis with anticoagulants that may minimize the occlusive and valve damage, particularly in the calf, and specific measures to avoid chronic edema in subsequent years, as described in A, below. Thrombolytic therapies of acute phlebitis may be of greater value than other anticoagulants in prevention of chronic venous insufficiency.

Treatment

A. General Measures: Bed rest, with the legs elevated to diminish chronic edema, is fundamental in the treatment of the acute complications of chronic venous insufficiency. Measures to control the tendency toward edema include (1) intermittent elevation of the legs during the day and elevation of the legs at night (kept above the level of the heart with pillows under the mattress); (2) avoidance of long periods of sitting or standing; and (3) the use of well-fitting, heavy-duty elastic supports worn from the mid foot to just below the knee during the day and evening if there is any tendency for swelling to develop.

B. Stasis Dermatitis: Eczematous eruption may be acute or chronic; treatment varies accordingly.

1. Acute weeping dermatitis–

a. Wet compresses for 1 hour four times daily of solutions containing boric acid, buffered aluminum acetate (Burow's solution), or isotonic saline.

b. Compresses are followed with a local corticosteroid such as 0.5% hydrocortisone cream in a water-soluble base. (Neomycin and nystatin may be incorporated into this cream.)

c. Systemic antibiotics are indicated only if active infection is present.

2. Subsiding or chronic dermatitis–

a. Continue hydrocortisone cream for 1–2 weeks or until no further improvement is noted. Cordran tape, a plastic tape impregnated with flurandrenolide, is a convenient way to apply both medication and dressing.

b. Zinc oxide ointment with ichthammol, 3%,

once or twice daily, cleaned off as desired with mineral oil.

    c. Broad-spectrum antifungal such as clotrimazole cream (1%) or miconazole cream (2%) may be used.

    3. Energetic treatment of chronic edema, as outlined in sections A and C, with almost complete bed rest is important during the acute phase of stasis dermatitis.

    C. Ulceration: Ulcerations are preferably treated with compresses of isotonic saline solution, which aid the healing of the ulcer or may help prepare the base for a skin graft. A lesion can often be treated on an ambulatory basis by means of a semirigid boot applied to the leg after much of the swelling has been reduced by a period of elevation. The pumping action of the calf muscles on the blood flow out of the lower extremity is enhanced by a circumferential nonelastic bandage on the ankle and lower leg. The boot must be changed every 1–2 weeks, depending to some extent on the amount of drainage from the ulcer. The ulcer, tendons, and bony prominences must be adequately padded. Special ointments on the ulcer are not necessary. The semirigid boot may be made with Unna's paste (Gelocast, Medicopaste) or Gauztex bandage (impregnated with a nonallergenic self-adhering compound). After the ulcer has healed, heavy below-the-knee elastic stockings are used in an effort to prevent recurrent edema and ulceration. Occasionally, the ulcer is so large and chronic that total excision of the ulcer, with skin graft of the defect, is the best approach. This is often combined with ligation of all incompetent perforating veins.

    D. Secondary Varicosities: Varicosities secondary to damage to the deep system of veins may in turn contribute to undesirable changes in the tissues of the lower leg. Varicosities should occasionally be removed and the incompetent veins connecting the superficial and deep system ligated, but the tendency toward edema will persist, because the chronic high venous pressure is usually not effectively lowered during walking by the procedure, and thus the measures outlined above (¶A) will be required for life. Varicosities can often be treated along with edema by elastic stockings and other nonoperative measures, and only about 15–20% require surgery. If the obstructive element in the deep system appears to be severe, B-mode ultrasonography, bidirectional Doppler velocity studies, or phlebography may be of value in mapping out the areas of venous obstruction or incompetence in the deep system as well as the number and location of the damaged perforating veins. A decision about whether to treat with surgery may be influenced by such a study; if the varicosities furnish the chief route of venous return, they should not be removed. Venous valvular reconstructive surgery is now in an investigative stage.

Prognosis

Individuals with chronic venous insufficiency often have recurrent problems, particularly if measures to counteract persistent venous hypertension, edema, and secondary tissue changes are not conscientiously adhered to throughout life. Additional episodes of acute thrombophlebitis may occur, and in reliable patients permanent anticoagulation is a reasonable therapeutic objective.

SUPERIOR VENA CAVAL OBSTRUCTION

Partial or complete obstruction of the thin-walled superior vena cava is a relatively rare condition that is usually secondary to the neoplastic or inflammatory process in the superior mediastinum. The most frequent causes are (1) neoplasms, such as lymphomas, primary malignant mediastinal tumors, or carcinoma of the lung with direct extension (over 80%); (2) chronic fibrotic mediastinitis, either of unknown origin or secondary to tuberculosis, histoplasmosis, or pyogenic infections; (3) thrombophlebitis, often by extension of the process from the axillary or subclavian vein into the innominate vein and vena cava and often associated with catheterization of these veins for central venous pressure measurements or for hyperalimentation; (4) aneurysm of the aortic arch; and (5) constrictive pericarditis.

Clinical Findings

    A. Symptoms and Signs: The onset of symptoms is acute or subacute. Symptoms include swelling of the neck and face, headache, dizziness, visual disturbances, stupor, and syncope. There is progressive obstruction of the venous drainage of the head, neck, and upper extremities. The cutaneous veins of the upper chest and lower neck become dilated, and flushing of the face and neck develops. Brawny edema of the face, neck, and arms occurs later, and cyanosis of these areas then appears. Cerebral and laryngeal edema ultimately results in impaired function of the brain as well as respiratory insufficiency. Bending over or lying down accentuates the symptoms; sitting quietly is generally preferred. The manifestations are more severe if the obstruction develops rapidly and if the azygos junction or the vena cava between that vein and the heart is obstructed.

    B. Laboratory Findings: The venous pressure is elevated (often > 20 cm of water) in the arm and is normal in the leg. Since lung cancer is a common cause, bronchoscopy is often performed; transbronchial biopsy, however, is relatively contraindicated because of venous hypertension and the risk of bleeding.

    C. Imaging: Chest radiographs and a CT scan will define the location and often the nature of the obstructive process, and phlebography will map out the extent and degree of the venous obstruction and the collateral circulation. Doppler ultrasound can demonstrate the presence of collaterals, and MRI may delineate the site of thrombosis as well as the nature of the cause. Brachial venography or radionuclide scanning following intravenous injection of technetium Tc 99m pertechnetate demonstrates a block to the flow of contrast material into the right heart and enlarged collateral veins. These techniques also allow estimation of blood flow around the occlusion as well as serial evaluation of the response to therapy.

Treatment

Though empiric therapy for neoplasm is occasionally warranted, the clinician should be aware of benign causes, especially histoplasmosis.

Urgent treatment for neoplasm consists of (1) cautious use of intravenous diuretics and (2) mediastinal irradiation, starting within 24 hours, with a treatment plan designed to give a high daily dose but a short total course of therapy to rapidly shrink the local tumor even further. Intensive combined therapy will palliate the process in up to 90% of patients. In patients with a subacute presentation, radiation therapy alone usually suffices. Chemotherapy is added if lymphoma or small-cell carcinoma is diagnosed.

Surgical procedures to bypass the obstruction are complicated by bleeding relating to high venous pressure. In cases secondary to mediastinal fibrosis or pericardial constriction, excision of the fibrous tissue around the great vessels may reestablish flow.

Prognosis

The prognosis depends upon the nature and degree of obstruction and its speed of onset. Slowly developing forms secondary to fibrosis may be tolerated for years. A high degree of obstruction of rapid onset secondary to cancer is often fatal in a few days or weeks because of increased intracranial pressure and cerebral hemorrhage, but treatment of the tumor with radiation and chemotherapeutic drugs may result in significant palliation.

Sculier JP, Feld R: Superior vena cava obstruction syndrome: Recommendations for management. Cancer Treat Rev 1985;12:209.

DISEASES OF THE LYMPHATIC CHANNELS

LYMPHANGITIS & LYMPHADENITIS

Essentials of Diagnosis

- Red streak from wound or area of cellulitis toward regional lymph nodes, which are usually enlarged and tender.
- Chills, fever, and malaise may be present.

General Considerations

Lymphangitis and lymphadenitis are common manifestations of a bacterial infection that is usually caused by hemolytic streptococci or staphylococci (or by both organisms) and usually arises from an area of cellulitis, generally at the site of an infected wound. The wound may be very small or superficial, or an established abscess may be present, feeding bacteria into the lymphatics. The involvement of the lymphatics is often manifested by a red streak in the skin extending in the direction of the regional lymph nodes, which are, in turn, generally tender and enlarged. Systemic manifestations include fever, chills, and malaise. The infection may progress rapidly, often in a matter of hours, and may lead to septicemia and even death.

Clinical Findings

A. Symptoms and Signs: Throbbing pain is usually present in the area of cellulitis at the site of bacterial invasion. Malaise, anorexia, sweating, chills, and fever of 37.8–40 °C (100–104 °F) develop rapidly. The red streak, when present, may be definite or may be very faint and easily missed, especially in dark-skinned patients. It is not usually tender or indurated, as is the area of cellulitis. The involved regional lymph nodes may be significantly enlarged and are usually quite tender. The pulse is often rapid.

B. Laboratory Findings: Leukocytosis with a left shift is usually present. Later, a blood culture may be positive, most often for staphylococcal or streptococcal species. Culture and sensitivity studies on the wound exudate or pus may be helpful in treatment of the more severe or refractory infections but are often difficult to interpret because of skin contaminants.

Differential Diagnosis

Lymphangitis may be confused with superficial thrombophlebitis, but the erythematous reaction associated with thrombosis overlies the induration of the inflammatory reaction in and around the thrombosed vein. Venous thrombosis is not associated with lymphadenitis, and a wound of entrance with the secondary cellulitis is generally absent. Superficial thrombophlebitis frequently arises as a result of intravenous therapy, particularly when the needle or catheter is left in place for more than 2 days; if bacteria have also been introduced, suppurative thrombophlebitis may develop.

Cat-scratch fever should be considered when lymphadenitis is present in which the nodes, though often very large, are relatively nontender. Exposure to cats is common, but the scratch may be forgotten by the patient.

It is extremely important to differentiate cellulitis from soft tissue infections that require early and aggressive incision and often resection of necrotic infected tissue, eg, acute streptococcal hemolytic gangrene, necrotizing fasciitis, gram-negative anaerobic cutaneous gangrene, and progressive bacterial synergistic gangrene. These are deeper infections that are more anatomically extensive; patients appear more seriously ill, and subcutaneous crepitus may be palpated or auscultated using the diaphragm with light pressure over the involved area.

Treatment

A. General Measures: Prompt treatment should include heat (hot, moist compresses or heating pad), elevation when feasible, and immobilization of the infected area. Analgesics may be prescribed for pain.

B. Specific Measures: Antibiotic therapy should always be instituted when local infection becomes invasive, as manifested by cellulitis and lymphangitis. Because the causative organism is so frequently the streptococcus, penicillin G is usually the drug of choice, although antistaphylococcal penicillins (eg, nafcillin) or cephalosporins are favored by some. If the patient is allergic to penicillin, erythromycin may be substituted. (See Chapter 37.)

C. Wound Care: Drainage of pus from an infected wound should be carried out, generally after the above measures have been instituted and only when it is clear that there is an abscess associated with the site of initial infection. An area of cellulitis should not be incised, because the infection may be spread by attempted drainage when pus is not present.

Prognosis

With proper therapy and particularly with the use of an antibiotic effective against the invading bacteria, control of the infection can usually be achieved in a few days. Delayed or inadequate therapy can still lead to overwhelming infection with septicemia.

LYMPHEDEMA

Essentials of Diagnosis

- Painless edema of one or both lower extremities, primarily in young women.

- Initially, pitting edema, which becomes brawny and often nonpitting with time.
- Ulceration, varicosities, and stasis pigmentation do not occur. There may be episodes of lymphangitis and cellulitis.

General Considerations

The underlying mechanism in lymphedema is impairment of the flow of lymph from an extremity. When due to congenital developmental abnormalities consisting of hypo- or hyperplastic involvement of the proximal or distal lymphatics, it is referred to as the primary form. The obstruction may be in the pelvic or lumbar lymph channels and nodes when the disease is extensive and progressive. The secondary form results when an inflammatory or mechanical obstruction of the lymphatics occurs from trauma, regional lymph node resection or irradiation, or extensive involvement of regional nodes by malignant disease or filariasis. Secondary dilation of the lymphatics that occurs in both forms leads to incompetence of the valve system, disrupting the orderly flow along the lymph vessels, and results in progressive stasis of a protein-rich fluid, with secondary fibrosis. Episodes of acute and chronic inflammation may be superimposed, with further stasis and fibrosis. Hypertrophy of the limb results, with markedly thickened and fibrotic skin and subcutaneous tissue and diminution in the fatty tissue.

Lymphangiography and radioactive isotope studies are often useful in defining the specific lymphatic defect.

Treatment

The treatment of lymphedema is often not very satisfactory. The majority of patients can be treated conservatively with some of the following measures: (1) The flow of lymph out of the extremity, with a consequent decrease in the degree of stasis, can be aided through intermittent elevation of the extremity, especially during the sleeping hours (foot of bed elevated 15–20 degrees, achieved by placing pillows beneath the mattress); the constant use of elastic bandages or carefully fitted heavy-duty elastic stockings; and massage toward the trunk—either by hand or by means of pneumatic pressure devices designed to milk edema out of an extremity. (The Wright linear pump delivers sequential pressure cycles that effectively milk fluid out of the foot and leg and then out of the thigh.) (2) Secondary cellulitis in the extremity should be avoided by means of good hygiene and treatment of any trichophytosis of the toes. Once an infection starts, it should be treated by adequate periods of rest, elevation, and antibiotics, with coverage of *Staphylococcus* and *Streptococcus*. Infection can be a serious and recurring problem and is often difficult to control. Intermittent prophylactic antibiotics may occasionally be necessary; dicloxacillin is a good choice. (3) Intermittent courses of diuretic therapy, especially in those with premenstrual or seasonal exacerbations. (4) In carefully selected cases, there are operative procedures that may give satisfactory functional results. Lymphaticovenous anastomosis using microsurgery has yielded some satisfactory cosmetic and functional results, particularly if lymph channels can be localized by lymphoscintigraphy and several lymphovenous anastomoses are made. This technique may replace the more deforming procedures and those aimed at introducing lymphatic bridges or lymphatic venous connections. Amputation is used as a last resort in very severe forms or when lymphangiosarcoma develops in the extremity.

Gloviczi P et al: Microsurgical lymphovenous anastomosis for treatment of lymphoedemas: A critical review. J Vasc Surg 1988;7:647.

HYPOTENSION & SHOCK

Essentials of Diagnosis

- Low systemic blood pressure and tachycardia.
- Peripheral hypoperfusion and, in most, vasoconstriction.
- Altered mental status.
- Oliguria or anuria.
- Metabolic acidosis in many.

General Considerations

Shock occurs when the circulation of arterial blood is inadequate to meet tissue metabolic needs. Treatment must be directed both at the manifestations of shock and at its cause.

Classification
(Table 12—1)

A. Hypovolemic Shock: Decreased intravascular volume resulting from loss of blood, plasma, or fluids and electrolytes may be obvious (eg, external hemorrhage) or subtle (eg, sequestration in a "third space," as in pancreatitis). Compensatory vasoconstriction temporarily reduces the size of the vascular bed and may temporarily maintain the blood pressure, but if fluid is not replaced, hypotension occurs, peripheral resistance increases, capillary and venous beds collapse, and the tissues become progressively more hypoxic. Even a moderate sudden loss of circulating fluids can result in severe damage to vital centers.

B. Cardiogenic Shock: Inadequate cardiac function may result from disorders of the heart muscle, valves, or the electrical pacing system. Shock associated with myocardial infarction or other serious

Table 12–1. Classification of shock by mechanism and common causes.[1]

Hypovolemic shock
  Loss of blood (hemorrhagic shock)
    External hemorrhage
      Trauma
      Gastrointestinal tract bleeding
    Internal hemorrhage
      Hematoma
      Hemothorax or hemoperitoneum
  Loss of plasma
    Burns
    Exfoliative dermatitis
  Loss of fluid and electrolytes
    External
      Vomiting
      Diarrhea
      Excessive sweating
      Hyperosmolar states (diabetic ketoacidosis, hyperosmolar nonketotic coma)
    Internal ("third spacing")
      Pancreatitis
      Ascites
      Bowel obstruction

Cardiogenic shock
  Dysrhythmia
    Tachyarrhythmia
    Bradyarrhythmia
  "Pump failure" (secondary to myocardial infarction or other cardiomyopathy)
  Acute valvular dysfunction (especially regurgitant lesions).
  Rupture of ventricular septum or free ventricular wall

Obstructive shock
  Tension pneumothorax
  Pericardial disease (tamponade, constriction)
  Disease of pulmonary vasculature (massive pulmonary emboli, pulmonary hypertension)
  Cardiac tumor (atrial myxoma)
  Left atrial mural thrombus
  Obstructive valvular disease (aortic or mitral stenosis)

Distributive shock
  Septic shock
  Anaphylactic shock
  Neurogenic shock
  Vasodilator drugs
  Acute adrenal insufficiency

[1]Reproduced, with permission, from Saunders CE, Ho MT (editors): *Current Emergency Diagnosis & Treatment*, 4th ed. Appleton & Lange, 1992.

cardiac disease still carries a very high mortality rate (75–80%).

C. Obstructive Shock: Obstruction of the systemic or pulmonary circulation, the aortic and mitral valves, or venous inflow, as in pericardial disease, may reduce cardiac output sufficiently to cause shock. Cardiac tamponade, tension pneumothorax, and massive pulmonary embolism are medical emergencies requiring prompt diagnosis and treatment. Tamponade calls for immediate echocardiography and pericardiocentesis. The prognosis for patients with massive pulmonary embolism is guarded despite therapy with anticoagulants or thrombolytics; surgical embolectomy adds little. A less common cause of obstructive shock is myxoma with pulmonary hypertension.

D. Distributive Shock: Reduction in systemic vascular resistance from such diverse causes as sepsis, anaphylaxis, or acute adrenal insufficiency may result in inadequate cardiac output despite normal circulatory volume.

1. Septic shock–Most commonly, vascular shock is due to gram-negative bacteremia (so-called septic shock). In overwhelming infection, there is an initial short period of vasoconstriction followed by vasodilation, with venous pooling of blood in the microcirculation. The mortality rate is high (40–80%). Responsible organisms are most commonly gram-negative rods (*Escherichia coli, Klebsiella, Proteus,* and *Pseudomonas*) as well as gram-positive cocci (*Staphylococcus, Streptococcus*) and gram-negative anaerobes (eg, *Bacteroides*). Septic shock occurs more often in the very young and the very old; in diabetes, hematologic cancers, and diseases of the genitourinary, hepatobiliary, and intestinal tracts; and in association with immunosuppressive therapy. Immediate precipitating factors may be urinary, biliary, or gynecologic manipulations.

Septic shock is suspected when a febrile patient has chills associated with hypotension. Early, the skin may be warm and the pulse full ("warm shock"). Hyperventilation results in respiratory alkalosis. The sensorium and urinary output are often initially normal, with classic signs of shock becoming manifest later. The symptoms and signs of the inciting infection are not invariably present.

The development of monoclonal antibodies to endotoxin has opened a potential new avenue of therapy. This is discussed in Chapter 32.

2. Neurogenic shock–Neurogenic or psychogenic factors, eg, spinal cord injury, pain, trauma, fright, gastric dilation, or vasodilator drugs, may also cause distributive shock due to reflex vagal stimulation with decreased cardiac output, hypotension, and decreased cerebral blood flow.

Diagnosis of Shock & Impending Shock

Shock may be impending if the following signs are present.

A. Hypotension: Hypotension in adults is traditionally defined as a systolic blood pressure of 90 mm Hg or less. However, some normal adults may have levels that low without ill effects, and some hypertensive persons develop shock with what would ordinarily be considered normal blood pressures.

B. Orthostatic Changes in Vital Signs: Patients who are not clearly hypotensive when tested in the supine position should have blood pressures measured and pulses counted while sitting up with the legs dangling. If no change occurs when this is done,

repeat the measurements with the patient standing. Three to 5 minutes between measurements are allowed to permit the pulse and blood pressure to stabilize. A drop in systolic pressure of 10–20 mm Hg or more associated with an increase in pulse rate of more than 15 beats/min suggests depleted intravascular volume. Some normovolemic patients with peripheral neuropathies or those taking certain medications (eg, some antihypertensive drugs) may demonstrate an orthostatic fall in blood pressure, but without associated increase in pulse rate.

C. Peripheral Hypoperfusion: Patients in shock often have cool or mottled extremities and weak or absent peripheral pulses.

D. Altered Mental Status: Patients may demonstrate normal mental status or may be restless, agitated, confused, lethargic, or comatose as a result of inadequate perfusion of the brain.

Treatment

Treatment depends upon prompt assessment of the cause, type, severity, and duration of shock as well as an accurate appraisal of underlying conditions that may influence the onset or maintenance of shock.

A. Position: The patient is placed in the Trendelenburg or supine position with legs elevated to maximize cerebral blood flow.

B. Oxygenation: Shock—especially septic shock—may result in hypoxia caused by pulmonary ventilation-perfusion mismatch or, in severe cases, by adult respiratory distress syndrome (see Chapter 9).

C. Analgesics: Severe pain is treated promptly with analgesic drugs. Morphine sulfate, 8–15 mg subcutaneously, is appropriate for severe pain; since subcutaneous absorption is poor in patients in shock, 4–8 mg slowly intravenously may be used as an alternative. Morphine should not be given to unconscious patients, to those who have head injuries, to those with severe hypotension or unstable blood pressure, or to those with respiratory depression.

D. Laboratory Studies: A complete blood count is obtained immediately, and a blood specimen is sent for typing and cross-matching. Electrolytes, blood glucose, and urinalysis are also important diagnostically. Arterial blood gases (or finger oximeter oxygen saturation) and electrolytes are obtained routinely.

E. Urine Flow: Both oliguric and nonoliguric renal failure may occur in shock. In the patient without preexisting renal disease, urine output is a reliable indication of organ perfusion. An indwelling catheter to monitor urine flow (which should be kept above 0.5 mL/kg/h) may be indicated. Urine flow of less than 25 mL/h indicates inadequate renal perfusion, which, if not corrected, can result in renal tubular necrosis.

F. Monitor Cardiac Rhythm: Periodic electrocardiography or continuous automated monitoring will permit early detection and prompt treatment of myocardial ischemia from hypoperfusion, and arrhythmias from similar causes or from electrolyte and acid-base disturbances.

G. Central Venous Pressure (CVP) or Pulmonary Capillary Wedge Pressure (PCWP): Monitoring of central venous pressure or pulmonary capillary wedge pressure is helpful in treating shock. Central venous pressure determination is relatively simple but is not as reliable as the pulmonary capillary wedge pressure (PCWP) measured by the Swan-Ganz catheter technique, which provides a better index of left ventricular function. Determination of PCWP is indicated in patients in whom there is uncertainty about the role of cardiac function in the genesis of shock or in myocardial infarction with shock. It is also useful in guiding volume resuscitation in shock patients with a history of heart disease or in such patients in whom pulmonary disease has produced high central venous pressure.

In central venous pressure determination, a catheter is inserted percutaneously (or by cutdown) through a major vein. Normal values range from 5 to 8 cm of water. A low central venous pressure suggests the need for fluid replacement. A high central venous pressure (above 15 cm of water) suggests volume expansion exceeding the upper limit of normal but also cardiac tamponade or bronchospasm. The PCWP catheter is inserted in a similar fashion, with localization of its tip determined by monitoring the morphology of the pressure tracing as it is advanced. A PCWP over 14 mm Hg may serve as a warning of impending pulmonary edema. Catheter insertion requires a skilled and experienced physician and is expensive; the catheter itself costs about $175.00. Surveillance for the catheter-induced complications of hemorrhage, sepsis, pneumothorax, arrhythmias, and pulmonary infarction is an important part of intensive care.

H. Volume Replacement: Initial or emergency needs may be determined by the history, general appearance, vital signs, and hematocrit. There is no simple technique by which to accurately judge the fluid requirements. An estimate of total fluid losses is an essential first step. Response to therapy—particularly the effect of carefully administered, gradually increasing amounts of intravenous fluids on the central venous pressure or PCWP—is a valuable index.

Selection of the proper fluid for restoration and maintenance of hemodynamic stability is often difficult and controversial. It will depend upon the type of fluid that has been lost (whole blood, plasma, water, electrolytes), associated medical problems, availability of the various replacement solutions, clinical and laboratory monitoring facilities, and, in some circumstances, expense. The most effective replacement fluid in case of hemorrhage is packed red cells with saline, but other available fluids should be given immediately pending return of laboratory studies.

Rapid volume replacement in blood loss will often prevent shock. If central venous pressure or PCWP is low and the hematocrit greater than 35%—and if there is no clinical evidence to suggest occult blood loss—blood volume should be supported with crystalloid solutions or colloids.

1. Crystalloid solutions–Isotonic (0.9%) sodium chloride solution 500–2000 mL, is given rapidly intravenously—ideally under central venous pressure or pulmonary capillary wedge pressure monitoring. The crystalloids are readily available for emergencies and mass casualties. They may obviate the need for blood or colloids. They are often effective, at least temporarily, when given in adequate doses.

2. Colloids–Colloids are high-molecular-weight substances that do not diffuse readily across normal capillary membranes. Colloidal solutions increase the plasma oncotic pressure and thus in theory can draw fluid from the interstitial space into the intravascular space to cause additional fluid volume expansion. Capillary membranes in the lungs are often damaged in the patient in shock, so that larger molecules may leak from the intravascular space into the interstitium and have an adverse effect on pulmonary function (adult respiratory distress syndrome).

a. Blood–Packed or frozen red cells are preferred to whole blood, since remaining blood products may be used for other purposes. The amount of blood given depends on the clinical course, the hematocrit, and hemodynamic findings.

Screening of blood donors for hepatitis B and C infection and for HIV has reduced the frequency of those infections following transfusion. The risk of AIDS infection from transfused blood is now estimated at approximately 1:40,000 in industrialized countries that screen appropriately. The risk for contracting hepatitis B is somewhat greater. Non-A, non-B hepatitis remains the commonest infectious complication of transfusion, with an incidence of 2–5%; this may decline with the advent of diagnostic tests for hepatitis C.

b. Plasma fractions–Group-specific frozen plasma is a satisfactory colloidal volume expander and occasionally can correct specific coagulation defects. Because of its expense, risk (same as blood transfusion), and relative ineffectiveness, however, its use should be limited. Unit-bagged plasma is preferable to pooled plasma. Albumin 5% in saline, albumin 25% in concentrate, or plasma protein fraction (containing 80–85% albumin) may be rapidly set up for emergencies, and blood typing is not required. These substances have been heat-treated to minimize the risk of infectious hepatitis.

c. Dextrans–Dextrans are high-molecular-weight polysaccharide colloids that are fairly effective plasma expanders. Because they can impair blood coagulation and interfere with blood typing and because they may cause anaphylactoid reactions, dextrans are used very infrequently now.

I. Vasoactive Drugs: Some adrenergic drugs can be useful in the adjunctive therapy of shock. *The adrenergic drugs should not be considered a primary form of therapy in shock.* Simple blood pressure elevation produced by the vasopressor drugs has little beneficial effect on the underlying disturbance, and in many instances the effect may be detrimental. Pressors are given only when hypotension persists after volume deficits are corrected and obstructive causes excluded or remedied.

1. Dopamine hydrochloride has an advantage over other adrenergic drugs because it has a beneficial effect on renal blood flow (at low dose) and because it increases cardiac output and blood pressure. Dopamine hydrochloride, 200 mg in 500 mL of sodium chloride injection USP (400 μg/mL), is given initially at a rate of 1–2 μg/kg/min. This dosage stimulates both the dopaminergic receptors, which increase the renal blood flow and urinary output, and the β-adrenergic cardiac receptors, which increase the cardiac output. If shock persists, gradually increasing doses of dopamine may be required. If dopamine alone fails to maintain adequate perfusion pressure, it may sometimes be necessary to use it in combination with another appropriate adrenergic drug.

Adverse reactions include ventricular arrhythmias, anginal pain, nausea and vomiting, headache, hypotension, azotemia, and rare cases of peripheral gangrene. Special care should be exercised when dopamine is used in the treatment of shock following myocardial infarction, because the drug's inotropic effect may increase myocardial oxygen demand. Dopamine should not be used in patients with pheochromocytoma or uncorrected tachyarrhythmias or in those who are receiving monoamine oxidase inhibitors.

2. Dobutamine, a synthetic catecholamine similar to dopamine but with greater inotropic effect, may be useful when filling pressures are high because of fluid overload or heart failure. Though dopamine at higher doses is a vasoconstrictor, dobutamine has no net effect on peripheral vascular resistance.

J. Corticosteroids: Corticosteroids are lifesaving in the treatment of shock associated with acute adrenal insufficiency (see Chapter 25). In other types of shock, however, corticosteroids are of no benefit.

K. Diuretics: Diuretics are not employed until volume deficits are corrected or obstructive causes remedied. There is no evidence that diuretics reduce the overall incidence of renal failure, though some believe they may convert oliguric renal insufficiency to a nonoliguric type.

L. Heparin: See Disseminated Intravascular Coagulation in Chapter 13.

M. Fluid and Electrolyte Balance: Abnormalities of fluid, electrolyte, and acid-base balance are addressed. There is growing evidence that vigorous treatment with sodium bicarbonate should not be used as standard therapy. Its use should be reserved for cases of acidosis that fail to respond to adequate fluid resuscitation.

N. Treatment of Cardiac Disorders: Digitalis glycosides are indicated only for those patients with preexisting or presenting evidence of cardiac failure or digitalis-responsive arrhythmias. Atropine may be of value in treating selected bradycardias. The use of vasopressor drugs in myocardial infarction is reserved for patients with hypotension and elevated left ventricular filling pressure. Continuous cardiac monitoring is required. The hemodynamic effectiveness of vasodilator drugs in reducing preload and outflow resistance in patients with left ventricular failure has been established, but the mortality rate of cardiogenic shock is unchanged.

Bone RC et al: A controlled clinical trial of high-dose methylprednisolone in the treatment of severe sepsis and septic shock. N Engl J Med 1987;317:653. (Most recent of several current studies concluding that steroids are of no benefit in the treatment of septic shock.)

Ognibene FD et al: Depressed left ventricular performance: Response to volume infusion in patients with sepsis and septic shock. Chest 1988;93:903. (Left ventricular stroke work index response to volume infusion was significantly less in septic shock, suggesting altered ventricular performance.)

REFERENCES

Moore WS (editor): *Vascular Surgery: A Comprehensive Review,* 2nd ed. Grune & Stratton, 1986.

Wilson SE, Williams RA (editors): *Vascular Surgery: Principles and Practice.* McGraw-Hill, 1987.

Blood

13

Charles A. Linker, MD

ANEMIAS

General Approach to Anemias

Anemia is present in adults if the hematocrit is less than 41% in males or 37% in females. In taking the history, congenital anemia may be suggested by the patient's personal and family history. Poor diet results in folic acid deficiency and may contribute to iron deficiency. Bleeding should always be considered in iron deficiency. Physical examination includes careful attention to signs of primary hematologic diseases (lymphadenopathy, hepatosplenomegaly, or bone tenderness). Mucosal changes such as a smooth tongue raise the possibility of megaloblastic anemia.

Anemias are classified according to their pathophysiologic basis, ie, whether related to diminished production or accelerated loss of red blood cells (Table 13–1); or according to cell size (Table 13–2). The diagnostic possibilities in microcytic anemia are iron deficiency, thalassemia, and anemia of chronic disease. A severely microcytic anemia (MCV < 70 fL) is always due either to iron deficiency or to thalassemia. Macrocytic anemia may be due to megaloblastic (folate or vitamin B_{12} deficiency) or nonmegaloblastic causes. A severely macrocytic anemia (MCV > 125 fL) is almost always due to megaloblastic causes; rare exceptions are the myelodysplastic syndromes, either before or after chemotherapy.

Wallerstein RO Jr.: Laboratory evaluation of anemia. West J Med 1987;146:443.

IRON DEFICIENCY ANEMIA

Essentials of Diagnosis

- Both pathognomonic: absent bone marrow iron stores or serum ferritin < 12 µg/L.
- Nearly always caused by bleeding in adults.
- Response to iron therapy.

General Considerations

Iron deficiency is the most common cause of anemia worldwide. The anemia is usually mild, but it may become moderate or even severe. It is important to make the diagnosis so that the underlying cause (usually gastrointestinal blood loss) can be identified and treated (Table 13–3).

Iron is necessary for the formation of heme and other enzymes. Total body iron ranges between 2 g and 4 g: approximately 50 mg/kg in men and 35 mg/kg in women. The majority (70–95%) of total body iron is present in hemoglobin in circulating red blood cells. One milliliter of packed red blood cells (not whole blood) contains approximately 1 mg of iron. In men, red blood cell volume is approximately 30 mL/kg. A 70-kg man will therefore have approximately 2100 mL of packed red blood cells and consequently 2100 mg of iron in his circulating blood. In women, the red cell volume is about 27 mL/kg; a 50-kg woman will thus have 1350 mg of iron circulating in her red blood cells. Only 200–400 mg of iron is present in myoglobin and nonheme enzymes. The amount of iron present in plasma is negligible. Aside from circulating red blood cells, the major location of iron in the body is the storage pool. Iron is deposited either as ferritin or as hemosiderin and is located largely in macrophages. The range for storage iron is wide (0.5–2 g); approximately 25% of women in the USA have none.

The average American diet contains 10–15 mg of iron per day. About 10% of this amount is absorbed. Absorption occurs in the stomach, duodenum, and upper jejunum. Dietary iron present as heme is efficiently absorbed (10–20%) but nonheme iron less so (1–5%), largely because of interference by phosphates, tannins, and other food constituents. Small amounts of iron—approximately 1 mg/d—are normally lost though exfoliation of skin and mucosal cells. There is no mechanism for increasing normal body iron losses.

Menstrual blood loss in women plays a major role in iron metabolism. The average monthly menstrual blood loss is approximately 50 mL, or about 0.7 mg/d. However, menstrual blood loss may be five times the average. In order to maintain adequate iron stores, women with heavy menstrual losses must ab-

Table 13–1. Classification of anemias by pathophysiology.

Decreased production
    Hemoglobin synthesis: Iron deficiency, thalassemia, anemia of chronic disease
    DNA synthesis: Megaloblastic anemia
    Stem cell: Aplastic anemia, myeloproliferative leukemia
    Bone marrow infiltration: Carcinoma, lymphoma
    Pure red cell aplasia
Increased destruction
    Blood loss
    Hemolysis (intrinsic)
        Membrane: Hereditary spherocytosis, elliptocytosis
        Hemoglobin: Sickle cell, unstable hemoglobin
        Glycolysis: Pyruvate kinase, etc
        Oxidation: G6PD deficiency
    Hemolysis (extrinsic)
        Immune: Warm antibody, cold antibody
        Microangiopathic: Thrombotic thrombocytopenic purpura, hemolytic-uremic syndrome, valve
        Infection: Clostridial
        Hypersplenism

Table 13–3. Causes of iron deficiency.

Deficient diet
Decreased absorption
Increased requirements
    Pregnancy
    Lactation
Blood loss
    Gastrointestinal
    Menstrual
    Blood donation
Hemoglobinuria
Iron sequestration
    Pulmonary hemosiderosis

sorb 3–4 mg of iron from the diet each day. This strains the upper limit of what may reasonably be absorbed, and women with menorrhagia of this degree will almost always become iron-deficient.

In general, iron metabolism is balanced between absorption of 1 mg/d and loss of 1 mg/d. Pregnancy may also upset the iron balance, since requirements increase to 2–5 mg of iron per day during pregnancy and lactation. Normal dietary iron cannot supply these requirements, and medicinal iron is needed during pregnancy and lactation.

It is possible to become iron-deficient because of dietary deficiency, though this is rare in adults. Decreased iron absorption can cause iron deficiency and is usually due to gastric surgery. Repeated pregnancy (especially with breast feeding) is a common cause of iron deficiency if increased requirements are not met with supplemental medicinal iron.

By far the most important cause of iron deficiency anemia is blood loss, especially gastrointestinal blood loss. Chronic aspirin use may cause chronic iron loss even without a documented structural lesion. Iron deficiency should prompt a search for a po-

Table 13–2. Classification of anemias by MCV.

Microcytic
    Iron deficiency
    Thalassemia
    Anemia of chronic disease
Macrocytic
    Megaloblastic
        Vitamin B_{12} deficiency
        Folate deficiency
    Nonmegaloblastic
        Myelodysplasia, chemotherapy
        Liver disease
        Increased reticulocytosis
        Myxedema
Normocytic
    Many causes

tential source of gastrointestinal bleeding unless another cause is identified. Other sources of blood loss include menorrhagia or other uterine bleeding and repeated blood donation.

Chronic hemoglobinuria may lead to iron deficiency, since more than 1 mg/d of iron can be lost by this route. The most common cause is traumatic hemolysis due to an abnormally functioning cardiac valve. Other causes of intravascular hemolysis (eg. paroxysmal nocturnal hemoglobinuria) should also be considered if hemoglobinuria is documented.

Rare causes of iron deficiency include sequestration of iron in pulmonary macrophages in the syndrome of idiopathic pulmonary hemosiderosis.

Clinical Findings

A. Symptoms and Signs: As a rule, the only symptoms of iron deficiency anemia are those of the anemia itself (easy fatigability, tachycardia, palpitations and tachypnea on exertion). Severe iron deficiency (uncommon in the USA) causes progressive skin and mucosal changes. These include a smooth tongue, brittle nails, and cheilosis. Advanced iron deficiency may cause dysphagia because of the formation of esophageal webs (Plummer-Vinson syndrome). Many iron-deficient patients develop pica, an unusual craving for specific foods (ice cubes, etc) that may or may not contain iron.

B. Laboratory Findings: Iron deficiency develops slowly and in stages. The first stage is depletion of iron stores. At this point, there is anemia and no changes in red blood cell size. The serum ferritin will become abnormally low. Ferritin values less than 30 μg/L nearly always indicate absent iron stores. The serum total iron-binding capacity (TIBC) rises.

After iron stores have been depleted, red blood cell formation will continue with deficient supplies of iron. Serum iron values will begin to fall to less than 30 μg/dL, and transferrin saturation will fall to less than 15%.

In the early stages, the MCV remains normal. Subsequently, the MCV falls and the blood smear shows hypochromic microcytic cells. With further progression, anisocytosis (variations in red blood cell size) followed by poikilocytosis (variation in shape of red cells) will develop. Severe iron deficiency will produce a bizarre peripheral blood smear, with severely hypochromic cells, target cells, hypochromic pencil-shaped cells, and occasionally small numbers of nucleated red blood cells. The platelet count is usually normal in mild iron deficiency anemia but is typically elevated in more severe cases.

Differential Diagnosis

Other causes of microcytic anemia include anemia of chronic disease, thalassemia, and (less commonly) sideroblastic anemia. Anemia of chronic disease is characterized by normal or increased iron stores in the bone marrow and a normal or elevated ferritin level. The TIBC is either normal or low. Thalassemia characteristically produces a greater degree of microcytosis for any given level of anemia than does iron deficiency. Red blood cell morphology on the peripheral smear becomes abnormal earlier in the evolution of anemia, and iron parameters should be normal.

Treatment

To make the diagnosis of iron deficiency anemia, one can either demonstrate an iron-deficient state or evaluate the response to a therapeutic trial of iron replacement.

Since the anemia itself is rarely life-threatening, the most important part of treatment is identification of the cause—especially a source of occult blood loss. Iron deficiency cannot be overcome by increasing dietary iron; medicinal iron is always required.

A. Oral Iron: There is no better treatment than ferrous sulfate, 325 mg three times daily, which provides 180 mg of iron daily of which 10–20 mg is usually absorbed (though absorption may exceed this amount in cases of severe deficiency). Although ferrous sulfate is optimally taken three times a day on empty stomach, compliance is often improved by introducing the medicine more slowly in a gradually escalating dose. Patients who cannot tolerate iron on an empty stomach should take it with food. An appropriate response is a return of the hematocrit level halfway toward normal within 3 weeks. It is advisable to see the patient after 3 weeks both to monitor the hematologic response and to answer questions about the medication that may improve compliance. In general, hematologic values return to normal after 2 months of treatment. Iron therapy should continue for 3–6 months after restoration of normal hematologic values in order to replenish iron stores. Failure of response to iron therapy is usually due to noncompliance, although occasional patients may absorb iron poorly. Other reasons for failure to respond include incorrect diagnosis (anemia of chronic disease, thalassemia) and ongoing gastrointestinal blood loss that exceeds the rate of new erythropoiesis.

B. Parenteral Iron: The indications are intolerance to oral iron, refractoriness to oral iron (poor absorption), gastrointestinal disease (usually inflammatory bowel disease) precluding the use of oral iron, and continued blood loss that cannot be corrected. Because of the possibility of severe and even fatal hypersensitivity reactions, parenteral iron therapy should be used only in cases of clinically significant documented iron deficiency after every reasonable attempt has been made to use oral therapy.

The dose may be calculated by estimating the decrease in volume of red blood cell mass and then supplying 1 mg of iron for each milliliter of volume of red blood cells below normal. One should then add approximately 1 g for storage iron. The total dose is typically 1.5–2 g. The entire dose may be given as an intravenous infusion over 4–6 hours. A test dose of a dilute solution is given first, and the patient should be observed closely during the entire infusion in a setting in which anaphylaxis can be treated.

Cook JD: Clinical evaluation of iron deficiency. Semin Hematol 1982;19:6.

ANEMIA OF CHRONIC DISEASE

Many chronic systemic diseases are associated with mild or moderate anemia. Common causes include chronic infection or inflammation, cancer, and liver disease. The anemia of chronic renal failure is somewhat different in pathophysiology and is usually more severe.

Red blood cell survival is modestly reduced, and the bone marrow fails to compensate adequately by increasing red blood cell production. Failure to increase red cell production is largely due to sequestration of iron within the reticuloendothelial system. Decrease in erythropoietin is rarely an important cause of underproduction of red cells except in renal failure, when decreased erythropoietin is the rule.

Clinical Findings

A. Symptoms and Signs: The clinical features are those of the anemia, which is usually modest. The diagnosis should be suspected in patients with known chronic diseases; it is confirmed by the findings of low serum iron, low TIBC, and normal or increased serum ferritin (or normal or increased bone marrow iron stores). In cases of significant anemia, coexistent iron deficiency or folic acid deficiency should be suspected. Decreased dietary intake of folate or iron is common in these ill patients, and many will also have ongoing gastrointestinal blood losses. Patients undergoing hemodialysis regularly lose both iron and folate during dialysis.

B. Laboratory Findings: The hematocrit rarely falls below 25% (except in renal failure). The MCV is usually normal but may be slightly reduced. Red blood cell morphology is nondiagnostic, and the reticulocyte count is neither strikingly reduced nor increased. Characteristically, both the serum iron values and the TIBC are reduced. Serum iron values may be unmeasurable, and transferrin saturation may be extremely low. A mistaken diagnosis of iron deficiency anemia may be made if overemphasis is placed on the reduced serum iron. A low serum iron and percentage saturation are diagnostic of iron deficiency only when the TIBC is also increased. In contrast to iron deficiency, serum ferritin values should be normal or increased. A serum ferritin value of less than 25 µg/L should suggest coexistent iron deficiency.

Treatment

In most cases no treatment is necessary. In some, however, red blood cell transfusions are required for symptomatic anemia. Purified recombinant erythropoietin has been shown to be safe and effective for treatment of the anemia of renal failure and other secondary anemias such as anemia related to cancer or inflammatory disorders (eg, rheumatoid arthritis). Erythropoietin is commercially available as epoetin alfa; however, it must be injected subcutaneously three or more times weekly and is very expensive. This agent should be used to alleviate anemia only when the patient is transfusion-dependent or when the quality of life is clearly improved by the hematologic response.

Krantz SB: Erythropoietin. Blood 1991;77:419.

THE THALASSEMIAS

Essentials of Diagnosis

- Microcytosis out of proportion to the degree of anemia.
- Positive family history or lifelong personal history of microcytic anemia.
- Abnormal red blood cell morphology with microcytes, acanthocytes, and target cells.
- In beta thalassemia, elevated levels of hemoglobin A_2 or F.

General Considerations

The thalassemias are hereditary disorders characterized by reduction in the synthesis of globin chains (alpha or beta). Reduced globin chain synthesis causes reduced hemoglobin synthesis and eventually produces a hypochromic microcytic anemia because of defective hemoglobinization of red blood cells. Thalassemias can be considered among the hypoproliferative anemias, the hemolytic anemias, and the anemias related to abnormal hemoglobin, since all of these factors may play a role.

Normal adult hemoglobin is primarily hemoglobin A, which represents approximately 98% of circulating hemoglobin. Hemoglobin A is formed from a tetramer—two alpha chains and two beta chains—and can be designated $\alpha_2\beta_2$. Two copies of the α-globin gene are located on chromosome 16, and there is no substitute for α-globin in the formation of hemoglobin. The β-globin gene resides on chromosome 11 adjacent to genes encoding the beta-like globin chains, delta and gamma. The tetramer of $\alpha_2\delta_2$ forms a hemoglobin A_2, which normally comprises 1–2% of adult hemoglobin. The tetramer $\alpha_2\gamma_2$ forms hemoglobin F, which is the major hemoglobin of fetal life but which comprises less than 1% of normal adult hemoglobin.

Alpha thalassemia is due primarily to gene deletion directly causing reduced α-globin chain synthesis (Table 13–4). Since all adult hemoglobins are alpha-containing, alpha thalassemia produces no change in the percentage distribution of hemoglobins A, A_2, and F. In severe forms of alpha thalassemia, excess beta chains may form a β_4 tetramer called hemoglobin H. Hemoglobin H has high oxygen affinity and delivers oxygen to tissues poorly. It is also unstable and subject to oxidative denaturation under conditions of infection or exposure to oxidative drugs (sulfonamides, etc).

Beta thalassemias are usually caused by point mutations rather than large deletions (Table 13–5). These mutations result in premature chain termination or in problems with transcription of RNA and ultimately result in reduced or absent β-globin chain synthesis. The molecular defects leading to beta thalassemia are numerous and heterogeneous. Defects that result in absent globin chain expression are termed β^0, whereas defects causing reduced synthesis are termed β^+. The reduced β-globin chain synthesis in beta thalassemia results in a relative increase in the percentages of hemoglobins A_2 and F compared to hemoglobin A, as the beta-like globins (gamma and delta) substitute for the missing beta chains. In the presence of reduced beta chains, the excess alpha chains are unstable and precipitate, leading to damage to red blood cell membranes. This damage causes marked intramedullary hemolysis (destruction of developing erythroid cells within the bone marrow) as well as hemolysis in the peripheral blood. The bone marrow becomes markedly hyperplastic under the drive of severe anemia and the ineffective erythropoiesis that results from destruction of the developing erythroid cells. This marked expansion of the erythroid

Table 13–4. Alpha thalassemia syndromes.

Alpha Globin Genes	Syndrome	Hematocrit	MCV
4	Normal	Normal	
3	Silent carrier	Normal	
2	Thalassemia minor	32–40%	60–75 fL
1	Hemoglobin H disease	22–32%	60–70 fL
0	Hydrops fetalis		

Table 13–5. Beta thalassemia syndromes.

	Beta Globin Genes	Hgb A	Hgb A$_2$	Hgb F
Normal	Homozygous β	97–99%	1–3%	< 1%
Thalassemia major	Homozygous β^0	0	4–10%	90–96%
	Homozygous β$^+$		4–10%	
Thalassemia intermedia	Homozygous β$^+$ (mild)	0–30%	0–10%	6–100%
Thalassemia minor	Heterozygous β^0	80–95%	4–8%	1–5%
	Heterozygous β$^+$	80–95%	4–8%	1–5%

element in the bone marrow causes severe bony deformities, osteopenia, and pathologic fractures.

Clinical Findings

A. Symptoms and Signs: The alpha thalassemia syndromes are seen primarily in persons from southeast Asia and China, and, less commonly, in blacks. Normally, adults have four copies of the α-globin chain. When three α-globin genes are present, the patient is hematologically normal and is called a silent carrier. When two α-globin genes are present, the patient is said to have alpha thalassemia trait, one form of thalassemia minor. These patients are clinically normal and have normal life expectancy and performance status. They have a very mild microcytic anemia. When only one α-globin chain is present, the patient has hemoglobin H disease. This is a chronic hemolytic anemia of variable severity (thalassemia minor or intermedia). Physical examination will reveal pallor and splenomegaly. Although affected individuals do not usually require transfusions, they may do so during periods of hemolytic exacerbation caused by infection or other stresses. When all four α-globin genes are deleted, the affected fetus is stillborn as a result of hydrops fetalis.

Beta thalassemia affects persons of Mediterranean origin (Italian, Greek) and to a lesser extent Chinese, other Asians, and blacks. Patients homozygous for beta thalassemia have the syndrome of thalassemia major. Affected children are normal at birth but during the first year of life develop severe anemia requiring transfusion. Signs of thalassemia typically develop after 6 months of age, because this is the time when hemoglobin synthesis switches from hemoglobin F to hemoglobin A. Numerous clinical problems ensue, including growth failure, bony deformities (abnormal facial structure, pathologic fractures), hepatosplenomegaly, and jaundice. The clinical course has been modified significantly by transfusion therapy. Children with severe thalassemia may grow normally until puberty, when they experience hypogonadism, growth failure, and clinical consequences of iron overload from years of transfusion. The transfusional iron overload (hemosiderosis) results in cardiomyopathy, progressive hepatomegaly, and numerous endocrine dysfunctions. Death from

cardiac failure usually occurs between ages 20 and 30.

Patients homozygous for a milder form of beta thalassemia (allowing a higher rate of globin gene synthesis) may have the syndrome of thalassemia intermedia. These patients have chronic hemolytic anemia but usually do not require transfusions except under periods of stress. These patients develop iron overload because of increased gut absorption of iron and periodic transfusion. They survive into adult life but with hepatosplenomegaly and bony deformities.

Patients heterozygous for beta thalassemia have thalassemia minor. These patients have a mild microcytic anemia that is not clinically significant.

Prenatal diagnosis is available for couples at risk of producing a child with one of the severe thalassemia syndromes. Asian couples whose parents on both sides have alpha thalassemia trait are at risk of producing an infant with hydrops fetalis. Mediterranean people (and, less commonly, Chinese or blacks) with two parents heterozygous for beta thalassemia are at risk of producing a homozygous child. Genetic counseling should be offered, and the opportunity for prenatal diagnosis should be discussed.

B. Laboratory Findings:

1. Alpha thalassemia trait–Patients with two α-globin genes have mild anemia, with hematocrits between 28% and 40%. The MCV is strikingly low (60–75 fL) despite the modest degree of anemia, and the red blood count is usually normal. The peripheral blood smear shows mild abnormalities, including microcytes, hypochromia, occasional target cells, and acanthocytes (cells with irregularly spaced bulbous projections). The reticulocyte count and iron parameters are normal. Hemoglobin electrophoresis will show no increase in the percentage of hemoglobins A$_2$ or F and no hemoglobin H. Alpha thalassemia trait is usually diagnosed by exclusion in a patient with modest anemia, significant microcytosis, and no elevation of hemoglobins A$_2$ or F. Definitive diagnosis depends upon hemoglobin gene mapping demonstrating a reduced number of α-globin genes, but this procedure is unnecessary for clinical diagnosis.

2. Hemoglobin H disease–These patients have a variably severe hemolytic anemia, with hematocrits between 22% and 32%. The MCV is strikingly low

(69–70 fL). The peripheral blood smear is markedly abnormal, with hypochromia, microcytosis, target cells, and poikilocytosis. The reticulocyte count is elevated. Hemoglobin electrophoresis will show the presence of a fast migrating hemoglobin (hemoglobin H), which comprises 10–40% of the hemoglobin. A peripheral blood smear can be stained with supravital dyes to demonstrate the presence of hemoglobin H.

3. Beta thalassemia minor–Like patients with alpha thalassemia trait, these patients have a modest anemia with hematocrit between 28% and 40%. The MCV ranges from 55 to 75 fL, and the red blood cell count is usually normal. The peripheral blood smear is mildly abnormal, with hypochromia, microcytosis, and target cells. In contrast to alpha thalassemia, basophilic stippling may be present. The reticulocyte count may be normal or slightly elevated. Hemoglobin electrophoresis (using quantitative techniques) may show an elevation of hemoglobin A_2 to 4–8% and occasional elevations of hemoglobin F to 1–5%.

4. Beta thalassemia major–Beta thalassemia major produces a severe life-threatening anemia, and without transfusion the hematocrit may fall to less than 10%. The peripheral blood smear is bizarre, showing severe poikilocytosis, hypochromia, microcytosis, target cells, basophilic stippling, and nucleated red blood cells. Little or no hemoglobin A is present. Variable amounts of hemoglobin A_2 are seen, and the major hemoglobin present is hemoglobin F.

Differential Diagnosis

Mild forms of thalassemia must be differentiated from iron deficiency. Compared to iron deficiency anemia, patients with thalassemia have a lower MCV, a more normal red blood count, and a more abnormal peripheral blood smear at modest levels of anemia. Iron parameters are normal. The diagnosis of beta thalassemia can be shown by demonstrating increased levels of hemoglobin A_2 (or, less commonly, hemoglobin F), while the diagnosis of alpha thalassemia is made by exclusion. Severe forms of thalassemia may be confused with other hemoglobinopathies. The diagnosis will be made by hemoglobin electrophoresis.

Treatment

Patients with mild thalassemia (alpha thalassemia trait or beta thalassemia minor) are clinically normal and require no treatment. Most importantly, patients with microcytosis should be identified so that they will not be subjected to repeated evaluations for iron deficiency and inappropriately given supplemental iron. Patients with hemoglobin H disease should take folate supplementation and avoid medicinal iron and oxidative drugs such as sulfonamide drugs. They may occasionally need transfusion during pregnancy or under periods of stress. Patients with severe thalassemia should be maintained on a regular transfusion schedule and should receive folate supplementation. Splenectomy is occasionally performed when hypersplenism causes a marked increase in the transfusion requirement. Deferoxamine is routinely given as an iron-chelating agent to avoid or postpone hemosiderosis. Oral iron chelators are now undergoing testing in an investigational setting and may have a major impact.

Allogeneic bone marrow transplantation has been introduced as treatment for beta thalassemia major. Children who have not yet experienced iron overload and chronic organ toxicity do well, with long-term survival in more than 80% of cases.

Kazazian HH, Boehm CD: Molecular basis and prenatal diagnosis of β-thalassemia. Blood 1988;72:1107.

SIDEROBLASTIC ANEMIA

The sideroblastic anemias are a heterogeneous group of disorders in which hemoglobin synthesis is reduced because of failure to incorporate heme into protoporphyrin to form hemoglobin. Iron accumulates, particularly in the mitochondria. A Prussian blue stain of the bone marrow will reveal ringed sideroblasts, cells with iron deposits (in the mitochondrion) encircling the red cell nucleus. The disorder is usually acquired. Sometimes it represents a stage in evolution of a generalized bone marrow disorder (myelodysplasia) that may ultimately terminate in acute leukemia. Other important causes include chronic alcoholism, drug toxicity (antituberculous agents, chloramphenicol), and lead poisoning.

Patients have no specific clinical features other than those related to anemia. The anemia is usually moderate, with hematocrits of 20–30%, but transfusions may occasionally be required. Although the MCV is usually normal or slightly increased, it may occasionally be low, leading to confusion with iron deficiency. The peripheral blood smear characteristically shows a dimorphic population of red blood cells, one normal and one hypochromic. It is the presence of hypochromic cells on peripheral smear combined with a low MCV that may raise the consideration of iron deficiency. In cases of lead poisoning, coarse basophilic stippling of the red cells is seen.

The diagnosis is made by examination of the bone marrow. Characteristically, there is marked erythroid hyperplasia, a sign of ineffective erythropoiesis (expansion of the erythroid compartment of the bone marrow that does not result in the production of reticulocytes in the peripheral blood). The iron stain of the bone marrow shows a generalized increase in iron stores and the presence of ring sideroblasts. Other characteristic laboratory features include a high serum iron and a high transferrin saturation. In the presence of lead poisoning, serum lead levels will be elevated.

When lead toxicity is causative, it may be treated with chelation therapy. Occasional patients will respond to pharmacologic doses of folate or pyridoxine, but most patients do not respond to therapy. Occasionally, the anemia is so severe that support with red cell transfusion is required. These patients usually do not respond to erythropoietin therapy.

Cazzola M et al: Natural history of idiopathic refractory sideroblastic anemia. Blood 1988;71:305.

VITAMIN B$_{12}$ DEFICIENCY

Essentials of Diagnosis
- Macrocytic anemia.
- Macro-ovalocytes and hypersegmented neutrophils on peripheral blood smear.
- Serum vitamin B$_{12}$ level less than 100 pg/mL.

General Considerations

Vitamin B$_{12}$ belongs to the family of cobalamins and serves as a cofactor for two important reactions in humans. As methylcobalamin, it serves as a cofactor for methionine synthetase in the conversion of homocysteine to methionine. As adenosylcobalamin, it serves as a cofactor for the conversion of methylmalonyl-CO to succinyl-CO. All vitamin B$_{12}$ comes from the diet, and vitamin B$_{12}$ is present in all foods of animal origin. The daily absorption of vitamin B$_{12}$ is 5 µg.

After being ingested, vitamin B$_{12}$ becomes bound to intrinsic factor, a protein secreted by gastric parietal cells. Other cobalamin-binding proteins (called R factors) compete with intrinsic factor for vitamin B$_{12}$. Vitamin B$_{12}$ bound to R factors cannot be absorbed. The vitamin B$_{12}$-intrinsic factor complex travels through the intestine and is absorbed in the terminal ileum by cells with specific receptors for the complex. It is then transported through plasma and stored in the liver. Three plasma transport proteins have been identified. Transcobalamins I and III (differing only in carbohydrate structure) are secreted by white blood cells. Although approximately 90% of plasma vitamin B$_{12}$ circulates bound to these proteins, only transcobalamin II is capable of transporting vitamin B$_{12}$ into cells. The liver contains 2000–5000 µg of stored vitamin B$_{12}$. Since daily losses are 3–5 µg/d, the body usually has sufficient stores of vitamin B$_{12}$ so that vitamin B$_{12}$ deficiency develops more than 3 years after vitamin B$_{12}$ absorption ceases.

Since vitamin B$_{12}$ is present in all foods of animal origin, dietary vitamin B$_{12}$ deficiency is extremely rare and seen only in vegans—strict vegetarians who avoid all dairy products as well as meat and fish (Table 13–6). Abdominal surgery may lead to vitamin B$_{12}$ deficiency in several ways. Gastrectomy will eliminate that site of intrinsic factor production; blind loop syndrome will cause competition for vitamin B$_{12}$

Table 13–6. Causes of vitamin B$_{12}$ deficiency.

Dietary deficiency (rare)
Decreased production of intrinsic factor
Pernicious anemia
Gastrectomy
Competition for vitamin B$_{12}$ in gut
Blind loop syndrome
Fish tapeworm (rare)
Decreased ileal absorption of vitamin B$_{12}$
Surgical resections
Crohn's disease
Transcobalamin II deficiency (rare)

by bacterial overgrowth in the lumen of the intestine; and surgical resection of the ileum will eliminate the site of vitamin B$_{12}$ absorption. Rare causes of vitamin B$_{12}$ deficiency include fish tapeworm (*Diphyllobothrium latum*) infection, in which the parasite uses luminal vitamin B$_{12}$, and severe Crohn's disease, causing sufficient destruction of the ileum to retard vitamin B$_{12}$ absorption.

The most common cause of vitamin B$_{12}$ deficiency is that associated with **pernicious anemia.** This is a hereditary autoimmune disorder historically seen in patients of Scandinavian or northern European ancestry but now increasingly recognized in young black and Hispanic women. Although the disease is hereditary, it is rarely manifested before age 35. Pernicious anemia produces a number of clinical findings in addition to vitamin B$_{12}$ deficiency. Atrophic gastritis is invariably present and results in histamine-fast achlorhydria. These patients may also have a number of other autoimmune diseases, including IgA deficiency, as well as polyglandular endocrine insufficiency. Over time, the atrophic gastritis is associated with an increased risk of gastric carcinoma.

Clinical Findings

A. Symptoms and Signs: The hallmark of vitamin B$_{12}$ deficiency is megaloblastic anemia. The anemia may be severe, with hematocrits as low as 10–15%. The megaloblastic state also produces changes in mucosal cells, leading to glossitis, as well as other vague gastrointestinal disturbances such as anorexia and diarrhea. Vitamin B$_{12}$ deficiency also leads to a complex neurologic syndrome. Peripheral nerves are usually affected first, and patients complain initially of paresthesias. The posterior columns next become impaired, and patients complain of difficulty with balance. In more advanced cases, cerebral function may be altered as well, and on occasion dementia and other neuropsychiatric changes may precede hematologic changes.

On examination, patients are usually pale and may be mildly icteric. Neurologic examination will reveal decreased vibration and position sense.

B. Laboratory Findings: The megaloblastic state produces an anemia of variable severity that on occasion may be very severe. The MCV is usually strikingly elevated, between 110 and 140 fL. However, it is possible to have vitamin B_{12} deficiency with a normal MCV. Occasionally, the normal MCV may be explained by coexistent thalassemia or iron deficiency, but in other cases the reason for the normal MCV is obscure. Patients with neurologic signs or symptoms that suggest possible vitamin B_{12} deficiency should be thoroughly evaluated for the possibility of that deficiency despite a normal MCV and the absence of anemia. The peripheral blood smear is usually strikingly abnormal, with anisocytosis and poikilocytosis. A characteristic finding is the macro-ovalocyte, but numerous other abnormal shapes are usually seen. Because of the strikingly abnormal red blood cell morphology, it is often mistakenly assumed that the anemia is hemolytic. The neutrophils are hypersegmented. Typical features include a mean lobe count greater than four or the finding of six-lobed neutrophils. The reticulocyte count is reduced. Because vitamin B_{12} deficiency affects all hematopoietic cell lines, in severe cases the white blood cell count and platelet count are reduced, and pancytopenia is present.

Bone marrow morphology is characteristically abnormal. Marked erythroid hyperplasia is present as a response to defective red blood cell production (ineffective erythropoiesis). Characteristic megaloblastic changes in the erythroid series include abnormally large cell size and asynchronous maturation of the nucleus and cytoplasm—ie, cytoplasmic maturation continues while impaired DNA synthesis causes retarded nuclear development. In the myeloid series, giant metamyelocytes are characteristically seen.

Other laboratory abnormalities include elevated serum LDH and a modest increase in indirect bilirubin. These two findings are a reflection of intramedullary destruction of developing abnormal erythroid cells.

The diagnosis of vitamin B_{12} deficiency is made by finding an abnormally low vitamin B_{12} serum level. Whereas the normal vitamin B_{12} level is 150–350 pg/mL, most patients with overt vitamin B_{12} deficiency will have serum levels less than 100 pg/mL. The Schilling test is used to document the decreased absorption of oral vitamin B_{12} characteristic of pernicious anemia. Initially, a large intramuscular dose of vitamin B_{12} is given to saturate plasma transport proteins. Radiolabeled vitamin B_{12} is given orally, and a 24-hour urine collection is performed to determine how much vitamin B_{12} is absorbed and subsequently excreted. Normally, more than 7% of an administered dose is present in the urine; most patients with impaired absorption will have less than 3% of the dose present in the urine. The second stage of the Schilling test is to administer radiolabeled vitamin B_{12} together with intrinsic factor. If pernicious anemia (a lack of intrinsic factor) is the case of vitamin B_{12} deficiency, the combined use of vitamin B_{12} and intrinsic factor should correct the abnormally low absorption. However, the full-blown megaloblastic state causes abnormalities in intestinal epithelium that may lead to generalized malabsorption. In these cases, the second stage of the Schilling test will remain abnormal until the intestinal mucosal defect is first corrected by vitamin B_{12} replacement (in approximately 2 months). If the deficiency is caused by bacterial overgrowth in a blind loop, a course of antibiotics will reverse the abnormal second stage of the Schilling test.

Differential Diagnosis

Vitamin B_{12} deficiency should be differentiated from folic acid deficiency, the other common cause of megaloblastic anemia, in which red blood cell folate is low while vitamin B_{12} levels are normal. The distinction between vitamin B_{12} deficiency and myelodysplasia (the other common cause of macrocytic anemia with abnormal morphology) is based on the characteristic morphology and the low vitamin B_{12} level.

It should be emphasized that any neurologic signs or symptoms suggestive of vitamin B_{12} deficiency should be evaluated for that disorder even in the absence of anemia or macrocytosis.

Treatment

Patients with pernicious anemia cannot absorb oral vitamin B_{12} and require parenteral therapy. Intramuscular injections of 200 µg are adequate for each dose. Replacement is usually given daily for the first week, weekly for the first month, and then monthly for life. It should be stressed that pernicious anemia is a lifelong disorder and that if patients discontinue their monthly therapy, the vitamin deficiency will recur.

Patients respond to therapy with an immediate improvement in their sense of well-being. Hypokalemia may complicate the first several days of therapy, particularly if the anemia is severe. A brisk reticulocytosis occurs in 5–7 days, and the hematologic picture normalizes in 2 months. Central nervous system symptoms and signs are reversible if they are of relatively short duration (less than 6 months), but they may be permanent if treatment is not initiated promptly.

Lindenbaum J et al: Neuropsychiatric disorders caused by cobalamin deficiency in the absence of anemia or macrocytosis. N Engl J Med 1988;318:1720. (Documents the existence of this phenomenon.)
Stabler SP et al: Clinical spectrum and diagnosis of cobalamin deficiency. Blood 1990;76:871.

FOLIC ACID DEFICIENCY

Essentials of Diagnosis
- Macrocytic anemia.
- Macro-ovalocytes and hypersegmented neutrophils on peripheral blood smear.

- Normal serum vitamin B_{12} levels.
- Reduced folate levels in red blood cells or serum.

General Considerations

Folic acid is the term commonly used for pteroylmonoglutamic acid. In its reduced form of tetrahydrofolate, it serves as an important mediator of many reactions involving one-carbon transfers. Important reactions include the conversion of homocysteine to methionine and of deoxyuridylate to thymidylate, an important step in DNA synthesis.

Folic acid is present in most fruits and vegetables (especially citrus fruits and green leafy vegetables) and daily requirements of 50–100 µg/d are usually met in the diet. Total body stores of folate are approximately 5000 µg, enough to supply requirements for 2–3 months.

By far the most common cause of folate deficiency is inadequate dietary intake (Table 13–7). Alcoholics, anorectic patients, elderly persons who do not eat fresh fruits and vegetables, and persons who overcook their food are candidates for folate deficiency. Reduced folate absorption is rarely seen, since absorption occurs from the entire gastrointestinal tract. However, drugs such as phenytoin or sulfasalazine may interfere with folate absorption. Folic acid requirements are increased in pregnancy, hemolytic anemia, and exfoliative skin disease, and in these cases the increased requirements (five to ten times normal) may not be met by a normal diet. Patients with increased folate requirements should receive supplementation with 1 mg/d of folic acid.

Clinical Findings

A. Symptoms and Signs: The clinical features are similar to those of vitamin B_{12} deficiency, with megaloblastic anemia and megaloblastic changes in mucosa. However, there are none of the neurologic abnormalities associated with vitamin B_{12} deficiency.

B. Laboratory Findings: The megaloblastic anemia is identical to that resulting from vitamin B_{12} deficiency (see above). However, the serum vitamin B_{12} level is normal. In contrast, the serum folic acid level is low, usually less than 3 ng/mL. The red blood cell folate level is more reliable and has replaced serum folate as the appropriate test. A red blood cell

Table 13–7. Causes of folate deficiency.

Dietary deficiency
Decreased absorption
   Tropical sprue
   Drugs: Phenytoin, sulfasalazine
Increased requirement
   Chronic hemolytic anemia
   Pregnancy
   Exfoliative skin disease
Loss: Dialysis
Inhibition of reduction to active form
   Methotrexate

folate level of less than 150 ng/mL is diagnostic of folate deficiency.

Differential Diagnosis

The megaloblastic anemia of folate deficiency should be differentiated from vitamin B_{12} deficiency by the finding of a normal vitamin B_{12} level and a reduced serum folate or red blood cell folate level. Alcoholics, who often have folate deficiency, may also have anemia of liver disease. This latter macrocytic anemia does not cause megaloblastic morphologic changes but rather produces target cells in the peripheral blood. Patients with HIV-related illnesses being treated with zidovudine frequently develop macrocytosis but do not manifest typical megaloblastic morphology. Hypothyroidism is also associated with mild macrocytosis.

Treatment

Folic acid deficiency is treated with folic acid, 1 mg/d orally. The response is similar to that seen in the treatment of vitamin B_{12} deficiency, with rapid improvement and a sense of well-being, reticulocytosis in 5–7 days, and total correction of hematologic abnormalities within 2 months. Large doses of folic acid may produce hematologic responses in cases of vitamin B_{12} deficiency but will allow neurologic damage to progress.

PURE RED CELL APLASIA

Adult acquired pure red cell aplasia is extremely rare. It appears to be an autoimmune disease in which an IgG antibody specifically attacks erythroid precursors. A congenital form (Diamond-Blackfan syndrome) has been identified. In adults, the disease is usually idiopathic. However, cases have been seen in association with systemic lupus erythematosus, chronic lymphocytic leukemia, lymphomas, or thymoma. Some drugs (phenytoin, chloramphenicol) may cause red cell aplasia. Transient episodes of red cell aplasia are probably common in response to viral infections, especially parvovirus infections, but also in viral hepatitis. However, these acute episodes will go unrecognized unless the patient has a chronic hemolytic disorder, in which case the hematocrit may fall precipitously.

Clinically, the only signs are those of anemia, unless the patient has an associated autoimmune or lymphoproliferative disorder. The anemia is often severe and is normochromic. Reticulocytes are very low or absent. Red blood cell morphology is normal, and the myeloid and platelet lines are unaffected. The bone marrow is normocellular. All elements present are normal, but erythroid precursors are markedly reduced or absent. In some cases, chest imaging studies will reveal a thymoma.

The disorder should be distinguished from aplastic

anemia (in which the marrow was generally hypocellular and other cell lines are affected) and from myelodysplasia. This latter disorder is recognized by the presence of morphologic abnormalities that should not be present in pure red cell aplasia.

If the thymoma is present, resection results in amelioration of anemia in some instances. In cases associated with autoimmune disorders, immunosuppressive treatment with cyclophosphamide or prednisone (or both) is indicated. Idiopathic cases have usually responded best to cyclosphosphamide treatment. High-dose intravenous immune globulin has produced excellent responses in a small number of cases. The duration of response remains to be determined, and more experience is needed before this treatment can be generally recommended. Antithymocyte globulin, useful in aplastic anemia, has also been reported to be of value. Possible offending drugs should be stopped.

McGuire WA et al: Treatment of antibody-mediated pure red cell aplasia with high-dose intravenous gammaglobulin. N Engl J Med 1987;317:1004.

HEMOLYTIC ANEMIAS

The hemolytic anemias are a group of disorders in which red blood cell survival is reduced, either episodically or continuously. The bone marrow has the ability to increase erythroid production up to eightfold in response to reduced red cell survival, so anemia will be present only when the ability of the bone marrow to compensate is outstripped. This will occur when red cell survival is extremely short or when the ability of the bone marrow to compensate is impaired for some second reason.

Since red blood cell survival is normally 120 days, in the absence of red cell production the hematocrit will fall at the rate of approximately 1/100 of the hematocrit per day, which translates to a decrease in the hematocrit reading of approximately 3% per week. For example, a fall of hematocrit from 45% to 36% over 3 weeks' time need not indicate hemolysis, since this rate of fall would result simply from cessation of red blood cell production. If the hematocrit is falling at a faster rate than that due to decreased production, blood loss or hemolysis is the cause.

Reticulocytosis is an important clue to the presence of hemolysis, since in most hemolytic disorders the bone marrow will respond with increased red blood cell production. However, hemolysis can be present without reticulocytosis when a second disorder (infection, folate deficiency) is superimposed on hemolysis; in these circumstances, the hematocrit will fall rapidly. However, reticulocytosis also occurs during recovery from hypoproliferative anemia or bleeding. Hemolysis is correctly diagnosed (when bleeding is excluded) when the hematocrit is either falling or stable despite reticulocytosis.

Hemolytic disorders are generally classified according to whether the defect is intrinsic to the red cell or due to some external factor (Table 13–8). Intrinsic defects have been described in all components of the red blood cell, including the membrane, glycolytic and other enzymes, and hemoglobin. Most of these disorders are hereditary. The vast majority of hemolytic anemias due to external factors are the immune hemolytic anemias.

Certain laboratory features are common to all the hemolytic anemias. Haptoglobin, a normal plasma protein that binds and clears hemoglobin released into plasma, may be depressed in hemolytic disorders. However, haptoglobin levels are influenced by many factors and, by themselves, are not a reliable indicator of hemolysis. When intravascular hemolysis occurs, transient hemoglobinemia occurs. Hemoglobin is filtered through the glomerulus and usually reabsorbed by tubular cells. Hemoglobinuria will be present only when the capacity for reabsorption of hemoglobin by these cells is exceeded. In the absence of hemoglobinuria, evidence for prior intravascular hemolysis is the presence of hemosiderin in shed renal tubular cells (positive urine hemosiderin). With severe intravascular hemolysis, hemoglobinemia and methemalbuminemia may be present. Hemolysis increases the indirect bilirubin, and the total bilirubin may rise to as high as 4 mg/dL. Bilirubin levels higher than this indicate some degree of hepatic dysfunction. Serum LDH levels are strikingly elevated in cases of microangiopathic hemolysis (thrombotic thrombocytopenic purpura, hemolytic-uremic syndrome) and may be elevated in other hemolytic anemias. Iron levels are usually not affected by hemolysis, since the iron from sequestered red cells is recycled through the reticuloendothelial system. Only causes of intravascular hemolysis will lead to iron deficiency due to hemoglobinemia.

Table 13–8. Classification of hemolytic anemias.

Intrinsic
    Membrane defects: Hereditary spherocytosis, hereditary elliptocytosis, paroxysmal nocturnal hemoglobinuria
    Glycolytic defects: Pyruvate kinase deficiency, severe hypophosphatemia
    Oxidation vulnerability: G6PD deficiency, methemoglobinemia
    Hemoglobinopathies: Sickle syndromes, unstable hemoglobins, methemoglobinemia

Extrinsic
    Immune: Autoimmune, lymphoproliferative disease, drug toxicity
    Microangiopathic: Thrombotic thrombocytopenic purpura, hemolytic-uremic syndrome, disseminated intravascular coagulation, valve hemolysis, metastatic adenocarcinoma, vasculitis
    Infection: *Plasmodium, Clostridium, Borrelia*
    Hypersplenism
    Burns

HEREDITARY SPHEROCYTOSIS

Essentials of Diagnosis
- Positive family history.
- Splenomegaly.
- Spherocytes and increased reticulocytes on peripheral blood smear.
- Negative Coombs test.

General Considerations
Hereditary spherocytosis is a disorder of the red blood cell membrane, leading to chronic hemolytic anemia. Normally, the red blood cell is a biconcave disk with a diameter of 7–8 μm. The red blood cells must be both strong and deformable—strong to withstand the stress of circulating for 120 days and deformable so as to pass through capillaries 3 μm in diameter and splenic fenestrations in the cords of the red pulp of approximately 2 μm. The red blood cell skeleton, made up primarily of the proteins spectrin and actin, gives the red cells these characteristics of strength and deformability.

The membrane defect in hereditary spherocytosis has not been defined but is most likely an abnormality in spectrin, the protein providing most of the scaffolding for the red blood cell membranes. The result is a decrease in surface-to-volume ratio that results in a spherical shape of the cell. These spherical cells are less deformable and unable to pass through 2-μm fenestrations in the splenic red pulp. Hemolysis takes place because of trapping of red blood cells within the spleen.

Clinical Findings
A. Symptoms and Signs: Hereditary spherocytosis is an autosomal dominant disease of variable severity. It is often diagnosed during childhood, but milder cases may be discovered incidentally late in adult life. Anemia may or may not be present, since the bone marrow may be able to compensate for shortened red cell survival. Severe anemia (aplastic crisis) may occur when bone marrow compensation is impaired by infection or folate deficiency. Chronic hemolysis may cause jaundice and pigment gallstones, leading to attacks of cholecystitis. Examination may reveal icterus and a palpable spleen.

B. Laboratory Findings: The anemia is of variable severity, and the hematocrit may be normal. Reticulocytosis is always present. The peripheral blood smear shows the presence of spherocytes, small cells that have lost their central pallor. Spherocytes usually make up only a small percentage of red blood cells on the peripheral smear. Hereditary spherocytosis is the only important disorder associated with increased MCHC, often greater than 36 g/dL. As with other hemolytic disorders, there may be an increase in indirect bilirubin. The Coombs test is negative.

The presence of spherocytes may be confirmed by the osmotic fragility test. Spherocytes are red cells that have lost some membrane surface and are abnormally vulnerable to swelling induced by hypotonic media. Increased osmotic fragility merely reflects the presence of spherocytes and does not distinguish hereditary spherocytosis from other spherocytic hemolytic disorders such as autoimmune hemolytic anemia.

Treatment
These patients should receive uninterrupted supplementation with folic acid, 1 mg/d. The treatment of choice is splenectomy, which will not correct the membrane defect or correct the spherocytosis but will eliminate the site of hemolysis. In very mild cases discovered late in adult life, splenectomy may not be necessary.

Friedman EW: Hereditary spherocytosis in the elderly. Am J Med 1988;84:513.

HEREDITARY ELLIPTOCYTOSIS

Hereditary elliptocytosis is a congenital disorder of the red blood cell membrane and probably is due to abnormalities in spectrin tetramer formation. The disorder is autosomal dominant and of variable severity. In the most common form of hereditary elliptocytosis, the mild hemolytic disorder is well compensated, and there is little or no anemia. However, more severe varieties do produce anemia, splenomegaly, and pigment gallstones.

In the common mild variety, the hallmark of the disorder is the elliptical shape of the majority of red blood cells on peripheral blood smear. Reticulocytosis may be present. In the rare severe varieties of the disorder (hereditary pyropoikilocytosis), the peripheral blood smear is extremely bizarre; and in addition to elliptocytes, microspherocytes and a variety of unusually shaped red cells are present.

No treatment is usually indicated. Severe variants are treated with splenectomy and folate supplementation.

PAROXYSMAL NOCTURNAL HEMOGLOBINURIA

Paroxysmal nocturnal hemoglobinuria is an acquired clonal stem cell disorder that results in abnormal sensitivity of the red blood cell membrane to lysis by complement. The defect involves both increased binding of C3b and increased vulnerability to lysis by complement, and is expressed as a deficiency in proteins normally linked to the cell by phosphoinositol. Paroxysmal nocturnal hemoglobinuria is a very rare disorder and should be suspected in confusing cases of hemolytic anemia.

The best screening test for paroxysmal nocturnal hemoglobinuria is the sucrose hemolysis test. The diagnosis can be confirmed by Ham's (acidified serum) test.

Clinical Findings

A. Symptoms and Signs: The anemia is of variable severity and may be severe. Classically, patients report episodic hemoglobinuria resulting in reddish brown urine. Hemoglobinuria may be present in the first morning urine, since the mild respiratory acidosis of sleep leads to enhanced complement activity. In addition to anemia, these patients are prone to thrombosis, especially mesenteric and hepatic vein thromboses. The reason for thrombus formation is unclear but may be related to platelet activation by complement. As this is a stem cell disorder, paroxysmal nocturnal hemoglobinuria may progress either to aplastic anemia or to acute myelogenous leukemia.

B. Laboratory Findings: Anemia is of variable severity, and reticulocytosis may or may not be present. Abnormalities on the blood smear are nondiagnostic and may include macro-ovalocytes. As with other hemolytic disorders, haptoglobin may be decreased or absent. Since the episodic hemolysis in paroxysmal nocturnal hemoglobinuria is intravascular, the finding of urine hemosiderin is a useful test. Serum LDH is characteristically elevated. Iron deficiency is commonly present and is related to chronic iron loss from hemoglobinuria, since hemolysis is primarily intravascular.

The white blood cell count and platelet count may be decreased. A decreased leukocyte alkaline phosphatase—evidence for qualitative abnormality in the myeloid series—is good evidence for paroxysmal nocturnal hemoglobinuria. Bone marrow morphology is variable and may show either hypoplasia or erythroid hyperplasia.

Research laboratories may be helpful in confirming the disorder by functional and antigenic assays.

Treatment

Iron replacement is often indicated for treatment of iron deficiency. This may improve the anemia but may also cause a transient increase in hemolysis. For unclear reasons, prednisone is effective in decreasing hemolysis, and some patients can be managed effectively with alternate-day steroids. In severe cases, allogeneic bone marrow transplantation has been used to correct the disorder.

Ware RE, Hall SE, Rosse WF: Paroxysmal nocturnal hemoglobinuria with onset in childhood and adolescence. N Engl J Med 1991;325:991.

PYRUVATE KINASE DEFICIENCY

The red blood cell obtains 90% of its energy from anaerobic glycolysis. Defects in glycolytic enzymes produce a chronic hemolytic anemia because of depletion of ATP. Severe hypophosphatemia may result in hemolysis for the same reason.

Pyruvate kinase deficiency is a very rare autosomal recessive disorder that causes chronic hemolytic anemia, usually with onset in childhood. In addition to the anemia, splenomegaly and pigment gallstones may be present. The red blood cell smear is normal, and the diagnosis is made by specific enzyme assays available only in specialized laboratories. Splenectomy is the treatment of choice.

Valentine WN, Tanaka KR, Paglia DE: Hemolytic anemias and erythrocyte enzymopathies. Ann Intern Med 1985;103:245. (Review of a complex topic.)

GLUCOSE-6-PHOSPHATE DEHYDROGENASE DEFICIENCY

Essentials of Diagnosis

- X-linked recessive disorder seen commonly in American black men.
- Episodic hemolysis in response to oxidant drugs or infection.
- Minimally abnormal peripheral blood smear.
- Reduced levels of G6PD between hemolytic episodes.

General Considerations

Glucose-6-phosphate dehydrogenase (G6PD) deficiency is a hereditary enzyme defect that causes episodic hemolytic anemia because of decreased ability of red blood cells to deal with oxidative stresses. The hexose monophosphate shunt is not an important source of energy generation in red cells but is important in generating reduced glutathione, which protects hemoglobin from oxidative denaturation. The first step in this pathway is the generation of NADPH by the action of G6PD on glucose 6-phosphate. NADPH serves as a cofactor for glutathione reductase in generating reduced glutathione, which detoxifies hydrogen peroxide. In the absence of reduced glutathione, hemoglobin may become oxidized. Oxidized hemoglobin denatures and forms precipitates called Heinz bodies. These Heinz bodies cause membrane damage, which leads to removal of these cells by the spleen.

Numerous types of G6PD enzymes have been described. The normal type found in Caucasians is designated G6PD-B. Most American blacks have G6PD-A, which is normal in function. Ten to 15 percent of American blacks have the variant G6PD designated A−, in which there is only 15% of normal enzyme activity, and enzyme activity declines rapidly as the red blood cell ages past 40 days, a fact that explains many of the clinical findings in this disorder. Many other G6PD variants have been described, including some Mediterranean variants with extremely low enzyme activity.

Clinical Findings

G6PD deficiency is an X-linked recessive disorder affecting 10–15% of American black males. Female carriers are rarely affected—only when an unusually high percentage of cells producing the normal enzyme are inactivated.

A. Symptoms and Signs: Patients are usually healthy, without chronic hemolytic anemia or splenomegaly. Hemolysis occurs as a result of oxidative stress on the red blood cells, generated either by infection or exposure to certain drugs. Common drugs initiating hemolysis include primaquine, quinidine, quinine, sulfonamides, and nitrofurantoin. When hemolysis occurs, the patient may become jaundiced and have dark urine. Even with continuous use of the offending drug, the hemolytic episode is self-limited because older red blood cells (with low enzyme activity) are removed and replaced with a population of young red blood cells with adequate functional levels of G6PD.

Severe G6PD deficiency (as in Mediterranean variants) may produce a chronic hemolytic anemia, and hemolytic crises may be severe or even fatal.

B. Laboratory Findings: Between hemolytic episodes, the blood is normal. During episodes of hemolysis, there is reticulocytosis and increased serum indirect bilirubin. The red blood cell smear is not diagnostic but may reveal a small number of "bite" cells—cells that appear to have had a bite taken out of their periphery. This in fact indicates pitting of hemoglobin aggregates by the spleen. Heinz bodies may be demonstrated by staining a peripheral blood smear with crystal violet. (They are not visible on the usual Wright-stained blood smear.) Specific enzyme assays for G6PD may reveal a low level. Results for G6PD assays may be misleading if they are performed shortly after a hemolytic episode when the enzyme-deficient cohort of cells has been removed and replaced with a young cohort with nearly normal enzyme activity. In these cases, the enzyme assays should be repeated weeks after hemolysis has resolved. In severe cases of G6PD deficiency, enzyme levels are always low.

Treatment

No treatment is necessary except to avoid known oxidant drugs.

Valentine WM, Tanaka KR, Paglia DE: Hemolytic anemias and erythrocyte enzymopathies. Ann Intern Med 1985;103:245.

SICKLE CELL ANEMIA & RELATED SYNDROMES

Essentials of Diagnosis

- Irreversibly sickled cells on peripheral blood smear.
- Positive family history and lifelong history of hemolytic anemia.
- Recurrent painful episodes.
- Hemoglobin S is the major hemoglobin seen on electrophoresis.

General Considerations

Sickle cell anemia is an autosomal recessive disorder in which an abnormal hemoglobin (hemoglobinopathy) leads to chronic hemolytic anemia with a variety of severe clinical consequences. The disorder is a classic example of disease caused by a point mutation in DNA. A single DNA base change leads to an amino acid substitution of valine for glutamine in the sixth position on the β-globin chain. The abnormal beta chain is designated β^s and the tetramer of $\alpha_2\beta^s_2$ is designated hemoglobin S.

When in the deoxy form, hemoglobin S forms polymers that damage the red blood cell membrane. Both polymer formation and early membrane damage are reversible. However, red blood cells that have undergone repeated sickling are damaged beyond repair and become irreversibly sickled cells.

The rate of sickling is influenced by a number of factors, most importantly by the concentration of hemoglobin S in the individual red blood cell. Red cell dehydration makes the cell quite vulnerable to sickling. Sickling is also strongly influenced by the presence of other hemoglobins within the cell. Hemoglobin F cannot participate in polymer formation, and its presence markedly retards sickling. Other factors that increase sickling are those which lead to formation of deoxyhemoglobin S, eg, acidosis and hypoxemia, either systemic or locally in tissues.

Prenatal diagnosis is now available for couples at risk of producing a child with sickle cell anemia. DNA from fetal cells can be directly examined, and the presence of the sickle cell mutation can be accurately and definitively diagnosed. Genetic counseling should be made available to such couples.

Clinical Findings

A. Symptoms and Signs: The hemoglobin S gene is carried in 8% of American blacks, and one birth out of 400 in American blacks will produce a child with sickle cell anemia. The disorder has its onset during the first year of life, when hemoglobin F levels fall as a signal (of unknown nature) is sent to the bone marrow to switch from γ-globin to β-globin production.

Chronic hemolytic anemia produces jaundice, pigment gallstones, splenomegaly, and poorly healing ulcers over the lower tibia. The chronic anemia may become life-threatening when severe anemia is produced by hemolytic or aplastic crises. Aplastic crises occur when the ability of the bone marrow to compensate is reduced by viral or other infection or by folate deficiency. Hemolytic crises may be related to splenic sequestration of sickled cells (primarily in childhood, before the spleen has been infarcted) or with coexistent disorders such as G6PD deficiency.

Acute painful episodes due to acute vaso-occlusion may occur spontaneously or be provoked by infection, dehydration, or hypoxia. Clusters of sickled red cells occlude the microvasculature of the organs involved. These episodes last hours to days and produce acute pain and low-grade fever. Common sites of acute painful episodes include the bones (especially the back and long bones) and the chest. Acute vaso-occlusion may also cause strokes and priapism. Vaso-occlusive episodes are not associated with increased hemolysis.

Repeated episodes of vascular occlusion affect a large number of organs, especially the heart and liver. Ischemic necrosis of bone occurs, rendering the bone susceptible to osteomyelitis due to staphylococci or (less commonly) salmonellae. In adult life, the spleen is infarcted. Infarction of the papillae of the renal medulla causes renal tubular concentrating defects and gross hematuria. Retinopathy is often present and may lead to blindness.

These patients are prone to delayed puberty and may rarely have an increased incidence of infection. Infections are related to hyposplenism as well as to defects in the alternative pathway of complement.

On examination, patients are often chronically ill and jaundiced. There is hepatomegaly, but the spleen is not palpable in adult life. The heart is enlarged, with a hyperdynamic precordium and systolic murmurs. Nonhealing ulcers of the lower leg and retinopathy may be present.

Sickle cell anemia becomes a chronic multisystem disease, with death from organ failure commonly occurring between ages 20 and 40.

B. Laboratory Findings: Chronic hemolytic anemia is present. The hematocrit is usually 20–30%. The peripheral blood smear is characteristically abnormal, with irreversibly sickled cells comprising 5–50% of red cells. Other findings include reticulocytosis (10–25%), nucleated red blood cells,

and hallmarks of hyposplenism such as Howell-Jolly bodies and target cells. The white blood cell count is characteristically elevated to 12,000–15,000/μL, and thrombocytosis may occur. Indirect bilirubin levels are high and haptoglobin is absent.

Most clinical laboratories offer a screening test for sickle cell hemoglobin, and the diagnosis of sickle cell anemia is then confirmed by hemoglobin electrophoresis (Table 13–9). Hemoglobin S has an abnormal migration pattern on electrophoresis and will usually comprise 85–98% of hemoglobin. In homozygous S disease, no hemoglobin A will be present. Hemoglobin F levels are variably increased, and high hemoglobin F levels are associated with a more benign clinical course.

Treatment

No specific treatment is available for the primary disease. However, both longevity and quality of life may be improved by comprehensive medical management by a concerned physician. Patients are maintained chronically on folic acid supplementation and should not routinely be given transfusions. Transfusions are indicated for aplastic or hemolytic crises and during the third trimester of pregnancy.

When acute painful episodes occur, precipitating factors should be identified and infections treated if present. The patient should be kept well hydrated, and oxygen should be given if the patient is hypoxic. Otherwise, treatment is supportive (hydration and analgesics).

Acute vaso-occlusive crises can be treated with exchange transfusion. Exchange transfusions are primarily indicated for the treatment of intractable crises, priapism, and stroke and as a preventive measure for patients undergoing general anesthesia. Hypertransfusion should be avoided because of the potential for further sickling by oxygen steal by the transfused red cells from those that are sickled.

Cytotoxic agents such as hydroxyurea have been shown to increase hemoglobin F levels (by stimulating erythropoiesis in more primitive erythroid precursors). Clinical trials are being conducted to evaluate whether this will ameliorate clinical disease. Pending results of these studies, the use of hydroxyurea cannot be recommended.

Table 13–9. Hemoglobin distribution in sickle cell syndromes.

Genotype	Diagnosis	Hgb A	Hgb S₃	Hgb A₂	Hgb F
AA	Normal	97–99%	0	1–2%	< 1%
AS	Sickle trait	60%	40%	1–2%	< 1%
SS	Sickle cell anemia	0	85–98%	1–3%	5–15%
SB⁰ thal	Sickle B thalassemia	0	70–80%	3–5%	10–20%
SB⁺ thal	Sickle B thalassemia	10–20%	60–75%	3–5%	10–20%
AS, α thalassemia	Sickle trait	70–75%	25–30%	1–2%	< 1%

Francis RB, Johnson CS: Vascular occlusion in sickle cell disease: Current concepts and unanswered questions. Blood 1991;77:1405. (Good review of the controversies.)

Goldberg MA et al: Treatment of sickle cell anemia with hydroxyurea and erythropoietin. N Engl J Med 1990; 323:366.

SICKLE CELL TRAIT

Patients with the heterozygous genotype (AS) have sickle cell trait. These persons are clinically normal and have acute painful episodes only under extreme conditions such as vigorous exertion at high altitudes (or in unpressurized aircraft). The patients are hematologically normal, with no anemia and normal red blood cells on peripheral blood smear. They may, however, have a defect in renal tubular function, causing an inability to concentrate the urine, and experience episodes of gross hematuria. A screening test for sickle hemoglobin will be positive, and hemoglobin electrophoresis will reveal that approximately 40% of hemoglobin is hemoglobin S (Table 13–9).

No treatment is necessary. These patients should be considered normal in all respects.

SICKLE THALASSEMIA

Patients with homozygous sickle cell anemia and alpha thalassemia have a somewhat milder form of hemolysis because of a slower rate of sickling related to reduced hemoglobin concentration (MCHC) within the red blood cell.

Patients who are double heterozygotes for sickle cell anemia and beta thalassemia are clinically affected with sickle cell syndromes. Sickle β^0 thalassemia is clinically very similar to homozygous SS disease. Vaso-occlusive crises may be somewhat less severe, and the spleen is usually not infarcted. Hematologically, the MCV is usually low-in contrast to the normal MCV of sickle cell anemia—and the smear usually reveals fewer irreversibly sickled cells. Hemoglobin electrophoresis (Table 13–9) reveals no hemoglobin A but will show an increase in hemoglobin A_2 which is not present in sickle cell anemia.

Sickle β^+ thalassemia is a milder disorder than homozygous SS disease, with fewer crises. The spleen is usually palpable. The hemolytic anemia is less severe, and the hematocrit is usually 30–38%, with reticulocytes of 5–10%. Hemoglobin electrophoresis shows the presence of some hemoglobin A.

HEMOGLOBIN C DISORDERS

Hemoglobin C is formed by a single amino acid substitution at the same site of substitution as in sickled hemoglobin but with lysine instead of valine substituted for glutamine at the β_6 position. Hemoglobin C is nonsickling but may participate in polymer formation in association with hemoglobin S. Homozygous hemoglobin C disease produces a mild hemolytic anemia with splenomegaly, mild jaundice, and pigment gallstones. The peripheral blood smear shows numerous target cells as well as occasional cells with rectangular crystals of hemoglobin C. Persons heterozygous for hemoglobin C are clinically normal.

Patients with hemoglobin SC disease are double heterozygotes for beta S and beta C. These patients, like those with sickle β^+ thalassemia, have a milder hemolytic anemia and milder clinical course than those with homozygous SS disease. There are fewer vaso-occlusive events, and the spleen remains palpable in adult life. However, persons with hemoglobin SC disease have more retinopathy and more ischemic necrosis of bone than those with SS disease. The hematocrit is usually 30–38%, with 5–10% reticulocytes and few irreversibly sickled cells on the blood smear. Target cells are more numerous than in SS disease. Hemoglobin electrophoresis will show approximately 50% hemoglobin C, 50% hemoglobin S, and no increase in hemoglobin F levels.

UNSTABLE HEMOGLOBINS

Unstable hemoglobins are prone to oxidative denaturation even in the presence of a normal G6PD system. The disorder is autosomal dominant and of variable severity. Most patients have a mild chronic hemolytic anemia with splenomegaly, mild jaundice, and pigment gallstones. Less severely affected patients are not anemic except under conditions of oxidative stress.

The diagnosis is made by the finding of Heinz bodies and a normal G6PD level. Hemoglobin electrophoresis is usually normal, since these hemoglobins characteristically do not have a change in their migration pattern. These hemoglobins can be shown to precipitate in isopropanol. Usually no treatment is necessary. Patients with chronic hemolytic anemia should receive folate supplementation and avoid known oxidative drugs. In rare severe cases, splenectomy may be required.

AUTOIMMUNE HEMOLYTIC ANEMIA

Essentials of Diagnosis

- Acquired anemia caused by IgG autoantibody.
- Spherocytes and reticulocytosis on peripheral blood smear.
- Positive Coombs test.

General Considerations

Autoimmune hemolytic anemia is an acquired disorder in which an IgG autoantibody is formed that binds to the red blood cell membrane. The antibody is most commonly directed against a basic component of the Rh system and is present on virtually all human red blood cells. When IgG antibodies coat the red blood cell, the Fc portion of the antibody is recognized by macrophages (with Fc receptor) present in the spleen and other portions of the reticuloendothelial system. The interaction between splenic macrophage and the antibody-coated red blood cell results in removal of red blood cell membrane and the formation of a spherocyte because of the decrease in surface-to-volume ratio of the red blood cell. These spherocytic cells have decreased deformability and become trapped in the red pulp of the spleen because of their inability to squeeze through the 2-μm fenestrations. When large amounts of IgG are present on red blood cells, complement may be fixed. Direct lysis of cells is rare, but the presence of C3b on the surface of red blood cells allows Kupffer cells in the liver to participate in the hemolytic process because of the presence of C3b receptors on Kupffer cells.

Approximately half of all cases of autoimmune hemolytic anemia are idiopathic. The disorder may also be seen in association with systemic lupus erythematosus, chronic lymphocytic leukemia, or diffuse lymphomas. It must be distinguished from drug-induced hemolytic anemia. Methyldopa commonly stimulates the production of an autoantibody with the same specificity as that in idiopathic autoimmune hemolytic anemia. Other drugs (penicillin, quinidine) become associated with the red blood cell membrane, and the antibody is directed against the membrane-drug complex.

The Coombs antiglobulin test forms the basis for diagnosis of these immune hemolytic disorders. The Coombs reagent is a rabbit IgM antibody raised against human IgG or human complement. The direct Coombs test is performed by mixing the patient's red blood cells with the Coombs reagent and looking for agglutination, which indicates the presence of antibody on the red blood cell surface. The indirect Coombs test is performed by mixing the patient's serum with a panel of type O red blood cells. After incubation of the test serum and panel red blood cells, the Coombs reagent is added. Agglutination in this system indicates the presence of free antibody in the patient's serum. Because the traditional Coombs test relies on visible agglutination as an end point, the test is not very sensitive and will not detect immune hemolytic anemias in which only a small amount of IgG is present on red blood cells. More sensitive tests (micro-Coombs) are now available.

Clinical Findings

A. Symptoms and Signs: Autoimmune hemolytic anemia typically produces an anemia of rapid onset that may be life-threatening in severity. Patients complain of fatigue and may present with angina or congestive heart failure. On examination, jaundice and splenomegaly are usually present. If the patient has an underlying disorder such as systemic lupus erythematosus or chronic lymphocytic leukemia, features of these diseases may be present.

B. Laboratory Findings: The anemia is of variable severity but may be severe, with hematocrit of less than 10%. Reticulocytosis is usually present, and spherocytes are seen on the peripheral blood smear. In cases of severe hemolysis, the stressed bone marrow may also release nucleated red blood cells. As with other hemolytic disorders, indirect bilirubin is increased. Approximately 10% of patients with autoimmune hemolytic anemia have coincident immune thrombocytopenia (Evans's syndrome).

The direct Coombs test is positive, and the indirect Coombs test may or may not be positive. A positive indirect Coombs test indicates the presence of a large amount of autoantibody that has saturated binding sites in the red blood cell and consequently appears in the serum. A patient with acquired spherocytic hemolytic anemia that may be of the autoimmune variety who has a negative Coombs test should be tested with a micro-Coombs test (which is necessary to make the diagnosis in approximately 10% of cases). Because the patient's serum usually contains the autoantibody, it may be difficult to obtain a compatible crossmatch with donor's cells. Suitable donors may be selected by special laboratory methods.

Treatment

Initial treatment is with prednisone, 1–2 mg/kg/d in divided doses. If anemia is life-threatening, transfusions should be given cautiously. Most transfused blood will survive no more poorly than the patient's own red blood cells. However, because of difficulty in performing the cross-match, it is possible that incompatible blood will be given, and patients must be monitored carefully during transfusion. Decisions regarding transfusions should be made in consultation with a hematologist (or blood bank physician). If prednisone is ineffective or if the disease recurs on tapering the dose of prednisone to an acceptable chronic dose, splenectomy should be performed. Patients with autoimmune hemolytic anemia refractory to prednisone and splenectomy may be treated with a variety of immunosuppressive agents.

High-dose intravenous immune globulin (500 mg/kg daily for 1–4 days) may be highly effective in controlling hemolysis. However, the benefit is short-lived (1–3 weeks), and the drug is very expensive. Treatment with IGIV should be given only in emergency situations or when prednisone is contraindicated.

The long-term prognosis for patients with this disorder is good. Splenectomy is often successful in controlling or at least ameliorating the disorder.

Besa EC: Rapid transient reversal of anemia and long-term effects of maintenance intravenous immunoglobulin for autoimmune hemolytic anemia in patients with lymphoproliferative diseases. Am J Med 1988;84:691.

COLD AGGLUTININ DISEASE

Essentials of Diagnosis
- Increased reticulocytes and spherocytes on peripheral blood smear.
- Coombs test positive only for complement.
- Positive cold agglutinin test.

General Considerations
Cold agglutinin disease is an acquired hemolytic anemia due to an IgM autoantibody usually directed against the I antigen on red blood cells. These IgM autoantibodies characteristically will not react with cells at 37 °C but only at lower temperatures. Since the blood temperature (even in the most peripheral parts of the body) rarely goes lower than 20 °C, only antibodies active at higher temperatures than this will produce clinical effects. In the cooler parts of the body (fingers, nose, ears), agglutination of red blood cells by the IgM antibodies will transiently occur. Hemolysis results indirectly from attachment of IgM, which in the cooler parts of the circulation binds and fixes complement. When the red blood cell returns to a warmer temperature, the IgM antibody dissociates, leaving complement on the cell. Lysis of cells rarely occurs. Rather, C3b present on the red cells is recognized by Kupffer cells (which have receptors for C3b), and red blood cell sequestration ensues.

Most cases of chronic cold agglutinin disease are idiopathic. Others occur in association with Waldenström's macroglobulinemia, in which a monoclonal IgM paraprotein is produced. Acute postinfectious cold agglutinin disease occurs following mycoplasmal pneumonia or infectious mononucleosis (with antibody directed against antigen i rather than I).

Clinical Findings
A. Symptoms and Signs: In chronic cold agglutinin disease, symptoms related to red blood cell agglutination occur on exposure to cold, and patients may complain of mottled or numb fingers or toes. Hemolytic anemia is rarely severe, but episodic hemoglobinuria may occur on exposure to cold. The hemolytic anemia in acute postinfectious syndromes is rarely severe.

B. Laboratory Findings: Mild anemia is present with reticulocytosis and spherocytes. The direct Coombs test will be positive for complement only. Occasionally, a micro-Coombs test is necessary to reveal bound complement (low-titer cold agglutinin disease). Bedside cold agglutinin studies are often falsely positive or falsely negative and should be confirmed by the clinical laboratory.

Treatment
Treatment is largely symptomatic, based on avoiding exposure to cold. Patients with severe involvement may be treated with alkylating agents such as chlorambucil. Splenectomy is ineffective, since hemolysis takes place in the liver. Prednisone is ineffective in reducing Kupffer cell function.

High-dose intravenous immunoglobulin (2 g/kg) may be effective temporarily. Interferon may be of benefit for some patients.

MICROANGIOPATHIC HEMOLYTIC ANEMIAS

The microangiopathic hemolytic anemias are a group of disorders in which red blood cell fragmentation takes place. The anemia is intravascular, producing hemoglobinemia, hemoglobinuria, and, in severe cases, methemalbuminemia. The hallmark of the disorder is the finding of fragmented red blood cells (schistocytes, helmet cells) on the peripheral blood smear.

These fragmentation syndromes can be caused by a variety of disorders (Table 13–8). Thrombotic thrombocytopenic purpura is the most important of these and is discussed below. Clinical features of the fragmentation syndromes are variable and depend on the underlying disorder. Coagulopathy and thrombocytopenia are variably present.

Chronic microangiopathic hemolytic anemia (such as is present with a malfunctioning cardiac valve prosthesis) may cause iron deficiency anemia because of continuous low-grade hemoglobinuria.

HEMOLYSIS RELATED TO INFECTION

Clostridial infections may cause severe intravascular hemolysis, presumably because of the action of a clostridial toxin on the red blood cell membrane. Malaria may cause intravascular hemolysis because of parasitism of red blood cells; falciparum malaria causes the severest form (blackwater fever). Other infections associated with hemolysis are bartonellosis and babesiosis.

APLASTIC ANEMIA

Essentials of Diagnosis
- Pancytopenia.
- No abnormal cells seen.
- Hypocellular bone marrow.

General Considerations

All hematopoietic cells are derived from a pluripotent stem cell that gives rise to precursors of erythroid, myeloid, and platelet forms. Injury to or suppression of this hematopoietic stem cell will result in pancytopenia—reduction in all three hematopoietic cell lines (red blood cells, neutrophils, and platelets). Aplastic anemia is a condition of bone marrow failure that arises from injury to or abnormal expression of the stem cell. The bone marrow becomes hypoplastic, and pancytopenia develops.

There are a number of causes of aplastic anemia (Table 13–10). Direct stem cell injury may be caused by radiation, chemotherapy, toxins, or pharmacologic agents. Systemic lupus erythematosus may rarely cause suppression of the hematopoietic stem cell by an IgG autoantibody directed against the stem cell. However, the most common pathogenesis of aplastic anemia appears to be autoimmune suppression of hematopoiesis by a T cell-mediated cellular mechanism.

Clinical Findings

A. Symptoms and Signs: Patients come to medical attention because of the consequences of bone marrow failure. Anemia leads to symptoms of weakness and fatigue; neutropenia causes vulnerability to bacterial infections; and thrombocytopenia results in mucosal and skin bleeding. Physical examination may reveal signs of pallor, purpura, and petechiae. Other abnormalities such as hepatosplenomegaly, lymphadenopathy, or bone tenderness should *not* be present, and their presence should lead one to question the diagnosis of aplastic anemia.

B. Laboratory Findings: The hallmark of aplastic anemia is pancytopenia. However, early in the evolution of aplastic anemia, only one or two cell lines may be reduced.

Anemia may be severe and is always associated with decreased reticulocytes. Red blood cell morphology is remarkable. The MCV is usually normal but occasionally may be increased. Neutrophils and platelets are reduced in number, and no immature or abnormal forms are seen. The bone marrow aspirate and the bone marrow biopsy appear hypocellular, with only scant amounts of normal hematopoietic progenitors. No abnormal cells are seen.

Table 13–10. Causes of aplastic anemia.

Congenital (rare)
"Idiopathic" (probably autoimmune)
Systemic lupus erythematosus
Chemotherapy, radiotherapy
Toxins: Benzene, toluene, insecticides
Drugs: Chloramphenicol, phenylbutazone, gold salts, sulfonamides, phenytoin, carbamazepine, quinacrine, tolbutamide
Posthepatitis
Pregnancy
Paroxysmal nocturnal hemoglobinuria

Differential Diagnosis

The diagnosis of aplastic anemia is made in cases of pancytopenia with a hypocellular marrow biopsy containing no abnormal cells. Aplastic anemia must be differentiated from other causes of pancytopenia (Table 13–11). Myelodysplastic disorders or acute leukemia may occasionally be confused with aplastic anemia. These are differentiated by the presence of morphologic abnormalities or increased blasts. Hairy cell leukemia has been misdiagnosed as aplastic anemia and should be recognized by a high incidence of splenomegaly and by the presence of abnormal lymphoid cells on the bone marrow biopsy. Pancytopenia in the presence of a normocellular bone marrow is usually due to systemic lupus erythematosus, disseminated infection, or hypersplenism. Isolated thrombocytopenia may occur early as aplastic anemia develops and be confused with immune thrombocytopenia.

Treatment

Mild cases of aplastic anemia may be treated with supportive care. Red blood cell transfusions and platelet transfusions are given as necessary, and antibiotics are used to treat infections.

Severe aplastic anemia is defined by the presence of neutrophils less than 500/μL, platelets less than 20,000/μL, reticulocytes less than 1%, and bone marrow cellularity less than 20%. When this constellation of features is present (or three of the four), the median survival without treatment is approximately 3 months, and only 20% of patients survive for 1 year. The treatment of choice for young adults (under age 40) who have HLA-matched siblings is allogeneic bone marrow transplantation. The best results are achieved in younger patients who have not had blood transfusions. Prior transfusion increases the risk of graft rejection, apparently because of sensitization to antigens present on hematopoietic progenitors. Young patients may tolerate severe anemia and thrombocytopenia and should not be transfused unless severely symptomatic. These patients and their siblings should be promptly HLA-typed and referred for further evaluation by a hematologist.

For adults over age 40 or those without HLA-matched siblings, the treatment of choice for severe

Table 13–11. Causes of pancytopenia.

Bone marrow disorders
  Aplastic anemia
  Myelodysplasia
  Acute leukemia
  Myelofibrosis
  Infiltrative disease: Lymphoma, myeloma, carcinoma, hairy cell leukemia
  Megaloblastic anemia
Nonmarrow disorders
  Hypersplenism
  Systemic lupus erythematosus
  Infection: Tuberculosis, AIDS, leishmaniasis, brucellosis

aplastic anemia is immunosuppression with anti-thymocyte globulin (ATG). ATG is a horse serum containing polyclonal antibodies against human T cells. The success of this form of treatment has helped confirm the notion that most cases of aplastic anemia are immunologically mediated rather than caused by irreversible stem cell injury. ATG is given in the hospital over 5–8 days in conjunction with transfusion and antibiotic support. Responses usually occur in 4–12 weeks. Responses to ATG are usually only partial, but the blood counts rise high enough to give patients a safe and transfusion-free life. Cyclosporine is another effective form of immuno-suppressive treatment, and the combination of cyclosporine plus ATG appears to be more effective than ATG alone.

For patients in whom neutropenia is the dominant abnormality, the myeloid growth factors G-CSF (filgastrim) or GM-CSF (sargramostim) may be effective in raising the neutrophil count and decreasing infections. However, they will not benefit other cell lines or provide definitive treatment.

Androgens have been widely used in the past, with a low response rate. However, a few patients can be maintained successfully with this form of treatment. One regimen is oxymetholone, 2–3 mg/kg orally daily. In the rare syndrome of systemic lupus erythematosus causing humorally mediated aplastic anemia, the combination of plasmapheresis and high-dose prednisone may be successful.

Children with severe aplastic anemia who lack HLA-identical siblings may be treated effectively with allogeneic bone marrow transplantation using matched but unrelated donors.

Course & Prognosis

Patients with severe aplastic anemia have a rapidly fatal illness if left untreated. Allogeneic bone marrow transplantation is highly successful in young adults with HLA-matched siblings. For this group of patients, the durable complete response rate is 80%. For older adults or those who have previously been exposed to blood products, long-term survival rates are between 40% and 70%. ATG treatment leads to partial response in approximately 60% of adults, and the long-term prognosis of responders appears to be very good. There is increasing evidence that some fraction of these nontransplanted patients may develop clonal hematologic disorders such as myelodysplasia after many years of follow-up.

NEUTROPENIA

Neutropenia exists when the neutrophil count falls below 1500/μL. However, blacks and other specific population groups may normally have neutrophil counts as low as 1200/μL. The neutropenic patient is increasingly vulnerable to infection by gram-positive and gram-negative bacteria and by fungi. The risk of infection is related to the severity of neutropenia. Patients with "chronic benign neutropenia" are free of infection for years despite very low neutrophil levels.

A variety of bone marrow disorders and non-marrow conditions may cause neutropenia (Table 13–12). All the causes of aplastic anemia (Table 13–10) and pancytopenia (Table 13–11) may cause neutropenia. Isolated neutropenia is often due to an idiosyncratic reaction to a drug, and agranulocytosis (complete absence of neutrophils in the peripheral blood) is almost always due to a drug reaction or to exposure to a variety of chemicals (eg, pesticides). In these cases, examination of the bone marrow shows virtual absence of myeloid precursors, with other cell lines undisturbed. Pure white cell aplasia is a rare condition in which an autoantibody is formed against myeloid progenitors. Felty's syndrome—neutropenia associated with seropositive nodular rheumatoid arthritis—is another cause. Neutropenia in the presence of a normal bone marrow may be due to immunologic peripheral destruction, sepsis, or hypersplenism.

Clinical Findings

Neutropenia results in stomatitis and in infections. Infections are usually due to gram-positive or gram-negative aerobic bacteria or to fungi such as *Candida* or *Aspergillus*. The most common infections are septicemia, cellulitis, and pneumonia. In the presence of severe neutropenia, the usual signs of inflammatory response to infection may be absent. Nevertheless, fever in the neutropenic patient should always be assumed to be of infectious origin.

Table 13–12. Causes of neutropenia.

Bone marrow disorders
Aplastic anemia
Pure white cell aplasia
Congenital (rare)
Cyclic neutropenia
Drugs: Sulfonamides, chlorpromazine, procainamide, penicillin, cephalosporins, cimetidine, methimazole, phenytoin, chlorpropamide
Benign chronic
Peripheral disorders
Hypersplenism
Sepsis
Immune
Felty's syndrome

Treatment

Potential causative drugs are discontinued. Infections are treated with many combinations of broad-spectrum antibiotics, but particular attention should be paid to enteric gram-negative bacteria. Combined treatment with aminoglycosides and a semisynthetic penicillin is commonly used, but third-generation cephalosporins such as ceftazidime are effective as single-agent therapy, obviating the need for an aminoglycoside.

When Felty's syndrome leads to repeated bacterial infections, splenectomy is the treatment of choice. Splenectomy usually leads to healing of leg ulcers and to reduction in the rate of infection whether or not the neutrophil count rises.

The prognosis of patients with neutropenia depends on the underlying cause. Most patients with drug-induced agranulocytosis can be supported with broad-spectrum antibiotics and will recover completely. The myeloid growth factors G-CSF (filgastrim) and GM-CSF (sargramostim) may be useful in shortening the duration of neutropenia associated with chemotherapy and can often correct neutropenia from other causes such as myelosuppressive medications.

Crawford J et al: A reduction by granulocyte colony stimulating factor of fever and neutropenia induced by chemotherapy in patients with small cell lung cancer. N Engl J Med 1991;325:164.

LEUKEMIAS & OTHER MYELOPROLIFERATIVE DISORDERS

Myeloproliferative disorders are due to acquired clonal abnormalities of the hematopoietic stem cell. Since the stem cell gives rise to myeloid, erythroid, and platelet cells, one sees qualitative and quantitative changes in all these cell lines. In some disorders (chronic myelogenous leukemia), specific characteristic chromosomal changes are seen. In others, although the disorder is presumed to be related to a defect in DNA, no characteristic cytogenetic abnormalities are seen.

Classically, the myeloproliferative disorders produce characteristic syndromes with well-defined clinical and laboratory features (Tables 13–13 and 13–14). However, these disorders are grouped together because the disease may evolve from one form into another and because hybrid disorders are commonly seen. All of the myeloproliferative disorders may progress to acute myelogenous leukemia.

POLYCYTHEMIA VERA

Essentials of Diagnosis

- Increased red blood cell mass.
- Splenomegaly.
- Normal arterial oxygen saturation.
- Usually elevated white blood count and platelet count.

General Considerations

Polycythemia vera is an acquired myeloproliferative disorder that causes overproduction of all three hematopoietic cell lines, most prominently the red blood cells. The hematocrit is elevated (at sea level) when values exceed 54% in males or 51% in females (Table 13–15).

When the hematocrit is elevated, the red blood cell mass should be measured to determine whether true polycythemia or relative polycythemia exists. Normal values for red blood cell mass are 26–34 mL/kg in men and 21–29 mL/kg in women. Relative ("spurious") polycythemia characteristically presents in middle-aged men who are overweight and hypertensive; the hematocrit is almost always less than 60%.

If the red blood cell mass is increased, one must determine whether the increase is primary or secondary. Primary polycythemia (polycythemia vera) is a bone marrow disorder characterized by autonomous overproduction of erythroid cells. Erythroid production is independent of erythropoietin, and the serum erythropoietin level is low. In vitro, erythroid progenitor cells grow without added erythropoietin, a finding not seen in normal individuals.

Polycythemia vera is a relatively common disorder. Sixty percent of patients are male, and the median age at presentation is 60. Polycythemia vera rarely occurs in adults under age 40.

Clinical Findings

A. Symptoms and Signs: Most patients present with symptoms related to expanded blood volume and increased blood viscosity. Common complaints include headache, dizziness, tinnitus, blurred vision, and fatigue. Generalized pruritus, especially that occurring following a warm shower or bath, may be a striking symptom and is related to histamine release from the increased number of basophils present. Patients may also initially complain of epistaxis. This is probably related to engorgement of mucosal blood

Table 13–13. Classification of myeloproliferative disorders.

Myeloproliferative syndromes
Polycythemia vera
Myelofibrosis
Essential thrombocytosis
Chronic myeloid leukemia
Myelodysplastic syndromes
Acute myeloid leukemia

Table 13–14. Laboratory features of myeloproliferative disorders.

	White Count	Hematocrit	Platelet Count	Red Cell Morphology
Chronic myeloid leukemia	↑↑	N	N or ↑	N
Myelofibrosis	N or ↓ or ↑	N or ↓	↓ or N or ↑	Abn
Polycythemia vera	N or ↑	↑	N or ↑	N
Essential thrombocytosis	N or ↑	N	↑↑	N

vessels in combination with abnormal hemostasis due to qualitative abnormalities in platelet function.

Physical examination reveals plethora and engorged retinal veins. The spleen is palpably enlarged in 75% of cases, but splenomegaly is nearly always present when imaged. Less commonly, the liver is mildly enlarged.

Thrombosis is the most common complication of polycythemia vera and the major cause of morbidity and death in this disorder. Thrombosis appears to be related to increased blood viscosity and abnormal platelet function. Uncontrolled polycythemia leads to a very high incidence of thrombotic complications of surgery, and elective surgery should be deferred until the condition has been treated. Paradoxically, in addition to thrombosis, increased bleeding also occurs. There is a high incidence of peptic ulcer disease as well as gastrointestinal bleeding. Overproduction of uric acid may lead to gout.

B. Laboratory Findings: The hallmark of polycythemia vera is a hematocrit above normal, at times greater than 60%. Red blood cell morphology is normal. The white blood count is characteristically elevated to 10,000–20,000/µL and the platelet count is variably elevated, sometimes with counts exceeding 1,000,000/µL. Platelet morphology is usually normal, but large hypogranular forms may be seen. White blood cells are usually normal, but basophilia is frequently present. By definition, the red blood cell mass is elevated.

The bone marrow is hypercellular, with panhyperplasia of all hematopoietic elements. A characteristic finding is increased numbers of megakaryocytes. Iron stores are usually absent from the bone marrow, having been transferred to the increased circulating red blood cell mass. Iron deficiency may result from chronic gastrointestinal blood loss. Bleeding may lower the hematocrit to the normal range (or lower), creating diagnostic confusion.

Table 13–15. Causes of polycythemia.

Spurious polycythemia
Secondary polycythemia
   Hypoxia: Cardiac disease, pulmonary disease, high altitude
   Carboxyhemoglobin: Smoking
   Renal lesions
   Erythropoietin-secreting tumors (rare)
   Abnormal hemoglobins (rare)
Polycythemia vera

Vitamin B_{12} levels are strikingly elevated because of increased levels of transcobalamin III (secreted by white blood cells). The leukocyte alkaline phosphatase is characteristically elevated as a marker of qualitative abnormalities in the myeloid line. Uric acid levels may be increased. There is no characteristic chromosomal abnormality in this disorder.

Although red blood cell morphology is usually normal at presentation, microcytosis, hypochromia, and poikilocytosis may result from iron deficiency following treatment by phlebotomy (see below). Progressive hypersplenism may also lead to elliptocytosis.

Differential Diagnosis

Spurious polycythemia, in which an elevated hematocrit is due to contracted plasma volume rather than increased red cell mass, may be related to diuretic use or may occur without obvious cause.

A secondary cause of polycythemia should be suspected if splenomegaly is absent and the high hematocrit is not accompanied by increases in other cell lines. Arterial oxygen saturation should be measured to determine if hypoxia is the cause. A smoking history should be taken and carboxyhemoglobin levels measured when indicated. A renal sonogram may be indicated to look for an erythropoietin-secreting cyst or tumor. A positive family history should lead to investigation for congenital high-oxygen-affinity hemoglobin.

Polycythemia vera should be differentiated from other myeloproliferative disorders (Table 13–14). Marked elevation of the white blood count above 30,000/µL should lead to consideration of chronic myelogenous leukemia. This disorder is confirmed by the finding of a low leukocyte alkaline phosphatase and by the presence of the Philadelphia chromosome. Abnormal red blood cell morphology and nucleated red blood cells in the peripheral blood should lead to the consideration of myelofibrosis. This condition is diagnosed by bone marrow biopsy showing fibrosis of the marrow. Essential thrombocytosis is diagnosed when the platelet count is strikingly elevated and the red blood cell count is normal.

Treatment

The treatment of choice is phlebotomy. One unit of blood (approximately 500 mL) is removed weekly until the hematocrit is less than 45%; the hematocrit is maintained at less than 45% by repeated phlebotomy as necessary. Because repeated phlebotomy produces iron deficiency, the requirement for phlebotomy should gradually decrease. It is important to avoid medicinal iron supplementation, as this can thwart the goals of a phlebotomy program. It is not necessary to manipulate the diet to decrease iron intake. Patients will usually feel much better as soon as the hematocrit is lowered. Maintaining the hematocrit at normal levels has been shown to decrease the incidence of thrombotic complications.

Occasionally, myelosuppressive therapy is indicated. Indications include a high phlebotomy requirement, marked thrombocytosis, and intractable pruritus. Although there is no proof, most hematologists believe that reduction of the platelet count to less than 700,000/µL will reduce the risk of thrombotic complications that are the major cause of morbidity and mortality in this disorder. Alkylating agents and radiophosphorus (^{32}P) have been shown to increase the risk of conversion of this disease to acute leukemia and should generally be avoided. Hydroxyurea is now being widely used when myelosuppressive therapy is indicated because of the presumption that it will not be leukemogenic. Busulfan may also be used. Interferon has recently been shown to have some ability to control the disease.

The role of antiplatelet agents such as aspirin in preventing thrombotic complications is controversial. High doses of aspirin (325 mg three times daily) plus dipyridamole (25 mg three times daily) cause a marked increase in gastrointestinal bleeding and should not be given routinely. However, antiplatelet treatment may be warranted in selected patients who have recurrent thromboses despite control of their platelet counts with myelosuppressive therapy. One aspirin tablet daily (325 mg) may be effective therapy.

Allopurinol may be indicated for hyperuricemia. Antihistamine therapy with diphenhydramine and cimetidine may be helpful for control of pruritus.

Prognosis

Polycythemia is an indolent disease with median survival of 11–15 years. The major cause of morbidity and mortality is arterial thrombosis. Over time, polycythemia vera may convert to myelofibrosis or to chronic myelogenous leukemia. In approximately 10% of cases, the disorder progresses to acute myelogenous leukemia, which is usually refractory to therapy.

Berk PD et al: Therapeutic recommendations in polycythemia vera based on Polycythemia Vera Study Group protocols. Semin Hematol 1986;23:132. (Results of a national trial establishing current standards of care.)

MYELOFIBROSIS

Essentials of Diagnosis

- Teardrop poikilocytosis on peripheral smear.
- Leukoerythroblastic blood picture; giant abnormal platelets.
- Hypercellular bone marrow with reticulin or collagen fibrosis.

General Considerations

Myelofibrosis (myelofibrosis with myeloid metaplasia, agnogenic myeloid metaplasia) is a myeloproliferative disorder characterized by fibrosis of the bone marrow, splenomegaly, and a leukoerythroblastic peripheral blood picture with teardrop poikilocytosis. It is widely believed that fibrosis occurs in response to increased secretion of platelet-derived growth factor (PDGF). In response to bone marrow fibrosis, extramedullary hematopoiesis (hematopoietic cell development outside the bone marrow) takes place in the liver, spleen, and lymph nodes. In these sites, mesenchymal cells responsible for fetal hematopoiesis can be reactivated.

Clinical Findings

A. Symptoms and Signs: Myelofibrosis develops in adults over age 50 and is usually insidious in onset. Patients most commonly present with fatigue related to their anemia or abdominal fullness related to splenomegaly. Uncommon presentations include bleeding and bone pain. On examination, splenomegaly is almost invariably present and is sometimes massive. The liver is enlarged in more than half of cases.

Later in the course of the disease, progressive bone marrow failure takes place as the marrow becomes progressively more fibrotic. Anemia becomes severe, and red cell transfusion becomes necessary. Progressive thrombocytopenia leads to bleeding. The spleen continues to enlarge, which leads to early satiety. Painful episodes of splenic infarction may occur. Late in the course, the patient becomes cachectic and may experience severe bone pain, especially in the lower legs. Hematopoiesis in the liver leads to portal hypertension with ascites, esophageal varices, and eventually liver failure.

B. Laboratory Findings: Patients are almost invariably anemic at presentation. The white blood count is variable—either low, normal, or elevated—and may be increased to 50,000/µL. The platelet count is variable. The peripheral blood smear is characteristic, consisting of significant poikilocytosis with numerous teardrop forms. Immature myeloid and erythroid forms are present (leukoerythroblastic blood picture). Nucleated red blood cells are present and the myeloid series is less strikingly shifted, with immature forms including a small percentage of promyelocytes or myeloblasts. Platelet morphology may be bizarre, and giant degranulated platelet forms (megakaryocyte fragments) may be seen. The triad of teardrop poikilocytosis, leukoerythroblastic blood, and giant abnormal platelets is almost diagnostic of myelofibrosis.

The bone marrow usually cannot be aspirated (dry tap), though early in the course of the disease it is hypercellular, with a marked increase in megakaryocytes. Fibrosis at this stage is detected only by a silver stain demonstrating increased reticulin fibers. Later, biopsy reveals more severe fibrosis, with eventual replacement of hematopoietic precursors by collagen. There is no characteristic chromosomal abnormality.

Differential Diagnosis

A leukoerythroblastic blood picture from other causes may be seen in response to severe infection or inflammation. However, teardrop poikilocytosis and giant abnormal platelet forms will not be present. Bone marrow fibrosis may be seen in metastatic carcinoma, Hodgkin's disease, and hairy cell leukemia. These disorders are diagnosed by characteristic tissue morphology.

Myelofibrosis is distinguished from other myeloproliferative disorders by the characteristic constellation of findings (Table 13–14). Chronic myelogenous leukemia is diagnosed when there is marked elevation of the white blood count, a low leukocyte alkaline phosphatase, normal red blood cell morphology, and the presence of the Philadelphia chromosome. Polycythemia vera is characterized by an elevated hematocrit, and patients with essential thrombocytosis should have normal red blood cells.

Treatment

There is no specific treatment for this disorder. Anemic patients are supported with red blood cells in transfusion. Androgens such as oxymetholone or testosterone help reduce the transfusion requirement in one-third of cases but are poorly tolerated by women. Recombinant erythropoietin (epoetin alfa) has been reported to be of value in a small number of cases. Splenectomy is not routinely performed but is indicated for splenic enlargement that causes recurrent painful episodes, severe thrombocytopenia, or an unacceptably high red blood cell transfusion requirement. Interferon may have a role in treatment, but this requires further study.

Course & Prognosis

It is often hard to date the onset of myelofibrosis, but the median survival from time of diagnosis is approximately 5 years. End-stage myelofibrosis is a wasting illness characterized by generalized debility, liver failure, and bleeding from thrombocytopenia. Some cases may terminate in acute myelogenous leukemia.

Demory JL: Cytogenetic studies and their prognostic significance in agnogenic myeloid metaplasia: A report on 47 cases. Blood 1988;72:855.

Silver RT: Interferon in the treatment of myeloproliferative disease. Semin Hematol 1990;27:6.

CHRONIC MYELOGENOUS LEUKEMIA

Essentials of Diagnosis

- Markedly elevated white blood count.
- Markedly left-shifted myeloid series with a low percentage of promyelocytes and blasts.
- Presence of Philadelphia chromosome.

General Considerations

Chronic myelogenous leukemia is a myeloproliferative disorder characterized by overproduction of myeloid cells. These myeloid cells retain the capacity for differentiation, and normal bone marrow function is retained during the early phases. The disease usually remains stable for years and then transforms to a more overtly malignant disease.

Chronic myelogenous leukemia is associated with a characteristic chromosomal abnormality, the Philadelphia chromosome, and was the first disease associated with a specific karyotypic abnormality. The Philadelphia chromosome is now recognized to be a reciprocal translocation between the long arms of chromosomes 9 and 22. A large portion of 22q is translocated to 9q, and a smaller piece of 9q is moved to 22q. This translocation is thought to be pathogenically significant, based on recent evidence that oncogene activation occurs. The portion of 9q that is translocated contains *abl*, a proto-oncogene that is the cellular homologue of the Ableson murine leukemia virus. The *abl* gene is received at a specific site on 22q, the break point cluster (bcr). The fusion gene bcr-*abl* produces a novel protein that differs from the normal transcript of the *abl* gene in that it possesses tyrosine kinase activity (a characteristic activity of transforming genes).

Usually at the time of diagnosis, the Philadelphia chromosome-positive clone dominates and may be the only one detected. However, a normal clone is present and may express itself either in vivo, after certain forms of therapy, or in vitro, in long-term bone marrow cultures. Approximately 5% of cases of chronic myelogenous leukemia are Philadelphia chromosome-negative. In almost all cases, although the characteristic karyotype is not seen at the light microscopic level, molecular studies demonstrate translocation of *abl* to 22q. In other cases of Philadelphia-negative chronic myelogenous leukemia, the disease is atypical and is better described as chronic myelomonocytic leukemia. Philadelphia chromosome-negative disease has a poor prognosis.

Early chronic myelogenous leukemia ("chronic phase") does not behave like a malignant disease.

Normal bone marrow function is retained, white blood cells differentiate, and, despite some qualitative abnormalities (low leukocyte alkaline phosphatase), the neutrophils combat infection normally. However, chronic myelogenous leukemia is inherently unstable, and the disease progresses to accelerated phase and finally after several years, to blast crisis. This progression of the disease is often associated with added chromosomal defects superimposed on the Philadelphia chromosome. Blast crisis chronic myelogenous leukemia is an overtly malignant process that becomes indistinguishable from acute leukemia.

Clinical Findings

A. Symptoms and Signs: Chronic myelogenous leukemia is a disorder of middle age (median age at presentation is 42 years). Patients usually present with fatigue, night sweats, and low-grade fever related to the hypermetabolic state caused by overproduction of white blood cells. At other times, the patient complains of abdominal fullness related to splenomegaly, or an elevated white blood count is discovered incidentally. Rarely, the patient will present with a clinical syndrome related to leukostasis with blurred vision, respiratory distress, or priapism. The white blood count in these cases is usually greater than 500,000/μL.

On examination, the spleen is enlarged (often markedly so), and sternal tenderness may be present as a sign of marrow overexpansion.

Acceleration of the disease is often associated with fever in the absence of infection, bone pain, and splenomegaly. In blast crisis, patients may experience bleeding and infection related to bone marrow failure.

B. Laboratory Findings: The hallmark of chronic myelogenous leukemia is an elevated white blood count; the median white blood count at diagnosis is 150,000/μL. The peripheral blood is characteristic. The myeloid series is left-shifted, with mature forms dominating and with cells usually present in proportion to their degree of maturation. Blasts are usually less than 5%. Basophilia of granulocytes may be present. The peripheral blood smear gives the impression that the bone marrow has spilled over into the blood. At presentation, the patient is usually not anemic. Red blood cell morphology is normal, and nucleated red blood cells are rarely seen. The platelet count may be normal or elevated (sometimes to strikingly high levels). Platelet morphology is usually normal, but abnormally large forms may be seen.

The bone marrow is hypercellular, with markedly left-shifted myelopoiesis. Myeloblasts comprise less than 5% of marrow cells.

The leukocyte alkaline phosphatase score is invariably low and is a sign of qualitative abnormalities in neutrophils. The vitamin B_{12} level is usually markedly elevated because of increased secretion of trans-

cobalamin III. Uric acid levels may be high.

The Philadelphia chromosome is almost invariably present and may be detected in either the peripheral blood or the bone marrow. The bcr-*abl* gene may be reliably detected in peripheral blood by molecular techniques (Southern blot) and is well enough established to substitute for cytogenetics if the only question is whether the Philadelphia chromosome is present.

With progression to the accelerated and blast phases, progressive anemia and thrombocytopenia occur, and the percentage of blasts in the blood and bone marrow increases. Blast phase chronic myelogenous leukemia is diagnosed when blasts comprise more than 30% of bone marrow cells.

Differential Diagnosis

Early chronic myelogenous leukemia must be differentiated from the reactive leukocytosis associated with infection, inflammation, or cancer. In these reactive disorders, the white blood count is usually less than 50,000/μL, splenomegaly is absent, the leukocyte alkaline phosphatase is normal or increased, and the Philadelphia chromosome is not present. If one is in doubt whether leukocytosis is due to chronic myelogenous leukemia or a reactive condition, the patient should be observed, since there is no advantage to early therapy for asymptomatic patients.

Chronic myelogenous leukemia must be distinguished from other myeloproliferative disease (Table 13–14). The hematocrit should not be elevated, the red blood cell morphology should be normal, and nucleated red blood cells should be rare or absent. Definitive diagnosis is made by finding the Philadelphia chromosome or bcr-*abl*.

Treatment

Treatment is usually not indicated even with white blood counts over 200,000/μL, since the majority of circulating cells are mature myeloid cells that are smaller and more deformable than primitive leukemic blasts. In the rare instances in which symptoms result from extreme hyperleukocytosis (priapism, respiratory distress, visual blurring, altered mental status), leukapheresis should be performed on an emergency basis in conjunction with myelosuppressive therapy.

The usual treatment is palliative and improves the patient's sense of well-being without altering the natural history of the disease. Myelosuppressive therapy consists of giving either busulfan or hydroxyurea in combination with allopurinol. When busulfan is used, the usual dose is 4–8 mg daily for 4–8 weeks. One aims to lower the white count to 10,000–20,000/μL. Busulfan has a notoriously prolonged duration of action, and because of resultant difficulties with neutropenia, hydroxyurea is more commonly used. The initial dose is usually 2–4 g/d orally, and the maintenance dose varies between 0.5 and 2 g/d as necessary to maintain the white blood count at 5000–10,000/μL. Hydroxyurea must be given without interruption, since the white blood count will rise within days after discontinuing this medication. The response to hydroxyurea is usually gratifying. The white blood count decreases, the spleen decreases in size, and the patient becomes asymptomatic. Most patients in the chronic phase of chronic myelogenous leukemia will have no symptoms either from the disease or their chemotherapy.

Recombinant alpha interferon has been used in the treatment of the chronic phase with good results. Sixty to 70 percent of patients have a good hematologic response. The role of interferon therapy for chronic myelogenous leukemia, however, remains controversial. Interferon, unlike other palliative agents, has the ability to suppress the Philadelphia chromosome and to allow cytogenetically normal cells to appear. This biologic effect may be complete (5–10% of cases) or partial (15–30% of cases). It usually occurs after 1 year (6–18 months) of treatment. Patients who respond in this way benefit with improved survival. Whether all patients should be treated with this expensive and symptom-producing drug is currently being debated.

Although the response to myelosuppressive therapy of the chronic phase is gratifying, the treatment is only palliative, and the disease is invariably fatal. The only available curative therapy is allogeneic bone marrow transplantation. This treatment is available for adults under age 55 who have HLA-matched siblings. Approximately 60% of adults have long-term disease-free survival following bone marrow transplantation and appear to be cured of their disease. The best results (70–80% success rate) are obtained in patients under age 40 who are transplanted within 1 year after initial diagnosis. All young patients should be given the opportunity for allogeneic bone marrow transplantation in the chronic phase if they have suitable bone marrow donors. For young patients without sibling donors, HLA-matched unrelated donors may be located through computer-based registries of volunteer bone marrow donors. Results are inferior to those achieved with matched sibling transplants but offer a cure rate of 30–50% for patients with an otherwise invariably fatal disease.

Blast crisis of chronic myelogenous leukemia is a notoriously difficult form of acute leukemia to treat. Lymphoid blast crisis (present in one-third of cases) should be identified because chemotherapy for this disorder is less toxic and more effective. Therapy with daunorubicin, vincristine, and prednisone (used in treatment of acute lymphoblastic leukemia) will lead to remission—usually short-lived—in 70% of these cases.

Course & Prognosis

Median survival is 3–4 years. Once the disease has progressed to the accelerated or blast phase, survival is measured in months. Approximately 60% of young adults who have successful allogeneic bone marrow transplantation appear to be cured.

McGlave P: Bone marrow transplants in chronic myelogenous leukemia: An overview of determinants of survival. Semin Hematol 1990;27:23.

Talpaz M et al: Interferon alpha produces sustained cytogenetic responses in chronic myelogenous leukemia: Philadelphia chromosome positive patients. Ann Intern Med 1991;114:532.

MYELODYSPLASTIC SYNDROMES

Essentials of Diagnosis

- Cytopenias with a hypercellular bone marrow.
- Morphologic abnormalities in two or more hematopoietic cell lines.

General Considerations

The myelodysplastic syndromes are a group of acquired clonal disorders of the hematopoietic stem cell. They are characterized by the constellation of cytopenias, a hypercellular marrow, and a number of morphologic and cytogenetic abnormalities. The disorders are usually idiopathic but may be seen after cytotoxic chemotherapy—especially procarbazine for Hodgkin's disease and melphalan for multiple myeloma or ovarian carcinoma.

Despite the presence of adequate numbers of hematopoietic progenitor cells, "ineffective hematopoiesis" occurs, resulting in various cytopenias. Ultimately, the disorder may evolve into frank acute myelogenous leukemia, and the term "preleukemia" has been used to describe these disorders. Although no specific chromosomal abnormality is seen in myelodysplasia, there are frequently abnormalities involving the long arm of chromosome 5 (which contains a number of genes encoding both growth factors and receptors involved in myelopoiesis) as well as deletions of chromosomes 5 and 7.

Myelodysplasia encompasses several heterogeneous syndromes. Those without excess bone marrow blasts are termed "refractory anemia," with or without ringed sideroblasts. Those with excess blasts are diagnosed as "refractory anemia with excess blasts" (RAEB 5–19% blasts) and "refractory anemia with excess blasts in transition"(RAEB-T 20–29% blasts). Those with a proliferative syndrome including peripheral blood monocytosis greater than 1000/μL are termed chronic myelomonocytic leukemia (CMML).

Clinical Findings

A. Symptoms and Signs: Patients are usually over age 60. Many are diagnosed while asymptomatic because of the finding of abnormal blood counts. Patients usually present with fatigue, infection, or bleeding related to bone marrow failure. The course may be indolent, and the disease may present as a wasting illness with fever, weight loss, and general debility. On examination, splenomegaly may be present in combination with pallor, bleeding, and various signs of infection.

B. Laboratory Findings: Anemia may be severe and may require transfusion support. The MCV is normal or increased, and macro-ovalocytes may be seen on the peripheral blood smear. The reticulocyte count is usually reduced. The white blood cell count is usually normal or reduced, and neutropenia is common. The neutrophils may exhibit morphologic abnormalities, including deficient numbers of granules or a bilobed nucleus (Pelger-Huet). The myeloid series may be left-shifted, and small numbers of promyelocytes or blasts may be seen. The platelet count is normal or reduced, and hypogranular platelets may be present.

The bone marrow is characteristically hypercellular. Erythroid hyperplasia is common, and signs of abnormal erythropoiesis include megaloblastic features, nuclear budding, or multinucleated erythroid precursors. The Prussian blue stain may demonstrate ringed sideroblasts. The myeloid series is often left-shifted, with variable increases in blasts. Deficient or abnormal granules may be seen. A characteristic abnormality is the presence of dwarf megakaryoctyes with a unilobed nucleus.

Differential Diagnosis

In subtle cases, cytogenetic evaluation of the bone marrow may help distinguish this clonal disorder from other causes of cytopenias. As the number of blasts increase in the bone marrow, myelodysplasia is arbitrarily separated from acute myelogenous leukemia by the presence of less than 30% blasts.

Treatment

Patients affected primarily by anemia are best supported with red blood cell transfusions. Patients with severe neutropenia or thrombocytopenia or those with marked constitutional symptoms may be treated with low-dose chemotherapy, although results of such treatment are poor. Erythropoietin (epoetin alfa) reduces the red cell transfusion requirement in some patients. The myeloid growth factors C-CSF (filgastrim) and GM-CSF (sargramostim) reliably raise the neutrophil count and reduce the incidence of infections. However, they do not usually benefit other cell types and appear not to change the course of the disease.

Young patients (under age 55) with matched sibling donors can be successfully treated with ablative chemotherapy and allogeneic bone marrow transplantation. Cure rates are approximately 30–50%

Course & Prognosis

Myelodysplasia is an ultimately fatal disease. Patients most commonly succumb to infections or bleeding. The risk of transformation to acute myelogenous leukemia depends on the percentage of blasts in the bone marrow. Patients with refractory anemia may survive many years, and the risk of leukemia is low (< 10%). Those with excess blasts or CMML have short survivals (usually < 2 years) and have a higher (20–50%) risk of developing acute leukemia. The finding of deletions of chromosomes 5 and 7 is associated with a poor prognosis. Allogeneic bone marrow transplantation is the only definitive therapy, though its optimal timing given the wide spectrum of prognostic possibilities may be difficult to determine.

Cheson BD: The myelodysplastic syndromes: Current approaches to therapy. Ann Intern Med 1990;112:932.

Feneaux P et al: Prognostic factors in adult chronic myelomonocytic leukemia: An analysis of 107 cases. J Clin Oncol 1988;6:1417.

Sanz GF, Sanz MA, Vallespi T: Two regression models and a scoring system for predicting survival and planning treatment in myelodysplastic syndromes: A multivariate analysis of prognostic factors in 370 patients. Blood 1989;74:395.

ACUTE LEUKEMIA

Essentials of Diagnosis

- Cytopenias or pancytopenia.
- Bone marrow failure causing infection, bleeding, or fatigue.
- More than 30% blasts in the bone marrow.
- Blasts in peripheral blood in 90%.

General Considerations

Acute leukemia is a malignancy of the hematopoietic progenitor cell. The malignant cell loses its ability to mature and differentiate. These cells proliferate in an uncontrolled fashion and ultimately replace normal bone marrow elements. Most cases arise with no clear cause. However, radiation and some toxins (benzene) are clearly leukemogenic. In addition, a number of chemotherapeutic agents (especially procarbazine, melphalan, other alkylating agents, and etoposide) may cause leukemia. The leukemias seen after toxin or chemotherapy exposure often develop from a myelodysplastic prodrome and are associated with abnormalities in chromosomes 5 and 7. Although a number of other cytogenetic abnormalities are seen in certain types of acute leukemia, their exact role in pathogenesis remains unclear.

Most of the clinical findings in acute leukemia are due to bone marrow failure, which results from replacement of normal bone marrow elements by the malignant cell. Less common manifestations include direct organ infiltration (skin, gastrointestinal tract, meninges). Acute leukemia is one of the outstanding examples of a once invariably fatal disease that is now treatable and potentially curable with combination chemotherapy.

Acute lymphoblastic leukemia (ALL) comprises 80% of the acute leukemias of childhood. The peak incidence is between 3 and 7 years of age. However, ALL is also seen in adults and comprises approximately 20% of adult acute leukemias. Acute myelogenous leukemia (AML; acute nonlymphocytic leukemia [ANLL]) is chiefly an adult disease with a median age at presentation of 50 years and an increasing incidence with advanced age. However, it is also seen in young adults and children.

Clinical Findings

A. Symptoms and Signs: Most patients with acute leukemia present with an acute illness and have been ill only for days or weeks. Bleeding (usually due to thrombocytopenia) is usually in the skin and mucosal surfaces, manifested as gingival bleeding, epistaxis, or menorrhagia. Less commonly, widespread severe bleeding is seen in patients with disseminated intravascular coagulation (seen in acute promyelocytic leukemia and monocytic leukemia). Infection is due to neutropenia, with the risk of infection becoming high as the neutrophil count falls below 500/μL. Patients with neutrophil counts less than 100/μL almost invariably become infected within several days. The most common pathogens are gram-negative bacteria (E coli, Klebsiella, Pseudomonas) or fungi (Candida, Aspergillus). Common presentations include cellulitis, pneumonia, and perirectal infections. Septicemia in severely neutropenic patients can cause death within a few hours if treatment with appropriate antibiotics is delayed.

Patients may also seek medical attention because of gum hypertrophy and bone and joint pain. The most dramatic presentation is hyperleukocytosis, in which a markedly elevated circulating blast count (usually > 200,000/μL) leads to impaired circulation, presenting as headache, confusion, and dyspnea. Such patients require emergent leukapheresis and chemotherapy.

On examination, patients are usually pale and have purpura, petechiae, and various signs of infection. Stomatitis and gum hypertrophy may be seen in patients with monocytic leukemia. There is variable enlargement of the liver, spleen, and lymph nodes. Bone tenderness, particularly in the sternum and tibia, may be present.

B. Laboratory Findings: The hallmark of acute leukemia is the combination of pancytopenia with circulating blasts. However, blasts may be absent from the peripheral smear in as many as 10% of cases ("aleukemic leukemia").

The bone marrow is usually hypercellular and dominated by blasts. More than 30% blasts are required to make a diagnosis of acute leukemia.

A number of other laboratory abnormalities may be present. Hyperuricemia may be seen. If disseminated intravascular coagulation is present, the fibrinogen level will be reduced, the prothrombin time prolonged, and fibrin degradation products present. Patients with acute lymphoblastic leukemia (especially T cell) may have a mediastinal mass visible on chest radiograph. Patients with meningeal leukemia will have blasts present in the spinal fluid. This is seen in approximately 5% of cases at diagnosis and is more common in monocytic types of acute myelogenous leukemia.

Acute leukemia should be classified as either acute lymphoblastic or acute myelogenous leukemia, also called acute nonlymphocytic leukemia. Patients with acute myelogenous leukemia may have granules visible in the blast cells. The Auer rod, an eosinophilic needle-like inclusion in the cytoplasm, is pathognomonic of acute myelogenous leukemia. To confirm the myeloid nature of the cells, histochemical stains demonstrating myeloid enzymes such as peroxidase or chloroacetate esterase may be useful. Monocytic lineage can be demonstrated by the finding of butyrate esterase. Acute lymphoblastic leukemia should be considered when there is no morphologic or histochemical evidence of myeloid or monocytic lineage. The diagnosis is confirmed by demonstrating surface markers characteristic of primitive lymphoid cells. Terminal deoxynucleotidal transferase (TdT) is present in 95% of cases of acute lymphoblastic leukemia. A variety of monoclonal antibodies have been used to define other phenotypes of acute lymphoblastic leukemia. Primitive B lymphocyte antigens include CD10 and CD19. T cell acute lymphoblastic leukemia is diagnosed by the finding of CD2, CD5, and CD7.

Acute myelogenous leukemia is usually categorized on the basis of morphology and histochemistry as follows: Acute undifferentiated leukemia (M0), acute myeloblastic leukemia (M1), acute myeloblastic leukemia with differentiation (M2), acute promyelocytic leukemia (M3), acute myelomonocytic leukemia (M4), acute monoblastic leukemia (M5), erythroleukemia (M6), and megakaryoblastic leukemia (M7).

Acute lymphoblastic leukemia is most usefully classified by immunologic phenotype as follows: common, early B lineage, and T cell.

Differential Diagnosis

Acute myelogenous leukemia must be distinguished from other myeloproliferative disorders, chronic myelogenous leukemia, and myelodysplastic syndromes. It is important to distinguish acute leukemia from a left-shifted bone marrow that is recovering from a previous toxic insult. If the question is in doubt, a bone marrow study should be repeated in several days to see if maturation has taken place. Acute lymphoblastic leukemia must be distinguished from other lymphoproliferative disease such as chronic lymphocytic leukemia, lymphomas, and hairy cell leukemia. It may also be confused with the atypical lymphocytosis of mononucleosis. An experienced observer can distinguish these entities based on morphology.

Treatment

Most young patients with acute leukemia are treated with the objective of effecting a cure. The first step in treatment is to obtain complete remission, defined as normal peripheral blood with resolution of cytopenias, normal bone marrow with no excess in blasts, and normal clinical status. However, complete remission is not synonymous with cure, and leukemia will invariably recur if no further treatment is given.

Acute myelogenous leukemia is treated initially with intensive combination chemotherapy, including daunorubicin and cytarabine. Effective treatment produces aplasia of the bone marrow, which takes 2–3 weeks to recover. During this period, intensive supportive care, including transfusion and antibiotic therapy, is required. Once complete remission has been achieved, several different types of postremission therapy are potentially curative. Options include repeated intensive chemotherapy, high-dose chemoradiotherapy with allogeneic bone marrow transplantation, and high-dose chemotherapy with autologous bone marrow transplantation.

Acute lymphoblastic leukemia is treated initially with combination chemotherapy, including daunorubicin, vincristine, prednisone, and sometimes asparaginase. Remission induction therapy for acute lymphoblastic leukemia is less myelosuppressive than treatment for acute myelogenous leukemia and does not necessarily produce marrow aplasia. After achieving complete remission, patients receive central nervous system prophylaxis with cranial irradiation and intrathecal methotrexate so that meningeal sequestration of leukemic cells does not develop. As with acute myelogenous leukemia, patients may be treated with either chemotherapy or high-dose chemotherapy plus bone marrow transplantation.

Prognosis

Approximately 70–80% of adults with acute myelogenous leukemia under age 60 achieve complete remission. High-dose postremission chemotherapy leads to cure in 30–40% of these patients. Allogeneic bone marrow transplantation (for younger adults with HLA-matched siblings) is curative in approximately 60% of cases. Autologous bone marrow transplantation is a promising new form of therapy that may cure 40–70% of patients in first remission. Older adults with acute myelogenous leukemia achieve complete remission approximately 50% of the time. A selected older patient may be treated with intensive chemotherapy with curative intent.

Eighty percent of adults with acute lymphoblastic

leukemia achieve complete remission. Subsequent postremission chemotherapy is curative in 30–50% of adults. Acute lymphoblastic leukemia in children is much more responsive to therapy, with 95% achieving complete remission and 60–70% of these being cured with postremission treatment that is far less toxic than that necessary for adults.

Once leukemia has recurred ("relapsed") after initial chemotherapy, bone marrow transplantation (BMT) is the only curative option. Allogenic BMT can be used for those under age 55 with histocompatible sibling donors and is successful in 30–40% of cases. Autologous BMT may be curative in 30–50% of cases after a second remission is achieved.

Horowitz MM et al: Chemotherapy compared with bone marrow transplantation for adults with acute lymphoblastic leukemia in first remission. Ann Intern Med 1991;115:13.

Linker CA et al: Treatment of adult acute lymphoblastic leukemia with intensive cyclical chemotherapy: A follow-up report. Blood 1991;78:2814.

Linker CA: Treatment of acute leukemia in adults. Curr Opin Oncol 1992;4:53.

Phillips GL et al: High dose cytarabine and daunorubicin induction and post remission chemotherapy for the treatment of acute myelogenous leukemia in adults. Blood 1991;77:1429.

Schiller GJ et al: Bone marrow transplantation vs high dose cytarabine based consolidation chemotherapy for acute myelogenous leukemia in first remission. J Clin Oncol 1992;10:41.

CHRONIC LYMPHOCYTIC LEUKEMIA

Essentials of Diagnosis

- Lymphocytosis > 15,000/μL.
- "Mature" appearance of lymphocytes.

General Considerations

Chronic lymphocytic leukemia (CLL) is a clonal malignancy of B lymphocytes (rarely T lymphocytes). The disease is usually indolent, with slowly progressive accumulation of long-lived small lymphocytes. These cells are immunoincompetent and respond poorly to antigenic stimulation.

Chronic lymphocytic leukemia is manifested clinically by immunosuppression, bone marrow failure, and organ infiltration with lymphocytes. Immunosuppression, bone marrow failure, and infiltration of organs account for most clinical manifestation. Immunodeficiency is also related to inadequate antibody production by the abnormal B cells. With advanced disease, chronic lymphocytic leukemia may cause damage by direct tissue infiltration.

Clinical Findings

A. Symptoms and Signs: Chronic lymphocytic leukemia is a disease of the elderly, with 90% of cases occurring after age 50 and a median age at presentation of 65. Many patients will be incidentally discovered to have lymphocytosis. Others present with fatigue or lymphadenopathy. On examination, 80% of patients will have lymphadenopathy and half will have enlargement of the liver or spleen.

A prognostically useful staging system has been developed as follows: stage 0, lymphocytosis only; stage I, lymphocytosis plus lymphadenopathy; stage II, organomegaly; stage III, anemia; stage IV, thrombocytopenia.

Chronic lymphocytic leukemia usually pursues an indolent course but occasionally will present as a rapidly progressive disease. These patients usually have larger, less mature-appearing lymphocytes and are said to have "prolymphocytic" leukemia. In 5–10% of cases, chronic lymphocytic leukemia may be complicated by autoimmune hemolytic anemia or autoimmune thrombocytopenia. In approximately 5% of cases, while the systemic disease remains stable, an isolated lymph node will be transformed into an aggressive large cell lymphoma (Richter's syndrome).

B. Laboratory Findings: The hallmark of chronic lymphocytic leukemia is isolated lymphocytosis. The white blood count is usually greater than 20,000/μL and may be markedly elevated. Usually 75–98% of the circulating cells are lymphocytes. Lymphocytes appear small and "mature," with condensed nuclear chromatin, and are morphologically indistinguishable from normal small lymphocytes. The hematocrit and platelet count are usually normal at presentation. The bone marrow is variably infiltrated with small lymphocytes. The malignant cells weakly express surface immunoglobulin, and the monoclonal nature of the cells can be demonstrated by the finding of a single light chain type on the surface. The immunophenotype of CLL is unique in that it co-expresses B lymphocyte lineage markers such as CD19 with the T lymphocyte marker CD5. Other B cell malignancies do not express CD5.

Hypogammaglobulinemia is present in half of cases and becomes more common with advanced disease. In some instances, a small amount of IgM paraprotein is present in the serum. Pathologic changes in lymph nodes are the same as in diffuse small cell lymphocytic lymphoma.

Differential Diagnosis

Few syndromes can be confused with chronic lymphocytic leukemia. Viral infections producing lymphocytosis should be obvious from the presence of fever and other clinical findings. Other lymphoproliferative diseases such as Waldenström's macroglobulinemia, hairy cell leukemia, or lymphoma in the leukemic phase are distinguished on the basis of the morphology of circulating lymphocytes and bone marrow.

Treatment

Most cases of early indolent chronic lymphocytic leukemia require no specific therapy. Indications for treatment include progressive fatigue, troublesome lymphadenopathy, or the development of anemia or thrombocytopenia. These patients have either symptomatic and progressive stage II disease or stage III/IV disease. Initial therapy includes chlorambucil and prednisone. A common regimen is chlorambucil, 0.6–1 mg/kg, in combination with 4 days of prednisone every 3 weeks. Complications such as autoimmune hemolytic anemia or immune thrombocytopenia may be treated with high-dose prednisone but often require splenectomy for control. Fludarabine is a promising new agent which is useful in treating disease refractory to other agents. Whether fludarabine is superior to chlorambucil as initial therapy is currently being evaluated. Long-term side effects of fludarabine remain to be defined.

Prognosis

Median survival is approximately 6 years, and 25% of patients live more than 10 years. Patients with stage 0 or I disease have a median survival of 10 years. It is important to reassure these patients that despite the frightening diagnosis of "leukemia" they can live a normal life for many years. Patients with stage III or IV disease have a median survival of less than 2 years. Chronic lymphocytic leukemia is managed in palliative fashion. Patients with advanced disease benefit only briefly from intensive therapy.

Digheiro G et al: B-cell chronic lymphocytic leukemia: Present status and future directions. Blood 1991; 78:1901.

Foon KA, Rai KR, Gale RP: Chronic lymphocytic leukemia: New insights into biology and therapy. Ann Intern Med 1990;113:525.

French Cooperative Group on Chronic Lymphocytic Leukemia: Effects of chlorambucil and therapeutic decision in initial forms of chronic lymphocytic leukemia (stage A): Results of a randomized clinical trial on 612 patients. Blood 1990;75:1414.

HAIRY CELL LEUKEMIA

Essentials of Diagnosis

- Pancytopenia.
- Splenomegaly, often massive.
- Hairy cells present on blood smear and bone marrow biopsy.

General Considerations

Hairy cell leukemia, an uncommon form of leukemia, is an indolent cancer of B lymphocytes.

Clinical Findings

A. Symptoms and Signs: The disease characteristically presents in middle-aged men. The median age at presentation is 55 years, and there is a striking 5:1 male predominance. Most patients present with gradual onset of fatigue, but others complain of symptoms related to markedly enlarged spleen and still others come to attention because of infection.

On physical examination, splenomegaly is almost invariably present and may be massive. The liver is enlarged in half of cases, but lymphadenopathy is uncommon.

B. Laboratory Findings: The hallmark of hairy cell leukemia is pancytopenia. Anemia is nearly universal, and 75% of patients have thrombocytopenia and neutropenia as well. Nearly all patients have striking monocytopenia, which is encountered in almost no other condition. The "hairy cells" are usually present in small numbers on the peripheral blood smear and have a characteristic appearance with numerous cytoplasmic projections. Less commonly, a "leukemic form" of the disorder exists in which large numbers of hairy cells dominate the peripheral blood smear. The bone marrow is usually inaspirable (dry tap), and the diagnosis is made by characteristic morphology on bone marrow biopsy. The hairy cells have a characteristic histochemical staining pattern, with tartrate-resistant acid phosphatase (TRAP). On immunophenotyping, the cells co-express the antigens CD11c and CD22. Pathologic examination of the spleen shows marked infiltration of the red pulp with hairy cells. This is in marked contrast to the usual predilection of lymphomas to involve the white pulp of the spleen.

Hairy cell leukemia is usually an indolent disorder whose course is dominated by pancytopenia and recurrent infections, including mycobacterial infections.

Differential Diagnosis

Hairy cell leukemia should be distinguished from other lymphoproliferative diseases such as Waldenström's macroglobulinemia and non-Hodgkin's lymphomas. It also may be confused with other causes of pancytopenia, including hypersplenism due to any cause or paroxysmal nocturnal hemoglobinuria.

Treatment

The treatment of hairy cell leukemia has been dramatically changed by the development of new effective agents. The treatment of choice is with cladribine (2-chlorodeoxyadenosine; CdA). This is a relatively nontoxic drug that produces benefit in 95% of cases and complete remission in more than 80%. Responses are long-lasting, with few patients relapsing in the first few years. Another useful agent is deoxycoformycin. Interferon and splenectomy are rarely used now.

Course & Prognosis

The development of new effective therapies (inter-feron and deoxycoformycin) appears to have changed the prognosis of this disease. Formerly, median survival was 6 years, and only one-third of patients survived longer than 10 years. Although longer follow-up will be required, it now appears that most patients with hairy cell leukemia will live longer than 10 years. With current trends in treatment, the prognosis appears open-ended at this time.

Piro LD: 2-Chlorodeoxyadenosine treatment of lymphoid malignancies. (Editorial.) Blood 1992;79:843.

Saven A, Piro LD: Treatment of hairy cell leukemia. Blood 1992;79:1111.

LYMPHOMAS

NON-HODGKIN'S LYMPHOMAS

The non-Hodgkin's lymphomas are a heterogeneous group of cancers of lymphocytes. The disorders are variable in clinical presentation and course, varying from indolent disease to rapidly progressive devastating illnesses.

Results of studies using techniques of molecular biology have provided clues to the pathogenesis of these disorders. The best-studied example is Burkitt's lymphoma, in which a characteristic cytogenetic abnormality of translocation between the long arms of chromosomes 8 and 14 has been identified. The proto-oncogene c-*myc* is translocated from its normal position on chromosome 8 to the heavy chain locus on chromosome 14. Cells committed to B cell differentiation are likely to have enhanced expression of this heavy chain locus, and it is likely that overexpression of c-*myc* (in its new anomalous position) is related to malignant transformation. In the follicular lymphomas, translocations of a possible oncogene *bcl*-2 from chromosome 8 to the heavy chain locus on chromosome 14 may play a similar role.

Classification of the lymphomas is a controversial area still undergoing evolution. Recently, the National Cancer Institute has sponsored a "working formulation" that characterizes these lymphomas according to their biologic behavior, whether indolent or aggressive (Table 13–16).

Clinical Findings

A. Symptoms and Signs: Patients with indolent lymphomas usually present with painless lymphadenopathy, which may be isolated or widespread. Involved lymph nodes may be present in the retroperitoneum, mesentery, and pelvis. However, the indolent lymphomas are often disseminated at the

Table 13–16. Classification of lymphomas; "working formulation."

Low-grade
  Small lymphocytic
  Small lymphocytic, plasmacytoid
  Follicular, small cleaved cell
  Follicular mixed cell
Intermediate-grade
  Follicular large cell
  Diffuse small cleaved cell
  Diffuse mixed cell
  Diffuse large cell
High-grade
  Immunoblastic
  Small noncleaved (Burkitt's)
  Small noncleaved (non-Burkitt's)
  Lymphoblastic
  True histiocytic
Other
  Cutaneous T cell (mycosis fungoides)
  Adult T cell leukemia/lymphoma
  T γ lymphocytosis

time of diagnosis, and bone marrow involvement is frequent.

Patients with high-grade lymphomas may present with adenopathy or with constitutional symptoms such as fever, drenching night sweats, or weight loss. On examination, lymphadenopathy may be isolated, or extranodal sites of disease (skin, gastrointestinal tract) may be found. Patients with Burkitt's lymphoma frequently present with abdominal pain or abdominal fullness because of the predilection of the disease for the abdomen. Patients with HIV disease also have an increased incidence of non-Hodgkin's lymphoma; it may be isolated to the central nervous system in such individuals.

Once a pathologic diagnosis is established, the patient should be staged. Physical examination is supplemented by chest x-ray and CT scan of the abdomen and pelvis. The bone marrow should be biopsied, and—in selected cases such as high-risk morphology—a lumbar puncture should be performed.

B. Laboratory Findings: The peripheral blood is usually normal, but a number of lymphomas may present in a "leukemic" phase. In these situations, the distinction between leukemia and lymphoma is arbitrary, as the malignant cell has the same characteristics. Examples of the diseases that may present as lymphoma or leukemia are small cell lymphoma (chronic lymphocytic leukemia), small cell plasmacytic lymphoma (Waldenström's macroglobulinemia), follicular small cleaved cell lymphoma (lymphosarcoma cell leukemia), cutaneous T cell lymphoma (Sézary syndrome), lymphoblastic lymphoma (T cell acute lymphoblastic leukemia), and Burkitt's lymphoma (B cell acute lymphoblastic leukemia).

Bone marrow involvement is usually manifested as paratrabecular lymphoid aggregates. In some high-grade lymphomas, the meninges may be involved and the spinal fluid may contain malignant cells. The chest radiograph may show a mediastinal mass in lymphoblastic lymphoma.

The serum LDH level is useful in evaluating the extent of disease and the aggressiveness of tumor behavior, with higher levels indicating more widespread disease.

The diagnosis of lymphoma is made by tissue biopsy. Needle aspiration may yield suspicious results, but usually a lymph node biopsy (or biopsy of involved extranodal tissue) is required.

Treatment

The indolent lymphomas are usually not curable and are approached with palliative therapy. If patients are asymptomatic, no initial treatment may be necessary. However, in 1–3 years, the disease will usually progress and require treatment. Treatment decisions are individualized depending on the patient's age and performance status and the extent of disease. Initial therapy is based on the alkylating agents. Appropriate regimens include chlorambucil, 0.6–1 mg/kg every 3 weeks, or combination therapy with cyclophosphamide, vincristine, and prednisone (CVP). Patients with more aggressive or resistant disease may require more intensive therapy. Those with apparently localized disease may be treated initially with local radiation.

Patients with high-grade lymphomas should be treated with curative intent. Irradiation is occasionally used for localized disease (supplemented by brief intensive chemotherapy), but the mainstay of therapy is combination chemotherapy. The traditional treatment regimen has been cyclophosphamide, doxorubicin, vincristine, and prednisone (CHOP). It remains to be proved that newer and more intensive regimens produce superior results. For patients with high-risk aggressive lymphomas, autologous bone marrow transplant may increase the likelihood of cure.

Patients who relapse following initial response have been successfully treated with intensive chemotherapy and autologous bone marrow transplantation.

Prognosis

The median survival of patients with indolent lymphomas is 6–8 years. These diseases ultimately become refractory to chemotherapy. This often occurs at the time of histologic progression of the disease to a more aggressive form of lymphoma. The prognosis of patients with high-grade lymphomas depends on their response to chemotherapy. Depending on the initial pathologic subtype and initial bulk of disease, these patients are variably curable.

With appropriate therapy, approximately 50% of patients with disseminated large-cell lymphomas may be cured. Results are better in those who are young, are in good clinical, condition, and have less advanced stages of disease. Salvage therapy with autologous bone marrow transplantation may be effective in 50% of cases if the disease is still responsive to chemotherapy and the patient comes to transplant in good condition and with minimal tumor bulk.

Coiffier B et al: Prognostic factors in aggressive malignant lymphomas: Description and validation of prognostic index that could identify patients requiring more intensive therapy. J Clin Oncol 1991;9:211.

Hoskins PJ et al: Prognostic variables in patients with diffuse large cell lymphoma treated with MACOP-B. J Clin Oncol 1991;9:220.

HODGKIN'S DISEASE

Essentials of Diagnosis
- Painless lymphadenopathy.
- Constitutional symptoms may be present.
- Pathologic diagnosis by lymph node biopsy.

General Considerations
Hodgkin's disease is a group of cancers characterized by Reed-Sternberg cells in an appropriate reactive cellular background. The nature of the malignant cell is a subject of controversy, but recent evidence suggests that it is of macrophage origin.

Clinical Findings
There is a bimodal age distribution, with one peak in the 20s and a second peak over age 50. Most patients present because of a painless mass, commonly in the neck. Others may seek medical attention because of constitutional symptoms such as fever, weight loss, or drenching night sweats, or because of generalized pruritus. An unusual symptom of Hodgkin's disease is pain in an involved lymph node following alcohol ingestion.

An important clinical feature of Hodgkin's disease is its tendency to arise within lymph node areas and to spread in an orderly fashion to contiguous areas of lymph nodes. Only late in the course of the disease will vascular invasion lead to widespread hematogenous dissemination.

The diagnosis is made by examination of lymph node tissue by an experienced hematopathologist. Hodgkin's disease is divided into several subtypes: lymphocyte predominance, nodular sclerosis, mixed cellularity, and lymphocyte depletion. Hodgkin's disease should be distinguished pathologically from other malignant lymphomas. It may also occasionally be confused with reactive lymph nodes seen in infectious mononucleosis, cat-scratch disease, or drug reactions (phenytoin).

Patients should initially undergo a "staging" evaluation to determine the extent of disease. The purpose of this evaluation is to determine whether localized treatment (radiotherapy) is indicated or if systemic chemotherapy must be given. The staging nomenclature is as follows: stage I, one lymph node region involved; stage II, involvement of two lymph node areas on one side of the diaphragm; stage III, lymph node region involved on both sides of the diaphragm; stage IV, disseminated disease with bone marrow or liver involvement. In addition, patients are designated stage A if they lack constitutional symptoms and stage B if significant weight loss, fever, or night sweats are present.

Treatment
Patients with localized disease (stages IA, IIA) are treated with radiation therapy. Patients with disseminated disease (IIIB, IV) are treated with aggressive combination chemotherapy. The treatment of choice appears to be Adriamycin (doxorubicin), bleomycin, vincristine, dacarbazine (ABVD) or ABVD alternating with mechlorethamine, Oncovin (vincristine), procarbazine, and prednisone (MOPP). The optimal management of patients with stages IIB or IIIA is controversial, but current evidence suggests an advantage to combination chemotherapy.

Prognosis
Virtually all patients with both localized and disseminated disease should be treated with curative intent. The prognosis of patients with stage IA or IIA disease treated by radiotherapy is excellent, with 10-year survival rates in excess of 80%. Patients with disseminated disease (IIIB, IV) have 5-year survival rates of (50–60%. Poorer results are seen in patients who are elderly, those who have bulky disease, and those with lymphocyte depletion or mixed cellularity on histologic examination. Patients whose disease recurs after initial radiotherapy treatment may still be curable with chemotherapy. Patients who relapse after initial chemotherapy may be cured with intensive therapy involving autologous bone marrow transplantation. Cure rates of 40–60% are seen in those who are still responsive to chemotherapy.

Armitage JO et al: Autologous bone marrow transplantation for patients with relapsed Hodgkin's disease. Am J Med 1991;91:605.

Longo DL et al: Radiation therapy vs combination chemotherapy in the treatment of early stage Hodgkin's disease: Seven year results of a prospective randomized trial. J Clin Oncol 1991;9:906.

Urba WJ, Longo DL: Hodgkin's disease. N Engl J Med 1992;326:678.

MULTIPLE MYELOMA

Essentials of Diagnosis
- Bone pain, often in the lower back.
- Monoclonal paraprotein by serum or urine protein electrophoresis or immunoelectrophoresis.

- Replacement of bone marrow by malignant plasma cells.

General Considerations

Multiple myeloma is a malignancy of plasma cells characterized by replacement of the bone marrow, bone destruction, and paraprotein formation. Myeloma is a complex disease that causes clinical signs and symptoms through a variety of mechanisms.

Replacement of the bone marrow (and perhaps humoral suppression of myelopoiesis) leads initially to anemia and later to general bone marrow failure. Bone destruction causes bone pain, osteoporosis, lytic lesions, and pathologic fractures. Hypercalcemia is common and appears to be mediated by osteoclast activating factor (OAF) or similar lymphokines. The malignant plasma cells can form tumors (plasmacytomas) that have a predilection for causing spinal cord compression.

The paraproteins secreted by the malignant plasma cells may cause problems in their own right. Very high paraprotein levels (either IgG or IgA) may cause the hyperviscosity syndrome, though this is more often caused by IgM in Waldenström's macroglobulinemia. The light chain component of the immunoglobulin may cause renal failure (often aggravated by hypercalcemia). Light chain components may be deposited in tissues as amyloid, worsening renal failure and causing a vast array of systemic symptoms.

Myeloma patients are prone to recurrent infections for a number of reasons, including neutropenia and the immunosuppressive effects of chemotherapy. Additionally, there is a failure of antibody production in response to antigen challenge, and myeloma patients are especially prone to infections with encapsulated organisms such as *Streptococcus pneumoniae* and *Haemophilus influenzae*.

Clinical Findings

A. Symptoms and Signs: Myeloma is a disease of older adults (median age at presentation, 60 years). The most common presenting complaints are those related to anemia, bone pain, and infection. Bone pain is most common in the back or ribs or may present as a pathologic fracture, especially of the femoral neck. Patients may also come to medical attention because of renal failure; spinal cord compression, or the hyperviscosity syndrome (mucosal bleeding, vertigo, nausea, visual disturbances, alterations in mental status). Occasionally, patients are diagnosed as having myeloma because of initial laboratory findings of hypercalcemia, proteinuria, elevated sedimentation rate, or abnormalities on serum protein electrophoresis.

Examination may reveal pallor, bone tenderness, and soft tissue masses. Patients may have neurologic signs related to neuropathy or spinal cord compression. Patients with amyloidosis may have an enlarged tongue, neuropathy, or congestive heart failure.

B. Laboratory Findings: Anemia is nearly universal. Red blood cell morphology is normal, but rouleau formation is common and may be marked. The neutrophil and platelet counts are usually normal at presentation. Only rarely will plasma cells be visible on peripheral smear (plasma cell leukemia).

The hallmark of myeloma is the finding of a paraprotein on serum protein electrophoresis (SPEP). The majority of patients will have a monoclonal spike visible in the beta or gamma globulin region. Immunoelectrophoresis (IEP) will reveal this to be a monoclonal protein. Approximately 15% of patients will have no demonstrable paraprotein in the serum. In these, IEP of the urine will reveal either complete immunoglobulin or light chains. Overall, approximately 60% of myeloma patients will have an IgG paraprotein, 25% an IgA, and 15% light chains only.

The bone marrow will be infiltrated by variable numbers of plasma cells ranging from 5% to 100%. Occasionally, the plasma cells may be morphologically indistinguishable from normal cells but more commonly will appear abnormal. Bone radiographs are important in establishing the diagnosis of myeloma. Lytic lesions are most commonly seen in the axial skeleton: skull, spine, proximal long bones, and ribs. At other times, only generalized osteoporosis is seen. The radionuclide bone scan is not useful in detecting bone lesions in myeloma, as there is usually no osteoblastic component.

Other laboratory features include hypercalcemia, renal failure, and an elevated erythrocyte sedimentation rate. Some patients have proximal renal tubular acidosis, with phosphaturia, glucosuria, and uricosuria. The urinalysis may reveal proteinuria, but the dipstick test (which detects primarily albumin) is unreliable for light chains. Often there is a narrow anion gap when the paraprotein is cationic. On occasion, the abnormal protein is cryoprecipitatable, resulting in positive studies for cryoglobulins.

Differential Diagnosis

When a patient is discovered to have a monoclonal paraprotein, the distinction between myeloma and benign monoclonal gammopathy must be made. Benign monoclonal gammopathy is present in 1% of all adults and 3% of adults over age 70. Thus, if one considers all patients with paraproteins, benign monoclonal gammopathy is far more common than myeloma. Most commonly, patients with benign monoclonal gammopathy will have a monoclonal IgG spike less than 2.5 g/dL, and the height of the spike remains stable. In approximately 25% of cases, benign monoclonal gammopathy progresses to overt malignant disease, but this may take years or even decades.

Myeloma is distinguished from benign monoclonal gammopathy by findings of replacement of the bone marrow, bone destruction, and progression over time. Although the height of the paraprotein spike should not be used by itself to distinguish benign from malignant disease, in practice all patients with IgG spikes greater than 3.5 g/dL prove to have myeloma. An IgA spike of greater than 2 g/dL is almost always due to myeloma. If there is doubt about whether paraproteinemia is benign or malignant, the patient should be observed without therapy, since there is no advantage to early treatment of asymptomatic multiple myeloma.

Myeloma should be distinguished from polyclonal hypergammaglobulinemia seen in reactive conditions. The distinction is made by finding the polyclonal as opposed to the monoclonal spike. Myeloma may also need to be distinguished from other malignant lymphoproliferative diseases such as Waldenström's macroglobulinemia, lymphomas, and primary amyloidosis.

Treatment

The goal of treatment of myeloma is usually palliation. Patients with minimal disease or in whom the diagnosis of malignancy is in doubt should be observed without treatment. Most commonly, patients require treatment at diagnosis because of bone pain or other symptoms related to the disease. In the past, standard therapy has been melphalan plus prednisone; more recently, combination chemotherapy with alkylating agents has been used. The optimal chemotherapy regimen has not been determined. The height of the paraprotein spike on SPEP is a useful marker for monitoring response to therapy. Patients who fail to respond to standard therapy may be effectively salvaged with low-dose continuous infusion therapy, the VAD (vincristine, Adriamycin [doxorubicin], dexamethasone) regimen.

A number of other ancillary measures are important in the treatment of myeloma. Localized radiotherapy may be useful for palliation of bone pain or for eradicating tumor at the site of pathologic fracture. Hypercalcemia should be treated aggressively and prolonged immobilization and dehydration avoided.

The only proved curative treatment for myeloma is allogeneic bone marrow transplantation. This can be offered to only a small fraction of myeloma patients because of the requirement for age under 55 years and a matched sibling donor. Autologous bone marrow transplantation is a promising treatment that can produce long disease-free and treatment-free survival times; its ultimate role is under study.

Prognosis

The median survival of patients with myelomas is 3 years. The prognosis is markedly affected by a number of prognostic features, with shorter survivals in those with high paraprotein spikes, renal failure, hypercalcemia, or extensive bony disease. Patients are said to have a "low tumor burden" if the IgG spike is less than 5 g/dL and there is no more than one lytic bone lesion and no evidence of severe anemia,

hypercalcemia, or renal failure. These patients have a median survival of 5–6 years. Conversely, patients with a "high tumor burden" have an IgG spike greater than 7 g/dL, hematocrit less than 25%, calcium greater than 12 mg/dL, or more than three lytic bone lesions. Median survival for this group is approximately 1 year.

Attal M et al: Intensive combined therapy for previously untreated aggressive myeloma. Blood 1992;79:1130.
Gregory WM, Richards MA, Malpas JS: Combination chemotherapy vs melphalan and prednisone in the treatment of multiple myeloma: An overview of published trials. J Clin Oncol 1992;10:334.
Mandelli F, Avvisati G, Tribalto M: Biology and treatment of multiple myeloma. Curr Opin Oncol 1992;4:73.

WALDENSTRÖM'S MACROGLOBULINEMIA

Essentials of Diagnosis

- Symptoms nonspecific: splenomegaly common on examination.
- Monoclonal IgM paraprotein.
- Infiltration of bone marrow by plasmacytic lymphocyte.
- Absence of lytic bone disease.

General Considerations

Waldenström's macroglobulinemia is a malignant disease of B cells that appear to be a hybrid of lymphocytes and plasma cells. These cells characteristically secrete an IgM paraprotein, and many clinical manifestations of the disease are related to this macroglobulin.

Clinical Findings

A. Symptoms and Signs: This disease characteristically presents insidiously in patients in their 60s or 70s. Patients usually present with fatigue related to anemia. Hyperviscosity of serum may be manifested in a number of ways. Mucosal and gastrointestinal bleeding is related to engorged blood vessels and platelet dysfunction. Other complaints include nausea, vertigo, and visual disturbances. Alterations in consciousness vary from mild lethargy to stupor and coma. The IgM paraprotein may also cause symptoms of cold agglutinin disease or peripheral neuropathy.

On examination, there may be hepatosplenomegaly or lymphadenopathy. The retinal veins are characteristically engorged. Purpura may be present. There should be no bone tenderness.

B. Laboratory Findings: Anemia is nearly universal, and rouleau formation is common. The anemia is related in part to expansion of the plasma volume by 50–100% due to the presence of the paraprotein. Other blood counts are usually normal. The abnormal plasmacytic lymphocyte usually appears in small numbers on the peripheral blood smear. The bone marrow is characteristically infiltrated by the plasmacytic lymphocytes.

The hallmark of macroglobulinemia is the presence of a monoclonal IgM spike seen on serum protein electrophoresis (SPEP) in the beta or gamma globulin region. The serum viscosity is usually increased above the normal of 1.4–1.8 times that of water. Symptoms of hyperviscosity usually develop when the serum viscosity is over four times that of water, and marked symptoms usually arise when the viscosity is over six times that of water. Because paraproteins vary in their physicochemical properties, there is no strict correlation between the concentration of paraprotein and serum viscosity. However, after a certain threshold, viscosity rises exponentially with small increments in paraprotein amounts.

The IgM paraprotein may cause a positive Coombs test or have cold agglutinin or cryoglobulin properties. If one suspects macroglobulinemia but the SPEP shows only hypogammaglobulinemia, one should repeat the test while taking special measures to maintain the blood at 37 °C, since the paraprotein may precipitate out at room temperature.

Bone radiographs are normal, and there is no evidence of renal failure.

Differential Diagnosis

Waldenström's macroglobulinemia is differentiated from benign monoclonal gammopathy by the finding of bone marrow infiltration. It is differentiated from chronic lymphocytic leukemia and multiple myeloma by bone marrow morphology and the finding of the characteristic IgM spike, and also on clinical grounds.

Treatment

Patients who present with marked hyperviscosity syndrome (stupor or coma) should be treated on an emergency basis with plasmapheresis. Pheresis will usually rapidly reduce the paraprotein level below the threshold required to produce symptoms. On a chronic basis, some patients can be managed with periodic plasmapheresis alone. Others are treated with intermittent chemotherapy with chlorambucil or cyclophosphamide. New agents such as fludarabine and cladribine have produced encouraging results.

Prognosis

Waldenström's macroglobulinemia is an indolent disease with a median survival rate of 3–5 years. However, patients may survive 10 years or longer.

Kantarjian HM et al: Fludarabine therapy in macroglobulinemic lymphoma. Blood 1990;75:1928.

DISORDERS OF HEMOSTASIS

Disorders of hemostasis may be due to defects in either platelet number or function or to problems in formation of a fibrin clot (coagulation). Bleeding due to platelet disorders is typically mucosal or skin bleeding. Common problems include epistaxis, gum bleeding, menorrhagia, gastrointestinal bleeding, purpura, and petechiae. Petechiae are seen almost exclusively in conditions of thrombocytopenia and not platelet dysfunction. Bleeding due to coagulopathy may occur as deep muscle hematomas as well as skin bleeding. Spontaneous hemarthroses are seen only in severe hemophilia.

IDIOPATHIC (AUTOIMMUNE) THROMBOCYTOPENIC PURPURA

Essentials of Diagnosis

- Isolated thrombocytopenia.
- Other hematopoietic cell lines normal.
- No systemic illness.
- Spleen not palpable.
- Normal bone marrow with normal or increased megakaryocytes.

General Considerations

Idiopathic thrombocytopenic purpura is an autoimmune disorder in which an IgG autoantibody is formed that binds to platelets. It is not clear which antigen on the platelet surface is involved. Although the antiplatelet antibody may bind complement, platelets are not destroyed by direct lysis. Rather, destruction takes place in the spleen, where splenic macrophages with Fc receptors bind to antibody-coated platelets. Since the spleen is the major site both of antibody production and platelet sequestration, splenectomy is highly effective.

Clinical Findings

A. Symptoms and Signs: Idiopathic thrombocytopenic purpura occurs commonly in childhood, frequently precipitated by viral infection and usually self-limited. In contrast, the adult form is usually a chronic disease and only infrequently follows a viral infection. It is a disease of young persons, with peak incidence between ages 20 and 50, and there is a 2:1 female predominance.

Patients are systemically well and not febrile. The presenting complaint is mucosal or skin bleeding. Common types of bleeding are epistaxis, oral bleeding, menorrhagia, purpura, and petechiae.

On examination, the patient appears well, and there are no abnormal findings other than those related to bleeding. An enlarged spleen should lead one to doubt the diagnosis. Common signs of bleeding are purpura, petechiae, and hemorrhagic bullae in the mouth.

B. Laboratory Findings: The hallmark of the disease is thrombocytopenia, which may be less than $10,000/\mu L$. Other counts are usually normal except for occasional mild anemia, which can be explained by bleeding or associated hemolysis. Peripheral blood cell morphology is normal except that platelets are slightly enlarged (megathrombocytes). These larger platelets are young platelets produced in response to enhanced platelet destruction. Approximately 10% of patients will have coexistent autoimmune hemolytic anemia, and in these cases one will see anemia, reticulocytosis, and spherocytes on peripheral smear. Red blood cell fragmentation should not be seen.

The bone marrow will appear normal, with a normal or increased number of megakaryocytes. Coagulation studies will be entirely normal. Tests now available to quantitate platelet-associated IgG may help in the diagnosis. At present, although these tests are highly sensitive (95%), they are very nonspecific, and 50% of all patients with thrombocytopenia from any cause may have increased levels of IgG on the platelet.

Differential Diagnosis

Thrombocytopenia may be produced either by abnormal bone marrow function or by peripheral destruction (Table 13–17). Although most bone marrow disorders produce abnormalities in addition to isolated thrombocytopenia, diagnoses such as myelodysplasia can only be excluded by examining the bone marrow. Most causes of thrombocytopenia resulting from peripheral destruction can be ruled out by initial evaluation. Disorders such as disseminated intravascular coagulation, thrombotic thrombocytopenic purpura, hemolytic-uremic syndrome, hyper-

Table 13–17. Causes of thrombocytopenia.

Bone marrow disorders
  Aplastic anemia
  Hematologic malignancies
  Myelodysplasia
  Megaloblastic anemia
  Chronic alcoholism
Nonmarrow disorders
  Immune disorders
    Idiopathic thrombocytopenic purpura
    Drug-induced
    Secondary
    Posttransfusion purpura
  Hypersplenism
  Disseminated intravascular coagulation
  Thrombotic thrombocytopenic purpura
  Hemolytic-uremic syndrome
  Sepsis
  Hemangiomas
  Viral infection, AIDS

splenism, and sepsis are easily excluded by the absence of systemic illness. Thus, patients with isolated thrombocytopenia with no other abnormal findings almost certainly have immune thrombocytopenia. Patients should be questioned regarding drug use, especially sulfonamides, quinidine, quinine, thiazides, cimetidine, gold, and heparin. Heparin is now the most common cause of drug-induced thrombocytopenia in hospitalized patients. Systemic lupus erythematosus and chronic lymphocytic leukemia are common causes of secondary idiopathic thrombocytopenic purpura.

Treatment

Few adults with idiopathic thrombocytopenic purpura will have spontaneous remissions, and most will require treatment. Initial treatment is with prednisone, 1–2 mg/kg/d. Prednisone works primarily by decreasing the affinity of splenic macrophages for antibody-coated platelets. High-dose prednisone therapy also reduces the binding of antibody to the platelet surface, and long-term therapy may decrease antibody production. Bleeding will often diminish within 1 day after beginning prednisone—even before the platelet count begins to rise. This effect has been attributed to enhanced vascular stability. The platelet count will usually begin to rise within a week, and responses are almost always seen within 3 weeks. About 80% of patients will respond, and the platelet count will usually return to normal. High-dose therapy should be continued until the platelet count is normal, and the dose should then be gradually tapered. In most patients, thrombocytopenia will recur if prednisone is completely withdrawn, and one aims to find a low prednisone dose that will maintain an adequate platelet count. It is not necessary for the platelet count to be entirely normal; the risk of bleeding is small with platelet counts above $50,000/\mu L$.

Splenectomy is the most definitive treatment for idiopathic thrombocytopenic purpura, and most adult patients will ultimately undergo splenectomy. High-dose prednisone therapy should not be continued indefinitely in an attempt to avoid surgery. Splenectomy is indicated if patients do not respond to prednisone initially or require unacceptably high doses to maintain an adequate platelet count. Other patients may be intolerant of prednisone or may simply prefer the surgical alternative. Splenectomy can be performed safely even with platelet counts less than $10,000/\mu L$. Approximately 80% of patients benefit from splenectomy with either complete or partial remission.

High-dose intravenous immunoglobulin, 400 mg/kg/d for 3–5 days, is highly effective in rapidly raising the platelet count. The response rate is approximately 90%, and the platelet count rises within 1–5 days. However, this treatment is very expensive (approximately $5000), and the beneficial effect lasts only 1–2 weeks. Immunoglobulin treatment should be reserved for emergency situations such as preparing a severely thrombocytopenic patient for surgery.

For patients who fail to respond to prednisone and splenectomy, danazol, 600 mg/d, has been used, with responses obtained in about half of cases. Immunosuppressive agents employed in refractory cases include vincristine, vinblastine infusions, azathioprine, and cyclophosphamide. In using any of these more toxic treatments, one must carefully balance the risks against the anticipated benefits.

Platelet transfusions are rarely used in the treatment of idiopathic thrombocytopenic purpura, since exogenous platelets will survive no better than the patient's own platelets and in many cases will survive less than a few hours. Platelet transfusion should be reserved for cases of life-threatening bleeding in which enhanced hemostasis for even an hour may be of benefit.

Prognosis

The prognosis for remission is good. In most cases, the disease is initially controlled with prednisone, and splenectomy offers definitive therapy for most patients. The major concern during the initial phases is cerebral hemorrhage, which becomes a risk when the platelet count is less than 5000/μL. These patients usually exhibit warning signs of mucosal bleeding. However, even at these very low platelet counts, fatal bleeding is rare. Chronic disease that has failed to respond to prednisone and splenectomy has a waxing and waning course over years and usually requires continued management.

Berchtold P, McMillan R: Therapy of chronic idiopathic thrombocytopenic purpura in adults. Blood 1989; 74:2309.
Samuels P et al: Estimation of the risk of thrombocytopenia in the offspring of pregnant women with presumed immune thrombocytopenic purpura. N Engl J Med 1990; 323:229.

THROMBOTIC THROMBOCYTOPENIC PURPURA

Essentials of Diagnosis

- Microangiopathic hemolytic anemia and thrombocytopenia.
- Elevated serum LDH.
- Neurologic abnormalities.
- Fever in the absence of infection.
- Normal coagulation tests.

General Considerations

Thrombotic thrombocytopenic purpura is an uncommon syndrome characterized by the triad of microangiopathic hemolytic anemia, thrombocytopenia, and neurologic abnormalities, as well as fever and renal abnormalities. The cause is unknown. A platelet-agglutinating factor has recently been identified in the plasma of these patients. Its role in pathogenesis remains controversial.

Thrombotic thrombocytopenic purpura is seen primarily in young adults between ages 20 and 50, and there is a slight female predominance. The syndrome is occasionally precipitated by estrogen use or pregnancy, and is increasingly encountered in association with HIV disease.

Clinical Findings

A. Symptoms and Signs: Patients come to medical attention because of anemia, bleeding, or neurologic abnormalities. The neurologic signs and symptoms are unusual in that they may wax and wane over minutes. Neurologic symptoms include headache, confusion, aphasia, and alterations in consciousness from lethargy to coma. With more advanced disease, one may see hemiparesis and seizures.

On examination, the patient appears acutely ill and is usually febrile. One may detect pallor, purpura, petechiae, and signs of neurologic dysfunction. Patients may have abdominal pain and tenderness due to pancreatitis.

B. Laboratory Findings: Anemia is universal and may be extremely severe. There is usually marked reticulocytosis and occasional circulating nucleated red blood cells. The hallmark is a microangiopathic blood picture with fragmented red blood cells (schistocytes, helmet cells, triangle forms) on the smear. One cannot make the diagnosis without significant red blood cell fragmentation. Thrombocytopenia is invariably present and may be severe. White blood cells may show increased band neutrophils.

Hemolysis may be manifested by increasing indirect bilirubin, absent haptoglobin, and occasionally hemoglobinemia and hemoglobinuria. In severe cases, methemalbuminemia may impart a brown color to the plasma. The LDH is usually markedly elevated in proportion to the severity of hemolysis. The Coombs test should be negative.

Coagulation tests (prothrombin time, partial thromboplastin time, fibrinogen) are normal. Elevated fibrin degradation products may be seen, as in other acutely ill patients. Renal insufficiency may be present, and the urinalysis may be abnormal.

Pathologically, one may see the characteristic hyaline thrombus in capillaries and small arteries.

Differential Diagnosis

The normal values of coagulation tests differentiate thrombotic thrombocytopenic purpura from disseminated intravascular coagulation (DIC). Other conditions causing microangiopathic hemolysis (Table 13–18) should be excluded. Evans's syndrome is characterized by the combination of autoimmune

Table 13–18. Causes of microangiopathic hemolytic anemia.

Thrombotic thrombocytopenic purpura
Hemolytic-uremic syndrome
Disseminated intravascular
coagulation
Prosthetic valve hemolysis
Metastatic adenocarcinoma
Malignant hypertension
Vasculitis

thrombocytopenia and autoimmune hemolytic anemia, but the peripheral smear will show spherocytes and not red blood cell fragments. Skin or muscle biopsy is usually not necessary for diagnosis but may be helpful when vasculitis is a consideration. Endocarditis may also closely simulate thrombotic thrombocytopenic purpura.

Treatment

Thrombotic thrombocytopenic purpura should be treated on an emergency basis with large-volume plasmapheresis. Sixty to 80 mL/kg of plasma should be removed and replaced with fresh-frozen plasma. Treatment should be continued daily until the patient is in complete remission. Prednisone and antiplatelet agents (aspirin and dipyridamole) have been used in addition to plasmapheresis, but their role is unclear.

Patients who do not respond to plasmapheresis or who have rapid recurrences require splenectomy. The combination of splenectomy, steroids, and dextran has been used with success.

Prognosis

With the advent of plasmapheresis, the formerly dismal prognosis of thrombotic thrombocytopenic purpura has been dramatically changed. Eighty to 90% of patients now recover completely. Neurologic abnormalities are almost always completely reversed. Most complete responses are durable, but in 10–20% of cases, the disease will be chronic and relapsing.

Shepard KV et al: Thrombotic thrombocytopenic purpura treated with plasmic exchange or exchange transfusions. West J Med 1991;154:410.

HEMOLYTIC-UREMIC SYNDROME

Essentials of Diagnosis

- Microangiopathic hemolytic anemia, thrombocytopenia, and renal failure.
- Elevated serum LDH.
- Normal coagulation tests.
- Absence of neurologic abnormalities.

General Considerations

Hemolytic-uremic syndrome is an uncommon disorder consisting of microangiopathic hemolytic anemia, thrombocytopenia, and renal failure due to

microangiopathy (with decreased glomerular filtration, proteinuria, and hematuria). The cause is unclear. The disease is similar to thrombotic thrombocytopenic purpura except that different vascular beds are involved. The pathogenesis of the two disorders is probably similar, and a platelet-agglutinating factor found in plasma may be involved. In children, hemolytic-uremic syndrome frequently occurs after a diarrheal illness secondary to infections with *Shigella, Salmonella, E coli* strain O157:H7, or viral agents. The mortality rate of this form is low (< 5%). In adults, this syndrome is frequently precipitated by estrogen use or pregnancy (especially postpartum) or occurs as a complication of malignant hypertension or renal transplantation. A familial (hereditary) type has been identified in which members of a family have recurrent episodes over several years.

Clinical Findings

A. Symptoms and Signs: Patients present with anemia, bleeding, or renal failure. The renal failure may or may not be oliguric. In contrast to thrombotic thrombocytopenic purpura, there are no neurologic manifestations other than those due to the uremic state.

B. Laboratory Findings: As in thrombotic thrombocytopenic purpura, there is microangiopathic hemolytic anemia and thrombocytopenia, but the thrombocytopenia is often less severe. The peripheral blood smear should show striking red blood cell fragmentation, and the diagnosis of hemolytic-uremic syndrome is untenable without this finding. The LDH is usually strikingly elevated in proportion to the severity of hemolysis, and the Coombs test is negative. Coagulation tests are normal with the exception of elevated fibrin degradation products.

Renal insufficiency is invariably present, and anuric renal failure requiring dialysis may be seen. Kidney biopsy will show endothelial hyaline thrombi in the afferent arterioles and glomeruli. Ischemic necrosis in the renal cortex may occur with obstruction from intravascular coagulation.

Differential Diagnosis

Disseminated intravascular coagulation is excluded by normal coagulation results. Other causes of microangiopathic hemolytic anemia (Table 13–18) should be considered. Occasionally, vasculitis or acute glomerulonephritis is considered, and in these cases renal biopsy may be necessary to establish the diagnosis if the platelet count will allow it.

Hemolytic-uremic syndrome is arbitrarily distinguished from thrombotic thrombocytopenic purpura by the consistent presence of renal failure and the lack of neurologic findings.

Treatment

In children, hemolytic-uremic syndrome is almost always self-limited and requires only conservative management of acute renal failure. In adults, however, without treatment, there is a high rate of permanent renal insufficiency and death. The treatment of choice (as in thrombotic thrombocytopenic purpura) is large-volume plasmapheresis with fresh-frozen replacement (exchange of up to 80 mL/kg), repeated daily until remission is achieved.

Prognosis

The prognosis of hemolytic-uremic syndrome in adults remains unclear. Without effective therapy, up to 40% of patients have died, and 80% have had chronic renal insufficiency. Early institution of aggressive therapy with plasmapheresis promises to be beneficial. Survival and correction of hematologic abnormalities is the rule, but restoration of renal function requires that treatment be initiated early.

Martin DL et al: The epidemiology and clinical aspects of the hemolytic uremic syndrome in Minnesota. N Engl J Med 1990;323:1161.
Siegler RL: Management of hemolytic uremic syndrome. J Pediatr 1988;112:1014.

CONGENITAL QUALITATIVE PLATELET DISORDERS

Bleeding disorders characterized by prolonged bleeding times despite a normal platelet count are called qualitative platelet disorders. Patients have a positive family history or lifelong personal history of the defect. The disorders may be classified as (1) von Willebrand's disease, a congenital disorder of a plasma protein necessary for platelet adhesion; and (2) congenital disorders intrinsic to the platelet (Table 13–19). When an intrinsic qualitative platelet disorder is suspected, platelet aggregation studies should be evaluated to make a specific diagnosis.

Table 13–19. Qualitative platelet disorders.

Congenital
Glanzmann's thrombasthenia
Bernard-Soulier syndrome
Storage pool disease
Acquired
Myeloproliferative disorders
Uremia
Drugs: Aspirin, anti-inflammatory agents
Autoantibody
Paraproteins
Acquired storage pool
Fibrin degradation products
Von Willebrand's disease

1. VON WILLEBRAND'S DISEASE

Essentials of Diagnosis

- Family history with autosomal dominant pattern of inheritance.
- Prolonged bleeding time, either at baseline or after challenge with aspirin.
- Reduced levels of factor VIII antigen or ristocetin cofactor.
- May have reduced levels of factor VIII coagulant activity.

General Considerations

Von Willebrand's disease is the most common congenital disorder of hemostasis. It is transmitted in an autosomal dominant pattern. It is a group of disorders characterized by deficient or defective von Willebrand factor (vWF), a protein that mediates platelet adhesion. Adhesion is a process separate from platelet aggregation. Platelets adhere to the subendothelium via vWF, which is bound to a specific receptor on the platelet composed of glycoprotein Ib (and missing in Bernard-Soulier syndrome). Platelets aggregate via fibrinogen, which binds to a different receptor composed of glycoproteins IIb and IIIa (deficient in Glanzmann's thrombasthenia). The platelet aggregation system is entirely normal in von Willebrand's disease.

Von Willebrand factor is synthesized in megakaryocytes and endothelial cells and circulates in plasma as multimers of varying size. Only the large multimeric forms are functional in mediating platelet adhesion. Von Willebrand factor has a separate function of binding the factor VIII coagulant protein and protecting it from degradation. The factor VIII coagulant protein (factor VIII:C), a protein encoded by a gene on the X chromosome, is the protein deficient in classic hemophilia. Any of the multimeric forms of vWF can bind and protect factor VIII:C. Von Willebrand's disease, which is primarily a disorder of platelet function, may secondarily cause a coagulation disturbance because of deficient levels of factor VIII:C. However, this coagulopathy is rarely severe.

There are several subtypes of von Willebrand's disease. The most common type (type I, 80% of all cases) is caused by a quantitative decrease in vWF. Type IIa is caused by a qualitative abnormality in protein that prevents multimer formation. Only small multimers are present, and both intermediate and large forms that mediate platelet adhesion are missing. Type IIb von Willebrand's disease is caused by a qualitative abnormality in the protein that causes rapid clearance of the large multimeric forms. Type III von Willebrand's disease is a rare autosomal recessive disorder in which vWF is nearly absent. Pseudo-von Willebrand disease is a rare disorder in which an abnormal platelet membrane has excessive avidity for the large multimeric forms of vWF, causing their clearance from plasma.

Clinical Findings

A. Symptoms and Signs: Von Willebrand's disease is a common disorder affecting both men and women. Most cases are mild. Most bleeding is mucosal (epistaxis, gingival bleeding, menorrhagia), but gastrointestinal bleeding may occur. In most cases, incisional bleeding occurs after surgery or dental extractions. Von Willebrand's disease is rarely as severe as hemophilia, and spontaneous hemarthroses do not occur.

The bleeding tendency is exacerbated by aspirin. Characteristically, bleeding decreases during pregnancy or estrogen use.

B. Laboratory Findings: Platelet number and morphology are normal, and the bleeding time is usually (not always) prolonged. The bleeding time should be ascertained whenever this diagnosis is considered and correlates most closely with the clinical bleeding tendency. When the bleeding time is normal, it is prolonged markedly by aspirin. Normal persons will prolong their bleeding time to a minor extent with aspirin but rarely out of the normal range. In the most common form of von Willebrand's disease (type I), vWF levels in plasma are reduced. This may be measured by factor VIII antigen, which measures the immunologic presence of vWF, or by ristocetin cofactor activity, which measures functional properties of vWF in mediating platelet adhesion.

When factor VIII antigen is reduced, one may also see a decrease in factor VIII coagulant (factor VIII:C) levels. When factor VIII:C levels are less than 25%, the partial thromboplastin time (PTT) will be prolonged. Platelet aggregation studies with standard agonists (ADP, collagen, thrombin) are normal, but platelet aggregation in response to ristocetin is usually subnormal.

In difficult cases, it may be helpful to assay directly the multimeric composition of vWF.

Differential Diagnosis

When patients present with a prolonged bleeding time, one must distinguish von Willebrand's disease from other qualitative platelet disorders (Table 13–19). Acquired qualitative platelet disorders can usually be diagnosed by recent onset of the bleeding tendency and other characteristic clinical features. Congenital intrinsic platelet disorders may present with a positive family history and lifelong history of bleeding episodes. Von Willebrand's disease is diagnosed by the finding of abnormal measurements of vWF and by normal results of platelet aggregation.

When patients present with a prolonged PTT, measurements of factor VIII:C will distinguish von Willebrand's disease from all disorders except hemophilia (Table 13–20). Hemophilia is diagnosed when factor VIII:C is reduced but all measurements of vWF (factor VIII antigen, ristocetin cofactor activity) are normal.

Table 13–20. Causes of prolonged partial thromboplastin time.

Congenital factor deficiencies
Contact factors
Factor XII
Factor XI
Factor IX
Factor VIII
Hemophilia
Von Willebrand's disease
Anticoagulants
Anti-VIII
Lupus
Heparin

Patients with a suspicious bleeding history but with normal bleeding time and PTT pose a diagnostic problem. On occasion, the postaspirin bleeding time can be used to unmask a bleeding disorder. At other times, one must perform further plasma assays of vWF to make the diagnosis. Von Willebrand's disease waxes and wanes in severity and may be difficult to diagnose, especially in a woman taking estrogens (which raise vWF levels).

It is often useful to distinguish between subtypes of von Willebrand's disease (Table 13–21), because only type I usually responds to desmopressin (DDAVP) and because type IIb may be aggravated by its use.

Treatment

The bleeding disorder is characteristically mild, and no treatment is routinely given other than avoidance of aspirin. However, patients often need to be prepared for surgical or dental procedures. The bleeding time is probably the best indicator of the likelihood of bleeding, and prophylactic therapy may be reasonably withheld if the procedure is minor and the bleeding time is normal.

Standard therapy for von Willebrand's disease has been transfusion of plasma cryoprecipitate. Each unit of cryoprecipitate will raise vWF levels approximately 3%, and thus 10–15 units of cryoprecipitate are commonly used to raise vWF levels by 30–50%. Factor VIII antigen levels decline, with a half-life of 12–18 hours, but the duration of corrected bleeding time is usually shorter than this. In some instances the prolonged bleeding time may be completely corrected. Factor VIII coagulant levels may remain elevated for 24–48 hours following cryoprecipitate infusion (unlike the 12–hour half-life of factor VIII:C in classic hemophilia), but these levels are not useful in determining therapy. When replacement therapy is indicated, cryoprecipitate should be given every 12 hours—or more frequently if the bleeding tendency is severe. Only the bleeding time correlates with bleeding risk, but it is impractical to perform this test frequently.

New factor VIII concentrates are now available that will probably replace cryoprecipitate as the treat-

Table 13–21. Types of Von Willebrand's disease.

	Bleeding Time	Factor VIII Antigen	Ristocetin Cofactor Activity	Factor VIII Coagulant Activity	Multimer
Type I	↑ or N	↓ or N	↓ or N	↓ or N	N
Type IIa	↑	↓ or N	0	↓ or N	Abn
Type IIb	↑	↓ or N	↓ or N	↓ or N	Abn
Type III	↑	0	0	0	...
Pseudo-vW disease	↑	↓ or N	↓ or N	↓ or N	Abn
Hemophilia A	N	N	N	↓	N

ment of choice for von Willebrand's disease. Some (not all) of these products now contain functional vWF and, unlike cryoprecipitate, do not transmit HIV or hepatitis. One appropriate product is Humate-P (Armour). The dose is 20–50 units/kg depending on disease severity.

Desmopressin acetate is useful for mild type I von Willebrand's disease. The dose is 0.3 μg/kg, after which vWF levels usually rise two- to threefold in 30–90 minutes. Desmopressin acetate appears to cause release of stored vWF from endothelial cells. The treatment can be given only every 24 hours as stores of vWF become depleted. The drug is not effective in type IIa von Willebrand's disease, in which no endothelial stores are present, and may be harmful in type IIb or may lead to thrombocytopenia and increased bleeding.

The antifibrinolytic agents aminocaproic acid and tranexamic acid are useful as adjunctive therapy during dental procedures. After either cryoprecipitate or desmopressin acetate, the patient is given 4 g orally every 4 hours for several days to reduce the likelihood of bleeding.

Prognosis

The prognosis is excellent. In most cases, the bleeding disorder is mild, and in the more serious cases replacement therapy is effective.

Rose EH, Aledort LM: Nasal spray desmopressin (DDAVP) for mild hemophilia A and Von Willebrand's disease. Ann Intern Med 1991;114:563.

2. DISORDERS INTRINSIC TO THE PLATELETS

Glanzmann's Thrombasthenia

This is a rare autosomal recessive intrinsic platelet disorder causing bleeding. Platelets are unable to aggregate because of lack of receptors (containing glycoproteins IIb and IIa) for fibrinogen, which forms the bridges between platelets during aggregation. Clinically, it is manifested chiefly as mucosal bleeding (epistaxis, gingival bleeding, menorrhagia) and

postoperative bleeding. The bleeding defect is of variable severity but may be severe.

Platelet numbers and morphology are normal, but the bleeding time is markedly prolonged. Platelets fail to aggregate in response to typical agonists (ADP, collagen, thrombin) but aggregate normally in response to ristocetin, which causes platelet clumping by a separate mechanism.

Patients are treated with platelet transfusions when necessary. Platelet transfusion therapy is limited by the tendency of these patients to develop multiple alloantibodies.

Bernard-Soulier Syndrome

This is a rare autosomal recessive intrinsic platelet disorder causing bleeding. Platelets cannot adhere to subendothelium because they lack receptors (composed of glycoprotein Ib) for von Willebrand factor, which mediates platelet adhesion. This is often a severe bleeding disorder with mucosal and postoperative bleeding.

Thrombocytopenia may be present, and platelets on smear are abnormally large. The bleeding time is markedly prolonged. Platelet aggregation is normal in response to standard agonists (collagen, ADP, thrombin), but platelets fail to aggregate in response to ristocetin. Measurements of von Willebrand factor in the plasma are normal. Patients are treated with platelet transfusion when necessary.

Storage Pool Disease

This is a group of mild bleeding disorders characterized by defective secretion of platelet granule contents (especially ADP) that stimulate platelet aggregation. Most patients are mildly affected and have increased bruising and postoperative bleeding.

Platelets are normal in number and morphology, but the bleeding time is slightly prolonged. In some cases, the baseline bleeding time is normal, but it becomes markedly prolonged after aspirin. There are variable abnormalities in platelet aggregation studies.

Most patients do not require treatment but should avoid aspirin. Platelet transfusions transiently correct the bleeding tendency. Some patients respond to infusions of cryoprecipitate, and some respond transiently to desmopressin acetate (DDAVP), 0.3 µg/kg.

George JN, Caen JP, Nurden AT: Glanzmann's thrombasthenia: The spectrum of clinical disease. Blood 1990; 75:1383.

ACQUIRED QUALITATIVE PLATELET DISORDERS

A number of acquired disorders lead to abnormal platelet function (Table 13–19).

Uremia

Uremia causes abnormal platelet function by unknown mechanisms. The severity of the bleeding tendency is roughly proportionate to the degree of renal insufficiency. Bleeding is most commonly mucosal and gastrointestinal and may occasionally be severe. Dialysis is effective in reducing the bleeding tendency but may not completely eliminate it. Patients appear to respond to transfusion with cryoprecipitate, ten units every 12 hours. Desmopressin acetate, 0.3 µg/kg every 24 hours, appears to be just as effective as cryoprecipitate.

Myeloproliferative Disorders

All the myeloproliferative disorders can produce abnormalities in platelet function. A number of biochemical abnormalities are present in these platelets, but the cause of the bleeding tendency is unclear. The severity of the bleeding tendency correlates roughly with the height of the platelet count, although conditions causing reactive thrombocytosis of normal platelets are not associated with abnormal function. Bleeding decreases when the platelet count is controlled with myelosuppressive therapy. In cases of life-threatening bleeding with high platelet counts, plateletpheresis may be necessary to control bleeding. Platelet transfusion will also be helpful temporarily.

Other Disorders

Aspirin causes a mild bleeding tendency by irreversibly acetylating cyclooxygenase, an enzyme that participates in platelet aggregation. The effect lasts for the life of the platelet and may be manifest for 7–10 days, although the major effect lasts only 3–5 days. The effect is not dose-dependent, and 65 mg of aspirin is sufficient.

Aspirin by itself does not cause significant bleeding, but it may unmask bleeding disorders such as mild von Willebrand's disease or mild thrombocytopenia. Certain antibiotics (ticarcillin, some cephalosporins) cause a mild bleeding tendency, presumably by coating the surface of platelets. Nonsteroidal anti-inflammatory drugs cause a transient aspirin-like effect.

Patients with autoantibodies against platelets may have prolonged bleeding times even in the absence of thrombocytopenia. Platelet-associated IgG levels should be high, and the bleeding tendency responds quickly to modest doses of prednisone such as 20 mg/d. Acquired storage pool disease refers to the circulation of "exhausted platelets" that have been stimulated to release their granule contents and hence are no longer functional. Such granule release occurs in response to cardiopulmonary bypass and severe vasculitis.

George JN, Shattil SJ: The clinical importance of acquired abnormalities of platelet function. N Engl J Med 1991;324:27.
Mannucci PM: Desmopressin: A nontransfusional form of treatment for congenital and acquired bleeding disorders. Blood 1988;72:1449.
Shemin D et al: Oral estrogens decrease bleeding time and improve clinical bleeding in patients with renal failure. Am J Med 1990;89:436.

HEMOPHILIA A

Essentials of Diagnosis

- X-linked recessive pattern of inheritance with only males affected.
- Low factor VIII coagulant activity.
- Normal factor VIII antigen.
- Spontaneous hemarthroses.

General Considerations

Hemophilia A (classic hemophilia, factor VIII deficiency hemophilia) is a hereditary disorder in which bleeding is due to deficiency of the coagulation factor VIII (VIII:C). In most cases, the factor VIII coagulant protein is quantitatively reduced, but in a small number of cases the coagulant protein is present by immunoassay but defective.

Hemophilia is a classic example of an X-linked recessive disease, and as a rule only males are affected. In rare instances, female carriers are clinically affected if their normal X chromosomes are disproportionately inactivated. Females may also become affected if they are the offspring of a hemophiliac father and carrier mother.

Hemophilia is classified as severe if factor VIII:C levels are less than 1%, moderate if levels are 1–5%, and mild if levels are greater than 5%. Families tend to breed true in the severity of hemophilia produced.

Clinical Findings

A. Symptoms and Signs: Hemophilia A is the most common severe bleeding disorder and after von Willebrand's disease is the most common congenital bleeding disorder overall. Approximately one in 10,000 males is affected. The bleeding tendency is related to factor VIII:C levels. Bleeding may occur anywhere. The most common sites of bleeding are into joints (knees, ankles, elbows), into muscles, and from the gastrointestinal tract. Spontaneous hemarthroses are so characteristic of severe hemophilia that they are almost diagnostic of the disorder. Patients with mild hemophilia bleed only in response to major trauma or surgery. Patients with moderately severe hemophilia bleed in response to mild trauma or surgery, and those with severe hemophilia bleed spontaneously.

Unfortunately, many hemophiliacs are now seropositive for HIV infection transmitted via factor VIII concentrate, and many have already developed AIDS. HIV-associated immune thrombocytopenia may aggravate the bleeding tendency.

B. Laboratory Findings: The partial thromboplastin time (PTT) is prolonged, and other measures of coagulation, including prothrombin time, bleeding time, and fibrinogen level, are normal. Levels of factor VIII:C are reduced, but measurements of von Willebrand factor are normal (Table 13–21).

If one mixes plasma from a hemophiliac patient with normal plasma, the PTT will become normal. Failure of the PTT to normalize in such a mixing test is diagnostic of the presence of a factor VIII inhibitor.

A low platelet count should raise a suspicion of HIV-associated immune thrombocytopenia.

Differential Diagnosis

The finding of a reduced factor VIII:C level will distinguish this disorder from other causes of prolonged PTT (Table 13–20). Clinically, factor VIII hemophilia is indistinguishable from factor IX hemophilia, and only specific factor assays can distinguish these disorders. In cases of mild hemophilia, the disorder needs to be distinguished from von Willebrand's disease by VIII:A assay, which shows normal levels of factor VIII antigen in the latter.

An important issue for the families of hemophiliac patients is identifying which females are carriers. Female carriers can usually be identified by the presence of low or normal levels of factor VIII:C with normal levels of factor VIII antigen.

Treatment

Patients with hemophilia should try to live as nearly normal lives as possible. Activities associated with a risk of trauma should be avoided, however, and aspirin should never be used.

Standard treatment is based on infusion of factor VIII concentrates, now heat-treated to reduce the likelihood of transmission of AIDS. Other purified factor VIII products are being produced, and recombinant factor VIII is being evaluated. The level of factor VIII one aims to achieve in plasma depends on the severity of the bleeding problem. In response to minor bleeding, it may be necessary only to raise factor VIII:C levels to 25% with one infusion. For moderate bleeding (such as deep muscle hematomas), it is adequate to raise the level initially to 50% and main-

tain the level at greater than 25% with repeated infusion for 2–3 days. When major surgery is to be performed, one raises the factor VIII:C level to 100% and then maintains the factor level at greater than 50% continuously for 10–14 days. Head injuries (with or without neurologic signs) should be emergently treated as though major bleeding were present.

The dose of factor VIII concentrate is calculated on the basis that one unit of factor VIII is the amount present in 1 mL of plasma. Plasma volume is 40 mL/kg, and the volume of distribution of factor VIII:C is 1.5 times the plasma volume. Thus, to raise the level 100%, the dose should be $40 \times 1.5 + 60$ units/kg, or approximately 4000 units. To raise the levels to 25% would require 1000 units. The half-life of factor VIII:C is approximately 12 hours. Thus, during major surgery, to achieve an initial level of 100% and maintain it continuously at greater than 50%, a dose of 60 units/kg (approximately 4000 units) initially followed by 30 units/kg (approximately 2000 units) every 12 hours should be adequate. During surgery, one should initially verify that these doses give the anticipated levels. If factor VIII levels fail to rise as expected, one should suspect an inhibitor. Patients with inhibitors require specialized therapy under direction of an experienced hematologist.

For mild hemophiliacs, desmopressin acetate, 0.3 μg/kg every 24 hours, may be useful in preparing for minor surgical procedures. Desmopressin acetate causes release of factor VIII:C and will raise the factor VIII:C levels two- to threefold for several hours. In the management of persistent bleeding following use of either desmopressin acetate or factor VIII concentrate, patients may be treated with aminocaproic acid (EACA; Amicar), 4 g orally every 4 hours for several days.

The ongoing care of patients with hemophilia should be coordinated with an orthopedic surgeon who can help manage the chronic joint deformities of these patients.

Prognosis

The prognosis of patients with hemophilia has been transformed by the availability of factor VIII replacement. The major limiting factors are disability from recurrent joint bleeding and viral infections (hepatitis B, AIDS) from recurrent transfusion. Approximately 15% of patients develop inhibitors to factor VIII, and these patents may die of bleeding because they cannot be adequately supported with factor VIII.

Brettler DB, Levine PH: Factor concentrates for treatment of hemophilia: Which one to choose? Blood 1989; 73:2067.

Furie B, Furie BC: Molecular basis of hemophilia. Semin Hematol 1990;27:270.

White GC, Shoemaker CB: Factor VIII gene and hemophilia A. Blood 1989;73:1.

HEMOPHILIA B

Essentials of Diagnosis

- X-linked recessive inheritance, with only males affected.
- Low levels of factor IX coagulant activity.
- Spontaneous hemarthroses.

General Considerations

Hemophilia B (Christmas disease, factor IX hemophilia) is a hereditary bleeding disorder due to deficiency of coagulation factor IX. Most commonly, factor IX is quantitatively reduced, but in one-third of cases an abnormally functioning molecule is immunologically present. Factor IX deficiency is one-seventh as common as factor VIII deficiency hemophilia but is otherwise clinically and genetically identical.

The PTT is prolonged, and factor IX levels are reduced when measured by specific factor assays. Other laboratory features are the same as for factor VIII hemophilia.

Treatment

Factor IX hemophilia is managed with factor IX concentrates. Factor VIII concentrates are ineffectual in this type of hemophilia; therefore it is imperative to distinguish between the two. The same dosing considerations apply as in factor VIII hemophilia, with the exception that the volume of distribution of factor IX is twice the plasma volume, so that 80 units/kg are necessary to achieve a 100% level. In addition, the half-life of factor IX is 18 hours. Thus, to maintain a patient through major surgery, the dosage should be 80 units/kg (approximately 6000 units) initially followed by 40 units/kg (3000 units) every 18 hours. Factor levels should be measured to ensure that expected levels are achieved and that an inhibitor is not present.

Unlike factor VIII concentrates, factor IX concentrates contain a number of other proteins, including activated coagulating factors that appear to contribute to a risk of thrombosis with recurrent usage of factor IX concentrates. Because of the risk of thrombosis, more care is needed in deciding to use these concentrates. Desmopressin acetate is not useful in this disorder.

Prognosis

The prognosis for these patients is the same as for those with factor VIII hemophilia.

OTHER CONGENITAL COAGULATION DISORDERS

Factor XI Deficiency

This disorder is seen primarily among Ashkenazi Jews and is autosomal recessive. The PTT may be markedly prolonged, and specific assays of factor XI will show reduced levels. This is usually a mild bleeding disorder manifested primarily by postoperative bleeding. Factor replacement is given with fresh-frozen plasma when necessary.

Afibrinogenemia

In this rare disorder, fibrinogen is absent and both prothrombin time and partial thromboplastin time are markedly prolonged. These patients may have a severe bleeding disorder similar to hemophilia. Fibrinogen is replaced with cryoprecipitate.

Other Coagulation Disorders

Bleeding disorders due to isolated deficiency of factors II, V, X, or VII are extremely rare. Deficiencies of factor XII and the contact pathway factors cause a markedly prolonged PTT but are not associated with any increased bleeding.

Factor XIII deficiency results in delayed bleeding after trauma or surgery. All coagulation tests are normal. The disorder is diagnosed by showing instability of the fibrin clot in 8-molar urea. Factor XIII is replaced with cryoprecipitate or plasma. A rare cause of bleeding is deficiency of the normal inhibitors of fibrinolytic activity: α_2-antiplasmin and plasminogen activator inhibitor.

Dieval J et al: A lifelong bleeding disorder associated with a deficiency of plasminogen activator inhibitor type 1. Blood 1991;77:528.

COAGULOPATHY OF LIVER DISEASE

Essentials of Diagnosis

- Prothrombin time more prolonged than PTT.
- No response to Vitamin K.

General Considerations

The liver is the site of synthesis of all the coagulation factors except factor VIII. As hepatic insufficiency develops, the vitamin K-dependent factors (factors II, VII, IX, X) and factor V are the first to be affected. Because of its rapid turnover (half-life 6 hours), factor VII levels are the first to decline. Conversely, fibrinogen levels are remarkably well conserved, and decreased fibrinogen synthesis does not occur unless liver disease is very severe.

Liver disease has a number of other effects on the hemostatic system. Increased fibrinolysis occurs because the liver synthesizes α_2-antiplasmin (the main inhibitor of fibrinolysis), which is responsible for the clearance of plasminogen activator. Biliary tract disease may lead to malabsorption of vitamin K, and congestive splenomegaly may produce mild thrombocytopenia. A variety of chronic liver diseases cause abnormal posttranslation modification of fibrinogen with resultant dysfibrinogenemia.

Clinical Findings

A. Symptoms and Signs: The coagulopathy of liver disease may lead to bleeding at any site. Excessive fibrinolysis may lead to oozing at venipuncture sites.

B. Laboratory Findings: Hepatic coagulopathy produces a more marked abnormality in the prothrombin time (PT) than in the partial thromboplastin time (PTT). Early in the course of liver disease, only the PT will become affected. Fibrinogen levels should be normal, and the thrombin time should be normal unless dysfibrinogenemia is present. The platelet count should be normal unless production is suppressed by acute alcohol ingestion or unless hypersplenism is present. The peripheral blood smear may show target cells.

Differential Diagnosis

Hepatic coagulopathy can be distinguished from vitamin K deficiency only by demonstrating the failure of vitamin K to correct the abnormal values. Liver disease is distinguished from disseminated intravascular coagulation by the normal fibrinogen level and lack of thrombocytopenia. End-stage liver disease almost invariably leads to some element of disseminated intravascular coagulation, and the disorders overlap (Tables 13–22 and 13–23).

Treatment

Long-term treatment of hepatic coagulopathy with factor replacement is usually ineffective. Fresh-frozen plasma is the treatment of choice, and volume overload will limit one's ability to maintain hemostatic factor levels. For example, to maintain factor levels greater than 25%, one must initially raise the level to 50% with 50% of the plasma volume (20 mL/kg) and then replace 10 mL/kg every 6 hours to maintain adequate factor VII levels. In average-sized persons, this will require transfusion of 1400 mL of plasma initially followed by 700 mL every 6 hours. Factor IX concentrates are contraindicated in liver disease because of their tendency to cause disseminated intravascular coagulation. If thrombocytopenia is present, platelet transfusion may be of some help,

Table 13–22. Causes of isolated prolonged prothrombin time.

Liver disease
Vitamin K deficiency
Warfarin therapy
Factor VII deficiency

Table 13–23. Causes of prolonged prothrombin time and partial thromboplastin time.

Liver disease
Vitamin K deficiency
Disseminated intravascular coagulation
Heparin
Warfarin
Isolated factor deficiencies (rare): II, V, X, I

but platelet recovery is usually disappointing because of hypersplenism.

Prognosis

The prognosis is that of the underlying liver disease.

VITAMIN K DEFICIENCY

Essentials of Diagnosis

- Prothrombin time more prolonged than PTT.
- Rapid correction with vitamin K replacement.
- Underlying dietary deficiency or antibiotic use.

General Considerations

Vitamin K plays a role in coagulation by acting as a cofactor for the posttranslational g-carboxylation of zymogens II, VII, IX, and X. The modified zymogens (with γ-carboxyglutamic acid residues) are able to bind to platelets in a calcium-dependent reaction and consequently better participate in the complex reactions that activate factors X and II. Without γ-carboxylation, these reactions on the platelet surface occur slowly and hemostasis is impaired.

Vitamin K is supplied in the diet primarily in leafy vegetables and endogenously from synthesis from intestinal bacteria. Factors that contribute to vitamin K deficiency include poor diet, malabsorption, and broad-spectrum antibiotics suppressing colonic flora. A characteristic setting for vitamin K deficiency is a postoperative patient who is not eating and who is receiving antibiotics. Body stores of vitamin K are small, and deficiency may develop in as little as 1 week.

Clinical Findings

A. Symptoms and Signs: There are no specific clinical features, and bleeding may occur at any site.

B. Laboratory Findings: The prothrombin time is prolonged to a greater extent than the PTT, and with mild vitamin K deficiency only the PT is defective (Tables 13–22 and 13–23). Fibrinogen level, thrombin time, and platelet count are not affected.

Differential Diagnosis

Vitamin K deficiency can be distinguished from hepatic coagulopathy only by assessing the response to vitamin K therapy. Surreptitious warfarin use will produce laboratory features indistinguishable from those of vitamin K deficiency.

Vitamin K deficiency is distinguished from disseminated intravascular coagulation by the normal platelet count and normal fibrinogen level in the former.

Treatment

Vitamin K deficiency responds rapidly to subcutaneous vitamin K, and a single dose of 15 mg will completely correct laboratory abnormalities in 12–24 hours.

Prognosis

The prognosis is excellent, as vitamin K deficiency can be completely corrected with replacement.

Furie B, Furie BC: Molecular basis of vitamin K-dependent gamma carboxylation. Blood 1990;75:1753.

DISSEMINATED INTRAVASCULAR COAGULATION (DIC)

Essentials of Diagnosis

- Hypofibrinogenemia, thrombocytopenia, fibrin degradation products, and prolonged prothrombin time.
- Underlying serious illness.
- Microangiopathic hemolytic anemia may be present.

General Considerations

Coagulation is usually confined to a localized area by the combination of blood flow and circulating inhibitors of coagulation, especially antithrombin III. If the stimulus to coagulation is too great, these control mechanisms can be overwhelmed, leading to the syndrome of disseminated intravascular coagulation. In pathophysiologic terms, disseminated intravascular coagulation can be thought of as the consequence of the presence of circulating thrombin (normally confined to a localized area). The effects of thrombin are to cleave fibrinogen to fibrin monomer, stimulate platelet aggregation, activate factors V and VIII, and release plasminogen activator, which generates plasmin. Plasmin in turn cleaves fibrin, generating fibrin degradation products, and further inactivates factors V and VIII. Thus, the excess thrombin activity produces hypofibrinogenemia, thrombocytopenia, depletion of coagulation factors, and fibrinolysis.

Disseminated intravascular coagulation can be caused by a number of serious illnesses, including sepsis (especially with gram-negative bacteria but possible with any widespread bacterial or fungal infection), severe tissue injury (especially burns and head injury), obstetric complications (amniotic fluid embolus, septic abortion, retained dead fetus), cancer

(acute promyelocytic leukemia, mucinous adenocarcinomas), and major hemolytic transfusion reactions.

Clinical Findings

A. Symptoms and Signs: Disseminated intravascular coagulation leads to both bleeding and thrombosis. Bleeding is far more common than thrombosis, but the latter may dominate if coagulation is activated to a far greater extent than fibrinolysis. Bleeding may occur at any site, but spontaneous bleeding and oozing at venipuncture sites or wounds are important clues to the diagnosis. Thrombosis is most commonly manifested by digital ischemia and gangrene, but catastrophic events such as renal-cortical necrosis and hemorrhagic adrenal infarction may occur. Disseminated intravascular coagulation may also secondarily produce microangiopathic hemolytic anemia.

Subacute disseminated intravascular coagulation is seen primarily in cancer patients and is manifested primarily as recurrent superficial and deep venous thromboses (Trousseau's syndrome).

B. Laboratory Findings: Disseminated intravascular coagulation produces a complex coagulopathy with the characteristic constellation of hypofibrinogenemia, elevated fibrin degradation products, thrombocytopenia, and a prolonged prothrombin time. Of the fibrin degradation products, the D-dimer is the most sensitive, since its cross-linking implies origin from fibrin in a clot. All fibrin degradation products are cleared by the liver and thus may be elevated in hepatic dysfunction. Hypofibrinogenemia is another important diagnostic laboratory feature, because few disorders (congenital hypofibrinogenemia, severe liver disease) will lower the fibrinogen level. In some cases of disseminated intravascular coagulation, when the patient's baseline fibrinogen level is markedly elevated, the initial fibrinogen level may be normal. However, since the half-life of fibrinogen is approximately 4 days, a noticeably falling fibrinogen level will confirm the diagnosis of disseminated intravascular coagulation.

Other laboratory abnormalities are variably present. The partial thromboplastin time may or may not be prolonged. In approximately one-fourth of cases, a microangiopathic hemolytic anemia is present, and fragmented red blood cells are seen on the peripheral smear. Antithrombin III levels may be markedly depleted. When fibrinolysis is activated, levels of plasminogen and α_2-antiplasmin may be low.

Subacute disseminated intravascular coagulation produces a very different laboratory picture. Thrombocytopenia and elevated D-dimer are usually the only abnormalities. Fibrinogen levels are normal, and the PTT may be normal.

Differential Diagnosis

Liver disease may prolong both the PT and PTT, but fibrinogen levels are usually normal, and the platelet count is usually normal or only slightly reduced. However, severe liver disease may be difficult to distinguish from disseminated intravascular coagulation. Vitamin K deficiency will not affect the fibrinogen level or platelet count and will be completely corrected by vitamin K replacement.

Sepsis may produce thrombocytopenia and digital ischemia, and coagulopathy may be present because of vitamin K deficiency. However, in these cases, the fibrinogen level should be normal.

Thrombotic thrombocytopenic purpura may produce fever and microangiopathic hemolytic anemia. However, fibrinogen levels and other coagulation tests should be normal.

Treatment

The primary focus should be the diagnosis and treatment of the underlying disorder that has given rise to disseminated intravascular coagulation. In many cases, disseminated intravascular coagulation will produce laboratory abnormalities with only mild clinical manifestations, and in these cases no specific therapy is required.

When the underlying cause of disseminated intravascular coagulation is rapidly reversible (such as in obstetric cases), replacement therapy alone may be indicated. The role of heparin in the treatment of disseminated intravascular coagulation is controversial. In some cases, when any increase in bleeding is unacceptable (neurosurgical procedures), heparin therapy is contraindicated. However, when disseminated intravascular coagulation is producing serious clinical consequences and the underlying cause is not rapidly reversible, heparin therapy may be necessary to control the syndrome. Such therapy is routinely used in the treatment of acute promyelocytic leukemia. In cases where disseminated intravascular coagulation causes thrombosis, heparin therapy is mandatory.

In replacement therapy, platelet transfusion should be used to maintain a platelet count greater than 30,000/μL, and 50,000/μL if possible. Fibrinogen is replaced with cryoprecipitate, and one should aim for a level of 150 mg/dL. One unit of cryoprecipitate usually raises the fibrinogen level by 6–8 mg/dL, so that 15 units of cryoprecipitate will raise the level from 50 to 150 mg/dL. Coagulation factor deficiency may require replacement with fresh-frozen plasma.

Heparin therapy must be used in combination with replacement therapy, since administering heparin on its own will lead to an unacceptable increase in bleeding. Heparin therapy usually requires a dose of 500–750 units per hour. Heparin cannot be effective if antithrombin III levels are markedly depleted. Antithrombin III levels should be measured, and fresh-frozen plasma should be used to raise levels to greater than 50%. In using heparin, it is not necessary to prolong the PTT. Successful therapy is indicated by a rising fibrinogen level. Fibrin degradation products will decline over 1–2 days. Improvement in the platelet count may lag as much as 1 week behind control of the coagulopathy.

In some cases, when disseminated intravascular coagulation is complicated by excessive fibrinolysis, even the combination of heparin and replacement therapy may not be adequate to control bleeding. In these cases, aminocaproic acid, 1 g intravenously per hour, or tranexamic acid, 10 mg/kg intravenously every 8 hours, should be added to decrease the rate of fibrinolysis, raise the fibrinogen level, and control bleeding. *Caution:* It must be emphasized that aminocaproic acid can *never* be used without heparin in disseminated intravascular coagulation, since fatal thrombosis may occur.

Prognosis

The prognosis is that of the underlying disease. Severe disseminated intravascular coagulation can be lethal.

Feinstein DI: Diagnosis and management of disseminated intravascular coagulation: The role of heparin therapy. Blood 1982;60:284.

ACQUIRED FACTOR VIII ANTIBODIES

Antibodies to factor VIII may develop either postpartum or with no underlying illness. Factor VIII antibodies also develop in 15% of patients with factor VIII hemophilia who have received infusions of plasma concentrates.

Acquired factor VIII antibodies usually produce a severe bleeding disorder. The PTT is prolonged, and the fibrinogen level, prothrombin time, and platelet count are not affected. A plasma mixing test will usually reveal the presence of an inhibitor by the failure of normal plasma to correct the prolonged PTT. However, the mixing test may require incubation for 2–4 hours to reveal the inhibitor. Factor VIII coagulant levels are low.

Factor VIII antibodies should be suspected in any acquired severe bleeding disorder associated with a prolonged PTT. Factor VIII antibodies are distinguished from lupus anticoagulants both by the presence of clinical bleeding and more importantly by the reduced factor VIII:C level. The diagnosis is confirmed by mixing tests and in vivo by the failure of factor VIII concentrates to raise the factor VIII:C levels by the expected amount.

The treatment of choice is cyclophosphamide, usually combined with prednisone. In the interim, aggressive factor VIII replacement may be necessary. Plasmapheresis to reduce inhibitor levels may be useful. Treatment of factor VIII antibodies is complex and should be done in consultation with a hematologist.

The prognosis of these patients is variable, and many die of overwhelming bleeding.

Lian EC et al: Combination immunosuppressive therapy after factor VIII infusion for factor VIII inhibitor. Ann Intern Med 1989;110:774.

HYPERCOAGULABLE STATES

In many cases, thrombosis is related to local factors causing stasis of blood flow or damage to a blood vessel. Common examples are deep venous thrombosis in the legs following prolonged sitting in one position and thrombosis in the femoral and iliac veins following hip surgery. However, in other cases a systemic disorder causes a general increase in the risk of thrombosis (Table 13–24).

Cancer is associated with an increased risk of both venous and arterial thrombosis. In some cases, low-grade disseminated intravascular coagulation appears to be responsible. In unusual cases, a unique cancer procoagulant stimulates the clotting system. Myeloproliferative disorders such as polycythemia vera, essential thrombocytosis, and paroxysmal nocturnal hemoglobinuria are associated with a high incidence of thrombosis, caused by qualitative platelet abnormalities. For the indolent diseases polycythemia vera and essential thrombocytosis, thrombosis is the major cause of morbidity and deaths. Venous thrombosis may occur in unusual locations such as the mesenteric, hepatic, or splenic venous beds. Arterial thrombosis occurs as well and may be manifested as large vessel occlusion (stroke, myocardial infarction) or as microvascular events with painful burning in the hands and feet.

Heparin is an uncommon but important cause of hypercoagulability. Heparin has been associated with thrombocytopenia in about 10% of treatment courses. Often the thrombocytopenia is modest and resolves spontaneously. However, in some cases severe thrombocytopenia occurs. It is most often in this set-ting that arterial thrombosis occurs as a complication. The arteries involved are often large ones, such as the iliac artery or even the aorta. It is imperative that heparin be discontinued in this setting, since continuing the drug almost always leads to a fatal outcome.

A number of congenital biochemical defects have also been associated with hypercoagulability (Table 13–24). A family history is usually present. The thromboses are almost always venous and may occur in the large veins of the abdomen. Thromboses often occur during early adulthood rather than in childhood and are often precipitated by factors such as trauma or pregnancy. Antithrombin III deficiency is by far the most common of these disorders. The diagnosis is made by demonstrating reduced levels of the factors in plasma. Dysfibrinogenemia is diagnosed by a prolonged reptilase time.

The syndrome of warfarin-induced skin necrosis may occur in patients with undiagnosed protein C deficiency. Protein C is vitamin K-dependent and has a shorter half-life than the coagulation proteins. Warfarin, by creating a vitamin K-dependent state, will transiently deplete protein C before it leads to anticoagulation. During the period of hypercoagulability due to unopposed protein C depletion, thrombosis of skin vessels may lead to infarction and necrosis. The syndrome can be prevented by the use of heparin for 5–7 days until warfarin induces anticoagulation.

Treatment

If a patient is recognized to be at increased risk of thrombosis, effective prophylactic therapy is usually available. Preoperatively, minidose heparin (5000 units every 8–12 hours) may be useful in reducing the risk of thrombosis in the perioperative period. The hypercoagulable state associated with cancer may benefit from treatment with heparin, 10,000 units subcutaneously every 12 hours. Warfarin is usually ineffective in preventing thrombosis in this situation, most likely because low-grade disseminated intravascular coagulation is the cause. In patients with myeloproliferative disease who have had symptoms of thrombosis, antiplatelet therapy may be helpful. However, such therapy should not be used indiscriminately, because these patients are also at increased risk of bleeding. For patients with erythromelalgia (painful redness and burning of the hands), aspirin, 325 mg daily, is almost always effective.

For patients with congenital biochemical defects such as deficiency of antithrombin III or the vitamin K-dependent proteins C and S, warfarin is effective and should probably be given for life. Family members should be screened for the presence of the defect so that their increased risk of thrombosis can be noted and acted upon.

Table 13–24. Causes of hypercoagulability.

Acquired
Cancer
Inflammatory disorders: Ulcerative colitis
Myeloproliferative disorders
Postoperative
Estrogens, pregnancy
Lupus anticoagulant
Heparin-induced thrombocytopenia
Anticardiolipin antibodies
Congenital
Antithrombin III deficiency
Protein C deficiency
Protein S deficiency
Dysfibrinogenemia
Abnormal plasminogen

Collen D, Lijene HR: Basic and clinical aspects of fibrinolysis and thrombolysis. Blood 1991;78:3114.

Furie B, Furie BC: Molecular and cellular biology of blood coagulation. N Engl J Med 1992;326:800.

Hirsh J: Heparin. N Engl J Med 1991;324:1565.

Hirsh J: Oral anti-coagulant drugs. N Engl J Med 1991;324:1865.

Menache D et al: Evaluation of safety, recovery, half-life and clinical efficacy of antithrombin III (human) in patients with hereditary anti-thrombin III deficiency. Blood 1990;75:33.

LUPUS ANTICOAGULANT

The lupus anticoagulant is an IgM or IgG immunoglobulin that produces a prolonged PTT by binding to the phospholipid used in the in vitro PTT assay. As such, it is a laboratory artifact and does not cause a clinical bleeding disorder. The "lupus anticoagulant" is seen in 5–10% of patients with systemic lupus erythematosus. More commonly, it is seen without an underlying disorder or in patients taking phenothiazines.

There is no bleeding defect unless a second disorder such as thrombocytopenia, hypoprothrombinemia, or a prolonged bleeding time is present. Paradoxically, the lupus anticoagulant has been associated with an increased risk of thrombosis and of recurrent spontaneous abortions.

The PTT is prolonged and fails to correct when the patient's plasma is mixed in a 1:1 dilution with normal plasma. The PT is either normal or slightly prolonged. The fibrinogen level and thrombin time are normal. The Russell viper venom (RVV) time is a more sensitive assay and is specifically designed to demonstrate the presence of a lupus anticoagulant. An antiphospholipid, the lupus anticoagulant, will cause a false-positive VDRL test for syphilis. A related autoantibody, anticardiolipin, can be detected by separate assays.

Lupus anticoagulant should be suspected in cases of a markedly prolonged PTT without clinical bleeding (other causes are factor XII or contact factor deficiency). The plasma mixing test will demonstrate the presence of an inhibitor by the failure of normal plasma to correct the PTT. When acquired factor VIII inhibitors are being considered, a factor VIII:C level may be measured; this will be normal in patients with lupus anticoagulant.

No specific treatment is necessary. Prednisone will usually rapidly eliminate the lupus anticoagulant, and it has been suggested that prednisone therapy reduces spontaneous abortions in this syndrome. It is not clear whether prednisone has any effect on the thrombotic tendency associated with lupus anticoagulant. Patients with thromboses should be treated with anticoagulation in standard doses. Because of the artificially prolonged PTT, heparin therapy is difficult to monitor properly. The dose of warfarin administered

may also be inadequate if the baseline PT is prolonged.

Asherson RA et al: The "primary" anti-phospholipid syndrome: Major clinical and serologic features. Medicine 1989;68:366.

Branch DW et al: Obstetric complications associated with the lupus anticoagulant. N Engl J Med 1985;313:1322.

Love PE, Santoro SA: Anti-phospholipid antibodies: Anticardiolipin and the lupus anticoagulant in systemic lupus erythematosus (SLE) and in non-SLE disorders: Prevalence and clinical significance. Ann Intern Med 1990;112:682.

BLOOD TRANSFUSIONS

RED BLOOD CELL TRANSFUSIONS

Red blood cell transfusions are given to raise the hematocrit levels in patients with anemia or to replace losses after acute bleeding episodes. Because of the inherent risks, blood transfusions should never be given to correct anemia when simpler measures such as administration of iron, folate, or vitamin B_{12} can be used instead. Several types of components containing red blood cells are available.

(1) Fresh whole blood: The major advantage of this component is the simultaneous presence of red blood cells, plasma, and fresh platelets. Fresh whole blood is never absolutely necessary, since all the above components are available separately. The major indications for use of whole blood are cardiac surgery or massive hemorrhage when more than ten units of blood are required in a 24-hour period.

(2) Packed red blood cells: Packed red cells are the component most commonly used to raise the hematocrit. Each unit has a volume of about 300 mL, of which approximately 200 mL consists of red blood cells. One unit of packed red cells will usually raise the hematocrit by approximately 4%. The expected rise in hematocrit can be calculated using an estimated red blood cell volume of 200 mL/unit and a total blood volume of about 70 mL/kg. For example, a 70-kg man will have a total blood volume of 4900 mL, and each unit of packed red blood cells will raise the hematocrit by 200 ÷ 4900 equals 4%.

(3) Leukopoor blood: Patients with severe leukoagglutinin reactions to packed red blood cells may require depletion of white blood cells and platelets from transfused units. White blood cells can be removed either by centrifugation or by washing. Preparation of leukopoor blood causes additional expense and leads to some loss of red cells.

(4) Frozen blood: Red blood cells can be frozen

and stored for up to 3 years, but the technique is cumbersome and expensive, and frozen blood should be used sparingly. The major application is for the purpose of maintaining a supply of rare blood types. Patients with very rare blood types may donate units for autologous transfusion should the need arise. Frozen red cells are also occasionally needed for patients with severe leukoagglutinin reactions or anaphylactic reactions to plasma proteins, since frozen blood has essentially all white blood cells and plasma components removed.

(5) Autologous packed red blood cells: Patients scheduled for elective surgery may donate blood for autologous transfusion. These units may be stored for up to 35 days.

Compatibility Testing

Before transfusion, the recipient's and the donor's blood are cross-matched to avoid hemolytic transfusion reactions. Although many antigen systems are present on red blood cells, only the ABO and Rh systems are specifically tested prior to all transfusions. The A and B antigens are the most important, because everyone who lacks one or both red cell antigens has isoantibodies against the missing antigen or antigens in his or her plasma. These antibodies activate complement and can cause rapid intravascular lysis of the incompatible red cells. In emergencies, type O blood can be given to any recipient, but only packed cells should be given to avoid transfusion of donor plasma containing anti-A or anti-B antibodies.

The other important antigen routinely tested for is the D antigen of the Rh system. Approximately 15% of the population lack this antigen. In patients lacking the antigen, anti-D antibodies are not naturally present, but the antigen is highly immunogenic. A recipient whose red cells lack D and who receives D-positive blood may develop anti-D antibodies that can cause severe lysis of subsequent transfusions of D-positive red cells.

Blood typing includes assay of recipient serum for unusual antibodies by mixing the serum with panels of red cells representing commonly occurring weak antigens. The screening is particularly important if the recipient has had previous transfusions.

Hemolytic Transfusion Reactions

Major hemolytic transfusion reactions are the most dread complication of transfusion and can be fatal. The most severe reactions are those involving mismatches in the ABO system. Most of these cases are due to clerical errors and mislabeled specimens. Hemolysis is rapid and intravascular, releasing free hemoglobin into the plasma. The severity of these reactions depends on the dose of red blood cells given. The most severe reactions are those seen in surgical patients under anesthesia. They will be unable to give early warning signs of myalgias and chills.

Hemolytic transfusion reactions caused by minor antigen systems are typically less severe. The hemolysis usually takes place at a slower rate and is extravascular. Sometimes these transfusion reactions may be delayed for 5–10 days after transfusion. In such cases, the recipient has received blood containing an immunogenic action, and in the time since transfusion, a new alloantibody has been formed. The most common antigens involved in such reactions are Duffy, Kidd, Kell, and C and E loci of the Rh system.

A. Signs and Symptoms: Major hemolytic transfusion reactions cause fever and chills and severe backache and headache. In severe cases, there may be apprehension, dyspnea, hypotension, and vascular collapse. Such symptoms will usually lead to recognition of a transfusion reaction. *The transfusion must be stopped immediately!* In severe cases, disseminated intravascular coagulation or acute renal failure from tubular necrosis can occur, or both may occur.

Patients under general anesthesia will not give such signs, and the first indication may be oliguria and generalized bleeding.

B. Laboratory Findings and Management:
1. Identification of the recipient and of the blood should be checked. The donor transfusion bag with its pilot tube must be returned to the blood bank, and a fresh sample of the recipient's blood must accompany the donor bag for retyping of donor and recipient blood samples and for repeat of the cross-match.

2. The hematocrit will fail to rise by the expected amount. Coagulation studies will reveal evidence of renal failure and disseminated intravascular coagulation in severe cases. Hemoglobinuria will turn the plasma pink and eventually result in hemoglobinuria. In cases of delayed hemolytic reactions, the hematocrit will fall and the indirect bilirubin will rise. In these cases, the new offending alloantibody is easily detected in the patient's serum.

C. Treatment: If a hemolytic transfusion reaction is suspected, the transfusion should be stopped at once. A sample of anticoagulated blood from the recipient should be centrifuged to detect free hemoglobin in the plasma. If hemoglobinemia is present, the patient should be vigorously hydrated to prevent acute tubular necrosis. There is some evidence that forced diuresis with mannitol may help prevent renal damage.

Leukoagglutinin Reactions

Most transfusion reactions are not hemolytic but represent reactions to antigens present on white blood cells or platelets in patients who have been sensitized to the antigens through previous transfusions or pregnancy. Most commonly, patients will develop fever and chills within 12 hours after transfusion. In severe cases, cough and dyspnea may occur and the chest x-ray may show transient pulmonary infiltrates. Because no hemolysis is involved, the hematocrit rises by the expected amount despite the reaction.

Leukoagglutinin reactions may respond to acetaminophen and diphenhydramine. In severe cases, steroids may be of help. Patients with severe leukoagglutinin reactions may require transfusion of leukopoor red blood cells in the future.

Anaphylactic Reactions

Rarely, patients will develop hives or bronchospasm during a transfusion. These reactions are almost always due to plasma proteins rather than white blood cells. Patients who are IgA-deficient may develop these reactions because of antibodies to IgA. Patients with such reactions may require transfusion of washed or even frozen red blood cells to avoid future severe reactions.

Contaminated Blood

Rarely, blood is contaminated with gram-negative bacteria. Transfusion can lead to septicemia and shock from endotoxin. If this is suspected, the offending unit should be cultured and the patient treated with antibiotics as indicated.

Diseases Transmitted Through Transfusion

Despite the use of only volunteer blood donors and the routine screening of blood, transfusion-associated hepatitis remains a problem. All blood products (red blood cells, platelets, plasma, cryoprecipitate) can transmit viral diseases. All blood is routinely screened for hepatitis B surface antigen. In addition, blood banks routinely test for antibodies to HIV and to hepatitis core antigen. Because of specific screening, hepatitis B accounts for less than 10% of cases of transfusion-associated hepatitis. The most common form is non-A, non-B hepatitis. Overt hepatitis occurs at a rate of approximately 1% for each unit of blood transfused, and subclinical hepatitis probably occurs ten times as often. Methods of detecting non-A, non-B hepatitis have been developed and will probably be in clinical use within the year. This should markedly reduce the problem of transfusion-associated hepatitis. Because of more rigorous screening of blood associated with the recent recognition of the possibility of transfusion-associated AIDS, the risk of hepatitis may decrease in the future. It is currently estimated that with proper screening the risk of transmitting AIDS is less than 1:100,000 for each unit of blood transfused.

Platelet Transfusion

Platelet transfusions are indicated in cases of thrombocytopenia due to decreased platelet production. They are not useful in immune thrombocytopenia, since transfused platelets will last no longer than the patient's endogenous platelets. The risk of spontaneous bleeding rises when the platelet count falls to less than 20,000/µL, and the risk of life-threatening bleeding increases when the platelet count is less than 10,000/µL. Because of this, prophylactic platelet transfusions are often given at these very low levels. Platelet transfusions are also given prior to invasive procedures or surgery, and the goal should be to raise the platelet count to over 50,000/µL.

Platelets are most commonly derived from donated blood units. One unit of platelets (derived from 1 unit of blood) usually contains $5–7 \times 10^{10}$ platelets suspended in 35 mL of plasma. Ideally, 1 platelet unit will raise the recipient's platelet count by 10,000/µL, and transfused platelets will last for 2 or 3 days. However, responses are often suboptimal, with poor platelet increments and short survival times. This may be due to sepsis, splenomegaly, or alloimmunization. Most alloantibodies causing platelet destruction are directed at HLA antigens. Patients requiring long periods of platelet transfusion support should be monitored to document adequate responses to transfusions so that the most appropriate product can be used. Patients may benefit from HLA-matched platelets derived from either volunteer donors or family members, with platelets obtained by plateletpheresis. Recently, techniques of cross-matching platelets have been developed and appear to identify suitable platelet donors (nonreactive with the patient's serum) without the need for HLA typing. Such single-donor platelets usually contain the equivalent of six units of random platelets, or $30–50 \times 10^{10}$ platelets suspended in 200 mL of plasma. Ideally, these platelet concentrates will raise the recipient's platelet count by 60,000/µL. Preliminary reports suggest that leukocyte-depleted platelets may be less immunogenic and that their use may delay the onset of alloimmunization.

Granulocyte Transfusions

Granulocytes for transfusion may be procured by leukapheresis. Approximately $1–3 \times 10^{10}$ times granulocytes can be collected from the donor. However, this number of granulocytes represents less than 10% of normal daily granulocyte production, and granulocytes survive only for hours. There is usually no detectable increase in the number of recipient granulocytes after such transfusions. Hazards of granulocyte transfusions include transmission of CMV infection and severe leukoagglutinin reactions. Because of these considerations, prophylactic granulocyte transfusions are not used in severely neutropenic patients.

Granulocyte transfusions are seldom indicated. However, they may be beneficial in patients with profound neutropenia (< 100/µL) who have gram-negative sepsis or progressive soft tissue infection despite optimal antibiotic therapy. In these cases, it is clear that progressive infection is due to failure of host defenses. In such situations, daily granulocyte transfusions should be given and continued until the neutrophil count rises to above 500/µL. Such granulocytes must be derived from ABO-matched donors. Although HLA matching is not necessary, it is preferred, since patients with alloantibodies to donor white blood cells will have severe reactions and no benefit.

The donor cells usually contain some immunocompetent lymphocytes capable of producing graft-versus-host disease in HLA-incompatible hosts whose immunocompetence may be impaired. Irradiation of the units of cells with 1500 cGy will destroy the lymphocytes without harm to the granulocytes or platelets.

TRANSFUSION OF PLASMA COMPONENTS

Fresh-frozen plasma is available in units of approximately 200 mL. Fresh plasma contains normal levels of all coagulation factors (about 1 unit/mL). Fresh frozen plasma is used to correct coagulation factors deficiency and to treat thrombotic thrombocytopenic purpura.

Cryoprecipitate is made from fresh plasma. One unit has a volume of approximately 20 mL and contains approximately 250 mg of fibrinogen and between 80 and 100 units of factor VIII and von Willebrand factor. Cryoprecipitate is used to treat factor VIII deficiency and von Willebrand's disease and to supplement fibrinogen in cases of congenital deficiency of fibrinogen or disseminated intravascular coagulation. One unit of cryoprecipitate will raise the fibrinogen level by about 8 mg/dL.

Mollison PL: *Blood Transfusions in Clinical Medicine.* Blackwell, 1988.

REFERENCES

Jandl JH (editor): *Blood: Textbook of Hematology.* Little, Brown, 1987.

Williams WJ et al (editors): *Hematology,* 4th ed. McGraw-Hill, 1990.

Alimentary Tract

14

Kenneth R. McQuaid, MD, & C. Michael Knauer, MD

SYMPTOMS & SIGNS OF GASTROINTESTINAL DISEASE

NAUSEA & VOMITING

These intensely disagreeable symptoms may occur singly or concurrently and may be due to a wide variety of factors (see below). The pathophysiology of vomiting is not completely understood. Vomiting appears to involve two functionally distinct medullary centers: the vomiting center, which initiates and controls the act of emesis; and the chemoreceptor trigger zone, which is activated by many drugs and endogenous and exogenous toxins. The vomiting center may receive stimuli from the alimentary tract and other organs, from the cerebral cortex, from the vestibular apparatus, and from the chemoreceptor trigger zone. Two or more stimuli may coexist.

An oversimplified classification of causes of vomiting is as follows:

(1) Alimentary disorders: Irritation, inflammation, motility disorder, or mechanical disturbance at any level of the gastrointestinal tract.

(2) Hepatobiliary and pancreatic disorders.

(3) Acute systemic infection.

(4) Central nervous system disorders: Increased intracranial pressure, stroke, migraine, infection, toxins, radiation sickness.

(5) Labyrinthine disorders: Motion sickness, infection, Meniere's syndrome.

(6) Endocrine disorders: Diabetic acidosis, adrenocortical crisis, pregnancy, starvation, lactic acidosis.

(7) Genitourinary disorders: Uremia, infection, obstruction.

(8) Cardiovascular disorders: Acute myocardial infarction, congestive heart failure.

(9) Drugs: Morphine, meperidine, codeine, excess alcohol, anesthetics, anticancer drugs, many others.

(10) Psychologic disorders: Reaction to pain, fear, or displeasure, chronic anxiety reaction, anorexia nervosa, bulimia, psychosis.

Complications of vomiting include fluid and electrolyte disturbances, pulmonary aspiration of vomitus, gastroesophageal mucosal tear (Mallory-Weiss syndrome), malnutrition, and postemetic rupture of the esophagus (Boerhaave's syndrome).

Treatment

Simple acute vomiting such as occurs following dietary or alcoholic indiscretion or during morning sickness of early pregnancy may require little or no treatment. Avoiding known aggravating factors and taking simple corrective dietary measures usually suffice.

Severe or prolonged nausea and vomiting usually require careful medical management in the hospital. The following general measures may be used as adjuncts to specific medical or surgical treatment:

A. Fluids and Nutrition: Hypokalemia and metabolic alkalosis are common in patients with severe vomiting. Withhold food temporarily and give intravenously 5% dextrose in saline with appropriate KCl supplementation to maintain euvolemia. If vomiting continues, employ a nasogastric tube to intermittent suction for gastric decompression. When oral feedings are resumed, begin with dry foods in small quantities, eg, salted crackers, graham crackers. With "morning sickness," these foods may best be taken before arising. Later, change to frequent small feedings of simple palatable foods. Hot beverages (tea and clear broths) and cold beverages (iced tea and carbonated liquids, especially ginger ale) are tolerated quite early. Avoid lukewarm beverages.

B. Medical Measures: *Note:* Unless nausea and vomiting of pregnancy are severe or progressive, avoid using medication for this purpose. The possible teratogenic effects of many classes of drugs are now being investigated.

Antiemetic drugs are usually better for preventing vomiting, but they may be employed selectively if the cause of vomiting cannot be treated effectively. The drugs should be used cautiously to avoid masking the development of serious illness and should be avoided in pregnancy. The choice of drug treatment depends on the reasons for the vomiting, the needs of the patient, and the known pharmacology of the available drugs:

1. Antihistamines, eg, dimenhydrinate, 50 mg orally, intramuscularly, or by suppository every 4 hours—up to 400 mg/24 h—may be useful for patients with vestibular disorders eg, Meniere's syndrome, motion sickness..

2. Phenothiazines, eg, prochlorperazine, 5–10 mg orally or by deep intramuscular injection into the upper outer quadrants in buttock muscle three or four times daily, or 25 mg by suppository twice daily, may be preferred for vomiting caused by drugs, radiation sickness, or surgery.

3. Metoclopramide, 10 mg orally or intravenously, is particularly helpful for the nausea and vomiting of diabetic gastroparesis and for the prevention of the nausea and vomiting of cancer chemotherapy.

4. Dronabinol, which contains tetrahydrocannabinol (from marihuana), and nabilone, a synthetic cannabinoid, are useful in treatment of refractory vomiting induced by cancer chemotherapy.

5. Sedatives, alone or with anticholinergics, may be helpful in patients with psychogenic vomiting.

C. Psychotherapy: Attempt to determine the possible psychic basis of prolonged nausea and vomiting, but avoid aggressive psychotherapy during the acute phase of the illness. Hospitalization and restricted visiting may be necessary.

Hull FM: Gastrointestinal symptoms. J Clin Pharm Therap 1990;15:307. (Review of nausea and vomiting, with management of choice depending in part on the cause.)
Wickham R: Managing chemotherapy-related nausea and vomiting: The state of the art. Oncol Nursing Forum 1989;15:563. (Concepts of drug therapy emphasized in this more restricted patient group.)

HICCUP
(Singultus)

Hiccup, although usually transient and benign, may be caused by or associated with a wide range of disorders. Of importance are disease processes just above and below the diaphragm, such as (1) inflammation (pneumonia, esophagitis, subphrenic abscess, pancreatitis); (2) gastric distention; (3) neoplasms; (4) myocardial infarction or pericardial disease; (5) metabolic derangements (azotemia); (6) central nervous system disorders (infection, tumors); and (7) idiopathic disorders. Correction of potentially remediable causes will be most effective in the management of hiccup. Occasionally, hiccup is unilateral; this may have implications for therapy in refractory cases.

Treatment
Countless measures have been suggested for interrupting the rhythmic reflex that produces hiccup. At times, however, none of these may be successful, and the symptom may be so prolonged and severe as to jeopardize the patient's life.

A. Simple Home Remedies: These measures probably act by diverting the patient's attention; they consist of distracting conversation, fright, painful or unpleasant stimuli, or of having the patient perform such apparently purposeless procedures as breath holding, sipping ice water, or inhaling strong fumes. Swallowing a teaspoon of dry cane sugar may be effective.

B. Medical Measures:

1. Sedation—Any of the common sedative drugs may be effective, eg, diazepam, 5 mg orally, or alprazolam, 0.25 mg orally.

2. Stimulation of nasopharynx—A soft catheter introduced nasally to stimulate the nasopharynx and pharynx is often successful.

3. Local anesthetics—Viscous 2% lidocaine, 15 mL orally, may be of some use. General anesthesia may be tried in intractable cases.

4. Prokinetic drug—Metoclopramide, 10 mg intramuscularly, may be useful.

5. CO_2 inhalations—Have the patient rebreathe into a paper bag for 3–5 minutes, or give 10–15% CO_2 mixture by face mask for 3–5 minutes.

6. Tranquilizers—Phenothiazine drugs have been used successfully for prolonged hiccup, eg, chlorpromazine, 25–50 mg orally three times a day for 2–3 days; if symptoms persist, one may try 25–50 mg intramuscularly.

7. Antacids.

C. Surgical Measures: Various phrenic nerve operations, including bilateral phrenicotomy, may be indicated in extreme cases that fail to respond to all other measures and are considered to be a threat to life.

CONSTIPATION

The frequency of defecation and the consistency and volume of stools vary so greatly from individual to individual that it is often difficult to determine what is "normal." Familial, social, and dietary customs may help determine individual differences in bowel habits. Normal bowel movements may range in frequency from three to 12 stools per week, and the weights may range from 35 to 200 g of stool per day. The complaint of constipation often reflects the attitude of the patient with respect to the expected pattern of bowel movements. The patient should be considered to be constipated only if defecation is unexplainably delayed for days or if the stools are unusually hard, dry, and difficult to express. Constipation may result from repeatedly ignoring the urge to defecate because of unwillingness to interrupt social, recreational, or occupational activities.

Because there are many specific organic causes of constipation (see below), it is essential to explore such possibilities in patients with unexplained constipation. Be especially suspicious of organic causes when there have been sudden and unaccountable changes in bowel habits, or blood in the stools.

Causes of Constipation

(1) Dietary factors: Highly refined and low-fiber foods, inadequate fluids.

(2) Physical inactivity: Inadequate exercise, prolonged bed rest.

(3) Pregnancy.

(4) Advanced age (often multifactorial).

(5) Drugs: Analgesics (codeine, oxycodone (Percodan), anesthetics, antacids (aluminum and calcium salts), anticholinergics, anticonvulsants, antidepressants (tricyclics, monoamine oxidase inhibitors), antihypertensives (ganglionic blocking agents), antiparkinsonism drugs, antipsychotic drugs (phenothiazines), β-adrenergic blocking agents, bismuth salts, calcium channel blockers, diuretics, iron salts, laxatives and cathartics (chronic use), metallic intoxications (arsenic, lead, mercury), muscle relaxants, opiates.

(6) Metabolic abnormalities: Hypokalemia, hyperglycemia, uremia, porphyria, amyloidosis.

(7) Endocrine abnormalities: Hypothyroidism, hypercalcemia, panhypopituitarism, pheochromocytoma, glucagonoma.

(8) Lower bowel abnormality: (a) Colon: prediverticular disease, diverticulosis, diverticulitis of sigmoid colon, neoplasm, extrinsic obstruction, inflammatory disease, especially with stricture and motility disorders. **(b) Rectum:** Disturbances in the defecatory mechanism, rectal intussusception, aganglionosis, pelvic floor spasm, neoplasm, inflammation. **(c) Anus:** Stricture, fissure, neoplasm.

(9) Neurogenic abnormalities: Innervation disorders of the bowel wall (aganglionosis, autonomic neuropathy), spinal cord disorders (trauma, multiple sclerosis, tabes dorsalis), disorders of the splanchnic nerves (tumors, trauma), cerebral disorders (strokes, parkinsonism, neoplasm).

(10) Psychogenic disorders.

(11) Enemas (chronic use).

Diagnosis

The history is all-important in the evaluation of this problem. If the cause is not obvious (no tumors, no stricture, etc) and the patient does not respond to simple measures (see below), further workup may be indicated to determine whether the problem is decreased motility or "outlet obstruction."

A. Motility Disorders: Assess transit through the colon with radiopaque markers.

B. Obstruction: Barium enema to assess for a possible obstructing lesion or distal aganglionic segment, rectal biopsy to assess the presence of ganglion cells, defecography to assess for rectal intussuscep-

tion (usual mechanism for solitary rectal ulcer and pelvic floor relaxation), anorectal manometry.

C. Metabolic Disorders: Hypothyroidism and hypercalciuria should be considered.

Treatment

The patient should be told that a daily bowel movement is not essential to health or well-being and that many symptoms (eg, lack of "pep") attributed to constipation have no such relationship.

A. Reestablishment of Regular Evacuation: Cathartics and enemas should not be used for simple constipation, since they interfere with the normal bowel reflexes. If it seems inadvisable to withdraw such measures suddenly from a patient who has employed them for a long time, the milder laxatives and enemas (see below) can be used temporarily. Bulking agents (eg, psyllium seed, methylcellulose) can be used indefinitely. Cathartic and enema "addicts" often defy all medical measures, and treatment is especially difficult when there is a serious underlying psychiatric disturbance.

B. Diet: The diet may be modified to satisfy the following requirements:

1. Adequate volume–Often "constipation" is merely due to inadequate food intake.

2. Adequate bulk or residue–Food with high fiber content such as bran and raw fruits and vegetables may be helpful.

3. Vegetable irritants–Unless there is a specific contraindication (eg, intolerance), stewed or raw fruits (particularly prunes and figs) or vegetables may be of value, especially in the "atonic" type of constipation.

4. Adequate fluids–The patient should be encouraged to drink adequate quantities of fluids to permit passage of intestinal contents. Six to eight glasses of fluid per day, in addition to the fluid content of foods, are ordinarily sufficient. A glass of hot water taken one-half hour before breakfast seems to exert a mild laxative effect.

C. Laxatives: Laxatives may be classified as (1) stimulants (irritants), (2) bulk-forming agents, (3) osmotic laxatives, (4) wetting agents, and (5) lubricants. They are intended for temporary use on a selective basis by patients with simple constipation. Laxatives should *never* be given to patients with undiagnosed abdominal pain or when there is a possibility of intestinal obstruction or fecal impaction. Prolonged use of laxatives (other than bulk-forming agents) is seldom justified unless definitive therapy for specific disease is not possible. Chronic laxative use interferes with normal bowel motility and reflexes, thereby setting up a pattern for persistent constipation. Habitual use may also result in damage to the myenteric plexus of the colon and rectum. Melanosis coli is the result of chronic use (4 months or more) of anthracene cathartics (cascara, senna, aloe) and gives the rectocolonic mucosa a brown-black mosaic pattern appearance; it is probably not functionally important. There are no advantages—and there may be serious disadvantages—to mixing various laxatives.

1. Stimulant (irritant) laxatives–

a. Cascara sagrada aromatic fluid extract, a mild agent; 4–8 mL acts within 6–12 hours.

b. Bisacodyl (Dulcolax, etc), a mild to moderate laxative that stimulates sensory nerve endings of the colon to produce parasympathetic reflexes; 10–15 mg given orally acts within 6 hours. In suppository form it is usually effective in 15–60 minutes; particularly useful in patients with spinal cord injury.

c. Phenolphthalein, a potent over-the-counter laxative; 60–200 mg acts within 4–10 hours.

d. Glycerin suppository, a local irritant that stimulates the rectocolic reflex and lubricates hard fecal material; 3 g acts within 30 minutes.

2. Bulk-forming agents–

a. Psyllium hydrophilic mucilloid and methylcellulose (Metamucil, others), more than 14 g (one or two rounded teaspoonfuls) two or three times daily after meals in a full glass of water, provides increased bulk—a stimulus to colon motility. It is nonsystemic but may cause increased flatus. It is particularly useful in elderly patients and in those with irritable colon syndrome.

b. Unprocessed bran, one-fourth cup daily with cereal or in unsweetened applesauce.

3. Osmotic laxatives–

a. Milk of magnesia (magnesium hydroxide), 15–30 mL at bedtime, is a common mild-to-moderate generically available laxative. It should not be used by patients with impaired renal function, in whom hypermagnesemia may develop.

b. Citrate of magnesia, 120–240 mL. Avoid use for patients with renal impairment (see above).

c. Sodium phosphate, 4–8 g in cold water before breakfast.

d. Lactulose syrup, 15—60 mL daily (relatively expensive). Sorbitol is equally effective and inexpensive; the dosage is the same.

4. Wetting agents–Docusate sodium, 50–350 mg/d. This agent interferes with sodium resorption in the colon, leading (allegedly) to increased water content in stool. Docusate sodium is also an "irritant" that produces mucosal changes in the small bowel, but the effect of this action on stool character or frequency is unclear.

5. Lubricants–Liquid petrolatum (mineral oil), 15–30 mL per rectum, may help soften stool. Administration orally should be avoided because of risk of aspiration with resulting lipid pneumonia, and because petrolatum may interfere with intestinal absorption of fat-soluble vitamins.

D. Enemas: Because they interfere with restoration of a normal bowel reflex, enemas should ordinarily be used only as a temporary expedient in chronic constipation or fecal impaction. Infrequently, it may be necessary to administer enemas for prolonged periods.

1. Saline enema (nonirritating)–Warm physiologic saline solution, 500–2000 mL.

2. Warm tap water (irritating)–500–1000 mL.

3. Soapsuds (SS) enema (irritating)–75 mL of soap solution per liter of water.

4. Oil retention enema–180 mL of mineral oil or vegetable oil instilled in the rectum in the evening, retained overnight, and evacuated the next morning.

E. Surgery: For the rare patient in whom all medical and dietary measures fail and in whom constipation continues to severely affect enjoyment of life, left or subtotal colectomy may prove beneficial.

Pemberton J: Chronic constipation: Matching type to treatment. Contemp Intern Med (Sept) 1989, p 64. (Pathophysiology and management.)

Wald A, Hinds JP, Caruna BJ: Psychological and physiological characteristics of patients with severe idiopathic constipation. Gastroenterology 1989;97:932. (Management needs to be individualized.)

FECAL IMPACTION

Hardened or putty-like stools in the rectum or colon may interfere with the normal passage of feces; if the impaction is not removed manually, by enemas, or by surgery, it can cause partial or complete intestinal obstruction. The impaction may be due to organic causes (painful anorectal disease, tumor, or neurogenic disease of the colon) or to functional causes (bulk laxatives, antacids, residual barium from x-ray study, low-residue diet, starvation, drug-induced colonic stasis, or prolonged bed rest and debility). The patient may give a history of obstipation, but more frequently there is a history of watery diarrhea. There may be blood or mucus in the stool. Physical examination may reveal a distended abdomen, palpable "tumors" in the abdomen, and a firm stool in the rectum. The impaction may be broken up digitally or dislodged with a sigmoidoscope. Cleansing enemas (preferably in the knee-chest position) or, in the case of impaction higher in the colon, colonic irrigations may be of value. Daily oil retention enemas followed by digital fragmentation of the impaction and saline enemas may be necessary.

Wald A: Colorectal function and constipation in the elderly. Pract Gastroenterol 1989;13:36. (Stresses effect on quality of life. Management dependent on cause.)

GASTROINTESTINAL GAS
(Flatulence)

The amount of gastrointestinal gas varies considerably from individual to individual. Subjective estimates by patients may be at considerable variance from observed findings, which indicate the average to be 17 passages of flatus per 24 hours. Five gases—nitrogen and oxygen from swallowed air, and carbon dioxide, hydrogen, and methane produced in the gut—constitute more than 99% of gastrointestinal gas. Excessive belching or eructation is usually due to air swallowed during eating or drinking, or it may be due to a nervous habit of sucking in air; the latter may be severe.

Excessive passage of flatus per rectum is due largely to gases formed by bacterial fermentation of maldigested carbohydrates and cellulose in the intestine. Rectal gas consists predominantly of H_2, CO_2, and CH_4—all odorless; there is little objective information on the malodorous gases. Many problems of abdominal bloating or distention with pain appear to be caused by disordered bowel motility rather than by excessive gas. Since excessive gastrointestinal gas may be due to both functional and organic disease, complaints of unusual belching, bloating, and flatulence may require search for specific causes.

Treatment

A. Correction of Aerophagia: Anxiety states are often associated with deep breathing and sighing and consequent swallowing of considerable quantities of air. Chewing gum contributes to swallowing of air.

B. Correction of Physical Defects: These sometimes interfere with normal swallowing or breathing: (1) Structural deformities of the nose and nasopharynx, eg, nasal obstruction and adenoids. (2) Spatial defects of the teeth or ill-fitting dentures.

C. Diet: The diet should be nutritious as tolerated and enjoyed by the patient, but eliminate foods that may lead to excessive flatulence in susceptible individuals. An initial trial of a lactose-free diet is often rewarding.

D. Medications: Drugs (including charcoal, simethicone, and antiflatulence tablets) are generally unsatisfactory and may be only of placebo value. Anticholinergic-sedative drugs serve to diminish the flow of saliva (which is often excessive in some patients), thereby reducing the aerophagia that accompanies swallowing; bowel motility is reduced.

Strocchi A, Leavitt MD: Alleviating intestinal gas. Contemp Int Med 1991;Jan:28. (Physiology, pathophysiology, and management.)

DIARRHEA

Diarrhea is defined as an increase in the frequency, fluidity, and volume (> 200 g/d) of bowel movements. Normal bowel function varies from individual to individual, and the definition of diarrhea must take this variation into account. Factors influencing stool consistency are poorly understood; water content is not the sole determinant. Thus, the definition of diarrhea in a clinical sense is an increase in frequency or increased fluidity of bowel movements in a given individual. In pathophysiologic terms, diarrhea results from the passage of stools containing excess water, ie, from malabsorption or secretion of water. Although daily stool weight or water is probably the best single index to diarrhea, "small-volume diarrhea" with frequent evacuations of blood, mucus, or exudate is a syndrome often signifying disease of the distal colon.

Pathophysiology

A. Types of Diarrhea:

1. With excess fecal water–

a. Osmotic diarrhea–Excess water-soluble molecules in the bowel lumen cause osmotic retention of intraluminal water. *Examples:* Magnesium hydroxide, undigested disaccharides, surreptitious use of laxatives.

b. Secretory diarrhea–Excessive active ion secretion by the mucosal cells of the intestine. *Examples:* Cholera, toxigenic *Escherichia coli*, Zollinger-Ellison syndrome, carcinoid syndrome, vipoma.

c. Exudative disease–Abnormal mucosal permeability, with intestinal loss of serum proteins, blood, mucus, or pus.

d. Impaired contact between intestinal chyme and absorbing surface–Rapid transit, short bowel syndromes.

e. Motility disturbances–Diabetes mellitus, scleroderma, amyloidosis; may lead to bacterial overgrowth and maldigestion.

2. Without excess fecal water–Frequent small, painful evacuations are usually a result of disease of the left colon or rectum.

B. Causes of Diarrhea: Most diarrheal states are self-limited and pose no special diagnostic problem. The following list of the causes of diarrhea is indicative of the extensive diagnostic evaluation that may be required in patients with unexplained, profound, or chronic diarrhea.

1. Psychogenic disorders–"Nervous" diarrhea. Best characterized by the "pre-exam" diarrhea of students.

2. Drugs–Magnesium-containing antacids, antibiotics, laxatives, sorbitol (excess diet drinks, sugarless gum, etc), metoclopramide.

3. Intestinal infections–

a. Viral infections–Enterovirus, Norwalk virus.

b. Bacterial infections–Most common are *Campylobacter jejuni*, *Shigella*, *Salmonella*, and *Yersinia enterocolitica*.

c. Bacterial toxins–*Clostridium difficile*, enterotoxigenic *Escherichia coli*, *Staphylococcus*, *V parahaemolyticus*, and *V cholerae*.

4. Parasitic infections–*Giardia lamblia*, En-

tamoeba histolytica, Cryptosporidium, and *Isospora* are the most common.

5. Other intestinal factors–Fecal impaction, lactase deficiency (milk intolerance), antibiotic therapy, inflammatory bowel disease, catharsis habituation, vagotomy, carcinoma, heavy metal poisoning, gastrocolic fistula, and amyloidosis.

6. Cholestatic syndromes–Hepatitis and bile duct obstruction may result in steatorrhea and mild diarrhea.

7. Malabsorption states–Primary small bowel mucosal diseases (eg, celiac sprue), short small bowel states, and intestinal blind loop syndrome (eg, diverticula, afferent loop).

8. Pancreatic disease–Pancreatic insufficiency, diabetes mellitus, pancreatic endocrine tumors.

9. Reflex from other viscera–Pelvic disease (extrinsic to gastrointestinal tract).

10. Neurologic disease–Tabes dorsalis, diabetic neuropathy.

11. Metabolic disease–Hyperthyroidism, diabetes mellitus with neuropathy.

12. Immunodeficiency disease–IgA deficiency, AIDS.

13. Malnutrition–Marasmus, kwashiorkor.

14. Food allergy.

15. Dietary factors–Excessive fresh fruit intake, caffeine-containing foods.

16. Factitious–Surreptitious laxative ingestion.

17. Unknown.

Diagnosis

A specific diagnosis can often be made on the basis of the history and physical examination alone. Otherwise, it is based on examination of diarrheal material for polymorphonuclear cells, parasites, and culture for bacterial pathogens. This is best accomplished at sigmoidoscopy prior to preparation with a cleansing enema. Cotton swabs should not be used in making slides, since both polymorphonuclear cells and parasites cling to cotton. The presence of polymorphonuclear cells indicates an inflammatory process. Rectal biopsy may prove helpful, particularly when *Entamoeba histolytica* is being considered and there is colitis. These studies should be performed prior to barium studies and before starting treatment. Assay for *Clostridium difficile* is highly accurate with current techniques.

Treatment

A. Correct Physiologic Changes Induced by Diarrhea:

1. Acid-base disturbance, fluid loss.

2. Electrolyte depletion (hyponatremia, hypokalemia, hypocalcemia, hypomagnesemia).

3. Malnutrition, vitamin deficiencies.

4. Psychogenic disturbances (eg, fixation on gastrointestinal tract or anxiety regarding incontinence in cases of long-standing diarrhea).

B. Diet:

1. Acute severe–Food should be withheld for the first 24 hours or restricted to lukewarm clear liquids—a physiologic glucose and salt solution, sipped slowly as needed to replace large fluid and electrolyte losses, may be especially useful in patients with severe watery diarrhea. Frequent small soft feedings are added as tolerated. Milk and milk products are the last foods to be added, since temporary lactase deficiency frequently is present after an "insult" to the small intestine.

2. Convalescent–Food should be incorporated into the diets of patients convalescing from acute diarrhea as tolerated. Nutritious food, preferably all cooked, in small frequent meals, is usually well tolerated. *Avoid* raw vegetables and fruits, fried foods, bran, whole grain cereals, preserves, syrups, candies, pickles, relishes, spices, coffee, and alcoholic beverages.

3. Chronic diarrhea–Chronic diarrhea is due to many causes. Nutritional disturbances range from none to marked depletion of electrolytes, water, protein, fat, and vitamins. Treat specific disease when known (eg, gluten-free diet in celiac sprue and enzyme replacement in pancreatic insufficiency). Give fat-soluble vitamins (vitamins A, D, E, K) when steatorrhea is present. Some patients are so ill that they require parenteral alimentation, sometimes at home.

C. Antidiarrheal Agents: Antidiarrheal drugs must be used with great caution in inflammatory bowel disease and amebiasis because of the risk of "toxic" dilation of the colon. They should usually be avoided in bacillary dysentery, since they may prolong or worsen the course of the acute illness.

1. Bismuth subsalicylate (Pepto-Bismol)–Give 30 mL (or two tablets) up to eight times a day for symptomatic treatment of diarrhea. Remind the patient that this agent causes black stools and tongue and that it contains salicylates.

2. Narcotic analogues–Avoid with possible acute infectious diarrhea, as they may worsen and prolong the course.

a. Diphenoxylate with atropine, one tablet three or four times daily as needed. It is contraindicated in patients with obstructive jaundice or with pseudomembranous or endotoxin-induced colitis. It must be used cautiously in patients with advanced liver disease and in those who are addiction-prone or who are taking sedatives. Use concurrently with MAO inhibitors may precipitate a hypertensive crisis.

b. Loperamide, 4 mg initially, then 2 mg after each loose stool (maximum dose: 16 mg/d) is effective in acute and chronic diarrhea.

3. Narcotics–Narcotics must be avoided in chronic diarrheas unless there is intractable diarrhea, vomiting, and colic. Always exclude the possibility of acute surgical abdominal disease before administering opiates, especially incomplete obstruction and diverticulitis. Give any of the following:

a. Paregoric, 4–8 mL after liquid movements as needed or with bismuth.

b. Codeine phosphate, 15–60 mg subcutaneously, if the patient is vomiting, after liquid bowel movements as needed.

c. Strong opiates–Morphine should be reserved for selected patients with severe acute diarrhea who fail to respond to more conservative measures.

4. Anticholinergic drugs, particularly when used in combination with sedatives, exert a mild antiperistaltic action in acute and chronic diarrheas associated with anxiety tension states. It may be necessary to administer the various drugs to a point near toxicity in order to achieve the desired effect.

D. Special Situations:

1. Clonidine, 1 mg patch, for managing diarrhea associated with diabetes, cryptosporidia, etc.

2. Octreotide acetate–Starting dose is 50 mg subcutaneously once or twice a day for patients with diarrhea due to carcinoid tumor, vipoma, AIDS, and perhaps diabetes. Dosage may have to go as high as 150 mg subcutaneously three times a day to be effective.

E. Psychotherapy: Source cases of chronic diarrhea are of psychogenic origin. A survey of anxiety-producing mechanisms should be made in all patients with this complaint. Antidepressant drug therapy may be useful, particularly since many of these agents have an anticholinergic effect.

F. Prophylaxis: Traveler's diarrhea, most commonly due to enterotoxigenic *E coli* or *Shigella,* can frequently be prevented with the prophylactic use of doxycycline or trimethoprim-sulfamethoxazole. However, the low incidence and moderate morbidity among travelers to developing countries probably do not warrant the risks of prophylactic treatment of all travelers.

Black RE: Epidemiology of traveler's diarrhea and relative importance of various pathogens. Rev Infect Dis 1990; 12(Suppl 1):73. (Geographic characteristics, epidemiology, and frequencies. Enterotoxigenic *E coli* accounts for 42% in Latin America.

Field M, Rao MR, Chang EB: Intestinal electrolyte transport and diarrheal disease. (Two parts.) N Engl J Med 1989;321:800, 879. (Rational approach to management.)

Guerrant RL, Bobak DA: Bacterial and protozoal gastroenteritis. N Engl J Med 1991;325:327. (Current review, with algorithm for diagnosis and management.)

Ogbounaya KI: Diabetic diarrhea: Pathophysiology, diagnosis, and management. Arch Intern Med 1990;150:262. (Clonidine and somatostatin analogues in treatment.)

GASTROINTESTINAL BLEEDING

1. UPPER GASTROINTESTINAL BLEEDING

Depending on the clinical situation, upper gastrointestinal bleeding may be characterized by coffee-ground emesis (blood that has been in contact with hydrochloric acid), bright red hematemesis, bright red blood per rectum (rapid transit), melena, or Hemoccult-positive stool.

Etiology

The major causes of gastrointestinal bleeding are listed below in approximate order of frequency.

(1) Gastroduodenal erosions or ulcers secondary to aspirin, NSAIDS, or alcohol (history is important).

(2) Peptic ulceration—duodenal, gastric, or esophageal. (History is of utmost importance, remembering that symptoms often clear with onset of bleeding.)

(3) Esophagitis (associated with heartburn, reflux of gastric contents, dysphagia, or odynophagia).

(4) Mallory-Weiss syndrome (usually preceded by retching, vomiting, coughing, or some other mode of sudden Valsalva maneuver).

(5) Esophageal or gastric varices (usually with a history and clinical evidence of chronic liver disease and portal hypertension, eg, hepatosplenomegaly, prominent abdominal veins, spider angiomas).

(6) Neoplasms such as leiomyoma, cancer.

(7) Vascular lesions such as Dieulafoy's erosions, angiodysplasia.

(8) Drugs such as warfarin, heparin.

Clinical Findings

The clinical picture depends on the acuteness of hemorrhage and its cause.

A. Massive Bleeding: Rapid loss of blood may occur to the point of clinical hypovolemia. The patient often presents with acute bright red hematemesis or profuse melena or with maroon stools. Hypotension, tachycardia, postural symptoms, and increased bowel sounds are frequently present.

B. Subacute Bleeding: Melena may be present for a few days with or without recurring coffee-ground emesis. There may be mild postural hypotension or a feeling of weakness.

C. Chronic Bleeding: In cases of chronic gastrointestinal bleeding there may be absence of overt bleeding or only intermittent bleeding but with increasing weakness, paleness, and even shortness of breath, particularly on exertion.

Diagnostic Evaluation

Verify bleeding with nasogastric tube and by rectal examination for blood.

A. Laboratory Studies: One should order a

baseline complete blood count, urinalysis, serum electrolytes, and BUN/creatinine ratio. An increased BUN is indicative of an increased amount of blood in the gastrointestinal tract, especially if the creatinine is normal.

1. Liver tests—Assess the presence of liver disease when clinically appropriate.

2. Coagulation studies—Determine the prothrombin time and platelet count and in occasional cases a partial thromboplastin time when there is a history of excessive bleeding such as with past dental or gynecologic procedures.

B. Endoscopy:

1. For massive bleeders, endoscopy should be performed emergently for both diagnosis and possible therapy as soon as the patient is reasonably stable.

2. For subacute bleeders and for bleeders currently not active, endoscopy should be performed, but it can be done on an urgent but scheduled basis.

3. For chronic bleeders, one can schedule endoscopy, and if it is not clear that hemorrhage is from the upper gastrointestinal tract, anoscopy and colonoscopy may be indicated as well.

C. Imaging Studies: If upper gastrointestinal endoscopy does not reveal the bleeding site, selective angiography should be considered if the bleeding persists. Arteriography may not be successful if the bleeding is less than 1 mL/min. Radionuclide scanning with technetium Tc 99m red cell labeling has also been advocated. Upper gastrointestinal film series may be useful in certain clinical settings when bleeding has abated.

Management

The patient with massive bleeding should be managed by the primary care physician, a gastroenterologist, and a surgeon from the outset. Hospitalization is required, with charting of fluid intake, urine output, and temperature. A large-bore nasogastric tube should be inserted to verify the source of hemorrhage and to remove the gastric contents prior to diagnostic or therapeutic endoscopy. If bleeding continues and hypotension persists, monitor and treat for shock (see Chapter 12). Insert a Foley catheter and two large-bore intravenous lines (at least 18-gauge). Blood is obtained immediately for complete blood count and cross-matching of at least four units of packed red blood cells. In interpreting the hematocrit, it should be kept in mind that after acute blood loss, a period of 12–24 hours may be required for equilibration of body fluids. In the interim, the hematocrit may not accurately reflect the extent of blood loss. Frequent determination of vital signs, especially those associated with postural changes, is helpful in estimating acute blood loss. In the hypotensive patient, replacement therapy is started immediately with normal saline, and packed red blood cells are given as clinically indicated to replace blood loss. Fresh-frozen plasma may be given to expand blood volume but

otherwise should be given in a ratio of one unit per five units packed red blood cells.

Aqueous vasopressin in 5% glucose in water by intravenous drip at a rate of 0.2–0.4 units/min may cause temporary arterial vasoconstriction and lowering of the portal venous pressure for variceal bleeding. Its efficacy is unproved. Water-soluble vitamin K (menadiol sodium diphosphate), 5–10 mg intramuscularly, is given empirically if hepatobiliary disease is suspected.

A. Blood Replacement: Treatment of shock by transfusion with red blood cells or fresh-frozen plasma (or both) is begun without delay. The objective of blood replacement is to correct shock and restore blood volume. The amount of blood required is estimated on the basis of vital signs, measured losses, central venous pressure, and renal perfusion as measured by urine output. While a patient is actively bleeding, at least six units of packed red blood cells should be available for emergency transfusion; rapid administration will usually control shock. When blood pressure and pulse rate have been restored to relatively normal levels and clinical signs of hypovolemia are no longer present, the rate of transfusion can be slowed. The total volume of red blood cells given is determined by the course of the disease. A poor response usually means continued bleeding (see below) or inadequate replacement. Venous pressure or pulmonary artery wedge pressure measurement is useful in selected patients in gauging adequacy of blood replacement and detecting overtransfusion and congestive heart failure. Rarely is it necessary to transfuse to a hematocrit of more than 25–26%.

B. Medical Measures: These are dependent on the diagnosis.

1. Massive and active bleeding—The patient with massive active bleeding should be managed by endoscopy for diagnosis and for therapy where indicated with such modalities as sclerotherapy, heater probe, or injection therapy.

2. Subacute or chronic bleeding—

a. General measures—Initial nasogastric tube placement to assess bleeding is indicated. If endoscopy is planned for the next day, the patient must be kept NPO until that is accomplished.

b. Diet—Depending on the diagnosis and the clinical situation, the patient may be started on a liquid diet for the first 24 hours and, if well tolerated, rapidly advanced to an appropriate diet for that individual.

c. Acid reduction—For the patient with a nasogastric tube in place, antacids such as aluminum hydroxide or magnesium hydroxide mixtures can be administered in a dose of 30 mL hourly by mouth to protect the distal esophagus from reflux and to help neutralize gastric contents not suctioned by the tube. For patients considered to be bleeding from esophagitis, gastritis, or ulcers, the use of an H_2 antagonist (cimetidine, 300 mg intramuscularly or intravenously every 6–8 hours; famotidine, 20 mg intravenously every 12 hours; or ranitidine, 50 mg intramuscularly or intravenously every 6–8 hours) is appropriate. For the nonfasting patient with ulcer disease, the H_2 receptor antagonists, antacids, and sucralfate are equally efficacious in inducing healing. Therapeutic doses of antacids 1 and 3 hours after meals and at bedtime may cause diarrhea.

There is no evidence that antacid therapy of any type is useful in stopping acute upper gastrointestinal bleeding.

C. Indications for Emergency Operation: Emergency surgery to stop active bleeding should be considered under any of the following circumstances:

1. When endoscopic therapeutic intervention has been unsuccessful.

2. When the patient has received six units of packed red blood cells or more but shock is not controlled or recurs promptly.

3. When acceptable blood pressure and hematocrit cannot be maintained with a maximum of two units of packed red blood cells every 8 hours.

4. When bleeding is slow but persists more than 2–3 days.

5. When bleeding stops initially but recurs while the patient is receiving adequate medical treatment.

6. When the patient is over age 60. The death rate from exsanguination in spite of conservative measures is greater in those over age 60 and in those who have shock or recurrent hemorrhage.

7. Some patients will have a pigmented protuberance—often called a "visible vessel"—in an ulcer base on endoscopy. About half of these patients will have uncontrolled or recurrent bleeding during the hospital stay and will require further endoscopic hemostatic therapy or surgery.

Prognosis

The overall mortality rate of about 14% indicates the seriousness of massive upper gastrointestinal hemorrhage. Fatality rates vary greatly, depending upon the cause of bleeding and the presence of other serious systemic disease. The overall operative mortality rate for emergency surgery to stop bleeding is high, and best results are obtained when bleeding can be controlled medically and surgery deferred until the patient has recovered from the effects of bleeding. Hemorrhage from duodenal ulcer causes death in about 3% of treated cases, whereas in bleeding varices the mortality rate may be as high as 50%.

Changchien CS et al: Different implications of stigmata of recent hemorrhage in gastric and duodenal ulcers. Dig Dis Sci 1988;33:400. (Clinical refinements on basis of endoscopic criteria.)

Hamilton FA et al: Endoscopy in bleeding ulcer. Gastrointest Endosc 1990;(36 Suppl Sep/Oct)36:1. (Proceedings of the NIH Consensus Conference, April 1989.)

Levy M et al: Major upper gastrointestinal tract bleeding: Relation to the use of aspirin and other nonnarcotic analgesics. Arch Intern Med 1988;148:281. (Increased risk.)

Wilcox CM, Truss CD: Gastrointestinal bleeding in patients receiving long-term anticoagulant therapy. Am J Med 1988;84:683. (Role of prothrombin time in diagnosis.)

2. LOWER GASTROINTESTINAL BLEEDING

Lower gastrointestinal bleeding may be characterized by bright red blood on toilet tissue, separated from formed stool, mixed in with stool, or associated with diarrheal stool, depending in large part on the cause. Bleeding is frequently occult and uncommonly is massive.

Etiology

A. Anal: Hemorrhoidal origin is most common. Other causes include anal fissure (associated with painful bowel movements) and, uncommonly, anal carcinoma.

B. Neoplasms: Hemoccult-positive stool with or without iron deficiency anemia is the classic presentation for cancer of the colon, especially right-sided. Benign polyps of the colon may present similarly or with blood-streaked stools.

C. Inflammatory: The major causes, especially when associated with diarrhea, are bacterial infection (*Shigella, Campylobacter, Salmonella*), parasitic infection (*Entamoeba histolytica*), and inflammatory bowel disease (chronic ulcerative colitis; less commonly, Crohn's disease).

D. Upper Gastrointestinal Source: Peptic ulcer, neoplasms, aortoduodenal fistula, and even esophageal varices may initially present as lower gastrointestinal bleeding.

E. Diverticulosis: Diverticulosis is a common cause of sudden, painless bright red or maroon blood per rectum, particularly in the elderly. Bleeding due to this cause usually stops spontaneously, but it may be massive.

F. Vascular Disorders: Angiodysplasia, bowel ischemia, colonic varices, aortoenteric fistula, and hereditary telangiectasia must be considered in appropriate clinical settings.

G. Coagulopathies: Blood coagulation disorders secondary to anticoagulants, blood dyscrasias, and even azotemia may be manifested by lower gastrointestinal bleeding.

Clinical Findings

The clinical presentation varies with the cause and acuteness of bleeding. In massive bleeding—most commonly due to diverticulosis—large volumes of bright red or maroon clots passed per rectum may lead to hypotension. Subacute bleeding is often intermittent and is most characteristically seen as bloody diarrhea associated with infections or inflammatory bowel disease.

Chronic bleeding tends to be occult, as seen with right-sided colonic neoplasms; or may appear as intermittent passage of bright red blood due to any of the causes listed above.

Diagnostic Evaluation

Verify the presence of bleeding and place a nasogastric tube if necessary to confirm that the source is not in the upper gastrointestinal tract.

A. Laboratory Studies: As for upper gastrointestinal bleeding.

B. Endoscopy: (For massive or subacute bleeding.) Sigmoidoscopy of the unprepared bowel should be part of the physical examination to evaluate for acute colitis and hemorrhoidal bleeding. Sigmoidoscopy offers a good opportunity for collecting specimens for culture, for examination for parasites, and even for biopsies depending on the clinical picture. Colonoscopy may be called for after the patient is stable and appropriately prepared if sigmoidoscopy has not identified the source or if the diagnosis is still obscure.

C. Imaging: Imaging studies are the same as for upper gastrointestinal bleeding. If Meckel's diverticulum is being considered, Tc 99m pertechnetate scintigraphy can be used to localize ectopic gastric mucosa with an accuracy of 90%.

Management & Prognosis

If there is massive bleeding, one must correct volume deficits as indicated. Patients with diarrhea should be kept NPO (and supported with parenteral fluids) to help decrease bowel motility.

Blood losses should be replaced with packed red cells as clinically indicated.

Specific treatment depends upon the cause, and the source of bleeding must be identified. In cases of major bleeding, surgical consultation should be sought from the outset.

The prognosis depends on the cause and the magnitude of bleeding.

Potter GD, Sellin JH: Lower gastrointestinal bleeding. Gastroenterol Clin North Am 1988;17:341. (Emphasizes diverticulosis and angiodysplasia as most common source.)

Richter JM et al: Angiodysplasia: Natural history and efficacy of therapeutic interventions. Dig Dis Sci 1989; 34:1542. (Rebleeding common, especially in the elderly.)

DISEASES OF THE PERITONEUM

ACUTE PERITONITIS

Essentials of Diagnosis

- Abdominal pain, vomiting, fever, and prostration.
- Abdominal rigidity and diffuse or local tenderness (often rebound).
- Later, abdominal distention and paralytic ileus.
- Leukocytosis.

General Considerations

Localized or generalized peritonitis is the most important complication of a wide variety of acute abdominal disorders. Peritonitis may be caused by infection or chemical irritation. Perforation or necrosis of the gastrointestinal tract is the usual source of infection. Chemical peritonitis occurs in acute pancreatitis and in the early stages of gastroduodenal perforation. Spontaneous bacterial peritonitis may occur in decompensated cirrhotic patients with ascites, especially those with ascitic protein content of less than 1.1 g/dL. Sclerosing peritonitis may be associated with neoplastic disease and certain drugs (eg, beta-blockers, methysergide).

Clinical Findings

A. Systemic Reaction: Malaise, prostration, nausea, vomiting, septic fever, leukocytosis, and electrolyte imbalance are usually seen in proportion to the severity of the process. If infection is not controlled, toxemia is progressive, and septic shock may develop.

B. Abdominal Signs:

1. Pain and tenderness–Depending upon the extent of involvement, pain and tenderness may be localized or generalized. Abdominal pain on coughing, rebound tenderness referred to the area of peritonitis, and tenderness to light percussion over the inflamed peritoneum are characteristic. Pelvic peritonitis is associated with rectal and vaginal tenderness.

2. Muscle rigidity–The muscles overlying the area of inflammation usually become spastic. When peritonitis is generalized (eg, after perforation of a peptic ulcer), marked rigidity of the entire abdominal wall may develop immediately. Rigidity is frequently diminished or absent in the late stages of peritonitis, in severe toxemia, and when the abdominal wall is weak.

3. Paralytic ileus–Intestinal motility is markedly inhibited by peritoneal inflammation. Diminished to absent peristalsis and progressive abdominal distention are the cardinal signs. Vomiting occurs as a result of pooling of gastrointestinal secretions and gas, most of which is swallowed air.

C. Imaging: Abdominal films show gas and fluid collections in both large and small bowel, usually with generalized rather than localized dilation. The bowel walls, when shown in relief by the gas patterns, may appear to be thickened, indicating the presence of edema or peritoneal fluid. A gentle barium enema will determine whether large bowel obstruction is present or not.

D. Diagnostic Abdominal Tap: Recovery of ascitic fluid for amylase and protein measurements, culture, and cytologic examination—to include absolute number of polymorphonuclear neutrophils—is useful.

Differential Diagnosis

Peritonitis, which may present a highly variable clinical picture, must be differentiated from acute intestinal obstruction, acute cholecystitis with or without choledocholithiasis, pancreatitis, renal colic, gastrointestinal hemorrhage, lower lobe pneumonias, porphyria, periodic fever, hysteria, black widow spider bite, and central nervous system disorders (eg, tabes dorsalis).

Complications

The most frequent sequela of peritonitis is abscess formation in the pelvis, in the subphrenic space, between the leaves of the mesentery, or elsewhere in the abdomen. Antibiotic therapy may mask or delay the appearance of localizing signs of abscess. When fever, leukocytosis, toxemia, or ileus fails to respond to the general measures outlined for the management of peritonitis, a collection of pus should be suspected. This will usually require percutaneous ultrasound-guided or surgical drainage. Liver abscess and pylephlebitis are rare complications. Adhesions may cause early or, more frequently, late intestinal obstruction.

Treatment

The measures employed in peritonitis as outlined below are generally applicable as supportive therapy in most acute abdominal disorders. The objectives are (1) to control infection, (2) to minimize the effects of paralytic ileus, and (3) to correct fluid, electrolyte, and nutritional disorders.

A. Specific Measures: Operative procedures to close perforations, to remove sources of infection such as gangrenous bowel or an inflamed appendix, or to drain abscesses are frequently required. A localized abscess can often be managed by ultrasound-guided percutaneous catheter placement and drainage.

B. General Measures: No matter what specific operative procedures are employed, their ultimate success will often depend upon the care with which the following general measures are performed:

1. Bed rest in the medium Fowler (semisitting) position is preferred.

2. Nasogastric suction with a sump tube is started to prevent gastrointestinal distention. Suction is continued until peristaltic activity returns and the patient begins passing flatus.

3. Give nothing by mouth. Oral intake can be resumed slowly after nasogastric suction is discontinued.

4. Fluid and electrolyte therapy and parenteral feeding are required.

5. Narcotics and sedatives should be used liberally to ensure comfort and rest.

6. Antibiotic therapy–Initial antibiotic therapy should be broad-spectrum, aimed at covering aerobic and anaerobic enteric flora. When cultures are available, antibiotics are chosen according to sensitivity studies.

7. Blood transfusions are used as needed to control anemia.

8. Septic shock, if it develops, requires intensive treatment.

Prognosis

If the cause of peritonitis can be corrected, the infection, accompanying ileus, and metabolic derangement can usually be managed successfully.

Akriviadis EA, Runyon BA: Utility of an algorithm in differentiating spontaneous from secondary bacterial peritonitis. Gastroenterology 1990;98:127. (Useful in differentiating infected ascites due to gut perforation from spontaneous bacterial peritonitis.)

PERIODIC DISEASE
(Benign Paroxysmal Peritonitis, Familial Mediterranean Fever, Periodic Fever, Recurrent Polyserositis)

Periodic disease is a heredofamilial disorder of unknown pathogenesis, probably metabolic, characterized by recurrent episodes of abdominal or chest pain, fever, and leukocytosis. It is usually restricted to people of Mediterranean ancestry, primarily Armenians, Sephardic Jews, and Arabs and to some extent people of Egypto-Arabic origin living in Turkey, Greece, and Italy. The disease suggests surgical peritonitis, probably serositis, and the acute attacks are recurrent, self-limited, and not fatal. Secondary amyloidosis (serum amyloid protein A-derived) may occur, and death may result from renal or cardiac failure. Acute episodes may be precipitated by emotional upsets, alcohol, or dietary indiscretion. Treatment is symptomatic and supportive. A low-fat diet may reduce the number and severity of attacks. Daily administration of colchicine, 0.6–1.8 mg, strikingly reduces the number of attacks.

Ben-Chetrit E, Levy M: Colchicine prophylaxis in familial Mediterranean fever: Reappraisal after 15 years. Semin Arthritis Rheum 1991;20:241. (Colchicine is effective and safe in preventing flares of familial Mediterranean fever and amyloidosis.)

DISEASES OF THE ESOPHAGUS

EVALUATION OF ESOPHAGEAL DISORDERS

Symptoms

The clinical history is extremely important in the diagnosis of esophageal disease. Heartburn, dysphagia, and odynophagia virtually always indicate a primary esophageal disorder.

A. Heartburn: Heartburn (pyrosis) is the feeling of substernal burning, often radiating to the neck. Caused by the reflux of acidic (or, rarely, alkaline) material into the esophagus, it is highly specific for gastroesophageal reflux disease.

B. Dysphagia: Difficulties in swallowing may arise from problems in transferring the food bolus from the oropharynx to the upper esophagus (oropharyngeal dysphagia) or from impaired transport of the bolus through the body of the esophagus (esophageal dysphagia). A careful history usually leads to the correct diagnosis.

1. Oropharyngeal dysphagia–The oropharyngeal phase of swallowing is a complex process requiring elevation of the tongue, closure of the nasopharynx, relaxation of the upper esophageal sphincter, closure of the airway, and pharyngeal peristalsis. A brain stem medullary swallowing center integrates cranial nerves V, VII, IX, X, and XII. A variety of mechanical and neuromuscular conditions can disrupt this process (Table 14–1). Oropharyngeal dysphagia is characterized by coughing, choking, and regurgitation that occurs immediately upon initiating swallowing. Liquids are more difficult to swallow than soft foods. There may be associated dysphonia, dysarthria, or other neurologic symptoms.

2. Esophageal dysphagia–Esophageal dysphagia may be caused by **mechanical lesions** obstructing the esophagus or by **motility disorders** (Table 14–2). Patients with mechanical obstruction experience dysphagia, primarily for solids. This is recurrent, predictable, and, if the lesion progresses, will worsen as the lumen narrows. Patients with motility disorders have dysphagia for both solids and liquids. It is episodic, unpredictable, and nonprogressive or progresses at a slow rate.

C. Odynophagia: Odynophagia is sharp substernal pain on swallowing that may limit oral intake. It usually reflects severe erosive disease. It is most commonly associated with infectious esophagitis due to *Candida,* herpesviruses, or cytomegalovirus, especially in immunocompromised patients. It may also be caused by corrosive injury due to caustic ingestions and by pill-induced ulcers.

Diagnostic Studies

A. Upper Endoscopy: Endoscopy is the study of choice for evaluating persistent heartburn, odynophagia, and structural abnormalities detected on barium esophagography. In addition to direct visualization, it allows biopsy of mucosal abnormalities and dilation of strictures.

B. Videoesophagography: Oropharyngea dysphagia is best evaluated with rapid sequence videoesophagography conducted by an experienced radiologist or speech pathologist.

C. Barium Esophagography: Patients with esophageal dysphagia are evaluated first with a radiographic barium study to differentiate between mechanical lesions and esophageal motility disorders. It provides limited information about esophageal motility. In patients in whom there is a high suspicion of a mechanical lesion, many clinicians will proceed to endoscopic evaluation without a barium study.

Table 14–1. Causes of oropharyngeal dysphagia.

Neurologic disorders
  Brain stem cerebrovascular accident, mass lesion
  Pseudobulbar palsy
  Amyotrophic lateral sclerosis, multiple sclerosis, poliomyelitis
  Myasthenia gravis
Muscular disorders
  Myopathies, polymyositis
  Hypothyroidism
Motility disorders
  Upper esophageal sphincter dysfunction
Structural defects
  Zenker's diverticulum
  Malignancy, surgery, radiation to oropharynx

Table 14–2. Causes of esophageal dysphagia.

	Clues

Mechanical obstruction
  Schatzki's ring
  Peptic stricture
  Esophageal cancer
  Rare: webs, mediastinal tumor, cervical osteophytes
	(Solid foods, not liquids.) Intermittent, not progressive. Progressive; chronic heartburn. Progressive; age over 50.

Motility disorders
  Achalasia
  Scleroderma
 	
  Diffuse esophageal spasm
 	
  Others: nonspecific disorders, hypertensive lower esophageal sphincter
	(Solids or liquids.) Progressive. Chronic heartburn; Raynaud's syndrome Intermittent, not progressive; may have chest pain.

D. Esophageal Manometry: Esophageal motility is best studied using manometric techniques. A small pressure-sensing catheter assembly is passed nasally into the esophagus, allowing manometric assessment of the lower and upper esophageal sphincters and esophageal body. It is the optimal study for evaluating dysphagia in patients in whom endoscopy or barium study has excluded a mechanical obstruction.

E. Ambulatory Esophageal pH Monitoring: Esophageal pH may be monitored continuously by means of a small pH probe passed transnasally and attached to a portable pH recording device. The probe and recorder are worn by the patient for up to 24 hours. The recording can be analyzed to determine the amount of gastroesophageal acid reflux and whether a patient's symptoms correlate with documented reflux.

INFLAMMATORY ESOPHAGEAL CONDITIONS

1. GASTROESOPHAGEAL REFLUX DISEASE

Essentials of Diagnosis

- Heartburn; may be exacerbated by meals, bending, or recumbency.
- Clinical diagnosis; typical uncomplicated cases do not require diagnostic studies.
- Endoscopy demonstrates abnormalities in < 50% of patients.
- Barium esophagography seldom helpful.

General Considerations

"Gastroesophageal reflux disease" is the term applied to the symptoms or tissue damage caused by the reflux of gastric contents (usually acidic) into the esophagus. It is extremely common, with one-third of adults reporting occasional heartburn and 10% complaining of daily symptoms. It is this more symptomatic group that is likely to seek medical attention. Most patients have mild disease. A few patients develop esophageal mucosal damage (reflux esophagitis) or more severe complications.

Several factors, either alone or in combination, may contribute to gastroesophageal reflux disease.

A. Incompetent Lower Esophageal Sphincter: In most patients, reflux occurs during spontaneous, transient relaxations of the lower esophageal sphincter, even though the baseline lower esophageal sphincteric pressures (10–30 mm Hg) are adequate. Patients with more severe involvement (especially those with strictures or Barrett's esophagus) generally have an incompetent lower esophageal sphincter (< 10 mm Hg), resulting in free reflux or stress reflux during abdominal straining, lifting, or bending.

B. Irritant Effects of Refluxate: Esophageal mucosal damage is related to the potency of the refluxate and the amount of time it is in contact with the mucosa. Acidic gastric fluid (pH < 3.9) is extremely caustic to the esophageal mucosa and is the major injurious agent in the majority of cases. In a few patients, reflux of bile or pancreatic secretions may be contributory.

C. Abnormal Esophageal Clearance: Acid refluxate normally is cleared and neutralized by esophageal peristalsis and salivary bicarbonate. During sleep, swallowing-induced peristalsis is infrequent, prolonging acid exposure. One-third of patients with severe gastroesophageal reflux disease also have diminished peristaltic clearance. Certain medical conditions such as Raynaud's phenomenon, CREST syndrome, and scleroderma, are frequently associated with diminished peristalsis. Conditions associated with impaired salivation such as Sjögren's syndrome, anticholinergic medications, and oral radiation therapy may exacerbate gastroesophageal reflux disease. Hiatal hernias are common and of no significance in asymptomatic people. They are present in over 90% of patients with severe erosive esophagitis, especially when complicated by the development of strictures or Barrett's esophagus. The hernia sac appears to retard esophageal acid clearance.

D. Delayed Gastric Emptying: Impaired gastric emptying due to gastroparesis or partial gastric outlet obstruction contributes to gastroesophageal reflux disease.

Clinical Findings

A. Symptoms and Signs: The typical symptom of gastroesophageal reflux disease is heartburn. This most often occurs 30–60 minutes after meals and upon reclining. Patients often report relief from taking antacids or baking soda. When this symptom is typical, the diagnosis is established with a high degree of reliability. The severity of heartburn is not correlated with the severity of esophageal tissue damage. In fact, some patients with severe esophagitis are almost asymptomatic. Patients may complain of regurgitation—the spontaneous reflux of sour or bitter gastric contents into the mouth. Less common symptoms include dysphagia, which may be due to abnormal peristalsis or the development of complications such as stricture or Barrett's metaplasia.

Gastroesophageal reflux disease may also be manifested by atypical symptoms such as asthma, chronic laryngitis, chronic cough, and atypical (noncardiac) chest pain.

Physical examination and laboratory data are normal in uncomplicated disease.

B. Special Examinations: Uncomplicated patients with typical symptoms of heartburn and regurgitation may be treated empirically for gastroesophageal reflux disease with antacids or H_2 receptor antagonists without the need for diagnostic studies. Further investigation is required in patients with complicated disease, patients with atypical symptoms, and patients unresponsive to empiric therapy.

1. Upper endoscopy–Upper endoscopy with biopsy is the standard procedure for documenting the type and extent of tissue damage in gastroesophageal reflux disease. Approximately 50–70% of patients with proved acid reflux will have visible mucosal abnormalities such as erythema and friability of the squamocolumnar junction and erosions. In addition, endoscopy can document the presence of Barrett's esophagus or peptic stricture. Esophageal abnormalities are graded on a scale of I (mild) to IV (severe erosions, stricture, or Barrett's esophagus). Endoscopy is normal in up to half of patients with reflux symptoms and does not exclude mild disease. Endoscopy is warranted in patients with severe reflux symptoms unresolved by empirical medical therapy. It is mandatory in complicated disease as suggested by dysphagia, hematemesis, guaiac-positive stools, or iron deficiency anemia.

2. Barium esophagography–This study plays a limited role in the evaluation of gastroesophageal reflux disease in most centers because of its limited ability to identify reflux or mucosal abnormalities. In patients with severe dysphagia, it is sometimes obtained prior to endoscopy to identify a stricture.

3. Ambulatory esophageal pH monitoring–Ambulatory pH monitoring is the standard procedure for documenting pathologic acid reflux. It is useful in patients suspected of having an atypical manifestation of gastroesophageal reflux, such as atypical chest pain, chronic cough, asthma, or laryngitis. Information is obtained about the frequency and duration of acid reflux and whether symptoms correlate with documented reflux episodes. In patients with reflux symptoms who have not responded to standard therapies, it can determine whether the patient has an abnormal amount of acid reflux. It is not needed in the vast majority of patients with acid gastroesophageal reflux disease.

C. Esophageal Manometry: This study should be obtained in reflux patients for whom surgical therapy is planned in order to determine the lower esophageal sphincteric pressure and the presence of adequate esophageal peristalsis.

Differential Diagnosis

Symptoms of gastroesophageal reflux disease may be similar to those of other diseases such as esophageal motility disorders, peptic ulcer, cholelithiasis, nonulcer dyspepsia, and angina pectoris. Reflux erosive esophagitis may be confused with pill-induced damage, radiation esophagitis, or infections (CMV, herpes, *Candida*).

Complications

A. Barrett's Esophagus: This is a condition in which the normal squamous epithelium of the esophagus is replaced by a metaplastic columnar epithelium containing goblet and columnar cells. Present in about 10% of patients with gastroesophageal reflux disease, it is believed to arise from chronic reflux-induced injury to the squamous epithelium. It is identified at endoscopy by its characteristic salmon-pink appearance, which contrasts with the yellow-white of the esophageal squamous mucosa. Barrett's esophagus invariably involves the most distal esophagus (at the gastroesophageal junction) and extends from one to several centimeters proximally in a circumferential or tongue-like fashion. Biopsies should be obtained to confirm the endoscopic diagnosis. Three types of columnar epithelium may be identified: gastric cardiac, gastric fundic, and specialized columnar (intestinal type). Only the specialized columnar type is of clinical significance.

Barrett's esophagus does not provoke specific symptoms. Rather, symptoms are a consequence of gastroesophageal reflux disease. Most patients have a long history of reflux symptoms, such as heartburn and regurgitation. Dysphagia due to impaired motility is common. Paradoxically, one-third of patients report minimal or no symptoms of gastroesophageal reflux disease, suggesting decreased acid sensitivity of Barrett's epithelium. Barrett's esophagus may be complicated by stricture formation or deep ulcerations, which can bleed.

Barrett's esophagus is indicative of severe gastroesophageal reflux disease and should be treated aggressively with H_2 antagonists or omeprazole to heal any active erosive esophagitis. Surgery may be desirable in some situations. Medical or surgical therapy may prevent progression of Barrett's esophagus, but there is no convincing evidence that regression occurs.

The most serious complication of Barrett's esophagus is esophageal adenocarcinoma, which may develops in up to 10% of patients. Virtually all adenocarcinomas of the esophagus and many such tumors of the gastric cardia arise from Barrett's metaplasia. Only the specialized columnar epithelium has significant malignant potential. Although still debated, most would recommend that patients with Barrett's esophagus should undergo endoscopic surveillance with mucosal biopsies every 2 years. Early adenocarcinoma should be resected. The management of patients with high-grade dysplasia is controversial. Close (3-month) endoscopic follow-up is urged; in some cases, surgery is warranted.

B. Peptic Stricture: Stricture formation occurs in about 10% of patients with esophagitis. It is manifested by the gradual development of solid food dysphagia, which progresses over months to years. Often there is a reduction in heartburn because the stricture acts as a barrier to reflux. Most strictures are located at the gastroesophageal junction. Strictures located above this level usually occur in the presence of Barrett's metaplasia. The barium swallow reveals a smooth circumferential narrowing of the esophageal lumen 1–4 cm in length. Endoscopy with biopsy is mandatory in all cases to differentiate peptic stricture from other benign or malignant causes of esophageal stricture (Schatzki's ring, esophageal carcinoma). Active erosive esophagitis is often present. Up to 90% of symptomatic patients are effectively treated with dilation. Bougienage is performed with tapered mercury-filled rubber (Maloney) dilators or with wire-guided tapered polyvinyl dilators. Endoscopically directed hydrostatic balloons may also be used. Dilation is continued over one to several sessions. A luminal diameter of 13–15 mm is usually sufficient to relieve dysphagia. Chronic reflux therapy with omeprazole or H_2 antagonists is usually required to decrease the likelihood of stricture recurrence. Some patients require intermittent stricture dilation to maintain luminal patency. Operative management is appropriate for strictures that do not respond to dilation.

Treatment

A. Medical Treatment: The treatment of gastroesophageal reflux disease may be approached in a stepwise fashion as outlined below.

1. Lifestyle modifications–Patients should avoid foods that affect lower esophageal sphincteric pressure or irritate the esophagus. These include fried or fatty foods, coffee, alcoholic beverages (especially red wine, brandy), tomato products, citrus juices, peppermint, cola drinks, and chocolate. Overeating should be avoided, as it potentiates lower esophageal sphincteric relaxation. Being overweight may exacerbate symptoms, and many patients note significant relief after weight loss. Patients should not lie down within 3 hours after eating (the period of greatest reflux). Elevation of the head of the bed on 6-inch blocks or by a wedge under the mattress reduces nocturnal reflux and enhances esophageal acid clearance.

2. Antacids–Occasional heartburn is effectively treated with antacids on an as-needed basis. A variety of different formulations are available. Commonly used preparations are Maalox TC liquid (10–15 mL) or Mylanta-II liquid (10–15 mL) or tablets (two to four), which afford rapid symptomatic relief. Gaviscon (two to four tablets) contains antacid and alginic acid, which floats like a foamy raft on the gastric pool and may decrease reflux when the patient is in the upright position. Use of Gaviscon may be superior to antacids alone. Antacids do not provide any significant healing of erosive esophagitis.

3. H_2-receptor antagonists–Patients with frequent symptoms who do not respond to lifestyle modifications are treated with H_2-receptor antagonists. Dosing twice daily is necessary in most patients. The initial doses are ranitidine, 150 mg twice daily; cimetidine, 400 mg two or three times daily; and famotidine, 20 mg twice daily. Most patients achieve dramatic symptomatic relief with these regimens, though prompt relapse usually occurs upon discontin-

uation of the drug. Lifelong therapy is required in most cases.

4. High-dose H_2 antagonists–Persistent symptomatology despite 4–8 weeks of H_2 antagonists warrants endoscopy to document the presence and severity of esophagitis. Patients with erosive esophagitis (grade II or higher) require more aggressive therapy. High-dosage H_2-receptor therapy (cimetidine, 800 mg twice daily; or ranitidine, 150 mg four times daily or 300 mg twice daily) heal 75% of cases of erosive esophagitis. These regimens are now FDA-approved.

5. Proton pump inhibitors (omeprazole)–In patients with erosive esophagitis confirmed by endoscopy who do not respond to H_2 antagonists, a 6- to 8-week course of omeprazole, 20–40 mg daily, is indicated. Over 90% of patients achieve dramatic symptomatic relief with complete healing of esophagitis. Because over 80% will relapse within 6 months after stopping omeprazole, patients should be maintained chronically on standard or high doses of H_2 antagonists.

In some cases, adequate symptomatic relief can only be achieved with chronic omeprazole therapy. Omeprazole is not approved for long-term treatment of gastroesophageal reflux disease because of unresolved concerns about its safety. In rats, omeprazole-induced hypergastrinemia caused the development of gastric enterochromaffin-like hyperplasia and carcinoid tumors after 2 years of therapy. However, clinical experience in patients taking omeprazole up to 5 years has not demonstrated toxicity. The risks and benefits of long-term therapy must be weighed separately for each patient.

6. Other agents–Prokinetic agents (metoclopramide, bethanechol) raise the lower esophageal sphincteric pressure and enhance gastric emptying. Although they are used by some clinicians to supplement H_2 antagonist therapy, the side effects and tachyphylaxis that develops after a few weeks limit their utility. Sucralfate has no role in the treatment of gastroesophageal reflux disease.

B. Unresponsive Disease: Patients with symptoms of gastroesophageal reflux disease who do not respond to H_2 antagonists and who do not have esophagitis at endoscopy should undergo ambulatory esophageal pH monitoring to confirm that their symptoms are truly reflux-related.

Approximately 10% of patients with erosive esophagitis fail to respond to standard doses of omeprazole. In such cases, a serum gastrin level should be obtained to exclude Zollinger-Ellison syndrome. Gastric acid secretory analysis should be performed to determine whether therapeutic failure is due to inadequate suppression of gastric acid secretion. If the gastric analysis confirms achlorhydria, the cause of esophagitis may be bile reflux or pill-induced disease.

C. Surgical Treatment: Surgery is indicated for

patients who fail or are noncompliant with medical therapy. It is also indicated in patients with difficult reflux-induced strictures requiring repeated dilation. In younger patients who require chronic omeprazole therapy, surgical therapy may be the preferable option. The most commonly performed procedure is Nissen fundoplication, which is successful in over 85% of cases. This operation may now be performed laparoscopically, enhancing its appeal. In some patients, the fundoplications break down after 5–15 years, resulting in a recurrence of symptoms. Esophageal manometry is performed preoperatively to assess the motility of the esophageal body; aperistalsis and severely decreased peristaltic amplitude are contraindications to surgery.

Prognosis

Gastroesophageal reflux disease is a lifelong condition in most patients. The overwhelming majority respond very well to medical management without complications and without need for surgery.

Hillman A et al: Cost and quality of alternative treatments for persistent gastroesophageal reflux disease. Arch Intern Med 1992;152:1467. (Decision tree analysis supports omeprazole as first-line agent rather than H$_2$ antagonist in patients with grade II esophagitis.)

Katz PO: Pathogenesis and management of gastroesophageal reflux disease. J Clin Gastroenterol 1991; 13(Suppl 2):S6.

Reid BJ: Barrett's esophagus and esophageal adenocarcinoma. Gastroenterol Clin North Am 1991;20:817.

Sontag S: The medical management of reflux esophagitis. Gastroenterol Clin North Am 1990;19:683.

Spechler SJ et al: Comparison of medical and surgical therapy for complicated gastroesophageal reflux disease in veterans. N Engl J Med 1992;326:786. (Randomized trial determined that surgery achieved better symptom control and healing of esophagitis than medical therapy with H$_2$ antagonists.)

INFECTIOUS ESOPHAGITIS

Essentials of Diagnosis

- Immunosuppressed patient.
- Odynophagia, dysphagia, and chest pain.
- Endoscopy with biopsy establishes diagnosis.

General Considerations

Infectious esophagitis occurs most commonly in immunosuppressed patients. Patients with AIDS, solid organ transplants, leukemia, lymphoma, and those receiving immunosuppressive drugs are at particular risk for opportunistic infections. *Candida albicans*, herpes simplex, and cytomegalovirus are the most common pathogens. *Candida* infection may also occur in patients who have uncontrolled diabetes and those being treated with systemic corticosteroids, chemotherapy, radiation therapy, or systemic antibi-

otic therapy. Herpes simplex can affect normal hosts, in which case the infection is generally self-limited.

Clinical Findings

A. Symptoms and Signs: The most common symptoms are odynophagia and dysphagia. Substernal chest pain occurs in some patients. Patients with candidal esophagitis are sometimes asymptomatic. Oral thrush is present in only 50% of patients with candidal esophagitis and 25–50% of patients with viral esophagitis and is therefore an unreliable indicator of the cause of esophageal infection. Patients with esophageal CMV infection may have infection at other sites such as the colon and retina. Oral ulcers (herpes labialis) are often associated with herpes simplex esophagitis.

B. Special Examinations: Treatment may be empiric. For diagnostic certainty, endoscopy with biopsy and cytologic brushings is preferred because of its high diagnostic accuracy. The endoscopic signs of candidal esophagitis are diffuse, linear, yellow-white plaques adherent to the mucosa. Cytomegalovirus esophagitis is characterized by one to several large, shallow, superficial ulcerations. Herpes esophagitis results in multiple, small, deep ulcerations.

Treatment

A. Candidal Esophagitis: Treatment depends on the immune status of the patient and the severity of the illness. Options include topical agents (nystatin, 500,000 units "swish and swallow" five times daily; clotrimazole troches, 10 mg five times daily), oral agents (ketoconazole, fluconazole), and intravenous agents (amphotericin B, fluconazole). Topical therapy is used initially in patients with a normal immune system. Initial therapy for immunocompromised patients (including AIDS) generally is with ketoconazole, 200–400 mg/d, or fluconazole, 100–200 mg/d, for 2–3 weeks. Although fluconazole is more expensive than ketoconazole, it is also more efficacious and does not require low gastric pH for absorption. Patients not responding to oral therapy are treated with low-dose amphotericin B, 0.1–0.3 mg/kg/d intravenously for 7 days.

B. Cytomegalovirus Esophagitis: Initial therapy is with ganciclovir, 5 mg/kg intravenously every 12 hours for 14–21 days. Neutropenia is a frequent dose-limiting side effect. If resolution of symptoms occurs, the drug may be discontinued. If the condition has improved but not resolved, full-dose therapy may be continued for an additional 2–3 weeks. In some cases (especially in patients with AIDS), continuous ganciclovir, 5 mg/kg intravenously daily, is required for suppressive therapy. Patients who either do not respond to or cannot tolerate ganciclovir are treated acutely with foscarnet, 60 mg/kg intravenously every 8 hours for 14–21 days.

C. Herpetic Esophagitis: Immune-competent patients may be treated symptomatically and generally do not require specific antiviral therapy. Immunosuppressed patients may be treated with oral acyclovir, 200 mg orally five times daily, or 5 mg/kg intravenously every 8 hours, usually for 7–10 days. Nonresponders require therapy with foscarnet, 40 mg/kg intravenously every 8 hours for 21 days.

Prognosis

Most patients with infectious esophagitis can be effectively treated with complete symptom resolution. Depending on the patient's underlying immunodeficiency, relapse of symptoms off therapy can raise difficulties. Chronic suppressive therapy is sometimes required.

Haulk AA et al: *Candida* esophagitis. Adv Intern Med 1991;36:307.

McBane RD, Gross JB: Herpes esophagitis: Clinical syndrome, endoscopic appearance, and diagnosis in 23 patients. Gastrointest Endosc 1991;37:600.

Nelson MR et al: Foscarnet in the treatment of cytomegalovirus disease in the acquired immunodeficiency syndrome. Am J Gastroenterol 1991;86:876.

Wilcox CM et al: Cytomegalovirus esophagitis in patients with AIDS. Ann Intern Med 1990;113:589.

PILL-INDUCED ESOPHAGITIS

A number of different medications may injure the esophagus, presumably through direct, prolonged mucosal contact. The most commonly implicated are the NSAIDs, potassium chloride pills, quinidine, and antibiotics. Because injury is most likely to occur if pills are swallowed without water or while supine, hospitalized or bed-bound patients are at greater risk. Symptoms include severe retrosternal chest pain, odynophagia, and dysphagia, often beginning several hours after taking a pill. These may occur suddenly and persist for days. Some patients (especially the elderly) have relatively little pain, presenting with dysphagia. Endoscopy may reveal one to several discrete ulcers that may be shallow or deep. Chronic injury may result in severe esophagitis with stricture, hemorrhage, or perforation. Healing occurs rapidly when the offending agent is eliminated.

Kikendall JW: Pill-induced esophageal injury. Gastroenterol Clin North Am 1991;20:835.

CAUSTIC ESOPHAGEAL INJURY

Caustic esophageal injury occurs from accidental (usually children) or deliberate (suicidal) ingestion of liquid or crystalline alkali (drain cleaners, etc) or acid. Ingestion is followed almost immediately by severe burning and varying degrees of chest pain, gagging, dysphagia, and drooling. Aspiration results in stridor and wheezing. Patients require urgent emergency room attention. Initial examination should be directed to circulatory status and to prompt assessment of airway status, including laryngoscopy. Subsequently, there should be a careful examination of the oral cavity, chest, and abdomen. Chest and abdominal radiographs are obtained looking for pneumonitis or free perforation. Initial treatment is supportive, with intravenous fluids and analgesics. Nasogastric lavage and oral antidotes may be dangerous and should generally not be administered. Most patients may be managed medically. Endoscopy is usually performed within the first 24 hours to assess the extent of injury. Many patients are discovered not to have any mucosal injury to the esophagus or stomach, allowing prompt discharge and psychiatric referral. Otherwise, endoscopic appearance does not accurately predict the likelihood of transmural injury and perforation. All patients with mucosal damage must therefore be observed carefully in the first 72 hours for signs of deterioration. Circumferential injury to the esophagus portends an increased risk of stricture formation. Previously, antibiotics and corticosteroids were used acutely in an effort to decrease the incidence of stricture formation, but these have not been found to be effective. Surgery is indicated for sepsis, shock, perforation, or progressive deterioration.

Kikendall JW. Caustic ingestion injuries. Gastroenterol Clin North Am 1991;20:847.

BENIGN ESOPHAGEAL LESIONS

1. MALLORY-WEISS SYNDROME (Mucosal Laceration of Gastroesophageal Junction)

Essentials of Diagnosis

- Hematemesis; usually self-limited.
- Prior history of vomiting, retching in 50%.
- Endoscopy establishes diagnosis.

General Considerations

Mallory-Weiss syndrome is characterized by a nonpenetrating mucosal tear at the gastroesophageal junction which is hypothesized to arise from events that suddenly raise transabdominal pressure, such as lifting, retching, or vomiting. Alcoholism is a strong predisposing factor. Mallory-Weiss tears appear to be responsible for approximately 5% of cases of upper gastrointestinal bleeding.

Clinical Findings

A. Symptoms and Signs: Patients usually present with hematemesis with or without melena. A history of antecedent retching, vomiting, or straining is obtained in about 50% of cases.

B. Special Examinations: As with other causes

of upper gastrointestinal hemorrhage, upper endoscopy should be performed after the patient has been appropriately resuscitated. The diagnosis is established by identification of a 0.5–4 cm linear mucosal tear usually located either at the gastroesophageal junction or, more commonly, just below the junction in the gastric mucosa.

Differential Diagnosis

At endoscopy, other potential causes of upper gastrointestinal hemorrhage are found in over 35% of patients with Mallory-Weiss tears, including peptic ulcer disease, erosive gastritis, arteriovenous malformations, and esophageal varices. Patients with underlying portal hypertension are at higher risk of continued or recurrent bleeding.

Treatment

Patients are initially treated as needed with fluid resuscitation and blood transfusions. Most patients stop bleeding spontaneously and require no therapy. Pharmacologic therapy with vasopressin or octreotide is of unproved benefit. Endoscopic hemostatic therapy is employed in patients who have continued, active bleeding. Injection with epinephrine (1:10,000) or cautery with a bipolar or heater probe coagulation device is effective in 90–95%. Angiographic arterial embolization or operative intervention is required in patients who fail endoscopic therapy.

Kovacs TO, Jensen DM: Endoscopic diagnosis and treatment of bleeding Mallory-Weiss tears. Gastroenterol Clin North Am 1991;1:387.

2. LOWER ESOPHAGEAL RING (Schatzki's Ring)

Schatzki's ring is a circumferential, thin, symmetric mucosal ring (< 4 mm in thickness) that occurs in the distal esophagus at the squamocolumnar junction. It is always associated with a hiatal hernia. Most are over 20 mm in diameter and are asymptomatic. Solid food dysphagia most often occurs with rings less than 13 mm in diameter. Characteristically, the dysphagia is intermittent and not progressive. Large, poorly chewed food boluses such as steak are most likely to cause dysphagia. Obstructing food boluses may pass by drinking extra liquids or are relieved by regurgitation. In some cases, an impacted bolus must be extracted endoscopically. Absence of gastroesophageal reflux symptoms and the nonprogressive nature of the dysphagia helps to distinguish Schatzki's ring from reflux-induced peptic strictures. Lower esophageal rings may be diagnosed by barium swallow or upper endoscopy.

The majority of symptomatic patients can be effectively and permanently treated with the passage of large (17–20 mm) bougie dilators, which disrupt the mucosal ring. A single dilation session usually suffices, but repeat dilations are sometimes necessary.

Goskreutz JL, Kim CH: Schatzki's ring: Long-term results following dilation. Gastrointest Endosc 1990;36:479.

3. ESOPHAGEAL WEBS

Webs are thin membranes of squamous mucosa that typically occur in the mid or upper esophagus. They are seldom circumferential. Webs may be asymptomatic or cause intermittent solid food dysphagia. An association with iron deficiency anemia (Plummer-Vinson syndrome) has been noted but is extremely rare. The diagnosis is established by barium esophagography or upper endoscopy. Symptomatic webs are effectively treated with bougienage.

4. ESOPHAGEAL DIVERTICULA

Zenker's Diverticulum

Zenker's diverticulum is a protrusion of pharyngeal mucosa that develops at the pharyngoesophageal junction between the inferior pharyngeal constrictor and the cricopharyngeus. The cause is uncertain. Symptoms of dysphagia and regurgitation tend to develop insidiously over years in middle-aged to elderly patients. Initial symptoms include vague oropharyngeal dysphagia with coughing or throat discomfort. As the diverticulum enlarges and retains food, patients may note halitosis, spontaneous regurgitation of undigested food, nocturnal choking, gurgling in the throat, or a protrusion in the neck. Complications include aspiration pneumonia, bronchiectasis, and lung abscess. The diagnosis is best established by a barium esophagogram. Endoscopy is unnecessary and potentially dangerous. Small asymptomatic diverticula may be observed.

Symptomatic patients require surgical diverticulectomy.

Esophageal Diverticula

Diverticula may occur in the mid or distal esophagus. These may arise secondary to motility disorders (diffuse esophageal spasm, achalasia) or may develop above esophageal strictures. Diverticula are seldom symptomatic, and treatment is directed at the underlying disorder.

Shay SS: Benign structural lesions of the esophagus. Gastroenterol Clin North Am 1991;20:673.

5. BENIGN ESOPHAGEAL NEOPLASMS

Benign tumors of the esophagus are quite rare. They are submucosal, the most common being leiomyoma. Most are asymptomatic and picked up incidentally on endoscopy or barium esophagography. Larger lesions can cause dysphagia. The major clinical importance of these lesions is to distinguish them from malignant neoplasms. At endoscopy, a smooth, sessile nodule is observed with normal overlying mucosal. Because the lesion is submucosal, endoscopic biopsies are generally nonrevealing. Endoscopic ultrasonography is extremely helpful to confirm the submucosal origin of the tumor.

MALIGNANT ESOPHAGEAL LESIONS (Cancer of the Esophagus)

Essentials of Diagnosis

- Progressive solid food dysphagia.
- Weight loss common.
- Endoscopy with biopsy establishes diagnosis.

General Considerations

Esophageal cancer usually develops in persons between 50 and 70 years of age. The overall ratio of men to women is 3:1. There are two histologic types: squamous cell carcinoma and adenocarcinoma. In the United States, squamous cell cancer is much more common in blacks than whites. Chronic alcohol and tobacco use are strongly associated with an increased risk of squamous cell carcinoma. The risk of cancer is also increased in patients with tylosis, achalasia, caustic-induced esophageal stricture, and other head and neck cancers. Adenocarcinoma is more common in whites and is increasing dramatically in incidence. The vast majority of adenocarcinomas develop as a complication of Barrett's metaplasia due to chronic gastroesophageal reflux. Thus, most adenocarcinomas arise in the distal third of the esophagus.

Clinical Findings

A. Symptoms and Signs: Unfortunately, most patients with esophageal cancer present with advanced, incurable disease. More than 90% of patients have solid food dysphagia, which progresses over weeks to months. Odynophagia is sometimes present. Significant weight loss is common. Local tumor extension into the tracheobronchial tree may result in a tracheoesophageal fistula, characterized by coughing on swallowing or pneumonia. Chest or back pain suggests mediastinal extension. Recurrent laryngeal involvement may produce hoarseness. Physical examination is often unrevealing. The presence of supraclavicular or cervical lymphadenopathy or of hepatomegaly implies metastatic disease.

B. Laboratory Findings: Laboratory findings are nonspecific. Anemia related to chronic disease or occult blood loss is common. Abnormal aminotransferase or alkaline phosphatase concentrations suggest hepatic or bony metastases. Hypoalbuminemia may result from malnutrition.

C. Imaging: Chest x-rays may show adenopathy, a widened mediastinum, pulmonary or bony metastases, or signs of tracheoesophageal fistula such as pneumonia. A barium esophagogram often is obtained by clinicians as the first study to evaluate dysphagia. The appearance of a polypoid, infiltrative, or ulcerative lesion is suggestive of carcinoma and requires endoscopic evaluation. However, even lesions felt to be benign by radiography warrant endoscopic evaluation.

D. Upper Endoscopy: Endoscopy with cytology and biopsy establishes the diagnosis of esophageal carcinoma with a high degree of reliability. In some cases, significant submucosal spread of the tumor may yield nondiagnostic mucosal biopsies. Repeated biopsy may be necessary.

Differential Diagnosis

Esophageal carcinoma must be distinguished from other causes of progressive dysphagia, including peptic stricture, achalasia, and adenocarcinoma of the gastric cardia with esophageal involvement. Benign-appearing peptic strictures should be biopsied at presentation to exclude occult malignancy.

Staging of Disease

After confirming the diagnosis of esophageal carcinoma, one should determine the stage of the disease, since doing so will influence the choice of therapy. After preoperative or intraoperative staging, patients can be classified into one of three categories: (1) resectable with curative intent, (2) resectable but not curable, and (3) not resectable and not curable. One's goal is to identify that small subset of patients who may benefit from curative resection while sparing the larger group of patients who will not benefit—and indeed may suffer—from such surgery.

Patients should undergo staging with chest and abdominal CT scanning. Endoscopic ultrasonography, not yet widely available, is superior to CT in demonstrating local tumor extension and local lymph node involvement. The presence of distant metastases, mediastinal or pleural invasion, or distant lymph node involvement excludes a curative resection.

Treatment

The approach to and treatment of esophageal cancer varies between institutions. Very few patients are candidates for curative surgical resections. In the remainder, the goal is local tumor control and palliation. This can be achieved by a variety of modalities.

A. Surgical Treatment: In the small number of patients in whom curative en bloc resections are possible, there is a 25–50% 3-year survival rate. Other patients with noncurable lesions may still be candidates for palliative resections, which may improve their ability to eat and may prevent local tumor complications but without improving overall survival. The utility of preoperative chemotherapy with radiation is under clinical investigation.

B. Radiation Therapy: Patients with unresectable disease or otherwise poor operative candidates are often referred for radiation therapy. Radiation therapy may provide significant short-term relief of local symptoms of dysphagia and pain.

C. Radiation and Chemotherapy: Combined therapy with radiation and chemotherapy appears to be superior to radiation therapy alone in patients with localized (ie, nonmetastatic) carcinoma in achieving local control and in overall survival. Clinical trials are ongoing. The most successful agents to date have been cisplatin and fluorouracil. Because the toxicity of this regimen is significantly greater than that of radiation alone, appropriate patient selection is critical.

D. Local Tumor Therapy: Palliation of dysphagia may be achieved by endoscopically guided dilation or laser therapy. In some patients, peroral placement of permanent plastic stents is useful.

Prognosis

The overall prognosis of esophageal carcinoma remains grim, with a 5-year survival rate of less than 10%.

Moses FM: Squamous cell carcinoma of the esophagus: Natural history, incidence, etiology, and complications. Gastroenterol Clin North Am 1991;20:703.

Bremner RM, DeMeester TR: Surgical treatment of esophageal carcinoma. Gastroenterol Clin North Am 1991; 20:743.

Herskovic A et al: Combined chemotherapy and radiotherapy compared with radiotherapy alone in patients with cancer of the esophagus. N Engl J Med 1992;326:1593. (Survival at 24 months in combined group was 38% versus 10% in radiotherapy group.)

ESOPHAGEAL MOTILITY DISORDERS

1. ACHALASIA

Essentials of Diagnosis

- Gradual, progressive dysphagia for solids and liquids.
- Regurgitation of undigested food.
- Barium esophagogram with "bird's beak" distal esophagus.
- Esophageal manometry confirms diagnosis.

General Considerations

Achalasia is an idiopathic motility disorder characterized by loss of peristalsis in the distal two-thirds (smooth muscle) of the esophagus and impaired relaxation of the lower esophageal sphincter. There appears to be denervation of the esophagus resulting from loss of ganglion cells in Auerbach's plexus and degeneration of the vagus nerve and dorsal motor nucleus.

Clinical Findings

A. Symptoms and Signs: Symptoms usually develop in patients between the ages of 25 and 60 years. Patients complain of the gradual onset of dysphagia for solid foods and, in the majority, of liquids also. Symptoms at presentation may have persisted for months to years. Substernal discomfort or fullness may be noted after eating. Many patients eat more slowly and adopt specific maneuvers such as lifting the neck or throwing the shoulders back in order to enhance esophageal emptying. Regurgitation of undigested food is common and may occur during meals or up to several hours later. Nocturnal regurgitation can provoke coughing or aspiration. Weight loss is common. Physical examination is unhelpful.

B. Imaging: Chest x-rays may show an air-fluid level in the enlarged, fluid-filled esophagus. Barium esophagography has characteristic findings, including esophageal dilation, loss of esophageal peristalsis, poor esophageal emptying, and a smooth, symmetric "bird's beak" tapering of the distal esophagus. Without treatment, the esophagus may become markedly dilated ("sigmoid esophagus").

C. Special Examinations: After esophagography, endoscopy is always performed to evaluate the distal esophagus and gastroesophageal junction in order to exclude a distal stricture or a submucosal infiltrating carcinoma. The diagnosis is confirmed by esophageal manometry. The typical manometric features are as follows: (1) Complete absence of peristalsis; swallowing results in simultaneous waves which are usually of low amplitude. (2) Incomplete lower esophageal sphincteric relaxation with swallowing. Whereas the normal sphincter relaxes by over 90%, relaxation with most swallows in patients with achalasia is less than 50%. In many patients, the baseline lower esophageal sphincteric pressure is quite elevated. (3) Intraesophageal pressures are greater than gastric pressures due to a fluid- and food-filled esophagus.

Differential Diagnosis

Primary or metastatic tumors can invade the gastroesophageal junction, resulting in a picture resembling that of achalasia, called "pseudoachalasia." Endoscopic ultrasonography and chest CT may be required to examine the distal esophagus in suspicious cases. Achalasia must be distinguished from other motility disorders such as diffuse esophageal spasm and scleroderma esophagus with a peptic stricture.

Treatment

Pharmacologic reduction of the lower esophageal

sphincteric pressure may be achieved with calcium channel blockers. Nifedipine, 10–20 mg sublingually 30 minutes before meals, results in significant short-term improvement in some patients with mild symptoms and a nondilated esophagus. Pharmacologic therapy is also used in patients with severe medical problems in whom other therapies are felt to be too risky.

Pneumatic dilation is the preferred initial method of therapy for most patients. Under fluoroscopic guidance, balloons ranging from 3 to 4 cm in size are positioned across the lower esophageal sphincter and inflated with the intention of disrupting the sphincter. Sixty to 75 percent of patients derive good to excellent relief of dysphagia. Perforation may occur in 6% of dilations, which may require operative intervention.

Surgical therapy is generally reserved for patients who have failed to improve after pneumatic dilation. A Heller myotomy of the lower esophageal sphincter results in excellent symptomatic relief in over 85% of patients. Although highly effective, this requires a laparotomy or thoracotomy. Gastroesophageal reflux may complicate myotomy. Recently, some centers have begun to perform myotomies thoracoscopically, reporting excellent results. Thoracoscopic surgery is minimally invasive and dramatically reduces the operative recovery time from 2–3 weeks to 2–3 days.

Prognosis

If treatment is provided before marked esophageal dilation develops, swallowing is near normal in most patients. The incidence of squamous cell carcinoma of the esophagus is increased in achalasia regardless of what therapy is given.

Elta GH, Kockman ML: Achalasia treatment: Is nifedipine a viable alternative? Gastroenterology 1992;102:1432. (Review of literature on pharmacotherapy.)
Goldenberg SP et al: Classic and vigorous achalasia: A comparison of manometric, radiographic and clinical findings. Gastroenterology 1991;101:743.
Richter JE: Surgery or pneumatic dilation for achalasia: A head-to-head comparison. Now are all the questions answered? Gastroenterology 1989;97:1340.

2. DIFFUSE ESOPHAGEAL SPASM

Diffuse esophageal spasm is an uncommon motility disorder characterized by intermittent dysphagia for solids and liquids which is generally nonprogressive. Periods of normal swallowing may alternate with periods of dysphagia, which is generally mild. Dysphagia may be provoked by stress, large boluses, or hot or cold liquids. Patients may also note anterior chest pain, which can be confused with angina pectoris but is not usually exertional. The pain is often unrelated to eating. Barium esophagography may detect simultaneous ("tertiary") contractions characterized as a "corkscrew" or "rosary bead" appearance. On esophageal manometry, intermittent simultaneous contractions (> 10% of swallows) are recorded along with periods of normal peristalsis.

Diffuse esophageal spasm is generally a mild condition that is not life-threatening. Therapy is directed at symptom reduction and reassurance. Nitrates (isosorbide dinitrate, 10–30 mg four times daily; nitroglycerin, 0.4 mg sublingually as needed) and calcium channel blockers (nifedipine, 10–30 mg four times daily; diltiazem, 60–90 mg four times daily) are reported to be effective, though no controlled trials have been conducted. Dilation with Maloney bougies provides symptomatic relief in some cases for unclear reasons. Rarely, a long surgical myotomy is required in debilitated patients.

Dalton CB et al: Diffuse esophageal spasm: A rare motility disorder not characterized by high-amplitude contractions. Dig Dis Sci 1991;36:1025.

3. SCLERODERMA ESOPHAGUS

Esophageal involvement is common in patients with progressive systemic sclerosis or the CREST syndrome, especially those who have Raynaud's phenomenon. Atrophy and fibrosis of the esophageal smooth muscle results in loss of lower esophageal sphincteric competency and markedly diminished esophageal peristaltic amplitude. Acid gastroesophageal reflux results that can cause a severe erosive esophagitis, sometimes resulting in the development of Barrett's esophagus or peptic stricture. Patients report heartburn or dysphagia. The dysphagia may be secondary to impaired peristalsis or may be due to peptic stricture. Barium esophagography demonstrates absent peristalsis in the distal esophagus and a patulous lower esophageal sphincter with free reflux. Esophageal manometry confirms a low or absent lower esophageal sphincteric pressure and markedly diminished peristaltic amplitude in the distal two-thirds of the esophagus. Aggressive therapy for the acid gastroesophageal reflux (see above) is given in order to prevent reflux complications. Peptic strictures may require dilation.

4. OTHER MOTILITY DISORDERS

A variety of other motility disorders have been characterized by manometry. These include nutcracker esophagus, hypertensive lower esophageal sphincter, and nonspecific motility abnormalities. These manometric findings are commonly identified in patients complaining of dysphagia or noncardiac chest pain. A cause-and-effect relationship between these manometric disorders and the patients' symptoms, however, is unproved. Symptomatic patients with these manometric abnormalities have a high incidence of psychiatric disorders, including depression, anxiety, panic disorder, and tendencies toward somatization and hypochondriasis. These esophageal manometric findings may represent markers of chronic psychologic stress and a clinical pain syndrome.

Langevin S, Castell D: Esophageal motility disorders and chest pain. Med Clin North Am 1991;75:1045.

CHEST PAIN OF UNDETERMINED ETIOLOGY

Patients with recurrent chest pain can pose a vexing clinical problem. Cardiac causes must be definitively excluded in patients with typical or atypical angina. These include coronary artery disease with ischemia, coronary spasm (Prinzmetal's angina), mitral valve prolapse, and a heretofore unappreciated entity, microvascular angina. The latter should be considered in patients with normal coronary angiograms who have abnormal exercise tolerance tests.

A variety of other rheumatologic, gastroenterologic, and psychiatric disorders may be associated with this syndrome. Chest wall and thoracic spine disease is easily diagnosed by a thorough physical examination. Gastroesophageal reflux may be a cause of chest pain in a significant subset (25%) of patients. Ambulatory pH monitoring is a useful test to determine whether there is a correlation between reflux episodes and chest pain events. Alternatively, an empiric trial of antireflux therapy with omeprazole, 20 mg daily for several weeks, may be diagnostic. Up to 35% of patients with recurrent chest pain of undetermined cause have an underlying panic disorder, which can be treated. Patients who have accompanying symptoms of dyspnea, tachycardia, sensation of smothering, sweating, fainting or dizziness, shaking, or fear of dying should be evaluated by a psychiatrist. Similarly, a significant number of patients have underlying depression, anxiety, and neuroticism that may benefit from pharmacologic or psychologic therapy. Finally, it is increasingly clear that a number of patients have a heightened visceral sensitivity to minor noxious stimuli such as intraesophageal balloon distention, intracardiac catheter manipulation, intraesophageal acid infusion, and intravenous edrophonium.

Cannon R et al: Pathophysiological dilemma of syndrome X. Circulation 1992;85:883.
Clouse R: Psychiatric disorders in patients with esophageal disease. Med Clin North Am 1991;75:1081.
Members of the AGA Patient Care Committee: Diagnosis of chest pain of esophageal origin. Dig Dis Sci 1990; 35:289.
Richter J: Gastroesophageal reflux as a cause of chest pain. Med Clin North Am 1991;75:1065.
Richter J: Practical approaches to the diagnosis of unexplained chest pain. Med Clin North Am 1991;75:1203.

DISEASES OF THE STOMACH & DUODENUM

GASTRITIS

The term gastritis is broad, vague, and surrounded by semantic confusion. Endoscopists employ the term to denote a number of gross mucosal features such as erythema, subepithelial hemorrhages, and erosions; to the pathologist, the term denotes histologic inflammation. For greater clarity in this clinical discussion, gastritis may be classified into three categories: (1) erosive or hemorrhagic gastritis; (2) nonerosive, nonspecific gastritis (chronic gastritis); and (3) specific types such as gastritis due to infection, granulomatous gastritis, eosinophilic gastritis, and Ménétrier's disease (hypertrophic gastropathy).

1. EROSIVE OR HEMORRHAGIC GASTRITIS

Essentials of Diagnosis
- Most commonly seen in critically ill patients or in alcoholics or patients taking NSAIDs.
- Often asymptomatic; may cause epigastric pain, nausea and vomiting.
- May cause hematemesis; usually not significant bleeding.

General Considerations
The most common causes of erosive gastritis are drugs (especially NSAIDs), alcohol, stress due to severe medical or surgical illness ("stress gastritis"), and portal hypertension ("portal gastropathy"). Uncommon causes include caustic ingestion and radiation. Erosive or hemorrhagic gastritis typically is diagnosed at endoscopy, often being performed because of epigastric pain or upper gastrointestinal bleeding. Endoscopic findings include subepithelial hemorrhages, petechiae, and erosion. These lesions are superficial, may vary in size and number, and may be focal or diffuse. There usually is no significant inflammation on histologic examination.

Clinical Findings
A. Symptoms and Signs: Erosive gastritis is

usually aymptomatic. Symptoms, when they occur, include anorexia, nausea, vomiting, and epigastric pain. There is poor correlation between these symptoms and the presence of endoscopic abnormalities. The most common clinical manifestation of erosive gastritis is upper gastrointestinal bleeding. This may present as hematemesis, "coffee grounds," blood in the aspirate of a patient being maintained on nasogastric suction, or melena. Because erosive gastritis is superficial, hemodynamically significant gastrointestinal bleeding is uncommon.

Physical examination may reveal epigastric tenderness, but the abdomen is otherwise benign. Rectal examination with fecal occult blood testing may confirm gastrointestinal blood loss.

B. Laboratory Findings: The laboratory findings may reflect the underlying disease process but are otherwise nonspecific. Hematocrit is low if significant bleeding has occurred.

C. Special Examinations: Upper endoscopy is the most sensitive method of diagnosis. Although bleeding from gastritis is usually insignificant, it cannot be distinguished on clinical grounds from more serious lesions such as peptic ulcers or esophageal varices. Hence, endoscopy is generally performed within 24 hours in patients with upper gastrointestinal bleeding to identify the bleeding source. An upper gastrointestinal series is less expensive than endoscopy but is insensitive for the diagnosis of gastritis.

Differential Diagnosis

Epigastric pain may be due to peptic ulcer, gastroesophageal reflux, gastric cancer, biliary tract disease, food poisoning, viral gastroenteritis, and nonulcer dyspepsia. With severe pain one should consider a perforated or penetrating ulcer, pancreatic disease, esophageal rupture, ruptured aortic aneurysm, ureteral colic, and myocardial infarction. Causes of upper gastrointestinal bleeding include peptic ulcer disease, esophageal varices, Mallory-Weiss tear, and arteriovenous malformations.

Specific Causes & Treatment

A. NSAID Gastritis: Although half of patients receiving NSAIDs on a chronic basis have gastritis at endoscopy, symptoms of dyspepsia develop in less than one-fourth. Furthermore, of patients with dyspepsia, up to half do not have significant mucosal abnormalities. Given the frequency of dyspeptic symptoms in patients receiving chronic NSAID therapy, it is neither feasible nor desirable to investigate all patients with dyspeptic symptoms. Symptoms may be improved by discontinuation of the agent, reduction to the lowest effective dose, administration with meals, or use of an alternative agent such as acetaminophen. Patients with persistent symptoms despite conservative measures or patients at high risk for NSAID-induced ulcers (see Peptic Ulcer Disease) should undergo diagnostic endoscopy. Those without significant NSAID ulceration may be treated symptomatically with sucralfate, 1 g four times daily, or with H_2 antagonists (cimetidine, 400 mg twice daily; ranitidine, 150 mg twice daily; famotidine, 20 mg twice daily). Upper gastrointestinal bleeding due to NSAID gastritis is generally not severe. If bleeding is severe, consideration should be given to administering platelets, since the patient's platelet function is impaired by aspirin for up to 5 days.

B. Alcoholic Gastritis: Erosive gastritis accounts for 20% of episodes of upper gastrointestinal bleeding in chronic alcoholics. These bleeding episodes are usually mild and respond to withdrawal of alcohol. Therapy with H_2 antagonists or sucralfate for 2–4 weeks is often prescribed.

C. Portal Hypertensive Gastropathy: Portal hypertension results in gastric mucosal and submucosal congestion of capillaries and venules. Bleeding from congestive gastropathy accounts for 25% of episodes of upper gastrointestinal bleeding in patients with portal hypertension. It may present suddenly with hematemesis or insidiously with iron deficiency anemia. Recurrent acute bleeding is common. Treatment with propranolol reduces the incidence of recurrent acute bleeding by lowering portal pressures. Patients without contraindications to beta-blockers should be started on propranolol, 20 mg twice daily. The dosage is increased gradually until the heart rate falls by 25% or below 55 beats/min. An average dose of propranolol is 60 mg twice daily. Patients who fail propranolol therapy may be successfully treated with portal decompressive procedures. Surgical portacaval shunts and radiologically placed transjugular intrahepatic portosystemic shunts (TIPS) control bleeding but are associated with a high incidence of hepatic encephalopathy.

D. Stress Gastritis: Stress-related mucosal erosions and subepithelial hemorrhages develop within 18 hours in the majority of critically ill patients. Clinically evident bleeding occurs in 16% of untreated patients but serious bleeding in less than 6%. Major risk factors include trauma, burns, hypotension, central nervous system injury, coagulopathy, sepsis, hepatic failure, renal failure, and mechanical ventilation. Patients with multiple risk factors have a higher risk of bleeding. Bleeding is associated with a higher mortality rate but is seldom the cause of death.

H_2 antagonists reduce the incidence of overt bleeding in the ICU when given prophylactically. Continuous infusions of H_2 antagonists at a dose sufficient to maintain intragastric pH > 4.0 should be given to all high-risk patients upon admission. Cimetidine (900–1200 mg), ranitidine (150 mg), or famotidine (20 mg) by continuous infusion over 24 hours is adequate in most patients. After 4–6 hours of infusion, the pH should be checked by nasogastric aspirate and the dose doubled if pH is < 4.0. Sucralfate suspension (1 g given every 4–6 hours) is comparable in efficacy to H_2 antagonists in the prevention of stress gastritis.

Furthermore, it may be associated with a lower incidence of nosocomial pneumonia and a lower overall mortality rate. Sucralfate may become the drug of choice for stress prophylaxis. Omeprazole should not be used in the ICU for prophylaxis owing to its unpredictable oral absorption in such patients.

Patients in whom stress gastritis results in overt bleeding should receive continuous infusions of H_2 antagonists at doses sufficient to maintain an intragastric pH of 5.0–7.0. Because bleeding is usually diffuse, endoscopic hemostasis techniques are not helpful. Operative intervention is rarely required and carries a high mortality rate.

E. Chronic Erosive Gastritis ("Varioliform Gastritis"): This is an idiopathic condition characterized by fluctuating abdominal pain, nausea, and vomiting. Biopsies reveal a lymphocytic gastritis. There is no established effective therapy.

Bresalier RS: The clinical significance and pathophysiology of stress-related gastric mucosal hemorrhage. J Clin Gastroenterol 1991;13(Suppl 2):S35.

Cook DJ et al: Stress ulcer prophylaxis in the critically ill: A meta-analysis. Am J Med 1991;91:519.

PerezDAyuso RM et al: Propranolol in prevention of recurrent bleeding from severe portal hypertensive gastropathy in cirrhosis. Lancet 1991;337:1431.

Soll AH: Nonsteroidal anti-inflammatory drugs and ulcers. West J Med 1992;157:465.

2. NONEROSIVE, NONSPECIFIC GASTRITIS (Chronic Gastritis)

The diagnosis of chronic gastritis is based upon histologic assessment of mucosal biopsies. Endoscopic findings are normal in many cases and do not reliably predict the presence of histologic inflammation. Chronic gastritis is divided into two types: type B, which involves mainly the antrum but may involve the entire stomach; and type A, which involves only the proximal acid-secreting portion of the stomach. The major cause of type B gastritis is a gram-negative bacterium, *Helicobacter pylori*. Pernicious anemia is the major cause of type A gastritis.

Chronic *Helicobacter pylori* Gastritis

The histologic diagnosis of *H pylori* gastritis is based upon endoscopic biopsies. The vast majority of infected people are asymptomatic. There is a strong association with the development of peptic ulcer disease.

H pylori is a spiral gram-negative rod that resides beneath the gastric mucus layer adjacent to epithelial cells. It causes chronic mucosal inflammation with lymphocytes and PMNs. The pathogenetic mechanisms of injury are not established. In the United States, the prevalence of *H pylori* infection increases with age 1% per year, rising from less than 10% in Caucasians under age 30 to over 50% in those over 60. The prevalence is higher in nonCaucasians and higher also in developing countries, and is inversely correlated with socioeconomic class. Transmission is from person to person, but the mode of spread is not known. In some patients, chronic inflammation progresses to gastric gland atrophy (atrophic gastritis) and to metaplasia of the gastric epithelium to intestinal type epithelium. Chronic *H pylori* gastritis with intestinal metaplasia is associated with a four- to sixfold increased risk of gastric adenocarcinoma.

Acute infection with *H pylori* causes a transient clinical illness characterized by nausea and abdominal pain that may last for several days and is associated with an acute histologic gastritis. After the symptoms resolve, the proportion of acutely infected patients who progress to chronic infection is unknown.

Chronic *H pylori* infection with gastritis is present in 30–50% of the population. The overwhelming majority of people do not develop symptoms or sequelae. *H pylori* infection is strongly associated with the development of peptic ulcer disease, which is discussed below. There is no significant evidence at this time that chronic *H pylori* gastritis causes dyspeptic symptoms in patients without ulcer disease ("nonulcer dyspepsia").

There are no specific laboratory abnormalities. Serum IgA and IgG antibodies to *H pylori* are detectable by ELISA and are highly sensitive. They are employed in epidemiologic studies and are thus far of limited clinical use.

At this time, established peptic ulcer disease is the only indication for investigating for *H pylori* infection. Direct identification of the organism requires endoscopic mucosal biopsy with histologic stains (silver, Giemsa, or H&E) or culture isolation. Histologic examination is more than 90% sensitive and specific and is the standard procedure for identification. *H pylori* produces a urease that converts transuded urea to ammonia. Endoscopic biopsies may be quickly tested for urease activity by placing them in a urea-containing medium with phenol red. Release of ammonia elevates the pH, producing a color change within 1–3 hours, and is presumptive evidence of *H pylori* infection. ^{13}C-urease breath tests may soon be clinically available that would provide a noninvasive way of screening for *H pylori* infection.

Successful eradication of *H pylori* infection may be achieved in over 85% of patients with a combination of two antibiotics and bismuth subsalicylate (Pepto-Bismol). Specific regimens are set forth in the section on peptic ulcer disease. After eradication, the chronic gastritis resolves. At present, the only indication for treating *H pylori* gastritis is in patients with recurrent peptic ulcer disease.

Correa P: Is gastric carcinoma an infectious disease? (Editorial.) N Engl J Med 1991;325:1170.

Graham DY et al: Epidemiology of *Helicobacter pylori* in an asymptomatic population in the United States. Gastroenterology 1991;100:1495.

Peterson SF: *Helicobacter pylori* and peptic ulcer disease. N Engl J Med 1991;324:1043.

Pernicious Anemia

Pernicious anemia is an autoimmune gastritis involving the fundic glands with resultant achlorhydria and vitamin B_{12} malabsorption. Fundic histology is characterized by severe gland atrophy. Parietal cell antibodies directed against the H^+-K^+ ATPase pump are present in 90% of patients. Achlorhydria leads to a pronounced hypergastrinemia (> 1000 pg/mL) due to loss of inhibition of gastrin cells. Hyperplasia of gastric enterochromaffin-like cells is common and attributable to hypergastrinemia. Three to 5 percent of patients develop small, multicentric gastric carcinoid tumors. Metastatic spread is uncommon in tumors less than 2 cm in diameter. Endoscopy with biopsy is indicated in patients with pernicious anemia at the time of diagnosis. Patients with dysplasia or small carcinoids require periodic endoscopic surveillance. Pernicious anemia is discussed in detail in Chapter 13.

Hirschowitz BI et al: Rapid regression of enterochromaffinlike cell gastric carcinoids in pernicious anemia after antrectomy. Gastroenterology 1992;102(4 Part 1):1409.

3. SPECIFIC TYPES OF GASTRITIS

A number of disorders are associated with specific histologic features in the gastric mucosa.

Infections

Acute infection with a variety of bacteria may produce a rare, life-threatening diffuse suppurative gastritis that requires surgical resection. Viral infection with CMV is commonly seen in patients with AIDS and after bone marrow or solid organ transplantation. Endoscopic findings include thickened gastric folds, petechiae, and ulcerations. Fungal infections with *Candida* may occur in immunocompromised patients. Larvae of the *Anisakis marina* parasite ingested in raw fish or sushi may become embedded in the gastric mucosa and produce severe abdominal pain. Pain persists for several days until the larvae die. Endoscopic removal of the larvae provides more rapid relief.

Granulomatous Gastritis

Chronic granulomatous inflammation may be caused by a variety of systemic diseases, including tuberculosis, syphilis, fungi, sarcoidosis, or Crohn's disease. These may be asymptomatic or associated with a variety of gastrointestinal complaints.

Eosinophilic Gastritis

This is a rare disorder in which eosinophils infiltrate the antrum and, sometimes, the proximal intestine. Infiltration may involve the mucosa, muscularis, or serosa. Peripheral eosinophilia is prominent. Symptoms include anemia from mucosal blood loss, abdominal pain, early satiety, and postprandial vomiting. Treatment with corticosteroids is beneficial in the majority of patients.

Ménétrier's Disease (Hypertrophic Gastropathy)

This is an idiopathic entity characterized by thickened gastric folds predominantly involving the body which are evident on upper gastrointestinal series and endoscopy. Patients complain of nausea, anorexia, epigastric pain, and diarrhea. Because of chronic protein loss, patients may develop severe hypoproteinemia and edema. Treatment is directed at symptoms. Gastric resection is required in severe cases.

PEPTIC ULCER DISEASE

Essentials of Diagnosis

- History of epigastric pain present in 80–90% of patients but is nonspecific. Relationship to meals is variable.
- 10–20% of patients present with ulcer complications without antecedent symptoms.
- Of NSAID-induced ulcers, 30–50% are asymptomatic.
- Ulcer symptoms characterized by rhythmicity and periodicity.
- Upper endoscopy with antral biopsy for *H pylori* is diagnostic procedure of choice in most patients.
- Gastric ulcer biopsy or documentation of complete healing necessary to exclude gastric malignancy.

General Considerations

Peptic ulcer is a break in the gastric or duodenal mucosa that arises when the normal mucosal defensive factors are impaired or are overwhelmed by aggressive luminal factors such as acid and pepsin. By definition, ulcers extend through the muscularis mucosae and are usually over 5 mm in diameter. In the United States, there are about 500,000 new cases per year of peptic ulcer and 4 million ulcer recurrences; the lifetime prevalence of ulcers in the adult population is approximately 10%. Ulcers occur five times more commonly in the duodenum, where over 95% are in the bulb or pyloric channel. In the stomach, benign ulcers are located most commonly in the antrum (60%) and at the junction of the antrum and body on the lesser curvature (25%).

Ulcers occur slightly more commonly in men than

in women (1.3:1). Although ulcers can occur in any age group, duodenal ulcers most commonly occur between the ages of 30 and 55, whereas gastric ulcers are more common between the ages of 55 and 70. Ulcers are more common in smokers and in patients receiving NSAIDs on a chronic basis (see below). Alcohol and dietary factors do not appear to cause ulcer disease. The role of stress is uncertain. The incidence of duodenal ulcer disease has been declining dramatically for the past 30 years, but the incidence of gastric ulcers appears to be increasing, perhaps as a result of the widespread use of NSAIDs.

Etiology

Three major causes of peptic ulcer disease are now recognized: NSAIDs, chronic *H pylori* infection, and acid hypersecretory states such as Zollinger-Ellison syndrome. NSAID- and *H pylori*-associated ulcers will be considered in the present section; Zollinger-Ellison syndrome will be discussed subsequently.

A. *H pylori*-Associated Ulcers: *H pylori* appears to be a necessary cofactor for the overwhelming majority of duodenal and gastric ulcers not associated with NSAIDs. Ninety to 95 percent of duodenal ulcer patients have associated *H pylori* gastritis. It is not known how chronic *H pylori* gastritis potentiates ulcers in the duodenum. The association with gastric ulcers is less clear, but *H pylori* is found in the majority in whom NSAIDs cannot be implicated. Overall, it is estimated that one in six infected patients will develop ulcer disease.

The natural history of peptic ulcer disease is well-defined. After standard therapies, 70–D85% of patients will have an endoscopically documented recurrence within 1 year. Half of these will be asymptomatic. In multiple trials, successful eradication of *H pylori* decreases the ulcer recurrence rate to less than 12% per year. At least some of these recurrences are due to NSAID use or failure to eradicate the organism. Although the pathogenetic mechanisms of ulcer formation by *H pylori* are unclear, its importance in ulcer formation is undeniable.

B. NSAID-Induced Ulcers: There is a 10–20% prevalence of gastric ulcers and a 2–5% prevalence of duodenal ulcers in chronic NSAID users. The relative risk of gastric ulcers is increased 40-fold, but the risk of duodenal ulcers is only slightly increased. Users of NSAIDs are at least three times more likely than non-users to suffer serious gastrointestinal complications from these ulcers such as bleeding, perforation, or death. It is noteworthy that gastric ulcers and duodenal ulcers cause about the same number of complications. Approximately 2.4% of chronic NSAID users will have a major complication within 1 year. Aspirin is the most ulcerogenic NSAID. The risk appears to be dose-related, with some risk even at doses as low as 325 mg every other day. A higher risk of NSAID complications is associated with higher NSAID dos-

age; with the first 3 months of administration; and with advanced age, a prior history of ulcer disease, concomitant corticosteroid administration, or serious medical illness. At equivalent anti-inflammatory doses, there is no clear evidence that any particular NSAIDs are safer than others.

H pylori does not increase the likelihood of development of NSAID-associated ulcers. It is increasingly apparent that NSAIDs may cause small intestinal ulcerations and perforations, colitis, and colonic strictures.

Clinical Findings

A. Symptoms and Signs: Epigastric pain (dyspepsia), the hallmark of peptic ulcer disease, is present in 80–90% of patients. However, this complaint is not sensitive or specific enough to serve as a reliable diagnostic criterion for peptic ulcer disease. The clinical history cannot accurately distinguish duodenal from gastric ulcers. Less than one-quarter of patients with dyspepsia have ulcer disease at endoscopy. Up to 20% of patients with ulcer complications such as bleeding have no antecedent symptoms ("silent ulcers"). In patients with NSAID-induced ulcers, up to half are asymptomatic. What is more troublesome is that up to 60% of patients with complications do not have prior symptoms.

Pain is typically well localized to the epigastrium and is not severe. It is described as gnawing, dull, aching, or "hunger-like." Classic features of peptic ulcer pain are rhythmicity and periodicity. Rhythmicity means that the pain fluctuates in intensity throughout the day and night. Approximately half of patients report relief of pain with food or antacids (especially duodenal ulcers) and a recurrence of pain 2–4 hours later. However, many patients deny any relationship to meals or report worsening of pain. Two-thirds of duodenal ulcers and one-third of gastric ulcers cause nocturnal pain that awakens the patient. A change from a patient's typical rhythmic discomfort to constant or radiating pain may reflect ulcer penetration or perforation. Most patients have symptomatic periods lasting up to several weeks with intervals of months to years in which they are pain-free (periodicity).

Nausea and anorexia may occur with gastric ulcers. Significant vomiting and weight loss are unusual with uncomplicated ulcer disease and suggest gastric outlet obstruction or gastric malignancy.

The physical examination is often unremarkable in uncomplicated peptic ulcer disease. Mild, localized epigastric tenderness to deep palpation may be present. Fecal occult blood testing may be positive in one-third of patients.

B. Laboratory Findings: Laboratory tests are normal in uncomplicated peptic ulcer disease but are frequently ordered to exclude ulcer complications or confounding disease entities. Anemia may occur with acute blood loss from a bleeding ulcer or less commonly from chronic blood loss. Leukocytosis suggests ulcer penetration or perforation. An elevated serum amylase in a patient with severe epigastric pain suggests ulcer penetration into the pancreas. A fasting serum gastrin level to screen for Zollinger-Ellison syndrome is obtained in some patients (see below).

C. Endoscopy: Upper endoscopy is the procedure of choice for the diagnosis of duodenal and gastric ulcers. In most cases, biopsies should be taken from the gastric antrum to assess for the presence of *H pylori* gastritis (see above). Duodenal ulcers are virtually never malignant and do not require biopsy. Three to 5 percent of benign-appearing gastric ulcers prove to be malignant. Hence, cytologic brushings and biopsies of the ulcer margin are almost always performed. All patients with gastric ulcers require follow-up endoscopy 12 weeks after the start of therapy to document complete healing.

D. Imaging: Barium upper gastrointestinal series is an acceptable alternative to screening of uncomplicated patients with dyspepsia. However, because it may incorrectly diagnose 20–30% of patients and has limited accuracy in distinguishing benign from malignant gastric ulcers, all gastric ulcers diagnosed by x-ray should be reevaluated with endoscopy after 8–12 weeks of therapy.

Differential Diagnosis

Peptic ulcer disease must be distinguished from other causes of epigastric distress. Gastroesophageal reflux, chronic cholecystitis, and biliary tract disease may all be manifested by epigastric discomfort. Over half of patients with dyspepsia have negative upper endoscopies and no obvious explanation for their complaints. These patients are classified as having "nonulcer dyspepsia" and can be extremely difficult to treat.

Severe epigastric pain is atypical for peptic disease unless complicated by perforation or penetration. Other causes include acute pancreatitis, acute cholecystitis or choledocholithiasis, esophageal rupture, ureteral colic, and ruptured aortic aneurysm.

Pharmacologic Agents
Used in Management of Peptic Ulcer

Several pharmacologic agents enhance the healing of peptic ulcers. Their pharmacology and mechanisms of action are discussed briefly here. Recommendations for their use are provided in subsequent sections.

A. Antisecretory Agents:

1. H₂-receptor antagonists–Four H_2 antagonists are available: cimetidine, ranitidine, famotidine, and nizatidine. These agents competitively inhibit histamine binding to the H_2 receptor on the gastric parietal cell, thereby reducing intracellular cAMP levels and acid secretion. They profoundly inhibit

basal acid output but are less effective at standard doses at inhibiting meal-stimulated acid secretion. Thus, administration of these drugs two to four times daily markedly raises the nocturnal pH but has only a modest impact upon the gastric daytime pH profile. Recently, once-daily nocturnal or evening dosing regimens of H_2 antagonists have demonstrated efficacy equivalent or superior to more frequent dosing in the healing of peptic ulcers. Equipotent doses of the agents are listed in Table 14–3.

The H_2 antagonists have an incidence of side effects of less than 3%. Differences in drug interactions are of clinical importance. Cimetidine inhibits hepatic P450 drug metabolism, raising the serum concentration of warfarin, theophylline, lidocaine, and phenytoin. Ranitidine binds P450 with only 10–20% of the avidity of cimetidine; famotidine and nizatidine have negligible effects. Cimetidine inhibits estradiol metabolism and dihydrotestosterone binding and may cause impotence or gynecomastia at higher doses. Central nervous system symptoms of headache, confusion, and lethargy may occur with all agents in 1% of patients, especially with intravenous administration.

2. Proton pump inhibitors (omeprazole)–Omeprazole is the first of a new line of antisecretory agents: the H^+-K^+ ATPase or "proton pump" inhibitors. This enzyme is the final step in the acid secretory process. Omeprazole is a prodrug and a weak base that is concentrated 10,000-fold in the acidified tubulovesicles of the parietal cell. After protonation, the active drug binds covalently to the proton pump, permanently inactivating it. Restoration of acid secretion requires synthesis of new pumps, which have a half-life of 18 hours. Thus, although the drug has a serum half-life of only 60 minutes, its duration of action exceeds 24 hours. Doses of 20 mg/d inhibit over 90% of 24-hour acid secretion, compared with 37–68% for standard doses of H_2 antagonists. Om-

Table 14–3. Treatment options for active peptic ulcer disease.

Active duodenal ulcer
H₂-receptor antagonists for 6–8 weeks
  Cimetidine, 800 mg at bedtime
  Ranitidine, 300 mg at bedtime
  Famotidine, 40 mg at bedtime
  Nizatidine, 300 mg at bedtime
Omeprazole, 20 mg daily for 4 weeks
Sucralfate, 1 g 4 times daily for 6–8 weeks
If *H pylori*-positive, H₂ antagonists for 6–8 weeks plus 2 weeks *H pylori* triple therapy (Table 14–4)
Active gastric ulcer
H₂-receptor antagonists for 8 weeks (as above)
Omeprazole, 20–40 mg daily for 8 weeks
Refractory ulcer
Omeprazole, 40 mg daily for 8 weeks
If *H pylori*-positive, treat with 2 weeks of *H pylori* triple therapy (Table 14–4)

494 / CHAPTER 14

eprazole should be administered once daily before breakfast.

Omeprazole is quite safe in short-term therapy. It inhibits a subset of P450 enzymes affecting warfarin and phenytoin metabolism. A rise in fasting gastrin above normal levels occurs in 10% of patients due to decreased acid feedback of antral G cells. These levels revert to normal within 2–4 weeks after stopping therapy and are of no clinical importance in short-term therapy. There remain serious concerns about the risks of long-term omeprazole therapy. In rats, chronic omeprazole produces profound hypergastrinemia, resulting in hyperplasia of enterochromaffin-like cells and carcinoid tumors. In humans, the risks of long-term omeprazole appear to be less, with no changes in enterochromaffin-like cells or carcinoids reported to date. Omeprazole is FDA-approved for only 4–8 weeks of therapy. Long-term use is unnecessary in peptic ulcer disease but is used in severe cases of gastroesophageal reflux disease. In these patients, gastrin levels should be monitored every 6–12 months and the drug terminated or decreased if levels rise above 500 pg/mL.

B. Agents Enhancing Mucosal Defense:

1. Sucralfate—Sucralfate is a complex salt of sucrose containing aluminum and sulfate. The negatively charged sulfate groups bind to positively charged proteins in the ulcer base, forming a protective barrier against acid, bile, and pepsin. In addition, sucralfate stimulates mucus and bicarbonate secretion, prostaglandin production, and mucosal blood flow and binds fibroblast growth factor. Sucralfate is unabsorbed and virtually devoid of systemic side effects. Constipation occurs in 2–3%. Aluminum toxicity has occurred rarely in patients with chronic renal failure.

2. Bismuth—Bismuth compounds in a variety of formulations have been used extensively to treat dyspepsia, peptic ulcer disease, and diarrhea. The only agent available in the USA is bismuth subsalicylate (Pepto-Bismol). Pepto-Bismol tablets contain 151 mg of bismuth and 102 mg salicylate. Bismuth appears to enhance mucosal protection by stimulating bicarbonate and prostaglandin production. Bismuth has a direct antibacterial action against *H pylori,* eradicating the organism in up to one-third of patients. Less than 1% of bismuth is absorbed and is renally excreted. Salicylate is freely absorbed but does not reach excessive levels at standard doses. These bismuth compounds have excellent safety profiles in short-term use. Darkening of the feces is expected. Encephalopathy is reported in overdoses or in protracted courses with high-dose therapy.

3. Prostaglandin analogues (misoprostol)— A variety of oral prostaglandin analogues have been developed, but only misoprostol is clinically available. These agents promote ulcer healing by stimulating mucus and bicarbonate secretion and by enhancing mucosal blood flow. At therapeutically ef- fective doses, they also inhibit acid secretion. Misoprostol causes a dose-related diarrhea that is often transient. Administration with meals may improve diarrhea. Misoprostol is contraindicated in pregnancy because it may stimulate uterine contractions and induce abortion.

4. Antacids—Until recently, antacids containing aluminum or magnesium were thought to exert their therapeutic effect by neutralization of gastric acidity. Recently, low-dose antacid regimens (120–240 mmol/d) have been proved to be just as effective as higher-dose antacid regimens or H_2 antagonists in ulcer healing. Low-dose aluminum-containing antacids appear to promote healing through stimulation of mucosal defense mechanisms—not by neutralization of gastric acidity. High-dose regimens (1000 mmol/d neutralizing capacity) result in significant diarrhea, hypophosphatemia, and hypermagnesemia. At low doses, diarrhea and constipation are infrequent.

Treatment

A. General Measures: Patients should be encouraged to eat balanced meals at regular intervals. There is no justification for bland or restrictive diets. High-fiber diets are associated with a lower incidence of ulcers and lower recurrence rates. Caffeinated and cola beverages are potent acid secretagogues, and their intake should be curtailed. Moderate alcohol intake does not appear to be harmful. Smoking retards the rate of ulcer healing and increases the frequency of recurrences and should be strongly discouraged. At present, a causal relationship between psychologic stress and ulcer disease is unproved.

B. Standard Therapies: A variety of effective therapeutic agents are available that appear to be equivalent in their ability to heal peptic ulcers. Drug selection rests upon factors such as cost, frequency of administration, patient acceptance, and side effects.

1. H_2-receptor antagonists—All H_2 antagonists are of proved efficacy in the treatment of duodenal and gastric ulcers. Until recently, peptic ulcer disease was treated with H_2 antagonists two to four times daily. For uncomplicated ulcer disease, these agents may now be administered once daily at bedtime for 6–8 weeks with equivalent efficacy. Approved doses are cimetidine, 800 mg; ranitidine, 300 mg; famotidine, 40 mg; and nizatidine, 300 mg. Complete pain relief usually occurs within 2 weeks. Duodenal ulcer healing rates of 85–90% are obtained after 6–8 weeks of therapy. Gastric ulcer healing rates may be delayed by 2–4 weeks compared with duodenal ulcers, but 8 weeks of therapy is sufficient in most patients.

2. Omeprazole—Omeprazole, 20 mg once daily, is highly effective in the treatment of duodenal ulcers. Compared with H_2 antagonists, it provides faster pain relief and heals over 90% of duodenal ulcers at 4 weeks. Although more expensive per pill than H_2 antagonists, it is less expensive to treat with four weeks of omeprazole than 6–8 weeks of H_2 antagonists. In gastric ulcers, omeprazole, 20–40 mg/d, heals over 90% of ulcers within 8 weeks. Although modestly superior to H$_2$ antagonists at 4 weeks, equivalent healing rates may be obtained with longer courses of H$_2$ antagonists.

3. Sucralfate–Sucralfate, 1 g four times daily, is equivalent in efficacy to H$_2$ antagonists in the treatment of duodenal ulcers. It also appears to be efficacious in gastric ulcers but has undergone far less study and is not currently approved. Whereas smoking retards ulcer healing rates in patients receiving H$_2$ antagonists, several trials have suggested that sucralfate overcomes the negative impact of smoking.

4. Antacids–Low-dose antacid regimens providing 120–240 mmol of acid-neutralizing capacity per day may be comparable to standard doses of H$_2$ antagonists in the healing of duodenal ulcers. This corresponds to three or four tablets four times daily of Maalox Plus or two tablets four times daily of Mylanta-II. However, antacids are seldom prescribed by physicians as sole therapy for active ulcers. Antacids are commonly administered in the first 2 weeks of ulcer therapy for additional symptomatic relief.

C. Maintenance Therapy: (Table 14–4.) Sixty to 80 percent of patients have an endoscopically documented recurrence within 12 months after completing a course of standard therapy. Males, smokers, and patients with a history of frequent recurrences are at greatest risk of recurrence. Continuous maintenance therapy with half-dose bedtime H$_2$ antagonists (cimetidine, 400 mg; ranitidine, 150 mg; famotidine, 20 mg) or with sucralfate, 1 g twice daily, reduces the symptomatic recurrence rate to 10–15% per year. Retrospective studies suggest that maintenance therapy reduces ulcer complications in all patients, including those with prior complications.

There is lack of unanimity among authorities as to how broadly maintenance therapy should be applied. For patients who are elderly, who have serious underlying medical problems, or who have had prior complications, chronic maintenance therapy is custom-

Table 14–4. Treatment options for prevention of peptic ulcer recurrence.

H pylori-associated
No chronic therapy; full-dose therapy for symptomatic recurrences
Chronic "maintenance therapy"
  Cimetidine, 400 mg at bedtime
  Ranitidine, 150 mg at bedtime
  Famotidine, 20 mg at bedtime
  Sucralfate, 1 g twice daily
H pylori eradication therapy ("triple therapy")
  Pepto-Bismol tablets, 2 orally 4 times daily for 2 weeks
  Tetracycline, 500 mg 4 times daily for 2 weeks
  Metronidazole, 250 mg 3 or 4 times daily for 2 weeks
NSAID-induced ulceration
  Misoprostol, 100–200 μg orally 4 times daily
  H$_2$-receptor antagonists (as above)–duodenal ulcers only

ary. Sixty percent of patients have mild disease with not more than one recurrence per year; these patients are not usually given maintenance therapy but instead should receive intermittent therapy for symptomatic recurrences. For patients with more frequent ulcer recurrences, chronic maintenance therapy is recommended. Increasingly, this subset is being treated with _H pylori_ eradication therapy in an attempt to cure the ulcer disease.

D. _H pylori_ Eradication Therapy: (Table 14–4.) It is now apparent that eradication of _H pylori_ dramatically alters the natural history of ulcer disease. Anti-_H pylori_ therapy accelerates ulcer healing and markedly decreases the incidence of ulcer recurrences. Compared with H$_2$ antagonists alone, the addition of antiD_H pylori_ therapy accelerates ulcer healing rates at 6–8 weeks by 10–15%. In addition, eradication therapy is effective in healing ulcers that are refractory to other agents. The most important observation, however, is that _H pylori_ eradication reduces ulcer recurrence rates to less than 12%, compared with a recurrence rate of 84% when standard ulcer therapies are employed. Recent studies report continued low recurrence rates 2–4 years after successful eradication.

Eradication of _H pylori_ has proved difficult, however. A variety of therapeutic regimens have been tested with various degrees of success. The most consistently successful regimens have used "triple therapy": a combination of two antibiotics with a bismuth-containing compound. A 14-day course of Pepto-Bismol, two tablets four times daily with meals, metronidazole, 250 mg three times daily with meals, and tetracycline, 500 mg four times daily, eradicates _H pylori_ in over 85–90% of patients and is relatively inexpensive ($50.00). At present, the only way of confirming successful eradication is by repeating endoscopy with antral biopsies 4 weeks after the completion of therapy, but this is unnecessary in most patients. Compliance with drug therapy appears to be the most important factor in achieving eradication. Side effects of nausea, vomiting, and diarrhea occur in 10–25% of patients during therapy, but most are able to complete the treatment course. The incidence of recurrent _H pylori_ infection appears to be low (< 5% per year).

The treatment of ulcer disease is presently in a state of great flux. The major clinical question at this time is whether anti-_H pylori_ therapy should be given to all ulcer patients with _H pylori_ or whether it should be restricted to those with more severe ulcer disease, ie, patients with two or more recurrences, patients with refractory ulcers, or patients with ulcers developing on maintenance therapy. Authorities presently advocate both approaches.

E. Treatment of NSAID-Associated Ulcers: In patients with NSAIDDinduced ulcers, the offending agent should be discontinued whenever possible. Both gastric and duodenal ulcers respond rapidly to the standard therapies outlined above once NSAIDs are withheld. In some patients with inflammatory disease, it may not be feasible to discontinue NSAIDs. In most cases, duodenal ulcers heal with standard doses of H_2 antagonists despite continuation of NSAID therapy. The healing rate of gastric ulcers, however, is markedly slowed by NSAIDs. Omeprazole, 40 mg/d, rapidly heals gastric ulcers despite NSAID therapy and is the preferred agent in this setting.

F. Prevention of NSAID-Associated Ulcers: (Table 14–4.) The prostaglandin analogue misoprostol is effective in the prevention of NSAID-induced gastric and duodenal ulcers and is the only agent approved by the FDA for this purpose. When coadministered with NSAIDs, misoprostol, 100–200 μg four times daily, reduces the incidence of peptic ulcers from over 20% to under 5%. H_2 antagonists and sucralfate have proved ineffective for the prophylactic therapy of gastric ulcers but do appear to be effective in preventing duodenal ulcers. Misoprostol is currently recommended for patients at high risk of developing NSAID-induced complications. These include the elderly (over age 60), those with serious underlying medical illnesses, those with prior gastrointestinal complications, and those taking chronic corticosteroids. These patients are better served, however, by avoiding NSAIDs entirely.

Refractory Ulcers

Ulcers that are truly refractory to medical therapy are now quite uncommon. Approximately 5–10% of ulcers are unhealed after 12 weeks of therapy with H_2 antagonists or sucralfate. Noncompliance is the most common cause of ulcer nonhealing. NSAIDs and cigarettes may retard ulcer healing and should be withheld. Fasting serum gastrin levels should be measured to exclude Zollinger-Ellison syndrome. Almost all refractory ulcers will heal with 8 weeks of omeprazole, 40 mg/d. Relapse rates after discontinuation of omeprazole are high, and for that reason most patients require maintenance ulcer therapy. In patients who are *H pylori*-positive, refractory ulcers may heal after *H pylori* eradication therapy.

Nonhealing gastric ulcers raise concerns that an undiagnosed gastric malignancy may be masquerading as a benign gastric ulcer. Repeat biopsies are mandatory after 2–3 months of therapy in all nonhealed gastric ulcers to exclude malignancy. These ulcers should be followed with serial endoscopies to verify complete healing. Persistent nonhealing gastric or duodenal ulcers should be referred for surgical therapy.

Agrawal NM et al: Misoprostol compared with sucralfate in the prevention of nonsteroidal anti-inflammatory drug-induced gastric ulcer. Ann Intern Med 1991;115:195.
Allison MC et al: Gastrointestinal damage associated with the use of nonsteroidal anti-inflammatory drugs. N Engl J Med 1992;327:749.
Bardhan KD: Omeprazole in the management of refractory duodenal ulcer. Scand J Gastroenterol 1989;24(Suppl 166):66.
Feldman R, Burton ME: Histamine$_2$-receptor antagonists (Two parts.) N Engl J Med 1990;323:1672, 1749.
Gorbach SL: Bismuth therapy in gastrointestinal diseases. Gastroenterology 1990;99:863.
Graham D et al: Effect of triple therapy (antibiotics plus bismuth) on duodenal ulcer healing. Ann Intern Med 1992; 115:266.
Graham D: Treatment of peptic ulcers caused by *Helicobacter pylori*. (Editorial.) N Engl J Med 1993;328:349.
Hentschel E et al: Effect of ranitidine and amoxicillin plus metronidazole on the eradication of *Helicobacter pylori* and the recurrence of duodenal ulcer. N Engl J Med 1993;328:308.
Maton PN: Omeprazole. N Engl J Med 1991;324:965.
McCarthy DM: Sucralfate. N Engl J Med 1991;325:1017.
McQuaid K, Isenberg J: Medical therapy of peptic ulcer disease. Surg Clin North Am 1992;72:285.
Talley NJ: Chronic peptic ulceration and nonsteroidal anti-Dinflammatory drugs: More to be said about NSAIDs? Gastroenterology 1992;102:1074.
Walen A et al: Effect of omeprazole and ranitidine on ulcer healing and relapse rates in patients with benign gastric ulcer. N Engl J Med 1989;320:69. (Confirms rapid gastric ulcer healing with omeprazole in patients continuing to take NSAIDs.)
Walsh J: *Helicobacter pylori:* Selection of patients for treatment. (Editorial.) Ann Intern Med 1992;116:770.

COMPLICATIONS OF PEPTIC ULCER DISEASE

1. GASTROINTESTINAL HEMORRHAGE

Essentials of Diagnosis

- Coffee ground emesis, hematemesis, melena, or hematochezia.
- Vital signs best indicator of volume status.
- Emergent upper endoscopy is diagnostic and therapeutic.

General Considerations

Approximately 50% of all episodes of upper gastrointestinal bleeding are due to peptic ulcers. Clinically significant bleeding occurs in 10–20% of ulcer patients. About 80% of patients stop bleeding spontaneously and generally have an uneventful recovery. Twenty percent of patients have more severe bleeding. The overall mortality rate for ulcer bleeding is 6–10%, but it is higher in the elderly or in patients with medical problems.

Clinical Findings

A. Symptoms and Signs: Up to 20% of patients have no antecedent symptoms of pain; this is particularly true of patients receiving NSAIDs. Common presenting signs include melena and h.. matemesis. Massive upper gastrointestinal bleeding or rapid gastrointestinal transit may result in hematochezia rather than melena; this may be misinterpreted as signifying a lower tract bleeding source. Nasogastric lavage that demonstrates "coffee grounds" or bright red blood confirms an upper tract source. Recovered nasogastric lavage fluid that is negative for blood does not exclude active bleeding from a duodenal ulcer.

The presence of postural changes in vital signs signifies a 15–20% loss in intravascular volume and is a better indicator of acute blood loss than the hematocrit, which may take 12–24 hours to equilibrate. Signs of severe gastrointestinal bleeding include shock or hemodynamic instability, continued bloody nasogastric lavage fluid, or hematochezia.

B. Laboratory Findings: The hematocrit may fall as a result of bleeding or expansion of the intravascular volume with intravenous fluids. The BUN may rise as a result of absorption of blood nitrogen from the small intestine and prerenal azotemia.

Treatment

The management of bleeding from the upper gastrointestinal tract is discussed elsewhere in this chapter. Specific issues pertaining to ulcer bleeding are described below.

A. Medical Therapy: Bleeding stops spontaneously within a few hours after admission in 80% of cases. Intravenous H_2-receptor antagonists are administered by continuous infusions at a dose sufficient to maintain the intragastric pH > 4.0. Starting doses are cimetidine, 37.5–50 mg/h; ranitidine, 6.25 mg/h; or famotidine, 1 mg/h. Doses should be doubled after 4–6 hours if the intragastric pH is < 4.0. Vasopressin and intravenous octreotide should not be used for ulcer bleeding.

B. Endoscopy: Endoscopy is the preferred diagnostic procedure in virtually all cases of upper gastrointestinal bleeding because of its high diagnostic accuracy, its ability to predict the likelihood of recurrent bleeding, and its capability for therapeutic intervention in high-risk lesions. In patients with severe bleeding, endoscopy is usually performed within 6–8 hours after admission once resuscitative efforts have been initiated and hemodynamic stability has been restored. Endoscopy is performed more urgently in patients with continued active bleeding.

The appearance of the ulcer base is predictive of the chance of rebleeding. Ulcers with a base that is clean or appear only as a flat red or black spot impose a less than 5% risk of significant bleeding. Such patients may be transferred quickly from the ICU, resume a normal diet, and begin oral medications. Conversely, ulcers with an adherent clot have a 33% chance and those with a visible vessel a 50% chance of significant rebleeding. Actively bleeding ulcers have a high probability of continuing to bleed.

Endoscopic therapy with a variety of hemostatic injection and coagulation techniques is now considered standard therapy for patients with clinical evidence of a major bleeding episode who have a visible vessel or active ulcer bleeding at endoscopy. Injection is performed into and around the ulcer vessel with epinephrine (1:10,000), ethanol, or saline. Coagulation may also be achieved with contact cautery probes such as the bipolar or heater probe. Using any of these injection or cautery modalities, successful hemostasis is achieved in 90% of actively bleeding lesions. Significant rebleeding occurs in 10–20% of cases. Endoscopic therapy decreases the number of transfusions required and the need for surgery. Less than 10% of patients treated with hemostatic therapy will require surgery.

C. Surgery: All patients with ulcer bleeding severe enough to warrant ICU admission or blood transfusion should be evaluated by a surgeon. Criteria for emergency surgery include the following: (1) Severe bleeding or rebleeding that cannot be controlled with two endoscopic hemostatic treatments. (2) Massive exsanguinating hemorrhage when resuscitative efforts have failed. (3) The need for more than six to eight units of blood in the first 24 hours, especially if endoscopic hemostasis is unsuccessful. (4) Slow, continuous bleeding for over 48 hours. The overall surgical mortality rate for emergency ulcer bleeding is less than 6%. The prognosis is much poorer, however, for patients over age 60, those with serious underlying medical illnesses, those with chronic renal failure, and those receiving multiple transfusions.

Surgery is also indicated in patients who have had two hospitalizations for ulcer hemorrhage and for patients developing ulcer bleeding despite chronic maintenance H_2 antagonist therapy.

2. ULCER PERFORATION

Perforations develop in 5% of ulcer patients, usually from ulcers on the anterior wall of the stomach or duodenum. The incidence of perforations may be increasing, perhaps as a consequence of using NSAIDs or crack cocaine. Consideration of Zollinger-Ellison disease should be made in patients who present with ulcer perforation. Perforation results in a chemical peritonitis that causes sudden, severe generalized abdominal pain that prompts most patients to seek immediate attention. Elderly or debilitated patients and those receiving chronic steroid therapy may experience minimal initial symptoms, presenting late with bacterial peritonitis, sepsis, and shock. On physical examination, patients appear ill, with a rigid, quiet abdomen and rebound tenderness. Hypotension is not a feature of early ulcer perforation but develops later after bacterial peritonitis has developed. If hypotension is present early with the onset of pain, one should consider other abdominal catastrophes such as a ruptured aortic aneurysm, mesenteric infarction, or acute pancreatitis. Leukocytosis is almost always present. A mildly elevated serum amylase (less than twice normal) is sometimes seen. Upright or decubitus films of the abdomen reveal free intraperitoneal air in 75% of cases, and in most cases this establishes the diagnosis without need for further studies. In the remainder of cases, adjacent omentum seals the perforation before significant leakage occurs. The absence of free air may lead to a misdiagnosis of pancreatitis, cholecystitis, or appendicitis. Upper gastrointestinal radiography with water-soluble contrast may be useful in this setting. Barium studies are contraindicated in patients with possible perforation.

The majority of patients with perforated ulcers should undergo emergency surgery. Closure of the perforation is performed with an omental patch. In most cases, proximal gastric vagotomy is performed to decrease the chance of ulcer recurrence. Although traditionally performed by laparotomy, vagotomy may now be done through a laparoscope.

The overall mortality rate in patients treated surgically is about 5%. Selected patients may be managed nonoperatively. Patients considered to be poor operative candidates and patients who present more than 24 hours after perforation who are stable and who have no evidence of leakage on gastroduodenography may be followed closely on fluids, nasogastric suction, and broad-spectrum antibiotics. If their condition deteriorates in the first 12–24 hours, they should be taken to the operating room. The mortality rate in medically treated patients is less than 5%.

3. ULCER PENETRATION

An ulcer located along the posterior wall of the duodenum or stomach may perforate into contiguous structures such as the pancreas, liver, or biliary tree. Patients complain of a change in the intensity and rhythmicity of their ulcer symptoms. The pain becomes more severe and constant, may radiate to the back, and is unresponsive to antacids or food. Physical examination and laboratory tests are nonspecific. Mild amylase elevations may sometimes occur. Endoscopy and barium xDray studies confirm the ulceration but are not diagnostic of an actual penetration. Patients should be placed on intravenous H_2 antagonists (as above) or omeprazole, 40 mg/d, and followed closely. Patients who fail to improve should be considered for surgical therapy.

4. GASTRIC OUTLET OBSTRUCTION

Gastric outlet obstruction occurs in 2% of patients with ulcer disease and is due to edema or cicatricial narrowing of the pylorus or duodenal bulb. Most patients have a prior known history of ulcer disease.

Obstruction is less commonly caused by gastric neoplasms or extrinsic duodenal obstruction by intraabdominal neoplasms. The most common symptoms are early satiety, vomiting, and weight loss. Early symptoms are epigastric fullness or heaviness after meals. Later, vomiting may develop that typically occurs one to several hours after eating and consists of partially digested food contents. Chronic obstruction may result in a grossly dilated, atonic stomach, severe weight loss, and malnutrition. Patients may develop dehydration, metabolic alkalosis, and hypokalemia. On physical examination, a succussion splash may be heard in the epigastrium. In most cases, nasogastric aspiration will result in evacuation of a large amount (> 200 mL) of foul-smelling fluid, which establishes the diagnosis. More subtle obstruction is diagnosed by a saline load test or by a nuclear gastric emptying study. Patients are treated initially with intravenous isotonic saline and KCl to correct fluid and electrolyte disorders, intravenous H_2 antagonists (doses given above), and nasogastric decompression of the stomach. Severely malnourished patients should receive total parenteral nutrition. Upper endoscopy is performed after 24–72 hours to define the nature of the obstruction and to exclude a gastric neoplasm. At 72 hours, all patients should be evaluated with a saline load test. A positive test consists of more than 400 mL of residual volume 30 minutes after instillation of 750 mL of normal saline into the stomach by nasogastric tube. Patients with a negative load test may be started on clear liquids and their diet advanced as tolerated. The remainder should remain on nasogastric suction for 5–7 days. Traditionally, patients unimproved after that time have been recommended for surgical treatment with vagotomy and either pyloroplasty or antrectomy. Recently, upper endoscopy with dilation of the gastric obstruction by hydrostatic balloons passed through the instrument has achieved success in two-thirds of patients. It may be reasonable to pursue dilation first in patients with milder symptoms, reserving surgery for those who fail to respond.

Cook DJ et al: Endoscopic therapy for acute nonvariceal upper gastrointestinal hemorrhage: A metaanalysis. Gastroenterology 1992;102:139.

Crofts TJ et al: A randomized trial of nonoperative treatment for perforated peptic ulcer. N Engl J Med 1989;320:970.

Krevsky B: Endoscopic management of gastric outlet obstruction. Gastroenterology 1991;101:553.

Stabile B: Current surgical management of duodenal ulcers. Surg Clin North Am 1992;72:335.

Therapeutic endoscopy and bleeding ulcers. (Consensus Conference.) JAMA 1989;262:1369.

ZOLLINGER-ELLISON SYNDROME
(Gastrinoma)

Essentials of Diagnosis

- Peptic ulcer disease; may be severe.
- Gastric acid hypersecretion.
- Diarrhea common.
- Gastrinoma; may be metastatic.
- Most sporadic; 25% with MEN I.

General Considerations

Zollinger-Ellison syndrome is caused by gastrin-secreting tumors (gastrinomas), which result in hypergastrinemia and acid hypersecretion. Less than 1% of peptic ulcer disease is caused by gastrinomas. Gastrinomas may arise in the pancreas (70%), duodenal wall (15–20%), or other ectopic sites (5–15%). Approximately 90% arise within the "gastrinoma triangle" bounded by the porta hepatis, the neck of the pancreas, and the third portion of the duodenum. Most gastrinomas are solitary or multifocal nodules that are potentially resectable. Over half of gastrinomas are malignant, and up to 40% of patients develop metastatic disease. Approximately 25% of patients have small multicentric gastrinomas associated with MEN I syndrome which are not resectable.

Clinical Findings

A. Symptoms and Signs: More than 90% of patients with Zollinger-Ellison syndrome develop peptic ulcers. In most cases, the symptoms are indistinguishable from other causes of peptic ulcer disease and therefore may go undetected for years. Ulcers usually are solitary and located in the duodenal bulb, but they may be multiple or occur more distally in the duodenum. Gastroesophageal reflux symptoms occur often. Diarrhea occurs in over half of patients, in some cases in the absence of peptic symptoms. Gastric acid hypersecretion can cause direct intestinal mucosal injury and pancreatic enzyme inactivation resulting in diarrhea, steatorrhea, and weight loss. Screening for Zollinger-Ellison syndrome with fasting gastrin levels should be obtained in patients with ulcers that are refractory to standard therapies, giant ulcers, ulcers located distal to the duodenal bulb, multiple duodenal ulcers, frequent ulcer recurrences, ulcers associated with diarrhea, ulcers occurring after ulcer surgery, and patients with ulcer complications. Ulcer patients with hypercalcemia or family histories of ulcers (suggesting MEN I) should also be screened.

B. Laboratory Findings: Patients with Zollinger-Ellison syndrome have fasting serum gastrin levels > 150 pg/mL. Levels should be obtained with patients not taking any H_2 antagonists for 24 hours and omeprazole for 6 days. To differentiate Zollinger-Ellison syndrome from other causes of hypergastrinemia, a secretin provocation test is subsequently performed. Secretin (2 CU/kg) is adminis-

tered by intravenous bolus with serum gastrin levels obtained 10 and 2 minutes before and 2, 5, 10, 15, 20, and 30 minutes after injection. A rise above basal gastrin of > 200 pg/mL is seen in 90% of patients. Elevated serum calcium suggests possible hyperparathyroidism and MEN I. Gastric acid secretory studies are generally performed to confirm acid hypersecretion. Most patients have a basal acid output exceeding 15 meq/h. A gastric pH > 3.0 excludes gastrinoma as a cause of hypergastrinemia.

C. Imaging: Imaging studies are performed in an attempt to localize the tumor and to determine whether there is metastatic disease. Preoperative localization can be extremely difficult. CT scanning and MRI detect only half of primary gastrinomas but a higher percentage of metastatic disease. When these noninvasive imaging studies are negative, selective abdominal angiography is performed and may detect an additional 15–30% of lesions. Nevertheless, there remain 20–50% of patients in whom tumors cannot be found despite these studies.

Differential Diagnosis

Zollinger-Ellison syndrome must be distinguished from other causes of hypergastrinemia. Atrophic gastritis with decreased acid secretion is detected by gastric secretory analysis. Other conditions such as routine peptic ulcer disease, antral G cell hyperfunction, and gastric outlet obstruction are associated with negative secretin stimulation tests.

Treatment

A. Metastatic Disease and MEN I: In these patients, gastrinoma resection is not attempted. Patients may have prolonged survival, though many die within 5 years. Initial therapy is directed at controlling the gastric acid hypersecretion. Omeprazole is given at a dose of 40–120 mg/d, which is titrated to achieve a basal acid output of < 10 meq/h. At this dose, there is complete symptomatic relief and ulcer healing. Chemotherapy has been disappointing in this disease but may be considered in patients with symptomatic metastases.

B. Localized Disease: Cure can only be achieved if gastrinoma is detected and removed before metastatic spread has occurred. Laparotomy should be considered in all patients in whom preoperative studies either fail to localize a tumor or suggest an isolated, resectable lesion. Careful operative palpation combined with intraoperative sonography can identify gastrinomas in the majority of patients. Cure is achieved in over 30% of cases—up to 90% in some series.

Howard TJ et al: Gastrinoma excision for cure. Ann Surg 1990;211:9.

Maton PN et al: Long-term efficacy and safety of omeprazole in patients with Zollinger-Ellison syndrome: A prospective study. Gastroenterology 1989;97:827.

Norton JA, Jensen RT: Unresolved surgical issues in the management of Zollinger-Ellison syndrome. World J Surg 1991;15:151.

BENIGN TUMORS OF THE STOMACH

Gastric epithelial polyps are usually detected incidentally at endoscopy. The majority are hyperplastic polyps, which are small, single or multiple, have no malignant potential, and do not require removal or endoscopic surveillance. Adenomatous polyps account for 10–20% of gastric polyps. They are usually solitary lesions. In rare instances they ulcerate, causing chronic blood loss. Because of their premalignant potential, endoscopic removal is indicated. Annual endoscopic surveillance is recommended to screen for further polyp development. Submucosal gastric polypoid lesions include leiomyoma and pancreatic rests.

MALIGNANT TUMORS OF THE STOMACH

1. GASTRIC ADENOCARCINOMA

Essentials of Diagnosis

- Dyspeptic symptoms with weight loss in patients over age 40.
- Iron deficiency anemia; occult blood in stools.
- Abnormality detected on upper gastrointestinal series or endoscopy.

General Considerations

Although gastric adenocarcinoma is the most common cancer (other than skin cancer) worldwide, its incidence has been decreasing steadily in the United States. The incidence is particularly high in native Japanese. Gastric cancer is uncommon in people under age 40 and is more common in men. Chronic atrophic gastritis with intestinal metaplasia—perhaps secondary to chronic *H pylori* infection—appears to be a strong risk factor for gastric cancer. Patients with pernicious anemia and with gastric resections over 15 years previously are also at increased risk. Although the majority of these cancers arise in the antrum, the incidence of tumors arising in the gastric cardia and fundus is increasing. Invasive tumors are manifested most commonly as polypoid or fungating intraluminal masses or as ulcerating lesions with irregular margins. Uncommonly, tumor may present as a linitis plastica lesion in which there is infiltration through the submucosa, resulting in thickened folds and a rigid, atonic stomach.

Clinical Findings

A. Symptoms and Signs: Gastric carcinoma is generally asymptomatic until the disease is quite advanced. Symptoms are nonspecific and are determined in part by the location of the tumor. Dyspepsia, vague epigastric pain, anorexia, early satiety, and weight loss are the presenting symptoms in most patients. Patients may derive initial symptomatic relief from over-the-counter remedies, further delaying diagnosis. Ulcerating lesions can lead to acute gastrointestinal bleeding with hematemesis or melena. Pyloric obstruction results in postprandial vomiting. Lower esophageal obstruction causes progressive dysphagia. Physical examination is rarely helpful. A gastric mass is seldom palpated. Signs of metastatic spread include a left supraclavicular lymph node (Virchow's node), an umbilical nodule (Sister Mary Joseph nodule), a rigid rectal shelf (Blumer's shelf), and ovarian metastases (Krukenberg tumor). Guaiac-positive stools may be detectable.

B. Laboratory Findings: Iron deficiency anemia due to chronic blood loss or anemia of chronic disease is common. Liver function test abnormalities may be present if there is metastatic liver spread. Other tumor markers are of no value.

C. Endoscopy: Upper endoscopy should be obtained in all patients over age 40 with new onset of epigastric symptoms. Endoscopy with cytologic brushings and biopsies of suspicious lesions is highly sensitive for detecting gastric carcinoma. It can be difficult to obtain adequate biopsy specimens in linitis plastica lesions. Because of the high incidence of gastric carcinoma in Japan, screening upper endoscopy is performed to detect early gastric carcinoma. Approximately 40% of tumors detected by screening are early, with a 5-year survival rate of over 60%. Screening programs are not recommended in this country.

D. Imaging: A barium upper gastrointestinal series is an acceptable alternative when endoscopy is not readily available but may not detect small or superficial lesions and cannot reliably distinguish benign from malignant ulcerations. Any abnormalities detected with this procedure require endoscopic confirmation.

Once a gastric cancer is diagnosed, preoperative evaluation is indicated to delineate the local extent of the primary tumor as well as nodal or distant metastases. Abdominal CT is valuable in identifying distant metastases and direct invasion of adjacent structures. Endoscopic ultrasound imaging is now available in many centers and is superior to CT in determining the depth of tumor penetration and nodal metastases.

Differential Diagnosis

Ulcerating gastric adenocarcinomas are distinguished from benign gastric ulcers by biopsies. Approximately 3% of gastric ulcers initially felt to be benign later prove to be malignant. To exclude malignancy, all gastric ulcers should be followed with endoscopy to complete healing, and nonhealing gastric ulcers should be resected. Infiltrative carcinoma with thickened gastric folds must be distinguished from lymphoma and other hypertrophic gastropathies such as Ménétrier's disease. Obtaining adequate biopsy specimens can be difficult, and an open, full-thickness biopsy is sometimes required.

Treatment

Surgical resection is the only available therapy with curative potential. Patients with localized disease without distant metastases or adjacent organ involvement who undergo a complete resection with curative intent have a 20–30% 5-year survival rate. There is no role at this time for adjuvant therapy after surgery with chemotherapy or radiation.

The majority of patients with gastric cancer present with advanced disease, and the prognosis is dismal. On the basis of preoperative and intraoperative evaluation, only 30% of patients have disease that is amenable to "curative" resection. In the remainder of patients, therapy is directed at palliation. Surgical palliative resection, where possible, is indicated in patients in whom survival for several months is expected. Patients developing obstruction require resection or a gastrojejunostomy bypass procedure. Tumor bleeding may be controlled with resection, radiation, or angiographic embolization. Chemotherapy does not improve survival and is not recommended outside of clinical protocols.

Ajan JA et al: Current strategies in the management of local, regional and metastatic gastric carcinoma. Cancer 1991; 67(Suppl 1):260.

Farley DR, Donahue JH: Early gastric cancer. Surg Clin North Am 1992;72:401. (Current options for diagnosis and treatment. Patients with early gastric cancer have an excellent survival rate.)

2. LYMPHOMA

Lymphomas account for less than 2% of gastric malignancies. These are almost always non-Hodgkin's lymphomas, predominantly of the diffuse histiocytic type. Gastric lymphoma is the most common type of extranodal non-Hodgkin's lymphoma. The clinical presentation and endoscopic appearance are similar to those of adenocarcinoma. Diagnosis is established by endoscopic biopsy.

Treatment is controversial. Patients with disease limited to the stomach (stage IE) should undergo surgical resection, but the role of adjuvant chemotherapy or radiation therapy is unclear. Patients with disease extending to local lymph nodes (stage II) or adjacent organs (stage III) or with distant spread of disease (stage IV) should undergo chemotherapy as the primary therapeutic modality. Surgical resection is added in some situations to decrease the risk of local complications such as perforation or bleeding during chemotherapy. Overall 5-year survival is 50% but may be 80% in patients with stage I or stage II disease.

Frazee RC, Roberts J: Gastric lymphoma treatment: Medical versus surgical. Surg Clin North Am 1992;72:423.

Sharma S et al: Primary gastric lymphoma: A prospective analysis of 12 cases and review of the literature. J Surg Oncol 1990;43:231.

CARCINOIDS

Gastric carcinoids are rare tumors that occur sporadically and in 3–5% of patients with Zollinger-Ellison syndrome and pernicious anemia due to chronic hypergastrinemia. They may be solitary or multicentric. Although they may secrete a variety of gut peptides, including serotonin, gastrin, pituitary hormones, and catecholamines, most are clinically silent and are detected incidentally at endoscopy. Symptom development generally reflects hepatic metastases. The majority are small, slow-growing, and benign in their behavior. Tumors larger than 2 cm in diameter have a greater potential for malignant spread and should be surgically excised. Small, solitary lesions may be removed endoscopically. Regression of small carcinoids occurs after antrectomy with resolution of hypergastrinemia.

Hirschowitz BI et al: Rapid regression of enterochromaffinlike cell gastric carcinoids in pernicious anemia after antrectomy. Gastroenterology 1992;102:1409.

DISEASES OF THE SMALL INTESTINE

REGIONAL ENTERITIS (Regional Ileitis, Granulomatous Ileocolitis, Crohn's Disease) (See also Inflammatory Bowel, below.)

Essentials of Diagnosis

- Insidious onset.
- Intermittent bouts of diarrhea, low-grade fever, and right lower quadrant pain.
- Fistula formation or right lower quadrant mass and tenderness (late finding).
- Radiographic evidence of abnormality of the terminal ileum.

General Considerations

Regional enteritis is a chronic inflammatory disease that may involve the alimentary tract anywhere from the mouth to the anus. The ileum is the principal site of the disease, either alone or in conjunction with the colon and jejunum. It generally occurs in young adults and runs an intermittent clinical course with mild to severe disability and frequent complications.

There is marked thickening of the submucosa with lymphedema, lymphoid hyperplasia, nonspecific granulomas, and often ulceration of the overlying mucosa. A marked lymphadenitis occurs in the mesenteric nodes. The inflammatory involvement tends to be transmural.

The cause is unknown. Genetic factors appear to play a role. There is a higher than normal incidence in monozygotic twins and a greater than random familial incidence. The most common familial pattern involves two or more affected siblings. Regional enteritis and chronic ulcerative colitis occur in the same families. The possibility of an infectious origin for regional enteritis has been raised by studies demonstrating transmission of an agent from tissues with regional enteritis into immunologically deficient mice and rabbits, but no agent to date has been substantiated.

Clinical Findings

A. Symptoms and Signs: The disease is characterized by exacerbations and remissions. Colicky or steady abdominal pain is present in the right lower quadrant or periumbilical area at some time during the course of the disease and varies from mild to severe. Diarrhea may occur, usually with intervening periods of normal bowel function or constipation. Patients with these symptoms are often diagnosed as having irritable or functional bowel disease. Fever may be low-grade or, rarely, spiking with chills. Anorexia, flatulence, malaise, and weight loss are present. Milk products and chemically or mechanically irritating foods may aggravate symptoms.

Abdominal tenderness is usually present, especially in the right lower quadrant, with signs of peritoneal irritation and an abdominal or pelvic mass in the same area. The mass is tender and varies from a sausage-like thickened intestine to matted loops of intestine.

Regional enteritis may pursue various clinical patterns. In certain instances, the course is indolent and the symptomatology mild. In other instances, the course is toxic, with fever, toxic erythema, arthralgia, anemia, etc. Still other patients pursue courses complicated by stricture or perforations of the bowel and suppurative complications of intra-abdominal perforation.

B. Laboratory Findings: There is usually a hypochromic (occasionally macrocytic due to vitamin B_{12} malabsorption) anemia and occult blood in the stool.

C. Imaging: The small bowel x-ray may show mucosal irregularity, ulceration, stiffening of the bowel wall, and luminal narrowing. Barium enema may show fissures or deep ulcers. Eccentric involvement, skipped areas of involvement, and strictures suggest Crohn's disease of the colon.

D. Special Examinations: Sigmoidoscopic examination may show an edematous hyperemic mucosa or a discrete ulcer when the colon is involved.

Differential Diagnosis

Acute regional enteritis may simulate acute appendicitis. Location in the terminal ileum requires differentiation from intestinal tuberculosis, *Yersinia enterocolitica* infection, lymphomas, and, in the immunodeficient patient, *Mycobacterium avium-intracellulare*. Regional enteritis involving the colon must be distinguished from idiopathic ulcerative colitis, amebic colitis, ischemic colitis, and infectious disease of the colon. The sigmoidoscopic and x-ray criteria distinguishing these various entities may not be absolute, and definitive diagnosis may require cultures, examinations of the stool for parasites, and biopsy in selected instances.

Complications

Ischiorectal and perianal fistulas occur frequently. Fistulas may occur to the bladder or vagina and even to the skin in the area of a previous scar. Mechanical intestinal obstruction may occur. Nutritional deficiency caused by malabsorption and maldigestion (the latter caused by a decreased bile salt pool) may produce a sprue-like syndrome. Generalized peritonitis is rare because perforation occurs slowly, is locally contained, or results in internal fistulization. The incidence of colorectal or small bowel cancer in regional enteritis patients is greater than in a control population, but less than for ulcerative colitis. Migratory peripheral synovitis and axial arthropathy indistinguishable from sporadic ankylosing spondylitis may occur.

Treatment & Prognosis

A. General Measures: The diet should be high in calories and vitamins and adequate in protein. Raw fruits and vegetables should be avoided in patients who have obstructive symptoms. These patients may benefit from a nonresidue, well-balanced diet to maintain nutrition until obstructive symptoms subside. Anemia, dehydration, diarrhea, and avitaminosis should be treated as indicated.

B. Antimicrobial Agents: In our present state of knowledge about this disease, antimicrobials are indicated only for specific infectious problems, ie, abscess, fistulas.

1. Sulfasalazine–Sulfasalazine, 2–8 g/d orally, has been shown to be effective, especially for disease involving the colon. The salicylate moiety of sulfasalazine, 5-aminosalicylic acid (mesalamine), appears to be of equal efficacy without the side effects attributable to the sulfapyridine portion of sulfasalazine.

2. Antibiotics–In cases of acute suppuration (manifested by tender mass, fever, leukocytosis), ampicillin, 2–4 g/d intravenously or orally, may be useful. Clindamycin or metronidazole (for anaerobes) and aminoglycosides are also effective. In cases where internal fistulization has led to a defunctionalized loop with bacterial overgrowth or where stricture formation has led to small bowel stasis with malabsorption, tetracycline, 1–2 g/d orally, may be valuable in combating bacterial overgrowth in the bowel and correcting absorptive malfunction.

3. Metronidazole–Metronidazole, 15 mg/kg/d in divided doses orally, is effective in colonic disease and for enterocutaneous fistulas, including perineal fistulas.

C. Adrenocortical Hormones: These agents are often of use in the diffuse form of the disease and are particularly helpful in the toxic forms (arthritis, anemia, toxic erythemas). The complications of long-term therapy can be minimized by administering the drug on an alternate-day schedule (eg, prednisone, 15–40 mg every other day) once the patient's clinical symptoms have been brought under control. In a national cooperative study, azathioprine (50–100 mg orally daily) proved to be of no value, though perhaps the observation period may have been too short. Mercaptopurine, the active metabolite of azathioprine, has a beneficial effect on the fistulas of Crohn's disease as well as on other features of the disease.

D. Other Medical Measures: When terminal ileal disease is present, vitamin B_{12} supplementation (100 μg subcutaneously per month) is often necessary. Calcium supplementation (0.5 g orally three times a day) in the form of calcium gluconate or Os-Cal will alleviate the frequent calcium deficiency seen in these patients and is also helpful in decreasing excessive oxalate absorption, resulting in lowered incidence of oxalate urinary tract stones.

E. Surgical Measures: Surgical treatment of this disease is best limited to the management of its complications. Resection of the small bowel, particularly the extensive resection often necessary in regional enteritis, leads to a "short bowel" syndrome (diminished absorptive surface), ie, malabsorption of vitamin B_{12} to varying degrees (loss of terminal ileum), hyperoxaluria, steatorrhea, osteomalacia, and macrocytic anemia (due to folic acid and vitamin B_{12} deficiency). Stricturoplasty may be helpful and preserve bowel. Short-circuiting operations may lead to blind loops (intestinal defunctionalization with bacterial overgrowth) with similar difficulties in absorption. When surgery is necessary in this disease, study of postsurgical bowel function is indicated to detect the possibility of impaired function.

Danzi JT: Extraintestinal manifestations of idiopathic inflammatory bowel disease. Arch Intern Med 1988; 148:297. (Incidence of 25–36%. May involve joints, eyes, skin, oral mucosa, and liver and may be associated with an increased incidence of cholelithiasis, nephrolithiasis, and amyloidosis.)

Dirks E et al: Clinical relapse of Crohn's disease under standardized conservative treatment and after excisional surgery. Dig Dis Sci 1989;34:1832. (Guidance for operation and benefits for selected patients.)

Drossman DA et al: Health status and health care use in persons with inflammatory bowel disease. Dig Dis Sci 1991;36:1746. (Crohn's patients have more psychologic difficulties. Despite everything, health status is quite good.)

Michelassi F et al: Primary and recurrent Crohn's disease: Experience with 1379 patients. Ann Surg 1991;214:230. (Large experience. Recurrence rate 20% at 5 years, 34% at 10 years.)

TUMORS OF THE SMALL INTESTINE

Benign and malignant tumors of the small intestine are rare. There may be no symptoms or signs, but bleeding or obstruction (or both) may occur. The obstruction consists of either an intussusception with the tumor in the lead or a partial or complete occlusion in the lumen by growth of the tumor. Bleeding may cause weakness, fatigability, light-headedness, syncope, pallor, sweating, tachycardia, and tarry stools. Obstruction causes nausea, vomiting, and abdominal pains. The abdomen is tender and distended, and bowel sounds are high-pitched and active. Malignant lesions produce weight loss and extraintestinal manifestations (eg, pain due to stretching of the liver capsule, flushing due to carcinoid). In the case of a duodenal carcinoma, a peptic ulcer syndrome may be present. A palpable mass is rarely found.

If there is bleeding, melena and hypochromic anemia occur. X-ray (small bowel series, preferably by enteroclysis) may show the tumor mass or dilation of the small bowel if obstruction is present; in the absence of obstruction, it is extremely difficult to demonstrate the mass.

Benign Tumors

Benign tumors may be symptomatic or may be incidental findings at operation or autopsy. Treatment consists of surgical removal.

Benign **adenomas** constitute 25% of all benign bowel tumors. **Lipomas** occur most frequently in the ileum; the presenting symptom is usually obstruction due to intussusception. **Leiomyomas** are usually associated with bleeding and may also cause intussusception. **Angiomas** behave like other small bowel tumors but have a greater tendency to bleed.

Multiple intestinal polyposis of the gastrointestinal tract (any level) associated with mucocutaneous pigmentation (Peutz-Jeghers syndrome) is a benign condition. Malignant change has been reported but is rare, and the entity becomes a problem only with complications such as obstruction or bleeding. The polyps are hamartomas, and the pigment is melanin. The pigment is most prominent over the lips and buccal mucosa.

Malignant Tumors

The treatment of malignant tumors and their complications is usually surgical.

Adenocarcinoma is the most common cancer of the small bowel, occurring most frequently in the duodenum and jejunum. Symptoms are due to obstructions or hemorrhage. The prognosis is very poor. **Lymphomas** are also first manifested by obstruction of bleeding. Perforation or malabsorption may also occur. Postoperative radiation therapy may occasionally be of value. **Sarcomas** occur most commonly in the mid small bowel and may first be manifested by mass, obstruction, or bleeding. The prognosis is guarded.

Carcinoid tumors arise from the argentaffin cells of the gastrointestinal tract. Ninety percent of these tumors occur in the appendix, and 75% of the remainder occur in the small intestine (usually the distal ileum). Carcinoids may arise in other sites, including the stomach, colon, bronchus, pancreas, and ovary. Most small bowel carcinoids do not produce carcinoid syndrome. The main problem is metastases. In general, carcinoid syndrome occurs only with malignant tumors that have metastasized. The tumor may secrete serotonin and bradykinin. The systemic manifestations may consist of (1) paroxysmal flushing and other vasomotor symptoms, (2) dyspnea and wheezing, (3) recurrent episodes of abdominal pain and diarrhea, and (4) symptoms and signs of right-sided valvular disease of the heart. The diagnosis is confirmed by finding elevated levels of 5-hydroxyindoleacetic acid in the urine. The primary tumor is usually small, and obstruction is unusual. The metastases are usually voluminous and surprisingly benign. Treatment is symptomatic and supportive; surgical excision may be indicated if the condition is recognized before widespread metastases have occurred. Response to treatment with serotonin antagonists has been irregular. Repeated administration of corticotropin or the corticosteroids may occasionally be of value. The prognosis for cure is poor, but long-term survival is not unusual.

Auger MJ, Allan NC: Primary ileocecal lymphoma. Cancer 1990;65:358. (Experience with 22 patients. Adequate initial surgery combined with chemotherapy appears to be optimal management.)

Sachs JR, Bralow SP: Primary malignancies of the small bowel. Intern Med 1989;10:120. (Rare, and diagnosed late.)

MECKEL'S DIVERTICULITIS

Meckel's diverticulum, a remnant of the omphalomesenteric duct, is found in about 2% of persons, more frequently in males. It arises from the ileum 60–90 cm from the ileocecal valve and may or may not have an umbilical attachment. Most are silent, but various abdominal symptoms may occur. The blind pouch may be involved by an inflammatory process similar to appendicitis; its congenital bands or inflammatory adhesions may cause acute intestinal obstruction; it may induce intussusception; or, in the 16% that contain heterotopic islands of gastric mucosa, it may form a peptic ulcer.

The symptoms and signs of the acute appendicitis-like disease and the acute intestinal obstruction caused by Meckel's diverticulitis cannot be differentiated from other primary processes except by exploration. Ulcer type distress, if present, is localized near the umbilicus or lower and, more importantly, is not relieved by alkalies or food. If ulceration has occurred, blood will be present in the stool. Massive gastrointestinal bleeding and perforation may occur. The presence of Meckel's diverticulum can frequently be determined in patients with gastric mucosa by a technetium radioisotope scan.

Meckel's diverticulitis should be resected, either for relief or for differentiation from acute appendicitis. Surgery is curative.

Farr CM et al: Bleeding Meckel's diverticulum in an adult. J Clin Gastroenterol 1989;11:208. (Nuclear red cell scan may be helpful. The disease may cause problems as late as the seventh decade.)

ACUTE ORGANIC SMALL INTESTINAL OBSTRUCTION

Essentials of Diagnosis

- Colicky abdominal pain, vomiting, constipation, borborygmus.
- Tender distended abdomen without peritoneal irritation.
- Audible high-pitched tinkling peristalsis or peristaltic rushes.
- Radiographic evidence of dilated loops of small intestine with or without fluid levels. Little or no leukocytosis.

General Considerations

Acute organic intestinal obstruction usually involves the small intestine, particularly the ileum. Major inciting causes are external hernia and postoperative adhesions. Less common causes are gallstones, neoplasms, granulomatous processes, intussusception, volvulus, internal hernia, and foreign bodies.

Clinical Findings

A. Symptoms and Signs: Colicky abdominal pain in the periumbilical area becomes more constant and diffuse as distention develops. Vomiting, at first of a reflex nature associated with the waves of pain, later becomes fecal in obstruction of the distal bowel. Borborygmus and consciousness of intestinal movement, obstipation, weakness, perspiration, and anxiety are often present. The patient is restless, changing position frequently with pain, and has sweating, tachycardia, and dehydration. Abdominal distention may be localized, with an isolated loop, but usually is generalized. The higher the obstruction, the less the distention; the longer the time of obstruction, the greater the distention. Audible peristalsis, peristaltic rushes with pain paroxysms, high-pitched tinkles, and visible peristalsis may be present. Moderate generalized abdominal tenderness may be present, and there are no signs of peritoneal irritation. Fever is absent or low-grade. A tender hernia may be present.

B. Laboratory Findings: Hemoconcentration may occur with true dehydration or may reflect sequestration of fluid in the obstructed loop or third space. Leukocytosis is absent or mild. Vomiting may cause electrolyte disturbances.

C. Imaging: Abdominal radiography reveals gas- and fluid-filled loops of bowel, and the gas does not progress downward on serial radiographs. Fluid levels may be visible.

Differential Diagnosis

The differential diagnosis includes other acute abdominal conditions such as inflammation and perforation of a viscus or renal or gallbladder colic. The absence of peritoneal signs, ie, rigidity and rebound tenderness, should aid in differentiating small bowel obstruction from ileus secondary to peritonitis, but the differential would then also include pseudo-obstruction. The absence of leukocytosis and the presence of high-pitched bowel sounds or intestinal rushes are also helpful. Similar also is mesenteric vascular disease and torsion of an organ (eg, ovarian cyst). In the late stages of obstruction it may be impossible to distinguish acute organic intestinal obstruction from the late stage of peritonitis with ileus.

Complications

Strangulation (necrosis of the bowel wall) occurs with impairment of the blood supply to the gut. Strangulation is difficult to determine clinically, but fever, marked leukocytosis, and signs of peritoneal irritation should alert the clinician to this possibility. Strangulation may lead to perforation, peritonitis, and sepsis. Strangulation increases the mortality rate of intestinal obstruction to about 25%.

Treatment

A. Supportive Measures:

1. Decompression of the intestinal tract by nasogastric suction should relieve vomiting, reduce intestinal distention, and prevent aspiration.

2. Correct fluid, electrolyte, and colloid deficits.

3. Give broad-spectrum antibiotics (gentamicin and ampicillin or clindamycin) if strangulation is suspected.

B. Surgical Measures: Complete obstruction of the intestine is treated surgically after appropriate supportive therapy. Strangulation is always a danger as long as obstruction persists, and fever, leukocytosis, peritoneal signs, or blood in the feces means that strangulation may have occurred and that immediate surgery is required.

If the bowel is successfully decompressed during the preoperative preparation period, with cessation of pain and passage of flatus and feces, surgery may be delayed. Otherwise, surgical relief of the obstruction is indicated. Surgery consists of relieving the obstruction and removing gangrenous bowel with reanastomosis.

Prognosis

Prognosis varies with the causative factor and the presence of strangulation.

Fabri PJ, Rosemurgy A: Reoperation for small intestinal obstruction. Surg Clin North Am 1991;71:131. (Adhesions are the commonest cause of small bowel obstruction in Western society.)

FUNCTIONAL OBSTRUCTION
(Adynamic Ileus, Paralytic Ileus)

Essentials of Diagnosis

- Continuous abdominal pain, distention, vomiting, and obstipation.
- History of a precipitating factor (surgery, peritonitis, pain, anticholinergic drugs, pneumonia, inferior myocardial infarction).
- Minimal abdominal tenderness; decreased to absent bowel sounds.
- X-ray evidence of gas and fluid in bowel.

General Considerations

Adynamic ileus is a neurogenic or muscular impairment of peristalsis that may lead to intestinal obstruction. It is a common disorder that may be due to a variety of intra-abdominal causes, eg, gastrointestinal surgery, peritoneal irritation (hemorrhage, ruptured viscus, pancreatitis, peritonitis), or anoxic organic obstruction. Drugs with anticholinergic properties, renal colic, vertebral fractures, spinal cord injuries, severe infections, uremia, diabetic coma, and electrolyte abnormalities (especially hypokalemia) also may cause adynamic ileus.

Clinical Findings

A. Symptoms and Signs: There is mild to moderate abdominal pain, continuous rather than colicky, associated with vomiting (which may later become fecal) and obstipation. Borborygmus is absent. Symptoms of the initiating condition may also be present (eg, fever; prostration due to ruptured viscus).

Abdominal distention is generalized and may be massive, with nonlocalized minimal abdominal tenderness and no signs of peritoneal irritation unless due to the primary disease. Bowel sounds are decreased to absent. Dehydration may occur after prolonged vomiting or from sequestration of fluid in bowel loops. Other signs of the initiating disorder may be present.

B. Laboratory Findings: With prolonged vomiting, hemoconcentration and electrolyte imbalance may occur. Leukocytosis, anemia, and elevated serum amylase may be present, depending upon the initiating condition.

C. Imaging: Radiography of the abdomen shows distended gas-filled loops of bowel in the small and large intestines and even in the rectum. There may be evidence of air-fluid levels in the distended bowel. When the underlying clinical problem is unclear, a barium enema and subsequent small bowel x-ray will rule out organic obstruction.

Differential Diagnosis

The symptoms and signs of obstruction with absent bowel sounds and a history of a precipitating condition leave little doubt about the diagnosis. It is important to make certain that the adynamic ileus is not secondary to an organic obstruction, especially anoxic, where conservative management is harmful and immediate surgery may be lifesaving.

Treatment

Most cases of adynamic ileus are postoperative and respond to restriction of oral intake with gradual liberalization of the diet as the bowel function returns. Severe and prolonged ileus may require gastrointestinal suction and complete restriction of oral intake. Parenteral restoration of fluids and electrolytes is essential in such instances. A rectal tube or even a colonoscope may be helpful to decompress a dilated colon. When conservative therapy fails, it may be necessary to operate for the purpose of decompressing the bowel by enterostomy or cecostomy and to rule out mechanical obstruction.

Those cases of adynamic ileus secondary to other disorders (eg, electrolyte imbalance, severe infection, intra-abdominal or back injury, pneumonitis) are managed as above plus by treatment of the primary disease.

Prognosis

The prognosis varies with that of the initiating disorder. Adynamic ileus may resolve without specific therapy when the cause is removed. Intubation with decompression is usually successful in causing return of function.

IDIOPATHIC INTESTINAL PSEUDO-OBSTRUCTION

This idiopathic disorder, usually seen in teenagers or young adults, is characterized by recurring symptoms of small bowel obstruction but no evidence of organic obstruction on x-ray or with surgical exploration. Ogilvie's syndrome, a similar problem, consists of primarily cecal dilation in older patients who are bedfast and often have chronic obstructive pulmonary disease. In both, all previously mentioned causes of functional obstruction are absent. The patient is treated with nasogastric suction, intravenous fluids, and parenteral nutrition as required; colonoscopic decompression or cecostomy may be necessary in Ogilvie's syndrome.

Strodel WE, Brothers T: Colonoscopic decompression of pseudo-obstruction and volvulus. Surg Clin North Am 1989;69:1327. (Good review of management.)

MALABSORPTION SYNDROMES (Primary Mucosal Disease)

Malabsorption syndromes may be associated with a wide variety of small intestine mucosal disease processes that have in common the malabsorption of nutrients by the gastrointestinal tract. These syndromes should be contrasted to states of maldigestion where intraluminal abnormalities result in failure to absorb nutrients, such as pancreatic insufficiency, bile salt deficiency, and a variety of postsurgical abnormalities. The clinical and laboratory manifestations are summarized in Table 14–5.

1. CELIAC SPRUE & TROPICAL SPRUE

Essentials of Diagnosis

- Bulky, pale, frothy, foul-smelling, greasy stools with increased fecal fat on chemical analysis of the stool.
- Weight loss and signs of multiple vitamin deficiencies. Impaired intestinal absorption of vitamins D, E, A, and K, as well as fat.
- Hypochromic or megaloblastic anemia; small bowel x-ray pattern that of small bowel dilation and dilution of barium.

General Considerations

Sprue syndromes are diseases of disturbed small intestine function characterized by impaired absorption, particularly of fats, and motor abnormalities. Celiac sprue responds to a gluten-free diet, whereas

Table 14–5. Clinical and laboratory manifestations of malabsorption.[1]

Manifestation	Laboratory Findings	Malabsorbed Nutrient
Steatorrhea (bulky, light-colored)	Increased fecal fat; decreased serum cholesterol	Fat
Diarrhea (increased fecal water)	Increased fecal fat or positive bile salt breath test	Fatty acids or bile salts
Weight loss; malnutrition (muscle wasting); weakness, fatigue	Increased fecal fat and nitrogen; decreased glucose and xylose absorption	Calories (fat, protein, carbohydrates)
Abdominal distention		
Iron deficiency anemia	Hypochromic anemia; low serum iron	Iron
Megaloblastic anemia	Macrocytosis; decreased vitamin B_{12} absorption (^{67}Co-labeled B_{12}); decreased serum vitamin B_{12} and folic acid activity (microbiologic assay)	Vitamin B_{12} or folic acid
Paresthesia; tetany; positive Trousseau and Chvostek signs	Decreased serum calcium, magnesium, and potassium	Calcium, vitamin D, magnesium, potassium
Bone pain; pathologic fractures; skeletal deformities	Osteoporosis; osteomalacia on x-ray	Calcium, protein
Bleeding tendency (ecchymoses, melena, hematuria)	Prolonged prothrombin time	Vitamin K
Edema	Decreased serum albumin; increased fecal loss of α_1-antitrypsin	Protein (or protein-losing enteropathy)
Nocturia; abdominal distention	Increased small bowel fluid on x-ray	Water
Milk intolerance (cramps, bloating, diarrhea)	Flat lactose tolerance test; decreased mucosal lactase levels	Lactose

[1]Modified from Bayless TM: Malabsorption in the elderly. Hosp Pract (Aug) 1979;14:57.

tropical sprue does not. The polypeptide gliadin is the offending substance in gluten. Although an infectious cause has not been conclusively demonstrated, tropical sprue behaves clinically like an infectious disease. It responds to folic acid and broad-spectrum antibiotics.

The clinical severity of sprue syndrome varies depending upon the extent of the lesion in the small intestine and the duration of the disease. Severe wasting, gastrointestinal protein loss, multiple vitamin deficiencies, and adrenal and pituitary deficiency may be associated with the severe forms of the disease. A flat intestinal mucosa without villi in the small intestine is noted, and some observers have described degenerative changes in the myenteric nerve plexuses. With the loss of villi, the microvilli are also lost, leading to disaccharidase deficiency, particularly lactase deficiency.

Rare secondary varieties of sprue syndrome in which the cause of the small intestine dysfunction is known include gastrocolic fistulas, obstruction of intestinal lacteals by lymphoma, Whipple's disease, extensive regional enteritis, and parasitic infections such as giardiasis, cryptosporidiosis, strongyloidiasis, and isosporiasis.

Clinical Findings

A. Tropical Sprue: Patients with tropical sprue are either residents of, or have had prolonged visits in, tropical regions. The main symptom is diarrhea; at first it is explosive and watery; later, stools are fewer and more solid and characteristically pale, frothy, foul-smelling, and greasy, with exacerbations on high-fat diet. Indigestion, flatulence, abdominal cramps, weight loss (often marked), pallor, asthenia, irritability, paresthesias, and muscle cramps may occur. Quiescent periods with or without mild symptoms may occur especially on leaving the tropics. Symptoms may appear years after the patient has left endemic areas.

Vitamin deficiencies cause glossitis, cheilosis, angular stomatitis, cutaneous hyperpigmentation, and dry, rough skin. Abdominal distention and mild tenderness are present. Edema occurs late.

Anemia is usually macrocytic, and, with blood loss or malabsorption of iron, may be hypochromic, microcytic, or mixed. The fecal fat is increased. Serum proteins, calcium, phosphorus, cholesterol, and prothrombin are low. Gastric hypochlorhydria is frequent. The pancreatic enzymes are normal.

Radiographs using nonflocculating barium show dilation of the intestine and occasionally excess fluid and gas.

B. Celiac Sprue: This disorder is characterized by defective absorption of fat, protein, carbohydrates, iron, and water. Absorption of fat-soluble vitamins A, D, and K is impaired. Osteomalacia may ensue. Protein loss from the intestine may occur. Elimination of gluten from the diet causes dramatic improvement. Gluten is found in wheat, barley, oats, and rye and is used as a filler in many prepared foods and medications. Diligent elimination of this substance from the diet is important in achieving remission.

In one-third of patients with celiac sprue, symptoms begin in early childhood. Symptoms may persist into adult life, but there is usually a latent phase of apparent good health. The anemia is usually hypochromic and microcytic. The complications of impaired absorption are more severe: infantilism, dwarfism, tetany, vitamin deficiency signs, and even rickets may be seen. The definitive diagnosis of steatorrhea requires quantitative measurement of fecal fat, preferably on a known fat intake, and a characteristic small bowel biopsy.

Patients presenting with dermatitis herpetiformis frequently have associated celiac sprue, usually symptomatic. Both the sprue and the dermatitis herpetiformis are responsive to a gluten-free diet—the latter only after many months, and rechallenge with gluten results in recurrence of the rash within weeks.

A small group of patients with apparent celiac sprue are nonresponsive to a gluten-free diet. On closer inspection of the small bowel mucosal biopsy, a collagenous layer is found between the surface absorptive cells and the lamina propria. No consistently helpful medical therapy has yet been found. Other causes of nonresponsiveness may include the development of lymphoma, ulcerative jejunoileitis, or perhaps a steroid-responsive lesion.

Differential Diagnosis

It is necessary to differentiate between the various causes of malabsorption to permit selection of specific therapy, if any. Anatomic abnormalities such as fistulas, blind loops, and jejunal diverticulosis may be found on radiography. Regional enteritis usually has a characteristic radiographic appearance but must be distinguished from intestinal tuberculosis and lymphoma. The small bowel x-ray appearance in Whipple's disease, nodular lymphoid hyperplasia, intestinal lymphoma, and amyloidosis is abnormal but not specific or diagnostic. In primary diseases of the small intestine, mucosal suction biopsy is the most effective way of making the diagnosis. The pathologic response in some diseases is patchy, and multiple specimens may be required. Pancreatic insufficiency due to obstruction may be diagnosed by low-volume output by the pancreas in response to intravenous administration of secretin.

Treatment

A. Tropical Sprue: Folic acid, 10–20 mg daily orally or intramuscularly for a few weeks, corrects diarrhea, anorexia, weight loss, glossitis, and anemia. Tetracycline, 250 mg orally four times daily, is given at the outset of treatment. When complete remission occurs, the patient may be maintained on 5 mg of folic acid daily. If the patient has achlorhydria, giving vitamin B_{12} intramuscularly should also be considered. Hypochromic anemia can be treated with oral iron. A high-calorie, high-protein, low-fat diet can be given.

B. Celiac Sprue: Strict elimination of gluten from the diet will lead to clinical recovery. If there is no response, inquire about other medications (many use gluten as a filler) and look for collagenous sprue. The diet must be gluten-free. In addition, the diet should be high in calories and protein and low in fat. Initially, the diet should also be lactose-free because of the loss of lactase-containing microvilli; once remission is induced, lactose-containing foods may be added. Prothrombin deficiency is treated by means of water-soluble vitamin K orally or, if urgent, parenterally. Treat hypocalcemia or tetany with calcium phosphate or gluconate, 2 g orally or intravenously (4.5–16 meq Ca^{2+} repeated as necessary to control tetany, infused slowly at a rate not to exceed 2 mL/min) three times daily, and vitamin D, 5000–20,000 units. Multiple vitamin supplements may also be advisable. Macrocytic anemia usually responds to vitamin B_{12}, 100 μg intramuscularly every month until the disease is in clinical remission.

Corticosteroids may be advantageous in certain patients with sprue, particularly the severely ill, since they increase the absorption of nitrogen, fats, and other nutrients from the gastrointestinal tract. They have a nonspecific effect in increasing appetite and inducing mild euphoria. Cortisol is best given in dosages of 100–300 mg/24 h intravenously and tapered off according to the patient's response.

Prognosis

With proper treatment, the response is good. Patients with celiac sprue have a late increased incidence of abdominal lymphoma and carcinomas. Patients who develop gastrointestinal symptoms while in remission on a gluten-free diet should be carefully evaluated for cancer.

Trier JS: Celiac sprue. (Medical Progress.) N Engl J Med 1991;325:1209.

2. DISACCHARIDASE DEFICIENCY

Lactase deficiency in the adult is common worldwide. It has been estimated from many studies that the incidence of lactase deficiency is 70–90% in Asians, blacks, Native Americans, and Mediterranean populations. The incidence of lactase deficiency in northern and western Europeans is 10–15%. Symptoms may vary from minor abdominal bloating, distention, flatulence, and discomfort to markedly severe diarrhea in response to even small amounts of lactose (including that in ice cream and some cheeses). The diagnosis, although often established clinically—by milk challenge or by a period of abstinence—is confirmed by a lactose tolerance test; marked diarrhea usually occurs with this test. Onset in the adult may follow gastroduodenal surgery and may be associated with regional enteritis. The primary mucosal diseases of the small intestine usually have associated lactase deficiency.

Intercurrent acute illnesses, such as viral and bacterial enteritis, particularly in children, will frequently injure the microvilli of the mucosal cells of the small intestine, resulting in temporary lactase deficiency.

Other congenital defects described thus far are sucrose-isomaltose and glucose-galactose intolerance. Secondary disaccharidase deficiencies have been described in patients with giardiasis, celiac disease, ulcerative colitis, short bowel syndrome, and cystic fibrosis and postgastrectomy. Removal of the offending sugar from the patient's diet will often result in remission. Lactase enzyme can be added to milk (eg, LactAid) or taken in capsule or chewable tablet form. Such products are usually well tolerated.

Dipalma J, Narvaez RM: Prediction of lactose malabsorption in referral patients. Dig Dis Sci 1988;33:303. (Clinical parameters are not very distinctive. Breath hydrogen lactase test is best for diagnosis.)

3. WHIPPLE'S DISEASE

Whipple's disease is an uncommon malabsorption disorder due to an infection of the gut with widespread systemic manifestations. Histologic examination of a small bowel mucosal biopsy specimen reveals characteristic large, foamy mononuclear cells filled with cytoplasmic material that gives a positive periodic acid-Schiff staining reaction. Electron microscopy reveals Whipple's bacilli in the intestines and in the eyes, heart, lungs, synovia, kidneys, and central nervous system. The disease occurs primarily in middle-aged men and is of insidious onset; without treatment, it is usually fatal. The manifestations include abdominal pain, diarrhea, steatorrhea, gastrointestinal bleeding, fever, lymphadenopathy, polyarthritis, edema, gray to brown skin pigmentation, and severe central nervous system manifestations. Anemia and hypoproteinemia are common.

Treatment programs are somewhat controversial but should be continued for at least 1 year and should include administration of agents that cross the blood-brain barrier. Current options are (1) trimethoprim-sulfamethoxazole (TMP-SMZ) alone, one double-strength capsule every 12 hours for 1 year; or (2) procaine penicillin, 600,000 units intramuscularly, plus streptomycin, 0.5 g intramuscularly, twice daily for 10 days, followed by TMP-SMZ as above. Reappearance of symptoms after or during therapy suggests emergence of resistant organisms, and the antibiotic should be changed.

Bai JC et al: Short-term treatment in Whipple's disease. J Clin Gastroenterol 1991;13:303. (Beware of relapses.

Differentiate from *Mycobacterium avium-intracellulare* infection of gastrointestinal tract.)

PROTEIN-LOSING ENTEROPATHY

Leakage of plasma proteins into the intestinal lumen is an integral phase of the metabolism of plasma proteins. In certain intestinal disease states, excessive protein loss into the intestinal lumen may be responsible for the hypoproteinemia that occurs. Excessive loss of plasma protein may be due to increased mucosal permeability to protein, inflammatory exudation, excessive cell desquamation, or direct leakage of lymph from obstructed lacteals. Gastrointestinal diseases associated with protein-losing enteropathy include all of the primary mucosal diseases of the small bowel, as well as gastric carcinoma, lymphoma, gastric rugal hypertrophy, parasitic infections, and others.

Treatment consists of management of the primary disorder.

APPENDICITIS

Essentials of Diagnosis
- Early periumbilical discomfort, followed by right lower quadrant abdominal pain and tenderness with signs of peritoneal irritation.
- Anorexia, nausea and vomiting, and constipation.
- Low-grade fever and mild polymorphonuclear leukocytosis.

General Considerations
Appendicitis is initiated by obstruction of the appendiceal lumen by a fecalith, inflammation, foreign body, or neoplasm. Obstruction is followed by infection, edema, and, frequently, infarction of the appendiceal wall. Intraluminal tension develops rapidly and tends to cause early mural necrosis and perforation. All ages and both sexes are affected, but appendicitis is more common in males between 10 and 30 years of age.

Appendicitis is one of the most frequent causes of acute surgical abdomen. The symptoms and signs usually follow a fairly stereotyped pattern, but appendicitis is capable of such protean manifestations that it should be considered in the differential diagnosis of every obscure case of intra-abdominal sepsis and pain.

Clinical Findings
A. Symptoms and Signs: An attack of appendicitis usually begins with epigastric or periumbilical pain associated with one or two episodes of vomiting. Within 2–12 hours, the pain shifts to the right lower quadrant, where it persists as a steady soreness that is aggravated by walking or coughing. There is an-

orexia, moderate malaise, and slight fever. Constipation is usual, but diarrhea occurs occasionally, as does nausea and vomiting.

At onset there are no localized abdominal findings. Within a few hours, however, progressive right lower quadrant tenderness can be demonstrated; careful examination will usually identify a single point of maximal tenderness. The patient can often place a finger precisely on this area, especially if asked to accentuate the soreness by coughing. Light percussion over the right lower quadrant is helpful in localizing tenderness. Rebound tenderness and spasm of the overlying abdominal muscles are usually present. Psoas and obturator signs, when positive, are strongly suggestive of appendicitis. Rectal tenderness is common and, in pelvic appendicitis, may be more definite than abdominal tenderness. Peristalsis is diminished or absent. Slight to moderate fever is present.

B. Laboratory Findings: Moderate leukocytosis (10,000–20,000/μL) with an increase in neutrophils is usually present. It is not uncommon to find microscopic hematuria and pyuria.

C. Imaging: There are no characteristic changes on plain films of the abdomen. However, visualization in the right lower quadrant of a radiopaque shadow consistent with fecalith in the appendix may heighten the suspicion of appendicitis. In uncertain cases, barium enemas are being used, as visualization of the entire appendix rules out acute appendicitis.

High-resolution real time sonography for the diagnosis of acute and complicated appendicitis has a sensitivity of 90% and a specificity of 98%, with an overall accuracy of 96%—the best yet achieved—and has reduced the incidence of negative laparotomy.

Factors That Cause Variations From the "Classic" Clinical Picture

A. Anatomic Location of Appendix: Abdominal findings are most definite when the appendix is in the iliac fossa or superficially located. When the appendix extends over the pelvic brim, abdominal signs may be minimal, greatest tenderness being elicited on rectal examination. Right lower quadrant tenderness may be poorly localized and slow to develop in retrocecal or retroileal appendicitis. Inflammation of a high-lying lateral appendix may produce maximal tenderness in the flank, and in the left lower quadrant in situs inversus. Bizarre locations of the appendix may rarely occur in association with a mobile or undescended cecum; in such cases, symptoms and signs may localize in the right upper or left lower quadrant.

B. Old Age: Elderly patients frequently have few or no prodromal symptoms. Abdominal findings may be unimpressive, with slight tenderness and negligible muscle guarding, until perforation occurs. Fever and leukocytosis may also be minimal or absent. When the white count is not elevated, a shift to the left is significant evidence of inflammation.

C. Obesity: Obesity frequently increases the difficulty of evaluation by delaying the appearance of abdominal signs and by preventing sharp localization.

D. Pregnancy: See discussion in Chapter 17.

Differential Diagnosis

Acute gastroenteritis is the disorder most commonly confused with appendicitis. In rare cases it either precedes or is coincident with appendicitis. Vomiting and diarrhea are more common. Fever and the white blood count may rise sharply and may be out of proportion to abdominal findings. Localization of pain and tenderness is usually indefinite and shifting. Hyperactive peristalsis is characteristic. Gastroenteritis frequently runs an acute course. A period of observation usually serves to clarify the diagnosis.

Mesenteric adenitis may cause signs and symptoms identical with appendicitis. Usually, however, there are some clues to the true diagnosis. Mesenteric adenitis is more likely to occur in children or adolescents; respiratory infection is a common antecedent; localization of right lower quadrant tenderness is less precise and constant; and true muscle guarding is infrequent. In spite of a strong suspicion of mesenteric adenitis, it is often safer to advise appendectomy than to risk a complication of appendicitis by delay.

Meckel's diverticulitis may mimic appendicitis. The localization of tenderness may be more medial, but this is not a reliable diagnostic criterion. Because operation is required in both diseases, the differentiation is not critical. When a preoperative diagnosis of appendicitis proves on exploration to be erroneous, it is essential to examine the terminal 150 cm of ileum for Meckel's diverticulitis and mesenteric adenitis.

Regional enteritis, amebiasis, acute ileitis due to *Yersinia pseudotuberculosis,* perforated duodenal ulcer, ureteral colic, acute salpingitis, mittelschmerz, ruptured ectopic pregnancy, and twisted ovarian cyst may also be confused with appendicitis. Right lower lobe pneumonia sometimes is associated with prominent right lower quadrant pain.

Complications

A. Perforation: Appendicitis may rarely subside spontaneously, but it is an unpredictable disease with a marked tendency (about 95%) to progression and perforation. Because perforation rarely occurs within the first 8 hours, diagnostic observation during this period is relatively safe. Signs of perforation include increasing severity of pain, tenderness, and spasm in the right lower quadrant followed by evidence of generalized peritonitis or of a localized abscess. Ileus, fever, malaise, and leukocytosis become more marked. If perforation with abscess formation or generalized peritonitis has already occurred when the patient is first seen, the diagnosis may be quite obscure.

The treatment of perforated appendicitis is appendectomy unless a well-localized right lower quadrant or pelvic abscess has already walled off the appendix. Supportive measures are as for acute peritonitis.

1. Generalized peritonitis–Clinical findings and treatment are discussed elsewhere in this chapter.

2. Appendiceal abscess–Malaise, toxicity, fever, and leukocytosis vary from minimal to marked. Examination discloses a tender mass in the right lower quadrant or pelvis. Pelvic abscesses tend to bulge into the rectum or vagina.

Abscesses usually become noticeable 2–6 days after onset, but antibiotic therapy may delay their appearance. Appendiceal abscess is occasionally the first and only sign of appendicitis and may be confused with neoplasm of the cecum, particularly in older persons, who may have little or no systemic reaction to the infection.

Treatment of early abscess is by intensive combined antibiotic therapy (eg, ampicillin, gentamicin, and metronidazole or clindamycin). On this regimen, the abscess will frequently resolve. Appendectomy should be performed 6–12 weeks later. A well-established progressive abscess in the right lower quadrant should be drained without delay. Pelvic abscess requires drainage when it bulges into the rectum or vagina and has become fluctuant.

B. Pylephlebitis: Suppurative thrombophlebitis of the portal system with liver abscess is a rare but highly lethal complication. It should be suspected when septic fever, chills, hepatomegaly, and jaundice develop after appendiceal perforation. Intensive combined antibiotic therapy with surgical drainage of the abscesses is indicated.

C. Other Complications: These include subphrenic abscess and other foci of intra-abdominal sepsis. Intestinal obstruction may be caused by adhesions.

Treatment

A. Preoperative Care:

1. Observation for diagnosis–Within the first 8–12 hours after onset, the symptoms and signs of appendicitis are frequently indefinite. Under these circumstances, a period of close observation is essential. The patient is placed at bed rest and given nothing by mouth. *Note:* Laxatives should not be prescribed when appendicitis or any form of peritonitis is suspected. Narcotic medications are avoided if possible, but sedation with tranquilizing agents is not contraindicated. Abdominal and rectal examinations, white blood count, and differential count are repeated periodically. Abdominal films and an upright chest film must be obtained as part of the investigation of all difficult diagnostic problems. In most cases of appendicitis, the diagnosis is clarified by localization of signs to the right lower quadrant within 12 hours after onset of symptoms.

2. Intubation–Preoperatively, a nasogastric tube is inserted if there is sufficient peritonitis or toxicity to indicate that postoperative ileus may be trouble-

some. In such patients the stomach is aspirated and lavaged if necessary, and the patient is sent to the operating room with the tube in place.

3. Antibiotics–In the presence of a marked systemic reaction with severe toxicity and high fever, preoperative administration of antibiotics (eg, the above-noted regimen, though many alternatives exist) is advisable.

B. Surgical Treatment: In uncomplicated appendicitis, appendectomy is performed as soon as fluid imbalance and other significant systemic disturbances are controlled. Little preparation is usually required. Early surgery has a mortality rate of a fraction of 1%. The morbidity and mortality rates associated with this disease reflect the occurrence of gangrene and perforation that occur when operation is delayed.

C. Emergency Nonsurgical Treatment: When surgical facilities are not available, treat as for acute peritonitis. On such a regimen, acute appendicitis may subside, and complications will be minimized.

Prognosis

With accurate diagnosis and early surgical removal, mortality and morbidity rates are minimal. Delay of diagnosis produces significant mortality and morbidity rates if complications occur.

Recurrent acute attacks may occur if the appendix is not removed. "Chronic appendicitis" does not exist.

Hoffman J, Rasmussen O: Aids in the diagnosis of acute appendicitis. Br J Surg 1989;76:774. (Most helpful are clinical observations, ultrasound, and barium enema.)
Schwerk WB et al: Acute and perforated appendicitis: Current experience with ultrasound aided diagnosis. World J Surg 1990;14:271. (Ultrasound is the current diagnostic technical procedure of choice.)

INTESTINAL TUBERCULOSIS
(Tuberculous Enterocolitis)

Gastrointestinal tuberculosis may occur anywhere along the gastrointestinal tract. Involvement of the intestine frequently complicates pulmonary tuberculosis but goes clinically unrecognized. Ingestion of milk containing tubercle bacilli is another means of infection. Many cases have neither association.

The mode of infection is by ingestion of tubercle bacilli, with the formation of ulcerating lesions in the intestine, particularly the ileocecal region, and involvement of the mesenteric lymph nodes; alternatively, reactivation of a primary intestinal focus may result in active intestinal tuberculosis.

Clinical Findings

Symptoms may be absent or minimal even with extensive disease. When present, they usually consist of fever, anorexia, nausea, flatulence, distention after eating, and food intolerance. There may be abdominal pain and mild to severe cramps, usually in the right lower quadrant and often after meals. Constipation may be present, but mild to severe diarrhea is more characteristic. Tuberculosis may involve the peritoneum. The disease of course is chronic and may be difficult to distinguish from inflammatory bowel disease, ameboma, or intestinal lymphoma or carcinoma.

Findings on abdominal examination are not characteristic, although there may be mild right lower quadrant tenderness. Fistula in ano may be evident. Weight loss occurs.

There are no characteristic laboratory findings. The presence of tubercle bacilli in the feces does not correlate with intestinal involvement.

Radiographic examination of the involved bowel reveals irritability and spasm, particularly in the cecal region; irregular hypermotility of the intestinal tract; ulcerated lesions and irregular filling defects, particularly in the right colon and ileocecal region; and usually pulmonary tuberculosis. Colonoscopy with biopsy may prove helpful in establishing the diagnosis.

Treatment & Prognosis

The prognosis varies with that of the pulmonary disease. The intestinal lesions usually respond to the same regimen as for pulmonary tuberculosis, ie, four drugs for 6–9 months (see Chapter 37). Operation may be required for intestinal obstruction or for diagnosis, though colonic lesions are readily accessible for endoscopic biopsy.

Pettengell KE et al: Gastrointestinal tuberculosis in patients with pulmonary tuberculosis. Q J Med 1990;74:303. (Twenty-eight percent of patients with cavitary pulmonary tuberculosis had proved intestinal involvement. An additional 18% had suspected involvement.)

DISEASES OF THE COLON & RECTUM

IRRITABLE BOWEL SYNDROME

Essentials of Diagnosis

- Abdominal pain relieved by defecation or associated with bowel habit change.
- At least two of the following:
  Altered stool frequency
  Altered stool form
  Altered stool passage
  Passage of mucus

General Considerations

Irritable bowel syndrome is a term denoting a clinical entity characterized by some combination of (1) abdominal pain; (2) altered bowel function, constipation, or diarrhea; (3) hypersecretion of colonic mucus; (4) dyspeptic symptoms (flatulence, nausea, anorexia); and (5) varying degrees of anxiety or depression. This common group of disorders has many names, eg, nervous indigestion, functional dyspepsia, pylorospasm, irritable colon, spastic "colitis," functional "colitis," mucous "colitis," intestinal neurosis, and laxative or cathartic "colitis."

Pathogenesis

Three main factors appear significant in the pathogenesis of irritable bowel syndrome. (1) Colonic motor activity: There is no abnormality of either motility or electrical activity of the colon specific to the irritable bowel syndrome. However, prediverticular disease can be frequently demonstrated and is characterized by increased width of the sigmoid circular muscles, increased segmentation, and increased nonpropulsive intraluminal pressures. Colonic motor activity is abnormally increased in patients with colonic pain, eg, after meals, after administration of cholecystokinin or cholinergic drugs, or after emotional stress. Altered small bowel motility may also occur and appears to be correlated with symptoms. (2) Psychologic stress: Many patients with irritable bowel syndrome exhibit colonic symptoms at times of stress. The changes in colonic function are common manifestations of emotional tension. The reaction, however, may be more severe in patients with irritable bowel. (3) Diet: A low-residue diet in some patients may be a prominent predisposing factor. Intolerance of lactose and other sugars may account for the irritable bowel syndrome in certain patients.

It is essential to eliminate the possibility of organic gastrointestinal disease. A history of "nervousness" and emotional disturbances can usually be obtained. Bowel consciousness and cathartic and enema habits are prominent features. There is a highly variable complex of gastrointestinal symptoms: nausea and vomiting, anorexia, foul breath, sour stomach, flatulence, cramps, and constipation or diarrhea; hysteria and depression are the most prevalent psychologic problems.

Nocturnal diarrhea, awakening the patient from a sound sleep, is frequently a result of organic disease of the bowel and is less prominent in irritable bowel syndrome.

Clinical Findings

Examination discloses variable abdominal tenderness, particularly along the course of the colon. Sigmoidoscopy often reveals marked spasm and mucus in the colonic lumen and will frequently provoke the patient's spontaneously occurring symptoms. Laboratory studies should include a complete blood count and stool examination to rule out the presence of occult blood, ova, parasites, and pathogenic bacteria. Gastrointestinal x-rays may show altered gastrointestinal motility without other evidence of abnormalities.

Treatment

A. Diet: No simple diet is applicable to all patients with irritable bowel syndrome. Patients at risk by history or racial background for lactose intolerance (Asians, blacks, Native Americans, Jews) may be helped by exclusion of milk and milk products. Many patients respond to an increase in dietary fiber (vegetables, fruits, grains) or can instead substitute a psyllium seed preparation or methylcellulose in a dose of one heaping teaspoon in a glass of water or juice twice daily.

Avoidance of gastrointestinal stimulants such as caffeine-containing beverages (coffee, "cokes," tea) may be beneficial.

B. General Measures: Anxiety-reducing measures such as a regular exercise program and periods of "quiet time" may prove helpful. Anticholinergic agents such as dicyclomine, 10–20 mg before meals, may occasionally help control symptoms.

C. Psychotherapy: Reassurance is important. The diagnosis of irritable bowel is often readily apparent on initial history taking, and it is better to make it the primary diagnosis, so inform the patient, and then rule out pertinent organic disease. If chronic anxiety appears to play a major role and is not resolved by simple measures, an antianxiety drug (eg, alprazolam, 0.25 mg two or three times daily) may be beneficial. For the depressed patient, antidepressants (eg, amitriptyline, 25–100 mg at bedtime, or doxepin, 25–150 mg at bedtime) will often ameliorate symptoms, in part because of the anticholinergic effects of these medications.

Hasler WL, Owyang C: Irritable bowel syndrome. In: *Textbook of Gastroenterology,* vol 2. Yamada T (editor). Lippincott, 1991.

INFECTIOUS COLITIS

Bacterial infections are common causes of acute colitis and are usually associated with fever, cramps, and diarrhea with tenesmus and often with blood in the stool. The most common causes are *Campylobacter jejuni, Shigella, Salmonella,* and *Yersinia enterocolitica.* (See Chapter 21.) Diarrhea due to the toxins of *E coli* (a common cause of "turista") should be considered, but this is a secretory diarrhea without evidence of colitis. Anal intercourse may be responsible for additional infectious diseases of the rectum, including gonorrhea, syphilis, lymphogranuloma venereum, condyloma latum, herpes simplex, and AIDS.

AIDS (see Chapter 30) is a multisystem disorder, and the impaired immune function of the intestinal tract makes it particularly vulnerable to damage because of the large number of potential pathogens usually found in the intestinal lumen. Diarrhea and weight loss may precede the other manifestations of AIDS. Rectal and jejunal biopsies may show histologic abnormalities in AIDS patients with diarrhea.

Sigmoidoscopy will usually reveal acute colitis with small ulcerations; a mucus smear will reveal a preponderance of polymorphonuclear neutrophils; and cultures may reveal the organism. Tuberculosis is an uncommon cause.

Acute and chronic colitis caused by parasites such as the protozoan *Entamoeba histolytica* is common worldwide and not uncommon in the USA. It may be clinically indistinguishable from other types of acute and chronic colitis; differentiation can often be made by smears of aspirates at sigmoidoscopy, multiple stool examinations, and, in patients with sigmoidoscopic abnormalities, mucosal biopsy. In chronic forms, the areas of involvement are most commonly the cecum, sigmoid colon, or rectum. The chronic form may mimic granulomatous colitis or neoplasm. Complications include local abscess, liver abscess, and fistula formation. For treatment, see Chapter 34.

Guerrant RL, Bobak DA: Bacterial and protozoal gastroenteritis . (Medical Progress.) N Engl J Med 1991;325:327.

ANTIBIOTIC-ASSOCIATED COLITIS

Antibiotic-associated colitis may occur during antibiotic usage or up to 2 weeks subsequent to usage. The disease usually subsides when the offending antibiotic is withdrawn, but it is potentially lethal, and diagnosis should be pursued.

Pseudomembranous colitis is characterized by profuse watery diarrhea with cramps, tenesmus, low-grade fever, and, rarely, blood per rectum. Current or recent antibiotic therapy is a usual part of the history. Almost all antibiotics have been implicated; clindamycin, ampicillin, and the cephalosporins are most common. Metronidazole is effective in treatment of pseudomembranous enterocolitis, but it has also been reported to be a cause of this disease. Uncommonly, the disease occurs without antibiotic usage. There is evidence for person-to-person spread.

Diarrhea occurs secondary to selective overgrowth of the bacterium *Clostridium difficile,* which produces a toxin that causes the lesion of pseudomembranous colitis. When pseudomembranous colitis is suspected but sigmoidoscopy appears negative, random biopsies may show the lesion. Diarrheal material obtained at sigmoidoscopy and looked at while fresh will almost always contain polymorphonuclear white cells. The laboratory diagnosis is dependent on assay for the toxin and has a sensitivity of approximately 67% and a specificity of 99%.

Physical findings may be minimal but can include a distended, tender abdomen with a dilated bowel. Sigmoidoscopy may reveal a pseudomembrane characterized by adherent plaques (mushroom caps) of exudate with intervening normal mucosa. Occasionally the exudate is confluent. When the pseudomembrane is stripped away, capillary type bleeding will occur from the denuded mucosa. In a few patients, routine sigmoidoscopy is normal but colonoscopy shows involvement of the sigmoid colon or more proximal areas, sometimes only the right colon is involved.

Metronidazole, 0.5 g orally three times a day for 7–10 days, is the drug of choice and is curative in about 90% of cases. For those infections not cleared by metronidazole, the much more expensive vancomycin at a dosage of 125 mg four times a day orally for 10 days is usually effective.

Complications of the untreated illness include dehydration with electrolyte imbalance, perforation, toxic megacolon, and death.

A similar colitis without pseudomembrane is clinically indistinguishable from pseudomembranous colitis and may be more common. It is usually (not always) *C difficile* toxin-related. Sigmoidoscopy and occasionally colonoscopy will show evidence of acute colitis, often right-sided. Ampicillin is often associated. All antibiotics should be withdrawn, and treatment should proceed as with pseudomembranous colitis if the toxin is demonstrated. Otherwise, treat expectantly.

Gerding DN: Epidemiology and management of *Clostridium difficile* disease. Contemp Int Med 1990;Sept:55.
McFarland LV et al: Nosocomial acquisition of *Clostridium difficile* infection. N Engl J Med 1989;320:204.
Silva J: Update on pseudomembranous colitis. (Medical Staff Conference.) West J Med 1989;151:644.

INFLAMMATORY BOWEL DISEASE

The term "chronic idiopathic inflammatory bowel disease" includes ulcerative colitis and Crohn's disease. Ulcerative colitis is a chronic, recurrent disease characterized by diffuse mucosal inflammation involving only the colon. Ulcerative colitis invariably involves the rectum and may extend proximally in a continuous fashion to involve part or all of the colon. Crohn's disease is a chronic, recurrent disease characterized by patchy transmural inflammation involving any segment of the gastrointestinal tract from the mouth to the anus.

Drug Therapies for Inflammatory Bowel Disease

Although ulcerative colitis and Crohn's disease appear to be distinct entities, the same pharmacologic agents are used to treat both. Despite intense research, there are still no specific therapies for these diseases. The mainstays of therapy remain 5-aminosalicylic acid derivatives, corticosteroids, and mercaptopurine.

A. 5-Aminosalicylic Acid: 5-ASA is a topically active agent that has a variety of anti-inflammatory effects. It is used in the active treatment of ulcerative colitis and Crohn's disease and during disease inactivity in order to maintain remission. It is readily absorbed from the small intestine but demonstrates minimal colonic absorption. A number of oral and topical compounds have been designed to deliver 5ASA to the colon or small intestine while minimizing absorption. Formulations of 5-ASA currently available are sulfasalazine, olsalazine, and mesalamine.

1. Sulfasalazine–Sulfasalazine consists of 5-ASA linked by an azo bond to a sulfapyridine moiety. It is largely unabsorbed in the small intestine. In the colon, bacterial azoreductases cleave 5-ASA from the sulfapyridine group. It is unclear whether the sulfapyridine group has any anti-inflammatory effects. One gram of sulfasalazine contains 400 mg of 5-ASA. The 5-ASA works topically and is largely unabsorbed. The sulfapyridine group, however, is absorbed and may cause side effects in 15–30% of patients. Dose-related side effects include nausea, headaches, leukopenia, oligospermia, and impaired folate metabolism. Allergic and idiosyncratic side effects are fever, rash, hemolytic anemia, neutropenia, worsened colitis, hepatitis, pancreatitis, and pneumonitis. Sulfasalazine is significantly less expensive than other 5–ASA agents.

2. Oral mesalamine agents–These 5–ASA agents are coated in various pH-sensitive resins or packaged in timed-release capsules. Mesalamine tablets dissolve at pH 7.0, releasing 5–ASA in the terminal small bowel and proximal colon. Pentasa (not yet available) releases 5–ASA slowly throughout the small intestine and colon. Side effects of these compounds are uncommon but include nausea, headache, pancreatitis, and nephropathy. Eighty percent of patients intolerant of sulfasalazine can tolerate 5-ASA.

3. Olsalazine–Olsalazine consists of two 5-ASA moieties linked by a diazo bond. Similar to sulfasalazine, it is not absorbed in the small intestine. In the colon, it is cleaved by bacteria, liberating the 5-ASA. Serious side effects are rare. A mild, dose-related secretory diarrhea that occurs in 20% of patients improves if the drug is administered with food.

4. Topical mesalamine–5-ASA is provided in the form of suppositories (500 mg) and enemas (4 g/60 mL). These formulations can deliver much higher concentrations of 5-ASA to the distal colon than oral compounds. Side effects are extremely uncommon.

B. Corticosteroids: A variety of intravenous, oral, and topical steroid formulations have been used in inflammatory bowel disease. They have utility in the short-term treatment of moderate to severe disease. However, long-term use is associated with serious, potentially irreversible side effects and is to be avoided. The agents, route of administration, duration of use, and tapering regimens employed are based more upon personal bias and experience than upon data from rigorous clinical trials. The most commonly used intravenous formulations have been hydrocortisone or methylprednisolone, which are given by continuous infusion or every 6 hours. Oral formulations are prednisone or methylprednisolone. Topical preparations are provided as hydrocortisone suppositories (100 mg), foam (90 mg) and enemas (100 mg).

C. Mercaptopurine: Mercaptopurine (6-MP) is used in 10–15% of patients with refractory Crohn's disease. Side effects occur in 10%, including pancreatitis, bone marrow suppression, infections, allergies, and, potentially, a higher risk of neoplasm. After therapy is started, complete blood counts should be obtained weekly for 1 month, then at least monthly.

Social Support for Inflammatory Bowel Disease

Inflammatory bowel disease is a lifelong illness that can have profound emotional and social impacts on the individual. Patients should be encouraged to become involved in the Crohn's and Colitis Foundation of America (CCFA). National headquarters may be contacted at 444 Park Avenue South, 11th Floor, New York, NY 10016–7374 ([212] 685–3440).

1. ULCERATIVE COLITIS

Essentials of Diagnosis

- Bloody diarrhea.
- Lower abdominal cramps and urgency.
- Anemia, low serum albumin.
- Negative stool cultures.
- Sigmoidoscopy is the key to diagnosis.

General Considerations

Ulcerative colitis is an idiopathic inflammatory condition that involves the mucosal surface of the colon, resulting in diffuse friability and erosions with bleeding. Approximately 50% of patients have disease confined to the rectosigmoid region (proctosigmoiditis); 30% extend to the splenic flexure (left-sided colitis); and less than 20% extend more proximally (extensive colitis). There is some correlation between disease extent and symptom severity. In the majority of patients, the extent of colonic involvement does not progress over time. In most patients,

the disease is characterized by periods of symptomatic flare-ups and remissions.

Clinical Findings

A. Symptoms and Signs: The clinical profile in ulcerative colitis is highly variable. Bloody diarrhea is the hallmark. On the basis of several clinical and laboratory parameters, it is clinically useful to classify patients as having mild, moderate, or severe disease (Table 14–6). Patients should be asked about stool frequency, the presence and amount of rectal bleeding, cramps, abdominal pain, fecal urgency, and tenesmus. Physical examination should focus upon the patient's volume status as determined by orthostatic blood pressure and pulse measurements and by nutritional status. On abdominal examination, the clinician should look for tenderness and evidence of peritoneal inflammation. Red blood may be present on digital rectal examination.

1. Mild to moderate disease–Patients with mild disease have a gradual onset of infrequent diarrhea (less than five movements per day) with intermittent rectal bleeding and mucus. Stools may be formed to loose in consistency. Because of rectal inflammation, there is fecal urgency and tenesmus. Left lower quadrant cramps relieved by defecation are common, but there is no significant abdominal tenderness. Patients with moderate disease have more severe diarrhea with frequent bleeding. Abdominal pain and tenderness may be present but are not severe. There may be mild fever, anemia, and hypoalbuminemia.

2. Severe disease–Patients with severe disease have more than six to ten bloody bowel movements per day, resulting in severe anemia, hypovolemia, and impaired nutrition with hypoalbuminemia. Abdominal pain and tenderness are present. "Fulminant colitis" is a subset of severe disease characterized by rapidly worsening symptoms with signs of toxicity.

3. Extracolonic manifestations–Ulcerative colitis is associated with extraintestinal manifestations in 25% of cases. Some extracolonic signs are associated with disease activity. These include erythema nodosum, pyoderma gangrenosum, episcler-

Table 14–6. Ulcerative colitis: Assessment of disease activity.

	Mild	Moderate	Severe
Stool frequency (per day)	<4	4–6	>6 (mostly bloody)
Pulse (beats/min)	<90	90–100	>100
Hematocrit (%)	Normal	30–40	<30
Weight loss (%)	None	1–10	>10
Temperature (F)	Normal	99–100	>100
ESR (mm/h)	<20	20–30	>30
Albumin (g/dL)	Normal	3–3.5	<3.0

itis, thromboembolic events, and an oligoarticular, nondeforming arthritis. In patients who are HLA B27-seropositive, there may be anterior uveitis or ankylosing spondylitis which is independent of colitis activity. Sclerosing cholangitis can occur in colitis patients even after total colectomy. Patients with this entity are at higher risk of developing cholangiocarcinoma.

B. Laboratory Findings: The degree of abnormality of the hematocrit, sedimentation rate, and serum albumin reflect disease severity.

C. Endoscopy: In acute colitis, the diagnosis is readily established by sigmoidoscopy. The mucosal appearance is characterized by edema, friability, mucopus, and erosions. Colonoscopy should not be performed in patients with severe disease because of the risk of perforation. After patients have been on therapy and the acute symptoms have improved, colonoscopy is sometimes performed to determine the extent of disease, which will dictate the need for subsequent cancer surveillance.

D. Imaging: Plain abdominal radiographs are obtained in patients with severe colitis to look for significant colonic dilation. Barium enemas are of little utility in the evaluation of acute ulcerative colitis and may precipitate toxic megacolon in patients with severe disease.

Differential Diagnosis

The initial presentation of ulcerative colitis is indistinguishable from other causes of colitis, clinically as well as endoscopically. Thus, the diagnosis of idiopathic ulcerative colitis is reached after excluding other known causes of colitis. Infectious colitis should be excluded by sending stool specimens for routine bacterial cultures (to exclude *Salmonella, Shigella,* and *Campylobacter*), ova and parasites (to exclude amebiasis), and stool toxin assay for *C difficile*. Mucosal biopsy can distinguish amebic colitis from ulcerative colitis. Enteroinvasive *E coli* and *E coli* O157:H7 will not be detected on routine bacterial cultures. CMV colitis occurs in immunocompromised patients (especially those with AIDS) and is diagnosed on mucosal biopsy. Gonorrhea, chlamydial infection, herpes, and syphilis are considerations in sexually active patients with proctitis. In elderly patients with cardiovascular disease, ischemic colitis may involve the rectosigmoid. A history of radiation to the pelvic region can result in proctitis months to years later. Crohn's disease involving the colon but not the small intestine may be confused with ulcerative colitis. In 10% of patients, a distinction between Crohn's disease and ulcerative colitis is not possible.

Treatment
(Table 14—7)

There is still no specific therapy for ulcerative colitis. Treatment is directed at symptomatic relief and

Table 14–7. Treatment of ulcerative colitis.

Distal colitis
Proctitis
  Mesalamine suppositories, 500 mg per rectum twice daily, or–
  Hydrocortisone foam, 90 mg per rectum daily, or–
  Hydrocortisone suppositories, 100 mg per rectum daily
Proctosigmoiditis
  Mesalamine enema, 4 g per rectum daily, or–
  Hydrocrotisone enema, 100 mg per rectum daily
Extensive colitis
Mild to moderate
  Sulfasalazine, 1.5–3 g orally twice daily, or–
  Mesalamine tablets (delayed release), 800 mg orally 3 times daily, or–
  Olsalazine, 0.75–1.5 g orally twice daily
  If no response after 2–4 weeks, add prednisone, 40–60 mg/d (taper by 5 mg/wk)
Severe
  Methylprednisolone, 48–60 mg IV daily

at suppression of inflammation. Without therapy, 75% per year of patients will have a disease relapse. Sulfasalazine, 1 g twice daily, decreases the relapse rate to less than 25%. Olsalazine, 500 mg twice daily, is effective in patients who cannot tolerate sulfasalazine. Therapy should be continued indefinitely in most patients.

There are two main treatment objectives: (1) to terminate the acute, symptomatic attack and (2) to prevent recurrence of attacks. The treatment of acute ulcerative colitis is dependent upon the extent of colonic involvement and the severity of illness.

Patients with mild to moderate disease should eat a regular diet, but caffeine and gas-producing vegetables are restricted. Fiber supplements decrease diarrhea and rectal symptoms (psyllium, 3.4 g twice daily; methylcellulose, 2 g twice daily; bran powder, 1 tbsp twice daily). Antidiarrheal agents should not be given in the acute phase of illness but are safe and helpful in patients with mild chronic symptoms. Loperamide (2 mg), diphenoxylate with atropine (one tablet), or tincture of opium (8–15 drops) may be given up to four times daily. Such remedies are particularly useful at nighttime and when taken prophylactically for occasions when patients may not have reliable access to toilet facilities.

A. Distal Colitis: Patients with disease confined to the rectum or rectosigmoid region generally have mild but distressing symptoms. Acute therapy is best approached with topical agents. Topical mesalamine is the drug of choice and is superior to topical corticosteroids. Mesalamine is administered as a suppository, 500 mg twice daily for proctitis, and as an enema, 4 g at bedtime for proctosigmoiditis, for 3–12 weeks, with 75% of patients improving. Topical steroids are a less expensive alternative to mesalamine but are also less effective. Hydrocortisone suppository or foam is prescribed for proctitis and hydrocortisone enema for proctosigmoiditis. Systemic effects from short-term use are very slight. It is not known whether combination therapy with mesalamine and hydrocortisone is advantageous. Patients with distal disease who fail to improve with topical therapy should be considered for systemic steroids or immunosuppressives as described below.

Patients whose acute symptoms resolve with acute therapy have an 80–90% chance of a symptomatic relapse within 1 year. Maintenance therapy with mesalamine suppositories (500 mg daily) or with oral agents (see below) reduce the relapse rate to less than 20% per year.

B. Mild to Moderate Colitis: Disease extending above the sigmoid colon is best treated with oral agents. The currently available agents—sulfasalazine, mesalamine, and olsalazine—result in symptomatic improvement in 50–75% of patients. These drugs appear to be comparable in efficacy, though olsalazine is not yet approved for treatment of active colitis. To minimize side effects, sulfasalazine is begun at a dose of 500 mg twice daily and increased gradually over 1–2 weeks to 1.5–2 g twice daily. Most patients improve within 3 weeks, though some require 2–3 months. Total doses of 5–6 g/d may have greater efficacy but are poorly tolerated. Because of their greater cost, olsalazine and mesalamine should be reserved for patients who are intolerant of sulfasalazine. Mesalamine, 800 mg three times daily, is approved for active disease. Higher doses of 1.2–1.6 g three times daily may be required in some patients. Olsalazine, 1 g two or three times daily, is not approved but also appears to be effective.

Patients with mild to moderate disease who fail to improve after 2–3 weeks of mesalamine therapy should have the addition of corticosteroid therapy. Topical therapy with hydrocortisone foam or enemas (80–100 mg twice daily) is tried first. Patients who fail to improve after 2 more weeks require systemic steroid therapy. Prednisone and methylprednisolone are most commonly used. Depending on the severity of illness, the initial oral dose of prednisone is 20–30 mg twice daily. Rapid improvement is observed in most cases. One can usually begin to taper prednisone after 2 weeks. Tapering of prednisone should proceed by no more than 5 mg/wk. After tapering to 15 mg/d, slower tapering is sometimes required. Complete tapering without symptomatic flare-ups is possible in the majority of patients.

C. Severe Colitis: About 10–15% of ulcerative colitis patients have a more severe course. Because they may deteriorate rapidly, hospitalization is generally required.

1. General measures–

a. Discontinue all oral intake. Total parenteral nutrition is indicated in patients with poor nutritional status.

b. Avoid all opiate or anticholinergic agents.

c. Restore circulating volume with fluids and blood as needed. Correct electrolyte abnormalities.

d. Perform frequent abdominal examinations to look for evidence of worsening distention or pain.

e. Obtain a plain abdominal radiograph on admission to look for evidence of colonic dilation.

f. Obtain surgical consultation in all patients with severe disease.

g. Send stools for bacterial (including *C difficile*) culture and examination for ova and parasites.

2. Corticosteroid therapy–Methylprednisolone, 48–80 mg, or hydrocortisone, 300 mg, is administered in four divided doses or by continuous infusion over 24 hours. Higher or "pulse" doses are of no benefit. Hydrocortisone enemas should also be administered twice daily as a drip, 100 mg over 30 minutes. In patients who have not previously received corticosteroids, administration of ACTH, 120 units/24 h, may be superior to corticosteroids. Approximately 50–75% of patients achieve remission with systemic steroids within 7–10 days. Once symptomatic improvement has occurred, oral fluids are reinstituted. If well tolerated, the patient is then converted to oral predisone (as described for moderate disease).

3. Cyclosporine–In limited trials, cyclosporine benefited over 75% of patients with severe colitis who had not improved after 7–10 days of corticosteroids. Further trials are in progress.

4. Surgical therapy–Patients with severe disease who fail to improve after 7–10 days of corticosteroid therapy are unlikely to respond to continued steroids, and surgery is recommended. Patients with fulminant disease or toxic megacolon who worsen or fail to improve within 48–72 hours should undergo surgery to prevent perforation. If operation is performed before perforation, the mortality rate should be extremely low.

D. Fulminant Colitis and Toxic Megacolon: A subset of patients with severe disease have a more "fulminant" course with rapid progression of symptoms over 1–2 weeks and signs of severe toxicity. These patients appear quite ill, with prominent hypovolemia, transfusion requiring hemorrhage, and abdominal distention with tenderness. They are at a higher risk of perforation or development of toxic megacolon and must be followed closely. Broad-spectrum antibiotics should be administered to cover anaerobes and gram-negative bacteria.

Toxic megacolon develops in less than 2% of cases of ulcerative colitis. It is characterized by colonic dilation of more than 6 cm on plain films with signs of toxicity. In addition to the therapies outlined above, nasogastric suction should be initiated. Patients should be instructed to roll from side to side and onto the abdomen in an effort to decompress the distended colon. Serial abdominal plain films should be obtained to look for worsening dilation or ischemia.

Risk of Colon Cancer

In ulcerative colitis patients with disease proximal

to the sigmoid colon, there is a markedly increased risk of developing colon carcinoma. In patients who have had colitis for more than 10 years, the risk of developing colon cancer increases approximately 0.5–1% per year. Colonoscopies are recommended every 1–2 years in patients with extensive colitis, beginning 8–10 years after diagnosis. At colonoscopy, multiple random biopsies are taken as well as biopsies of mass lesions to look for dysplasia or carcinoma. Because of the relatively high incidence of concomitant carcinoma in patients with dysplasia, colectomy is recommended.

Surgery in Ulcerative Colitis

Surgery is required in 25% of patients. Severe hemorrhage, perforation, and documented carcinoma are absolute indications for surgery. Surgery is indicated also in patients with fulminant colitis or toxic megacolon that does not improve within 48–72 hours, (as outlined above); in patients with dysplasia on surveillance colonoscopy; and in patients with refractory disease requiring chronic steroids to control symptoms.

Although total proctocolectomy provides a complete cure of the disease, most patients seek to avoid it out of concern for the impact it may have upon their bowel function, their self-image, and their social interactions. After complete colectomy, patients may have a standard ileostomy with an external appliance, a continent ileostomy, or an internal ileal pouch which is anastomosed to the anal canal (ileoanal anastomosis). The latter maintains intestinal continuity, thereby obviating an ostomy. Under optimal circumstances, patients have five to seven loose bowel movements per day without incontinence.

Prognosis

Ulcerative colitis is a lifelong disease characterized by exacerbations and remissions. For most patients, the disease is readily controlled by medical therapy without need for surgery. The majority never require hospitalization. A subset of patients with more severe disease will require surgery, which results in complete cure of their disease. Properly managed, most ulcerative colitis patients lead close to normal productive lives.

Jewell DP, Phil D: Corticosteroids for the management of ulcerative colitis and Crohn's disease. Gastroenterol Clin North Am 1989;18:21.

Kohler LW et al: Quality of life after proctocolectomy: A comparison of Brooke ileostomy, Kock pouch and ileal pouch-anal anastomosis. Gastroenterology 1991;101:679.

Lichtiger S, Present DH: Preliminary report: Cyclosporine in treatment of severe ulcerative colitis. Lancet 1990:336:16.

Nugent FW et al: Cancer surveillance in ulcerative colitis. Gastroenterology 1991;100:1241.

Podolsky DK: Inflammatory bowel disease. (Two parts.) N Engl J Med 1991;325:928, 1008.

2. CROHN'S DISEASE

Essentials of Diagnosis

- Insidious onset.
- Intermittent bouts of low-grade fever, diarrhea, and right lower quadrant pain.
- Right lower quadrant mass and tenderness.
- Perianal disease with abscess, fistulas.
- Radiographic evidence of ulceration, stricturing, or fistulas of the small intestine or colon.

General Considerations

Crohn's disease is an idiopathic inflammatory process that can affect any portion of the alimentary tract from the mouth to the anus. One-third of cases involve only the small bowel, most commonly the terminal ileum (ileitis). About half of cases involve the small bowel and colon, most often the terminal ileum and adjacent proximal ascending colon (ileocolitis). In 15–20% of cases, the colon alone is affected. Unlike ulcerative colitis, Crohn's disease is a transmural process that can result in mucosal inflammation and ulceration, stricturing, fistulous development, and abscess formation.

Clinical Findings

A. Symptoms and Signs: Because of the variable location of involvement and severity of inflammation, Crohn's disease may present with a variety of symptoms and signs. In eliciting the history, the clinician should take particular note of fevers, the patient's general sense of well-being, the presence of abdominal pain, the number of liquid bowel movements per day, and prior surgical resections. Physical examination should focus upon the patient's temperature, weight, and nutritional status, the presence of abdominal tenderness or an abdominal mass, rectal examination, and extraintestinal manifestations. Most commonly, there is one or a combination of the following clinical constellations.

1. Chronic inflammatory disease—This is the most common presentation and is often seen in patients with ileitis or ileocolitis. Patients report low-grade fever, malaise, weight loss, and loss of energy. There may be diarrhea, which is nonbloody and often intermittent. Cramping or steady right lower quadrant or periumbilical pain is present. Physical examination reveals focal tenderness, usually in the right lower quadrant. A palpable, tender mass may be present in the lower abdomen which represents thickened or matted loops of inflamed intestine.

2. Intestinal obstruction—Narrowing of the small bowel may occur as a result of inflammation, spasm, or fibrotic stenosis. Patients report postprandial bloating, cramping pains, and loud borborygmi.

This sometimes occurs in patients with active inflammatory symptoms (as above). More commonly, however, it occurs later in the disease from chronic fibrosis without other systemic symptoms or signs of inflammation.

3. Fistulization with or without infection–A subset of patients develop sinus tracts that penetrate through the bowel and form fistulas to a number of locations. Fistulas to the mesentery are usually asymptomatic but can result in intra-abdominal or retroperitoneal abscesses manifested by fevers, chills, a tender abdominal mass, and leukocytosis. Fistulas from the colon to the small intestine or stomach can result in bacterial overgrowth with diarrhea, weight loss, and malnutrition. Fistulas to the bladder or vagina produce recurrent infections. Enterocutaneous fistulas usually occur at the site of surgical scars.

4. Perianal disease–One-third of patients with either large or small bowel involvement develop perianal disease manifested by anal fissures, perianal abscesses, and fistulas. This can be a distressing problem.

5. Extraintestinal manifestations–The extracolonic manifestations described above with ulcerative colitis may also be seen with Crohn's disease, particularly Crohn's colitis. Other problems may also arise. Oral aphthous lesions are common. There is an increased prevalence of gallstones due to malabsorption of bile salts from the terminal ileum. Nephrolithiasis with urate or calcium oxalate stones may occur.

B. Laboratory Findings: There is a poor correlation between laboratory studies and the patient's clinical picture. Laboratory values may reflect inflammatory activity or nutritional complications of disease. A complete blood count and serum albumin should be obtained in all patients. Anemia may reflect chronic inflammation, mucosal blood loss, iron deficiency, or vitamin B_{12} malabsorption secondary to terminal ileal inflammation or resection. Leukocytosis may reflect inflammation or abscess formation or may be secondary to corticosteroid therapy. Hypoalbuminemia may be due to intestinal protein loss (protein-losing enteropathy), malabsorption, or chronic inflammation. The sedimentation rate or C-reactive protein level is elevated in many patients during active inflammation. Stool specimens are sent for examination for routine pathogens, ova and parasites, and *C difficile* toxin.

C. Special Diagnostic Studies: In most patients, the initial diagnosis of Crohn's disease is based upon a compatible clinical picture with supporting radiographic findings. An upper gastrointestinal series with small bowel follow-through is obtained in all patients. Suggestive findings include ulcerations, strictures, and fistulas. To evaluate the colon, a barium enema or colonoscopy is obtained. Colonoscopy offers the advantage of obtaining mucosal biopsies of the colon or terminal ileum. Typical endoscopic findings include aphthoid ulcers, linear or stellate ulcers, strictures, and segmental involvement with areas of normalDappearing mucosa adjacent to inflamed mucosa. In 10% of cases, it may be impossible to distinguish ulcerative colitis from Crohn's disease. The presence of granulomas on biopsy are seen in less than 25% of patients but are highly suggestive of Crohn's disease.

Complications

A. Abscess: The presence of a tender abdominal mass with fever and leukocytosis suggests an abscess. Emergent CT of the abdomen is necessary to confirm the diagnosis. Patients should be given broad-spectrum antibiotics and, if malnourished, maintained on TPN. Percutaneous drainage or surgery is usually required.

B. Obstruction: Small bowel obstruction may develop secondary to active inflammation or chronic fibrotic stricturing, often acutely precipitated by dietary indiscretion. Patients should be given intravenous fluids with nasogastric suction for several days. Systemic steroids are indicated in patients with signs or symptoms of active inflammation but are unhelpful in patients with inactive, fixed disease. Patients unimproved on medical management require surgical resection of the stenotic area or stricturoplasty.

C. Fistulas: The majority of enteromesenteric and enteroenteric fistulas are asymptomatic and require no specific therapy. Most symptomatic fistulas require surgical therapy, particularly when there is evidence of intestinal stricturing below the fistula. Medical therapy is effective in a subset of patients and is usually tried before surgery. Many fistulas close temporarily in response to TPN but recur when oral feedings are resumed. Mercaptopurine heals fistulas in 30–40% of patients but requires 3–6 months.

D. Perianal Disease: Patients with fissures, fistulas, and skin tags have perianal discomfort that is treated conservatively with sitz baths and cotton pads to absorb drainage. Control of diarrhea is important. Metronidazole, 250 mg three or four times daily, and mercaptopurine may help some patients with perianal disease. Surgical treatment of perianal fistulas is unnecessary and to be avoided in most patients. Patients with abscesses require conservative surgical incision and drainage.

E. Carcinoma: Patients with colonic Crohn's disease are at increased risk of developing colon carcinoma. Screening colonoscopy is recommended by some authorities.

F. Hemorrhage: Unlike ulcerative colitis, severe hemorrhage is unusual in Crohn's disease.

G. Malabsorption: Malabsorption may arise from bacterial overgrowth in patients with enterocolonic fistulas, strictures and stasis, extensive jejunal inflammation, and prior surgical resections.

Differential Diagnosis

Chronic cramping abdominal pain and diarrhea are typical of both irritable bowel syndrome and Crohn's disease, but x-ray examinations are normal in the former. Acute fever and right lower quadrant pain may resemble appendicitis or *Yersinia enterocolitica* enteritis. Intestinal lymphoma causes fever, pain, weight loss, and abnormal small bowel radiographs that may mimic Crohn's disease. Patients with undiagnosed AIDS may present with fever and diarrhea. Segmental colitis may be caused by tuberculosis, *Entamoeba histolytica, Chlamydia,* or ischemic colitis. Diverticulitis with abscess formation may be difficult to distinguish acutely from Crohn's disease.

Treatment of Active Disease

Crohn's disease is a chronic lifelong illness characterized by exacerbations and periods of remission. As no specific therapy exists, current treatment is directed toward symptomatic improvement and controlling the disease process. The treatment must address the specific problems of the individual patient.

A. Nutrition:

1. Diet–Patients should eat a well-balanced diet. Because lactose intolerance is common, a trial off dairy products is warranted. Patients with mainly colonic involvement benefit from fiber supplementation. Conversely, patients with obstructive symptoms should be placed on a low-roughage diet, ie, no raw fruits or vegetables, popcorn, nuts, etc. Resection of more than 100 cm of terminal ileum results in fat malabsorption. A low-fat diet with medium-chain triglyceride supplementation is used.

2. Enteral therapy–Enteral therapy with elemental diets (eg, Vivonex) for 4 weeks is as effective as corticosteroids in inducing remission, but the relapse rate after return to a normal diet is high.

3. Total parenteral nutrition–TPN is used short-term in patients with active disease and severe malnutrition; in patients with fistulas while medical therapy is being introduced; and preoperatively to improve nutritional status. It is required long-term in a small subset of patients with extensive intestinal resections resulting in short bowel syndrome with malnutrition.

B. Symptomatic Medications:

1. Antidiarrheals–Chronic diarrhea may respond dramatically to antidiarrheal agents. Loperamide (2–4 mg), diphenoxylate with atropine (one tablet), and tincture of opium (8–15 drops) may be given as needed up to four times daily. Patients with active terminal ileal disease or terminal ileal resection of less than 100 cm may benefit from cholestyramine (2–4 g) or colestipol (5 g) once or twice daily to bind malabsorbed bile salts.

2. Antispasmodics–Propantheline (15 mg), dicyclomine (10–20 mg), or L-hyoscyamine (0.125 mg) given before meals may reduce abdominal cramps. Patients should discontinue these agents at the first sign of intestinal obstruction.

C. Specific Drug Therapy:

1. 5-ASA agents–Sulfasalazine, 1.5–2 g twice daily, is effective in reducing clinical signs of disease activity in patients with colonic involvement but confers little benefit in small intestine disease. Unlike sulfasalazine, the new mesalamine compounds release 5-ASA in the distal small bowel, offering theoretical advantages. Their efficacy in active Crohn's disease is under investigation.

2. Corticosteroids–Corticosteroids dramatically suppress the acute clinical signs and symptoms in most patients with both small and large bowel disease. However, steroids do not appear to alter the underlying disease diathesis. Prednisone, 40–60 mg/d, is generally administered to patients with an active flare-up of Crohn's disease. After improvement at 2–3 weeks, tapering proceeds at 5 mg/wk until a dosage of 20 mg/d is being given. Thereafter, very slow tapering of 2.5 mg/wk or every other week is recommended. Some patients cannot be completely withdrawn from steroids without experiencing a symptomatic flare-up. Chronic low steroid doses (2.5–10 mg/d) are often required. These may be associated with serious complications such as aseptic necrosis of the hips, osteoporosis, cataracts, growth retardation in children, diabetes, and hypertension. For these reasons, chronic steroids are to be avoided where possible.

Patients with more severe disease manifested by severe weight loss or malnutrition should be hospitalized and treated with intravenous steroids (as described for ulcerative colitis). In patients with a tender, palpable inflammatory abdominal mass, a CT scan of the abdomen should be obtained prior to administering steroids in order to rule out an abscess. Even if no abscess is identified, steroids should be administered cautiously along with broad-spectrum antibiotics.

3. Mercaptopurine–Mercaptopurine (6-MP) is indicated in patients with unresponsive disease, those receiving chronic steroid therapy, and those with symptomatic fistulas. It permits reduction or elimination of steroids in over 75% and fistulous closing in 30–40%. Therapy is initiated at a dosage of 50 mg/d. Blood counts should be monitored weekly for the first month, then monthly. The mean time to symptomatic response is 3–6 months, so this option is not suitable for acute exacerbations.

Maintenance of Remission

Crohn's disease is characterized by recurrent symptomatic flare-ups and remissions. Chronic administration of sulfasalazine and corticosteroids has not been shown to prevent disease recurrence. However, preliminary studies demonstrate that mesalamine, 800 mg three times daily, delays clinical relapse.

Indications for Surgery

Over half of patients will require at least one surgical procedure. The main indications for surgery are intractability to medical therapy, intraDabdominal abscess, massive bleeding, and obstruction with fibrous stricture. Patients with active inflammation who are unresponsive to medical therapy or who require chronic prednisone in doses exceeding 15 mg/d may achieve dramatic relief from limited surgical excision for 5–15 years before disease recurs.

Prognosis

With proper medical and surgical treatment, the majority of patients are able to cope with this chronic disease and its complications and lead productive lives. Few patients die as a direct consequence of the disease.

O'Brien JJ et al: Use of azathioprine or 6-mercaptopurine in the treatment of Crohn's disease. Gastroenterology 1991;101:39.

Prantera C et al: Oral 5-aminosalicylic acid (Asacol) in the maintenance treatment of Crohn's disease. Gastroenterology 1992;103:363.

Rijk MC et al: Sulphasalazine and prednisone compared with sulphasalazine for treating active Crohn disease. Ann Intern Med 1991;114:445. (The use of prednisone resulted in faster initial improvement, but at 16 weeks there was no significant difference.)

Singleton J: Enteral feeding versus drug therapy in Crohn's disease: A continuing story. Gastroenterology 1991; 101:1127. (Enteral feeding is used as primary therapy by many clinicians in Europe. This editorial summarizes the controversies.)

DIVERTICULAR DISEASE OF THE COLON

Essentials of Diagnosis

- Intermittent, cramping left lower abdominal pain.
- Constipation or alternating constipation and diarrhea.
- Tenderness in the left lower quadrant.
- X-ray evidence of diverticula, thickened interhaustral folds, narrowed lumen.

General Considerations

Diverticula of the colon occur with increasing frequency after age 40—5% in the fifth decade and 50% in the ninth decade. Although diverticula may occur throughout the gut, excluding the rectum, they are most common in the high-pressure areas of the colon (eg, sigmoid). They tend to dissect along the course of the nutrient vessels, and they consist of a mucosal layer and the serosa. The inflammatory complication, diverticulitis, probably affects 10–20% of patients at some time.

Inflammatory changes in diverticulitis vary from mild polymorphonuclear infiltration in the wall of the sac to extensive inflammatory change in the surrounding area (peridiverticulitis), with perforation or abscess formation. The changes are comparable to those that occur in appendicitis.

Clinical Findings

A. Symptoms and Signs: Left lower quadrant pain may be steady and severe and last for days or may be cramping and intermittent and relieved by a bowel movement. Constipation is usual, but diarrhea may occur. Occult blood is found in the stool in about 20% of cases. Diverticulosis coli (without inflammation) is the most common cause of colonic hemorrhage; lower gastrointestinal hemorrhage is uncommon in diverticulitis.

B. Laboratory Findings: Noncontributory in uncomplicated diverticular disease.

C. Imaging: Barium enema reveals diverticula and in some cases spasm, interhaustral thickening, or narrowing of the colonic lumen. In the patient with suspected diverticulitis, barium enema, if done, must be done carefully because of the probable presence of at least a closed perforation. CT scanning may show evidence of pericolic inflammation or abscess.

Complications

Diverticulitis is a complication of diverticular disease in which gross or microscopic perforation of the diverticulum has occurred. The clinical manifestations vary with the extent of the inflammatory process and may include pain, signs of peritoneal irritation, chills, fever, sepsis, ileus, and partial or complete colonic obstruction. Peritonitis and abscess formation may also occur. Urinary frequency and dysuria are associated with bladder involvement in the inflammatory process. Fistula formation usually involves the bladder (usually vesicosigmoid, with pneumaturia a characteristic symptom) but may also be to the skin, perianal area, or small bowel. The white blood count shows polymorphonuclear leukocytosis. Red and white blood cells may be seen in the urine and, with fistula, numerous bacteria. Blood and urine cultures may be positive.

Differential Diagnosis

The constrictive lesion of the colon seen on x-ray or at sigmoidoscopy must be differentiated from carcinoma of the colon. The appearance of a short lesion with abrupt transition to normal bowel suggests carcinoma. Colonoscopy with biopsy can be very useful in these instances.

Treatment

The treatment of uncomplicated diverticular disease consists primarily of increasing bulk in the diet by means of the following: (1) high-residue diet; (2) unprocessed bran, 1/4 cup daily in fruit juice or muffins; or (3) bulk additives such as psyllium hydrophilic mucilloid (Metamucil, others) or methylcellulose. Other measures that may be helpful are

(1) stool softeners such as docusate sodium (Colace, others), 240 mg/d; and (2) anticholinergic drugs (eg, dicyclomine, 10–20 mg before meals three times a day) to decrease "spasm" in the sigmoid colon.

The treatment of acute diverticulitis requires antibiotic therapy. Agents should be selected with the intention of eradicating aerobic and anaerobic intestinal flora, eg, combinations of broad-spectrum penicillins, cephalosporins, aminoglycosides, and clindamycin or metronidazole.

Recurrent attacks of diverticulitis or the presence of perforation, fistula formation, or abscess formation requires surgical resection of the involved portion of the colon.

Massive diverticular hemorrhage usually stops spontaneously. Adequate blood replacement and careful endoscopic and barium studies are indicated to rule out other causes of bleeding. In certain instances, selective arteriography may localize the site of the bleeding and make it possible to control the bleeding with vasopressin. Operation may be required for uncontrolled bleeding.

Diverticulitis most typically occurs in the left colon; hemorrhage is most often noted to originate from right-sided diverticula.

Prognosis

The usual case is mild and responds well to dietary measures and antibiotics.

Cheskin LJ et al: Diverticular disease in the elderly. Gastroenterol Clin North Am 1990;19:31. (Current concepts of diagnosis and management.)

ANGIODYSPLASIA OF THE COLON

Angiodysplasia is a disorder characterized by abnormal clusters of arterioles and dilated vascular spaces and veins in the submucosa and mucosa. Angiodysplasia of the colon as a cause of acute and chronic lower gastrointestinal bleeding is being increasingly recognized. It is seen chiefly in patients over age 50 (most of them over 70) with a prevalence of approximately 2% and is characterized by painless, usually self-limited intermittent rectal bleeding. The bleeding is usually of dark red blood but may be occult. There may be tarry stools. Up to 30% of patients have a history of surgery for gastrointestinal bleeding—eg, vagotomy and pyloroplasty, gastrectomy. Most lesions of angiodysplasia are in the cecum and right colon.

Treatment

A. Medical Treatment: The patient must be stabilized with fluids and packed red cells as clinically dictated and then evaluated for bleeding diatheses. To rule out an upper gastrointestinal site, upper endoscopy should be seriously considered even when the gastric aspirate is negative for blood and positive for bile. The sequence of additional evaluation is controversial, partly depending upon the resources available, but would include the following:

1. Technetium-labeled red cell scan to attempt to localize the site of bleeding. This is more sensitive than angiography; it has been shown to identify bleeding at a rate of 0.05 mL/min in experimental settings and at a rate of 0.5 mL/min clinically.

2. Colonoscopy after appropriate cleansing of the colon. In some studies, over 80% of patients with angiographically proved angiodysplasia are identified in this way.

3. Angiography provides definitive diagnosis at centers where experts with the procedure are available.

B. Surgical Treatment: The major options are cautery or sclerosis of the vascular lesion via colonoscopy, or surgical resection.

Imperiale TF, Ransohoff DF: Aortic stenosis, idiopathic gastrointestinal bleeding, and angiodysplasia: Is there an association? Gastroenterology 1988;95:1670. (Probably not.)
Hemingway AP: Angiodysplasia: Current concepts. Postgrad Med J 1988;64:259. (Commonest single cause of obscure gastrointestinal bleeding in the elderly. Usually colonic. Diagnosis is by colonoscopy and angiography.)

POLYPS OF THE COLON & RECTUM (Intestinal Polyps)

Adenomatous polyps of the colon and rectum are common benign neoplasms that are usually asymptomatic but may cause painless rectal bleeding. They may be single or multiple, occur most frequently in the sigmoid and rectum, and are found incidentally in about 9% of autopsies. The incidence of polyps increases with age. The diagnosis is established by sigmoidoscopy, double contrast barium enema, and colonoscopy. When a polyp is found in the rectum, the colon should be studied by x-ray or colonoscopy.

Whether polyps are precancerous is an important question. Pedunculated adenomatous polyps less than 1 cm in diameter have very slight malignant potential and can usually be managed by simple polypectomy through the colonoscope. Larger adenomatous polyps impose a greater cancer risk and must be removed. Pedunculated adenomatous polyps less than 1 cm in diameter have a less than 1% chance of being malignant. Adenomatous polyps greater than 1 cm impose a cancer risk of 2–10% or more, risks increasing with increased size of the polyp. Most of these polyps can be removed at colonoscopy. Villous adenomas are usually sessile and become malignant in 10% of cases if they are 2 cm in diameter or less and in up to 50% of cases if they are larger. These too require removal, which can often be accomplished with the colonoscope; if not, surgical resection is required. Because colonic polyps tend to recur and because of their malignant potential, colonoscopic surveillance should be scheduled at 1 year postpolypectomy. If no polyps are found at that time, a repeat examination is indicated 2 years later unless clinically indicated sooner. For polyps removed by colonoscopic polypectomy that are determined to be malignant, the sufficiency of polypectomy as the sole treatment is determined by the histologic characteristics of the cancer and the extent of invasion of the stalk and the mucosa.

There are several familial polyp syndromes, some of which have a strong predilection for carcinoma. These need to be identified and treated and genetic counseling provided. For polyps with high malignant potential, colectomy with ileostomy or ileoproctostomy—after stripping of the rectal mucosa—is indicated.

Burt RW, Samowitz WS: The adenomatous polyp and the hereditary polyposis syndromes. Gastroenterol Clin North Am 1988;17:657. (Good review to include cancer risks.)

Ransohoff DF et al: Colonoscopic surveillance after polypectomy: Consideration of cost effectiveness. Ann Intern Med 1991;114:177. (A thoughtful look at costs and benefits.)

Russel JB et al: When is polypectomy sufficient treatment for colorectal cancer in a polyp? Ann Surg 1990; 160:665. (Adequate when polyp less than 1.5 cm and cancer did not go through muscularis mucosae.)

CANCER OF THE COLON & RECTUM

Essentials of Diagnosis

- Most colon cancers are asymptomatic.
- Altered bowel function (constipation) and bright red rectal bleeding in distal lesions.
- Blood in the feces, unexplained anemia, weight loss in right-sided carcinomas.
- Palpable mass involving colon or rectum valuable when present.
- Endoscopic or radiographic evidence of neoplasm.

General Considerations

Carcinoma is the only common cancer of the colon and rectum. Lymphoma, carcinoid, melanoma, fibrosarcoma, and other types of sarcoma occur rarely. The treatment of all is essentially the same.

Carcinoma of the colon and rectum accounts for about 15% of cancer deaths, second only to cancer of the lung. Predisposing causes are listed in Table 14–8. Males are affected slightly more commonly than females. The highest incidence is in patients about 50 years of age, but occasional cases have been reported in younger persons and even in children.

Table 14–8. Factors associated with increased risk of colonic cancer.

Standard Risk	High Risk[1]
After age 40 (both men and women)	Rectocolonic polyps (familial polyposis, villous polyps, adenomatous polyps, history of juvenile polyps) Cancer elsewhere in the body Familial history of colon cancer Ulcerative colitis Granulomatous colitis Immunodeficiency disease

[1]Listed in approximate decreasing frequency or importance.

Previously reported distribution of cancer of the large bowel was approximately 16% in the cecum and ascending colon, 5% in the transverse colon, 9% in the descending colon, 20% in the sigmoid, and 50% in the rectum; many observers believe the incidence of more proximal lesions is increasing. The techniques and frequency of screening for colon cancer are controversial; they should be modified depending on the patient and the patient's family history (see Chapter 1 concerning screening).

Many lesions of the rectum and colon lie within reach of the examining finger or sigmoidoscope and therefore can be biopsied on the first visit.

Clinical Findings

Symptoms vary depending upon whether the lesion is in the right or the left side of the colon. In either case, a persistent change in the customary bowel habits should invariably alert the physician to investigate the colon. Bright red blood per rectum is a cardinal diagnostic point. Hemoccult-positive stool is a more subtle and frequent presentation.

An acute abdominal emergency may be precipitated by perforation or colonic obstruction (due to circumferential narrowing, not intussusception). The diagnosis of rectal and colonic cancer may be established by endoscopic or radiologic examination of the large bowel. The presence of polyps of the left colon or rectum requires careful examination of the right colon. The incidence of synchronous lesions in this setting is 20–30%. About 5% of colon cancer patients have multiple primaries.

A. Carcinoma of the Right Colon: Because the fecal stream is fluid and the bowel lumen large in the right half of the colon, symptoms of obstruction occur less frequently than in left-sided tumors. Vague abdominal discomfort is often the only initial complaint. This may progress to cramp-like pain, occasionally simulating cholecystitis or appendicitis. Secondary anemia with associated weakness and weight loss is found in half of patients with right colon lesions. The stools are usually positive for occult blood but rarely show gross blood. The patient is likely to have diarrhea. The first indication of cancer may be the discovery of a palpable mass in the right lower quadrant.

B. Carcinoma of the Left Colon: Obstructive symptoms predominate, particularly increasing constipation. There may be short bouts of diarrhea. Occasionally the first sign is acute colonic obstruction. A small amount of bright red blood with bowel movements is common, and anemia is found in about 20% of cases. At times a mass is palpable. About half of patients give a history of weight loss.

Differential Diagnosis

Diverticulitis is usually associated with fever and has a different x-ray appearance. Functional bowel distress may also simulate cancer of the colon symptomatically, as may hemorrhoids. Other causes of iron deficiency anemia also merit consideration.

Treatment

Treatment is primarily surgical and determined by the Dukes stage of the carcinoma: Dukes A (mucosal involvement only) and Dukes B disease (local invasion but without penetration of the serosa) have high cure rates following surgical resection. For patients with Dukes C disease (involvement of regional lymph nodes), surgical en bloc resection plus adjuvant chemotherapy with fluorouracil and levamisole provides a 60% 4-year survival rate. Patients with Dukes D disease (distant metastases), resection of the primary lesion is usually indicated for palliation. Occasionally, surgical pursuit of single metastases to the liver is warranted.

Radiation therapy appears useful for rectal carcinomas.

Prognosis

Over 90% of patients with carcinoma of the colon and rectum are suitable for either curative or palliative resection, with an operative mortality rate of 3–6%. The overall 5-year survival rate after resection is about 50%. If the lesion is confined to the bowel and there is no evidence of lymphatic or blood vessel invasion, the 5-year survival rate is 60–70%. Local recurrence of carcinoma in the anastomotic suture line or wound area occurs in 10–15% of cases. The incidence of local recurrence can be decreased if special precautions are taken at operation to avoid implantation of malignant cells. Early identification of resectable local recurrence of a new neoplasm depends upon careful follow-up with sigmoidoscopy and barium enema every 6 months for 2 years and yearly thereafter. Carcinoembryonic antigen (CEA) is also a marker for detection of recurrent tumor (levels increase) in patients with falls to normal levels after resection and may prove useful if monitored at 6-month intervals.

Enblad G et al: Relationship between age and survival in cancer of the colon and rectum with special reference to patients less than 40 years of age. Br J Surg 1990;77:611. (Prognosis appears to be the same.)

Krook JE et al: Effective surgical adjuvant therapy for high risk rectal carcinoma. N Engl J Med 1991;324:709. (Postoperative radiation plus systemic fluorouracil regimen improves outcome.)

Lieberman DA: Colon cancer screening: The dilemma of positive screening tests. Arch Intern Med 1990;150:740. (Reviews different strategies.)

Moertel CG et al: Levamisole and fluorouracil B for adjuvant therapy of resected colon carcinoma. N Engl J Med 1990;322:352. (Beneficial regimen for those with Dukes C cancers.)

Riff ER, DeLaan K, Garewal GS: The role of sigmoidoscopy for asymptomatic patients: Results of three annual screening sigmoidoscopies, polypectomy and subsequent surveillance colonoscopy in a primary care setting. Cleve Clin J Med 1990;57:131. (Reinforces the concept of the index polyp as an indication for colonoscopy.)

ANORECTAL DISEASES

HEMORRHOIDS

Essentials of Diagnosis

- Rectal bleeding, protrusion, and vague discomfort.
- Mucoid discharge from rectum.
- Characteristic findings on external anal inspection or anoscopic examination.

General Considerations

Internal hemorrhoids are varices of the portion of the venous hemorrhoidal plexus that lies submucosally just proximal to the dentate margin. External hemorrhoids arise from the same plexus but are located subcutaneously immediately distal to the dentate margin. There are three primary internal hemorrhoidal masses; right anterior, right posterior, and left lateral. Three to five secondary hemorrhoids may be present between the three primaries. Straining at stool, constipation, prolonged sitting, and anal infection are contributing factors and may precipitate complications such as thrombosis. The diagnosis is suspected on the history of protrusion, anal pain, or bleeding and is confirmed by proctologic examination.

Carcinoma of the colon or rectum not infrequently aggravates hemorrhoids or produces similar complaints. Polyps may be present as a cause of bleeding that is wrongly attributed to hemorrhoids. For these reasons, the treatment of hemorrhoids is always preceded by sigmoidoscopy and barium enema. When portal hypertension is suspected as a causative factor, investigations for liver disease should be carried out. Hemorrhoids that develop during pregnancy or parturition tend to subside thereafter and should be treated conservatively unless persistent.

Clinical Findings

The symptoms of hemorrhoids are usually mild and remittent, but a number of disturbing complications may develop and call for active medical or surgical treatment. These complications include pruritus; incontinence; recurrent protrusion requiring manual replacement by the patient; fissure, infection, or ulceration; prolapse and strangulation; and secondary anemia due to chronic blood loss. Carcinoma has been reported to develop very rarely in hemorrhoids.

Treatment

Conservative treatment suffices in most instances of mild hemorrhoids, which may improve spontaneously or in response to a high-roughage diet, psyllium seed preparation, or nonirritating laxatives to produce soft stools. Local pain and infection are managed with warm sitz baths and insertion of a soothing anal suppository two or three times daily. Prolapsed or strangulated hemorrhoids may be treated conservatively by gentle reduction with a lubricated gloved finger; by rubber band ligation, thermal (infrared) technique, or cryosurgery; or by surgical resection.

For severe symptoms or complications, complete internal and external hemorrhoidectomy is advisable and is a highly satisfactory procedure when properly done. Excision of a single external hemorrhoid, evacuation of a thrombosed pile, and the injection treatment of internal hemorrhoids fall within the scope of office practice. Injection therapy is effective, but there is a recurrence rate of more than 50%.

Evacuation of Thrombosed External Hemorrhoid

This condition is caused by the rupture of a vein at the anal margin, forming a clot in the subcutaneous tissue. The patient complains of a painful lump, and examination shows a tense, tender, bluish mass covered with skin. If the patient is seen after 24–48 hours when the pain is subsiding—or if symptoms are minimal—hot sitz baths are prescribed. If discomfort is marked, removal of the clot is indicated. With the patient in the lateral position, the area is prepared with antiseptic, and 1% lidocaine is injected intracutaneously around and over the lump. An ellipse of skin is then excised and the clot evacuated. A dry gauze dressing is held in place for 12–24 hours by taping the buttocks together, and daily sitz baths are then begun.

Leibach JR, Cerda JJ: Hemorrhoids: Modern treatment methods. Hosp Med (Aug) 1991;53. (An update on when and how to treat.)

CRYPTITIS & PAPILLITIS

Anal pain and burning of brief duration with defecation is suggestive of cryptitis and papillitis. Digital and anoscopic examination reveals hypertrophied papillae and indurated or inflamed crypts. Treatment consists of adding bulk agents, such as psyllium seed preparations, to the diet; sitz baths; and anal suppositories containing hydrocortisone after each bowel movement. Some recommend local application of 5% phenol in oil or carbolfuchsin compound to the crypts. If these measures fail, surgical excision of involved crypts and papillae should be considered.

ANORECTAL INFECTIONS

Anorectal infections are seen chiefly in homosexual men and can be divided into two clinical syndromes: proctitis and proctocolitis.

Proctitis

Proctitis is characterized by anorectal pain, mucopurulent or bloody discharge, tenesmus, constipation, and an inflamed, often mucopurulent rectal mucosa. The most common pathogens are *Neisseria gonorrhoeae*, chlamydiae, and herpesvirus. The diagnosis can be made on sigmoidoscopy, with specimens obtained for Gram's stain and culture as well as by biopsy. Syphilis may cause proctitis, with a chancre appearing 2–6 weeks after anal intercourse. Secondary syphilis may be characterized by condyloma latum, which must be differentiated from anal warts.

The differential diagnosis should include traumatic proctitis.

Treatment depends upon the cause.

Proctocolitis

Proctocolitis implies involvement beyond the rectum to include at least the sigmoid colon. The causes may include those of proctitis, but more commonly are due to *Shigella, Campylobacter,* or amebiasis. Symptoms usually include diarrhea, abdominal cramping, and fever—in addition to the symptoms of proctitis.

Ulcerative colitis and granulomatous colitis must be considered in the differential diagnosis.

Treatment depends upon the specific bacteriologic diagnosis.

RECTAL PROLAPSE & SOLITARY ULCER

Rectal prolapse is a not uncommon problem, particularly among the elderly, and is associated with a long history of constipation and straining. The support structures of the anorectal area have usually become weakened, leading to rectal intussusception with straining. An early manifestation may be solitary rectal ulcer—a painful condition with ulcerogenesis apparently secondary to the intussusception.

Management consists of surgical correction of the lax support system.

Bartolo DC: Anorectal disease. Curr Opin Gastroenterol 1990;6:65.
Wald A: Disorders of defecation and fecal incontinence. Cleve Clin J Med 1989;56:45. (Physiologically based review.)

FISSURA IN ANO
(Anal Fissure)

Acute fissures represent linear disruption of the anal epithelium due to various causes. They usually clear if bowel movements are kept regular and soft (eg, with a bulk agent, bran, or psyllium seed preparation). The local application of a mild styptic such as 1–2% silver nitrate or 1% gentian violet solution may be of value.

Chronic fissure is characterized by (1) acute pain during and after defecation; (2) spotting of bright red blood at stool, with occasional more abundant bleeding; (3) tendency to constipation through fear of pain; and (4) the late occurrence of a sentinel pile, a hypertrophied papilla, and spasm of the anal canal (usually very painful on digital examination). Regulation of bowel habits with use of bran or psyllium seed preparation in the diet or use of stool softeners, sitz baths, or anal suppositories (eg, Anusol) twice daily should be tried. If these measures fail, the fissure, sentinel pile, or papilla and the adjacent crypt must be excised surgically. Postoperative care is along the lines of the preoperative treatment.

ANAL ABSCESS

Perianal abscess should be considered the acute stage of an anal fistula until proved otherwise. The abscess should be adequately drained as soon as localized. Hot sitz baths may hasten the process of localization. The patient should be warned that the fistula may persist after drainage of the abscess. It is painful and fruitless to search for the internal opening of a fistula in the presence of acute infection. The presence of an anal abscess should alert the clinician to the possibility of inflammatory bowel disease, especially Crohn's disease.

FISTULA IN ANO

About 95% of all anal fistulas arise in an anal crypt, and they are often preceded by an anal abscess. If an anal fistula enters the rectum above the pectinate line and there is no associated disease in the crypts, granulomatous colitis, regional ileitis, rectal tuberculosis, lymphogranuloma venereum, cancer, or foreign body should be considered in the differential diagnosis.

Acute fistula is associated with a purulent discharge from the fistulous opening. There is usually local itching, tenderness, or pain aggravated by bowel movements. Recurrent anal abscess may develop. The involved crypt can occasionally be located anoscopically with a crypt hook. Probing the fistula should be gentle because false passages can be made with ease, and in any case demonstration of the internal opening by probing is not essential to the diagnosis.

Treatment is by surgical incision or excision of the fistula under general anesthesia. If a fistula passes deep to the entire anorectal ring, so that all the muscles must be divided in order to extirpate the tract, a two-stage operation must be done to prevent incontinence.

ANAL CONDYLOMAS
(Genital Warts)

These wart-like papillomas of the perianal skin and anal canal flourish on moist, macerated surfaces, particularly in the presence of purulent discharge. They are not true tumors but are infectious and autoinoculable, probably owing to a sexually transmitted papovavirus. They must be distinguished from condylomata lata caused by syphilis. The diagnosis of the latter rests on a positive serologic test for syphilis or discovery of *Treponema pallidum* on darkfield examination.

Treatment consists of cautious accurate application of liquid nitrogen or 25% podophyllum resin in tincture of benzoin to the lesion (with bare wooden or cotton-tipped applicator sticks to avoid contact with uninvolved skin). The compound should be washed off after 2–4 hours. Condylomas in the anal canal are treated through the anoscope and the painted site dusted with powder to localize the application and minimize discomfort. Electrofulguration under local anesthesia is useful if there are numerous lesions. Local cleanliness and the frequent use of a talc dusting powder are essential.

Condylomas tend to recur. The patient should be observed for several months and advised to report promptly if new lesions appear.

BENIGN ANORECTAL STRICTURES

Traumatic

Acquired stenosis is usually the result of surgery or trauma that denudes the epithelium of the anal canal. Hemorrhoid operations in which too much skin is removed or which are followed by infection are the commonest cause. Constipation, ribbon stools, and pain on defecation are the most frequent complaints.

Stenosis predisposes to fissure, low-grade infection, and, occasionally, fistula.

Prevention of stenosis after radical anal surgery is best accomplished by local cleanliness, hot sitz baths, and gentle insertion of the well-lubricated finger twice weekly for 2–3 weeks beginning 2 weeks after surgery. When stenosis is chronic but mild, graduated anal dilators of increasing size may be inserted daily by the patient. For marked stenosis, a plastic operation on the anal canal is advisable.

Inflammatory

Lymphogranuloma venereum and granuloma inguinale are discussed in Chapter 32.

Sohn N: The rectum in AIDS. Pract Gastroenterol 1988; 12:50. (Delineates the many old and new rectal problems seen in these patients.)

ANAL INCONTINENCE

Obstetric tears, anorectal operations (particularly fistulotomy), and neurologic disturbances are the most frequent causes of anal incontinence. Diarrhea due to any cause or fecal impaction may contribute to incontinence. When incontinence is due to surgery or trauma, surgical repair of the divided or torn sphincter is indicated. Repair of anterior childbirth lacerations should be delayed for 6 months or more. In those with manometrically demonstrated decreased anal sphincter tone, biofeedback therapy has been moderately successful in achieving continence.

Wald A: Disorders of defecation and fecal incontinence. Cleve Clin J Med 1989;56:491. (Good review of therapeutic options—pharmacologic, behavioral, and surgical.)

SQUAMOUS CELL CARCINOMA OF THE ANUS

These tumors are relatively rare, comprising only 1–2% of all cancers of the anus and large intestine. Bleeding, pain, and local tumor are the commonest symptoms. The lesion is often confused with hemorrhoids or other common anal disorders. These tumors tend to become annular, invade the sphincter, and spread upward into the rectum; they are encountered regularly in AIDS patients.

Except for very small lesions (which can be adequately excised locally), treatment is by combined abdominoperineal resection. Radiation therapy is reserved for palliation and for patients who refuse or cannot withstand operation. Metastases to the inguinal nodes are treated by radical groin dissection when clinically evident. The 5-year survival rate after resection is about 50%.

REFERENCES

Kirsner JB, Shorter RG: *Inflammatory Bowel Disease,* 3rd ed. Lea & Febiger, 1988.
Smith PD et al: Gastrointestinal infections in AIDS: NIH conference. Ann Intern Med 1992;116:63.

Yamada T et al: *Textbook of Gastroenterology,* 2 vols. Lippincott, 1991.

Liver, Biliary Tract, & Pancreas

Lawrence S. Friedman, MD, & C. Michael Knauer, MD

JAUNDICE
(Icterus)

Since antiquity, a yellowish appearance of the skin and scleras has been recognized as a manifestation of liver disease. Jaundice is evidence of accumulation of bilirubin—a red pigment product of heme metabolism—in the body tissues; it has extrahepatic as well as hepatic causes. Hyperbilirubinemia may be due to abnormalities in the formation, transport, metabolism, and excretion of bilirubin. Total serum bilirubin is normally 0.2–1.2 mg/dL, and jaundice may not be clinically recognizable until levels are about 3 mg/dL.

Pathophysiologically, jaundice may result from predominantly unconjugated or conjugated bilirubin in the serum (Table 15–1). Unconjugated hyperbilirubinemia may result from overproduction of bilirubin because of hemolysis; impaired hepatic uptake of bilirubin due to certain drugs; or impaired conjugation of bilirubin by glucuronide, as in neonatal jaundice normally found between the second and fifth days of life, Gilbert's syndrome, which is due to mild decreases in glucuronyl transferase, or Crigler-Najjar syndrome, due to moderate decreases or absence of glucuronyl transferase. Predominantly conjugated hyperbilirubinemia may result from impaired excretion of bilirubin from the liver due to hepatocellular disease, drugs, sepsis, and hereditary disorders such as Dubin-Johnson syndrome or extrahepatic biliary obstruction. Features of some hyperbilirubinemic syndromes are summarized in Table 15–2. The term "cholestasis" or "cholestatic jaundice" is often used when conjugated hyperbilirubinemia results from obstruction to bile flow in the absence of hepatocellular damage.

Frank B et al: Clinical evaluation of jaundice: A guideline of the Patient Care Committee of the American Gastroenterological Association. JAMA 1989;262:3031.

Gollan JL (editor): Pathobiology of bilirubin and jaundice. Semin Liver Dis 1988;8:105.

Manifestations of Diseases
Associated With Jaundice

A. Unconjugated Hyperbilirubinemia: Weakness or abdominal or back pain may occur with acute hemolytic crises. There is normal stool and urine color, mild jaundice, indirect (unconjugated) hyperbilirubinemia with no bilirubin in the urine, and splenomegaly in hemolytic disorders, except in sickle cell anemia. Hepatomegaly is variable.

B. Conjugated Hyperbilirubinemia:

1. Hereditary cholestatic syndromes or intrahepatic cholestasis–The patient may be asymptomatic; the intermittent cholestasis is often accompanied by pruritus, light-colored stools, and, occasionally, malaise.

2. Hepatocellular disease–Malaise, anorexia, low-grade fever, and right upper quadrant discomfort are frequent. Dark urine, jaundice, and amenorrhea occur. An enlarged, tender liver; vascular spiders; palmar erythema; ascites; gynecomastia; sparse body hair; fetor hepaticus; and asterixis may be present, depending on the cause, severity, and chronicity of liver dysfunction.

C. Biliary Obstruction: There is colicky right upper quadrant pain, weight loss (carcinoma), jaundice, dark urine, and light-colored stools. Symptoms and signs may be intermittent owing to a stone or to carcinoma of the ampulla or junction of the intrahepatic ducts. Occult blood in the stools suggests cancer. Hepatomegaly, visible and palpable gallbladder (Courvoisier's sign), ascites, rectal (Blumer's) shelf, and weight loss also suggest cancer. Fever and chills suggest cholangitis.

Diagnostic Methods for Evaluation of Liver Disease & Jaundice (Table 15–3)

A. Laboratory Studies: Elevated serum aminotransferase levels (AST, ALT) result from hepatocellular necrosis or inflammation; ALT is more specific for the liver than AST, but an AST level at least twice that of the ALT is typical of alcoholic liver injury. Elevated alkaline phosphatase levels suggest cholestasis or infiltrative liver disease (eg, tumor, abscess, granulomas). Alkaline phosphatase elevations of hepatic rather than bone, intestinal, or placental origin are suggested by concomitant elevation of γ-glutamyl transpeptidase or 5'-nucleotidase levels.

B. Liver Biopsy: Percutaneous liver biopsy is the definitive study for determining the cause and extent of hepatocellular dysfunction or infiltrative liver

Table 15–1. Classification of jaundice.

Type of Hyperbilirubinemia	Location and Cause
Unconjugated hyperbilirubinemia (predominant indirect-acting bilirubin)	Increased bilirubin production (eg, hemolytic anemias, hemolytic reactions, hematoma, infarction). Impaired bilirubin uptake and storage (eg, posthepatitis hyperbilirubinemia, Gilbert's syndrome, drug reactions).
Conjugated hyperbilirubinemia (predominant direct-acting bilirubin)	**HEREDITARY CHOLESTATIC SYNDROMES** Impaired glucuronyl transferase activity (eg, Crigler-Najjar syndrome, Gilbert's syndrome). Faulty excretion of bilirubin conjugates (eg, Dubin-Johnson syndrome, Rotor's syndrome). **HEPATOCELLULAR DYSFUNCTION** Biliary epithelial damage (eg, hepatitis, hepatic cirrhosis). Intrahepatic cholestasis (eg, certain drugs, biliary cirrhosis, sepsis, postoperative jaundice). Hepatocellular damage or intrahepatic cholestasis resulting from miscellaneous causes (eg, spirochetal infections, infectious mononucleosis, cholangitis, sarcoidosis, lymphomas, industrial toxins). **BILIARY OBSTRUCTION** Choledocholithiasis, biliary atresia, carcinoma of biliary duct, sclerosing cholangitis, choledochal cyst, external pressure on common duct, pancreatitis, pancreatic neoplasms.

Table 15–2. Uncommon hyperbilirubinemic disorders.

	Nature of Defect	Type of Hyperbilirubinemia	Clinical and Pathologic Characteristics
Constitutional hepatic dysfunction (Gilbert's syndrome)	Glucuronyl transferase deficiency	Unconjugated (indirect) bilirubin	Benign, asymptomatic hereditary jaundice. Hyperbilirubinemia increased by 24- to 36-hour fast. No treatment required. Prognosis excellent.
Crigler-Najjar syndrome			Severe, nonhemolytic hereditary jaundice of neonates. Type I cases sustain CNS damage (kernicterus). Milder cases (type II) may persist into adult life and may benefit from treatment with phenobarbital.
Familial chronic idiopathic jaundice (Dubin-Johnson syndrome)	Faulty excretory function of liver cells (hepatocytes)	Conjugated (direct) bilirubin	Benign, asymptomatic hereditary jaundice. Gallbladder does not visualize on oral cholecystography. Liver darkly pigmented on gross examination. Biopsy shows centrilobular brown pigment. Prognosis excellent.
Rotor's syndrome			Similar to Dubin-Johnson syndrome but liver is not pigmented and the gallbladder is visualized on oral cholecystography. Prognosis excellent.
Benign intermittent cholestasis	Cholestasis of uncertain pathogenesis, often on a familial basis	Unconjugated plus conjugated (total) bilirubin	Benign intermittent idiopathic jaundice, itching, and malaise. Onset in early life and may persist for lifetime. Alkaline phosphatase increased. Cholestasis found on liver biopsy. (Biopsy is normal during remission.) Prognosis excellent.
Recurrent jaundice of pregnancy			Benign cholestatic jaundice of unknown cause, usually occurring in the third trimester of pregnancy. Itching, gastrointestinal symptoms, and abnormal liver excretory function tests. Cholestasis noted on liver biopsy. Prognosis excellent, but recurrence with subsequent pregnancies or use of birth control pills is characteristic.

Table 15–3. Liver function tests: Normal values and changes in two types of jaundice.

Tests	Normal Values	Hepatocellular Jaundice	Uncomplicated Obstructive Jaundice

Bilirubin
  Direct
  Indirect
	0.1–0.3 mg/dL
	0.2–0.7 mg/dL
		Increased
		Increased
			Increased
			Increased

Urine bilirubin	None	Increased	Increased
Serum albumin/total protein	Albumin, 3.5–5.5 g/dL Total protein, 6.5–8.4 g/dL	Albumin decreased	Unchanged
Alkaline phosphatase	30–115 IU/L	Increased (+)	Increased (++++)
Prothrombin time	INR[1] of 1.0–1.4. After vitamin K, 10% increase in 24 hours	Prolonged if damage severe and does not respond to parenteral vitamin K	Prolonged if obstruction marked, but responds to parenteral vitamin K
ALT, AST	ALT, 5–35 IU/L; AST, 5–40 IU/L	Increased in hepatocellular damage, viral hepatitis	Minimally increased

[1]INR = International Normalized Ratio.

disease. In patients with suspected metastatic disease or a hepatic mass, liver biopsy should be performed under ultrasound or CT guidance.

C. Imaging: Demonstration of dilated bile ducts by ultrasonography or CT scan indicates biliary obstruction (80–90% sensitivity). Ultrasonography, CT scan, and MRI can be used to demonstrate hepatomegaly, intrahepatic tumors, and changes of portal hypertension. Ultrasonography can detect gallstones with a sensitivity of 95%.

If obstructive jaundice is suspected on the basis of clinical and laboratory findings, endoscopic retrograde cholangiopancreatography (ERCP) or percutaneous transhepatic cholangiography (PTC) can identify the cause, location, and extent of biliary obstruction. PTC is preferred when a proximal cholangiocarcinoma is suspected. Complications of PTC may include fever, bacteremia, bile peritonitis, and intraperitoneal hemorrhage. ERCP requires a skilled endoscopist and may be utilized to demonstrate pancreatic or ampullary causes of jaundice, to carry out papillotomy and stone extraction, or to insert a stent through an obstructing lesion. Complications of ERCP include pancreatitis in 2–4% of cases, cholangitis, and bleeding or duodenal perforation after papillotomy.

Bennett WF, Bova JG: Review of hepatic imaging and a problem-oriented approach to liver masses. Hepatology 1990;12:761. (Available imaging techniques and algorithms for their use.)

Borsch G et al: Clinical evaluations, ultrasound, cholescintigraphy and endoscopic retrograde cholangiography in cholestasis: A prospective comparative clinical study. J Clin Gastroenterol 1988;10:185. (Clinical evaluation and ultrasound had a probability of correctness of 92.6%, with little added by further tests.)

Gollan JL et al: Pathobiology of bilirubin and jaundice. Semin Liver Dis 1988;8:105.

Malchow-Miller A et al: A decision tree for early differentiation between obstructive and non-obstructive jaundice. Scand J Gastroenterol 1988;23:391. (Correctly classified in about 90%.)

Sherman KE: Alanine aminotransferase in clinical practice: A review. Arch Intern Med 1991;151:260. (The ins and outs of ALT.)

Tygstrup N: Assessment of liver function: Principles and practice. J Gastroenterol Hepatol 1990;5:468. (Includes descriptions of newer quantitative tests of liver function such as aminopyrine breath test, caffeine clearance, and galactose elimination capacity.)

DISEASES OF THE LIVER

VIRAL HEPATITIS

Essentials of Diagnosis

- Anorexia, nausea, vomiting, malaise, symptoms of upper respiratory throat infection or flu-like syndrome, aversion to smoking.
- Fever, enlarged and tender liver, jaundice.
- Normal to low white cell count; abnormal liver tests, especially markedly elevated aminotransferases early in the course.
- Liver biopsy shows characteristic hepatocellular necrosis and mononuclear infiltrate but is rarely indicated.

General Considerations

Hepatitis can be caused by many drugs and toxic agents as well as by numerous viruses, the clinical manifestations of which may be quite similar. The development of serologic tests has made possible the identification of a growing number of specific viruses causing viral hepatitis. The more common of these are (1) hepatitis A virus (HAV); (2) hepatitis B virus (HBV); (3) hepatitis C virus (HCV; formerly non-A, non-B hepatitis virus); (4) hepatitis D virus (delta agent); (5) hepatitis E virus (an enterically transmitted hepatitis seen in epidemic form in Asia, North Africa, and Mexico); and (6) less commonly or in immunocompromised hosts, cytomegalovirus, Epstein-Barr virus, and herpes simplex virus.

A. Hepatitis A: (Figure 15–1.) HAV is a 27-nm RNA enterovirus that may cause epidemics or sporadic cases of hepatitis. Transmission of the virus is usually by the fecal-oral route, and spread is enhanced by crowding and poor sanitation. Common source outbreaks may result from contaminated water or food. The excretion of hepatitis A virus (HAV) occurs up to 2 weeks prior to clinical illness. HAV is rarely demonstrated in feces after the first week of illness. Blood and stools are infectious during the incubation period (2–6 weeks) and early illness until peak aminotransferase levels are achieved. The mortality rate for hepatitis A is low, and fulminant hepatitis A is uncommon. Chronic hepatitis does not occur and there is no carrier state. Clinical illness is more severe in adults than in children, in whom hepatitis A is often asymptomatic.

Antibody to hepatitis A (anti-HAV) appears early in the course of the illness. Both IgM and IgG anti-HAV are detectable in serum soon after the onset of the illness. Peak titers of IgM anti-HAV occur during the first week of clinical disease and usually disappear within 3–6 months. Detection of IgM anti-HAV is an excellent test for demonstration of acute hepatitis A. Peak titers of IgG anti-HAV occur after 1 month of the disease and may persist for years. The presence of IgG anti-HAV indicates (1) previous exposure to HAV, (2) noninfectivity, and (3) immunity to recurring HAV infection.

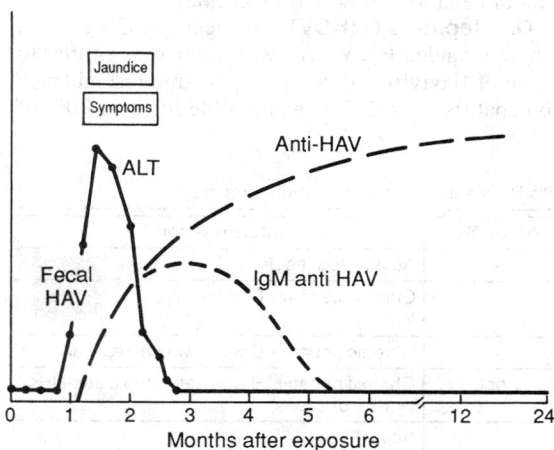

Figure 15–1. The typical course of acute type A hepatitis. (HAV, hepatitis A antigen; anti-HAV, antibody to hepatitis A virus; ALT, alanine aminotransferase.) (Reproduced, with permission, from Schafer DF, Hoofnagle JH: View Dig Dis 1982;14:5.)

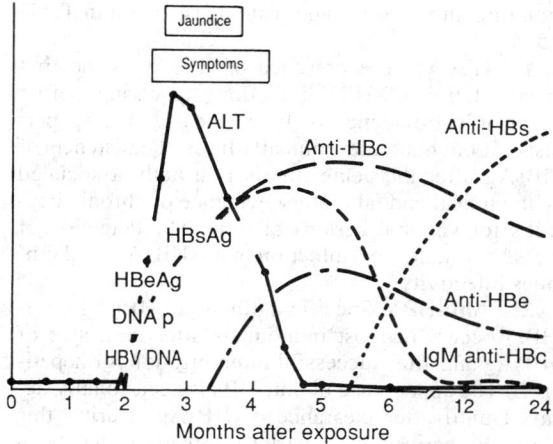

Figure 15–2. The typical course of acute type B hepatitis. (HBsAg, hepatitis B surface antigen; anti-HBs, antibody to HBsAg; HBeAg, hepatitis B e antigen; anti-HBe, antibody to HBeAg; anti-HBc, antibody to hepatitis B core antigen; DNA p, DNA polymerase; ALT, alanine aminotransferase.) (Reproduced, with permission, from Hoofnagle JH, Schafer DF: Semin Liver Dis 1986;6:1.)

B. Hepatitis B: (Figure 15–2) Hepatitis B virus (HBV) is a 42-nm hepadnavirus with a partially double-stranded DNA genome, inner core protein (hepatitis B core antigen, HBcAg) and outer surface coat (hepatitis B surface antigen, HBsAg). HBV is usually transmitted by inoculation of infected blood or blood products. HBsAg-positive mothers may transmit HBV to their neonates at the time of delivery; the risk of chronic infection in the infant is as high as 90%. HBsAg has been found in most body secretions, and the disease can be spread by sexual contact. Hepatitis B virus (HBV) is highly prevalent in homosexuals and intravenous drug abusers. Other groups at high risk include patients and staff at hemodialysis centers, physicians, dentists, nurses, and personnel working in clinical and pathology laboratories and blood banks. The incubation period of hepatitis B is 6 weeks to 6 months but may be prolonged by the administration of hepatitis B immune globulin. Clinical features of hepatitis A and B are similar; however, the onset in hepatitis B tends to be more insidious and the aminotransferase levels higher. The risk of fulminant hepatitis is less than 1%, with a mortality rate of over 60%. Following acute hepatitis B, HBV infection may persist in 1–2% of immunocompetent adults and a higher percentage of immunocompromised adults or children. Persons with chronic hepatitis B, particularly when HBV infection is acquired early in life, are at substantial risk of cirrhosis and hepatocellular carcinoma (up to 25–40%).

There are three distinct antigen-antibody systems that relate to HBV infection and a variety of circulating markers that are useful in diagnosis. Interpretation of common serologic patterns is shown in Table 15–4.

1. HBsAg–The presence of HBsAg is the first manifestation of HBV infection, appearing before biochemical evidence of liver disease. HBsAg persists throughout the clinical illness. Persistence of HBsAg after the acute illness is usually associated with clinical and laboratory evidence of chronic hepatitis for variable periods of time. The detection of HBsAg establishes infection with HBsAg and implies infectivity.

2. Anti-HBs–Specific antibody to HBsAg (anti-HBs) occurs in most individuals after clearance of HBsAg and after successful immunization for hepatitis B. The appearance of anti-HBs is occasionally delayed until after clearance of HBsAg. During this serologic gap (window period), infectivity has been demonstrated. Development of anti-HBs signals recovery from HBV, noninfectivity, and protection from recurrent HBV infection.

3. Anti-HBc–IgM anti-HBc appears shortly after HBsAg is detected. (HBcAg itself does not appear free in serum.) Its presence in the setting of acute hepatitis indicates a diagnosis of acute hepatitis B, and it fills the serologic gap in patients who have cleared HBsAg but do not yet have detectable anti-HBs. IgM anti-HBc can persist for 3–6 months or more. IgM anti-HBc may also reappear during flares of previously inactive chronic hepatitis B. IgG anti-HBc also appears during acute hepatitis B but persists indefinitely, whether the patient recovers (with the appearance of anti-HBs in serum) or develops chronic hepatitis B (with persistence of HBsAg).

4. HBeAg–HBeAg is a soluble protein found only in HBeAg-positive sera. It represents a secretory form of HBcAg that appears during the incubation period shortly after the detection of HBsAg as early as the fourth week of illness. HBeAg indicates viral replication and infectivity. Persistence of HBeAg in serum beyond 3 months suggests an increased likelihood of chronic hepatitis B. Disappearance of HBeAg is often followed by the appearance of anti-HBe, signifying diminished viral replication.

5. HBV DNA–The presence of HBV DNA in serum, now detectable by a commercial "dot" hybridization assay—generally parallels the presence of HBeAg, though HBV DNA is a more precise marker of viral replication and infectivity. In Mediterranean countries, a frequent variant form of HBV is characterized by severe chronic active hepatitis and the presence of HBV DNA without HBeAg in serum because of a mutation that prevents synthesis of HBeAg in infected hepatocytes.

C. Delta Agent (Hepatitis D): The delta agent is a defective RNA virus that causes hepatitis only in association with hepatitis B infection and specifically only in the presence of HBsAg; it is cleared when the latter is cleared.

Clinically, the delta agent may co-infect with HBV, aggravate previously existing chronic hepatitis B, or cause acute hepatitis in asymptomatic HBsAg carriers. When acute hepatitis D is coincident with an acute HBV infection, the infection is generally similar in severity to acute hepatitis B alone. In chronic active hepatitis B, superinfection by the delta agent appears to carry a more severe prognosis, often resulting in fulminant hepatitis or chronic active hepatitis that progresses rapidly to cirrhosis. Vertical transmission of this agent appears to be much less frequent than that of HBV. The delta agent is endemic in some areas, such as Mediterranean countries, where up to 80% of HBV carriers may be superinfected with it. In the USA, infection occurs primarily among intravenous drug users. Diagnosis is by detection of antibody to hepatitis D antigen in serum.

At present, hepatitis D is best prevented by prevention of hepatitis B (eg, HBV vaccine).

D. Hepatitis C (HCV): The hepatitis C virus is a single-stranded RNA virus with properties similar to those of flavivirus. It bears no genomic resemblance to hepatitis B or D. It is responsible for over 80% of

Table 15–4. Common serologic patterns in hepatitis B virus infection and their interpretation.

HBsAg	Anti-HBs	Anti-HBc	HBeAg	Anti-HBe	Interpretation
+	–	IgM	+	–	Acute hepatitis B
+	–	IgG[1]	+	–	Chronic hepatitis B with active viral replication
+	–	IgG	–	+	Chronic hepatitis B with low viral replication
+	+	IgG	+ or –	+ or –	Chronic hepatitis B with heterotypic anti-HBs (≈ 10% of cases)
–	–	IgM	+ or –	–	Acute hepatitis B
–	+	IgG	–	+ or –	Recovery from hepatitis B (immunity)
–	+	–	–	–	Vaccination (immunity)
–	–	IgG	–	–	False-positive; less commonly, infection in remote past

[1]Low levels of IgM anti-HBc may also be detected.

cases of posttransfusion hepatitis and many cases of sporadic hepatitis. Only 4% of cases of hepatitis C are attributable to blood transfusions; 40% of cases are related to intravenous drug use. The risk of sexual and maternal-neonatal transmission is small, and the source of infection in many patients is uncertain. The incubation period averages 6–7 weeks, and clinical illness is often mild, usually asymptomatic, and characterized by waxing and waning aminotransferase elevations and a high rate (> 50%) of chronic hepatitis. Hepatitis C may be a pathogenic factor in cryoglobulinemia, glomerulonephritis, and Sjögren's syndrome.

Diagnosis of hepatitis C is based on a second-generation enzyme immunoassay that detects antibodies to structural and nonstructural (enzyme) proteins expressed by different regions of the HCV genome (C200, C33c, C22-3). Limitations of the enzyme immunoassay include low sensitivity for the diagnosis of acute hepatitis C (false-negatives) and low specificity in healthy blood donors and some persons with elevated gamma globulin levels (false-positives). In these situations, a diagnosis of hepatitis C may be confirmed by use of a supplemental recombinant immunoblot assay (RIBA) that detects antibodies to four HCV antigens embedded on nitrocellulose (5-1-1, C100-3, C33c, C22). Most RIBA-positive persons are potentially infectious, as confirmed in research laboratories by use of polymerase chain reaction to detect HCV RNA. Testing of donated blood for HCV (as well as with surrogate markers of HCV—elevated ALT, anti-HBc) has helped reduce the risk of transfusion-associated hepatitis C from 10% a decade ago to 1% today.

E. Hepatitis E (HEV): Formerly termed enterically transmitted non-A, non-B hepatitis, HEV is a 29- to 32-nm RNA virus thought to be a calicivirus and responsible for waterborne hepatitis outbreaks in India, Burma, Afghanistan, Algeria, and Mexico. Illness is self-limited (no carrier state) with a high mortality rate (10–20%) in pregnant women.

F. Miscellaneous Causes: Other viral agents that cause hepatitis include Epstein-Barr virus and cytomegalovirus. About 15–20% of cases of transfusional hepatitis are not caused by HCV.

Clinical Findings

The clinical picture of viral hepatitis is extremely variable, ranging from asymptomatic infection without jaundice to a fulminating disease and death in a few days.

A. Symptoms:

1. Prodromal phase–The speed of onset varies from abrupt to insidious, with general malaise, myalgia, arthralgia, easy fatigability, upper respiratory symptoms (nasal discharge, pharyngitis), and severe anorexia out of proportion to the degree of illness. A distaste for smoking, paralleling anorexia, may occur early. Nausea and vomiting are frequent, and diarrhea or constipation may occur. Skin rashes, arthritis, or serum sickness may be seen early in acute hepatitis B. Fever is generally present but is rarely over 39.5 °C (103.1 °F) save in occasional cases of hepatitis A. Defervescence often coincides with the onset of jaundice. Chills or chilliness may mark an acute onset.

Abdominal pain is usually mild and constant in the right upper quadrant or right epigastrium and is often aggravated by jarring or exertion. (On rare occasions, upper abdominal pain may be severe enough to simulate cholecystitis or cholelithiasis.)

2. Icteric phase–Clinical jaundice occurs after 5–10 days but may appear at the same time as the initial symptomatology. Most patients never develop clinical icterus. With the onset of jaundice, there is often an intensification of the prodromal symptoms, followed by progressive clinical improvement.

3. Convalescent phase–There is an increasing sense of well-being, return of appetite, and disappearance of jaundice, abdominal pain and tenderness, and fatigability.

4. Course and complications–The acute illness usually subsides rapidly over a 2- to 3-week period with complete clinical and laboratory recovery by 9 weeks in hepatitis A and by 16 weeks in hepatitis B and hepatitis C. In 5–10% of cases, the course may be more protracted, and less than 1% will have an acute fulminant course.

B. Signs: Hepatomegaly—rarely marked—is present in over half of cases. Liver tenderness is usually present. Splenomegaly is reported in 15% of patients, and soft, enlarged lymph nodes—especially in the cervical or epitrochlear areas—may occur. Signs of general toxemia vary from minimal to severe.

C. Laboratory Findings: The white cell count is normal to low, especially in the preicteric phase. Large atypical lymphocytes, such as are found in infectious mononucleosis, may occasionally be seen. Mild proteinuria is common, and bilirubinuria often precedes the appearance of jaundice. Acholic stools are often present during the initial icteric phase. Blood and urine studies reflect hepatocellular damage with often strikingly elevated AST or ALT values. Bilirubin and alkaline phosphatase are elevated and, in a minority of patients, remain so after aminotransferase levels have normalized. Cholestasis is occasionally marked in acute hepatitis A. The prothrombin time may be prolonged in severe hepatitis and is a useful prognostic factor.

Differential Diagnosis

The differential diagnosis of hepatitis includes other viral diseases such as infectious mononucleosis, cytomegalovirus infection, and herpes simplex virus infection; spirochetal diseases such as leptospirosis and secondary syphilis; brucellosis; rickettsial diseases such as Q fever; drug-induced liver disease; and shock liver (ischemic hepatitis). Occasionally, chronic active hepatitis (see below) may have an acute onset mimicking acute viral hepatitis. Rarely, metastatic cancer of the liver may present with a hepatitis-like picture.

The prodromal phase of viral hepatitis must be distinguished from other infectious disease such as influenza, upper respiratory infections, and the prodromal stages of the exanthematous diseases. Occasionally. cholestasis may be prominent in viral hepatitis and mimic obstructive jaundice.

Prevention

Strict isolation of patients is not necessary, but hand washing after bowel movements is required. Thorough hand washing by medical attendants who come into contact with contaminated utensils, bedding, or clothing is essential. Careful handling of disposable needles—including not recapping used needles—is important for medical personnel. Screening of donated blood for HBsAg, anti-HBc, anti-HCV, and elevated ALT (a "surrogate" marker of HCV) has reduced the risk of transfusion-associated hepatitis markedly. In addition, all pregnant women should undergo testing for HBsAg. Unnecessary transfusions and commercially obtained blood should be avoided.

A. Immune Globulin: Immune globulin should be routinely given to all *close* (eg, household) personal contacts of patients with hepatitis A. The recommended dose of 0.02 mL/kg intramuscularly has been found to be protective for hepatitis A if administered during the incubation period. It is also desirable that individuals traveling to or residing in endemic regions receive immune globulin within 2 weeks after arrival; if staying more than 2 months, the recommended dose is 5 mL for adults. In the event of prolonged residence, a second dose should be given after 5–6 months. A hepatitis A vaccine should be available commercially in the near future.

B. Hepatitis B Immune Globulin: Hepatitis B immune globulin may be protective if given in large doses within 7 days of exposure and again at 30 days (adult dose is 0.06 mL/kg body weight). At present, this preparation is recommended for individuals exposed to hepatitis B surface antigen-contaminated material via the mucous membranes or through breaks in the skin. Persons who have had sexual contact with patients with acute hepatitis B surface antigen-positive disease should also receive hepatitis B hyperimmune globulin. Hepatitis B immune globulin is also indicated for newborn infants of HBsAg-positive mothers; give 0.5 mL intramuscularly shortly after birth. In addition to immune hepatitis B globulin in the above clinical situation, the vaccine series should be promptly initiated (see below).

C. Hepatitis B Vaccine: The currently used vaccine is recombinant-derived. Recipients should have a negative serologic test for HBsAg and HBcAb. Until recently, the vaccine was targeted to persons at high risk, including renal dialysis patients and attending personnel, patients requiring repeated transfusions, spouses of HBsAg-positive individuals, male homosexuals, intravenous drug abusers, newborns of HBsAg-positive mothers, entering medical and nursing students as well as all medical technologists. Because this strategy failed to lower the incidence of hepatitis B, the CDCP has recommended universal vaccination of infants and children in the USA. Over 90% of recipients of the vaccine mount protective antibody to hepatitis B. The dose for adults is 1 mL initially and 1 mL again at 1 and 6 months; for greatest reliability of absorption, the deltoid muscle is the preferred site of injection. The newborn and pediatric dose is one-half the adult dose. Postimmunization anti-HBs titers need to be checked to ascertain response. Protection appears to be excellent even if the titer wanes—at least up to 9 years.

Treatment

Bed rest is recommended only on an as-needed basis during the acute initial phase of the disease, when symptoms are most severe. However, return to normal activity during the convalescent period should be gradual. If nausea and vomiting are pronounced or if oral intake is substantially decreased, intravenous administration of 10% glucose solution is indicated. If the patient shows signs of impending coma, protein should be restricted until clinical improvement takes place. In general, dietary management consists of giving palatable meals as tolerated, without overfeeding. Patients with acute hepatitis should avoid strenuous physical exertion, alcohol, and hepatotoxic agents. While the administration of small doses of oxazepam is safe (not metabolized or excreted by the liver), it is recommended that morphine sulfate be avoided.

In controlled studies, corticosteroids have demonstrated no benefit in patients with viral hepatitis, including those with fulminant hepatitis. Preliminary trials suggest some benefit from interferon in acute hepatitis C (decreased risk of chronic hepatitis C), but further study is required.

Prognosis

The clinical course, morbidity, and mortality of viral hepatitis may vary considerably. In most cases, clinical recovery is complete in 3–16 weeks. Laboratory evidence of liver dysfunction may persist for a longer period, but most such patients recover completely. The overall mortality rate is less than 1%, but the rate is reportedly higher in older people.

Hepatitis A does not progress to chronic liver disease, though hepatitis A may persist for up to 1 year, and clinical and biochemical relapses may occur before full recovery. The mortality rate is less than 0.2%. Less than 10% of hepatitis B patients and as many as 50% of hepatitis C patients develop chronic liver disease (see below). The mortality rate for acute hepatitis B is 0.1–1%, and it is even higher for superimposed hepatitis D. For unknown reasons, the mortality rate for hepatitis E is especially high in pregnant women (10–20%).

Chronic hepatitis, characterized by elevated aminotransferase levels for more than 6 months, occurs in 5–10% of patients with hepatitis B and 50% of those with hepatitis C. Some patients with chronic hepatitis develop chronic active hepatitis with cirrhosis; this occurs in up to 30% of those with chronic hepatitis C and 40% of those with chronic hepatitis B. These patients are also at risk for hepatocellular carcinoma.

Alter HJ: Descartes before the horse: I clone, therefore I am: the hepatitis C virus in current perspective. Ann Intern Med 1991;115:644. (Account of the discovery of hepatitis C virus and review of epidemiology and diagnosis.)

Alter HJ et al: Detection of antibody to hepatitis C virus in prospectively followed transfusion recipients with acute and chronic non-A, non-B hepatitis. N Engl J Med 1989;321:1494. (Evidence that hepatitis C is responsible for most cases of posttransfusion hepatitis.)

Carman WF, Thomas HC: Genetic variation in hepatitis B virus. Gastroenterology 1992;102:711.

Carson JL et al: The risks of blood transfusion: The relative influence of acquired immunodeficiency syndrome and non-A, non-B hepatitis. Am J Med 1992;92:45. (Non-A, non-B accounts for 97% of transfusion-related deaths.)

Dienstag JL (editor): Viral hepatitis. Semin Liver Dis 1991;11:73.

Estabon JI et al: Evaluation of antibodies to hepatitis C virus in a study of transfusion-associated hepatitis. N Engl J Med 1990;323:1107. (Screening of blood donors for anti-HCV antibody should prevent half of cases of posttransfusion hepatitis.)

Gust ID, Feinstone SM: Hepatitis A. Prog Liver Dis 1990;9:371.

Hepatitis B virus: A comprehensive strategy for eliminating transmission in the U.S. through universal childhood vaccination. MMWR 1991;40 RR 13 :1.

CLINICAL VARIANTS OF VIRAL HEPATITIS

Cholestatic Hepatitis

In occasional cases of acute hepatitis A, cholestasis is the dominant manifestation of the disease. The course tends to be more prolonged than that of ordinary hepatitis. The symptoms are often extremely mild, but jaundice is deeper and pruritus is often present. Laboratory tests of liver function indicate hyperbilirubinemia, bilirubinuria, and elevated alkaline phosphatase and cholesterol. Differentiation of this type of hepatitis from extrahepatic obstruction may be difficult. Ultrasonography should be performed to exclude biliary dilation. Rarely, percutaneous transhepatic cholangiography or endoscopic retrograde cholangiography may be necessary to exclude biliary obstruction.

Fulminant Hepatitis

Hepatitis may take a rapidly progressive course terminating in death in less than 10 days. Up to 50% of cases of fulminant viral hepatitis are due to hepatitis B—in some cases detectable only by molecular techniques (polymerase chain reaction). Most of the remainder are due to hepatitis A or unknown viruses. In endemic areas, hepatitis D and hepatitis E may cause fulminant hepatitis. Hepatitis C appears to be a rare cause of fulminant hepatitis. Extensive necrosis of large areas of the liver gives the typical pathologic picture of acute liver atrophy. Toxemia, gastrointestinal symptoms, and hemorrhagic phenomena are common. Hepatic encephalopathy and coagulopathy are invariable. Jaundice may be absent or minimal, but laboratory tests show severe hepatocellular damage. A more insidious (subfulminant) course is occasionally seen, characterized by progressive clinical deterioration over an 8- to 24-week period, leading to encephalopathy and then usually to death.

The treatment of fulminant hepatitis is directed toward those metabolic abnormalities associated with severe liver cell dysfunction. They include coagulation defects; disordered fluid, electrolyte, and acid-base balance; hypoglycemia; and nitrogenous intoxication. Monitoring of the patient, with vigorous correction of the deficits noted, provides the hope that some patients will survive who might otherwise succumb before liver regeneration can occur. Early transfer to a liver transplantation center is essential. Extradural sensors may be placed to monitor intracranial pressure.

Adrenocorticosteroids, exchange transfusions, and perfusions through pig and baboon livers have not proved effective. The mortality rate of fulminant hepatitis with severe encephalopathy is as high as 80%. Emergency liver transplantation has been associated with an 80% survival rate at 1 year.

Capocaccia L, Angelo M: Fulminant hepatic failure: Clinical features, etiology, epidemiology and current management. Dig Dis Sci 1991;36:775.

Martin PP, Pappas C: Fulminant hepatic failure. Dig Dis 1990;8:138. (Pathophysiology and management.)

CHRONIC HEPATITIS

Chronic hepatitis is defined as a chronic inflammatory reaction of the liver of more than 6 months' duration, as demonstrated by persistently abnormal serum aminotransferase levels and characteristic histologic findings. The causes of chronic hepatitis include HBV, HCV, and HDV. Idiopathic chronic active hepatitis is an autoimmune disease associated with a variety of circulating autoantibodies. Additionally, chronic hepatitis may be associated with certain medications, including methyldopa and isoniazid. Wilson's disease, α_1-antiprotease (α_1-antitrypsin) deficiency, hemochromatosis, and alcoholic liver disease can also present as chronic hepatitis.

1. CHRONIC PERSISTENT HEPATITIS

Chronic persistent hepatitis generally represents an essentially benign condition with a good prognosis. The diagnosis is confirmed by liver biopsy, which may show portal tract infiltration with primarily mononuclear cells and occasional areas of focal inflammation in the parenchyma. The boundary between portal tracts and parenchyma remains sharp, and there is little or no "piecemeal necrosis" (a process in which the liver cells are gradually destroyed and replaced by fibrous tissue septa). The architecture of the hepatic lobule remains intact. The symptomatology varies from the asymptomatic state to various vague manifestations including fatigability, anorexia, malaise, and lassitude. Physical examination is usually normal. Laboratory findings are those of intermittent or persistent elevations of aminotransferase levels, usually in the range of two or three times normal.

Liver biopsy establishes the diagnosis of chronic persistent hepatitis. The prognosis is generally excellent, but recent studies suggest that chronic persistent hepatitis B or C may in occasional cases slowly progress to cirrhosis, and treatment with interferon alfa-2b should be considered (see below).

2. CHRONIC ACTIVE HEPATITIS

Chronic active hepatitis is characterized by piecemeal necrosis, an inflammatory process at the interface of the portal area and the liver lobule. In severe cases, piecemeal necrosis may be associated with considerable hepatic fibrosis and ultimately with cirrhosis; aminotransferase levels may be very high. In very mild cases, it may be difficult to distinguish this entity from chronic persistent hepatitis. Liver biopsies repeated at varying intervals may be necessary to make the distinction as well as to monitor therapy.

Clinical Findings & Diagnosis

A. Idiopathic (Autoimmune) Chronic Active Hepatitis: This is generally a disease of young people, particularly young women. However, the disease can occur at any age. The onset is usually insidious, but about 25% of cases present as an acute attack of hepatitis. Although the serum bilirubin is usually increased, 20% of these patients have anicteric disease. Examination often reveals a healthy-appearing young woman with multiple spider nevi, cutaneous striae, acne, and hirsutism. Amenorrhea may be a feature of this disease. Extrahepatic features include arthritis, Sjögren's syndrome, thyroiditis, nephritis, and Coombs-positive hemolytic anemia. In classic idiopathic (autoimmune) chronic active hepatitis, 20–50% of patients are positive for antinuclear antibody (ANA) and 40–80% for smooth muscle antibody. Serum gamma globulin levels are typically elevated (up to 5–6 g/dL). Markers for hepatitis B are absent.

B. Chronic Active Hepatitis B: Chronic active hepatitis B affects chiefly males. It may be noted as a continuum of acute hepatitis or may be diagnosed on evaluation of persistently elevated aminotransferase levels.

In the more active form, HBeAg and HBV DNA are present, indicative of active viral replications. IgM anti-HBc is also present in about 70%. In some patients, clinical and biochemical improvement coincides with disappearance of HBeAg and HBV DNA from serum, appearance of anti-HBe, and integration of the HBV genome into the host genome in infected hepatocytes. There are increased risks for the development of cirrhosis and hepatocellular carcinoma in these patients.

C. Delta Agent in Hepatitis B: Acute delta infection superimposed on chronic HBV infection may result in severe acute hepatitis or severe chronic active hepatitis. The latter may progress rapidly to cirrhosis, which may be fatal. The diagnosis is confirmed by detection of anti-HDV in serum.

D. Chronic Active Hepatitis C: This type occurs in up to 50% or more of patients with posttransfusion hepatitis and in sporadic cases. It is clinically indistinguishable from chronic active hepatitis due to other causes and may actually be the most common. The diagnosis is confirmed by detection of anti-HCV by second-generation enzyme immunoassay (EIA). In occasional cases of suspected chronic hepatitis C but a negative EIA, the diagnosis may be confirmed by a positive recombinant immunoblot assay (RIBA).

Treatment

Prolonged or enforced bed rest has not been shown to be beneficial. Activity should be modified according to the patient's symptoms. The diet should be well balanced, without specific limitations other than sodium or protein restrictions as dictated by water retention or encephalopathy.

Prednisone with or without azathioprine has been shown to decrease the serum bilirubin, aminotransferase, and gamma globulin levels and reduce the piecemeal necrosis in patients with idiopathic (autoimmune) chronic active hepatitis. Symptomatic patients with serum aminotransferase levels elevated tenfold (or fivefold if the serum globulins are elevated at least twofold) are candidates for therapy. The mortality rate in patients treated with corticosteroids is significantly reduced.

Prednisone or an equivalent drug is given initially in doses of 30 mg orally daily with azathioprine or mercaptopurine, 50 mg/d orally. Azathioprine at doses of more than 1.5 mg/kg body weight for a prolonged period imposes a significant hazard of bone marrow suppression, but doses of 50 mg/d are well tolerated and permit the use of lower corticosteroid doses. Nevertheless, complete blood counts should be monitored weekly for the first 8 weeks of therapy and at less frequent intervals subsequently. The dose of prednisone is lowered from 30 mg/d after 1 week to 20 mg/d and again after 2 weeks to 15 mg/d. Ultimately, a maintenance dose of 10 mg/d is achieved. While symptomatic improvement is often prompt, biochemical improvement is more gradual, with normalization of serum aminotransferase levels after 6–12 months in many cases. Histologic resolution of inflammation may take up to 18–24 months, the recommended time for repeat liver biopsy. Failure of aminotransferase levels to normalize invariably predicts lack of histologic resolution.

The response rate to therapy with prednisone and azathioprine is as high as 80–90%. Cirrhosis, however, does not reverse with therapy and may even develop after apparent biochemical and histologic remission (absence of inflammation). Once remission is achieved, therapy may be withdrawn, but the subsequent relapse rate is 50–90%. Relapses may again be treated in the same manner as the initial episode, with again an expected remission rate of 80–90%. After successful treatment of a relapse, the patient may be kept indefinitely on azathioprine 50 mg and the lowest dose of prednisone needed to maintain normal aminotransferase levels.

Patients with chronic hepatitis B and active viral replication (HBeAg and HBV DNA in serum; elevated aminotransferase levels) may be treated with recombinant human interferon alfa-2b in a dose of 5 million units a day intramuscularly for 4 months. About 40% of treated patients will respond with normalization of aminotransferase levels, disappearance of HBeAg and HBV DNA from serum, and appearance of anti-HBe. Moreover, over 60% of these responders may eventually clear HBsAg from serum and liver, develop anti-HBs in serum, and thus be cured of the infection. Relapses are uncommon in such complete responders.

Recombinant human interferon alfa-2b in a dose of 3 million units three times a week for 24 weeks has been shown to induce biochemical and histologic improvement in up to 50% of patients with chronic hepatitis C. After stopping the medication at 24 weeks, only 30–50% of the treated responders will maintain the improvement. Experience with this agent is still limited, treatment is costly, and side effects, which include flu-like symptoms, are almost universal; more serious side effects, ie, psychiatric symptoms (irritability, depression), thyroid dysfunction, and bone marrow suppression, are less common. Interferon is contraindicated in patients with decompensated cirrhosis due to chronic hepatitis B, profound cytopenias, psychiatric disease, and autoimmune diseases.

Prognosis

The course of chronic active hepatitis is variable and unpredictable. Untreated idiopathic chronic active hepatitis has a 5-year mortality rate of 50%, which decreases markedly with treatment. The sequelae of chronic active hepatitis secondary to hepatitis B include cirrhosis, liver failure, and hepatocellular carcinoma. Up to 40–50% of patients with chronic active hepatitis B and cirrhosis die within 5 years after onset of symptoms. Whether therapy with interferon will alter the natural history remains to be determined. Chronic hepatitis C is an indolent, often subclinical disease that may lead to cirrhosis and hepatocellular carcinoma after decades. The impact of interferon also remains to be seen.

DiBisceglie AM, Hoofnagle JH: Therapy of chronic hepatitis C with alpha-interferon: The answer? Or more questions? Hepatology 1991;13:601. (Thoughtful editorial. More information and better techniques still needed.)

Hay JE et al: The nature of unexplained chronic aminotransferase elevations of a mild to moderate degree in asymptomatic patients. Hepatology 1989;9:193. (Only histopathology will differentiate.)

Hoofnagle JH: Type D (delta) hepatitis. JAMA 1989;261:1321. (Inexorably linked to hepatitis B. Review of clinical course and markers.)

Maddrey WC: Chronic hepatitis. Dis Mon (Feb) 1993;39:53. (Definition, etiology, diagnosis, pathogenesis, and management.)

Marcellin P et al: Recombinant human alpha-interferon in patients with chronic non-A, non-B hepatitis: A multicentered randomized controlled trial from France. Hepatology 1991;13:393. (Three million units intramuscularly three times a week has long-term effectiveness in 50% of those [35–50%] who responded to the initial 6 months of treatment.)

Meyer zum Büschenfelde K-H (editor): Autoimmune hepatitis. Semin Liver Dis 1991;11:183.

ALCOHOLIC HEPATITIS

Alcoholic hepatitis is an acute or chronic inflammation of the liver that occurs as a result of parenchymal necrosis induced by alcohol abuse and is a precursor of alcoholic cirrhosis.

While alcoholic hepatitis is often a reversible disease, it is the most common cause of cirrhosis in the USA. This is especially significant, since cirrhosis ranks among the most common causes of death of adults in this country. Alcoholic hepatitis does not develop in all chronic heavy drinkers; the exact prevalence and incidence are not known but have been estimated to be about 8–15%. Women appear to be more susceptible than men, in part because of lower gastric mucosal alcohol dehydrogenase levels.

Alcoholic hepatitis usually occurs after years of excessive drinking. Although it may not develop in many patients even after several decades of alcohol abuse, it appears in a few individuals within a year of excessive drinking. Over 80% of patients with alcoholic hepatitis were drinking 5 years or more before developing any symptoms that could be attributed to liver disease. In general, the longer the duration of drinking (10–15 or more years) and the larger the alcoholic consumption (usually more than 120 g of alcohol per day, which is equal to 8 oz of 100-proof whiskey, 30 oz of wine, or 100 oz of beer (eight 12-oz cans), the greater the probability of developing alcoholic hepatitis and cirrhosis. It is also important to realize that while drinking large amounts of alcoholic beverages is essential for the development of alcoholic hepatitis, drunkenness is not. In drinking individuals, the rate of ethanol metabolism can be sufficiently high to permit the consumption of large quantities of spirits without raising the blood alcohol level over 80 mg/dL, the concentration at which the conventional breath analyzer begins to detect ethanol.

The role of deficiencies in vitamins and calories in the development of alcoholic hepatitis or in the progression of this lesion to cirrhosis are not understood.

Only liver biopsy can establish the diagnosis with certainty, since any of the manifestations of alcoholic hepatitis can be seen in other types of alcoholic liver disease such as fatty liver or cirrhosis, as well as liver disease due to other causes.

Clinical Findings

A. Symptoms and Signs: Alcoholic hepatitis is usually seen after a recent period of heavy drinking. That history in addition to complaints of anorexia and nausea and the demonstration of hepatomegaly and jaundice strongly suggest the diagnosis. Abdominal pain and tenderness, splenomegaly, ascites, fever, and encephalopathy support the diagnosis. The clinical presentation of alcoholic hepatitis can vary from an asymptomatic patient with an enlarged liver to a critically ill individual who dies quickly.

B. Laboratory Findings: Anemia is variable and usually macrocytic. Leukocytosis with shift to the left is common and is seen more frequently in patients with severe disease. Leukopenia is occasionally seen and disappears after cessation of drinking. About 10% of patients have thrombocytopenia that appears related to a direct toxic effect of alcohol on megakaryocyte production.

AST is usually elevated but rarely above 300 units/mL. AST is almost invariably greater than ALT, often by a factor of 2–5 or more. Serum alkaline phosphatase is generally elevated, but rarely more than three times the normal value. Serum bilirubin is increased in 60–90% of patients. Serum bilirubin levels greater than 10 mg/dL and marked prolongation of the prothrombin time ($\geq$ 6 seconds above control) indicate severe disease with a mortality rate as high as 50%. The serum albumin is depressed, and the gamma globulin level is elevated in 50–75% of

individuals with alcoholic hepatitis even in the absence of cirrhosis.

Liver biopsy is usually diagnostic and demonstrates macrovesicular fat, PMN infiltration, and Mallory bodies (alcoholic hyaline). Micronodular cirrhosis may be present as well.

C. Special Procedures: Ultrasound is often helpful in ruling out biliary obstruction or to assess for subclinical ascites. CT scanning with intravenous contrast or MRI may be indicated in selected cases to evaluate patients for collateral vessels, space-occupying lesions of the liver, or concomitant disease of the pancreas.

Differential Diagnosis

Alcoholic hepatitis may be closely mimicked by diseases of the hepatobiliary tree such as cholecystitis and cholelithiasis. A history of chronic insobriety and recent debauch is helpful but far from conclusive. Percutaneous liver biopsy, if there is no contraindication, is a reliable means of differentiation; alternatively, various imaging procedures may indicate primary biliary tract disease. The clinical, biochemical, and histologic picture of alcoholic hepatitis may be mimicked by certain drugs such as amiodarone.

Complications

Clinical deterioration and worsening abdominal pain and tenderness may result in the unfortunate decision to perform laparotomy. The postoperative mortality rate of acutely ill patients with alcoholic hepatitis is far greater than that of those who are operated on for intra- or extrahepatic cholestasis. This is related to the poor nutritional status of these patients and the compromised synthesizing function of the liver. Ascites may develop during the course of alcoholic hepatitis and should resolve as the hepatitis improves; diuretics are not generally indicated. Bleeding due to coagulopathy is a potential complication.

Treatment

A. General Measures: Discontinue all alcoholic beverages. During periods of anorexia, every effort should be made to provide sufficient amounts of carbohydrate and calories to reduce endogenous protein catabolism and to support gluconeogenesis and prevent hypoglycemia. Although the clinical value of intravenous hyperalimentation has not been established, the judicious administration of parenteral fluids is most important. Caloric intake is gratifyingly improved by the use of palatable liquid formulas during the transition period between totally intravenous alimentation and normal feeding. The administration of vitamins, particularly folic acid and thiamin, is indicated, especially when deficiencies are noted.

B. Corticosteroids: Several studies have shown that methylprednisolone, 32 mg/d for 1 month, is beneficial in patients with alcoholic hepatitis and either encephalopathy or greatly elevated bilirubin concentrations and prolonged prothrombin times. Propylthiouracil, which reverses the hypermetabolic state associated with alcoholic hepatitis, has shown some promise in early trials. Insulin and glucagon may stimulate hepatic regeneration but may cause fatal hypoglycemia and cannot be recommended.

Prognosis

A. Short-Term: When the prothrombin time is short enough to permit performance of liver biopsy without risk, the 1-year mortality rate is 7.1%, rising to 18% if there is progressive prolongation of that parameter during hospitalization. Individuals in whom the prothrombin time is so prolonged that liver biopsy cannot be attempted have a 42% mortality rate at 1 year. Other unfavorable prognostic factors are a serum bilirubin greater than 10 mg/dL, hepatic encephalopathy, and azotemia.

B. Long-Term: In the USA, the mortality rate over a 3-year period of persons who recover from acute alcoholic hepatitis is ten times greater than that of average individuals of comparable age. The histologically severe form of the disease is associated with continued excessive mortality rates after 3 years, whereas the death rate is not increased after the same period in those whose liver biopsies show only mild alcoholic hepatitis. Complications of portal hypertension (ascites, varices) following recovery from acute alcoholic hepatitis also suggest a poor long-term prognosis.

The most important prognostic consideration is the indisputable fact that continued excessive drinking is associated with reduction of life expectancy in these individuals. The prognosis is indeed poor if the patient is unable to abstain from drinking.

Carithers RL Jr et al: Methylprednisolone therapy in patients with severe alcoholic hepatitis: A randomized multicenter trial. Ann Intern Med 1989;110:685. (Striking decrease in short-term mortality rate.)
Maddrey WC: Alcoholic hepatitis: Clinicopathologic features and therapy. Semin Liver Dis 1988;8:91.
Ramond MJ et al: A randomized trial of prednisolone in patients with severe alcoholic hepatitis. N Engl J Med 1992;326:507. (Improves short-term survival in patients with severe disease—encephalopathy or profound coagulopathy.)

DRUG- & TOXIN-INDUCED LIVER DISEASE

The continuing synthesis, testing, and introduction of new drugs into clinical practice has resulted in an increase in toxic reactions of many types. Many widely used therapeutic agents may cause hepatic injury. The diagnosis of drug-induced liver injury is not always easy. Drug-induced liver disease can mimic viral hepatitis or biliary tract obstruction. In any patient with liver disease, the clinician must inquire carefully about the use of potentially hepatotoxic drugs or exposure to hepatotoxins. Drug toxicity may be categorized on the basis of pathogenesis or histologic appearance.

Direct Hepatotoxic Group

The liver lesion caused by this group of drugs is characterized by (1) dose-related severity, (2) reproducibility in experimental animals, (3) a latent period following exposure, and (4) susceptibility in all individuals. Examples include acetaminophen, alcohol, carbon tetrachloride, chloroform, heavy metals, mercaptopurine, phosphorus, tetracyclines, valproic acid, and vitamin A.

Idiosyncratic Reactions

Reactions of this type are sporadic, not related to dose, and occasionally associated with features suggesting an allergic reaction, such as fever and eosinophilia. In some cases, toxicity results directly from a metabolite that is produced only in certain individuals on a genetic basis. Examples include amiodarone, aspirin, chloramphenicol, dantrolene, halothane, isoniazid, ketoconazole, methyldopa, oxazacillin, phenylbutazone, phenytoin, pyrazinamide, quinidine, and streptomycin.

Cholestatic Reactions

There are two general categories that differ in clinical presentation and histopathologic features. These reactions are dose-dependent, but marked differences in individual susceptibility exist:

A. Noninflammatory: Probable direct effect of agent on bile secretory mechanisms and on inflammatory reactions: azathioprine, mercaptopurine, mestranol, methyltestosterone, norethandrolone.

B. Inflammatory: Inflammation of portal areas, with allergic features, eg, eosinophilia: chlorothiazide, chlorpromazine, chlorpropamide, erythromycin estolate, penicillamine, prochlorperazine, promazine, sulfadiazine, thiouracils.

Chronic Active Hepatitis

Clinically and histologically indistinguishable from idiopathic chronic active hepatitis: aspirin, dantrolene, isoniazid, methyldopa, nitrofurantoin, oxyphenisatin, sulfonamides.

Miscellaneous Reactions

A. Fatty Liver:

1. Large fatty inclusions–Alcohol, amiodarone, corticosteroids, methotrexate.

2. Small cytoplasmic droplets–Tetracyclines, valproic acid.

B. Granulomas: Allopurinol, quinidine, phenylbutazone, phenytoin.

C. Fibrosis and Cirrhosis: Methotrexate.

D. Peliosis Hepatis: Anabolic steroids (fluoxymesterone), azathioprine, oral contraceptive steroids.

E. Neoplasms: Oral contraceptive steroids (hepatic adenoma); vinyl chloride (angiosarcoma).

Kaplowitz N (editor): Recent advances in drug metabolism and hepatotoxicity. Semin Liver Dis 1990;10:235.

FATTY LIVER

It was formerly believed that malnutrition rather than ethanol was responsible for steatosis (fatty metamorphosis) of the liver in the alcoholic. More recently, it has become clear that ethanol is hepatotoxic in the absence of malnutrition. Nevertheless, inadequate diets—specifically, those deficient in choline, methionine, and dietary protein—can produce fatty liver (kwashiorkor) in children, and malnutrition may contribute to liver damage caused by ethanol.

Other nonalcoholic causes of steatosis are obesity (the commonest cause), starvation, diabetes mellitus, corticosteroids, poisons (carbon tetrachloride and yellow phosphorus), endocrinopathies such as Cushing's syndrome, hyperlipidemia, and total parenteral nutrition. (Microvesicular steatosis may result from Reye's syndrome, valproic acid, high-dose tetracycline, or acute fatty liver of pregnancy.)

There are apparently at least five factors, acting in varying combinations, that are responsible for the accumulation of fat in the liver: (1) increased mobilization of fatty acids from peripheral adipose depots; (2) decreased utilization or oxidation of fatty acids by the liver; (3) increased hepatic fatty acid synthesis; (4) increased esterification of fatty acids into triglycerides; and (5) decreased secretion or liberation of fat from the liver.

Liver function studies may show mildly elevated aminotransferase and alkaline phosphatase levels. Increased hepatic fat is readily demonstrated on MRI. Percutaneous liver biopsy is diagnostic but seldom needed.

Treatment consists of removing or modifying the offending factor.

Prognosis depends on the underlying condition.

Gauthier M et al: Reye's syndrome: A reappraisal of diagnosis in 49 presumptive cases. Am J Dis Child 1989;143:1181.
Mabie WC: Acute fatty liver of pregnancy. Crit Care Clin 1991;7:799.
Powell EE et al: The natural history of nonalcoholic steatohepatitis: A follow-up study of forty-two patients. Hepatology 1990;11:74. (A probable cause of "cryptogenic cirrhosis.")

CIRRHOSIS

Cirrhosis is the end result of hepatocellular injury that leads to both fibrosis and nodular regeneration throughout the liver. Cirrhosis is a serious and irreversible disease and was the ninth leading cause of death in the USA in 1989, with an incidence of 9:100,000 per year, over 65% of cases alcohol-related. The clinical features of cirrhosis result from hepatic cell dysfunction, portosystemic shunting, and portal hypertension.

The histopathology of cirrhosis may change with the passage of time in any one patient. Terms such as "portal" and "postnecrotic" cirrhosis refer not so much to separate disease states with different causes as to different expressions of hepatic injury.

The most common histologic classification divides cirrhosis into micronodular, mixed, and macronodular forms. It is important, however, to remember that these are descriptive terms rather than separate diseases and that each form may be seen in the same patient at different stages of his or her disease.

(1) Micronodular cirrhosis is the form in which the regenerating nodules are no larger than the original lobules, ie, approximately 1 mm in diameter or less. It has been suggested that this feature results from the persistence of the offending agent (alcohol), a substance that prevents regenerative growth.

(2) Macronodular cirrhosis is characterized by larger nodules, which can measure several centimeters in diameter and often contain central veins. This form corresponds more or less to postnecrotic (posthepatitic) cirrhosis but does not necessarily follow episodes of massive necrosis and stromal collapse.

(3) Mixed macro- and micronodular cirrhosis signifies that the features of cirrhosis are variable. In any case, the configuration of the liver is determined by the mixture of liver cell death and regeneration as well as the deposition of fat, iron, and fibrosis.

There does exist a limited relationship between the histologic form of cirrhosis and etiology and prognosis. For example, alcoholics who continue to drink tend to have micronodular cirrhosis. The presence of fatty micronodular cirrhosis is strongly suggestive of chronic alcoholism. On the other hand, there is a higher incidence of hepatocellular carcinoma in macronodular than in micronodular cirrhosis. This propensity to malignancy is perhaps related either to increased regenerative activity in the liver in macronodular cirrhosis or to the long period required for the process to develop.

Clinical Findings

A. Symptoms and Signs: Micronodular (Laennec's) cirrhosis may cause no symptoms for long periods, both at onset and later in the course (compensated phase). The onset of symptoms may be insidious or, less often, abrupt. Weakness, fatigability, and weight loss are common. In advanced cirrhosis, anorexia is usually present and may be extreme, with associated nausea and occasional vomiting. Abdominal pain may be present and is related either to hepatic enlargement and stretching of Glisson's capsule or to the presence of ascites. Menstrual abnormalities (usually amenorrhea), impotence, loss of libido, sterility, and painfully enlarged breasts in men may occur. Hematemesis is the presenting symptom in 15–25%.

In 70% of cases, the liver is enlarged, palpable, and firm if not hard and has a blunt or nodular edge; and the left lobe may predominate. Skin manifestations consist of spider nevi (usually only on the upper half of the body), palmar erythema (mottled redness of the thenar and hypothenar eminences), telangiectases of exposed areas, and evidence of vitamin deficiencies (glossitis and cheilosis). Weight loss, wasting, and the appearance of chronic illness are present. Jaundice—usually not an initial sign—is mild at first, increasing in severity during the later stages of the disease. Ascites, pleural effusion, peripheral edema, and purpuric lesions are late findings. Precoma (sleep reversal, asterixis, tremor, dysarthrias, delirium, and drowsiness) and coma also occur very late except when precipitated by an acute hepatocellular insult or an episode of gastrointestinal bleeding. Fever may be present in 35% on presentation and usually reflects a complication such as alcoholic hepatitis, spontaneous bacterial peritonitis, cholangitis, or some other intercurrent event. Clinical splenomegaly is present in 35–50% of cases. The superficial veins of the abdomen and thorax may be dilated and reflect the intrahepatic obstruction to portal blood flow, as do rectal varices and hemorrhoids.

B. Laboratory Findings: Laboratory abnormalities are either absent or minimal in latent or quiescent cirrhosis. Anemia, a frequent finding, is often macrocytic; causes include suppression of erythropoiesis by alcohol as well as folate deficiency, hemolysis, hypersplenism, and insidious or overt blood loss from the gastrointestinal tract. The white cell count may be low, elevated, or normal, reflecting hypersplenism or infection; thrombocytopenia may be secondary to alcoholic marrow suppression, sepsis, folate deficiency, or splenic sequestration. Coagulation abnormalities may also be a result of failure of synthesis of clotting constituents in the liver.

Blood chemical studies show primarily hepatocellular injury and dysfunction, reflected by elevations of AST, alkaline phosphatase, and bilirubin. Serum albumin is low; gamma globulin is increased.

Liver biopsy may show inactive cirrhosis (fibrosis with regenerative nodules) with no specific features to suggest the underlying cause. Alternatively, there may be additional features of alcoholic liver disease, chronic active hepatitis, or other specific causes of cirrhosis.

C. Imaging: Plain films of the abdomen may re-

veal hepatic or splenic enlargement. Barium studies of the upper gastrointestinal tract may reveal the presence of esophageal or gastric varices, though endoscopy is more sensitive. Ultrasound is helpful for determining the presence of occult ascites, liver size, or hepatic nodules, including small hepatocellular carcinomas. Together with Doppler studies, ultrasound is increasingly used to evaluate patency of the splenic, portal, and hepatic veins, but splenoportography is still the standard procedure. Hepatic nodules may be characterized further by CT scan with intravenous bolus contrast injection or MRI along with serum alpha-fetoprotein levels. Nodules suspicious for malignancy may be biopsied under ultrasound or CT guidance.

D. Special Examinations: Esophagogastroscopy demonstrates or confirms the presence of varices and detects specific causes of bleeding in the esophagus, stomach, and proximal duodenum. Laparoscopy may be helpful in judging the type of cirrhosis present though it is usually unnecessary for clinical purposes.

Differential Diagnosis

As previously noted, differentiation of one type of cirrhosis from another can be difficult, but determining the cause is important both for prognostic and, potentially, therapeutic reasons. Hemochromatosis may be associated with "bronzing" of the skin, arthritis, heart failure, and diabetes mellitus; greater than 50% saturation of serum transferrin or an elevated serum ferritin level will add to the suspicion for hemochromatosis, and special staining for iron and quantitation of the iron on liver biopsy will confirm the diagnosis. Primary biliary cirrhosis occurs more frequently in women and is associated with marked pruritus, significant elevation of alkaline phosphatase, elevated immunoglobulin (IgM) and cholesterol levels, and antimitochondrial antibodies. Congestive heart failure and constrictive pericarditis may lead to hepatic fibrosis ("cardiac cirrhosis") complicated by ascites and may be mistaken for cirrhosis.

Complications

Upper gastrointestinal tract bleeding may occur from varices, portal hypertensive gastropathy, or gastroduodenal ulcer. Hemorrhage may be massive, resulting in fatal exsanguination or portosystemic encephalopathy. Liver failure may be precipitated by alcoholism, surgery, and infection. Carcinoma of the liver and portal vein thrombosis occur more frequently in patients with cirrhosis but are still uncommon. Hepatic Kupffer cell (reticuloendothelial) dysfunction and decreased opsonic activity lead to an increased risk of systemic infection.

Treatment

A. General Measures: The most important principle of treatment is abstinence from alcohol. The diet should be palatable, with adequate calories and protein (75–100 g/d) and, if there is fluid retention, sodium restriction. In the presence of hepatic precoma or coma, protein intake should be reduced. Vitamin supplementation is desirable.

B. Special Problems:

1. Ascites and edema due to sodium retention, hypoproteinemia, and portal hypertension–Diagnostic paracentesis is usually indicated. Abdominal paracentesis is rarely associated with serious complications such as bleeding, infection, or bowel perforation even in patients with severe coagulopathy.

In some patients, there is a rapid diminution of ascites on bed rest and dietary sodium restriction alone. In individuals with severe fluid retention or those who are considered to have "intractable" ascites, the urinary excretion of sodium is usually less than 10 meq/L. Mechanisms postulated to explain sodium retention in cirrhosis include portal hypertension (increased hydrostatic pressure), hypoalbuminemia (decreased oncotic pressure), peripheral vasodilation with resulting increases in renin and angiotensin levels, and impaired liver inactivation of aldosterone and increased aldosterone secretion secondary to increased renin production. Free water excretion is also impaired in cirrhosis, and hyponatremia may develop. In all patients with cirrhotic ascites, dietary sodium intake may initially be restricted to 400–800 mg/d; the intake of sodium may be liberalized slightly after diuresis ensues. Restriction of fluid intake (800–1000 mL/d) is required for patients with hyponatremia (serum sodium < 130 meq/L).

a. Restoration of plasma proteins–This is dependent upon improving liver function and serves as a practical index of recovery. Therapeutic use of albumin intravenously is of little value.

b. Diuretics–Spironolactone should be used in patients who do not respond to salt restriction alone. After starting with 50 mg twice daily and monitoring the aldosterone antagonist effect, reflected by an increase in the urinary sodium concentration, the dose may be increased by 100 mg every 3 days (up to a maximal conventional single daily dose of 400 mg/d, though higher doses have been used) until diuresis is achieved, typically preceded by a rise in the urinary sodium concentration. Monitoring for hyperkalemia is important. Diuresis may be augmented by the addition of small doses of a potent agent such as furosemide. This potent diuretic, however, will maintain its effect even with a falling glomerular filtration rate, with resultant prerenal azotemia. The dose of furosemide ranges from 40 to 120 mg/d, and the drug should be administered with careful monitoring of blood pressure, urine output, mental status, and serum electrolytes, especially potassium.

The goal of weight loss in the ascitic patient without associated peripheral edema should be no more than 1–1.5 lb/d.

c. Large-volume paracentesis–In patients with massive ascites and respiratory compromise, ascites refractory to diuretics, or intolerable diuretic side effects, large-volume paracentesis (4–6 L) is effective; when this is done, it is safest to give intravenous albumin concomitantly at a dosage of 8–10 g/L of ascites fluid removed to protect the intravascular volume. Large-volume paracentesis can be repeated daily until ascites is largely resolved. The procedure is expensive (albumin is $15.00 per gram), but it may decrease the need for hospitalization. If possible, diuretics should be continued in the hope of preventing recurrent ascites.

d. Peritoneovenous shunts–Peritoneovenous shunts have been advocated for use in patients with refractory ascites or hepatorenal syndrome. These shunts may be effective but carry a considerable complication rate: disseminated intravascular coagulation in 65% of patients (25% symptomatic; 5% severe), bacterial infections in 4–8%, congestive heart failure in 2–4%, and variceal bleeding from sudden expansion of intravascular volume. Recently, transjugular intrahepatic portosystemic shunts (TIPS) have also shown benefit in patients with severe ascites (see below).

2. Hepatic encephalopathy–Hepatic encephalopathy is a state of disordered central nervous system function resulting from failure of the liver to detoxify noxious agents of gut origin because of hepatocellular dysfunction and portosystemic shunting. Ammonia is the most readily identified toxin but is not solely responsible for the disturbed mental status. Enhanced sensitivity of central nervous system neurons to the inhibitory neurotransmitter γ-aminobutyric acid (GABA) is thought to be a pathogenic factor. Bleeding into the intestinal tract may significantly increase the amount of protein in the bowel and may precipitate rapid development of liver coma. Other factors that may precipitate hepatic encephalopathy include alkalosis, potassium deficiency induced by diuretics, narcotics, hypnotics, and sedatives; medications containing ammonium or amino compounds; paracentesis with attendant hypovolemia; and hepatic or systemic infection.

Dietary protein should be withheld during acute episodes. Gastrointestinal bleeding should be controlled if possible and blood purged from the gastrointestinal tract. This can be accomplished with 120 mL of magnesium citrate by mouth or nasogastric tube every 3–4 hours until the stool is free of gross blood or with administration of lactulose.

Lactulose, a nonabsorbable synthetic disaccharide, is digested by bacteria in the colon to short-chain fatty acids, resulting in acidification of colon contents. This acidification favors the formation of ammonium ion in the $NH_4^+ \leftrightarrow NH_3$ equation; NH_4^+ is not absorbable, whereas NH_3 is absorbable and thought to be neurotoxic. Lactulose also leads to a change in bowel flora so that less ammonia-forming organisms are present. When given orally, the initial dose of lactulose for acute hepatic encephalopathy is 30 mL three or four times daily. The dose should be titrated so that no more than two or three soft stools per day are produced. When rectal use is indicated because of the patient's inability to take medicines orally, the dose is 300 mL of lactulose in 700 mL of saline or sorbitol as a retention enema for 30–60 minutes; it may be repeated every 4–6 hours.

The ammonia-producing intestinal flora may also be controlled with neomycin sulfate, 0.5–1 g orally every 6 hours for 5–7 days. Side effects of neomycin include diarrhea, malabsorption, superinfection, ototoxicity, and nephrotoxicity, usually only after prolonged use. Alternative antibiotics are vancomycin, 1 g orally twice daily, or metronidazole, 250 mg orally three times daily.

Avoid narcotics, tranquilizers, and sedatives metabolized or excreted by the liver. If agitation is marked, oxazepam, 10–30 mg, which is not metabolized by the liver, may be given cautiously by mouth or by nasogastric tube.

3. Anemia–For iron deficiency anemia, give ferrous sulfate, 0.3 g enteric-coated tablets, one tablet three times daily after meals. Folic acid, 1 mg/d orally, is indicated in the treatment of macrocytic anemia associated with alcoholism.

4. Hemorrhagic tendency–A bleeding tendency due to hypoprothrombinemia may be treated with vitamin K preparations. This treatment is ineffective in the presence of severe hepatic disease when other coagulation factors are deficient. Transfusions with packed red blood cells may be necessary to replace blood loss. Correcting the prolonged prothrombin time in these situations requires large volumes of fresh-frozen plasma, and the effect is transient; for that reason, plasma infusions are not indicated unless there is active bleeding or before an invasive procedure. Phytonadione, 5 mg orally daily, seldom helps but is often tried.

5. Hemorrhage from esophageal varices–For active variceal bleeding, attempts should be made to sclerose the bleeding varices transendoscopically. If this procedure cannot be performed or is not successful, bleeding can often be controlled by use of the quadruple-lumen (Minnesota) tube. Unfortunately, there is a high incidence of recurrent variceal bleeding after balloon tamponade has been discontinued. Intravenous vasopressin, 0.4 units/min, may also stop variceal bleeding; nitroglycerin may be given concurrently by intravenous infusion, sublingually, or by patch to minimize vasoconstrictive side effects. Octreotide acetate, 250 µg/h intravenously, is at least as effective as vasopressin but with little toxicity. While drug therapy may stop bleeding, there is no effect on survival. Injection sclerotherapy has proved to be quite effective (> 80%) in stopping the acute episode of variceal bleeding. The advantages of this technique are simplicity and avoidance of a major surgical procedure in a poor-risk patient. Repeated injections may be necessary. Recently, perendoscopic band ligation of varices has been used for the same indications as sclerotherapy but with lower complication rates (ulcers, strictures). If bleeding cannot be controlled by sclerotherapy or variceal band ligation, emergency surgical decompression of portal hypertension may be considered in selected patients. Morbidity and mortality rates are substantially lower when surgical shunting procedures are performed electively than when performed on an urgent basis and when the patient's Child classification is A or B (see Table 15–5). Transjugular intrahepatic portosystemic shunt (TIPS) is a promising alternative to surgical shunting in selected cases. The technique involves insertion of a prosthetic shunt between a branch of the hepatic vein and portal vein over a catheter inserted via the internal jugular vein. Complications include hepatic encephalopathy, infection, and shunt occlusion, and the long-term patency rate is unknown.

After the patient has been stabilized for 3–5 days after an acute episode of variceal bleeding, propranolol can be given in an attempt to lower the portal pressure. The dosage is usually 20–80 mg twice daily, with the goal of reducing the pretreatment resting pulse by 25% but not below 60/min. There is increasing evidence that propranolol (and atenolol) decrease the frequency of bleeding both in those who have bled and those who are at risk of bleeding from varices or portal hypertensive gastropathy. Prophylactic

Table 15–5. Child's criteria for hepatic functional reserve.[1]

	A Minimal	B Moderate	C Advanced
Serum bilirubin (mg/dL)	<2.0	2.0–3.0	>3.0
Serum albumin (g/dL)	>3.5	3.0–3.5	<3.0
Ascites	None	Easily controlled	Poorly controlled
Neurologic disorder	None	Minimal	Advanced, "coma"
Nutrition	Excellent	Good	Poor, "wasting"

[1]Modified, with permission, from Child CG III, Turcotte J: In: *The Liver and Portal Hypertension.* Child CG III (editor). Saunders, 1965.

sclerotherapy is of uncertain benefit—clearly less efficacious than propranolol. Prophylactic propranolol is indicated for patients with very large (grade 3 or 4) varices or those with red "wales" (varices on varices), signifying a high bleeding risk.

6. Spontaneous bacterial peritonitis–This occurs in cirrhotic patients with ascites. Abdominal pain, increasing ascites, fever, and progressive encephalopathy suggest the possibility, though symptoms may be mild. Paracentesis reveals an ascitic fluid with, most commonly, a total white cell count of more than 300 cells/μL with more than 250 PMNs/μL and a protein concentration of 1 g/dL or less. Cultures of ascites give the highest yield—80–90% positive—when aerobic and anaerobic blood culture bottles are inoculated at the bedside. Common organisms found are *E coli* and pneumococci. Pending culture results, if there are 250 or more PMNs/μL, intravenous antibiotic therapy should be initiated with cefotaxime, 2 g intravenously every 6 hours. The mortality rate is high. In survivors, recurrent peritonitis may be prevented by norfloxacin, 400 mg orally twice daily.

7. Hepatorenal syndrome–Hepatorenal syndrome is characterized by azotemia, oliguria, hyponatremia, low urinary sodium, and hypotension in a patient with end-stage liver disease. It is diagnosed only when other causes of renal failure have been excluded. The cause is unknown; histologically, the kidneys are normal. Death is commonly due to complicating infection or hemorrhage.

C. Liver Transplantation: Liver transplantation is indicated in selected cases of irreversible, progressive chronic liver disease, fulminant hepatic failure, and certain metabolic diseases in which the metabolic defect is in the liver. Contraindications include sepsis, malignancy (except small hepatocellular carcinomas in a cirrhotic liver), advanced cardiopulmonary disease (except pulmonary arteriovenous shunting due to portal hypertension and cirrhosis), AIDS, and lack of patient understanding. Alcoholics should be abstinent for 6 months. Liver transplantation should be considered in patients with worsening functional status, rising bilirubin, decreasing albumin, worsening coagulopathy, refractory ascites, recurrent variceal bleeding, or worsening encephalopathy. Five-year survival rates as high as 70% are now reported. Hepatocellular carcinoma, hepatitis B, and Budd-Chiari syndrome may recur in the transplanted liver, but other chronic liver diseases do not. Immunosuppression is achieved with cyclosporine, corticosteroids, and azathioprine and may be complicated by infections, renal failure, and neurologic disorders as well as graft rejection, vascular occlusion, or bile leaks.

Prognosis

The prognosis in advanced cirrhosis has shown little change over the years. Factors determining survival include the patient's ability to stop the intake of alcohol as well as the Child class (Table 15–5). In established cases with severe hepatic dysfunction, only 50% survive 2 years and 35% survive 5 years. Hematemesis, jaundice, and ascites are unfavorable signs.

Burroughs AK: Somatostatin and octreotide for variceal bleeding. J Hepatol 1991;13:1. (Safer and as effective as vasopressin in stopping acute bleeding, but neither drug has been shown to influence survival.)

Conn HO: Transjugular intrahepatic portal-systemic shunts: The state of the art. Hepatology 1993;17:148. (Comprehensive review of a promising approach to varices and ascites. Results of long-term trials are awaited.)

Cosimi AB: Update on liver transplantation. Transplant Proc 1991; 23:2083.

Groszmann RJ, Grace ND (editors): Complications of portal hypertension: Esophagogastric varices and ascites. Gastroenterol Clin North Am 1992:21:1.

Henderson JM et al: Endoscopic variceal sclerosis compared with distal splenorenal shunt to prevent recurrent variceal bleeding in cirrhosis: A prospective randomized trial. Ann Intern Med 1990;112:262. (Most representative of current wisdom.)

Pagliaro L et al: Prevention of first bleeding in cirrhosis: A meta-analysis of randomized trials of nonsurgical treatment. Ann Intern Med 1992;117:59. (Propranolol is preferred over variceal sclerotherapy to prevent initial hemorrhage from large varices.)

Runyon BA, Antillon MR, Montano AA: Effect of diuresis vs. therapeutic paracentesis on ascitic fluid, opsonic activity and serum complement. Gastroenterology 1989: 97:158. (Suggests diuresis may be a more physiologic approach to treatment.)

Runyon BA: Spontaneous bacterial peritonitis: An explosion of information. Hepatology 1988;8:171.

Soriano G et al: Selective intestinal decontamination prevents spontaneous bacterial peritonitis. Gastroenterology 1991:100:477. (In those with low ascitic fluid protein levels, prophylactic norfloxacin appears to decrease the incidence.)

Stanley MM et al: Peritoneovenous shunting as compared with medical treatment in patients with alcoholic cirrhosis and massive ascites. N Engl J Med 1989;321:1632. (Alleviates ascites more rapidly, but survival is not affected.)

Stiegmann GV et al: Endoscopic sclerotherapy as compared with endoscopic ligation for bleeding esophageal varices. N Engl J Med 1992:236:1527. (Ligation associated with fewer side effects and lower mortality rate.)

Westaby D et al: A controlled trial of oral propranolol compared with injection sclerotherapy for the long-term management of variceal bleeding. Hepatology 1990;11:353. (Suggests equal efficacy in preventing recurrent bleeding.)

Wiesner RH et al: Hepatic allograft rejection: new developments in terminology, diagnosis, prevention, and treatment. Mayo Clin Proc 1993;68:69. (New immunosuppressant FK 506 is often effective in rejection unresponsive to standard therapy but is at least as nephrotoxic as cyclosporine when used long-term.)

BILIARY CIRRHOSIS

1. PRIMARY BILIARY CIRRHOSIS

Primary biliary cirrhosis is a chronic disease of the liver manifested by cholestasis. It is insidious in onset, occurs usually in women aged 40–60, and is often detected by the chance finding of elevated alkaline phosphatase levels. The disease is progressive and complicated often by steatorrhea, xanthomatous neuropathy, osteoporosis, osteomalacia, and portal hypertension.

Clinical Findings
A. Symptoms and Signs: Many patients are asymptomatic for years. The onset of clinical illness is insidious and is heralded by pruritus. Jaundice usually occurs within 2 years of onset of pruritus. Physical examination reveals hepatosplenomegaly. Xanthomatous lesions may occur in the skin and tendons and around the eyelids.

B. Laboratory Findings: Hemograms are normal early in the disease. Liver function tests reflect cholestasis with elevation of alkaline phosphatase, cholesterol, and, in later stages, bilirubin. Antimitochondrial antibodies are present in 95% of patients.

Differential Diagnosis
The disease must be differentiated from chronic biliary tract obstruction (stone or stricture), carcinoma of the bile ducts, cholestatic liver disease associated with inflammatory bowel disease, sarcoidosis, and in some cases chronic active hepatitis.

Treatment
Treatment is symptomatic. Cholestyramine (4 g) or colestipol (5 g) in water or juice three times daily may be beneficial for the pruritus. Rifampin has been of benefit also in some studies, but not others. Opiate antagonists show promise in the treatment of pruritus. Deficiencies of vitamins A, K, and D may occur if steatorrhea is present and may be further aggravated when cholestyramine or colestipol is administered. Replacement dosages of these vitamins must be individualized. Calcium supplementation (500 mg three times daily) may be helpful to prevent osteomalacia but is of uncertain benefit in osteoporosis. Penicillamine, corticosteroids, and azathioprine have proved to be of no benefit. Colchicine (0.6 mg twice daily), methotrexate (15 mg/wk), and ursodeoxycholic acid (10–15 mg/kg/d) have had some reported benefit in preliminary studies. Liver transplantation for advanced primary biliary cirrhosis has become one of the major success stories for this treatment modality.

Bodenheimer H Jr, Schaffner F, Pezzullo J: Evaluation of colchicine therapy in primary biliary cirrhosis. Gastroenterology 1988;95:124. (Shows some promise.)

deCaestecker JS et al: Ursodeoxycholic acid in chronic liver disease. Gut 1991;32:1061. (Improves liver tests in early primary biliary cirrhosis. Effect on long-term survival uncertain.)

Esquivel CO et al: Transplantation for primary biliary cirrhosis. Gastroenterology 1988;94:1207. (The most rewarding group of patients for liver transplant.)

MacKay IR, Gershwin ME (editors): Primary biliary cirrhosis: Current knowledge, perspectives, and future directions. Semin Liver Dis 1989;9:149.

2. SECONDARY BILIARY CIRRHOSIS

Secondary biliary cirrhosis follows chronic obstruction to bile flow. Superimposed infection may hasten the process. Bile flow is most commonly impaired in an extrahepatic site by calculus, neoplasm, stricture, or biliary atresia.

Clinical Findings
A. Symptoms and Signs: The clinical presentation is usually that of the underlying cause of the cholestasis (eg, carcinoma of the pancreas, choledocholithiasis, choledochal cysts).

B. Laboratory Findings: Hemograms are normal except insofar as they reflect the inciting lesion (eg, cholangitis associated with choledocholithiasis). Liver function tests reflect cholestasis with elevated alkaline phosphatase and bilirubin. Antimitochondrial antibodies are absent.

C. Imaging: Ultrasound may reveal dilated ducts (especially intrahepatic), hilar or pancreatic masses, and occasionally common duct stones. Either CT scan or MRI is more accurate than ultrasound for lesions of the pancreas.

The site of obstruction and often the cause are determined by endoscopic retrograde cholangiography (ERCP) or percutaneous transhepatic cholangiography. Selection of one or the other is dictated by the expertise available and the anticipated problem: For choledocholithiasis, ERCP is clearly the procedure of choice, since papillotomy with stone extraction can usually be accomplished and is therapeutic. Either method allows placement of stents, fine-needle aspiration, brushings for cytologic examination, and biopsy. For balloon dilation of ductal strictures, ERCP is preferable.

Geenen DJ et al: Endoscopic therapy for benign bile strictures. Gastrointest Endosc 1989;35:367. (Twenty-two of 25 patients benefited.)

Oren R et al: Localized primary sclerosing cholangitis mimicking a cholecystectomy stricture relieved by an endoprosthesis. Postgrad Med J 1991;67:482. (Led to improvement for 2 years.)

HEMOCHROMATOSIS

Hemochromatosis is an autosomal recessive disease with linkage to HLA-A3 and HLA-B14 or HLA-A3 and HLA-B7. It is characterized by increased accumulation of iron as hemosiderin in the liver, pancreas, heart, adrenals, testes, pituitary, and kidneys. Eventually the patient may develop hepatic, pancreatic, and cardiac insufficiency. The disease usually occurs in males and is rarely recognized before the fifth decade. The clinical disease appears in affected women 10–20 years postmenopause.

Clinical Findings

Clinical manifestations include arthropathy, hepatomegaly and evidence of hepatic insufficiency (late finding), occasional skin pigmentation (slate gray due to iron and brown due to melanin), cardiac enlargement with or without heart failure or conduction defects, diabetes mellitus with its complications, and impotence in the male. Bleeding from esophageal varices may occur, and in patients who develop cirrhosis, there is a 15–20% incidence of hepatic carcinoma. The disease should be considered in those with a family history and in patients with unexplained mild liver test abnormalities.

Laboratory findings include mildly abnormal liver tests (AST, alkaline phosphatase), an elevated plasma iron with greater than 50% saturation of the transferrin, and an elevated serum ferritin. CT and MRI may show changes consistent with iron overload of the liver, but these techniques are not sensitive enough for screening asymptomatic persons. The liver biopsy characteristically shows extensive iron deposition in hepatocytes and usually in bile ducts, vessel walls and supporting tissues. Diagnosis is confirmed by determination of the hepatic iron content on a liver biopsy specimen.

Treatment

Early diagnosis and treatment in the precirrhotic phase of hemochromatosis is of great importance. Treatment consists initially of weekly phlebotomies of 500 mL of blood (about 250 mg of iron), continued for up to 2–3 years to achieve depletion of iron stores. This process is monitored by hematocrit and serum iron determinations. When iron store depletion is achieved, maintenance phlebotomies (every 2–4 months) are continued. The chelating agent, deferoxamine, administered intramuscularly to patients with hemochromatosis, has been shown to produce urinary excretion of up to 5–18 g of iron per year. This rate of urinary excretion compares favorably with the rate of 10–20 g of iron removed annually by weekly or biweekly phlebotomies. The treatment, however, is painful—given in a dosage of 0.5–1 g intramuscularly daily or 20–40 mg subcutaneously over an 8- to 24-hour period with a constant infusion pump until the desired goal is reached—and

not always practical. Active treatment of the complications of hemochromatosis—arthropathy, diabetes, heart and liver disease, and hypopituitarism—is important.

Available data indicate that the course of the disease may be favorably altered by phlebotomy therapy. In precirrhotic patients, cirrhosis may be prevented. There appear to be fewer cardiac conduction defects and lower insulin requirements with these treatments. Family members should be screened with serum iron studies and, in siblings, HLA typing.

Adams PC et al: Clinical presentation of hemochromatosis: A changing scene. Am J Med 1991;90:445. (Family screening leads to early diagnosis at a presymptomatic stage.)

Smith LH Jr: Overview of hemochromatosis. West J Med 1990;153:296.

WILSON'S DISEASE

Wilson's disease (hepatolenticular degeneration) is a rare autosomal recessive disorder that usually occurs between the first and third decades. The condition is characterized by excessive deposition of copper in the liver and brain.

Awareness of the entity is important, since it may masquerade as chronic active hepatitis, psychiatric disorder, or neurologic disease. It is potentially reversible, and appropriate therapy will prevent neurologic and hepatic damage.

The major physiologic aberration in Wilson's disease is excessive absorption of copper from the small intestine and decreased excretion of copper by the liver, resulting in increased tissue deposition, especially in the liver, brain, cornea, and kidney. Serum ceruloplasmin, the plasma copper-carrying protein, is low. Urinary excretion of copper is high.

Clinical Findings

Wilson's disease tends to present as liver disease in adolescents and neuropsychiatric disease in young adults, but there is great variability. The diagnosis should always be considered in any child or young adult with hepatitis, splenomegaly with hypersplenism, hemolytic anemia, portal hypertension, and neurologic or psychiatric abnormalities. Wilson's disease should also be considered in persons under 40 years of age with chronic active hepatitis or acute fulminant hepatitis.

The neurologic manifestations are related to basal ganglia dysfunction and are characterized by rigidity or parkinsonian tremor. Hepatic involvement may range from elevated liver tests to cirrhosis and portal hypertension. The pathognomonic sign of the condition is the Kayser-Fleischer ring, which represents fine pigmented granular deposits in Descemet's membrane in the cornea close to the endothelial surface. Scattering and reflection of light by these deposits give rise to the typically brownish or gray-green appearance of the ring. The ring is usually most marked at the superior and inferior poles of the cornea. It can frequently be seen with the naked eye and almost invariably by slit lamp examination. It may be absent in patients with hepatic manifestations only but is invariably present in those with neuropsychiatric disease.

The diagnosis is based on demonstration of increased urinary copper excretion (> 100 μg/24 h) or low serum ceruloplasmin levels (< 20 μg/dL), and elevated hepatic copper concentration (> 100 μg/g of dry liver). Early in the course of Wilson's disease, the serum alkaline phosphatase appears to be lower than for matched normals. Liver biopsy may show acute or chronic active hepatitis or cirrhosis.

Treatment

Early treatment is essential for removal of copper before it can produce neurologic or hepatic damage. Oral penicillamine (0.75–2 g/d in divided doses) is the drug of choice, making possible urinary excretion of chelated copper. Pyridoxine, 50 mg per week, is added, since penicillamine is an antimetabolite of this vitamin. If penicillamine treatment cannot be tolerated because of gastrointestinal, hypersensitivity, or autoimmune reactions, consider the use of trientine, 250–500 mg three times a day. Early in the treatment phase, restriction of dietary copper (shellfish, organ foods, legumes are rich in copper) may be of value. Oral zinc acetate, 50 mg three times a day, promotes fecal copper excretion and may be used as maintenance therapy after decoppering with a chelating agent or as first-line therapy in presymptomatic or pregnant patients.

Treatment should continue indefinitely. The prognosis is good in patients who are effectively treated before liver or brain damage has occurred. Family members, especially siblings, require screening with serum ceruloplasmin, liver function tests, and slit-lamp examination.

Stremmel W et al: Wilson's Disease: Clinical presentation, treatment and survival. Ann Intern Med 1991;115:720. (Long-term treatment with D-penicillamine can relieve symptoms and improve prognosis.)

Yarze JC et al: Wilson's disease: Current status. Am J Med 1992;92:643.

Yuzbasiyan-Gurkan V et al: Diagnosis and characterization of presymptomatic patients with Wilson's disease and the use of molecular genetics to aid in the diagnosis. J Lab Clin Med 1991;118:458. (Important approach to preventing the clinical ravages of this disease in potentially susceptible patients.)

HEPATIC VEIN OBSTRUCTION (Budd-Chiari Syndrome)

This uncommon disorder is due to occlusion of the hepatic veins from a variety of causes. Many cases are associated with polycythemia vera or other myeloproliferative diseases, which may be subclinical. Hepatovenous obstructions may be associated with caval webs, right-sided heart failure or constrictive pericarditis, use of birth control pills, neoplasms causing hepatic vein occlusions, paroxysmal nocturnal hemoglobinuria, and pregnancy. Some cytotoxic agents and pyrrolizidine alkaloids ("bush teas") may cause hepatic veno-occlusive disease (occlusion of terminal venules), which mimics Budd-Chiari syndrome clinically.

Clinical manifestations may include tender, painful hepatic enlargement; jaundice; splenomegaly; and ascites. With advanced disease, bleeding varices and hepatic coma may be evident. Hepatic imaging studies may show prominent caudate lobes, since its venous drainage may not come from the hepatic vein. Caval venogram can delineate caval webs and occluded hepatic veins. Percutaneous liver biopsy frequently shows a characteristic central lobular congestion.

Ascites should be treated with fluid and salt restriction and diuretics and efforts made to find treatable causes. Surgical compression (mesocaval or mesoatrial shunt) of the congested liver may be required. Liver transplantation is considered in patients with marked hepatocellular dysfunction. Patients often require lifelong anticoagulation and treatment of the underlying myeloproliferative disease.

Jamieson NV et al: Liver transplantation for Budd-Chiari syndrome, 1976–1990. Ann Chir 1991;45:362. (Procedure of choice in those with underlying end-stage liver disease. One-year survival rate of 69%.)

McDermott WV, Ridker PM: The Budd-Chiari syndrome and hepatic veno-occlusive disease: Recognition and treatment. Arch Surg 1990;125:525. (Remember pyrrolizidine alkaloids contained in *Crotalaria* and *Senecio* as etiologic possibilities.)

Ohnishi K et al: Budd-Chiari syndrome: Diagnosis with duplex sonography. Am J Gastroenterol 1990;85:165. (An accurate noninvasive technique.)

Orloff MJ et al: Treatment of Budd-Chiari syndrome due to inferior vena cava occlusion by combined portal and vena caval decompression. Am J Surg 1992;163:137. (Vascular decompression is the treatment of choice in most.)

NONCIRRHOTIC PORTAL HYPERTENSION

Noncirrhotic portal hypertension must be considered in the differential diagnosis of splenomegaly or upper gastrointestinal bleeding due to esophageal or gastric varices and normal liver function. This syndrome may be due to portal vein obstruction, splenic vein obstruction (gastric varices without esophageal varices), schistosomiasis, noncirrhotic intrahepatic portal sclerosis, or arterial-portal vein fistula. Angiography of the portal system is confirmatory, as is needle biopsy of the liver, particularly for schistosomiasis and noncirrhotic intrahepatic portal sclerosis. Other than for splenomegaly, the physical findings are not remarkable, and the endoscopic findings are those of esophageal or gastric varices. The liver tests are usually normal, but there may be findings of hypersplenism.

If splenic vein thrombosis is the cause, splenectomy is curative. In other cases, sclerotherapy is initiated for variceal bleeding, and portosystemic shunting is reserved for sclerotherapy failures.

Valla D et al: Etiology of portal vein thrombosis in adults: A prospective evaluation of primary myeloproliferative disorders. Gastroenterology 1988;94:1063. (Thirty-three patients with portal vein thrombosis, about half due to myeloproliferative disorders.)

HEPATIC ABSCESS

1. PYOGENIC ABSCESS

There are five ways in which the liver can be invaded by bacteria: (1) by way of the portal vein; (2) by way of ascending cholangitis in the common duct; (3) by way of the hepatic artery, secondary to bacteremia; (4) by direct extension from an infectious process; and (5) by traumatic implantation of bacteria through the abdominal wall.

Despite the use of antimicrobial drugs, 10% of cases of liver abscess are secondary to appendicitis. Another 10% have no demonstrable cause and are classified as idiopathic. At present, ascending cholangitis is the most common cause of hepatic abscess in the USA. Bacterial infection of the hepatobiliary tree is more likely to accompany obstruction by stone than obstruction by carcinoma of the head of the pancreas. The most frequently encountered organisms are *Escherichia coli, Proteus vulgaris, Enterobacter aerogenes,* and multiple anaerobic species.

Hepatic candidiasis is being reported with increasing frequency, particularly in immunocompromised patients.

Clinical Findings

Clinically, fever is almost always present and may antedate other symptoms or signs. Pain is prominent and is localized to the right hypochondrium or epigastric area. Jaundice, tenderness in the right upper abdomen, and either steady or swinging fever are the chief physical findings.

Laboratory examination reveals leukocytosis with a shift to the left. Chest roentgenograms will usually reveal elevation of the diaphragm if the abscess is on the right side. Left-sided abscess does not produce significant diaphragmatic elevation. Ultrasound or CT scan may reveal the presence of intrahepatic defects. Hepatic candidiasis is seen usually in the setting of systemic candidiasis, and on CT scan the characteristic appearance is that of multiple "bulls-eyes," but imaging studies may be negative in neutropenic patients. Liver function studies are nonspecifically abnormal.

Treatment

Treatment should consist of antimicrobial agents (a third-generation cephalosporin and metronidazole) that are effective against coliform organisms and anaerobes. If adequate response to therapy is not rapid, needle or surgical drainage should be undertaken. Failure to recognize and treat the condition is attended by mortality rates of about 60% in patients with multiple abscesses. Hepatic candidiasis often responds to intravenous amphotericin B (total dose of 2–9 g).

Stain SC et al: Pyogenic liver abscess: Modern treatment. Arch Surg 1991;126:991. (Antibiotics and percutaneous catheter drainage is the treatment of choice.)
Thaler M et al: Hepatic candidiasis in cancer patients: The evolving picture of the syndrome. Ann Intern Med 1988;108:88. (Requires more than 2 g total dose of amphotericin B—perhaps as much as 9 g.)
Webb TH et al: Liver abscess. Hosp Physician (April) 1989, p 46.

2. AMEBIC LIVER ABSCESS

Amebic abscess is more common as a primary presentation than is pyogenic abscess. Usual symptoms and signs, which may have been present for 1–30 days, are right upper quadrant pain, often with associated fever, and right pleuritic chest pain. Associated dysentery is uncommon, but 20% of patients will have had a significant recent diarrheal episode. Usually there is a history of travel to endemic areas.

Clinical Findings

Physical examination discloses fever in most cases, toxic appearance of varying degree, and a tender palpable liver with marked "punch" tenderness. Right lung base abnormalities and localized intercostal tenderness are common. Acute amebic appendicitis is not an uncommon precursor.

Laboratory findings usually consist of mild to moderate anemia, moderate leukocytosis with a shift to the left, and slightly abnormal liver tests. Serologic amebic gel diffusion tests or indirect hemagglutination tests for *Entamoeba histolytica* are positive in 95% of patients but may be nondiagnostic on presentation, with a marked rise in titer over the subsequent 3–4 weeks.

An elevated right hemidiaphragm is frequently seen on chest radiograph. Ultrasonography, CT scan, or MRI is helpful in delineating the location and number of abscesses. Most are in the right lobe.

Treatment

Metronidazole, 750 mg three times per day orally for 5–10 days, is the drug of choice. Occasionally, a second course is necessary. In the acutely toxic patient, percutaneous needle aspiration and decompression of the abscess bring about a greater feeling of well-being and also allow for demonstration of the ameba in over 50% of cases. Following completion of treatment for the abscess, the patient needs to take iodoquinol, 650 mg three times a day after meals for 20 days (for adults), to eradicate the intestinal cyst phase of amebiasis.

Fever usually subsides rapidly once treatment is initiated. The hepatic defect may persist for over 6 months.

Complications include rupture of the abscess transcutaneously, into the peritoneal cavity, pleural space, lungs, or pericardium, with a significant associated mortality rate if undiagnosed. Rarely, distal embolization has been reported.

Lyche KD et al: Pleuropulmonary manifestations of hepatic amebiasis. West J Med 1990;153:273. (Pleuropulmonary manifestations resolve with amebicidal treatment of hepatic abscess.)
Maltz G et al: Amebic liver abscess: A 15 year experience. Am J Gastroenterol 1991;86:704. (A predominantly male disease.)

NEOPLASMS OF THE LIVER

1. HEPATOCELLULAR CARCINOMA

Neoplasms of the liver that arise from parenchymal cells are called hepatocellular carcinomas; those that originate in the ductular cells are called cholangiocarcinomas.

Hepatocellular carcinomas are associated with cirrhosis in general and hepatitis B or C in particular. In Africa and Asia, hepatitis B is of major etiologic significance, whereas in western countries and Japan hepatitis C and alcoholic cirrhosis are the most common causes. Other associations include hemochromatosis, aflatoxin exposure, α_1-antiprotease (α_1-antitrypsin) deficiency, and tyrosinemia.

Histologically, hepatocellular carcinoma is made up of cords or sheets of cells that roughly resemble the hepatic parenchyma. Blood vessels such as portal or hepatic veins are commonly involved by tumor.

The presence of a hepatocellular carcinoma may be unsuspected until there is deterioration in the condition of a cirrhotic patient who was formerly stable. Cachexia, weakness, and weight loss are associated symptoms. The sudden appearance of ascites, which may be bloody, suggests portal or hepatic vein thrombosis by tumor or bleeding from the necrotic tumor. In the chronic HBsAg carrier, surveillance for the development of hepatocellular carcinoma should be considered and has been practiced in endemic areas with regular alpha-fetoprotein testing and ultrasonography. In the United States, experience with surveillance has been sporadic and of uncertain benefit.

Physical examination is positive for tender enlargement of the liver, with an occasionally palpable mass. In Africa, young patients typically present with a rapidly expanding abdominal mass. Auscultation may reveal a bruit over the tumor or a friction rub when the process has extended to the surface of the liver.

Laboratory tests may reveal leukocytosis, as opposed to the leukopenia that is frequently encountered in cirrhotic patients. A normal or elevated hematocrit may be found, owing to elaboration of erythropoietin by the tumor. Sudden and sustained elevation of the serum alkaline phosphatase in a patient who was formerly stable is a common finding. Hepatitis B surface antigen is present in a majority of cases in endemic areas, whereas in the United States anti-HCV is found in up to 40% of cases. Alpha-fetoprotein levels are elevated in up to 60% of patients with hepatocellular carcinoma. Cytologic study of ascitic fluid rarely reveals malignant cells.

Arteriography is frequently diagnostic, revealing a tumor "blush" that reflects the highly vascular nature of the tumor. Almost as helpful is CT scanning when done with and without intravenous contrast or MRI to characterize the location and vascularity of the tumor. Liver biopsy is diagnostic.

Attempts at surgical resection are usually fruitless if concomitant cirrhosis is present and if the tumor is multifocal. Surgical resection of solitary hepatocellular carcinomas may result in cure if the unaffected liver is normal. Chemotherapy has not been shown to prolong life, but chemoembolization via the hepatic artery may be palliative. Recent success has also been achieved by injection of small tumors (< 3 cm) with absolute ethanol.

2. MISCELLANEOUS LIVER NEOPLASMS

Benign and malignant neoplasms have been encountered in women taking oral contraceptives. Two distinct entities with characteristic clinical, radiologic, and histopathologic features have been described. **Focal nodular hyperplasia** occurs at all ages but is questionably related to oral contraceptives. It is usually asymptomatic and hypervascular on CT scan or MRI. Microscopically, focal nodular hyperplasia consists of hyperplastic units of hepatocytes with a centrally placed "stellate" scar containing proliferating bile ducts. **Liver cell adenoma** occurs most commonly in the third and fourth decades of life; the clinical presentation is often one of acute abdominal disease due to necrosis of the tumor with hemorrhage. The tumor is hypovascular and reveals a cold defect on liver scan. Grossly, the cut surface appears structureless. As seen microscopically, the liver cell adenoma consists of sheets of hepatocytes without portal tracts or central veins. The only physical finding in focal nodular hyperplasia or liver cell adenoma is a palpable abdominal mass in some cases. Liver function is usually normal. Treatment of focal nodular hyperplasia is resection in the symptomatic patient. The prognosis is excellent. Liver cell adenoma often undergoes necrosis and rupture; resection is advised. Regression of benign hepatic tumors may follow cessation of oral contraceptives.

The most common benign neoplasm of the liver is the cavernous hemangioma, often an incidental finding on CT scan. This lesion must be differentiated from other space-occupying intrahepatic lesions, usually by MRI. Fine-needle biopsy may be necessary to differentiate these lesions and does not appear to carry an increased risk. They rarely require treatment.

DiBisceglie AM et al: Hepatocellular carcinoma. Ann Intern Med 1988;108:390. (Surgery offers the only hope at present. Best results are with small asymptomatic single neoplasms.)

Regan LS: Screening for hepatocellular carcinoma in high-risk individuals: A clinical review. Arch Intern Med 1989;149:1741. (Emphasizes adjusting intensity of screening to the degree of risk of hepatocellular carcinoma.)

Simonetti RG et al: Hepatitis C virus infection as a risk factor for hepatocellular carcinoma in patients with cirrhosis: A case control study. Ann Intern Med 1992;116:97. (Hepatitis B, hepatitis C, and cirrhosis are all independent risk factors.)

DISEASES OF THE BILIARY TRACT

CHOLELITHIASIS
(Gallstones)

Gallstones are more common in women than in men and increase in incidence in both sexes and all races with aging. Data indicate that in the USA over 10% of men and 20% of women have gallstones by age 65 and that the total exceeds 20 million people. Although gallstones are less common in black people, cholelithiasis attributable to hemolysis has been encountered in over a third of individuals with sickle cell anemia. Native Americans of both the Northern and Southern Hemispheres have a high rate of cholesterol cholelithiasis, probably because of a genetic predisposition. As many as 75% of Pima women over the age of 25 years have cholelithiasis. The incidence of gallstones is also high in individuals with certain diseases such as regional enteritis. Approximately one-third of individuals with inflammatory involvement of the terminal ileum have gallstones due to disruption of bile salt resorption that results in decreased solubility of the bile. The incidence of cholelithiasis is also increased in patients with diabetes mellitus. Pregnancy is associated with an increased risk of gallstone and of symptomatic gallbladder disease.

Classification of Gallstones

The simplest classification of gallstones is according to chemical composition: stones containing predominantly cholesterol and stones containing predominantly calcium bilirubinate. The latter comprise less than 20% of the stones found in Europe or the USA but 30–40% of stones found in Japan.

Three compounds comprise 80–95% of the total solids dissolved in bile: conjugated bile salts, lecithin, and cholesterol. Cholesterol is a neutral sterol; lecithin is a phospholipid; and both are almost completely insoluble in water. However, bile salts are able to form multimolecular aggregates (micelles) or vesicles that solubilize cholesterol in an aqueous solution. Bile salts alone are relatively inefficient in solubilizing cholesterol (approximately 50 molecules of bile salt are necessary to solubilize 1 molecule of cholesterol), but the solubilization of lecithin in bile salt solutions results in a mixed micelle that is seven times more efficient in the solubilization of cholesterol. Precipitation of cholesterol microcrystals may come about because of increased biliary secretion of cholesterol, defective formation of vesicles, an excess of factors promoting the nucleation of cholesterol crystals (or deficiency of antinucleating factors), or delayed emptying of the gallbladder.

Treatment

Cholelithiasis is frequently asymptomatic and is discovered fortuitously in the course of routine radiographic study, operation, or autopsy.

There is generally no known need for prophylactic cholecystectomy in an asymptomatic person.

Operation is usually indicated for symptomatic cholelithiasis. "Symptomatic" cholelithiasis may be quite diverse in its presentation but usually includes right upper quadrant discomfort and colicky pain. There must be careful consideration of other sources of the symptoms.

Cheno- and ursodeoxycholic acids are bile salts

that on oral administration are able to cause dissolution of some cholesterol stones. Chenodeoxycholic acid may induce diarrhea and mild liver test abnormalities, and ursodeoxycholic acid is expensive. They are most effective in patients with a functioning gallbladder, as determined by gallbladder visualization on oral cholecystography (represents not more than 15% of patients with gallstones), and in the management of multiple small "floating" gallstones. These agents may be most efficacious in terms of safety, cost, and rapidity of stone dissolution when used in combination at a dosage of 7 mg/kg body weight of each daily in two divided doses. Alternatively, ursodeoxycholic acid, 8–13 mg/kg/d, may be given. Dissolution of gallstones may require 2 years or longer. In half of patients, gallstones recur within 5 years after treatment is stopped. Obesity may induce resistance to therapy. Intermittent therapy is ineffective.

Lithotripsy as a treatment modality for cholelithiasis has had some success in a limited number of patients. This procedure requires concomitant treatment with cheno- or ursodeoxycholic acid (or both). The best candidates are patients with single radiolucent stones < 20 mm in diameter and a functioning gallbladder.

Laparoscopic cholecystectomy has become the treatment of choice for symptomatic gallbladder disease. The minimal trauma to the abdominal wall makes it possible for patients to go home the day after the procedure and to return to work in days (instead of weeks for those with open cholecystectomy). This procedure is suitable in most patients, including those with acute cholecystitis. If problems are encountered, the surgery can be converted to the conventional open cholecystectomy. Bile duct injuries occur in 0.1% of cases done by experienced surgeons.

Nervi F et al: Influence of legume intake on biliary lipids and cholesterol saturation in young Chilean men. Gastroenterology 1989;96:825. (Legume intake a risk factor.)
NIH Consensus Development Panel on Gallstones and Laparoscopic Cholecystectomy. Gallstones and laparoscopic cholecystectomy. JAMA 1993;269:1018.
Podda M et al: Efficacy and safety of a combination of chenodeoxycholic acid and ursodeoxycholic acid for gallstone dissolution. Gastroenterology 1989;96:222. (Combinations appear better.)
Ponchon T et al: Gallstone disappearance after extracorporeal lithotripsy and oral bile dissolution. Gastroenterology 1989;97:457. (Procedure works; moderate number of complications, and additional procedures required. Need to be very selective.)
The Southern Surgeons Club: A prospective analysis of 1518 laparoscopic cholecystectomies. N Engl J Med 1991;324:1073. (Appears to be the procedure of choice for most.)
Strasberg SM, Clavien PDA: Cholecystolithiasis: Lithotherapy for the 1990s. Hepatology 1992:16:820. (Indications and cost-effectiveness of bile acid therapy,
extracorporeal shock wave lithotripsy, laparoscopic cholecystectomy, and open cholecystectomy.)

ACUTE CHOLECYSTITIS

Essentials of Diagnosis
- Steady, severe pain and tenderness in the right hypochondrium or epigastrium.
- Nausea and vomiting.
- Fever and leukocytosis.

General Considerations
Cholecystitis is associated with gallstones in over 90% of cases. It occurs when a calculus becomes impacted in the cystic duct and inflammation develops behind the obstruction. Vascular abnormalities of the bile duct or pancreatitis may rarely produce cholecystitis in the absence of gallstones. Acalculous cholecystitis should be considered when unexplained fever or right upper quadrant pain occurs within 2–4 weeks of major surgery or in a critically ill patient who has had no oral intake for a prolonged period. Primarily as a result of ischemic changes secondary to distention, gangrene may develop, with resulting perforation. Although generalized peritonitis is possible, the leak usually remains localized and forms a chronic, well-circumscribed abscess cavity.

Clinical Findings
A. Symptoms and Signs: The acute attack is often precipitated by a large or fatty meal and is characterized by the relatively sudden appearance of severe, minimally fluctuating pain which is localized to the epigastrium or right hypochondrium and which in the uncomplicated case may gradually subside over a period of 12–18 hours. Vomiting occurs in about 75% of patients and in half of instances affords variable relief. Right upper quadrant abdominal tenderness is almost always present and is usually associated with muscle guarding and rebound pain. A palpable gallbladder is present in about 15% of cases. Jaundice is present in about 25% of cases and, when persistent or severe, suggests the possibility of choledocholithiasis. Fever is usually present.

B. Laboratory Findings: The white count is usually high (12,000–15,000/μL). Total serum bilirubin values of 1–4 mg/dL may be reported even in the absence of common duct obstruction. Serum aminotransferase and alkaline phosphatase are often elevated—the former as high as 300 IU/mL, or even higher when associated with ascending cholangitis. Serum amylase may also be moderately elevated.

C. Imaging: Films of the abdomen may show radiopaque gallstones in 15% of cases. ^{99m}Tc hepatobiliary imaging (using iminodiacetic acid compounds), also known as the HIDA scan, is useful in demonstrating an obstructed cystic duct, which is the cause of acute cholecystitis in most patients. This test is reliable if the bilirubin is under 5 mg/dL (98% sensitivity and 81% specificity for acute cholecystitis). Right upper quadrant abdominal ultrasound may show the presence of gallstones but is not specific for acute cholecystitis (67% sensitivity, 82% specificity).

Differential Diagnosis

The disorders most likely to be confused with acute cholecystitis are perforated peptic ulcer, acute pancreatitis, appendicitis in a high-lying appendix, perforated colonic carcinoma or diverticulum of the hepatic flexure, liver abscess, hepatitis and pneumonia with pleurisy on the right side. The definite localization of pain and tenderness in the right hypochondrium, with radiation around to the infrascapular area, strongly favors the diagnosis of acute cholecystitis. True cholecystitis without stones raises the question of polyarteritis nodosa (rarely).

Complications

A. Gangrene of the Gallbladder: Continuation or progression of right upper quadrant abdominal pain, tenderness, muscle guarding, fever, and leukocytosis after 24–48 hours suggests severe inflammation and possible gangrene of the gallbladder. Necrosis may occasionally develop without definite signs in the obese, diabetic, elderly, or immunosuppressed patient.

B. Cholangitis: Cholangitis classically presents with Charcot's triad, namely, fever and chills, right upper quadrant pain, and jaundice. Although 95% of patients who present with this picture will have common duct stones, only a minority have common duct stones that will present in this manner.

Treatment

Acute cholecystitis will usually subside on a conservative regimen (withholding of oral feedings, intravenous alimentation, analgesics, and antibiotics). Meperidine may be preferable to morphine for pain because of less spasm of the sphincter of Oddi. Cholecystectomy can be performed within 2–3 days after hospitalization in most cases or can be scheduled for 6–8 weeks later in patients who are poor risks for early surgery. If, as occasionally happens, recurrent acute symptoms develop during this waiting period, cholecystectomy or cholecystostomy (in poor-risk patients) is indicated without delay. If nonsurgical treatment has been elected, the patient (especially if diabetic or elderly) should be watched carefully for evidence of gangrene of the gallbladder or cholangitis.

Operation is mandatory when there is evidence of gangrene or perforation. It is usually best to defer surgery, if possible, in the presence of acute pancreatitis, and ERCP with papillotomy should be performed when pancreatitis due to choledocholithiasis is severe or when there is cholangitis.

Prognosis

Mild acute cholecystitis usually subsides, but recurrences are common. Symptomatic cholecystitis is a definite indication for surgery. Persistence of symptoms after removal of the gallbladder (postcholecystectomy syndrome) implies either mistaken diagnosis, functional bowel disorder, technical error, retained or recurrent common bile duct stone, or spasm of the sphincter of Oddi (see below).

Hickman MS, Schwesinger WH, Page CP: Acute cholecystitis in the diabetic: A case-control study of outcome. Arch Surg 1988;123:409. (Infectious complications postoperatively are greater in diabetics; sepsis is the major cause of death.)

Hidalgo LA et al: The influence of age on early surgical treatment of cholecystitis. Surg Gynec Obstet 1989;169:393. (Mortality rate not different in those over 60 compared with those under 60.)

Williamson RCN: Progress report: Acalculous disease of the gallbladder. Gut 1988;29:860.

Zeman RK, Garra BS: Gallbladder imaging: The state of the art. Gastroenterol Clin North Am 1991;20:127. (HIDA 98% sensitive, 81% specific for acute cholecystitis. Ultrasound 67% and 82%, respectively.)

CYSTIC DUCT SYNDROMES

Precholecystectomy

A small group of patients (mostly women) has been reported in whom right upper quadrant abdominal pain occurs frequently following meals. Conventional radiographic study of the upper gastrointestinal tract and gallbladder—including intravenous cholangiography—is unremarkable. However, using cholecystokinin (CCK) as a gallbladder stimulant, contraction and evacuation of the viscus does not take place, as usually occurs in the 3- to 5-minute period after injection of the hormone. Instead, the gallbladder assumes a "golf ball" configuration, and biliary type pain is reproduced. At the time of cholecystectomy, the gallbladders are often enlarged and cannot be emptied by manual compression. Anatomic and histologic examination of the operative specimens reveals obstruction of the cystic ducts either because of fibrotic stenosis at their proximal ends or because of adhesions and kinking. Additional diagnostic considerations are ampullary spasm and biliary dyskinesia (see below).

Postcholecystectomy

Following cholecystectomy, a variable group of patients complain of continuing symptoms, ie, right upper quadrant pain, flatulence, and fatty food intolerance. The persistence of symptoms in this group of patients suggests the possibility of an incorrect diagnosis prior to cholecystectomy, eg, esophagitis, pancreatitis, radiculopathy, or functional bowel disease. It is important to rule out the possibility of choledocholithiasis or common duct stricture as a cause for persistent symptoms in the postoperative period.

Pain has been associated with dilatation of the cystic duct remnant, neuroma formation in the ductal wall, foreign body granuloma, or traction on the common duct by a long cystic duct. The clinical presentation of colicky pain, chills, fever, or jaundice should suggest biliary tract disease, including spasm of the ampulla of Vater. Liver tests for cholestasis, abdominal ultrasonography, or retrograde cholangiography may be necessary to rule out biliary tract disease. Biliary manometry during ERCP may be helpful, demonstrating elevated baseline sphincter of Oddi pressures. Endoscopic sphincterotomy or surgical sphincteroplasty with common duct exploration for stones and removal of the cystic duct remnant may be necessary.

Csendes A et al: Mirizzi syndrome and cholecystobiliary fistula: A unifying classification. Brit J Surg 1989; 76:1139. (Compression of the common bile duct by a stone impacted in the gallbladder neck.)
Steinberg WM: Sphincter of Oddi dysfunction: A clinical controversy. Gastroenterology 1988;95:1409. (Reviews the controversies. Controlled trials of therapy are still needed.)

CHRONIC CHOLECYSTITIS

The most common disorder that results from cholelithiasis is chronic cholecystitis, characterized pathologically by varying degrees of chronic inflammation on gross inspection or microscopic examination of the gallbladder. In about 4–5% of cases, the villi of the gallbladder undergo polypoid enlargement due to deposition of cholesterol that may be visible to the naked eye ("strawberry gallbladder," cholesterolosis). In other instances, adenomatous hyperplasia of all or part of the gallbladder wall may be so marked as to give the appearance of a myoma (pseudotumor). Calculi are usually present. The diagnosis of chronic cholecystitis is often erroneously applied to collections of symptoms that are only vaguely or indirectly related to gallbladder dysfunction.

Clinical Findings
A. Symptoms and Signs:
1. Pain–Chronic cholecystitis may be associated with discrete bouts of right hypochondriac and epigastric pain that is either steady or intermittent. Discomfort is usually persistent, but, if intermittent, the height of pain may be separated by 15- to 60-minute intervals.

The onset of pain may be abrupt, with maximum intensity and plateau reached within 15 minutes to 1 hour. Attacks of biliary colic may persist for as long as several hours or be as brief as 15–20 minutes, the

average duration being about 1 hour. Pain referral to the interscapular area or shoulder is occasionally noted.

Fatty food intolerance, belching, flatulence, a sense of epigastric heaviness, upper abdominal pain of varying intensity, and pyrosis are often erroneously considered to be suggestive of cholelithiasis and cholecystitis but are usually not relieved by cholecystectomy.

2. Physical examination–Physical examination is nonspecific, revealing abdominal tenderness which may be localized to the right hypochondrium and epigastric area but which may also be diffuse. Hydrops of the gallbladder results when acute cholecystitis subsides but cystic duct obstruction persists, producing distention of the gallbladder with a clear mucoid fluid. The gallbladder in that circumstance is palpable in the right upper abdomen. The presence of jaundice supports the diagnosis of cholecystitis with choledocholithiasis.

B. Laboratory Findings: Routine laboratory studies (white count, liver function tests, amylase) are often normal or minimally elevated.

C. Imaging: Films of the abdomen taken prior to oral cholecystography may reveal opacification of the gallbladder caused by high concentrations of calcium carbonate (limy bile) or radiopaque stones. Nonvisualization of the gallbladder implies cholecystitis (95% accuracy) provided there is radiologic evidence that the oral contrast material has been absorbed and excreted. Technical reasons for nonvisualization must be excluded: failure to ingest the dye, vomiting or diarrhea, gastric outlet obstruction or esophageal stricture, intestinal malabsorption, abnormal location of the gallbladder, liver disease (including preicteric hepatitis), Dubin-Johnson syndrome, fat-free diet prior to cholecystography, and previous cholecystectomy.

Ultrasound examination of the gallbladder is a useful means of detecting stones. The sensitivity of diagnosis of cholelithiasis (but not cholecystitis) is high (96%) and the incidence of false-positive results low (2%).

Differential Diagnosis
When nonspecific symptoms are present, it is necessary to consider gastroduodenal ulcer disease, chronic relapsing pancreatitis, irritable bowel syndrome, and malignant neoplasms of the stomach, pancreas, hepatic flexure, or gallbladder. Barium enema and upper gastrointestinal series complement cholecystography. Microscopic examination of bile obtained by biliary drainage is occasionally helpful in confirming calculous disease of the gallbladder. (The test is valid only in the absence of hepatic disease.)

Complications
The presence of cholelithiasis with chronic cholecystitis may be associated with acute exacerbations

of gallbladder inflammation, common duct stone, cholecystenteric fistulization, pancreatitis, and, rarely, carcinoma of the gallbladder. Calcified (porcelain) gallbladder has a high association with gallbladder carcinoma and is an indication for cholecystectomy.

Treatment

Surgical treatment is the same as for acute cholecystitis. If indicated, cholangiography can be performed during laparoscopic cholecystectomy. Choledocholithiasis can also be excluded by either pre- or postoperative ERCP.

Prognosis

The overall mortality rate of cholecystectomy is less than 1%, but hepatobiliary tract surgery is a more formidable procedure in the elderly, in whom the mortality rate is 5–10%. A technically successful surgical procedure in an appropriately selected patient is generally followed by complete cessation of symptoms.

Ramond MJ et al: Sensitivity and specificity of microscopic examination of gallbladder bile for gallstone recognition and identification. Gastroenterology 1988;95:1339. (Presence of crystals in gallbladder bile is highly predictive of gallstone disease.)

The Southern Surgeons Club: A prospective analysis of 1518 laparoscopic cholecystectomies. N Engl J Med 1991;124:1073. (Results similar to those of conventional cholecystectomy with much shorter convalescence.)

CHOLEDOCHOLITHIASIS

Essentials of Diagnosis

- Often a history of biliary colic or jaundice.
- Sudden onset of severe right upper quadrant or epigastric pain, which may radiate to the right scapula or shoulder.
- Occasional patients present with painless jaundice.
- Nausea and vomiting.
- Fever, often followed by hypothermia and gramnegative shock, jaundice, and leukocytosis.
- Abdominal films may reveal gallstones.

General Considerations

About 15% of patients with gallstones have choledocholithiasis. The percentage rises with age, and the incidence in elderly people may be as high as 50%. Common duct stones usually originate in the gallbladder but may also form spontaneously in the common duct postcholecystectomy. The stones are frequently "silent" as no symptoms result unless there is obstruction.

Clinical Findings

A. Symptoms and Signs: A history suggestive of biliary colic or prior jaundice can usually be obtained. Biliary colic results from rapid increases in common bile duct pressure due to obstructed bile flow. The additional features that suggest the presence of a common duct stone are (1) frequently recurring attacks of right upper abdominal pain that is severe and persists for hours: (2) chills and fever associated with severe colic; and (3) a history of jaundice associated with episodes of abdominal pain. The combination of pain, fever (and chills), and jaundice represents **Charcot's triad** and denotes the classic picture of cholangitis. The presence of altered sensorium, lethargy, and septic shock connotes acute suppurative cholangitis accompanied by pus in the obstructed duct and represents an endoscopic emergency.

Hepatomegaly may be present in calculous biliary obstruction, and tenderness is usually present in the right hypochondrium and epigastrium. Usually there are no specific physical findings.

B. Laboratory Findings: Bilirubinuria and elevation of serum bilirubin are present if the common duct is obstructed; levels commonly fluctuate. Serum alkaline phosphatase elevation is especially suggestive of obstructive jaundice. Not uncommonly, serum amylase elevations are present because of secondary pancreatitis. On occasion, acute obstruction of the bile duct produces a transient striking increase in serum aminotransferase levels (> 1000 units/L). Prolongation of the prothrombin time occurs when there is prolonged interruption of the flow of bile to the intestine. When extrahepatic obstruction persists for more than a few weeks, differentiation of obstruction from chronic cholestatic liver disease becomes progressively more difficult.

C. Imaging: Ultrasonography, CT scan, and radionuclide imaging may demonstrate dilated bile ducts and impaired bile flow. Percutaneous transhepatic cholangiography or endoscopic retrograde cholangiography (ERCP) provides the most direct and accurate means of determining the cause, location, and extent of obstruction. If the obstruction is thought to be due to a stone, ERCP is the procedure of choice because it permits papillotomy with stone extraction.

Differential Diagnosis

The most common cause of obstructive jaundice is common duct stone. Next in frequency is carcinoma of the pancreas, ampulla of Vater, or common duct. Metastatic carcinoma involving porta hepatis lymph nodes (usually from the gastrointestinal tract) and direct extension of gallbladder cancer are other important causes of obstructive jaundice. Chronic cholestatic liver diseases (primarily biliary cirrhosis, sclerosing cholangitis) must be considered. Hepatocellular jaundice can usually be differentiated by the history, clinical findings, and liver tests, but liver biopsy is necessary on occasion.

Complications

A. Biliary Cirrhosis: Common duct obstruction lasting longer than 30 days results in liver damage leading to cirrhosis. Hepatic failure with portal hypertension occurs in untreated cases.

B. Hypoprothrombinemia: Patients with obstructive jaundice or liver disease may bleed excessively as a result of prolonged prothrombin times. In contrast to hepatocellular dysfunction, hypoprothrombinemia due to obstructive jaundice will respond to 10 mg of parenteral vitamin K or water-soluble oral vitamin K (phytonadione, 5 mg) within 24–36 hours.

Treatment

Common duct stone in a patient with cholelithiasis is usually treated by cholecystectomy and choledochostomy. In the postcholecystectomy patient with choledocholithiasis, endoscopic papillotomy with stone extraction is preferable to transabdominal surgery. Lithotripsy, external or endoscopic, may be a therapeutic consideration for large stones.

A. Preoperative Preparation: Emergency intervention is rarely necessary unless severe ascending cholangitis is present. Liver function should be evaluated thoroughly. Prothrombin time should be restored to normal by parenteral administration of vitamin K preparations (see above). Nutrition should be restored by a high-carbohydrate, high-protein diet and vitamin supplementation. Cholangitis, if present, should be controlled with antimicrobials—eg, mezlocillin, 3 g intravenously every 4 hours, plus either metronidazole, 500 mg intravenously every 8 hours (if no prior manipulation of duct), or gentamicin, 2 mg/kg intravenously as loading dose, plus 1.5 mg/kg every 8 hours adjusted for renal function (if prior manipulation of duct)—but more urgent decompression may be required.

B. Indications for Common Duct Exploration: At every operation for cholelithiasis, the advisability of exploring the common duct must be considered. Operative cholangiography via the cystic duct is a very useful procedure for demonstrating common duct stones.

1. Preoperative findings suggestive of choledocholithiasis include a history (or the presence) of obstructive jaundice; frequent attacks of biliary colic; cholangitis; a history of pancreatitis; and a preoperative cholangiogram showing stone, obstruction, or dilatation of the duct.

2. Operative findings of choledocholithiasis are palpable stones in the common duct; dilatation or thickening of the wall of the common duct; gallbladder stones small enough to pass through the cystic duct; and pancreatitis.

3. For the patient with a T tube and a common duct stone, manipulation with various special instruments via the T tube or T tube sinus tract is often successful in extracting the stone.

4. For the poor-risk patient, endoscopic sphincterotomy has become the treatment of choice even if cholecystectomy for cholelithiasis is considered too risky.

C. Postoperative Care:

1. Antibiotics–Postoperative antibiotics are not administered routinely after biliary tract surgery. Cultures of the bile are always taken at operation. If biliary tract infection was present preoperatively or is apparent at operation, ampicillin (500 mg every 6 hours intravenously) with gentamicin or a third-generation cephalosporin is administered postoperatively until the results of sensitivity tests on culture specimens are available.

2. Management of the T-tube–Following choledochostomy, a simple catheter or T tube is placed in the common duct for decompression. A properly placed tube should drain bile at the operating table and continuously thereafter; otherwise, it should be considered blocked or dislocated. The volume of bile drainage varies from 100 to 1000 mL daily (average, 200–400 mL). Above-average drainage may be due to obstruction at the ampulla (usually by edema).

3. Cholangiography–A T-tube cholangiogram should be done on about the seventh or eighth postoperative day. If the cholangiogram shows no stones in the common duct and the opaque medium flows freely into the duodenum, the tube is clamped overnight and removed by simple traction the following day. A small amount of bile frequently leaks from the tube site for a few days.

Bonar S et al: Recurrent cholangitis secondary to Oriental cholangiohepatitis. J Clin Gastroenterol 1989;11:464. (Part of the differential diagnosis of cholangitis in Southeast Asia.)

Greig JD, Krukowski ZH, Matheson NA: Surgical morbidity and mortality in 129 patients with obstructive jaundice. Br J Surg 1988;75:216. (Results suggest that preoperative biliary drainage is of little benefit.)

Kozarek RA (editor): Endoscopic approach to biliary stones. Gastrointest Endosc Clin North Am 1991;1:1.

Lai ECS et al: Acute cholangitis: Endoscopic drainage or emergency surgery? Surgery 1990;107:268. (Either procedure controls the sepsis. Unclear which is preferable.)

Siegman-Igra Y et al: Septicemia from biliary tract infection. Arch Surg 1988;123:366. (Gram-negative rods— *E coli, Klebsiella-Enterobacter*—account for 70% of cases of sepsis of biliary tract origin. Recommend ampicillin and gentamicin as initial treatment.)

BILIARY STRICTURE

Benign biliary strictures are the result of surgical trauma in about 95% of cases. The remainder are caused by blunt external injury to the abdomen, pancreatitis, or erosion of the duct by a gallstone.

Signs of injury to the duct may or may not be recognized in the immediate postoperative period. If complete occlusion has occurred, jaundice will develop rapidly; but more often a tear has been accidentally made in the duct, and the earliest manifestation of injury may be excessive or prolonged loss of bile from the surgical drains. Bile leakage may predispose to localized infection, which in turn accentuates scar formation and the ultimate development of a fibrous stricture.

Cholangitis is the most common syndrome produced by stricture. Typically, the patient experiences episodes of pain, fever, chills, and jaundice within a few weeks to months after cholecystectomy. With the exception of jaundice during an attack of cholangitis and right upper quadrant abdominal tenderness, physical findings are usually not significant.

Serum alkaline phosphatase is usually elevated. Hyperbilirubinemia is variable, fluctuating during exacerbations and usually remaining in the range of 5–10 mg/dL. Blood cultures may be positive during an episode of cholangitis. Percutaneous transhepatic cholangiography or endoscopic retrograde cholangiopancreatography can be valuable in demonstrating the stricture, permitting biopsy and cytologic specimens, and allowing dilation and stent placement.

Differentiation from cholangiocarcinoma may require surgical exploration. Operative treatment of a stricture frequently necessitates performance of choledochojejunostomy or hepaticojejunostomy to reestablish bile flow into the intestine.

Biliary stricture is not a benign condition, since significant hepatocellular disease will inevitably occur if it is allowed to continue uncorrected. The death rate for untreated stricture ranges from 10% to 15%.

Standfield NJ et al: Benign non-traumatic inflammatory strictures of the extrahepatic biliary system. Br J Surg 1989;76:849. (Do well with surgical correction.)

Venu RP et al: A new guidewire technique for biliary strictures. Gastrointest Endosc 1991;37:553. (Fairly technical but short, pertinent bibliography.)

PRIMARY SCLEROSING CHOLANGITIS

Primary sclerosing cholangitis is a rare nonspecific inflammatory reaction of unknown cause involving both the intra- and extrahepatic biliary ducts. It is characterized by a diffuse inflammation of the biliary tract leading to fibrosis and strictures of the biliary system. The disease is closely associated with ulcerative colitis, which is present in approximately two-thirds of patients with primary sclerosing cholangitis; however, only 1% of patients with ulcerative colitis develop clinically significant sclerosing cholangitis. Patients with primary sclerosing cholangitis often (60–80%, versus 25% for controls) have the histocompatible antigen HLA-B8, suggesting that genetic

factors may play an etiologic role. Primary sclerosing cholangitis may occur at any period of life but is most common in males aged 20–40.

The diagnosis of primary sclerosing cholangitis is made by endoscopic retrograde cholangiography and biliary obstruction by a stone or tumor. In a minority of cases, the disease is confined to small intrahepatic bile ducts, ERCP is normal, and the diagnosis is suggested by liver biopsy. In general, the diagnosis of primary sclerosing cholangitis cannot be made after biliary surgery or intrahepatic artery chemotherapy, which may result in bile duct injury. Cholangiocarcinoma may complicate the course of primary sclerosing cholangitis in 10–15% of cases and may be difficult to diagnose by cytologic examination or biopsy because of false-negative results. In patients with AIDS, sclerosing cholangitis may result from infections caused by CMV, *Cryptosporidium,* or *Microsporidium.*

Clinically, the disease presents as progressively obstructive jaundice, frequently preceded by malaise, pruritus, anorexia, and indigestion. Some patients are diagnosed in a presymptomatic phase because of an elevated alkaline phosphatase. Treatment with corticosteroids and broad-spectrum antimicrobial agents has been employed with inconsistent and unpredictable results. Ursodeoxycholic acid and methotrexate are experimental therapies. Surgical intervention is in part dependent on the stage of the disease. In patients without cirrhosis on liver biopsy, careful evaluation of the biliary tree may make balloon dilation of localized strictures a good option. If there is a major stricture, stenting is a possibility. For those with cirrhosis and clinical decompensation, liver transplantation is the procedure of choice. Actuarial survival rates with liver transplantation for this disease are 71% at 1 year, 57% at 3 years.

The prognosis is poor, with few individuals living more than a few years after the appearance of symptoms.

Case Records of the Massachusetts General Hospital: Weekly clinicopathological exercises. A 17-year-old boy with autoimmune hemolytic anemia and abnormal liver function. N Engl J Med 1991;324:180.

LaRusso NF et al (editors): Primary sclerosing cholangitis. Semin Liver Dis 1991;11:1.

CARCINOMA OF THE BILIARY TRACT

Carcinoma of the gallbladder occurs in approximately 2% of all people operated on for biliary tract disease. It is notoriously insidious, and the diagnosis is usually made unexpectedly at surgery. Spread of the cancer—by direct extension into the liver or to the peritoneal surface—may be the initial manifestation.

Carcinoma of the extrahepatic bile ducts accounts

for 3% of all cancer deaths in the USA. It affects both sexes equally but is more prevalent in individuals age 50–70. Tumors often arise at the confluence of the hepatic ducts (Klatskin tumors). The incidence of carcinoma in those with choledochal cysts has been reported to be 2–8%. There is an increased incidence in patients with chronic nonspecific ulcerative colitis. In southeast Asia, infection of the bile ducts with helminths (*Clonorchis sinensis, Fasciola hepatica*) is associated with chronic cholangitis and an increased risk of cholangiocarcinoma.

Clinical Findings

Progressive jaundice is the most common and usually the first sign of obstruction of the extrahepatic biliary system. Pain is usually present in the right upper abdomen and radiates into the back. Anorexia and weight loss are common and frequently associated with fever and chills. Rarely, hematemesis results from erosion of tumor into a blood vessel (hemobilia). Fistula formation between the biliary system and adjacent organs may also occur. The course is usually one of rapid deterioration, with death occurring within a few months.

Physical examination will reveal profound jaundice. A palpable gallbladder with obstructive jaundice usually is said to signify malignant disease (Courvoisier's law); however, this clinical generalization has been proved to be accurate only about 50% of the time. Hepatomegaly is usually present and is associated with liver tenderness. Ascites may occur with peritoneal implants. Pruritus and skin excoriations are common.

Laboratory examination reveals predominantly conjugated hyperbilirubinemia, with total serum bilirubin values ranging from 5 to 30 mg/dL. There is usually concomitant elevation of the alkaline phosphatase and serum cholesterol. AST is normal or minimally elevated.

The most helpful diagnostic studies before surgery are either percutaneous transhepatic or endoscopic retrograde cholangiography with biopsy and cytologic specimens. One or both of these procedures may be required in order to define the pathologic anatomy of the ductal obstruction.

Treatment

In young and fit patients, curative surgery may be attempted if the tumor is well localized. If the tumor is unresectable at laparotomy, cholecystoduodenostomy or T tube drainage of the common duct can be performed. In poor surgical risks, palliation can be achieved by placement of a stent via the endoscopic or percutaneous transhepatic route. The prognosis is poor, with few patients surviving for more than 6 months after surgery.

Chao TC, Greager JA: Primary carcinoma of the gallbladder. J Surg Oncol 1991;46:215. (Late diagnosis a problem. Five-year survival rate is 5.4%.)
Ishikawa O et al: The difference in malignancy between pedunculated and sessile polypoid lesions of the gallbladder. Am J Gastroenterol 1989;84:1386. (Thirteen percent of pedunculated and 33% of sessile lesions were malignant.)
Lygidakis NJ, Van Der Heyde MN (editors): Klatskin tumors. Semin Liver Dis 1990;10:85.
Nesbit GM et al: Cholangiocarcinoma: Diagnosis and evaluation of resectability by CT and sonography as procedures complementary to cholangiography. Am J Roentgenol 1988;151:933.

DISEASES OF THE PANCREAS

ACUTE PANCREATITIS

Essentials of Diagnosis

- Abrupt onset of dull epigastric pain, often with radiation to the back.
- Nausea, vomiting, sweating, weakness.
- Abdominal tenderness and distention, fever.
- Leukocytosis, elevated serum amylase, elevated serum lipase.
- History of previous episodes, often related to alcohol intake.

General Considerations

Acute pancreatitis is thought to result from "escape" of activated pancreatic enzymes from acinar cells into surrounding tissues. Most cases are related to biliary tract disease or heavy alcohol intake. Among the numerous other causes or associations are hypercalcemia, hyperlipidemias (types I, IV, and V), abdominal trauma (including surgery), drugs (including sulfonamides and thiazides), vasculitis, viral infections, and ERCP. The exact pathogenesis is not known but may include edema or obstruction of the ampulla of Vater with resultant reflux of bile into pancreatic ducts or direct injury to the acinar cells. In patients with pancreas divisum, a congenital anomaly in which the dorsal and ventral pancreatic ducts fail to fuse, acute pancreatitis may result from stenosis of the minor papilla with obstruction to flow from the accessory pancreatic duct.

Pathologic changes vary from acute edema and cellular infiltration to necrosis of the acinar cells, hemorrhage from necrotic blood vessels, and intra- and extrapancreatic fat necrosis. All or part of the pancreas may be involved.

Clinical Findings

A. Symptoms and Signs: Epigastric abdominal pain, generally abrupt in onset, is steady and severe and often made worse by walking and lying supine and better by sitting and leaning forward. The pain usually radiates into the back but may radiate to the right or left. Nausea and vomiting are usually present. Severe weakness, sweating, and anxiety are noted in severe attacks. There may be a history of alcohol intake or a heavy meal immediately preceding the attack, or a history of milder similar episodes or biliary colic in the past.

The abdomen is tender mainly in the upper abdomen, most often without guarding, rigidity, or rebound. The abdomen may be distended, and bowel sounds may be absent in associated paralytic ileus. Fever of 38.4–39 °C (101.1–102.2 °F), tachycardia, hypotension (even true shock), pallor, and a cool clammy skin are often present. Mild jaundice is common. Occasionally, an upper abdominal mass may be present. Acute renal failure (usually prerenal) may occur early in the course of acute pancreatitis.

B. Assessment of Severity: Ranson's criteria are generally used in assessing the severity of acute alcoholic pancreatitis on presentation (pancreatitis due to other causes has similar criteria). When three or more of the following criteria are present on admission, a severe course can be predicted:

1. Age over 55 years.
2. White blood cell count over 16,000/μL.
3. Blood glucose over 200 mg/dL.
4. Base deficit over 4 meq/L.
5. Serum LDH over 350 IU/L.
6. AST over 250 IU/L.

Development of the following in the first 48 hours indicates a worsening prognosis:

1. Hematocrit drop of more than ten percentage points.
2. BUN rise greater than 5 mg/dL.
3. Arterial PO_2 of less than 60 mm Hg.
4. Serum calcium of less than 8 mg/dL.
5. Estimated fluid sequestration of more than 6 L.

Mortality rates correlate with the number of criteria present:

Number of Criteria	Mortality Rate
0–2	1%
3–4	16%
5–6	40%
7–8	100%

C. Laboratory Findings: Findings of leukocytosis (10,000–30,000/μL), proteinuria, casts (25% of cases), glycosuria (10–20% of cases), hyperglycemia, and elevated serum bilirubin may be present. Blood urea nitrogen and serum alkaline phosphatase may be elevated and coagulation tests abnormal. Decrease in serum calcium may reflect saponification and correlates well with severity of disease. Levels lower than 7 mg/dL (when serum albumin is normal)

are associated with tetany and an unfavorable prognosis.

Serum amylase and lipase are elevated within 24 hours in 90% of cases, and return to normal is variable depending on the severity of disease. In those who develop ascites or left pleural effusions, amylase content is high and suggests the underlying cause.

D. Imaging: Plain radiographs of the abdomen may show gallstones, a "sentinel loop" (a segment of air-filled small intestine most commonly in the left upper quadrant), the "colon cutoff sign" (a gas-filled segment of transverse colon abruptly ending at the area of pancreatic inflammation), or linear focal atelectasis of the left lower lobe of the lungs with or without pleural effusion. These findings suggest acute pancreatitis but are not diagnostic. CT scan is useful in demonstrating an enlarged pancreas, in detecting pseudocysts, and in determining the extent of a phlegmon (swollen mass of inflamed pancreatic tissue) as well as differentiating pancreatitis from other possible intra-abdominal catastrophes. Dynamic bolus CT is of particular value in identifying areas of pancreatic necrosis that may require surgical debridement; the presence of a fluid collection correlates with an increased mortality rate. Ultrasonography is less reliable, because the echoes are deflected by the gas-distended small intestine frequently associated with pancreatitis.

E. Electrocardiographic Findings: ST–T wave changes may occur, but they usually differ from those of myocardial infarction. Abnormal Q waves do not occur as a result of pancreatitis.

Differential Diagnosis

Acute pancreatitis may be difficult to differentiate from an acutely perforated duodenal ulcer. Pancreatitis may be the presenting clinical picture of choledocholithiasis, with or without cholangitis, and of a penetrating duodenal ulcer, and may result from mumps virus infection or ERCP or may occur postoperatively owing to surgical manipulation in the area of the pancreas. Serum amylase may also be elevated in high intestinal obstruction, in mumps not involving the pancreas (salivary amylase), in ectopic pregnancy, after administration of narcotics, and after abdominal surgery. Other conditions to be differentiated are acute cholecystitis, acute intestinal obstruction, leaking aortic aneurysm, renal colic, and acute mesenteric vascular insufficiency or thrombosis.

Complications

Intravascular volume depletion secondary to leakage of fluids in the pancreatic bed and ileus with fluid-filled loops of bowel may result in prerenal azotemia and even acute tubular necrosis without overt shock. This usually occurs within 24 hours of the onset of acute pancreatitis and lasts 8–9 days. Some patients require peritoneal dialysis or hemodialysis.

One of the most serious complications of acute

pancreatitis is adult respiratory distress syndrome (ARDS); cardiac dysfunction may be superimposed. It usually occurs 3–7 days after the onset of pancreatitis in patients who have required large volumes of fluid and colloid to maintain blood pressure and urine output. Most patients with ARDS require assisted respiration with positive end-expiratory pressure.

Pancreatic abscess is a suppurative process in necrotic tissue, characterized by with rising fever, leukocytosis, and localized tenderness and epigastric mass 2–3 weeks into the course of acute pancreatitis. This may be associated with a left-sided pleural effusion or an enlarging spleen secondary to splenic vein thrombosis.

Pseudocysts, encapsulated fluid collections with high enzyme content, commonly appear in pancreatitis when CT scans are used to monitor the evolution of an acute attack. Although the natural history of pseudocysts is still not well delineated, it appears that those less than 6 cm in diameter often resolve spontaneously. Pseudocysts most commonly are within or adjacent to the pancreas but can present anywhere (eg, mediastinal, retrorectal), by extension along anatomic planes. Pseudocysts are multiple in 14% of cases. Pseudocysts may become secondarily infected, necessitating drainage as for an abscess. Erosion of the inflammatory process into a blood vessel can result in a major hemorrhage into the cyst.

Chronic pancreatitis develops in about 10% of cases. Permanent diabetes mellitus and exocrine pancreatic insufficiency occur uncommonly after a single acute episode.

Treatment

A. Management of Acute Disease: In most patients, acute pancreatitis is a mild disease that subsides spontaneously within several days. The pancreatic rest program includes withholding food and liquids by mouth, bed rest, and, in those with moderately severe pain or ileus, nasogastric suction. Pain is controlled with meperidine, up to 100–150 mg intramuscularly every 3–4 hours as necessary. In those with severe hepatic or renal dysfunction, the dose may need to be reduced. Other narcotics may be used if pain control is not achieved, but they may cause greater smooth muscle contraction (spasm of the ampulla of Vater).

In more severe pancreatitis, there may be considerable leakage of fluids, necessitating large amounts of intravenous fluids to maintain intravascular volume. Saline is chiefly used, but fresh-frozen plasma or serum albumin may be necessary. With colloid solutions, there may be an increased risk of developing adult respiratory distress syndrome. If shock persists after adequate volume replacement (including packed red cells), pressors may be required. For the patient requiring a large volume of parenteral fluids, central venous pressure and blood gases should be monitored at regular intervals.

Calcium gluconate must be given intravenously if there is evidence of hypocalcemia with tetany. Antibiotics should be reserved for specific infections. Cultures of blood, urine, sputum, and pleural effusion (if present) and needle aspirations of areas of pancreatic necrosis (with CT guidance) should be obtained. Proved or suspected infections should be treated with appropriate antibiotics.

The patient with severe pancreatitis requires attention in an intensive care unit. Close follow-up of blood count, hematocrit, serum electrolytes, serum calcium, serum creatinine, and arterial blood gases is mandatory.

B. Treatment of Complications and Follow-Up: No fluid or foods should be given orally until the patient is largely free of pain and has bowel sounds. Clear liquids are then given, and a gradual progression to a regular low-fat diet is pursued, guided by the patient's tolerance and by the absence of pain. Pancreatitis complicated by prolonged ileus (24 hours or more), abdominal distention, or vomiting requires nasogastric suction until they subside, along with parenteral nutrition. Intravenous fluids are given as needed to replace lost fluids, electrolytes, and blood.

A surgeon should be consulted in all cases of suspected acute pancreatitis. If the diagnosis is in doubt and investigations indicate a strong possibility of a serious surgically correctable lesion (eg, perforated peptic ulcer, common duct stone), exploration is indicated. When acute pancreatitis is unexpectedly found on exploratory laparotomy, it is usually wise to close without intervention of any kind. If the pancreatitis appears mild and cholelithiasis is present, cholecystostomy or cholecystectomy may be justified.

Aggressive surgery and enteral or parenteral hyperalimentation may increase survival in patients with pancreatic necrosis. Initially, enterostomy tubes and drainage are established. Subsequent surgery is performed to debride necrotic pancreas and surrounding tissue. Peritoneal lavage has not been shown to improve survival in severe acute pancreatitis. Late septic complications are unaffected.

The development of a pancreatic abscess is an indication for prompt drainage, usually through the flank. Pseudocysts may require drainage, when infected or associated with persisting pain, pancreatitis, or common duct obstruction. Diagnosis of infection in a pseudocyst may be difficult; empirical broad-spectrum antibiotics are initiated—a third-generation cephalosporin and metronidazole, 15 mg/kg,d—and the decision to explore surgically or drain percutaneously is mainly a clinical one.

Prognosis

Recurrences are common in alcoholic pancreatitis. The mortality rate for severe acute pancreatitis (> three Ranson criteria) is high, especially when hepatic, cardiovascular, or renal impairment is present.

Adler J, Barkin JS: Management of pseudocysts, inflammatory masses and pancreatic ascites. Gastroenterol Clin North Am 1990;19:863.

Gumaste V et al: Serum lipase: A better test to diagnose acute alcoholic pancreatitis. Am J Med 1992;92:239. (No overlap of values in patients with image-proved pancreatitis and asymptomatic alcoholics as opposed to a 45% overlap in amylase values.)

Hodgdon AK, Wolfson AB: Pancreatitis. Emerg Med Clin 1990;8:873. (Causes, clinical presentation, and initial management.)

Kelly TR, Wagner DA: Gallstone pancreatitis: A prospective randomized trial of the timing of surgery. Surgery 1988;104:600. (Best after pancreatitis has subsided.)

Levine SA, Feinsilver SH, Fein AM: What to do when pancreatitis causes pleuropulmonary complications. J Crit Illness 1990;5:715. (Occult hypoxemia may be the first sign of acute lung injury.)

Pisters PWT, Ranson JHC: Nutritional support for acute pancreatitis. Surg Gynecol Obstet 1992;175:275.

CHRONIC PANCREATITIS

Chronic pancreatitis occurs most often in patients with alcoholism, hereditary pancreatitis, severe malnutrition, or untreated hyperparathyroidism, or it may be idiopathic. Progressive fibrosis and destruction of functioning glandular tissue occur as a result. Pancreaticolithiasis and obstruction of the duodenal end of the pancreatic duct are often present. (Acute pancreatitis recurring after cholecystectomy for cholelithiasis should raise the suspicion of a retained or newly developed common duct stone.)

Differentiation of chronic from recurrent pancreatitis is important in that recurrent pancreatitis is initiated by a specific event (eg, alcoholic binge, passage of a stone), whereas chronic pancreatitis is a self-perpetuating disease characterized by pain and pancreatic exocrine or endocrine insufficiency.

Clinical Findings

A. Symptoms and Signs: Persistent or recurrent episodes of epigastric and left upper quadrant pain with referral to the upper left lumbar region are typical. Anorexia, nausea, vomiting, constipation, flatulence, and weight loss are common. Abdominal signs during attacks consist chiefly of tenderness over the pancreas, mild muscle guarding, and paralytic ileus. Attacks may last only a few hours or as long as 2 weeks; pain may eventually be almost continuous. Steatorrhea (as indicated by bulky, foul, fatty stools) may occur late in the course.

B. Laboratory Findings: Serum amylase, lipase, and bilirubin may be elevated during acute attacks; normal amylase does not exclude the diagnosis, however. Glycosuria may be present. Excess fecal fat may be demonstrated on chemical analysis of the stool; pancreatic insufficiency may be confirmed by a bentiromide (NBT-PABA) test or secretin stimulation test.

C. Imaging: Plain films often show calcifications due to pancreaticolithiasis and mild ileus. Right upper quadrant ultrasound may reveal cholelithiasis, and upper gastrointestinal series may demonstrate a widened duodenal loop. Endoscopic retrograde cholangiopancreatography may show dilated ducts, intraductal stones, strictures, or pseudocyst.

Complications

Narcotic addiction is common. Other frequent complications include diabetes mellitus, pancreatic pseudocyst or abscess, cholestatic liver disease with or without jaundice, common bile duct stricture, steatorrhea, malnutrition, and peptic ulcer.

Treatment

Correctable coexistent biliary tract disease should be treated surgically.

A. Medical Measures: A low-fat diet should be prescribed. Alcohol is forbidden because it frequently precipitates attacks. Anticholinergics (eg, propantheline, 15 mg before meals three times daily) may be helpful. Narcotics should be avoided if possible. Steatorrhea is treated with pancreatic supplements that are selected on the basis of their high lipase activity. The usual dose is 30,000 units of lipase in capsules given before, during, and after meals (Table 15–6). Concurrent administration of sodium bicarbonate or H_2 receptor antagonists (eg, ranitidine, 150 mg twice daily) decreases the inactivation of lipase by acid and may thereby further decrease steatorrhea. In selected cases of alcoholic pancreatitis and in cystic fibrosis, enteric-coated microencapsulated preparations may also offer an advantage. Pain secondary to idiopathic chronic pancreatitis may be benefited by the use of pancreatic enzymes. Treat associated diabetes as for any other insulinopenic patient. Every effort is made to manage the disease medically.

Table 15–6. Selected pancreatic enzyme (pancrelipase) preparations.[1]

Product	Enzyme Content Per Unit Dose		
	Lipase	Amylase	Protease
Conventional preparations			
Viokase	8,000	30,000	30,000
Ilozyme	11,000	30,000	30,000
Cotazyme	8,000	30,000	30,000
Enteric-coated microencapsulated preparations			
Pancrease	4,000	25,000	20,000
Pancrease MT16	16,000	48,000	48,000
Cotazyme-S	5,000	20,000	20,000

[1]Adapted from Morrow JD: Topics in clinical pharmacology: Pancreatic enzyme replacement therapy. Am J Med Sci 1989; 198:357.

B. Surgical Treatment: Surgery may be indicated in chronic pancreatitis for internal drainage of persistent pseudocysts, to treat other complications, or, rarely, to attempt to relieve pain. The objectives of surgical intervention are to eradicate biliary tract disease, ensure a free flow of bile into the duodenum, and eliminate obstruction of the pancreatic duct. When obstruction of the duodenal end of the duct can be demonstrated by endoscopic retrograde cholangiopancreatography, dilatation of the duct or resection of the tail of the pancreas with implantation of the distal end of the duct by pancreaticojejunostomy may be successful. When the pancreatic duct is diffusely dilated, anastomosis between the longitudinally split duct and a defunctionalized limb of jejunum (Puestow procedure) is associated with relief of pain in 75% of cases. In advanced cases, subtotal or total pancreatectomy may be considered as a last resort with variable results and a high rate of pancreatic insufficiency.

Prognosis

This is a serious disease and often leads to chronic invalidism. The prognosis is best in patients with recurrent acute pancreatitis caused by a remediable condition such as chronic cholecystitis and cholelithiasis, choledocholithiasis, stenosis of the sphincter of Oddi, or hyperparathyroidism. Medical management of the hyperlipidemias frequently associated with the condition may also prevent recurrent attacks. In alcoholic pancreatitis, pain relief is most likely when a dilated pancreatic duct can be decompressed. In patients with disease not amenable to decompressive surgery, addiction to narcotics is a frequent outcome of treatment.

Karanjic ND, Reber HA: The cause and management of the pain of chronic pancreatitis. Gastroenterol Clin North Am 1990;19:895. (Mechanisms of pain and indications for surgical management.)

Levy P et al: Mortality factors associated with chronic pancreatitis: Unidimensional and multidimensional analysis of a medical-surgical series of 240 patients. Gastroenterology 1989;96:1165. (Alcohol abstinence appears to have a favorable influence.)

Li Y et al: Exocrine pancreatic function tests: A review. Can J Gastroenterol 1989;3:153. (The standard is measurement of pancreatic secretory volume and bicarbonate concentration in response to a secretagogue such as secretin; simpler screening tests include the bentiromide [N-benzoyl-L-tyrosyl-p-aminobenzoic acid] test, in which urinary concentrations of PABA correlate with breakdown of the orally administered test substrate by pancreatic chymotrypsin.)

Maguire S, Goodchild MC: Enzyme contents of pancreatic extract preparations: Are they optimal? Drugs 1992; 44:685. (All currently available preparations are degraded in an acid pH; an acid-stable preparation is under development.)

Nealon WT et al: Operative drainage of the pancreatic duct delays functional impairment in patients with chronic pancreatitis: A prospective analysis. Ann Surg 1988; 208:321. (A consideration.)

CARCINOMA OF THE HEAD OF THE PANCREAS & THE PERIAMPULLARY AREA

Essentials of Diagnosis

- Obstructive jaundice (may be painless).
- Enlarged gallbladder (may be painful).
- Upper abdominal pain with radiation to back, weight loss, and thrombophlebitis are usually late manifestations.

General Considerations

Carcinoma is the commonest neoplasm of the pancreas. About 75% are in the head and 25% in the body and tail of the organ. Carcinomas involving the head of the pancreas, the ampulla of Vater, the common bile duct, and the duodenum are considered together, because they are usually indistinguishable clinically; of these, carcinomas of the pancreatic head constitute over 90%. They comprise 3% of all cancers and 5% of cancer deaths.

Clinical Findings

A. Symptoms and Signs: Pain is present in over 70% of cases and is often vague, diffuse, and located in the epigastrium. Radiation of pain into the back is common and sometimes predominates. Sitting up and leaning forward may afford some relief, and this usually indicates that the lesion has spread beyond the pancreas and is inoperable. The pain is rarely confused with biliary colic. Diarrhea, as a relatively early symptom, is seen occasionally. Migratory thrombophlebitis is a rare sign. Jaundice and weight loss are common but late findings. An uncommon occurrence is that jaundice associated with a palpable gallbladder is indicative of obstruction by neoplasm (Courvoisier's law), but there are frequent exceptions. In addition, a hard, fixed, occasionally tender mass may be present.

B. Laboratory Findings: There may be mild anemia. Glycosuria, hyperglycemia, and impaired glucose tolerance or true diabetes mellitus are found in 10–20% of cases. The serum amylase or lipase level is occasionally elevated. Liver function tests may suggest obstructive jaundice. Steatorrhea in the absence of jaundice is uncommon. Occult blood in the stool is suggestive of carcinoma of the ampulla of Vater. CA19–9, with a sensitivity of 70% and a specificity of 87%, has not proved sensitive enough for early detection; increased values are also found in acute and chronic pancreatitis and cholangitis.

C. Imaging: With carcinoma of the head of the pancreas, the upper gastrointestinal series may show a widening of the duodenal loop, mucosal abnormalities in the duodenum ranging from edema to invasion or ulceration, or spasm or compression. Ultrasound is not reliable because of interference by intestinal gas. CT or MRI may detect a mass in over 80% of cases of proved pancreatic cancer. CT scan and MRI are most helpful in delineating the extent of pancreatic mass and allowing for percutaneous fine-needle aspiration of the mass for cytologic studies. Selective celiac and superior mesenteric arteriography may be most helpful by demonstrating vessel invasion by tumor, a finding that would interdict attempts at surgical resection. Endoscopic retrograde cholangiopancreatography may clarify an ambiguous CT or MRI study by delineating the pancreatic duct system or confirming an ampullary or biliary neoplasm. With obstruction of the splenic vein, splenomegaly or gastric varices are present, the latter delineated by an upper gastrointestinal series, endoscopy, or angiography.

Treatment

Abdominal exploration is usually necessary when cytologic diagnosis cannot be made or if resection is to be attempted, which includes about 30% of patients. Radical pancreaticoduodenal resection is indicated for lesions strictly limited to the head of the pancreas, periampullary zone, and duodenum. When resection is not feasible, cholecystojejunostomy or endoscopic stenting is performed to relieve jaundice. A gastrojejunostomy is also done if duodenal obstruction is expected to develop later. Combined irradiation and chemotherapy may be used for palliation of unresectable cancer confined to the pancreas. However, chemotherapy has been disappointing in metastatic pancreatic cancer.

Prognosis

Carcinoma of the head of the pancreas has a poor prognosis. Reported 5-year survival rates range from 2.3% to 5.2%. Lesions of the ampulla have a better prognosis, with reported 5-year survival rates of 20–40% after resection. The reported operative mortality rate of radical pancreaticoduodenectomy is 10–15%.

Freeny PC et al: Pancreatic ductal adenocarcinoma: Diagnosis and staging with dynamic CT. Radiology 1988;166:125. (Correct diagnosis in 91%, false-positive in 8%, and false-negative in 2% of 174 patients. More accurate than angiography for staging.)

Kamisawa T et al: Carcinoma of the ampulla of Vater: Expression of cancer-associated antigens inversely correlated with prognosis. Am J Gastroenterol 1988;83:1118. (Tissue CEA immunoreactivity may correlate with mean survival.)

Pleskow DK et al: Evaluations of a serologic marker, CA19–9, in the diagnosis of pancreatic cancer. Ann Intern Med 1989;110:704. (Has 70% sensitivity, 87% specificity, and negative predictive value of 92%.)

CARCINOMA OF THE BODY & TAIL OF THE PANCREAS

About 25% of pancreatic cancers arise in the body or tail. There are no characteristic findings in the early stages. The initial symptoms are vague epigastric or left upper quadrant distress. Anorexia and weight loss usually occur. Later, pain becomes more severe and frequently radiates through to the left lumbar region. A mass in the mid or left epigastrium may be palpable. The spontaneous development of thrombophlebitis may suggest an occult pancreatic cancer. If suspected, the diagnosis can often be supported by CT scanning or MRI and confirmed by percutaneous aspiration of the mass for cytologic analysis. Surgical exploration is sometimes necessary for diagnosis. The tumor is usually widespread by the time of diagnosis. Resection is rarely feasible, and cure is rarer still. The response to fluorouracil has been disappointing.

Trede M et al: Survival after pancreatoduodenectomy: 118 consecutive resections without an operative mortality. Ann Surg 1990;211:447. (Thirty-six percent 5-year actuarial survival in those with radical resection.)

REFERENCES

Schiff L: *Diseases of the Liver,* 6th ed. Lippincott, 1987.

Sherlock S, Dooley J: *Diseases of the Liver and Biliary System,* 9th ed. Lippincott/Blackwell, 1993.

Sleisenger MH, Fordtran JS (editors): *Gastrointestinal Disease: Pathophysiology, Diagnosis, Management,* 4th ed. Saunders, 1989.

Smith PD et al: Gastrointestinal infections in AIDS: NIH conference. Ann Intern Med 1992;116:63.

Steinberg WM (guest editor): Diseases of the pancreas. Gastroenterol Clin North Am 1990;19:783.

Yamada T et al: *Textbook of Gastroenterology.* Lippincott, 1991.

Zakim D, Boyer TD: *Hepatology: A Textbook of Liver Disease,* 2nd ed. Saunders, 1990.

Breast

16

Armando E. Giuliano, MD

CARCINOMA OF THE FEMALE BREAST

Essentials of Diagnosis

- Higher incidence in women who have delayed childbearing, those with a family history of breast cancer, and those with a personal history of breast cancer or some types of mammary dysplasia.
- Early findings: Single, nontender, firm to hard mass with ill-defined margins; mammographic abnormalities and no palpable mass.
- Later findings: Skin or nipple retraction; axillary lymphadenopathy; breast enlargement, redness, edema, pain; fixation of mass to skin or chest wall.
- Late findings: Ulceration; supraclavicular lymphadenopathy; edema of arm; bone, lung, liver, brain, or other distant metastases.

COMMON SIGNS & SYMPTOMS

The most common sign and symptom of breast disease is a palpable mass. This is usually found by the patient and may lead to the diagnosis of either benign or malignant disease. A palpable mass may be smooth and rubbery (ie, a fibroadenoma or tense cyst) or may be firm and irregular (ie, a carcinoma). While many patients complain of breast pain, this is not commonly associated with a serious disease and usually is due to underlying fibrocystic changes in a premenopausal woman. However, some patients who complain of pain are found to have a malignancy. Most commonly, patients have diffuse nodularity associated with pain leading to the clinical diagnosis of fibrocystic disease. Benign and malignant breast disease may present as nipple discharge or even erosion or an eczema-like rash of the nipple. Most nipple discharge is associated with benign duct ectasia or cysts. A bloody discharge can be a sign of a malignancy but is usually a sign of a benign intraductal papilloma. Nipple erosion or even an eczema-like rash can be related to an underlying malignancy, as in Paget's disease. More diffuse skin changes can also be seen in benign and malignant conditions. Erythema and edema may signify underlying mastitis or advanced or inflammatory carcinoma. Breast tenderness is associated most commonly with fibrocystic disease, but when accompanied by erythema and edema it signifies mastitis. Local skin dimpling (indentation) or nipple retraction may be a sign of benign fibrocystic disease or a past mastitis but may signify an underlying malignancy. Rarely, a malignancy may present with palpable adenopathy and no abnormality within the breast itself.

A malignancy may be very obvious, presenting with a mass, adenopathy, and skin involvement, or may be a subtle thickening in a portion of the breast with no other identifiable abnormality. While the overwhelming majority of patients with complaints related to their breasts will have benign conditions, most breast symptoms and signs may be due to an associated or underlying malignancy and warrant workup and follow-up care.

DIAGNOSTIC TESTS

The most reliable diagnostic test for breast cancer is **open excisional biopsy.** When the sample is properly taken by the surgeon and examined by the pathologist, such a test should give no false-negative and no false-positive results.

Large-needle (core needle) biopsy is an accepted diagnostic technique in which a core of tissue is removed with a large cutting needle. As in the case of any needle biopsy, the main problem is sampling error due to improper positioning of the needle, giving rise to a false-negative test result.

Fine-needle aspiration cytology is a useful technique whereby cells from a breast tumor are aspirated with a small (usually 22-gauge) needle and examined by the pathologist. This technique can be performed easily with no morbidity and is much less expensive than excisional or open biopsy. The main disadvantages are that it requires a pathologist skilled in the cytologic diagnosis of breast cancer and that it is subject to sampling problems, particularly because deep lesions may be missed. The incidence of false-positive diagnoses is extremely low, perhaps 1–2%. The rate of false-negative diagnoses with fine-needle aspiration biopsy is as high as 10% in some series. Most experienced clinicians would not leave a dominant mass in the breast even when fine-needle aspiration cytology is negative unless the clinical diagnosis, breast imaging studies, and cytologic studies were all in agreement.

Ultrasonography is performed chiefly to differentiate cystic from solid lesions and is not diagnostic of malignancy. Ultrasonography may show an irregular mass within a cyst in the rare case of intracystic carcinoma. If a tumor is palpable and clinically feels like a cyst, an 18-gauge needle can be used to aspirate the fluid and make the diagnosis of cyst. If a cyst is aspirated and the fluid is nonbloody, it does not have to be examined cytologically. If the mass does not recur, no further diagnostic test is necessary. Nonpalpable mammographic densities that appear benign should be investigated with ultrasound to determine whether the lesion is cystic or solid.

When a suspicious abnormality is identified by mammography alone and cannot be palpated by the clinician, the patient should undergo **mammographic localization biopsy.** This is performed by obtaining a mammogram in two perpendicular views and placing a needle or hook-wire near the abnormality so that the surgeon can use the metal needle or wire as a guide during operation to locate the lesion. After mammography confirms the position of the needle in relation to the lesion, an incision is made and the subcutaneous tissue is dissected until the needle is identified. Using the films as a guide, the abnormality can then be localized and excised. It often happens that the abnormality cannot even be palpated through the incision—this is the case with microcalcifications—and it is thus essential to obtain a mammogram of the specimen to document that the lesion was excised. At that time, a second marker needle can further localize the lesion for the pathologist.

Computerized stereotactic modifications have recently been added to mammographic units in order to localize abnormalities and perform needle biopsy without surgery. Under mammographic guidance, a biopsy needle can be inserted into the lesion in the mammographer's suite, and a core of tissue for histologic examination or cells for cytology can be examined. Some studies suggest that the false-negative rate may be too high to justify this technique. However, continued trials of new stereotactic equipment may permit mammographic localization biopsies to be done accurately without surgical excision.

INCIDENCE & RISK FACTORS

The breast is the most common site of cancer in women, and cancer of the breast is second only to lung cancer as a cause of death from cancer among women. The probability of developing breast cancer increases throughout life. The mean and the median age of women with breast cancer is between 60 and 61 years.

There will be about 182,000 new cases of breast cancer and about 46,000 deaths from this disease in women in the USA in 1994. At the present rate of incidence, the American Cancer Society predicts that one of every eight or nine American women will develop breast cancer during her lifetime. Women whose mothers or sisters had breast cancer are more likely to develop the disease than others. Risk is increased in patients whose mothers' or sisters' breast cancers occurred before menopause or was bilateral and in those with a family history of breast cancer in two or more first-degree relatives. However, there is no history of breast cancer among female relatives in over 90% of breast cancer patients. Nulliparous women and women whose first full-term pregnancy was after age 35 have a slightly higher incidence of breast cancer than multiparous women. Late menarche and artificial menopause are associated with a lower incidence of breast cancer, whereas early menarche (under age 12) and late natural menopause (after age 50) are associated with a slight increase in risk of developing breast cancer. Mammary dysplasia (fibrocystic disease of the breast), when accompanied by proliferative changes, papillomatosis, or atypical epithelial hyperplasia, is associated with an increased incidence of cancer. A woman who has had cancer in one breast is at increased risk of developing cancer in the other breast. Women with cancer of the uterine corpus have a breast cancer risk significantly higher than that of the general population, and women with breast cancer have a comparably increased endometrial cancer risk. In the USA, breast cancer is more common in whites than in nonwhites. The incidence of the disease among nonwhites (mostly blacks), however, is increasing, especially in younger women. In general, rates reported from developing countries are low, whereas rates are high in developed countries, with the notable exception of Japan. Some of the variability may be due to underreporting in the developing countries, but a real difference probably exists. Dietary factors, particularly increased fat content, may account for some differences in incidence. Oral contraceptives do not appear to increase the risk of breast cancer. There is some evidence that administration of estrogens to postmenopausal women may result in a slightly increased risk of breast cancer, but only with higher, long-term doses of estrogens. Other studies suggest that women with a family history of breast cancer who take postmenopausal estrogens or those who take estradiol or unconjugated estrogens do slightly increase their risk of breast cancer. Alcohol consumption may increase the risk of breast cancer slightly.

Women who are at greater than normal risk of developing breast cancer (Table 16–1) should be identi-

Table 16–1. Factors associated with increased risk of breast cancer.[1]

Race	White
Age	Older
Family History	Breast cancer in mother or sister (especially bilateral or premenopausal)
Previous medical history	Endometrial cancer Some forms of mammary dysplasia Cancer in other breast
Menstrual history	Early menarche (under age 12) Late menopause (after age 50)
Pregnancy	Late first pregnancy

[1]Normal lifetime risk in white women = 1 in 8 or 9.

fied by their physicians, taught the techniques of breast self-examination, and followed carefully. Screening programs involving periodic physical examination and mammography of asymptomatic high-risk women increase the detection rate of breast cancer and improve the survival rate by as much as 30%. Unfortunately, most women who develop breast cancer do not have significant identifiable risk factors, and analysis of epidemiologic data has failed to identify women who are not at significant risk and would not benefit from screening. Therefore, virtually all women over about age 35 are at sufficient risk of breast cancer so that they could benefit from screening. The cost-benefit ratio of screening programs to society as a whole is unclear. Less expensive screening techniques such as single-view mammography and the use of mobile vans are being investigated in an attempt to reduce the cost of widespread screenings. Recently, the NSAB began actually comparing tamoxifen with placebo for patients who show no evidence of breast cancer but who are at high risk for its occurrence. This controversial trial may identify a pharmacologic means of preventing the disease in young women.

EARLY DETECTION OF BREAST CANCER

Screening Programs

A number of mass screening programs consisting of physical and mammographic examination of the breasts of asymptomatic women have been conducted. Such programs frequently identify more than six cancers per 1000 women. About 80% of these women have negative axillary lymph nodes at the time of surgery, whereas only 45% of patients found in the course of usual medical practice have uninvolved axillary nodes. Detecting breast cancer before it has spread to the axillary nodes greatly increases the chance of survival, and about 85% of such women will survive at least 5 years.

Both physical examination and mammography are necessary for maximum yield in screening programs, since about 35–50% of early breast cancers can be discovered only by mammography and another 40% can be detected only by palpation. About one-third of the abnormalities detected on screening mammograms will be found to be malignant when biopsy is performed. Women 20–40 years of age should have a breast examination as part of routine medical care every 2–3 years. Women over age 40 should have yearly breast examinations. The sensitivity of mammography varies from approximately 60% to 90%. This sensitivity depends on several factors, including patient age (breast density), tumor size, location, and mammographic appearance. In young women with dense breasts, mammography is less sensitive than in older woman with fatty breasts, in whom mammography can detect nearly 90% of malignancies. Smaller tumors, particularly those without calcifications, are more difficult to detect, especially in dense breasts. The lack of sensitivity in young women is leading to questions concerning the value of mammography for screening in women 40–50 years of age. The specificity of mammography varies from about 30% to 40% for nonpalpable mammographic abnormalities to 85% to 90% for clinically evident malignancies.

The American College of Radiology and the American Cancer Society have published guidelines regarding use of mammography in asymptomatic women. A baseline mammogram should be performed on all women between ages 35 and 40 years. Women aged 40–49 years should have a mammogram every 1–2 years. Annual mammograms are indicated for women age 50 years or older. The US Preventive Services Task Force recommends mammography screening every 1 or 2 years for women aged 50–75 and physical examination annually for women over age 40. High-risk women—those whose mothers or sisters had bilateral or premenopausal breast cancer, those who have had cancer of one breast, and those with histologic abnormalities associated with subsequent cancer (eg, atypical epithelial hyperplasia, papillomatosis, lobular carcinoma in situ)—should have a yearly mammogram and twice-yearly physical examinations. The usefulness of screening mammography in young women without identifiable risk factors is not yet of proved value. However, in a recent large study of women under age 50, nearly half of all cancers were detected by mammography alone. Critics of screening question whether early detection actually improves survival sufficiently to justify its cost. Mammographic parenchymal patterns are not a reliable predictor of the risk of developing breast cancer.

Ductography is useful to evaluate the cause of nipple discharge. In this study, the radiologist injects contrast medium into the discharging duct and obtains a mammogram. The injected duct may contain a filling defect (most commonly an intraductal papilloma) or may have a dilated or cystic appearance in patients with duct ectasia or fibrocystic disease. Malignancy may appear as an abrupt obstruction or filling defect.

Other modalities of breast imaging have been investigated. Automated breast ultrasonography is very useful in distinguishing cystic from solid lesions but should be used only as a supplement to physical examination and mammography in screening for breast cancer. Diaphanography (transillumination of the breasts) and thermography are of no proved screening value.

Self-Examination

All women over age 20 should be advised to examine their breasts monthly. Premenopausal women should perform the examination 7–8 days after the menstrual period. The breasts should be inspected initially while standing before a mirror with the hands at the sides, overhead, and pressed firmly on the hips to contract the pectoralis muscles. Masses, asymmetry of breasts, and slight dimpling of the skin may become apparent as a result of these maneuvers. Next, in a supine position, each breast should be carefully palpated with the fingers of the opposite hand. Physicians should instruct women in the technique of self-examination and advise them to report at once for medical evaluation if a mass or other abnormality is noted.

Some women discover small breast lumps more readily when their skin is moist while bathing or showering.

Most women do not practice self-examination, and its value is controversial. Clearly, however, it is not harmful and may be beneficial.

Mammography

Mammography is the most useful technique for the detection of early breast cancer. The two methods of mammography in common use are ordinary film screen radiography and xeroradiography. From the standpoint of diagnosing breast cancer, the two methods give comparable results. Using film screen techniques, it is now possible to perform a high-quality mammogram while delivering less than 0.4 cGy to the mid breast per view, and for this reason film screen mammography has largely replaced the xeromammographic technique, which delivers more radiation.

Mammography is the only reliable means of detecting breast cancer before a mass can be palpated in the breast. Slowly growing breast cancers can be identified by mammography at least 2 years before reaching a size detectable by palpation.

Calcifications are the most easily recognized mammographic abnormality. The most common mammographic abnormalities associated with carcinoma of the breast are clustered polymorphic microcalcifications. Such calcifications are usually at least five to eight in number, aggregated in one part of the breast and differing from each other in size and shape, often including branched or V- or Y-shaped configurations. There may be an associated mammographic mass density or, at time, only a mass density with no calcifications. Such a density usually has irregular or ill-defined borders and may lead to architectural distortion within the breast. A small mass or architectural distortion, particularly in a dense breast, may be subtle and difficult to detect.

Indications for mammography are as follows: (1) to evaluate each breast when a diagnosis of potentially curable breast cancer has been made, and at yearly intervals thereafter; (2) to evaluate a questionable or ill-defined breast mass or other suspicious change in the breast; (3) to search for an occult breast cancer in a woman with metastatic disease in axillary nodes or elsewhere from an unknown primary; (4) to screen women prior to cosmetic operations or prior to biopsy of a mass, to examine for an unsuspected cancer; (5) to screen at regular intervals a selected group of women who are at high risk for developing breast cancer (see above); and (6) to follow those women with breast cancer who have been treated with breast-conserving surgery and radiation.

Patients with a dominant or suspicious mass must undergo biopsy despite mammographic findings. The mammogram should be obtained prior to biopsy so that other suspicious areas can be noted and the contralateral breast can be checked. Mammography is never a substitute for biopsy, because it may not reveal clinical cancer in a very dense breast, as may be seen in young women with mammary dysplasia, and may not reveal medullary type cancers.

CLINICAL FINDINGS & DIAGNOSIS

The patient with breast cancer usually presents with a lump in the breast. When the history is taken, special note should be made of breast cancer risk factors, the temporal relationship of mass to menstrual cycle, and previous breast problems. Clinical evaluation should include assessment of the local lesion and a search for evidence of metastases in regional nodes or distant sites. After the diagnosis of breast cancer has been confirmed by biopsy, additional studies are often needed to complete the search for distant metastases or an occult primary in the other breast. Then, before any decision is made about treatment, all the available clinical data are used to determine the extent or stage of the patient's disease.

Symptoms

The presenting complaint in about 70% of patients with breast cancer is a lump (usually painless) in the breast. About 90% of breast masses are discovered by the patient herself. Less frequent symptoms are breast pain; nipple discharge; erosion, retraction, enlargement, or itching of the nipple; and redness, generalized hardness, enlargement, or shrinking of the breast. Rarely, an axillary mass or swelling of the arm may be the first symptom. Back or bone pain, jaundice, or weight loss may be the result of systemic metastases, but these symptoms are rarely seen on initial presentation.

Signs

The relative frequency of carcinoma in various anatomic sites in the breast is shown in Figure 16–1.

Inspection of the breast is the first step in physical examination and should be carried out with the patient sitting, arms at sides and then overhead. Abnormal variations in breast size and contour, minimal nipple retraction, and slight edema, redness, or retraction of the skin can be identified. Asymmetry of the breasts and retraction or dimpling of the skin can often be accentuated by having the patient raise her arms overhead or press her hands on her hips in order to contract the pectoralis muscles. Axillary and supraclavicular areas should be thoroughly palpated for enlarged nodes with the patient sitting (Figure 16–2). Palpation of the breast for masses or other changes should be performed with the patient both seated and supine with the arm abducted (Figure 16–3). Some authorities recommend palpation with a rotary motion of the examiner's fingers as well as a horizontal stripping motion.

Breast cancer usually consists of a nontender, firm or hard lump with poorly delineated margins (caused by local infiltration). Slight skin or nipple retraction is an important sign. Minimal asymmetry of the breast may be noted. Very small (1–2 mm) erosions of the nipple epithelium may be the only manifestation of Paget's carcinoma. Watery, serous, or bloody

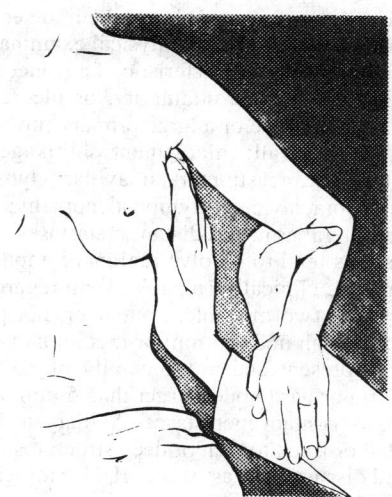

Figure 16–2. Palpation of axillary region for enlarged lymph nodes.

discharge from the nipple is an occasional early sign but is more often associated with benign disease.

A lesion smaller than 1 cm in diameter may be difficult or impossible for the examiner to feel and yet may be discovered by the patient. She should always be asked to demonstrate the location of the mass; if the physician fails to confirm the patient's suspicions, the examination should be repeated in 1 month, preferably 1–2 weeks after the onset of menses. During the premenstrual phase of the cycle, increased innocuous nodularity may suggest neoplasm or may obscure an underlying lesion. If there is any question regarding the nature of an abnormality under these circumstances, the patient should be asked to return after her period. Thirty-five to 50 percent of women with cancers detected during orga-

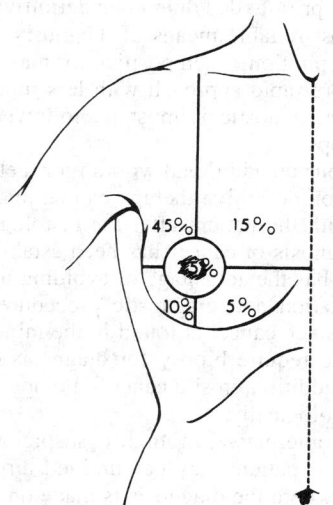

Figure 16–1. Frequency of breast carcinoma at various anatomic sites.

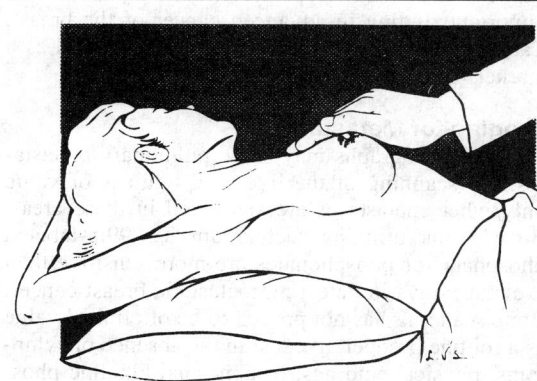

Figure 16–3. Palpation of breasts. Palpation is performed with the patient supine and arm abducted.

nized screening programs have them detected by mammography only and not physical examination.

The following are characteristic of advanced carcinoma: edema, redness, nodularity, or ulceration of the skin; the presence of a large primary tumor; fixation to the chest wall; enlargement, shrinkage, or retraction of the breast; marked axillary lymphadenopathy; supraclavicular lymphadenopathy; edema of the ipsilateral arm; and distant metastases.

Metastases tend to involve regional lymph nodes, which may be clinically palpable. With regard to the axilla, one or two movable, nontender, not particularly firm lymph nodes 5 mm or less in diameter are frequently present and are generally of no significance. Firm or hard nodes larger than 5 mm in diameter usually contain metastases. Axillary nodes that are matted or fixed to skin or deep structures indicate advanced disease (at least stage III). Histologic studies show that microscopic metastases are present in about 30% of patients with clinically negative nodes. On the other hand, if the examiner thinks that the axillary nodes are involved, that impression will be borne out by histologic section in about 85% of cases. The incidence of positive axillary nodes increases with the size of the primary tumor and with the local invasiveness of the neoplasm.

In most cases no nodes are palpable in the supraclavicular fossa. Firm or hard nodes of any size in this location or just beneath the clavicle (infraclavicular nodes) are suggestive of metastatic cancer and should be biopsied. Ipsilateral supraclavicular or infraclavicular nodes containing cancer indicate that the tumor is in an advanced stage (stage IV). Edema of the ipsilateral arm, commonly caused by metastatic infiltration of regional lymphatics, is also a sign of advanced (stage IV) cancer.

Laboratory Findings

A consistently elevated sedimentation rate may be the result of disseminated cancer. Liver or bone metastases may be associated with elevation of serum alkaline phosphatase. Hypercalcemia is an occasional important finding in advanced cancer of the breast. Carcinoembryonic antigen (CEA) may be used as a marker for recurrent breast cancer.

Imaging for Metastases

Chest radiographs may show pulmonary metastases. CT scanning of the liver and brain is of value only when metastases are suspected in these areas. Bone scans utilizing technetium Tc 99m-labeled phosphates or phosphonates are more sensitive than skeletal x-rays in detecting metastatic breast cancer. Bone scanning has not proved to be of clinical value as a routine preoperative test in the absence of symptoms, physical findings, or abnormal alkaline phosphatase levels. The frequency of abnormal findings on bone scan parallels the status of the axillary lymph nodes on pathologic examination. Bone scan should be performed for patients with symptoms and for those with elevated calcium or alkaline phosphatase levels.

Biopsy

The diagnosis of breast cancer depends ultimately upon examination of tissue removed by biopsy. Treatment should never be undertaken without an unequivocal histologic diagnosis of cancer. The safest course is biopsy examination of all suspicious masses found on physical examination and, in the absence of a mass, of suspicious lesions demonstrated by mammography. About 30% of lesions thought to be definitely cancer prove on biopsy to be benign, and about 15% of lesions believed to be benign are found to be malignant. These findings demonstrate the fallibility of clinical judgment and the necessity for biopsy. Dominant masses or suspicious nonpalpable mammographic findings must be biopsied. A breast mass should not be followed without histologic diagnosis, except perhaps in the premenopausal woman with a nonsuspicious mass presumed to be fibrocystic disease. A lesion such as this could be observed through one or two menstrual cycles. However, if the mass does not completely resolve during this time, it must be biopsied. Figures 16–4 and 16–5 present algorithms for management of breast masses in pre- and postmenopausal patients.

The simplest method is needle biopsy, either by aspiration of tumor cells (fine-needle aspiration cytology) or by obtaining a small core of tissue with a Vim-Silverman or other special needle. A nondiagnostic needle biopsy or fine-needle aspiration should be followed by open biopsy, because false-negative needle biopsies may occur in 5–10% of cancers. False-positive results occur rarely (< 1%).

Open biopsy under local anesthesia as a separate procedure prior to deciding upon definitive treatment is the most reliable means of diagnosis. Needle biopsy or aspiration, when positive for malignancy, offers a more rapid approach with less morbidity, but when nondiagnostic it must be followed by excisional biopsy.

Decisions on additional workup for metastatic disease and on definitive therapy can be made and discussed with the patient after the histologic or cytologic diagnosis of cancer has been established. This approach has the advantage of avoiding unnecessary hospitalization and diagnostic procedures in many patients, since cancer is found in the minority of patients who require biopsy for diagnosis of a breast lump. In addition, in situ cancers are not easily diagnosed cytologically.

As an alternative in highly suspicious circumstances, the patient may be admitted directly to the hospital, where the diagnosis is made on frozen section of tissue obtained by open biopsy under general anesthesia. If the frozen section is positive, the surgeon could proceed immediately with operation. This

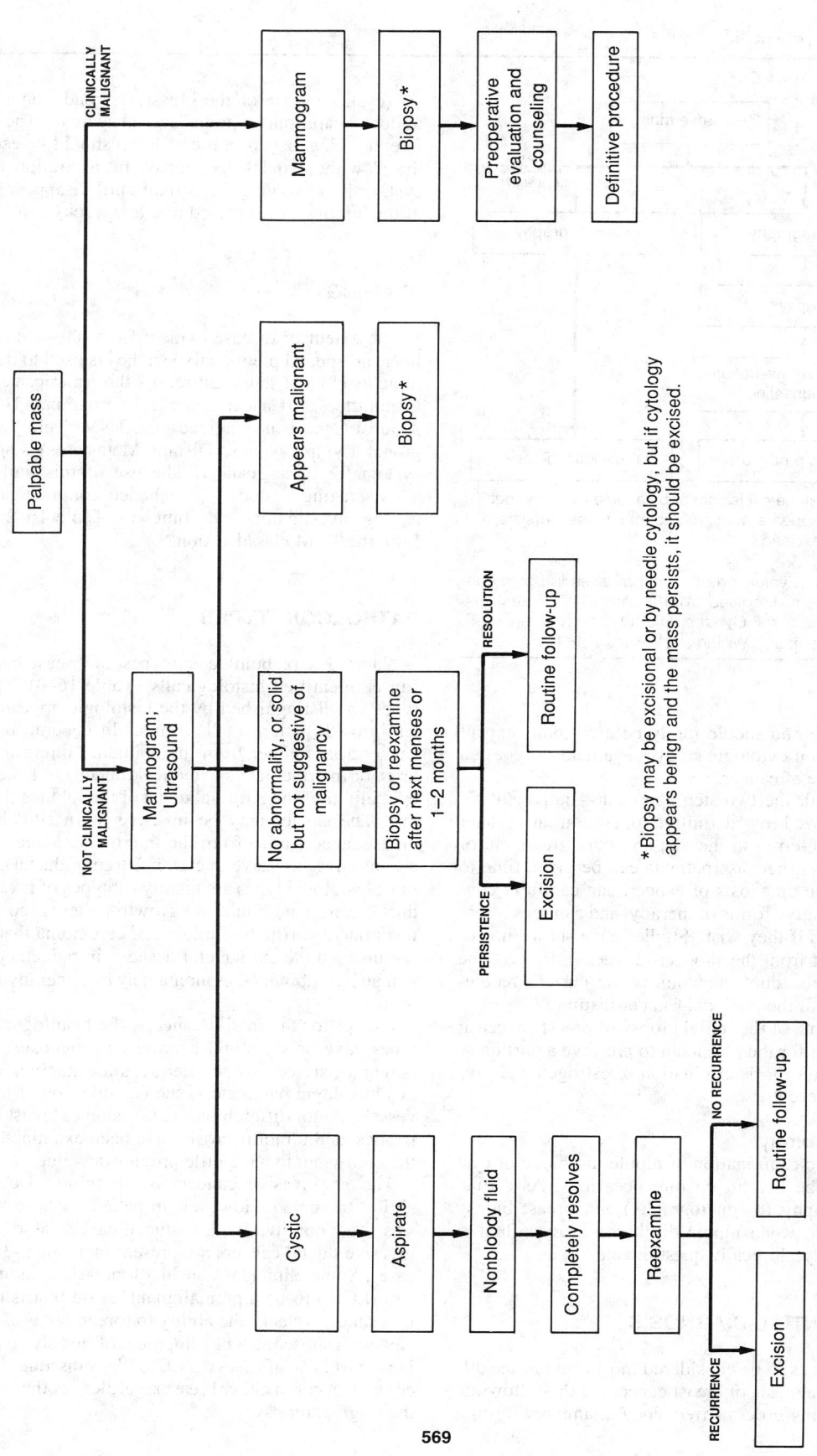

Figure 16–4. Evaluation of breast masses in premenopausal women. (Modified from Giuliano AE: Breast disease. In: *Practical Gynecologic Oncology*. Berek JS, Hacker NF [editors]. Williams & Wilkins, 1989.)

*Biopsy may be excisional or by needle cytology, but if cytology appears benign and the mass persists, it should be excised.

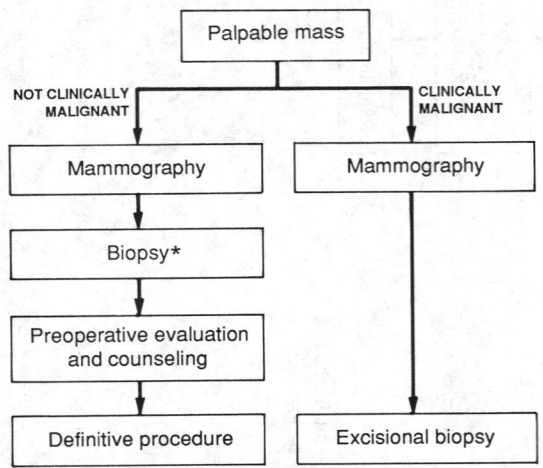

* Biopsy may be excisional or by needle cytology, but if cytology appears benign and the mass persists, it should be excised.

Figure 16–5. Evaluation of breast masses in postmenopausal women. (Modified from Giuliano AE: Breast disease. In: *Practical Gynecologic Oncology.* Berek JS, Hacker NF [editors]. Williams & Wilkins, 1989.)

one-step method should rarely be used today except perhaps when cytologic study has already suggested the presence of cancer.

In general, the two-step approach—outpatient biopsy followed by definitive operation at a later date—is preferred in the diagnosis and treatment of breast cancer, because patients can be given time to adjust to the diagnosis of cancer, can carefully consider alternative forms of therapy, and can seek a second opinion if they wish. Studies have shown no adverse effect from the short (1–2 weeks) delay of the two-step procedure, and this is the current recommendation of the National Cancer Institute.

At the time of the initial biopsy of breast cancer, it is important for the physician to preserve a portion of the specimen for determination of estrogen and progesterone receptors.

Other Cytology

Cytologic examination of nipple discharge or cyst fluid may be helpful on rare occasions. As a rule, mammography (or ductography) and breast biopsy are required when nipple discharge or cyst fluid is bloody or cytologically questionable.

DIFFERENTIAL DIAGNOSIS

The lesions to be considered most often in the differential diagnosis of breast cancer are the following, in descending order of frequency: mammary dyspla-

sia (cystic disease of the breast), fibroadenoma, intraductal papilloma, lipoma, and fat necrosis. The differential diagnosis of a breast lump should be established without delay by biopsy, by aspiration of a cyst, or by observing the patient until disappearance of the lump within a period of a few weeks.

STAGING

The extent of disease evident from physical findings and special preoperative studies is used to determine its clinical stage. Currently, the American Joint Committee on Cancer and the International Union Against Cancer have agreed on a TNM (Tumor, Regional Lymph Nodes, Distant Metastases) staging system for breast cancer. The use of this uniform TNM staging system will enhance communication among investigators and clinicians. Table 16–2 sets forth the TNM classification.

PATHOLOGIC TYPES

Numerous pathologic subtypes of breast cancer can be identified histologically (Table 16–3). These types are distinguished by the histologic appearance and growth pattern of the tumor. In general, breast cancer arises either from the epithelial lining of the large or intermediate-sized ducts (ductal) or from the epithelium of the terminal ducts of the lobules (lobular). The cancer may be invasive or in situ. Most breast cancers arise from the intermediate ducts and are invasive (invasive ductal, infiltrating ductal), and most histologic types are merely subtypes of invasive ductal cancer with unusual growth patterns (colloid, medullary, scirrhous, etc). Ductal carcinoma that has not invaded the extraductal tissue is intraductal or in situ ductal. Lobular carcinoma may be either invasive or in situ.

Except for the in situ cancers, the histologic subtypes have only a slight bearing on prognosis when outcomes are compared after accurate staging. Various histologic parameters, such as invasion of blood vessels, tumor differentiation, invasion of breast lymphatics, and tumor necrosis have been examined, but they too seem to have little prognostic value.

The noninvasive cancers by definition lack the ability to spread. However, in patients whose biopsies show noninvasive intraductal cancer, associated invasive ductal cancers are present in about 1–3% of cases. Some clinicians consider lobular carcinoma in situ (LCIS) to be a premalignant lesion that is not a true cancer. It lacks the ability to spread but is associated with subsequent development of invasive cancer in at least 20% of cases. In LCIS, the subsequent cancer may occur in either breast regardless of the side of the original biopsy.

Table 16–2. TNM staging for breast cancer.[1]

Stage	T	N	M
0	Tis	N0	M0
I	T1	N0	M0
IIA	T0	N1	M0
	T1	N1	M0
	T2	N0	M0
IIB	T2	N1	M0
	T3	N0	M0
IIIA	T0	N2	M0
	T1	N2	M0
	T2	N2	M0
	T3	N1, N2	M0
IIIB	T4	Any N	M0
	Any T	N3	M0
IV	Any T	Any N	M1

Tumor Size (T)

TX	Primary tumor cannot be assessed.
T0	No evidence of primary tumor.
Tis	Carcinoma in situ; intraductal carcinoma, lobular carcinoma in situ, or Paget's disease of the nipple with no tumor.
T1	Tumor 2 cm or less in greatest dimension. T1a 0.5 cm or less in greatest dimension. T1b More than 0.5 cm but not more than 1 cm in greatest dimension. T1c More than 1 cm but not more than 2 cm in greatest dimension.
T2	Tumor more than 2 cm but not more than 5 cm in greatest dimension.
T3	Tumor more than 5 cm in greatest dimension.
T4	Tumor of any size with direct extension to chest wall or skin.

Regional Lymph Nodes (N)

NX	Regional lymph nodes cannot be assessed (eg, previously removed).
N0	No regional lymph node metastases.
N1	Metastasis to movable ipsilateral lymph node(s).
N2	Metastasis to ipsilateral axillary lymph node(s) fixed to one another or to other structures.
N3	Metastasis to ipsilateral internal mammary lymph node(s).

Distant Metastases (M)

MX	Presence of distant metastasis cannot be assessed.
M0	No distant metastasis.
M1	Distant metastasis (includes metastasis to ipsilateral supraclavicular lymph node[s]).

[1]American Joint Committee on Cancer: *Manual for Staging of Cancer,* 3rd ed. Lippincott, 1988.

Table 16–3. Histologic types of breast cancer.

	Percent Occurrence
Infiltrating ductal (not otherwise specified)	70–80
Medullary	5–8
Colloid (mucinous)	2–4
Tubular	1–2
Papillary	1–2
Invasive lobular	6–8
Noninvasive	4–6
Intraductal	2–3
Lobular in situ	2–3
Rare cancers	<1
Juvenile (secretory)	...
Adenoid cystic	...
Epidermoid	...
Sudoriferous	...

SPECIAL CLINICAL FORMS OF BREAST CANCER

Paget's Carcinoma

The basic lesion is usually an infiltrating ductal carcinoma, usually well differentiated. The nipple epithelium is infiltrated, but gross nipple changes are often minimal, and a tumor mass may not be palpable. The first symptom is often itching or burning of the nipple, with superficial erosion or ulceration. The diagnosis is established by biopsy of the erosion.

Paget's carcinoma is not common (about 1% of all breast cancers), but it is important because it appears innocuous. It is frequently diagnosed and treated as dermatitis or bacterial infection, leading to unfortunate delay in detection. When the lesion consists of nipple changes only, the incidence of axillary metastases is about 5%, and the prognosis is excellent. When a breast tumor is also present, the incidence of axillary metastases rises, with an associated marked decrease in prospects for cure by surgical or other treatment.

Inflammatory Carcinoma

This is the most malignant form of breast cancer and constitutes less than 3% of all cases. The clinical findings consist of a rapidly growing, sometimes painful mass that enlarges the breast. The overlying skin becomes erythematous, edematous, and warm. Often there is no distinct mass, since the tumor infiltrates the involved breast diffusely. The diagnosis should be made when the redness involves more than one-third of the skin over the breast and biopsy shows invasion of the subdermal lymphatics. The inflammatory changes, often mistaken for an infectious process, are caused by carcinomatous invasion of the dermal lymphatics, with resulting edema and hyperemia. If the physician suspects infection but the lesion does not respond rapidly (1–2 weeks) to antibiotics, biopsy examination must be performed. Metastases tend to occur early and widely, and for this reason inflammatory carcinoma is rarely curable. Mastectomy is seldom, if ever, indicated. Radiation, hormone therapy, and anticancer chemotherapy are the measures most likely to be of value.

Breast Cancer Occurring During Pregnancy or Lactation

Only 1–2% of breast cancers occur during pregnancy or lactation. Breast cancer complicates approximately one in 3000 pregnancies. The diagnosis is frequently delayed, because physiologic changes in the breast may obscure the true nature of the lesion. This results in a tendency of both patients and physicians to misinterpret the findings and to procrastinate in deciding on biopsy. When the neoplasm is confined to the breast, the 5-year survival rate after mastectomy is about 70%. Axillary metastases are already present in 60–70% of patients, and for them the 5-year survival rate after mastectomy is only 30–40%. Pregnancy (or lactation) is not a contraindication to operation, and treatment should be based on the stage of the disease as in the nonpregnant (or nonlactating) woman. Overall survival rates have improved, since cancers are now diagnosed in pregnant women earlier than in the past.

Bilateral Breast Cancer

Clinically evident simultaneous bilateral breast cancer occurs in less than 1% of cases, but there is a 5–8% incidence of later occurrence of cancer in the second breast. Bilaterality occurs more often in women under age 50 and is more frequent when the tumor in the primary breast is lobular. The incidence of second breast cancers increases directly with the length of time the patient is alive after her first cancer—about 0.5% per year.

In patients with breast cancer, mammography should be performed before primary treatment and at regular intervals thereafter, to search for occult cancer in the opposite breast. Routine biopsy of the opposite breast is usually not warranted.

Noninvasive Cancer

Noninvasive cancer can occur within the ducts (ductal carcinoma in situ) or lobules (lobular carcinoma in situ). While ductal carcinoma in situ behaves as an early malignancy, lobular carcinoma in situ would perhaps be better called lobular neoplasia. Ductal carcinoma in situ tends to be unilateral and most likely progresses to invasive cancer. Approximately 40–60% of women who have ductal carcinoma in situ treated with biopsy alone will develop invasive cancer within the same breast. Lobular carcinoma in situ, however, appears to be more of a risk factor calling attention to the probability of developing invasive cancer in either breast. Approximately 20% of women with lobular carcinoma in situ will develop invasive cancer (usually ductal). This invasive cancer occurs with equal frequency in either breast.

The treatment of intraductal lesions is controversial. Ductal carcinoma can be treated with total mastectomy or breast conservation with wide excision with or without radiation therapy. Lobular carcinoma in situ is probably best managed with careful observation. However, patients who are unwilling to accept the increased risk of breast cancer may be offered bilateral total mastectomy. Axillary metastases are rare.

HORMONE RECEPTOR SITES

The presence or absence of estrogen and progesterone receptors in the cytoplasm of tumor cells is of paramount importance in managing all patients with breast cancer, especially those with recurrent or metastatic disease. They are of proved value in determining adjuvant therapy and therapy for patients with advanced disease. Up to 60% of patients with metastatic breast cancer will respond to hormonal manipulation if their tumors contain estrogen receptors. However, fewer than 5% of patients with metastatic, ER-negative tumors can be successfully treated with hormonal manipulation.

Progesterone receptors may be an even more sensitive indicator than estrogen receptors of patients who may respond to hormonal manipulation. Up to 80% of patients with metastatic progesterone receptor-positive tumors seem to respond to hormonal manipulation. Receptors probably have no relationship to response to chemotherapy.

Some studies suggest that estrogen receptors are of prognostic significance. Patients whose primary tumors are receptor-positive have a more favorable course than those whose tumors are receptor-negative.

Receptor status is not only valuable for the management of metastatic disease but may help in the selection of patients for adjuvant therapy. Some studies suggest that adjuvant hormonal therapy (tamoxifen) for patients with receptor-positive tumors and adjuvant chemotherapy for patients with receptor-negative tumors may improve survival rates even in the absence of lymph node metastases (see Adjuvant Therapy, p 574).

Estrogen and progesterone receptor assays should be done routinely for every breast cancer at the time of initial diagnosis. Small tumors with insufficient tissue volume for quantitative assay may be examined by immunohistochemistry. The value of this assay technique remains to be proved. Receptor status may change after hormonal therapy, radiotherapy, or chemotherapy. The specimen requires special handling, and the laboratory should be prepared to process the specimen correctly.

CURATIVE TREATMENT

Treatment may be curative or palliative. Curative treatment is advised for clinical stage I and stage II disease (Table 16–2). Patients with locally advanced (stage III) tumors may be cured with multimodality therapy, but in most cases palliation is all that can be expected. Palliative treatment is appropriate for all patients with stage IV disease and for previously treated patients who develop distant metastases or who have unresectable local cancers.

The growth potential of tumors and host resistance factors vary over a wide range from patient to patient and may be altered during the course of the disease. The doubling time of breast cancer cells ranges from several weeks in a rapidly growing lesion to nearly a year in a slowly growing one. Assuming that the rate of doubling is constant and that the neoplasm originates in one cell, a carcinoma with a doubling time of 100 days may not reach clinically detectable size (1 cm) for about 8 years. On the other hand, rapidly growing cancers have a much shorter preclinical course and a greater tendency to metastasize to regional nodes or more distant sites by the time a breast mass is discovered.

The relatively long preclinical growth phase and the tendency of breast cancers to metastasize have led many clinicians to believe that breast cancer is a systemic disease at the time of diagnosis. Although it may be true that breast cancer cells are released from the tumor prior to diagnosis, variations in the host-tumor relationship may prohibit the growth of disseminated disease in many patients. For this reason, a pessimistic attitude concerning the management of localized breast cancer is not warranted, and many patients can be cured with proper treatment.

Choice of Primary Therapy

The extent of disease and its biologic aggressiveness are the principal determinants of the outcome of primary therapy. Clinical and pathologic staging help in assessing extent of disease (Table 16–2), but each is to some extent imprecise. Other factors such as DNA flow cytometry, tumor grade, hormone receptor assays, and oncogene amplification may be of prognostic value but are not important in determining the type of local therapy. Since about two-thirds of patients eventually manifest distant disease regardless of the form of primary therapy, there is a tendency to think of breast carcinoma as being systemic in most patients at the time they first present for treatment.

There is a great deal of controversy regarding the optimal method of primary therapy of stage I, II, and III breast carcinoma, and opinions on this subject have changed considerably in the past decade. Legislation initiated in California and Massachusetts and now adopted in numerous states requires physicians to inform patients of alternative treatment methods in the management of breast cancer.

Breast-Conserving Therapy

The results of the Milan trial and a large randomized trial conducted by the National Surgical Adjuvant Breast Project (NSABP) in the USA showed that disease-free survival rates were similar for patients treated by partial mastectomy plus axillary dissection followed by radiation therapy and for those treated by modified radical mastectomy (total mastectomy plus axillary dissection). All patients whose axillary nodes contained tumor received adjuvant chemotherapy.

In the NSABP trial, patients were randomized to three treatment types: (1) "lumpectomy" (removal of the tumor with *confirmed* tumor-free margins) plus whole breast irradiation, (2) lumpectomy alone, and (3) total mastectomy. All patients underwent axillary lymph node dissection. Some patients in this study had tumors as large as 4 cm with (or without) palpable axillary lymph nodes. The lowest local recurrence rate was among patients treated with lumpectomy and postoperative irradiation; the highest was among patients treated with lumpectomy alone. However, no statistically significant differences were observed in overall or disease-free survival among the three treatment groups. This study shows that lumpectomy and axillary dissection with postoperative radiation therapy is as effective as modified radical mastectomy for the management of patients with stage I and stage II breast cancer. A high local failure rate (nearly 40% at 8 years) was seen for lumpectomy without radiation therapy.

The results of these and other trials have demonstrated that much less aggressive surgical treatment of the primary lesion than has previously been thought necessary gives equivalent therapeutic results and may preserve an acceptable cosmetic appearance.

Tumor size is a major consideration in determining the feasibility of breast conservation. The lumpectomy trial of the NSABP randomized patients with tumors as large as 4 cm. To achieve an acceptable cosmetic result, the patient must have a breast of sufficient size to enable excision of a 4 cm tumor without considerable deformity. Therefore, large size is only a relative contraindication. Subareolar tumors are also difficult to excise without considerable deformity. Clinically detectable multifocality is a relative contraindication to breast-conserving surgery, as is fixation to the chest wall or skin or involvement of the nipple or overlying skin. However, the patient and not the surgeon should be the judge of what is cosmetically acceptable; some patients would prefer breast deformity rather than complete absence of the breast or even reconstruction.

It is important to recognize that axillary dissection

is valuable both in planning therapy and in staging cancer. Operation is extremely effective in preventing axillary recurrences. In addition, lymph nodes removed during the procedure can be pathologically assessed. This assessment is essential for the planning of adjuvant therapy, which is often recommended.

Current Recommendations

A recent NIH consensus statement argues that breast-conserving surgery with radiation is the preferred form of treatment for patients with early-stage breast cancer. However, this technique has still not gained wide acceptance by physicians or patients. Despite the numerous randomized trials comparing breast conserving surgery and radiation therapy to mastectomy, breast-conserving surgery appears underutilized and mastectomy remains the more common treatment. In a recent survey, only 25% of patients in the United States with stage I or II breast cancer were treated with breast-conserving surgery and radiation therapy, compared with 75% treated with mastectomy. This seems to vary by region of the country, ranging from 15% in the South Central United States to approximately 30% in the Pacific Region.

Modified radical mastectomy (total mastectomy plus axillary lymph node dissection) has been the standard therapy for most patients with breast cancer. This operation removes the entire breast, overlying skin, nipple, and areolar complex as well as the underlying pectoralis fascia with the axillary lymph nodes in continuity. It offers the same overall survival and local control rates as does lumpectomy with axillary dissection and postoperative radiation therapy. The major advantage of modified radical mastectomy is that radiation therapy is usually not necessary. The disadvantage, of course, is the psychologic trauma associated with breast loss. Radical mastectomy, which removes the underlying pectoralis muscle, should be performed rarely if at all. Axillary node dissection is not indicated for noninfiltrating cancers, because nodal metastases are rarely present.

Preoperatively, full discussion with the patient regarding the rationale for operation and various alternative forms of treatment is essential. Breast-conserving surgery and radiation should be offered whenever possible, since most patients would prefer to save the breast. Breast reconstruction should be discussed with patients who choose or require mastectomy, and the option of simultaneous mastectomy with immediate reconstruction should be discussed. Time spent preoperatively in educating the patient and her family about these matters is time well spent.

Adjuvant Therapy

Chemotherapy or hormonal therapy is advocated for most patients with curable breast cancer. The objective of adjuvant therapy is to eliminate the occult metastases responsible for late recurrences while they are microscopic and theoretically most vulnerable to anticancer agents.

Numerous clinical trials with various adjuvant chemotherapeutic regimens have been completed. The most extensive clinical experience to date is with the CMF regimen (cyclophosphamide, methotrexate, and fluorouracil). Cyclophosphamide can be given either orally, in a dose of 100 mg/m^2 daily for 14 days; or intravenously, in a dose of 600 mg/m^2 on days 1 and 8. Methotrexate is given intravenously, 40 mg/m^2 on days 1 and 8; and fluorouracil is given intravenously, 600 mg/m^2 on days 1 and 8. This cycle is repeated every 4 weeks. Some clinicians prefer to give the drugs on 1 day only every 3 weeks. There appears to be no obvious advantage except that patient compliance is assured when the cyclophosphamide is give intravenously. The regimen should be continued for 6 months in patients with axillary metastases. Premenopausal women with positive axillary nodes definitely benefit from adjuvant chemotherapy. The recurrence rate in premenopausal patients who received no adjuvant chemotherapy was more than 1½ times that of those who received such therapy. No therapeutic effect with CMF has been shown in postmenopausal women with positive nodes, perhaps because therapy was modified so often in response to side effects that the total amount of drugs administered was less than planned. Other trials with different agents support the value of adjuvant chemotherapy; in some studies, postmenopausal women benefit as well.

Adjuvant chemotherapy can be offered confidently to premenopausal women with metastases in axillary lymph nodes, but the use of adjuvant chemotherapy in postmenopausal women and patients with negative axillary lymph nodes is more controversial. While postmenopausal women benefit from chemotherapy, selection of patients must take into account other common health problems that older women may have and the effects of chemotherapy on the patient's overall health. Tamoxifen can be given with few side effects even in the elderly. Tamoxifen appears to increase bone density and favorably affect lipid and lipoprotein profiles, which may explain the observed decreased mortality rate from coronary artery disease seen in patients taking tamoxifen.

The addition of hormones may improve the results of adjuvant therapy. For example, tamoxifen has been shown to enhance the beneficial effects of melphalan and fluorouracil in postmenopausal women whose tumors are ER-positive. Tamoxifen alone in a dosage of 10 mg orally twice a day has been the recommended treatment for postmenopausal women with ER-positive tumors. However, a recent NSABP trial showed that tamoxifen plus chemotherapy (Adriamycin [doxorubicin] plus cyclophosphamide [AC] or prednisone plus Adriamycin plus fluorouracil [PAF]) lowered recurrence rates more than tamoxifen alone in postmenopausal women with ER-positive tumors.

The length of time adjuvant therapy must be administered remains uncertain. Several studies suggest that shorter treatment periods may be as effective as longer ones. For example, one study compared 6 versus 12 cycles of postoperative CMF and found 5-year disease-free survival rates to be comparable. One of the earliest adjuvant trials used a 6-day perioperative regimen of intravenous cyclophosphamide alone; follow-up at 15 years shows a 15% improvement in disease-free survival rates for treated patients, suggesting that short-term therapy may be effective.

Patients with negative nodes have not been treated with adjuvant therapy until recently. Several studies of adjuvant therapy in node-negative women have now been published and show a beneficial effect of adjuvant chemotherapy or tamoxifen in delaying recurrence, but as of yet no effect has been seen on survival. A number of protocols, including CMF—cyclophosphamide, methotrexate, and fluorouracil—with leucovorin rescue as well as tamoxifen alone have increased disease-free survival times. The magnitude of this improvement is about one-third, ie, a group of women with an estimated 30% recurrence rate would have a 20% recurrence rate after adjuvant systemic therapy. Quality of life while receiving chemotherapy does not appear to be greatly altered.

The current recommendations for adjuvant chemotherapy can be summarized as follows (Tables 16–4 and 16–5):

(1) Premenopausal women with positive lymph nodes and either ER-positive or ER-negative tumors should be treated with adjuvant combination chemotherapy.

(2) Premenopausal women with negative nodes whose tumors are ER-positive benefit from tamoxifen; premenopausal women with negative axillary nodes whose tumors are ER-negative benefit from combination chemotherapy.

(3) Postmenopausal patients with positive lymph nodes and positive hormone receptor tumors should receive tamoxifen.

(4) Postmenopausal patients with positive lymph nodes whose tumors are ER-negative benefit from adjuvant combination chemotherapy.

Table 16–4. Adjuvant chemotherapy for premenopausal women. (Summary of NIH Consensus Conference June 18–21, 1990.)

Nodal Involvement	Estrogen Receptors	Adjuvant Systemic Therapy
Yes	Positive	Combination chemotherapy
Yes	Negative	Combination chemotherapy
No	Positive	Tamoxifen[1]
No	Negative	Combination chemotherapy[1]

[1]Effect on overall survival not yet demonstrated.

Table 16–5. Adjuvant chemotherapy for postmenopausal women. (Summary of NIH Consensus Conference June 18–21, 1990.)

Nodal Involvement	Estrogen Receptors	Adjuvant Systemic Therapy
Yes	Positive	Tamoxifen
Yes	Negative	Combination chemotherapy[1]
No	Positive	Tamoxifen[1]
No	Negative	Combination chemotherapy[1]

[1]Effect on overall survival not yet clearly demonstrated.

(5) Postmenopausal women with negative axillary nodes whose tumors are ER-positive may benefit from adjuvant tamoxifen; postmenopausal women with negative axillary lymph nodes whose tumors are ER-negative may benefit from adjuvant chemotherapy.

A 1990 consensus statement from the NIH on early-stage breast cancer recommends (1) that all patients who are candidates for clinical trials be offered the opportunity to participate, and (2) that node-negative patients who are not candidates for clinical trials ". . . should be made aware of the benefits and risks of adjuvant systemic therapy. The decision to use adjuvant treatment should follow a thorough discussion with the patient regarding the likely risk of recurrence without adjuvant therapy, the expected reduction in risk with adjuvant therapy, toxicities of therapy, and its impact on quality of life." In practice, most medical oncologists are currently using systemic adjuvant therapy for patients with early-stage breast cancer. Other prognostic factors being used to determine the patient's risks are tumor size, estrogen and progesterone receptor status, nuclear grade, histologic type, proliferative rate, and oncogene expression. Table 16–6 summarizes these prognostic factors. The assumption is made that patients with node-negative aggressive tumors should receive ad-

Table 16–6. Prognostic factors in node-negative breast cancer.

Prognostic Factor	Increased Recurrence	Decreased Recurrence
Size	T3 T2	T1 T0
Hormone receptors	Negative	Positive
DNA flow cytometry	Aneuploid	Diploid
Histologic grade	High	Low
Tumor labeling index	<3%	>3%
S phase fraction	>5%	<5%
Lymphatic or vascular invasion	Present	Absent
Cathepsin D	High	Low
HER–*neu* oncogene	High	Low
Epidermal growth factor receptor	High	Low

juvant therapy. However, the role of adjuvant therapy for these patients is still unclear because of the short follow-up in the node-negative studies and the lack of an observed effect on survival to date.

Important questions remaining to be answered are the timing and duration of adjuvant chemotherapy, which chemotherapeutic agents should be applied for which subgroups of patients, how best to coordinate adjuvant chemotherapy with postoperative radiation therapy, the use of combinations of hormonal therapy and chemotherapy, and the value of prognostic factors other than hormone receptors in predicting response to adjuvant therapy. Adjuvant systemic therapy is not currently indicated for patients with small nonpalpable tumors (ie, tumors that cannot be quantitatively tested for hormonal receptors) and those with negative lymph nodes who have had favorable DNA studies.

PALLIATIVE TREATMENT

This section covers palliative therapy of disseminated disease incurable by surgery (stage IV).

Radiotherapy

Palliative radiotherapy may be advised for locally advanced cancers with distant metastases in order to control ulceration, pain, and other manifestations in the breast and regional nodes. Irradiation of the breast and chest wall and the axillary, internal mammary, and supraclavicular nodes should be undertaken in an attempt to cure locally advanced and inoperable lesions when there is no evidence of distant metastases. A small number of patients in this group are cured in spite of extensive breast and regional node involvement. Adjuvant chemotherapy should be considered for such patients.

Palliative irradiation is of value also in the treatment of certain bone or soft tissue metastases to control pain or avoid fracture. Radiotherapy is especially useful in the treatment of isolated bony metastasis and chest wall recurrences.

Hormone Therapy

Disseminated disease may respond to prolonged endocrine therapy such as administration of hormones (eg, estrogens, androgens, progestins; see Table 16–7); ablation of the ovaries, adrenals, or pituitary; or administration of drugs that block hormone receptor sites (eg, antiestrogens) or drugs that block the synthesis of hormones (eg, aminoglutethimide). Hormonal manipulation is usually more successful in postmenopausal women. If treatment is based on the presence of estrogen receptor protein in the primary tumor or metastases, however, the rate of response is nearly equal in premenopausal and postmenopausal women. A favorable response to hormonal manipulation occurs in about one-third of patients with metastatic breast cancer. Of those whose tumors contain estrogen receptors, the response is about 60% and perhaps as high as 80% for patients whose tumors contain progesterone receptors as well. Because only 5–10% of women whose tumors do not contain estrogen receptors respond, they should not receive hormonal therapy except in unusual circumstances such as an elderly patient who could not tolerate chemotherapy.

Since the quality of life during a remission induced by endocrine manipulation is usually superior to a remission following cytotoxic chemotherapy, it is usually best to try endocrine manipulation first in cases where the estrogen receptor status of the tumor is unknown. However, if the estrogen receptor status is unknown but the disease is progressing rapidly or involves visceral organs, endocrine therapy is rarely successful, and introducing it may waste valuable time.

In general, only one type of systemic therapy should be given at a time unless it is necessary to irradiate a destructive lesion of weight-bearing bone while the patient is on another regimen. The regimen should be changed only if the disease is clearly progressing but not if it appears to be stable. This is especially important for patients with destructive bone metastases, since minor changes in the status of these lesions are difficult to determine radiographically. A plan of therapy that would simultaneously minimize

Table 16–7. Commonly used hormonal agents for management of metastatic breast cancer.

Drug	Action	Usual Oral Dose	Major Side Effects
Tamoxifen (Nolvadex)	Antiestrogen	10 mg twice daily	Hot flushes, uterine bleeding, thrombophlebitis, rash
Diethylstilbestrol (DES)	Estrogen	5 mg 3 times daily	Fluid retention, uterine bleeding, thrombophlebitis, nausea
Megestrol acetate (Megace)	Progestin	40 mg 4 times daily	Fluid retention
Aminoglutethimide (Cytadren)[1]	Aromatase inhibitor	250 mg 4 times daily	Adrenal suppression, skin rashes, neurologic reactions

[1]Used with hydrocortisone.

toxicity and maximize benefits is often best achieved by hormonal manipulation.

The choice of endocrine therapy depends on the menopausal status of the patient. Women within 1 year of their last menstrual period are considered to be premenopausal, while women whose menstruation ceased more than a year ago are postmenopausal. The initial choice of therapy is referred to as primary hormonal manipulation; subsequent endocrine treatment is called secondary or tertiary hormonal manipulation.

A. The Premenopausal Patient:

1. Primary hormonal therapy–The potent antiestrogen tamoxifen is the endocrine treatment of choice in the premenopausal patient. Tamoxifen is usually given orally in a dose of 10 mg twice a day. At least two randomized clinical trials have now shown no significant difference in survival or response between tamoxifen therapy and bilateral oophorectomy. Most physicians prefer to use tamoxifen rather than perform oophorectomy, since it can be given with little morbidity and few side effects. Controversy continues about whether a response to tamoxifen is predictive of probable success with other forms of endocrine manipulation.

Bilateral oophorectomy is a reasonable alternative for primary hormonal manipulation in premenopausal women. It can be achieved rapidly and safely by surgery or, if the patient is a poor operative risk, by irradiation of the ovaries. Ovarian radiation therapy should be avoided in otherwise healthy patients, however, because of the high rate of complications and the longer time necessary to achieve results. Oophorectomy presumably works by eliminating estrogens, progestins, and androgens, which stimulate growth of the tumor. The average remission is about 12 months.

2. Secondary or tertiary hormonal therapy– Although patients who do not respond to tamoxifen or oophorectomy should be treated with cytotoxic drugs, those who respond and then relapse may subsequently respond to another form of endocrine treatment (Table 16–7). The initial choice for secondary endocrine manipulation has not been clearly defined. Adrenalectomy or hypophysectomy induces regression in approximately 30–50% of patients who have previously responded to oophorectomy. However, these procedures are rarely performed now.

Patients who respond initially to oophorectomy but subsequently relapse should receive tamoxifen. If this treatment fails, use of aminoglutethimide or megestrol acetate should be considered. Aminoglutethimide is an inhibitor of adrenal hormone synthesis and, when combined with a corticosteroid, provides a therapeutically effective "medical adrenalectomy." Megestrol is a progestational agent. Both drugs cause less morbidity and mortality than surgical adrenalectomy; can be discontinued once the patient improves; and are not associated with the many problems of postsurgical hypoadrenalism, so that patients who require chemotherapy are more easily managed.

B. The Postmenopausal Patient:

1. Primary hormonal therapy–Tamoxifen, 10 mg twice daily, is now the initial therapy of choice for postmenopausal women with metastatic breast cancer amenable to endocrine manipulation. It has fewer side effects than diethylstilbestrol, the former therapy of choice, and is just as effective. The main side effects of tamoxifen are nausea, vomiting, and skin rash. Rarely, it may induce hypercalcemia.

2. Secondary or tertiary hormonal therapy– Postmenopausal patients who do not respond to primary endocrine manipulation should be given cytotoxic drugs such as cyclophosphamide, methotrexate, and fluorouracil (CMF) or Adriamycin (doxorubicin) and cyclophosphamide (AC). Postmenopausal women who respond initially to tamoxifen but later manifest progressive disease could be given diethylstilbestrol or megestrol acetate. Some authorities use aminoglutethimide. Megestrol has fewer side effects than either aminoglutethimide or diethylstilbestrol. Androgens have many side effects and should rarely be used. In general, hypophysectomy or adrenalectomy is rarely necessary.

Chemotherapy

Cytotoxic drugs should be considered for the treatment of metastatic breast cancer (1) if visceral metastases are present (especially brain or lymphangitic pulmonary); (2) if hormonal treatment is unsuccessful or the disease has progressed after an initial response to hormonal manipulation; or (3) if the tumor is ER-negative. The most useful single chemotherapeutic agent to date is doxorubicin (Adriamycin), with a response rate of 40–50%. Single agents are rarely used. The remissions tend to be brief, and in general, experience with single-agent chemotherapy in patients with disseminated disease has not been encouraging.

Combination chemotherapy using multiple agents has proved to be more effective, with objectively observed favorable responses achieved in 60–80% of patients with stage IV disease. Various combinations of drugs have been used, and clinical trials are continuing in an effort to improve results and reduce undesirable side effects. Doxorubicin (40 mg/m^2 intravenously on day 1) and cyclophosphamide (200 mg/m^2 orally on days 3–6) produce an objective response in about 85% of patients so treated. Other chemotherapeutic regimens have consisted of various combinations of drugs, including cyclophosphamide, vincristine, methotrexate, and fluorouracil, with response rates ranging up to 60–70%. Prior adjuvant chemotherapy does not seem to alter response rates in patients who relapse. Few new drugs or combinations of drugs have been sufficiently effective in breast cancer to warrant wide acceptance.

Recently, high-dose chemotherapy and autologous bone marrow transplantation have aroused widespread interest for the treatment of metastatic breast cancer. With this technique, the patient receives high doses of cytotoxic agents. These cause severe side effects, including bone marrow suppression, for which the patient subsequently undergoes autologous bone marrow transplantation. Reported complete response rates are as high as 30–35%—considerably better than what can be achieved with conventional chemotherapy. However, median survival times and overall survival rates do not appear to be significantly different from those reported with conventional chemotherapy. No randomized controlled clinical trial has been published that compares high-dose chemotherapy followed by bone marrow transplantation with conventional chemotherapy. A study is under way to evaluate these two options in a controlled prospective manner. High-dose chemotherapy with autologous bone marrow transplantation is an exciting modality with promise for the future, but the procedure is probably best regarded as experimental at present. Some studies are currently examining the technique in an adjuvant setting for patients at extremely high risk of recurrence of breast cancer.

Malignant Pleural Effusion

This condition develops at some time in almost half of patients with metastatic breast cancer (see Chapter 9).

PROGNOSIS

The stage of breast cancer is the single most reliable indicator of prognosis (Table 16–8). Patients with disease localized to the breast and no evidence of regional spread after microscopic examination of the lymph nodes have by far the most favorable prognosis. Estrogen and progesterone receptors appear to be an important prognostic variable, because patients with hormone receptor-negative tumors and no evidence of metastases to the axillary lymph nodes have a much higher recurrence rate than do patients with

Table 16–8. Approximate survival (%) of patients with breast cancer by TNM stage.

TNM Stage	Five Years	Ten Years
0	95	90
I	85	70
IIA	75	50
IIB	70	40
IIIA	55	30
IIIB	30	30
IV	5	2
All	65	30

hormone receptor-positive tumors and no regional metastases. The histologic subtype of breast cancer (eg, medullary, lobular, comedo) seems to have little, if any, significance in prognosis once these tumors are truly invasive. Flow cytometry of tumor cells to analyze DNA index and S-phase frequency aid in prognosis. Tumors with marked aneuploidy have a poor prognosis (Table 16–6). "Her 2-*neu* oncogene amplification, epidermal growth factor receptors, and cathepsin D may have some prognostic value, but few data exist as to their usefulness."

Most patients who develop breast cancer will ultimately die of that disease. The mortality rate of breast cancer patients exceeds that of age-matched normal controls for nearly 20 years. Thereafter, the mortality rates are equal, although deaths that occur among breast cancer patients are often directly the result of tumor. Five-year statistics do not accurately reflect the final outcome of therapy.

When cancer is localized to the breast, with no evidence of regional spread after pathologic examination, the clinical cure rate with most accepted methods of therapy is 75–90%. Exceptions to this generalization may be related to the hormonal receptor content of the tumor, tumor size, host resistance, or associated illness. Patients with small estrogen and progesterone receptor-positive tumors and no evidence of axillary spread probably have a 5-year survival rate of nearly 90%. When the axillary lymph nodes are involved with tumor, the survival rate drops to 40–50% at 5 years and probably less than 25% at 10 years. In general, breast cancer appears to be somewhat more malignant in younger than in older women, and this may be related to the fact that fewer younger women have ER-positive tumors.

FOLLOW-UP CARE

After primary therapy, patients with breast cancer should be followed for life for at least two reasons: to detect recurrences and to observe the opposite breast for a second primary carcinoma. About 10% of patients will develop a contralateral primary malignancy. Local and distant metastases occur most frequently within the first 3 years. During this period, the patient is examined every 3–4 months. Thereafter, examination is done every 6 months until 5 years postoperatively and then every 6–12 months. Special attention is given to the remaining breast, because of the increased risk of developing a second primary. The patient should examine her own breast monthly, and a mammogram should be obtained annually. In some cases, metastases are dormant for long periods and may appear up to 10–15 years or longer after removal of the primary tumor. Estrogen and progestational agents are rarely used for a patient free of disease after treatment of primary breast cancer, particularly if the tumor was hormone receptor-positive. However, studies have failed to show an adverse effect of hormonal agents in patients who are free of disease. Indeed, even pregnancy has not been clearly associated with shortened survival of patients rendered disease-free—yet most oncologists are reluctant to advise a young patient with breast cancer that she may become pregnant.

Local Recurrence

The incidence of local recurrence correlates with tumor size, the presence and number of involved axillary nodes, the histologic type of tumor, and the presence of skin edema or skin and fascia fixation with the primary. About 8% of patients develop local recurrence on the chest wall after total mastectomy and axillary dissection. When the axillary nodes are not involved, the local recurrence rate is 5%, but the rate is as high as 25% when they are involved. A similar difference in local recurrence rate was noted between small and large tumors. Factors that affect the rate of local recurrence in patients who had partial mastectomies are not yet determined. However, early studies show that such things as multifocal cancer, in situ tumors, positive resection margins, chemotherapy, and radiotherapy are important.

Chest wall recurrences usually appear within the first 2 years but may occur as late as 15 or more years after mastectomy. Suspect nodules should be biopsied. Local excision or localized radiotherapy may be feasible if an isolated nodule is present. If lesions are multiple or accompanied by evidence of regional involvement in the internal mammary or supraclavicular nodes, the disease is best managed by radiation treatment of the entire chest wall including the parasternal, supraclavicular, and axillary areas.

Local recurrence after mastectomy usually signals the presence of widespread disease and is an indication for bone and liver scans, posteroanterior and lateral chest x-rays, and other examinations as needed to search for evidence of metastases. Most patients with locally recurrent tumor will develop distant metastases within 2 years. When there is no evidence of metastases beyond the chest wall and regional nodes, irradiation for cure or complete local excision should be attempted. Patients with local recurrence may be cured with local resection or radiation. After partial mastectomy, however, local recurrence does not have as serious a prognostic significance. However, those patients who do develop a breast recurrence have a worse prognosis than those who do not. It is speculated that the ability of a cancer to recur locally after radiotherapy is a sign of aggressiveness associated with distant disease rather than a cause of it. Completion of the mastectomy should be done for local recurrence after partial mastectomy; overall survival does not appear to be altered. Systemic chemotherapy or hormonal treatment should be used for postmenopausal women who develop disseminated disease or those in whom local recurrence occurs following total mastectomy.

Edema of the Arm

Significant edema of the arm occurs in about 5% after modified radical mastectomy and about 10–30% of patients after radical mastectomy. Edema of the arm is less frequent after modified radical mastectomy than after radical mastectomy and occurs more commonly if radiotherapy has been given or if there was postoperative infection. Early trials suggest that partial mastectomy with radiation to the axillary lymph nodes is followed by chronic edema of the arm in 10–20% of patients. To avoid this complication, many authorities advocate axillary lymph node sampling rather than complete axillary dissection. However, since axillary dissection is a more accurate staging operation than axillary sampling, we recommend axillary dissection, with removal of at least level I and II lymph nodes, in combination with partial mastectomy. Judicious use of radiotherapy, with treatment fields carefully planned to spare the axilla as much as possible, can greatly diminish the incidence of edema.

Late or secondary edema of the arm may develop years after treatment, as a result of axillary recurrence or of infection in the hand or arm, with obliteration of lymphatic channels. Infection in the arm or hand on the dissected side should be treated promptly with antibiotics, rest, and elevation. When edema develops, careful examination of the axilla should be done to detect a regional recurrence. If there is no sign of recurrence, the swollen extremity should be treated with rest and elevation. A mild diuretic may be helpful for a few weeks. If there is no improvement, a compressor pump should be used to decrease the swelling, and the patient should then be fitted with an elastic glove or sleeve. Most patients are not bothered enough by mild edema to wear an uncomfortable glove or sleeve and will treat themselves with elevation alone. Rarely, edema may be severe enough to interfere with use of the limb.

Breast Reconstruction

Breast reconstruction, with the implantation of a prosthesis, is usually feasible after standard or modified radical mastectomy. Reconstruction should probably be discussed with patients prior to mastectomy, because it offers an important psychologic focal point for recovery. However, most patients who are initially interested in reconstruction decide later that they no longer wish to undergo the procedure. Reconstruction is not an obstacle to the diagnosis of recurrent cancer. The most common breast reconstruction has been implantation of a silicone gel prosthesis in the subpectoral plane between the pectoralis minor and pectoralis major muscles. Recently, the Food and Drug Administration has placed a moratorium on the use of silicone gel implants because of possible leakage of silicone and associated autoimmune disorders. This remote possibility should not prevent the cancer patient from having a reconstruction. Most plastic surgeons currently would place a saline-filled prosthesis rather than a silicone gel implant. Alternatively, autologous tissue can be used for reconstruction. The most popular autologous technique currently is the trans-rectus abdominis muscle flap (TRAM flap), which is done by rotating the rectus abdominis muscle with attached fat and skin cephalad to make a breast mound. A latissimus dorsi flap can be swung from the back but offers less fullness than the TRAM flap and is therefore less acceptable cosmetically. All patients who undergo mastectomy should be offered the option of breast reconstruction.

Risks of Pregnancy

Data are insufficient to determine whether interruption of pregnancy improves the prognosis of patients who are discovered during pregnancy to have potentially curable breast cancer and who receive definitive treatment. Theoretically, the increasingly high levels of estrogen produced by the placenta as the pregnancy progresses could be detrimental to the patient with occult metastases of hormone-sensitive breast cancer. Moreover, occult metastases are present in most patients with positive axillary nodes, and treatment by adjuvant chemotherapy would be potentially harmful to the fetus. Under these circumstances, interruption of early pregnancy seems reasonable, with progressively less rationale for the procedure as term approaches. Obviously, the decision must be highly individualized and will be affected by many factors, including the patient's desire to have the baby and the generally poor prognosis when axillary nodes are involved.

Equally problematic and important is the advice regarding future pregnancy (or abortion in case of pregnancy) to be given to women of child-bearing age who have had a mastectomy or other definitive treatment for breast cancer. Under these circumstances, one must assume that pregnancy will be harmful if occult metastases are present, although this has not been demonstrated. Patients whose tumors are ER-negative probably would not be affected by pregnancy. A number of studies have shown no adverse effect of pregnancy on survival of pregnant women who have had breast cancer.

In patients with inoperable or metastatic cancer (stage IV disease), induced abortion is usually advisable because of the possible adverse effects of hormonal treatment, radiotherapy, or chemotherapy upon the fetus.

General

American College of Radiology et al: Standards for breast-conservation treatment. CA 1992;42:134.

Baines CJ: Breast self-examination. Cancer 1989;64:2661.

Bassett LW et al: The prevalence of carcinoma in palpable vs. impalpable, mammographically detected lesions. Am J Roentgenol 1991;157:21.

Bassett LW, Giuliano AE, Gold RH: Staging for breast carcinoma. Am J Surg 1989;157:250.

Bornstein BA et al: Results of treating ductal carcinoma in situ of the breast with conservative surgery and radiation therapy. Cancer 1991;67:7.

Bulens P et al: Breast conserving treatment of Paget's disease. Radiother Oncol 1990;17:305.

Callahan R et al: Somatic mutations and human breast cancer: A status report. Cancer 1992;69;1582.

Clayton F, Hopkins CL: Pathologic correlates of prognosis in lymphnode-positive breast carcinomas. Cancer 1993;71:1780.

Donegan WL, Padrta B: Combined therapy for inflammatory breast cancer. Arch Surg 1990;125:578.

Donovan AJ: Bilateral breast cancer. Surg Clin North Am 1990;70:1141.

Dorr FA: Prognostic factors observed in current clinical trials. Cancer 1993;71:2163.

Dupont WD, Page DL: Menopausal estrogen replacement therapy and breast cancer. Arch Intern Med 1991;151;67.

Elliott RL et al: Steriotaxic needle localization and biopsy of occult breast lesions: first years experience. Amn Surg 1992;58:126.

Fisher B et al: DNA flow cytometric analysis of primary operable breast cancer: Relation of ploidy and S-phase fraction to outcome of patients in NSABP B 04. Cancer 1991;68:1465.

Fisher B et al: Eight-year results of a randomized clinical trial comparing total mastectomy and lumpectomy with or without irradiation in the treatment of breast cancer. N Engl J Med 1989;320:822.

Fisher B et al: Significance of ipsilateral breast tumour recurrence after lumpectomy. Lancet 1991;338:327.

Fisher ER et al: Pathologic findings from the National Surgical Adjuvant Breast Project (protocol 4): Discriminants for 15 year survival. Cancer 1993;71:2141.

Harris JR et al: Breast Cancer. (Three parts.) N Engl J Med 1992;327:319, 390, 473.

Harris JR et al: Conservative surgery and radiotherapy for early breast cancer. Cancer 1990;66:1427.

Henrich JB: The postmenopausal estrogen/breast cancer controversy. JAMA 1992;268:1900.

Henson DE, Ries LA: Progress in early breast cancer detection. Cancer 1990;65(9 Suppl):2155.

Holm LE et al: Treatment failure and dietary habits in women with breast cancer. J Natl Cancer Inst 1993;85:32.

Isola J: Cathepsin D expression detected by immunohistochemistry has independent prognostic value in axillary node-negative breast cancer. J Clin Oncol 1993;11:36.

Kinne DW: Staging and follow-up of breast cancer patients. Cancer 1991;67(Suppl 4):1196.

Kopald KH et al: The pathology of nonpalpable breast cancer. Am Surg 1990;56:782.

Layfield LJ et al: Mammographically guided fine-needle aspiration biopsy of non-palpable breast lesions: Can it replace open biopsy? Cancer 1991;68:2007.

Lazovich D et al: Underutilization of breast-conserving

surgery with radiation therapy among women with stage I or II breast cancer. JAMA 1991;266:3433.

Leis HP Jr: Concepts regarding breast biopsies. Breast Dis 1991;4:223.

Lichter AS: Lumpectomy and radiation: Improving the outcome. J Clin Oncol 1992;10:349.

McDivitt RW et al: Histologic types of benign breast disease and the risk for breast cancer. Cancer 1992; 69:1408.

Mesko TW et al: Risk factors for breast cancer. Compr Ther 1990;16:3.

Moore MP et al: Inflammatory breast cancer. Arch Surg 1991;126:304.

Morrison AS: Review of evidence on the early detection and treatment of breast cancer. Cancer 1989;64(12 Suppl):2651.

Nattinger AB et al: Geographic variation in the use of breast-conserving treatment for breast cancer. N Engl J Med 1992;326:1102.

Rosner D et al: Ductal carcinoma in situ with microinvasion: A curable entity using surgery alone without need for adjuvant therapy. Cancer 1991;67:1498.

Senie RT et al: Obesity at diagnosis of breast carcinoma influences duration of disease-free survival. Ann Intern Med 1992;116:26.

Stotter AT et al: The role of limited surgery with radiation and primary treatment of ductal in situ breast cancer. Int J Radiat Oncol Biol Phys 1990;18:283.

Vetrani A et al: Fine-needle aspiration biopsies of breast masses: An additional experience with 1153 cases (1985–1988) and a meta-analysis. Cancer 1992; 69:736.

Vicini FA et al: The optimal extent of resection for patients with stages I or II breast cancer treated with conservative surgery and radiotherapy. Ann Surg 1991;214:200.

Wazer DE et al: Factors influencing cosmetic outcome and complication risk after conservative surgery and radiotherapy for early-stage carcinoma. J Clin Oncol 1992;10:356.

Witzig TE et al: DNA ploidy and percent S-phase as prognostic factors in node-positive breast cancer: Results from patients enrolled in two prospective randomized trials. J Clin Oncol 1993;11:351.

Zavertnik JJ et al: Cost effective management of breast cancer. Cancer 1992;69:1979.

Mammography

Feig SA, Ehrlich SM: Estimation of radiation risks from screening mammography: Recent trends and comparison with expected benefits. Radiology 1990;174(3 Part 1):638.

Harris RP et al: Mammography and age: Are we targeting the wrong women? A community survey of women and physicians. Cancer 1991;67:2010.

Hindle WH: Screening mammography reports: toward clear concise clinical descriptions. West J Med 1992; 157:152.

Holleb AI: Review of breast cancer screening guidelines. Cancer 1992;69:1911.

McLelland R: Screening mammography. Cancer 1991; 67(4 Suppl)1129.

Nattinger AB et al: Screening mammography for older women: a case of mixed messages. Arch Intern Med 1992;152:922.

Hormone Receptors

Ferno M et al: Estrogen and progesterone receptor analyses in more than 4000 human breast cancer samples: A study with special reference to age at diagnosis and stability of analyses. (From the Southern Swedish Breast Cancer Study Group.) Acta Oncol 1990; 29:129.

Hawkins RA et al: Does the estrogen receptor concentration of a breast cancer change during systemic therapy? Br J Cancer 1990;61:877.

Lerner LJ, Jordan CV: Development of antiestrogens and their use in breast cancer. Cancer Res 1990;50:4177.

Lundy J et al: The use of fine-needle aspirates of breast cancers to evaluate hormone-receptor status. Arch Surg 1990;125:174.

Pertschuk LP et al: Steroid hormone receptor immunohistochemistry and amplification of c-myc protooncogene. Cancer 1993;71:162.

Robertson JFR et al: Comparison of two oestrogen receptor assays in the prediction of the clinical course of patients with advanced breast cancer. Br J Cancer 1992;65:727.

Adjuvant Systemic Therapy

Bagdade JD et al: Effects of tamoxifen treatment on plasma lipids and lipoprotein lipid composition. J Clin Endocrinol Metab 1990;70:1132.

Buzdar AU et al: Is chemotherapy effective in reducing the local failure rate in patients with operable breast cancer? Cancer 1990;65:394.

Carbone PP: Breast cancer adjuvant therapy. Cancer 1990;66:1378.

Castiglione M et al: Adjuvant systematic therapy for breast cancer in the elderly: Competing causes of mortality. J Clin Oncol 1990;8:519.

Cooper MR: The role of chemotherapy for node-negative breast cancer. Cancer 1991;67:1744.

Davidson NE, Abeloff MD: Adjuvant systemic therapy in women with early-stage breast cancer at high risk for relapse. J Natl Cancer Inst 1992;84:301.

DeGregorio MW: Is tamoxifen chemo prevention worth the risk in healthy women? J NIH Res 1992;4:84.

DeVita VT Jr: Breast cancer therapy: Exercising all our options. (Editorial.) N Engl J Med 1989;320:527.

Early Breast Cancer Trialists' Collaborative Group: Systemic treatment of early breast cancer by hormonal cytotoxic or immune therapy: 133 randomized trials involving 31,000 recurrences and 24,000 deaths among 75,000 women. Lancet 1992;339:1, 71.

Fisher B et al: A randomized clinical trial evaluating sequential methotrexate and fluorouracil in the treatment of patients with node-negative breast cancer who have estrogen receptor-negative tumors. N Engl J Med 1989;320:473.

Fisher B et al: A randomized clinical trial evaluating tamoxifen in the treatment of patients with node-negative breast cancer who have estrogen receptor-positive tumors. N Engl J Med 1989;320:479.

Fisher ER et al: Pathologic findings from the National Surgical Adjuvant Breast and Bowel Projects (NSABP): Prognostic discriminants for 8-year survival for node-negative invasive cancer patients. Cancer 1990;65 (9 Suppl): 2121.

Fornander T et al: Long term adjuvant tamoxifen in early

breast cancer: Effect on bone mineral density in postmenopausal women. J Clin Oncol 1990;8:1019.

Levine MN et al: A bedside decision instrument to elicit a patient's preference concerning adjuvant chemotherapy for breast cancer. Ann Intern Med 1992; 17:53.

Ludwig Breast Cancer Study Group: Prolonged disease-free survival after one course of perioperative adjuvant chemotherapy for node-negative breast cancer. N Engl J Med 1989;320:491.

McGuire WL: Adjuvant therapy of node-negative breast cancer. (Editorial.) N Engl J Med 1989;320:525.

Mueller CB, Lesperance ML: NSABP trials of adjuvant chemotherapy for breast cancer: A further look at the evidence. Ann Surg 1991;214:206.

National Institutes of Health: Clinical Alert. National Institutes of Health Consensus Development Conference Statement: Adjuvant chemotherapy for breast cancer. Vol 8, No. 16, 1990.

Recht A et al: Integration of conservative surgery, radiotherapy, and chemotherapy for the treatment of early-stage, node-positive breast cancer: sequencing, timing, and outcome. J Clin Oncol 1991;9:1662.

Treatment of Advanced Breast Cancer

Buzdar AU: Current status of endocrine treatment of carcinoma of the breast. Semin Surg Oncol 1990;6:77.

Christman K et al: Chemotherapy of metastatic breast cancer in the elderly: The Piedmont Oncology Association Experience. JAMA 1992;268:57.

Eddy DM: High-dose chemotherapy with autologous bone marrow transplantation for the treatment of metastatic breast cancer. J Clin Oncol 1992;10:657.

Henderson IC et al: Comprehensive management of disseminated breast cancer. Cancer 1990;66:1439.

Hillner BE et al: Efficacy and cost-effectiveness of autologous bone marrow transplantation in metastatic breast cancer: Estimate using decision analysis while awaiting clinical trial results. JAMA 1992;267:2055.

Ingle JN: Principles of therapy in advanced breast cancer. Hematol Oncol Clin North Am 1989;3:743.

Nemoto T et al: Aminoglutethimide in patients with metastatic breast cancer. Cancer 1989;63:1673.

Perez DJ et al: A randomized comparison of single-agent doxorubicin and epirubicin as first-line cytotoxic therapy in advanced breast cancer. J Clin Oncol 1991; 9:2148.

Price JE: The biology of metastatic breast cancer. Cancer 1990;66(6 Suppl):1313.

Rose C, Mouridsen HT: Endocrine management of advanced breast cancer. Hormone Res 1989;32(Suppl 1):189.

Swain SM et al: Fluorouracil and high dose leucovorin in previously treated patients with metastatic breast cancer. J Clin Oncol 1989;7:890.

Turken S et al: Effects of tamoxifen on spinal bone density in women with breast cancer. J Natl Cancer Inst 1989;81:1086.

CARCINOMA OF THE MALE BREAST

Essentials of Diagnosis

- A painless lump beneath the areola in a man usually over 50 years of age.
- Nipple discharge, retraction, or ulceration may be present.

General Considerations

Breast cancer in men is a rare disease; the incidence is only about 1% of that in women. The average age at occurrence is about 60—somewhat older than the commonest presenting age in women. The prognosis, even in stage I cases, is worse in men than in women. Blood-borne metastases are commonly present when the male patient appears for initial treatment. These metastases may be latent and may not become manifest for many years. As in women, hormonal influences are probably related to the development of male breast cancer. There is a high incidence of both breast cancer and gynecomastia in Bantu men, theoretically owing to failure of estrogen inactivation by a damaged liver associated with vitamin B deficiency.

Clinical Findings

A painless lump, occasionally associated with nipple discharge, retraction, erosion, or ulceration, is the chief complaint. Examination usually shows a hard, ill-defined, nontender mass beneath the nipple or areola. Gynecomastia not uncommonly precedes or accompanies breast cancer in men. Nipple discharge is an uncommon presentation for breast cancer in men, as it is in women. However, nipple discharge in a man is an ominous finding associated with carcinoma in nearly 75% of cases.

Breast cancer staging is the same in men as in women. Gynecomastia and metastatic cancer from another site (eg, prostate) must be considered in the differential diagnosis of a breast lesion in a man. Biopsy settles the issue.

Treatment

Treatment consists of modified radical mastectomy in operable patients, who should be chosen by the same criteria as women with the disease. Irradiation is the first step in treating localized metastases in the skin, lymph nodes, or skeleton that are causing symptoms. Examination of the cancer for hormone receptor proteins may prove to be of value in predicting response to endocrine ablation. Adjuvant chemotherapy is used for the same indications as in breast cancer in women.

Since breast cancer in men is frequently a disseminated disease, endocrine therapy is of considerable importance in its management. Castration in advanced breast cancer is the most successful palliative measure and more beneficial than the same procedure in women. Objective evidence of regression may be seen in 60–70% of men who are castrated—approximately twice the proportion in women. The average duration of tumor growth remission is about 30 months, and life is prolonged. Bone is the most frequent site of metastases from breast cancer in men (as in women), and castration relieves bone pain in most patients so treated. The longer the interval between mastectomy and recurrence, the longer the tumor growth remission following castration. As in women, there is no correlation between the histologic type of the tumor and the likelihood of remission following castration.

Tamoxifen (10 mg orally twice daily) is becoming increasingly popular and should replace castration as the initial therapy for metastatic disease. However, little clinical experience is available with tamoxifen in male breast cancers. Aminoglutethimide (250 mg orally four times a day) should replace adrenalectomy in men as it has in women. Corticosteroid therapy alone has been considered to be efficacious but probably has no value when compared with major endocrine ablation.

Estrogen therapy—5 mg of diethylstilbestrol three times daily orally—may be effective as secondary hormonal manipulation after medical adrenalectomy (with aminoglutethimide). Androgen therapy may exacerbate bone pain. Castration and tamoxifen are the main therapeutic resources for advanced breast cancer in men at present. Chemotherapy should be administered for the same indications and using the same dosage schedules as for women with metastatic disease.

Prognosis

The prognosis of breast cancer is poorer in men than in women. The crude 5- and 10-year survival rates for clinical stage I breast cancer in men are about 58% and 38%, respectively. For clinical stage II disease, the 5- and 10-year survival rates are approximately 38% and 10%. The survival rates for all stages at 5 and 10 years are 36% and 17%.

Donegan WL: Cancer of the breast in men. CA 1991; 41:539.

Guinee VF et al: The prognosis of breast cancer in males. Cancer 1993;71:154.

Jaiyesimi IA et al: Carcinoma of the male breast. Ann Intern Med 1992;117:771.

Ribeiro G, Swindell R: Adjuvant tamoxifen for male breast cancer. Br J Cancer 1992;65:252.

OTHER BREAST DISORDERS

MAMMARY DYSPLASIA
(Fibrocystic Disease)

Essentials of Diagnosis

- Rapid fluctuation in the size of the masses is common.
- Frequently, pain occurs or increases and size increases during premenstrual phase of cycle.
- Most common age is 30–50. Rare in postmenopausal women.

General Considerations

This disorder, also known as fibrocystic disease or chronic cystic mastitis, is the most frequent lesion of the breast. It is common in women 30–50 years of age but rare in postmenopausal women; this suggests that it is related to ovarian activity. Estrogen hormone is considered a causative factor. The term "mammary dysplasia," or "fibrocystic disease," is imprecise and encompasses a wide variety of pathologic entities. These lesions are always associated with benign changes in the breast epithelium, some of which are found so commonly in normal breasts that they are probably variants of normal breast histology but have unfortunately been termed a "disease."

The microscopic findings of fibrocystic disease include cysts (gross and microscopic), papillomatosis, adenosis, fibrosis, and ductal epithelial hyperplasia. Although mammary dysplasia has generally been considered to increase the risk of subsequent breast cancer, only the variants in which proliferation of epithelial components is demonstrated represent true risk factors.

Clinical Findings

Mammary dysplasia may produce an asymptomatic lump in the breast that is discovered by accident, but pain or tenderness often calls attention to the mass. There may be discharge from the nipple. In many cases, discomfort occurs or is increased during the premenstrual phase of the cycle, at which time the cysts tend to enlarge. Fluctuation in size and rapid appearance or disappearance of a breast tumor are common in cystic disease. Multiple or bilateral masses are common, and many patients will give a history of a transient lump in the breast or cyclic breast pain.

Differential Diagnosis

Pain, fluctuation in size, and multiplicity of lesions are the features most helpful in differentiation from carcinoma. However, if a dominant mass is present, the diagnosis of cancer should be assumed until disproved by biopsy. Final diagnosis often depends on biopsy. Mammography may be helpful, but the breast tissue in these young women is usually too radiodense to permit a worthwhile study. Sonography is useful in differentiating a cystic from a solid mass.

Treatment

Because mammary dysplasia is frequently indistinguishable from carcinoma on the basis of clinical findings, suspicious lesions should be biopsied. Fine-needle aspiration cytology may be used, but if a suspicious mass that is nonmalignant on cytologic examination does not resolve over several months, it must be excised. Surgery should be conservative, since the primary objective is to exclude cancer. Simple mastectomy or extensive removal of breast tissue is rarely, if ever, indicated for mammary dysplasia.

When the diagnosis of mammary dysplasia has been established by previous biopsy or is practically certain because the history is classic, aspiration of a discrete mass suggestive of a cyst is indicated. The patient is reexamined at intervals thereafter. If no fluid is obtained or if fluid is bloody, if a mass persists after aspiration, or if at any time during follow-up a persistent lump is noted, biopsy examination should be performed.

Breast pain associated with generalized mammary dysplasia is best treated by avoiding trauma and by wearing (night and day) a brassiere that gives good support and protection. Hormone therapy is not advisable, because it does not cure the condition and has undesirable side effects. Danazol (100–200 mg twice daily orally), a synthetic androgen, has been used for patients with severe pain. This treatment suppresses pituitary gonadotropins, and androgenic effects (acne, edema, hirsutism) usually make this treatment intolerable; it should therefore be reserved for the unusual severe case.

The role of caffeine consumption in the development and treatment of fibrocystic disease is controversial. Some studies suggest that eliminating caffeine from the diet is associated with improvement. Many patients are aware of these studies and report relief of symptoms after giving up coffee, tea, and chocolate. Similarly, many women find vitamin E (400 IU daily) helpful. However, these observations have been difficult to confirm and are anecdotal.

Prognosis

Exacerbations of pain, tenderness, and cyst formation may occur at any time until the menopause, when symptoms usually subside, except in patients receiving estrogens. The patient should be advised to examine her own breasts each month just after menstruation and to inform her physician if a mass appears. The risk of breast cancer in women with mammary dysplasia showing proliferative or atypical changes in the epithelium is higher than that of women in general. Follow-up examinations at regular intervals should therefore be arranged.

Dogliotti L, Orlandi R, Angeli A: The endocrine basis of benign breast disorders. World J Surg 1989;13:674.

Dupont WD et al: Influence of exogenous estrogens, proliferative breast disease, and other variables on breast cancer risk. Cancer 1989;63:948.

London SJ et al: A prospective study of benign breast disease and the risk of breast cancer. JAMA 1992;267:941.

Maddox PR, Mansel RE: Management of breast pain and nodularity. World J Surg 1989;13:699.

McDivitt RW et al: Histologic types of benign breast disease and the risk for breast cancer. Cancer 1992;69:1408.

Page DL, Dupont WD: Anatomic markers of human premalignancy and risk of breast cancer. Cancer 1990;66(6 Suppl):1326.

FIBROADENOMA OF THE BREAST

This common benign neoplasm occurs most frequently in young women, usually within 20 years after puberty. It is somewhat more frequent and tends to occur at an earlier age in black than in white women. Multiple tumors in one or both breasts are found in 10–15% of patients.

The typical fibroadenoma is a round, firm, discrete, relatively movable, nontender mass 1–5 cm in diameter. The tumor is usually discovered accidentally. Clinical diagnosis in young patients is generally not difficult. In women over 30, cystic disease of the breast and carcinoma of the breast must be considered. Cysts can be identified by aspiration. Fibroadenoma does not normally occur after the menopause, but postmenopausal women may occasionally develop fibroadenoma after administration of estrogenic hormone.

Treatment is by excision under local anesthesia as an outpatient procedure, with pathologic examination of the specimen.

Cystosarcoma phyllodes is a type of fibroadenoma with cellular stroma that tends to grow rapidly. This tumor may reach a large size and if inadequately excised will recur locally. The lesion is rarely malignant. Treatment is by local excision of the mass with a margin of surrounding breast tissue. The treatment of malignant cystosarcoma phyllodes is more controversial. In general, complete removal of the tumor and a rim of normal tissue should avoid recurrence. Since these tumors may be large, simple mastectomy is sometimes necessary to achieve complete control.

Dent DM, Cant PJ: Fibroadenoma. World J Surg 1989; 13:706.

Hart J et al: Practical aspects in the diagnosis and management of cystosarcoma phyllodes. Arch Surg 1988; 123:1079.

Hindle WH, Alonzo LJ: Conservative management of breast fibroadenomas. Am J Obstet Gynecol 1991; 164:1647.

Yu H et al: Risk factors for fibroadenoma: A case-control study in Australia. Am J Epidemiol 1992;135:247.

NIPPLE DISCHARGE

In order of increasing frequency, the following are the commonest causes of nipple discharge in the nonlactating breast: carcinoma, intraductal papilloma, and mammary dysplasia with ectasia of the ducts. The important characteristics of the discharge and some other factors to be evaluated by history and physical examination are as follows:

(1) Nature of discharge (serous, bloody, or other).
(2) Association with a mass or not.
(3) Unilateral or bilateral.
(4) Single duct or multiple duct discharge.
(5) Discharge is spontaneous (persistent or intermittent) or must be expressed.
(6) Discharge produced by pressure at a single site or by general pressure on the breast.
(7) Relation to menses.
(8) Premenopausal or postmenopausal.
(9) Patient taking contraceptive pills, or estrogen for postmenopausal symptoms.

Unilateral, spontaneous serous or serosanguineous discharge from a single duct is usually caused by an intraductal papilloma or, rarely, by an intraductal cancer. In either case, a mass may not be palpable. The involved duct may be identified by pressure at different sites around the nipple at the margin of the areola. Bloody discharge is more suggestive of cancer but is usually caused by a benign papilloma in the duct. Cytologic examination may identify malignant cells, but negative findings do not rule out cancer, which is more likely in women over age 50. In any case, the involved duct—and a mass if present—should be excised. Ductography may identify a filling defect prior to excision of the duct system.

In premenopausal women, spontaneous multiple duct discharge, unilateral or bilateral, most marked just before menstruation, is often due to mammary dysplasia. Discharge may be green or brownish. Papillomatosis and ductal ectasia are usually seen on biopsy. If a mass is present, it should be removed.

Milky discharge from multiple ducts in the nonlactating breast may occur in certain syndromes (Chiari-Frommel, Argonz-Del Castillo [Forbes-Albright]), presumably as a result of increased secretion of pituitary prolactin. Serum prolactin and TSH levels should be obtained to search for a pituitary tumor or hypothyroidism. Drugs of the chlorpromazine type and contraceptive pills may also cause milky discharge that ceases on discontinuance of the medication.

Oral contraceptive agents may cause clear, serous, or milky discharge from a single duct, but multiple duct discharge is more common. The discharge is more evident just before menstruation and disappears on stopping the medication. If it does not and is from a single duct, exploration should be considered.

Purulent discharge may originate in a subareolar abscess and require excision of the abscess and related lactiferous sinus.

When localization is not possible and no mass is palpable, the patient should be reexamined every week for 1 month. When unilateral discharge persists, even without definite localization or tumor, exploration must be considered. The alternative is careful follow-up at intervals of 1–3 months. Mammography should be done. Cytologic examination of nipple discharge for exfoliated cancer cells may be helpful in diagnosis.

Chronic unilateral nipple discharge, especially if bloody, is an indication for resection of the involved ducts.

Leis HP Jr: Management of nipple discharge. World J Surg 1989;13:736.
Takeda T et al: Nipple discharge cytology and mass screening for breast cancer. Acta Cytol 1990;34:21.

FAT NECROSIS

Fat necrosis is a rare lesion of the breast but is of clinical importance because it produces a mass, often accompanied by skin or nipple retraction, that is indistinguishable from carcinoma. Trauma is presumed to be the cause, though only about half of patients give a history of injury to the breast. Ecchymosis is occasionally seen near the tumor. Tenderness may or may not be present. If untreated, the mass associated with fat necrosis gradually disappears. As a rule, the safest course is to obtain a biopsy. The entire mass should be excised, primarily to rule out carcinoma. Fat necrosis is common after segmental resection and radiation therapy.

BREAST ABSCESS

During nursing, an area of redness, tenderness, and induration not infrequently develops in the breast. The organism most commonly found in these abscesses is *Staphylococcus aureus*. In the early stages, the infection can often be reversed while nursing is continued from that breast by administering an antibiotic such as dicloxacillin or oxacillin, 250 mg four times daily for 7–10 days (see Puerperal Mastitis, Chapter 17). If the lesion progresses to form a localized mass with local and systemic signs of infection, an abscess is present and should be drained, and nursing should be discontinued.

A subareolar abscess may develop (rarely) in young or middle-aged women who are not lactating. These infections tend to recur after incision and drainage unless the area is explored in a quiescent interval with excision of the involved lactiferous duct or ducts at the base of the nipple. Except for the subareolar type of abscess, infection in the breast is very rare unless the patient is lactating. In the nonlactating breast, inflammatory carcinoma must always be considered. Therefore, findings suggestive of abscess in the nonlactating breast are an indication for incision and biopsy of any indurated tissue.

REFERENCES

Bland KI, Copeland EM III: *The Breast: Comprehensive Management of Benign and Malignant Diseases.* Saunders, 1991.

Kopans DD: *Breast Imaging.* Lippincott, 1989.

Benson EA: Management of breast abscesses. World J Surg 1989;13:753.

Edmiston CE Jr et al: The nonpuerperal breast infection: Aerobic and anaerobic microbial recovery from acute and chronic disease. J Infect Dis 1990;162:695.

Ragaz J, Ariel IM: *High Risk Breast Cancer.* Springer-Verlag, 1989.

Gynecology & Obstetrics

17

H. Trent MacKay, MD, MPH, & Arthur T. Evans, MD

GYNECOLOGY

ABNORMAL PREMENOPAUSAL BLEEDING

Normal menstrual bleeding lasts an average of 4 days (range, 1–7 days), with a mean blood loss of 35 mL. Blood loss of over 80 mL per cycle is abnormal and frequently produces anemia. Excessive bleeding, often with the passage of clots, may occur at regular menstrual intervals **(menorrhagia)** or irregular intervals **(dysfunctional uterine bleeding).** When there are fewer than 21 days between the onset of bleeding episodes, the cycles are likely to be anovular. **Ovulation bleeding,** a single episode of spotting between regular menses, is quite common. Heavier or irregular intermenstrual bleeding warrants investigation.

Clinical Findings
A. Symptoms and Signs: The diagnosis of the disorders underlying the bleeding usually depends upon (1) a careful description of the duration and amount of flow, related pain, and relationship to the last menstrual period (LMP); (2) a history of pertinent illnesses; (3) a history of all medications the patient has taken in the past month, so that possible inhibition of ovulation or endometrial stimulation can be assessed; and (4) a careful pelvic examination to look for pregnancy, uterine myomas, adnexal masses, infection, or evidence of endometriosis.

B. Laboratory Studies: Cervical smears should be obtained as needed for cytologic and culture studies. Blood studies should include measurements of hemoglobin, hematocrit, white blood cell count and differential, sedimentation rate, and platelet count. Urinalysis and measurement of blood sugar levels should be performed to rule out diabetes. A test for pregnancy and studies of thyroid function and blood clotting should be considered in the clinical evaluation. Tests for ovulation in cyclic menorrhagia include basal body temperature records, serum progesterone measured 1 week before the expected onset of menses, and analysis of an endometrial biopsy specimen for secretory activity shortly before the onset of menstruation.

C. Imaging: Pelvic ultrasound may be useful to diagnose intrauterine or ectopic pregnancy, subserous or intrauterine myomas, endometriosis, or adnexal masses that may be related to abnormal bleeding. Hysterosalpingography can outline endometrial polyps, submucous myomas, or uterine synechiae. MRI can definitively diagnose submucous myomas and adenomyosis.

D. Cervical Biopsy and Endometrial Curettage: Biopsy, curettage, or aspiration of the endometrium and curettage of the endocervix are often necessary to diagnose the cause of bleeding. These and other invasive gynecologic diagnostic procedures are described in Table 17–1, Polyps, tumors, and submucous myomas are commonly identified in this way. If cancer of the cervix is a possibility, multiple quadrant biopsies (or colposcopically directed biopsies) and endocervical curettage are indicated as first steps.

E. Hysteroscopy: Hysteroscopy can visualize endometrial polyps, submucous myomas, and exophytic endometrial cancers. It is useful immediately before D&C.

Treatment
Premenopausal patients with abnormal uterine bleeding include those with submucous myomas, infection, early abortion, or pelvic neoplasms. The history, physical examination, and laboratory findings should identify such patients, who require definitive therapy depending upon the cause of the bleeding. A large group of patients remains, most of whom have dysfunctional uterine bleeding on a hormonal basis.

Dysfunctional uterine bleeding is usually caused by overgrowth of endometrium due to estrogen stimulation without adequate progesterone to stabilize growth; this occurs in anovular cycles. Anovulation associated with high estrogen levels commonly occurs in teenagers, in women aged late 30s to late 40s, and in extremely obese women or those with polycystic ovaries. The use of exogenous estrogen without added progestin is another common cause. Prolonged low levels of unopposed estrogen can cause

Table 17–1. Common gynecologic diagnostic procedures.

Colposcopy
Visualized of cervical, vaginal, or vulvar epithelium under 5–50× magnification to identify abnormal areas requiring biopsy. Used to identify genital warts on males as well as females. An office procedure.

D&C
Dilation of the cervix and curettage of the entire endometrial cavity, using a metal curet or suction cannula and often using forceps for the removal of endometrial polyps. Performed to diagnose endometrial disease and to stop heavy bleeding. Can usually be done in the office under local anesthesia.

Endometrial biopsy
Removal of one or more areas of the endometrium by means of a curet or small aspiration device without cervical dilation. Less accurate diagnostically than D&C. An office procedure performed under local anesthesia.

Endocervical curettage
Removal of endocervical epithelium with a small curet for diagnosis of cervical dysplasias and cancer. An office procedure performed under local anesthesia.

Hysteroscopy
Visual examination of the uterine cavity with a small fiberoptic endoscope passed through the cervix. Biopsies, excision of myomas, and other procedures can be performed. Can be done in the office under local anesthesia or in the operating room under general anesthesia.

Hysterosalpingography
Injection of radiopaque dye through the cervix to visualize the uterine cavity and oviducts. Mainly used in diagnosis of infertility.

Laparoscopy
Visualization of the abdominal and pelvic cavity through a small fiberoptic endoscope passed through a subumbilical incision. Permits diagnosis, tubal sterilization, and treatment of many conditions previously requiring laparotomy. General anesthesia is usually used.

spotting; high levels can result in profuse or prolonged bleeding.

Such bleeding can usually be treated hormonally; progestins, which limit and stabilize endometrial growth, are generally effective. Office D&C is usually not necessary in women under age 40. Medroxyprogesterone acetate, 10 mg/d, or norethindrone acetate, 5 mg/d, should be given for 10–14 days starting on day 15 of the cycle, following which withdrawal bleeding (so-called medical curettage) will occur. The treatment is repeated for several cycles; it can be reinstituted if amenorrhea or dysfunctional bleeding recurs. In young women who are bleeding actively, oral contraceptives can be given four times daily for 5–7 days; after withdrawal bleeding occurs, pills are taken in the usual dosage for three cycles. In cases of intractable heavy bleeding, danazol in doses of 200 mg four times daily is sometimes used to create an atrophic endometrium. This drug generally stops bleeding and will allow the patient to build up her hemoglobin for a few months prior to definitive surgery. Alternatively, a GnRH agonist can be used to create a temporary cessation of menstruation by ovarian suppression. Symptoms of hypoestrinism are common and occur early in treatment, while use be-

yond 6 months is associated with significant osteopenia that is reversible after therapy is terminated. Two preparations are available at this time: long-acting injectable leuprolide acetate and the nasal spray nafarelin.

In cases of heavy bleeding, intravenous conjugated estrogens, 25 mg every 4 hours for three or four doses, can be used, followed by oral estrogen for 1 week or a combination oral contraceptive. This will thicken the endometrium and control the bleeding. If the abnormal bleeding is not controlled by hormonal treatment, a D&C is necessary to check for incomplete abortion, polyps, submucous myomas, or endometrial cancer. In women over age 40, a D&C or careful endometrial biopsy is generally indicated to rule out neoplasm before beginning hormonal therapy.

Endometrial ablation through the hysteroscope with laser photocoagulation or electrocautery is currently being used; this technique is designed to reduce or prevent any future menstrual flow.

Nonsteroidal anti-inflammatory drugs (ibuprofen, naproxen, mefenamic acid, etc) will often reduce blood loss in menorrhagia, even that associated with an IUD.

Prolonged use of a progestin, as in a minipill, in injectable contraceptives, or in the therapy of endometriosis, can also lead to intermittent bleeding, sometimes severe. In this instance, the endometrium is atrophic and fragile. If bleeding occurs, it should be treated with estrogen as follows: ethinyl estradiol, 20 μg, or conjugated estrogens, 1.25 mg/d for 7 days.

It is useful for the patient and the physician to discuss stressful situations or life-styles that may contribute to anovulation and dysfunctional bleeding, such as prolonged emotional turmoil or excessive use of drugs or alcohol.

Cowan BD, Morrison JC: Management of abnormal genital bleeding in girls and women. N Engl J Med 1991; 324:1710.

POSTMENOPAUSAL VAGINAL BLEEDING

Vaginal bleeding that occurs 6 months or more following cessation of menstrual function should be investigated. The most common causes are atrophic endometrium, endometrial proliferation, hyperplasia, or cancer; cervical cancer; and administration of estrogens in a noncyclic manner or without added progestin. Other causes include atrophic vaginitis, trauma, endometrial polyps, trophic ulcers of the cervix associated with prolapse of the uterus, and blood dyscrasias. Uterine bleeding is usually painless, but pain will be present if the cervix is stenotic, if bleeding is severe and rapid, or if infection or torsion or extrusion of a tumor is present. The patient may report a single episode of spotting or profuse bleeding for days or months.

Diagnosis

The vulva and vagina should be inspected for areas of bleeding, ulcers, or neoplasms. A cytologic smear of the cervix and vaginal pool should be taken; this may disclose exfoliated neoplastic cells. An unstained wet mount of vaginal fluid in saline and potassium hydroxide may reveal white blood cells, infective organisms, or basal epithelial cells indicative of a low estrogen effect. Endocervical curettage and sampling by aspiration of the endometrium should be performed next, and careful search for endometrial polyps should be made. The tissue obtained may reveal polyps, endometrial hyperplasia (with or without an atypical glandular pattern), or cancer.

Vaginal probe sonography can be used to measure endometrial thickness (< 5 mm indicating atrophy, > 15 mm indicating hypertrophy).

Treatment

Aspiration curettage (with polypectomy if indicated) will frequently be curative. If simple endometrial hyperplasia is found, give cyclic progestin therapy (medroxyprogesterone acetate, 10 mg/d, or norethindrone acetate, 5 mg/d) for 21 days of each month for 3 months. A repeat D&C or endometrial biopsy can then be performed, and if tissues are normal and estrogen replacement therapy is reinstituted, a progestin should be prescribed (as above) for the last 10–14 days of each estrogen cycle, followed by 5 days with no hormone therapy, so that the uterine lining will be shed. If endometrial hyperplasia with atypical cells or carcinoma of the endometrium is found, hysterectomy is necessary.

Granberg S et al: Endometrial thickness as measured by endovaginal ultrasonography for identifying endometrial abnormality. Am J Obstet Gynecol 1991;64:47. (Could eliminate the need for many curettage procedures.)

PREMENSTRUAL SYNDROME
(Premenstrual Tension)

The premenstrual syndrome is a recurrent, variable cluster of troublesome physical and emotional symptoms that develop during the 7–14 days before the onset of menses and subside when menstruation occurs. The syndrome intermittently affects about one-third of all premenopausal women, primarily those 25–40 years of age. In about 10% of affected women, the syndrome may be recurrent and severe. Although not every woman experiences all the symptoms or signs at one time, many describe bloating, breast pain, ankle swelling, a sense of increased weight, skin disorders, irritability, aggressiveness, depression, inability to concentrate, libido change, lethargy, and food cravings.

The pathogenesis of premenstrual syndrome is still uncertain. Psychosocial factors may play a role. Suppression of ovarian function with a GnRH agonist has been shown to diminish all symptoms during therapy. Suppression of ovulation with the oral contraceptive is sometimes helpful, but the patient often complains that she still has premenstrual syndrome.

It is obvious that further investigation and well-controlled therapeutic studies of this heterogeneous syndrome will be necessary for rational treatment. Current treatment methods are mainly empiric. The physician should provide the best support possible for the patient's emotional and physical distress. This includes the following:

(1) Careful evaluation of the patient, with understanding, explanation, and reassurance, is of first importance.

(2) Advise the patient to keep a daily diary of all symptoms for 2–3 months, to help in evaluating the timing and characteristics of the syndrome. If her symptoms occur throughout the month rather than in the 2 weeks before menses, she may be depressed or may have other emotional problems in addition to premenstrual syndrome. Psychotherapy and self-help groups are helpful for many women or couples.

(3) A diet emphasizing complex carbohydrates (whole grains, vegetables, and fruits) can be recommended. Foods high in sugar content and alcohol should be avoided to minimize reactive hypoglycemia. Salt intake should be restricted to reduce fluid retention. Use of caffeine should be minimized whenever tension and irritability predominate.

(4) A variety of vitamins and minerals in relatively high doses have been suggested for this syndrome, but none have proved useful in double-blind studies, and some have undesirable side effects. If a supplement is desired, use a single daily dose of a multivitamin-multimineral containing the RDA for these substances.

(5) A program of regular conditioning exercise, such as jogging, has been found to decrease depression, anxiety, and fluid retention premenstrually in several studies.

(6) Natural progesterone taken daily or by vaginal suppositories in doses of 50–400 mg daily during the luteal phase is widely used for premenstrual syndrome. Double-blind studies have not confirmed its efficacy, nor has the safety of this treatment been evaluated.

(7) Danazol (100–200 mg daily during the luteal phase) has been reported to be helpful, as has mefenamic acid (250 mg four times daily in the luteal phase). Short-acting benzodiazepines have also been used, but the potential for addiction to these drugs makes their use problematic in this recurrent disorder.

Rapkin AJ (editor): Premenstrual syndrome. Clin Obstet Gynecol 1992;35:585. (A series of articles on diagnosis and treatment.)

Rubinow DR: The premenstrual syndrome. New views. JAMA 1992;268:1908. (Review of current knowledge on etiology.)

DYSMENORRHEA

1. PRIMARY DYSMENORRHEA

Primary dysmenorrhea is menstrual pain associated with ovular cycles in the absence of pathologic findings. The pain usually begins within 1–2 years after the menarche and may become more severe with time. The frequency of cases increases up to age 20 and then decreases with age and markedly with parity. Fifty to 75 percent of women are affected at some time, and 5–6% have incapacitating pain.

Primary dysmenorrhea is low, midline, wave-like, cramping pelvic pain often radiating to the back or inner thighs. Cramps may last for 1 or more days and may be associated with nausea, syncope, diarrhea, headache, and flushing. The pain is produced by uterine vasoconstriction, anoxia, and sustained contractions mediated by prostaglandins.

Clinical Findings

The pelvic examination is normal between menses; examination during menses may produce discomfort, but there are no pathologic findings.

Treatment

Nonsteroidal anti-inflammatory drugs (ibuprofen, ketoprofen, mefenamic acid, naproxen) are generally helpful. Drugs should be started at the onset of bleeding to avoid inadvertent drug use during early pregnancy. Medication should be continued on a regular basis for 2–3 days. Ovulation can be suppressed and dysmenorrhea usually prevented by oral contraceptives.

2. SECONDARY DYSMENORRHEA

Secondary dysmenorrhea is menstrual pain for which an organic cause exists. It usually begins well after menarche, sometimes even as late as the third or fourth decade of life.

Clinical Findings

The history and physical examination commonly suggest endometriosis or pelvic inflammatory disease. Other causes may be submucous myoma, IUD use, cervical stenosis with obstruction, or blind uterine horn (rare).

Diagnosis

Laparoscopy is often needed to differentiate endometriosis from pelvic inflammatory disease. Submucous myomas can be detected most reliably by MRI but also by hysterogram, by hysteroscopy, or by passing a sound or curette over the uterine cavity during D&C. Cervical stenosis may result from induced abortion, creating crampy pain at the time of expected menses with no blood flow; this is easily cured by passing a sound into the uterine cavity after administering a paracervical block.

Treatment

A. Specific Measures: Periodic use of analgesics, including the nonsteroidal anti-inflammatory drugs given for primary dysmenorrhea, may be beneficial, and oral contraceptives may give relief, particularly in endometriosis and chronic salpingitis. Danazol and GnRH agonists are effective in the treatment of endometriosis.

B. Surgical Measures: If disability is marked or prolonged, laparoscopy or exploratory laparotomy is usually warranted. Definitive surgery depends upon the degree of disability and the findings at operation.

Dawood MY: Dysmenorrhea. Clin Obstet Gynecol 1990; 33:168.

VAGINITIS

Inflammation and infection of the vagina are common gynecologic problems, resulting from a variety of pathogens, allergic reactions to vaginal contraceptives or other products, or the friction of coitus. The normal vaginal pH is 4.5 or less, and *Lactobacillus* is the predominant organism. At the time of the midcycle estrogen surge, clear, elastic, mucoid secretions from the cervical os are often profuse. In the luteal phase and during pregnancy, vaginal secretions are thicker, white, and sometimes adherent to the vaginal walls. These normal secretions can be confused with vaginitis by concerned women.

Clinical Findings

When the patient complains of vaginal irritation, pain, or unusual discharge, a careful history should be taken, noting the onset of the menstrual period; recent sexual activity; use of contraceptives, tampons, or douches; and the presence of vaginal burning, pain, pruritus, or unusually profuse or malodorous discharge. The physical examination should include careful inspection of the vulva and speculum examination of the vagina and cervix. The cervix is cultured for gonococcus or *Chlamydia* if applicable. A specimen of vaginal discharge is examined under the microscope in a drop of normal saline solution to look for trichomonads, bacteria, white blood cells, and clue cells (stippled or granulated epithelial cells whose cell borders are obscured by bacteria; see Bacterial Vaginosis, below). Discharge from the vaginal walls should be inspected in a drop of 10% potassium hydroxide to search for *Candida*. The vaginal pH can be tested; it is frequently greater than 4.5 in infections due to trichomonads and bacterial vaginosis. A bimanual examination to look for evidence of pelvic infection should follow.

A. Candida albicans: Pregnancy, diabetes, and use of broad-spectrum antibiotics or corticosteroids predispose to *Candida* infections. Heat, moisture, and occlusive clothing also contribute to the risk. Pruritus, vulvovaginal erythema, and a white curd-like discharge that is not malodorous are found. Microscopic examination with 10% potassium hydroxide reveals filaments and spores. Cultures with Nickerson's medium may be used if *Candida* is suspected but not demonstrated.

B. Trichomonas vaginalis: This protozoan flagellate infects the vagina, Skene's ducts, and lower urinary tract in women and the lower genitourinary tract in men. It is transmitted through coitus. Pruritus and a malodorous frothy, yellow-green discharge occur, along with diffuse vaginal erythema and red macular lesions on the cervix in severe cases. Motile organisms with flagella are seen by microscopic examination of a wet mount with saline solution.

C. Bacterial Vaginosis: This condition is considered to be a polymicrobial disease which is not sexually transmitted. An overgrowth of *Gardnerella* and other anaerobes is often associated with increased malodorous discharge without obvious vulvitis or vaginitis. The discharge is grayish and sometimes frothy, with a pH of 5.0–5.5. An amine-like ("fishy") odor is present if a drop of discharge is alkalinized with 10% potassium hydroxide. On wet mount in saline, epithelial cells are covered with bacteria to such an extent that cell borders are obscured (clue cells). Vaginal cultures are generally not useful in diagnosis.

D. Atrophic Vaginitis: In the absence of estrogen stimulation, the vulvar and vaginal tissues shrink, the vaginal walls become thin and dry, and rugal folds disappear. Tenderness and pruritus, with resulting dysuria and dyspareunia, may occur. Fissures and ulcerations of tissue with spotting or bleeding may result from coitus. The wet mount will reveal predominantly parabasal cells.

E. Condylomata Acuminata (Genital Warts): Warty growths on the vulva, perianal area, vaginal walls, or cervix are caused by various types of the human papillomavirus. They are sexually transmitted. Pregnancy and immunosuppression favor growth. Vulvar lesions may be obviously wart-like or may be diagnosed only after application of 4% acetic acid (vinegar) and colposcopy, when they appear whitish, with prominent papillae. Fissures may be present at the fourchette. Vaginal lesions may show diffuse hypertrophy or a cobblestone appearance.

Cervical lesions may be visible only by colposcopy after pretreatment with 4% acetic acid. These lesions are believed to be related to dysplasia and cervical cancer. Vulvar cancer is also currently considered to be associated with the human papillomavirus.

Treatment

A. Candida albicans: Treatment with butaconazole, clotrimazole, terconazole, or miconazole cream or suppositories nightly for 3–7 days is generally effective. Tioconazole ointment and a 500-mg clotrimazole tablet are also effective as single-dose treatment. Single-dose treatments should be reserved for mild, uncomplicated cases and multi-day regimens for severe or complicated candidal vaginitis. Recurrent vulvovaginal candidiasis may be treated with ketoconazole, 100 mg orally once daily, for up to 6 months.

B. Trichomonas vaginalis: Treatment of both partners simultaneously is necessary; metronidazole, 2 g as a single dose or 500 mg for 7 days, is usually employed. In the case of treatment failure, the patient should be retreated with metronidazole, 500 mg twice a day for 7 days. If repeated failure occurs, treat with a single dose of 2 g of metronidazole once daily for 3–5 days. If this is not effective in eradicating the organisms, laboratory sensitivity tests can be arranged with the Centers for Disease Control and Prevention in Atlanta. Metronidazole should be avoided in the first trimester of pregnancy.

C. Bacterial Vaginosis: Recommended regimens include metronidazole, 500 mg twice daily for 7 days, or metronidazole as a single dose of 2 g. The single-dose regimen is slightly less efficacious than the 7-day regimen but is probably equally effective in actual clinical practice as compliance with the single-dose regimen is better. Alternative regimens include clindamycin vaginal cream (2%) once daily for 7 days, metronidazole gel (0.75%) twice daily for 5 days, or clindamycin, 300 mg orally twice daily for 7 days.

D. Atrophic Vaginitis: Treatment consists of oral hormone replacement therapy or local applications of estrogen cream. Conjugated estrogen cream, one-eighth applicatorful (0.3 mg of conjugated estrogens), applied daily for 1 week and then every other day, will relieve most symptoms of dyspareunia with minimal systemic effects. Testosterone propionate cream 1% is helpful for individuals unable to use estrogen. For symptomatic relief, this treatment must be maintained indefinitely.

E. Condylomata Acuminata: A variety of modalities are available for treatment. Treatment for small vulvar warts is with podophyllum resin 25% in tincture of benzoin (do not use during pregnancy or on bleeding lesions) or 50–90% trichloroacetic acid, carefully applied to avoid the surrounding skin. The pain of trichloroacetic acid application can be lessened by a sodium bicarbonate paste applied immediately after treatment. Podophyllum resin must be washed off after 2–4 hours. Podofilox, an active lignan from the crude podophyllum resin, can be safely and comfortably applied by the patient. Freezing with liquid nitrogen or a cryoprobe and electrocautery are also effective. Vaginal warts may be treated with cryotherapy with liquid nitrogen, trichloroacetic acid, or podophyllum resin. Extensive warts may require treatment with CO_2 laser under local or general anesthesia. Interferon is not recommended because it is very expensive and no more effective than other therapies. Therapy with fluorouracil has not been studied in controlled trials, frequently causes local irritation, and is not recommended. Treatment of sex partners is not necessary for management of genital warts, since the role of reinfection appears to be a small one.

Greenberg MD et al: A double-blind, randomized trial of 0.5% podofilox and placebo for the treatment of genital warts in women. Obstet Gynecol 1991;77:735.

Haseltine FP, Horowitz BJ (moderators): Vulvovaginitis: Causes and therapies. Am J Obstet Gynecol 1991; 165:1163.

Sexually transmitted diseases: Treatment guidelines. MMWR Morb Mortal Wkly Rep 1989;38:38.

CERVICITIS

Infection of the cervix must be distinguished from physiologic ectopy of columnar epithelium, which is common in young women. True cervicitis is characterized by a red edematous cervix with purulent, often blood-streaked discharge and tenderness on cervical motion. The infection may follow tears during delivery or abortion or may result from a sexually transmitted pathogen such as *Neisseria gonorrhoeae, Chlamydia,* or herpesvirus (which presents with vesicles and ulcers on the cervix during a primary herpetic infection). Yellow mucopurulent endocervical secretions and the presence of ten or more polymorphonuclear leukocytes per high dry field are suggestive of chlamydial infection.

Mucopurulent cervicitis is an insensitive predictor of either gonorrheal or chlamydial infection and in addition has a low positive predictive value. Presumptive antibiotic treatment of mucopurulent cervicitis is not indicated unless there is a high prevalence of either *N gonorrhoeae* or *Chlamydia* in the population. (See Chapter 32 for discussion.) Three months after treatment, approximately 20% of women will have persistent or recurrent mucopus in the cervix, not explained by relapse or reinfection. This may be related to cervical ectopy and an inflammatory reaction caused by columnar cell contact with the vaginal environment.

Paavonen J et al: Randomized treatment of mucopurulent cervicitis with doxycycline or amoxicillin. Am J Obstet Gynecol 1989;161:128.

CYST & ABSCESS OF BARTHOLIN'S DUCT

Gonorrhea and other infections often involve Bartholin's duct, causing obstruction of the gland. Drainage of secretions is prevented, leading to pain, swelling, and abscess formation. The infections usually resolve and pain disappears, but stenosis of the duct outlet with distention often persists. Reinfection causes recurrent tenderness and further enlargement of the duct.

The principal symptoms are periodic painful swelling on either side of the introitus and dyspareunia. A fluctuant swelling 1–4 cm in diameter in the inferior portion of either labium minus is a sign of occlusion of Bartholin's duct. Tenderness is evidence of active infection.

Pus or secretions from the gland should be cultured for gonorrhea, *Chlamydia,* and other pathogens and treated accordingly (see Chapter 32); frequent warm soaks may be helpful. If an abscess develops, aspiration or incision and drainage are the simplest forms of therapy, but the problem may recur. Marsupialization, incision and drainage with the insertion of an indwelling Word catheter, or laser treatment will establish a new duct opening.

EFFECTS OF EXPOSURE TO DIETHYLSTILBESTROL IN UTERO

Between 1947 and 1971, diethylstilbestrol (DES) was widely used in the USA for diabetic women during pregnancy and to treat threatened abortion. It is estimated that 2–3 million fetuses were exposed. A relationship between fetal DES exposure and clear cell carcinoma of the vagina was later discovered, and a number of other related anomalies have since been noted. In one-third of all exposed women, there are changes in the vagina (adenosis, septa), cervix (deformities and hypoplasia of the vaginal portion of the cervix), or uterus (T-shaped cavity). In males exposed to DES in utero, testicular and epididymal abnormalities and an increase in oligospermia (although not carcinoma) have been reported.

At present, all exposed women are advised to have an initial colposcopic examination to outline vaginal and cervical areas of abnormal epithelium, followed by cytologic examination of the vagina (all four quadrants of the upper half of the vagina) and cervix at yearly intervals. Lugol's iodine stain of the vagina and cervix will also outline areas of metaplastic squamous epithelium.

Many women are not aware of having been exposed to DES. Therefore, in the age groups at risk (25–45), examiners should pay attention to structural changes of the vagina and cervix that may signal the possibility of DES exposure and indicate the need for follow-up.

The incidence of clear cell carcinoma is approximately one in 1000 exposed women, and the incidence of cervical and vaginal intraepithelial neoplasia (dysplasia and carcinoma in situ) is twice as high as in unexposed women. DES daughters have more difficulty conceiving and have an increased incidence of early abortion, ectopic pregnancy, and premature births. In addition, mothers treated with DES in pregnancy appear to have a small increase in the incidence of breast cancer, beginning 20 years after exposure.

Bernstein J et al: Development of cervical and vaginal squamous cell neoplasia as a late consequence of in utero exposure to diethylstilbestrol. Obstet Gynecol Survey 1988;43:15.
Linn S et al: Adverse outcomes of pregnancy in women exposed to diethylstilbestrol in utero. J Reprod Med 1988; 33:3.

CERVICAL INTRAEPITHELIAL NEOPLASIA (CIN; Dysplasia of the Cervix)

The squamocolumnar junction of the uterine cervix represents an area of active squamous cell proliferation. In childhood, this junction is located on the exposed vaginal portion of the cervix. At puberty, because of hormonal influence and possibly because of changes in the vaginal pH, the squamous margin begins to encroach on the single-layered, mucus-secreting epithelium, creating an area of metaplasia (transformation zone). Factors associated with coitus (see Prevention, below) may lead to cellular abnormalities, which over a period of time can result in the development of squamous cell dysplasia or cancer. There are varying degrees of dysplasia (Table 17–2), defined by the degree of cellular atypia; all types must be observed and treated if they persist or become more severe. At present, the malignant potential of a specific lesion cannot be predicted. Some lesions remain stable for long periods of time; some regress; and others advance.

Clinical Findings

There are no specific signs or symptoms of cervical intraepithelial neoplasia. The presumptive diagnosis is made by cytologic screening of an asymptomatic population with no grossly visible cervical changes. All visibly abnormal cervical lesions should be biopsied.

Table 17–2. Classification systems for Papanicolaou smears.

Numerical	Dysplasia	CIN	Bethesda System
1	Benign	Benign	Normal
2	Benign with inflammation	Benign with inflammation	Normal
3	Mild dysplasia	CIN I	Low-grade SIL
3	Moderate dysplasia	CIN II	High-grade SIL
3	Severe dysplasia	CIN III	High-grade SIL
4	Carcinoma in situ		
5	Invasive cancer	Invasive cancer	Invasive cancer

CIN = cervical intraepithelial neoplasia; SIL = squamous intraepithelial lesion.

Diagnosis

A. Cytologic Examination (Papanicolaou Smear): Specimens should be taken from a nonmenstruating patient, spread on a single slide, and fixed. A specimen should be obtained from the squamocolumnar junction with a wooden or plastic spatula and from the endocervix with a cotton swab or nylon brush.

Cytologic reports from the laboratory may describe findings in one of several ways (see Table 17–2). While use of class I–IV is decreasing, the CIN classification continues to be used along with a description of abnormal cells, including evidence of human papillomavirus (HPV). A new term, "squamous intraepithelial lesions (SIL)," low-grade or high-grade, will be used increasingly. Cytopathologists consider a Pap smear to be a medical consultation and will recommend further diagnostic procedures, treatment for infection, and comments on factors that prevent adequate evaluation of the specimen. Cervical cytologic testing to determine the presence of HPV and its subtypes is expensive and does not provide clinically useful information.

B. Colposcopy: Viewing the cervix with 10–20 × magnification allows for assessment of the size and margins of an abnormal transformation zone and determination of extension into the endocervical canal. The application of 3–5% acetic acid (vinegar) dissolves mucus, and the acid's desiccating action sharpens the contrast between normal and actively proliferating, thickened squamous epithelium. Abnormal changes include white patches and vascular atypia, which indicate areas of greatest cellular activity. Paint the cervix with Lugol's solution (strong iodine solution [Schiller's test]). Normal squamous epithelium will take the stain; nonstaining squamous epithelium should be biopsied. (The single-layered, mucus-secreting endocervical tissue will not stain either but can readily be distinguished by its darker pink, shinier appearance.)

C. Biopsy: Colposcopically directed punch biopsy and endocervical curettage are office procedures. If colposcopic examination is not performed, the normal-appearing cervix shedding atypical cells can be evaluated by endocervical curettage and multiple punch biopsies of nonstaining squamous epithelium or tissue from each quadrant of the cervix.

Microscopic examination of biopsy specimens will diagnose the degree of cellular atypia suggested by the cytologic examination. Endocervical curettage will confirm the presence of abnormalities in the endocervical canal. Data from both procedures are important in deciding on treatment.

Prevention

Current data suggest that cervical infection with the human papillomavirus (HPV) is associated with a high percentage of all cervical dysplasias and cancers. There are over 60 recognized HPV subtypes, of which types 6 and 11 tend to cause mild dysplasias, while types 16, 18, 31, and others cause higher grade cellular changes. Herpes simplex virus may play a synergistic role but is not believed to be a major etiologic agent in human genital cancers.

Cervical cancer almost never occurs in virginal women; it is epidemiologically related to the number of sexual partners a woman has had and the number of other female partners a male partner has had. Use of the diaphragm or condom has been associated with a protective effect. Long-term oral contraceptive users develop more dysplasias and cancers of the cervix than users of other forms of birth control, and smokers are also more at risk. Preventive measures therefore include the following:

(1) Sexually active women should undergo regular cytologic screening to detect abnormalities.

(2) Women should limit the number of sexual partners.

(3) Use of a diaphragm by the woman or condom by the man will protect the cervix.

(4) Women should stop smoking.

(5) If a cytologic abnormality is found, the woman should consider using a diaphragm or ask her male partner to use a condom.

Treatment

Treatment varies depending on the degree and extent of cervical intraepithelial neoplasia. Biopsies should always precede treatment.

A. Cauterization or Cryosurgery: The use of either hot cauterization or freezing (cryosurgery) is effective for noninvasive small lesions visible on the cervix without endocervical extension.

B. CO_2 Laser: This well-controlled method minimizes tissue destruction. It is colposcopically directed and requires special training. It may be used with large visible lesions. In current practice it in-

volves the vaporization of the transformation zone on the cervix and the distal 5–7 mm of endocervical canal.

C. Loop Resection: When the CIN is clearly visible in its entirety, a wire loop can be used for excisional biopsy. Cutting and hemostasis are effected with a low-voltage electrosurgical machine (Bovie). This newly defined office procedure with local anesthesia is quick and uncomplicated.

D. Conization of the Cervix: Conization allows for complete histopathologic assessment and generally results in excision of the lesion. It should be reserved for cases of severe dysplasia or cancer in situ (CIN III), particularly those with endocervical extension. The procedure can be performed with the scalpel or CO_2 laser.

E. Follow-Up: Because recurrence is possible—especially in the first 2 years after treatment—and because the false-negative rate of a single cervical cytologic test is 20%, close follow-up is imperative. Vaginal cytologic examination should be repeated at 3-month intervals. After 2 years, yearly examinations suffice.

The Bethesda system for reporting cervical and vaginal cytologic diagnoses: Report of the 1991 Bethesda workshop. J Fam Pract 1992;35:98.

Wright TC Jr et al: Treatment of cervical intraepithelial neoplasia using the loop electrosurgical excision procedure. Obstet Gynecol 1992;79:173.

CARCINOMA OF THE UTERINE CERVIX

Essentials of Diagnosis

- Abnormal uterine bleeding and vaginal discharge.
- Cervical lesion may be visible on inspection as a tumor or ulceration.
- Vaginal cytology usually positive; must be confirmed by biopsy.

General Considerations

Cancer appears first in the intraepithelial layers (the preinvasive stage, or carcinoma in situ). Preinvasive cancer (CIN III) is a common diagnosis in women 25–40 years of age and is etiologically related to infection with the human papillomavirus. Two to 10 years are required for carcinoma to penetrate the basement membrane and invade the tissues. After invasion, death usually occurs in 3–5 years in untreated or unresponsive patients.

Clinical Findings

A. Symptoms and Signs: The most common signs are metrorrhagia, postcoital spotting, and cervical ulceration. Bloody or purulent, odorous, nonpruritic discharge appears after invasion. Bladder and rectal dysfunction or fistulas and pain are late symptoms. Anemia, anorexia, and weight loss are signs of advanced disease.

B. Cervical Biopsy and Endocervical Curettage, or Conization: These procedures are necessary steps after a positive Papanicolaou smear to determine the extent and depth of invasion of the cancer. Even if the smear is positive, treatment is never justified until definitive diagnosis has been established through biopsy studies.

C. "Staging," or Estimate of Gross Spread of Cancer of the Cervix: The depth of penetration of the malignant cells beyond the basement membrane is a reliable clinical guide to the extent of primary cancer within the cervix and the likelihood of secondary to metastatic cancer. It is customary to stage cancers of the cervix under anesthesia as shown in Table 17–3. Further assessment may be carried out by abdominal and pelvic CT scanning or MRI.

Complications

Metastases to regional lymph nodes occur with increasing frequency from stage I to stage IV. Paracervical extension occurs in all directions from the cervix. The ureters are often obstructed lateral to the cervix, causing hydroureter and hydronephrosis and consequently impaired kidney function. Almost two-thirds of patients with untreated carcinoma of the cervix die of uremia when ureteral obstruction is bilateral. Pain in the back and in the distribution of the lumbosacral plexus is often indicative of neurologic involvement. Gross edema of the legs may be indicative of vascular and lymphatic stasis due to tumor.

Pelvic infections may complicate cervical carcinoma. Vaginal fistulas to the rectum and urinary tract are severe late complications. Incontinence of urine and feces is a major late complication, particularly in debilitated individuals.

Hemorrhage is the cause of death in 10–20% of patients with extensive invasive carcinoma.

Treatment

A. Emergency Measures: Vaginal hemorrhage originates from gross ulceration and cavitation in stage II–IV cervical carcinoma. Ligation and suturing of the cervix are usually not feasible, but ligation of the uterine or hypogastric arteries may be lifesaving when other measures fail. Styptics such as negatol, Monsel's solution, or acetone are effective, although delayed sloughing may result in further bleeding. Wet vaginal packing is helpful. Irradiation usually controls bleeding.

B. Specific Measures:

1. Noninvasive uterine carcinoma (stage 0)– In women over age 40 who have completed childbearing, total hysterectomy is the treatment of choice. In a younger woman who wishes to retain her uterus, acceptable alternatives include cervical conization or, in experienced hands, ablation of the lesion with cryotherapy or laser. Close follow-up with Papanicolaou smears every 4 months for 1 year and every 6 months for another year is necessary after cryotherapy or laser.

2. Invasive carcinoma–Microinvasive carcinoma (stage IA) is treated with simple, extrafascial

Table 17–3. International classification of cancer of the cervix.[1]

Preinvasive carcinoma	
Stage 0	Carcinoma in situ, intraepithelial carcinoma.
Invasive carcinoma	
Stage I	Carcinoma strictly confined to the cervix (extension to the corpus should be disregarded).
IA	Preclinical carcinomas of the cervix, ie, those diagnosed only by microscopy.
	IA1 Minimal microscopically evident stromal invasion.
	IA2 Lesions detected microscopically that can be measured. The upper limits of the measurement should not show a depth of invasion of >5 mm taken from the base of the epithelium, either surface or glandular, from which it originates; and a second dimension, the horizontal spread, must not exceed 7 mm. Larger lesions should be classified as stage IB.
Stage II	Carcinoma extends beyond the cervix but has not extended to the pelvic wall. The carcinoma involves the vagina but not as far as the lower third.
IIA	No obvious parametrial involvement.
IIB	Obvious parametrial involvement.
Stage III	Carcinoma has extended to the pelvic wall. On rectal examination, there is no cancer-free space between the tumor and the pelvic wall. The tumor involves the lower third of the vagina. All cases with hydronephrosis or nonfunctioning kidney unless known to be due to other causes.
IIIA	No extension onto the pelvic wall. Vaginal involvement, but not the lower third.
IIIB	Extension onto the pelvic wall and/or hydronephrosis or nonfunctioning kidney.
Stage IV	Carcinoma extended beyond the true pelvis or clinically involving the mucosa of the bladder or rectum. Do not allow a case of bullous edema as such to be allotted to stage IV.
IVA	Spread of growth to adjacent organs (ie, rectum or bladder with positive biopsy from those organs).
IVB	Spread of growth to distant organs.

[1]International Federation of Gynecology and Obstetrics: *Annual Report on the Results of Treatment in Gynecological Cancer,* vol 20. FIGO, 1988.

hysterectomy. Stage IB and stage IIA cancers may be treated with either radical hysterectomy or radiation therapy. Stage IIB and stage III and IV cancers must be treated with radiation therapy. Because radical surgery results in fewer long-term complications than irradiation and may allow preservation of ovarian function, it may be the preferred mode of therapy in younger women without contraindications to major surgery.

Prognosis

The overall 5-year relative survival rate for carcinoma of the cervix is 68% in white women and 55% in black women in the United States. Survival rates are inversely proportionate to the stage of cancer: stage 0, 99–100%; stage I, 76%; stage II, 55%; stage III, 31%; stage IV, 7%.

CARCINOMA OF THE ENDOMETRIUM (Corpus or Fundal Cancer)

Adenocarcinoma of the uterine corpus is the second most common cancer of the female genital tract. It occurs most often in women 50–70 years of age. Many patients with this problem will have taken unopposed estrogen in the past; their increased risk appears to persist for 10 or more years after stopping the drug. Obesity, nulliparity, diabetes, and polycystic ovaries with prolonged anovulation and the extended use of tamoxifen for the treatment of breast cancer are also risk factors.

Abnormal bleeding is the presenting sign in 80% of cases. Pyometra or hematometra may be due to carcinoma of the endometrium. Pain occurs late in the disease, with metastases or infection.

Papanicolaou smears of the cervix occasionally show atypical endometrial cells but are an inconsistent diagnostic tool. Endocervical and endometrial curettage is the only reliable means of diagnosis. Adequate specimens of each can usually be obtained during an office procedure performed following local anesthesia (paracervical block) and sedation. Simultaneous hysteroscopy can be a valuable addition in order to find localized growth or polyps within the uterine cavity. Recently, vaginal ultrasonography has been used to determine the thickness of the endometrium as an indication of hypertrophy and possible neoplastic change.

Pathologic assessment is important in differentiating hyperplasias, which often can be treated with cyclic oral progestins.

Prevention

Prompt D&C for patients who report abnormal menstrual bleeding or postmenopausal uterine bleeding will reveal many incipient as well as clinical cases of endometrial cancer. Postmenopausal women taking estrogens or younger women with prolonged anovulation can be given oral progestins for 13 days at the end of each estrogen cycle in order to promote periodic shedding of the uterine lining; this has been associated with a decreased incidence of uterine adenocarcinoma.

Staging

Examination under anesthesia, fractional D&C, chest x-ray, intravenous urography, cystoscopy, sigmoidoscopy, and MRI will help determine the extent of the disease and its appropriate treatment. The staging is based on the surgical and pathologic evaluation.

Treatment

Treatment consists of total hysterectomy and bilateral salpingo-oophorectomy. Peritoneal material for cytologic examination is routinely taken. Preliminary external irradiation or intracavitary radium therapy is indicated if the cancer is poorly differentiated or if the uterus is definitely enlarged in the absence of myomas. If invasion deep into the myometrium has occurred or if sampled preaortic lymph nodes are positive for tumor, postoperative irradiation is indicated.

Palliation of advanced or metastatic endometrial adenocarcinoma may be accomplished with large doses of progestins, eg, medroxyprogesterone, 400 mg intramuscularly weekly, or megestrol acetate, 80–160 mg daily orally.

Prognosis

With early diagnosis and treatment, the 5-year survival is 80–85%.

Creasman WT: New gynecologic cancer staging. Obstet Gynecol 1990;75:287.
Rubin GL et al: Estrogen replacement therapy and the risk of endometrial cancer: Remaining controversies. Am J Obstet Gynecol 1990;162:148.

CERVICAL POLYPS

Cervical polyps commonly occur after the menarche and are occasionally noted in postmenopausal women. The cause is not known, but inflammation may play an etiologic role. The principal symptoms are discharge and abnormal vaginal bleeding. However, abnormal bleeding should not be ascribed to a cervical polyp without sampling the endocervix and endometrium. The polyps are visible in the cervical os on speculum examination.

Cervical polyps must be differentiated from polypoid neoplastic disease of the endometrium, small submucous pedunculated myomas, and endometrial polyps. Cervical polyps rarely contain malignant foci.

Treatment

Cervical polyps can generally be removed in the

office by avulsion. If the cervix is soft, patulous, or definitely dilated and the polyp is large, surgical D&C is required (especially if the pedicle is not readily visible). Exploration of the cervical and uterine cavities with the polyp forceps and curette may reveal multiple polyps. All tissue removed should be submitted for microscopic examination.

MYOMA OF THE UTERUS
(Fibroid Tumor, Fibromyoma)

Essentials of Diagnosis
- Irregular enlargement of the uterus (may be asymptomatic).
- Heavy or irregular vaginal bleeding, dysmenorrhea.
- Acute and recurrent pelvic pain if the tumor becomes twisted on its pedicle or infarcted.
- Symptoms due to pressure on neighboring organs (large tumors).

General Considerations
Myoma is the most common benign neoplasm of the female genital tract. It is a discrete, round, firm, often multiple uterine tumor composed of smooth muscle and connective tissue. The most convenient classification is by anatomic location: (1) intramural, (2) submucous, (3) subserous, (4) intraligamentous, (5) parasitic (ie, deriving its blood supply from an organ to which it becomes attached), and (6) cervical. A submucous myoma may become pedunculated and descend through the cervix into the vagina.

Clinical Findings
A. Symptoms and Signs: In nonpregnant women, myomas are frequently asymptomatic. However, they can cause urinary frequency, dysmenorrhea, heavy bleeding (often with anemia), or other complications due to the presence of an abdominal mass. Occasionally, degeneration occurs, causing intense pain. Infertility may be due to a myoma that significantly distorts the uterine cavity.

In pregnant women, myomas occasionally cause additional hazards: abortion, malpresentation, failure of engagement, premature labor, localized pain (from red degeneration or torsion), dystocia, ineffectual labor, and postpartum hemorrhage.

B. Laboratory Findings: Hemoglobin levels may be decreased as a result of blood loss, but in rare cases polycythemia is present, presumably as a result of the production of erythropoietin by the myomas.

C. Imaging: Ultrasonography will confirm the presence of uterine myomas and can be used sequentially to monitor growth. When multiple subserous or pedunculated myomas are being followed, ultrasonography is important to exclude ovarian masses. MRI delineates intramural and submucous myomas accurately and can diagnose adenomyosis. Hystero-graphy or hysteroscopy can also confirm cervical or submucous myomas.

Differential Diagnosis
Irregular myomatous enlargement of the uterus must be differentiated from the similar but symmetric enlargement that may occur with uterine pregnancy or adenomyosis. Subserous myomas must be distinguished from ovarian tumors. Leiomyosarcoma is an unusual tumor occurring in 0.5% of women operated on for symptomatic myoma. It is very rare under the age of 40 and increases in incidence thereafter.

Treatment
A. Emergency Measures: If the patient is markedly anemic as a result of long, heavy menstrual periods, preoperative treatment with depot medroxyprogesterone acetate or danazol will slow or stop bleeding, and medical treatment of anemia can be given prior to surgery. Emergency surgery is required for acute torsion of a pedunculated myoma. The only emergency indication for myomectomy during pregnancy is torsion; abortion is not an inevitable result.

B. Specific Measures:

1. Nonpregnant women–In women who are not pregnant, small asymptomatic myomas should be observed at 6-month intervals. Elective myomectomy can be done to preserve the uterus. Myomas do not require surgery on an urgent basis unless they cause significant pressure on the ureters, bladder, or bowel or severe bleeding leading to anemia or unless they are undergoing rapid growth. Cervical myomas larger than 3–4 cm in diameter or pedunculated myomas that protrude through the cervix must be removed. Submucous myomas can be removed using a hysteroscope and laser or resection instruments.

GnRH analogues are being used preoperatively for 2- to 3-month periods to induce reversible hypogonadism, which reduces the size of myomas, suppresses their further growth, and reduces surrounding vascularity. These effects are often desirable before myomectomy or hysterectomy. Regrowth of myomas occurs within several months after termination of GnRH.

2. Pregnant patients–If the uterus is no larger than a 6-month pregnancy by the fourth month of gestation, an uncomplicated course may be anticipated. If the mass (especially a cervical tumor) is the size of a 5- or 6-month pregnancy by the second month, abortion will probably occur. If possible, defer myomectomy or hysterectomy until 6 months after delivery, at which time involution of the uterus and regression of the tumor will be complete.

C. Surgical Measures: Surgical measures available for the treatment of myoma are myomectomy and total or subtotal abdominal or vaginal hysterectomy. Myomectomy is the treatment of choice during the childbearing years. The ovaries should be preserved if possible in women under age 50.

Prognosis

Surgical therapy is curative. Future pregnancies are not endangered by myomectomy, although cesarean delivery may be necessary after wide dissection with entry into the uterine cavity.

Benagiano G, Morini A, Primiero FM: Fibroids: Overview of current and future treatment options. Br J Obstet Gynaecol 1992;99(Suppl 7):18.

Leibson S et al: Leiomyosarcoma in a series of hysterectomies performed for presumed uterine leiomyomas. Am J Obstet Gynecol 1990;162:968.

CARCINOMA OF THE VULVA

Essentials of Diagnosis

- History of genital warts.
- History of prolonged vulvar irritation, with pruritus, local discomfort, or slight bloody discharge.
- Early lesions may suggest or include nonneoplastic epithelial disorders.
- Late lesions appear as a mass, an exophytic growth, or a firm, ulcerated area in the vulva.
- Biopsy is necessary to make the diagnosis.

General Considerations

The vast majority of cancers of the vulva are squamous lesions that classically have occurred in women over 50 years of age. Several subtypes (particularly 6, 16, and 18) of the human papillomavirus have been identified in some but not all vulvar cancers. As with squamous cell lesions of the cervix, dysplasias of varying severity are now recognized on the vulva. A grading system of vulvar intraepithelial neoplasia (VIN) from mild dysplasia to carcinoma in situ has been established.

Differential Diagnosis

Biopsy is essential for the diagnosis of vulvar cancer and should be performed with any localized atypical vulvar lesion, including white patches. Multiple skin-punch specimens can be taken in the office under local anesthesia, with care to include tissue from the edges of each lesion sampled.

Benign vulvar disorders that must be excluded in the diagnosis of carcinoma of the vulva include chronic granulomatous lesions (eg, lymphogranuloma venereum, syphilis), vulvar nodulations, condylomas, hidradenoma, or neurofibroma. Kraurosis, lichen sclerosus and other associated leukoplakic changes in the skin should be biopsied. The likelihood that a superimposed vulvar cancer will develop in a woman with a nonneoplastic epithelial disorder (vulvar dystrophy) ranges from 1% to 5%.

Treatment

A. General Measures: Early diagnosis and treatment of irritative or other predisposing or contributing causes to carcinoma of the vulva should be pursued. A 7:3 combination of betamethasone and crotamiton is particularly effective for itching. After an initial response, fluorinated steroids should be replaced with hydrocortisone because of their skin atrophying effect. Testosterone propionate (1–2% in petrolatum) offers the best results in lichen sclerosus and can be used chronically in decreasing amounts and frequency.

B. Surgical Measures:

1. In situ squamous cell carcinoma of the vulva and small, invasive basal cell carcinoma of the vulva should be excised with a wide margin. If the squamous carcinoma in situ is extensive or multicentric, laser therapy or superficial surgical removal of vulvar skin may be required. In this way, the clitoris and uninvolved portions of the vulva may be spared. Skin grafting may be necessary, but mutilating vulvectomy is avoided.

2. Invasive carcinoma confined to the vulva without evidence of spread to adjacent organs or to the regional lymph nodes will necessitate radical vulvectomy and inguinal lymphadenectomy if the patient is able to withstand surgery. Debilitated patients may be candidates for palliative irradiation only.

Prognosis

Patients with vulvar carcinoma 3 cm in diameter or less without inguinal lymph node metastases who can sustain radical surgery have about a 90% chance of a 5-year arrest of the cancer. If the lesion is greater than 3 cm and has metastasized, the likelihood of 5-year survival is less than 25%.

Crum CP: Carcinoma of the vulva: Epidemiology and pathogenesis. Obstet Gynecol 1992;79:448.

Shafi MI et al: Vulval intraepithelial neoplasia: Management and outcome. Br J Obstet Gynaecol 1989;96:1339.

ENDOMETRIOSIS

Aberrant growth of endometrium outside the uterus, particularly in the dependent parts of the pelvis and in the ovaries, is a common cause of abnormal bleeding and secondary dysmenorrhea. This condition is known as endometriosis. Its causes, pathogenesis and natural course are poorly understood. The prevalence in the USA is 2% among fertile women and three- to fourfold greater than that in the infertile. Depending on the location and extent of the endometrial implants, infertility, dyspareunia, or rectal pain with bleeding may result. Aching pain tends to be constant, beginning 2–7 days before the onset of menses, and becomes increasingly severe until flow slackens. Pelvic examination may disclose tender indurated nodules in the cul-de-sac, especially if the examination is done at the onset of menstruation.

Endometriosis must be distinguished from pelvic

inflammatory disease, ovarian neoplasms, and uterine myomas. In general, only in salpingitis and endometriosis are the symptoms aggravated by menstruation. Bowel invasion by endometrial tissue may produce clinical findings, including blood in the stool, that must be distinguished from bowel neoplasm. Differentiation in these instances depends upon proctosigmoidoscopy and biopsy.

Ultrasound examination will often reveal complex fluid-filled masses that cannot be distinguished from neoplasms. Barium enema may delineate colonic involvement of endometriosis. The clinical diagnosis of endometriosis is presumptive and must be confirmed by laparoscopy or laparotomy.

Treatment

A. Medical Treatment: The goal of medical treatment is to preserve the fertility of women wanting future pregnancies, ameliorate symptoms, and simplify future surgery or make it unnecessary. Medications are designed to inhibit ovulation over 4–9 months and lower hormone levels, thus preventing cyclic stimulation of endometriotic implants and decreasing their size. The optimum duration of therapy is not clear, and the relative merits in terms of pregnancies, side effects, and long-term risks and benefits show insignificant differences when compared with each other, with surgery (including laser surgery), and, in mild cases, with placebo.

1. The GnRH analogues nafarelin nasal spray and long-acting injectable leuprolide acetate used for 6 months suppress ovulation. Side effects of hypoestrinism may occur, including hot flashes and vaginal dryness.

2. Danazol is used for 6–9 months in the lowest dose necessary to suppress menstruation, usually 200–400 mg twice daily. Side effects are androgenic and include decreased breast size, weight gain, acne, and hirsutism.

3. Combination estrogen-progestin oral contraceptives, one daily continuously for 6–9 months. Increase the dose only with the onset of breakthrough bleeding.

4. Medroxyprogesterone acetate, 100 mg intramuscularly every 2 weeks for four doses; then 100 mg every 4 weeks; add oral estrogen or estradiol valerate, 30 mg intramuscularly, for breakthrough bleeding. Use for 6–9 months.

5. Low-dose oral contraceptives can be given for 21 days out of each 28; prolonged suppression of ovulation will often inhibit further stimulation of residual endometriosis, especially if taken after one of the therapies mentioned above.

6. Analgesics, with or without codeine, may be needed during menses. Nonsteroidal anti-inflammatory drugs may be helpful.

B. Surgical Measures: The surgical treatment of moderately extensive endometriosis depends upon the patient's age and symptoms and her desire to preserve reproductive function. If the patient is under 35, resect the lesions, free adhesions, and suspend the uterus. At least 20% of patients so treated can become pregnant, although some must undergo surgery again if the disease progresses. If the patient is over 35 years old, is disabled by pain, and has involvement of both ovaries, bilateral salpingo-oophorectomy and hysterectomy will probably be necessary.

Foci of endometriosis can be treated at laparoscopy by bipolar coagulation or laser vaporization. Because pelvic endometriosis can take forms other than the classic powder burns and hemorrhagic cysts, a meticulous survey of the peritoneum is required.

Prognosis

The prognosis for reproductive function in early or moderately advanced endometriosis is good with conservative therapy. Bilateral ovariectomy is curative for patients with severe and extensive endometriosis with pain. Following hysterectomy and oophorectomy, estrogen replacement therapy is indicated.

Shaw RW: Treatment of endometriosis. Lancet 1992; 340:1267.

VAGINAL HERNIAS
(Cystocele, Rectocele, Enterocele)

Cystocele, rectocele, and enterocele are vaginal hernias commonly seen in multiparous women. Cystocele is a hernia of the bladder wall into the vagina, causing a soft anterior fullness. Cystocele may be accompanied by urethrocele, which is not a hernia but a sagging of the urethra following its detachment from the symphysis during childbirth. Rectocele is a herniation of the terminal rectum into the posterior vagina, causing a collapsible pouch-like fullness. Enterocele is a vaginal vault hernia containing small intestine, usually in the posterior vagina and resulting from a deepening of the pouch of Douglas. Enterocele may also accompany uterine prolapse or follow hysterectomy, when weakened vault supports or a deep unobliterated cul-de-sac containing intestine protrudes into the vagina. One or more of the three types of hernias often occur in combination.

Supportive measures include a high-fiber diet. Weight reduction in obese patients and limitation of straining and lifting are helpful. Pessaries may reduce cystocele, rectocele, or enterocele temporarily and are helpful in women who do not wish surgery or are chronically ill.

The only cure for symptomatic cystocele, rectocele, or enterocele is corrective surgery. The prognosis following an uncomplicated procedure is good.

UTERINE PROLAPSE

Uterine prolapse most commonly occurs as a delayed result of childbirth injury to the pelvic floor (particularly the transverse cervical and uterosacral ligaments). Unrepaired obstetric lacerations of the levator musculature and perineal body augment the weakness. Attenuation of the pelvic structures with aging and congenital weakness can accelerate the development of prolapse.

In slight prolapse, the uterus descends only part way down the vagina; in moderate prolapse, the corpus descends to the introitus and the cervix protrudes slightly beyond; and in marked prolapse (procidentia), the entire cervix and uterus protrude beyond the introitus and the vagina is inverted. Inability to walk comfortably because of protrusion or discomfort from the presence of a vaginal mass is an indication that surgical treatment should be considered.

Treatment

The type of surgery depends upon the extent of prolapse and the patient's age and her desire for menstruation, pregnancy, and coitus. The simplest, most effective procedure is vaginal hysterectomy with appropriate repair of the cystocele and rectocele. If the patient desires pregnancy, a partial resection of the cervix with plication of the cardinal ligaments can be attempted. For elderly women who do not desire coitus, partial obliteration of the vagina is surgically simple and effective. Abdominal uterine suspension or ventrofixation will fail in the treatment of prolapse.

A well-fitted vaginal pessary (eg, inflatable doughnut type, Gellhorn pessary) may give relief if surgery is refused or contraindicated.

PELVIC INFLAMMATORY DISEASE
(PID; Salpingitis, Endometritis)

Essentials of Diagnosis

- Lower abdominal adnexal and cervical motion tenderness.
- Cervical or vaginal discharge.
- Laboratory evidence of cervical infection with *Neisseria gonorrhoeae* or *Chlamydia trachomatis*.
- Tubo-ovarian abscess on sonography or laparoscopic abnormalities consistent with pelvic inflammatory disease.

General Considerations

Pelvic inflammatory disease is a polymicrobial infection of the upper genital tract associated with the sexually transmitted organisms *N gonorrhoeae* and *C trachomatis* as well as endogenous organisms, including anaerobes, *H influenzae*, enteric gram-negative rods, and streptococci. It is most common in young, nulliparous, sexually active women with mul-

tiple partners. Other risk markers include nonwhite race, douching, and smoking. The use of oral contraceptives or barrier methods of contraception may provide significant protection.

Tuberculous salpingitis is rare in the USA but more common in developing countries; it is characterized by pelvic pain and irregular pelvic masses not responsive to antibiotic therapy. It is not sexually transmitted.

Clinical Findings

A. Symptoms and Signs: Patients with pelvic inflammatory disease may have lower abdominal pain, chills and fever, menstrual disturbances, purulent cervical discharge, and cervical and adnexal tenderness. Right upper quadrant pain (Fitz-Hugh and Curtis syndrome) may indicate an associated perihepatitis. However, diagnosis of PID is complicated by the fact that many women may have subtle or mild symptoms, not readily recognized as PID. Women with lower abdominal, adnexal, or cervical motion tenderness should be considered to have PID and be treated with antibiotics unless there is a competing diagnosis such as ectopic pregnancy or appendicitis.

B. Laboratory Findings: The white blood cell count and sedimentation rate are not consistently elevated. Gram stain and culture of endocervical discharge or material obtained by culdocentesis may be valuable guides to therapy. The presence of plasma cells in an endometrial biopsy strongly suggests upper tract infection. Definitive diagnosis can usually be made by laparoscopy.

C. Imaging Studies: Pelvic ultrasound may help to distinguish pelvic masses associated with PID from those of endometriosis, uterine myomas, ovarian cysts or tumors, and ectopic pregnancy. Ultrasound may also be used for guidance of catheters for direct percutaneous drainage of pelvic abscesses.

Differential Diagnosis

Appendicitis, ectopic pregnancy, septic abortion, hemorrhagic or ruptured ovarian cysts or tumors, twisted ovarian cyst, degeneration of a myoma, and acute enteritis must be considered. Pelvic inflammatory disease is more likely to occur when there is a history of pelvic inflammatory disease, recent sexual contact, recent onset of menses, or an IUD in place or if the partner has a sexually transmitted disease. Acute pelvic inflammatory disease is highly unlikely when recent intercourse has not taken place or an IUD is not being used. A sensitive serum pregnancy test should be obtained to rule out ectopic pregnancy. Culdocentesis will differentiate hemoperitoneum (ruptured ectopic pregnancy or hemorrhagic cyst) from pelvic sepsis (salpingitis, ruptured pelvic abscess, or ruptured appendix). Pelvic and vaginal ultrasound is helpful in the differential diagnosis of ectopic pregnancy of over 6 weeks. Laparoscopy is often utilized to diagnose pelvic inflammatory disease, and it is imperative if the diagnosis is not certain or if the patient has not responded to antibiotic therapy after 48 hours. The appendix should be visualized at laparoscopy to rule out appendicitis. Cultures obtained at the time of laparoscopy are often specific and helpful.

Treatment

A. Hospitalization: Patients with acute pelvic inflammatory disease should be admitted for intravenous antibiotic therapy if: (1) the diagnosis is uncertain and surgical emergencies such as appendicitis or ectopic pregnancy cannot be ruled out; (2) a pelvic abscess is suspected; (3) the patient is pregnant; (4) the patient is an adolescent; (5) the patient is unable to follow or tolerate an outpatient regimen; (6) the patient has failed to respond clinically to outpatient therapy; (7) clinical follow-up within 72 hours cannot be arranged; (8) the patient is HIV-positive. Many experts recommend that all patients with acute PID be hospitalized for intravenous antibiotic therapy.

B. Antibiotics: Early treatment with appropriate antibiotics effective against N gonorrhoeae, C trachomatis, and the endogenous organisms listed above is essential to prevent long-term sequelae. The sexual partner should be examined and treated appropriately.

Two inpatient regimens have been shown to be effective in the treatment of acute pelvic inflammatory disease: (1) Cefoxitin, 2 g intravenously every 6 hours, or cefotetan, 2 g every 12 hours, plus doxycycline, 100 mg intravenously or orally every 12 hours. This regimen is continued for at least 48 hours after the patient shows significant clinical improvement. Doxycycline, 100 mg twice daily, should be continued to complete a total of 14 days therapy. (2) Clindamycin, 900 mg intravenously every 8 hours, plus gentamicin intravenously in a loading dose of 2 mg/kg followed by 1.5 mg/kg every 8 hours. This regimen is continued for at least 48 hours after the patient shows significant clinical improvement and is followed by either clindamycin, 450 mg four times daily, or doxycycline, 100 mg twice daily, to complete a total of 14 days of therapy.

Two outpatient regimens are recommended: (1) Ofloxacin, 400 mg orally twice daily for 14 days, plus either clindamycin, 450 mg orally four times daily, or metronidazole, 500 mg orally twice daily, for 14 days. (2) Either a single dose of cefoxitin, 2 g intramuscularly, with probenecid, 1 g orally, or ceftriaxone, 250 mg intramuscularly, plus doxycycline, 100 mg orally twice daily, for 14 days.

C. General Measures: Bed rest in a semi-Fowler position and adequate fluid intake are recommended. Pain is controlled with mild analgesics. Sexual intercourse should be avoided until recovery is complete, often for 2–3 months. Subsequent use of a condom or a diaphragm with spermicide and avoid-

ance of coitus during menses may reduce the risk of reinfection.

D. Surgical Measures: Tubo-ovarian abscesses may require surgical excision or transcutaneous or transvaginal aspiration. Unless rupture is suspected, institute high-dose antibiotic therapy in the hospital, and monitor therapy with ultrasound. In 70% of cases, antibiotics are effective; in 30%, there is inadequate response in 48–72 hours, and intervention is required. Unilateral adnexectomy in the presence of unilateral abscess is acceptable. Hysterectomy and bilateral salpingo-oophorectomy may be necessary for overwhelming infection or in cases of chronic disease with intractable pelvic pain.

Prognosis

One-fourth of women with acute disease develop long-term sequelae, including repeated episodes of infection, chronic pelvic pain, dyspareunia, ectopic pregnancy, or infertility. The risk of infertility increases with repeated episodes of salpingitis: it is estimated at 10% after the first episode, 25% after a second episode, and 50% after a third episode.

Sexually transmitted disease guidelines. Centers for Disease Control and Prevention, 1993.

Wølner-Hanssen P et al: Association between vaginal douching and acute pelvic inflammatory disease. JAMA 1990;263:1936.

OVARIAN TUMORS

Ovarian tumors are common forms of neoplastic disease in women. Most are benign, but some are malignant. The wide range of types and patterns of ovarian tumors is due to the complexity of ovarian embryology and differences in tissue of origin. Most systems of classification utilize largely the tumor histogenesis, but there may be advantages to employing other criteria such as clinical behavior—functional and nonfunctional, cystic or solid—and always macroscopic or microscopic appearance (Table 17–4).

The incidence of ovarian cancer is increased in women with breast cancer or a family history of ovarian cancer in a first-degree relative.

The history and physical examination may be supplemented by selected imaging studies to define the status of the pelvis by ultrasound and MRI: evaluate other sites by upper and lower intestinal studies and intravenous urography. Laparoscopy is often useful for preoperative evaluation. Neither serial CA 125 blood level measurement nor pelvic ultrasound has been found to be a satisfactory screening test for early ovarian cancer.

Treatment

Small unilocular tumors (as determined by ultrasound) in premenopausal women can be observed for

Table 17–4. Ovarian functional and neoplastic tumors.

Tumor	Incidence	Size	Consistency	Menstrual Irregularities	Endocrine Effects	Potential for Malignancy	Special Remarks
Follicle cysts	Rare in childhood; frequent in menstrual years; never in postmenopausal years.	< 6 cm, often bilateral.	Moderate	Occasional	Occasional anovulation with persistently proliferative endometrium.	0	Often disappear after a 2-month regimen of oral contraceptives.
Corpus luteum cysts	Occasional, in menstrual years.	4–6 cm, unilateral.	Moderate	Occasional delayed period	Prolonged secretory phase.	0	Functional cysts. Intraperitoneal bleeding occasionally.
Theca lutein cysts	Occurs with hydatidiform mole, choriocarcinoma; also with gonadotropin or clomiphene therapy.	To 4–5 cm, multiple, bilateral. (Ovaries may be ≥ 20 cm in diameter.)	Tense	Amenorrhea	hCG elevated as a result of trophoblastic proliferation.	0	Functional cysts. Hematoperitoneum or torsion of ovary may occur. Surgery to be avoided.
Inflammatory (tubo-ovarian abscess)	Concomitant with acute salpingitis.	To 15–20 cm, often bilateral.	Variable, painful	Menometrorrhagia	Anovulation usual.	0	Unilateral removal indicated if possible.
Endometriotic cysts	Never in preadolescent or postmenopausal years. Most common in women age 20–40 years.	To 10–12 cm, occasionally bilateral.	Moderate to softened	Rare	0	Very rare	Associated pelvic endometriosis. Medical treatment or conservative surgery recommended.
Teratoid tumors: Benign teratomas (dermoid cysts)	Childhood to postmenopause.	< 15 cm; 15% are bilateral.	Moderate to softened	0	0	Rare	Torsion can occur. Partial oophorectomy recommended.
Malignant teratomas	< 1% of ovarian tumors. Usually in infants and young adults.	> 20 cm, unilateral.	Irregularly firm	0	Occasionally, hCG elevated.	All	Unresponsive to any therapy.

Tumor	Frequency/Age	Size/Laterality	Consistency	Menstrual Changes	Hormones	Malignancy	Comments
Cystadenoma, cystadenocarcinoma	Common in reproductive years.	Serous: < 25% cm, 33% bilateral. Mucinous: up to 1 meter, 10% bilateral.	Moderate to softened; Moderate to softened	0	0	> 50% for serous. About 5% for mucinous.	Peritoneal implants often occur with serous tumors, rarely occur with mucinous tumors. If mucinous tumor is ruptured, pseudomyxoma peritonei may occur.
Endometrioid carcinoma	15% of ovarian carcinomas.	Moderate, 13% bilateral.	Firm	0	0	All	Adenocarcinoma of endometrium coexists in 15–30% of cases.
Fibroma	< 5% of ovarian tumors.	Usually < 15 cm.	Very firm	0	0	Rare	Ascites in 20% (rarely, pleural fluid).
Arrhenoblastoma	Rare. Average age 30 years or more.	Often small (< 10 cm), unilateral.	Firm to softened	Amenorrhea	Androgens elevated.	< 20%	Recurrences are moderately sensitive to irradiation.
Theca cell tumor (thecoma)	Uncommon.	< 10 cm, unilateral.	Firm	Occasionally irregular periods	Estrogens or androgens elevated.	< 1%	
Granulosa cell tumor	Uncommon. Usually in prepubertal girls or women older than 50 years.	May be very small.	Firm to softened	Menometrorrhagia	Estrogens elevated.	15–20%	Recurrences are moderately sensitive to irradiation.
Dysgerminoma	About 1–2% of ovarian tumors.	< 30 cm, bilateral in one-third of cases.	Moderate to softened	0	...	All	Very radiosensitive.
Brenner tumor	About 1% of ovarian tumors.	< 30 cm, unilateral.	Firm	0	...	Very rare	> 50% occur in postmenopausal years.
Secondary ovarian tumors	10% of fatal malignant disease in women.	Varies, often bilateral.	Firm to softened	Occasional	Very rare (thyroid, adrenocortical origin).	All	Bowel or breast metastases to ovary common.

a few months. A 2-month trial of suppression of ovulation with oral contraceptives usually causes functional cysts to disappear. If ultrasound suggests septation or solid components, a neoplasm is more likely, and surgical exploration should be prompt; with calcification, a benign teratoma is likely. Whenever possible in young women, ovarian cystectomy rather than total removal of the ovary is desirable. An enlarged ovary in a postmenopausal woman should be evaluated promptly. If ultrasound study shows enlargement to twice the size of the contralateral ovary, surgery is indicated. Small (< 5 cm in diameter), thin-walled, unilocular ovarian cysts in postmenopausal women are unlikely to be malignant (2%) and can be followed for growth by serial ultrasound examinations.

The initial surgery is the optimum time for a complete evaluation of the extent of the tumor and for its definitive treatment. Operations for suspected ovarian cancer should be performed at hospitals with facilities for performing frozen section biopsy and by personnel familiar with extended surgery, including bowel and bladder procedures.

Treatment for ovarian cancer is surgery (excision or debulking of any visible neoplasia, hysterectomy and bilateral oophorectomy (5–7% occult bilaterality), appendectomy, omentectomy, selective lymphadenectomy) and chemotherapy.

Prognosis

The prognosis for benign ovarian tumors after surgical removal is excellent. The outlook for ovarian cancer, unless diagnosed in the earliest stages, is poor. The CA 125 blood test can be used to follow the possibility of recurrence after surgery or the response to chemotherapy.

Andolf E, Jorgensen C, Astedt B: Ultrasound examination for detection of ovarian carcinoma in risk groups. Obstet Gynecol 1990;75:106.

Goldstein SR et al: The postmenopausal cystic adnexal mass: The potential role of ultrasound in conservative management. Obstet Gynecol 1989;73:8.

PERSISTENT ANOVULATION
(Polycystic Ovary Syndrome, Stein-Leventhal Syndrome)

Essentials of Diagnosis

- Chronic anovulation.
- Infertility.
- Elevated plasma testosterone and LH values and a reversed FSH/LH ratio.
- Hirsutism (in 70% of patients).

General Considerations

Polycystic ovary syndrome is a common endocrine disorder affecting 2–5% of women of reproductive age. The primary lesion is unknown. These patients have a relatively steady state of high estrogen, androgen, and LH levels, rather than the fluctuating condition seen in ovulating women. Increased levels of estrone come from obesity (conversion of ovarian and adrenal androgens to estrone in body fat) or from excessive levels of androgens seen in some women of normal weight. The high estrone levels are believed to cause a suppression of pituitary FSH and a relative increase in LH. Constant LH stimulation of the ovary results in anovulation, multiple cysts, and theca cell hyperplasia with excess androgen output. The polycystic ovary has a thickened, pearly white capsule and may not be enlarged.

Women with Cushing's syndrome, congenital adrenal hyperplasia, and androgen-secreting adrenal tumors also tend to have high circulating androgen levels and anovulation with polycystic ovaries.

Clinical Findings

Polycystic ovary syndrome is manifested by hirsutism (70% of cases), obesity (40%), and virilization (20%). Fifty percent of patients have amenorrhea, 30% have abnormal uterine bleeding, and 20% have normal menstruation. Additionally, they show insulin resistance and hyperinsulinemia when infused with glucose. The patients are generally infertile, although they may ovulate occasionally. They have an increased long-term risk of cancer of the breast and endometrium because of unopposed estrogen secretion.

Differential Diagnosis

Anovulation in the reproductive years may also be due to (1) premature menopause (high FSH and LH levels); (2) rapid weight loss or extreme physical exertion (normal FSH and LH levels for age); (3) discontinuation of oral contraceptives (anovulation for 6 months or more occasionally occurs); (4) pituitary adenoma with elevated prolactin (galactorrhea may or may not be present); (5) hyper- or hypothyroidism. Always check FSH, LH, prolactin, TSH, testosterone, and dehydroepiandrosterone sulfate (DHEAS) levels when amenorrhea has persisted for 6 months or more without a diagnosis. A 10-day course of progestin (eg, medroxyprogesterone acetate, 10 mg/d) will cause withdrawal bleeding if estrogen levels are high. This will aid in the diagnosis and prevent endometrial hyperplasia. In long-term anovular patients over age 35, it is wise to search for an estrogen-stimulated cancer with mammography and endometrial aspiration.

Treatment

In obese patients with polycystic ovaries, weight reduction is often effective; a decrease in body fat will lower the conversion of androgens to estrone and thereby help to restore ovulation.

If the patient wishes to become pregnant, clomiphene or other drugs can be employed for ovulatory stimulation. Ovulation can also be restored in some patients with dexamethasone, 0.5 mg each night. Wedge resection of the ovary is often successful in restoring ovulation and fertility, although this procedure is used less commonly now that medical treatments are available.

If the patient does not desire pregnancy, give medroxyprogesterone acetate, 10 mg/d for the first 10 days of each month. This will ensure regular shedding of the endometrium so that hyperplasia will not occur. If contraception is desired, a low-dose combination oral contraceptive can be used; this is also useful in controlling hirsutism, for which treatment must be continued for 6–12 months before results are seen.

Hirsutism may be managed with epilation and electrolysis. Dexamethasone, 0.5 mg each night, is helpful in women with excess adrenal androgen secretion. If hirsutism is severe, some patients will elect to have a hysterectomy and bilateral oophorectomy followed by estrogen replacement therapy. Spironolactone, an aldosterone antagonist, is also useful for hirsutism in doses of 25 mg three or four times daily.

Goldzieher JW, Young RW: Selected aspects of polycystic ovarian disease. Endocrinol Metab Clin North Am 1992;1:141.

URINARY INCONTINENCE

Occasional loss of urine under a variety of circumstances occurs in 40% of women. Urinary frequency, nocturia, and urgency are sometimes associated with incontinence. A careful history of drinking and voiding habits, amount of leakage and timing of leakage, and evidence of urinary tract infection will help in diagnosis. The normal bladder holds up to 500 mL, and voiding generally occurs every 2–3 hours while awake.

Women with stress incontinence following childbirth have urethras displaced downward from the normal position above the urogenital diaphragm. Sudden increases in intra-abdominal pressure are transmitted to the otherwise normally functioning bladder but not to the prolapsed urethra, and so urine tends to leak at that moment. Estrogen-deprived postmenopausal women have similar urine loss due to decreased tone of the urethra and surrounding tissue.

Clinical aspects and treatment are discussed in Chapter 2.

Wall LL:Diagnosis and management of urinary incontinence due to detrusor instability. Obstet Gynec Surv 1990;45(Suppl):S1.

PAINFUL INTERCOURSE (Dyspareunia)

Questions related to sexual functioning should be asked as part of the reproductive history. Two helpful questions are, "Are you sexually active?" and "Are you having any sexual difficulties at this time?" The physician should be able to provide basic sex counseling and should allow adequate time for a discussion of problems related to sexuality, personal relationships, contraception, and fears of pregnancy.

Painful intercourse may be caused by vulvovaginitis; vaginismus; an incompletely stretched hymen; insufficient lubrication of the vagina; vaginal atrophy; endometriosis; or tumors or other pathologic conditions. During the pelvic examination, the patient should be placed in a half-sitting position and given a hand-held mirror and then asked to point out the site of pain and describe the type of pain.

Etiology

A. Vulvovaginitis: Vulvovaginitis is inflammation or infection of the vagina. Areas of marked tenderness in the vulvar vestibule without visible inflammation occasionally show lesions resembling small condylomas on colposcopy. For a detailed discussion of vaginitis, see that section of this chapter.

B. Vaginismus: Vaginismus is voluntary or involuntary contraction of muscles around the introitus. It results from fear, pain, sexual trauma, or having learned negative attitudes toward sex during childhood.

C. Remnants of the Hymen: The hymen is usually adequately stretched during initial intercourse, so that pain does not occur subsequently. In some women, the pain of initial intercourse may produce vaginismus. In others, a thin or thickened rim or partial rim of hymen remains after several episodes of intercourse, causing pain.

D. Insufficient Lubrication of the Vagina: Insufficient vaginal lubrication may be due to inadequate time for sexual arousal or to low estrogen effect during lactation or following menopause. When estrogen levels are normal (as evidenced by the occurrence of menstrual periods or the presence of moist, healthy-appearing vaginal mucosa with rugal folds), dyspareunia is probably due to inadequate sexual arousal prior to coitus. Low estrogen levels are evidenced by decreased introital diameter, dry vaginal mucosa, fewer rugal folds, and thinned, reddened epithelium.

E. Infection, Endometriosis, Tumors, or Other Pathologic Conditions: Pain occurring with deep thrusting during coitus is usually due to acute or chronic infection of the cervix, uterus, or adnexa; endometriosis; adnexal tumors; or adhesions resulting from prior pelvic disease or operation. Careful history taking and a pelvic examination will generally help in the differential diagnosis.

F. Dyspareunia Due to Unknown Cause: Occasionally, no organic cause of pain can be found. These patients may have psychosexual conflicts or a history of childhood sexual abuse.

Treatment

A. Vulvovaginitis: Lesions resembling warts on colposcopy or biopsy should be treated in the appropriate way (see Vaginitis). The sexual partner should also be treated to prevent recurrence. Irritation from spermicides may be a factor. The couple may be helped by a discussion of noncoital techniques to achieve organism until the infection subsides.

B. Vaginismus: Sexual counseling and education on anatomy and sexual functioning may be appropriate. The patient can be instructed in self-dilation, using a lubricated finger or test tubes of graduated sizes. Before coitus (with adequate lubrication) is attempted, the patient—and then her partner—should be able to easily and painlessly introduce two fingers into the vagina. Penetration should never be forced, and the woman should always be the one to control the depth of insertion during dilation or intercourse.

C. Remnants of the Hymen: In rare situations, manual dilation of a remaining hymen under general anesthesia is necessary. Surgery should be avoided.

D. Insufficient Lubrication of the Vagina: If inadequate sexual arousal is the cause, sexual counseling for the woman—and her partner if possible—is helpful. Lubricants may be used during sexual foreplay. For women with low plasma estrogen levels, use of a lubricant during coitus is sometimes sufficient. If not, use conjugated estrogen cream, one-eighth applicatorful daily for 10 days and then every other day. Using the applicator or a finger, the patient can apply the cream directly to the most tender area, usually the hymenal ring. Testosterone cream 1–2% in a water-soluble base is also helpful.

E. Infection, Endometriosis, Tumors, or Other Pathologic Conditions: Medical treatment of acute cervicitis, endometritis, or salpingitis and temporary abstention from coitus usually relieve pain. Hormonal or surgical treatment of endometriosis may be helpful. Dyspareunia resulting from chronic pelvic inflammatory disease or any condition causing extensive adhesions or fixation of pelvic organs is difficult to treat without extirpative surgery. Couples can be advised to try coital positions that limit deep thrusting and to use manual and oral sexual techniques.

F. Dyspareunia Due to Unknown Cause: Colposcopy in discrete areas of pain without obvious lesions may be useful to rule out papilloma virus infections. Biopsies should be taken if there is an identifiable lesion. Supportive, understanding discussion may be helpful. Small amounts of topical remedies such as 1% testosterone cream, estrogen cream, or topical lidocaine gel may relieve pain. Resolution

of psychosexual problems or problems relating to traumatic sexual experiences may be necessary.

Bachman GA, Leiblum SR, Grill J: Brief sexual inquiry in gynecologic practice. Obstet Gynecol 1989;73:425.

Mann MS et al: Vulvar vestibulitis: Significant clinical variables and treatment outcome. Obstet Gynecol 1991; 79:122.

Reiter RC et al: Correlation between sexual abuse and somatization in women with somatic and nonsomatic chronic pain. Am J Obstet Gynecol 1991;165:104.

INFERTILITY

A couple is said to be infertile if pregnancy does not result after 1 year of normal sexual activity without contraceptives. About 14% of couples are infertile; the incidence of infertility increases with age. The male partner contributes to about 40% of cases of infertility. A combination of factors is common. Couples whose infertility is unexplained after evaluation have a 34% chance of conceiving within 6 months and a 76% chance by 2 years. At some time in their reproductive life, 24% of women attempting to conceive experience an episode of subfertility.

Diagnostic Survey

During the initial interview, the physician can present an overview of infertility and discuss a plan of study. Separate private consultations are then conducted, allowing appraisal of psychosexual adjustment without embarrassment or criticism. Pertinent details (eg, sexually transmitted disease or prior pregnancies) must be obtained. The ill effects of excess caffeine, cigarettes, alcohol, and other recreational drugs on fertility in both men and women should be discussed. Prescription drugs that impair male potency should be noted. The gynecologic history should include queries regarding the menstrual pattern. The present history includes use and types of contraceptives, douches, libido, sex techniques, frequency and success of coitus, and correlation of intercourse with time of ovulation. Family history includes repeated abortions and maternal DES use.

General physical and genital examinations are performed on both partners. Basic laboratory studies include complete blood count, urinalysis, cervical culture for *Chlamydia,* serologic test for syphilis, rubella antibody determination, and thyroid function tests. Tay-Sachs screening should be offered if both parents are Jews and sickle cell screening if both parents are black. Screening mammography can also be offered to women over 35.

The woman is instructed to chart her basal body temperature orally daily on arising and to record on a graph episodes of coitus and days of menstruation. Self-performed urine tests for the midcycle LH surge can be used to enhance temperature observations relating to ovulation.

The man is instructed to bring a complete ejaculate for analysis. Sexual abstinence for at least 3 days before the semen is obtained is emphasized. A clean, dry, wide-mouthed bottle for collection is preferred. Condoms should not be employed, as the protective powder or lubricant may be spermicidal. Semen should be examined within 1–2 hours after collection. Semen is considered normal with the following minimum values; volume, 3 mL; concentration, 20 million sperm per milliliter; motility, 50% after 2 hours; and normal forms, 60%. If the sperm count is abnormal, further evaluation includes a search for exposure to environmental and workplace toxins, alcohol or drug abuse, and hypogonadism.

A. First Testing Cycle: A postcoital test (Sims-Huhner test) is scheduled for just before ovulation (eg, day 12 or 13 in an expected 28-day cycle). Pre-ovulation timing can be enhanced by serial urinary LH tests or repeated measurement of ovarian follicle growth by ultrasound. The patient is examined within 6 hours after coitus. The cervical mucus should be clear, elastic, and copious owing to the influence of the preovular estrogen surge. (The mucus is scantier and more viscid before and after ovulation.) A good spinnbarkeit (stretching to a fine thread 4 cm or more in length) is desirable. A small drop of cervical mucus should be obtained from within the cervical os and examined under the microscope. The presence of five or more active sperm per high-power field constitutes a satisfactory postcoital test. If no spermatozoa are found, the test should be repeated (assuming that active spermatozoa were present in the semen analysis). Sperm agglutination and sperm immobilization tests should be considered if the sperm are immotile or show ineffective tail motility.

The presence of more than three white blood cells per high-power field in the postcoital test suggests cervicitis in the woman or prostatitis in the man. When estrogen levels are normal, the cervical mucus dried on the slide will form a fern-like pattern when viewed with a low-power microscope. This type of mucuš is necessary for normal sperm transport.

The serum progesterone level should be measured at the midpoint of the secretory phase (21st day); a level of 10–20 ng/mL confirms adequate luteal function.

B. Second Testing Cycle: Hysterosalpingography using an oil dye is performed within 3 days following the menstrual period. This x-ray study will demonstrate uterine abnormalities (septa, polyps, submucous myomas) and tubal obstruction. A repeat x-ray film 24 hours later will confirm tubal patency if there is wide pelvic dispersion of the dye. This test has been associated with an increased pregnancy rate by some observers. If the woman has had prior pelvic inflammation, give tetracycline, 2 g/d, beginning immediately before and for 7 days after the x-ray study.

C. Further Testing:

1. Gross deficiencies of sperm (number, motility, or appearance) require repeat analysis. Zona-free hamster egg penetration tests are available to evaluate the ability of human sperm to fertilize an egg.

2. Obvious obstruction of the uterine tubes requires assessment for microsurgery or in vitro fertilization.

3. Absent or infrequent ovulation requires additional laboratory evaluation. Elevated FSH and LH levels indicate ovarian failure causing premature menopause. Elevated LH levels in the presence of normal FSH levels confirm the presence of polycystic ovaries. Elevation of blood prolactin (PRL) levels suggests pituitary microadenoma.

4. Major histocompatibility antigen typing of both partners will confirm human leukocyte antigen-B locus homozygosity, which is found in greater than expected numbers among couples with unexplained infertility.

5. Ultrasound monitoring of folliculogenesis may reveal the occurrence of unruptured luteinized follicles.

6. Endometrial biopsy in the luteal phase associated with simultaneous serum progesterone levels will rule out luteal phase deficiency.

D. Laparoscopy: Approximately 25% of women whose basic evaluation is normal will have findings on laparoscopy explaining their infertility (eg, peritubal adhesions, endometriotic implants).

Treatment

A. Medical Measures: Fertility may be restored by appropriate treatment in many patients with endocrine imbalance, particularly those with hypo- or hyperthyroidism. Antibiotic treatment of cervicitis is of value. After 6 months of condom protection during intercourse, an antigen-antibody reaction will usually resolve, and sperm agglutination or immobilization should cease to be a problem.

Women who engage in vigorous athletic training often have low sex hormone levels; fertility improves with reduced exercise and some weight gain.

B. Surgical Measures: Excision of ovarian tumors or ovarian foci of endometriosis can improve fertility. Microsurgical relief of tubal obstruction due to salpingitis or tubal ligation will reestablish fertility in a significant number of cases. In special instances of cornual or fimbrial block, the prognosis with newer surgical techniques has become much better. Peritubal adhesions or endometriotic implants often can be treated via laparoscopy or via laparotomy immediately following laparoscopic examination if prior consent has been obtained.

With varicocele in the male, sperm characteristics are often improved following surgical treatment.

C. Induction of Ovulation:

1. Clomiphene citrate–Clomiphene citrate stimulates gonadotropin release, especially LH. Consequently, plasma estrone (E_1) and estradiol (E_2) also rise, reflecting ovarian follicle maturation. If E_2 rises sufficiently, an LH surge occurs to trigger ovulation.

After a normal menstrual period or induction of withdrawal bleeding with progestin, give 50 mg of clomiphene orally daily for 5 days. If ovulation does not occur, increase the dose to 100 mg orally daily for 5 days. If ovulation still does not occur, repeat the course with 150 and then 200 mg daily for 5 days and add chorionic gonadotropin, 10,000 units intramuscularly, 7 days after clomiphene.

The rate of ovulation following this treatment is 90% in the absence of other infertility factors. The pregnancy rate is high. Twinning occurs in 5% of these patients, and three or more fetuses are found in rare instances (< 0.5% of cases). An increased incidence of congenital anomalies has not been reported. Painful ovarian cyst formation occurs in 8% of patients and may warrant discontinuation of therapy.

In the presence of increased androgen production (DHEA-S > 200 μg/dL), the addition of dexamethasone, 0.5 mg, or prednisone, 5 mg, at bedtime, improves the response to clomiphene. Dexamethasone should be discontinued after pregnancy is confirmed.

2. Bromocriptine–Use only if PRL levels are elevated and there is no withdrawal bleeding following progesterone administration (otherwise use clomiphene). The usual dose is 2.5 mg twice daily. To minimize side effects (nausea, diarrhea, dizziness, headache, fatigue), bromocriptine should be taken with meals. Begin with 2.5 mg once daily and increase to two or three times daily in increments of 1.25 mg. The drug is discontinued once pregnancy has occurred.

3. Human menopausal gonadotropins (hMG)–hMG is indicated in cases of hypogonadotropism and most other types of anovulation (exclusive of ovarian failure). Because of the complexities, laboratory tests, and expense associated with this treatment, patients who require hMG for the induction of ovulation should be referred to a specialist. Hypothalamic amenorrhea unresponsive to clomiphene will be reliably and successfully treated with subcutaneous pulsatile gonadotropin-releasing hormone (GnRH). Use of this substance will avoid the dangerous ovarian complications and the 25% incidence of multiple pregnancy associated with hMG.

4. Ovarian wedge resection–Wedge resection is indicated rarely and only when medical measures are not effective.

D. Treatment of Endometriosis: See p 599.

E. Treatment of Low Midluteal Progesterone Levels: Midluteal progesterone levels of less than 10 ng/mL can be treated with one of the following regimens:

1. Progesterone suppositories, 50 mg twice daily on days 17–31 of the ovarian cycle. If the woman becomes pregnant, continue for 8 weeks.

2. Clomiphene (see above) can also be used for luteal phase insufficiency.

F. Treatment of Inadequate Transport of Sperm:

1. Cervical mucus will provide better transport following administration of 0.3 mg of conjugated equine estrogens from days 5 to 15 of the ovarian cycle (ovulation may be delayed).

2. Intrauterine insemination of concentrated washed sperm has been used to bypass a poor cervical environment associated with scant or hostile cervical mucus. The sperm must be handled by sterile methods, washed in sterile saline or tissue culture solutions, and centrifuged. A small amount of fluid (0.5 mL) containing the sperm is then instilled into the uterus.

G. Artificial Insemination in Azoospermia: If azoospermia is present, artificial insemination by a donor usually results in pregnancy, assuming female function is normal. Both partners must consent to this method. The use of frozen sperm is currently preferable to fresh sperm because the frozen specimen can be held pending cultures and blood test results for sexually transmitted diseases, including AIDS.

H. New Reproductive Technologies—In Vitro Fertilization-Embryo Transfer (IVF-ET): This technique is becoming a standard approach to fertility problems involving severe tubal disease, in couples with unexplained long-term infertility, and where the male is oligospermic. A highly organized team of specialists in reproductive function and sophisticated technology are required for successful results. Ultrasound-guided aspiration of oocytes has replaced laparoscopic retrieval in most cases. Two or three embryos are placed to maximize the chances of implantation. Cryopreservation of excess embryos has allowed repeated transfers if the initial attempt fails. Women with transmissible genetic diseases or those with premature ovarian failure are potential recipients of donated frozen embryos. Use of donor oocytes or embryos from younger women improves the results of IVF-ET in women over 40.

Data collected in 1990 showed that the in vitro fertilization pregnancy rate was 19% of completed transfer cycles, with 14% of these pregnancies resulting in living children with no excess of anomalies. Variations in the standard transcervical placement of embryos now include gamete or zygote intra-fallopian tube transfer (GIFT; ZIFT).

Prognosis

The prognosis for conception and normal pregnancy is good if minor (even multiple) disorders can be identified and treated; poor if the causes of infertility are severe, untreatable, or of prolonged duration (over 3 years).

It is important to remember that in the absence of severe causes of infertility (azoospermia, prolonged amenorrhea, or bilateral tubal obstruction), 30% of couples will achieve a pregnancy within 3 years. Most of these successes will be unrelated to therapy. Offering appropriately timed information about adoption is considered part of a complete infertility regimen.

Jaffe SB, Jewelewicz R: The basic infertility investigation. Fertil Steril 1991;56:599.
Medical Research International, Society for Assisted Reproductive Technology, The American Fertility Society: In vitro fertilization-embryo transfer (IVF-ET) in the United States: 1990 results from the IVF-ET registry. Fertil Steril 1992;57:15.

CONTRACEPTION

Voluntary control of childbearing benefits women, men, and the children born to them. Contraception should be available to all women and men of reproductive ages. Education about contraception and access to contraceptive pills or devices are especially important for sexually active teenagers and for women following childbirth or abortion.

Education about sexually transmitted disease, especially AIDS, should be given to all sexually active people, along with information that condoms with spermicide offer a high degree of protection (but not complete protection) to both sexes against sexually transmitted disease as well as pregnancy. The worldwide AIDS epidemic should cause a significant shift toward the use of condoms plus spermicide.

DaVanzo J, Parnell AM, Foege WH: Health consequences of contraceptive use and reproductive patterns. JAMA 1991;265:2692.

1. ORAL CONTRACEPTIVES

Combined Oral Contraceptives

A. Efficacy and Methods of Use: Oral contraceptives (birth control pills) have a theoretical failure rate of less than 0.5% if taken absolutely on schedule and a typical failure rate of 3%. Their primary mode of action is suppression of ovulation. The pills are initially started on the first or fifth day of the ovarian cycle and taken daily for 21 days, followed by 7 days of placebos or no medication, and this schedule is then continued for each cycle. The pills are often initially started on the first Sunday after the onset of menses, to help patients remember their starting day and to avoid menses on the weekend. If a pill is missed at any time, two pills should be taken the next day, and another method of contraception should be used for the rest of the cycle (eg, condoms or foam). A backup method should also be used during the first cycle if the pills are started later than the fifth day. Taking low-dose oral contraceptives is no longer

contraindicated in women aged 35–50 who are non-smokers and have no complicating conditions. Regular blood pressure checks, mammography, and blood tests for lipids and hyperglycemia are indicated.

B. Benefits of Oral Contraceptives: Besides offering convenient, effective contraception, there are noncontraceptive advantages to oral contraceptives. Menstrual flow is lighter, resultant anemia is less common, and dysmenorrhea is relieved for most women. Functional ovarian cysts generally disappear with oral contraceptive use, and new cysts do not occur. Pain with ovulation and postovulatory aching are relieved. The risk of ovarian and endometrial cancer is decreased. The risks of salpingitis and ectopic pregnancy may be diminished. Acne is usually improved. The frequency of developing myomas is lower in long-term users (> 4 years).

C. Selection of an Oral Contraceptive: Most clinicians first prescribe 30–35 μg of estrogen combined with 1 mg or less of progestin. This low dose of estrogen provides highly effective contraception but is also associated with more spotting, breakthrough bleeding, and missed menstrual periods than higher doses, and the patient should be warned of these side effects. Patients taking pills containing more than 50 μg of estrogen should be switched to lower doses, since many adverse side effects of the pill are dose-related. The progestins vary in potency and androgenicity. When hirsutism or acne is a problem, it is best to use ethynodiol diacetate or norethindrone. When breakthrough bleeding or dysfunctional bleeding occurs, many clinicians use a compound with norgestrel. Low-dose oral contraceptives currently used in the USA are shown in Table 17–5.

D. Drug Interactions: Several drugs interact with oral contraceptives to decrease their efficacy by causing induction of microsomal enzymes in the liver, by increasing sex hormone-binding globulin, and by other mechanisms. Some commonly prescribed drugs in this category are the anticonvulsants phenytoin, phenobarbital (and other barbiturates), primidone, and carbamazepine and the antituberculous drug rifampin. Women taking these drugs should use another means of contraception for maximum safety.

E. Contraindications and Adverse Effects: Oral contraceptives have been associated with many adverse effects; they are contraindicated in some situations and should be used with caution in others (Table 17–6).

1. Myocardial infarction–The risk of heart attack is higher with use of oral contraceptives, particularly with pills containing 50 μg of estrogen or more. Age over 44 years; cigarette smoking; obesity; or the presence of hypertension, diabetes, or hypercholesterolemia increases the risk. Young non-smoking women have minimal increased risk. Smokers over age 40 and women with other cardiovascular risk factors should use other methods of birth control.

Table 17–5. Commonly used low-dose oral contraceptives.

Name	Type	Progestin	Estrogen (Ethinyl Estradiol)
Lo/Ovral	Combination	0.3 mg dl-norgestrel	30 µg
Nordette and Levlen	Combination	0.15 mg levonorgestrel	30 µg
Norinyl 1/35 and Ortho-Novum 1/35	Combination	1 mg norethindrone	35 µg
Loestrin 1.5/30	Combination	1.5 mg norethindrone acetate	30 µg
Demulen 1/35	Combination	1 mg ethynodiol diacetate	35 µg
Brevicon and Modicon	Combination	0.5 mg norethindrone	35 µg
Ovcon 35	Combination	0.4 mg norethindrone	35 µg
Ortho-Cept and Desogen	Combination	0.15 mg desogestrel	30 µg
Tricyclen	Triphasic	0.15 mg norgestimate (days 1–7)	35 µg
		0.215 mg norgestimate (days 8–14)	
		0.25 mg norgestimate (days 15–21)	
Ortho-novum 777	Triphasic	0.5 mg norethindrone (days 1–7)	35 µg
		0.75 mg norethindrone (days 8–14)	
		1 mg norethindrone (days 15–21)	
Tri-Norinyl	Triphasic	0.5 mg norethindrone (days 1–7)	35 µg
		1 mg norethindrone (days 8–16)	
		0.5 mg norethindrone (days 17–21)	
Triphasil and Tri-Levlen	Triphasic	0.05 mg levonorgestrel (days 1–6)	30 µg
		0.0075 mg levonorgestrel (days 7–11)	40 µg
		0.125 mg levonorgestrel (days 12–21)	30 µg
Micronor and Nor-QD	Progestin-only minipill	0.35 mg norethindrone to be taken continuously	
Ovrette	Progestin-only minipill	0.075 mg dl-norgestrel to be taken continuously	

2. Thromboembolic disease–An increased rate of fatal and nonfatal venous thromboembolism is found in oral contraceptive users, especially if the dose of estrogen is 50 µg or more. Women who develop thrombophlebitis should stop using this method, as should those at risk of thrombophlebitis because of surgery, fracture, serious injury, or immobilization.

3. Cerebrovascular disease–A small increased risk of hemorrhagic stroke and subarachnoid hemorrhage and a substantial increase in the risk of

Table 17–6. Contraindications to use of oral contraceptives.

Absolute contraindications
  Pregnancy
  Thrombophlebitis or thromboembolic disorders (past or present)
  Stroke or coronary artery disease (past or present)
  Cancer of the breast (known or suspected)
  Undiagnosed abnormal vaginal bleeding
  Estrogen-dependent cancer (known or suspected)
  Benign or malignant tumor of the liver (past or present)
Relative contraindications
  Age over 35 years and heavy cigarette smoking (>15 cigarettes daily)
  Cervical intraepithelial neoplasia
  Migraine or recurrent persistent, severe headache
  Hypertension
  Cardiac or renal disease
  Diabetes
  Gallbladder disease
  Cholestasis during pregnancy
  Active hepatitis or infectious mononucleosis
  Sickle cell disease (S/S or S/C type)
  Surgery, fracture, or serious injury
  Lactation
  Significant psychologic depression

thrombotic stroke has been found; smoking is associated with increased risk. Women who develop warning symptoms such as severe headache, blurred or lost vision, or other transient neurologic disorders should stop using oral contraceptives. Women with hypertension should not use the pill.

4. Carcinoma–A relationship between long-term (3–4 years) oral contraceptive use and occurrence of cervical dysplasia and cancer has been found in various studies. No confirmed relationship has been found between use of oral contraceptives and cancer of the breast. Birth control pills appear to protect against endometrial and ovarian cancer. Rarely, oral contraceptives have been associated with the development of benign or malignant hepatic tumors; this may lead to rupture of the liver, hemorrhage, and death. The risk increases with higher dosage, longer duration of use, and older age.

5. Gallbladder disease–There is an increased risk of gallbladder disease and subsequent cholecystectomy for cholesterol stones in pill users.

6. Metabolic disorders–A decrease in glucose tolerance and an increase in triglyceride levels is seen in pill takers, and women with diabetes using this method should be carefully monitored.

7. Hypertension–Oral contraceptives may cause hypertension in some women; the risk is increased with longer duration of use and older age. Women who have or develop hypertension should use other contraceptive methods.

8. Headache–Migraine or other vascular headaches may occur or worsen with pill use. If severe or frequent headaches develop while using this method, it should be discontinued.

9. Amenorrhea—Postpill amenorrhea lasting a year or longer occurs occasionally, sometimes with galactorrhea. PRL levels should be checked; if elevated, a pituitary prolactinoma may be present.

10. Disorders of lactation—Combined oral contraceptives can impair the quantity and quality of breast milk and should therefore not be given before the infant is weaned. Progestin-only minipills can be used during lactation.

11. Other disorders—Depression may occur or be worsened with oral contraceptive use. Fluid retention may occur. Asthma may be worsened. Patients who had cholestatic jaundice during pregnancy may develop it while taking birth control pills. Contact lens use may become more difficult.

F. Minor Side Effects: Nausea and dizziness may occur in the first few months of pill use. A weight gain of 2–5 lb commonly occurs. Spotting or breakthrough bleeding between menstrual periods may occur, especially if a pill is skipped or taken late; this may be helped by switching to a pill of slightly greater potency (see ¶C, above). Missed menstrual periods may occur, especially with low-dose pills. A pregnancy test should be performed if pills have been skipped or if two or more menstrual periods are missed. Depression, fatigue, and decreased libido can occur. Chloasma may occur, as in pregnancy, and is increased by exposure to sunlight.

Progestin Minipill

A. Efficacy and Methods of Use: Formulations containing 0.35 mg of norethindrone or 0.075 mg of norgestrel are available in the USA. Their efficacy is slightly lower than that of combined oral contraceptives, with failure rates of 1–4% being reported. The minipill is believed to prevent conception by causing thickening of the cervical mucus to make it hostile to sperm, alteration of ovum transport (which may account for the higher rate of ectopic pregnancy with these pills), and inhibition of implantation. Ovulation is inhibited inconsistently with this method. The minipill is begun on the first day of a menstrual cycle and then taken continuously for as long as contraception is desired.

B. Advantages: The low dose and absence of estrogen make the minipill safe during lactation; it may increase the flow of milk. It is often tried by women who want minimal doses of hormones and by patients who are over age 35. The minipill can be used by women with uterine myomas or sickle cell disease (S/S or S/C). Like the combined pill, the minipill decreases the likelihood of pelvic inflammatory disease by its effect on cervical mucus.

C. Complications and Contraindications: Minipill users often have bleeding irregularities (eg, prolonged flow, spotting, or amenorrhea); such patients may need monthly pregnancy tests. Ectopic pregnancies are more frequent, and complaints of abdominal pain should be investigated with this in mind. The absolute contraindications and many of the relative contraindications listed in Table 17–6 apply to the minipill. Exceptions are mentioned in ¶B, above. Minor side effects of combination oral contraceptives such as weight gain and mild headache may also occur with the minipill.

Thorogood M et al: Fatal stroke and use of oral contraceptives: Findings from a case-control study. Am J Epidemiol 1992;136:35. (A large case-control study of stroke in users of lowdose oral contraceptives.)

Williams RS: Benefits and risks of oral contraceptive use. Postgrad Med 1992:92;155. (Risks and benefits of pill use.)

2. CONTRACEPTIVE INJECTIONS & IMPLANTS (Long-Acting Progestins)

The injectable progestin medroxyprogesterone acetate was recently approved for contraceptive use in the USA. There is extensive worldwide experience with this method over the past 2 decades. The medication is given as a deep intramuscular injection of 150 mg every 3 months and has a contraceptive efficacy of 99.7%. Common side effects include irregular bleeding, amenorrhea, weight gain, and headache. Bone mineral loss may occur. Users commonly have irregular bleeding initially and subsequently develop amenorrhea. Ovulation may be delayed after the last injection. Contraindications are similar to those for the minipill.

The other available long-acting progestin is the Norplant system, a contraceptive implant containing levonorgestrel. The system consists of six small Silastic capsules that are inserted subcutaneously in the inner aspect of the upper arm. They release daily and provide highly effective contraception for 5 years. In the first year of use, Norplant is 99.8% effective. Contraceptive effectiveness drops slightly in succeeding years, but even in the fifth year it is more effective than the combination pill. The most common side effects include irregular bleeding and spotting, amenorrhea, headache, acne, and weight gain. Irregular bleeding is the most common reason for discontinuation. Hormone levels drop rapidly after removal of the implants, and there is no delay in the return of fertility. Contraindications are similar to those for the minipill. Insertion of the implants requires a minor surgical procedure under local anesthesia. Removal is also done under local anesthesia and may be more difficult than insertion.

3. INTRAUTERINE DEVICES (IUDs)

The only IUDs currently manufactured in the USA are the Progestasert (which secretes progesterone into the uterus) and the Copper T380A. Some all-plastic IUDs (Lippes Loop) are also still in use. Failure rates of most IUDs are 1–2%; the mechanism of action is thought to be related to impaired fertilization due to effects on sperm motility and to abnormal development in the oviduct of those ova that may have been fertilized.

The all-plastic IUDs do not need to be replaced at a specific time, and some women use them for 10 years or more. The copper-bearing IUDs must be replaced every 8 years for maximum efficacy. The progesterone-secreting IUDs must be replaced yearly but have the advantage of causing decreased cramping and menstrual flow.

The IUD is often an excellent contraceptive method for parous women with one sexual partner. It is less desirable for young nulliparas because of the greater threat of pelvic inflammatory disease in young women and the possible impairment of future fertility.

Insertion

Insertion can be performed during or after the menses, at midcycle to prevent implantation, or later in the cycle if the patient has not become pregnant. Most clinicians wait for 6–8 weeks postpartum before inserting an IUD. When insertion is performed during lactation, there is greater risk of uterine perforation or embedding of the IUD. Insertion immediately following abortion is acceptable if there is no sepsis and if follow-up insertion a month later will not be possible; otherwise, it is wise to wait until 4 weeks postabortion. Because of the risk of pelvic inflammation, a single prophylactic dose of doxycycline 1 hour before insertion is often used.

Contraindications & Complications

Contraindications to use of IUDs are outlined in Table 17–7.

A. Pregnancy: An IUD can be inserted within 5 days following a single episode of unprotected midcycle coitus as a postcoital contraceptive. An IUD

Table 17–7. Contraindications to IUD use.

Absolute contraindications
  Pregnancy
  Acute or subacute pelvic inflammatory disease or purulent
    cervicitis
Relative contraindications
  Past history of pelvic inflammatory disease or ectopic
    pregnancy
  Multiple sexual partners
  Nulliparous woman concerned about future fertility
  Lack of available follow-up care
  Menorrhagia or severe dysmenorrhea
  Cervical or uterine neoplasia
  Abnormal size or shape of uterus, including myomas
    distorting cavity
  Valvular heart disease
  Diabetes

should not be inserted into a pregnant uterus. If pregnancy occurs as an IUD failure, there is a greater chance of spontaneous abortion if the IUD is left in situ (50%) than if it is removed (25%). Spontaneous abortion with an IUD in place is associated with a high risk of severe sepsis, and death can occur rapidly. Women using an IUD who become pregnant should have the IUD removed if the string is visible. It can be removed at the time of abortion if this is desired. If the string is not visible and the patient wants to continue the pregnancy, she should be informed of the serious risk of sepsis and, occasionally, death with such pregnancies. She should be informed that any flu-like symptoms such as fever, myalgia, headache, or nausea warrant immediate medical attention for possible septic abortion.

Since the ratio of ectopic to intrauterine pregnancies is increased among IUD wearers, clinicians should search for adnexal masses in early pregnancy and should always check the products of conception for placental tissue following abortion.

B. Pelvic Infection: There is an increased risk of pelvic infection during the first month following insertion. The subsequent risk of pelvic infection appears to be primarily related to the risk of acquiring sexually transmitted infections. The risk of infection at the time of insertion may be reduced by the use of antibiotic prophylaxis such as 200 mg of doxycycline. The threat of sexually transmitted pelvic infection can be essentially eliminated by limiting the use of the IUD to parous women with a single sexual partner. The use of IUDs by young nulliparas is undesirable because of the increased risk of sexually transmitted disease and the threat to future fertility.

C. Menorrhagia or Severe Dysmenorrhea: The IUD can cause heavier menstrual periods, bleeding between periods, and more cramping, so it is generally not suitable for women who already suffer from these problems. However, progesterone-secreting IUDs can be tried in these cases, as they often cause decreased bleeding and cramping with menses. Nonsteroidal anti-inflammatory drugs are also helpful in decreasing bleeding and pain in IUD users.

D. Complete or Partial Expulsion: Spontaneous expulsion of the IUD occurs in 10–20% of cases during the first year of use. Remove any IUD if the body of the device can be seen or felt in the cervical os.

E. Missing IUD Strings: If the transcervical tail cannot be seen, this may signify unnoticed expulsion, perforation of the uterus with abdominal migration of the IUD, or simply retraction of the string into the cervical canal or uterus owing to movement of the IUD or uterine growth with pregnancy. Once pregnancy is ruled out, one should probe for the IUD with a sterile sound or forceps designed for IUD removal, after administering a paracervical block. If the IUD cannot be detected, pelvic ultrasound will demonstrate the IUD if it is in the uterus. Alternatively, obtain anteroposterior and lateral x-rays of the pelvis with another IUD or a sound in the uterus as a marker, to confirm an extrauterine IUD. If the IUD is in the abdominal cavity, it should generally be removed by laparoscopy or laparotomy. Open-looped all-plastic IUDs such as the Lippes Loop can be left in the pelvis without danger, but ring-shaped IUDs may strangulate a loop of bowel and copper-bearing IUDs may cause tissue reaction and adhesions.

Perforations of the uterus are less likely if insertion is performed slowly, with meticulous care taken to follow directions applicable to each type of IUD.

Farley TMM et al: Intrauterine devices and pelvic inflammatory disease: An international perspective. Lancet 1992;339:785. (Definitive study of the risk.)

4. DIAPHRAGM & CERVICAL CAP

The diaphragm (with contraceptive jelly) is a safe and effective contraceptive method with features that make it acceptable to some women and not others. Failure rates range from 2% to 20%, depending on the motivation of the woman and the care with which the diaphragm is used. The advantages of this method are that it has no systemic side effects and gives significant protection against pelvic infection and cervical dysplasia as well as pregnancy. The disadvantages are that it must be inserted near the time of coitus and that pressure from the rim predisposes some women to cystitis after intercourse.

The cervical cap (with contraceptive jelly) is similar to the diaphragm but fits snugly over the cervix only (the diaphragm stretches from behind the cervix to behind the pubic symphysis). The cervical cap is more difficult to insert and remove than the diaphragm. The main advantages are that it can be used by women who cannot be fitted for a diaphragm because of a relaxed anterior vaginal wall or by women who have discomfort or develop repeated bladder infections with the diaphragm.

Because of the small risk of toxic shock syndrome, a cervical cap or diaphragm should not be left in the vagina for over 12–18 hours, nor should these devices be used during the menstrual period (see above).

5. CONTRACEPTIVE SPONGE, FOAM, CREAM, JELLY, & SUPPOSITORY

These products are available without prescription, are easy to use, and are fairly effective, with reported failure rates of 2–30%. All contain the spermicides nonoxynol 9 or octoxynol 9, which also have some virucidal and bactericidal activity. Spermicides may alter the vaginal bacterial flora and allow overgrowth of E coli with an increased risk of bacteriuria. The contraceptive sponge is inserted before intercourse and can be used for repeated acts of intercourse but should not be left in the vagina for longer than 12–18 hours, because of the risk of toxic shock syndrome (see Chapter 29). The sponge is more effective in nulliparous women than in parous women. Foams, creams, jellies, and suppositories also have the advantages of being simple to use and easily available. Their disadvantage is a slightly higher failure rate than with the diaphragm or condom.

Hooten TM et al: *Escherichia coli* bacteriuria and contraceptive method. JAMA 1991;265:64.

6. CONDOM

The male sheath of latex or animal membrane affords good protection against pregnancy—equivalent to that of a diaphragm and spermicidal jelly; latex (but not animal membrane) condoms also offer protection against sexually transmitted disease and cervical dysplasia. Men and women seeking protection against HIV transmission are advised to use a latex condom along with spermicide during vaginal or rectal intercourse. When a spermicide such as vaginal foam is used with the condom, the failure rate approaches that of oral contraceptives. Condoms coated with spermicide are now available in the USA. The disadvantages of condoms are dulling of sensation and spillage of semen due to tearing, slipping, or leakage with detumescence of the penis.

A female condom has been approved for marketing by the FDA. The reported failure rate in preventing pregnancy (26%) is somewhat higher than other barrier methods. However, it is the only female-controlled method that offers significant protection from both pregnancy and sexually transmitted diseases.

Rietmeijer CAM et al: Condoms as physical and chemical barriers against human immunodeficiency virus. JAMA 1988;259:1851.

7. CONTRACEPTION BASED ON AWARENESS OF FERTILE PERIODS

There is renewed interest in methods to identify times of ovulation and avoidance of unprotected intercourse at that time as a means of family planning. These methods are most effective when the couple restricts intercourse to the postovular phase of the cycle or uses a barrier method at other times. Women benefit from learning to identify their fertile periods. Well-instructed, motivated couples may achieve low pregnancy rates with fertility awareness, but in many field trials, the pregnancy rates were as high as 20%.

"Symptothermal" Natural Family Planning

The basis for this approach is patient-observed increase in clear elastic cervical mucus, brief abdominal midcycle discomfort ("mittelschmerz"), and a sustained rise of the basal body temperature about 2 weeks after onset of menstruation. Unprotected intercourse is avoided from shortly after the menstrual period, when fertile mucus is first identified, until 48 hours after ovulation, as identified by a sustained rise in temperature and the disappearance of clear elastic mucus.

Calendar Method

After the length of the menstrual cycle has been observed for at least 8 months, the following calculations are made: (1) The first fertile day is determined by subtracting 18 days from the shortest cycle; (2) the last fertile day is determined by subtracting 11 days from the longest cycle. For example, if the observed cycles run from 24 to 28 days, the fertile period would extend from the sixth day of the cycle (24 minus 18) through the 17th day (28 minus 11).

Basal Body Temperature Method

This method indicates the safe time after ovulation has passed. The temperature must be taken immediately upon awakening, before any activity. A slight drop in temperature often occurs 1–1½ days before ovulation, and a rise of about 0.4 °C (0.7 °F) occurs 1–2 days after ovulation. The elevated temperature continues throughout the remainder of the cycle. The second day after the rise marks the end of the fertile period.

Queenan JT et al: (editors): Natural family planning: Current knowledge and new strategies for the 1990s. Proceedings of a conference. Am J Obstet Gynecol 1991; 165:1977.

8. POSTCOITAL CONTRACEPTION

If unprotected intercourse occurs in midcycle and the woman is certain she has not inadvertently become pregnant earlier in the cycle, the following regimens are effective in preventing implantation. The failure rate is less than 1.5%. These methods should be started within 72 hours after coitus. (1) Ethinyl estradiol, 2.5 mg twice daily for 5 days. (2) Ovral (50 µg of ethinyl estradiol with 0.5 mg of norgestrel, two tablets at once followed by two tablets 12 hours later. Antinausea medication may be necessary with these regimens. Bleeding should occur within 3–4 weeks. If pregnancy occurs, abortion is advisable because of fetal exposure to possibly teratogenic doses of sex steroids.

IUD insertion within 5 days after one episode of unprotected midcycle coitus will also prevent pregnancy; copper-bearing IUDs have been tested for this purpose. The disadvantage of this method is possible infection, especially in rape cases; the advantage is ongoing contraceptive protection if this is desired in a patient for whom the IUD is a suitable choice.

9. ABORTION

Since the legalization of abortion in the USA in 1973, the related maternal mortality rate has fallen markedly, because illegal and self-induced abortions have been replaced by safer medical procedures. Abortions in the first trimester of pregnancy are performed by vacuum aspiration under local anesthesia. A similar technique, dilatation and evacuation, is often used in the second trimester, with general or local anesthesia. Techniques utilizing intra-amniotic instillation of hypertonic saline solution or prostaglandins are also occasionally used after 18 weeks from the LMP but are more difficult for the patient. Abortions are rarely performed after 20 weeks from the LMP. It is currently believed that fetal viability begins at about 24 weeks. Legal abortion has a mortality rate of 1:100,000. Rates of morbidity and mortality rise with length of gestation. Currently in the USA, 90% of abortions are performed before 12 weeks' gestation and only 3–4% after 17 weeks. Every effort should be made to continue the trend toward earlier abortion.

Complications resulting from abortion include retained products of conception (often associated with infection and heavy bleeding) and unrecognized ectopic pregnancy. Immediate analysis of the removed tissue for placenta can exclude or corroborate the diagnosis of ectopic pregnancy. Women presenting with fever, bleeding, or abdominal pain after abortion should be examined; use of broad-spectrum antibiotics and reaspiration of the uterus are frequently necessary. Hospitalization is advisable if acute salpingitis requires intravenous administration of antibiotics. Complications following illegal abortion often need emergency care for hemorrhage, septic shock, or uterine perforation.

Rh immune globulin should be given to all Rh-negative women following abortion. Contraception should be thoroughly discussed and contraceptive supplies or pills provided at the time of abortion. In women with a past history of pelvic inflammatory disease, prophylactic antibiotics are indicated: A one-dose regimen is doxycycline, 300 mg orally 1 hour before the procedure, or aqueous penicillin G, 1 million units intravenously 30 minutes before. In the second trimester, use cefazolin, 1 g intravenously 30 minutes before the procedure. Many clinics prescribe tetracycline, 500 mg four times daily for 5 days after the procedure for all patients.

Long-term sequelae of repeated induced abortions

have been studied, but as yet there is no consensus on whether there are increased rates of fetal loss or premature labor. It is felt that such adverse sequelae can be minimized by performing early abortion with minimal cervical dilatation or by the use of *Laminaria* to induce gradual cervical dilatation.

An oral abortifacient, mifepristone (RU 486), 600 mg as a single dose followed in 36–48 hours by a prostaglandin vaginally or intramuscularly, is 95% successful in spontaneously terminating pregnancies of up to 8 weeks' duration with minimum complications. The drug acts as an antihormone to progesterone and glucocorticoids without producing adrenal insufficiency. It may find clinical use in the treatment of Cushing's disease, meningiomas, breast cancer with progesterone receptors, endometriosis, and certain viral infections as well as promoting cervical ripening to induce labor. Currently available in some European countries, it is not approved for use in the USA.

Silvestre L et al: Voluntary interruption of pregnancy with mifepristone (RU 486) and a prostaglandin analogue: A large scale experience. N Eng J Med 1990;322:645.

10. STERILIZATION

In the USA, sterilization is the most popular method of birth control for couples who want no more children. Although sterilization is reversible in some instances, reversal surgery in both men and woman is costly, complicated, and not always successful. Therefore, patients should be counseled carefully before sterilization and should view the procedure as final.

Vasectomy is a safe, simple procedure in which the vas deferens is severed and sealed through a scrotal incision under local anesthesia. Long-term follow-up studies on vasectomized men show no excess risk of heart disease, cancer, or immune system problems.

Female sterilization is currently performed via laparoscopic bipolar electrocoagulation or plastic ring application on the uterine tubes or via minilaparotomy with Pomeroy tubal resection. The advantages of laparoscopy are minimal postoperative pain, small incisions, and rapid recovery. The advantages of minilaparotomy are that it can be performed with standard surgical instruments under local or general anesthesia. However, there is more postoperative pain and a longer recovery period. Failure rates after tubal sterilization are approximately 0.5%; this fact should be discussed with women preoperatively. There are recent reports that menstrual irregularities may increase after sterilization by unipolar tubal coagulation, but probably not after other techniques.

RAPE

Rape, or sexual assault, is legally defined in different ways in various jurisdictions. Physicians and emergency room personnel who deal with rape victims should be familiar with the laws pertaining to sexual assault in their own state. From a medical and psychologic viewpoint, it is essential that persons treating rape victims recognize the nonconsensual and violent nature of the crime. About 95% of reported rape victims are women. Penetration may be vaginal, anal, or oral and may be by the penis, hand, or a foreign object. The absence of genital injury does not imply consent by the victim. The assailant may be unknown to the victim or may be an acquaintance or even the spouse.

"Unlawful sexual intercourse," or statutory rape, is intercourse with a female before the age of majority even with her consent.

Rape represents an expression of anger, power, and sexuality on the part of the rapist. The rapist is usually a hostile man who uses sexual intercourse to terrorize and humiliate a woman. Women neither secretly want to be raped, nor do they expect, encourage, or enjoy rape.

Rape involves severe physical injury in 5–10% of cases and is always a terrifying experience in which most victims fear for their lives. Consequently, all victims suffer some psychologic aftermath. Moreover, some may acquire sexually transmissible disease or become pregnant.

Because rape is a personal crisis, each patient will react differently. The rape-trauma syndrome comprises two principal phases:

(1) Immediate or acute: Shaking, sobbing, and restless activity may last from a few days to a few weeks. The patient may experience anger, guilt, shame, and fear of revenge or may repress these emotions. Reactions vary depending on the victim's personality and the circumstances of the attack.

(2) Late or chronic: Problems related to the attack may develop weeks or months later. The lifestyle and work patterns of the individual may change. Sleep disorders or phobias often develop. Loss of self-esteem can rarely lead to suicide.

Physicians and emergency room personnel who deal with rape victims should work with community rape crisis centers whenever possible to provide ongoing supportive, skilled counseling.

General Office Procedures

The physician who first sees the alleged rape victim should be empathetic. Begin with a statement such as, "This is a terrible thing that has happened to you. I want to help."

(1) Secure written consent from the patient, guardian, or next of kin for gynecologic examination; for photographs if they are likely to be useful as evidence; and for notification of police. If police are to be notified, do so, and obtain advice on the transfer of evidence.

(2) Obtain and record the history in the patient's own words. The sequence of events, ie, the time, place, and circumstances, must be included. Note the date of the LMP, whether or not the woman is pregnant, and the time of the most recent coitus prior to the sexual assault. Note the details of the assault such as body cavities penetrated, use of foreign objects, and number of assailants.

Note whether the victim is calm, agitated, or confused (drugs or alcohol may be involved). Record whether the patient came directly to the hospital or whether she bathed or changed her clothing. Record findings but do not issue even a tentative diagnosis lest it be erroneous or incomplete.

(3) Have the patient disrobe while standing on a white sheet. Hair, dirt, and leaves; underclothing; and any torn or stained clothing should be kept as evidence. Scrape material from beneath fingernails and comb pubic hair for evidence. Place all evidence in separate clean paper bags or envelopes and label carefully.

(4) Examine the patient, noting any traumatized areas that should be photographed. Examine the body and genitals with a Wood light to identify semen, which fluoresces; positive areas should be swabbed with a premoistened swab and air-dried in order to identify PSA from prostatic secretions. Colposcopy can be used to identify small areas of trauma from forced entry especially at the posterior fourchette.

(5) Perform a pelvic examination, explaining all procedures and obtaining the patient's consent before proceeding gently with the examination. (In children, general anesthesia may be necessary during the pelvic examination or for repair of vaginal lacerations.) Use a narrow speculum lubricated with water only. Collect material with sterile cotton swabs from the vaginal walls and cervix and make two air-dried smears on clean glass slides. Swab the mouth (around molars and cheeks) and anus in the same way, if appropriate. Label all slides carefully. Collect secretions from the vagina, anus, or mouth with a premoistened cotton swab, place at once on a slide with a drop of saline, and cover with a coverslip. Look for motile or nonmotile sperm under high, dry magnification, and record the percentage of motile forms.

(6) Perform appropriate laboratory tests as follows. Culture the vagina, anus, or mouth (as appropriate) for *N gonorrhoeae* and *Chlamydia*. Perform a Papanicolaou smear of the cervix, a wet mount for *T vaginalis,* a baseline pregnancy test, and VDRL test. A confidential test for HIV antibody can be obtained if desired by the patient and repeated in 2–4 months if initially negative. Repeat the pregnancy test if the next menses is missed, and repeat the VDRL test in 6 weeks. Obtain blood (10 mL without anticoagulant) and urine (100 mL) specimens if there is a history of forced ingestion or injection of drugs or alcohol.

(7) Transfer clearly labeled evidence, eg, laboratory specimens, directly to the clinical pathologist in charge or to the responsible laboratory technician, in the presence of witnesses (never via messenger), so that the rules of evidence will not be breached.

Treatment

(1) Give analgesics or tranquilizers if indicated.

(2) Administer tetanus toxoid if deep lacerations contain soil or dirt particles.

(3) Give ceftriaxone, 125 mg intramuscularly, to prevent gonorrhea. In addition, give metronidazole, 2 g as a single dose, and doxycycline, 100 mg twice daily for 7 days to treat chlamydial infection. Incubating syphilis will probably be prevented by these medications, but the VDRL test should be repeated 6 weeks after the assault.

(4) Prevent pregnancy by using one of the methods discussed under Postcoital Contraception, if necessary (see above).

(5) Vaccinate against hepatitis B.

(6) Make sure the patient and her family and friends have a source of ongoing psychologic support.

Green WM: *Rape: The Evidential Examination and Management of the Adult Female Victim.* Lexington Books, 1988.

Young WE et al: Sexual assault: Review of a national protocol for forensic and medical evaluation. Obstet Gynecol 1992;80:878. (Controversial issues in assessment of the rape victim.)

MENOPAUSAL SYNDROME

Essentials of Diagnosis

- Cessation of menses due to aging or to bilateral oophorectomy.
- Elevation of FSH and LH levels.
- Hot flushes and night sweats (in 80% of women).
- Decreased vaginal lubrication; thinned vaginal mucosa with or without dyspareunia.

General Considerations

The term "menopause" refers to the final cessation of menstruation, either as a normal part of aging or as the result of surgical removal of both ovaries. In a broader sense, as the term is commonly used, it denotes a 1- to 3-year period during which a woman adjusts to a diminishing and then absent menstrual flow and the physiologic changes that may be associated—hot flushes, night sweats, and vaginal dryness or soreness with coitus.

The average age at menopause in Western societies today is 51 years. Premature menopause is defined as ovarian failure and menstrual cessation before age

40; this often has a genetic or autoimmune basis. Surgical menopause due to bilateral oophorectomy is common and can cause more severe symptoms owing to the sudden rapid drop in sex hormone levels.

There is no objective evidence that cessation of ovarian function is associated with severe emotional disturbance or personality changes. However, mood changes towards depression and anxiety can occur at this time. Additionally, the time of menopause often coincides with other major life changes, such as departure of children from home, a midlife identity crisis, or divorce. These events, coupled with a sense of the loss of youth, may exacerbate the symptoms of menopause and cause psychologic distress.

Clinical Findings

A. Symptoms and Signs:

1. Cessation of menstruation–Menstrual cycles generally become irregular as menopause approaches. Anovular cycles occur more often, with irregular cycle length and occasional menorrhagia. Menstrual flow usually diminishes in amount owing to decreased estrogen secretion, resulting in less abundant endometrial growth. Finally, cycles become longer, with missed periods or episodes or spotting only. When no bleeding has occurred for one year, the menopausal transition can be said to have occurred. Any bleeding after this time warrants investigation by endometrial curettage or aspiration to rule out endometrial cancer.

2. Hot flushes–Hot flushes (feelings of intense heat over the trunk and face, with flushing of the skin and sweating) occur in 80% of women as a result of the decrease in ovarian hormones. Hot flushes can begin before the cessation of menses. An increase in pulsatile release of gonadotropin-releasing hormone from the hypothalamus is believed to trigger the hot flushes by affecting the adjacent temperature-regulating area of the brain. Hot flushes are more severe in women who undergo surgical menopause. Flushing is more pronounced late in the day, during hot weather, after ingestion of hot foods or drinks, or during periods of tension. Occurring at night, they often cause sweating and insomnia and result in fatigue on the following day.

3. Dyspareunia–With decreased estrogen secretion, thinning of the vaginal mucosa and decreased vaginal lubrication occur and may lead to dyspareunia. The introitus decreases in diameter. Pelvic examination reveals pale, smooth vaginal mucosa and a small cervix and uterus. The ovaries are not normally palpable after the menopause. Continued sexual activity will help prevent tissue shrinkage; use of lubricants, estrogen or testosterone cream, or oral estrogen therapy can prevent or relieve pain.

4. Osteoporosis–Osteoporosis may occur as a late sequela of menopause (see Chapter 22).

B. Laboratory Findings: Vaginal cytologic examination will show a low estrogen effect with predominantly parabasal cells. Serum FSH and LH levels are elevated.

Treatment

A. Natural Menopause: Education and support from health providers, midlife discussion groups, and reading material will help most women having difficulty adjusting to the menopause. Physiologic symptoms can be treated as follows:

1. Vasomotor symptoms–Give conjugated estrogens, 0.3 mg or 0.625 mg; estradiol, 0.5 or 1 mg; or estrone sulfate, 0.625 mg; or estradiol can be given transdermally (Estraderm) as skin patches that are changed twice weekly and secrete 0.05–0.1 mg of hormone daily. When either form of estrogen is used, add a progestin (medroxyprogesterone acetate) to prevent endometrial hyperplasia or cancer. The hormones can be given in several differing regimens. Give estrogen on days 1–25 of each calendar month, with 5–10 mg of medroxyprogesterone acetate added on days 14–25. Withhold hormones from day 26 until the end of the month, when the endometrium will be shed, producing a light, generally painless monthly period. Alternatively, give the estrogen along with 2.5 mg of medroxyprogesterone acetate daily, without stopping. This regimen causes some initial bleeding or spotting, but within a few months it produces an atrophic endometrium that will not bleed. If the patient has had a hysterectomy, a progestin need not be used. Explain to the patient that hot flushes will probably return if the hormone is discontinued. When women wish to stop hormone therapy, the dose should be tapered.

Clonidine, an α-adrenergic agonist, has been found to be effective in reducing hot flashes when given orally or transdermally in doses of 100–150 μg daily. Side effects include dry mouth, drowsiness, and blood pressure decrease, but the effects are usually mild at these low dosages. Natural methods to decrease the severity of hot flashes include daily exercise, electroacupuncture, relaxation practices, and avoiding caffeine and alcohol.

2. Dyspareunia–This problem can be treated with hormone therapy as outlined above. Alternatively, topical use of hormone creams in small doses will often relieve pain with minimal systemic absorption. Use Premarin or Estrace vaginal cream, one-eighth applicatorful (0.3 mg of conjugated estrogen) nightly for 7–10 nights. Thereafter, use every other night or twice weekly. Testosterone propionate 1–2% in a vanishing cream base used in the same manner is also effective if estrogen is contraindicated. A bland lubricant such as unscented cold cream or water-soluble gel can be helpful at the time of coitus.

3. Osteoporosis–Women should ingest at least 800 mg of calcium daily throughout life. Nonfat or low-fat milk products, calcium-fortified orange juice, green leafy vegetables, corn tortillas, and canned sardines or salmon consumed with the bones are good dietary sources. In addition, 1 g of elemental calcium should be taken as a daily supplement at the time of the menopause and thereafter; calcium supplements should be taken with meals to increase their absorption. Vitamin D, 400 IU/d from food, sunlight, or supplements, is necessary to enhance calcium absorption. A daily program of energetic walking and exercise to strengthen the arms and upper body helps maintain bone mass.

Women most at risk for osteoporotic fractures should consider hormone replacement therapy. This includes Caucasian and Asian women, especially if they have a family history of osteoporosis; are thin, short, cigarette smokers, and physically inactive; or have had a low calcium intake in adult life. The dosage is usually the same as for treatment of vasomotor symptoms. Etidronate, a diphosphonate used in Paget's disease, has recently been shown to increase spinal bone mass and decrease the incidence of new vertebral fractures. It is given in a dosage of 400 mg daily for 2 weeks four times a year. Calcitonin by daily injection or nasal spray and calcitriol—the activated form of vitamin D—are also under study for the prevention and treatment of osteoporosis.

B. Surgical Menopause: The abrupt hormonal decrease resulting from oophorectomy generally results in severe vasomotor symptoms and rapid onset of dyspareunia and osteoporosis unless treated. Estrogen replacement is generally started immediately after surgery. Conjugated estrogen, 1.25 mg, estrone sulfate, 1.25 mg, or estradiol, 2 mg, is given for 25 days of each month. After age 45–50 years, this dose can be tapered to 0.625 mg of conjugated estrogen or equivalent.

C. Advantages and Risks of Hormone Therapy: Long-term estrogen therapy has been shown to decrease a woman's risk of fatal heart attack, probably by decreasing LDL cholesterol, increasing HDL cholesterol, and increasing the elasticity of blood vessel walls. Progestins counteract some but not all of these favorable effects. Estrogen helps to prevent osteoporosis, hot flashes, and dyspareunia and may elevate mood. The risks of estrogen include a probable small increase in breast cancer, especially in women with a close family history of the disease. Endometrial cancer can occur unless adequate progestin is used. Since estrogen doubles the risk of gallbladder disease necessitating cholecystectomy, its use in women with gallstones or a history of cholecystitis is unwise. Estrogen may cause the growth of uterine myomas, which otherwise shrink after the menopause.

American College of Physicians: Guidelines for counseling postmenopausal women about preventive hormone therapy. Ann Intern Med 1992;117:1038. (This and Grady et al [see below] are companion articles that address in detail the risks and benefits of hormone replacement therapy and make specific recommendations about its use.)

Clisham PR et al: Comparison of continuous versus sequential estrogen and progestin therapy in postmenopausal women. Obstet Gynecol 1991;77:241. (Bleeding patterns were similar, but adverse lipid effects occurred with continuous therapy with high-dose medroxyprogesterone.)

Grady D et al: Hormone therapy to prevent disease and prolong life in postmenopausal women. Ann Intern Med 1992;117:1016.

OBSTETRICS

DIAGNOSIS & DIFFERENTIAL DIAGNOSIS OF PREGNANCY

It is advantageous to diagnose pregnancy as promptly as possible when a sexually active woman misses a menstrual period or has symptoms suggestive of pregnancy. In the event of a desired pregnancy, prenatal care can begin early, and potentially harmful medications and activities, such as drug and alcohol use, smoking, and occupational chemical exposure, can be halted. In the event of an unwanted pregnancy, counseling about termination of the pregnancy can be provided at an early stage.

Pregnancy Tests

All urine or blood pregnancy tests rely on the detection of hCG produced by the placenta. hCG levels increase shortly after implantation, double approximately every 48 hours, reach a peak at 50–75 days, and fall to lower levels in the second and third trimesters. Laboratory and home pregnancy tests now use monoclonal antibodies specific for hCG. These tests are performed on urine or serum and are accurate at the time of the missed period or shortly after it.

Compared with intrauterine pregnancies, ectopic pregnancies may show lower levels of hCG, which level off or fall in serial determinations. Quantitative assays of hCG repeated at 48- to 72-hour intervals are used in the diagnosis of ectopic pregnancy, as well as in cases of molar pregnancy, threatened abortion, and missed abortion. Comparison of hCG levels between laboratories may be misleading in a given patient because different international standards produce results that vary by a factor of two.

Manifestations of Pregnancy

The following symptoms and signs are usually due to pregnancy, but none are diagnostic. A record of the time and frequency of coitus is helpful for diagnosing and dating a pregnancy.

A. Symptoms: Amenorrhea, nausea and vomiting, breast tenderness and tingling, urinary frequency and urgency, "quickening" (noted at about the 18th week), weight gain.

B. Signs (in Weeks From LMP): Breast changes (enlargement, vascular engorgement, colostrum), abdominal enlargement, cyanosis of vagina and cervical portion (about the seventh week), softening of the cervix (seventh week), softening of the cervicouterine junction (eighth week), generalized enlargement and diffuse softening of the corpus (after eighth week).

The uterine fundus is palpable above the pubic symphysis by 12–15 weeks from the LMP and reaches the umbilicus by 20–22 weeks. Fetal heart tones can be heard by Doppler at 10–12 weeks of gestation and by 20 weeks with an ordinary fetoscope.

Differential Diagnosis

The nonpregnant uterus enlarged by myomas can be confused with the gravid uterus, but it is usually very firm and irregular. An ovarian tumor may be found midline, displacing the nonpregnant uterus to the side or posteriorly. Ultrasonography and a pregnancy test will provide accurate diagnosis in these circumstances.

ESSENTIALS OF PRENATAL CARE

The first prenatal visit should occur as early as possible after the diagnosis of pregnancy and should include the following.

History

Age, ethnic background, occupation. Onset of LMP and its normality, possible conception dates, bleeding after LMP, medical history, all prior pregnancies (duration, outcome, and complications), symptoms of present pregnancy. Use of drugs, alcohol, tobacco, caffeine, nutritional habits (Table 17–8). Family history of congenital anomalies and heritable diseases.

Physical Examination

Height, weight, blood pressure, general physical examination. Abdominal and pelvic examination: (1) estimate uterine size or measure fundal height; (2) evaluate bony pelvis for symmetry and adequacy; (3) evaluate cervix for structural anatomy, infection, effacement, dilation; (4) detect fetal heart sounds by ultrasound after 6 weeks or with Doppler device after 10 weeks.

Laboratory Tests

Urinalysis, culture of a clean-voided midstream urine sample, complete blood count with red cell indices, serologic test for syphilis, rubella antibody titer, blood group, Rh type, atypical antibody screening, and HBsAg evaluation. Human immunodeficiency virus (HIV) screening should be offered to all

Table 17–8. Common drugs that are teratogenic or fetotoxic.[1]

Alcohol	Anticonvulsants
Amebicides	Aminoglutethimide, ethotoin, phenytoin, paramethadione, trimethadione, valproic acid
Carbarsone	
Analgesics and antipyretics	
Aspirin and other salicylates (in third trimester); narcotics (prolonged use)	Antidiabetics
	Oral hypoglycemics
	Antihypertensives
Antibiotics	Diazoxide, thiazide diuretics, reserpine
Aminoglycosides, chloramphenicol, tetracycline, trimethoprim, sulfonamides (in third trimester)	Antineoplastics
	All agents
	Antithyroid drugs
	Radioiodine, propylthiouracil, methimazole
Antifungal drugs	Disulfiram (Antabuse)
Griseofulvin, ketoconazole	Ergotamine
Antiparasitic drugs	Hormones
Lindane, mebendazole, Fansidar (sulfadoxine and pyrimethamine), and others	Estrogens, diethylstilbestrol, progestins, androgens
	Isotretinoin (Accutane)
Antiviral drugs	Nonsteroidal anti-inflammatory drugs in third trimester
Amantadine, ribavirin, and others	
Anticoagulants	Psychoactive drugs
Warfarin, dicumarol and other coumarin derivatives	Lithium, benzodiazepines, amitriptyline
	Tobacco smoking

[1]Additional drugs are also contraindicated during pregnancy. Evaluate any drug for its need and its potential adverse effects. Further information on any drug can be obtained by telephoning the drug manufacturer or by calling the Massachusetts Teratogen Information Service ([617] 787–4957).

pregnant women. If indicated clinically, cervical cultures are obtained for *Neisseria gonorrhoeae* and *Chlamydia*, along with a Papanicolaou smear of the cervix. Hemoglobin electrophoresis for anemic women of black or Mediterranean ancestry (Hb S, C, F) and for Asian women (Hb A_2). Tuberculosis skin testing is increasingly indicated. Genetic counseling with the option of chorionic villus sampling or genetic amniocentesis should be offered to all women who will be 35 years of age or older at delivery and those who have had prior offspring with chromosomal abnormalities. Tay-Sachs blood screening is offered to Jewish women with Jewish partners.

Pregnant women who work in medical-dental health care or the public safety field and those who are household contacts of a hepatitis B virus carrier or a hemodialysis patient and are HBsAg-negative at prenatal screening are at high risk of acquiring hepatitis B. They should be vaccinated during pregnancy.

Advice to Patients

(1) Prenatal care should begin early and with adherence to a schedule of regular prenatal visits:

0–28 weeks: every 4 weeks
28–36 weeks: every 2 weeks
36 weeks on: weekly

(2) Diet:

    (a) Eat a balanced diet containing the major food groups.

    (b) Take prenatal vitamins with iron and folic acid.

    (c) Expect to gain 20–40 lb. Do not diet to lose weight during pregnancy.

    (d) Decrease caffeine intake to 0–1 cup of coffee, tea, or cola daily.

    (e) Avoid eating raw or rare meat, and wash hands after handling raw rare meat.

    (f) Eat fresh fruits and vegetables and wash them before eating.

(3) Do not take medications unless prescribed or authorized by your physician.

(4) Abstain from alcohol, tobacco, and all street drugs. No safe level of alcohol intake has been established for pregnancy. Women who smoke should quit or at least reduce the number of cigarettes smoked per day to as few as possible.

(5) Avoid x-rays unless essential and approved by a physician. Always inform the dentist or physician that you are pregnant.

(6) Obtain adequate rest each day.

(7) Abstain from strenuous physical work or activities, particularly when heavy lifting or weight bearing is required.

(8) Exercise regularly at a mild to moderate level. Avoid exhausting or hazardous exercises or new athletic training programs during pregnancy. Heart rate should be kept below 140 beats/min during exercise.

(9) Enroll with your partner in a childbirth preparation class well before your due date.

(10) Avoid situations where there are chemical or radiation hazards.

(11) Avoid excessive heat in hot tubs or saunas.

(12) Avoid handling cat feces or cat litter. Wear gloves when gardening.

Tests & Procedures

A. Each Visit: Weight, blood pressure, fundal height, fetal heart rate, urine specimen for protein and glucose. Review patient's concerns about pregnancy, health, and nutrition.

B. 6–12 Weeks: Confirm uterine size and growth by pelvic examination. Document fetal heart tones (audible at 10–12 weeks of gestation by Doppler). Chorionic villus sampling between 8 and 12 weeks when indicated.

C. 12–18 Weeks: Genetic counseling for women 35 years or older at EDC, or those with a family history of congenital anomalies, a previous child with a chromosomal abnormality, metabolic disease, or neural tube defect. Amniocentesis is performed as indicated and requested by the patient.

D. 12–24 Weeks: Fetal ultrasound examination when indicated to determine pregnancy dating or evaluate fetal anatomy. An earlier examination provides the most accurate dating, while a later examination demonstrates fetal anatomy in greater detail. The best compromise is at 18–20 weeks of gestation.

E. 16–20 Weeks: Maternal serum alpha-fetoprotein testing is offered to all women. In some states, such testing is mandatory.

F. 20–24 Weeks: Instruct patient in signs and symptoms of preterm labor and rupture of membranes.

G. 24 Weeks to Delivery: Ultrasound examination is performed as indicated. Typically, fetal size and growth are evaluated when fundal height is 2 cm less than or more than expected for gestational age. In multiple pregnancies, ultrasound should be performed every 4 weeks to evaluate for discordant growth.

H. 26–28 Weeks: Screening for gestational diabetes by a 50-g glucose load (Glucola) and a 1-hour post-Glucola blood glucose determination. A blood glucose concentration less than 140 mg/dL is normal. Abnormal values should be followed up with a 3-hour glucose tolerance test unless the Glucola screen value is great than 200 mg/dL, in which case the diagnosis is established.

I. 28 Weeks: Repeat antibody testing for Rh-negative, unsensitized patients. If still Rh antibody-negative, Rh_o (D) immune globulin is administered.

J. 28–32 Weeks: Repeat the complete blood count to evaluate for anemia of pregnancy.

K. 28 Weeks to Delivery: Determination of fetal position and presentation. Question the patient at each visit for signs or symptoms of preterm labor or rupture of membranes. Assess maternal perception of fetal movement at each visit. Antepartum fetal testing is performed as medically indicated.

L. 36 Weeks to Delivery: Repeat HIV testing and cervical cultures for *N gonorrhoeae* in at-risk patients. Cultures for group B streptococcus are performed only in selected-risk patients. Discuss with the patient the indicators of onset of labor, admission to hospital, management of labor and delivery, and options for analgesia and anesthesia. Weekly cervical examinations are not necessary unless indicated for assessment of status for labor. Elective delivery (whether by induction or cesarean section) prior to 39 weeks of gestation requires confirmation of fetal lung maturity.

M. 41 Weeks and Beyond: Cervical examination to determine probability of successful induction of labor. Based on this, induction of labor is undertaken if the cervix is favorable; if unfavorable, antepartum fetal testing is begun.

Friedman JM et al: Potential human teratogenicity of frequently prescribed drugs. Obstet Gynecol 1990;75:594.

MRC Working Party: Medical research council European trial of chorionic villus sampling. Lancet 1991;337:1491.

Rosen MG, Merkatz IR, Hill JG: Caring for our future: A report by the expert panel on the content of prenatal care. Obstet Gynecol 1991;77:782.

NUTRITION IN PREGNANCY

Nutrition in pregnancy significantly affects maternal health and infant size and well-being. Pregnant women should have nutrition counseling early in prenatal care and access to supplementary food programs if they lack funds for adequate nutrition. Counseling should stress abstention from alcohol, smoking, and drugs. Caffeine and artificial sweeteners should be used only in small amounts. "Empty calories" should be avoided, and the diet should contain the following foods: protein foods of animal and vegetable origin, milk and milk products, whole-grain cereals and breads, and fruits and vegetables—especially green leafy vegetables.

Weight gain in pregnancy should be 20–40 lb, which includes the added weight of the fetus, placenta, and amniotic fluid and of maternal reproductive tissues, fluid, blood, increased fat stores, and increased lean body mass. Maternal fat stores are a caloric reserve for pregnancy and lactation; weight restriction in pregnancy to avoid developing such fat stores may affect the development of other fetal and maternal tissues and is not advisable. Obese women can have adequateDsized infants with less weight gain (15–20 lb) but should be encouraged to eat high-quality foods. Normally, a pregnant woman gains 2–5 lb in the first trimester and slightly less than 1 lb/wk thereafter. She needs approximately an extra 200–300 kcal/d (depending on energy output) and 30 g/d of additional protein for a total protein intake of about 75 g/d. Appropriate caloric intake in pregnancy helps prevent the problems associated with low birth weight.

Rigid salt restriction is not necessary. While the consumption of highly salted snack foods and prepared foods is not desirable, 2–3 g/d of sodium is permissible. The increased calcium needs of pregnancy (1200 mg/d) can be met with milk, milk products, green vegetables, soybean products, corn tortillas, and calcium carbonate supplements.

The increased need for iron and folic acid should be met from foods as well as vitamin and mineral supplements. (See section on anemia in pregnancy.) Megavitamins should not be taken in pregnancy, as they may result in fetal malformation or disturbed metabolism. However, a balanced prenatal supplement containing 30–60 mg of elemental iron, 0.5–0.8 mg of folate, and the recommended daily allowances of various vitamins and minerals is widely used in the USA and is probably beneficial to many women with marginal diets. There is evidence that periconceptional vitamin supplements—particularly folic acid—decrease the risk of neural tube defects in the fetus. Lactovegetarians and ovolactovegetarians do well in pregnancy; vegetarian women who eat neither eggs nor milk products should have their diets assessed for adequate calories and protein and should

take oral vitamin B_{12} supplements during pregnancy and lactation.

Institute of Medicine, National Academy of Sciences: *Nutrition During Pregnancy.* Part I, *Weight Gain;* Part II, *Nutrient Supplements.* National Academy Press, 1990.
Wald N et al: Prevention of neural tube defects: Results of the medical research council vitamin study. Lancet 1991;338:131.

TRAVEL DURING PREGNANCY

During an otherwise normal low-risk pregnancy, travel can be planned most safely between the 18th and 32nd weeks. Commercial flying in pressurized cabins does not pose a threat to the fetus. An aisle seat in the nonsmoking section will allow frequent walks. Adequate fluids should be taken during the flight.

It is not advisable to travel to endemic areas of yellow fever in Africa or Latin America or to areas of Africa or Asia where chloroquine-resistant falciparum malaria is a hazard, since complications of malaria are more common in pregnancy.

Ideally, all immunizations should precede pregnancy. Live virus products are contraindicated (measles, rubella, yellow fever). Inactivated poliovaccine (Salk) can be used instead of the oral vaccine. Vaccines against pneumococcal pneumonia and meningococcal meningitis can be used, but their safety during pregnancy has not been conclusively proved.

Pooled gamma globulin to prevent hepatitis A is safe and does not carry a risk of HIV transmission. Chloroquine can be used for malaria prophylaxis in pregnancy, and proguanil is also safe.

Water should be purified by boiling, since iodine purification may provide more iodine than is safe during pregnancy.

Do not use prophylactic antibiotics or bismuth subsalicylate during pregnancy to prevent diarrhea. Use oral rehydration fluids, and treat bacterial diarrhea with erythromycin or ampicillin if necessary.

Barry M, Bia F: Pregnancy and travel. JAMA 1989; 261:728.

VOMITING OF PREGNANCY
(Morning Sickness)
& HYPEREMESIS GRAVIDARUM
(Pernicious Vomiting of Pregnancy)

Morning or evening nausea and vomiting usually begin soon after the first missed period and cease after the fourth to fifth months of gestation. At least half of women, most of them primiparas, complain of nausea and vomiting during early pregnancy. This problem exerts no adverse effects on the pregnancy and does not presage other complications, though it is particularly common with multiple pregnancy and hydatidiform mole. The cause of vomiting during pregnancy is believed to be high estrogen levels.

Persistent, severe vomiting during pregnancy—hyperemesis gravidarum—can be disabling and require hospitalization. Dehydration, acidosis, and nutritional deficiencies may develop with protracted vomiting. Thyroid dysfunction can be associated with hyperemesis gravidarum, so it is advisable to determine TSH and free T_4 values in these patients.

Treatment

A. Mild Nausea and Vomiting of Pregnancy: Reassurance and dietary advice are all that is required in most instances. Because of possible teratogenicity, drugs used during the first half of pregnancy should be restricted to those of major importance to life and health. Antiemetics, antihistamines, and antispasmodics are generally unnecessary to treat nausea of pregnancy. Vitamin B_6 (pyridoxine), 50–100 mg/d orally, is nontoxic and may be helpful in some patients.

B. Hyperemesis Gravidarum: Hospitalize the patient in a private room at bed rest. Give nothing by mouth for 48 hours, and maintain hydration and electrolyte balance by giving appropriate parenteral fluids and vitamin supplements as indicated. Rarely, total parenteral nutrition may become necessary. As soon as possible, place the patient on a dry diet consisting of six small feedings daily with clear liquids 1 hour after eating. Prochlorperazine rectal suppositories may be useful. After in-patient stabilization, the patient can be maintained at home even if she requires intravenous fluids in addition to her oral intake.

Sahakian V et al: Vitamin B_6 is effective therapy for nausea and vomiting of pregnancy: A randomized, double-blind placebo-controlled study. Obstet Gynecol 1991;78:33.

SPONTANEOUS ABORTION

Abortion is defined as termination of gestation before the 20th week of pregnancy. About three-fourths of spontaneous abortions occur before the 16th week; of these, three-fourths occur before the eighth week. Almost 20% of all clinically recognized pregnancies terminate in spontaneous abortion.

More than 60% of spontaneous abortions result from chromosomal defects due to maternal or paternal factors; about 15% are caused by maternal trauma, infections, dietary deficiencies, diabetes mellitus, hypothyroidism, or anatomic malformations. There is no reliable evidence that abortion may be induced by psychic stimuli such as severe fright, grief, anger, or anxiety. In about one-fourth of cases, the cause of abortion cannot be determined. Currently there is no evidence that video display terminals or associated electromagnetic fields are related to an increased risk of spontaneous abortion.

It is important to differentiate women with a history of incompetent cervix from those with more typical early abortion and those with premature labor or rupture of the membranes. Characteristically, incompetent cervix presents as "silent" cervical dilation (ie, with minimal uterine contractions) between 16 and 28 weeks of gestation. Women with incompetent cervix often present with significant cervical dilation (2 cm or more) and minimal symptoms. When the cervix reaches 4 cm or more, active uterine contractions or rupture of the membranes may occur secondary to the degree of cervical dilation. This does not change the primary diagnosis. Factors that predispose to incompetent cervix are a history of incompetent cervix with a previous pregnancy; cervical conization or surgery; cervical injury; DES exposure; and anatomic abnormalities of the cervix. Prior to pregnancy or during the first trimester, there are no methods for determining whether the cervix will eventually be incompetent. After 14–16 weeks, ultrasound may be used to evaluate the internal anatomy of the lower uterine segment and cervix for the funneling and shortening abnormalities indicative of cervical incompetence.

Clinical Findings

A. Symptoms and Signs:

1. Threatened abortion–Bleeding or cramping occurs, but the pregnancy continues. The cervix is not dilated.

2. Inevitable abortion–The cervix is dilated, but passage of the products of conception has not occurred. Bleeding and cramping persist, and passage of the products of conception is considered inevitable.

3. Complete abortion–The fetus and placenta are completely expelled. Pain ceases, but spotting may persist.

4. Incomplete abortion–Some portion of the products of conception (usually placental) remain in the uterus. Only mild cramps are reported, but bleeding is persistent and often excessive.

5. Missed abortion–The pregnancy has ceased to develop, but the conceptus has not been expelled. Symptoms of pregnancy disappear. There is a brownish vaginal discharge but no free bleeding. Pain does not develop. The cervix is semifirm and slightly patulous; the uterus becomes smaller and irregularly softened; the adnexa are normal.

B. Laboratory Findings: Pregnancy tests show low or falling levels of hCG. A complete blood count should be obtained if bleeding is heavy. Determine Rh type, and give Rh_o (D) immune globulin if the type is Rh-negative. All tissue recovered should be assessed by a pathologist.

C. Ultrasonographic Findings: The gestational sac can be identified at 5–6 weeks from the LMP, a fetal pole at 6 weeks, and fetal cardiac activity at 6–7 weeks. Serial observations are often required to evaluate changes in size of the embryo. A small, irregular sac without a fetal pole is diagnostic of inevitable abortion.

Differential Diagnosis

The bleeding that occurs in abortion of a uterine pregnancy must be differentiated from the abnormal bleeding of an ectopic pregnancy and anovular bleeding in a nonpregnant woman. The passage of hydropic villi in the bloody discharge is diagnostic of the abortion of a hydatidiform mole.

Treatment

A. General Measures:

1. Threatened abortion–Place the patient at bed rest for 24–48 hours followed by gradual resumption of usual activities, with abstinence from coitus and douching. Hormonal treatment is contraindicated. Antibiotics should be used only if there are signs of infection.

2. Missed or inevitable abortion–This calls for counseling regarding the fate of the pregnancy and planning for its elective termination at a time chosen by the patient and physician. Insertion of a laminaria to dilate the cervix followed by aspiration is the method of choice. Prostaglandin vaginal suppositories are an effective alternative.

B. Surgical Measures:

1. Incomplete abortion–Prompt removal of any products of conception remaining within the uterus is required. Analgesia and a paracervical block are useful, followed by uterine exploration with ovum forceps or uterine aspiration.

2. Cerclage and restriction of activities–These are the treatment of choice for incompetent cervix. A 5-mm Mersilene band is used to create a purse-string type of stitch around the cervix, using either the McDonald or Shirodkar method. Cerclage should be undertaken with caution when there is advanced cervical dilation or membranes are prolapsed into the vagina. Rupture of the membranes and infection are specific contraindications to cerclage. Cervical cultures for *N gonorrhoeae, Chlamydia,* and group B streptococci should be obtained before or at the time of cerclage.

Wilcox AJ et al: Incidence of early loss of pregnancy. N Engl J Med 1988;319:189.

RECURRENT (HABITUAL) ABORTION

Recurrent, or habitual, abortion has been defined for years as the loss of three or more previable (< 500 g) pregnancies in succession. Recurrent or chronic abortion occurs in about 0.4–0.8% of all pregnancies. Ab-

normalities related to repeated abortion can be identified in approximately half of the couples. If a woman has lost three previous pregnancies without identifiable cause, she still has a 70–80% chance of carrying a fetus to viability. If she has aborted four or five times, the likelihood of a successful pregnancy is 65–70%.

Recurrent abortion is a clinical rather than pathologic diagnosis. The clinical findings are similar to those observed in other types of abortion (see above).

Treatment

A. Preconception Therapy: Preconception therapy is aimed at detection of maternal or paternal defects that may contribute to abortion. A thorough general and gynecologic examination is essential. Polycystic ovaries should be ruled out. Cervical cultures should be prepared for *Chlamydia,* herpesvirus, and cytomegalovirus and endometrial cultures for *Ureaplasma urealyticum* and *Toxoplasma gondii,* A random blood glucose test and thyroid function studies (including thyroid antibodies) should be done. Lupus anticoagulant detection and an antinuclear antibody test are indicated if there is a history of a lupus-like syndrome. Endometrial tissue should be examined in the postovulation stage of the cycle to determine the adequacy of the response of the endometrium to hormones. The competency of the cervix must be determined and hysteroscopy or hysterography used to exclude submucous myomas and congenital anomalies. Chromosomal (karyotype) analysis of both partners rules out balanced translocations (found in 5% of infertile couples).

Recent experiments have focused on the major histocompatibility complex (MHC) of chromosome 6, which carries HLA loci and other genes that may influence reproductive success. Many couples who experience habitual abortion share a significant number of HLA antigens, and some women demonstrate a lack of maternal antibody response to paternal lymphocytes, which is customarily found in normal women after successful childbearing. Centers where HLA typing can be performed will identify couples whose unusual gene sharing may play a role in habitual abortion. The immunologic approach of enhancing maternal antibody response to paternal lymphocytes is still experimental.

B. Postconception Therapy: Provide early prenatal care and schedule frequent office visits. Complete bed rest is justified only for bleeding or pain. Empiric steroid sex hormone therapy is contraindicated.

Prognosis

The prognosis is excellent if the cause of abortion can be corrected.

Infante-Rivard C et al: Lupus anticoagulants, anti-cardiolipin antibodies, and fetal loss: A case-control study. N Engl J Med 1991;325:1063.

Stirrat GM: Recurrent miscarriage: I. Definition and epidemiology. Lancet 1990;336:673.

Stirrat GM: Recurrent miscarriage: II. Clinical associations, causes and management. Lancet 1990:336:728.

ECTOPIC PREGNANCY

Any pregnancy arising from implantation of the ovum outside the cavity of the uterus is ectopic. Ectopic implantation occurs in about one out of 150 live births. About 98% of ectopic pregnancies are tubal. Other sites of ectopic implantation are the peritoneum or abdominal viscera, the ovary, and the cervix. Any condition that prevents or retards migration of the fertilized ovum to the uterus can predispose to an ectopic pregnancy, including a history of infertility, pelvic inflammatory disease, ruptured appendix, and prior tubal surgery. Combined intra- and extra-uterine pregnancy (heterotopic) may occur rarely. In the USA, undiagnosed or undetected ectopic pregnancy is currently the most common cause of maternal death in pregnancies with abortive outcomes.

Clinical Findings

A. Symptoms and Signs: The cardinal symptoms and signs of tubal pregnancy are (1) amenorrhea or irregular bleeding and spotting, followed by (2) pelvic pain, and (3) pelvic (adnexal) mass formation. They may be acute or chronic.

1. Acute (40 %)–Severe lower quadrant pain occurs in almost every case. It is sudden in onset, lancinating, intermittent, and does not radiate. Backache is present during attacks. Shock occurs in about 10%, often after pelvic examination. At least two-thirds of patients give a history of abnormal menstruation; many have been infertile.

2. Chronic (60 %)–Blood leaks from the tubal ampulla over a period of days, and considerable blood may accumulate in the peritoneum. Slight but persistent vaginal spotting is reported, and a pelvic mass can be palpated. Abdominal distention and mild paralytic ileus are often present.

B. Laboratory Findings: Blood studies may show anemia and slight leukocytosis. Quantitative serum pregnancy tests will show levels generally lower than expected for normal pregnancies of the same duration. If pregnancy tests are followed over a few days, there may be a slow rise or a plateau rather than the doubling every 2 days associated with normal early intrauterine pregnancy or the falling levels that occur with spontaneous abortion.

C. Imaging: Ultrasonography can reliably demonstrate a gestational sac 6 weeks from the LMP and a fetal pole at 7 weeks if located in the uterus. An empty uterine cavity raises a strong suspicion of extrauterine pregnancy, which can occasionally be revealed by endovaginal ultrasound.

D. Special Examinations: Aspiration of the pouch of Douglas (culdocentesis) with an 18-gauge spinal needle will confirm hemoperitoneum. Laparoscopy to confirm an ectopic pregnancy is of great value prior to laparotomy.

Differential Diagnosis

Clinical and laboratory findings suggestive or diagnostic of pregnancy will distinguish ectopic pregnancy from many acute abdominal illnesses such as acute appendicitis, acute pelvic inflammatory disease, ruptured corpus luteum cyst or ovarian follicle, and urinary calculi. Uterine enlargement with clinical findings similar to those found in ectopic pregnancy is also characteristic of an aborting uterine pregnancy or hydatidiform mole. Ectopic pregnancy should be suspected when postabortal tissue examination fails to reveal placenta. They must take steps for immediate diagnosis, including prompt microscopic tissue examination, ultrasonography, and serial hCG titers every 48 hours. Patients must be warned of possible ectopic pregnancy problems and followed very closely.

Treatment

The patient is hospitalized if there is a reasonable likelihood of ectopic pregnancy. Blood is typed and cross-matched. Ideally, diagnosis and operative treatment should precede frank rupture of the tube and intra-abdominal hemorrhage.

Surgical treatment is definitive. Generally, salpingectomy will be required if the tube has ruptured. If the condition of the patient permits, assessment of the other tube is important at the time of laparotomy. Patency of the contralateral tube can be established by the injection of indigo carmine into the uterine cavity with appropriate compression of the lower uterine segment.

When the ectopic pregnancy is unruptured, it can be removed by salpingostomy via the laparoscope. Methotrexate—given systemically or by local injection into the ectopic pregnancy—is being used experimentally.

Iron therapy for anemia may be necessary during convalescence. Give Rh$_o$ (D) immune globulin to Rh-negative patients.

Prognosis

Repeat tubal pregnancy occurs in about 12% of cases. This should not be regarded as a contraindication to future pregnancy, but the patient requires careful observation and early ultrasound confirmation of an intrauterine pregnancy.

Ory SJ: New options for diagnosis and treatment of ectopic pregnancy. JAMA 1992;267:534.

Stabile I, Grudzinskas JG: Ectopic pregnancy: A review of

incidence, etiology and diagnostic aspects. Obstet Gynecol Surv 1990;45:335.

PREECLAMPSIA-ECLAMPSIA

Preeclampsia-eclampsia can occur any time after 20 weeks of gestation and up to 6 weeks postpartum. It is a disease unique to pregnancy, with the only cure being delivery of the fetus and placenta. Approximately 7% of pregnant women in the United States develop preeclampsia-eclampsia. Primiparas are most frequently affected; however, the incidence of preeclampsia-eclampsia is increased with multiple pregnancies, chronic hypertension, diabetes, renal disease, collagen-vascular and autoimmune disorders, and gestational trophoblastic disease. Uncontrolled eclampsia is a significant cause of maternal death. Five percent of women with preeclampsia progress to eclampsia.

The basic cause of preeclampsia-eclampsia is not known. Epidemiologic studies suggest an immunologic cause for preeclampsia, since it occurs predominantly in women who have had minimal exposure to sperm (having used barrier methods of contraception) or have new consorts; in primigravidas; and in women both of whose parents have similar HLA antigens. Recent laboratory investigations suggest that it is an endothelial disorder resulting from poorly perfused placenta, which releases a factor—perhaps lipid peroxide—that injures the endothelium and causes a shift in prostacyclin-thromboxane balance that tends to activate coagulation and increases sensitivity to pressors. Although placental changes are initiated in the first trimester, the problem is not recognized clinically until the second half of pregnancy. Before the syndrome is clinically manifest, there is generalized vasospasm, causing increased total peripheral resistance and reduction of plasma volume and blood flow. The longer vasospasm continues, the greater the likelihood of associated pathologic changes in maternal organs, including the placenta, with consequent adverse effects on the fetus.

None of the interventions recommended to reduce the incidence or severity of the process have proved to be of significant value when studied objectively, including diuretics, dietary restriction or enhancement, sodium restriction, and vitamin-mineral supplements. The only cure is termination of the pregnancy at a time as favorable as possible for fetal survival in the light of the medical condition of the mother.

Recent clinical investigations suggest that low-dose aspirin (100 mg daily starting in the third trimester) reduces the incidence of preeclampsia in women at high risk for developing the problem. A similar study on women who already had mild pregnancy-induced hypertension showed that aspirin was not curative in those instances.

The search for a test reliably predicting which women will be at risk during pregnancy is focusing on altered platelet function or a possible growth factor related to abnormal endothelial changes at the placental site.

Definition

Preeclampsia is defined as the presence of the triad of elevated blood pressure, proteinuria, and edema during pregnancy. Eclampsia occurs with the addition of seizures to this triad. The three abnormalities of preeclampsia-eclampsia are defined as follows:

A. Blood Pressure: An elevation of at least 30 mm Hg systolic or 15 mm Hg diastolic (or both) over baseline values established prior to 20 weeks of gestation. In the absence of baseline values, blood pressures of 140/90 mm Hg or more (in the absence of chronic hypertension) after 20 weeks of gestation are abnormal. An alternative definition is a 20 mm Hg increase in mean arterial pressure (MAP) or an absolute MAP of 105 mm Hg alone:

$$MAP = \frac{\text{Systolic BP} + (2 \times \text{Diastolic BP})}{3}$$

All abnormal blood pressure readings must be confirmed with two separate readings at least 6 hours apart.

B. Proteinuria: At least 0.3 G/24 h as determined by 24-hour urine collection.

C. Edema: Clinically apparent fluid retention, or increase in weight of 5 lb or more in 1 week. The edema may involve the upper extremities and face rather than just the lower extremities.

Classically, the presence of all three elements is required for the diagnosis of preeclampsia-eclampsia. Clinically, however, there is a great deal of variation in presentation. Hypertension occurs most frequently, but proteinuria or edema may be the initially dominant abnormality. Subtle elevations in blood pressure that meet the 30/15 mm Hg criteria but with the reading still under 140/90 mm Hg are significant but may be overlooked. The absence of one or two components does not exclude the diagnosis of preeclampsia-eclampsia, and many women with the disorder are asymptomatic early. Diagnosis at an early stage thus requires careful attention to details and a high index of suspicion.

Clinical Findings

Clinically, the severity of preeclampsia-eclampsia can be measured with reference to the six major sites in which it exerts its effects: the central nervous system, the kidneys, the liver, the hematologic and vascular systems, and the fetal-placental unit. By evaluating each of these areas for the presence of mild to moderate versus severe preeclampsia-eclampsia, the degree of involvement can be assessed, and an appropriate management plan can be formulated that is integrated with gestational age assessment (Table 17–9.)

A. Preeclampsia:

1. Mild to moderate—Precise differentiation between mild and moderate preeclampsia-eclampsia is difficult because the abnormalities that define the disease are quite variable and fail to accurately predict progression to more severe disease. Consequently, these two forms of the disease are frequently considered together clinically as is done here. Symptoms are generally minimal or mild. With mild preeclampsia, patients usually have few complaints, and the diastolic blood pressure is less than 90–100 mm Hg. Edema is usually more pronounced with moderate disease, and blood pressures are in the range of 90–110 mm Hg. The platelet count is over 100,000/μL, antepartum fetal testing is reassuring, central nervous system irritability is minimal, epigastric pain is not present, and liver enzymes are not excessively elevated.

2. Severe—Symptoms are more dramatic and persistent. The blood pressure is often quite high, with readings over 160/110 mm Hg. The use of antihypertensive medications (usually to reduce blood pressure to levels < 160/110 mm Hg) indicates the presence of severe preeclampsia. Thrombocytopenia

Table 17–9. Indicators of mild to moderate versus severe preeclampsia-eclampsia.

Site	Indicator	Mild to Moderate	Severe
Central nervous system		Hyperreflexia Headache	Seizures Blurred vision Scotomas Headache Clonus Irritability
Kidney	Proteinuria	<4 g/24 h	>4 g/24 h or catheterized urine with 4+ protein
	Urine output	>20–30 mL/h	<20–30 mL/h
Liver	AST, ALT, LDH	Normal	Elevated Epigastric pain Ruptured liver
Hematologic	Platelets Hemoglobin and hematocrit	>100,000/μL Normal range	<100,000/μL Elevated
Vascular	Blood pressure Retina	<160/110 mm Hg Arteriolar spasm	>160/110 mm Hg Retinal hemorrhages
Fetal-placental unit	Growth retardation Oligohydramnios Fetal distress	Absent May be present Absent	Present Present Present

(platelet counts < 100,000/μL) may be present and progress to disseminated intravascular coagulation. The HELLP syndrome (hemolysis, elevated liver enzymes, low platelets) is a form of severe preeclampsia.

B. Eclampsia: The occurrence of seizures defines eclampsia. It is a manifestation of severe central nervous system involvement. The other abnormal findings of severe preeclampsia are also observed with eclampsia.

Differential Diagnosis

Preeclampsia-eclampsia can mimic and be confused with many other diseases, including (among many others) chronic hypertension, chronic renal disease, primary seizure disorders, gallbladder and pancreatic disease, idiopathic or thrombotic thrombocytopenic purpura, and hemolytic uremic syndrome. It must always be considered as a disease of exclusion in any pregnant women beyond 20 weeks of gestation. It is particularly difficult to diagnose when preexisting chronic disease is present, such as chronic hypertension. Uric acid values can be quite helpful in such situations, since hyperuricemia is uncommon in pregnancy except with gout, renal failure, or preeclampsia-eclampsia. The first two are relatively rare and easy to diagnose. Since uric acid levels decrease in pregnancy due to the increase in blood volume, a value exceeding 5–6 mg/dL with a serum creatinine less than 1 mg/dL is virtually diagnostic of preeclampsia-eclampsia.

Treatment

A. Preeclampsia: Early recognition is the key to treatment. This requires careful attention to the details of prenatal care—especially subtle changes in blood pressure and weight. The objectives are to prolong pregnancy either to term or to fetal lung maturity while preventing progression to severe disease and eclampsia. The critical factors are the gestational age of the fetus, fetal pulmonary maturity status, and the severity of maternal disease. Preeclampsia-eclampsia at 36 weeks or more of gestation is managed by delivery regardless of how mild or severe the disease is judged to be. Prior to 36 weeks, severe preeclampsia-eclampsia requires delivery except in unusual circumstances associated with extreme fetal prematurity, in which case prolongation of pregnancy may be attempted. Epigastric pain, thrombocytopenia, and visual disturbances are strong indications for delivery of the fetus. For mild to moderate preeclampsia-eclampsia, bed rest is the cornerstone of therapy. This increases central blood flow to the kidneys, heart, brain, liver, and placenta and may stabilize or even improve the degree of preeclampsia-eclampsia for a period of time.

Bed rest may be attempted at home or in the hospital. Prior to making this decision, the physician should evaluate the six sites of involvement listed above and make an assessment about the severity of disease.

1. Home management–Home management with bed rest may be attempted for patients with mild preeclampsia and a stable home situation. This requires homemaking assistance, rapid access to the hospital, a reliable patient, and the ability to obtain frequent blood pressure readings. A home health nurse can often provide frequent home visits and assessment.

2. Hospital care–Hospitalization is required for women with moderate or severe preeclampsia or those with unreliable home situations. Regular assessment of blood pressure, reflexes, urine protein, and fetal heart tones and activity are required. A complete blood count, platelet count, and electrolyte panel including liver enzymes should be checked every 1 or 2 days. A 24-hour urine collection for creatinine clearance and total protein should be obtained on admission and repeated as indicated. Sedatives and narcotics should be avoided because of their fetal central nervous system depressant effect, which interferes with fetal testing. Magnesium sulfate is not used until the diagnosis of severe preeclampsia-eclampsia is made or labor or delivery occurs.

Fetal evaluation should be obtained as an integral part of the workup. If the patient is being admitted to the hospital, fetal testing must be performed on the same day to make certain that the fetus is stable and safe. This may be done by fetal heart rate testing with nonstress or stress testing or by biophysical profile. A regular schedule of fetal surveillance must then be followed. Daily fetal kick counts can be recorded by the patient herself. Consideration should be given to amniocentesis to evaluate fetal lung maturity status if hospitalization occurs at 30–37 weeks of gestation. If immaturity is not present, steroids (betamethasone or dexamethasone) can be administered. Fetuses between 26 and 30 weeks of gestation can be presumed to be immature and given steroids.

The method of delivery is determined by the maternal and fetal status. Cesarean section is reserved for the usual fetal indications.

B. Eclampsia:

1. Emergency care–If the patient is convulsing, she is turned on her side to prevent aspiration and to improve blood flow to the placenta. A padded tongue blade or plastic airway is inserted between the teeth. Fluid or food is aspirated from the glottis or trachea. The seizure may be stopped by giving an intravenous bolus of either magnesium sulfate, 4 g, or diazepam, 5–10 mg, over 4 minutes or until the seizure stops. A continuous intravenous infusion of magnesium sulfate is then started at a rate of 3 g/h unless the patient is known to have significantly reduced renal function. Magnesium blood levels are then checked every 4–6 hours and the infusion rate adjusted to maintain a therapeutic blood level. Deep tendon reflexes, the respiratory rate and depth, and urine output are checked

hourly to monitor for magnesium toxicity, which can be reversed with calcium gluconate.

2. General care–The occurrence of eclampsia necessitates delivery once the patient is stabilized. It is important, however, that assessment of the status of the patient and fetus take place first. Continuous fetal monitoring must be performed and blood typed and cross-matched quickly. A urinary catheter is inserted to monitor urine output, and blood is sent for complete blood count, platelets, liver enzymes, uric acid, creatinine or urea nitrogen, and electrolytes. If hypertension is present with diastolic values over 110 mm Hg, antihypertensive medications should be administered to reduce the diastolic blood pressure to 90–100 mm Hg. Lower blood pressures than this may induce placental insufficiency through reduced perfusion. Hydralazine given in 5- to 10-mg increments intravenously every 20 minutes is frequently used to lower blood pressure. Nifedipine, 10 mg sublingually or orally, or labetalol can also be used.

3. Delivery–Except in unusual circumstances, delivery is mandated once eclampsia has occurred. Vaginal delivery may be attempted if the patient has already been in active labor or the cervix is quite favorable *and* the patient is clinically stable. The rapidity with which delivery must be achieved depends on the fetal and maternal status following the seizure and the availability of laboratory data on the patient. Oxytocin may be used to induce or augment labor. Regional analgesia or anesthesia is acceptable. Cesarean section is used for the usual obstetric indications or when rapid delivery is necessary for maternal or fetal indications.

4. Postpartum–Magnesium sulfate infusion should be continued until preeclampsia-eclampsia has begun to resolve postpartum. This may take 1–7 days. The most reliable indicator of this is the onset of diuresis with urine output of over 100–200 mL/h. When this occurs, magnesium sulfate can be discontinued. Late-onset preeclampsia-eclampsia can occur during the postpartum period. It is usually manifested by either hypertension or seizures. Treatment is the same as prior to delivery—ie, with magnesium sulfate—though other antiseizure medications can be used since the fetus is no longer present.

Cunningham FG, Lindheimer MD: Hypertension in pregnancy. (Current Concepts.) N Engl J Med 1992;326:927.

Fenakel K et al: Nifedipine in the treatment of severe preeclampsia. Obstet Gynecol 1991;77:331.

Imperiale TF, Petrulis AS: A meta-analysis of low-dose aspirin for the prevention of pregnancy-induced hypertensive disease. JAMA 1991;266:260.

TROPHOBLASTIC NEOPLASIA

Gestational trophoblastic neoplasia is a spectrum of disease that includes hydatidiform mole, invasive mole, and choriocarcinoma. Cytogenetics has demonstrated that complete hydatidiform moles develop from androgenetic conceptions, which are almost always euploid (46 chromosomes). Partial moles are from conceptions in which sets of paternal chromosomes exceed maternal sets and thus are generally polyploid (23 × 3 or more chromosomes). Partial moles generally show evidence of an embryo or gestational sac, are slower-growing and less symptomatic, and are often present clinically as a missed abortion. Partial moles tend to follow a benign course, while complete moles have a greater tendency to become choriocarcinomas.

The highest rates of gestational trophoblastic neoplasia occur in some developing countries, with rates of 1:125 pregnancies in certain areas of the Orient. In the USA, the frequency is 1:1500 pregnancies. Risk factors include low socioeconomic status, a history of mole, and age below 18 or above 40. Approximately 10% of women require further treatment after evacuation of the mole; 5% develop choriocarcinoma.

Clinical Findings

A. Symptoms and Signs: Excessive nausea and vomiting occur in over one-third of patients with hydatidiform mole. Uterine bleeding, beginning at 6–8 weeks, is observed in virtually all instances and is indicative of threatened or incomplete abortion. In about one-fifth of cases, the uterus is larger than would be expected in a normal pregnancy of the same duration. Intact or collapsed vesicles may be passed through the vagina. These grape-like clusters or enlarged villi are diagnostic. Bilaterally enlarged cystic ovaries are sometimes palpable. They are the result of ovarian hyperstimulation due to excess of hCG.

Preeclampsia-eclampsia, frequently of the fulminating type, may develop during the second trimester of pregnancy, but this is unusual.

Choriocarcinoma may be manifested by continued or recurrent uterine bleeding after evacuation of a mole or following a delivery, abortion, or ectopic pregnancy. The presence of an ulcerative vaginal tumor, pelvic mass, or evidence of distant metastatic tumor may be the presenting observation. The diagnosis is established by pathologic examination of curettings or by biopsy.

B. Laboratory Findings: A serum hCG β-subunit value above 40,000 mIU/mL or a urinary hCG value in excess of 100,000 IU/24 h increases the likelihood of hydatidiform mole, though such values are occasionally seen with a normal pregnancy (eg, in multiple gestation).

C. Imaging: Ultrasound has virtually replaced all other means of preoperative diagnosis of hydatidiform mole. The multiple echoes indicating edematous villi within the enlarged uterus and the absence of a fetus and placenta are pathognomonic. A preoperative chest film is indicated to rule out pulmonary metastases of trophoblast.

Treatment

A. Specific (Surgical) Measures: Empty the uterus as soon as the diagnosis of hydatidiform mole is established, preferably by suction. Do not resect ovarian cysts or remove the ovaries; spontaneous regression of theca lutein cysts will occur with elimination of the mole.

If malignant tissue is discovered at surgery or during the follow-up examination, chemotherapy is indicated.

Thyrotoxicosis indistinguishable clinically from that of thyroid origin may occur. Surgical removal of the mole promptly corrects the thyroid overactivity.

B. Follow-Up Measures: Effective contraception (preferably birth control pills) should be prescribed. Weekly quantitative hCG level measurements are initially required. Moles show a progressive decline in hCG. After two negative weekly tests (< 5 mIU/mL), the interval may be increased to monthly for 6 months and then to every 2 months for a year. If levels plateau or begin to rise, the patient should be evaluated by repeat chest film and D&C before the initiation of chemotherapy.

C. Antitumor Chemotherapy: For low-risk patients with a good prognosis, give methotrexate, 0.4 mg/kg intramuscularly over a 5-day period, or dactinomycin, 10–12 μg/kg/d intravenously over a 5Dday period (see Chapter 5). Refer patients with a poor prognosis to a tumor center, where multiple-agent chemotherapy probably will be given. The side effects—anorexia, nausea and vomiting, stomatitis, rash, diarrhea, and bone marrow depression—usually are reversible in about 3 weeks and can be ameliorated by the administration of folic acid. Repeated courses of methotrexate 2 weeks apart generally are required to destroy the trophoblast and maintain a zero chorionic gonadotropin titer, as indicated by hCG β-subunit determination.

D. Supportive Measures: Prescribe oral contraceptives (if acceptable) or another reliable birth control method to avoid the hazard and confusion of elevated hCG from a new pregnancy. hCG levels should be negative for a year before pregnancy is again attempted. In the pregnancy following a mole, the hCG level should be checked 6 weeks postpartum.

Prognosis

A 5-year arrest after courses of chemotherapy, even when metastases have been demonstrated, can be expected in at least 85% of cases of choriocarcinoma.

THIRD-TRIMESTER BLEEDING

Five to ten percent of women have vaginal bleeding in late pregnancy. The physician must distinguish between placental causes (placenta previa, placental abruption, vasa previa) and nonplacental causes (infection, disorders of the lower genital tract, systemic disease). The approach to bleeding in late pregnancy should be conservative and expectant unless fetal distress or risk of maternal hemorrhage occurs.

The patient should be hospitalized and placed at bed rest with continuous fetal monitoring. A complete blood count should be obtained and two to four units of blood typed and cross-matched. If an ultrasound examination has been performed earlier in the pregnancy, it may be possible to exclude placenta previa as a cause. If not, one should be performed to determine placental location. A speculum and digital pelvic examination is done only after ultrasound study has ruled out placenta previa. Continuous electronic fetal monitoring is required to exclude fetal distress. Uterine contractions, pain, or tenderness, if present, often indicate associated abruptio placentae. A negative ultrasound, however, does not exclude it. If vaginal bleeding is profuse and the uterus painful or contracting, the patient is prepared for cesarean section, and blood is available when the vaginal examination is performed.

If the patient is less than 36 weeks of gestation, continued hospitalization and bed rest may be necessary, especially with placenta previa during the initial 7–10 days following vaginal bleeding. If the patient has close proximity to the hospital and accessibility to strict bed rest, as well as complete resolution of bleeding and uterine contractions, home management may be considered. She must be well instructed and counseled regarding the risks. Patients with vaginal bleeding at less than 36 weeks of gestation should also be considered for amniocentesis to test for fetal lung maturity. Steroid therapy is indicated at less than 34 weeks if fetal lung immaturity is present.

Patients with placenta previa should be offered phlebotomy for autologous blood banking.

McVay PA et al: Safety and use of autologous blood donation during the third trimester of pregnancy. Am J Obstet Gynecol 1989;160:1479.

MEDICAL CONDITIONS COMPLICATING PREGNANCY

Anemia

Plasma volume increases 50% during pregnancy, while red cell volume increases 25%, causing lower hemoglobin and hematocrit values, which are maximally changed around the 24th week. Anemia in pregnancy is often defined as a hemoglobin measurement below 10 g/dL or hematocrit below 30%. Anemia is very common in pregnancy, causing fatigue, anorexia, dyspnea, and edema. Prevention through optimal nutrition and iron and folic acid supplementation is desirable.

A. Iron Deficiency Anemia: Many women enter pregnancy with low iron stores resulting from heavy menstrual periods, previous pregnancies, breast feeding, or poor nutrition. It is difficult to meet the increased requirement for iron through diet, and anemia often develops unless iron supplements are given. Red cells may not become hypochromic and microcytic until the hematocrit has fallen significantly. When this occurs, a serum iron level below 40 µg/dL, and a transferrin saturation less than 10% suggest iron deficiency anemia. Treatment consists of a diet containing iron-rich foods and 60 mg of elemental iron (eg, 300 mg of ferrous sulfate) three times a day with meals. Iron is best absorbed if taken with a source of vitamin C (raw fruits and vegetables, lightly cooked greens). All pregnant women should take daily iron supplements.

B. Folic Acid Deficiency Anemia: Folic acid deficiency anemia is the main cause of macrocytic anemia in pregnancy, since vitamin B_{12} deficiency anemia is rare in the childbearing years. The daily requirement doubles from 400 µg to 800 µg in pregnancy. Twin pregnancies, infections, malabsorption, and use of anticonvulsant drugs such as phenytoin can precipitate folic acid deficiency. The anemia may first be seen in the puerperium owing to the increased need for folate during lactation.

The diagnosis is made by finding macrocytic red cells and hypersegmented neutrophils in a blood smear. However, blood smears in pregnancy may be difficult to interpret, since they frequently show iron deficiency changes as well. Because the deficiency is hard to diagnose and folate intake is inadequate in some socioeconomic groups, 0.8–1 mg of folic acid is given as a supplement in pregnancy; the dose in established deficiency is 1–5 mg/d.

Good sources of folate in food are leafy green vegetables, orange juice, peanuts, and beans. Cooking and storage of food destroy folic acid. Strict vegetarians who eat no eggs or milk products should take vitamin B_{12} supplements during pregnancy and lactation.

C. Sickle Cell Anemia: Women with sickle cell anemia are subject to serious complications in pregnancy. The anemia becomes more severe, and crises may occur more frequently. Complications include infections, bone pain, pulmonary infarction, congestive heart failure, and preeclampsia. There is an increased rate of spontaneous abortion and higher maternal and perinatal mortality rates. Newer methods of intensive medical treatment have improved the outcome for mother and fetus. Frequent transfusions of packed cells or leukocyte-poor washed red cells lower the level of hemoglobin S and elevate the level of hemoglobin A; this minimizes the severity of anemia and the risk of sickle cell crises.

A patient with sickle cell disease or sickle trait may wish to undergo first-trimester chorionic villus biopsy or second-trimester amniocentesis to determine whether the abnormality has been passed on to the fetus. Genetic counseling should be offered, and elective sterilization and therapeutic abortion should be available if desired. IUDs and oral contraceptives are contraindicated, but progestin-only contraceptives may be used. Women with sickle cell trait alone usually have an uncomplicated gestation. Sickle cell-hemoglobin C disease in pregnancy is similar to sickle cell anemia and is treated similarly.

Asthma

The effect of pregnancy on asthma is unpredictable. About 50% of patients have no change, 25% improve, and 25% get worse. For acute attacks of bronchospasm, subcutaneous epinephrine is the treatment of choice. For mild episodes, theophylline or ephedrine can be used; cromolyn for prevention is also considered safe. For severe cases, 5–7 days of prednisone (30–50 mg/d) can be helpful, with inhaled beclomethasone dipropionate being used to permit a gradual decrease in oral corticosteroids.

AIDS During Pregnancy

In the USA at present, 80% of women with AIDS are intravenous drug users or partners of drug users. Prostitutes, women partners of hemophiliacs and bisexual men, and recipients of HIV-contaminated blood transfusions (1978–1985) represent smaller groups of infected women. The prevalence of AIDS among heterosexual women without identified risks is estimated to be 0.02%. Asymptomatic infection is not associated with a decreased pregnancy rate or increased risk of adverse pregnancy outcomes. There is no evidence that pregnancy causes AIDS progression.

The rates of transplacental transmission of AIDS have varied from 10% to 40%, apparently related to the stage of the mother's illness. Most cases of transmission occur close to or at delivery. HIV-infected women should be advised not to breast-feed their infants.

Appropriate counseling of HIV antibody-positive pregnant women includes the option of pregnancy termination.

Obstetric caregivers should meticulously observe the established protocols for skin and eye protection against blood and internal secretions, particularly at the time of delivery.

Sperling RS et al: Treatment options for human immunodeficiency virus-infected pregnant women. Obstet Gynecol 1992;79:443.

Diabetes Mellitus

During pregnancy, there is increased tissue resistance to insulin with resultant increased levels of blood insulin as well as glucose and triglycerides. These changes result from placental lactogen and elevated estrogen and progesterone. Although pregnancy does not appear to alter the long-term conse-

quences of diabetes, retinopathy and nephropathy may appear or become worse during pregnancy. The White classification of diabetes during pregnancy (Table 17–10) has allowed description and comparison of diabetic pregnant women.

Even in carefully managed diabetics, the incidence of hydramnios, preeclampsia-eclampsia, infections, and prematurity is increased. Infants of diabetic women are larger than those of nondiabetic women. There is an increase in the number of third-trimester fetal deaths and a high rate of neonatal deaths. There is general agreement that the outcome of diabetic pregnancies is best among women managed by teams of experienced clinicians.

Prepregnancy metabolic evaluation of diabetic women is essential. Fasting and preprandial glucose values are lower in normal pregnant women; thus, the range of euglycemia is 60–80 mg/dL fasting and before meals. This is the target for good diabetic control during pregnancy. Glycosylated hemoglobin (HbA_{1c}) levels determine the quality of glucose control. Fair to good control is generally associated with levels of HbA_{1c} less than 8–9%. Euglycemia should be established before conception and maintained with patient-performed blood glucose monitoring at home four times daily and frequent small meals (six per day). Perinatal problems for mother and newborn are decreased by fastidious diabetic control.

Attempts are under way to decrease the number of congenital anomalies associated with diabetic pregnancies. Prepregnancy evaluation and adjustment of insulin control based on glycosylated hemoglobin will maintain strict euglycemia in early pregnancy when organogenesis is occurring. The use of a continuous insulin pump is currently limited to women with difficult, brittle diabetes. The timing of delivery is dictated by the quality of diabetic control, the presence or absence of medical complications, and fetal

Table 17–10. Modified White classification of diabetes mellitus.[1]

Class A: Chemical diabetes diagnosed *before pregnancy;* managed by diet *alone;* any age of onset or duration.

Class B: Insulin treatment necessary *before* pregnancy; onset after age 20; duration of less than 10 years.

Class C: Onset at age 10–19; or duration of 10–19 years.

Class D: Onset before age 10; or duration of 20 or more years; or chronic hypertension; or background retinopathy.

Class F: Renal disease.

Class H: Coronary artery disease.

Class R: Proliferative retinopathy.

Class T: Renal transplant.

[1]Reproduced, with permission, from Pernoll ML (editor): *Current Obstetric & Gynecologic Diagnosis & Treatment,* 7th ed. Appleton & Lange, 1991.

Table 17–11. Screening and diagnostic criteria for gestational diabetes mellitus.

Screening for gestational diabetes

1. 50-g oral glucose load, administered between the 24th and 28th weeks, without regard to time of day or time of last meal, to all pregnant women who have not been identified as having glucose intolerance before the 24th week.
2. Venous plasma glucose measured 1 hour later.
3. Value of 140 mg/dL (7.8 mmol/L) or above in venous plasma indicates the need for a full diagnostic glucose tolerance test.

Diagnosis of gestational diabetes mellitus

1. 100-g oral glucose load, administered in the morning after overnight fast lasting at least 8 hours but not more than 14 hours, and following at least 3 days of unrestricted diet (>150 g carbohydrate) and physical activity.
2. Venous plasma glucose is measured fasting and at 1, 2, and 3 hours. Subject should remain seated and not smoke throughout the test.
3. Two or more of the following venous plasma concentrations must be equaled or exceeded for positive diagnosis: fasting, 105 mg/dL (5.8 mmol/L); 1 hour, 190 mg/dL (10.6 mmol/L); 2 hours, 165 mg/dL (9.2 mmol/L); 3 hours, 145 mg/dL (8.1 mmol/L).

status. The goal is to achieve 39 weeks and then proceed with delivery. Confirmation of lung maturity is necessary only for delivery at 38 weeks of pregnancy or earlier. Cesarean sections are performed for obstetric indications.

Because 15% of patients with gestational diabetes require insulin during pregnancy and because the infants of gestational diabetics have some risks similar to those of infants of diabetic mothers (particularly macrosomia), screening of all pregnant women for glucose intolerance has been recommended between the 24th and 28th weeks of pregnancy (Table 17–11). Gestational diabetes should be evaluated 6–8 weeks postpartum by a 2-hour oral glucose tolerance test (75 g glucose load).

Kitzmiller J et al: Preconception care of diabetes: Glycemic control prevents congenital deformities. JAMA 1991; 265:731.

Heart Disease

Most cases of heart disease complicating pregnancy in the USA are congenital, with 5% of maternal deaths due to heart disease. Normal pregnancy causes a faster pulse, an increase of cardiac output of more than 30%, and a rise in plasma volume greater than red cell mass with relative hemodilution. Both vital capacity and oxygen consumption rise only slightly.

For practical purposes, the functional capacity of the heart is the best single measurement of cardiopulmonary status.

Class I: Ordinary physical activity causes no discomfort (perinatal mortality rate about 5%).

Class II: Ordinary activity causes discomfort and slight disability (perinatal mortality rate 10–15%).

Class III: Less than ordinary activity causes discomfort or disability; patient is barely compensated (perinatal mortality rate about 35%).

Class IV: Patient decompensated; any physical activity causes acute distress (perinatal mortality rate over 50%).

In general, patients with class I or class II functional disability (80% of pregnant women with heart disease) do well obstetrically, with four-fifths of maternal deaths due to heart disease occur in women with class III or class IV disability. Congestive failure is the usual cause of death. Most deaths occur in the early puerperium. Pregnancy is contraindicated in Eisenmenger's complex; in primary pulmonary hypertension; in severe mitral stenosis with secondary pulmonary hypertension; and in Marfan's syndrome, in which the aorta is prone to dissection and rupture. In addition, pregnancy is poorly tolerated in patients with aortic stenosis, aortic coarctation, tetralogy of Fallot, and active rheumatic carditis.

Therapeutic abortion and elective sterilization should be offered to patients with significant cardiac disease. Cesarean section should be performed only for obstetric indications. Appropriate antibiotic prophylaxis against infective endocarditis is indicated after delivery or termination of pregnancy.

Herpes Genitalis
(See also Chapter 6.)

Infection of the lower genital tract by herpes simplex virus type 2 (HSV-2) is a common sexually transmitted disease of potential seriousness to pregnant women and their newborn infants. Although up to 20% of women in an obstetric practice may have antibodies to HSV-2, a history of the infection is unreliable and the incidence of neonatal infection is low (1:20,000–1:3000 live births). Most infected neonates are born to women with no symptoms, signs, or history of infection.

Cesarean section is indicated at the time of labor if there are prodromal symptoms, active genital lesions, or a positive cervical culture obtained within the preceding week. Abdominal delivery is protective to the baby up to 4 hours after rupture of the membranes and perhaps longer.

Women who have had *primary* herpes infection late in pregnancy are at high risk of shedding virus at delivery. They should be screened by means of weekly cultures during the last month of pregnancy, because the neonatal attack rate is 50%.

Women with a history of recurrent genital herpes have a neonatal attack rate of 5% and should be followed by clinical observation and culture of any suspicious lesions. Since asymptomatic viral shedding is not predictable by antepartum cultures, current recommendations do not include routine cultures in individuals with a history of herpes without active disease. However, when labor begins, vulvar and cervical inspection and cultures should be performed, with prompt treatment of a newborn after a positive culture.

For treatment, see Chapter 37. The safety of acyclovir in pregnancy has not been established.

Prober CG et al: Use of routine viral cultures at delivery to identify neonates exposed to herpes simplex virus. N Engl J Med 1988;318:887.

Hypertensive Disease

Hypertensive disease in women of childbearing age is usually essential, but less common causes should be looked for: coarctation of the aorta, pheochromocytoma, aldosteronism, and renovascular and renal hypertension.

Preeclampsia is superimposed on 20% of pregnancies in hypertensive women and appears earlier, is more severe, and is more often associated with intrauterine growth retardation. It may be difficult to determine whether or not hypertension in a pregnant woman precedes or derives from the pregnancy if she is not examined until after the 20th week. Serum uric acid can help differentiate, since it is elevated with preeclampsia and normal in chronic hypertension. If hypertension persists for 6–8 weeks postpartum, essential hypertension is likely.

Pregnant women with chronic hypertension require medication only if the diastolic pressure is sustained at or above 100 mm Hg. For initiation of treatment, methyldopa is still the drug of choice. Start with 250 mg orally twice daily and increase in divided doses as needed to as much as 3 g daily. One should strive to keep the diastolic pressure between 80 and 100 mm Hg.

If a hypertensive woman is being managed successfully by medical treatment when she registers for antenatal care, one may generally continue the antihypertensive medication. Diuretics are usually discontinued in pregnancy and ACE inhibitors replaced by another drug.

Continued use of antihypertensive medications in preeclampsia remains controversial. This should be attempted only with significant fetal prematurity, absence of fetal compromise, and close supervision of the patient.

Therapeutic abortion may be indicated in cases of severe hypertension during pregnancy. If pregnancy is allowed to continue, the risk to the fetus must be assessed periodically in anticipation of early delivery. An early second-trimester ultrasound examination will confirm the duration of pregnancy, and follow-up examinations after 28 weeks will evaluate intrauterine growth retardation.

Dekker GA, van Geijn HP: Hypertensive disease in pregnancy. Curr Opin Obstet Gynecol 1992;4:10.

Maternal Hepatitis B Carrier State

There are an estimated 200 million chronic carriers of hepatitis B virus worldwide. Among these people there is an increased incidence of chronic active hepatitis, cirrhosis, and hepatocellular carcinoma. The frequency of the hepatitis B carrier state varies from 1% in the USA and Western Europe to 35% in parts of Africa and Asia. All pregnant women should be screened for hepatitis B surface antigen (HBsAg). Transmission of the virus to the baby after delivery is likely if both surface antigen and e antigen are positive. Vertical transmission can be blocked by the immediate postdelivery administration to the newborn of 0.5 mL of hepatitis B immunoglobulin and hepatitis B vaccine intramuscularly. The vaccine dose is repeated at 1 and 6 months of age.

Centers for Disease Control: Hepatitis B virus: A comprehensive strategy for eliminating transmission in the United States through universal childhood vaccination: Recommendations of the Immunization Practices Advisory Committee. MMWR Morb Mortal Wkly Rep 1991;40 RR 13:1.

Seizure Disorders

Women contemplating pregnancy who have not had a seizure for 5 years should consider a prepregnancy trial of withdrawal from seizure medication. Those with recurrent epilepsy should use a single drug with blood level monitoring. Trimethadione and valproate are contraindicated during pregnancy; phenytoin is also considered teratogenic and should not be used unless absolutely necessary. Phenobarbital is considered the drug of choice. Serum levels should be measured at least monthly and dosage adjustments made to keep serum levels in the low normal therapeutic range. Pregnant women taking these drugs should receive vitamin supplements, including folic acid and vitamin D, throughout pregnancy. Vitamin K, 20 mg/d, is administered during the last month to help prevent bleeding problems in the newborn, who are at risk of bleeding tendencies due to decreased levels of clotting factors. Such infants should receive an injection of vitamin K_1, 1 mg given subcutaneously immediately after delivery, and should have clotting studies 2–4 hours later. Breast feeding is not contraindicated.

Yerby MS: Problems and management of the pregnant woman with epilepsy. Epilepsia 1987;28(Suppl 3):529.

Syphilis, Gonorrhea, & *Chlamydia trachomatis* Infection
(See also Chapters 32 and 33.)

These sexually transmitted diseases have significant consequences for mother and child. Untreated syphilis in pregnancy will cause late abortion or transplacental infection with congenital syphilis. Gonorrhea will produce large-joint arthritis by hematogenous spread as well as newborn eye damage. Maternal chlamydial infections are largely asymptomatic but are manifested in the newborn by inclusion conjunctivitis and, at age 2–4 months, by pneumonia. The diagnosis of each can be reliably made by appropriate laboratory tests, which should be included in all prenatal care. The sexual partners of women with sexually transmitted diseases should be identified and treated also if that can be done.

Thyrotoxicosis

Thyrotoxicosis during pregnancy may result in fetal anomalies, late abortion, or preterm labor and fetal hyperthyroidism with goiter. Thyroid storm in late pregnancy or labor is a life-threatening emergency.

Radioactive isotope therapy must never be given during pregnancy. The thyroid inhibitor of choice is propylthiouracil, which acts to prevent further thyroxine formation by blocking iodination of tyrosine. There is a 2 to 3-week delay before the pretreatment hormone level begins to fall. The initial dose of propylthiouracil is 100–150 mg three times a day; the dose is lowered as the euthyroid state is approached. It is desirable to keep thyroxine in the high normal range during pregnancy. A maintenance dose of 100 mg/d minimizes the chance of fetal hypothyroidism and goiter. Elective thyroidectomy is recommended by some in preference to medical management during and even after pregnancy (see Chapter 25).

Recurrent postpartum thyroiditis is a newly recognized entity occurring 3–6 months after delivery. A hyperthyroid state of 1–3 months' duration is followed by hypothyroidism, sometimes misdiagnosed as depression. Microsomal thyroid antibodies and thyroglobulin antibodies are present. Recovery is spontaneous in over 90% of cases after 3–6 months.

Tuberculosis

The diagnosis of tuberculosis in pregnancy is made by history taking, physical examination, and skin testing, with special attention to women from ethnic groups with a high prevalence of the disease (such as women from southeast Asia). Chest films should not be obtained as a routine screening measure in pregnancy but should be used only in patients with a skin test conversion or with suggestive findings in the history and physical examination. Abdominal shielding must be used if a chest film is obtained.

If adequately treated, tuberculosis in pregnancy has an excellent prognosis. There is no increase in spontaneous abortion, fetal problems, or congenital anomalies in patients receiving antituberculosis chemotherapy.

Treatment is with isoniazid and ethambutol or isoniazid and rifampin. Because isoniazid therapy may

result in vitamin B_6 deficiency, a supplement of 50 mg/d of vitamin B_6 should be given simultaneously. Streptomycin, ethionamide, and most other antituberculous drugs should be avoided in pregnancy.

Urinary Tract Infection

The urinary tract is especially vulnerable to infections during pregnancy because the altered secretions of steroid sex hormones and the pressure exerted by the gravid uterus upon the ureters and bladder cause hypotonia and congestion and predispose to urinary stasis. Labor and delivery and urinary retention postpartum also may initiate or aggravate infection. *Escherichia coli* is the offending organism in over two-thirds of cases.

From 2% to 8% of pregnant women have asymptomatic bacteriuria, which some believe to be associated with an increased risk of prematurity. It is estimated that 20–40% of these women will develop pyelonephritis during pregnancy.

A first-trimester urine culture is indicated in women with a history of recurrent or recent episodes of urinary tract infection. If the culture is positive, treatment should be initiated as a prophylactic measure. Sulfisoxazole, nitrofurantoin, penicillins, and cephalosporins are acceptable medications for 7–10 days. Sulfonamides should not be given in the third trimester. If bacteriuria returns, suppressive medication (one daily dose of an appropriate antibiotic) for the remainder of the pregnancy is indicated. Acute pyelonephritis requires hospitalization for intravenous administration of antibiotics until the patient is afebrile; this is followed by a full course of oral antibiotics.

SURGICAL COMPLICATIONS DURING PREGNANCY

Elective major surgery should be avoided during pregnancy. Normal uncomplicated pregnancy does not alter operative risk except as it may interfere with the diagnosis of abdominal disorders and increase the technical problems of intra-abdominal surgery. Abortion is not a serious hazard after operation unless peritoneal sepsis or other significant complication occurs. During the first trimester, congenital anomalies may be induced in the developing fetus by hypoxia. Thus, the second trimester is usually the optimal time for operative procedures.

The second trimester is usually the optimal time for elective operative procedures.

Appendicitis

Appendicitis occurs in about one of 5000 pregnancies. Diagnosis is difficult, since the appendix is carried high and to the right, away from McBurney's point, as the uterus enlarges, and localization of pain does not usually occur. Nausea, vomiting, fever, and leukocytosis occur regularly. Any right-sided abdominal pain associated with these symptoms should arouse the suspicion. In at least 20% of obstetric patients, the diagnosis of appendicitis is not made until rupture occurs and peritonitis has become established. Such a delay may lead to premature labor or abortion. With early diagnosis and appendectomy, the prognosis is good for mother and baby.

Carcinoma of the Breast

Cancer of the breast (see also Chapter 16) is diagnosed approximately once in 3500 pregnancies. Pregnancy may accelerate the growth of cancer of the breast, and delay in diagnosis affects the outcome of treatment more significantly. Inflammatory carcinoma is an extremely virulent type of breast cancer that occurs most commonly during lactation. Prepregnancy mammography should be encouraged for women over age 35 who are anticipating a pregnancy.

Breast enlargement during pregnancy obscures parenchymal masses, and breast tissue hyperplasia decreases the accuracy of mammography. Any discrete mass should be evaluated by aspiration to verify its cystic structure, with fine-needle biopsy if it is solid. A definitive diagnosis may require excisional biopsy under local anesthesia. If breast biopsy confirms the diagnosis of cancer, surgery should be done regardless of the stage of the pregnancy. If spread to the regional glands has occurred, irradiation or chemotherapy should be considered. Under these circumstances, the alternatives are termination of an early pregnancy and delay of therapy for fetal maturation.

Choledocholithiasis, Cholecystitis, & Idiopathic Cholestasis of Pregnancy

Severe choledocholithiasis and cholecystitis are not common during pregnancy. When they do occur, it is usually in late pregnancy or in the puerperium. About 90% of patients with cholecystitis have gallstones; 90% of stones will be visualized by ultrasonography. Symptomatic relief may be all that is required.

Gallbladder surgery in pregnant women should be attempted only in extreme cases (eg, obstruction), because it increases the perinatal mortality rate to about 15%. Cholecystostomy and lithotomy may be all that is feasible during advanced pregnancy, cholecystectomy being deferred until after delivery. On the other hand, withholding surgery may result in necrosis and perforation of the gallbladder and peritonitis. Cholangitis due to impacted common duct stone requires surgical removal of gallstones and establishment of biliary drainage. Endoscopic retrograde cholangiopancreatography and endoscopic retrograde sphincterotomy can be performed safely in pregnant women if precautions are taken to minimize exposure to radiation.

Idiopathic cholestasis of pregnancy is due to a hereditary metabolic (hepatic) deficiency aggravated by the high estrogen levels of pregnancy. It causes intrahepatic biliary obstruction of varying degrees. The rise in bile acids is sufficient in the third trimester to cause severe, intractable, generalized itching and sometimes clinical jaundice. There may be mild elevations in blood bilirubin and alkaline phosphatase levels. The fetus is generally unaffected, although an increased prematurity rate has been reported. Resins such as cholestyramine (4 g three times a day) absorb bile acids in the large bowel and relieve pruritus but are difficult to take and may cause constipation. Their use requires vitamin K supplementation. The disorder is relieved once the infant has been delivered, but it recurs in subsequent pregnancies and sometimes with the use of oral contraceptives.

Ovarian Tumors

The most common adnexal mass in early pregnancy is the corpus luteum, which may become cystic and enlarge to 6 cm in diameter. Any persistent mass over 6 cm should be evaluated by ultrasound examination; unilocular cysts are likely to be corpus luteum cysts, whereas septated or semisolid tumors are likely to be neoplasms. The incidence of malignancy in ovarian masses over 6 cm diameter is 2.5%. Ovarian tumors may undergo torsion and cause abdominal pain and nausea and vomiting and must be differentiated from appendicitis, other bowel disease, and ectopic pregnancy. Patients with suspected ovarian cancer should be referred to a gynecologic oncologist to determine whether the pregnancy can progress to fetal viability or whether treatment should be instituted without delay.

Allen JR, Helling TS, Langenfeld M: Intra-abdominal surgery during pregnancy. Am J Surg 1989;158:567.
Mazze R, Kallen B: Reproductive outcome after anesthesia and operation during pregnancy: A registry study of 5405 cases. Am J Obstet Gynecol 1989;161:1178.

PREVENTION OF HEMOLYTIC DISEASE OF THE NEWBORN (Erythroblastosis Fetalis)

The antibody anti-Rh_o (D) is responsible for most severe instances of hemolytic disease of the newborn (erythroblastosis fetalis). About 15% of whites and much lower proportions of blacks and Asians are Rh_o (D)negative. If an Rh_o (D)-negative woman carries an Rh_o (D)-positive fetus, she may develop antibodies against Rh_o (D) when fetal red cells enter her circulation at delivery (or during abortion, ectopic pregnancy, abruptio placentae, or other antepartum bleeding problems). This antibody, once produced, remains in the woman's circulation and poses the threat of hemolytic disease for subsequent Rh-positive fetuses.

Passive immunization against hemolytic disease of the newborn is achieved with Rh_o (D) immune globulin, a purified concentrate of antibodies against Rh_o (D) antigen. The Rh_o (D) immune globulin is given within 72 hours after delivery (or spontaneous or induced abortion or ectopic pregnancy). The antibodies in the immune globulin destroy fetal Rh-positive cells so that the mother will not produce anti-Rh_o (D). During her next Rh-positive gestation, erythroblastosis will be prevented. The usual dose of Rh_o (D) immune globulin for prevention of isoimmunization is one vial (300 mg) intramuscularly.

It has recently been demonstrated that a rare Rh-negative woman will become sensitized by small fetomaternal bleeding episodes in the early third trimester. An additional safety measure is the administration of the immune globulin at the 28th week of pregnancy. The antibody molecules are too large to pass through the placenta and affect an Rh-positive fetus. The maternal clearance of the globulin is slow enough that protection will continue for 12 weeks.

Mild to moderate degrees of hemolytic disease continue to occur in association with Rh subgroups (C, c, or E) or Kell, Kidd, and other factors. Therefore, atypical antibodies should be checked in the third trimester of all pregnancies.

Rodeck CH, Letsky E: How the management of erythroblastosis fetalis has changed. Brit J Obstet Gynecol 1989;96:759.

PREVENTION OF PRETERM (PREMATURE) LABOR

Preterm (premature) labor is labor that begins before the 37th week of pregnancy; it is responsible for 85% of neonatal illnesses and deaths. The onset of labor is a result of a complex sequence of biologic events involving regulatory factors that are still poorly understood. The most significant risk factors for the onset of preterm labor are a past history of preterm delivery, premature rupture of the membranes, urinary tract infection, or exposure to diethylstilbestrol. In the current pregnancy, multiple gestation and abdominal or cervical surgery are especially important. To estimate the clinical risk, see Table 17–12.

Low rates of preterm delivery are associated with success in educating patients to identify regular, frequent uterine contractions and in alerting medical and nursing staff to evaluate these patients early and initiate treatment if cervical changes can be identified. Cessation of work or physical activities that seem related to increased uterine activity is mandatory. Resting at home will often suffice to slow contractions. Portable lightweight monitors of uterine contractions permit a woman to record uterine activity at will or on a schedule and to transmit the data by telephone to a central terminal for analysis.

In more acute situations, intravenous magnesium sulfate in doses similar to those used for the treatment of preeclampsia is an effective tocolytic and can be used before intravenous beta-adrenergic drugs are initiated. Magnesium sulfate is given as a 4- or 6-g bolus, followed by a continuous infusion of 2–3 g/h. The rate may be increased by 1 g/h every 1½–2 hours until contractions cease or a blood magnesium concentration of 6–8 mg/dL is reached. Magnesium levels are determined every 4–6 hours to monitor the therapeutic blood level. After contractions have ceased for 24–48 hours, magnesium can be stopped and the situation reassessed.

Uterine smooth muscle is largely under sympathetic nervous system control, and stimulation of β_2 receptors relaxes the myometrium. Consequently, inhibition of uterine contractility often can be accomplished by the administration of beta-adrenergic drugs such as ritodrine or terbutaline.

Ritodrine can be administered by intravenous infusion in lactated Ringer's solution, beginning at a rate of 50 mg/min and increasing by 50 mg/min every 20 minutes until contractions cease or become less frequent than every 10 minutes or until an infusion rate of 350 mg/min is reached. After 1 hour of satisfactory tocolysis, the infusion rate can be decreased by 50 mg/min every 30 minutes to a rate that continues inhibition. If labor recurs, the step-up and step-down regimen can be reinstituted. Oral therapy is started 30 minutes before stopping intravenous ritodrine and is continued in a dose of 10–20 mg every 4–6 hours. A dose-related elevation of heart rate of 20–40 beats/min may occur. An increase of systolic blood pressure up to 10 mm Hg is likely, and the diastolic pressure may fall 10–15 mm Hg during the infusion. Nonetheless, cardiac output increases considerably. Transient elevation of blood glucose, insulin, and fatty acids together with slight reduction of serum potassium have been reported. Fetal tachycardia may be slight or absent. No drug-caused perinatal deaths have been reported. Maternal side effects requiring dose limitation are tachycardia ($\geq$ 120 beats/min), palpitations, and nervousness. Fluids should be limited to 2500 mL/24 h. Serious side effects (pulmonary edema, chest pain with or without electrocardiographic changes) are often idiosyncratic, not dose-related, and warrant termination of therapy.

One must identify cases in which untimely delivery is the sole threat to the life or health of the infant. An effort should be made to eliminate (1) maternal conditions that compromise the intrauterine environment and make premature birth the lesser risk, eg, preeclampsia-eclampsia; (2) fetal conditions that either are helped by early delivery or render attempts to stop premature labor meaningless, eg, severe erythroblastosis fetalis; and (3) clinical situations in which it is likely that an attempt to stop labor will be futile, eg, ruptured membranes, cervix fully effaced and dilated more than 3 cm, strong labor in progress.

Table 17–12. Risk of preterm delivery.[1]

Score[2]	Socioeconomic Status	Past History	Daily Habits	Current Pregnancy	
				Mother	Fetus
1	2 children at home. Low socioeconomic status	One first trimester abortion. Less than 1 year since last birth.	Work outside home.	Unusual fatigue.	...
2	Under 20 years of age. Over 40 years of age. Single parent.	Two first trimester abortions.	More than 10 cigarettes per day.	Less than 12 lb weight gain by 32 weeks. Albuminuria. Hypertension. Bacteriuria.	...
3	Very low socioeconomic status. Malnourished. Shorter than 150 cm (5 ft). Weighs less than 45 cm (100 lb).	Three first trimester abortions.	Unusual anxiety. Heavy work. Long, tiring travel. Long commute distance.	Weight loss of 2 kg. Febrile illness. Leiomyomas.	Head engaged before 34 weeks.
4	Under 18 years of age.	Pyelonephritis.	...	Uterine bleeding after 12 weeks. Effacement or dilation of cervix before 36 weeks. Uterine irritability.	...
5	...	Uterine anomaly. Second trimester abortion. Cone biopsy.	...	Placenta previa. Hydramnios.	...
10	...	Premature delivery. DES exposure. Repeated second trimester abortion.	...	Abdominal surgery. Cervical surgery.	Twins. Small-for-dates fetus.

[1]Modified and reproduced, with permission, from Zuspan FK, Quilligan EJ (editors): *Practical Manual of Obstetric Care.* Mosby, 1982. (Modified from Creasy R: Personal communication.)
[2]Score is computed by addition of the number of points given any item in any column. 0–5 = minimal risk; 6–9 = moderate risk; 10 or more = high risk.

In pregnancies of less than 34 weeks' duration, betamethasone (12 mg intramuscularly repeated in 24 hours) is administered to hasten fetal lung maturation and permit delivery 48 hours after initial treatment when prolongation of pregnancy is contraindicated.

Besinger RE, Niebyl JR: The safety and efficacy of tocolytic agents for the treatment of preterm labor. Obstet Gynecol Surv 1990;45:415.
Katz M, Goodyear K, Creasey RK: Early signs and symptoms of preterm labor. Am J Obstet Gynecol 1990; 162:1150.

LACTATION

Breast feeding should be encouraged by educative measures throughout pregnancy and the puerperium. Mothers should be told the benefits of breast feeding—it is emotionally satisfying, promotes mother-infant bonding, is economical, and gives significant immunity to the infant. The period of amenorrhea associated with frequent and consistent breast feeding provides good birth control until menstruation begins at 6–12 months postpartum or the intensity of breast feeding diminishes. If the mother must return to work, even a brief period of nursing is beneficial. Transfer of immunoglobulins in colostrum and breast milk protects the infant against many systemic and enteric infections. Macrophages and lymphocytes transferred to the infant from breast milk play an immunoprotective role. The intestinal flora of breast-fed infants inhibits the growth of pathogens. Breast-fed infants have fewer bacterial and viral infections, less severe diarrhea, fewer allergy problems, and less subsequent obesity than bottle-fed infants.

Frequent breast feeding on an infant demand schedule enhances milk flow and successful breast feeding. Mothers breast feeding for the first time need help and encouragement from physicians, nurses, and other nursing mothers. Milk supply can be increased by increased suckling and increased rest.

Nursing mothers should have a fluid intake of over 2 L/d. The United States RDA calls for 21 g of extra protein (over the 44 g/d baseline for an adult woman) and 550 extra kcal/d in the first 6 months of nursing.

Table 17–13. Common drugs or substances to be used cautiously or not at all by nursing mothers.[1] (Additional drugs are also contraindicated during pregnancy and lactation. Evaluate any drug for its need and its potential adverse effects.)

Drugs or Substances	Effect on Nursing Infant
Alcohol	No harmful effects unless taken in excess, when it can be associated with decreased linear growth and sedation.
Antibiotics	
Aminoglycosides	Not advised; will alter infant's bowel flora.
Nitrofurantoin	May cause hemolytic anemia in infant with glucose-6-phosphate dehydrogenase (G6PD) deficiency.
Tetracycline	Effects are dose-related; amount infant receives from milk is too small to cause discoloration of teeth. Safe.
Chloramphenicol[2]	Neonate may be unable to conjugate the drug; potential harm to bone marrow, leading to anemia, shock, and death.
Sulfonamides[2]	May cause jaundice in the neonatal period; may cause hemolytic anemia in infant with glucose-6-phosphate dehydrogenase (G6PD) deficiency.
Metronidazole	Nursing may be resumed 48 hours after last dose.
Anticoagulants	
Phenindione[2]	Can use heparin or warfarin instead.
Antihistamines	Contraindicated because of increased sensitivity of newborns and infants to antihistamines.
Antineoplastics[2]	Suspend nursing if these drugs are taken.
Antithyroids	
Thiouracil;[2] methimazole[2]	Contraindicated; may cause goiter or agranulocytosis.
Propylthiouracil	Considered safe.
Cardiac drugs	
Quinidine[2]	Contraindicated; may cause arrhythmia in infant.
Cimetidine,[2] ranitidine	Concentrated in breast milk; may suppress gastric acidity and cause central nervous system stimulation.
Ergot alkaloids	
Ergotamine (in doses to treat migraine)[2]	Causes vomiting, diarrhea, convulsions. May suppress lactation.
Bromocriptine[2]	Suppresses lactation.
Gold salts[2]	Contraindicated.
Hormones	
Oral contraceptives	Contraindicated; may cause reduction of milk supply. Progestin-only minipill may be used.
Laxatives	
Cascara, senna	Can cause diarrhea in infant.
Lithium carbonate[2]	Contraindicated because of toxicity.
Nicotine	Increased respiratory disease in infants exposed to smoke.
Radioactive materials for testing[2]	
^{67}Ga	Insignificant amount excreted in milk; no nursing for 2 weeks.
^{125}I	Discontinue nursing for 48 hours.
^{131}I	After a test dose, nursing may be resumed after 24–36 hours; after a treatment dose, nursing may be resumed after 2–3 weeks.
^{99m}Tc	Discontinue nursing for 72 hours (half-life, 6 hours).
Sedatives and tranquilizers	Can cause sedation in infant. Benzodiazepines should be avoided.
Other drugs	
Caffeine	Irritability, poor sleep pattern with large amounts.
Cannabis;[2] cocaine;[2] polyhalogenated biphenyls[2] (eg, PCBs, PBBs); D-lysergic acid[2] (LSD)	Contraindicated; may interfere with mother's caretaking abilities and nutrition.

[1]Modified and reproduced, with permission, from Sahu S: Drugs and the nursing mother. Am Fam Physician (Dec) 1981;24:137.
[2]Absolutely contraindicated.

Calcium intake should be 1200 mg/d. Continuation of a prenatal vitamin and mineral supplement is wise. Strict vegetarians who eschew both milk and eggs should always take vitamin B_{12} supplements during pregnancy and lactation.

Effects of Drugs in a Nursing Mother

Drugs taken by a nursing mother may accumulate in milk and be transmitted to the infant. The amount of a drug entering the milk depends on the drug's lipid solubility, mechanism of transport, and degree of ionization (Table 17–13).

Suppression of Lactation

A. Mechanical Suppression: The simplest and safest method of suppressing lactation after it has started is to gradually transfer the baby to a bottle or a cup over a 3-week period. Milk supply will decrease with decreased demand, and minimal discomfort ensues. If nursing must be stopped abruptly, the mother should avoid nipple stimulation, refrain from expressing milk, and use a snug brassiere. Ice packs and analgesics can be helpful. If suppression is desired before nursing has begun, use this same technique. Engorgement will gradually recede over a 2 to 3-day period.

B. Hormonal Suppression: Oral and long-acting injections of hormonal preparations are available to suppress lactation. They are all effective if begun at the time of delivery but have occasional side effects—increased thromboembolic episodes (estrogens), hair growth (androgens), changes in blood pressure, and temporary emotional changes (bromocriptine).

1. Suppression with estrogens—Ethinyl estradiol, 0.05 mg, is administered as follows:

a. Four tablets (0.2 mg) twice daily on the first postpartum day.

b. Three tablets (0.15 mg) twice daily on the second day.

c. Two tablets (0.1 mg) twice daily on the third day.

d. One tablet (0.05 mg) twice daily on the fourth to seventh days.

2. Suppression with estrogen and androgens—Testosterone enanthate, 180 mg/mL, and estradiol valerate, 8 mg/mL, 2 mL injected intramuscularly immediately after delivery, are very effective.

3. Suppression with bromocriptine—Bromocriptine, 2.5 mg orally twice daily with meals for 10–14 days, will suppress lactation in women who do not wish to nurse their infants or after stillbirth or abortion. Rebound lactation may occur when the drug is discontinued. The drug should not be started until 4 hours postpartum, when vital signs are stable. Postural hypotension, nausea, headache, dizziness, nasal congestion, and mild constipation have been noted as side effects. These symptoms can be allayed by reducing the dose of the drug temporarily. Hypertension, seizures, strokes, and myocardial infarctions have also been reported in a small number of women. Because of this possibility, the drug should not be used in patients with pregnancy-induced hypertension and should be discontinued if severe headache or visual disturbances occur. Blood pressure should be monitored carefully throughout the duration of bromocriptine use.

Watson DL et al: Bromocriptine mesylate for lactation suppression: A risk for postpartum hypertension. Obstet Gynecol 1989;74:573.

PUERPERAL MASTITIS (See also Chapter 16.)

Postpartum mastitis occurs sporadically in nursing mothers shortly after they return home, or it may occur in epidemic form in the hospital. *Staphylococcus aureus* is usually the causative agent. Inflammation is generally unilateral, and women nursing for the first time are more often affected.

Mastitis frequently begins within 3 months after delivery and may start with a sore or fissured nipple. There is obvious cellulitis in an area of breast tissue, with redness, tenderness, local warmth, and fever. Treatment consists of antibiotics effective against penicillin-resistant staphylococci (dicloxacillin or a cephalosporin) and regular emptying of the breast by nursing followed by expression of any remaining milk by hand or with a mechanical suction device.

If the mother begins antibiotic therapy before suppuration begins, infection can usually be controlled in 24 hours. If delay is permitted, breast abscess can result. Incision and drainage are required for abscess formation. Despite puerperal mastitis, the baby usually thrives without prophylactic antimicrobial therapy.

REFERENCES

Callen P: *Ultrasonography in Obstetrics and Gynecology,* 2nd ed. Saunders, 1988.

Cunningham FG, Macdonald PC, Gant NF: *Williams Obstetrics,* 18th ed. Appleton & Lange, 1989.

Gleicher N (editor): *Principles and Practices of Medical*

Therapy in Pregnancy, 2nd ed. Appleton & Lange, 1992.

Hatcher RA et al: *Contraceptive Technology, 1990–1992,* 15th rev ed. Irvington, 1990.

Kaplan HS et al: *The Evaluation of Sexual Disorders: Psychological and Medical Aspects.* Brunner-Mazel, 1983.

Pernoll M, Benson RC (editors): *Current Obstetric & Gynecologic Diagnosis & Treatment,* 7th ed. Appleton & Lange, 1991.

Ryan KJ, Berkowitz R, Barbieri RL: *Kistner's Gynecology: Principles and Practice,* 5th ed. Year Book, 1990.

Scott JR et al: *Danforth's Obstetrics and Gynecology,* 6th ed. Lippincott, 1990.

Speroff L, Glass R, Kase N: *Clinical Gynecologic Endocrinology and Infertility,* 4th ed. Williams & Wilkins, 1989.

Worthington-Roberts BS, Vermeersch J, Williams SL: *Nutrition in Pregnancy and Lactation,* 4th ed. Mosby, 1989.

18 Allergic & Immunologic Disorders

Daniel C. Adelman, MD, & Abba Terr, MD

A wide variety of diseases are associated with disordered immune responses. Knowledge of immunoglobulin structure and function and of the cellular basis of immunity has resulted in a better understanding of these disorders. Diseases of immunity are usually caused by pathologic imbalances resulting from either excesses or deficiencies of immunocompetent cells or their products that disrupt normal homeostasis. This chapter provides a brief overview of basic and clinical immunology as an approach to the patient with an allergic or immunologic disease.

IMMUNOGLOBULINS & ANTIBODIES

IMMUNOGLOBULIN STRUCTURE & FUNCTION

Immunoglobulins, which represent about 25% of plasma proteins, are specialized molecules that possess antibody activity. The basic unit of all immunoglobulins consists of four polypeptide chains linked by disulfide bonds. There are two identical heavy chains (MW 55,000–70,000) and two identical light chains (MW about 23,000). Both heavy and light chains have a C-terminal constant (C) region and an N-terminal variable (V) region. A hypervariable portion of the V regions of heavy and light chains folded together in a three-dimensional conformation form the combining site, which is responsible for the specific interaction with antigen.

Antibodies contain one of five classes of heavy chains (γ, α, μ, δ, ε) and one of two types of light chains (κ and λ). Either type of light chain can be associated with each of the heavy chain classes. Approximately 60% of human immunoglobulins have κ light chains, and 40% have λ light chains. About 10 million different antibody specificities are thought to exist in a given individual.

Immunoglobulin Classes

A. Immunoglobulin M (IgM): IgM is made up of five identical basic immunoglobulin units. These units are connected to one another by disulfide bonds and a small polypeptide known as the J chain. The molecular weight of IgM is about 900,000. The IgM molecule is found predominantly in the intravascular compartment and on the surface of B lymphocytes and does not normally cross the placenta. IgM antibody predominates early in immune responses; carbohydrate antigens such as blood group substances stimulate IgM.

B. Immunoglobulin A (IgA): IgA is present in blood and in relatively high concentrations in saliva, colostrum, tears, and secretions of the bronchi and gastrointestinal tract. Serum IgA is a single immunoglobulin unit, whereas secretory IgA is made up of two units connected to each other by a J chain. A 70,000-MW molecule called secretory component is attached to the Fc portion. It is necessary to transport IgA into the lumens of exocrine glands, and it confers resistance to enzymatic destruction. Secretory IgA plays an important role in host defense against viral and bacterial infections by blocking transport of microbes across mucosa.

C. Immunoglobulin G (IgG): IgG is a single immunoglobulin unit of MW 150,000 that comprises about 85% of total serum immunoglobulins. IgG is distributed in the extracellular fluid and is the only immunoglobulin that normally crosses the placenta. IgG binds complement via an Fc receptor present in the constant region of the heavy chain. IgG binds to the surface of cells and microbes, which allows them to be phagocytosed or killed by cytotoxic cells.

D. Immunoglobulin E (IgE): IgE is present in serum in very low concentrations as a single immunoglobulin unit with heavy chains. Approximately 50% of patients with allergic diseases have increased serum IgE levels. IgE is a skin-sensitizing or reaginic antibody by virtue of attachment to mast cells. The specific interaction between antigen and IgE bound to the surface of mast cells results in the release of inflammatory products such as histamine, leukotrienes, proteases and chemotactic factors. These mediators can result in bronchospasm, vasodilation, smooth muscle contraction, and chemoattraction of other inflammatory and immune cells.

E. Immunoglobulin D (IgD): IgD is present in

the serum in very low concentrations as a single basic immunoglobulin unit with eavy chains. IgD is found on the surface of most B lymphocytes in association with IgM, where it probably serves as a receptor for antigen.

Goodman JW: Immunoglobulins: Structure and function. In: *Basic & Clinical Immunology,* 7th ed. Stites DP, Terr AI (editors). Appleton & Lange, 1991.
Hasemann CA, Capra JD: Immunoglobulins: Structure and function. In: *Fundamental Immunology,* 2nd ed. Paul WE (editor). Raven Press, 1989.

Immunoglobulin Genes

Genes that code for immunoglobulin light and heavy chain molecules undergo rearrangements in the DNA of B cells, which result in the synthesis and expression of the highly diverse group of immunoglobulin molecules. Clonal rearrangements of immunoglobulin genes in B cells are useful for determining the lineage of many leukemias and lymphomas.

Parlsow TG: Immunoglobulin genetics. In: *Basic & Clinical Immunology,* 7th ed. Stites DP, Terr AI (editors). Appleton & Lange, 1991.

Tests for Immunoglobulins

Immunoglobulin levels can be elevated or reduced in a large number of diseases. In some diseases, particularly gammopathies (see below), increased serum immunoglobulins, especially monoclonal types, are critical for diagnosis. In other diseases such as chronic liver diseases, chronic infection, or idiopathic inflammatory states, polyclonal increases in immunoglobulins are incidental or of unknown significance. If immunodeficiency is suspected in the presence of recurrent bacterial infections, measurement of serum immunoglobulins provides an essential test of B cell and plasma cell function. In acquired immune deficiencies such as AIDS, with many recurrent infections, paradoxical increases in immunoglobulins may occur.

Antibodies and immunoglobulins can be measured in three ways: (1) by quantitative and qualitative determinations of serum immunoglobulins; (2) by determination of isohemagglutinin and febrile agglutinin titers; and (3) by determination of antibody titers following immunization with tetanus toxoid, diphtheria toxoid, or pertussis vaccines. The first method tests for the presence of serum immunoglobulins but not for the functional adequacy of the immunoglobulins. The second method tests for functional antibodies that are present in the serum of almost all individuals as a consequence of exposure to blood group substances or infection. The third method examines functional antibody activity in the serum after intentional immunization. Commonly used clinical tests of antibody immunity, for many diseases, are protein

electrophoresis, immunoelectrophoresis, and quantitative immunoglobulin determinations.

Protein Electrophoresis & Immunoelectrophoresis

Protein electrophoresis is a screening test to measure semiquantitatively various proteins in body fluids, usually serum or urine. Proteins are electrically separated on a strip of cellulose acetate on the basis of charge into albumin, α_1, α_2, β, and γ globulins. The relative concentration of gamma globulins that contains nearly all immunoglobulins is determined with protein stains. This test is useful to screen for diseases with excess or deficiency of immunoglobulins.

Immunoelectrophoresis is used to identify the specific immunoglobulin class in a body fluid. Serum, for example, is separated electrophoretically and then reacted with appropriate antisera directed against IgG, IgA, or IgM. The resulting patterns produced allow identification of abnormal immunoglobulins such as myeloma (M) proteins. This method is also useful in differentiation of monoclonal from polyclonal increases in immunoglobulins. It is only semiquantitative and thus cannot be used to determine immunoglobulin levels precisely, eg, in Waldenström's macroglobulinemia.

Another similar technique called immunofixation electrophoresis has to a large extent replaced immunoelectrophoresis. With this technique, serum proteins are separated electrophoretically in a gel and then immunoprecipitated in situ with monospecific antisera. Those proteins not precipitated are then washed away and the remaining immunoprecipitation bands revealed by protein staining. This method has the advantages of more rapid results and slightly higher resolution of low levels of monoclonal immunoglobulin chains. If protein electrophoresis is normal despite suspicion of an M protein, immunoelectrophoresis or immunofixation electrophoresis of both serum and concentrated urine should be performed because of the greater sensitivity of these tests.

Quantitative Immunoglobulin Determinations: Radial Diffusion & Nephelometry Techniques

Quantitative determinations of serum IgG, IgA, and IgM levels can be made using the radial diffusion technique. Circular wells are cut in a gel plate impregnated with a specific antiserum directed against a single human immunoglobulin class. The radius or diameter of the circular precipitin ring is proportionate to the concentration of serum immunoglobulin. The precise immunoglobulin level is determined by comparing the diameter of the unknown serum to that of a standard containing known levels of immunoglobulins.

Determinations of the serum concentrations of

IgM, IgG, and IgA can also be made accurately and rapidly by nephelometry. This method employs an instrument to measure the turbidity produced by the interaction of immunoglobulin and anti-immunoglobulin complexes. It is much more rapid than radial diffusion and is useful for measuring a wide spectrum of serum proteins. The measurement of immunoglobulin levels alone does not distinguish monoclonal immunoglobulins, as does the immunoelectrophoresis or immunofixation electrophoresis procedure.

IgD levels have no recognized clinical use, and IgE levels must be measured with more sensitive techniques such as radioimmunoassay or enzyme-linked immunoassay.

Stites DP, Rodgers RP: Clinical laboratory tests for detection of antigens and antibodies. In: *Basic & Clinical Immunology,* 7th ed. Stites DP, Terr AI (editors). Appleton & Lange, 1991.

DISEASES OF IMMUNOGLOBULIN OVERPRODUCTION (Gammopathies)

The monoclonal gammopathies include those disease entities in which there is a disproportionate proliferation of a single clone of immunoglobulin-forming cells that produce a homogeneous heavy chain, light chain, or complete molecule. The amino acid sequence of the variable (V) regions is fixed, and only one type (κ or λ) of light chain is produced. Polyclonal gammopathies result from proliferation of many B cell clones, which results in a diffuse increase of immunoglobulins.

Benign Monoclonal Gammopathy

The diagnosis is made upon finding a homogeneous (monoclonal) immunoglobulin (with either κ or λ chains but not both) in immunoelectrophoresis of the serum. The incidence of homogeneous serum immunoglobulins increases with age and may approach 3% in persons 70 years of age or older. As many as 20% of individuals with apparently benign monoclonal gammopathies will eventually develop lymphoid malignancies or multiple myelomas. Therefore, indefinite follow-up is recommended. Parameters that suggest a favorable prognosis in "benign" monoclonal gammopathy include the following: (1) concentration of homogeneous immunoglobulin less than 2 g/dL, (2) no significant increase in the concentration of the homogeneous immunoglobulin from the time of diagnosis, (3) no decrease in the concentration of normal immunoglobulins, (4) absence of a homogeneous light chain in the urine, and (5) normal hematocrit and serum albumin concentration.

Multiple Myeloma (See also Chapter 12.)

This disease is characterized by the overproduction and spread of neoplastic plasma cells throughout the bone marrow. Myeloma cells sometimes express molecules of early B cell or myelomonocytic lineages. Rarely, extraosseous plasmacytomas may be found. Anemia, hypercalcemia, increased susceptibility to infection, and bone pain are frequent. Diagnosis depends upon the presence of the following: (1) radiographic findings of osteolytic lesions or diffuse osteoporosis, (2) the presence of a homogeneous serum immunoglobulin (myeloma protein) or a single type of light chain in the urine (Bence Jones proteinuria), and (3) finding of an abnormal plasma cell infiltrate in the bone marrow biopsy (see Chapter 12). There is an approximate correlation between the incidence of immunoglobulin type in myeloma and the normal serum concentration of the immunoglobulin involved. That is, IgG>IgA>IgD>IgE. IgM myeloma does not occur for all practical purposes.

Waldenström's Macroglobulinemia

Waldenström's macroglobulinemia is characterized by a proliferation of abnormal lymphoid cells that have morphologic features of both B cells and plasma cells. These cells secrete a homogeneous macroglobulin (IgM) detectable by immunoelectrophoresis. Monoclonal light chains are present in 10% of cases. Clinical manifestations depend upon the physicochemical characteristics of the macroglobulin. Raynaud's phenomenon and peripheral vascular occlusions are associated with cold-insoluble proteins (cryoglobulins). Retinal hemorrhages, visual impairment, and transient neurologic deficits are common with high-viscosity serum. Bleeding diatheses or hemolytic anemia can occur when the macroglobulin complexes with coagulation factors or binds to the surface of red blood cells.

Amyloidosis

Amyloidosis is a group of disorders manifested by impaired organ function from infiltration of tissues with insoluble protein fibrils or proteins complexed with polysaccharides. Variations in composition of the fibrils can be largely correlated with the clinical syndromes (Table 18–1). Amyloid occurs in a primary form or in company with plasmacytosis in bone marrow or lymphoid tissues. The protein fibrils in these entities are composed of immunoglobulin light chains or fragments of light chains, particularly the V region. This form of amyloid has been designated AL.

A nonimmunoglobulin protein (AA) is the major component of amyloid fibrils that form secondary to infection (osteomyelitis, tuberculosis), inflammation, rheumatoid arthritis, Hodgkin's disease, regional enteritis, renal cell carcinoma, leprosy, and intravenous

Table 18–1. Classification of amyloidosis.[1]

	Clinical Type	Common Sites of Deposition
Familial	Amyloid polyneuropathy (Portuguese, dominant inheritance)	Peripheral nerves, viscera
	Familial Mediterranean fever (recessive)	Liver, spleen, kidneys, adrenals
Generalized	Primary	Tongue, heart, gut, skeletal and smooth muscles, nerves, skin, ligaments
	Associated with plasma cell dyscrasia	Liver, spleen, kidneys, heart, adrenals
	Secondary (infection, inflammation, etc)	Any site
	Chronic hemodialysis	Skin
Localized	Lichen amyloidosis	Skin
	Endocrine-related (eg, thyroid medullary carcinoma, diabetes mellitus, Addison's disease)	Endocrine organ (thyroid)
Senile	Also localized	Heart, brain, pancreas

[1]Modified and reproduced, with permission, from Stites DP et al (editors): *Basic & Clinical Immunology*, 7th ed. Appleton & Lange, 1991.

drug abuse. The hereditary systemic amyloidosis associated with familial Mediterranean fever is composed of AA protein. This protein is derived from the acute-phase reactant SAA (serum amyloid-associated).

Symptoms and signs of amyloid infiltration are related to malfunction of the organ involved, (eg, nephrotic syndrome, chronic renal failure, cardiomyopathy, cardiac conduction defects, intestinal malabsorption, intestinal obstruction, carpal tunnel syndrome, macroglossia, peripheral neuropathy, end-organ insufficiency of endocrine glands, respiratory failure, obstruction to ventilation, and capillary damage with ecchymosis). Amyloidosis due to deposition of β_2-microglobulin in joints and bones occurs in chronic hemodialysis patients. Table 18–1 lists organs characteristically involved with each type of amyloid.

The diagnosis of amyloidosis is based on suspicion, family history, and preexisting long-standing infection or debilitating illness. Microscopic examination of biopsy (eg, gingival, renal, rectal) or surgical specimens is diagnostic. Amyloid binds Congo red dye in tissues and emits apple green fluorescence with ultraviolet light. Fine-needle biopsy of subcuta-

neous abdominal fat is a simple and reliable method for diagnosing secondary systemic amyloidosis.

Treatment of localized amyloid "tumors" is by surgical excision. There is no effective treatment of systemic amyloidosis, and death usually occurs within 1–3 years. Patients who develop renal failure requiring dialysis have a median survival of less than 1 year, and usually die due to extrarenal progression of their systemic amyloidosis. Treatment of the predisposing disease may cause a temporary remission or slow the progress of the disease, but it is unlikely that the established metabolic process is altered. Patients with amyloid due to plasma cell dyscrasia may occasionally respond to treatment with melphalan and prednisone. Colchicine is of use in familial Mediterranean fever. Early and adequate treatment of pyogenic infections may prevent secondary amyloidosis.

Heavy Chain Disease
(α, γ, μ)

These are rare disorders in which the abnormal serum and urine protein is a part of a homogeneous α, γ, or μ heavy chain. The clinical presentation is more typical of lymphoma than multiple myeloma, and there are no destructive bone lesions. Gamma chain disease presents as a lymphoproliferative disorder commonly with autoimmune features or in the context of a lymphoid malignancy. Alpha chain disease is frequently associated with severe diarrhea and infiltration of the lamina propria of the small intestine with abnormal plasma cells. Mu chain disease is associated with chronic lymphocytic leukemia.

Gandara DR, Mackenzie MR: Differential diagnosis of monoclonal gammopathy. Med Clin North Am 1988; 72:1155.

Gertz MA, Kyle RA, O'Fallon WM: Dialysis support of patients with primary systemic amyloidosis. Arch Intern Med 1992;152:2245.

Gertz MA, Kyle RA: Primary systemic amyloidosis: A diagnostic primer. Mayo Clin Proc 1989;64:1505.

Kyle RA, Bayrd EA: *The Monoclonal Gammopathies: Multiple Myeloma and Related Plasma Cell Disorders.* Thomas, 1976.

Stone MJ: Amyloidosis: A final common pathway for protein deposition in tissues. Blood 1990;75:531.

CELLULAR IMMUNITY

CELLS INVOLVED IN IMMUNITY

Development of T & B Lymphocytes

Lymphocytes interact with antigens via specific receptors and thereby initiate immune responses. In birds, two lines of lymphocytes exist: one derived from the thymus and the other from the bursa of Fabricius. The thymus-derived cells are involved in cellular immune responses; the bursa-derived cells are involved in antibody responses. In mammals, T lymphocytes are analogous to the thymus-derived cells in birds and B lymphocytes (bone marrow-derived cells) are analogous to the bursa-derived cells.

Both T and B lymphocytes are derived from precursor or stem cells in the marrow. Precursors of T cells migrate to the thymus, where they develop some of the functional and cell surface characteristics of mature T cells. Clones of autoreactive T cells are eliminated, and mature antigen reactive T cells then migrate to the peripheral lymphoid tissues and enter the pool of long-lived lymphocytes that recirculate from the blood to the lymph.

B cell maturation has antigen-independent and antigen-dependent stages. Antigen-independent maturation includes development from precursor cells in the marrow through the virgin B cell (a cell that has not been exposed to antigen previously) found in the peripheral lymphoid tissues. The production and maturation of virgin B cells are ongoing processes even in adult animals. Antigen-dependent maturation occurs following the interaction of antigen with virgin B cells. The final products of B cell development are circulating long-lived memory B cells and plasma cells that secrete copious amounts of specific antibody. Mature B cells in the periphery are found predominantly in primary follicles and germinal centers of the lymph nodes and spleen.

Subpopulations of T Cells

T lymphocytes are heterogeneous with respect to their cell surface features (Table 18–2) and functional characteristics. At least four subpopulations of T cells are now recognized.

A. Helper-Inducer T Cells: These cells help to amplify the production of antibody-forming cells from B lymphocytes after interaction with antigen. Helper T cells also amplify the production of effector T cells that mediate cytotoxicity. The several different functions of these T cells may reflect various stages of development rather than unique or separate lineages of these lymphocytes. Recently, two subsets of helper T cells have been identified on the basis of their pattern of cytokine production. The subsets are called T_H1 cells (which produce interleukin 2 and interferon gamma), and T_H2 cells (which produce interleukins 4, 5, and 6). These subsets of helper cells are important in combating infections and in the generation of allergic responses to allergens.

B. Cytotoxic or Killer T Cells: These cells are generated after mature T cells interact with certain antigens such as those present on the surface of foreign cells. These cells are responsible for organ graft rejection and for killing of virally infected cells and some tumor cells.

C. Suppressor T Cells: These cells suppress the

Table 18–2. Selected surface antigens detected by monoclonal antibodies on T and B cells.

Cluster of Differentiation	Antibody Designation	Distribution
CD2	Leu-5	Pan T cell marker, NK cells
CD3	Leu-4, OKT3	TcR-associated antigen
CD4	Leu-3, T4	Mature helper-inducer T cells
CD8	Leu-2, T8	Cytotoxic-suppressor T cells
CD19	B4	Pan B cell marker
CD25	Tac	One chain in the IL-2 receptor; seen on activated T cells and some B and NK cells
CD45RA	2H4	"Naive" CD4 and CD8 T cells; some B cells and monocytes
CD45RO	UCH-1	"Memory" CD4 and CD8 T cells

formation of antibody-forming cells from B lymphocytes. Suppressor T cells are regarded as regulatory cells that modulate antibody formation. Cell-mediated immunity (ie, organ graft rejection) is also regulated by suppressor cells.

D. Suppressor-Inducer T Cells: These cells, which have helper cell (not suppressor cell) surface antigens, amplify the development of suppressor T cells.

Identification of T Cell Subpopulations With Monoclonal Antibodies

Monoclonal antibodies to T cell subpopulations are produced by immunizing animals with human T cells and then fusing the spleen cells of the animal with mouse myeloma cells to develop hybridoma cell lines. These hybridoma lines secrete monoclonal antibodies that identify cell surface antigens common to all human T cells (Table 18–2). The term CD (cluster of differentiation) is used to designate various lymphocyte types. Lymphocytes stained with fluorescent monoclonal antibodies are enumerated by microscopy or flow cytometry. About 75% of the peripheral blood lymphocytes of normal individuals are T cells; 50% are helper-inducer T cells, and 25% are suppressor or cytotoxic T cells.

Changes in the number or ratio of various T cell subsets occur in a wide variety of clinical conditions. For example, the ratio of helper to suppressor (H/S) cells in healthy individuals is about 1.6–2.2. In many acute viral infections, this ratio falls temporarily both as a result of decrease in helper/inducer cells and of increase in suppressor/cytotoxic cells. In AIDS and related HIV infections, H:S ratios are nearly always reduced (probably irreversibly) by the destructive effects of this lymphotropic virus. Among other clinical applications of the enumeration of these cells are the diagnosis of some immunodeficiencies, phenotyping of leukemias and lymphomas, and monitoring of immunologic changes following organ transplantation.

Cytokines

Many T cell functions are mediated by cytokines, which are humoral factors secreted by lymphocytes among numerous other cells. Cytokines are secreted when cells are activated by antigens or other cytokines. Table 18–3 lists some examples of cytokines and their functions. The cytokines can be functionally organized into groups according to their major activities: (1) those that promote and mediate natural immunity, such as IL-1, IL-6, interferon (IFN)-γ, and IL-8; (2) those that support allergic inflammation, such as IL-4, which acts to promote IgE production, IL-3, -4, -9, and -10, which act to promote mast cell growth, and IL-3, IL-5, and granulocyte-macrophage colony stimulating factor (GM-CSF), which promote the growth of eosinophils; (3) those that exert lymphocyte regulatory activity, such as IL-10 (produced by the T_H2 helper T cell, and IFN-γ, which is produced by the T_H1 T helper cell; and (4) those that act as hematopoietic growth factors (IL-7 and GM-CSF). This complicated network of interacting cytokines functions to modulate and regulate cellular function so that the host may survive in an otherwise hostile environment.

Therapeutically, cytokines are being used experimentally both to evaluate immune function and to treat disease. Receptors for IL-2 circulate in blood and are a measure of generalized immune stimulation. IL-2 in combination with autologous lymphocytes has been tested as an anti-cancer treatment in selected patients with limited success. Aldesleukin is now available and approved for treatment of metastatic renal cell carcinoma in adults.

T Cell Antigen Receptors

T cells interact with several different types of cells during the regulation and mediation of immune responses. These interactions include presentation of antigens to T cells by macrophages or other cells, T cell-induced differentiation of B cells into antibody-secreting cells, and T cell killing of a variety of other cells. In all of these cell-cell interactions, T cells recognize foreign antigens on the surface of the target cell in association with other cell surface antigens that are coded for by the major histocompatibility gene complex of the non-T cell. T cells have cell surface receptors that recognize at least two different molecules; one recognition site binds to any single foreign antigen (viral, bacterial, etc.), and the other binds to major histocompatibility antigens. An example of this "dual recognition" is observed in the killing of virus-infected target cells by cytolytic T cells. Cytolytic T cells taken from humans immunized to a given virus will kill virus-infected target cells if the target cells carry the same histocompatibility antigens as the immunized host.

The structure of T cell antigen receptors and the genes that encode these glycoproteins have been de-

Table 18–3. Major sources and activities of selected cytokines.

Cytokine	Primary Cellular Source	Primary Biologic Activity
IL-1	Macrophages	Immunologic and inflammatory mediator; acute phase reactant; augments immune responses.
IL-2	T lymphocytes	Promotes T lymphocyte activation, growth.
IL-3	T lymphocytes	Hematopoietic growth factor, "multicolony stimulating factor."
IL-4	T lymphocytes	T and B lymphocyte, mast cell growth factor; promotes IgE isotype switching.
IL-5	T lymphocytes	B cell growth factor; promotes IgA production; promotes eosinophil growth and differentiation.
IL-6	Macrophages, T lymphocytes	B cell differentiation factors; acute phase reactant.
IL-7	Stromal cells of the spleen and thymus	Growth factor for very early B and T lymphocytes.
TNF	Macrophages, T cells, mast cells, NK cells	Overlaps activity with IL-1 but has more antitumor activity.
IFN-α IFN-β IFN-γ	B lymphocytes, macrophages Fibroblasts, epithelial cells T lymphocytes	Antiviral and antitumor activities; activates macrophages; enhances cytotoxic lymphocyte and NK activity.
GM-CSF	T lymphocytes, fibroblasts, endothelial cells	Growth factor for granulocytes, macrophage and eosinophil colonies; activates neutrophil phagocytgosis; enhances eosinophil-mediated cytotoxicity; promotes basophil histamine release.

Key: IL = interleukin; GM-CSF = granulocyte-macrophage colony-stimulating factor; NK = natural killer cells.

fined. The antigen recognition structure is a complex of two molecules, one containing variable α and β or γ and δ chains and the other the monomorphic T3 (CD3) molecule. Genes encoding the β chain have homology to immunoglobulin genes. Clonal rearrangement of T cell receptor genes proceeds during T cell development to generate diversity for antigen recognition in a fashion similar to that of immunoglobulin genes in B cells. T cell receptor gene rearrangements have been used to identify T cell leukemias, lymphomas, and mycosis fungoides, a rare malignant neoplasm of the skin.

Arai K et al: Cytokines: coordinators of immune and inflammatory responses. Ann Rev Biochem 1990;59:783.
Goverman J, Parnes JR: The T cell receptor. In: *Basic & Clinical Immunology,* 7th ed. Stites DP, Terr AI (editors). Appleton & Lange, 1991.

B Lymphocytes

B cells express different classes of surface molecules in (Table 18–2). The majority of B cells express both IgM and IgD on the surface and are derived from pre-B cells found mainly in the bone marrow. Pre-B cells contain intracytoplasmic IgM but do not express surface immunoglobulin. Patients with X-linked hypogammaglobulinemia frequently show a developmental arrest at the stage of the pre-B cell. The majority of patients with acquired hypogammaglobulinemia have a block of transition from the mature B cell to the plasma cell. Thus, most patients with this disease have normal numbers of circulating mature B cells but reduced numbers of plasma cells.

B cells have been commonly identified by other surface markers in addition to immunoglobulins. These include the receptor for the Fc piece of immunoglobulins, B cell-specific antigens CD19 and CD20, and surface antigens coded for by the HLA-D genetic region in humans (Table 18–2). All mature B cells bear surface immunoglobulin that is the antigen-specific receptor. The major role of B cells is differentiation to antibody-secreting plasma cells. However, B cells may also release cytokines and function as antigen-presenting cells.

Other Cells Involved in Immune Responses

A. Macrophages: Macrophages are involved in the ingestion, processing and presentation of particulate antigens for interaction with lymphocytes. They play an important role in T and B lymphocyte cooperation in the induction of antibody responses. In addition, they are effector cells for certain types of tumor immunity.

B. NK (Natural Killer) Cells: These lymphocytic cells, which are indirectly related to the T cell lineage, can kill a wide spectrum of target cells. They are recognized by the presence of specific surface antigens and Fc receptors. Many appear as large granular lymphocytes. Their role in host defense is probably the killing of virally infected cells and tumor cells in the absence of prior sensitization and without MHC restriction.

Lanier L: Cells of the immune response. In: *Basic & Clinical Immunology,* 7th ed. Stites DP, Terr AI (editors). Appleton & Lange, 1991.
Robertson MJ, Ritz J: Biology and clinical relevance of human natural killer cells. Blood 1990;76:2421.

TESTS FOR CELLULAR IMMUNITY

Techniques for Identification & Human B & T Cells

A. B Cells: Cell surface characteristics usually found on B but not T cells include the following: (1) easily detectable surface immunoglobulin, (2) specific antigens (CD19, CD20), (3) a receptor for the Fc portion of immunoglobulins that have been aggregated or complexed with antigen, and (4) DR antigens (Table 18–2).

These surface markers are detected with monoclonal antibodies conjugated to various fluorochromes either by microscopy or flow cytometry.

B. T Cells: T cell markers include surface antigens identified by specific monoclonal antibodies. Monoclonal antisera have been used in both immunofluorescence staining and in vitro cytotoxicity assays to identify T cell subsets (Table 18–2). T cells can also be detected in tissue sections or suspensions using enzyme-labeled antibodies that produce colors on incubation with chromogenic substrates. Approximately 75% of human peripheral blood lymphocytes are T cells, and up to 20% are B cells. The remainder are NK cells.

C. Flow Cytometry: Flow cytometers are instruments that accurately measure the size, density, and multiple colors of immunofluorescent monoclonal antibodies on human lymphocytes. Thousands of cells can be analyzed individually for the presence of all these parameters at once. This method greatly improves the accuracy, speed, and precision of identifying human T and B cells in the clinical laboratory.

Procedures for Testing Cell-Mediated Immunity, or T Cell Function

A. Skin Testing: Cell-mediated immunity can be assessed qualitatively by evaluating skin reactivity following intradermal injection of a battery of antigens to which humans are frequently sensitized (ie, streptokinase, streptodornase, purified protein derivative, Trichophyton, Dermatophyton, or Candida). Intradermal injections of 0.1 mL of recommended test strengths are observed for maximal induration and erythema at 24 and 48 hours. A positive reaction varies in size with particular antigens but is generally at least 10 mm in diameter. Anergy or lack of skin reactivity to all of these substances usually indicates a depression of cell-mediated immunity. Delayed hypersensitivity skin tests depend on complex interactions of T cells, macrophages, and other immunoreactants; thus, failure to respond cannot specifically identify a defect in a particular cell type.

B. In Vitro Stimulation of Peripheral Blood Lymphocytes With Mitogens or Antigens: T lymphocytes are transformed to blast cells upon short-term incubation with mitogens such as phytohemagglutinin or recall antigens in vitro. T cell activation can be determined quantitatively by following the cellular uptake of ^{3}H-thymidine introduced into the culture medium. The in vitro uptake of ^{3}H-thymidine by human peripheral blood lymphocytes indicates T cell function and correlates well with other manifestations of cell-mediated immunity as measured by delayed hypersensitivity skin tests. These functional tests can detect abnormalities in T cells despite normal or slightly reduced cell counts, particularly following bone marrow transplantation or in congenital immunodeficiency diseases. Stimulation of transplant recipients' lymphocytes or donor lymphocytes (the mixed lymphocyte reaction) is critical test for determining histocompatibility, especially in renal and bone marrow transplantation.

APPLICATIONS OF T & B CELL TESTS

Immunodeficiency Diseases

Thymic hypoplasia is associated with a marked decrease in the number of T cells in the peripheral blood. On the other hand, the absence of B cells in the blood is frequently found in X-linked hypogammaglobulinemia. Marked reduction of both T and B cells occurs in severe combined immunodeficiency disease (SCID). Typing of blood T and B cells can aid in the diagnosis of these diseases in early childhood. Patients with HIV infection and particularly the acquired immunodeficiency syndrome (AIDS) have reduced numbers of T cells and reduced T helper-to-suppressor ratios.

Lymphoproliferative Diseases

A marked increase in the number of peripheral blood lymphocytes that bear immunoglobulin of a single heavy chain class and light chain type represents a monoclonal proliferation of cells. Blood lymphocytes from almost all patients with chronic lymphocytic leukemia and non-Hodgkin's lymphoma with blood involvement show this abnormality. On the other hand, lymphocytosis secondary to viral or bacterial infection is associated with a normal percentage of B cells and the usual distribution of immunoglobulin classes on the cell surface.

Lymphocytic leukemias can be classified by

phenotyping T and B cells, with implications for prognosis and, sometimes, treatment. Monitoring various T cell subsets is also useful in following patients with organ transplants.

Stites DP: Clinical laboratory methods for detection of cellular immunity. In: *Basic & Clinical Immunology,* 7th ed. Stites DP, Terr AI (editors). Appleton & Lange, 1991.

IMMUNOLOGIC DEFICIENCY DISEASES

The primary immunologic deficiency diseases include congenital and acquired disorders of humoral immunity (B cell function) or cell-mediated immunity (T cell function). Most of these diseases are rare and since they are genetically determined, occur primarily in children.

Classification

Some immunodeficiency disorders affect adults, and several are discussed below. The WHO classification of immunodeficiency disorders more often affecting adults includes the following:

(1) Common variable immunodeficiency (see below).
(2) Selective IgA deficiency (see below).
(3) X-linked immunodeficiency with hyper-IgM.
(4) Immunodeficiency with normal serum globulins or hyperimmunoglobulinemia.
(5) Immunodeficiency with thymoma.
(6) Acquired immunodeficiency syndrome (AIDS) (see below).

Ammann AJ, Frank M: Immunodeficiency disorders. In: *Basic & Clinical Immunology,* 7th ed. Stites DP, Terr AI (editors). Appleton & Lange, 1991.
Stiehm ER: *Immunologic Disorders in Infants and Children,* 3rd ed. Saunders, 1989.

COMMON VARIABLE IMMUNODEFICIENCY

Onset is typically late in adolescence or early in adulthood. Increased susceptibility to pyogenic infections is the hallmark of the disease, which if left untreated often leads to recurrent sinusitis and pneumonia progressing to bronchiectasis. Patients may also develop a sprue-like syndrome with diarrhea, steatorrhea, malabsorption, protein-losing enteropathy, and hepatosplenomegaly.

Arthritis of the type associated with congenital

hypogammaglobulinemia and autoimmune diseases may occur. Serum IgG levels are usually less than 250 mg/dL; serum IgA and IgM levels are subnormal. Lymph nodes may be enlarged in these patients, yet biopsies show marked reduction in plasma cells. Noncaseating granulomas are frequently found in the spleen, liver, lungs, or skin. There is an increased propensity for the development of B cell neoplasms, gastric carcinomas, and skin cancers.

The cause of the panhypogammaglobulinemia in the overwhelming majority of common variable immunodeficiency patients is an intrinsic B cell defect in antibody production. In a small number of patients, excessive suppressor T cell activity which inhibits B cells—or helper T cell activity inadequate to assist B cells to make antibody—has been identified. The absolute B cell count in the peripheral blood in most patients, despite the underlying cellular defect, is normal. A subset of these patients have concomitant T cell immunodeficiency with increased numbers of activated CD8 cells, splenomegaly, and decreased delayed-type hypersensitivity. Therapy at present is similar to that of congenital hypogammaglobulinemia, with infusions of 300–400 mg/kg of intravenous immune globulin at about monthly intervals. Such therapy is effective in decreasing the incidence of (or preventing) potentially life-threatening infections. It is important that the diagnosis be firmly established, because the yearly cost of monthly infusions can be in excess of $20,000–$30,000.

SELECTIVE IMMUNOGLOBULIN A DEFICIENCY

Selective IgA deficiency is the most common primary immunodeficiency disorder and is characterized by the absence of serum IgA with normal levels of IgG and IgM; its prevalence is about 1:700 to 1:500 individuals. Some cases of IgA deficiency may spontaneously remit. When IgG$_2$ subclass deficiency occurs in combination with IgA deficiency, recurrent infections are common. Occasionally, a sprue-like syndrome with steatorrhea has been associated with an isolated IgA deficit. Treatment with commercial immune globulin is ineffective, since IgA and IgM are present only in small quantities in these preparations. Frequent infusions of plasma (containing IgA) are hazardous, since anti-IgA antibodies may develop, resulting in systemic anaphylaxis or serum sickness.

ACQUIRED IMMUNODEFICIENCY SYNDROME (AIDS)
(See also Chapter 30.)

AIDS is a chronic retroviral infection with human immunodeficiency virus (HIV) that produces severe, life-threatening T cell defects. In addition to reduction of CD4 (helper T cells), there is an increase in CD8 (suppressor/cytotoxic T cells), most of which have a cytotoxic phenotype.

B cell function is altered so that many infected individuals have marked hypergammaglobulinemia, and AIDS patients fail to respond normally to antigens when immunized. Autoantibodies and circulating immune complexes are present. Most infected individuals progress from health to AIDS over several years. The immunologic determinants of the clinical fate of persons infected with HIV are unknown.

In AIDS, immunologic tests reveal a severe selective deficiency of T lymphocyte function and number, with little alteration in B lymphocyte numbers. Patients are frequently anergic. In vitro tests of peripheral blood T cell function such as proliferative responses to antigens and mitogens are markedly reduced or absent. The absolute lymphocyte count is severely decreased (frequently < 500 cells/μL), and the ratio of helper to suppressor/cytotoxic T cells is considerably lower than normal. Although T cell depletion in HIV infection is a consequence of destruction of CD4 cells by the virus, other mechanisms to deplete T cells and suppress immune responses are also operative. The immunologic changes that occur in asymptomatic HIV seropositive individuals are usually not as marked as those in AIDS patients.

Fauci AS et al: Immunopathogenic mechanisms in human immunodeficiency virus (HIV) infection. Ann Intern Med 1991;114:678.
Ho DD, Mudgil T, Alam M: Quantitation of HIV type I in the blood of infected persons. N Engl J Med 1989;321:1621.
What science knows about AIDS. Sci Am (Oct) 1988;259.

SECONDARY IMMUNODEFICIENCY

Deficiencies in T cell immunity, antibody immunity, or both have been associated with many diseases. Two examples of altered immunity secondary to underlying disease are discussed below.

Immunodeficiency Associated With Sarcoidosis

The immunodeficiency associated with sarcoidosis is characterized by a partial deficit in T cell function with intact or increased B cell function. Patients with sarcoidosis often are relatively nonreactive to intradermal injections of common antigens. However, complete lack of skin reactivity is infrequent. A positive reaction to purified protein derivative is usually noted during active infection with *Mycobacterium tuberculosis*. Serum immunoglobulin levels are normal or high, and specific antibody formation is generally normal.

Immunodeficiency Associated With Hodgkin's Disease

A moderate to severe deficit in T cell function with intact B cell function is frequently found in Hodgkin's disease. Only 10–20% of patients with Hodgkin's disease show skin reactivity to common antigens, as compared to 70–90% of controls. Many patients show depressed responses to in vitro stimulation of peripheral blood lymphocytes with phytohemagglutinin. Serum immunoglobulins are normal, and specific antibody formation is intact except in agonal cases.

The clinical significance of depressed cell-mediated immunity in Hodgkin's disease is difficult to evaluate, since most patients are treated with potent immunosuppressive agents. Nevertheless, frequent infections with herpes zoster and *Cryptococcus* are probably related to immunodeficiency associated with the underlying disease.

Buckley RH: Immunodeficiency disease. JAMA 1992; 268:2797.(A concise review of the major immunodeficiency diseases, including a practical approach to the patient with recurrent infections).

Shearer WT, Anderson DC: The secondary immunodeficiencies. In: *Immunologic Disorders in Infants and Children,* 3rd ed. Stiehm ER (editor). Saunders, 1989.

AUTOIMMUNITY

Autoimmune diseases cannot be explained by a solitary cause or mechanism. Small amounts of autoantibodies are normally produced and may have physiologic roles in cellular interactions. The major theories regarding the development of autoimmune disease are (1) release of normally sequestered antigens, (2) the presence of abnormal clones, (3) shared antigens between the host and microorganisms, and (4) defects in helper or suppressor T cell function. A genetic susceptibility is also a likely determinant of autoimmune disease. In nearly all autoimmune diseases, multiple mechanisms of autoimmunity are operative and the exact underlying causes are unknown.

Cell-Mediated Autoimmunity

Certain autoimmune diseases are mediated by T cells that have become specifically immunized to autologous tissues. Cytotoxic or killer T cells generated by this aberrant immune response attack and injure specific organs in the absence of serum autoantibodies.

Diminished suppressor T cell activity results in disordered regulation of immune responses and may promote overactivity of other autoreactive mechanisms. The immune damage in systemic (non-organ-specific) specific diseases such as systemic lupus erythematosus may be in part due to such a mechanism.

Antibody-Mediated Autoimmunity

Several autoimmune diseases have been shown to be caused by autoantibodies in the absence of cell-mediated autoimmunity. The autoimmune hemolytic anemias, idiopathic thrombocytopenia, and Goodpasture's syndrome appear to be mediated solely by autoantibodies directed against autologous cell membrane constituents. In these diseases, antibody attaches to cell membranes, fixes complement, and the ensuing inflammatory reaction severely injures the cells.

The existence of anti-receptor antibodies that compete with or mimic various physiologic agonists for cellular receptors is a specific autoimmune mechanism in several diseases. In Graves' disease, antibodies are present that bind to thyroid cells' TSH receptors and thereby stimulate thyroid hormone production. In rare instances of type I diabetes mellitus, anti-insulin receptor antibodies cause insulin resistance in peripheral target tissues. In contrast, the anti-islet cell antibodies that are usually found in type I diabetes produce insulin deficiency by destroying islet cells in the pancreas. In myasthenia gravis, antibodies to acetylcholine receptors of the myoneural junction block neuromuscular transmission and thereby produce muscle weakness.

Immune Complex Disease

In this group of diseases (systemic lupus erythematosus, rheumatoid arthritis, some drug-induced hemolytic anemias and thrombocytopenias), autologous tissues are injured as "innocent bystanders." Autoantibodies are not directed against cellular components of the target organ but rather against autologous or heterologous antigens in the serum. The resultant antigen-antibody complexes bind nonspecifically to autologous membranes (eg, glomerular basement membrane) and fix complement. Fixation and subsequent activation of complement components produce a local inflammatory response that results in tissue injury.

Steinberg AD: Mechanisms of disordered immune regulation. In: *Basic & Clinical Immunology,* 7th ed. Stites DP, Terr AI (editors). Appleton & Lange, 1991.

AUTOIMMUNE DISEASES (See also Chapter 19.)

The diagnosis and treatment of specific autoimmune diseases are described elsewhere in this book. Autoantibodies associated with certain autoimmune diseases may not be implicated in the pathogenesis of tissue injury but are thought instead to be by-products of the injury (eg, autoimmune thyroiditis and anti-thyroglobulin antibody).

TESTS FOR AUTOANTIBODIES ASSOCIATED WITH AUTOIMMUNE DISEASES

Assays for autoantibodies are similar to those used for detection of antibodies to foreign antigens. Four commonly used methods are discussed below.

Many of the autoantibodies are not specific for a single disease entity (eg, antinuclear antibody, rheumatoid factor). Tests for the latter autoantibodies are best used when the clinical diagnosis is uncertain, in that a negative result makes the diagnosis of certain autoimmune diseases unlikely. For example, a negative antinuclear antibody test makes the diagnosis of systemic lupus erythematosus unlikely, since this antibody is detected in the serum of more than 95% of lupus patients. The disease associations of several autoantibodies are summarized in Table 18–4.

Agglutination of Antigen-Coated Red Blood Cells

Red cells (human, sheep, etc) are incubated with tannic acid or other chemicals so that the cell surface becomes "sticky." The red cells are subsequently incubated with purified specific antigen (eg, thyroglobulin), which is adsorbed to the cell surface. The antigen-coated cells are suspended in the patient's serum, and antibody is detected by red cell agglutination. Antigen-coated latex particles are substituted for red cells in the latex fixation tests.

Enzyme-Linked Immunoassays (ELISA)

Antibodies to various tissue antigens can be readily detected by ELISA tests. Extracted and purified antigens are fixed to a plastic microtiter well or beads. Patient's serum is added, and excess proteins are removed by washing and centrifugation. A second antibody coupled to an enzyme (eg, alkaline phosphatase) is added. The enzyme's substrate is then added, and color forms that is measured in a spectrophotometer. This test can also be adapted to antigen detection by placing the antibody on the plastic surface. ELISA assays are very widely applied in clinical laboratory testing.

Immunofluorescence Microscopy

This technique is most frequently used for detection of antinuclear antibody. Frozen sections of mouse liver or other substrates are cut and placed on glass slides. A patient's serum is placed over the sections and washed away. Fluorescein-conjugated rabbit anti-human immunoglobulin is then applied and washed. Antinuclear antibody specifically binds to the nucleus, and the fluorescein conjugate binds to the human antibody. Fluorescence of the cell nucleus observed by fluorescence microscopy indicates a positive test.

Complement Fixation

Specific antigen, unknown serum, and complement are reacted together. Sheep red blood cells coated with anti-sheep cell antibody are subsequently added to the above reaction mixture for 30 minutes at 37 °C. Lysis of sheep cells indicates that complement is present (attaches to sheep cell surface). Lack of lysis indicates that complement has been fixed by the interaction of antibody in the unknown serum with the specific antigen. Lack of lysis is a positive test for the presence of specific antibody.

Treatment of Autoimmune Diseases

Therapy of autoimmune diseases involves a variety of approaches. Suppression of production of autoantibodies with corticosteroids and cytotoxic agents is often effective. Anti-inflammatory drugs such as aspirin, NSAIDs, colchicine, and corticosteroids relieve tissue damage from immune complexes. Plasmapheresis to remove offending autoantibodies and circulating immune complexes, when combined with cytotoxic drugs, has been useful in some diseases. All of these modalities are directed at symptoms, since the underlying cause of these disorders remains unknown.

Condemi JJ: The autoimmune diseases. JAMA. 1992; 268:2882. (A review of the immunologic features of autoimmune diseases and selected disorders.)

Rose NR, Mackay IR (editors): *The Autoimmune Diseases II.* Academic Press, 1992. (A comprehensive presentation by experts.)

IMMUNOGENETICS & TRANSPLANTATION

GENETIC CONTROL OF THE IMMUNE RESPONSE

The ability to mount a specific immune response is under the direct control of genes closely associated on the same chromosome with the structural genes for the major transplantation antigens. The major transplantation antigens are the cell surface glycoproteins (found on most cells of the body), which elicit the strongest transplantation rejection reaction when tissues are exchanged between two members of a particular species. These molecules function to present antigens to various immunocompetent cells. In humans, this genetic region has been designated the

Table 18–4. Autoantibodies: Associations with connective tissue diseases.[1]

Suspected Disease State	Test	Primary Disease Association (Sensitivity, Specificity)	Other Disease Associations	Comments
CREST[2] syndrome	Anticentromere antibody	CREST (70–90%, high)	Scleroderma (10–15%), Raynaud's disease (10–30%)	Predictive value of a positive test is >95% for scleroderma or related disease (CREST, Raynaud's). Diagnosis of CREST is made clinically.
Systemic lupus erythematosus (SLE)	Antinuclear antibody (ANA)	SLE (>95%, low)	Rheumatoid arthritis (30–50%), discoid lupus, scleroderma (60%), drug-induced lupus (100%), Sjögren's syndrome (80%), miscellaneous inflammatory disorders.	Often used as a screening test; a negative test virtually excludes SLE; a positive test, while nonspecific, increases posttest probability of SLE. Titer does not correlate with disease activity.
	Anti-double-stranded-DNA (anti-ds-DNA)	SLE (60–70%, high)	Lupus nephritis, rarely rheumatoid arthritis, connective tissue disease, usually in low titer.	Predictive value of a positive test is >90% for SLE if present in high titer; a decreasing titer may correlate with worsening renal disease. Titer generally correlates with disease activity.
	Anti-Smith antibody (anti-Sm)	SLE (30–40%, high)		SLE-specific. A positive test substantially increases posttest probability of SLE. Test rarely indicated.
Mixed connective tissue disease (MCTD)	Anti-ribonucleoprotein antibody (RNP)	Scleroderma (20–30%, low), MCTD (95–100%, low)	SLE (30%), Sjögren's syndrome, rheumatoid arthritis (10%), discoid lupus (20–30%).	A negative test essentially excludes MCTD; a positive test in high titer, while nonspecific, increases posttest probability of MCTD.
Rheumatoid arthritis	Rheumatoid factor (RF)	Rheumatoid arthritis (50–90%)	Other rheumatic diseases, chronic infections, some malignancies, some healthy individuals, elderly patients.	Titer does not correlate with disease activity.
Scleroderma	Anti-Scl-70 antibody	Scleroderma (15–20%, low)		Predictive value of a positive test is >95% for scleroderma.
Sjögren's syndrome	Anti-SS-A/Ro antibody	Sjögren's (60–70%, low)	SLE (30–40%), rheumatoid arthritis (10%), subacute cutaneous lupus, vasculitis.	Useful in counseling women of childbearing age with known connective tissue disease, since a positive test is associated with a small but real risk of neonatal SLE and congenital heart block.
Wegener's granulomatosis	Anti-neutrophil cytoplasmic antibody (ANCA)	Wegener's granulomatosis (systemic necrotizing vasculitis) (56–96%, high)	Crescentic glomerulonephritis or other systemic vasculitis (eg, polyarteritis nodosa).	Ability of this assay to reflect disease activity remains unclear.

[1]Modified, with permission, from Harvey AM et al (editors): *The Principles and Practice of Medicine,* 22nd ed. Appleton & Lange, 1988; White RH, Robbins DL: Clinical significance and interpretation of antinuclear antibodies. West J Med 1987;147:210; and Tan EM: Autoantibodies to nuclear antigens (ANA): Their immunobiology and medicine. Adv Immunol 1982,33:167.
[2]CREST = calcinosis, Raynaud's phenomenon, esophageal dysmotility, sclerodactyly, and telangiectasia.

human leukocyte antigen (HLA) complex because these antigens were first detected on peripheral blood lymphocytes. The complex includes antigens HLA-A, -B, -C, -DR and others, each with many alleles.

The HLA region has been localized to chromosome 6, and the order of the different HLA loci is shown in Figure 18–1. Most (98%) of the time, the HLA complex is inherited intact as two haplotypes (one from each parent), and within any particular family, therefore, the number of different combinations found will be fairly small; (eg, siblings have a 1:4 chance of being HLA-identical). In contrast, the number of antigen combinations among unrelated individuals is huge, resulting in probabilities of fewer

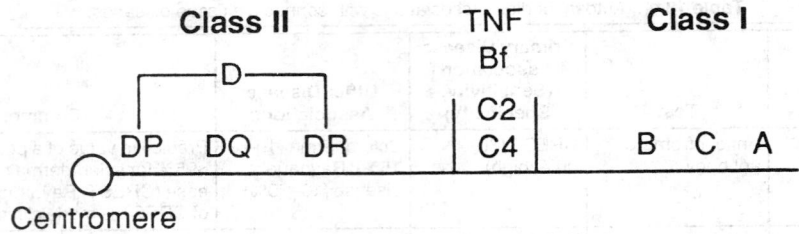

Figure 18–1. Genetic map of the HLA region. The centromere is to the left. (Bf, C2, and C4 are genes for components of the complement system. TNF is the tumor necrosis factor gene.)

than one in several thousand, depending upon the phenotype involved, of finding HLA-compatible individuals in a random donor pool. This is particularly important when compatible donors are needed for allosensitized patients requiring platelet transfusions or organ transplantation. Family members have the highest likelihood of being compatible donors, whereas HLA compatibility between two unrelated individuals has a very low probability. HLA-A and -B typing or cross-matching is utilized for selection of compatible donors for platelet transfusions to allosensitized, thrombocytopenic recipients. Typing for these class I antigens as well as for HLA-D antigens is important in determining compatibility for organ transplantation. Typing for HLA markers is of value in studying associations between the HLA system and genetic control of disease susceptibility.

In the genetic region determining the major transplantation antigen complex, there are genes determining the ability to mount a specific immune response. These are called immune response, or Ir, genes. Although the exact mechanism of action of Ir genes is not yet known, it is clear that they affect the ability to recognize foreign antigens and to initiate the development of T and B cell immunity to these antigens. Genes with such a strong effect on specific immune responsiveness might be expected to have major effects on resistance or susceptibility to a wide variety of infectious, neoplastic, and autoimmune diseases.

Schwartz BD: The human major histocompatibility HLA complex. In: *Basic & Clinical Immunology*, 7th ed. Stites DP, Terr AI (editors). Appleton & Lange, 1991.

HLA TYPING

The standard method for detecting HLA-A, -B, and -C antigens is that of lymphocyte microcytotoxicity. Lymphocytes isolated from peripheral blood or lymph nodes are added to each well of a typing tray that has been preloaded with sera containing the appropriate cytotoxic alloantibody. After allowing for the alloantibodies to bind to target lymphocytes,

complement is added. Those cells to which antibody has been specifically bound will have complement activated at the cell surface, resulting in cell death or lysis. By addition of a vital dye (eg, eosin, fluorescein diacetate, or trypan blue), viable and nonviable cells can be distinguished. It is thus possible to type for all of the known HLA-A, -B, and -C specificities. At present, the best sources of alloantisera are parous women, 10–30% of whom become sensitized during pregnancy to paternal antigens carried by the fetus. A few antibodies are also provided by individuals allosensitized by other causes (eg, transfusion or transplantation, and a few monoclonal antibodies are also used).

Typing for the class II antigens HLA-DR and -DQ is performed as described above, except that separated B lymphocytes are used as targets rather than unseparated peripheral blood lymphocytes. Antigens of the HLA-D and -DP series are detected by in vitro cellular reactivity. Lymphocytes of one individual will undergo DNA synthesis and proliferation upon encountering lymphocytes from another individual possessing foreign HLA-D antigens. Donor cells are irradiated or treated with mitomycin to ablate their immune responsiveness. These "stimulator" cells are then mixed with peripheral blood lymphocytes of the recipient (responder) in this mixed leukocyte reaction (MLR) culture. A responder lacking the stimulator's D antigen will respond by brisk DNA synthesis and proliferation that can readily be measured by DNA incorporation of tritiated thymidine. Responders possessing the D antigen of the donor will remain nonreactive.

HLA-DP antigens are identified by an extension of the MLR called primed lymphocyte typing. Following priming stimulation in a first MLR, the responder cells are restimulated in a secondary MLR by a different stimulator cell. If the two stimulator cells share the same DP antigen not possessed by the responder, the responder cells will demonstrate a brisk proliferative response.

Although technically demanding and requiring viable lymphoid cells and experienced laboratories, HLA typing is available at most large medical centers or blood banks.

Colombe BW: Histocompatibility testing. In: *Basic & Clinical Immunology,* 7th ed. Stites DP, Terr AI (editors). Appleton & Lange, 1991.

CLINICAL TRANSPLANTATION

Organ transplants are commonly used in the treatment of many diseases. The main limitations to their more widespread use are the scarcity of donor organs and the expense of these procedures. Failure to achieve completely successful grafts is primarily due to histoincompatibility and lack of totally safe and effective immunosuppressive regimens to halt rejection. Great care in avoiding transmission of infectious agents (eg, HIV, HBV, HCV, CMV) from donor to recipient requires extensive pre-transplant serologic testing.

Kidney Transplantation

End-stage renal disease is the indication for kidney transplantation. Kidneys from living related donors who are HLA-identical and also red blood cell ABO-matched have 90% survival at 1 year; less identical grafts have a somewhat lower survival rate. Transplants with matched cadaver kidney donors survive nearly as long, especially if the recipient does not contain antibodies to donor antigens. A positive cross-match by cytotoxicity testing between recipient serum and donor cells is considered a contraindication to that transplant. Donor screening is performed in all cases to avoid transmission of HIV and other infectious agents. Pretreatment of recipients with blood transfusions from the donor appears to extend graft survival even longer. Graft rejection is manifested by diminishing renal function and is treated with immunosuppressive drugs, especially cyclosporine (see below).

Heart Transplantation

The indication for heart transplantation is end-stage cardiac disease clearly refractory to medical treatment. Donors and recipients are matched by excluding anti-HLA antibodies in the recipient, since there is rarely time for HLA typing. Rejection is diagnosed by endomyocardial biopsy and treated with immunosuppressants, particularly cyclosporine. Five-year survival is as high as 80% at selected centers.

Lung Transplantation

Lung transplantation is most often combined with heart transplantation because of the poorer results achieved with lung grafts alone. Combined heart-lung transplants have a one year survival of approximately 65%, whereas for single lung transplants, survival is approximately 60%.

Liver Transplantation

The major indications for liver transplantation are severe liver dysfunction as manifested by synthetic or regulatory abnormalities which are likely to progress to death within 2 years, and the absence of serious systemic complications of hepatic failure. Children with developmental defects (eg, extrahepatic biliary atresia, inborn errors of metabolism) are typical recipients. The indications for liver transplantation in adults in selected cases includes, chronic active hepatitis (although the risk of recurrent disease in the graft is substantial), primary biliary cirrhosis, sclerosing cholangitis and inborn errors of metabolism. Recipients are selected on the basis of ABO matching and organ size. HLA typing has not achieved practical results. One-year survival rates range between 70% and 85%.

Pancreas & Islet Cell Transplants

Although these procedures currently are largely experimental, the indications are pancreatic insufficiency and, in some cases, diabetes mellitus. Clinical results have improved, with 1-year graft survival at selected centers of up to 80%.

Bone Marrow Transplantation

Leukemia, aplastic anemia, and congenital immunologic defects are currently the main indications for marrow transplants. Irradiation and immunosuppressive drugs are used to prepare recipients. Close HLA matching is essential for successful bone marrow transplantation. Graft-versus-host disease caused by attack of donor cells on histoincompatible host cells may be fatal. This occurs more commonly in adults, which limits the use of histoincompatible bone marrow transplantation in this age group. Autologous marrow harvested during disease-free periods has been used successfully for marrow reconstitution in selected patients. Infections during the period of emerging immune competence can also present life-threatening problems.

The success rates of bone marrow transplantation depend most upon the underlying disease and the associated risk of relapse (in cases of leukemia), the level of matching between donor and recipient and thus the likelihood of graft-versus-host disease, the age of the recipient (over the age of 30 years, the incidence of graft-versus-host disease increases), and the complications associated with conditioning (veno-occlusive liver disease and infection). Overall, the success rates are about 60–70% in aplastic anemia, 40–75% survival at 1 year in various forms of leukemia, and extremely variable in immunologic deficiency diseases.

Other Organs & Tissues

Transplantation of other organs or tissues (ie, skin, cornea, bone, and heart valves) is now routine surgical procedures. Much further research remains to be done on transplantation of other organs, particularly neural tissue.

Garovoy MR et al: Clinical transplantation. In: *Basic & Clinical Immunology,* 7th ed. Stites DP, Terr AI (editors). Appleton & Lange, 1991.

Takemoto S et al: Survival of nationally shared, HLA-matched kidney transplants from cadaveric donor. The UNOS Scientific Renal Transplant Registry. N Engl J Med 1992;327:834. (Report of a prospective trial from all US transplantation centers on nationwide shipment of cadaveric organs to HLA-A, -B, and DR matched recipients.)

MECHANISM OF ACTION OF IMMUNOSUPPRESSIVE DRUGS

Therapies that suppress immune or inflammatory responses are used commonly to treat recipients of organ transplants and patients with autoimmune diseases or neoplasms. The most frequently used drugs and their modes of action are briefly summarized below. Many new drugs with potent immunosuppressive actions and reduced toxicities are under development and in clinical trials

Corticosteroids

This group of drugs has potent anti-inflammatory and direct effects on immunocompetent cells. Corticosteroids inhibit cell-mediated immune responses more severely than antibody responses. T helper cells are preferentially reduced owing to redistribution. Neutrophils are increased owing to demargination and bone marrow release. Monocytes and eosinophils are reduced. These cellular changes result in reduced inflammatory responses. Disruption of the interaction between T cells and macrophages appears to be an important mechanism, and corticosteroids have been shown to block the activation of T cells by interleukin-1 (IL-1) derived from macrophages. In addition, corticosteroids inhibit the expression of class II histocompatibility antigens on the macrophage surface, thereby interfering with presentation of antigen to T cells.

Cytotoxic Drugs

The most frequently used cytotoxic drugs are azathioprine and cyclophosphamide. Azathioprine is a derivative of mercaptopurine, an antagonist of purine synthesis. Azathioprine is a phase-specific drug that kills rapidly replicating cells. It inhibits proliferation of both T and B cells as well as macrophages. Cyclophosphamide is an alkylating agent that damages cells by cross-linking DNA. Although this cycle-specific drug is most effective in killing cells going through the mitotic cycle, it can also cause intermitotic cell injury and death. Cyclophosphamide can inhibit both T and B cell immunity as well as inflammation. Azathioprine and cyclophosphamide are effective inhibitors of the production of serum antibodies.

Antimetabolites

The most commonly used antimetabolite is methotrexate, an inhibitor of folic acid synthesis. Methotrexate inhibits rapidly proliferating cells in S phase and suppresses both cell-mediated and humoral immunity as well as inflammation.

Cyclosporine

This cyclic polypeptide derived from a fungus has been used recently as an immunosuppressive drug in organ transplant recipients. Cyclosporine interferes with the secretion of interleukin-2 (IL-2) by T lymphocytes. Since IL-2 is necessary for T cell replication, this drug is a potent inhibitor of T cell proliferation and thereby inhibits T cell-mediated immune responses. Little effect has been shown on direct B cell immune responses or on inflammation. Its toxic effects are primarily on renal and hepatic function.

FK 506

A new drug being developed for use in transplantation, FK 506, is a macrolide and has potent anti-T cell properties and a mode of action similar to that of cyclosporine. Like cyclosporine, FK 506 inhibits IL-2 and interferon-γ production and T cell activation. Clinical trials are under way in kidney, liver, and heart transplantation.

Goodwin J: Anti-inflammatory drugs. In: *Basic & Clinical Immunology,* 7th ed. Stites DP, Terr AI (editors). Appleton & Lange, 1991.

Winkelstein A: Immunosuppressive therapy. In: *Basic & Clinical Immunology,* 7th ed. Stites DP, Terr AI (editors). Appleton & Lange, 1991.

ASSOCIATIONS BETWEEN HLA ANTIGENS & SPECIFIC DISEASES

In humans, very striking associations are observed between particular HLA antigens and specific diseases. These facts are important in relating HLA to diseases: HLA antigen frequencies vary substantially among different ethnic groups, and therefore control populations must be carefully selected. Appropriate statistical corrections must be made to compensate for the large number of antigens tested. Accurate clinical definition of disease is necessary to avoid diluting an HLA-disease association by mixing together diseases that are pathogenetically different but clinically similar. If the disease studied has a fatal outcome, then the proper disease phase must be selected to demonstrate associations. Some quantitative measure of strength of association is necessary to compare different HLA-disease relationships.

Table 18–5 is a partial list of HLA-disease associations. Studies have revealed that the strongest association is between HLA-B27 and ankylosing spondylitis, which holds in all ethnic groups but is more striking in Japanese people than in Caucasians studied. Other spondyloarthropathies (eg, Reiter's syndrome, arthritis following Salmonella or Yersinia infection) are also strongly associated with B27, suggesting that despite apparently different causes the pathogeneses of these diseases share some common factor related to the B27 marker. B27 is not specific for all arthritis; eg, rheumatoid arthritis associates not with that antigen but with DR4. Furthermore, disease associations are not restricted to B and DR: eg, psoriasis vulgaris is associated with a C locus antigen and acute lymphocytic leukemia with an A locus antigen. In diabetes mellitus, heterozygote individuals possess both the DR3 and the DR4 antigens and have a relative risk of 33, far greater than expected by simple addition of risks for DR3 plus DR4. It also appears that a single mechanism may associate with different antigens in different ethnic groups. Among Caucasians studied in whom the Dw12 antigen is almost absent, Dw3 is associated with Graves' disease. Among Japanese people where Dw3 is almost completely lacking, Dw12 is associated with Graves' disease.

Sometimes combinations of antigens exhibit disease associations. This suggests either interaction among different genes affecting susceptibility or unusual linkage between the known HLA genes and some nearby gene actually responsible for the disease susceptibility.

Paul WE, Fathman GG, Metzger H (editors): Annu Rev Immunol 1984–present. (Annual entire issue.)
Schwartz BD: The human major histocompatibility HLA complex. In: *Basic & Clinical Immunology*, 7th ed. Stites DP, Terr AI (editors). Appleton & Lange, 1991.
Tiwari JL, Terasaki PI: *HLA and Disease Associations.* Springer, 1985.
Williamson AR, Turner MW: *Essential Immunogenetics.* Blackwell, 1987.

ALLERGIC DISEASES

Allergy is the most common form of immunologic disease. It is defined as an immunologically mediated reaction to a foreign antigen (allergen), causing tissue inflammation and organ dysfunction. The disease can be local or systemic. Because the allergen is foreign (ie, environmental), the skin and respiratory tract are the organs most frequently involved in allergic disease. Allergic reactions may also localize to the vasculature, gastrointestinal tract, or other visceral organs. Anaphylaxis and serum sickness are systemic forms of allergy.

Table 18–5. HLA and disease associations.

Disease	Antigen	Frequency		Relative Risk
		Patients (%)	Controls (%)	
Ankylosing spondylitis				
Caucasians	B27	89	4–13	69.1
Japanese	B27	85	<1	207
Reiter's disease	B27	80	9	37
Salmonella arthritis	B27	60–92	8–14	30
Rheumatoid arthritis	DR4	68	25	3.8
Psoriasis vulgaris	Cw6	27	4	8.5
Graves' disease				
Caucasians	Dw3	56	25	3.7
Japanese	Dw12	48	16	5
Diabetes mellitus	DR3 heterozygotes			3
Diabetes mellitus	DR4 heterozygotes			3.6
Diabetes mellitus	DR3/DR4 heterozygotes			33
Acute lymphocytic leukemia	A2	83	44	6
Systemic lupus erythematosus	DR4	73	33	5
Narcolepsy	DR2	100	34	358

CLASSIFICATION

Allergic diseases can be classified according to (1) the immunologic mechanism involved in pathogenesis, (2) the organ system affected, and (3) the nature and source of the allergen. An immunologic classification is preferred, because it serves as a rational basis for diagnosis and treatment.

Immunologic Mechanisms

The two major pathways of immunologically induced inflammation involve the reaction of the antigen with T cells and with B cell products (antibodies). Of the five immunoglobulin classes of antibodies, only three, IgG, IgM, and IgE, are known to be involved in hypersensitivity reactions. Classification of the hypersensitivity disorders helps elucidate the underlying pathogenic mechanism of clinical symptoms. The Gell and Coombs classification of the hypersensitivity diseases is as follows: Type I, IgE-mediated reactions (ie, allergic rhinitis, asthma, anaphylaxis); Type II, antibody-antigen mediated hypersensitivity reactions (ie, hemolytic anemia or Rh hemolytic disease; Type III, antigen-antibody complex mediated hypersensitivity (ie, serum sickness and Arthus reactions); and Type IV, cell mediated reactions. Unlike the first three, Type IV reactions are mediated by helper T lymphocytes, not by antibodies (ie, contact dermatitis, tuberculin reactions).

A. Type I, or IgE-Mediated (Immediate) Hypersensitivity: IgE antibodies occupy receptor sites on mast cells. Within minutes after exposure to the allergen, vasoactive and inflammatory mediators are activated and released from the mast cell, causing vasodilation, visceral smooth muscle contraction, and mucus secretory gland stimulation. Other mediators induce a late-phase inflammatory response that appears several hours later. There are two clinical subgroups of IgE-mediated allergy: atopy and anaphylaxis.

1. Atopy—Atopy is a group of diseases (allergic rhinitis, allergic asthma, atopic dermatitis, and allergic gastroenteropathy), that occur in certain persons with an inherited tendency to develop IgE antibodies to multiple common organic environmental allergens. The reaction is localized to a susceptible target organ, but more than one of these diseases may occur simultaneously in an allergic individual. There is a strong familial tendency involving complex genetic factors.

2. Anaphylaxis—Certain allergens, especially drugs, insect venom, and foods, may induce an IgE antibody response that causes a generalized release of mediators from mast cells, resulting in systemic anaphylaxis. This disease is characterized by (1) hypotension or shock from widespread vasodilation, (2) bronchospasm, (3) gastrointestinal and uterine muscle contraction, and (4) urticaria or angioedema. The condition is potentially fatal and is thus a medical emergency. Unlike atopy, sensitivities are rarely multiple. The condition affects either nonatopic or atopic persons. Urticaria and angioedema are cutaneous forms of anaphylaxis, but they are much more common. Like anaphylaxis, they are usually caused by a drug, food, or insect venom. These disorders are generally benign unless extensive enough to cause hypotension or unless angioedema obstructs the larynx or hypopharynx, causing respiratory obstruction.

B. Type II, Antibody-Mediated (Cytotoxic) Hypersensitivity: Cytotoxic reactions involve the binding of either IgG or IgM antibody to cell-bound antigens. Antibody binding to antigen results in activation of the complement cascade and the destruction of the cell to which the antigen is bound. Examples of tissue injury by this mechanism include immune hemolytic anemia and Rh hemolytic disease in the newborn. Autoimmune hyperthyroidism in which thyroid stimulating antibodies stimulate the thyroid tissue, or TSH binding inhibitory antibodies that inhibit the binding of TSH to its receptor are also type II reactions, though cytolysis is not a component of these reactions.

C. Type III, (Immune Complex-Mediated) Hypersensitivity: Antibodies of the IgG or IgM isotype can form complexes with the allergen and thereby activate complement to generate mediators of inflammation. Under conditions of high concentrations of both allergen and antibody, the clinical manifestations of disease include the Arthus reaction, a localized cutaneous and subcutaneous inflammatory response to injected allergen; serum sickness, a systemic disease characterized by fever, arthralgias, and dermatitis; and an acute form of hypersensitivity pneumonitis from inhalation of the allergen.

D. Type IV, T Cell-Mediated Hypersensitivity (Delayed Hypersensitivity, Cell-Mediated Hypersensitivity): The most common expression of T cell-mediated allergy is "allergic" contact dermatitis, in which the allergen causes dermal inflammation on direct contact with the skin. The dermatitis appears after a latent period of 1–2 days from the time of contact. Hypersensitivity pneumonitis (extrinsic allergic alveolitis) in its chronic form is predominantly a pulmonary T cell-mediated disease.

Organ System

Patients present to the physician with symptoms and physical findings that may be either localized or generalized. Knowledge of the organs involved may help to determine the type of allergy and the nature of the allergen (see Table 18–6).

Allergens & Antigens

Although any exogenous (environmental) material can theoretically be allergenic, certain ones are encountered more frequently than are others. For diagnostic purposes, it is convenient to classify them by route of exposure.

Table 18–6. Allergic diseases classified according to the involved organ or tissue.

Organ or Tissue	Disease	Mechanism			
		T Cell	IgE	Immune Complex	Uncertain
Skin	Allergic contact dermatitis	•			
	Atopic dermatitis		•		
	Urticaria and angioedema		•		
	Arthus reaction			•	
	Generalized drug eruption				•
	Fixed drug eruption				•
Upper respiratory tract	Allergic rhinitis		•		
Bronchi	Asthma		•		
	Allergic bronchopulmonary aspergillosis		•	•	
Alveoli	Hypersensitivity pneumonitis				
	Acute			•	
	Chronic	•			
Eyes	Allergic conjunctivitis		•		
Gastrointestinal tract	Allergic gastroenteropathy		•		
Liver	Hepatic drug reaction				•
Kidney	Allergic interstitial nephritis				•
Systemic	Anaphylaxis		•		
	Serum sickness			•	

A. Inhalants: Pollens, mold spores, animal products (danders, saliva, urine), house dust, and insect and arthropod emanations (especially the house dust mite) are the usual allergens that cause atopic disease. The house dust mite (*Dermatophagoides* spp) may be the most prevalent allergen for atopic allergy worldwide. Its importance in allergic asthma and atopic dermatitis has been confirmed in a number of recent studies. Hypersensitivity pneumonitis (see Chapter 9) can be caused by many airborne organic dusts, microorganisms, some organic chemicals, and by some drugs such as minocycline. Occasionally, the allergens causing contact dermatitis may reach the skin via atmospheric fumes. Immunologic analysis of bronchoalveolar lymphocytes from patients with drug-induced hypersensitivity pneumonitis suggests a central role for T lymphocytes in the pathogenesis of this disease.

B. Ingestants: Foods cause allergic gastroenteropathy and may cause atopic dermatitis, asthma, anaphylaxis, and urticaria or angioedema. Allergic reactions to drugs are most commonly urticaria and anaphylaxis. Drug-induced nonurticarial dermatitis or fixed drug eruptions are suspected to be allergic in origin, though the immunologic mechanism is uncertain. Serum sickness is usually caused by injected foreign protein (eg, antilymphocyte globulin), but mild reactions may occur after oral administration of drugs.

C. Injectants: Drugs, Hymenoptera venom, and injected atopic allergens account for most cases of anaphylaxis and acute urticaria or angioedema.

D. Contactants: Plant oils, cosmetics and perfumes, nickel in jewelry or on buckles and undergarment fasteners, hair dyes, topical medications including their additives, and occupational chemicals are the most common causes of T-cell-mediated (type IV) contact dermatitis.

Occasionally, urticaria or anaphylaxis may be induced by direct skin contact with the allergen. In recent years, the number of cases of anaphylaxis and urticaria from contact with gloves, catheters, dental dams, and other medical devices has increased dramatically. These disorders are caused by allergy to a protein in the latex and affect both patients and health care workers.

Guillon JM et al: Minocycline-induced cell-mediated hypersensitivity pneumonitis. Ann Intern Med 1992; 117:476. (Case study in which immunologic analysis of the phenotype and function of alveolar lymphocytes from serial bronchoalveolar lavage in a patient with drug-induced hypersensitivity pneumonitis.)

Middleton E, Reed C, Ellis E (editors): *Allergy: Principles and Practice,* 3rd ed. Mosby, 1988.

Sampson HA, Metcalfe DD: Food allergies. JAMA. 1992;268:2840. (Review of the pathophysiology and clinical manifestations and diagnosis of the IgE and non-IgE mediated hypersensitivity reactions to foods.)

Terr AI: Mechanisms of hypersensitivity. In: *Basic & Clinical Immunology,* 7th ed. Stites, DP, Terr, AI (editors). Appleton & Lange, 1991.

DIAGNOSIS

Virtually all of the clinical manifestations of allergy can also occur in the absence of an immunologic mechanism. For example, non-allergic (intrinsic) asthma is triggered by the nonimmunologic "irritant" effect of inhaled dusts and fumes, weather changes, stress, etc: irritant contact dermatitis is the result of physical or chemical damage to the skin; and anaphylactoid reactions are produced nonimmunologically by iodinated radiologic contrast media, by some drugs, and by physical exercise. Therefore, the diagnosis of allergy requires answers to the following three questions: (1) What is the nature of the disease? (2) Is the disease caused by allergy? (3) What specific allergens (one or several) are responsible?

A thorough history is essential. It must include details of symptomatology and a survey of allergens associated with home, work, hobbies, habits, and medications. Physical examination will reveal evidence of active disease if the patient is examined during a period of allergen exposure. Radiologic or other imaging studies may be necessary to supplement the physical examination. In some cases, physiologic testing such as pulmonary function tests is required to establish the diagnosis of a specific disease, but these procedures do not identify an allergic cause of that disease.

Tests of Specific Immune Responses

"Allergy tests" reveal an immune response to a particular allergen. To confirm a diagnosis of allergic disease, evidence of an immune response (ie, a positive test result) must be correlated with the history before one can conclude that the allergen caused the illness. The type of immune response must be consistent with the nature of the disease, for example, IgE antibody causes allergic rhinitis but not allergic contact dermatitis.

A. IgE Antibody Tests: IgE antibodies are detected by in vivo (skin tests) or in vitro methods.

1. Skin tests–Epicutaneous or cutaneous allergen testing produces a localized pruritic wheal and erythema which is maximal at 15–20 minutes. It is used most commonly in the diagnosis of allergic respiratory disease (rhinitis and asthma). Standard sets of allergen extracts are available commercially for pollens, fungi, animal danders, dust, and dust mites. The pollen and mold allergens must be appropriate to the patient's geographic area.

To avoid a systemic reaction, most allergists perform epicutaneous (prick) testing first, followed by selected intradermal tests to allergens that were negative by prick testing. Special allergenic extracts can be prepared for other allergens where indicated. Skin testing for food allergy is appropriate only if the patient has symptoms consistent with IgE-mediated allergy within 2 hours after eating the suspect food.

Skin testing to drugs is reliable for protein drugs (eg, heterologous serum, insulin), not for haptenic drugs (low-molecular-weight organic compounds). An important exception is penicillin, which will frequently, but not always, elicit a positive wheal-and-erythema skin test in patients with anaphylactic allergy to penicillin. The combination of skin testing with the major and minor metabolic determinants of penicillin (the minor determinants are not available commercially, although may be synthesized and are often available at academic medical centers) and assessment of the severity and type of previous penicillin allergic reaction may allow the designation of patients into high and low risk groups for subsequent reactions. The negative predictive value of skin tests for IgE-mediated reactions to subsequently administered penicillin is good. Little prospective data are available for determining the cross reactivity between the cephalosporin antibiotics and penicillins. There appears to be no allergic cross-reactivity between the monobactam antibiotics (aztreonam) and the penicillins and no adverse reactions have been reported in patients with true IgE-mediated penicillin reactions administered a monobactam antibiotic. A high degree of cross reactivity exists between the penicillin and the carbapenem, imipenem, and this drug should only be given to the penicillin allergic patient with the same degree of caution as if the patient were to receive penicillin.

Some drugs, notably opiates, cause non-immunologic release of mast cell mediators and thereby give universal wheal-and-erythema reactions. A negative diluent control test is essential. A positive control with histamine or a histamine liberator, such as morphine, is desirable.

Skin testing is preferred to in vitro methods (discussed below) because it detects the presence of IgE antibody in tissue and shows biologic activity. It is convenient, inexpensive, and provides an immediate result. Any drug with antihistamine effect must be withdrawn prior to testing. Extensive active dermatitis may limit the availability of skin for testing. There is an exceedingly small risk of inducing a systemic reaction when skin testing is conducted properly. Skin testing for anaphylactic reactions to Hymenoptera venom or a drug is performed by serial titration, starting with extremely dilute solutions to avoid a systemic reaction. Some physicians use serial titration of inhalant allergens in testing for atopic diseases.

2. In vitro tests of IgE antibody–IgE antibodies can be detected in serum by radioallergosorbent test (RAST) or enzyme-linked immunosorbent assay (ELISA). Protein allergens are covalently linked to the immunosorbent. Haptenic allergens must first be coupled to a nonallergenic protein carrier such as human serum albumin, which is then linked to the immunosorbent. Many of the usual atopic allergens are not available commercially for RAST or ELISA testing.

In vitro tests detect allergen-specific antibody in serum. Since IgE-mediated allergy is caused by IgE antibodies bound to mast cells (not by IgE antibodies in the circulation), in vitro tests generally are less sensitive than skin tests for diagnostic use. They are not affected by antihistamine therapy, but they can give false-positive results in patients with high total serum IgE and false-negative results in patients treated with immunotherapy who have significant allergen-specific IgG antibodies. There is no risk of a systemic reaction. The test is significantly more expensive than skin testing, and results are not immediately available. The RAST or ELISA method is particularly useful for detecting IgE antibodies to certain occupational chemicals or potentially toxic allergens.

The total IgE level in serum is higher on average in atopic patients than it is in nonatopic individuals. There is considerable overlap, so that it is not a satisfactory screening test for atopy.

B. Tests for Immune Complex Allergic Diseases: The IgG antibody may be present in sufficient quantity in serum to be detected by the precipitin-in-gel method. ELISA will detect antibodies present in lesser amounts. Reduced serum levels of C3, C4, or CH_{50} may be evidence of complement activation.

C. Tests for T Cell-Mediated Hypersensitivity: Cell-mediated immunity or hypersensitivity is detected by intradermal (tuberculin-type) skin tests which elicit 48-hour inflammatory induration or by patch testing in the diagnosis of allergic contact dermatitis. The patch test is performed by topical application of the suspected contactant allergen. A positive test at 48–72 hours consists of erythema, swelling, and papules. Concentrations of allergens for patch testing must be screened in nonallergic subjects to avoid false-positive irritant responses.

Cell-mediated hypersensitivity can be detected in vitro by exposing peripheral blood mononuclear cells to allergen to detect the release of cytokines or inhibition of cell migration, but such tests are rarely useful for diagnosis.

Provocation Tests

Occasionally, direct allergen challenge of the target organ or tissue under controlled conditions is required for definitive diagnosis. Such challenges may be bronchial, nasal, conjunctival, oral, or cutaneous. A positive test confirms that the reaction can be caused by the test substance, but it does not prove that an immunologic mechanism is responsible.

A. Bronchoprovocation Testing: An aerosolized solution of the allergen is delivered by inhalation through a dosimeter in graded increasing dosages. The response in FEV_1 or FEV_1/FVC is measured by spirometry, and the provoking dose (PD_{20}) producing a 20% fall in FEV_1 is determined. This test should be done in a facility where the patient can be monitored for 24 hours after allergen inhalation because of the possibility of a late-phase response. Bronchoprovocation is not necessary in the routine diagnosis of allergic asthma, but it may be helpful in some cases of occupational asthma.

Provocation testing should not be performed if there is a suspicion that the patient might develop a systemic anaphylactic reaction to the test.

"Natural" provocation field testing can be done by having the patient make serial determinations of peak expiratory flow rate (PEFR) using a portable peak flowmeter during periods of natural exposure to a suspected airborne allergen.

Bronchial provocation with exercise or with inhalation of methacholine, histamine, or cold air is a test for the nonspecific bronchial hyperirritability of asthma. These procedures do not detect allergic sensitivities.

B. Nasal Provocation Testing: This procedure is similar to bronchial provocation except that the allergen is inhaled through the nose and change in nasal airway resistance is measured. The procedure is complicated by significant excursions of nasal airway resistance that occur normally.

C. Conjunctival Provocation: A drop of allergen extract is instilled into one conjunctival sac. An allergic reaction produces itching, conjunctival injection, swelling, and tearing within minutes. The control contralateral eye is not affected. The method is unpleasant and therefore rarely used.

D. Oral Provocation: In most cases of suspected allergy to a food or drug, double-blind placebo-controlled oral challenge is the definitive test. For a positive test, the reported clinical findings must be reproduced. Freeze-dried foods in large opaque capsules provide a sufficient dose of allergen for testing.

Adelman D: Epitomes: Important Advances in Allergy and Immunology. Penicillin allergy. West J Med 1991; 154:456.

AMA Council on Scientific Affairs: In vitro testing for allergy: Report II. JAMA 1987;258:1639.

AMA Council on Scientific Affairs: In vivo diagnostic testing and immunotherapy for allergy. (Two parts.) JAMA 1987;258:1363, 1508.

Lin RY: A perspective on penicillin allergy. Arch Intern Med. 1992;152:930.

Sogn DD et al: Results of the National Institute of Allergy and Infectious Diseases Collaborative Clinical Trial to test the predictive value of skin testing with major and minor penicillin derivatives in hospitalized adults. Arch Intern Med 1992;152:1025.

Terr AI: In vitro tests for immediate hypersensitivity. Ann Rev Med 1988;39:135.

Townley RJ, Hopp RJ: Inhalation methods for the study of airway responsiveness. J Allergy Clin Immunol 1987; 80:111.

MANAGEMENT

Allergic disease management requires both symptomatic therapy and allergen-specific treatment. General measures for treating each of the diseases are presented elsewhere in this book. This section will discuss only the management of the allergic causes.

The three basic principles of allergy management are: (1) avoidance of the allergen, (2) symptomatic therapy, and (3) immunotherapy.

Avoidance Therapy

Avoidance is the most effective treatment for any allergic condition, and it should always be considered in addition to pharmacologic and immunologic treatment. Avoidance of allergen exposure may or may not reduce the underlying immunologic sensitivity to that allergen. Success requires accurate diagnosis of the causative allergens in each case.

A. Pollens: Remaining indoors in air-conditioned environments will avoid exposure to pollens, but this is not a long-term practical solution.

B. Animal Danders: If the allergy is slight, the patient may benefit from merely keeping the animal out of the bedroom; usually, however, it is necessary to remove the animal from the home altogether.

C. House Dust and Dust Mites: The mattress and pillows should be encased in dust-proof material, and the bedroom floor should be uncarpeted. The room should be dusted frequently. Electronic air purifiers are of unproved effectiveness. Acaricides to eliminate dust mites are under investigation.

D. Mold Spores: Out of doors, mold spores are unavoidable. Indoor mold contamination can be controlled by repairing leaks and cleaning mold buildup on sinks, shower curtains, pipes, etc.

E. Insect Stings: Sensitive patients should not walk barefoot outdoors, because yellow jackets nest in the ground. Wasp nests and beehives should not be disturbed. Garbage cans should be well covered, and outdoor eating should be avoided.

F. Drugs: It is necessary to avoid all cross-reacting drugs. Allergy to penicillin or to sulfonamides often encompass most if not all penicillin or sulfonamide derivatives, respectively. Rarely, a patient exquisitely sensitive to penicillin may react to penicillin in milk products, which then must be avoided.

G. Foods: Most persons with well-documented food allergy are allergic to one or a small number of foods, so that avoidance is rarely a problem. Persons with peanut anaphylaxis can have a fatal reaction to ingestion of a minute amount of the food. The presence of peanut can be unsuspected in some foods, so that the patient must be vigilant in restaurants or at parties. Soy-based formulas are available for infants with milk allergy.

H. Contactants: Patients with poison ivy or other plant oil allergy must learn to identify and avoid contact with the plant. In California, poison oak allergen is often transmitted to human skin by pets. Nickel-containing jewelry, buckles, etc., can be coated with clear nail polish. Protective clothing and gloves may be necessary for occupational contact dermatitis.

Drug Therapy

Pharmacotherapy of the immune response to reduce the allergic manifestations is achieved with drugs that alter the inflammatory phase.

A. IgE-Mediated Allergy: Three classes of drugs are useful for IgE-mediated diseases, based on (1) inhibition of release of mediators from mast cells, (2) inhibition of the action of mediators on their target cells, and (3) reversal of the vascular and inflammatory responses in the target tissues.

1. Cromolyn–Numerous studies show that pretreatment with this drug prevents the response to allergen by "stabilizing" the mast cell, though the specific molecular mechanism of action is unknown. Cromolyn is effective only when applied directly to the involved organ, and its action is short-lived. It is available as a bronchial inhaler (Intal) or a nasal spray (Nasalcrom). Dosage is usually four times daily on a continuous maintenance schedule as long as there is exposure to the allergen. Not all patients respond, but the drug has very few side effects and a wide margin of safety. Recently, a high-dose oral form of the drug has been released for use in treating systemic mastocytosis, but its effectiveness in preventing food-induced allergic gastroenteropathy is not known.

2. Antimediator drugs–Of the numerous mediators released from mast cells by reaction of allergen with IgE antibody, histamine is the only one that can be effectively blocked by drugs currently available. Antihistamine drugs are competitive inhibitors for the histamine receptors. Those that inhibit H1 receptors are used to treat IgE-mediated allergy. There are a number of such drugs on the market (Table 18–7), but their use is limited by side effects, primarily sedation and dryness. Rare complications are convulsions and tachyarrhythmias. Terfenadine and astemizole are nonsedating and have prolonged action. Rare complications of antihistamine overdosage, especially for those two drugs, are ventricular tachyarrhythmias and QT interval prolongation. Concomitant use of ketoconazole or macrolide antibiotics with terfenadine or astemizole may precipitate QT prolongation, torsades de pointes, other ventricular arrhythmias, cardiac arrest and death.

Antihistamine therapy is particularly helpful in allergic rhinitis and in urticaria, but it is not effective in all patients. It does not alleviate asthma, though it is not contraindicated in that disease when used to treat a concomitant rhinitis or pruritus. The antipruritic effect of antihistamines may be a useful adjunct in treatment of eczematous diseases. Intramuscular or intravenous antihistamines are used as adjunctive treatment of systemic anaphylaxis.

3. Sympathomimetic drugs–Adrenergic agonists are used for both α-adrenergic (vasoconstricting) and β-adrenergic (bronchodilating) properties. Injected epinephrine is initial therapy in anaphylaxis, because it has both effects and acts rapidly. Alpha-

Table 18–7. H$_1$ antihistamines.

Chemical Class	Representative Drugs	Usual Daily Dosage	Approximate Wholesale Price for 1 Month of Treatment
Ethanolamine	Diphenhydramine Clemastine	25–50 mg every 4–6 hours 0.34–2.68 mg every 12 hours	$8.20 $22.96
Ethylenediamine	Tripelennamine	25–50 mg every 4–6 hours	$7.44
Alkylamine	Brompheniramine	4 mg every 4–6 hours, or 8–12 mg of SR form every 8–12 hours	$3.76 $18.76
	Chlorpheniramine	4 mg every 4–6 hours, or 8–12 mg of SR form every 8–12 hours	$4.90 $5.38
	Triprolidine	2.5 mg every 4–6 hours	$5.04
Phenothiazine	Promethazine	25 mg at bedtime	$7.30
Piperazine	Hydroxyzine	25 mg every 6–8 hours	$3.80
Piperidines	Terfenadine (nonsedating) Astemizole (nonsedating) Azatadine Cyproheptadine	60 mg every 12 hours 10 mg/d 1–2 mg every 12 hours 4 mg every 6–8 hours	$45.84 $44.58 $81.68 $2.46

adrenergic agonists are used orally as nasal decongestants and conjunctivally as vasoconstrictors in allergic rhinitis and conjunctivitis, respectively. Beta-adrenergic drugs are primarily used for reversal of acute asthma, and they can be given by aerosol, by metered-dose inhaler, or orally. Recent epidemiologic studies suggest that regular multiple-dose daily β-drenergic drugs given by inhalation as primary treatment of chronic asthma may worsen disease morbidity, so "as-needed" dosing is now recommended by many specialists. The main side effect is muscle tremor, especially when the drug is taken orally, but tolerance usually develops with continued use.

4. Theophylline—This drug is used as a bronchodilator. Its mechanism of action is unknown, but it may involve inhibition of the bronchodilating effect of endogenous adenosine, liberated during the allergic reaction. If that is true, theophylline could be classified as an antimediator drug. Long-term continuous dosing with slow-release oral preparations to achieve a blood level of 10–20 μg/mL is effective for some asthmatic patients.

5. Glucocorticoids—These drugs have a therapeutic role in virtually all types of allergic diseases because of their anti-inflammatory action, rather than by their immunosuppressive effects. They are extremely effective, but they do not modify the underlying disease. Their use in allergy treatment requires close attention to side effects and toxicity. Corticosteroid drugs are available in oral, intramuscular, intravenous, intranasal, and bronchial inhalational forms, as eye drops, and in topical formulations for dermatologic use. Short-term systemic burst therapy is indicated for treatment of severe asthma, allergic contact dermatitis, and acute exacerbations of hypersensitivity pneumonitis and allergic bronchopulmonary aspergillosis. Steroid eye drops are for short-term treatment of acute allergic conjunctivitis, but the patient must be monitored for signs of corneal ulceration, keratitis, and glaucoma. Corticosteroid nasal spray is effective and probably safe for long-term use, but epistaxis can occur and nasal septal perforation is a possible complication. Flunisolide, beclomethasone, and triamcinolone are similarly efficacious, often requiring only a single daily dose after an initial period of therapy with four doses daily for 1 week. Long-term high-dose inhaled corticosteroid therapy for asthma is currently considered an important aspect of management of the inflammatory phase of the disease. Systemic absorption may occur. Oral candidiasis is a complication that is usually prevented by immediate mouth washing after each application. Topical steroid therapy is the primary treatment of atopic dermatitis. It may be effective in very mild cases of contact dermatitis.

6. Treatment of anaphylaxis—This is a medical emergency that demands immediate recognition and treatment to prevent death or morbidity from respiratory obstruction, circulatory failure, or both.

At the first suspicion of anaphylaxis, aqueous epinephrine 1:1000 in a dose of 0.2–0.5 mL (0.2–0.5 mg) is injected subcutaneously or intramuscularly. Repeated injections can be given every 20–30 minutes when necessary. Intracardiac injection of 1:10,000 concentration may be necessary for the patient in shock.

The definitive therapy of anaphylactic shock is the rapid intravenous infusion of large volumes of fluids (saline, lactated Ringer's, plasma, colloid solutions, or plasma expanders) to replace loss of intravascular plasma into tissues. Other vasopressor drugs (dopamine, dobutamine, norepinephrine, phenylephrine) may be necessary if the patient is refractory to epinephrine.

Airway obstruction may be caused by edema of the

larynx and hypopharynx or by bronchospasm. The former is treated by maintenance of an airway with endotracheal intubation or tracheostomy and oxygen. Bronchospasm responds to subcutaneous epinephrine or terbutaline. Inhalation of selective β_2-adrenergic agonists such as albuterol or terbutaline and intravenous administration of theophylline are given for bronchospasm.

Antihistamines (H_1 and H_2 receptor antagonists) are most useful as adjuvant therapy for alleviating the cutaneous manifestations of urticaria or angioedema and pruritus and for the gastrointestinal and uterine smooth muscle spasms. Corticosteroids will not reverse respiratory obstruction or shock even when given intramuscularly or intravenously, but these drugs may be helpful in moderating later sequelae of the vascular damage. Long-term combined oral antihistamine-prednisone therapy has been shown to reduce the number and severity of attacks in patients with frequent life-threatening episodes of idiopathic anaphylaxis.

There may be a clinical "late-phase" IgE response in anaphylaxis, as there is in atopy. Since this begins some hours after exposure to the allergen and after subsidence of the immediate-phase response, all patients with anaphylaxis should be monitored for up to 24 hours.

Anaphylaxis in a patient being treated with β-adrenergic blocker drugs is a special problem because of refractoriness to epinephrine and selective β-adrenergic agonists. Higher than usual doses of these drugs may be required for the desired effect; using glucagon in those patients taking beta-blockers may be additionally beneficial.

B. Immune Complex Allergic Diseases:

1. Serum sickness—This disease is self-limited, so treatment is usually conservative and symptomatic only. Aspirin will relieve the arthralgias. Antihistamines and topical steroids will control the dermatitis. Corticosteroid therapy is rarely necessary. Because the disease is usually free of long-term sequelae, these drugs should be given in dosages sufficient to just control symptoms.

2. Allergic bronchopulmonary aspergillosis—Patients with this disease have asthma complicated by periodic episodes of *Aspergillus* bronchitis and pneumonitis. Every effort should be made to prevent the development of bronchiectasis. Attacks characterized by dyspnea, cough, fever, pulmonary infiltrates, and elevated total serum IgE are treated promptly with prednisone, 1 mg/kg/d, for 2 weeks or longer to clear the infiltrates, after which the drug is slowly tapered. For those patients requiring chronic maintenance steroid therapy, a low dose of systemic corticosteroid is probably more reliable than inhaled beclomethasone.

3. Hypersensitivity pneumonitis—Acute exacerbations are treated with systemic steroids until they resolve fully.

C. T Cell-Mediated Hypersensitivity: Allergic contact dermatitis is treated with systemic steroids and topical emollients.

D. Radiocontrast Media Reactions: Reactions to radiocontrast media do not appear to be mediated by IgE antibodies, yet clinically are similar to anaphylaxis. These anaphylaxis-like events are referred to as anaphylactoid reactions. If a patient has had an anaphylactoid reaction to conventional radiocontrast media, then the risk for a second reaction upon reexposure may be as high as 30%. The management of patients experiencing radiocontrast media reactions includes the use of the lower osmolar radiocontrast media (which are associated with fewer anaphylactoid reactions), and by prophylactic pretreatment with prednisone, diphenhydramine and ephedrine. The use of the lower-osmolality radiocontrast media in combination with the pretreatment regimen decreases the incidence of reactions to less than 1%.

Immunotherapy

Treatment of atopy, especially allergic rhinitis, by the repeated long-term injection of allergen has been shown in many controlled clinical trials to be an effective method for reducing or eliminating symptoms and signs of the allergic disorder.

A. Procedure: Based on the clinical evaluation, a sterile aqueous solution of the allergen or allergens responsible for the individual patient's disease is administered repeatedly by subcutaneous injection in increasing doses once or twice a week until a maintenance dose is reached. The maintenance dose is determined individually based on improvement in symptoms and signs of the allergic disease and without systemic or excessive local reactions to the injected allergen. Thereafter, the same maintenance dose is injected every 2–4 weeks for several years. It is essential that the patient be monitored closely for correct diagnosis, proper dose, efficacy, and side effects.

B. Immunologic Effects: The term "allergen immunotherapy" is usually used instead of "desensitization," because the immunologic basis for this form of treatment is currently unknown. Nevertheless, certain immunologic changes can be induced by these injections. Circulating levels of IgE antibodies specific to the injected allergens increase slightly during the first few months, then decrease, eventually to substantially lower levels than before treatment. Seasonal rises in IgE antibodies to pollens are blunted or eliminated. IgG "blocking" antibody is produced. Changes in regulatory T cells favoring suppression of IgE antibody production have been reported. All of these effects are allergenically specific.

C. Clinical Effects: Most patients with allergic rhinitis caused by pollen become more tolerant to natural pollen exposure during successive seasons while on immunotherapy; some become completely asymptomatic, while a few patients derive no benefit. A beneficial response may or may not persist after treatment is stopped. Clinical effects, like the immunologic responses, are specific for the injected allergens only.

D. Adverse Effects: Reactions to treatment may be local or systemic. Localized immediate and late-phase skin reactions occur at injection sites. These are not harmful, but the dose must be adjusted to avoid excessively large or prolonged local reactions. Immediate systemic reactions or anaphylaxis are a potential problem with each injection and must be prevented by careful monitoring of dosage. The patient must remain for at least 20 minutes after each injection visit at the treatment facility where drugs and equipment for treating anaphylaxis are available. Exacerbation of the patient's allergic manifestations (rhinitis, asthma, eczema) also calls for reducing the subsequent dosage.

No long-term adverse immunologic or non-immunologic consequences of aqueous allergen extract immunotherapy are known.

E. Indications: This treatment is recommended for patients with severe allergic rhinitis who respond poorly to drug therapy and whose allergens are not avoidable. It is also used for allergic asthma, though there are few definitive clinical trials in that disease. There is no current evidence for an effect on atopic dermatitis. Inhalant allergens only are used. Food allergy is treated by avoidance.

Immunotherapy of systemic anaphylaxis to Hymenoptera venom has been shown to be extremely effective. Duration of treatment to achieve permanent immunity is currently under investigation. The current recommendations for continued protection are that venom immunotherapy should be continued indefinitely, until conclusive data are available. Risk factors for recurrent allergic reactions to insect stings if immunotherapy is discontinued include: a presenting history of a severe systemic reactions and systemic reactions to the therapy.

Short-course desensitization for IgE allergy to certain drugs, especially penicillin and insulin, has been successful in many cases. This is usually accomplished by a course of injections of increasing doses over a period of hours rather than the weeks or months as required for atopic disease treatment. Oral, injected, or topical desensitization for contact dermatitis has been attempted without evidence yet that it is efficacious.

Norman PS: Immunotherapy for nasal allergy (Symposium). J Allergy Clin Immunol 1988;81:992.

Ohman JL Jr: Allergen immunotherapy in asthma: Evidence for efficacy. J Allergy Clin Immunol 1989;84:133.

Terr AI: Desensitization. In: *Basic & Clinical Immunology,* 7th ed. Stites DP, Terr AI (editors). Appleton & Lange, 1991.

Valentine MD: Anaphylaxis and stinging insect hypersensitivity. JAMA 1992;268:2830. (Clinical management.)

Arthritis & Musculoskeletal Disorders

David B. Hellmann, MD

DIAGNOSIS & EVALUATION

Examination of the Patient

The diagnosis of a rheumatic disease can often be made in the office or at the bedside by history and physical examination. In general, the two clinical clues most helpful for diagnosis are the joint pattern and the presence or absence of extra-articular manifestations. The joint pattern is defined by answering three questions: (1) Is inflammation present? (2) How many joints are involved? and (3) What specific joint sites are affected? Joint inflammation is manifested by redness, warmth, swelling, and morning stiffness of at least 30 minutes' duration. Both the number of affected joints and the specific sites of involvement help determine the differential diagnosis (Table 19–1). Some diseases—gout, for example—are characteristically monarticular, whereas other diseases, such as rheumatoid arthritis, are chiefly polyarticular (Table 19–1). The location of joint involvement can also be distinctive. Only two diseases cause prominent involvement of the distal interphalangeal joint (DIP): osteoarthritis and psoriatic arthritis. As will be detailed in the discussion of specific diseases, the presence or absence of extra-articular manifestations such as fever, rash, nodules, or neuropathy helps narrow the differential diagnosis (see Table 19–1).

Laboratory procedures complete the evaluation, most commonly including sedimentation rate, tests for rheumatoid factor and antinuclear or other antibodies, synovial fluid analysis, and x-rays of affected joints. These studies are important for diagnosis and as a baseline for judging the results of therapy.

Arthrocentesis & Examination of Joint Fluid

Synovial fluid examination (Table 19–2) may provide specific diagnostic information in joint disease. Contraindications to arthrocentesis include infection of the overlying skin, coagulopathy, bleeding disorder, or inability of the patient to cooperate. Most large joints are easily aspirated (Figure 19–1).

A. Types of Studies: When synovial fluid is examined, the following studies should be included:

1. Gross examination–If fluid is green or purulent, a Gram's stain is indicated. If grossly bloody, consider a bleeding disorder, trauma, or "traumatic tap."

2. Microscopic examination–

a. Cell count and differential–Collect 2–5 mL in a heparinized tube. The red and white cells are counted, using the same equipment and technique as for a standard white count. Differential counts are performed on thin smears with Wright's stain.

b. Crystals–Compensated polarized light microscopy identifies the existence and type of crystals. The demonstration of urate or calcium pyrophosphate crystals is most important diagnostically.

3. Culture–Collect 1 mL of fluid in a sterile culture tube and perform routine bacterial cultures as well as special studies for gonococci, tubercle bacilli, or fungi when indicated.

B. Interpretation: (See Table 19–2.) Synovial fluid studies are not diagnostic unless a specific organism is identified in the culture or urate crystals of gout or calcium pyrophosphate crystals of pseudogout are demonstrated. There is considerable overlap in the cytologic and biochemical values obtained in different diseases (see Table 19–3). These studies do make possible, however, a differentiation according to severity of inflammation. The synovial fluid white blood cell and differential count have the greatest sensitivity and specificity. Inflammatory joint fluids have more than 3000 white blood cells per microliter, of which 50% or more are polymorphonuclear neutrophils (Table 19–2). Noninflammatory disease fluids have fewer than 3000/μL and less than 25% polymorphonuclear neutrophils. Synovial fluid glucose and protein levels usually change in relation to the degree of inflammation (Table 19–2) but add little information and, therefore, should not be ordered.

Shmerling RH et al: Synovial fluid tests: What should be ordered? JAMA 1990;264:1009. (Sensitivity and specificity of synovial fluid tests in distinguishing inflammatory from noninflammatory diseases: synovial white

Table 19–1. Diagnostic value of the joint pattern.

Characteristic	Status	Representative Disease
Inflammation	Present	Rheumatoid arthritis, systemic lupus erythematosus, gout
	Absent	Osteoarthritis
Number of involved joints	Monoarticular	Gout, trauma, septic arthritis, Lyme disease
	Oligoarticular (2–4 joints)	Reiter's disease, psoriatic arthritis, inflammatory bowel disease
	Polyarticular (≥ 5 joints)	Rheumatoid arthritis, systemic lupus erythematosus
Site of joint involvement	Distal interphalangeal	Osteoarthritis, psoriatic arthritis (not rheumatoid arthritis)
	Metacarpal phalangeal, wrists	Rheumatoid arthritis, systemic lupus erythematosus (not osteoarthritis)
	First metatarsal phalangeal	Gout, osteoarthritis

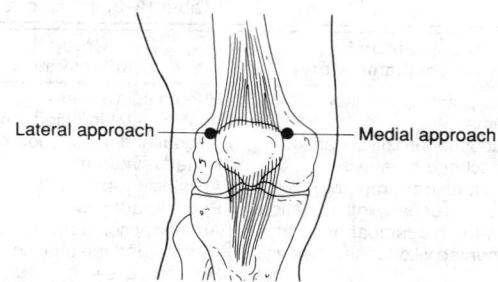

Figure 19–1. Aspiration of the knee joint. The knee joint—the most commonly aspirated joint—can be entered either medially or laterally. The patient should be supine, with the leg fully extended. Apply pressure on the side of the joint opposite to the puncture site to assist in directing the needle toward the bulging synovium. From the lateral approach, the needle (held parallel to the examining table) is directed medially, just beneath the patella, into the suprapatellar space. From the medial approach, the needle (held parallel to the examining table) is introduced between the patella and the medial condyle and advanced upward and laterally, beneath the patella and into the joint space. (Reproduced, with permission, from: Detmer W et al: *Pocket Guide to Diagnostic Tests.* Appleton & Lange 1992.)

blood cell count [sensitivity 0.84, specificity 0.84], percentage of polymorphonuclear cells [sensitivity 0.75, specificity 0.92], glucose [sensitivity 0.20, specificity 0.84], protein [sensitivity 0.52 specificity, 0.56].)

GENERAL PRINCIPLES IN MANAGEMENT OF PATIENTS WITH CHRONIC ARTHRITIS

Education & Emotional Factors

Chronic diseases such as rheumatoid arthritis destroy the belief—harbored by most people in good health—that individuals have control over their lives. This feeling of helplessness is often more frightening and disabling than the disease process itself. Therefore, the physician should explain the disease, describe the normal fluctuations of the disease process, and indicate how decisions about therapy will be made. Most patients think of "treatment" as a brief course of antibiotic or other drug followed by rapid recovery. The concept of chronic disease control and empiric treatment employing different agents in series must be explained if the patient is to have confidence in the physician. In addition, general information about the prognosis can be helpful in alleviating fear, since most patients have an excessively negative view of what is in store for them.

At some point, the patient's spouse should be in-

Table 19–2. Examination of joint fluid.

Measure	Normal	Group I (Noninflammatory)	Group II (Inflammatory)	Group III (Septic)
Volume (mL) (knee)	< 3.5	Often > 3.5	Often > 3.5	Often > 3.5
Clarity	Transparent	Transparent	Translucent-opaque	Opaque
Color	Clear	Yellow	Yellow to opalescent	Yellow to green
WBC (per μL)	< 200	200–3000	3000–50,000	> 50,000[1]
Polymorphonuclear leukocytes (%)	< 25%	< 25%	50% or more	75% or more[1]
Culture	Negative	Negative	Negative	Usually positive
Glucose (mg/dL)	Nearly equal to serum	Nearly equal to serum	> 25, lower than serum	< 25, much lower than serum

[1]Counts are lower with infections caused by organisms of low virulence or if antibiotic therapy has been started.

Table 19–3. Differential diagnosis by joint fluid groups.[1]

Group I (Noninflammatory)	Group II (Inflammatory)	Group III (Purulent)	Hemorrhagic
Degenerative joint disease Trauma[2] Osteochondritis dissecans Osteochondromatosis Neuropathic arthropathy[2] Subsiding or early inflammation Hypertrophic osteoarthropathy[3] Pigmented villonodular synovitis[2]	Rheumatoid arthritis Acute crystal-induced synovitis (gout and pseudogout) Reiter's syndrome Ankylosing spondylitis Psoriatic arthritis Arthritis accompanying ulcerative colitis and regional enteritis Rheumatic fever[3] Systemic lupus erythematosus[3] Progressive systemic sclerosis (scleroderma)[3] Tuberculosis Mycotic infections	Pyogenic bacterial infections	Hemophilia or other hemorrhagic diathesis Trauma with or without fracture Neuropathic arthropathy Pigmented villonodular synovitis Synovioma Hemangioma and other benign neoplasm

[1]Reproduced from Rodnan GP (editor): Primer on the rheumatic diseases, 7th ed. JAMA 1973;224(Suppl):662.
[2]May be hemorrhagic.
[3]Group I or II.

vited to the office with the patient for a discussion of the problem and given an opportunity to ask questions. In this way, education of the family serves as a source of the emotional support so critical to the patient's long-term well-being.

Physical & Occupational Therapies

Physical and occupational therapists know about the nonpharmacologic treatments of arthritis (described below) and can effectively teach them to patients. Most patients are hungry for this type of practical information. The therapist should develop a program the patient can follow at home, with only periodic monitoring by the therapist. Physicians and patients should avoid considering physical therapy as something "done to the patient"; for maximal benefit, the patient must make a commitment to maintaining the program at home.

Systemic Rest

The amount of systemic rest required depends upon the presence and severity of inflammation. Complete bed rest may be desirable in patients with profound systemic and articular inflammation, as can occur in rheumatoid arthritis, systemic lupus erythematosus, or psoriatic arthritis. With mild inflammation, 2 hours of rest each day may suffice. In general, rest should be continued until significant improvement is sustained for at least 2 weeks; thereafter, the program may be liberalized. However, the increase of physical activity must proceed gradually and with appropriate support for any involved weight-bearing joints.

Articular Rest

Decrease of articular inflammation may be expedited by articular rest. Relaxation and stretching of the hip and knee muscles, to prevent flexion contractures, can be accomplished by having the patient lie in the prone position for 15 minutes several times daily in addition to nighttime rest. Sitting in a flexed position for prolonged periods is a poor form of joint rest. Appropriate adjustable supports provide rest for inflamed weight-bearing joints, relieve spasm, and may reduce deformities, soft tissue contracture, or instability of the ligaments. The supports must be removable to permit daily range of motion and exercise of the affected extremities (see below). When ambulation is started, care must be taken to avoid weight bearing, which may aggravate flexion deformities. This is accomplished with the aid of crutches or braces until the tendency toward contracture has subsided.

Exercise

Therapeutic exercises are designed to preserve joint motion, muscular strength, and endurance. Initially, for inflammatory disease, passive range of motion and isometric exercises (such as straight leg raising) are best tolerated. The buoyancy of water permits maximum isotonic and isometric exercise with no more stress on joints than active range of motion exercises. Although ideal for arthritic patients, the cost of hydrotherapy often precludes its use. As tolerance for exercise increases and the activity of the disease subsides, progressive resistance exercises may be introduced. Patients should follow the general rule of eliminating any exercise that produces increased pain 1 hour after the exercise has ended.

Heat & Cold

These are used primarily for their muscle-relaxing and analgesic effects. Radiant or moist heat is generally most satisfactory. The ambulatory patient will find warm tub baths convenient. Paraffin baths for the hands are inexpensive and help many patients to reduce morning stiffness. Exercise may be better performed after exposure to heat. Some patients derive more relief of joint pain from local application of cold.

Assistive Devices

Patients with significant hip or knee arthritis may benefit from having a raised toilet seat, a gripping bar, or a cane. Patients should be instructed to hold the cane in the hand opposite to the affected knee or hip, thus leaning away from the affected joint. Crutches or walkers may be needed for patients with more extensive disease.

Splints

Splints may provide joint rest, reduce pain, and prevent contracture, but certain principles should be adhered to.

(1) Night splints of the hands or wrists (or both) should maintain the extremity in the position of optimum function. The elbow and shoulder lose motion so rapidly that other local measures and corticosteroid injections are usually preferable to splints.

(2) The best "splint" for the hip is prone-lying for several hours a day on a firm bed. For the knee, prone-lying may suffice, but splints in maximum tolerated extension are frequently needed. Ankle splints are of the simple right-angle type.

(3) Splints should be applied for the shortest period needed, should be made of lightweight materials for comfort, and should be easily removable for range-of-motion exercises once or twice daily to prevent loss of motion.

(4) Corrective splints, such as those for overcoming knee flexion contractures, should be used under the guidance of a physician familiar with their proper use.

Note: Avoidance of prolonged sitting or knee pillows may decrease the need for splints.

Weight Loss

For overweight patients, achieving ideal body weight will reduce the wear and tear placed on arthritic joints of the lower extremities.

DEGENERATIVE & CRYSTAL-INDUCED ARTHRITIS

DEGENERATIVE JOINT DISEASE (Osteoarthritis)

Essentials of Diagnosis

- A degenerative disorder without systemic manifestations.

- Pain relieved by rest; morning stiffness brief. Articular inflammation minimal.
- X-ray findings: narrowed joint space, osteophytes, increased density of subchondral bone, bony cysts.
- Commonly secondary to other articular disease.

General Considerations

Osteoarthritis is the most common form of joint disease, sparing no age, race, or geographic area. At least 20 million adults in the USA suffer from the effects of this condition at any one time, and 90% of all people will have radiographic features of osteoarthritis in weight-bearing joints by age 40. Symptomatic disease also increases with age.

This arthropathy is characterized by degeneration of cartilage and by hypertrophy of bone at the articular margins. Inflammation is usually minimal. Hereditary and mechanical factors may be variably involved in the pathogenesis.

Degenerative joint disease is traditionally divided into two types: (1) primary, which most commonly affects the terminal interphalangeal joints (Heberden's nodes) and less commonly the proximal interphalangeal joints (Bouchard's nodes), the metacarpophalangeal and carpometacarpal joints of the thumb, the hip, the knee, the metatarsophalangeal joint of the big toe, and the cervical and lumbar spine; and (2) secondary, which may occur in any joint as a sequela to articular injury resulting from either intra-articular (including rheumatoid arthritis) or extra-articular causes. The injury may be acute, as in a fracture; or chronic, as that due to occupational overuse of a joint, metabolic disease (eg, hyperparathyroidism, hemochromatosis, ochronosis), or neurologic disorders (tabes dorsalis; see below).

Pathologically, the articular cartilage is first roughened and finally worn away, and spur formation and lipping occur at the edge of the joint surface. The synovial membrane becomes thickened, with hypertrophy of the villous processes; the joint cavity, however, never becomes totally obliterated, and the synovial membrane does not form adhesions. Inflammation is prominent only in occasional patients with acute interphalangeal joint involvement (Heberden's nodes).

Clinical Findings

A. Symptoms and Signs: The onset is insidious. Initially, there is articular stiffness, seldom lasting more than 15 minutes; this develops later into pain on motion of the affected joint and is made worse by prolonged activity and relieved by rest. Deformity may be absent or minimal; however, bony enlargement is occasionally prominent, and flexion contracture or valgus or varus deformity of the knee is not unusual. There is no ankylosis, but limitation of motion of the affected joint or joints is common. Coarse crepitus may often be felt in the joint. Joint effusion and other articular signs of inflammation are mild. There are no systemic manifestations.

B. Laboratory Findings: Elevated sedimentation rate and other laboratory signs of inflammation are not present.

C. Imaging: Radiographs may reveal narrowing of the joint space, sharpened articular margins, osteophyte formation and lipping of marginal bone, and thickened, dense subchondral bone. Bone cysts may also be present.

Differential Diagnosis

Because articular inflammation is minimal and systemic manifestations are absent, degenerative joint disease should seldom be confused with other arthritides. The distribution of joint involvement in the hands also helps distinguish osteoarthritis from rheumatoid arthritis: Osteoarthritis chiefly affects the distal and proximal interphalangeal joints and spares the wrist and metacarpophalangeal joints; rheumatoid arthritis chiefly involves the wrists and metacarpophalangeal joints and spares the distal interphalangeal joints. Furthermore, the joint enlargement is bony-hard and cool in osteoarthritis but spongy and warm in rheumatoid arthritis. Neurogenic arthropathy is easily distinguished by physical examination. Degenerative joint disease may coexist with any other type of joint disease. Furthermore, one must be cautious in attributing all skeletal symptoms to degenerative changes in joints, especially in the spine, where metastatic neoplasia, osteoporosis, multiple myeloma, or other bone disease may coexist.

Prevention

Weight reduction has been shown in women to reduce the risk of developing symptomatic knee osteoarthritis. Reduction in weight of approximately 12 lb cuts the risk in half.

Treatment

A. General Measures: Education, rest, diet, exercise, and physical therapy (reviewed above) are very important in the success of treatment of osteoarthritis. For patients with osteoarthritis of the knee, a supervised walking program improves functional status without aggravating the joint pain.

B. Analgesic and Anti-inflammatory Drugs: Salicylates or other nonsteroidal anti-inflammatory drugs (see Chapter 1) are indicated for the relief of pain. High doses of salicylates, as used in more inflammatory arthritides, are unnecessary. Acetaminophen is as effective as ibuprofen in the treatment of osteoarthritis of the knee.

C. Orthopedic Measures: Orthopedic measures to correct developmental anomalies, deformities, disparity in leg length, and severely damaged joint surfaces may be required (see above).

D. Surgical Measures: Total hip replacement provides excellent symptomatic and functional improvement when that joint is seriously afflicted, as usually indicated by severely restricted walking and pain at rest, particularly at night. Knee replacement is also an option, though the results are less impressive.

Prognosis

Marked disability is less common than in rheumatoid arthritis, but symptoms may be quite severe and limit activity considerably (especially with involvement of the hips, knees, and cervical spine). Proper treatment may relieve symptoms and improve function.

Bradley JD et al: Comparison of an anti-inflammatory dose of ibuprofen, an analgesic dose of ibuprofen, and acetaminophen in the treatment of patients with osteoarthritis of the knee. N Engl J Med 1991;325:87. (Acetaminophen is as effective as ibuprofen.)

Felson DT et al: Weight loss reduces the risk for symptomatic knee osteoarthritis in women: The Framingham study. Ann Intern Med 1992;116:535.

Kovar PA et al: Supervised fitness walking in patients with osteoarthritis of the knee: A randomized, controlled trial. Ann Intern Med 1992;116:529. (A program of patient education and supervised fitness walking can improve functional status.)

McCarthy GM, McCarty DJ: Effect of topical capsaicin in the therapy of painful osteoarthritis of the hands. J Rheumatol 1992;19:604. (In osteoarthritis but not in rheumatoid arthritis, topical capsaicin is better than placebo.)

CRYSTAL DEPOSITION ARTHRITIS

1. GOUTY ARTHRITIS

Essentials of Diagnosis

- Acute onset, usually monarticular, often involving the first metatarsophalangeal joint.
- Postinflammatory desquamation and pruritus.
- Hyperuricemia.
- Identification of urate crystals in joint fluid or tophi.
- Asymptomatic periods between acute attacks.
- With chronicity, urate deposits in subcutaneous tissue, bone, cartilage, joints, and other tissues.
- Dramatic therapeutic response to NSAIDs or colchicine.

General Considerations

Gout is a metabolic disease of heterogeneous nature, often familial, associated with abnormal amounts of urates in the body and characterized early by a recurring acute arthritis, usually monarticular, and later by chronic deforming arthritis.

Primary gout is a heritable metabolic disease in which hyperuricemia is usually due to overproduction or underexcretion of uric acid—sometimes both.

It is rarely due to a specifically determined genetic aberration (eg, Lesch-Nyhan syndrome). Secondary gout, which may have some latent heritable component, is related to acquired causes of hyperuricemia, eg, diuretic use, myeloproliferative disorders, multiple myeloma, hemoglobinopathies, chronic renal disease, and lead poisoning.

About 90% of patients with primary gout are men, usually over 30 years of age. In women the onset is usually postmenopausal. The characteristic histologic lesion is the tophus, a nodular deposit of monosodium urate monohydrate crystals, and an associated foreign body reaction. These may be found in cartilage, subcutaneous and periarticular tissues, tendon, bone, the kidneys, and elsewhere. Urates have been demonstrated in the synovial tissues (and fluid) during acute arthritis; indeed, the acute inflammation of gout is believed to be activated by the phagocytosis by polymorphonuclear cells of urate crystals with the ensuing release from the neutrophils of chemotactic and other substances capable of mediating inflammation. The precise relationship of hyperuricemia to acute gouty arthritis is still obscure, since chronic hyperuricemia is a frequent finding in people who never develop gout or uric acid stones (Table 19–4). Rapid fluctuations in serum urate levels, either increasing or decreasing, are important factors in precipitating acute gout. The mechanism of the late, chronic stage of gouty arthritis is better understood. This is characterized pathologically by tophaceous invasion of the articular and periarticular tissues, with structural derangement and secondary degeneration (osteoarthritis).

Uric acid kidney stones are present in 10–20% of patients with gouty arthritis. The term gouty nephropathy (or "gouty nephritis") refers to kidney disease due to sodium urate deposition in the renal interstitium. Uric acid stones are not related to its pathogenesis, and a relationship to renal insufficiency has not been established.

Unless there is a rapid breakdown of cellular nucleic acid following aggressive treatment of leukemia or lymphoma, uric acid-lowering drugs need not be instituted until arthritis, renal calculi, or tophi become apparent. Psoriasis, sarcoidosis, and diuretic drugs are commonly overlooked causes of hyperuricemia and may precipitate attacks in patients with gout. Asymptomatic hyperuricemia should not be treated.

Clinical Findings

A. Symptoms and Signs: The acute arthritis is characterized by its sudden onset, frequently nocturnal, either without apparent precipitating cause or following rapid fluctuations in serum urate levels from food and alcohol excess, surgery, infection, diuretics, chemicals (eg, meglumine diatrizoate, Urografin), or uricosuric drugs. The metatarsophalangeal joint of the great toe is the most susceptible joint ("podagra"), although others, especially those of the feet, ankles, and knees, are commonly affected. Hips and shoulders are rarely involved in gouty arthritis. More than one joint may occasionally be affected during the same attack; in such cases, the distribution of the arthritis is usually asymmetric. As the attack progresses, the pain becomes intense. The involved joints are swollen and exquisitely tender and the overlying skin tense, warm, and dusky red. Fever is common and may reach 39 °C (102.2 °F). Local desquamation and pruritus during recovery from the acute arthritis are characteristic of gout but are not always present. Tophi may be found in the external ears, hands, feet, olecranon, and prepatellar bursas. They are usually seen only after several attacks of acute arthritis.

Asymptomatic periods of months or years commonly follow the initial acute attack. Later, gouty arthritis may become chronic, with symptoms of progressive functional loss and disability. Gross deformities, due usually to tophaceous invasion, are seen. Signs of inflammation may be absent or superimposed.

B. Laboratory Findings: The serum uric acid is practically always elevated (> 7.5 mg/dL) unless uricopenic drugs are being given. During an acute attack, the erythrocyte sedimentation rate and white cell count are usually elevated. Examination of the material aspirated from a tophus shows the typical crystals of sodium urate and confirms the diagnosis. Further confirmation is obtained by identification of sodium urate crystals by compensated polariscopic examination of wet smears prepared from joint fluid aspirates. Such crystals are negatively birefringent

Table 19–4. Origin of hyperuricemia.[1]

Primary Hyperuricemia
A. Increased production of purine:
  1. Idiopathic.
  2. Specific enzyme defects (eg, Lesch-Nyhan syndrome, glycogen storage disease).
B. Decreased renal clearance of uric acid (idiopathic).

Secondary Hyperuricemia
A. Increased catabolism and turnover of purine:
  1. Myeloproliferative disorders.
  2. Lymphoproliferative disorders.
  3. Carcinoma and sarcoma (disseminated).
  4. Chronic hemolytic anemias.
  5. Cytotoxic drugs.
  6. Psoriasis.
B. Decreased renal clearance of uric acid:
  1. Intrinsic kidney disease.
  2. Functional impairment of tubular transport:
    a. Drug-induced (eg, thiazides, probenecid).
    b. Hyperlacticemia (eg, lactic acidosis, alcoholism).
    c. Hyperketoacidemia (eg, diabetic ketoacidosis, starvation).
    d. Diabetes insipidus (vasopressin-resistant).
    e. Bartter's syndrome.

[1]Modified from Rodnan GP: Gout and other crystalline forms of arthritis. Postgrad Med (Oct) 1975;58:6.

and needle-like and may be found free or in neutrophils.

C. Imaging: Early in the disease, radiographs show no changes. Later, punched-out areas in the bone (radiolucent urate tophi) are seen. When these are adjacent to a soft tissue tophus, they are diagnostic of gout.

Differential Diagnosis

Once the diagnosis of acute gouty arthritis is suspected, it is confirmed by the presence of hyperuricemia, dramatic response to NSAIDs or colchicine, local desquamation and pruritus as the edema subsides, and polariscopic examination of joint fluid. Acute gout is often confused with cellulitis. Appropriate bacteriologic studies should exclude acute pyogenic arthritis. Acute chondrocalcinosis (pseudogout) may be distinguished by the identification of calcium pyrophosphate crystals in the joint fluid, usually normal serum uric acid, the x-ray appearance of chondrocalcinosis, and the relative therapeutic ineffectiveness of colchicine.

Chronic tophaceous arthritis may rarely mimic chronic rheumatoid arthritis. In such cases, the diagnosis of gout is suggested by an earlier history of monarthritis and is established by the demonstration of urate crystals in the contents of a suspected tophus. Biopsy may be necessary to distinguish tophi from rheumatoid nodules. An x-ray appearance similar to that of gout may be found in rheumatoid arthritis, sarcoidosis, multiple myeloma, hyperparathyroidism, or Hand-Schüller-Christian disease. Chronic lead intoxication may result in attacks of gouty arthritis and renal insufficiency.

Treatment

A. Acute Attack: The most common mistake in managing gout is starting drug treatment for both the acute arthritis and the hyperuricemia simultaneously. Treatment must be separated by treating the acute arthritis first and hyperuricemia later. Sudden reduction of serum uric acid often precipitates further episodes of gouty arthritis. Treatment of hyperuricemia is more safely started once the acute gouty episode has resolved.

1. Nonsteroidal anti-inflammatory drugs– NSAIDs have become the treatment of choice for acute gout. Traditionally, indomethacin has been the most frequently used agent, but all of the other newer NSAIDs are probably equally effective. Indomethacin is initiated at a dosage of 50 mg every 8 hours and continued until the symptoms have resolved (usually 5–10 days). Active peptic ulcer disease, impaired renal function, and a history of allergic reaction to NSAIDs are contraindications to the use of these drugs.

2. Colchicine–Colchicine is also effective for acute gout but is less favored, since 80% of treated patients develop significant abdominal cramping, diarrhea, nausea, or vomiting. Colchicine is thought to work by inhibiting the chemotactic property of leukocytosis and thus interferes with the inflammatory response to urate crystals. Once a full chemotactic response has occurred (after the first 24–48 hours), colchicine loses its effectiveness. The dose is 0.5 or 0.6 mg by mouth every hour until pain is relieved or until nausea or diarrhea appears; the drug is then stopped. The usual total dose required is 4–8 mg. The incidence of gastrointestinal side effects of colchicine can be reduced by intravenous administration in an initial dose of 1–2 mg in 10–20 mL of saline solution. Use of intravenous colchicine, however, should be discouraged because of potential severe toxicity, including local pain, tissue damage from extravasation during injection, bone marrow suppression, disseminated intravascular coagulation, and death. Single intravenous doses should not exceed 2–3 mg; the total dose should not exceed 4–5 mg; and no additional colchicine should be given by mouth for 3 weeks. Dosages must be reduced in the presence of renal or hepatic disease or old age. Combined renal and hepatic disease contraindicates the use of intravenous colchicine. Intravenous administration of colchicine is rarely necessary and is inadvisable if the oral route can be used. Oral colchicine should not be used in patients with inflammatory bowel disease.

3. Corticosteroids–Corticosteroids often give dramatic symptomatic relief in acute episodes of gout and will control most attacks if continued long enough. Corticosteroids are best reserved for patients with acute gout who are unable to take oral NSAIDs. If the patient's gout is monarticular, intra-articular administration (eg, triamcinolone, 10–40 mg depending on the size of the joint) is most effective. For polyarticular gout, corticosteroids may be given intravenously (eg, methylprednisolone, 40 mg/d tapered off over 7 days) or orally (eg, prednisone, 40–60 mg/d tapered off over 7 days). It should be recognized that gouty and septic arthritis can coexist, even if rarely. Therefore, joint aspiration and Gram stain of synovial fluid should be performed before corticosteroids are given.

4. Analgesics–At times the pain of an acute attack may be so severe that analgesia is necessary before a more specific drug becomes effective. In these cases, codeine or meperidine may be given. Aspirin should be avoided (see below).

5. Bed rest is important in the management of the acute attack and should be continued for about 24 hours after the acute attack has subsided. Early ambulation may precipitate a recurrence.

Physical therapy is of little value during the acute attack, though hot or cold compresses to or elevation of the affected joints makes some patients more comfortable.

B. Management Between Attacks: Treatment during symptom-free periods is intended to minimize urate deposition in tissues, which causes chronic tophaceous arthritis, and to reduce the frequency and severity of recurrences.

1. Diet–It is important to avoid obesity, fasting, excessive alcohol, and dehydration. Rigid diets fail to influence the hyperuricemia or the course of gouty arthritis. Since dietary sources of purines contribute very little to the causation of the disease, restriction of foods high in purine (eg, kidney, liver, sweetbreads, sardines, anchovies, meat extracts) cannot be expected to contribute significantly to the management of the disease. Specific foods or alcoholic beverages that precipitate attacks should be avoided. A high liquid intake and, more importantly, a daily urinary output of 2 L or more will aid urate excretion and minimize urate precipitation in the urinary tract.

2. Avoidance of hyperuricemic medications–Diuretics such as hydrochlorothiazide and furosemide inhibit renal excretion of uric acid, thereby producing or increasing hyperuricemia. Whenever possible, these diuretics should be avoided in patients with gout. Similarly, low doses of aspirin also inhibit renal excretion of uric acid and aggravate hyperuricemia. Nicotinic acid is yet another medication that can produce hyperuricemia.

3. Colchicine–The decision to begin chronic pharmacologic treatment of gout should be based on an estimate of the likelihood of the patient's having another attack. A 43-year-old obese man who has had a single episode of gout and is willing to lose weight and stop taking low-dose aspirin is at low risk of another attack and therefore is unlikely to benefit from chronic medical therapy. In contrast, a 54-year-old man with mild chronic renal failure, a requirement for thiazide diuretic use, and a history of multiple attacks of gout is much more likely to benefit from pharmacologic treatment. In general, the higher the uric acid level and the more frequent the attacks of gout, the more likely it is that chronic medical therapy will be beneficial.

Daily colchicine use has two indications: (1) Colchicine can be used by itself to prevent future attacks of gout. The drug does not affect the uric acid level but reduces the frequency of attacks. For the person who has mild hyperuricemia and has had several attacks of gouty arthritis, chronic colchicine prophylaxis may be all that is needed to reduce substantially the chance of a future attack. The usual dose is 0.6 mg twice a day. Patients who have coexisting moderate renal insufficiency or heart failure should have the dose reduced to once a day in order to avoid the development of a mixed peripheral neuropathy and myositis that can complicate the use of higher doses. (2) Colchicine prophylaxis is also used when uricosuric drugs or allopurinol (see below) are started, to suppress the acute attacks that can be precipitated by abrupt changes in the serum uric acid level.

4. Reduction of serum uric acid–Indications include frequent acute arthritis not controlled by colchicine prophylaxis, tophaceous deposits, or renal damage. It is emphasized that hyperuricemia with infrequent attacks of arthritis may not require treatment; asymptomatic hyperuricemia should not be treated.

Two classes of agents may be used to lower the serum uric acid—the uricosuric drugs and allopurinol (neither is of value in the treatment of acute gout). The choice of one or the other depends on the result of a 24-hour urine uric acid determination. A value under 800 mg/d indicates undersecretion of uric acid, which is amenable to uricosuric agents. Patients with more than 800 mg of uric acid in a 24-hour urine collection are overproducers of uric acid who require allopurinol.

a. Uricosuric drugs–These drugs, by blocking tubular reabsorption of filtered urate and reducing the metabolic pool of urates, prevent the formation of new tophi and reduce the size of those already present. Furthermore, when administered concomitantly with colchicine, they may lessen the frequency of recurrences of acute gout. The indication for uricosuric treatment is the increasing frequency or severity of acute attacks. Uricosuric agents are ineffective in patients with renal insufficiency, as manifested by a serum creatinine of more than 2 mg/dL.

The following uricosuric drugs may be employed: (1) Probenecid, 0.5 g daily initially, with gradual increase to 1–2 g daily; or (2) sulfinpyrazone, 100 mg daily initially, with gradual increase to 200–400 mg daily. The maintenance dose is determined by observation of the serum uric acid response and the urinary uric acid response. Ideally, one attempts to maintain a normal serum urate level.

Hypersensitivity to either uricosuric drug in the form of fever and rash occurs in 5% of cases; gastrointestinal complaints occur in 10%.

Precautions with uricosuric drugs. It is important to maintain a daily urinary output of 2000 mL or more in order to minimize the precipitation of uric acid in the urinary tract. This can be further prevented by giving alkalinizing agents to maintain a urine pH of above 6.0. Uricosuric drugs are best avoided in patients with a history of uric acid lithiasis. Avoid using salicylates, since they antagonize the action of uricosuric agents.

b. Allopurinol–The xanthine oxidase inhibitor allopurinol promptly lowers plasma urate and urinary uric acid concentrations and facilitates tophus mobilization. The drug is of special value in uric acid overproducers; in tophaceous gout; in patients unresponsive to the uricosuric regimen; and in gouty patients with uric acid renal stones. It should be used cautiously in patients with renal insufficiency and is not indicated in asymptomatic hyperuricemia. The most frequent adverse effect is the precipitation of an acute gouty attack. However, the commonest sign of hypersensitivity to allopurinol (occurring in 5% of cases) is a pruritic rash that may progress to toxic epidermal necrolysis, a potentially fatal complication.

Vasculitis and severe hepatitis are other rare complications.

The daily dose is determined by the serum uric acid response. The initial dose of allopurinol is 100 mg/d for 1 week; the dose is increased if the serum uric acid is still high. A normal serum uric acid level is often obtained with a daily dose of 200–300 mg. Occasionally (and in selected cases) it may be helpful to continue the use of allopurinol with a uricosuric drug. Neither of these drugs is useful in acute gout.

C. Chronic Tophaceous Arthritis: Tophaceous deposits can be made to shrink and disappear altogether with allopurinol therapy. The treatment is essentially the same as that outlined for the intervals between acute attacks. Surgical excision of large tophi offers immediate mechanical improvement in selected deformities but is rarely required.

Prognosis

Without treatment, the acute attack may last from a few days to several weeks, but proper treatment quickly terminates the attack. The intervals between acute attacks vary up to years, but the asymptomatic periods often become shorter if the disease progresses. Chronic tophaceous arthritis occurs after repeated attacks of acute gout, but only after inadequate treatment. Although the deformities may be marked, only a small percentage of patients become bedridden. The younger the patient at the onset of disease, the greater the tendency to a progressive course. Destructive arthropathy is rarely seen in patients whose first attack is after age 50.

Patients with gout have an increased incidence of hypertension, renal disease (eg, nephrosclerosis, tophi, pyelonephritis), diabetes mellitus, hypertriglyceridemia, and atherosclerosis, although these relationships are not well understood.

Roubenoff RR: Gout and hyperuricemia. Rheumat Dis Clin North Am 1990;16:539.

Wallace SL et al.: Renal function predicts colchicine toxicity: Guidelines for the prophylactic use of colchicine in gout. J Rheumatol 1991;18:264. (Myopathy and neuropathy—potential complications of chronic colchicine, 0.6 mg twice daily—occurred only in patients with a creatinine clearance under 50 mL/min.)

Wernick R, Winkler C, Campbell S: Tophi as the initial manifestation of gout: Report of six cases and review of the literature. Arch Intern Med 1992;152:873.

2. CHONDROCALCINOSIS & PSEUDOGOUT (Calcium Pyrophosphate Dihydrate [PD] Deposition Disease)

The term chondrocalcinosis refers to the presence of calcium-containing salts in articular cartilage. It is most often first diagnosed radiologically. It may be familial and is commonly associated with a wide variety of metabolic disorders, eg, hemochromatosis, hyperparathyroidism, ochronosis, diabetes mellitus, hypothyroidism, Wilson's disease, and true gout. Pseudogout, most often seen in persons age 60 or older, is characterized by acute, recurrent and rarely chronic arthritis that usually involves large joints (principally the knees and the wrists) and is almost always accompanied by chondrocalcinosis of the affected joints. Identification of calcium pyrophosphate crystals in joint aspirates is diagnostic of pseudogout. With light microscopy, the rhomboid-shaped pseudogout crystals can usually be distinguished from the needle-shaped gout crystals. A red compensator is used for positive identification, since pseudogout crystals are blue when parallel and yellow when perpendicular to the axis of the compensator. Urate crystals give the exact opposite color pattern. A useful mnemonic is that "parallel," "yellow," and "allopurinol" all have double *l*'s. X-ray examination shows not only calcification (usually symmetric) of cartilaginous structures but also signs of degenerative joint disease (osteoarthritis). Unlike gout, pseudogout is usually associated with normal serum urate levels and is not dramatically improved by colchicine.

Treatment of chondrocalcinosis is directed at the primary disease, if present. Some of the nonsteroidal anti-inflammatory agents (salicylates, indomethacin, naproxen, and other drugs) are helpful in the treatment of acute episodes of pseudogout. Colchicine, 0.6 mg orally twice daily, appears to be more effective for prophylaxis than for acute attacks. Aspiration of the inflamed joint and intra-articular injection of triamcinolone, 10–40 mg, depending on the size of the joint, is also of value in resistant cases.

Jones AC et al: Diseases associated with calcium pyrophosphate deposition disease. Semin Arthritis Rheum 1992; 22:188. (Hemochromatosis, hyperparathyroidism, hypomagnesemia, and hypophosphatasia are associated with chondrocalcinosis and pseudogout.)

PAIN SYNDROMES

CERVICOBRACHIAL PAIN SYNDROMES

A large group of articular and extra-articular disorders is characterized by pain that may involve simultaneously the neck, shoulder girdle, and upper extremity. Diagnostic differentiation is often difficult. Some of these entities and clinical syndromes represent primary disorders of the cervicobrachial region; others are local manifestations of systemic disease. The clinical picture is further complicated when two or more of these conditions occur coincidentally.

Clinical Findings

A. Symptoms and Signs: Neck pain may be limited to the posterior neck region or, depending upon the level of the symptomatic joint, may radiate segmentally to the occiput, anterior chest, shoulder girdle, arm, forearm, and hand. It may be intensified by active or passive neck motions. The general distribution of pain and paresthesias corresponds roughly to the involved dermatome in the upper extremity. Radiating pain in the upper extremity is often intensified by hyperextension of the neck and deviation of the head to the involved side. Limitation of cervical movements is the most common objective finding. Neurologic signs depend upon the extent of compression of nerve roots or the spinal cord. Compression of the spinal cord may cause long-tract involvement resulting in paraparesis or paraplegia.

B. Imaging: The radiographic findings depend on the cause of the pain; many are completely normal. An early finding is loss of the normal anterior convexity of the cervical curve (loss of cervical lordosis). Comparative reduction in height of the involved disk space is a frequent finding. The most common late x-ray finding is osteophyte formation anteriorly, adjacent to the disk; other late changes occur around the apophyseal joint clefts, chiefly in the lower cervical spine. Computer-assisted myelography and MRI are valuable for demonstrating nerve root or spinal cord compression.

Differential Diagnosis & Treatment

The causes of neck pain include acute and chronic cervical strain or sprains, herniated nucleus pulposus, osteoarthritis, ankylosing spondylitis, rheumatoid arthritis, osteomyelitis, neoplasms, spinal stenosis, compression fractures, and functional disorders.

A. Acute or Chronic Cervical Musculotendinous Strain: Cervical strain is generally caused by mechanical postural disorders, overexertion, or injury (eg, whiplash). Acute episodes are associated with pain, decreased cervical spine motion, and paraspinal muscle spasm, resulting in stiffness of the neck and loss of motion. Muscle trigger points can often be localized. Management includes neck and head immobilization by traction, a cervical collar, and administration of analgesics. Gradual return to full activity is encouraged.

Patients with chronic symptoms often have few objective findings. Mechanical stress due to work or recreational activities is often implicated. Chronic pain, especially that radiating into the upper extremity, may require additional treatment such as bracing.

B. Herniated Nucleus Pulposus: Rupture or prolapse of the nucleus pulposus of the cervical disks into the spinal canal causes pain that radiates to the arms at the level of C6–7. When intra-abdominal pressure is increased by coughing, sneezing, or other movements, symptoms are aggravated, and cervical muscle spasm may often occur. Neurologic abnor-

malities may include decreased reflexes of the deep tendons of the biceps and triceps and decreased sensation and muscle atrophy or weakness in the forearm or hand. Cervical traction, bed rest, and other conservative measures are usually successful. Myelography or electromyography helps delineate lesions that may require surgical treatment (laminectomy, fusion).

C. Arthritic Disorders: Cervical spondylosis (degenerative arthritis) is a collective term describing degenerative changes that occur in the apophyseal joints and intervertebral disk joints, with or without neurologic signs. Osteoarthritis of the articular facets is characterized by progressive thinning of the cartilage, subchondral osteoporosis, and osteophytic proliferation around the joint margins. Degeneration of cervical disks and joints may occur in adolescents but is more common after age 40. Degeneration is progressive and is marked by gradual narrowing of the disk space, as demonstrated by x-ray. Osteocartilaginous proliferation occurs around the margin of the vertebral body and gives rise to osteophytic ridges that may encroach upon the intervertebral foramina and spinal canal, causing compression of the neurovascular contents. A large anterior osteophyte may occasionally cause dysphagia.

Ankylosing spondylitis is discussed below. Atlantoaxial subluxation may occur in patients with rheumatoid arthritis, regardless of the severity of disease. Inflammation of the synovial structures resulting from erosion and laxity of the transverse ligament can lead to neurologic signs of spinal cord compression. Treatment may vary from use of a cervical collar or more rigid bracing to operative treatment, depending on the degree of subluxation and neurologic progression. Surgical treatment may involve stabilization of the cervical spine.

D. Other Disorders: Osteomyelitis and neoplasms are discussed below. Osteoporosis is discussed in Chapter 25.

LOW BACK PAIN

The approach to the patient with nontraumatic low back pain is dictated by several observations. First, low back pain is exceedingly common, experienced at some time by up to 80% of the population. Second, the differential diagnosis of low back pain is broad and includes systemic diseases (eg, metastatic cancer), primary spine disease (eg, disk herniation, degenerative arthritis), and regional diseases (eg, aortic dissection) that refer pain to the low back. Third, a precise diagnosis cannot be made in the majority of cases. The frequent use of the terms "strain," "sprain," or "lumbago" underscores the common imprecision of diagnosis. Even when anatomic defects—such as vertebral osteophytes or a narrowed disk space—are present, clinical disease cannot be assumed since such "defects" are common in asymptomatic patients. Fourth, the great majority of patients will improve in 1–4 weeks with conservative therapy and need no evaluation beyond the initial history and physical examination. The diagnostic challenge, then, is to identify among the many sufferers of low back pain those few patients who require more extensive or urgent evaluation.

In practice this means identifying those patients who have "serious" disease, defined as (1) infection, (2) cancer, (3) inflammatory back disease such as ankylosing spondylitis, (4) important regional disease such as dissecting aortic aneurysm, or (5) significant or rapidly progressing neurologic deficits. If there is no evidence that the patient has any of these five problems, conservative therapy is called for.

1. CLINICAL APPROACH TO DIAGNOSIS

General History & Physical Examination

The single most common mistake in evaluating patients with low back pain is to concentrate on the back to the exclusion of a careful general history and physical examination. Yet it is in this very setting that the general history and physical examination are so important in detecting clues or "red flags" suggesting the presence of "serious" back disease. Low back pain is a final common pathway of many processes. The pain of vertebral osteomyelitis is not very different in quality and intensity from the pain due to back strain of the weekend gardener. The physician who concentrates on the back pain symptoms and neglects the general history risks missing the rare patient with low back pain needing further evaluation.

Specifically, the physician should note a history of smoking, weight loss, advanced age, and a history of cancer, all of which are risk factors for vertebral body metastasis. Vertebral body osteomyelitis most frequently occurs in adults with a history of recurrent urinary tract infections and is especially common in diabetics.

A history of peptic ulcer disease and prednisone therapy may be clues suggesting that a patient's refractory back pain is due to a perforated ulcer with retroperitoneal abscess. A history of rheumatic fever or other cardiac valvular lesions should raise concern that new back pain might represent endocarditis with microembolization of the vertebral bodies. Indeed, back pain is a not uncommon manifestation of endocarditis. A history of renal stones or neglected hypertension might indicate another serious cause of referred back pain.

The general physical examination is also of great importance, since elevated temperature or blood pressure, palpable lymph nodes, and abdominal, pelvic, or rectal masses would all be important indications that a patient's back pain has a serious cause.

History of the Back Pain

While most back pain is not distinctive, certain qualities of a patient's pain can indicate a specific diagnosis. **Sciatica,** characterized by low back pain radiating down the buttock and below the knee, suggest a herniated disk causing nerve root irritation. Other conditions—including sacroiliitis, facet joint degenerative arthritis, spinal stenosis, or irritation of the sciatic nerve from a wallet—can also cause sciatica.

The diagnosis of disk herniation is further suggested by physical examination (see below) and confirmed by imaging techniques. It should be emphasized that disk herniation can be asymptomatic, so that the mere presence of it on a scan does not always signify clinical disease.

Unrelenting low back pain at night, unrelieved by rest or the supine position, should suggest the possibility of malignancy, either vertebral body metastasis or a cauda equina tumor.

Symptoms of large or rapidly evolving **neurologic deficits** identify patients who need urgent evaluation for possible cauda equina tumor, epidural abscess, or, rarely, massive disk herniation. Severe neurologic symptoms with back pain are unusual and should prompt concern. Even with a herniated disk and nerve root impingement, pain is the most prominent symptom; numbness and weakness are less commonly reported and when present are of the magnitude consistent with compression of a single nerve root. Thus, symptoms of bilateral leg weakness (from multiple lumbar nerve root compressions) or of saddle area anesthesia, bowel or bladder incontinence, or impotence (indicating multiple sacral nerve root compressions) indicate an atypically large neurologic deficit requiring urgent evaluation.

Low back pain that **worsens with rest and improves with activity** is characteristic of ankylosing spondylitis or other seronegative spondyloarthropathies, especially when the onset is insidious and begins before age 40. Most degenerative back diseases produce precisely the opposite pattern, with rest alleviating and activity aggravating the pain.

Acute, **writhing** low back pain should suggest referred pain from an abdominal catastrophe such as an aortic dissection.

Low back pain associated with **pseudoclaudication** often indicates spinal stenosis. The typical patient is approximately 60 years old and is bothered less by back pain than by a discomfort occurring in the buttock, thigh, or leg that (like true claudication) is brought on by walking but (unlike claudication) can also be the elicited by prolonged standing. The discomfort is frequently bilateral. Classically, the pain is improved with rest or with flexion of the lumbar spine, which is why patients have less difficulty walking uphill than downhill. Some patients complain less about leg discomfort and more about an exercise-dependent weakness or unsteadiness of the legs—often described as "spaghetti legs" or the gait of a "drunken sailor."

Physical Examination of the Back

Although examination of the back usually does not suggest a specific cause, several physical findings should be sought because they do help identify those few patients who need more than just conservative management.

Neurologic examination of the lower extremities will detect the small deficits produced by disk disease and the large deficits complicating such problems as cauda equina tumors. A positive straight leg raising test indicates nerve root irritation. The examiner performs the test on the supine patient by passively raising the patient's leg. The test is positive if *radicular* pain is produced with the leg raised 60 degrees or less. The test is not specific but is 95% sensitive in patients with herniation at the L4–5 or L5–S1 level (the sites of 95% of disk herniations). It can be falsely negative, especially in patients with herniation above the L4–5 level.

The crossed straight leg sign is less sensitive but much more specific for disk herniation and is positive when raising the contralateral leg reproduces the sciatica.

Detailed examination of the sacral and lumbar nerve roots, especially L5 and S1, are essential for detecting neurologic deficits associated with back pain. Disk herniation produces deficits predictable for the site involved (Table 19–5). Deficits of multiple nerve roots suggest a cauda equina tumor, an epidural abscess, or some other important process that requires urgent evaluation and treatment.

Measurement of spinal motion in the patient with acute pain is rarely of diagnostic utility and usually simply confirms that pain limits motion. An exception to this general rule is that evidence of decreased range of motion in multiple regions of the spine (cervical, thoracic, and lumbar) indicates a diffuse spinal disease such as ankylosing spondylitis. But by the time the patient has such limits, the diagnosis is usually not a mystery.

If the back pain is not severe and does not itself limit motion, Schober's test of lumbar motion is helpful in early diagnosis of ankylosing spondylitis. To perform this test, two marks are made, one 10 cm above S1 and another 5 cm below. The patient then bends forward as far as possible, and the distraction between the points is measured. Normally, the points distract at least 5 cm. Anything less indicates reduced lumbar motion, which in the absence of severe pain is most commonly due to ankylosing spondylitis or other seronegative spondyloarthropathies.

Palpation of the spine usually does not yield diagnostic information. Point tenderness over a vertebral body is reported to suggest osteomyelitis, but this association appears much tighter in dusty textbooks than in living patients. A step-off noted between the spinous process of adjacent vertebral bodies may indicate spondylolisthesis, but the sensitivity of this finding is extremely low. Tenderness of the soft tissues overlying the greater trochanter of the hip is a manifestation of trochanteric bursitis.

Inspection of the spine is not often of value in identifying serious causes of low back pain. The classic posture of ankylosing spondylitis is a late finding. Scoliosis of mild degree is not associated with an increased risk of clinical back disease. Cutaneous neurofibromas can identify the very rare patient who has nerve root encasement.

Examination of the hips should be part of the complete examination. While hip arthritis usually produces groin pain, some patients have buttock or low back symptoms.

Further Examination

If the history and physical examination do not suggest the presence of infection, cancer, inflammatory back disease, major neurologic deficits, or pain referred from abdominal or pelvic disease, further evaluation can be eliminated or deferred while conservative therapy is tried. The great majority of patients will spontaneously improve with conservative care over 1–4 weeks.

Regular radiographs of the lumbosacral spine give 20 times the radiation dose of a chest x-ray and provide limited, albeit important, information. X-rays can provide evidence of vertebral body osteomyelitis, cancer, fractures, or ankylosing spondylitis. Degenerative changes in the lumbar spine are ubiquitous in patients over 40 and do not prove clinical disease. Plain x-rays have very low sensitivity or specificity for disk disease. Thus, plain x-rays are warranted early for patients suspected of having infection, cancer, fractures, or inflammation and in selected other patients who fail to improve after 2–4 weeks of conservative therapy.

MRI and CT scans provide exquisite anatomic detail but should be reserved for patients in whom the information would change therapy. Clearly, sophisticated imaging is needed urgently in any patient suspected of having an epidural mass or cauda equina tumor. On the other hand, sophisticated imaging is not needed early in the course of a patient suspected

Table 19–5. Neurologic testing of lumbosacral nerve disorders.

Nerve Root	Motor	Reflex	Sensory Area
L4	Dorsiflexion of foot	Knee jerk	Medial calf
L5	Dorsiflexion of great toe	None	Medial forefoot
S1	Eversion of foot	Ankle jerk	Lateral foot

of having a routine disk herniation. Since most such patients will improve over 4–6 weeks of conservative therapy, these imaging techniques should be reserved for patients who have failed conservative therapy and who are good surgical candidates. The relative merits of MRI versus CT scanning remain controversial.

Radionuclide bone scanning has limited utility in the evaluation of low back pain. It is most useful for early detection of vertebral body osteomyelitis or metastases. The bone scan is often normal in multiple myeloma.

Blood tests (eg, complete blood count, calcium, alkaline phosphatase, serum protein electrophoresis, sedimentation rate) and urinalysis should be performed early only on patients suspected of having serious disease. Electrophysiologic testing can be useful in confirming the diagnosis of spinal stenosis.

2. MANAGEMENT

While any management plan must be individualized, key elements of most conservative treatments for back pain include rest, analgesia, and education. Two days of bed rest is (on average) just as effective as 7 days in achieving relief of acute sciatica, but individual patients vary greatly. Analgesia can usually be provided with nonsteroidal anti-inflammatory drugs, but severe pain may require opiates. Rarely does the need for opiates extend beyond 1–2 weeks, and opiates are contraindicated in the management of chronic low back pain.

Limited evidence supports the use of "muscle relaxants" such as diazepam, cyclobenzaprine, carisoprodol, and methocarbamol. These drugs should also be limited to courses of 1–2 weeks. Their use should be avoided in older patients, who are at risk of falling. All patients should be taught how to protect the back in daily activities—ie, not to lift heavy objects, to use the legs rather than the back when lifting, to use a chair with arm rests, and to arise from bed by first rolling to one side and then using the arms to push to an upright position. Physical therapists are excellent sources for patient education.

The value of corsets or traction is dubious. Back exercises are contraindicated during acute pain, but extension exercises may have some value in preventing recurrences. The efficacy of epidural corticosteroid injections in treating sciatica is still being debated. Corticosteroid injections into facet joints are ineffective for chronic low back pain.

Surgical consultation is needed urgently for any patient with a large or evolving neurologic deficit. Surgery for disk disease is indicated when there is documentation of herniation by some imaging procedure, a consistent pain syndrome, and a consistent neurologic deficit that has failed to respond to 4–6 weeks of conservative therapy. Percutaneous lumbar discectomy, performed under local anesthesia, is a safe and effective alternative to laminectomy for selected patients. The percutaneous procedure is contraindicated in the presence of tumor, infection, spondylolisthesis, foraminal stenosis, or severe facet joint arthritis. With careful patient selection, percutaneous discectomy succeeds in 70–75% of cases.

Complaints of a tired and weak back with pain (not necessarily severe) and no objective findings may suggest a psychologic problem. Hysterical back pain may be severe and dramatically exaggerated. A history of domestic or work-related problems and observation of a flat affect with a bizarre reaction to treatment will further suggest the disorder. Treatment may include reassurance and judicious use of mild analgesics and sedatives.

The patient with compensatory back or neck pain may be interested in monetary gain, whereas the malingerer seeks a conscious real or imagined secondary gain. Subjective complaints in both types of patients are out of proportion to objective findings. The experienced clinician can often identify the malingerer or the patient with compensatory back or neck pain. These diagnostic impressions should not be conveyed to the patient. It is best to state simply that no organic disorder can be found that explains the patient's symptoms.

Carett S et al: A controlled trial of corticosteroid injections into facet joints for chronic low back pain. N Engl J Med 1991;325:1002. (Injections are of little value.)

Deyo RA, Rainville J, Kent DL: What can the history and physical examination tell us about low back pain? JAMA 1992;268:760. (Underlying systemic disease suggested by age over 50, history of cancer, unexplained weight loss, and failure to improve after 1 month.)

Deyo RA et al: Diagnostic imaging procedures for the lumbar spine. Ann Intern Med 1989;111:865. (Relative merits.)

Deyo RA et al: Herniated lumbar intervertebral disk. Ann Intern Med 1990;112:598. (Clinical picture and indications for surgery.)

Kambin P, Schaffer JL: Percutaneous lumbar discectomy: Prospective review of 100 patients and current practice. Clin Orthop 1989;238:24.

Shekelle PG et al: Spinal manipulation for low-back pain. Ann Intern Med 1992;117:590. (Spinal manipulation of modest benefit for acute, uncomplicated low back pain.)

THORACIC OUTLET SYNDROMES

Thoracic outlet syndromes include those disorders that result in compression of the neurovascular structures supplying the upper extremity. Patients often have a history of trauma to the head and neck areas.

Symptoms and signs may arise from intermittent or continuous pressure on elements of the brachial plexus and the subclavian or axillary vessels by a variety of anatomic structures of the shoulder girdle region. The neurovascular bundle can be compressed between the anterior or middle scalene muscles and a normal first thoracic rib or a cervical rib. Descent of the shoulder girdle may continue during adulthood and cause compression. Faulty posture, chronic illness, and occupation may be other predisposing factors. The components of the median nerve that encircle the axillary artery may cause compression and vascular symptoms. Sudden or repetitive strenuous physical activity may initiate "effort thrombosis" of the axillary or subclavian vein.

Pain may radiate from the point of compression to the base of the neck, the axilla, the shoulder girdle region, arm, forearm, and hand. Paresthesias are frequently present and are commonly distributed to the volar aspect of the fourth and fifth digits. Sensory symptoms may be aggravated at night or by prolonged use of the extremities. Weakness and muscle atrophy are the principal motor abnormalities. Vascular symptoms consist of arterial ischemia characterized by pallor of the fingers on elevation of the extremity, sensitivity to cold, and, rarely, gangrene of the digits or venous obstruction marked by edema, cyanosis, and engorgement.

Deep reflexes are usually not altered. When the site of compression is between the upper rib and clavicle, partial obliteration of subclavian artery pulsation may be demonstrated by abduction of the arm to a right angle with the elbow simultaneously flexed and rotated externally at the shoulder so that the entire extremity lies in the coronal plane. Neck or arm position has no effect on the diminished pulse, which remains constant in the subclavian steal syndrome.

Radiographic examination is helpful in differential diagnosis. Chest x-ray will identify patients with cervical rib. MRI with the arms held in different positions is useful in identifying sites of impaired blood flow. Intra-arterial or venous obstruction is confirmed by angiography. Determinations of the conduction velocities of the ulnar and other peripheral nerves of the upper extremity may help to localize the site of their compression.

Thoracic outlet syndrome must be differentiated from symptomatic osteoarthritis of the cervical spine, tumors of the cervical spinal cord or nerve roots, periarthritis of the shoulder, and other cervicobrachial pain syndromes.

Conservative treatment is directed toward relief of compression of the neurovascular bundle. The patient is instructed to avoid physical activities likely to precipitate or aggravate symptoms. Overhead pulley exercises are useful to improve posture. Shoulder bracing, although uncomfortable, provides a constant stimulus to improve posture. When lying down, the shoulder girdle should be bolstered by arranging pillows in an inverted "V" position.

Symptoms may disappear spontaneously or may be relieved by conservative treatment. Operative treatment is more likely to relieve the neurologic rather than the vascular component that causes symptoms.

SCAPULOHUMERAL CALCAREOUS TENDINITIS

Calcareous tendinitis of the shoulder joint is an acute or chronic inflammatory disorder of the capsulotendinous cuff (especially the supraspinatus portion) characterized by deposits of calcium salts among tendon fibers. It is a common cause of acute pain near the lateral aspect of the shoulder joint in men over age 30. The calcium deposit may be restricted to the tendon substance or may rupture into the overlying bursa.

Symptoms consist of pain (at times severe), tenderness to pressure, and restriction of shoulder joint motion.

Radiographic examination confirms the diagnosis and demonstrates the site of the lesion.

Calcareous tendinitis must be differentiated from other cervicobrachial pain syndromes, pyogenic arthritis, osteoarthritis, gout, Pancoast tumors, and tears of the rotator cuff.

The aim of treatment is to relieve pain and restore shoulder joint function. Pain is best treated by injection of the lesion with a local anesthetic with corticosteroid. After treatment, early recovery of shoulder joint function should be fostered by supervised exercises. NSAIDs are also effective. Acute symptoms occasionally subside after spontaneous rupture of the calcium deposit into the subacromial bursa. Chronic symptoms may be treated by analgesics, exercises, and injection of local anesthetics with 20–40 mg of triamcinolone; repeated injections should be avoided. Rarely, calcific deposits may require surgical evacuation.

When x-ray examination shows that a deposit has disappeared, recurrence of that deposit is rare. Symptoms of periarthritis may persist if shoulder joint motion is not completely regained.

Smith DL, Campbell SM: Painful shoulder syndromes: Diagnosis and management. J Gen Intern Med 1992;7:328.

SCAPULOHUMERAL PERIARTHRITIS (Adhesive Capsulitis, Frozen Shoulder)

Periarthritis of the shoulder joint is an inflammatory disorder primarily involving the soft tissues. The condition may be divided into a primary type, in which no obvious cause can be identified, and a secondary type associated with an organic lesion (eg, rheumatoid arthritis, osteoarthritis, fracture or dislocation). The primary type is most common among women after the fourth decade. It may be manifested as inflammation of the articular synovia, the tendons around the joint, the intrinsic ligamentous capsular bands, the paratendinous bursae (especially the subacromial), or the bicipital tendon sheath. Calcareous tendinitis and attritional disease of the rotator cuff, with or without tears, are incidental lesions.

The onset of pain, which is aggravated by extremes of shoulder joint motion, may be acute or insidious. Pain may be most annoying at night and may be intensified by pressure on the involved extremity when the patient sleeps in the lateral decubitus position. Tenderness upon palpation is often noted near the tendinous insertions into the greater tuberosity or over the bicipital groove. Although a sensation of stiffness may be noted only at onset, restriction of shoulder joint motion soon becomes apparent and is likely to progress unless effective treatment is instituted.

Pain can usually be controlled with nonsteroidal anti-inflammatory agents. Passive exercise of the shoulder by an overhead pulley mechanism should be repeated slowly for about 2 minutes four times daily. Forceful manipulation of the shoulder joint during this exercise should be avoided. Injection of tender areas with corticosteroids gives transitory relief. Operative treatment should be reserved for the occasional refractory case.

Ekelund AL, Rydell N: Combination treatment for adhesive capsulitis of the shoulder. Clin Orthop 1992;282:105. (Combination of distention-arthrography, local anesthetics, intra-articular steroids, and manipulation improves pain and range of motion.)

EPICONDYLITIS
(Tennis Elbow, Epicondylalgia)

Epicondylitis is a pain syndrome affecting the mid portion of the upper extremity; no single causative lesion has been identified. It has been postulated that chronic strain of the forearm muscles due to repetitive grasping or rotatory motions of the forearm causes microscopic tears and subsequent chronic inflammation of the common extensor or common flexor tendon at or near their respective osseous origins from the epicondyles.

Epicondylitis occurs most frequently in the dominant extremity during middle life. Pain is predominantly on the medial or lateral aspect of the elbow region, may be aggravated by grasping, and may radiate proximally into the arm or distally into the forearm. The point of maximal tenderness to pressure is 1–2 cm distal to the epicondyle but may also be present in the muscle bellies more distally. Resisted dorsiflexion or volar flexion of the wrist may accentuate the pain. X-ray examination generally reveals no significant change.

Treatment is directed toward relief of pain. Most symptoms can be relieved by rest and NSAIDs. An elastic bandage applied about the proximal forearm may ameliorate discomfort when the patient is grasping forcefully. Infiltration of "trigger points" by local anesthetic solutions with corticosteroids may be helpful. Operative treatment is reserved for severe, refractory cases.

Chop WM et al: Tennis elbow. Postgrad Med 1990;87:32.

FIBROSITIS

Essentials of Diagnosis

- Chronic widespread musculoskeletal pain syndrome with multiple tender points.
- Fatigue, headaches, numbness common.
- Most frequent in women aged 20–50.
- Objective signs of inflammation absent. No specific laboratory or diagnostic test.
- Partially responsive to exercise, amitriptyline.

General Considerations

Fibrositis (also called fibromyalgia), is one of the most common rheumatic syndromes in ambulatory general medicine. It shares many features with the chronic fatigue syndrome, namely, an increased frequency among women aged 20–50, absence of objective findings, and absence of diagnostic laboratory tests. While many of the clinical features of the two conditions overlap, musculoskeletal pain predominates in fibrositis whereas fatigue dominates the chronic fatigue syndrome.

The cause is unknown, but sleep disorders, hysteria, depression, and viral infections have all been proposed. Subtle histochemical abnormalities in muscle biopsies have been identified and await confirmation. Fibrositis can be a complication of hypothyroidism or rheumatoid arthritis.

Clinical Findings

A. Symptoms and Signs: The typical patient is a premenopausal woman with chronic aching pain and stiffness, frequently involving the entire body but with prominence of pain around the neck, shoulders, low back, and hips. Fatigue, sleep disorders, subjective numbness, chronic headaches, and irritable bowel symptoms are common. The patient feels incapable of performing normal activities, and even minor exertion aggravates pain and increases fatigue. Patients occasionally trace the onset of symptoms to an acute event or viral-like illness. Physical examination is normal except for "trigger points" of pain produced by palpation of various areas such as the trapezius, the medial fat pad of the knee, and the lateral epicondyle of the elbow.

B. Laboratory Findings: None.

Differential Diagnosis

Fibrositis is a diagnosis of exclusion. A detailed

history and physical examination can obviate the need for extensive laboratory testing. Rheumatoid arthritis and systemic lupus erythematosus virtually always present with objective physical findings or abnormalities on routine testing, including the erythrocyte sedimentation rate. Thyroid function tests are useful, since hypothyroidism can produce a secondary fibromyalgia syndrome. Polymyositis usually produces weakness rather than pain. The diagnosis of fibrositis probably should not be made in a patient over age 50 and should never be invoked to explain fever, weight loss, or any other objective signs. Polymyalgia rheumatica produces shoulder and girdle pain, is associated with anemia and an elevated sedimentation rate, and occurs after age 50.

Treatment

Patient education is of paramount importance. Patients can be comforted by the knowledge that they have a recognizable diagnosable syndrome that can be managed by means of specific though imperfect therapies and that the course is not progressive. Placebo-controlled trials have demonstrated modest efficacy of amitriptyline, chlorpromazine, or cyclobenzaprine. Amitriptyline is initiated at a dosage of 10 mg at bedtime and gradually increased to 40–50 mg depending on its efficacy and toxicity. Exercise programs are also beneficial. NSAIDs are generally ineffective. Opiates and corticosteroids are ineffective and should never be used to treat fibrositis.

Prognosis

Most patients have chronic symptoms. With treatment, however, many do eventually resume increased activities. Progressive or objective findings do not develop.

Wolfe F et al: The American College of Rheumatology 1990 criteria for the classification of fibromyalgia. Arthritis Rheum 1990;33:160. (The combination of widespread musculoskeletal pain and multiple trigger points is 88% sensitive and 81% specific for the diagnosis of fibromyalgia.)

CARPAL TUNNEL SYNDROME

Carpal tunnel syndrome is a common painful disorder caused by compression of the median nerve between the carpal ligament and other structures within the carpal tunnel (entrapment neuropathy). The volume of the contents of the tunnel can be increased by organic lesions such as synovitis of the tendon sheaths or carpal joints, recent or malhealed fractures, tumors, and occasionally congenital anomalies. Even though no anatomic lesion is apparent, flattening or even circumferential constriction of the median nerve may be observed during operative section of the ligament. The disorder may occur in pregnancy

and is seen in individuals with a history of repetitive use of the hands, and it may follow injuries of the wrists. A familial type of carpal tunnel syndrome has been reported in which no etiologic factor can be identified.

Carpal tunnel syndrome can also be a feature of many systemic diseases: rheumatoid arthritis and other rheumatic disorders (inflammatory tenosynovitis); myxedema, amyloidosis, sarcoidosis, and leukemia (tissue infiltration); acromegaly; hyperparathyroidism, hypocalcemia, and diabetes mellitus.

Clinical Findings

Pain in the distribution of the median nerve, which may be burning and tingling (acroparesthesia), is the initial symptom. Aching pain may radiate proximally into the forearm and occasionally proximally to the shoulder, neck, and chest. Pain is exacerbated by manual activity, particularly by extremes of volar flexion or dorsiflexion of the wrist. It may be most bothersome at night. Impairment of sensation in the median nerve distribution may not be apparent. Subtle disparity between the affected and opposite sides can be demonstrated by testing for two-point discrimination or by requiring the patient to identify different textures of cloth by rubbing them between the tips of the thumb and the index finger. Tinel's or Phalen's sign may be positive. (Tinel's sign is tingling or shock-like pain on volar wrist percussion; Phalen's sign, pain or paresthesia in the distribution of the median nerve when the patient flexes both wrists to 90 degrees with the dorsal aspects of the hands held in apposition for 60 seconds.) The carpal compression test, performed by applying direct pressure on the carpal tunnel, may be more sensitive and specific than the Tinel and Phalen tests. Muscle weakness or atrophy, especially of the abductor pollicis brevis, appears later than sensory disturbances. Useful special examinations include electromyography and determinations of segmental sensory and motor conduction delay. Distal median sensory conduction delay may be evident before motor delay.

Differential Diagnosis

This syndrome should be differentiated from other cervicobrachial pain syndromes, from compression syndromes of the median nerve in the forearm or arm, and from mononeuritis multiplex. When left-sided, it may be confused with angina pectoris.

Treatment

Treatment is directed toward relief of pressure on the median nerve. When a primary lesion is discovered, specific treatment should be given. When soft tissue swelling is a cause, elevation of the extremity may relieve symptoms. Splinting of the hand and forearm at night may be beneficial. Injection of corticosteroid into the carpal tunnel can alleviate symptoms in some patients, particularly those with synovitis of the wrist. To reduce the chance of nerve injury, this injection should be performed by a physician thoroughly familiar with the anatomy of the carpal tunnel.

Operative division of the volar carpal ligament gives lasting relief from pain, which usually subsides within a few days. Muscle strength returns gradually, but complete recovery cannot be expected when atrophy is pronounced.

Durkan JA: A new diagnostic test for carpal tunnel syndrome. J Bone Joint Surg [Am] 1991;73:535. (Direct pressure over the carpal tunnel—the carpal compression test—is more sensitive and specific than the Tinel and Phalen tests.)

Katz JN et al: The carpal tunnel syndrome: Diagnostic utility of the history and physical examination findings. Ann Intern Med 1990;112:321. (Tinel's sign or Phalen's sign had positive predictive value of approximately 0.50 and negative predictive value of 0.70.)

DUPUYTREN'S CONTRACTURE

This relatively common disorder is characterized by hyperplasia of the palmar fascia and related structures, with nodule formation and contracture of the palmar fascia. The cause is unknown, but the condition has a genetic predisposition and occurs primarily in white men over 50 years of age. The incidence of Dupuytren's contracture is higher among alcoholics and patients with chronic systemic disorders (eg, cirrhosis, diabetes, epilepsy, tuberculosis). The onset may be acute, but slowly progressive chronic disease is more common.

Dupuytren's contracture manifests itself by nodular or cord-like thickening of one or both hands, with the fourth and fifth fingers most commonly affected. The patient may complain of tightness of the involved digits, with inability to satisfactorily extend the fingers, and on occasion there is tenderness. The resulting functional and cosmetic problems may be extremely disabling. Fasciitis involving other areas of the body may lead to plantar fibromatosis (10% of patients) or Peyronie's disease (1–2%).

Periodic examination of patients in early stages of disease is recommended. If the palmar nodule is growing rapidly, injections of triamcinolone into the nodule may be of benefit. Surgical intervention is indicated in patients with significant flexion contractures, depending on the location, but recurrence is not uncommon.

Gonzalez SM, Gonzalez RI: Dupuytren's disease. West J Med 1990;152:430.

REFLEX SYMPATHETIC DYSTROPHY

Reflex sympathetic dystrophy is a syndrome of pain and swelling of an extremity accompanied by signs of trophic skin changes in the extremity (eg, skin atrophy, hyperhidrosis) and signs and symptoms of vasomotor instability. Any extremity can be involved, but the disorder most commonly occurs in the hand and is associated with ipsilateral restricted shoulder motion (shoulder-hand syndrome). The swelling in reflex sympathetic dystrophy is diffuse ("catcher's mitt hand") and not restricted to joints. Pain is often described as burning in quality. The **shoulder-hand variant** of reflex sympathetic dystrophy is common after neck or shoulder injuries or following myocardial infarction. Direct trauma to the hand or foot can also provoke this syndrome. Reflex sympathetic dystrophy can also develop after a knee injury or after arthroscopic knee surgery. There are no systemic symptoms, and x-rays reveal severe generalized osteopenia. The severe osteoporosis occurring in the posttraumatic variant of reflex sympathetic dystrophy is known as Sudeck's atrophy. Bone scans also show increased uptake. In a significant minority of cases, symptoms and findings are bilateral.

This syndrome should be differentiated from other cervicobrachial pain syndromes, rheumatoid arthritis, polymyositis, scleroderma, and gout.

In addition to specific treatment of the underlying disorder, treatment is directed toward restoration of function. For most patients, physical therapy is the cornerstone of treatment. Patients who have restricted shoulder motion may benefit from the treatment described for scapulohumeral periarthritis. In resistant cases, prednisone, 30–40 mg/d for 2 weeks and then tapered off over 2 weeks, may be effective. Stellate ganglion block can also be effective for reflex sympathetic dystrophy.

The prognosis depends in part upon the stage in which the lesions are encountered and the extent and severity of associated organic disease. Early treatment offers the best prognosis for recovery.

Ameratunga R, Daly M, Caughey DE: Metastatic malignancy associated with reflex sympathetic dystrophy. J Rheumatol 1989;16:406.

BURSITIS

Inflammation of the synovium-like cellular membrane overlying bony prominences may be secondary to trauma, infection, or arthritic conditions. The most common locations are the subdeltoid, olecranon, ischial, and prepatellar bursae. Clinically and anatomically, this syndrome can be differentiated from adjacent inflammatory disorders of tendons, and the attacks may suggest an arthritic process. On occasion, calcific deposits are noted on x-rays of the involved bursae.

Various methods of treatment have been used, including local heat, immobilization, analgesics, nonsteroidal anti-inflammatory agents, and local steroid injections. Infected bursae usually require surgical drainage or aspiration and antibiotic therapy.

McAfee JH, Smith DL: Olecranon and prepatellar bursitis: Diagnosis and treatment. West J Med 1988;149:607.

JOGGING INJURIES

The beneficial effects on cardiovascular function and the sense of well-being associated with aerobic activity have led to considerable enthusiasm for jogging and running. This has resulted in a large number of musculoskeletal injuries, which are estimated to occur in about 75% of runners. In addition, osteoporosis, hematuria, heat stroke, exercise-induced ectopy, and even death have occurred as consequences of running.

Many of the deleterious effects can be prevented by appropriate precautions, such as stretching exercises, proper footwear, avoidance of overexertion, and prompt attention to injuries. After an injury has healed, a graduated schedule for returning to training is necessary to avoid recurrence. Since injuries occur frequently in long-distance runners, it is most important that these individuals avoid overexertion, and, when early signs of injury appear, reduce the amount of distance run. The psychologic effects of complete inactivation in athletes whose identity is intimately tied to their sport should be recognized and addressed, since severe depression may develop in such circumstances.

Zarins B and Adams M: Knee injuries in sports. N Engl J Med 1988;318:950. (Epidemiology, biomechanics, diagnosis, and treatment of knee injuries in sports.)

AUTOIMMUNE DISEASES
(Collagen Diseases,
Connective Tissue Diseases)

The autoimmune disorders are a protean group of acquired diseases in which genetic factors appear to play a role. They have in common widespread immunologic and inflammatory alterations of connective tissue.

These illnesses share certain clinical features, and differentiation among them is often difficult because of this. Common findings include synovitis, pleuritis,

myocarditis, endocarditis, pericarditis, peritonitis, vasculitis, myositis, skin rash, alterations of connective tissues, and nephritis. Laboratory tests may reveal Coombs-positive hemolytic anemia, thrombocytopenia, leukopenia, immunoglobulin excesses or deficiencies, antinuclear antibodies (which include antibodies to many nuclear constituents, including DNA and extractable nuclear antigen), rheumatoid factors, cryoglobulins, false-positive serologic tests for syphilis, elevated muscle enzymes, and alterations in serum complement.

Although the autoimmune disorders are regarded as acquired diseases, their causes cannot be determined in most instances.

Some of the laboratory alterations that occur in this group of diseases (eg, false-positive serologic tests for syphilis, rheumatoid factor) occur in asymptomatic individuals. These changes may also be demonstrated in certain asymptomatic relatives of patients with connective tissue diseases, in older persons, in patients using certain drugs, and in patients with chronic infectious diseases.

RHEUMATOID ARTHRITIS

Essentials of Diagnosis

- Prodromal systemic symptoms of malaise, fever, weight loss, and morning stiffness.
- Onset usually insidious and in small joints; progression is centripetal and symmetric; deformities common.
- Radiographic findings: juxta-articular osteoporosis, joint erosions, and narrowing of the joint spaces.
- Rheumatoid factor usually present.
- Extra-articular manifestations: subcutaneous nodules, pleural effusion, pericarditis, lymphadenopathy, splenomegaly with leukopenia, and vasculitis.

General Considerations

Rheumatoid arthritis is a chronic systemic inflammatory disease of unknown cause, chiefly affecting synovial membranes of multiple joints. The disease has a wide clinical spectrum with considerable variability in joint and extra-articular manifestations. The prevalence in the general population is 1–2%; female patients outnumber males almost 3:1. The usual age at onset is 20–40 years, although rheumatoid arthritis may begin at any age. Susceptibility to rheumatoid arthritis is genetically determined. Virtually all patients have a class 2 human leukocyte antigen (HLA) with an identical five-amino-acid sequence.

The pathologic findings in the joint include chronic synovitis with pannus formation. The pannus erodes cartilage, bone, ligaments, and tendons. In the acute phase, effusion and other manifestations of inflammation are common. In the late stage, organization may result in fibrous ankylosis; true bony ankylosis is rare. In both acute and chronic phases, inflammation of soft tissues around the joints may be prominent and is a significant factor in joint damage.

The microscopic findings most characteristic of rheumatoid arthritis are those of the subcutaneous nodule. This is a granuloma with a central zone of fibrinoid necrosis, a surrounding palisade of radially arranged elongated connective tissue cells, and a periphery of chronic granulation tissue. Pathologic alterations indistinguishable from those of the subcutaneous nodule are occasionally seen in the myocardium, pericardium, endocardium, heart valves, visceral pleura, lungs, sclera, dura mater, spleen, and larynx as well as in the synovial membrane, periarticular tissues, and tendons. Nonspecific pericarditis and pleuritis are found in 25–40% of patients at autopsy. Additional nonspecific lesions associated with rheumatoid arthritis include inflammation of small arteries, pulmonary fibrosis, round cell infiltration of skeletal muscle and perineurium, and hyperplasia of lymph nodes. Secondary amyloidosis may also be present.

Clinical Findings

A. Symptoms and Signs: The clinical manifestations of rheumatoid disease are highly variable. The onset of articular signs of inflammation is usually insidious, with prodromal symptoms of malaise, weight loss, and vague periarticular pain or stiffness. Less often, the onset is acute, apparently triggered by a stressful situation such as infection, surgery, trauma, emotional strain, or the postpartum period. There is characteristically symmetric joint swelling with associated stiffness, warmth, tenderness, and pain. Stiffness is prominent in the morning and subsides during the day; its duration is a useful indicator of activity of disease. Stiffness may recur after daytime inactivity and may be much more severe after strenuous activity. Although any joint may be affected in rheumatoid arthritis, the proximal interphalangeal and metacarpophalangeal joints of the fingers as well as the wrists, knees, ankles, and toes are most often involved. Monarticular disease is occasionally seen early. Synovial cysts and rupture of tendons may occur. Entrapment syndromes are not unusual—particularly entrapment of the median nerve at the carpal tunnel of the wrist. Palmar erythema is noted occasionally, as are tiny hemorrhagic infarcts in the nail folds or finger pulps, which are signs of vasculitis. Twenty percent of patients have subcutaneous nodules, most commonly situated over bony prominences but also observed in the bursas and tendon sheaths. A small number of patients have splenomegaly and lymph node enlargement. Low-grade fever, anorexia, weight loss, fatigue, and weakness often persist; chills are rare. After months or years, thickening of the periarticular tissue, flexion deformities, subluxation, fibrosis, and ankylosis may occur. Atro-

phy of skin or muscle is common. Dryness of the eyes, mouth, and other mucous membranes is found especially in advanced disease (see Sjögren's Syndrome). Other ocular manifestations include episcleritis and scleromalacia, often due to scleral nodules. Pericarditis and pleural disease, when present, are frequently silent clinically. Aortitis is a rare late complication that can result in aortic regurgitation or rupture and is usually associated with evidence of rheumatoid vasculitis elsewhere in the body.

B. Laboratory Findings: Serum protein abnormalities are often present. Rheumatoid factor, an IgM antibody directed against other globulins, is present in the sera of more than 75% of patients. High titers of rheumatoid factor are commonly associated with severe rheumatoid disease. Titers may also be significantly elevated in a number of diverse conditions, including syphilis, sarcoidosis, infective endocarditis, tuberculosis, leprosy, and parasitic infections; in advanced age; and in asymptomatic relatives of patients with autoimmune diseases. Antinuclear antibodies are demonstrable in 20% of patients, though their titers are lower in rheumatoid arthritis than in systemic lupus erythematosus.

During both the acute and chronic phases, the erythrocyte sedimentation rate and the gamma globulins (most commonly IgM and IgG) are typically elevated. A moderate hypochromic normocytic anemia is common. The white cell count is normal or slightly elevated, but leukopenia may occur, often in the presence of splenomegaly (eg, Felty's syndrome). The platelet count is often elevated, roughly in proportion to the severity of overall joint inflammation. Joint fluid examination is valuable, reflecting abnormalities that are associated with varying degrees of inflammation. (See Tables 19–1 and 19–2.)

C. Imaging: Of all the laboratory tests, x-ray changes are the most specific for rheumatoid arthritis. X-rays, however, are not sensitive in that most of those taken during the first 6 months are read as normal. The earliest changes occur in the wrists or feet and consist of soft tissue swelling and juxta-articular demineralization. Later, diagnostic changes of uniform joint space narrowing and erosions develop. The erosions are often first evident at the ulnar styloid and at the juxta-articular margin, where the bony surface is not protected by cartilage. Diagnostic changes also occur in the cervical spine, with C1–2 subluxation, but these changes usually take several years to develop.

Differential Diagnosis

The differentiation of rheumatoid arthritis from other diseases of connective tissue can be difficult. However, certain clinical features are helpful. Rheumatic fever is characterized by the migratory nature of the arthritis, an elevated antistreptolysin titer, and a more dramatic and prompt response to aspirin; carditis and erythema marginatum may occur in adults, but chorea and subcutaneous nodules virtually never do. Butterfly rash, discoid lupus erythematosus, photosensitivity, alopecia, high titer to anti-DNA, renal disease, and central nervous system abnormalities point to the diagnosis of systemic lupus erythematosus. Degenerative joint disease (osteoarthritis) is not associated with constitutional manifestations, and the joint pain is characteristically relieved by rest, in contrast to the morning stiffness of rheumatoid arthritis. Signs of articular inflammation, prominent in rheumatoid arthritis, are usually minimal in degenerative joint disease. Osteoarthritis—in contrast to rheumatoid arthritis—spares the wrist and the metacarpophalangeal joints. While in the early years gouty arthritis is almost always intermittent and monarticular, in later years it can become a chronic polyarticular process that mimics rheumatoid arthritis. Gouty tophi can at times resemble rheumatoid nodules. The early history of intermittent monarthritis and the presence of synovial urate crystals are distinctive features of gout. Pyogenic arthritis can be distinguished by chills and fever, demonstration of the causative organism in joint fluid, and the frequent presence of a primary focus elsewhere, eg, gonococcal arthritis. Chronic Lyme disease typically involves only one joint, most commonly the knee, and is associated with positive serologic tests (see Chapter 33). Human parvovirus B19 infection in adults can occasionally mimic rheumatoid arthritis. The mean age at onset is 35–37; arthralgias are much more prominent than arthritis; and rash—on the cheeks, torso, or extremities—is common. The patients are rheumatoid factor-negative, do not have erosions, and have serologic evidence of recent human parvovirus B19 infection (ie, serum positive for anti-parvovirus B19 IgM antibody). Polymyalgia rheumatica occasionally causes polyarthritis in patients over age 50, but these patients remain rheumatoid factor-negative and have chiefly proximal muscle pain and stiffness. A variety of cancers produce paraneoplastic syndromes, including polyarthritis. One form is hypertrophic pulmonary osteoarthropathy most often produced by lung and gastrointestinal carcinomas, characterized by a rheumatoid-like arthritis associated with clubbing, periosteal new bone formation, and a negative rheumatoid factor. Diffuse swelling of the hands with palmar fasciitis has also been reported with a variety of cancers, especially ovarian carcinoma.

Treatment

A. Basic Program (Conservative Management): The primary objectives in treating rheumatoid arthritis are reduction of inflammation and pain, preservation of function, and prevention of deformity. To a large extent, patient satisfaction and the success of therapy depend on how effectively the physician utilizes the nonpharmacologic measures reviewed at the beginning of this chapter.

B. Nonsteroidal Anti-inflammatory Drugs (NSAIDs):

1. Aspirin–Aspirin is an effective anti-inflammatory antipyretic agent and the least expensive of the various drugs available to treat rheumatoid arthritis. It is usually the first drug employed unless there is some contraindication to its use. Patients under the age of 65 can start with 1 g three or four times per day. Aspirin, like alcohol, is metabolized at different rates in different people, so that the total dose of aspirin needed to achieve improvement varies considerably among individuals. Salicylate levels can be monitored, with the therapeutic range being 20–30 mg/dL; however, it is simpler and cheaper to increase the dose by 0.3–0.6 g each week until the patient experiences maximal improvement or toxicity. After the first week, the salicylate half-life increases to 15 hours, making less frequent dosing theoretically possible if not always preferred by patients. If tinnitus—one of the most common early manifestations of toxicity—occurs, the daily dose should be lowered by 0.6 or 0.9 g every 3 days until this symptom disappears. Many different preparations of aspirin are now available, including sustained-release forms. Enteric-coated aspirin is recommended because it decreases the high frequency of gastric ulceration seen with chronic use of plain or buffered aspirin. Nonacetylated forms of salicylates, such as salsalate, are probably equally effective at reducing gastric ulceration but are more expensive. Symptoms of gastric irritation may be lessened by the ingestion of salicylates with meals and by taking them with antacid. No salicylate should be used by patients with a history of allergy to aspirin or related products.

2. Other NSAIDs–If aspirin proves ineffective or if intolerable gastrointestinal effects occur, a trial of the newer NSAIDs is indicated. Because of a simpler dosage schedule for most of these agents, compliance may be better. A number of NSAIDs are available, including ibuprofen, fenoprofen, naproxen, tolmetin, sulindac, meclofenamate sodium, piroxicam, flurbiprofen, diclofenac, oxaprozin, nabumetone, and ketoprofen (see Table 1–9). In terms of efficacy for groups of patients, all of the nonsteroidal anti-inflammatory drugs—including aspirin—are equivalent. It is surprising, however, that individual patients may respond to one preparation but not to another.

In terms of toxicity, gastrointestinal side effects are most frequent. All the NSAIDs inhibit gastric prostaglandin E, a local hormone responsible for gastric mucosal cytoprotection. Consequently, these drugs can produce gastric ulceration and bleeding. There is no evidence that any of the newer nonsteroidals produce massive gastrointestinal bleeding any less frequently than does aspirin. But the newer NSAIDs are similar to enteric-coated aspirin in greatly reducing the frequency of gastric symptoms and gastric ulceration seen in patients chronically taking plain aspirin.

H_2 blockers and carafate do not reduce the frequency of gastric ulceration, only the dyspepsia. The efficacy of concomitant antacids has not been formally tested.

Only misoprostol, a synthetic analogue of prostaglandin E, reduces the incidence of gastric ulceration. Whether this drug will also decrease the risk of gastrointestinal hemorrhage is not yet known. Furthermore, the side effects—especially the diarrhea—of this agent limit its use in many patients, particularly the elderly.

NSAIDs can also affect the lower intestinal tract, causing perforation or aggravating inflammatory bowel disease.

The overall rate of bleeding with NSAID use in the general population appears to be low: 1:10,000 to 1:6000 users. The frequency of bleeding is increased by chronic use, concomitant use of corticosteroids or anticoagulants, the presence of rheumatoid arthritis, a history of peptic ulcer disease or alcoholism, and old age. Some reports suggest that each year 1:1000 patients with rheumatoid arthritis will require hospitalization for gastrointestinal NSAID-related bleeding or perforation. Thus, though the exact indications for misoprostol have not yet been determined, it should probably be reserved for patients who must take a nonsteroidal drug and have substantial risk factors for gastric bleeding. Misoprostol is an abortifacient and thus is contraindicated in patients who are or might become pregnant.

All of the NSAIDs, including aspirin, can produce renal toxicity, resulting in interstitial nephritis, nephrotic syndrome, reversible renal failure, and aggravation of baseline hypertension. Hyperkalemia due to hyporeninemic hypoaldosteronism may also be seen. The risk of renal toxicity is low but is increased by age over 60, a history of renal disease, congestive heart failure, ascites, and diuretic use.

Indomethacin is probably no more effective than the salicylates in rheumatoid arthritis, and its untoward effects are greater. Phenylbutazone is not advised for chronic therapy because of its toxicity.

C. Other Anti-inflammatory Drugs: If the patient fails to respond to the basic regimen with a reduction in morning stiffness, fatigue, and joint swelling, additional medications are added.

1. Antimalarials–Hydroxychloroquine sulfate (Plaquenil), is the antimalarial agent most often used against rheumatoid arthritis. It should be reserved for patients with mild disease, since only 25% will respond and in some of those cases only after 3–6 months of therapy. The advantage of hydroxychloroquine is its comparatively low toxicity. A dosage of 200–400 mg/d minimizes the likelihood of toxic reactions. The most important reaction, pigmentary retinitis causing visual loss, is fortunately rare when the dosage is kept low. Biannual ophthalmologic examinations are required when this drug is employed for long-term therapy. Other reactions include neuropathies and myopathies of both skeletal and cardiac muscle, which usually improve when the drug is withdrawn.

2. Methotrexate–Many now believe that methotrexate is the treatment of choice for patients with severe rheumatoid arthritis who fail to respond to NSAIDs. Methotrexate is generally well-tolerated and often produces a beneficial effect in 2–4 weeks—compared with the 2- to 6-month onset of action for drugs such as gold, penicillamine, and antimalarials. The usual dose is 7.5 mg of methotrexate orally once weekly. The most frequent side effects are gastric irritation and stomatitis. A severe, potentially life-threatening interstitial pneumonitis occurs rarely and usually responds to cessation of the drug and institution of corticosteroids. Hepatotoxicity with fibrosis and cirrhosis is another important toxic effect of methotrexate that fortunately appears to be very rare. Diabetes, obesity, and renal disease appear to increase the risk of hepatotoxicity. Liver function tests should be monitored, but because of their insensitivity, periodic liver biopsy is needed. In a patient with no risk factors for hepatotoxicity, liver biopsy is not needed initially but should be done after every 2.5–3 g of methotrexate. Cytopenia due to bone marrow suppression and infection are other important potential side effects. To date, methotrexate has not been shown to increase the risk of malignancy. While methotrexate is an effective medication, its toxicity and teratogenic potential are such that it should only be used by physicians thoroughly familiar with its effects.

3. Gold salts (chrysotherapy)–For patients who fail to improve on or who cannot tolerate methotrexate, treatment with gold salts may be effective. About 60% of patients may be expected to benefit from gold therapy, although complete remissions are uncommon. Their mode of action is not known.

a. Indications–Disease responding unfavorably to conservative management; erosive disease.

b. Contraindications–Previous gold toxicity; significant renal, hepatic, or hematopoietic dysfunction.

c. Preparations of choice–Intramuscular gold sodium thiomalate or aurothioglucose; oral auranofin. Intramuscular gold is used most often because it is more effective than oral gold.

d. Dosage–Intramuscular gold is given as a 10 mg test dose the first week and a 25 mg dose the second week before reaching the maintenance dose of 50 mg weekly, which is then continued (for up to 20 weeks) unless toxic reactions appear. If there is no response after 800 mg has been administered, the drug should be discontinued. If the response is good, a total dose of 1 g should be given, followed by a regimen of 50 mg every 2 weeks and, with continued improvement, every 3 and then every 4 weeks for an indefinite period.

The oral dose of auranofin is 3 mg twice daily until benefit or toxicity occurs.

e. Toxic reactions–About 32% of patients (range in various series: 4–55%) experience toxic reactions to gold therapy; the mortality rate is less than 0.4%. The manifestations of toxicity are similar to those of poisoning by other heavy metals (notably arsenic) and include dermatitis (mild to exfoliative, and pruritic), stomatitis, neutropenia, proteinuria, and nitritoid reactions (especially to gold thiomalate and presumably due to its vehicle). Auranofin causes side effects less frequently than intramuscular gold, though diarrhea is common. In order to prevent or reduce the severity of toxic reactions, gold should not be given to patients with any of the contraindicating disorders listed above. Periodic urinalyses and complete blood counts should be obtained.

If signs of toxicity appear, the drug should be withdrawn immediately. Severe toxicity may require corticosteroids for control, and failure to respond might then be an indication for the cautious use of penicillamine or dimercaprol (BAL) as chelating agents for the gold. Worsening of articular symptoms after the initial dose is often temporary and is not an indication for withdrawal of the drug. Patients so affected may ultimately respond favorably if treatment is continued.

4. Corticosteroids–Although corticosteroids usually produce an immediate and dramatic anti-inflammatory effect in rheumatoid arthritis, they may not alter the natural progression of the disease; furthermore, clinical manifestations of active disease commonly reappear when the drug is discontinued. The serious problem of untoward reactions resulting from prolonged corticosteroid therapy greatly limits its long-term use. Another disadvantage that might stem from the use of steroids lies in the tendency of the patient and the physician to neglect the less spectacular but proved benefits derived from general supportive treatment, physical therapy, and orthopedic measures.

Corticosteroids may be used on a short-term basis to tide patients over acute disabling episodes, to facilitate other treatment measures (eg, physical therapy), or to manage serious extra-articular manifestations (eg, pericarditis, perforating eye lesions). Corticosteroids may also be indicated for active and progressive disease that does not respond favorably to conservative management and when there are contraindications to or therapeutic failure of gold salts and penicillamine.

The least amount of steroid that will achieve the desired clinical effect should be given, but not more than 10 mg of prednisone or equivalent per day is appropriate for articular disease. Many patients do reasonably well on 5–7.5 mg daily. (The use of 1 mg tablets is to be encouraged.) When the steroids are to be discontinued, they should be phased out gradually on a planned schedule appropriate to the duration of treatment.

Intra-articular corticosteroids may be helpful if one or two joints are the chief source of difficulty. Intra-articular triamcinolone, 10–40 mg, may be given for symptomatic relief, but no more often than four times a year.

5. Sulfasalazine–This drug has become established as a second-line agent for rheumatoid arthritis, with an efficacy similar to that of gold and penicillamine. Sulfasalazine is usually introduced at a dosage of 1 g daily and then, after 1–2 weeks, increased to 2 g daily. Side effects occur in 10–25% and are serious in 2–5%. Because neutropenia and thrombocytopenia are the most frequent important side effects, patients taking sulfasalazine should have complete blood counts monitored frequently.

6. Azathioprine–This agent, like methotrexate, is an antimetabolite that is effective for severe rheumatoid arthritis not responsive to gold or antimalarials. The usual initial dose is 1 mg/kg, gradually increased as needed to a maximum of 2.5–3 mg/kg. Its potential for severe toxicity, including immunosuppression complicated by opportunistic infection, restricts its use to physicians experienced with the drug.

7. Penicillamine–Penicillamine may be used in patients with severe rheumatoid arthritis who have continuing rheumatic activity in spite of therapy with the agents discussed above. This agent may prove effective in a number of such patients, although toxicity is substantial. The mechanism of action is not understood. Up to one-half of patients experience some side effects such as oral ulcers, loss of taste, fever, rash, thrombocytopenia, leukopenia, and aplastic anemia. Proteinuria and nephrotic syndrome may occur. Immune complex diseases (eg, myasthenia gravis, systemic lupus erythematosus, polymyositis, Goodpasture's syndrome) appear to be induced by the drug. It should not be used during pregnancy.

If penicillamine is employed, one should start with small doses: 250 mg daily, increasing by 125 mg every 2–3 months up to a maximum of 0.75–1 g/d. Penicillamine is given between meals to enhance absorption. Careful monitoring for toxicity is essential.

D. Experimental Therapy: Cyclophosphamide, chlorambucil, cyclosporine, total lymph node irradiation, and monoclonal antibodies directed against T cell structures have been used with success in experimental studies. Only patients who fail to respond to all other measures should be considered for these treatments, which should be provided by physicians familiar with their toxicities.

E. Surgical Measures: See below.

Course & Prognosis

Determining the best initial treatment is difficult because patients suspected of having rheumatoid arthritis can follow two widely divergent courses. Of all patients who present with possible or probable rheumatoid arthritis, 50–75% experience remission within 2 years. These patients are often negative for rheumatoid factor, have good functional status even during disease activity, and are commonly seen in community practices but rarely in academic center practices. Clearly, conservative therapy makes good sense for this patient population.

For patients whose joint symptoms persist beyond 2 years the outcome is not so favorable. Patients in this group die, on average, 10–15 years earlier than people without rheumatoid arthritis. In fact, for patients who have persistent symptoms and poor functional status, the mortality curve resembles that for stage IV Hodgkin's disease or triple-vessel coronary artery disease. Factors that identify those at particular risk of early death include poor functional status, more than 30 inflamed joints, extra-articular manifestations (eg, rheumatoid lung disease), and low educational level. These patients, then, need aggressive therapy and probably need it early, since extensive bone damage can occur during the first 2 years. Recent studies suggest that patients at risk of developing severe disease can be identified by genotypes for HLA-DRB1 alleles. If so, then it will be possible to determine whether earlier institution of potent second-line agents such as methotrexate or use of agents in combination will improve the outcome in this unfortunate minority population.

Brooks PM, Day RO: Nonsteroidal anti-inflammatory drugs: Differences and similarities. N Engl J Med 1991;324:1716.

Epstein WV et al: Effect of parenterally administered gold therapy on the course of adult rheumatoid arthritis. Ann Intern Med 1991;114:437. (Patients receiving parenteral gold therapy for at least 2 years did not have a different outcome when compared with those not receiving such therapy.)

Felson DT, Anderson JJ, Meenan RF: The comparative efficacy and toxicity of second-line drugs in rheumatoid arthritis. Arthritis Rheum 1990;33:1449. (Oral gold least effective; intramuscular gold most toxic.)

Savage RL et al: Variation in the risk of peptic ulcer complications with nonsteroidal anti-inflammatory drug therapy. Arthritis Rheum 1993;36:84. (Risk of hemorrhage or perforation of peptic ulcer disease with NSAIDs increased fivefold. Piroxicam has higher risk than diclofenac, ketoprofen, or sulindac.)

Walt RP: Misoprostol for the treatment of peptic ulcer and anti-inflammatory-drug-induced gastroduodenal ulceration. N Engl J Med 1992;327:1575. (Routine prophylaxis with misoprostol is not justified.)

Weyand CM et al: The influence of HLA-DRB1 genes on disease severity in rheumatoid arthritis. Ann Intern Med 1992;117:801. (HLA-DRB1 alleles identify patients with severe disease.)

Whiting-O'Keefe QE, Fye KH, Sack KD: Methotrexate and histologic hepatic abnormalities: A meta-analysis. Am J Med 1991;90:711. (After 3 g, there is a 1:35 chance of advanced liver fibrosis.)

JUVENILE CHRONIC ARTHRITIS

Rheumatoid-like disease with onset before age 17 is referred to as juvenile chronic arthritis. Synovitis that persists for at least 6 weeks is the essential criterion of the diagnosis. Four forms are recognized:

(1) The **polyarticular form** resembles adult rheumatoid arthritis in joint distribution, seropositivity, and prognosis.

(2) The **oligoarticular form** affects chiefly young girls during the peak ages of 2–4, is negative for rheumatoid factor, has a good chance for complete remission, and may be associated with a positive ANA test, which in turn is associated with uveitis. Since the uveitis is often initially silent, all children with the oligoarticular form and a positive ANA test should be examined by an ophthalmologist.

(3) A third form is termed **systemic-onset disease,** or **Still's disease,** characterized by high spiking fevers that may antedate arthritis by months; a characteristic evanescent, salmon-colored morbilliform rash; and—commonly but not always—hepatosplenomegaly, lymphadenopathy, pleuropericarditis, anemia, and leukocytosis.

(4) The fourth form of juvenile chronic arthritis is a juvenile form of **ankylosing spondylitis** characterized initially by inflammatory arthritis involving a few peripheral joints, particularly in a lower extremity, that later extends to the spine.

Systemic-onset disease (Still's disease) can occur in adults and may present initially as fever of undetermined origin. While there is no diagnostic laboratory test, the constellation of signs and symptoms—especially the very characteristic rash—may suggest the diagnosis. The rash is often missed because it is present chiefly during episodes of fever, which characteristically occur during the night.

In many children with polyarticular chronic arthritis, the apophyseal joints of the cervical spine, especially C2–3, are affected. Abnormalities of bony growth and development are related to active disease and may be transient and reversible or, with chronic disease activity, may be irreversible and result in premature closure of epiphyses or ossification centers; micrognathia is one consequence.

The differential diagnosis of juvenile chronic arthritis includes leukemia or lymphoma, inflammatory bowel disease, and chronic infectious disease (eg, Lyme disease; see Chapter 33). Joint fluid examination, culture, serologic tests, and synovial biopsy may be useful in diagnosis.

The treatment of juvenile chronic arthritis must be individualized; in general, the approach to therapy is similar to that for adult rheumatoid arthritis.

Leak AM et al: A crossover study of naproxen, diclofenac and tolmetin in seronegative juvenile chronic arthritis. Clin Exp Rheum 1988;6:157. (Equally effective.)

Pouchot J et al: Adult Still's disease: Manifestations, disease course, and outcome in 62 patients. Medicine 1991;70:118. (Polyarthritis, foot joint arthritis, and rash predict a chronic course.)

SYSTEMIC LUPUS ERYTHEMATOSUS

Essentials of Diagnosis

- Occurs mainly in young women.
- Rash over areas exposed to sunlight.
- Joint symptoms in 90% of patients. Multiple system involvement.
- Depression of hemoglobin, white blood cells, platelets.
- Serologic findings: antinuclear antibody with high titer to native DNA.

General Considerations

Systemic lupus erythematosus (SLE) is an inflammatory autoimmune disorder that may affect multiple organ systems. Its clinical manifestations are thought to be secondary to the trapping of antigen-antibody complexes in capillaries of visceral structures. The clinical course may vary from a mild episodic disorder to a rapidly fulminating fatal illness.

Systemic lupus erythematosus is not uncommon. Figures from a large representative urban community population indicate a prevalence exceeding one in 2000 persons. About 85% of patients are women. Although the disease may occur at any age, most patients are between ages 10 and 50, with greatest clustering between 20 and 40. Blacks are affected more often than members of other races.

Before making a diagnosis of spontaneous SLE, it is imperative to ascertain that the condition has not been induced by a drug. A host of pharmacologic agents have been implicated as causing a lupus-like syndrome, but only a few cause the disorder with appreciable frequency (Table 19–6). Procainamide, hydralazine, and isoniazid are the most important and best studied of these drugs. While antinuclear antibody tests and other serologic findings become positive in many persons receiving these agents, in only a few do clinical manifestations occur.

Four features of drug-induced lupus separate it from spontaneously occurring disease: (1) the sex ratio is nearly equal; (2) nephritis and central nervous system features are not ordinarily present; (3) depressed serum complement and antibodies to native DNA are absent; and (4) the clinical features and most laboratory abnormalities often revert toward normal when the offending drug is withdrawn.

The familial occurrence of SLE has been repeatedly documented, and the disorder has involved identical twins in a number of instances. Aggregation of serologic features (positive antinuclear antibody, antibodies to DNA, hypergammaglobulinemia) is seen in asymptomatic family members, and the prevalence

Table 19–6. Drugs associated with lupus erythematosus.[1]

Definite association	Chlorpromazine Hydralazine Isoniazid	Methyldopa Procainamide Quinidine
Possible association	Acebutolol Atenolol Captopril Carbamazepine Cimetidine Ethosuximide Hydrazines Labetalol Levodopa Lithium Mephenytoin Methimazole Metoprolol	Nitrofurantoin Oxprenolol Penicillamine Phenelzine Phenytoin Pindolol Practolol Propranolol Propylthiouracil Sulfasalazine Sulfonamides Trimethadione
Unlikely association	Allopurinol Chlorthalidone Gold salts Griseofulvin Methysergide Oral contraceptives	Penicillin Phenylbutazone Reserpine Streptomycin Tetracyclines

[1]Modified and reproduced, with permission, from Hess EV Mongey AB: Drug-related lupus. Bull Rheum Dis 1991;40:1.

of other rheumatic diseases is increased among close relatives of patients. There is increased incidence of HLA-DR2 and -DR3 in lupus. Defective regulation of T cells, B cells, and humoral factors such as complement are all hypothesized to contribute to the pathogenesis of systemic lupus.

The diagnosis of SLE should be suspected in patients having a multisystem disease with serologic positivity (eg, antinuclear antibody, serologic test for syphilis). Differential diagnosis includes diseases that may present in a similar manner, such as rheumatoid arthritis, vasculitis, scleroderma, chronic active hepatitis, acute drug reactions, polyarteritis, and drug-induced lupus.

The diagnosis of SLE can be made with reasonable probability if four of the 11 criteria set forth in Table 19–7 are met. These criteria should be viewed as rough guidelines that do not supplant clinical judgment in the diagnosis of SLE.

Clinical Findings

A. Symptoms and Signs: The systemic feature include fever, anorexia, malaise, and weight loss. Most patients have skin lesions at some time; the characteristic "butterfly" rash affects fewer than half of patients. Other cutaneous manifestations are discoid lupus, typical fingertip lesions, periungual erythema, nail fold infarcts, and splinter hemorrhages. Alopecia is common. Mucous membrane lesions tend to occur during periods of exacerbation. Raynaud's phenomenon, present in about 20% of patients, often antedates other features of the disease.

Joint symptoms, with or without active synovitis, occur in over 90% of patients and are often the earliest manifestation. The arthritis is rarely deforming;

Table 19–7. Criteria for the classification of SLE.[1] (A patient is classified as having SLE if any 4 or more of 11 criteria are met.)

1. Malar rash
2. Discoid rash
3. Photosensitivity
4. Oral ulcers
5. Arthritis
6. Serositis
7. Renal disease
   a. > 0.5 g/d proteinuria, or
   b. ≥ 3 + dipstick proteinuria, or—
   c. Cellular casts
8. Neurologic disease
   a. Seizures, or—
   b. Psychosis (without other cause)
9. Hematologic disorders
   a. Hemolytic anemia, or—
   b. Leukopenia (< 400/µL), or—
   c. Lymphopenia (< 1500/µL), or—
   d. Thrombocytopenia (< 100,000/µL)
10. Immunologic abnormalities
    a. Positive LE cell preparation, or—
    b. Antibody to native DNA, or—
    c. Antibody to Sm, or—
    d. False-positive serologic test for syphilis
11. Positive antinuclear antibody (ANA)

[1]Modified and reproduced, with permission, from Tan EM et al: The 1982 revised criteria for the classification of systemic lupus erythematosus. Arthritis Rheum 1982;25:1271.

erosive changes are almost never noted on x-ray study. Subcutaneous nodules are rare.

Ocular manifestations include conjunctivitis, photophobia, transient blindness, and blurring of vision. Cotton-wool spots on the retina (cytoid bodies) represent degeneration of nerve fibers due to occlusion of retinal blood vessels.

Pleurisy, pleural effusion, bronchopneumonia, and pneumonitis are frequent. Restrictive lung disease is often demonstrated.

The pericardium is affected in the majority of patients. Cardiac failure may result from myocarditis and hypertension. Cardiac arrhythmias are common. Atypical verrucous endocarditis of Libman-Sacks is usually clinically silent but occasionally can produce acute or chronic valvular incompetence—most commonly mitral regurgitation—and can serve as a source of thrombotic emboli.

Abdominal pains, ileus, and peritonitis may result from vasculitis; the right colon is especially susceptible. Nonspecific reactive hepatitis or that induced by salicylates may alter liver function.

Neurologic complications of SLE include psychosis, organic brain syndrome, seizures, peripheral and cranial neuropathies, transverse myelitis, and strokes. Severe depression and psychosis are sometimes heightened by the administration of large doses of corticosteroids.

Several forms of glomerulonephritis may occur, including mesangial, focal proliferative, diffuse proliferative, and membranous. Some patients may also have interstitial nephritis. With appropriate therapy, the survival rate even for patients with serious renal disease (proliferative glomerulonephritis) is favorable.

Other clinical features include arterial and venous thrombosis, lymphadenopathy, splenomegaly, Hashimoto's thyroiditis, hemolytic anemia, and thrombocytopenic purpura.

B. Laboratory Findings: SLE is characterized by the production of many different autoantibodies (eg, positive Coombs) which in turn produce specific laboratory abnormalities (eg, hemolytic anemia) (Tables 19–8 and 19–9). Antinuclear antibody tests are sensitive but not specific for systemic lupus—ie, they are positive in virtually all patients with lupus but are positive also in many patients with nonlupus conditions such as rheumatoid arthritis, various forms of hepatitis, and interstitial lung disease (Tables 19–8 and 19–9). Antibodies to double-stranded DNA and to Sm are specific for systemic lupus but not sensitive, since they are present in only 60% and 30% of patients, respectively. Depressed serum complement—a finding suggestive of disease activity—often returns toward normal in remission. Anti-native DNA antibody levels also correlate with disease activity; anti-Sm levels do not.

Three types of antiphospholipid antibodies occur (Table 19–9): The first causes the biologic false-positive tests for syphilis; the second is the lupus anticoagulant, which despite its name is a risk factor for venous and arterial thrombosis and miscarriage. It is most commonly identified by prolongation of the activated partial thromboplastin time, though other phospholipid-dependent coagulation tests, such as Russell's viper venom time, are more sensitive. Anticardiolipin antibodies are the third type of antiphospholipid antibodies and may be a risk factor for fetal death in pregnant patients with lupus. A primary antiphospholipid antibody syndrome is diagnosed in patients who have recurrent venous or arterial occlusions in the presence of antiphospholipid antibodies but without specific features of SLE. Antibody titers to a wide variety of other cellular tissues and organ tissues may be observed.

Abnormality of urinary sediment is almost always found in association with renal lesions. Showers of red blood cells, with or without casts, and mild proteinuria are frequent during exacerbation of the disease; these usually abate with remission.

Treatment

Many patients with SLE have a benign form of the disease requiring only supportive care and need little or no medication. Emotional support, as described for rheumatoid arthritis, is especially important for patients with lupus. Patients with photosensitivity should be cautioned against sun exposure and should apply a protective lotion to the skin while out of doors. Skin lesions often respond to the local administration of corticosteroids. Joint symptoms can usu-

Table 19–8. Frequency (%) of autoantibodies in rheumatic diseases.

	ANA	Anti-Native DNA	Rheu-matoid Factor	Anti-Sm	Anti-Ro	Anti-La	Anti-SCL-70	Anti-Centro-mere	Anti-Jo-1	ANCA
Rheumatoid arthritis	30–60	0–5	72–85	0	0–5	0–2	0	0	0	0
Systemic lupus erythematosus	95–100	60	20	10–25	15–20	5–20	0	0	0	0–1
Sjögren's syndrome	95	0	75	0	60–70	60–70	0	0	0	0
Diffuse scleroderma	80–95	0	25–33	0	0	0	33	1	0	0
Limited scleroderma (CREST syndrome)	80–95	0	25–33	0	0	0	20	50	0	0
Polymyositis/dermatomyositis	80–95	0	33	0	0	0	10	0	20–30	0
Wegener's granulomatosis	0–15	0	50	0	0	0	0	0	0	93–96[1]

ANA = antinuclear antibodies; ANCA = anti-neutrophil cytoplasmic antibody.
[1]Frequency for generalized, active disease.

ally be alleviated by rest and full dosage with a salicylate or other NSAID. Every drug that may have precipitated the condition should be withdrawn if possible.

Antimalarials (hydroxychloroquine) may be helpful in treating the joint and skin features. When these are used, the dose should not exceed 400 mg/d, and biannual monitoring for retinal changes is necessary. Drug-induced neuropathy and myopathy may be erroneously ascribed to the underlying disease.

Corticosteroids are required for the control of certain serious complications. These include thrombocytopenic purpura, hemolytic anemia, myocarditis, pericarditis, convulsions, and nephritis. Forty to 60 mg of prednisone is often needed initially; however, the lowest dose of corticosteroid that controls the condition should be employed. Central nervous system lupus may require higher doses of corticosteroids than are usually given; however, steroid psychosis may mimic lupus cerebritis, in which case reduced doses are appropriate. In lupus nephritis, sequential studies of serum complement and antibodies to DNA

often permit early detection of disease exacerbation and thus prompt increase in corticosteroid therapy. Such studies also allow for lowering the dosage of the drugs and withdrawing them when they are no longer needed. Immunosuppressive agents such as cyclophosphamide, chlorambucil, and azathioprine are used in cases resistant to corticosteroids. The exact role of immunosuppressive agents is controversial. Cyclophosphamide improves renal survival. Overall patient survival, however, is no better than in the prednisone-treated group. Very close follow-up is needed to watch for potential side effects when immunosuppressants are employed; these agents should be given by physicians experienced in their use. The androgenic steroid danazol may be effective therapy for thrombocytopenia not responsive to corticosteroids. Anticoagulation, most commonly with warfarin, is prescribed for patients who have antiphospholipid antibodies and clotting of the arterial or venous systems. Systemic steroids are not usually given for arthritis, skin rash, leukopenia, or the anemia associated with chronic disease. Positive serologic findings in asymptomatic patients are not an indication for treatment.

Table 19–9. Percent frequency of laboratory abnormalities in systemic lupus erythematosus.[1]

Anemia	60
Leukopenia	40
Thrombocytopenia	30
Biologic false-positive tests for syphilis	25
Lupus anticoagulant	7
Anti-cardiolipin antibody	25
Direct Coombs-positive	30
Proteinuria	30
Hematuria	30
Hypocomplementemia	60
ANA	95–100
Anti-native DNA	50
Anti-Sm	20

[1]Modified and reproduced, with permission, from Hochberg MC et al: Systemic lupus erythematosus: A review of clinico-laboratory features and immunologic matches in 150 patients with emphasis on demographic subsets. Medicine 1985; 64:285.

Course & Prognosis

The prognosis for patients with systemic lupus appears to be considerably better than older reports implied. From both community settings and university centers, 10-year survival rates exceeding 85% are routine. In most patients, the illness pursues a mild chronic course, occasionally interrupted by disease activity. With time, the number and intensity of exacerbations decrease and the probability of major insult to visceral structures declines. After 5 years of disease, abnormal laboratory findings such as raised sedimentation rates and anti-DNA titers tend to become normal in many patients. However, there are some in whom the disease pursues a virulent course, leading to serious impairment of vital structures such as lung, heart, brain, or kidneys, and the disease may lead to death. With improved control of lupus activity and with increasing use of corticosteroids and immunosuppressive drugs, the mortality and morbidity patterns in lupus have changed. Infections—especially with opportunistic organisms—have become the leading cause of death, followed by active SLE, chiefly due to renal or central nervous system disease. Although such manifestations are more likely to be seen in the early phases of the illness, one must be alert to the possibility of their occurrence at any time. Accelerated atherosclerosis attributed, in part, to corticosteroid use, has been responsible for a rise in late deaths due to myocardial infarction. With more patients living longer, it has become evident that avascular necrosis of bone, affecting most commonly the hips and knees, is responsible for substantial morbidity. Still, it must be emphasized that the outlook for most patients with SLE has become increasingly favorable.

Boumpas DT et al: Controlled trial of pulse methylprednisolone versus two regimens of pulse cyclophosphamide in severe lupus nephritis. Lancet 1992;340:741.

The Canadian Hydroxychloroquine Study Group: A randomized study of the effect of withdrawing hydroxychloroquine sulfate in systemic lupus erythematosus. N Engl J Med 1991;324:150. (Hydroxychloroquine helps prevent mild and severe flares.)

Love PE, Santoro SA: Antiphospholipid antibodies: Anticardiolipin and the lupus anticoagulant in systemic lupus erythematosus and in non-SLE disorders. Ann Intern Med 1990;112:682. (A review of the evidence that antiphospholipid antibodies are risk factors for thrombosis, neurologic disease, thrombocytopenia, and fetal loss.)

Petri M et al: Coronary artery disease risk factors in the Johns Hopkins Lupus Cohort: Prevalence, recognition by patients, and preventive practices. Medicine 1992; 71:291. (Coronary artery disease present in 8%.)

Rosove MH, Brewer PMC: Antiphospholipid thrombosis: Clinical course after the first thrombotic event in 70 patients. Ann Intern Med 1992;117:303. (Half will have recurrent thrombotic episodes. Arterial events were followed by arterial events and venous events by venous events in 91% of instances. High-intensity warfarin [PTT > 1.5 times control] reduced thrombosis. Low-intensity warfarin [PTT < 1.3 times control] or aspirin did not.)

Steinberg AD et al: Systemic lupus erythematosus. Ann Intern Med 1991;115:548. (Review of pathogenesis.)

PROGRESSIVE SYSTEMIC SCLEROSIS (Scleroderma)

Essentials of Diagnosis

- Diffuse thickening of skin, with telangiectasia and areas of increased pigmentation and depigmentation.
- Raynaud's phenomenon in 90% of patients.
- Systemic features of dysphagia, hypomotility of gastrointestinal tract, pulmonary fibrosis, and cardiac and renal involvement.

General Considerations

Progressive systemic sclerosis is a chronic disorder characterized by diffuse fibrosis of the skin and internal organs. The causes of scleroderma are not known, but autoimmunity, fibroblast disregulation, and occupational exposure have been implicated. Symptoms usually appear in the third to fifth decades, and women are affected two to three times as frequently as men.

Scleroderma may be localized or systemic. Localized scleroderma—morphea, linear scleroderma—is not associated with visceral organ involvement and is therefore benign. Two forms of systemic scleroderma are generally recognized: diffuse (20% of patients) and limited (80%). Patients with limited systemic scleroderma frequently have calcinosis cutis, Raynaud's phenomenon, esophageal involvement, sclerodactyly, and telangiectasia (CREST syndrome). Patients with CREST syndrome differ from those with diffuse systemic scleroderma in having skin tightening limited to the hands and face (versus the trunk), a lower risk of renal involvement, a higher risk of pulmonary hypertension, and an overall better prognosis.

Rapid progression of visceral organ disease leading to death within a few years is much more common in diffuse systemic scleroderma than in CREST syndrome.

Clinical Findings

A. Symptoms and Signs: Most frequently, the disease makes its appearance in the skin, although visceral involvement may precede cutaneous alteration. Polyarthralgia and Raynaud's phenomenon (present in 90% of patients) are early manifestations. Subcutaneous edema, fever, and malaise are common. With time the skin becomes thickened and hidebound, with loss of normal folds. Telangiectasia, pigmentation, and depigmentation are characteristic. Ulceration about the fingertips and subcutaneous calcification are seen. Dysphagia due to esophageal dysfunction, which occurs in 90% of patients, results from abnormalities in motility and later from fibrosis. Fibrosis and atrophy of the gastrointestinal tract cause hypomotility, and malabsorption results from bacterial overgrowth. Large-mouthed diverticula occur in the jejunum, ileum, and colon. Diffuse pulmonary fibrosis and pulmonary vascular disease are reflected in low diffusing capacity and decreased lung compliance. Cardiac abnormalities include pericarditis, heart block, myocardial fibrosis, and right heart failure secondary to pulmonary hypertension. Hypertensive uremic syndrome, resulting from obstruction to smaller renal blood vessels, indicates a grave prognosis.

B. Laboratory Findings: Mild anemia is often present, and it is occasionally hemolytic because of mechanical damage to red cells from diseased small vessels. Elevation of the sedimentation rate and hypergammaglobulinemia are also common. Proteinuria and cylindruria appear in association with renal involvement. Antinuclear antibody tests are frequently positive (Table 19–8). The scleroderma antibody (SCL-70) is found in one-third of patients with diffuse scleroderma and in 20% of those with CREST syndrome; an anticentromere antibody is seen in 50% of those with CREST syndrome and in 1% of individuals with diffuse scleroderma (Table 19–8). Though these tests may be useful and of academic interest, their lack of sensitivity and (usually) specificity precludes cost-effective application in diagnosis.

Differential Diagnosis

Eosinophilic fasciitis is a rare disorder presenting with skin changes that appear to be like those in diffuse systemic scleroderma. The inflammatory abnormalities, however, are limited to the fascia rather than the dermis and epidermis. Patients with eosinophilic fasciitis are further distinguished from those with systemic scleroderma by the presence of peripheral blood eosinophilia, the absence of Raynaud's phenomenon, the good response to prednisone, and the increased risk of developing aplastic anemia.

The eosinophilia myalgia syndrome was first noted in 1989 in patients who ingested tryptophan, an essential amino acid that was sold—until banned by the Food and Drug Administration—as an over-the-counter remedy for insomnia and premenstrual symptoms. Weeks to months after beginning ingestion of tryptophan, affected patients developed a syndrome of eosinophilia greater than $1000/\mu L$, severe generalized myalgias, and cutaneous abnormalities ranging from hives to generalized swelling and induration of the arms and legs similar to that seen in scleroderma or eosinophilic fasciitis. Other common clinical manifestations have included pulmonary symptoms, fever, myopathy, lymphadenopathy, and ascending polyneuropathy. Besides eosinophilia, laboratory features include mild elevations of aldolase with normal creatine kinase levels and, frequently, positive ANA tests. Full-thickness biopsies reveal at times features of scleroderma and at other times evidence of fasciitis or myositis or small vessel vasculitis. While some patients improve after discontinuing tryptophan, others progress and have required corticosteroid therapy, which is not always effective. Deaths have been reported, especially from neurologic involvement. Therefore, anyone with a scleroderma or an eosinophilic fasciitis-like syndrome should be asked about tryptophan use.

Treatment

Treatment of progressive systemic sclerosis is symptomatic and supportive. Severe Raynaud's syndrome may respond to calcium channel blockers, eg, nifedipine, 30–60 mg/d. Patients with esophageal disease should take medications in liquid or crushed form. Esophageal reflux can be reduced and scarring prevented by avoiding late-night meals, elevating the head of the bed, and using antacids and H_2 blockers. Omeprazole, 20–40 mg/d, is the only drug that produces near-complete inhibition of gastric acid production, and it is remarkably effective for refractory esophagitis. Patients with delayed gastric emptying maintain their weight better if they eat small, frequent meals and remain upright for at least 2 hours after eating. Malabsorption due to bacterial overgrowth responds to antibiotics, eg, tetracycline, 500 mg four times daily. The hypertensive crises seen chiefly in diffuse systemic scleroderma can often be treated with angiotensin-converting enzyme inhibitors, eg, captopril, 37.5–75 mg/d in three divided doses. The ability of drugs to prevent the development of visceral disease is controversial. The best evidence, however imperfect, suggests that penicillamine in doses as for rheumatoid arthritis (see above) may be helpful for patients at high risk of developing early visceral involvement, ie, those with rapidly progressive diffuse systemic scleroderma. Prednisone has little or no role in the treatment of scleroderma.

The prognosis tends to be worse in blacks, in males, and in older patients. In most cases, death results from renal, cardiac, or pulmonary failure.

Barnett AJ, Miller MH, Littlejohn GO: A survival study of patients with scleroderma diagnosed over 30 years (1953–1983): The value of a simple cutaneous classification in the early stages of the disease. J Rheumatol 1988;15:276. (Ten-year survival, 71% with skin tightness limited to fingers but 21% with diffuse truncal skin involvement.)

Gimenez SA, Siegal SH: A 15-year prospective study of treatment of rapidly progressive systemic sclerosis with D-penicillamine. J Rheumatol 1991;18:1496. (Penicillamine improved the skin and prolonged survival in patients with early, rapidly progressive systemic sclerosis.)

Steen VD et al: Outcome of renal crisis in systemic sclerosis: Relation to availability of angiotensin converting enzyme inhibitors. Ann Intern Med 1990;113:352. (Dramatic improvement with these drugs.)

Weiner ES et al: Prognostic significance of anticentromere antibodies and anti-topoisomerase I antibodies in Raynaud's disease. Arthritis Rheum 1991;34:68. (A positive anticentromere antibody was associated with a 63-fold increased risk of developing a connective tissue disease.)

Wigley FM et al: Intravenous iloprost treatment of Raynaud's phenomenon and ischemic ulcers secondary to systemic sclerosis. J Rheumatol 1992;19:1407. (Iloprost, a prostacyclin analogue, helps heal digital ulcers.)

Varga J, Uitto J, Jimenez SA: The cause and pathogenesis of the eosinophilia-myalgia syndrome. Ann Intern Med 1992;116:140.

POLYMYOSITIS-DERMATOMYOSITIS

Essentials of Diagnosis

- Bilateral proximal muscle weakness (all cases).
- Heliotrope suffusion of upper eyelids, characteristic rash, papules over knuckles (many cases).
- Diagnostic tests: elevated CPK and other muscle enzymes, muscle biopsy, electromyogram.
- Increased incidence of malignancy, especially when rash is present and with late age of onset.

General Considerations

Polymyositis is a systemic disorder of unknown cause whose principal manifestation is muscle weakness. It is the most frequent primary myopathy in adults. When skin manifestations are associated with it, the entity is designated dermatomyositis. The true incidence is not known, since milder cases are frequently not diagnosed. The disease may affect persons of any age group, but the peak incidence is in the fifth and sixth decades of life. Women are affected twice as commonly as men. There is an increased risk of malignancy, especially in patients with dermatomyositis. The malignancy may be evident initially or may not become evident for months after the muscle disease presents.

Clinical Findings

A. Symptoms and Signs: Polymyositis may begin abruptly, although often it is gradual and progressive. The characteristic rash is dusky red and may be seen over the butterfly area of the face, neck, shoulders, and upper chest and back. Periorbital edema and a purplish (heliotrope) suffusion over the upper eyelids are typical signs. Subungual erythema, cuticular telangiectases, and scaly patches over the dorsum of the proximal interphalangeal and metacarpophalangeal joints (Gottron's sign) are highly suggestive. Muscle weakness chiefly involves proximal groups, especially of the extremities. Neck flexor weakness occurs in two-thirds of cases. Pain and tenderness of affected muscles are frequent but not universal, and Raynaud's phenomenon and joint symptoms may be associated. Atrophy and contractures occur late. Associated myocarditis is uncommon. Interstitial pulmonary disease, usually mild, is sometimes associated, and calcinosis may be observed, especially in children. Polymyositis may occur in association with Sjögren's syndrome, SLE, or scleroderma.

B. Laboratory Findings: Measurement of serum levels of muscle enzymes, especially creatine phosphokinase and aldolase, is most useful in diagnosis and in assessment of disease activity. Anemia is uncommon. The sedimentation rate is not appreciably elevated in half of the patients. Rheumatoid factor is found in a minority of patients. Antinuclear antibodies are present in many patients, and anti-Jo-1 antibodies are seen in the subset of patients who have associated interstitial lung disease (Table 19–8). Chest x-rays are usually normal, though interstitial fibrosis is occasionally seen. Electromyographic abnormalities consisting of polyphasic potentials, fibrillations, and high-frequency action potentials are helpful in establishing the diagnosis. None of the studies are specific. The search for an occult malignancy should begin with a careful history and physical examination and should include the cancer screening tests that would be routine for that patient (see Chapter 1). If these evaluations are unremarkable, then a more invasive or extensive laboratory evaluation is not cost-effective. No matter how extensive the initial screening, some malignancies will not become evident for months after the initial presentation.

C. Muscle Biopsy: Biopsy of clinically involved muscle, usually proximal, is the only specific diagnostic study. Findings include necrosis of muscle fibers associated with inflammatory cells, sometimes located near blood vessels. The muscle biopsy may, however, reveal little change in spite of significant muscle weakness owing to the patchy distribution of pathologic abnormalities.

Differential Diagnosis

Most endocrine diseases can be associated with proximal muscle weakness. This is particularly true for hyper- and hypothyroidism, and the latter is associated also with elevations of creatinine phosphokinase. Patients with polymyalgia rheumatica are over the age of 50 and—in contrast to patients with polymyositis—have much more pain than weakness. Disorders of the peripheral and central nervous systems (eg, chronic inflammatory polyneuropathy, multiple sclerosis, myasthenia gravis, Eaton-Lambert disease and amyotrophic lateral sclerosis) can produce weakness but are distinguished by characteristic neurologic signs and electromyographic abnormalities. Many drugs, including corticosteroids, alcohol, clofibrate, penicillamine, tryptophan, and hydroxychloroquine, can produce proximal muscle weakness. Recent reports have indicated that chronic use of colchicine at doses as low as 0.6 mg twice a day in elderly patients with mild to moderate renal insufficiency can produce a mixed neuropathy-myopathy that mimics polymyositis. The weakness and muscle enzyme elevation reverse with cessation of the drug. Lovastatin (Mevacor), a drug increasingly used to treat hypercholesterolemia, also can rarely produce myositis. Polymyositis can occur as a complication of HIV or HTLV-I infection and with zidovudine therapy as well. Inclusion body myositis is distinguished from polymyositis in that most patients are over 50 years old, have involvement of distal muscles, experience slow progression of disease over years, do not respond to prednisone, and have characteristic inclusion bodies in the muscle identifiable by electron microscopy.

Treatment

Most patients respond to corticosteroids. Often a daily dose of 40–60 mg or more of prednisone is required initially. The dose is then adjusted downward according to the response of sequentially observed serum levels of muscle enzymes. Long-term use of steroids is often needed, and the disease may recur or reemerge when they are withdrawn. Patients with an associated neoplasm have a poor prognosis, although remission may follow treatment of the tumor; steroids may or may not be effective in these patients. In patients resistant or intolerant to corticosteroids, therapy with methotrexate or azathioprine has been advised, but these agents should be used with caution in view of their adverse effects. Uncontrolled studies have suggested that intravenous gamma globulin may be effective, but the high cost of such therapy should restrict its use to experimental protocols. Leukapheresis and plasma exchange are ineffective for corticosteroid-resistant polymyositis.

Dalakas MC: Polymyositis, dermatomyositis, and inclusion-body myositis. N Engl J Med 1991;325:1487.
Miller FW et al: Controlled trial of plasma exchange and leukapheresis in polymyositis and dermatomyositis. N Engl J Med 1992;326:1380. (Plasma exchange and leukapheresis are ineffective.)
Sigurgeirsson B et al: Risk of cancer in patients with dermatomyositis or polymyositis: A population-based study. N Engl J Med 1992;326:363. (Dermatomyositis and perhaps polymyositis increase the risk of cancer.)

OVERLAP (OR MIXED) CONNECTIVE TISSUE DISEASE

Not infrequently, patients have features of more than one rheumatic disease. Special attention has been drawn to patients who have overlapping features of SLE, scleroderma, and polymyositis. Initially, these patients were thought to have a distinct entity ("mixed connective tissue disease") defined by a specific autoantibody to ribonuclear protein (RNP). More recent studies suggest that the concept of mixed connective tissue disease is flawed, since with time in many patients the manifestations evolve to one predominant disease, such as scleroderma, and since many patients with antibodies to RNP have clear-cut SLE. Therefore, "overlap connective tissue disease" is the preferred designation for patients having features of different rheumatic diseases.

SJÖGREN'S SYNDROME

Essentials of Diagnosis

- 90% of patients are women; the average age is 50 years.
- Dryness of eyes and dry mouth (sicca components)

are the most common features; they occur alone or in association with rheumatoid arthritis or other connective tissue disease.
- Rheumatoid factor and other autoantibodies common.
- Increased incidence of lymphoma.

General Considerations

Sjögren's syndrome, an autoimmune disorder, is the result of chronic dysfunction of exocrine glands in many areas of the body. It is characterized by dryness of the eyes, mouth, and other areas covered by mucous membranes and is frequently associated with a rheumatic disease, most often rheumatoid arthritis. The disorder is predominantly a disease of women, in a ratio of 9:1, with greatest incidence between age 40 and 60 years.

Disorders with which Sjögren's syndrome is frequently associated include rheumatoid arthritis, SLE, primary biliary cirrhosis, scleroderma, polymyositis, Hashimoto's thyroiditis, polyarteritis, and interstitial pulmonary fibrosis. When Sjögren's syndrome occurs without rheumatoid arthritis, HLA-DR2 and -DR3 antigens are present with increased frequency.

Clinical Findings

A. Symptoms and Signs: Keratoconjunctivitis sicca results from inadequate tear production caused by lymphocyte and plasma cell infiltration of the lacrimal glands. Symptoms include burning, itching, ropy secretions, and impaired tear production during crying. Parotid enlargement, which may be chronic or relapsing, develops in one-third of patients. Dryness of the mouth (xerostomia) leads to difficulty in speaking and swallowing and to severe dental caries. There may be loss of taste and smell. Desiccation may involve the nose, throat, larynx, bronchi, vagina, and skin.

Systemic manifestations include dysphagia, pancreatitis, pleuritis, neuropsychiatric dysfunction, and vasculitis; they may be related to the associated diseases noted above. Renal tubular acidosis (type I, distal) occurs in 20% of patients. Chronic interstitial nephritis, which may result in impaired renal function, may be seen. A glomerular lesion is rarely observed but may occur secondary to associated cryoglobulinemia.

A spectrum of lymphoproliferation ranging from benign to malignant may be found. Malignant lymphomas and Waldenström's macroglobulinemia occur 44 times more frequently than can be explained by chance alone.

B. Laboratory Findings: Laboratory findings include mild anemia, leukopenia, and eosinophilia. Rheumatoid factor is found in 70% of patients. Heightened levels of gamma globulin, antinuclear antibodies, and antibodies against RNA, salivary gland, lacrimal duct, and thyroid may be noted. Antibodies against cytoplasmic antigens SS-A (or Ro) and SS-B (or La) are found predominantly in Sjögren's syndrome alone, whereas antibodies against salivary ducts and the RANA antigen are found in Sjögren's syndrome in association with rheumatoid arthritis (Table 19–8). When SS-A antibodies are present, extraglandular manifestations of Sjögren's syndrome are far more common.

Useful ocular diagnostic tests include the Schirmer test, which measures the quantity of tears secreted. Labial biopsy, a simple procedure, is the only specific diagnostic technique and has minimal risk; if lymphoid foci are seen, the diagnosis is confirmed. Biopsy of the parotid gland should be reserved for patients with atypical presentations such as unilateral gland enlargement.

Treatment & Prognosis

Treatment is symptomatic and supportive. Artificial tears applied frequently will relieve ocular symptoms and avert further desiccation. The mouth should be kept well lubricated. Atropine drugs and decongestants decrease salivary secretions and should be avoided. A program of oral hygiene is essential in order to preserve dentition. If there is an associated rheumatic disease, its treatment is not altered by the presence of Sjögren's syndrome.

The disease is usually benign and may be consistent with a normal life span; it is influenced mainly by the nature of the associated disease.

St Clair EW: Sjögren's syndrome and autoimmunity. Concepts Immunopathol 1992;8:161.

VASCULITIS SYNDROMES

The vasculitis syndromes are a heterogeneous group of disorders characterized by the pathologic features of inflammation and necrosis of blood vessels. The cause of most forms of vasculitis is not known. Hepatitis B is strongly associated with some cases of polyarteritis, hepatitis C with cryoglobulinemia, and other infections have been implicated, eg, the vasculitis that occurs in bacterial endocarditis. Drug reactions—especially to penicillins, sulfonamides, and allopurinol—can produce serum sickness associated with vasculitis. No common pathogenic link has been identified for these disorders, though the deposition of immune complexes in the vascular system occurs in many.

Although vasculitis is seen in multiple disorders, only the major vasculitides will be discussed here.

POLYARTERITIS NODOSA

Essentials of Diagnosis

- Clinical findings depend on arteries involved.
- Affects kidneys, muscles, joints, nerves, heart, gastrointestinal tract in most patients; cutaneous and pulmonary involvement unusual but possible.
- Manifestations of fever, hypertension, abdominal pain, livedo reticularis, mononeuritis multiplex, anemia, hematuria, elevated sedimentation rate.
- Diagnostic confirmation by biopsy or angiogram.

General Considerations

Polyarteritis is characterized by focal or segmental lesions of blood vessels, especially arteries of small to medium size, resulting in a variety of clinical presentations depending upon the specific site of the blood vessel involved. The pathologic hallmark of the disease is acute necrotizing inflammation of the arterial media, with fibrinoid necrosis and extensive inflammatory cell infiltration of all coats of the vessel and surrounding tissue. Aneurysmal dilatations occur; hemorrhage, thrombosis, and fibrosis may lead to occlusion of the lumen. Arterial lesions may be seen in all stages—acute, healing, and healed. Such vascular lesions may involve virtually every organ of the body but are especially prominent in the kidney, heart, liver, gastrointestinal tract, muscle, and testes.

The cause of polyarteritis is unknown. Hepatitis B has been strongly implicated, with 30–50% of patients having serologic evidence of the infection. In addition, immune complexes consisting in part of hepatitis B antigens have been identified in the serum and in the inflamed vessels of some patients. It is not surprising, therefore, that polyarteritis nodosa is more common in intravenous drug abusers and in other groups who have a high prevalence of hepatitis B infection. Yet at least half of patients with polyarteritis have no evidence of hepatitis B infection. Polyarteritis may occur at any age but is more frequent in young adults, and men are affected three times as frequently as women.

Clinical Findings

A. Symptoms and Signs: The clinical onset may be abrupt, often accompanied by fever, chills, and tachycardia. Arthralgia and myositis with muscle tenderness are prominent. A wide variety of cutaneous abnormalities develop. Livedo reticularis is most common; vasculitic involvement causing skin ulcers is less common. Occlusion of retinal vessels results in cotton-wool spots (cytoid bodies). Hypertension occurs in half of patients and renal involvement in more than 80%. The renal lesion is a segmental necrotizing glomerulonephritis with extracapillary proliferation, often with localized intravascular coagulation. Abdominal pain and nausea and vomiting are common. Infarction due to the arteritis compromises the function of major viscera and may lead to cholecystitis, appendicitis, and intestinal obstruction. Cardiac involvement is manifested by pericarditis, myocarditis, and arrhythmias; myocardial infarction secondary to coronary vasculitis also occurs. Multiple asymmetric neuropathies occur as a result of vasculitis of the vasa nervorum. Polyarteritis is an occasional cause of fever of unknown origin.

B. Laboratory Findings: Laboratory findings include proteinuria, hematuria, and cylindruria. Most patients manifest anemia and leukocytosis. Eosinophilia is more frequently encountered in association with pulmonary lesions, which may represent a different disease process (Churg-Strauss vasculitis), though overlap is not universal. The sedimentation rate is almost always elevated. Rheumatoid factor, antinuclear antibody, positive serologic test for syphilis, and increased serum concentration of gamma globulin are neither sensitive nor specific. Serum complement is often normal or elevated. Serologic tests for hepatitis B, such as HBsAg and HBeAg, are positive in 30–50%.

The role of anti-neutrophil cytoplasmic antibodies (ANCA) in the diagnosis of polyarteritis is not yet fully defined. A cytoplasmic pattern (C-ANCA) is produced by antibodies to a proteinase and is seen chiefly in patients with Wegener's granulomatosis (see above). A perinuclear pattern (P-ANCA) is caused by antibodies specific for myeloperoxidase and is found chiefly in patients with systemic polyarteritis or with vasculitis limited to the kidney (microscopic polyarteritis). Neither pattern is absolutely specific. The sensitivity of ANCA as a marker for polyarteritis is not yet determined. Therefore, the diagnosis of polyarteritis requires histopathologic confirmation.

C. Biopsy and Angiography: Biopsy of symptomatic sites (such as muscle, nerve, or testicle) is sensitive (70%) and specific (97%), with low morbidity and virtually no associated deaths. If these biopsies are negative or if there is no symptomatic site, the patient should undergo visceral angiography to look for characteristic aneurysmal dilatation of the renal, mesenteric, or hepatic arteries. Visceral angiography has sensitivity and specificity similar to those of biopsy of symptomatic sites, but angiography can produce complications such as a rise in creatinine and, rarely, death.

Treatment

Corticosteroids in high doses (up to 60 mg of prednisone daily) may control fever and constitutional symptoms and heal vascular lesions. Immunosuppressive agents, especially cyclophosphamide, appear to improve the survival of patients when given with steroids. These drugs may be required for long periods, and relapses are not infrequent when they are withdrawn.

Prognosis

Without treatment, the 5-year survival rate is 20%. Corticosteroids alone improve the 5-year survival to 50%. With corticosteroids and immunosuppressive drugs, the 5-year survival has improved to 80–90%.

Albert DA, Rimon D, Silverstein MD: The diagnosis of polyarteritis nodosa. Arthritis Rheum 1988;31:1117. (Best initial strategy: biopsy symptomatic site or perform visceral angiogram.)

Hellmann DB et al: Mononeuritis multiplex: The yield of evaluations for occult rheumatic diseases. Medicine 1988;67:145. (Simultaneous onset of systemic symptoms and mononeuritis multiplex is highly suggestive of polyarteritis.)

Jarrousse LG et al: Longterm followup after treatment of polyarteritis nodosa and Churg-Strauss angiitis with comparison of steroids, plasma exchange, and cyclophosphamide to steroids and plasma exchange: A prospective randomized trial of 71 patients. J Rheumatol 1991;18:567. (Cyclophosphamide appeared to be more effective but more toxic. Overall, there was no difference between the 10-year survival rates of the two groups.)

POLYMYALGIA RHEUMATICA & GIANT CELL ARTERITIS

Polymyalgia rheumatica, a disorder affecting middle-aged or elderly persons, is rare before age 50. The disease often develops abruptly, with pain and stiffness of the pelvis and shoulder girdle in association with fever, malaise, and weight loss. Anemia and a markedly elevated sedimentation rate are almost always present. The course is generally limited to 1–2 years.

Polymyalgia rheumatica bears a close relationship to giant cell arteritis. The two conditions often coexist, but each may occur independently; when they coexist, the clinical manifestations of polymyalgia rheumatica almost always precede those of giant cell arteritis. The importance of diagnosing arteritis lies in the risk of blindness due to obstruction of the posterior ciliary and ophthalmic arteries; this may occur unless treatment is given. Suggestive symptoms of arteritis include unilateral throbbing headache, scalp sensitivity, visual symptoms, and jaw claudication, but arteritis may be present without local symptoms. Indeed, 40% of patients will have nonclassic presentations with respiratory tract problems (most frequently dry cough), mononeuritis multiplex (most frequently with painful paralysis of a shoulder), or fever of unknown origin.

In the presence of headache and other symptoms suggestive of cranial arteritis, therapy with prednisone, 60 mg daily, is initiated immediately to prevent blindness, and temporal artery biopsy is promptly obtained. How quickly the histologic changes in the temporal artery resolve after initiation of therapy is unclear, but biopsies obtained within

5–7 days after initiation of therapy should be reliable. An adequate biopsy specimen (3–5 cm in length) is essential, because the disease tends to be segmental; bilateral biopsies add 10–20% to the yield. Ten to 15 percent of patients have vasculitis of other major arteries. Prednisone should be continued in a dosage of 60 mg/d for 1–2 months before tapering. When only the symptoms of polymyalgia rheumatic are present, temporal artery biopsy is not necessary. Furthermore, polymyalgia—in the absence of arteritis—responds quickly (1–5 days) and dramatically to smaller doses of prednisone (10–15 mg daily). If such a response does not occur, the diagnosis of polymyalgia rheumatica should be questioned.

In adjusting the dosage of steroid, the erythrocyte sedimentation rate is a useful but not absolute guide to disease activity. Blindness rarely occurs when the ESR has reached the normal range. The drug may be discontinued when disease activity ceases, although the disorder may recur and in some patients remains active for years. Chronic infectious disease such as bacterial endocarditis, which have systemic symptoms similar to those of polymyalgia rheumatica, should always be excluded before corticosteroids are started. Multiple myeloma and other malignant disorders should also be considered as causes of anemia and a markedly elevated sedimentation rate.

Hellmann DB: Immunopathogenesis, diagnosis, and treatment of giant cell arteritis, temporal arteritis, polymyalgia rheumatica, and Takayasu's arteritis. Curr Opin Rheumatol (Jan) 1993;5:25. (Review of recent literature.)

Hellmann DB: Occult manifestations of giant cell arteritis. Medical Grand Rounds 1989;2:296.

Jund JW, Mock D: Temporal arteritis with normal erythrocyte sedimentation rates presenting as occipital neuralgia. Arthritis Rheum 1991;34:217. (Occipital pain was the presenting manifestation in 17% of patients, several of whom had sedimentation rates of less than 40 mm/h.)

WEGENER'S GRANULOMATOSIS

Wegener's granulomatosis is a rare disorder characterized by vasculitis, necrotizing granulomatous lesions of both upper and lower respiratory tract, and glomerulonephritis. Without treatment it is invariably fatal, most patients surviving less than a year after diagnosis. It occurs most commonly in the fourth and fifth decades of life and affects men and women with equal frequency.

Clinical Findings

A. Symptoms and Signs: The disorder presents as a febrile illness with weakness, malaise, and weight loss. Symptoms include those of purulent sinusitis and rhinitis; polyarthralgia may also be present. Dyspnea, cough, chest pain, and hemoptysis may dominate the clinical picture. Ulcerations of the nasal septum are noted on physical examination. X-ray of the chest often reveals nodular pulmonary lesions, frequently cavitating; histologic examination of the lesions shows necrotizing vasculitis with granuloma formation. Although limited forms of Wegener's granulomatosis have been described in which the kidney is spared, severe progressive renal disease usually ensues and results in rapid deterioration of renal function. In such cases the urinary sediment invariably contains red cells, with or without white cells, and red cell casts. Renal biopsy discloses a segmental necrotizing glomerulonephritis with multiple crescents; this is characteristic but not diagnostic. Granulomas are observed in 10%.

B. Laboratory Findings: Laboratory studies show anemia (occasionally microangiopathic), leukocytosis, and a rapid sedimentation rate. Over 90% of patients with active Wegener's granulomatosis will have a positive ANCA. C-ANCA is more common in these patients, but P-ANCA occurs also (see above). Since other diseases—including Takayasu's arteritis, lymphomatoid granulomatosis, cutaneous vasculitis, polyarteritis nodosa, and necrotizing glomerular nephritis—can produce either pattern of ANCA, the diagnosis of Wegener's syndrome rests on histologic grounds.

Treatment

It is essential that the diagnosis be made early, since treatment may be lifesaving; lung tissue is preferred, as findings are more often specific than in tissue from nasal mucosal biopsy. Remissions have been induced in up to 75% of patients treated with cyclophosphamide. Unfortunately, half of the patients who achieve remission eventually have a recurrence of the disease. Most patients also have serious morbidity from the disease or its treatment. The risk of cancer—particularly bladder cancer and lymphoma—is increased in patients treated with cyclophosphamide. The cyclophosphamide must be given daily by mouth; intermittent high-dose intravenous cyclophosphamide is less effective. Corticosteroids are usually of limited value. Preliminary studies suggest that methotrexate, 20 mg/wk, may be as effective as oral cyclophosphamide for patients who do not have immediately life-threatening disease. The value of trimethoprim-sulfamethoxazole (one double-strength table twice daily) is under investigation.

Hoffman G et al: Treatment of Wegener's granulomatosis with intermittent high-dose intravenous cyclophosphamide. Am J Med 1990;89:403.

Hoffman GS et al: The treatment of Wegener's granulomatosis with glucocorticoids and methotrexate. Arthritis Rheum 1992;35:1322. (Open study of 29 patients suggests methotrexate, 20 mg/wk, is effective when the disease is not immediately life-threatening.)

Hoffman GS et al: Wegener granulomatosis: An analysis of 158 patients. Ann Intern Med 1992;116:488. (A sobering review of the complications of the disease and its treatment. Eighty-six percent of patients had serious morbidity from irreversible features of the disease, and 46% had serious adverse effects of therapy. Cyclophosphamide was associated with a 2.4-fold increase in all malignancies, a 33-fold increase in bladder cancers, and an 11-fold increase in lymphomas.)

Nolle B et al: Anticytoplasmic autoantibodies: Their immunodiagnostic value in Wegener granulomatosis. Ann Intern Med 1989;111:28. (Highly specific [98–99%]). Sensitivity was 93–96% for generalized active disease, 60–67% for active regional disease, and 32–40% for disease in remission.)

CRYOGLOBULINEMIA

Vasculitis secondary to cryoglobulinemia is uncommon but should be considered when patients present with palpable purpura on the lower extremities, glomerulonephritis (reflected by hematuria, proteinuria, and red blood cell casts), and peripheral neuropathy. Abnormal liver function tests, abdominal pain, cardiac disease, and pulmonary disease may also occur. The diagnosis is based on a compatible clinical picture and a positive serum test for cryoglobulins. Type II (monoclonal antibody with rheumatoid factor activity) and type III (polyclonal antibody with rheumatoid factor activity) cryoglobulins are most common in patients with vasculitis. Type I cryoglobulin (a monoclonal protein that does not have rheumatoid factor activity) is more commonly seen in lymphoproliferative disease associated with a hyperviscosity syndrome. Although the cause of cryoglobulinemia in vasculitis is unknown, the majority of patients have evidence of hepatitis C infection. Prednisone and immunosuppressive drugs are, at best, moderately effective for visceral complications such as renal insufficiency and neuropathy.

Agnello V, Chung RT, Kaplan LM: A role for hepatitis C virus infection in type II cryoglobulinemia. N Engl J Med 1992;327:1490. (Forty-two percent had hepatitis C antibodies and 84% had hepatitis C RNA.)

HENOCH-SCHÖNLEIN PURPURA

This is a form of purpura of unknown cause; the underlying pathologic feature is vasculitis, which principally affects small blood vessels. Although the disease is predominantly seen in children, adults are also affected. Hypersensitivity to aspirin and food and drug additives has been reported. The purpuric skin lesions are typically located on the lower extremities but may also be seen on the hands, arms, and trunk. Localized areas of edema, especially common on the dorsal surfaces of the hands, are frequently observed. Joint symptoms are present in the vast majority of patients, the knees and ankles being most commonly involved. Abdominal pain secondary to vasculitis of the intestinal tract is often associated with gastrointestinal bleeding. Hematuria signals the presence of a renal lesion that is usually reversible, although it occasionally may progress to renal insufficiency. Biopsy of the kidney reveals segmental glomerulonephritis with crescents and mesangial deposition of IgA and, sometimes, IgG. Aside from an elevated sedimentation rate, most laboratory findings are noncontributory; the platelet count is normal or elevated.

The disease is usually self-limited, lasting 1–6 weeks, and subsides without sequelae if renal involvement is not severe. There is no effective treatment, although immunosuppressive drugs have met with some success in the nephropathy of this disorder.

Goldstein AR et al: Long-term follow-up of childhood Henoch-Schönlein nephritis. Lancet 1992;339:280. (Proteinuria and hypertension can develop long after the initial episode of nephritis and are particularly likely to emerge during pregnancy.)

Michel BA et al: Hypersensitivity vasculitis and Henoch-Schönlein purpura: A comparison between the two disorders. J Rheumatol 1992;19:721. (Presence of palpable purpura, bowel angina, gastrointestinal bleeding, hematuria, or age at onset less than 20 favors Henoch-Schönlein purpura.)

SERONEGATIVE SPONDYLOARTHROPATHIES

The diseases included under this heading are noted for onset usually before age 40, inflammatory arthritis of either the spine or the large peripheral joints, uveitis in a significant minority, a strong association with HLA-B27, and the absence of autoantibodies in the serum.

ANKYLOSING SPONDYLITIS

Essentials of Diagnosis

- Chronic low backache in young adults.
- Progressive limitation of back motion and of chest expansion.
- Transient (50%) or permanent (25%) peripheral arthritis.
- Diagnostic x-ray changes in sacroiliac joints.
- Uveitis in 20–25%. Accelerated erythrocyte sedimentation rate and negative serologic tests for rheumatoid factor.
- HLA-B27 usually positive.

General Considerations

Ankylosing spondylitis is a chronic inflammatory disease of the joints of the axial skeleton, manifested clinically by pain and progressive stiffening of the spine. The age at onset is usually in the late teens or early 20s. The incidence is greater in males than in females, and symptoms are more prominent in men, and ascending involvement of the spine is more likely to occur.

Clinical Findings

A. Symptoms and Signs: The onset is usually gradual, with intermittent bouts of back pain that may radiate down the thighs. As the disease advances, symptoms progress in a cephalad direction and back motion becomes limited, with the normal lumbar curve flattened and the thoracic curvature exaggerated. Atrophy of the trunk muscles is common. Chest expansion is often limited as a consequence of costovertebral joint involvement. Radicular symptoms due to the cauda equina syndrome may occur years after onset of the disease. In advanced cases, the entire spine becomes fused, allowing no motion in any direction. Transient acute arthritis of the peripheral joints occurs in about 50% of cases, and permanent changes in the peripheral joints—most commonly the hips, shoulders, and knees—are seen in about 25%.

Spondylitic heart disease, characterized chiefly by atrioventricular conduction defects and aortic insufficiency, occurs in 3–5% of patients with long-standing severe disease. Nongranulomatous anterior uveitis is associated in as many as 25% of cases and may be a presenting feature. Pulmonary fibrosis of the upper lobes, with progression to cavitation and bronchiectasis mimicking tuberculosis, may occur, characteristically long after the onset of skeletal symptoms. Constitutional symptoms similar to those of rheumatoid arthritis are absent in most patients.

B. Laboratory Findings: The erythrocyte sedimentation rate is elevated in 85% of cases, but serologic tests for rheumatoid factor are characteristically negative. There may be leukocytosis and anemia.

HLA-B27 is found in 90% of patients with ankylosing spondylitis, as opposed to 6–8% among unaffected individuals. These figures are lower in blacks. HLA-B27 is found with greater than normal frequency in some other rheumatic diseases such as Reiter's syndrome, psoriasis, and inflammatory bowel disease. HLA-B27 is also more frequent in patients who have anterior uveitis alone. The incidence of B27 positivity is highest in ankylosing spondylitis. Because of the noted incidence of this antigen in the normal population, it is not an absolutely specific diagnostic test.

Persons with other rheumatic diseases such as rheumatoid arthritis, degenerative joint disease (osteoarthritis), and gout do not show a higher than normal incidence of HLA-B27.

C. Imaging: The earliest radiographic changes are usually in the sacroiliac joints. In the first few months of the disease process, the sacroiliac changes may be detectable only by CT scanning. Later, erosion and sclerosis of these joints are evident on regular radiographs. Later, involvement of the apophyseal joints of the spine, ossification of the annulus fibrosus, calcification of the anterior and lateral spinal ligaments, and squaring and generalized demineralization of the vertebral bodies may occur. The term "bamboo spine" has been used to describe the late radiographic changes.

Additional x-ray findings include periosteal new bone formation on the iliac crest, ischial tuberosities and calcanei, and alterations of the pubic symphysis and sternomanubrial joint similar to those of the sacroiliacs. Radiologic changes in peripheral joints, when present, tend to be asymmetric and lack the demineralization and erosions seen in rheumatoid arthritis.

Differential Diagnosis

Although rheumatoid arthritis may ultimately involve the spine, it does so characteristically in the cervical region, usually sparing the sacroiliac joints. Other features that differentiate ankylosing spondylitis from rheumatoid arthritis are the rare involvement of the small joints of the hands and feet, the absence of subcutaneous nodules, and the negative serologic tests for rheumatoid factor in spondylitis. The history and physical findings of ankylosing spondylitis serve to distinguish this disorder from other causes of low back pain such as disk disease, osteoporosis, soft tissue trauma, and tumors. The single most valuable distinguishing radiologic sign of ankylosing spondylitis is the appearance of the sacroiliac joints, although a similar pattern may be seen in Reiter's syndrome and in the arthritis associated with inflammatory intestinal diseases and psoriasis. A spondyloarthropathy associated with hidradenitis suppurativa has been described in blacks. In ankylosing hyperostosis (diffuse idiopathic skeletal hyperostosis [DISH], Forestier's disease), there is exuberant osteophyte formation. The osteophytes are thicker and more anterior than the syndesmophytes of ankylosing spondylitis, and the sacroiliac joints are not affected. The x-ray appearance of the sacroiliac joints in spondylitis should be distinguished from that in osteitis condensans ilii. In some geographic areas and in persons with appropriate occupations, brucellosis and fluoride poisoning may be important in the differential diagnosis.

Treatment

A. Basic Program: The general principles of managing chronic arthritis (see above) apply equally well to ankylosing spondylitis. The importance of postural and breathing exercises should be stressed.

B. Drug Therapy: The nonsteroidal anti-inflammatory agents are employed in the treatment of this disorder. Of these, indomethacin appears to be the most effective, though it is not unreasonable to begin therapy with aspirin. The dosage of indomethacin is usually 25–50 mg three times a day, but the least amount should be used that will provide symptomatic improvement. Agents such as naproxen, fenoprofen, tolmetin, sulindac, piroxicam, and other newer NSAIDs are valuable alternatives and may even be used as primary therapy. Indomethacin may produce a variety of untoward reactions, including headache, giddiness, nausea and vomiting, peptic ulcer, renal insufficiency, depression, and psychosis.

C. Physical Therapy: See above.

Prognosis

Spontaneous remissions and relapses are common and may occur at any stage. Occasionally, the disease progresses to ankylosis of the entire spine. In general, the functional prognosis is good unless the hips are seriously involved and consequently ankylosed.

Guillemin F et al: Long-term disability and prolonged sick leaves as outcome measuring in ankylosing spondylitis. Arthritis Rheum 1990;33:1001. (Long-term disability more common with male gender, onset before age 26, and more than two peripheral joints affected.)
Maugars Y et al: Corticosteroid injection of the sacroiliac joint in patients with seronegative spondyloarthropathy. Arthritis Rheum 1992;35:564. (Very good response in 79%.)

PSORIATIC ARTHRITIS

Essentials of Diagnosis

- Psoriasis precedes onset of arthritis in 80% of cases.
- Arthritis usually asymmetric, with "sausage" appearance of fingers and toes; resembles rheumatoid arthritis; rheumatoid factor is absent from serum.
- Sacroiliac joint involvement common; ankylosing spondylitis may be associated.
- X-ray findings: osteolysis; pencil-in-cup deformity; relative lack of osteoporosis; bony ankylosis; asymmetric sacroiliitis and atypical syndesmophytes.

General Considerations

In 15–20% of patients with psoriasis, arthritis coexists. The patterns or subsets of arthritis that may accompany psoriasis include the following:

(1) Joint disease that resembles rheumatoid arthritis in which polyarthritis is symmetric. Usually, fewer joints are involved than in rheumatoid arthritis, and rheumatoid factor is absent from the serum.

(2) An oligoarticular form that may lead to considerable destruction of the affected joints.

(3) A pattern of disease in which the distal interphalangeal joints are primarily affected. Early, this may be monarticular, and often the joint involvement is asymmetric. Pitting of the nails and onycholysis are frequently associated.

(4) A severe deforming arthritis (arthritis mutilans) in which osteolysis is severe.

(5) A spondylitic form with sacroiliitis and spinal involvement predominating; 45% of these patients are HLA-B27 positive.

Clinical Findings

A. Symptoms and Signs: Although psoriasis usually precedes the onset of arthritis, in 20–25% of patients the arthritis precedes the skin disease. Arthritis is at least five times more common in patients with severe skin disease than in those with only mild skin findings. Occasionally, however, patients may have a single patch of psoriasis (typically hidden in the scalp, gluteal cleft, or umbilicus) and are unaware of it. Thus, a detailed search for cutaneous lesions is essential in patients with arthritis of new onset. Also, the psoriatic lesions may have cleared when arthritis appears—in such cases, the history is most useful. Nail pitting, a residue of previous psoriasis, is sometimes the only clue.

B. Laboratory Findings: Laboratory studies show an elevation of the sedimentation rate, but rheumatoid factor is not present. Uric acid levels may be high, reflecting the active turnover of skin affected by psoriasis. There is a correlation between the extent of psoriatic involvement and the level of uric acid, but gout is no more common than in patients without psoriasis. Desquamation of the skin may also reduce iron stores.

C. Imaging: Radiographic findings are most helpful in distinguishing the disease from other forms of arthritis. There are marginal erosions of bone and irregular destruction of joint and bone, which, in the phalanx, may give the appearance of a sharpened pencil. Fluffy periosteal new bone may be marked, especially at the insertion of muscles and ligaments into bone. Such changes will also be seen along the shafts of metacarpals, metatarsals, and phalanges. Paravertebral ossification occurs, which may be distinguished from ankylosing spondylitis by the absence of ossification in the anterior aspect of the spine.

Treatment

Treatment regimens are symptomatic. Nonsteroidal anti-inflammatory drugs are useful. Antimalarials may exacerbate the psoriasis. Gold therapy is often effective. In resistant cases, methotrexate has been used with some success, but it should be employed only by those fully conversant with its use. Successful treatment of the skin lesions commonly—though not invariably—is accompanied by an improvement in peripheral articular symptoms.

Espinoza LR et al: Psoriatic arthritis: Clinical response and side effects to methotrexate therapy. J Rheumatol 1992;19:872. (Thirty-seven of 40 patients had an excellent or good response.)

Palit J et al: A multicentre double-blind comparison of auranofin, intramuscular gold thiomalate, and placebo in patients with psoriatic arthritis. Br J Rheumatol 1990; 29:280. (Intramuscular gold was safe and more effective than auranofin [oral gold].)

REITER'S SYNDROME

Reiter's syndrome is a clinical tetrad of unknown cause consisting of urethritis, conjunctivitis (or, less commonly, uveitis), mucocutaneous lesions, and arthritis. It occurs most commonly in young men. It may follow (within days or weeks) infection with *Chlamydia, Campylobacter, Salmonella,* or *Yersinia* and is usually accompanied by a systemic reaction, including fever. The arthritis is most commonly asymmetric and frequently involves the large weight-bearing joints (chiefly the knee and ankle); sacroiliitis or ankylosing spondylitis is observed in at least 20% of patients, especially after frequent recurrences. The mucocutaneous lesions may include balanitis, stomatitis, and keratoderma blenorrhagicum, resembling pustular psoriasis with involvement of the skin and nails. Carditis and aortic regurgitation may occur. While most signs of the disease disappear within days or weeks, the arthritis may persist for several months or even years. The test for HLA-B27 is positive in 80% of white patients and 50–60% of blacks. (See Chapter 18 for further discussion of HLA-B27.) Characteristically, the initial attack is self-limited and terminates spontaneously.

Recurrences involving any combination of the clinical manifestations are common and are sometimes followed by permanent sequelae, especially in the joints. X-ray signs of permanent or progressive joint disease may be seen in the sacroiliac as well as the peripheral joints.

Reiter's syndrome must be distinguished from gonococcal arthritis, especially when conjunctivitis has been mild or overlooked. Rheumatoid arthritis, idiopathic ankylosing spondylitis, and psoriatic arthritis must also be considered. Reiter's syndrome appears to be more common in patients infected with HIV and may precede or follow AIDS.

Treatment is symptomatic. Antibiotics are ineffective. As in psoriatic arthritis, the most useful drugs are the NSAIDs.

Rahman MU et al: Molecular evidence for the presence of *Chlamydia* in the synovium of patients with Reiter's syndrome. Arthritis Rheum 1992;35:521. (Seven of nine patients had chlamydial RNA molecules in synovium.)

ARTHRITIS & INFLAMMATORY INTESTINAL DISEASES

Arthritis is a common complication of ulcerative colitis, regional enteritis, and Whipple's disease. Occasionally, such joint disease is indistinguishable from rheumatoid arthritis and may represent a coincidence of the two disorders. More commonly, however, intestinal arthritis is asymmetric, affects large joints, parallels the course of the bowel disease, and rarely results in residual deformity. Articular symptoms may be prominent enough to cause the patient to overlook intestinal symptoms. Ankylosing spondylitis, which may accompany inflammatory bowel disease, is indistinguishable from idiopathic ankylosing spondylitis and usually runs a course separate from bowel disease activity.

The synovitis is pathologically nonspecific. Rheumatoid factor is usually negative and HLA-B27 is often positive, and its presence may predispose to the development of spondylitis. Treatment of intestinal arthritis involves control of intestinal inflammation and use of supportive anti-inflammatory drugs; that of ankylosing spondylitis is the same as for idiopathic ankylosing spondylitis.

About 15% of patients who have jejunoileal bypass surgery for morbid obesity develop an inflammatory symmetric polyarticular disorder. The arthritis is usually acute in onset and nonmigratory and may affect the small as well as the large joints. The sedimentation rate is elevated, and antinuclear antibody and rheumatoid factor tests may be positive. Nonsteroidal anti-inflammatory agents are often effective, although some patients require prednisone.

Ratain JS, Hellmann DB: Colitic arthritis and spondylitis. In: *Current Management of Inflammatory Bowel Disease.* Bayless T (editor). Decker, 1989. (Reviews presentations and treatments.)

Weiner SR et al: Rheumatic manifestations of inflammatory bowel disease. Semin Arthritis Rheum 1991;20:353.

RELAPSING POLYCHONDRITIS

This is a rare disease of unknown cause characterized by inflammatory destructive lesions of cartilaginous structures, principally the ears, nose, trachea, and larynx. It may be associated either with other immunologic disorders such as SLE, rheumatoid arthritis, or Hashimoto's thyroiditis or with cancers, especially multiple myeloma. The disease, which is usually episodic, affects males and females equally. The cartilage is painful, swollen, and tender during an attack and subsequently becomes atrophic, resulting in permanent deformity. Biopsy of the involved cartilage shows inflammation and chondrolysis. Noncartilaginous manifestations of the disease include fever, episcleritis, uveitis, deafness, aortic insufficiency, and rarely immune complex-mediated renal disease. In 85% of patients, an arthropathy is seen that tends to be migratory, asymmetric, and seronegative, affecting both large and small joints and the parasternal articulation.

Corticosteroid therapy is often effective. Dapsone may also be effective, sparing the need for chronic high-dose corticosteroid treatment. Involvement of the tracheobronchial tree, leading to its collapse, may cause death if tracheostomy is not done promptly.

Lipnick RN, Fink CW: Acute airway obstruction in relapsing polychondritis: Treatment with pulse methylprednisolone. J Rheumatol 1991;18:98. (Report of two cases.)

PALINDROMIC RHEUMATISM

Palindromic rheumatism is a disease of unknown cause characterized by frequent recurring attacks (at irregular intervals) of acutely inflamed joints. Periarticular pain with swelling and transient subcutaneous nodules may also occur. The attacks cease within several hours to several days. The knee and finger joints are most commonly affected, but any peripheral joint may be involved. Systemic manifestations other than fever do not occur. Although hundreds of attacks may take place over a period of years, there is no permanent articular damage. Laboratory findings are usually normal. Palindromic rheumatism must be distinguished from acute gouty arthritis and an atypical, acute onset of rheumatoid arthritis.

Symptomatic treatment with NSAIDs is usually all that is required during the attacks. Hydroxychloroquine may be of value in preventing recurrences.

Youssef W, Yan A, Russell AS: Palindromic rheumatism: A response to chloroquine. J Rheumatol 1991;18:35.

INFECTIOUS ARTHRITIS*

NONGONOCOCCAL ACUTE BACTERIAL (SEPTIC) ARTHRITIS

Essentials of Diagnosis

- Sudden onset of acute arthritis, usually monarticular, most often in large weight-bearing joints and wrists.
- Chills and fever. Joint fluid findings often diagnostic. Previous joint damage or intravenous drug abuse common risk factors.

*Lyme disease is discussed in Chapter 33.

- Infection with causative organisms commonly found elsewhere in body.

General Considerations

Nongonococcal acute bacterial arthritis is a disease of an abnormal host. The key risk factors are persistent bacteremia (eg, intravenous drug abuse, endocarditis) and damaged joints (eg, rheumatoid arthritis). *Staphylococcus aureus* is the most common cause of nongonococcal septic arthritis, followed by group A and group B streptococci. Gram-negative septic arthritis, once rare, has become more common, especially in intravenous drug abusers and in other immunocompromised hosts. *Escherichia coli* and *Pseudomonas aeruginosa* are the most common gram-negative isolates in adults.

The widespread use of arthroscopy and prosthetic joint surgery has also increased the frequency of septic arthritis. In the latter conditions, *Staphylococcus epidermidis* is the usual offending organism. Pathologic changes include varying degrees of acute inflammation, with synovitis, effusion, abscess formation in synovial or subchondral tissues, and, if treatment is not adequate, articular destruction.

Clinical Findings

A. Symptoms and Signs: The onset is usually sudden, with acute pain, swelling, and heat of one joint—most frequently the knee. Other commonly affected sites are the hip, wrist, shoulder, and ankle. Unusual sites, such as the sternoclavicular or sacroiliac joint, can be involved in intravenous drug abusers. Chills and fever are common but are absent in up to 20% of patients. Infection of the hip usually does not produce gross swelling but results in groin pain greatly aggravated by walking.

B. Laboratory Findings: Blood cultures are positive in approximately 50% of patients. The leukocyte count of the synovial fluid may be greater than 100,000/μL, with 90% or more polymorphonuclear cells. Synovial fluid glucose is usually low. Gram stain of the synovial fluid is positive in 75% of staphylococcal infections and in 50% of gram-negative infections.

C. Imaging: Radiographs are usually normal early in the disease, but evidence of demineralization may be present within days of onset. Bony erosions and narrowing of the joint space followed by osteomyelitis and periostitis may be seen within 2 weeks.

Differential Diagnosis

The septic course with chills and fever, the acute systemic reaction, the joint fluid findings, evidence of infection elsewhere in the body, and the evidence of response to appropriate antibiotics are diagnostic of bacterial arthritis. Gout and pseudogout are excluded by the failure to find crystals on synovial fluid analysis. Acute rheumatic fever and rheumatoid arthritis commonly involve many joints; Still's disease may mimic septic arthritis, but laboratory evidence of infection is absent. Pyogenic arthritis may be superimposed on other types of joint disease, notably rheumatoid arthritis, and must be excluded (by joint fluid examination) in any apparent acute relapse of the primary disease, particularly when a joint has been needled or one is more strikingly inflamed than the others.

Treatment

Prompt systemic antibiotic therapy of any septic arthritis should be based on the best clinical judgment of the causative organism and the results of smear and culture of joint fluid, blood, urine, or other specific sites of potential infection. If the organism cannot be determined clinically, treatment should be started with bactericidal antibiotics effective against staphylococci, pneumococci, and gram-negative organisms.

Frequent (even daily) local aspiration is indicated when synovial fluid rapidly reaccumulates and causes symptoms. Immediate surgical drainage is reserved for septic arthritis of the hip, because that site is inaccessible to repeated aspiration. For most other joints, surgical drainage is used only if medical therapy fails over 2–4 days to improve the fever and the synovial fluid volume, white blood count, and culture results. Pain can be relieved with local hot compresses and by immobilizing the joint with a splint or traction. Rest, immobilization, and elevation are used at the onset of treatment. Early active motion exercises within the limits of tolerance will hasten recovery.

Prognosis

With prompt antibiotic therapy, functional recovery is usually good. Bony ankylosis and articular destruction commonly occur if treatment is delayed or inadequate.

Ho G: Bacterial arthritis. Curr Opin Rheumatol (Aug) 1991;3:603.

Mozen PH, Zell SC: Sternoclavicular bacterial arthritis. West J Med 1988;148:310.

Vyskocil JJ et al: Pyogenic infection of the sacroiliac joint: Case reports and review of the literature. Medicine 1992;70:188. (Major predisposing factors include intravenous drug use, trauma, or infection in another location.)

GONOCOCCAL ARTHRITIS

Essentials of Diagnosis

- Prodromal migratory polyarthralgias.
- Tenosynovitis most common sign.
- Purulent monarthritis in 50%.
- Characteristic skin rash.
- Most common in young women during menses or pregnancy.
- Symptoms of urethritis frequently absent.
- Dramatic response to antibiotics.

General Considerations

Disseminated gonococcal infection is the most common cause of infectious arthritis in large urban areas. In contrast to nongonococcal bacterial arthritis, gonococcal arthritis chiefly occurs in otherwise healthy individuals. Host factors, however, influence the expression of the disease: gonococcal arthritis is two to three times more common in women than in men, is especially common during menses and pregnancy, and is rare after age 40. Gonococcal arthritis is also common in male homosexuals, whose high incidence of asymptomatic gonococcal pharyngitis and proctitis predisposes them to disseminated gonococcal infection. Some of the signs of disseminated gonococcal infection may result from an immunologic reaction to nonviable fragments of the organism's cell wall; this may explain the frequent inability to culture organisms from skin and joint lesions. Recurrent disseminated gonococcal infection should prompt evaluation for a congenital deficiency of complement components, especially C7 and C8.

Clinical Findings

A. Symptoms and Signs: One to 4 days of migratory polyarthralgias involving the wrist, knee, ankle, or elbow is the most common initial course. Thereafter, two patterns emerge, one (60% of patients) characterized by tenosynovitis and the other (40%) by purulent monarthritis, most frequently involving the knee. Less than half of patients have fever, and less than one-fourth have any genitourinary symptoms. Most patients will have asymptomatic but highly characteristic skin lesions that usually consist of two to ten small necrotic pustules distributed over the extremities, especially the palms and soles.

B. Laboratory Findings: The peripheral blood leukocyte count averages 10,400 cells/μL and is elevated in less than one-third of patients. The synovial fluid white blood cell count, however, averages over 50,000 cells/μL. The synovial fluid Gram stain is positive in one-fourth of cases and culture in less than half. Positive blood cultures are seen in 40% of patients with tenosynovitis and virtually never in patients with suppurative arthritis. Urethral, throat, and rectal cultures should be done in all patients, since they are often positive in the absence of local symptoms. Culturing *Neisseria gonorrhoeae* is facilitated by rapid transport to the microbiology laboratory, inoculation on chocolate agar, and incubation in carbon dioxide.

C. Imaging: Radiographs are usually normal or show only soft tissue swelling.

Differential Diagnosis

Reiter's syndrome can also produce acute monarthritis in a young person but is distinguished by negative cultures, sacroiliitis, and failure to respond to antibiotics. Lyme disease involving the knee is less acute, does not show positive cultures, and may be preceded by known tick exposure and characteristic rash. The synovial fluid analysis will exclude gout, pseudogout, and nongonococcal bacterial arthritis. Rheumatic fever and sarcoidosis can produce migratory tenosynovitis but have other distinguishing features. Infective endocarditis with septic arthritis can mimic disseminated gonococcal infection.

Treatment

In most cases, patients suspected of having gonococcal arthritis should be admitted to the hospital to confirm the diagnosis and to start treatment. While outpatient treatment has been recommended in the past, the rapid rise in gonococci resistant to penicillin makes initial inpatient treatment necessary. Approximately 4–5% of all gonococcal isolates produce a β-lactamase that confers penicillin resistance. An additional 15–20% of gonococcal species have chromosomal mutations that result in relative resistance to penicillin. Therefore, the new recommendations for initial treatment of gonococcal arthritis are to give ceftriaxone, 1 g intravenously daily for 7–10 days. If the diagnosis of gonococcal arthritis and penicillin sensitivity are confirmed, amoxicillin, 500 mg orally four times a day, can be given on an outpatient basis to complete a 10- to 14-day course.

Prognosis

Generally, gonococcal arthritis responds dramatically in 24–48 hours after initiation of antibiotics so that daily joint aspirations are rarely needed. Complete recovery is the rule.

Keat A: Sexually transmitted arthritis syndromes. Med Clin North Am 1990;74:1617.

Livneh A, Sewell KL, Barland P: Chronic gonococcal arthritis. J Rheumatol 1989;16:245. (Case report of low-grade gonococcal arthritis of 30½ months' duration, showing that gonococcal arthritis can rarely cause chronic monarthritis.)

RHEUMATIC MANIFESTATIONS OF HIV INFECTION

Infection with human immunodeficiency virus (HIV) has been associated with various rheumatic disorders, most commonly Reiter's syndrome or reactive arthritis or arthralgias and more rarely myositis, psoriatic arthritis, Sjögren's syndrome, or vasculitis (see Chapter 30). It is possible that these disorders stem directly from HIV infection itself or from the many other infections that occur in immunodeficient patients. The rheumatic syndromes can follow or precede by several months the diagnosis of acquired AIDS. Thus, HIV infection must be considered as a possible cause of Reiter's syndrome, and Reiter's syndrome should be considered a possible early manifestation of HIV infection. The lower extremity joints, especially the knees and ankles, are most commonly affected. Often, as in classic Reiter's syndrome, Achilles tendon inflammation (enthesopathy) or knee periarthritis is a prominent and distinguishing feature. Many patients respond to NSAIDs, though a few are unresponsive and develop progressive deformities. The use of immunosuppressive agents, however, is contraindicated in these immunodeficient patients.

Berman A et al: Rheumatic manifestations of human immunodeficiency virus infection. Am J Med 1988;85:59. (Prospective evaluation of 101 patients: arthralgias in 35, Reiter's syndrome in ten, psoriatic arthritis in two, myositis in two, and vasculitis in one.)

Espinoza LR et al: Rheumatic manifestations associated with human immunodeficiency virus infection. Arthritis Rheum 1989;32:1615. (Review of the literature.)

VIRAL ARTHRITIS

Arthritis may be a manifestation of many viral infections. It is generally mild and of short duration, and it terminates spontaneously without lasting ill effects. Mumps arthritis may occur in the absence of parotitis. Rubella arthritis, which occurs more commonly in adults than in children, may appear immediately before, during, or soon after the disappearance of the rash. Its usual polyarticular and symmetric distribution mimics that of rheumatoid arthritis. However, the seronegative tests for rheumatoid factor and the rising rubella titers in convalescent serum help to confirm the diagnosis. Post-rubella vaccination arthritis may have its onset as long as 6 weeks following vaccination and occurs in all age groups. In adults, arthritis may follow infection with human parvovirus B19.

Polyarthritis may be associated with type B hepatitis and typically occurs before the onset of jaundice; it may occur in anicteric hepatitis as well. Urticaria or other types of skin rash may be present. Indeed, the clinical picture may be indistinguishable from that of serum sickness. Serum transaminase levels are elevated, and hepatitis B surface antigen is most often present. Serum complement levels are usually low during active arthritis and become normal after remission of arthritis. False-positive tests for rheumatoid factor, when present, disappear within several weeks. The arthritis is mild; it rarely lasts more than a few weeks and is self-limiting and without deformity.

Naides SJ et al: Rheumatologic manifestations of human parvovirus B19 infection in adults. Arthritis Rheum 1990;33:1297. (21 patients with parvovirus-related arthritis. Mean age 35–37; arthralgias > arthritis; rash in the majority, usually responsive to NSAIDS.)

INFECTIONS OF BONES

Direct microbial contamination of bones results from open fracture, surgical procedures, gunshot wounds, diagnostic needle aspirations, and therapeutic or self-administered drug injections.

Indirect or secondary infections are first noticed in other areas of the body and extend to bones by hematogenous routes.

ACUTE PYOGENIC OSTEOMYELITIS

Essentials of Diagnosis

- Fever and chills associated with pain and tenderness of involved bone.
- Aspiration of involved bone is usually diagnostic.
- Culture of blood or lesion tissue is essential for precise diagnosis.
- Radiographs early in the course are typically negative.

General Considerations

Initial bone infections are indirectly seeded by a single strain of pyogenic bacteria about 95% of the time. About 75% of hematogenous acute infections of bone are due to staphylococci; group A hemolytic streptococci are the next most common pathogens. Vertebral osteomyelitis, due to more indolent organisms, is being encountered with increasing frequency in elderly patients. Among intravenous drug abusers, gram-positive organisms (eg, *Staphylococcus aureus*) and Enterobacteriaceae (eg, *Escherichia coli*) account for 80% of cases of osteomyelitis. Infections of bone due to trauma are often polymicrobial.

Salmonellae cause many cases of bacteremia associated with sickle cell disease. Among patients with hemoglobinopathies, osteomyelitis is caused by salmonellae almost ten times as often as by other pyogenic bacteria. In otherwise healthy patients with salmonellosis, bone lesions are likely to be solitary. In typhoid fever, however, infections of bones occur as a complication in less than 1% of cases. (See Salmonellosis, Chapter 32.)

Bone infection is an uncommon complication of brucellosis, but the clinical picture when it does occur is characteristic. Bone lesions most commonly occur in the lumbar spine or sacroiliac joints.

Clinical Findings

A. Symptoms and Signs: The onset of acute osteomyelitis in adults is less likely to be striking than the sudden and alarming presentation often seen in children. Generalized toxic symptoms of bacteremia may be absent, and vague or evanescent local pain may be the earliest manifestation. Tenderness may be present or absent, depending upon the extent and duration of bone involvement.

B. Laboratory Findings: Aspiration of bone and periosteum to recover organisms for culture is necessary for accurate diagnosis. Blood cultures are frequently positive, particularly when systemic symptoms are prominent, in which case the white count and sedimentation rate are often elevated.

With infections due to *Salmonella* or *Brucella,* significant rising serologic agglutination titers support a tentative diagnosis during the acute stage. Culture of material from the osteoid focus is specific.

C. Imaging: Early findings may include soft tissue swelling, loss of tissue planes, and periarticular demineralization of bone. About 2 weeks after onset of symptoms, erosion of bone and alteration of cancellous bone appear, followed by periostitis. Radionuclide imaging is especially sensitive, becoming positive within 1–2 days after onset of acute osteomyelitis. CT scans and MRI are also more sensitive than conventional radiographs and are particularly helpful in demonstrating the extent of soft tissue involvement. When osteomyelitis involves the vertebrae, it commonly traverses the disk space—a finding that is not observed in tumor.

Differential Diagnosis

Acute hematogenous osteomyelitis should be distinguished from suppurative arthritis, rheumatic fever, and cellulitis. More subacute forms must be differentiated from tuberculous or mycotic infections of bone and Ewing's sarcoma or from metastatic tumor (vertebral osteomyelitis).

Complications

Inadequate treatment of bone infections results in chronicity of infection, and this possibility is increased by delay in diagnosis and treatment. Extension to adjacent bone or joints may complicate acute osteomyelitis. Recurrence of bone infections often results in anemia, weight loss, weakness, and, rarely, amyloidosis or nephrotic syndrome. Pseudoepitheliomatous hyperplasia, squamous cell carcinoma, or fibrosarcoma may occasionally arise in persistently infected tissues.

Treatment

Cultures and antibiotic sensitivity studies should determine the choice of antibiotic agents; the initial selection of drug is based on clinical assessment of the most probable cause. Oral therapy with ciprofloxacin, 750 mg twice daily for 6–8 weeks, has been shown to be as effective as standard parenteral antibiotic therapy for chronic osteomyelitis in adults with susceptible organisms. Open or closed drainage of the local lesion is important when prompt clinical response to initial treatment does not occur. Analgesics, rest, immobilization, and elevation of the part should be used from the beginning of treatment.

Prognosis

If sterility of the lesion is achieved within 2–4 days, a good result can be expected in most cases if there is no compromise of the patient's immune system. However, progression of the disease to a chronic form may occur. It is especially common in the lower extremities and in patients in whom circulation is impaired (eg, diabetics). Surgical saucerization, excision of bone, and debridement of healthy tissues are often necessary.

Gentry LO, Rodriguez GG: Oral ciprofloxacin compared with parenteral antibiotics in the treatment of osteomyelitis. Antimicrob Agents Chemother 1990;34:40. (Ciprofloxacin, 750 mg twice a day for 56 days, was as effective as parenteral antibiotics given for 47 days.)

Mader JT, Cantrell JS, Calhoun J: Oral ciprofloxacin compared with standard parenteral antibiotic therapy for chronic osteomyelitis in adults. J Bone Joint Surg [Am] 1990;72:104.

MYCOTIC INFECTIONS OF BONES & JOINTS

Fungal infections of the skeletal system are usually secondary to a primary infection in another organ, frequently the lungs (see Chapter 36). Although skeletal lesions have a predilection for the cancellous extremities of long bones and the bodies of vertebrae, the predominant lesion—a granuloma with varying degrees of necrosis and abscess formation—does not produce a characteristic clinical picture.

Differentiation from other chronic focal infections depends upon culture studies of synovial fluid or tissue obtained from the local lesion. Serologic tests provide presumptive support of the diagnosis.

1. COCCIDIOIDOMYCOSIS

Coccidioidomycosis of bones and joints is usually secondary to primary pulmonary infection. Arthralgia with periarticular swelling, especially in the knees and ankles, occurring as a nonspecific manifestation of systemic coccidioidomycosis, should be distinguished from actual bone or joint infection. Osseous lesions commonly occur in cancellous bone of the vertebrae or near the ends of long bones. These lesions are initially osteolytic and thus may mimic metastatic tumor or myeloma.

The precise diagnosis depends upon recovery of *Coccidioides immitis* from the lesion or histologic examination of tissue obtained by open biopsy. Rising titers of complement-fixing antibodies provide further evidence of the disseminated nature of the disease.

Ketoconazole, 400 mg/d for 6–12 months, has become the treatment of choice for bone and joint coccidioidomycosis. It is important to exclude concomitant meningeal infection, for which ketoconazole is ineffective. Chronic infection may require operative excision of infected bone and soft tissue; amputation may be the only solution for stubbornly progressive infections. Immobilization of joints by plaster casts and avoidance of weight bearing provide benefit. Synovectomy, joint debridement, and arthrodesis are reserved for more advanced joint infections.

2. HISTOPLASMOSIS

Focal skeletal or joint involvement in histoplasmosis is rare and generally represents dissemination from a primary focus in the lungs. Skeletal lesions may be single or multiple and are not characteristic.

TUBERCULOSIS OF BONES & JOINTS

Essentials of Diagnosis

- A disease of children, the elderly, or those with HIV infection.
- In most cases, a single site of bone or joint is infected.
- Spine—especially lower thoracic—or knee most common sites.
- Chest x-ray abnormal in less than half.

General Considerations

Most tuberculous infections in the USA are caused by the human strain of *Mycobacterium tuberculosis* (see Chapter 9). Infection of the musculoskeletal system is caused by hematogenous spread from a primary lesion of the respiratory tract; it may occur shortly after primary infection or may be seen years later as a reactivation disease. Tuberculosis of the thoracic or lumbar spine (Pott's disease) may be associated with an active lesion of the genitourinary tract or may occur as an isolated finding. It is usually a disease of children in developing nations and of the elderly in the United States. Tuberculous osteomyelitis secondary to cutaneous inoculation has been reported.

Clinical Findings

A. Symptoms and Signs: The onset of symptoms is generally insidious and not accompanied by general manifestations of fever, sweating, toxicity, or prostration. Pain may be mild at onset, is usually worse at night, and may be accompanied by stiffness. As the disease process progresses, limitation of joint motion becomes prominent because of muscle contractures and destruction of the joint. The knee is the most commonly involved peripheral joint. Symptoms of pulmonary tuberculosis may also be present.

Local findings during the early stages may be limited to tenderness, soft tissue swelling, joint effusion, and increase in skin temperature about the involved area. As the disease progresses without treatment, muscle atrophy and deformity become apparent. Abscess formation with spontaneous drainage externally leads to sinus formation. Progressive destruction of bone in the spine may cause a gibbus, especially in the thoracolumbar region.

B. Laboratory Findings: The precise diagnosis rests upon recovery of the acid-fast organism from joint fluid, pus, or tissue specimens. Biopsy of the bony lesion, synovium, or a regional lymph node may demonstrate the characteristic histopathologic picture of caseating necrosis and giant cells.

C. Imaging: There is a latent period between the onset of symptoms and the initial positive radiographic finding. The earliest changes of tuberculous arthritis are those of soft tissue swelling and distention of the capsule by effusion. Subsequently, bone atrophy causes thinning of the trabecular pattern, narrowing of the cortex, and enlargement of the medullary canal. As joint disease progresses, destruction of cartilage, both in the spine and in peripheral joints, is manifested by narrowing of the joint cleft and focal erosion of the articular surface, especially at the margins. Extensive destruction of joint surfaces causes deformity. As healing takes place, osteosclerosis becomes apparent around areas of necrosis and sequestration. Where the lesion is limited to bone, especially in the cancellous portion of the metaphysis, the x-ray picture may be that of single or multilocular cysts surrounded by sclerotic bone. As intraosseous foci expand toward the limiting cortex and erode it, subperiosteal new bone formation takes place. When bony tuberculosis is suspected, a chest film may be helpful in revealing characteristic pulmonary abnormalities even in the absence of symptoms.

Differential Diagnosis

Tuberculosis of the musculoskeletal system must be differentiated from all subacute and chronic infections, rheumatoid arthritis, gout, and, occasionally, osseous dysplasia. In the spine, metastatic tumor may be suggested.

Complications

Destruction of bones or joints may occur in a few weeks or months if adequate treatment is not provided. Deformity due to joint destruction, abscess formation with spread into adjacent soft tissues, and sinus formation are common. Paraplegia is the most serious complication of spinal tuberculosis. As healing of severe joint lesions takes place, spontaneous fibrous or bony ankylosis follows.

Treatment
(See also Chapter 37.)

A. General Measures: General care is especially important when prolonged recumbency is necessary; skillful nursing care must be provided.

B. Chemotherapy: Combinations of antituberculosis agents (eg, isoniazid, 300 mg/d, and rifampin, 600 mg/d, for 9 months) are recommended. The emergence of drug-resistant organisms, noted chiefly in Chicago and New York, has increased the need for sensitivity testing. Cure without need for surgical intervention may be effected in most cases, even with extensive disease.

C. Surgical Measures: In acute infections where synovitis is the predominant feature, treatment can be conservative, at least initially. Immobilization by splint or plaster, aspiration, and chemotherapy may suffice to control the infection. This treatment is especially desirable for the management of infections of large joints of the lower extremities in children during the early stage of the infection. Synovectomy may be valuable for less acute hypertrophic lesions that involve tendon sheaths, bursae, or joints.

Garrido G et al: A review of peripheral tuberculous arthritis. Semin Arthritis Rheum 1988;18:142. (Ninety percent monarticular, knee most common site; 21% with extra-articular tuberculosis; fever in 10%; normal hematocrit and white blood cell count in 66%.)

Messner RP: Arthritis due to tuberculosis, fungal infections, and parasites. Curr Opin Rheumatol (Aug) 1991;3:617.

TUMORS & TUMOR-LIKE LESIONS OF BONE

Essentials of Diagnosis

- Persistent pain, swelling, or tenderness of a skeletal part. Pathologic ("spontaneous") fractures.
- Suspicious areas of bony enlargement, deformity, radiodensity, or radiolucency on x-ray.
- Histologic evidence of bone neoplasm on biopsy specimen.

General Considerations

Primary tumors of bone are relatively uncommon in comparison with secondary or metastatic neoplasms. They are, however, of great clinical significance because of the possibility of cancer and because some of them grow rapidly and metastasize widely.

Although tumors of bone have been categorized classically as primary or secondary, there is some disagreement about which tumors are primary to the skeleton. Tumors of mesenchymal origin that reflect skeletal tissues (eg, bone, cartilage, and connective tissue) and tumors developing in bones that are of hematopoietic, nerve, vascular, fat cell, and notochordal origin should be differentiated from secondary malignant tumors that involve bone by direct extension or hematogenous spread. Because of the great variety of bone tumors, it is difficult to establish a satisfactory simple classification of bone neoplasms.

Clinical Findings

Persistent skeletal pain and swelling, with or without limitation of motion of adjacent joints or spontaneous fracture, are indications for prompt clinical, x-ray, laboratory, and possibly biopsy examination. X-rays may reveal the location and extent of the lesion and certain characteristics that may suggest the specific diagnosis. The so-called classic x-ray findings of certain tumors (eg, punched-out areas of the skull in multiple myeloma, "sun ray" appearance of osteogenic sarcoma, and "onion peel" effect of Ewing's sarcoma), although suggestive, are not pathognomonic. Even histologic characteristics of the tumor, when taken alone, cannot provide infallible information about the nature of the process. The age of the patient, the duration of complaints, the site of involvement and the number of bones involved, and the presence or absence of associated systemic disease—as well as the histologic characteristics—must be considered collectively for proper management.

The possibility of benign developmental skeletal abnormalities, metastatic neoplastic disease, infections (eg, osteomyelitis), posttraumatic bone lesions, or metabolic disease of bone must always be kept in mind. If bone tumors occur in or near the joints, they may be confused with the various types of arthritis, especially monarticular arthritis.

Specific Bone Tumors

Tumors arising from osteoblastic connective tissue include osteoid osteoma and osteogenic sarcoma. Osteoid osteomas are benign tumors of children and adolescents that should be surgically removed. Osteogenic sarcomas usually involve the knees or long bones and are treated by resection and chemotherapy, with improving survival in recent years. Fibrosarcomas, which are derived from nonosteoblastic connective tissue, have an outlook similar to that of the osteogenic sarcomas. Tumors derived from cartilage include enchondromas, chondromyxoid fibromas, and chondrosarcomas. Histologic examination is confirmatory in this group, and the outlook with appropriate curettement or surgery is generally good.

Other bone tumors include giant cell tumors (osteoclastomas), chondroblastomas, and Ewing's sarcoma. Of these, chondroblastomas are almost always benign. About 50% of giant cell tumors are benign, while the rest may be frankly malignant or recur after excision. Ewing's sarcoma, which affects children, adolescents, and young adults, has a 50% mortality rate in spite of chemotherapy, irradiation, and surgery.

Treatment

Although prompt action is essential for optimal treatment of certain bone tumors, accurate diagnosis is required because of the great potential for harm that may result either from temporization or from radical or ablative operations or unnecessary irradiation.

Smith LM, Cox RS, Donaldson SS: Second cancers in long-term survivors of Ewing's sarcoma. Clin Orthop 1992;274:275. (The risk of developing a second cancer at 5 years is 8%.)

NEUROGENIC ARTHROPATHY (Charcot's Joint)

Neurogenic arthropathy is joint destruction resulting from loss or diminution of proprioception, pain, and temperature perception. Although traditionally associated with tabes dorsalis, it is more frequently seen in diabetic neuropathy, syringomyelia, spinal cord injury, pernicious anemia, leprosy, and peripheral nerve injury. Prolonged administration of hydrocortisone by the intra-articular route may also cause Charcot's joint. As normal muscle tone and protective reflexes are lost, a marked secondary degenerative joint disease ensues; this results in an enlarged, boggy, painless joint with extensive erosion of cartilage, osteophyte formation, and multiple loose joint bodies. X-ray changes may be degenerative or hypertrophic in the same patient.

Treatment is directed against the primary disease; mechanical devices are used to assist in weight bearing and prevention of further trauma. In some instances, amputation becomes unavoidable.

ARTHRITIS IN SARCOIDOSIS

The frequency of arthritis among patients with sarcoidosis is variously reported between 10% and 35%. It is usually acute in onset, but articular symptoms may appear insidiously and often antedate other manifestations of the disease. Knees and ankles are most commonly involved, but any joint may be affected. Distribution of joint involvement is usually polyarticular and symmetric. The arthritis is commonly self-limiting after several weeks or months; infrequently, the arthritis is recurrent or chronic. Despite its occasional chronicity, the arthritis is rarely associated with joint destruction or significant deformity. Although sarcoid arthritis is often associated with erythema nodosum, the diagnosis is contingent upon the demonstration of other extra-articular manifestations of sarcoidosis and, notably, biopsy evidence of non-caseating granulomas. In chronic arthritis, x-ray shows rather typical changes in the bones of the extremities with intact cortex and cystic changes.

Treatment of arthritis in sarcoidosis is usually symptomatic and supportive. Colchicine may be of value. A short course of corticosteroids may be effective in patients with severe and progressive joint disease.

Enzenauer RJ, West SG: Sarcoidosis in autoimmune disease. Semin Arthritis Rheum 1992;22:1. (Sarcoidosis is an uncommon complication of various autoimmune diseases, including SLE, rheumatoid arthritis, and Sjögren's syndrome.)

OTHER RHEUMATIC DISORDERS

BEHÇET'S SYNDROME

Named after the Turkish dermatologist who first described it, this disease of unknown cause is characterized by recurrent oral and genital ulcers, uveitis, seronegative arthritis, and central nervous system abnormalities. Other features include ulcerative skin lesions, erythema nodosum, thrombophlebitis, and vasculitis. Arthritis occurs in about two-thirds of patients, most commonly affecting the knees and ankles. Keratitis, uveitis—often with hypopyon (pus in the anterior chamber)—and optic neuritis are observed. The ocular involvement is often fulminant and may result in blindness. Involvement of the central nervous system often results in serious disability or death. Findings include cranial nerve palsies, convulsions, encephalitis, mental disturbances, and spinal cord lesions. Leukocytosis and a rapid sedimentation rate are common.

The clinical course may be chronic but is often characterized by remissions and exacerbations. Corticosteroids, azathioprine, chlorambucil, and cyclosporine have been used with beneficial results. Oral base corticosteroids may be of some help for oral ulcerations.

Yazici H et al: A controlled trial of azathioprine in Behçet's syndrome. N Engl J Med 1990;322:281. (More effective than placebo in preventing uveitis.)

OSTEOGENESIS IMPERFECTA
(Fragilitas Ossium, Brittle Bones)

Osteogenesis imperfecta is a heritable disorder of connective tissue usually transmitted as an autosomal dominant, although some cases may be autosomal recessive. Two recognized clinical types may occur: osteogenesis imperfecta congenita (fetal type), in which fractures occur in utero and skeletal deformities are apparent at birth; and osteogenesis imperfecta tarda, in which fractures and deformities occur after birth. Fragility of bones is the single most obvious diagnostic criterion. Clearness or blue coloration of the scleras, conduction deafness, and spinal deformities (scoliosis and kyphosis) are often present. Milder cases of the late form may simulate idiopathic juvenile or menopausal osteoporosis. Unfortunately, there is no treatment for the inadequate formation of osteoid.

RHEUMATIC MANIFESTATIONS
OF CANCER

Rheumatologic syndromes may be the presenting manifestations for a variety of cancers. Dermatomyositis in adults, for example, is not infrequently associated with cancer. Middle-aged or older patients with polyarthritis that mimics rheumatoid arthritis but is associated with new onset of clubbing and periosteal new bone formation should be suspected of having hypertrophic pulmonary osteoarthropathy, a disorder commonly associated with both malignant diseases (eg, lung and intrathoracic cancers) and non-malignant ones (eg, cyanotic heart disease, cirrhosis, and lung abscess). Palmar fasciitis is characterized by bilateral palmar swelling and finger contraction and may be the first indication of cancer, particularly ovarian carcinoma. Occasionally, occult cancers produce a polymyalgia rheumatica-like syndrome that uncharacteristically does not respond to low doses of corticosteroids. Palpable purpura due to leukocytoclastic vasculitis may be the presenting complaint in myeloproliferative disorders. Hairy cell leukemia can be associated with medium-sized vessel vasculitis such as polyarteritis nodosa. Acute leukemia can produce joint pains that are disproportionately severe in comparison to the minimal swelling and heat that are present. Rheumatic manifestations of myelodysplastic syndromes include cutaneous vasculitis, lupus-like syndromes, neuropathy, and episodic intense arthritis. Erythromelalgia, a painful warmth and redness of the extremities that (unlike Raynaud's) improves with cold exposure or with elevation of the extremity, is often associated with myeloproliferative diseases.

Kraus A, Alarcon-Segovia D: Erythermalgia, erythromelalgia, or both? Conditions neglected by rheumatologists. J Rheumatol 1993;20:1. (Reviews the association with myeloproliferative diseases and the efficacy of aspirin.)

AVASCULAR NECROSIS OF BONE

Avascular necrosis of bone is a complication of corticosteroid use, trauma, SLE, pancreatitis, alcoholism, gout, sickle cell disease, infiltrative diseases (eg, Gaucher's disease), and caisson disease. The most commonly affected sites are the proximal and distal femoral heads, leading to hip or knee pain. Many patients with hip disease actually first present with referred knee pain. Physical examination will disclose that it is internal rotation of the hip—not movement of the knee—that is painful. Other commonly affected sites include the ankle, shoulder, and elbow. Initially, plain x-rays are often normal; MRI, CT scan, and bone scan are all more sensitive techniques. Treatment involves avoidance of weight bearing on the affected joint for several weeks at least. The merit of surgical core decompression is controversial.

Mankin HJ: Nontraumatic necrosis of bone (osteonecrosis). N Engl J Med 1992;326:1473.

SOME ORTHOPEDIC PROCEDURES FOR ARTHRITIC JOINTS

Synovectomy

This procedure has been used for over 50 years to attempt to retard joint destruction by invasive synovial pannus of rheumatoid arthritis. However, its prophylactic effect has not been documented, and inflammation of regenerated synovial membrane occurs. Thus, the only indication for synovectomy is intractable pain in an isolated joint, most commonly the knee.

Joint Replacement
(See also Total Joint Arthroplasty, below.)

Total hip replacement has been highly successful. Infection, the major complication, is uncommon. The long-term effects of replacement of the knee—and more recently the ankle, shoulder, and other joints—have not been fully determined.

Arthroplasty

Realignment and reconstruction of the knee, wrist, and small joints of the hand are feasible in a small number of selected patients.

Tendon Rupture

This is a fairly common complication in rheumatoid arthritis and requires immediate orthopedic referral. The most common sites are the finger flexors and extensors, the patellar tendon, and the Achilles tendon.

Arthrodesis

Arthrodesis (fusion) is being used less now than formerly, but a chronically infected, painful joint may be an indication for this surgical procedure.

Total Joint Arthroplasty

In the last 2 decades, remarkable progress has been made in the replacement of severely damaged joints with prosthetic materials. At present, artificial joint replacement is primarily indicated to relieve pain and only secondarily to restore function. Many patients who have minimal pain, therefore, even with marked destruction of the joint on radiographic examination, are not suitable candidates for joint replacement.

Success of the replacement depends upon the amount of physical stress to which the prosthetic components are subjected. Vigorous impact activity, even with the most advanced biomaterials and design, will result in failure of the prosthesis with time. Revision operations are technically more difficult, and the results may not be as good as with the primary procedure. The patient, therefore, must understand the limitations of joint replacement and the consequences of unrestrained joint usage.

A. Total Hip Arthroplasty: Hip replacement was originally designed for use in patients over 65 years of age with severe osteoarthritis. In these patients—usually less active physically—the prosthesis not only functioned well but outlasted the patients. Severe arthritis that fails to respond to conservative measures remains the principal indication for hip arthroplasty. Hip arthroplasty may also be indicated in younger patients severely disabled by painful hip disease (eg, rheumatoid arthritis), since in such cases it can be assumed that stress on the prosthetic joint will not be great. Contraindications to the operation include active infection and neurotrophic joint disease. Serious complications may occur in about 1% of patients and include thrombophlebitis, pulmonary embolization, sepsis, and dislocation of the joint. Extensive experience has now been accumulated, and the results are generally successful in properly selected patients.

B. Total Knee Arthroplasty: The indications and contraindications for total knee arthroplasty are similar to those for hip arthroplasty, but experience with the artificial knee is not as extensive. Results are slightly better in osteoarthritis patients than in those with rheumatoid arthritis. Knee arthroplasty is probably not advisable in younger individuals. Complications are similar to those with hip arthroplasty. The failure rate of knee arthroplasty is slightly higher than that of hip arthroplasty.

C. Total Arthroplasty: Prostheses are now available for total arthroplasty of every major joint of the extremities, but experience with joints other than the hip and the knee has been limited.

Harris WH, Sledge CB: Total hip and total knee replacement. (2 parts.) N Engl J Med 1990;323:725, 801. (A thorough review.)

REFERENCES

McCarty DJ, Koopman WJ, Hollander JL: *Arthritis and Allied Conditions: A Textbook of Rheumatology,* 12th ed. Lea & Febiger, 1993.

Payan DG: Nonsteroidal anti-inflammatory drugs; nonopiate analgesics; drugs used in gout. In: *Basic & Clinical Pharmacology,* 5th ed. Katzung BG (editor). Appleton & Lange, 1992.

Stites DP, Terr AI (editors): *Basic & Clinical Immunology,* 7th ed. Appleton & Lange, 1991.

Fluid & Electrolyte Disorders $\quad$ 20

Maxine A. Papadakis, MD

DIAGNOSIS OF FLUID & ELECTROLYTE DISORDERS

Alterations in Body Fluid Volume

Changes in body fluid volume can usually be determined by the physical examination.

A. Volume Overload: Volume overload is manifested by (1) peripheral edema or (2) heart failure from circulatory overload.

B. Volume Depletion: Volume depletion is evident by (1) excessive thirst, (2) dry mucous membranes, and, if severe, (3) circulatory compromise from decreased intravascular volume with resting tachycardia, orthostatic hypotension, or shock.

Alterations in Electrolyte Concentration

Morbidity and mortality from electrolyte disorders are mainly due to disturbances in the central nervous system. Patients may be asymptomatic, have cognitive impairment and organic brain syndrome, or develop lethargy, weakness, confusion, delirium, and seizures. Often these symptoms are mistaken for primary neurologic or metabolic disorders. Measurement of electrolytes (sodium, potassium, chloride, bicarbonate, calcium, magnesium, and phosphorus) is indicated for any patient with even vague neuromuscular symptoms.

Approach to the Patient

A. History: The following information should be elicited:

1. For volume overload–

a. Recent increase in weight.

b. Edema or ascites.

c. Symptoms of heart failure.

d. Increased dietary sodium intake.

e. Change in medication (eg, nonsteroidal anti-inflammatory agents, diuretic agents, medication noncompliance).

2. For volume depletion–

a. Gastrointestinal losses from vomiting or diarrhea.

b. Urinary losses from administration of diuretics, renal disease, diabetes mellitus or insipidus.

c. Dehydration from inadequate oral intake associated with altered mental status.

d. Excessive insensible loss from skin associated with sweating or fever.

B. Physical Examination: The physical examination should determine if significant volume depletion or expansion has occurred (see above). Documentation of recent change in body weight is very useful.

C. Evaluation and Treatment: Treatment of fluid and electrolyte disorders is based on (1) assessment of total body water and its distribution, (2) electrolyte concentrations, and (3) serum osmolality.

1. Body water–Table 20–1 shows the sex difference in total body water and the decrease in total body water that occurs with aging.

2. Electrolytes–Table 20–2 shows the reference ranges for serum electrolytes.

3. Serum osmolality–The reference range for serum osmolality is 285–295 mosm/kg. It can be calculated from the following formula:

$$\text{Osmolality} = 2(Na^+ \text{ mmol/L}) + \text{Glucose mmol/L} + \text{BUN mmol/L}$$

$$\text{or} = 2(Na^+ \text{meq/L}) + \frac{\text{Glucose mg/dL}}{18} + \frac{\text{BUN mg/dL}}{2.8}$$

(1 mosm of glucose equals 180 mg/L, and 1 mosm of urea nitrogen equals 28 mg/L).

Solute concentration is usually expressed in terms of osmolarity. The number of particles in solution (either molecules or ions) determines the number of milliosmols. Each particle has a unit value of 1, so if a substance ionizes, each ion contributes the same amount as a nonionizable molecule. For example, glucose in solution is nonionizable. Therefore, 1 mmol of glucose has an osmolar concentration of 1 mosm/L. One mmol of NaCl, however, forms two ions in water (one Na^+ and one Cl^-) and has an osmolar concentra-

Table 20–1. Total body water (as percentage of body weight) in relation to age and sex.

Age	Male	Female
18–40	60%	50%
40–60	60–50%	50–40%
Over 60	50%	40%

tion of roughly 2 mosm/L. Osmole per kilogram of water is termed osmolality; osmole per liter of solution is termed osmolarity. At the solute concentration of body fluids, the two measurements correspond so closely that they are interchangeable.

TREATMENT OF SPECIFIC FLUID, ELECTROLYTE, & ACID-BASE DISORDERS

DISORDERS OF SODIUM CONCENTRATION

Hyponatremia is defined as a serum sodium concentration less than 130 meq/L and is the most common electrolyte abnormality observed in a general hospitalized population, seen in about 2% of patients. The differential diagnosis and therapy for the hyponatremic patient depend on volume status.

Pseudohyponatremia may arise from the following conditions:

(1) Hyperglycemia is the most common cause of pseudohyponatremia. Technically, this is not pseudohyponatremia, since the sodium concentration does indeed fall, which it does not in pseudohyponatremia. When blood glucose becomes acutely elevated, water is drawn from the cells to the extracellular space, diluting the serum sodium level. The plasma sodium

Table 20–2. Normal serum chemistry concentrations and SI conversions.[1]
(P = plasma, S = serum, B = blood)

Current metric units × Conversion factor = SI units
SI units ÷ Conversion factor = Current metric units

Component	Conventional Units	SI Units	Conversion Factor	Mass Conversion
Bicarbonate [S]	24–28 meq/L	24–28 mmol/L	1.00	61 mg = 1 meq
Calcium [S]	8.5–10.3 mg/dL	2.1–2.6 mmol/L	0.2495	40 mg = 1 mmol
Calcium, ionized [S]	4.25–5.25 mg/dL; 2.1–2.6 meq/L	1.05–1.3 mmol/L	0.2495	
Chloride [S or P]	96–106 meq/L	96–106 mmol/L	1.00	35 mg = 1 meq
CO_2 content [S or P]	24–29 meq/L	24–29 mmol/L	1.00	
Creatinine [S or P]	0.6–1.2 mg/dL	50–110 mmol/L	88.40	
Glucose [S or P]	65–110 mg/dL	3.6–6.1 mmol/L	0.05551	
Lactate [B, venous; special handling]	4–16 mg/dL	0.44–1.8 mmol/L	0.1110	
Magnesium [S or P]	1.8–3 mg/dL	0.75–1.25 mmol/L	0.4114	24 mg = 1 mmol
Osmolality [S]	280–296 mosm/kg water	280–296 mmol/kg water	1.00	
Oxygen arterial PO_2(PaO_2)	80–100 mm Hg (sea level)	10.67–13.33 kPa (sea level)		
$PaCO_2$ [B, arterial]	35–45 mm Hg	4.7–6.0 kPa		
pH (reaction) [B, arterial]	7.35–7.45 ([H^+])	44.7–45.5 mmol/L		
Phosphorus, inorganic [S, fasting]	3–4.5 mg/dL	1–1.5 mmol/L	0.3229	31 mg = 1 mmol
Potassium [S or P]	3.5–5 meq/L	3.5–5 mmol/L	1.00	39 mg = 1 meq
Sodium [S or P]	136–145 meq/L	136–145 mmol/L	1.00	23 mg = 1 meq
Urea nitrogen [S or P]	8–20 mg/dL	2.9–7.1 mmol/L	0.3570	

[1]Data modified from Young DS: Implementation of SI units for clinical laboratory data. Ann Intern Med 1987;106:114.

level falls 1.6 meq/L for every 100 mg/dL rise in glucose concentration over 200 mg/dL.

(2) Hyperlipidemia and hyperproteinemia: In these disorders, the marked increases in lipids and proteins occupy a disproportionately large portion of the plasma volume. Decreased volume of water results, so that the sodium concentration in total plasma volume is decreased. However, the sodium concentration in the plasma water is normal.

1. HYPONATREMIA WITH HYPOVOLEMIA

Hyponatremia with decreased extracellular fluid volume occurs in the setting of renal or extrarenal volume loss. Total body sodium is decreased. In order to increase intravascular volume, antidiuretic hormone (ADH) secretion increases, and free water is retained. The drive to replenish intravascular volume supersedes the drive to maintain osmolality; losses of salt and water have been partially replaced by water alone.

Urine sodium helps distinguish renal from nonrenal causes of hyponatremia. Urine sodium exceeding 20 meq/L is consistent with renal salt wasting (diuretics, ACE inhibitors, mineralocorticoid deficiency, salt-losing nephropathy). Hyponatremia in AIDS patients may be due to a relative mineralocorticoid deficiency. Urine sodium less than 10 meq/L or fractional excretion of sodium less than 1% (unless diuretics have been given) implies avid sodium retention by the kidney to compensate for extrarenal fluid losses from vomiting, diarrhea, sweating, or third-spacing, as with ascites. Fractional excretion of sodium can be calculated using untimed "spot" urine samples with simultaneously obtained plasma samples for sodium (Na^+) and creatinine (Cr):

$$FENa^+ = \frac{(U/P)Na^+}{(U/P)Cr} \times 100$$

Treatment

Treatment consists of replacement of lost volume with isotonic saline or lactated Ringer's injection. Corticosteroids can be used empirically if hypocortisolism is considered in the differential diagnosis. See Adrenocortical Hypofunction in Chapter 25 for diagnosis (by means of the cosyntropin stimulation test) and treatment of hypocortisolism.

2. HYPONATREMIA WITH VOLUME OVERLOAD

Hyponatremia with increased extracellular fluid volume is seen in edema-associated disorders such as congestive heart failure, cirrhosis, and nephrotic syndrome. Total body sodium is increased, yet effective circulating volume is sensed as inadequate by baroreceptors. ADH secretion occurs, which results in a greater retention of water.

The **urine sodium** concentration is generally less than 10 meq/L unless the patient has been taking diuretics, which may cause greater sodium excretion.

Treatment

A. Water Restriction: The treatment of hyponatremia is that of the underlying condition (eg, improving cardiac output in congestive heart failure) and water restriction (to < 1–2 L of water daily).

B. Diuretics: To hasten excretion of water and salt, use of diuretics may be indicated. Since diuretics may cause hyponatremia, the hyponatremic patient must be cautioned not to increase free water intake or the hyponatremia may worsen. Therapy with demeclocycline (see below) in cirrhosis appears to increase the risk of renal failure, and for that reason the drug should not be used.

C. Hypertonic (3%) Saline: Hypertonic saline administration may be dangerous in this volume-overloaded state and is not routinely recommended. In patients with severe hyponatremia (serum sodium < 110 meq/L) and central nervous system symptoms, judicious administration of small amounts (100–200 mL) of 3% saline with diuretics may be necessary. Emergency dialysis should also be considered.

3. HYPONATREMIA WITH EUVOLEMIA

In this setting, determinations of urine osmolality along with urine sodium are useful for appropriate diagnosis.

Clinical Syndromes

A. Syndrome of Inappropriate ADH Secretion (SIADH): Increased ADH secretion is physiologic in hypovolemic states, and for that reason the diagnosis of SIADH can only be made if the patient is euvolemic. In SIADH, release of ADH occurs without osmolality-dependent or volume-dependent physiologic stimulation. Conditions associated with SIADH include malignant neoplasms, pulmonary and central nervous systems processes, and certain drugs. The following characteristics are seen in SIADH: (1) hyponatremia; (2) decreased plasma osmolality (< 285 mosm/kg) with inappropriately increased urine osmolality (> 300 mosm/kg); (3) normal thyroid and adrenal function (see Chapter 25 for thyroid function tests and cosyntropin stimulation test); and (4) urine sodium over 20 meq/L to compensate for slight increase in volume expansion from ADH secretion and maintain the balance between sodium intake and excretion. The slight expansion of extracellular volume is not large enough to cause clinical hypervolemia, hypertension, or edema since the factors that control sodium excretion are preserved. Other changes frequently seen in this dilutional state include low blood urea nitrogen (BUN) (< 10 mg/dL) and low plasma uric acid level (< 4 mg/dL). A high BUN suggests a volume-contracted state, which precludes making the diagnosis of SIADH.

B. Postoperative Hyponatremia: Severe postoperative hyponatremia can develop in 2 days or less after elective surgery in healthy patients, especially premenopausal women. Most have received excessive postoperative hypotonic fluid in the setting of elevated ADH levels related to pain or surgery. Patients awake normally from general anesthesia but within 2 days develop nausea, headache, seizures and even respiratory arrest. Serum sodium levels may be less than 110 meq/L.

C. Hypothyroidism: Hyponatremia is not commonly caused by hypothyroidism, but it can occur with serum sodium levels as low as 103 meq/L. Water retention (dilutional hyponatremia) is the cause, probably both from inappropriately elevated ADH levels and from nonhormonal alterations in the handling of water by the kidneys.

D. Psychogenic Polydipsia: Marked excess free water intake (generally > 10 L/d) may produce hyponatremia. Euvolemia is maintained through the renal excretion of sodium. Urine sodium is therefore generally elevated (> 20 meq/L), but unlike SIADH, levels of ADH are suppressed. Urine osmolality is appropriately low (< 300 mosm/kg) as the increased free water is excreted. Hyponatremia from high bursts of ADH can occur in manic-depressive patients who have excess free water intake.

E. Beer Potomania: Excessive chronic intake of beer (generally at least 4 L daily) can cause hyponatremia as low as 100 meq/L. This disorder occurs primarily in patients with cirrhosis, who have elevated levels of ADH and decreased glomerular filtration rates. Beer generally has a very low content of sodium (< 10 meq/L), and hyponatremia develops through retention of free water (beer).

F. Idiosyncratic Diuretic Reaction: In addition to hyponatremia that develops from volume contraction due to diuretic therapy (see above), a less common, but severe, diuretic-induced (generally thiazide) hyponatremia can occur in euvolemic patients. This syndrome is most often seen in healthy elderly women (over 70 years old). Serious symptoms often develop after only a few days of therapy. The mechanism for the hyponatremia appears to be a combination of excessive renal sodium loss and water retention. ACE inhibitors can cause central polydipsia and increased antidiuretic hormone secretion, both of which can cause severe, symptomatic hyponatremia. Patients given ACE inhibitors who develop polydipsia should have their serum Na$^+$ levels checked.

Treatment

A. Symptomatic Hyponatremia: Symptomatic hyponatremia is usually seen in patients with SIADH. Serum sodium levels are generally under 115 meq/L. If there are central nervous system symptoms, hyponatremia should be rapidly treated at any level of serum sodium concentration.

1. Rate and degree of correction–Brain damage, including central pontine myelinolysis, may occur from overly rapid correction of serum sodium (to levels above 135 meq/L within the initial 48 hours of therapy or elevation of serum sodium by more than 25 meq/L within the first 24 hours of therapy). A reasonable approach is to increase the serum sodium concentration by 0.5–1 meq/L/h, aiming not to exceed 130 meq/L in the first 48 hours. This compromise level is above the critical level of 120 meq/L but guards against overcorrection.

2. Saline plus furosemide–Hypertonic (3%) saline with furosemide is indicated for symptomatic hyponatremic patients. If one administers 3% saline without a diuretic to a patient with SIADH, the serum sodium concentration may not change. The excess sodium may be excreted in the urine, because such patients are euvolemic and in sodium balance. If one adds furosemide (0.5–1 mg/kg intravenously), however, the kidney cannot concentrate urine even in the presence of high levels of ADH. Infusion of 3% saline is accompanied by excretion of isotonic urine with a net loss of free water. The sodium concentration of 3% saline is 513 meq/L, and the osmolality is 1026 mosm/kg. In order to determine how much 3% saline to administer, one must measure a spot urinary Na$^+$ after a furosemide diuresis has begun. The excreted Na$^+$ is replaced with 3% saline, empirically begun at 50–75 mL/h and then adjusted based on urinary output and urinary sodium. For example, after administration of furosemide, urine volume excretion may be 400 mL/h and sodium concentration is 100 meq/L. The excreted Na$^+$ is 40 meq/h, which is replaced with 78 mL/h of 3% saline (40 meq/h divided by 513 meq/L). Free water loss is the difference between urine volume excreted and 3% saline infused, or 322 mL (400 mL – 78 mL). A rise in plasma sodium concentration of 1.5 meq/L/h can be expected. Spot measurements of urinary sodium and plasma sodium should be done approximately every 4 hours. The necessity for careful monitoring and measurement of input and output may require that the patient be in an intensive care unit.

B. Asymptomatic Hyponatremia:

1. Water restriction—Water intake should be restricted to 0.5—1 L/d. Gradual increase of serum sodium will occur over days.

2. Normal saline–Normal saline with furosemide may be used in asymptomatic patients whose serum sodium is less than 120 meq/L. Replace urinary sodium and potassium losses as above.

3. Demeclocycline– Demeclocycline (300–600

mg twice daily) is useful for patients who cannot adhere to water restriction or need additional therapy. Onset of action may require 1 week.

Ayus JC, Wheeler JM, Arieff AI: Postoperative hyponatremic encephalopathy in menstruant women. Ann Intern Med 1992;117:891. (When hyponatremic encephalopathy develops, premenopausal women are about 25 times more likely to die or have permanent brain damage).

Arieff AI, Ayus JC: Treatment of symptomatic hyponatremia: Neither haste nor waste. (Editorial.) Crit Care Med 1991;19:748.

Friedman E et al: Thiazide-induced hyponatremia: Reproducibility by single-dose rechallenge and an analysis of pathogenesis. Ann Intern Med 1989;110:24. (Useful discussion of an idiosyncratic reaction.)

Papadakis MA, Arieff AI: Hyponatremia and hypernatremia in liver disease. In: *The Kidney in Liver Disease.* Epstein M (editor). Williams & Wilkins, 1988. (Review of sodium abnormalities in liver disease. Hyponatremia is extremely common. Hypernatremia is usually iatrogenic from lactulose therapy.)

4. HYPONATREMIA IN AIDS

Hyponatremia is seen in up to 50% of patients hospitalized for AIDS and in 20% of ambulatory AIDS patients. If hyponatremia is present at the time of hospital admission, it is just as likely to be due to hypovolemic gastrointestinal losses as to euvolemic SIADH. However, if hyponatremia develops after hospital admission, most patients have euvolemic SIADH. Infrequently, hypovolemic hyponatremia is due to adrenal insufficiency, isolated mineralocorticoid deficiency with hyporeninemic hypoaldosteronism, or an HIV-specific impairment in renal sodium conservation. Hyponatremia from adrenal insufficiency, generally associated with hyperkalemia, may coexist with hypokalemia if the patient also has diarrhea. Adrenal function can be tested with corticotropin stimulation to determine the adequacy of serum cortisol response (see Chapter 25). Patients with isolated hyporeninemic hypoaldosteronism have normal cortisol responses to corticotropin but have decreased serum aldosterone levels. The mortality rate in hospitalized hyponatremic AIDS patients is nearly twice that of normonatremic patients.

Tang WW et al: Hyponatremia in hospitalized patients with the acquired immunodeficiency syndrome (AIDS) and the AIDS-related complex. Am J Med 1993;94:169. (This common disorder is frequently associated with gastrointestinal losses or SIADH and an increased mortality rate.)

5. HYPERNATREMIA

Hypernatremia (serum sodium > 145 meq/L) is a common clinical finding and is present in about 2% of patients over 60 years of age in a general hospital population. Hypernatremia can develop from excess water loss, frequently accompanied by an impaired thirst mechanism (eg, dehydration, lactulose therapy in cirrhosis, or diabetes insipidus). Hypokalemia, hypercalcemia, or sickle cell anemia can cause nephrogenic diabetes insipidus. Rarely, excessive sodium intake may cause hypernatremia (eg, accidental intravascular injection of hypertonic saline used for induction of abortion or use of large doses of sodium bicarbonate therapy during cardiac arrest). Since total body sodium content is the major determinant of extracellular fluid volume, one must determine if the hypernatremia is accompanied by a normal, decreased, or increased extracellular fluid volume.

Clinical Findings

A. Symptoms and Signs: Usually there is thirst (unless hypothalamic lesions are the cause), weight loss, tachycardia and hypotension, and oliguria. Fever, delirium, and coma may be seen with severe hyperosmolality.

B. Laboratory Findings: Urine osmolality measures the kidney's ability to conserve water.

1. Urine osmolality greater than 400 mosm/kg–Renal water-conserving ability is functioning.

a. Nonrenal losses–Hypernatremia will develop if water ingestion fails to keep up with hypotonic losses from excessive sweating, exertional losses from the respiratory tract, or through stool water. Lactulose causes an osmotic diarrhea with loss of free water.

b. Renal losses–While diabetic hyperglycemia can cause pseudohyponatremia (see above), progressive volume depletion from the osmotic diuresis of glycosuria can result in hypernatremia. Osmotic diuresis can occur with the use of mannitol or urea.

2. Urine osmolality less than 250 mosm/kg–A dilute urine with osmolality less than 250 mosm/kg with hypernatremia is characteristic of diabetes insipidus. Nephrogenic diabetes insipidus, seen with lithium or demeclocycline therapy or after relief of prolonged urinary tract obstruction, results from renal insensitivity to ADH.

Treatment

Treatment of hypernatremia is directed toward correcting the cause of the fluid loss and replacing water and, as needed, electrolytes. In response to increases in plasma osmolality, brain cells synthesize solutes—or idiogenic osmoles—which increase osmotic flow of water back into the brain cells to regulate brain cell volume. This begins 4–6 hours after dehydration and takes several days to reach a steady state. If hypernatremia is too rapidly corrected, the osmotic imbalance may cause water to preferentially enter brain cells, causing cerebral edema and potentially severe neurologic impairment. Fluid therapy should be administered over a 48-hour period, aiming for a decrease in serum sodium of 1 meq/L/h (1 mmol/L/h). Potassium and phosphate may be added as indicated by serum levels. Plasma electrolytes should be monitored frequently, usually every 4 hours. As soon as possible, oral intake should be resumed.

A. Choice of Type of Fluid for Replacement:

1. Hypernatremia with hypovolemia–Severe hypovolemia should be treated with isotonic (0.9%) saline to restore the volume deficit and to treat the hyperosmolality, since the osmolality of isotonic saline (308 mosm/kg) is often lower than that of the patient. This should be followed by 0.45% saline to replace any remaining free water deficit. Milder volume deficit may be treated with 0.45% saline and 5% dextrose in water.

2. Hypernatremia with euvolemia–Water drinking or 5% dextrose and water will result in excretion of excess sodium in the urine. If GFR is decreased, diuretics will increase urinary sodium excretion but may impair renal concentrating ability, increasing the quantity of water that needs to be replaced.

3. Hypernatremia with hypervolemia–Treatment consists of providing water as 5% dextrose in water to reduce hyperosmolality, but this will expand vascular volume. Simultaneously, loop diuretics such as furosemide (0.5–1 mg/kg) should be administered intravenously to remove the excess sodium. In severe renal insufficiency, hemodialysis may be necessary.

B. Calculation of Water Deficit: When calculating fluid replacement, both the deficit and the maintenance requirements should be added to each 24-hour replacement regimen.

1. Acute hypernatremia–In acute dehydration without much solute loss, free water loss is similar to the weight loss. Initially, 5% dextrose in water may be employed. As correction of water deficit progresses, therapy should continue with 0.45% saline with dextrose.

2. Chronic hypernatremia–Water deficit is calculated to restore normal osmolality for total body water. The volume of water required can be determined as follows: Calculate current total body water (TBW) (Table 20–1). TBW correlates with muscle mass and therefore decreases with advancing age, cachexia, and dehydration and is lower in women than in men. Current TBW equals 0.4–0.6 of current body weight. $[Na^+]$ = measured serum Na^+.

$$\text{Volume in liters to be replaced} =$$

$$\text{Current TBW} \times \frac{[Na^+]-140}{140}$$

Oh MS, Carroll HJ: Disorders of sodium metabolism: Hypernatremia and hyponatremia. Crit Care Med 1992;20:94. (Pathogenesis, diagnosis, and treatment.)

HYPEROSMOLAR DISORDERS

1. HYPEROSMOLALITY WITH ONLY TRANSIENT OR NO SIGNIFICANT SHIFT IN WATER

Urea and alcohol are two substances that readily cross cell membranes and can produce hyperosmolality. Urea may be administered acutely in large doses to "draw" water from cells, but the effect is transient, as is the diuresis, and urea soon equilibrates throughout body water. Alcohol quickly equilibrates between intracellular and extracellular water, adding 22 mosm/L for every 1000 mg/L. The hyperosmolality does not produce significant difficulty, but in any condition of stupor or coma in which measured osmolality exceeds that calculated from values of serum Na^+ and glucose and BUN, alcohol should be considered as a possible explanation of the discrepancy (osmolar gap). Methanol or ethylene glycol ingestion also causes osmolar gap characterized by severe metabolic acidosis.

2. HYPEROSMOLALITY ASSOCIATED WITH SIGNIFICANT SHIFTS IN WATER

Increased concentrations of solutes that do not readily enter cells produce a shift of water from the intracellular space to effect a true intracellular dehydration. Sodium and glucose are the solutes commonly involved.

Clinical symptoms are mainly referred to the central nervous system. The severity of symptoms depends on the degree of hyperosmolality and how rapidly it developed. In acute hyperosmolality, symptoms of somnolence and confusion can appear when the osmolality exceeds 320–330 mosm/L, and coma, respiratory arrest, and death may occur when the osmolality exceeds 340–350 mosm/L.

Gennari FJ: Serum osmolality: Uses and limitations. (Medical Intelligence.) N Engl J Med 1984;310:102.

DISORDERS OF POTASSIUM CONCENTRATION

1. HYPOKALEMIA

A total body deficit of about 350 meq occurs for each 1 meq/L decrement in serum potassium concentration below a level of 4 meq/L. However, changes in blood pH and hormones (insulin, β-adrenergic agonists, and aldosterone) independently affect serum potassium levels (Table 20–3).

Table 20–3. Changes in serum potassium concentration attributable to arterial blood pH changes.[1]

	ΔpH	$\Delta[K^+]$ (meq/L)
Metabolic acidosis		
Mineral (HCl)	$\downarrow$0.1	$\uparrow$0.7
Organic (ketoacidosis or lactic acidosis)	$\downarrow$0.1	0
Respiratory acidosis	$\downarrow$0.1	$\uparrow$0.1
Metabolic alkalosis	$\uparrow$0.1	$\downarrow$0.3
Respiratory alkalosis	$\uparrow$0.1	$\downarrow$0.2

[1]Reproduced, with permission, from Cogan MG: *Fluid and Electrolytes: Physiology and Pathophysiology.* Appleton & Lange, 1991.

Clinical Findings

A. Symptoms and Signs: Muscular weakness, fatigue, and muscle cramps are frequent complaints in mild to moderate hypokalemia. Smooth muscle involvement may result in constipation or ileus. Flaccid paralysis, hyporeflexia, tetany, and rhabdomyolysis may be seen with severe hypokalemia (< 2.5 meq/L).

B. Laboratory Findings: The ECG shows decreased amplitude and broadening of T waves, prominent U waves, depressed ST segments, and, in more severe deficits, atrioventricular block and finally cardiac arrest. (Hypokalemia increases the likelihood of digitalis toxicity.)

Treatment

The safest way to treat mild to moderate deficiency is with oral potassium, which is rapidly absorbed (Table 20–4). Liquid potassium chloride has an unpleasant taste and may be better tolerated if added to fruit juice. Rarely, enteric-coated or slow-release tablets or capsules of potassium chloride can cause peptic ulceration. Potassium content of foods is shown in Table 20–5.

Intravenous potassium replacement is indicated for patients with severe hypokalemia and in those who cannot take oral supplementation. If the serum potassium level is greater than 2.5 meq/L and there are no electrocardiographic abnormalities characteristic of hypokalemia, potassium can be given at a rate of 10 meq/L/h by peripheral intravenous line in concentrations that should never exceed 40 meq/L. For severe deficiency, potassium may be given through a peripheral intravenous line at rates up to 40 meq/L/h. Continuous electrocardiographic monitoring is indicated, and the serum potassium level should be checked every 3–6 hours.

Occasionally, hypokalemia may be refractory to potassium replacement. Magnesium deficiency may impair potassium correction. Repletion of magnesium is indicated.

Kruse JA, Carlson RW: Rapid correction of hypokalemia using concentrated intravenous potassium chloride infu-

Table 20–4. Oral potassium replacement.[1]

LIQUIDS			
Amount	meq of K^+	Anion	Names
15 mL	10	Cl$^-$	5% potassium chloride
15 mL	20	Cl$^-$	10% potassium chloride (Kaochlor 10%, Kaochlor S-F, Kay Ciel, Klor-10%, SK-potassium)
15 mL	40	Cl$^-$	20% potassium chloride (Kaon-Cl 20%, SK-potassium chloride)
15 mL	20	Gluconate$^-$	Potassium gluconate (Kaon, My-K Elixir)
POWDERS			
Packet	15	Cl$^-$	(K-Lor)
Packet	20	Cl$^-$	Potassium chloride (Kato, Kay Ciel, K-Lor)
Packet	25	Cl$^-$	(K-Lyte/Cl)
TABLETS			
One	8	Cl$^-$	(Slow-K)
One	8	Cl$^-$	(Micro-K Extencaps)
One	10	Cl$^-$	(K-Dur 10)
One	20	Cl$^-$	(K-Dur 20)

[1]Modified from Cogan MG: *Fluid and Electrolytes: Physiology and Pathophysiology.* Appleton & Lange, 1991.

sions. Arch Intern Med: 1990;150:613. (Useful clinical tool for rapid potassium replacement.)

Whang R, Whang DD, Ryan MP: Refractory potassium repletion. A consequence of magnesium deficiency. Arch Intern Med 1992;152:40. (Reviews magnesium and potassium interactions. In patients with both deficiencies, magnesium repletion is necessary to replete potassium.)

2. HYPERKALEMIA

Many cases of hyperkalemia are spurious or associated with acidosis (Table 20–6). The common practice of repeatedly clenching and unclenching a fist during venipuncture may raise the potassium concentration by 1–2 meq/L by causing local release of potassium from forearm muscles.

Intracellular potassium shifts to the extracellular fluid in hyperkalemia associated with acidosis. Serum potassium concentration rises about 0.7 meq/L for every decrease of 0.1 pH unit during acidosis (Table 20–3). In the absence of acidosis, serum potassium concentration rises about 1 meq/L when there is a a total body potassium excess of 50–200 meq/L. However, the higher the serum potassium concentration, the smaller the excess necessary to raise the potassium levels further.

Table 20–5. Potassium content of foods.

	Very High (12–20 meq)	High (5–12 meq)
Beans (½ cup or as stated)	Garbanzo beans Soy beans	Kidney beans Lima beans Navy beans Pinto beans
Fruit (½ cup or as stated)	Papaya (one medium)	Apricots (3 halves) Banana (6 inch) Cantaloupe (¼ inch slice) Honeydew melon (¼ inch slice) Orange (3 inch diameter) Orange juice Pear (one large) Prunes (4) Prune juice Rhubarb
Vegetables (½ cup or as stated)		Artichoke (one) Avocado (¼) Brussels sprouts Carrot (7½ inch) Chard Ketchup (1 tbsp) Potato (one baked, one broiled, 10 fries, ½ cup mashed) Pumpkin Spinach Tomato (one) Tomato or vegetable juice

Table 20–6. Causes of hyperkalemia.

Spurious
Leakage from erythrocytes if separation of serum from clot is delayed
Thrombocytosis, with release of K^+ from platelets (plasma K^+ not affected)
Marked leukocytosis
Repeated fist clenching during phlebotomy, with release of K^+ from forearm muscles
Specimen drawn from arm with K^+ infusion

Decreased excretion
Renal failure, acute and chronic
Severe oliguria due to severe dehydration or shock
Renal secretory defects (may or may not have frank renal failure): renal transplant, interstitial nephritis, SLE, sickle cell disease, amyloidosis, obstructive uropathy
Adrenocortical insufficiency
Hyporeninemic hypoaldosteronism (often with long-term diabetes mellitus) or selective hypoaldosteronism (some patients with AIDS)
Drugs that inhibit potassium excretion (spironolactone, triamterene, ACE inhibitors, NSAIDs)

Shift of K^+ from tissues
Massive release of intracellular K^+ in burns, rhabdomyolysis, crush injury, hemolysis, severe infection, internal bleeding, vigorous exercise
Metabolic acidosis
Insulin deficiency (metabolic acidosis may not be apparent)
Hyperkalemic periodic paralysis
Drugs: succinylcholine, arginine, digitalis toxicity, β-adrenergic antagonists

Excessive intake of K^+
Overtreatment with K^+, orally or parenterally

Clinical Findings

The elevated K^+ concentration interferes with normal neuromuscular function to produce weakness and flaccid paralysis; abdominal distention and diarrhea may occur. Electrocardiography is not a sensitive method for detecting hyperkalemia, since nearly half of patients with a serum potassium level greater than 6.5 meq/L will not manifest electrocardiographic changes. When electrocardiographic changes of hyperkalemia occur, the ECG reflects impaired conduction by peaked T waves of increased amplitude, atrial arrest, widening of the QRS, and biphasic QRS–T complexes (Figure 20–1). The heart rate may be slow; ventricular fibrillation and cardiac arrest are terminal events.

Treatment
(Table 20–7)

First confirm that the elevated level of serum K^+ is genuine (Table 20–6). Potassium concentration can be measured in plasma rather than in serum to avoid leakage of potassium out of cells into the serum of the blood sample in the course of clotting. Treatment consists of withholding potassium and giving cation exchange resins by mouth or enema. Sodium polystyrene sulfonate, 40–80 g/d in divided doses, is usually effective. Emergent treatment of hyperkalemia is indicated if cardiac toxicity or muscular paralysis is present or if the hyperkalemia is severe (serum potassium > 6.5–7.0 meq/L) even in the absence of electrocardiographic changes. Insulin plus 10–50% glucose may be employed to deposit K^+ with glycogen in the liver, and Ca^{2+} may be given intravenously as an an-

ECG:

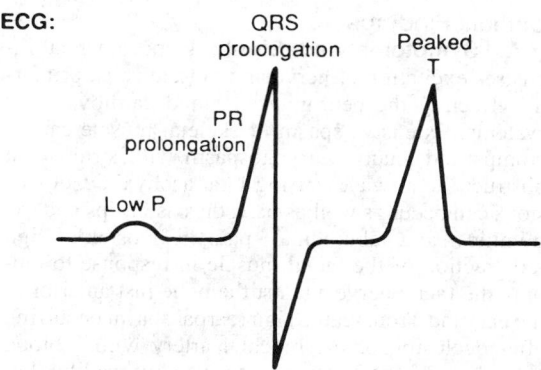

Figure 20–1. Electrocardiographic changes in hyperkalemia. (Reproduced, with permission, from Cogan MG: *Fluid and Electrolytes: Physiology and Pathophysiology.* Appleton & Lange, 1991.)

tagonist ion. Transcellular shifts of potassium can also be mediated by β_2-adrenergic stimulation. Albuterol, a nebulized β_2 agonist, is effective in decreasing serum potassium in patients on hemodialysis. For such patients, nebulized albuterol can reduce serum K^+ 0.5–1.0 meq/L within 30 minutes after administration, and this effect is sustained for at least 2 hours. Albuterol and insulin are probably equally efficacious in lowering potassium in uremic patients, and the hypokalemic effects of coadministration of the two drugs (with glucose) are additive and appear not to be a hazard. Sodium bicarbonate can be given intravenously as an emergency measure in severe hyperkalemia; the increase in blood pH results in a shift of K^+ into cells. Hemodialysis or peritoneal dialysis may be required to remove K^+ in the presence of protracted renal insufficiency. Therapy of the precipitating event proceeds concurrently.

Allon M, Copkney C: Albuterol and insulin for treatment of hyperkalemia in hemodialysis patients. Kidney Int 1990;38:869. (Albuterol and insulin are equally efficacious, and both drugs given together—with glucose—have an additive effect and appear to be safe.)

Don BR et al. Pseudohyperkalemia caused by fist clenching

Table 20–7. Treatment of hyperkalemia.[1]

EMERGENCY					
Modality	**Mechanism of Action**	**Onset**	**Duration**	**Prescription**	**K^+ Removed From Body**
Calcium	Antagonizes cardiac conduction abnormalities	0–5 minutes	1 hour	Calcium gluconate 10%, 5–30 mL IV; or calcium chloride 5%, 5–30 mL IV	0
Bicarbonate	Distributes K^+ into cells	15–30 minutes	1–2 hours	NaHCO$_3$, 44–88 meq (1–2 ampules) IV	0
Insulin	Distributes K^+ into cells	15–60 minutes	4–6 hours	Regular insulin, 5–10 units IV, plus glucose 50%, 25 g (1 ampule) IV	0
Albuterol	Distributes K^+ into cells	15–30 minutes	2–4 hours	Nebulized albuterol, 10–20 mg in 4 mL normal saline, inhaled over 10 minutes	0

NONEMERGENCY				
Modality	**Mechanism of Action**	**Duration of Treatment**	**Prescription**	**K^+ Removed From Body**
Loop diuretic	↑Renal K^+ excretion	0.5–2 hours	Furosemide, 40–160 mg IV or orally with or without NaHCO$_3$, 0.5–3 meq/kg daily	Variable
Sodium polystyrene sulfonate (Kayexalate)	Ion exchange resin binds K^+	1–3 hours	Oral: 15–30 g in 20% sorbitol (50–100 mL). Rectal: 50 mg in 20% sorbitol	0.5–1 meq/g
Hemodialysis	Extracorporeal K^+ removal	48 hours	Blood flow ≥200–300 mL/min. Dialysate [K^+] = 0.	200–300 meq
Peritoneal dialysis	Peritoneal K^+ removal	48 hours	Fast exchange, 3–4 L/h	200–300 meq

[1]Modified and reproduced, with permission, from Cogan MG: *Fluid and Electrolytes: Physiology and Pathophysiology.* Appleton & Lange, 1991.

during phlebotomy. N Engl J Med 1990;322:1290. (Releases potassium from forearm.)

Wrenn KD, Slovis CM, Slovis BS: The ability of physicians to predict hyperkalemia from the ECG. Ann Emerg Med 1991;20:1229 (Electrocardiography is only about 60% sensitive for serum potassium above 6.5 meq/L.)

DISORDERS OF CALCIUM CONCENTRATION

Calcium constitutes about 2% of body weight, but only about 1% of the total body calcium is in solution in body fluid. In the plasma, calcium is present as a nondiffusible complex with protein (33%); as a diffusible but undissociated complex with anions such as citrate, bicarbonate, and phosphate (12%); and as ionized calcium (55%). The normal total plasma (or serum) calcium concentration is 8.5–10.3 mg/dL. It is the ionized calcium that is necessary for muscle contraction and nerve function.

1. HYPOCALCEMIA

Important causes of hypocalcemia are listed in Table 20–8.

Hypocalcemia is seen commonly in critically ill patients. Twenty percent of previously normocalcemic patients with gram-negative bacterial sepsis have hypocalcemia, which is a marker for increased mortality. Hypocalcemia in these patients is due to acquired defects in the parathyroid-vitamin D axis. The hypocalcemia frequently results in hypotension, which responds to calcium replacement therapy. Hypocalcemia in pancreatitis is a marker for severe disease (see Chapter 15).

Table 20–8. Causes of hypocalcemia.

Decreased intake or absorption
  Malabsorption
  Small bowel bypass, short bowel
  Vitamin D deficit (decreased absorption, decreased production of 25-hydroxyvitamin D or 1,25-dihydroxyvitamin D)
Increased loss
  Chronic renal insufficiency
  Diuretic therapy
Endocrine disease
  Hypoparathyroidism (genetic, acquired; including hypo- and hypermagnesemia)
  Sepsis
  Pseudohypoparathyroidism
  Calcitonin secretion with medullary carcinoma of the thyroid
Physiologic causes
  Associated with decreased serum albumin
  Decreased end-organ response to vitamin D
  Hyperphosphatemia
  Induced by aminoglycoside antibiotics, plicamycin, loop diuretics, foscarnet

Clinical Findings

A. Symptoms and Signs: Hypocalcemia increases excitation of nerve and muscle cells, primarily affecting the neuromuscular and cardiovascular systems. Extensive spasm of skeletal muscle causes cramps and tetany. Laryngospasm with stridor can obstruct the airway, causing fatal asphyxia. Convulsions can occur as well as paresthesias of lips and extremities and abdominal pain. Chvostek's sign (contraction of the facial muscle in response to tapping the facial nerve against the bone just anterior to the ear) and Trousseau's sign (carpal spasm occurring after occlusion of the brachial artery with a blood pressure cuff for 3 minutes) are usually readily elicited. Prolongation of the QT interval predisposes to the development of arrhythmias, especially heart block and ventricular fibrillation. Hypotension and heart failure can occur. In chronic hypoparathyroidism, cataracts and calcification of basal ganglia of the brain may appear. (See Hypoparathyroidism, Chapter 25.)

B. Laboratory Findings: Serum Ca^{2+} is low (< 8.5 mg/dL). The level of serum Ca^{2+} must be correlated with the simultaneous concentration of serum albumin: When albumin concentration is depressed, serum Ca^{2+} concentration is also depressed in a ratio of 0.8–1 mg of Ca^{2+} to 1 g of albumin. Serum phosphate is usually elevated. Serum Mg^{2+} is commonly low, and hypomagnesemia reduces tissue responsiveness to parathyroid hormone. In respiratory alkalosis, total serum calcium is normal but ionized calcium is low, which can be measured by use of a Ca^{2+}-sensitive electrode. The ECG shows a prolonged QT interval.

Treatment*
(Table 20–9)

A. Severe, Symptomatic Hypocalcemia: In the presence of tetany, arrhythmias, or seizures, calcium gluconate 10% (10–20 mL) administered intravenously over 10–15 minutes is indicated. Because of the short duration of the acute infusion, subsequent calcium infusion is usually required. Ten to 15 milligrams of calcium per kilogram body weight, or six to eight 10-mL vials of 10% calcium gluconate (558–744 mg of calcium), is added to 1 L of D_5W and infused over 4–6 hours. By monitoring the serum calcium level frequently (every 4–6 hours), the physician should adjust the infusion rate to maintain the serum calcium level at 7–8.5 mg/dL.

B. Asymptomatic Hypocalcemia: Oral calcium and vitamin D preparations (Table 25–12) are used. Calcium carbonate is well tolerated and less expensive than many other calcium tablets. The low serum Ca^{2+} associated with low serum albumin con-

---

*See also Chapter 25 for discussion of the treatment of hypoparathyroidism.

Table 20–9. Treatment of hypocalcemia.

Modality	Amount of Ca^{2+}	Onset	Dose
Intravenous calcium Calcium gluconate 10%	93 mg (4.7 meq) per 10 mL	Immediate	93–186 mg over 10–15 minutes; then 10–15 mg/kg over 4–6 hours
Oral calcium Calcium carbonate (generic, Os-Cal, Biocal, Caltrate, Tums)	40% elemental calcium: 250 mg/624 mg tablet or 500 mg/1250 mg tablet or 600 mg/1500 mg tablet	<1 hour	250–500 mg calcium 4 times a day
Vitamin D preparations	See Table 25–12.		

centration does not require replacement therapy. If serum Mg^{2+} is low, therapy must include replacement of magnesium, which by itself usually will correct hypocalcemia.

Zaloga GP: Hypocalcemia in critically ill patients. Crit Care Med 1992;20:251. (Hypocalcemia causes hypotension, cardiac arrhythmias, or neuromuscular insufficiency.)

2. HYPERCALCEMIA

Important causes of hypercalcemia are listed in Table 20–10.

Clinical Findings

A. Symptoms and Signs: Anorexia, nausea and vomiting, constipation, polyuria, muscle weakness with hyporeflexia, tremor, lethargy, and confusion are common. Stupor, coma, and azotemia ensue. Ventricular extrasystoles and idioventricular rhythm may occur and can be accentuated by digitalis.

B. Laboratory Findings: A significant eleva-

Table 20–10. Causes of hypercalcemia.

Increased intake or absorption
  Milk-alkali syndrome
  Vitamin D or vitamin A excess
Endocrine disorders
  Primary hyperparathyroidism (adenoma, hyperplasia, carcinoma)
  Secondary hyperparathyroidism (renal insufficiency, malabsorption)
  Acromegaly
  Adrenal insufficiency
Neoplastic diseases
  Tumors producing PTH-related proteins (ovary, kidney, lung)
  Metastases to bone
  Lymphoproliferative disease, including multiple myeloma
  Secretion of prostaglandins and osteolytic factors
Miscellaneous causes
  Thiazide diuretic-induced
  Sarcoidosis
  Paget's disease of bone
  Hypophosphatasia
  Immobilization
  Familial hypocalciuric hypercalcemia
  Complications of renal transplantation
  Iatrogenic

tion of serum Ca^{2+} is seen; the level must be interpreted in relation to the serum albumin level (see Hypocalcemia). Serum phosphate may or may not be low, depending on the cause. The ECG shows a shortened QT interval.

Treatment

Because symptomatic hypercalcemia is associated with a high mortality rate, treatment must be started promptly. Until the primary disease can be brought under control, renal excretion of calcium with resultant decrease in serum Ca^{2+} concentration should be promoted. Excretion of Na^+ is accompanied by excretion of Ca^{2+}; therefore, inducing natriuresis by giving saline with furosemide is the emergency treatment of choice. In dehydrated patients with normal cardiac and renal function, 0.45% saline or 0.9% saline can be given rapidly (250–500 mL/h). Intravenous furosemide (20–40 mg every 2 hours) prevents volume overload and enhances Ca^{2+} excretion. Thiazides can actually worsen hypercalcemia (as can furosemide if inadequate saline is given). Replacement of K^+ and Mg^{2+} is usually necessary. See Chapter 5 for a discussion of the treatment of hypercalcemia of malignancy; and see Chapter 25 for a a discussion of the treatment of hypercalcemia of hyperparathyroidism.

Strewler GJ, Nissenson RA: Hypercalcemia in malignancy. West J Med 1990;153:635. (Review of pathogenesis.)

DISORDERS OF PHOSPHORUS CONCENTRATION

Eighty percent of the phosphorus in the body is combined with calcium in bones and teeth. Only 10% is incorporated into a variety of organic compounds, and 10% is combined with proteins, lipids, carbohydrates, and other compounds in muscle and blood. Organic phosphate is the principal intracellular anion; inorganic phosphate comprises only a small fraction of intracellular phosphorus.

Phosphate compounds are integral agents in energy transfer and in the metabolism of carbohydrate, protein, and fat. Phosphate serves as the principal urinary buffer (HPO_4^{2-}, H_2PO^{4-}), constituting most of titratable acidity.

Renal tubular reabsorption of filtered phosphate is reduced (phosphate excretion increased) by parathyroid hormone, expansion of extracellular fluid volume, increased intake of sodium, hypercalcemia, calcitonin, glucocorticoids, and growth hormone.

Phosphorus metabolism and homeostasis are intimately related to calcium metabolism. See sections on metabolic bone disease in Chapter 25.

1. HYPOPHOSPHATEMIA

Hypophosphatemia may occur in the presence of normal phosphate stores. Serious depletion of body phosphate stores may exist with low, normal, or high concentrations of phosphorus in serum. Leading causes of hypophosphatemia are listed in Table 20–11.

Clinical Findings

A. Symptoms and Signs: Acute, severe hypophosphatemia (0.1–0.2 mg/dL) can lead to acute hemolytic anemia with increased erythrocyte fragility, impaired oxygen delivery to tissues, increased susceptibility to infection from impaired chemotaxis of leukocytes, and platelet dysfunction with petechial hemorrhages. Rhabdomyolysis, encephalopathy (irritability, confusion, dysarthria, seizures, and coma), and heart failure are uncommon but serious manifestations.

Chronic severe depletion may be manifested by anorexia, pain in muscles and bones, and fractures.

B. Laboratory Findings: In acute symptomatic hypophosphatemia, serum phosphorus is less than 1 mg/dL. Evidence of anemia due to hemolysis may be present (eg, elevated serum lactate dehydrogenase). Rhabdomyolysis results in elevated serum creatine kinase (which contains mostly the MM fraction but also some MB fraction) and, in many cases, myoglobin in the urine. Other values vary according to the cause. In chronic depletion, radiographs and biopsies of bones show changes resembling those of osteomalacia.

Treatment
(Table 20–12)

Treatment is best directed toward prophylaxis by including phosphate in repletion and maintenance fluids. A rapid decline in calcium levels can occur with parenteral administration of phosphate; therefore, when possible, oral replacement of phosphate is preferable. For parenteral alimentation, 620 mg (20 mmol) of phosphorus is required for every 1000 nonprotein kcal to maintain phosphate balance and to ensure anabolic function. A daily ration for prolonged parenteral fluid maintenance is 620–1240 mg (20–40 mmol) of phosphorus. For asymptomatic hypophosphatemia (serum phosphorus 0.7–1 mg/dL), an infusion should provide 279–310 mg (9–10 mmol)/12 h until the serum phosphorus exceeds 1 mg/dL. A magnesium deficit often coexists and should be treated simultaneously. In administering phosphate-containing solutions, serum creatinine must be assessed and serum calcium monitored to guard against production of hypocalcemia.

For oral use, phosphate salts are available in skim milk (approximately 1 g [33 mmol]/L). Tablets or capsules of mixtures of sodium and potassium phosphate may be given to provide 0.5–1 g (18–32 mmol) per day.

Contraindications to therapy with phosphate salts include hypoparathyroidism, renal insufficiency, tissue damage and necrosis, and hypercalcemia.

Singhal PC et al: Prevalence and predictors of rhabdomyolysis in patients with hypophosphatemia. Am J Med 1992;92:458. (Hypophosphatemia, a common cause of rhabdomyolysis, may be masked because of the ongoing rhabdomyolysis.)

Yu GC, Lee DB: Clinical disorders of phosphorus metabolism. West J Med 1987;147:569.

Table 20–11. Causes of hypophosphatemia.

Diminished supply or absorption
   Starvation
   Parenteral alimentation with inadequate phosphate content
   Malabsorption syndrome, small bowel bypass
   Absorption blocked by oral aluminum hydroxide or bicarbonate
   Vitamin D-deficient and vitamin D-resistant osteomalacia

Increased loss
   Hyperparathyroidism (primary or secondary)
   Hyperthyroidism
   Renal tubular defects permitting excessive phosphaturia (congenital, induced by monoclonal gammopathy, heavy metal poisoning)
   Hypokalemic nephropathy
   Inadequately controlled diabetes mellitus

Intracellular shift of phosphorus
   Administration of glucose, fructose (transient)
   Anabolic steroids, estrogen, oral contraceptives
   Respiratory alkalosis
   Salicylate poisoning

Electrolyte abnormalities
   Hypercalcemia
   Hypomagnesemia
   Metabolic alkalosis

Abnormal losses followed by inadequate repletion
   Diabetes mellitus with acidosis, particularly during aggressive therapy
   Recovery from starvation or prolonged catabolic state
   Chronic alcoholism, particularly during restoration of nutrition; associated with hypomagnesemia
   Respiratory alkalosis
   Recovery from severe burns

Table 20–12. Treatment of hypophosphatemia.[1]

Preparation and Dosage	Phosphorus Content	Na$^+$ Content	K$^+$ Content
Intravenous: 2–7.5 mg/kg over 6–8 hours			
Sodium phosphate	93 mg/mL	4 meq/L	0
Potassium phosphate	93 mg/mL	0	4 meq/L
Oral: 250–500 mg 4 times daily			
Neutral sodium-potassium phosphate (neutra-Phos, K-Phos-Neutral, Uro-KP-Neutral)	250 mg/cap or tab or 250 mg/75 mL	6–13 meq/tab	1–7 meq/tab
Potassium phosphate (Neutra-Phos-K, K-Phos)	125 or 250 mg/cap or tab or 125 or 250 mg/75 mL	0	4–14 meq/tab
Sodium phosphate (Fleet's Phospho-Soda)	129 mg/mL	5 meq/L	0
Rectal:			
Sodium phosphate (Fleet's Enema)	43 mg/mL	1.6 meq/mL	0

[1]Reproduced, with permission, from Cogan MG: *Fluid and Electrolytes: Physiology and Pathophysiology.* Appleton & Lange, 1991.

2. HYPERPHOSPHATEMIA

Causes of hyperphosphatemia are given in Table 20–13. Growing children normally have serum phosphate levels higher than those of adults.

Clinical Findings

A. Symptoms and Signs: The clinical manifestations are those of the underlying disorders (eg, chronic renal failure, hypoparathyroidism).

B. Laboratory Findings: Serum phosphate is increased. Other blood chemistry values are those characteristic of the underlying disease.

Treatment

Treatment is that of the underlying disease and of acute onset of hypocalcemia. In acute and chronic renal failure, dialysis will reduce serum phosphate, but high-flux dialysis is more effective than conventional dialysis. Absorption of phosphate can be reduced by administration of calcium carbonate, 0.5–1.5 g three times daily with meals (500 mg tablets). This approach is preferred to the traditional use of aluminum hydroxide because of increased awareness of aluminum toxicity.

Table 20–13. Causes of hyperphosphatemia.

Endocrine disease
  Excessive growth hormone (acromegaly)
  Hypoparathyroidism associated with low calcium
  Pseudohypoparathyroidism associated with low calcium
Decreased excretion
  Chronic renal insufficiency
  Acute renal failure
Catabolic states; tissue destruction
  Stress or injury, rhabdomyolysis (especially if renal insufficiency exists)
  Chemotherapy of malignant disease, particularly lymphoproliferative disease
Excessive intake or absorption
  Laxatives or enemas containing phosphate
  Hypervitaminosis D

DISORDERS OF MAGNESIUM CONCENTRATION

About 50% of total body magnesium exists in the insoluble state in bone. Only 5% is present as extracellular cation; the remaining 45% is contained in cells as intracellular cation. The normal plasma concentration is 1.5–2.5 meq/L, with about one-third bound to protein and two-thirds existing as free cation. Excretion of magnesium ion is via the kidney.

Magnesium is an important activator ion, participating in the function of many enzymes involved in phosphate transfer reactions. Magnesium exerts physiologic effects on the nervous system resembling those of calcium. Magnesium acts directly upon the myoneural junction.

Altered concentration of Mg^{2+} in the plasma usually provokes an associated alteration of Ca^{2+}. Hypermagnesemia suppresses secretion of parathyroid hormone with consequent hypocalcemia. Severe and prolonged magnesium depletion impairs secretion of PTH with consequent hypocalcemia. Hypomagnesemia may impair end-organ response to PTH as well.

1. HYPOMAGNESEMIA

Causes of hypomagnesemia are given in Table 20–14. Nearly half of hospitalized patients in whom serum electrolytes are ordered have unrecognized hypomagnesemia. Twenty to 60 percent of critically ill patients have hypomagnesemia, which may predispose them to arrhythmias and sudden death. Common causes include use of large volumes of intravenous fluids, diuretics, cisplatin in cancer patients (with concomitant hypokalemia), and administration of nephrotoxic agents such as aminoglycosides and amphotericin B.

Clinical Findings

A. Symptoms and Signs: Common symptoms are weakness, muscle cramps, and tremor. There is

Table 20–14. Causes of hypomagnesemia.

Diminished absorption or intake
  Malabsorption, chronic diarrhea, laxative abuse
  Prolonged gastrointestinal suction
  Small bowel bypass
  Malnutrition
  Alcoholism
  Parenteral alimentation with inadequate Mg^{2+} content
Increased loss
  Diabetic ketoacidosis
  Diuretic therapy
  Diarrhea
  Hyperaldosteronism, Bartter's syndrome
  Associated with hypercalciuria
  Renal magnesium wasting
Unexplained
  Hyperparathyroidism
  Postparathyroidectomy
  Vitamin D therapy
  Induced by aminoglycoside antibiotics, cisplatin, ampho-
    tericin B

marked neuromuscular and central nervous system hyperirritability, with tremors, athetoid movements, jerking, nystagmus, and a positive Babinski response. There may be hypertension, tachycardia, and ventricular arrhythmias. Confusion and disorientation may be prominent features.

B. Laboratory Findings: The serum Mg^{2+} is low. Hypocalcemia and hypokalemia are often present. The ECG shows a prolonged QT interval, particularly due to lengthening of the ST segment.

Treatment

Treatment consists of the use of intravenous fluids containing magnesium as chloride or sulfate, 240–1200 mg/d (10–50 mmol/d) during the period of severe deficit, followed by 120 mg/d (5 mmol/d) for maintenance. Magnesium sulfate may also be given intramuscularly in a dosage of 200–800 mg/d (8–33 mmol/d) in four divided doses. Serum levels must be monitored and dosage adjusted to keep the concentration from rising above 2.5 mmol/L. K^+ and Ca^{2+} may be required as well. Magnesium oxide, 250–500 mg by mouth two to four times daily, is useful for repleting stores in those with chronic hypomagnesemia.

Ryzen E, Rude RK: Low intracellular magnesium in patients with acute pancreatitis and hypocalcemia. West J Med 1990;152:145.

Salem M, Munoz R, Chernow B: Hypomagnesemia in critical illness: A common and clinically important problem. Crit Care Clin 1991;7:225. (Emphasizes that hypomagnesemia is a common and reversible cause of morbidity in critically ill patients.)

Whang R, Ryder KW: Frequency of hypomagnesemia and hypermagnesemia: Requested vs. routine. JAMA 1990; 263:3063. (Most magnesium abnormalities are not recognized by physicians. Authors advocate routine measurement of this electrolyte.)

2. HYPERMAGNESEMIA

Magnesium excess is almost always the result of renal insufficiency and the inability to excrete what has been taken in from food or drugs, especially antacids.

Clinical Findings

A. Symptoms and Signs: Muscle weakness, mental obtundation, and confusion are characteristic manifestations. Weakness—even flaccid paralysis—and fall in blood pressure are evident on examination. There may be respiratory muscle paralysis or cardiac arrest.

B. Laboratory Findings: Serum Mg^{2+} is elevated. In the common setting of renal insufficiency, concentrations of BUN and of serum creatinine, phosphate, and uric acid are elevated; serum K^+ may be elevated. Serum Ca^{2+} is often low. The ECG shows increased PR interval, broadened QRS complexes, and elevated T waves.

Treatment

Treatment is directed toward alleviating renal insufficiency. Calcium acts as an antagonist to Mg^{2+} and may be given intravenously as calcium chloride, 500 mg or more at a rate of 100 mg (4.5 mmol)/min. Hemodialysis or peritoneal dialysis may be indicated.

Van Hook JW: Endocrine crises. Hypermagnesemia. Crit Care Clin 1991;7:215.

Whang R, Ryder KW: Frequency of hypomagnesemia and hypermagnesemia: Requested vs routine. JAMA 1990; 263:3063.

ACID-BASE DISORDERS

In order to assess a patient's acid-base status, measurement of arterial pH, partial pressure of carbon dioxide (PCO_2), and plasma bicarbonate (HCO_3^-) is needed. Blood gas analyzers directly measure pH and PCO_2, and the HCO_3^- value is calculated from the Henderson-Hasselbalch equation:

$$pH = 6.1 + \log \frac{[HCO_3^-]}{0.03 \times PCO_2}$$

The total venous CO_2 measurement is a more direct determination of HCO_3^-. Because of the dissociation characteristics of carbonic acid (H_2CO_3) at body pH, dissolved CO_2 is almost exclusively in the form of HCO_3^-, and for clinical purposes the total carbon dioxide content is equivalent ($\pm$ 3 meq/L) to the HCO_3^- concentration:

$$H^+ + HCO_3^- \leftrightarrow H_2CO_3 \leftrightarrow CO_2 + H_2O$$

The syringe used for taking blood arterial blood gas determinations should be coated with 1 mL of heparin (1000 units/mL) as an anticoagulant, but excessive heparin artificially lowers the PCO_2 and HCO_3^- derived from that sample. Customarily, arterial—rather than venous—blood gases are measured because it is believed that venous blood provides unreliable information. Certainly, arterial blood is needed for accurate measurement of PO_2. But if precise measurements of oxygenation are not needed or if oxygen saturation obtained from the pulse oximeter is adequate, venous blood gases generally provide useful information for assessment of acid-base balance and can be used interchangeably with arterial blood gases since the arteriovenous differences in pH and PCO_2 are small and relatively constant. Venous blood pH is usually only 0.03–0.04 units lower than that of arterial blood, and venous blood PCO_2 is only 7 or 8 mm Hg higher. Calculated HCO_3^- concentration in venous blood is at most 2 meq/L higher than that of arterial blood. An important exception to the rule of interchangeability between arterial and venous blood gases for determination of acid-base balance is during cardiopulmonary arrest. In this setting, arterial pH may be 7.41 and venous pH 7.15. Arterial blood PCO_2 can be 32 mm Hg with a venous blood PCO_2 of 74 mm Hg. Further work will determine if clinicians should monitor both venous and arterial blood during cardiopulmonary resuscitation as a more accurate reflection of acid-base status.

There are two fundamental types of acid-base disorders: respiratory and metabolic. Primary respiratory disorders affect blood acidity by causing changes in PCO_2, and primary metabolic disorders are caused by disturbances in the HCO_3^- concentration. The primary disturbances are usually accompanied by compensatory changes, but these changes do not fully compensate for the primary acid-base disorders even if the disorders are chronic. Therefore, if the pH is less than 7.40, the primary process is acidosis (either respiratory or metabolic). If the pH is higher than 7.40, the primary process is either respiratory or metabolic alkalosis. The presence of one disorder with its appropriate compensatory change is a simple disorder.

Mixed Acid-Base Disorders.

The presence of more than one simple disorder (not compensatory) is a mixed disorder. Double or triple disorders can coexist but not quadruple ones, since simultaneous respiratory acidosis and alkalosis are not possible.

Clinicians frequently find it difficult to decide if a mixed disorder is present. One useful scheme is to determine if the degree of compensation for the primary disorder is appropriate (Table 20–15). In respiratory disorders, if the magnitude of compensation in HCO_3^- level differs from that which is predicted, the patient has a mixed disorder. Therefore, superimposed metabolic acidosis will decrease HCO_3^- to lower than the predicted level, and a metabolic alkalosis will increase HCO_3^- over the predicted value. For example, a patient with chronic respiratory acidosis and PCO_2 of 60 mm Hg should have a HCO_3^- of 35 meq/L (assuming that normal HCO_3^- is 28 meq/L). If the HCO_3^- is 25 meq/L, a superimposed metabolic acidosis exists, and if the HCO_3^- is 45 meq/L, there is a superimposed metabolic alkalosis. Using data from Table 20–15, similar calculations can be made for primary metabolic disorders.

Relman AS: "Blood gases": Arterial or venous? N Engl J Med 1986;315:188. (Editorial promoting the use of venous blood gases for assessment of acid-base status in most settings.)

1. RESPIRATORY ACIDOSIS

Respiratory acidosis results from decreased alveolar ventilation and subsequent hypercapnia. Pulmonary as well as nonpulmonary disorders can cause hypoventilation (Table 20–16). The clinician must be mindful of readily reversible causes of respiratory acidosis, especially that due to narcotic-induced central nervous system depression.

Acute respiratory failure is associated with severe

Table 20–15. Primary acid-base disorders and expected compensation.

Disorder	Primary Defect	pH	Compensatory Response	Magnitude of Compensation
Respiratory				
Acidosis				
Acute	$\uparrow PCO_2$	$\downarrow pH$	$\uparrow HCO_3^-$	$\uparrow$1 meq HCO_3^- per 10 mm Hg $\uparrow PCO_2$
Chronic	$\uparrow PCO_2$	$\downarrow pH$	$\uparrow HCO_3^-$	$\uparrow$3.5 meq HCO_3^- per 10 mm Hg $\uparrow PCO_2$
Alkalosis				
Acute	$\downarrow PCO_2$	$\uparrow pH$	$\downarrow HCO_3^-$	$\downarrow HCO_3^-$ 2 meq/L per 10 mm Hg $\downarrow PCO_2$
Chronic	$\downarrow PCO_2$	$\uparrow pH$	$\downarrow HCO_3^-$	$\downarrow HCO_3^-$ 5 meq/L per 10 mm Hg $\downarrow PCO_2$
Metabolic				
Acidosis	$\downarrow HCO_3^-$	$\downarrow pH$	$\downarrow PCO_2$	$\downarrow PCO_2$ 1.3 mm Hg per $\downarrow$1 meq HCO_3^-
Alkalosis	$\uparrow HCO_3^-$	$\uparrow pH$	$\uparrow PCO_2$	$\uparrow PCO_2$ 0.7 mm Hg per $\uparrow$1 meq HCO_3^-

Table 20–16. Causes of respiratory acidosis.[1]

Acute	Chronic
Airway obstruction Aspiration of foreign body or vomitus Laryngospasm Generalized bronchospasm Obstructive sleep apnea	**Airway obstruction** Chronic obstructive lung disease (bronchitis, emphysema)
Respiratory center depression General anesthesia Sedative overdosage Cerebral trauma or infarction Central sleep apnea	**Respiratory center depression** Chronic sedative overdosage Primary alveolar hypoventilation (Ondine's curse) Obesity-hypoventilation syndrome (Pickwickian syndrome) Brain tumor Bulbar poliomyelitis
Circulatory catastrophes Cardiac arrest Severe pulmonary edema	
Neuromuscular defects High cervical cordotomy Botulism, tetanus Guillain-Barré syndrome Crisis in myasthenia gravis Familial hypokalemic periodic paralysis Hypokalemic myopathy Polymyositis Drugs or toxic agents (eg, curare, succinylcholine, aminoglycosides, organophosphorus)	**Neuromuscular defects** Polymyositis Multiple sclerosis Muscular dystrophy Amyotrophic lateral sclerosis Diaphragmatic paralysis Myxedema Myopathic disease
Restrictive defects Pneumothorax Hemothorax Flail chest Severe pneumonitis Infant respiratory distress syndrome (hyaline membrane disease) Adult respiratory distress syndrome **Mechanical hypoventilation**	**Restrictive defects** Kyphoscoliosis, spinal arthritis Fibrothorax Hydrothorax Interstitial fibrosis Decreased diaphragmatic movement (eg, ascites) Prolonged pneumonitis Obesity

[1]Adapted from Madias NE, Cohen JJ: Respiratory acidosis. In: *Acid/Base.* Cohen JJ, Kassirer JP (editors). Little, Brown, 1982.

acidosis and only a small increase in the plasma bicarbonate. After 6–12 hours, the primary increase in PCO_2 evokes a renal compensatory response to generate more HCO_3^-, which tends to ameliorate the respiratory acidosis. This usually takes several days to complete. In acute respiratory acidosis, the serum HCO_3^- level should increase by 1 meq/L for each increment of 10 mm Hg in PCO_2 (Table 20–15).

Chronic respiratory acidosis is generally seen in patients with underlying lung disease, such as chronic obstructive disease. In chronic respiratory acidosis, the serum bicarbonate level should increase by 3.5 meq/L for each increment of 10 mm Hg PCO_2. Urinary excretion of acid in the form of NH_4^+ and Cl^- ions results in the characteristic hypochloremia of chronic respiratory acidosis. When chronic respiratory acidosis is corrected suddenly, especially in patients who receive mechanical ventilation, there is a 2- to 3-day lag in renal bicarbonate excretion, resulting in posthypercapnic metabolic alkalosis.

Clinical Findings

A. Symptoms and Signs: With acute onset, there is somnolence and confusion, and myoclonus with asterixis may be seen. Coma from CO_2 narcosis ensues. Severe hypercapnia increases cerebral blood flow and cerebrospinal fluid pressure. Signs of increased intracranial pressure (papilledema, pseudotumor cerebri) may be seen.

B. Laboratory Findings: Arterial pH is low, and PCO_2 is increased. Serum HCO_3^- is elevated, but not enough to completely compensate for the hypercapnia. If the disorder is chronic, hypochloremia is seen.

Treatment

Since drug overdose is an important reversible cause of acute respiratory acidosis, administration of naloxone, 0.04–2 mg intravenously (see Chapter 39) should be considered in all such patients if no obvious cause for respiratory depression is present. In all forms of respiratory acidosis, treatment is directed at the underlying disorder to improve ventilation. Mechanical ventilation may be necessary (see Chapter 9 for treatment of respiratory failure).

2. RESPIRATORY ALKALOSIS

Respiratory alkalosis, or hypocapnia, occurs when hyperventilation reduces the PCO_2, which increases the pH. The most common cause of respiratory alkalosis is hyperventilation syndrome (Table 20–17). Symptoms in acute respiratory alkalosis are related to

Table 20–17. Causes of respiratory alkalosis.[1]

Hypoxia
  Decreased inspired oxygen tension
  High altitude
  Ventilation-perfusion inequality
  Hypotension
  Severe anemia
CNS-mediated disorders
  Voluntary hyperventilation
    Anxiety-hyperventilation syndrome
  Neurologic disease
  Cerebrovascular accident (infarction, hemorrhage)
  Infection
  Trauma
  Tumor
  Pharmacologic and hormonal stimulation
    Salicylates
    Dinitrophenol
    Nicotine
    Xanthines
    Pressor hormones
    Pregnancy (progesterone)
  Hepatic failure
  Gram-negative septicemia
  Recovery from metabolic acidosis
  Heat exposure
Pulmonary disease
  Interstitial lung disease
  Pneumonia
  Pulmonary embolism
  Pulmonary edema
Mechanical overventilation

[1]Adapted from Gennar FJ, Kassirer JP: Respiratory alkalosis. In: *Acid/Base.* Cohen JJ, Kassirer JP (editors). Little, Brown, 1982.

decreased cerebral blood flow induced by the disorder. The physiologic state of pregnancy is chronic respiratory alkalosis, probably from progesterone stimulation of the respiratory center, with an average PCO_2 of 30 mm Hg.

Determination of appropriate compensatory changes in the HCO_3^- is useful to sort out the presence of an associated metabolic disorder (see above under Mixed Acid-Base Disorders). As in respiratory acidosis, the changes in HCO_3^- values are greater if the respiratory alkalosis is chronic (Table 20–15). In acute respiratory alkalosis, HCO_3^- decreases 2 meq/L for every 10 mm Hg fall in PCO_2. In chronic respiratory alkalosis, there is a compensatory decrease in renal acid excretion. Serum HCO_3^- decreases by 5 meq/L for every 10 mm Hg drop in PCO_2. While serum HCO_3^- is frequently below 15 meq/L in metabolic acidosis, it is unusual to see such a low level in respiratory alkalosis, and its presence would imply a superimposed (noncompensatory) metabolic acidosis.

Clinical Findings

A. Symptoms and Signs: In acute cases (hyperventilation), there is light-headedness, anxiety, paresthesias, numbness about the mouth, and a tingling sensation in the hands and feet. Tetany occurs in more severe alkalosis from a fall in Ca^{2+}. In chronic cases, symptomatic findings are those of the primary disease.

B. Laboratory Findings: Arterial blood pH is elevated, and PCO_2 is low. Serum bicarbonate is decreased in chronic respiratory alkalosis.

Treatment

Treatment is directed toward the underlying cause. In acute hyperventilation syndrome from anxiety, rebreathing into a paper bag will increase the PCO_2. Sedation may be necessary if the maneuver does not terminate the attack. Rapid correction of chronic respiratory alkalosis may result in metabolic acidosis as PCO_2 is increased in the setting of previous compensatory decrease in HCO_3^-.

3. METABOLIC ACIDOSIS

The hallmark of metabolic acidosis is decreased HCO_3^-, seen also in respiratory alkalosis (see above), but the pH distinguishes between the two disorders. Calculation of the anion gap is extremely useful in determining the cause of the metabolic acidosis even though, physiologically, electrical neutrality rather than an anion gap exists (Table 20–18). The anion

Table 20–18. Anion gap acidosis.[1]

Decreased (<6 meq)
  Hypoalbuminemia (decreased unmeasured anion)
  Plasma cell dyscrasias
    Monoclonal protein (cationic paraprotein) (accompanied by chloride and bicarbonate)
Increased (>12 meq)
  Metabolic anion
    Diabetic ketoacidosis
    Alcoholic keotacidosis
    Lactic acidosis
    Renal insufficiency (PO_4^{3-}, SO_4^{2-})
    Starvation
    Metabolic alkalosis (increased number of negative charges on protein)
  Drug or chemical anion
    Salicylate intoxication
    Sodium carbenicillin therapy
    Methanol (formic acid)
    Ethylene glycol (oxalic acid)
Normal (6–12 meq)
  Loss of HCO_3^-
  Diarrhea
  Pancreatic fluid loss
  Ileostomy (unadapted)
  Carbonic anhydrase inhibitors
  Chloride retention
  Renal tubular acidosis
  Ileal loop bladder
  Administration of HCl equivalent
  NH_4Cl
  Arginine and lysine in parenteral nutrition

[1]Reference ranges for anion gap may vary based on differing laboratory methods.

gap represents the difference between readily measured anions and cations (Figure 20–2).

In plasma,

$$Na^+ + Unmeasured\ cations = HCO_3^- + Cl^- + Unmeasured\ anions$$

$$Anion\ gap = (Na^+) - (HCO_3^- + Cl^-)$$

The major unmeasured cations are calcium (5 meq/L), magnesium (2 meq/L), gamma globulins, and potassium (4 meq/L). The major unmeasured anions are negatively charged albumin (2 meq/L per g/dL), phosphate (2 meq/L), sulfate (1 meq/L), lactate (1–2 meq/L), and other organic anions (3–4 meq/L). Traditionally, the normal anion gap has been 12 ± 4 meq/L. With the new generation of autoanalyzers (Bechman ASTRA analyzer), the reference range may be lower (6 ± 1 meq/L), primarily from an increase in Cl^- values. Despite its usefulness, the serum anion gap can be misleading. Non-acid base disorders that may contribute to an error in anion gap interpretation include hypoalbuminemia (see below), hyperviscosity or hyperlipidemia (displacement by lipids falsely lowers Na^+ and Cl^- levels, but the absolute change in the Na^+ is more than that in the Cl^-, therefore lowering the anion gap), antibiotic administration (eg, carbenicillin is an unmeasured anion; polymyxin is an unmeasured cation), hypernatremia, or hyponatremia.

Decreased Anion Gap

Decreased anion gap can occur because of a decrease in unmeasured anions or an increase in unmeasured cations.

A. Decreased Unmeasured Anions: If the sodium concentration remains normal but HCO_3^- and Cl^- increase, the anion gap will decrease. This is seen when there are decreased unmeasured anions, especially in hypoalbuminemia. For every 1 g/dL decline in serum albumin, a 2 meq/L decrease in anion gap will occur. The new reference range for anion gap diminishes the usefulness of a low anion gap categorization except to detect an increased anion gap acidosis mimicking a normal anion gap acidosis.

B. Increased Unmeasured Cations: If the sodium concentration falls because of addition of unmeasured cations but HCO_3^- and Cl^- remain unchanged, the anion gap will decrease (Figure 20–2). This is seen in (1) severe hypercalcemia, hypermagnesemia, or hyperkalemia; (2) IgG myeloma, where the immunoglobulin is cationic; and (3) lithium toxicity.

Increased Anion Gap Acidosis (Increased Unmeasured Anions)

The hallmark of this disorder is that metabolic acidosis (thus low HCO_3^-) is associated with normal serum Cl^-, so that the anion gap increases. Pseudometabolic acidosis is caused by underfilling Vacutainer tubes. If 1 mL of blood is put into a 10-mL red-top Vacutainer tube, a significant decline in HCO_3^- with an increase in anion gap occurs. Normochloremic metabolic acidosis generally results from addition to the blood of nonchloride acids such as lactate, acetoacetate, β-hydroxybutyrate, and exogenous toxins. An exception is uremia, with underexcretion of organic acids and anions.

A. Lactic Acidosis: Lactic acid is formed from pyruvate in anaerobic glycolysis. Therefore, most of the lactate is produced in tissues with high rates of glycolysis, such as gut (responsible for over 50% of lactate production), skeletal muscle, brain, skin, and erythrocytes. Normally, lactate levels remain low (1 meq/L) because of metabolism of lactate principally by the liver through gluconeogenesis or oxidation via the Krebs cycle. Furthermore, the kidneys metabolize about 30% of lactate.

In lactic acidosis, lactate levels are at least 4–5 meq/L but commonly 10–30 meq/L. The mortality rate exceeds 50%. There are two basic types of lactic acidosis, both associated with increased lactate production and decreased lactate utilization. Type A is characterized by hypoxia or decreased tissue perfusion, whereas in type B there is no clinical evidence of hypoxia. Type A (hypoxic) lactic acidosis is the

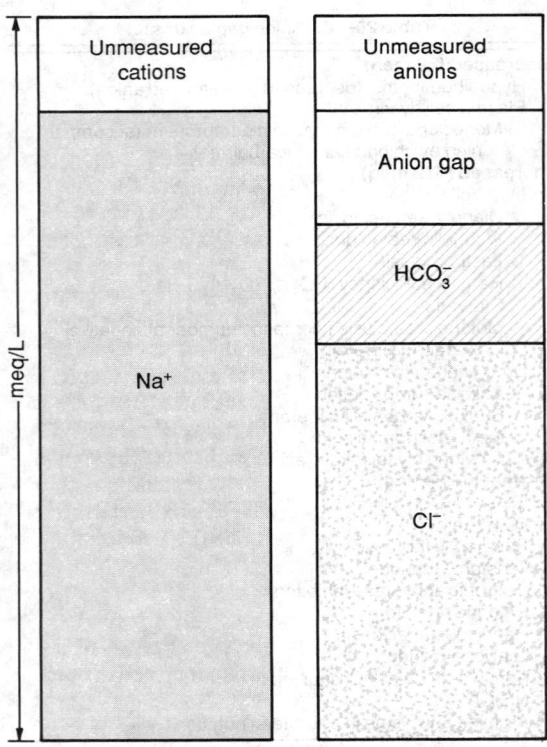

Figure 20–2. Composition of ions in plasma.

more common type, resulting from poor tissue perfusion; cardiogenic, septic, or hemorrhagic shock; or carbon monoxide poisoning. These conditions not only cause lactic acid production to increase peripherally but, more importantly, hepatic metabolism of lactate to decrease as liver perfusion declines. In addition, severe acidosis impairs the ability of the liver to extract the perfused lactate.

Type B lactic acidosis may be due to metabolic causes, such as diabetes, ketoacidosis, liver disease, renal failure, infection, leukemia, or lymphoma; or may occur as a result of toxicity from ethanol, methanol, salicylates, isoniazid, or phenformin. It is postulated that tissue oxygen utilization is impaired. Recently, the association of AIDS with type B lactic acidosis has been described. These patients do not have AIDS-related lymphoma as a cause of lactic acidosis.

Idiopathic lactic acidosis, usually in debilitated patients, has an extremely high mortality rate. (For treatment of lactic acidosis, see Chapter 26).

B. Diabetic Ketoacidosis: See Chapter 26 and the section below on normal anion gap acidosis.

C. Alcoholic Ketoacidosis: This is a common disorder of chronically malnourished patients who consume large quantities of alcohol daily. Most of these patients have mixed acid-base disorders (10% have a triple acid-base disorder). While decreased HCO_3^- is usual, half the patients may have normal or alkalemic pH. The three types of metabolic acidosis seen in alcoholic ketoacidosis are the following: (1) Ketoacidosis due to β-hydroxybutyrate and acetoacetate excess. (2) Lactic acidosis: Alcohol metabolism increases the NADH:NAD ratio, causing increased production and decreased utilization of lactate. Moderate to severe elevations of lactate (> 6 mmol/L) are seen with concomitant disorders such as sepsis, pancreatitis, or hypoglycemia. (3) Hyperchloremic acidosis from bicarbonate loss in the urine associated with ketonuria. Metabolic alkalosis occurs from volume contraction and vomiting. Respiratory alkalosis results from alcohol withdrawal, pain, or associated disorders such as sepsis or liver disease. Half of the patients have either hypoglycemia or hyperglycemia. When serum glucose levels are greater than 250 mg/dL, the distinction from diabetic ketoacidosis is difficult. The diagnosis of alcoholic ketoacidosis is supported by absence of a diabetic history and by no evidence of glucose intolerance after initial therapy.

D. Toxins: (See also Chapter 39.) Multiple toxins and drugs can increase the anion gap by increasing endogenous acid production. Examples include methanol (metabolized to formic acid), ethylene glycol (glycolic and oxalic acid), and salicylates (salicylic acid and lactic acid), which can cause a mixed disorder of metabolic acidosis with respiratory alkalosis.

E. Uremic Acidosis: At glomerular filtration rates below 20 mL/min, the inability to excrete H^+ with retention of acid anions such as PO_4^{3-} and SO_4^{2-} result in an anion gap acidosis, which rarely is severe. The unmeasured anions "replace" HCO_3^- (which is consumed as a buffer). Hyperchloremic normal anion gap acidosis may be seen in milder cases of renal insufficiency.

Normal Anion Gap Acidosis
(Table 20–19)

The hallmark of this disorder is that the low HCO_3^- of metabolic acidosis is associated with hyperchloremia, so that the anion gap remains normal. The most common causes are gastrointestinal HCO_3^- loss and defects in renal acidification (renal tubular acidoses). The urinary anion gap can differentiate between these two common causes (see below).

A. Gastrointestinal HCO_3^- Loss: Bicarbonate is secreted in multiple areas in the gastrointestinal tract. Small bowel and pancreatic secretions contain large amounts of HCO_3^-. Therefore, diarrhea or pancreatic drainage can result in HCO_3^- loss because of increased HCO_3^- secretion and decreased absorption. Hyperchloremia occurs because the ileum and colon secrete HCO_3^- in a one-to-one exchange for Cl^- by countertransport. The resultant volume contraction causes increased Cl^- retention by the kidney in the setting of decreased anion, HCO_3^-. Patients with ureterosigmoidostomies can develop hyperchloremic metabolic acidosis because the colon secretes HCO_3^- in the urine in exchange for Cl^-.

B. Renal Tubular Acidosis: In renal tubular acidosis, the defect is either inability to excrete H^+ or inadequate generation of new HCO_3^-. Four discrete types can be differentiated by the clinical setting, urinary pH, urinary anion gap (see below), and serum K^+ level.

1. Classic distal renal tubular acidosis (type I)–This disorder is characterized by hypokalemic hyperchloremic metabolic acidosis and is due to selective deficiency in H^+ secretion in the distal nephron. Despite acidosis, urinary pH cannot be acidified and is always above 5.5. Urinary excretion of $NH_4^+Cl^-$ is decreased, and the urinary anion gap is positive (see below). Enhanced K^+ excretion occurs probably because there is less competition from H^+ in the distal nephron transport system. Furthermore, as a response to renal salt wasting, hyperaldosteronism occurs. Nephrocalcinosis and nephrolithiasis frequently accompany this disorder.

2. Proximal renal tubular acidosis (type II)–Proximal renal tubular acidosis is a hypokalemic hyperchloremic metabolic acidosis due to a selective defect in the proximal tubule's ability to adequately reabsorb filtered HCO_3^-. Carbonic anhydrase inhibitors (acetazolamide) can cause proximal renal tubular acidosis. About 90% of filtered HCO_3^- is absorbed by the proximal tubule. The distal nephron has a limited ability to absorb HCO_3^- but becomes overwhelmed and does not function adequately when there is in-

Table 20–19. Hyperchloremic, normal anion gap metabolic acidoses.[1]

Renal Defect	GFR	Serum [K+]	Proximal H+ Secretion[2]	Distal H+ Secretion		Urinary Anion Gap	Treatment
				Minimal Urine pH	Urinary NH4+ Plus Titratable Acid		
Gastrointestinal HCO3− loss	↓	↓	Normal	<5.5	↑↑	Negative	Na+, K+, and HCO3− as required
Renal tubular acidosis							
I. Classic distal	Distal H+ secretion	↓	Normal	>5.5	↓	Zero or positive	NaHCO3 (1–3 meq/kg/d)
II. Proximal	Proximal H+ secretion	↓	↓[3]	<5.5	Normal	Zero or positive	NaHCO3 or KHCO3 (10–15 meq/kg/d), thiazide
III. Glomerular insufficiency	NH3 production	↓	Normal	Normal	<5.5	Normal	Zero or positive	NaHCO3 (1–3 meq/kg/d)
IV. Hyporeninemic hypoaldosteronism	Distal Na+ reabsorption, K+ secretion, and H+ secretion	↓	↑	Normal	<5.5	↓	Zero or positive	Fludrocortisone (0.1–0.5 mg/d), dietary K+ restriction, furosemide (40–160 mg/d), NaHCO3 (1–3 meq/kg/d)

[1]Reproduced, with permission, from Cogan MG: *Fluid and Electrolytes: Physiology and Pathophysiology.* Appleton & Lange, 1991.
[2]HCO3− reabsorption during HCO3− loading.
[3]Fractional excretion of bicarbonate > 15% during bicarbonate loading; usually associated with Fanconi's syndrome.

creased delivery. Eventually, distal delivery of filtered HCO_3^- declines because the plasma HCO_3^- level has dropped as a result of progressive urinary HCO_3^- wastage. When the plasma HCO_3^- level drops to 15–18 meq/L, delivery of HCO_3^- drops to the point where the distal nephron is no longer overwhelmed and can regain function. At that point, bicarbonaturia disappears, and urinary pH can be acidified. Thiazide-induced volume contraction can be used to decrease distal HCO_3^- delivery and improve bicarbonaturia and renal acidification. The increased delivery of HCO_3^- to the distal nephron also increases K^+ secretion, and hypokalemia results. If proximal renal tubular acidosis exists with other defects in absorption of the proximal tubule, glucosuria, aminoaciduria, phosphaturia, and uricaciduria will occur (Fanconi's syndrome).

3. Renal tubular acidosis of glomerular insufficiency (type III)–When GFR decreases to 20–30 mL/min, ability to generate adequate NH_3 is impaired, with subsequent decreased $NH_4^+Cl^-$ excretion. A normokalemic, hyperchloremic metabolic acidosis ensues. Further reduction in GFR results in increased anion gap acidosis of uremia (see above).

4. Hyporeninemic hypoaldosteronemic renal tubular acidosis (type IV)–Type IV is the only type characterized by hyperkalemic, hyperchloremic acidosis. The defect is aldosterone deficiency or antagonism, which impairs distal nephron Na^+ reabsorption and K^+ and H^+ excretion. Renal salt wasting is frequently present. Relative hypoaldosteronism from hyporeninemia is most commonly found in diabetic nephropathy, tubulointerstitial renal diseases, and hypertensive nephrosclerosis. In patients with these disorders, caution must be taken when using drugs that can exacerbate the hyperkalemia, such as angiotensin-converting enzyme inhibitors, which will further reduce aldosterone levels, and aldosterone receptor blockers such as spironolactone.

C. Dilutional Acidosis: Rapid dilution of plasma volume by 0.9% NaCl may cause a mild hyperchloremic acidosis. Greatest retention of NaCl occurs in a volume-contracted state.

D. Recovery From Diabetic Ketoacidosis: Anion gap acidosis is the acid-base disturbance generally ascribed to diabetic ketoacidosis:

$$H^+ + B^- + NaHCO_3 \leftrightarrow CO_2 + NaB + H_2O$$

where B^- is β-hydroxybutyric acid or acetoacetic acid.

However, during the recovery phase of diabetic ketoacidosis, anion gap acidosis can be transformed into hyperchloremic acidosis. The mechanism for this is as follows: As GFR increases from NaCl therapy of diabetic ketoacidosis, the retention of Cl^- causes a mild decrease in anion gap from dilution (see above). More importantly, the increased GFR causes ketone salts (NaB) to be excreted. The kidney reabsorbs ketone anions poorly but can compensate for the loss of anions (and therefore Na^+) by increasing the reabsorption of Cl^-.

E. Posthypocapnia: In prolonged respiratory alkalosis, HCO_3^- decreases and Cl^- increases from decreased renal $NH_4^+Cl^-$ excretion (Table 20–15). If the respiratory alkalosis is corrected quickly, PCO_2 will increase acutely but HCO_3^- will remain low until the kidneys can generate new HCO_3^-, which generally takes several days. The increased PCO_2 with low HCO_3^- causes metabolic acidosis.

F. Hyperalimentation: Hyperalimentation fluids may contain amino acid solutions that acidify when metabolized, such as arginine hydrochloride and lysine hydrochloride.

Urinary Anion Gap to Assess Hyperchloremic Metabolic Acidosis

Increased renal $NH_4^+Cl^-$ excretion to enhance H^+ removal is a normal physiologic response to metabolic acidosis. NH_3 reacts with H^+ to form NH_4^+, which is accompanied by the anion Cl^- for excretion.

$$Cl^- + NH_3 + H^+ \rightarrow NH_4Cl$$

Urinary anion gap from a random urine sample ($[Na^+ + K^+] - Cl^-$) reflects the ability of the kidney to excrete NH_4Cl and aids in the distinction between gastrointestinal and renal causes of hyperchloremic acidosis. If the cause of the metabolic acidosis is gastrointestinal HCO_3^- loss (diarrhea), renal acidification ability remains normal and NH_4Cl excretion increases in response to the acidosis. The urinary anion gap is negative (eg, –30 meq/L). If the cause is distal renal tubular acidosis, the urinary anion gap is positive (eg, +25 meq/L), since the basic lesion in the disorder is inability of the kidney to excrete H^+ and thus increase NH_4Cl excretion. Urinary pH may not as readily differentiate between the two causes. Despite acidosis, if volume depletion from diarrhea causes inadequate Na^+ delivery to the distal nephron and therefore decreased exchange with H^+, urinary pH may not be lower than 5.3. Potassium depletion, which can accompany diarrhea (and surreptitious laxative abuse), may also impair renal acidification. Thus, when volume depletion is present, the urinary anion gap is a better measurement of ability to acidify the urine than urinary pH.

Clinical Findings

A. Symptoms and Signs: Symptoms of metabolic acidosis are mainly those of the underlying disorder. Compensatory hyperventilation is an important clinical sign and may be misinterpreted as a primary respiratory disorder; when severe, Kussmaul respirations (deep, regular, sighing respirations) are seen.

B. Laboratory Findings: Blood pH, serum HCO_3^-, and PCO_2 are decreased. Anion gap may be normal (hyperchloremic) or increased (normochloremic). Hyperkalemia may be seen (see above).

Treatment

A. Increased Anion Gap Acidosis: Treatment is aimed at the underlying disorder, such as insulin and fluid therapy for diabetes and appropriate volume resuscitation to restore tissue perfusion. The metabolism of lactate will produce HCO_3^- to restore HCO_3^- and increase pH. The use of supplemental HCO_3^- is indicated for treatment of hyperkalemia (Table 20–7) and some forms of normal anion gap acidosis but has been controversial for treatment of increased anion gap metabolic acidosis. Administration of large amounts of HCO_3^- may have deleterious effects, including hypernatremia and hyperosmolality. Furthermore—and paradoxically—intracellular pH may decrease while cardiac output, blood pressure, and tissue perfusion decline, which may exacerbate lactic acidosis. Oxygen release by hemoglobin decreases because the oxygen dissociation curve is shifted to the right. HCO_3^- therapy should probably not be used if the metabolic acidosis is associated with hypoxia but is most likely beneficial if the metabolic acidosis is secondary to gastrointestinal HCO_3^- loss or renal tubular acidosis. Small doses (50–100 meq) of $NaHCO_3$ may be indicated for arterial pH less than 7.20 in the absence of hypoxia.

B. Normal Anion Gap Acidosis: (Table 20–19.) Each 650 mg tablet of $NaHCO_3$ tablet contains 8 meq of HCO_3^-. Citrate, which is converted to HCO_3^-, is often better tolerated than HCO_3^- but is more expensive. Bicitra (500 mg sodium citrate and 334 mg citric acid per teaspoon) yields the equivalent of 1 meq $NaHCO_3$/mL. The usual adult dose is 10–30 mL dissolved in 1–3 ounces of water after meals and at bedtime.

Arieff AI: Managing metabolic acidosis: Update of the sodium bicarbonate controversy. J Crit Illness 1993;8:224. (Favors the use of HCO_3^- in metabolic acidosis only if tissue hypoxia is absent, such as with diarrhea, hyperkalemia, or renal tubular acidoses.)

Battle DC et al: The use of the urinary anion gap in the diagnosis of hyperchloremic metabolic acidosis. N Engl J Med 1988;318:594. (The urinary anion gap can distinguish between renal or gastrointestinal causes of hyperchloremic metabolic acidosis.)

Chattha G et al: Lactic acidosis complicating the acquired immunodeficiency syndrome. Ann Intern Med 1993; 118:37. (This occurs in the absence of hypoxia.)

Mizock BA, Falk JL: Lactic acidosis in critical illness. Crit Care Med 1992;20:80.

Oh MS, Carroll HJ, Uribarri J: Mechanism of normochloremic and hyperchloremic acidosis in diabetic ketoacidosis. Nephron 1990;54:1. (Controversial causes of transition of normochloremic acidosis to hyperchloremic acidosis during the recovery phase of diabetic ketoacidosis.)

Salem MM, Mujais SK: Gaps in the anion gap. Arch Intern Med 1992;152:1625. (Pitfalls in use of anion gap.)

Wrenn KD et al: The syndrome of alcoholic ketoacidosis. Am J Med 1991;91:119. (Multifactorial disorder of ketoacidosis, volume depletion, alcohol withdrawal, sepsis, and liver disease.)

4. METABOLIC ALKALOSIS

Classification

Metabolic alkalosis is characterized by high HCO_3^-. The high HCO_3^- is seen also in chronic respiratory acidosis (see above), but pH differentiates the two disorders. It is useful to classify the causes of metabolic alkalosis into two groups based on "saline responsiveness" or urinary Cl⁻, which are markers for volume status (Table 20–20). Saline-responsive metabolic alkalosis is a sign of extracellular volume contraction, and saline-unresponsive alkalosis implies a volume-expanded state. It is rare for a compensatory increase in PCO_2 to exceed 55 mm Hg. A higher value implies a superimposed respiratory acidosis.

A. Saline-Responsive Metabolic Alkalosis: Saline-responsive metabolic alkalosis is by far the more common disorder. It is characterized by normotensive extracellular volume contraction and hypokalemia. Less frequently, hypotension or orthostatic hypotension may be seen. In vomiting or nasogastric suction, for example, loss of acid (HCl) initiates the alkalosis, but volume contraction from loss of Cl⁻ sustains the alkalosis. Volume contraction sustains metabolic alkalosis because the decline in GFR causes avid renal Na⁺ and HCO_3^- reabsorption. Since there is Cl⁻ depletion from loss of HCl, NaCl, and KCl from the stomach, the available anion is HCO_3^-, whose reabsorption is increased proximally. Renal Cl⁻ reabsorption (as well as Na⁺) reabsorption is high, and the urinary Cl⁻ is therefore low (10–20 meq/L). In alkalosis, bicarbonaturia with Na⁺ excreted as the accompanying cation may occur even if volume depletion is present. Therefore, urinary Cl⁻ is preferred to urinary Na⁺ as a measure of extracellular volume. An exception to the usefulness of urinary Cl⁻ is in patients who have recently received diuretics. Their urine may contain high Na⁺ and Cl⁻ despite extracellular volume contraction. If diuretics are discontinued, the urinary Cl⁻ will decrease.

Metabolic alkalosis is generally associated with hypokalemia, due partly to secondary hyperaldosteronism from volume depletion, which further worsens the metabolic alkalosis. Repletion of KCl is important to reverse the disorder.

1. Contraction alkalosis–Diuretics can acutely decrease extracellular volume from urinary loss of NaCl and water. There is no associated bicarbonaturia, so that body HCO_3^- content remains normal. However, plasma HCO_3^- increases because of extracellular fluid contraction—the reverse of what occurs in dilutional acidosis.

2. Posthypercapnia alkalosis–In chronic re-

Table 20–20. Metabolic alkalosis.[1]

Saline-Responsive (U_{Cl} <10 meq/d)	Saline-Unresponsive (U_{Cl} >10 meq/d)

Excessive body bicarbonate content
  Renal alkalosis
    Diuretic therapy
    Poorly reabsorbable anion therapy: Carbenicillin, penicillin,
      sulfate, phosphate
    Posthypercapnia
  Gastrointestinal alkalosis
    Gastric alkalosis
    Intestinal alkalosis: Chloride diarrhea
  Exogenous alkali
    $NaHCO_3$ (baking soda)
    Sodium citrate, lactate, gluconate, acetate
    Transfusions
    Antacids
Normal bicarbonate content
  "Contraction alkalosis"
	Excess body bicarbonate content
	  Renal alkalosis
	    Normotensive
	      Bartter's syndrome
	      Severe potassium depletion
	      Refeeding alkalosis
	      Hypercalcemia and hypoparathyroidism
	    Hypertensive
	      Endogenous mineralocorticoids
	        Primary aldosteronism
	        Hyperreninism
	        Adrenal enzyme deficiency: 11- and 17-hydroxylase
	        Liddle's syndrome
	      Exogenous mineralocorticoids
	        Licorice
	        Carbenoxolone
	        Chewing tobacco

[1]Reproduced, with permission, from Narins RG et al: Diagnostic strategies in disorders of fluid, electrolyte and acid-base homeostasis. Am J Med 1983;72:496.

spiratory acidosis, compensatory increases in HCO_3^- occur (Table 20–15). Hypercapnia also directly affects the proximal tubule to decrease NaCl reabsorption, which can cause extracellular volume depletion. If PCO_2 is corrected rapidly, as with mechanical ventilation, metabolic alkalosis will ensue until adequate bicarbonaturia occurs. Hypovolemia will inhibit bicarbonaturia until Cl^- is repleted. Many patients with chronic respiratory acidosis receive diuretics, which further exacerbates the metabolic alkalosis.

B. Saline-Unresponsive Alkalosis:

1. Hyperaldosteronism–Primary hyperaldosteronism causes expansion of extracellular volume with hypertension. Metabolic alkalosis with hypokalemia results from the renal mineralocorticoid effect. In an attempt to decrease extracellular volume, high levels of NaCl are excreted, and for that reason the urinary Cl^- is high (> 20 meq/L). Therapy with NaCl will only increase volume expansion and hypertension and will not treat the underlying problem of mineralocorticoid excess.

2. Alkali administration with decreased GFR–Despite large ingestions of HCO_3^-, enhanced bicarbonaturia almost always prevents a patient with normal renal function from developing metabolic alkalosis. However, with renal insufficiency, urinary excretion of bicarbonate is inadequate. If large amounts of HCO_3^- or metabolizable salts of organic acids such as sodium lactate, sodium citrate, or sodium gluconate are consumed, as with intensive antacid therapy, metabolic alkalosis will occur. In milk-alkali syndrome, large and sustained ingestion of absorbable antacids and milk causes renal insufficiency from hypercalcemia. Decreased GFR prevents appropriate bicarbonaturia from the ingested alkali, and metabolic alkalosis occurs. Volume contraction from renal hypercalcemic effects further exacerbates the alkalosis.

Clinical Findings

A. Symptoms and Signs: There are no characteristic symptoms or signs. Weakness and hyporeflexia occur if serum K^+ is markedly low. Tetany and neuromuscular irritability occur rarely.

B. Laboratory Findings: The arterial blood pH and bicarbonate are elevated. The arterial PCO_2 is increased. Serum potassium and chloride are decreased. There may be an increased anion gap.

Treatment

Mild alkalosis is generally well tolerated. Severe or symptomatic alkalosis (pH > 7.60) requires urgent treatment.

A. Saline-Responsive Metabolic Alkalosis: Therapy for saline-responsive metabolic alkalosis is aimed at correction of extracellular volume deficit. Depending on the degree of hypovolemia, adequate amounts of 0.9% NaCl and KCl should be administered. Discontinuation of diuretics and administration of H_2-blockers in patients whose alkalosis is due to nasogastric suction can be useful. If impaired pulmonary or cardiovascular status prohibits adequate volume repletion, acetazolamide, 250–500 mg intravenously every 4–6 hours, can be used. Administration of acid can be used as emergency therapy. HCl, 0.1 mol/L, is infused via a central vein (the solution is sclerosing). Dosage is calculated to decrease the HCO_3^- level by one-half over 2–4 hours, assuming a HCO_3^- volume of distribution (L) of 0.5 × body

Table 20–21. Daily maintenance rations for average adult (60–100 kg) requiring parenteral fluids.

Glucose	100–200 g
Na^+	80–120 meq
K^+	80–120 meq
Water	2500 mL

Table 20–22. Electrolyte concentrations of commonly used intravenous crystalloid solutions.[1]

	Osmolality (mosm/kg H$_2$O)	Na$^+$ (meq/L)	Cl$^-$ (meq/L)	Glucose (g/L)
Isotonic				
0.9% saline	308	154	154	0
D$_5$0.9% saline	560	154	154	50
Ringer's lactate[2]	273	130	109	0
Hypotonic				
D$_5$W	252	0	0	50
D$_5$0.22% saline	320	34	34	50
0.45% saline	154	77	77	0
D$_5$0.45% saline	405	77	77	50

[1]Modified and reproduced, with permission, from Cogan MG: *Fluid and Electrolytes: Physiology and Pathophysiology.* Appleton & Lange, 1991.
[2]Also contains 28 meq/L lactate (which is converted to HCO$_3^-$), 4 meq/L K$^+$, and 2 meq/L Ca^{2+}.

weight (kg). Patients with marked renal insufficiency may require dialysis.

B. Saline-Unresponsive Metabolic Alkalosis: Therapy for saline-unresponsive metabolic alkalosis includes surgical removal of a mineralocorticoid-producing tumor and blockage of aldosterone effect with an angiotensin-converting enzyme inhibitor or with spironolactone.

Cogan MG: *Fluid & Electrolytes. Physiology & Pathophysiology.* Appleton & Lange, 1991.
Haber RJ: A practical approach to acid-base disorders. West J Med 1991;155:146.
Narins RG, Emmett M: Simple and mixed acid-base disorders: A practical approach. Medicine 1980;59:161.
Narins RG et al: Diagnostic strategies in disorders of fluid, electrolyte and acid-base homeostasis. Am J Med 1982;72:496.

FLUID MANAGEMENT

Most of those who require water and electrolyte intravenously are relatively normal people who cannot take orally what they require for maintenance. Table 20–21 shows that the range of tolerance for water and electrolytes (homeostatic limits) permits reasonable latitude in therapy provided normal renal function exists to accomplish the final regulation of volume and concentration.

An average adult whose entire intake is parenteral would require for maintenance 2500–3000 mL of 5% dextrose in 0.2% saline solution (34 meq Na$^+$ plus 34 meq Cl$^-$/L). To each liter, 30 meq of KCl could be added. In 3 L, the total chloride intake would be 192 meq, which is easily tolerated. Table 20–22 sets forth the composition of commonly used crystalloid solutions. Guidelines for gastrointestinal fluid losses are shown in Table 20–23.

In situations requiring maintenance or maintenance plus replacement of fluid and electrolyte by parenteral infusion, the total daily ration should be

Table 20–23. Replacement guidelines for sweat and gastrointestinal fluid losses.

	Average Electrolyte Composition				Replacement Guidelines per Liter Lost				
	Na$^+$ (meq/L)	K$^+$ (meq/L)	Cl$^-$ (meq/L)	HCO$_3^-$ (meq/L)	0.9% saline (mL)	0.45% saline (mL)	D$_5$W (mL)	KCl (meq/L)	7.5% NaHCO$_3$ (45 meq HCO$_3^-$/amp)
Sweat	30–50	5	50			500	500	5	
Gastric secretions	20	10	10			300	700	20	
Pancreatic juice	130	5	35	115		400	600	5	2 amps
Bile	145	5	100	25	600		400	5	0.5 amp
Duodenal fluid	60	15	100	10		1000		15	0.25 amp
Ileal fluid	100	10	60	60		600	400	10	1 amp
Colonic diarrhea[1]	140	10	85	60		1000		10	1 amp

[1]In the absence of diarrhea, colonic fluid Na$^+$ levels are low (40 meq/L).

administered continuously over the 24-hour period in order to ensure the best utilization by the patient.

If parenteral fluids are the only source of water, electrolyte, and calories for longer than a week, more complex fluids containing amino acids, lipid, trace metals, and vitamins may be indicated. (See Total Parenteral Nutrition, Chapter 28.)

REFERENCES

Brenner BM, Rector FC Jr (editors): *The Kidney,* 4th ed. Saunders, 1990.

Cogan MG: *Fluid and Electrolytes: Physiology and Pathophysiology.* Appleton & Lange, 1991.

Rose BD: *Clinical Physiology of Acid-Base & Electrolyte Disorders,* 3rd ed. McGraw-Hill, 1989.

21

Genitourinary Tract

Joseph C. Presti, Jr., MD, Marshall L. Stoller, MD, & Peter R. Carroll, MD

UROLOGIC EVALUATION

HISTORY

Systemic Manifestations

Fever when associated with other symptoms of a urinary tract infection (see below) helps to localize the site of infection. In the female, high fevers and irritative voiding symptoms typically occur in acute pyelonephritis. Fevers are not typical of uncomplicated cystitis. In the male, a febrile urinary tract infection implies acute pyelonephritis, acute prostatitis, or acute epididymitis. Fever may also be seen in hypernephroma.

Weight loss and malaise also may be associated with tumor or disease states associated with chronic renal failure. In the pediatric population exhibiting "failure to thrive," one must exclude underlying urologic disorders.

Pain

Pain in the genitourinary tract is usually associated with distention of a hollow viscus (ureteral obstruction, urinary retention) or the capsule of an organ (acute prostatitis, acute pyelonephritis). Pain may be local or referred. Pain associated with malignancy is usually a late manifestation and indicative of advanced disease.

A. Renal Pain: Pain of renal origin is usually located in the ipsilateral costovertebral angle. It may radiate to the umbilicus and may be referred to the ipsilateral testicle in men or the labium in women. In infection, the pain is typically constant, whereas in obstruction it may come and go. Nausea and vomiting may result from reflex stimulation of the celiac ganglion. Patients with intraperitoneal pathology will typically lie motionless to avoid pain, while patients with renal disease will move about to try to find a more comfortable position.

B. Ureteral Pain: Ureteral pain is usually acute and a result of obstruction. Distention of the ureter and possibly the renal capsule along with hyperperistalsis and spasm of the smooth muscle of the ureter may result in two different pain patterns. The distention may cause a constant dull ache, while the spasms result in colic. The site of obstruction may sometimes be determined by the site of pain. Upper ureteral obstruction may result in pain referred to the scrotum in males or to the labium in females. Midureteral obstruction may cause pain in the lower quadrant and thus may be confused with appendicitis in right-sided ureteral obstruction or diverticulitis in left-sided ureteral obstruction. Lower ureteral obstruction may cause inflammation of the ureteral orifice and thus be associated with symptoms of vesical irritability.

C. Vesical Pain: Acute urinary retention results in severe suprapubic discomfort. Chronic urinary retention is usually painless despite tremendous vesical distention. Suprapubic pain not related to the act of micturition is rarely vesical in origin. Acute cystitis pain is usually referred to the distal urethra and is associated with the act of micturition.

D. Prostatic Pain: Prostatic pain is usually associated with inflammation and is located in the perineum. This pain may radiate to the lumbosacral spine, inguinal canals, or lower extremities. Because of its location near the bladder neck, inflammatory processes of the prostate may result in irritative voiding complaints.

E. Penile Pain: Pain in the flaccid penis is usually secondary to inflammatory processes caused by sexually transmitted diseases or paraphimosis, a condition of the uncircumcised male in which the retracted foreskin is trapped behind the glans penis, resulting in vascular congestion and painful swelling of the glans. Pain in the erect penis may be due to Peyronie's disease (fibrous plaque of the tunica albuginea, resulting in painful curvature of the erect penis) or to priapism (prolonged painful erection necessitating immediate intervention).

F. Testicular Pain: Acute conditions such as trauma, torsion of the testis or one of its appendices, or epididymo-orchitis cause acute pain within the scrotum with radiation to the ipsilateral groin. Chronic pain produced by a varicocele or hydrocele usually results in a dull "heaviness" without radiation. Disorders of the kidney, retroperitoneal structures, or inguinal canal may result in pain referred to the testis.

Hematuria

Gross hematuria in adults should be considered a sign of malignancy until proved otherwise.

The character of the hematuria may give a clue to the site of origin. **Initial hematuria,** the presence of blood at the beginning of the urinary stream which clears during the stream, implies an anterior (penile) urethral source. **Terminal hematuria,** the presence of blood at the end of the urinary stream, implies a bladder neck or prostatic urethral source. **Total hematuria,** the presence of blood throughout the urinary stream, implies a bladder or upper tract source.

Associated symptoms may give important clues as to the cause of hematuria. Hematuria associated with renal colic may imply a ureteral stone, yet the passage of blood clots from a bleeding renal tumor may mimic this scenario. Severe irritative voiding symptoms in a young woman may suggest an acute bacterial infection and associated hemorrhagic cystitis, yet the same scenario in an older woman or in any male must raise concerns for neoplasm. In any situation, if urine cultures are negative or symptoms fail to resolve after appropriate therapy, further evaluation is warranted. In the absence of other symptoms, gross hematuria may be more indicative of neoplasm, yet other disorders such as staghorn calculi, glomerulonephropathies, or polycystic kidney disease must be considered.

Irritative Voiding Symptoms

Urgency is the strong, sudden desire to void. It may be observed in inflammatory conditions such as cystitis or in hyperreflexic neuropathic conditions such as neurogenic bladders resulting from upper motor neuron lesions. **Dysuria** (painful urination) is usually associated with inflammation. The pain is typically referred to the tip of the penis in men or to the urethra in women. **Frequency** is the increased number of voids during the daytime, and **nocturia** is nocturnal frequency. Adults normally void five or six times a day and once or not at all during the nighttime hours. Increased numbers of voidings may result from increased urinary output or decreased functional bladder capacity. Diabetes mellitus, diabetes insipidus, excess fluid ingestion, and diuretics (including caffeine and alcohol) are a few of the causes of increased urinary output. Decreased functional bladder capacities may result from bladder outlet obstruction (increased residual urine volume results in a lower functional capacity), neurogenic bladder disorders (spasticity and reduced compliance), extrinsic bladder compression (uterine fibroids, radiation-induced fibrosis, pelvic neoplasms), or psychologic factors (anxiety).

Obstructive Voiding Symptoms

Hesitancy is a delay in the initiation of micturition. It results from the increased time required for the bladder to attain the high pressures necessary to exceed that of the urethra in the obstructed setting. **Decreased force of stream** results from the high resistance the bladder faces and is often associated with a decrease in caliber of the stream. **Intermittency** and **postvoid dribbling** are interruption of the urinary stream and the uncontrolled release of the terminal few drops of urine, respectively. Obstructive symptoms are most commonly due to benign prostatic hyperplasia, urethral stricture, or neurogenic bladder disorders. Less commonly, they may result from prostatic or urethral carcinoma or a foreign body.

Incontinence

Urinary incontinence is the involuntary loss of urine. The history permits subclassification into one of four categories of incontinence. Such a distinction is necessary, as the workup and treatment vary with each of the categories. With **total incontinence,** patients lose urine at all times and in all positions. **Stress incontinence** is the loss of urine associated with activities which result in an increase in intra-abdominal pressure (coughing, sneezing, lifting, exercising). The uncontrolled loss of urine which is preceded by a strong urge to void is known as **urge incontinence.** Chronic urinary retention may result in **overflow incontinence.**

Other Symptoms

Hematospermia, the presence of blood in the ejaculate, usually results from inflammation of the prostate or seminal vesicles. Blood in the initial portion of the ejaculate implicates the prostate, whereas terminal hematospermia implies a seminal vesicle origin.

Pneumaturia, the presence of gas in the urine, is almost always secondary to a fistula between the bladder and the gastrointestinal tract. Diverticulitis, carcinoma of the bladder or sigmoid colon, and regional enteritis are some of the more common underlying causes.

Urethral discharge is the most common symptom of sexually transmitted diseases. Dysuria and urethral itching are commonly seen in association with the discharge. A bloody urethral discharge, especially in an elderly patient, suggests urethral carcinoma.

Cloudy urine may be secondary to a urinary tract infection, yet in the absence of infection it is commonly a result of an alkaline urinary pH. Such conditions result in phosphate crystal precipitation. Chyluria, the presence of lymph in the urine, results from a fistula between the urinary tract and the lymphatic system. Filariasis, tuberculosis, and retroperitoneal tumors are some of the possible causes of this rare symptom.

PHYSICAL EXAMINATION

General Examination

Inspection of the skin may reveal pallor associated with anemia. Cachexia may be seen in malignancy. Gynecomastia occurs in testicular carcinomas or may occur as a treatment-related complication of hormonal therapy in prostatic cancer. Hypertension can be a result of renovascular disease or adrenal cancer. In the pediatric age group, gross deformity of the external ear may be associated with ipsilateral renal anomalies.

Detailed Examination

A. Kidney: Because of the liver, the right kidney is lower than the left. The lower pole of the right kidney may be palpable in thin patients, yet the left kidney is usually not palpable unless abnormally enlarged. To palpate the kidney, one hand is placed posteriorly in the costovertebral angle to push the kidney anteriorly, while the second hand is placed anteriorly under the costal margin. With inspiration, the kidney may be palpated between the two hands. In the pediatric population, a palpable flank mass may be transilluminated to distinguish between a cystic or hydronephrotic kidney from one with a solid mass.

Auscultation of the upper abdominal quadrants in hypertensive patients may reveal a systolic bruit associated with renal artery stenosis or an arteriovenous malformation.

Patients presenting with flank pain should be tested for hyperesthesia of the overlying skin by pin testing, as this may be secondary to nerve root irritation and radiculitis rather than being of renal origin.

B. Bladder: The normal adult bladder is not palpable unless it is filled with at least 150 mL of urine. Percussion is better than palpation in diagnosing the distended bladder. Dullness is perceived over the full bladder and changes to tympany over the air-filled bowel.

Bimanual examination under anesthesia is critical in the evaluation of patients with bladder neoplasms. In the male, the bladder is palpated between the abdominal wall and the rectum while in the female it is palpated between the abdominal wall and the vagina. This is the best means of assessing vesical mobility and thus resectability.

C. Penis: The foreskin must be retracted in the uncircumcised male to permit inspection of the urethral meatus and glans. The position of the urethral meatus, the presence of urethral discharge, inflammation, penile tumor, and other skin lesions must be noted. In **phimosis,** the foreskin cannot be retracted over the glans. In **paraphimosis,** the foreskin has been left retracted behind the glans, resulting in painful engorgement and edema of the glans. If not attended to, this may result in glandular ischemia. Congenital anomalies of position of the urethral meatus are called **hypospadias** when the meatus is lo-

cated on the ventral aspect of the penis, scrotum, or perineum and **epispadias** when it is located on the dorsal aspect of the penis. A thick yellow urethral discharge is seen in gonococcal urethritis, whereas a thin clear or white discharge is noted in nongonococcal urethritis. Palpation of the dorsal penile shaft for plaques of Peyronie's disease and of the ventral surface for urethral tumors should be performed.

D. Scrotum and Its Contents: The most common referral to the urologist involving the scrotum is for evaluation of a scrotal mass. It is thus critical to determine whether the lesion resides within the testicle or whether it is related to the epididymis or cord structures. The testes are palpated between the fingertips of both hands. Normal testes measure 6×4 cm and are rubbery in consistency. The epididymis normally rests posterolateral to the testis and varies in its degree of testicular attachment. Masses arising from within the testes are usually malignant, while those arising from the epididymis and spermatic cord structures are usually benign. Transillumination is critical to the evaluation of any scrotal mass and will distinguish between solid and cystic lesions.

The differential diagnosis of scrotal masses includes both benign and malignant processes. The history and physical examination can make the diagnosis in the majority of cases. Tumors of the testis are usually painless, firm, solid lesions within the substance of the testis. These lesions do not transilluminate.

Acute epididymitis is an acute infectious process of the epididymis and is associated with painful enlargement of the epididymis. Fever and irritative voiding symptoms are common. In advanced states, the infection can spread to the testis, making the distinction between the epididymis and the testicle difficult on physical examination. The entire scrotal contents may be painful on palpation, yet relief may be offered to the supine patient by elevation of the scrotum above the pubic symphysis (Prehn's sign).

A **hydrocele** is a collection of fluid between the two layers of the tunica vaginalis. The diagnosis is readily made by transillumination. Careful evaluation of the testis is necessary, as approximately 10% of testicular tumors may have an associated hydrocele.

A **varicocele** is engorgement of the internal spermatic veins above the testis. These almost always occur on the left side as the left spermatic vein empties into the left renal vein while the right spermatic vein empties into the inferior vena cava. Varicoceles should diminish in size or disappear with the patient in the supine position. The sudden onset of a right varicocele should raise the question of a retroperitoneal malignancy resulting in obstruction of the right spermatic vein.

Torsion of the testis typically occurs in the 10- to 20-year age group and presents with the acute onset of pain and swelling within the testis. Examination may reveal a painful testis that may have a "high lie" in relation to the other testis. The acute onset, lack of voiding symptoms, and the different age distribution may help distinguish it from epididymitis.

Torsion of the appendices of the testis or epididymis may be indistinguishable from torsion of the testis. On occasion a small palpable lump on the superior pole of the testis or epididymis is discernible that may appear blue when the skin is pulled tautly over it ("blue dot sign").

E. Rectal Examination in the Male: Rectal examinations should be performed with the patient bent over the examining table or in the knee-chest position. Inspection for anal pathology (fissures, warts, carcinoma, hemorrhoids) should be performed. Upon insertion of the finger, anal tone can be estimated and a bulbocavernosus reflex can be elicited. As the anal and urinary sphincter derive from a common innervation, important clues to neurogenic disorders may be obtained. The entire prostate is then examined, with attention being directed toward size and consistency. The normal prostate is approximately 4 × cm. Normal consistency is that of the contracted thenar eminence with the thumb opposed to the little finger. Rubbery enlargement of the prostate is noted in benign prostatic hyperplasia. Induration may be perceived with carcinoma but also with chronic inflammation. The remainder of the rectum is then examined to exclude primary rectal disease.

F. Pelvic Examination in the Female: Examination of the introitus should include inspection for atrophic changes, ulcers, discharge, and warts. The urethral meatus can be inspected for caruncles and palpated for tumors or diverticula. Bimanual examination of the bladder, uterus, and adnexa should be performed with two fingers in the vagina and one hand on the abdomen, and attention is directed toward abnormal masses.

URINALYSIS

Collection of Specimens

In the male patient, a clean-catch urine is obtained in separate aliquots. Such a scheme may permit localization of disease. The first 5–10 mL is collected and represents the urethral specimen (VB-1, or voided bladder 1). An aliquot of the midstream specimen (VB-2) represents the bladder and upper urinary tracts. If necessary, the prostate is then massaged and the expressed prostatic secretions are collected. If no fluid is obtained, the next 2–3 mL of urine are collected (VB-3), which reflects the prostate.

Dipstick Urinalysis

A. pH: Dipsticks use two indicators, methyl red and bromthymol blue, which provide a pH range from 5.0 to 9.0. Urinary pH may be helpful in the diagnosis and treatment of some urologic conditions. Alkaline urine in a patient with a urinary tract infec-

tion suggests the presence of a urea-splitting organism, most commonly *Proteus mirabilis,* though some strains of *Klebsiella, Pseudomonas, Providencia,* and *Staphylococcus* may also produce urease. Acidic urine in a patient with urolithiasis suggests uric acid or cystine stones. The inability to acidify the urine below a pH of 5.5 despite acid loading is indicative of renal tubular acidosis.

B. Protein: Dipsticks using bromphenol blue can detect protein in concentrations exceeding 10 mg/dL. It measures albumin and is not sensitive for the light chain of immunoglobulins (Bence Jones proteins). False-positive results are seen in urine containing numerous leukocytes or epithelial cells. Persistently elevated urinary protein levels may indicate glomerulonephropathy or other problems and require further evaluation.

C. Urobilinogen and Bilirubin: Urobilinogen is formed from the catabolism of conjugated bilirubin in the gut by bacteria, and the majority is cleared by the liver. Normally, only 1–4 mg of urobilinogen is excreted in the urine per day. Hemolytic processes or hepatocellular disease can lead to increased urinary levels, while complete biliary obstruction or broad-spectrum antibiotics that alter the gut bacterial flora may result in absent urinary urobilinogen. Unconjugated bilirubin is not filtered by the glomerulus, while only 1% of conjugated bilirubin is filtered. Normally no bilirubin is detected by urinary dipstick, since only concentrations greater than 0.4 mg/dL. are detectable. Conditions manifesting elevated conjugated bilirubin in the serum will result in higher urinary levels. Ascorbic acid may cause false-negative results, while phenazopyridine may cause false-positive results.

D. Glucose and Ketones: Only small amounts of glucose are normally excreted in the urine, and these levels are below the sensitivity of the dipstick. Any positive finding requires medical evaluation to exclude diabetes mellitus. The test is specific for glucose and does not cross-react with any other sugars. Ascorbic acid or elevated ketones may result in false-negative results.

Ketones are not normally found in the urine, but fasting, postexercise states, and pregnancy may result in elevated urinary ketones. Diabetics often demonstrate elevated urinary ketone levels prior to an elevation in serum levels. False-positive results may occur in dehydration or in the presence of levodopa metabolites, mesna (sodium mercaptoethanesulfonate), and other sulfhydryl-containing compounds.

E. Nitrites: Normally, the urine does not contain nitrites. Many gram-negative bacteria can reduce nitrate to nitrite, which is thus an indicator of bacteriuria. However, the low sensitivity of the test requires clarification. Adequate numbers of bacteria must be present (10^5 organisms/mL), nitrates must be available in the urine, and the bacteria must be in contact with the urine for a sufficient time (usually 4 hours).

Therefore, the first morning voided sample is preferable. False-negative results may be due to non-nitrate-reducing organisms, frequent urination, dilute or acidic urine (pH < 6.0), and the presence of urobilinogen. False-positive results are usually secondary to contaminated specimens, so that bacteria are indeed present in the sample yet not present in the urinary tract.

F. Leukocyte Esterase: Leukocyte esterase is an enzyme produced by white cells. The dipstick test is thus a means of detecting leukocytes in the urine, which is thus suggestive but not diagnostic for bacteria. False-positive tests result from specimen contamination. False-negative tests result from high specific gravity, glycosuria, the presence of urobilinogen, and medications, including rifampin, phenazopyridine, and ascorbic acid.

G. Blood: The urinary dipstick for blood measures intact erythrocytes, free hemoglobin, and myoglobin. False-positive results in women may occur as a result of contamination at collection with menstrual blood. Concentrated urine may also cause a false-positive result, as patients normally excrete 1000 erythrocytes per milliliter of urine. Vigorous exercise and vitamins or foods associated with high oxidant levels may also give a false-positive result. High ascorbic acid levels may give a false-negative result.

Microscopic Urinalysis

A. Leukocytes: The presence of more than five leukocytes per high-power field is considered significant pyuria. Leukocytes in the urine are indicative of injury to the urinary tract, which may or may not be due to infection. Other causes of pyuria include calculous disease, stricture disease, neoplasm, glomerulonephropathy, or interstitial cystitis. Leukocyte counts will vary by the state of hydration, method of collection, and degree of injury to the urinary tract.

B. Erythrocytes: The presence of more than five erythrocytes per high-power field is considered significant and warrants further investigation. The appearance of the red cells sometimes gives a clue to their origin within the urinary tract. Dysmorphic (irregularly shaped) cells have an uneven distribution of hemoglobin and cytoplasm. Such cells tend to favor glomerular origin and have dysmorphic features as a consequence of passage through the nephron. Red cells that are round, with evenly distributed hemoglobin, are epithelial in origin and suggest disease along the epithelial lining of the urinary tract. All patients with hematuria require further diagnostic workup (see below); morphology, though of interest, is not of sufficient accuracy to allow firm diagnostic conclusions.

C. Epithelial Cells: The presence of squamous epithelial cells in the urinary sediment is indicative of contamination and thus requires a repeat collection. Transitional epithelial cells are occasionally noted in normal urinary sediment, but if present in large num-bers or clumps they cause concern about possible neoplasm. Experienced cytopathologists are necessary to confirm the finding.

D. Bacteria and Yeasts: The identification of organisms in an uncontaminated specimen implies infection, which must be confirmed by culture. The presence of several organisms per high-power field usually correlates with a culture count of 10^5 organisms per milliliter. Gram staining may further aid in characterizing the organism. *Candida albicans* is the most common yeast seen in the urine, and characteristic budding and clumps are typically observed.

E. Casts: Casts are formed in the distal tubules and collecting ducts as a result of Tamm-Horsfall mucoprotein precipitation. Casts tend to congregate near the edges of the coverslip and are detected best in a fresh specimen viewed under low power. If devoid of cells, hyaline casts are formed. Casts with entrapped red cells are indicative of glomerulonephritis or vasculitis. Leukocyte casts are suggestive of pyelonephritis. Epithelial casts in small numbers are considered normal, but in large numbers they suggest intrinsic renal disease. Granular casts result from degeneration of other cellular casts and also suggest intrinsic renal disease.

F. Crystals: Uric acid, oxalate, and cystine crystals are more often precipitated in acid urine, while phosphate crystals are more commonly seen in alkaline urine. The presence of uric acid, phosphate, and oxalate crystals can be seen in normal patients as well as in stone-formers. Cystine crystals, with a characteristic hexagonal benzene ring shape, are seen only in patients with cystinuria and are thus pathologic.

de Caestecker MP et al: Localization of hematuria by red cell analyzers and phase contrast microscopy. Nephron 1989;52:170.

Hinman F Jr: Differential diagnosis of flank pain. Probl Urol 1989;3:179.

Lowe FC, Brendler CB: Evaluation of the urologic patient. In: *Campbell's Urology,* 6th ed. Walsh PC et al (editors). Saunders, 1992.

Pels RJ et al: Dipstick urinalysis screening of asymptomatic adults for urinary tract disorders. II. Bacteriuria. JAMA 1989;262:1221.

Woolhandler S et al: Dipstick urinalysis screening of asymptomatic adults for urinary tract disorders. I. Hematuria and proteinuria. JAMA 1989;262:1215.

EVALUATION OF HEMATURIA

Evaluation begins with a history and physical examination. If gross hematuria occurs, a description of the timing (initial, terminal, total) may give a clue to the localization of disease. Associated symptoms (ie, renal colic, irritative voiding symptoms, constitutional symptoms) should be investigated. Drug ingestion and associated medical problems may also provide diagnostic clues. Anticoagulants, analgesic abuse (papillary necrosis), cyclophosphamide (chemical cystitis), antibiotics (interstitial nephritis), diabetes mellitus, sickle cell trait or disease (papillary necrosis), a history of stone disease, or malignancy should all be investigated.

Physical examination should emphasize signs of systemic disease (fever, rash, lymphadenopathy, abdominal or pelvic masses) as well as signs of medical renal disease (hypertension, volume overload). Urologic evaluation may demonstrate an enlarged prostate, flank mass, or urethral disease.

Initial laboratory investigations include a urinalysis and urine culture. Proteinuria and casts suggest renal origin. Irritative voiding symptoms, bacteriuria, and a positive urine culture in the female suggests urinary tract infection, but follow-up urinalysis is important after treatment to ensure resolution of the hematuria.

Further evaluation includes urinary cytology, upper tract imaging, and cystoscopy. Cytology assists in the diagnosis of neoplasm, and three voided samples are recommended to maximize sensitivity. Upper tract imaging (usually an intravenous urogram) may identify neoplasms of the kidney or ureter as well as identifying benign conditions such as urolithiasis, obstructive uropathy, papillary necrosis, medullary sponge kidney, or polycystic kidney disease. The role of ultrasonographic evaluation of the urinary tract for hematuria is unclear. While it may provide adequate information for the kidney, its sensitivity in detecting ureteral disease may be lower. In addition, its higher degree of operator dependence may further confound the issue. Cystoscopy can assess for bladder or urethral neoplasm, benign prostatic enlargement, and radiation or chemical cystitis. For gross hematuria, cystoscopy is ideally performed while the patient is actively bleeding to allow better localization (ie, lateralize to one side of the upper tracts, bladder, or urethra).

It is estimated that the cause of the hematuria will be identified in 70% of patients following this evaluation. The remainder may have a form of glomerulonephritis or vascular abnormality. Repeat evaluation is warranted so as to avoid a missed malignancy; however, the ideal frequency of such evaluations is not defined. Urinary cytology can be repeated in 3–6 months, and cystoscopy and upper tract imaging may be repeated in 1 year.

Abuelo JG: Evaluation of hematuria. Urology 1983;21:215.
Messing EM et al: Urinary tract cancers found by home screening with hematuria dipsticks in healthy men over 50 years of age. Cancer 1989;64:2361.

URINARY TRACT INFECTIONS

Urinary tract infections are among the most common entities encountered in medical practice. In acute infections, a single pathogen is usually found, whereas two or more pathogens are often seen in chronic infections. Coliform bacteria are responsible for most nonnosocomial, uncomplicated urinary tract infections, with *E coli* being the most common. Such infections typically are sensitive to a wide variety of orally administered antibiotics and respond quickly. Nosocomial infections often are due to more resistant pathogens and may require parenteral antibiotics. Renal infections are of particular concern because if they are inadequately treated, loss of renal function may result. Previously, a colony count $> 10^5$/mL was considered the criterion for urinary tract infection. However, it is now recognized that up to 50% of women with symptomatic infections have lower counts. In addition, the presence of pyuria correlates poorly with the diagnosis of urinary tract infection, and thus urinalysis alone is not adequate for diagnosis. With respect to treatment, soft tissue infections (pyelonephritis, prostatitis) require intensive therapy for 3–4 weeks, while mucosal infections (cystitis) may require 1–3 days of therapy.

Classification & Pathogenesis

First infections—ie, first documented infections—in young women tend to be uncomplicated. **Unresolved bacteriuria** occurs when the urinary tract is never sterilized during therapy. This may result from bacterial resistance to therapy, noncompliance, mixed infections with organisms having different susceptibilities, renal insufficiency, or the rapid emergence of resistance from an initially sensitive organism. **Persistent bacteriuria** occurs when the urinary tract is initially sterilized during therapy but a persistent source of infection in contact with the urinary tract remains. This may result from infected stones, chronic pyelonephritis or prostatitis, vesicoenteric or vesicovaginal fistulas, obstructive uropathy, foreign bodies, or urethral diverticula. **Reinfections** occur when new infections with new pathogens occur following successful treatment.

Ascending infection from the urethra is the most common route. Women are particularly at risk for urinary tract infections because the female urethra is short and the vagina becomes colonized with bacteria. Sexual intercourse is a major precipitating factor in young women. Pyelonephritis most commonly results from ascent of infection up the ureter. **Hematogenous spread** to the urinary tract is uncommon, with the exceptions being tuberculosis and cortical renal abscesses. **Lymphogenous spread** is rare. **Di-**

rect extension from other organs may occur, especially from intraperitoneal abscesses in inflammatory bowel disease or pelvic inflammatory disease.

Susceptibility Factors

A. Bacterial Virulence Factors: Over 90% of first infections are caused by *E coli*. While there are over 150 strains of *E coli*, most infections are caused by only five serogroups (O1, O4, O6, O18, and O75). It appears that strains implicated in infection have a higher degree of bacterial adherence, which is mediated by the bacterial fimbriae or pili. A relationship between the type of fimbriae and the type of infection exists. P-fimbriated strains of *E coli* are associated with pyelonephritis in normal urinary tracts, whereas strains without P fimbriae are associated with pyelonephritis only when vesicoureteral reflux is present.

B. Host Susceptibility Factors:

1. Bladder and upper tract factors–Intrinsic defense mechanisms in the bladder include efficient emptying of the bladder with voiding, which decreases colony counts; a protective glycosaminoglycan layer, which interferes with bacterial adherence; and the antimicrobial properties of urine (high osmolality and extremes of pH). The presence of vesicoureteral reflux, diminished renal blood flow, or intrinsic renal disease may increase the likelihood of upper tract involvement.

2. Female-specific factors–The anatomically short female urethra facilitates the ascent of organisms from the introitus into the bladder. Women with recurrent urinary tract infections have more adhesin receptors on their genitourinary mucosa and therefore have more binding sites for pathogens. Women whose mucosal secretions lack fucosyltransferase activity ("nonsecretors") are more prone to urinary tract infections. The lack of this enzyme results in lack of expression of the A, B, and H blood group antigens that normally may mask some of the bacterial adhesin receptors, making these receptors more available for pathogen binding.

3. Male-specific factors–A higher incidence of urinary tract infections in the uncircumcised male in comparison to the circumcised male has been observed. The mucosal surface of the foreskin has a propensity for colonization with P-fimbriated bacteria in a fashion analogous to that of the female introitus. The prostate in normal males secretes zinc, which is a potent antibacterial agent and thus prevents ascending infection. Lower zinc levels are seen in prostatic secretions of men with bacterial prostatitis.

Prevention of Reinfections

Prophylactic antibiotic therapy is given to prevent recurrence after treatment of urinary tract infection. The two most common urologic indications are children with vesicoureteral reflux and women with recurrent cystitis. Only the latter will be addressed here.

Women who have more than three episodes of cystitis per year are considered candidates for prophylaxis. Prior to institution of therapy, a thorough urologic evaluation is warranted to exclude any anatomic abnormality (stones, reflux, fistula, etc). Only selected antimicrobial agents are effective in prophylaxis. To be successful, the agent must eliminate pathogenic bacteria from the fecal or introital reservoirs and not cause bacterial resistance. Single dosing at bedtime or at the time of intercourse is the recommended schedule. The three most commonly used agents for prophylaxis are trimethoprim-sulfamethoxazole (40 mg/200 mg), nitrofurantoin (100 mg), and cephalexin (250 mg).

ACUTE PYELONEPHRITIS

Essentials of Diagnosis

- Fever.
- Flank pain.
- Irritative voiding symptoms.
- Positive urine culture.

General Considerations

Acute pyelonephritis is an infectious inflammatory disease involving the kidney parenchyma and renal pelvis. Gram-negative bacteria are the most common causative agents including *E coli, Proteus, Klebsiella, Enterobacter,* and *Pseudomonas.* Gram-positive bacteria are less commonly seen, including *Streptococcus faecalis* and *Staphylococcus aureus.* The infection usually ascends from the lower urinary tract—with the exception of *S aureus,* which usually is spread by a hematogenous route.

Clinical Findings

A. Symptoms and Signs: Symptoms include fever, flank pain, shaking chills, and irritative voiding symptoms (urgency, frequency, dysuria). Nausea and vomiting and diarrhea are not uncommon. Young children may have fever and abdominal discomfort. Signs include fever and tachycardia. Costovertebral angle tenderness is usually pronounced.

B. Laboratory Findings: Complete blood count shows leukocytosis and a left shift. Urinalysis shows pyuria, bacteriuria, and varying degrees of hematuria. White cell casts may be seen. Urine culture demonstrates heavy growth of the offending agent.

C. Imaging: In complicated pyelonephritis, renal ultrasound may show hydronephrosis from a stone or other source of obstruction.

Differential Diagnosis

Acute intra-abdominal disease such as appendicitis, cholecystitis, pancreatitis, or diverticulitis must be distinguished from pyelonephritis. A normal urinalysis is seen in gastrointestinal disorders, and abnormal liver function tests or elevated amylase levels will assist in the differentiation. Lower lobe pneumonia is distinguishable by the pleuritic chest pain and abnormal chest radiograph.

In the male patient, the main differential diagnosis for a febrile urinary tract infection includes acute epididymitis, acute prostatitis, and acute pyelonephritis. Physical examination and the location of the pain should permit this distinction.

Treatment

Severe infections or complicating factors require hospital admission. Urine and blood cultures are obtained to identify the causative agent and to determine antimicrobial sensitivity. Intravenous ampicillin and an aminoglycoside are initiated prior to obtaining sensitivity results. In the outpatient setting, trimethoprim-sulfamethoxazole or quinolones may be initiated (Table 21–1). Antibiotics are adjusted according to sensitivities. Fevers may persist for up to 72 hours; failure to respond warrants radiographic imaging (ultrasound) to exclude complicating factors that may require prompt intervention. Catheter drainage may be necessary in the face of urinary retention, and nephrostomy drainage required if there is ureteral obstruction. In inpatients, intravenous antibiotics are maintained for 24 hours after the patient defervesces, and oral antibiotics are then given to complete a 3-week course of therapy. Follow-up urine cultures are mandatory upon the completion of treatment.

Prognosis

With prompt diagnosis and appropriate treatment, acute pyelonephritis carries a good prognosis. Complicating factors, underlying renal disease, and increasing patient age may lead to a less favorable outcome.

ACUTE CYSTITIS

Essentials of Diagnosis

- Irritative voiding symptoms.
- Patient usually afebrile.
- Positive urine culture.

General Considerations

Acute cystitis is an infection of the bladder most commonly due to the coliform bacteria (especially *E coli*) and occasionally gram-positive bacteria (enterococci). Viral cystitis due to adenovirus is sometimes seen in children but is rare in adults. The route of infection is typically ascending from the urethra.

Clinical Findings

A. Symptoms and Signs: Irritative voiding symptoms are common (frequency, urgency, dysuria) as well as suprapubic discomfort. Women may demonstrate gross hematuria. Symptoms in women may often appear following sexual intercourse. Physical examination may elicit suprapubic tenderness, but examination is often unremarkable. Systemic toxicity is absent.

B. Laboratory Findings: Urinalysis shows pyuria and bacteriuria and varying degrees of hematu-

Table 21–1. Empiric therapy for urinary tract infections.

Diagnosis	Antibiotic	Route	Duration
Acute pyelonephritis	Ampicillin, 1 g every 6 hours, and gentamicin, 1 mg/kg every 8 hours	IV	21 days
	Trimethoprim-sulfamethoxazole, 160/800 mg every 12 hours	Orally	21 days
	Ciprofloxacin, 750 mg every 12 hours	Orally	21 days
Chronic pyelonephritis	Same as acute pyelonephritis but duration of therapy is 3–6 months.		
Acute cystitis	Trimethoprim-sulfamethoxazole, 160/800 mg every 12 hours	Orally	1–3 days
	Cephalexin, 250–500 mg every 6 hours	Orally	1–3 days
	Ciprofloxacin, 250–500 mg every 12 hours	Orally	1–3 days
	Norfloxacin, 400 mg every 12 hours	Orally	1–3 days
Acute bacterial prostatitis	Same as for acute pyelonephritis		21 days
Chronic bacterial prostatitis	Trimethoprim-sulfamethoxazole, 160/800 mg every 12 hours	Orally	1–3 months
	Ciprofloxacin, 250–500 mg every 12 hours	Orally	1–3 months
Acute epididymitis Sexually transmitted	Ceftriaxone, 250 mg as single dose, plus doxycycline, 100 mg every 12 hours	IM Orally	10 days
Non-sexually transmitted	Same as chronic bacterial prostatitis.		3 weeks

ria. The degree of pyuria and bacteriuria does not necessarily correlate with the severity of symptoms. Urine culture is positive for the offending organism, but colony counts exceeding 10^5/mL are not essential for the diagnosis.

C. Imaging: Follow-up imaging is warranted only if pyelonephritis, recurrent infections, or anatomic abnormalities are suspected.

Differential Diagnosis

In women, infectious processes such as vulvovaginitis and pelvic inflammatory disease can usually be distinguished by pelvic examination and urinalysis. Children may have vulvar or urethral irritation from detergents or bubble bath. In men, urethritis and prostatitis may be distinguished by physical examination (urethral discharge or prostatic tenderness). Cystitis in males is rare and implies a pathologic process such as infected stones, prostatitis, or chronic urinary retention requiring further investigation.

Noninfectious causes of cystitis-like symptoms include pelvic irradiation, chemotherapy (cyclophosphamide), bladder carcinoma, interstitial cystitis, voiding dysfunction disorders, and psychosomatic disorders.

Treatment

Uncomplicated cystitis in women can be treated with short-term antimicrobial therapy, which consists of single-dose therapy or 1–3 days of therapy. Trimethoprim-sulfamethoxazole or cephalexin is often effective (Table 21–1). Because uncomplicated cystitis is rare in men, elucidation of the underlying problem with appropriate investigations is warranted. Hot sitz baths or urinary analgesics (phenazopyridine) may provide symptomatic relief.

Prognosis

Infections typically respond rapidly to therapy, and failure to respond suggests resistance to the selected drug or anatomic abnormalities requiring further investigation.

ACUTE BACTERIAL PROSTATITIS

Essentials of Diagnosis
- Fever.
- Irritative voiding symptoms.
- Perineal or suprapubic pain; exquisite tenderness common on rectal examination.
- Positive urine culture.

General Considerations

Acute bacterial prostatitis is usually caused by gram-negative rods, especially *E coli* and *Pseudomonas* species and less commonly by gram-positive organisms (eg, *Enterococcus*). The most likely routes of infection include ascent up the urethra and reflux of infected urine into the prostatic ducts. Lymphatic and hematogenous routes are probably rare.

Clinical Findings

A. Symptoms and Signs: Perineal, sacral, or suprapubic pain, fever, and irritative voiding complaints are common. Varying degrees of obstructive symptoms may occur as the acutely inflamed prostate swells, which may lead to urinary retention. High fevers and a warm and tender prostate are detected on examination. Care should be taken in performing a gentle rectal examination, as vigorous manipulations may result in septicemia. Prostatic massage is contraindicated.

B. Laboratory Findings: Complete blood count shows leukocytosis and a left shift. Urinalysis shows pyuria, bacteriuria and varying degrees of hematuria. Urine cultures will demonstrate the offending pathogen.

Differential Diagnosis

Acute pyelonephritis or acute epididymitis should be distinguishable by the location of pain as well as by physical examination. Acute diverticulitis is occasionally confused with acute prostatitis; however, the history and urinalysis should permit clear distinction. Urinary retention from benign or malignant prostatic enlargement is distinguishable by initial or follow-up rectal examination (Table 21–1).

Treatment & Prognosis

Hospitalization is usually required and parenteral antibiotics (ampicillin and aminoglycoside) should be initiated until organism sensitivities are available (Table 21–1). After the patient is afebrile for 24–48 hours, appropriate oral antibiotics are used to complete 4–6 weeks of therapy. Effective oral agents include trimethoprim-sulfamethoxazole and quinolones, depending upon sensitivities. If urinary retention develops, urethral catheterization or instrumentation is contraindicated, and a percutaneous suprapubic tube is required. Follow-up urine culture and examination of prostatic secretions should be performed after the completion of therapy to ensure eradication.

Prognosis

With effective treatment, chronic bacterial prostatitis is rare.

CHRONIC BACTERIAL PROSTATITIS

Essentials of Diagnosis
- Irritative voiding symptoms.
- Perineal or suprapubic discomfort, often dull and poorly localized.
- Positive expressed prostatic secretions and culture.

General Considerations

Although chronic bacterial prostatitis may evolve from acute bacterial prostatitis, many men have no history of acute infection. Gram-negative rods are the most common etiologic agents, but only one gram-positive organism *(Enterococcus)* is associated with chronic infection. Routes of infection are the same as discussed for acute infection.

Clinical Findings

A. Symptoms and Signs: Clinical manifestations are variable. Some patients are asymptomatic, but most have varying degrees of irritative voiding symptoms. Low back and perineal pain is not uncommon. Many patients report a history of urinary tract infections. Physical examination is often unremarkable, though the prostate may feel normal, boggy, or indurated.

B. Laboratory Findings: Urinalysis is normal unless a secondary cystitis is present. Expressed prostatic secretions demonstrate increased numbers of leukocytes (> 10/hpf), especially lipid-laden macrophages. However, this finding is consistent with inflammation and is not diagnostic of bacterial prostatitis. Culture of the secretions or VB-3 is necessary to make the diagnosis.

C. Imaging: Imaging tests are not necessary, though pelvic radiographs or transrectal ultrasound may demonstrate prostatic calculi.

Differential Diagnosis

Chronic urethritis may mimic chronic prostatitis, though cultures of the fractionated urine will localize the source of infection. Cystitis may be secondary to prostatitis, yet again fractionated urine samples should localize the infection. Anal disease may share some of the symptoms of prostatitis, but physical examination should permit a distinction between the two (Table 21–2).

Treatment

Few antimicrobial agents attain therapeutic intraprostatic levels in the absence of acute inflammation. Trimethoprim does diffuse into the prostate, and trimethoprim-sulfamethoxazole is associated with the best cure rates (Table 21–1). Other effective agents include carbenicillin, erythromycin, cephalexin, and, more recently, the quinolones. The optimal duration of therapy remains controversial, ranging from 6 to 12 weeks. Symptomatic relief may be provided by anti-inflammatory agents (indomethacin, ibuprofen) and hot sitz baths.

Prognosis

Chronic bacterial prostatitis is difficult to cure, but its symptoms and tendency to cause recurrent urinary tract infections can be controlled by suppressive antibiotic therapy.

NONBACTERIAL PROSTATITIS

Essentials of Diagnosis

- Irritative voiding symptoms.
- Perineal or suprapubic discomfort, similar to that of chronic bacterial prostatitis.
- Positive expressed prostatic secretions, but culture is negative.

General Considerations

Nonbacterial prostatitis is the most common of the prostatitis syndromes, and its cause is unknown. Speculation implicates chlamydiae, mycoplasmas, *Ureaplasma,* and viruses, but no substantial proof exists. Nonbacterial prostatitis is believed to represent a noninfectious inflammatory disorder. Some investigators believe that it is an autoimmune disease. Nonbacterial prostatitis is thus a diagnosis of exclusion.

Clinical Findings

A. Symptoms and Signs: The clinical presentation is identical to that of chronic bacterial prostatitis; however, no history of urinary tract infections is present.

B. Laboratory Findings: Increased numbers of leukocytes are seen on expressed prostatic secretions, but all cultures are negative.

Differential Diagnosis

The major distinction is from chronic bacterial

Table 21–2. Clinical characteristics of prostatitis and prostatodynia syndromes.

Findings	Acute Bacterial Prostatitis	Chronic Bacterial Prostatitis	Nonbacterial Prostatitis	Prostatodynia
Fever	+	–	–	–
Urinalysis	+	–	–	–
Expressed prostatic secretions	Contraindicated	–	–	–
Bacterial culture	+	+	–	–

Key: + = finding present or laboratory test positive
    – = finding absent or laboratory test negative

prostatitis. The absence of a history of urinary tract infection and of positive cultures makes the distinction (Table 21–2). In older men with irritative voiding symptoms and negative cultures, the possibility of bladder cancer must be excluded. Urinary cytologic examination and cystoscopy are warranted.

Treatment

Because of the uncertainty regarding the etiology of nonbacterial prostatitis, a trial of antimicrobial therapy directed against *Ureaplasma, Mycoplasma,* or *Chlamydia* is warranted. Erythromycin or minocycline can be initiated for 14 days yet should only be continued if a favorable clinical response ensues. Some symptomatic relief may be obtained with anti-inflammatory agents or sitz baths. Dietary restrictions are not necessary unless the patient relates a history of symptom exacerbation by certain substances such as alcohol, caffeine, and perhaps certain foods.

Prognosis

Annoying, recurrent symptoms are common, but serious sequelae have not been identified.

PROSTATODYNIA

Prostatodynia is a noninflammatory disorder that affects young and middle-aged men and has variable causes. The term prostatodynia is a misnomer, as the prostate is actually normal. Causes include voiding dysfunction and pelvic floor musculature dysfunction.

Clinical Findings

A. Symptoms and Signs: Symptoms are the same as those seen with chronic prostatitis, yet there is no history of urinary tract infection. Additional symptoms may include hesitancy and interruption of flow. Patients may relate a lifelong history of voiding difficulty. Physical examination is unremarkable, but increased anal sphincter tone and paraprostatic tenderness may be observed.

B. Laboratory Findings: Urinalysis is normal. Expressed prostatic secretions show normal numbers of leukocytes. Urodynamic testing may show signs of dysfunctional voiding (detrusor contraction without urethral relaxation, high urethral pressures, spasms of the urinary sphincter).

Differential Diagnosis

Normal urinalysis will distinguish it from acute infectious processes. Examination of expressed prostatic secretions is crucial to distinguish this entity from prostatitis syndromes (Table 21–2).

Treatment

Bladder neck and urethral spasms can be treated by α-blocking agents. Pelvic floor muscle dysfunction may respond to diazepam and biofeedback techniques. Sitz baths may contribute to symptomatic relief.

Prognosis

Prognosis is variable depending upon the specific cause.

ACUTE EPIDIDYMITIS

Essentials of Diagnosis

- Fever.
- Irritative voiding symptoms.
- Painful enlargement of epididymis.

General Considerations

Most cases of acute epididymitis are infectious and can be divided into one of two categories that have different age distributions and etiologic agents. Sexually transmitted forms typically occur in men under age 40, are associated with urethritis, and result from *C trachomatis* or *N gonorrhoeae*. Non-sexually transmitted forms typically occur in older men, are associated with urinary tract infections and prostatitis, and are caused by gram-negative rods. The route of infection is probably via the urethra to the ejaculatory duct and then down the vas deferens to the epididymis.

Clinical Findings

A. Symptoms and Signs: Symptoms may follow acute physical strain (heavy lifting) or trauma or sexual activity. Associated symptoms of urethritis (pain at the tip of the penis and urethral discharge) or cystitis (irritative voiding symptoms) may occur. Pain develops in the scrotum and may radiate along the spermatic cord or to the flank. Fever and scrotal swelling is usually apparent. Early in the course, the epididymis may be distinguishable from the testis; however, later the two may appear as one enlarged, tender mass. The prostate may be tender on rectal examination.

B. Laboratory Findings: Complete blood count shows leukocytosis and a left shift. In the sexually transmitted variety, Gram staining of a smear of urethral discharge may be diagnostic of gram-negative intracellular diplococci *(N gonorrhoeae)*. White cells without visible organisms on urethral smear represent nongonococcal urethritis, and *C trachomatis* is the most likely pathogen. In the non-sexually transmitted variety, urinalysis shows pyuria, bacteriuria, and varying degrees of hematuria. Urine cultures will demonstrate the offending pathogen.

C. Imaging: Scrotal ultrasound may aid in the diagnosis if examination is difficult because of the presence of a large hydrocele or because questions exist regarding the diagnosis.

Differential Diagnosis

Tumors generally cause painless enlargement of the testis. Urinalysis is negative, and examination reveals a normal epididymis. Scrotal ultrasound is helpful to define the pathology. Testicular torsion usually occurs in prepubertal males but is occasionally seen in young adults. Acute onset of symptoms and a negative urinalysis favors torsion. Prehn's sign (elevation of the scrotum above the pubic symphysis improves pain from epididymitis) may be helpful but is not completely reliable. Torsion of one of the testicular or epididymal appendages also usually occurs in prepubertal males, and the history and urinalysis are most helpful in making the distinction.

Treatment

Bed rest with scrotal elevation is important in the acute phase. Treatment is directed towards the identified pathogen (Table 21–1). The sexually transmitted variety is treated with 10–21 days of antibiotics, and the sexual partner must be treated as well. Non-sexually transmitted forms are treated for 21–28 days with appropriate antibiotics, at which time evaluation of the urinary tract is warranted to identify underlying disease.

Prognosis

Prompt treatment usually results in a favorable outcome. Delayed or inadequate treatment may result in epididymo-orchitis, decreased fertility, or abscess formation.

Berger RE et al: Case-control study of men with suspected chronic idiopathic prostatitis. J Urol 1989;141:328.

Doble A et al: The role of *Chlamydia trachomatis* in chronic abacterial prostatitis: A study using ultrasound guided biopsy. J Urol 1989;141:332.

Meares EM Jr: Acute and chronic prostatitis: Diagnosis and treatment. Infect Dis Clin North Am 1987;1:855.

Sheinfeld J et al: Association of the Lewis blood-group phenotype with recurrent urinary tract infections in women. N Engl J Med 1989;320:773.

Stamm WE et al: Urinary tract infections: From pathogenesis to treatment. J Infect Dis 1989;159:400.

URINARY STONE DISEASE

Stone disease in the United States is increasing in incidence and is estimated to afflict 240,000–720,000 Americans per year. Men are more frequently affected by urolithiasis than women, with a ratio of 4:1. Initial presentation predominates in the third and fourth decades. The ratio of men to women approaches parity in the sixth and seventh decades.

There are five major types of urinary stones: calcium oxalate, calcium phosphate, struvite, uric acid, and cystine. The most common types are composed of calcium. Most urinary stones are radiopaque. Uric acid stones can be radiolucent yet frequently are composed of a combination of uric acid and calcium oxalate and thus are radiopaque. Cystine stones frequently have a ground-glass appearance.

Geographic factors contribute to the development of stones. In developing countries, children—especially prepubescent boys—are prone to bladder calculi. In industrialized countries, most calculi are seen in adults as renal or ureteral stones. Areas of high humidity and elevated temperatures appear to be contributing factors, and the incidence of symptomatic ureteral stones is greatest during hot summer months.

Diet and fluid intake may be important factors in the development of urinary stones. Excess intake of calcium, oxalate, and purines can increase the incidence of stones in predisposed individuals. Additionally, water or other fluid intake is important in preventing urolithiasis. Persons in sedentary occupations have a higher incidence of stones than manual laborers.

Genetic factors may contribute to urinary stone formation. Cystinuria is an autosomal recessive disorder. Homozygous individuals have markedly increased excretion of cystine and frequently have numerous recurrent episodes of urinary stones despite attempts to optimize medical treatment. Renal tubular acidosis appears to be transmitted as a hereditary trait, and urolithiasis occurs in up to 75% of patients affected with this disorder.

Clinical Findings

A. Symptoms and Signs: Obstructing urinary stones usually present with acute colic. Pain usually occurs suddenly, is localized to the flank, is usually severe, and may be associated with nausea and vomiting. Patients are constantly moving—in sharp contrast to those with an acute abdomen. The pain may occur episodically and may radiate anteriorly over the abdomen. As the stone progresses down the ureter, the pain may be referred into the ipsilateral testis or labium. If the stone becomes lodged at the ureterovesical junction, patients will complain of marked urinary urgency and frequency. Stone size does not correlate with the severity of the symptoms.

B. Laboratory Findings: Urinalysis usually reveals microscopic or gross hematuria. However, the absence of microhematuria does not exclude urinary stones. Infection must be excluded, because the combination of infection and urinary tract obstruction requires prompt intervention as described below. Urinary pH is a valuable clue as to the cause of the possible stone. Persistent urinary pH below 5.0 is suggestive of uric acid or cystine stones, both relatively radiolucent as seen on plain films of the abdomen. In contrast, a persistent pH above 7.5 is suggestive of a struvite infection stone, radiopaque on plain films.

C. Imaging: A plain film of the abdomen and renal ultrasound examination will diagnose most stones. Stones suspected of being located at the ureterovesical junction can be imaged with ultrasonography with the aid of the acoustic window of a full bladder. When the diagnosis remains uncertain, intravenous urography is indicated.

Medical Treatment & Prevention

To reduce the recurrence rate of urinary stones, one must attempt to achieve a stone-free status. Small stone fragments may serve as a nidus for future stone development. Selected patients must be thoroughly evaluated and followed in a stone clinic to reduce stone recurrence rates. If no medical treatment is provided after surgery, stones will recur in 50% of patients within 5 years. Of greatest importance in reducing stone recurrence is an increased fluid intake. Absolute volumes are not targeted, yet doubling previous fluid intake is recommended. Patients are encouraged to ingest fluids during meals, 2 hours after each meal (when the body is most dehydrated), and prior to going to sleep in the evening—enough to awaken the patient to void during the night. Increasing fluids only during daylight hours may not dilute a supersaturated urine and thus initiate a new stone.

A. Calcium Nephrolithiasis:

1. Hypercalciuric—Hypercalciuric calcium nephrolithiasis (> 200 mg/24 h) can be caused by absorptive, resorptive, and renal disorders.

Absorptive hypercalciuria is secondary to increased absorption of calcium at the level of the small bowel, predominantly in the jejunum, and can be further subdivided into types I, II, and III. Type I absorptive hypercalciuria is independent of calcium intake. There is increased urinary calcium on a regular or even a calcium-restricted diet. Treatment is centered upon decreasing bowel absorption of calcium. Cellulose phosphate, a chelating agent, is an effective form of therapy. It binds to the calcium and impedes small bowel absorption due to its increased bulk. Cellulose phosphate does not change the intestinal transport mechanism. It should be given with meals so it will be available to bind to the calcium. Taking this chelating agent prior to bedtime is ineffective. Growing children or postmenopausal women should not be treated. It is interesting, however, that there is no change in bone density after long-term use. Inappropriate use without a metabolic evaluation may result in a negative calcium balance and a secondary parathyroid stimulation. Long-term use may result in hypomagnesemia and secondary hyperoxaluria.

Thiazide therapy is an alternative to cellulose phosphate in the treatment of type I absorptive hypercalciuria. Thiazides have no impact on intestinal absorption. This therapy results in increased bone density of approximately 1% per year. This stabilizes over time. Thiazides have limited long-term utility as they lose their hypocalciuric effect with continued therapy.

Type II absorptive hypercalciuria is diet-dependent. Decreasing calcium intake by 50% (approximately 400 mg/d) will decrease the hypercalciuria to normal values (150–200 mg/24 h). There is no specific medical therapy.

Type III absorptive hypercalciuria is secondary to a renal phosphate leak. This results in increased vitamin D synthesis and secondarily increased small bowel absorption. This can be readily reversed by orthophosphates. Orthophosphates (0.5 g three times per day) do not change intestinal absorption but rather inhibit vitamin D synthesis.

Resorptive hypercalciuria is secondary to hyperparathyroidism. The stigmas of this disease can make the diagnosis obvious, including hypercalcemia, hypophosphatemia, hypercalciuria, and an elevated parathyroid hormone value. Appropriate surgical resection of the adenoma cures the disease and the urinary stones. Medical management is invariably a failure.

Finally, in renal hypercalciuria, the renal tubules are unable to efficiently deal with a calcium load, and hypercalciuria results. Spilling calcium in the urine results in secondary hyperparathyroidism. Serum calcium is normal. Hydrochlorothiazides are effective long-term therapy in patients with this disorder.

2. Hyperuricosuric—Hyperuricosuric calcium nephrolithiasis is secondary to dietary excesses or uric acid metabolic defects. Both disorders can be treated with purine dietary restrictions or allopurinol therapy (or both). In contrast to uric acid nephrolithiasis, hyperuricosuric calcium stones will maintain a urinary pH greater than 5.5. Monosodium urates absorb inhibitors and promote heterogeneous nucleation. Hyperuricosuric calcium nephrolithiasis is probably secondary to epitaxy, or heterogeneous nucleation. In such situations, similar crystal structures (ie, uric acid and calcium oxalate) can grow together with the aid of a protein matrix infrastructure.

3. Hyperoxaluric—Hyperoxaluric calcium nephrolithiasis is usually due to primary intestinal disorders. Patients usually present with a history of chronic diarrhea frequently associated with inflammatory bowel disease or steatorrhea. Increased bowel fat combines with intraluminal calcium to form a soap-like product. Calcium is therefore unavailable to bind to oxalate, which is then freely and rapidly absorbed. A small increase in oxalate absorption will significantly increase stone formation. If the diarrhea or steatorrhea cannot be effectively curtailed, oral calcium supplements should be given with meals. Emphasis on encouraging increased fluid intake is required for these patients as for all stone-formers.

4. Hypocitraturic—Hypocitraturic calcium nephrolithiasis is secondary to chronic diarrhea, type I (distal tubule) renal tubular acidosis, and chronic hydrochlorothiazide treatment and in rare case is idiopathic. It is frequently associated with other forms of calcium stone formation. Citrate appears to bind to calcium in solution, thereby decreasing available calcium for stone formation. Potassium citrate supplements may be effective. The potassium will supplement the frequent hypokalemic states, and citrate will help to correct the acidosis.

B. Uric Acid Calculi: The average urinary pH is 6.4. Uric acid stone-formers frequently have urinary pH values less than 5.5. The pK of uric acid is 5.75, at which point half of the uric acid is ionized as a urate salt and is soluble, while the other half is insoluble. Increasing the pH above 6.5 dramatically increases solubility and can effectively dissolve large calculi. Patients with uric acid calculi should be given nitrazine pH paper with which to monitor the effectiveness of their urinary alkalinization. Other contributing factors include hyperuricemia, myeloproliferative disorders, malignancy with increased uric acid production, and uricosuric medications. If hyperuricemia is present, allopurinol should be instituted. Although pure uric acid stones are relatively radiolucent, most have some calcium components and can be visualized on plain abdominal radiographs. Renal ultrasonography is a helpful adjunct for appropriate diagnosis and long-term management.

C. Struvite Calculi: Struvite stones are synonymous with magnesium-ammonium-phosphate stones. They are commonly seen in women with recurrent urinary tract infections recalcitrant to appropriate antibiotics. They rarely form as ureteral stones. Frequently they are discovered as a large staghorn calculi forming a cast of the renal collecting system. These stones are radiodense. Urinary pH is high, usually above 7.0–7.5. These stones are formed secondary to urease-producing organisms, including *Proteus, Pseudomonas, Providencia,* and less commonly *Klebsiella.* These frequently large stones are relatively soft and amenable to percutaneous nephrolithotomy. Appropriate perioperative antibiotics are required. These stones can recur rapidly, and efforts

should be taken to render the patient stone-free. Postoperative irrigation through nephrostomy tubes can eliminate small fragments. Acetohydroxamic acid is an effective urease inhibitor. However, because of gastrointestinal side effects, it is poorly tolerated by most patients.

D. Cystine Calculi: Cystine stones are a result of abnormal excretion of cystine, ornithine, lysine, and arginine. Cystine is the only amino acid that becomes insoluble in urine. These stones are particularly difficult to manage medically. Prevention is centered around increased fluid intake, alkalinization of the urine above pH 7.5 (monitored with nitrazine pH paper), and a variety of medications including penicillamine and tiopronin.

Metabolic Evaluation

Stone analysis should be performed on recovered stones. Much controversy exists in deciding which patients need a thorough metabolic evaluation for stone disease. Uncomplicated first-time stone-formers should probably undergo blood screening for abnormalities of serum calcium, phosphate, electrolytes, and uric acid as a baseline.

More extensive evaluation is required in recurrent stone-formers or patients with a family history of stone disease. A 24-hour urine collection on a random diet should ascertain volume, urinary pH, and calcium, uric acid, oxalate, and citrate excretion. A second collection on a restricted calcium (400 mg/d), sodium (100 meq/d), and oxalate diet is undertaken to subcategorize patients, if necessary. Serum PTH and calcium load tests can be performed at a third visit. Table 21–3 demonstrates the diagnostic criteria for the hypercalciuric states.

Surgical Treatment

Forced intravenous fluids will not push stones down the ureter. Effective peristalsis requires coaptation of the ureteral walls. Massive diuresis is counterproductive and will exacerbate the pain. Appropriate pain medications are required. Associated fever may

Table 21–3. Diagnostic criteria of different types of hypercalciuria.

	Absorptive Type I	Absorptive Type II	Absorptive Type III	Resorptive	Renal
Serum					
Calcium	N	N	N	+	N
Phosphorus	N	N	–	–	N
PTH	N	N	N	+	+
Vitamin D	N	N	+	+	+
Urinary calcium					
Fasting	N	N	+	+	+
Restricted	+	N	+	+	+
After calcium load	+	+	+	+	+

Key: + = elevated
– = low
N = normal

represent infection, which is a medical emergency. Fever in association with upper tract obstruction requires prompt drainage by a ureteral catheter or a percutaneous nephrostomy tube. Antibiotics alone in the face of impending or florid urosepsis are unsatisfactory.

A. Ureteral Stones: Impediment to urine flow by ureteral stones usually occurs at three sites: (1) at the ureteropelvic junction, (2) at the crossing of the ureter over the iliac vessels, and finally (3) as the ureter enters the bladder at the ureterovesical junction. Prediction of spontaneous stone passage is difficult. Stones less than 6 mm in diameter as seen on a plain abdominal radiograph will usually pass spontaneously. Conservative observation with appropriate pain medications is appropriate for the first few months. If spontaneous stone passage has failed, therapeutic intervention is required. Distal ureteral stones are best managed either with ureteroscopic stone extraction or in situ extracorporeal shock wave lithotripsy (ESWL). Ureteroscopic stone extraction involves placement of a small endoscope per urethram. Under direct vision, basket extraction or fragmentation followed by extraction is performed. Complications during endoscopic retrieval increase as the duration of conservative observation increases beyond 2 months. Indications for earlier intervention include severe pain unresponsive to medications, fever, persistent nausea and vomiting requiring intravenous hydration, social requirements requiring return to work, or anticipated remote travel. Most upper tract stones that enter the bladder can exit the urethra with minimal discomfort.

In situ ESWL, an alternative, utilizes an external energy source that is focused upon the stone. This focused energy is additive, resulting in minimal tissue insult except at the focus where the stone is positioned with the aid of fluoroscopy or ultrasonography. This can be performed under monitored anesthesia care as an outpatient procedure and usually results in stone fragmentation. It requires time for the stone fragments to pass spontaneously. Women of childbearing age should not be treated with ESWL for stone in the lower ureter, as the impact upon the ovary is unknown.

Proximal and midureteral stones—those above the inferior margin of the sacroiliac joint—can be treated with ESWL or ureteroscopy. ESWL can be delivered directly to the stone in situ, or the stones can be pushed back into the renal pelvis (via a retrograde ureteral catheter) to allow for a more capacious surrounding space and thus for more efficient fragmentation. To help ensure adequate drainage after ESWL, a double J ureteral stent is frequently placed. Double J stents do not ensure passage of stone fragments after ESWL. Occasionally, stone fragments will obstruct the ureter. Conservative management will usually result in spontaneous resolution with eventual passage of the stone fragments. If this is unsuccess-

ful, adequate proximal drainage through a percutaneous nephrostomy tube will facilitate passage. In rare instances, ureteroscopic extraction will be required.

B. Renal Stones: Renal stones less than 3 cm in diameter are best treated with ESWL. Stones located in the inferior calix frequently result in suboptimal stone-free rates as measured at 3 months by x-ray. Such stones and others of larger diameter are best treated via percutaneous nephrolithotomy. Perioperative antibiotic coverage should be given on the basis of preoperative urine cultures.

Pak CY: Etiology and treatment of urolithiasis. Am J Kidney Dis 1991;18:624.

URINARY INCONTINENCE

Urinary incontinence is most common in the elderly. Its prevalence varies from 5 $ to 15% in the community to perhaps more than 50% in long-term care facilities. The normal urinary bladder can store relatively large volumes of urine at low pressures. Continence is dependent upon a compliant reservoir and sphincteric efficiency that has two components: the involuntary smooth muscle of the bladder neck and the voluntary skeletal muscle of the external sphincter.

Classification

Urinary incontinence occurs when urine leaks involuntarily and can be classified into one of four categories as described in the following paragraphs.

A. Total Incontinence: With total incontinence, patients lose urine at all times and in all positions. Total incontinence results when sphincteric efficiency is lost (previous surgery, nerve damage, cancerous infiltration) or when an abnormal connection between the urinary tract and the skin exists that bypasses the urinary sphincter (vesicovaginal or ureterovaginal fistulas). In the pediatric setting, congenital anomalies such as ectopic ureters also must be considered.

B. Stress Incontinence: Stress incontinence is the loss of urine associated with activities that result in an increase in intra-abdominal pressure (coughing, sneezing, lifting, exercising). Patients do not leak in the supine position. Laxity of the pelvic floor musculature—most commonly seen in the multiparous woman or in patients who have undergone pelvic surgery—results in urethral sphincteric insufficiency.

C. Urge Incontinence: The uncontrolled loss of urine that is preceded by a strong, unexpected urge to void is known as urge incontinence. It is unrelated to position or activity and is indicative of detrusor hyperreflexia or sphincter dysfunction. Inflammatory conditions or neurogenic disorders of the bladder are commonly associated with urge incontinence.

D. Overflow Incontinence: Chronic urinary retention may result in overflow incontinence. Incontinence results from the chronically distended bladder receiving an additional increment of urine, so that intravesical pressure just exceeds the outlet resistance, allowing a small amount of urine to dribble out.

Clinical Findings

A. Symptoms and Signs: The history is the most important step in the evaluation of urinary incontinence. It may be supplemented with a voiding diary prepared by the patient. Physical examination is important to exclude fistula for cases of total incontinence, neurologic abnormalities in cases of urge incontinence (spasticity, flaccidity, rectal sphincter tone), or the distended bladder in cases of overflow incontinence. Rectal examination will reveal the general function of the pelvic floor. Normal anal tone suggests an intact external sphincter. A tender levator ani suggests an overfacilitated pelvic floor. A lax sphincter suggests a lower motor neuron lesion. The bulbocavernosus reflex further confirms the integrity of the lower motor neurons. This reflex is confirmed by feeling an anal contraction in response to pressure on the glans penis or the clitoris.

B. Laboratory Findings: Urinalysis and urine culture are important to exclude urinary tract infection in cases of urge incontinence. Abnormal renal function may be detected in cases of overflow incontinence. Cystograms may demonstrate fistula sites. Lateral stress cystograms may show descensus of the bladder neck (descent of bladder neck more than 1.5 cm on straining view) in cases of stress incontinence. Those suspected of overflow incontinence can have postvoid residual urine volume assessed by urethral catheterization or ultrasonography.

C. Special Tests: Urinary continence depends upon both bladder and sphincteric mechanisms; dysfunction of either component may result in incontinence. Urodynamic evaluation can assess both bladder and sphincteric function. Such testing is indicated in patients with moderate to severe incontinence, those suspected of having neurologic disease, and those with urge incontinence when infection and neoplasm have been excluded.

Bladder capacity, accommodation, sensation, voluntary control, contractility, and response to pharmacologic intervention can be assessed by cystometry. Cystometry is performed by filling the bladder with water or CO_2 and simultaneously recording intravesical pressure.

During filling, the normal bladder has the ability to maintain a low pressure. As volume increases, compliance increases. Normal sensation is first appreciated with volumes less than 150 mL. There is a strong sensation prior to micturition. Normal capacity in an adult bladder is 350–500 mL. Micturition is consciously initiated starting with pelvic floor relaxation followed by a sustained bladder contraction. Normal bladder function will empty the bladder completely. Uninhibited contractions during the normal filling phase are abnormal and are usually associated with a strong urge to void. Causes of decreased urinary capacity include incontinence, infections, interstitial cystitis, radiation damage, upper motor neuron lesions, and postoperative changes. Increased bladder capacity is seen with chronic urinary tract obstruction; congenital defects, as with megacystis; lower motor neuron lesions; and sensory neuropathies.

Responses to routine medications during cystometry will help confirm a diagnosis and facilitate appropriate therapy. Lack of an appropriate detrusor contraction may be secondary to poor bladder muscle function or inadequate filling. Myogenic function can be assessed with bethanechol chloride, a parasympathomimetic drug. Lack of response to intravenous bethanechol suggests intrinsic muscle damage. In contrast, an exaggerated response is suggestive of a lower motor neuron lesion.

Sphincteric function assessment is necessary in the evaluation of urinary incontinence. More formal evaluation of the urinary sphincter may be performed using urethral profilometry, electromyography, or combined video studies.

Treatment

A. Total Incontinence: True incontinence is due to anatomic abnormalities, either congenital or acquired. Congenital defects, including bladder exstrophy, ectopic ureteral orifices, and urethral diverticula, and acquired lesions such as vesicovaginal fistulas require surgical correction. Sphincter injuries following prostatectomy may be managed by surgical reconstruction (bladder neck reconstruction), periurethral Teflon or collagen injections, or placement of an artificial urinary sphincter.

B. Stress Incontinence: In patients with stress urinary incontinence, the bladder neck will descend below the midportion of the pubic symphysis when viewed on a lateral stress cystogram. Urodynamic investigations usually reveal a shortened functional urethral length, decreased urethral closure pressure, minimal augmentation of closure pressure with stress activities, decreased urethral pressure and length when assuming an upright position, and decreased closure pressure with bladder filling.

If hypoestrogenism of the vagina or urethra is discovered, topical estrogen creams applied locally are indicated. Mild cases can be treated medically with agents directed at increasing urethral resistance (phenylpropanolamine, 50 mg orally daily). Surgical treatment is centered upon placing the bladder neck into an appropriate anatomic location, allowing increased intra-abdominal pressure to be transmitted to both the bladder and the bladder neck. These procedures also lengthen the urethra. Transvaginal or suprapubic (culpocystourethropexy) approaches can pull the bladder neck into proper position. Surgery is usually corrective.

C. Urge Incontinence: The etiology of urge urinary incontinence includes urethral or detrusor instability or a combination of these mechanisms. Treatment is medical rather than surgical. Effective agents include antispasmodic medication (oxybutinin, 5 mg orally three times daily), anticholinergic medication (propantheline 15 mg orally three times daily), or tricyclic antidepressants (imipramine, 25–75 mg orally at bedtime). Alternative experimental treatments include nerve stimulation and acupuncture.

D. Overflow Incontinence: Placement of a urethral catheter is both diagnostic and therapeutic in the acute setting. Further treatment must address the underlying disease. Elderly men with benign prostatic hyperplasia can be treated with medical therapy, prostatectomy, or newer less invasive procedures (see below). Patients with urethral strictures can be treated with a direct internal urethrotomy or open urethroplasty. Neurogenic causes (external sphincteric spasticity) may be managed with intermittent catheterization regimens with or without pharmacotherapy.

Leach G: Evaluation and treatment of urinary incontinence. Urol Clin North Am 1991;18:175.

Resnick MN, Yalla SV, Laurino E: The pathophysiology of urinary incontinence in the elderly. N Engl J Med 1989;320:1.

Resnick MN: Initial evaluation of the incontinent patient. J Am Geriatr Soc 1990;38:311.

MALE ERECTILE DYSFUNCTION & SEXUAL DYSFUNCTION

Impotence is defined as the consistent inability to maintain an erect penis with sufficient rigidity to allow sexual intercourse. This condition is thought to affect 10 million American men, and its incidence is age-related. Approximately 25% of all men older than age 65 suffer from this disorder. Most cases of male erectile disorders have an organic rather than a psychogenic cause. Normal male erection is a neurovascular phenomenon relying on an intact autonomic and somatic nerve supply to the penis, smooth and striated musculature of the corpora cavernosa and pelvic floor, and arterial inflow supplied by the paired pudendal arteries. Erection is precipitated and maintained by an increase in arterial flow, active relaxation of the smooth muscle elements of the sinusoids within the corporal bodies of the penis, and an increase in venous resistance. Contraction of the bulbocavernosus and ischiocavernosus muscles results in further rigidity of the penis. The neurotransmitters that initiate the process have not been identified with certainty, though nitric oxide, vasoactive intestinal polypeptide, acetylcholine, and prostaglandins have all been postulated to initiate or contribute to male erection.

Male sexual dysfunction may be manifested in a variety of ways, and the history is critical to the proper classification and subsequent treatment. Androgens have a strong influence on the sexual desire of men. A **loss of libido** may indicate androgen deficiency on the basis of either hypothalamic, pituitary or testicular disease. Serum testosterone and gonadotropin levels may help localize the site of disease. **Loss of erections** may result from arterial, venous, neurogenic, or psychogenic causes. Concurrent medical problems may damage one or more of the mechanisms. In addition, many medications, especially antihypertensives, are associated with erectile dysfunction. It is important to determine whether the patient ever had any normal erections, such as early morning or during sleep. If normal erections do occur, an organic cause is unlikely. The gradual loss of erections over a period of time is more suggestive of an organic cause. The **loss of emission** (lack of antegrade seminal fluid during ejaculation) may result from several underlying disorders. **Retrograde ejaculation** may occur as a result of mechanical disruption of the bladder neck, especially following transurethral resection of the prostate or sympathetic denervation as a result of medications, diabetes mellitus, or radical pelvic or retroperitoneal surgery. Androgen deficiency may also result in lack of emission by decreasing the amount of prostatic and seminal vesicle secretions. If libido and erection are intact, the **loss of orgasm** is usually of psychologic origin. **Premature ejaculation** is usually an anxiety-related disorder and rarely has an organic cause. The history may elucidate the presence of a new partner, unreasonable expectations about performance, or emotional disorders.

Clinical Findings

A. Symptoms and Signs: Impotence should be clearly distinguished from problems of ejaculation, libido, and orgasm. The degree of the dysfunction (whether chronic, occasional, or situational) as well as its timing should be noted. The history should include inquiries about hyperlipidemia, hypertension, neurologic disease, diabetes mellitus, renal failure, and adrenal and thyroid disorders. Trauma to the pelvis or pelvic or peripheral vascular surgery also identifies patients at increased risk of impotence. A complete recording of drug use should be made, since about 25% of all cases of sexual dysfunction may be drug-related. The use of alcohol, tobacco, and recreational drugs should be recorded as well, since each is associated with an increased risk of sexual dysfunction.

During the physical examination, secondary sexual characteristics should be assessed. Neurologic and peripheral vascular examination should be performed. Motor and sensory examination should be performed as well as palpation and quantification of lower extremity vascular pulsations. The genitalia should be examined, noting the presence of penile scarring or plaque formation (Peyronie's disease) and any abnormalities in size or consistency of either testicle. Examination of the prostate is an essential feature of the urologic examination in all adult patients.

B. Laboratory Findings: Laboratory evaluation is limited and should consist of a complete blood count, urinalysis, lipid profile, determination of serum testosterone, glucose, and prolactin. Patients with abnormalities of testosterone or prolactin require further evaluation with measurement of serum FSH and LH, and endocrinologic consultation is advised.

C. Special Tests: Further testing is based on the patient's goals. Patients who will accept only noninvasive forms of therapy may be offered medical therapy or a vacuum constriction device, as described below. Most patients undergo further evaluation with direct injection of vasoactive substances into the penis. Such substances (prostaglandin E_1, papaverine, or a combination of drugs) will induce erections in men with intact vascular systems. Patients who respond with a rigid erection require no further vascular evaluation. However, organic and psychogenic impotence can be differentiated by use of nocturnal penile tumescence testing, where the frequency as well as the rigidity of erections are recorded by a simple device attached to the penis before sleep. Patients with psychogenic impotence will have nocturnal erections of adequate frequency and rigidity.

Additional vascular testing is indicated in patients who fail to achieve an erection with injection of vasoactive substances on serial attempts using increasing doses or combination of drugs and who would consider vascular reconstructive surgery. The diameter and flow in the cavernous arteries can be assessed using duplex ultrasound. Patients with poor arterial inflow in the absence of known peripheral vascular disease (as in patients who have sustained pelvic trauma) are candidates for pelvic arteriography before planned arterial reconstruction. Patients with normal arterial inflow should be suspected of suffering from venous leak. Further testing in this group would include cavernosometry (measurement of flow required to maintain erection) and cavernosography (contrast study of the penis to determine site and extent of venous leak).

Treatment

The vast majority of men suffering from erectile dysfunction can be managed successfully with one of the approaches outlined below. Men who do not suffer from organic dysfunction will probably benefit from behaviorally oriented sex therapy.

A. Medical Treatment: Testosterone injections (200 mg intramuscularly every 3 weeks) are offered to men with documented androgen deficiency who have undergone endocrinologic evaluation as described and in whom prostatic cancer has been excluded.

B. Vacuum Constriction Device: The vacuum constriction device is a cylindric device that draws the penis into an erect state by inducing a vacuum within the cylinder. Once adequate tumescence has been achieved, a rubber constriction device or band is placed around the proximal penis to prevent loss of erection, and the cylinder is removed. Such devices are suitable for patients with venous disorders of the penis and those who fail to achieve an adequate erection with injection of vasoactive substances. Complications are rare.

C. Injection Therapy: Direct injection of vasoactive substances into the penis is an acceptable form of treatment for most men with impotence. These injections are performed using a tuberculin syringe .The base and lateral aspect of the penis is used as the injection site to avoid injury to the superficial blood supply located anteriorly. Complications are rare and include dizziness, local pain, fibrosis, and infection. A prolonged erection requiring aspiration of blood and injection of epinephrine and phenylephrine to achieve detumescence occurs very rarely.

D. Penile Prostheses: Prosthetic devices may be implanted directly into the paired corporal bodies. Such prostheses may be rigid, malleable, hinged, or inflatable. Each is manufactured in a variety of sizes and diameters. Inflatable models may result in a more cosmetic appearance but may be associated with a greater likelihood of mechanical failure.

E. Vascular Reconstruction: Patients with disorders of the arterial system are candidates for various forms of arterial reconstruction, including endarterectomy and balloon dilation for proximal arterial occlusion and arterial bypass procedures utilizing arterial (epigastric) or venous (deep dorsal vein) segments for distal occlusion. Patients with disorders of venous occlusion may be managed with ligation of certain veins (deep dorsal or emissary veins) or the crura of the corpora cavernosa. Experience with vascular reconstructive procedures is still limited, and many patients so treated still fail to achieve a rigid erection.

Lue TF: Physiology of erection and pathophysiology of impotence. In: *Campbell's Urology,* 6th ed. Walsh PC et al (editors). Saunders, 1992.

Morley JE, Kaiser FE: Impotence: The internist's approach to diagnosis and treatment. Adv Intern Med 1993; 38:151.

BENIGN PROSTATIC HYPERPLASIA

Essentials of Diagnosis
- Decreased force and caliber of the urinary stream.
- Nocturia.
- High postvoid residual urine volume.
- Azotemia and urinary retention on occasion.

General Considerations
Benign prostatic hyperplasia is a common disorder, and its incidence is age-related. Its histologic prevalence in autopsy studies rises from approximately 20% in men aged 41–50 years to over 80% in men older than 80 years. Although clinical evidence of disease occurs less commonly, symptoms of prostatic obstruction are also age-related. At age 55, approximately 25% of men report obstructive voiding symptoms. At age 75 years, 50% of men will complain of a decrease in the force and caliber of their urinary stream.

The cause is not completely understood but seems to be multifactorial and under endocrine control. The prostate is composed of both stromal and epithelial elements, and each—alone or in combination—can give rise to hyperplastic nodules and the symptoms associated with hyperplasia of the organ. Indeed, both elements are targets of medical management schemes. Whereas prostatic cancers originate in the peripheral zone of the prostate, benign prostatic hyperplasia originates in the periurethral and transition zones. The natural history is quite variable, and a large number of affected patients may note either improvement or stabilization of their symptoms with time.

Clinical Findings
A. Symptoms and Signs: Benign prostatic hyperplasia may be associated with both obstructive and irritative voiding symptoms. Obstructive symptoms include decreased force and caliber of the urinary stream, an intermittent stream, and urinary hesitancy. Irritative symptoms, which may be a consequence of bladder dysfunction, include urinary frequency, nocturia, and urgency. Symptoms may be quantitated by various scoring schemes, which may aid in selecting patients for various forms of treatment and assessing their response to such treatment. Digital rectal examination may reveal either focal or uniform enlargement of the prostate. Focal areas of induration may represent malignant rather than benign prostatic growth, and further evaluation (transrectal ultrasound and possible biopsy) is indicated in such patients. The volume of the prostate estimated on digital rectal examination should not direct therapy, because the size of the prostate estimated in this

manner may not correlate with either the symptoms or signs of the disorder or the need for treatment. Examination of the lower abdomen should be performed to assess for a distended bladder consistent with urinary retention, which may occur silently in the absence of severe symptoms. A limited neurologic examination should be performed assessing the sacral nerve roots.

B. Laboratory Findings: Serum urea nitrogen and creatinine may be elevated in patients with high postvoid residual volumes and impairment of renal function. Urinalysis should be performed to exclude associated infection or hematuria. Prostate-specific antigen is often measured in order to increase the sensitivity of prostatic cancer detection.

C. Imaging: Intravenous urography was at one time performed routinely in the evaluation of men with signs or symptoms of prostatic hypertrophy. Elevation of the bladder base, trabeculation and thickening of the bladder, diverticular formation, elevation of the distal ureters, and poor emptying are commonly observed. Evidence of hydronephrosis occurs less commonly. However, intravenous urography is normal in the majority of patients and should be reserved for those with hematuria or when there upper urinary tract disease is suspected. A plain film of the abdomen may reveal urinary tract calculi, and ulrasonography can be used to assess bladder or upper tract changes described earlier. In addition, prostate volume can be determined. However, routine imaging is not necessary in patients with mild to moderate symptoms and a normal urinalysis, serum creatinine, and physical examination.

D. Urodynamic Evaluation: Uroflowmetry is the most commonly performed and perhaps the most useful urodynamic technique for the assessment of benign prostatic hypertrophy. The maximum urinary flow rate is most commonly recorded, and such a measurement is only reliable if the total volume voided exceeds 150 mL. Most urologists agree that a peak flow rate less than 10 mL per second is indicative of infravesical obstruction. More detailed urodynamic evaluation is indicated in patients with signs or symptoms of hyperplasia and known neurologic disorders; in very young patients; and in those with primarily irritative, rather than obstructive, symptoms.

E. Cystourethroscopy: Cystourethroscopy is an invasive procedure and should be performed when the diagnosis is uncertain and, on occasion, when patients are being evaluated for newer forms of treatment. When prostatectomy is indicated, cystourethrography should be performed immediately before the procedure.

Differential Diagnosis
The symptoms so commonly associated with benign prostatic hypertrophy may be produced by other disorders that may also cause bladder outlet obstruc-

tion: urethral stricture, bladder neck contracture, bladder calculi, and cancers of the prostate or bladder. Urinary tract infection, which may lead to irritative voiding symptoms, should be excluded. Neurologic disease can lead to voiding disorders and should be considered in patients with a history of such diseases and in those with an abnormal neurologic examination.

Treatment

Indications for treatment have not been well defined. Absolute indications for treatment include recurrent urinary retention, azotemia, hydronephrosis, and urinary incontinence as a result of bladder outlet obstruction; recurrent urinary tract infection associated with increased residual urine volume; and severe hematuria. Patients with significant symptoms that impact on their perceived quality of life are also candidates for treatment. At present it appears that prostatectomy is most likely to restore a normal voiding pattern in patients with urinary retention and severe complications of hyperplasia. Management of patients with moderate to severe symptoms but no serious sequelae remains controversial. Such patients should be advised of all options and they should actively participate in the selection of initial therapy.

A. Medical Treatment: Prostatic enlargement may be a product of stromal or epithelial hyperplasia. Medical management may target either or both elements. It appears that prostatic androgen levels play at least a permissive role in benign hypertrophy, and therapies that reduce their levels will reduce prostatic size and improve obstructive symptoms. Androgen deprivation may be induced at various levels along the hypothalamic-pituitary-testicular axis (Table 21–4). Methods that reduce circulating levels of testosterone will result in loss of libido and sexual function,

however. The human prostate and bladder base contains both α_1 and α_2 adrenoceptors, and the prostate will show a contractile response to such agonists. The contractile properties of the prostate are mediated primarily by α_1 receptors. Alpha blockade has been shown to result in both objective and subjective degrees of improvement in the symptoms and signs of benign prostatic hypertrophy in some patients (Table 21–5). Side effects of such therapy are related to the antagonism of α_2 adrenoceptors, whereas efficacy is related to antagonism of α_1 adrenoceptors. In placebo-controlled trials, both use of finasteride and selective α_1 blockade seems to benefit a small to moderate number of patients with respect to improvements in symptom score, urinary flow rates, and residual urine volumes. The long-term benefits of such therapy are unknown at present.

B. Surgical Treatment: Removal of obstructing adenomatous prostatic tissue can be accomplished either through an incision or transurethrally. Transurethral resection is associated with a low mortality rate (0.1%), a moderate morbidity rate (18%), and a very high likelihood of both objective and symptomatic improvement in the symptoms and signs of benign prostatic hypertrophy. Retrograde ejaculation is a common occurrence after this procedure. Complications occur uncommonly and include bladder neck contracture (2.7%), urethral stricture disease (2.5%), and incontinence (1.7%). Repeat resection is necessary in less than 10% of men who undergo transurethral prostatectomy. Transurethral resection has come under more intense scrutiny for several reasons. It is the second most common surgical procedure in men over age 60, and its costs have escalated in recent years. The relative risk of death may be higher in patients undergoing transurethral compared to open prostatectomy. Reasons for this discrepancy are not known. In addition, other treatment options are available that are perhaps associated with less morbidity. Whether alternative treatment methods will prove to be equivalent or superior to transurethral prostatectomy for the long-term control of benign prostatic hypertrophy is not known.

Patients with symptoms and signs of benign prostatic hypertrophy associated with smaller glands—especially in younger men—may benefit from transurethral incision of the prostate. No tissue is resected, antegrade ejaculation is usually maintained, and the

Table 21–4. Androgen ablation and blockade for benign prostatic hyperplasia.

Agent	Action	Effects
LHRH agonists (leuprolide, buserelin, nafarelin)	Inhibit pituitary luteinizing hormone secretion; decrease testosterone and dihydrotestosterone.	Impotence, loss of libido; hot flushes, gynecomastia.
Progestational agents (megestrol acetate, hydroxyprogesterone caproate)	Inhibit pituitary LH secretion; decrease testosterone and dihydrotestosterone.	Impotence, loss of libido.
Antiandrogens (flutamide)	Androgen receptor inhibition.	Gynecomastia, diarrhea; libido maintained.
5α-Reductase inhibitors (finasteride)	Decreases dihydrotestosterone.	Libido maintained.

Table 21–5. Alpha$_1$ blockade for benign prostatic hyperplasia.

Agent	Action	Dose
Phenoxybenzamine	Alpha$_1$ and alpha$_2$ blockade	5–10 mg twice daily
Prazosin	Alpha$_1$ blockade	1–5 mg twice daily
Terazosin	Alpha$_1$ blockade	1–10 mg daily
Doxazosin	Alpha$_1$ blockade	1–8 mg daily

procedure can usually be performed on an outpatient basis.

C. Other Treatment Methods: A variety of minimally invasive procedures have been developed and are currently being evaluated for the management of benign prostatic hypertrophy. Balloon dilation is easily performed, but its effects seem to be transitory. Neodymium-YAG laser energy can be delivered to obstructing tissue using right-angle delivery fibers. Laser energy may be applied under visual or ultrasound guidance. Prostatic tissue may be desiccated using either transurethral or transrectal application of microwave hyperthermia. Self-retaining intraurethral stents have been developed. The use of laser energy, microwave hyperthermia, and stents is still investigational, and their use for the treatment of benign prostatic hypertrophy is the subject of several ongoing trials.

Barry MJ et al: Watchful waiting vs. immediate transurethral resection for symptomatic prostatism. JAMA 1988; 259:3010.
Lepor H, Walsh PC (editors): Benign prostatic hyperplasia. Urol Clin North Am 1990;7(3):1.

MALIGNANT URINARY TRACT DISORDERS

CANCER OF THE PROSTATE

Essentials of Diagnosis
- Prostatic induration on digital rectal examination or elevation of PSA.
- Most often asymptomatic.
- Systemic symptoms (weight loss, bone pain) in 20% of patients.

General Considerations
Prostatic cancer is the most common cancer detected in American men. In 1992, more than 160,000 American men were found to have prostatic cancer, and 35,000 men died of the disease. However, the clinical incidence of the disease does not match the prevalence noted at autopsy. At autopsy, more than 40% of men over 50 years of age are found to have prostatic carcinoma. Most such occult cancers are small and contained within the prostate gland. Few are associated with regional or distant disease. The incidence of prostatic cancer increases with age. Whereas 30% of men age 60–69 will have disease, the autopsy incidence increases to 67% in men aged 80–89 years. Interestingly, the prevalence of prostatic cancer in autopsy specimens from men around the world varies little. However, the clinical incidence is considerably different (high in North America and European countries, intermediate in South America, and low in the Far East), suggesting that environmental or dietary differences among populations may be important for prostatic cancer growth. A 50-year-old American man has a lifetime risk of 40% for latent cancer, 9.5% for developing clinically apparent cancer, and a 2.9% risk of death due to prostatic cancer. Black men with a family history of prostatic cancer and perhaps men who have undergone vasectomy are at an increased risk of developing the disease

The incidence of prostatic cancer is increasing in this country, partly due to wider application of detection techniques (transrectal ultrasound and PSA testing). The goal of a screening effort should be to detect and treat only those prostatic carcinomas most likely to cause morbidity or mortality if left untreated. Detection of latent, nonprogressive cancers would expose patients to unnecessary treatment and its attendant complications and costs. Whether screening for prostatic cancer will result in a decrease in yearly mortality rates due to the disease is unknown and the subject of much debate.

Clinical Findings
A. Symptoms and Signs: Most prostatic cancers are detected in asymptomatic men who are found to have focal nodules or areas of induration within the prostate at the time of digital rectal examination. Depending on the patient population being evaluated, detection rates using digital rectal examination will vary from 2% to 7%. Unfortunately, most cancers detected by digital rectal examination are advanced (stages T3 or metastatic).

Rarely, patients present with signs of urinary retention (palpable bladder) or neurologic symptoms as a result of epidural metastases and cord compression. Obstructive voiding symptoms are most often due to benign prostatic hyperplasia, which occurs in the same age group. However, large or locally extensive prostatic cancers can cause obstructive voiding symptoms. Lymph node metastases can lead to lower extremity lymphedema. As the axial skeleton is the most common site of metastases, patients may present with back pain or pathologic fractures.

B. Laboratory Findings:
1. Serum tumor markers–Prostate-specific antigen (PSA) is a glycoprotein produced only in the cytoplasm of benign and malignant prostate cells. The serum level correlates with the volume of both benign and malignant prostatic tissue.. Measurement of PSA may be useful in detecting and staging prostatic cancer, monitoring response to treatment, and detecting recurrence well before it becomes obvious clinically. As a first-line screening test, PSA will be elevated in approximately 10–15% of men self referred for screening. Approximately 20–25% of men with intermediate degrees of elevation (4.1–10 ng/mL; normal < 4 ng/mL) will be found to have

prostatic cancer. Almost two-thirds of those with elevations greater than 10 ng/mL will have prostatic cancer. Patients with intermediate levels of PSA will usually have localized and therefore potentially curable cancers. However, it should be remembered that approximately 20% of patients who undergo radical prostatectomy for localized prostatic cancer will have normal levels of PSA.

In untreated patients with prostatic cancer, the level of PSA correlates with the volume and stage of the disease. Whereas most organ-confined cancers are associated with PSA levels less than 10 ng/mL, more advanced disease (seminal vesicle invasion, lymph node involvement, or occult distant metastases) is more common in patients with PSA levels in excess of 40 ng/mL. Approximately 98% of patients with metastatic prostatic cancer will have elevated PSA. However, there are occasional cancers which are localized despite substantial elevations in PSA. Therefore, treatment decisions in patients with untreated cancers cannot be made on the basis of PSA testing alone. A rising level of PSA after treatment is consistent with progressive disease whether it be locally recurrent or metastatic.

Until the advent of PSA testing, serum acid phosphatase was the standard serum tumor marker used in the evaluation of patients with localized and metastatic prostatic cancer. Because PSA is more sensitive than serum acid phosphatase, it has largely replaced its use. However, an elevated serum acid phosphatase is more predictive of metastatic disease than an elevated PSA, and for this reason it is still used by some. Serum acid phosphatase levels will be normal in approximately 25% of patients with metastatic disease.

2. Miscellaneous laboratory testing–Patients in urinary retention or those with ureteral obstruction due to locally or regionally advanced prostatic cancers may present with elevations in serum urea nitrogen or creatinine. Patients with bony metastases may have elevations in alkaline phosphatase or hypercalcemia. Laboratory and clinical evidence of disseminated intravascular coagulation can occur in patients with advanced prostatic cancers.

3. Prostatic biopsy–Transrectal ultrasound-guided biopsy seems to be a better method for detection of prostatic cancer than finger-guided biopsy. The use of a spring-loaded, 18-gauge biopsy needle has allowed transrectal biopsy to be performed with little patient discomfort and low attendant morbidity. The specimen preserves glandular architecture and allows for accurate grading as described below. Taking biopsy specimens from the apex, midportion, and base of the prostate is recommended by some and should be considered in patients with significant elevations in PSA but a normal digital rectal examination. Patients with abnormalities of the seminal vesicles can have guided biopsies of these structures performed to allow for detection of local tumor invasion. Aspiration biopsies of the prostate, though accurate and associated with low morbidity, have been used rarely since the introduction of the spring-loaded biopsy device but should be considered in patients at an increased risk of bleeding.

C. Imaging: Modern transrectal ultrasound instrumentation provides high-definition images of the prostate. Transrectal ultrasonography has been used largely for the staging of prostatic carcinomas. In addition, transrectal ultrasound-guided—rather than digitally guided—biopsy of the prostate may be a more accurate way to investigate suspicious lesions. Most prostatic cancers are hypoechoic. Transrectal ultrasonography should not be used as a first-line screening tool because of its expense, its low specificity (and therefore high biopsy rate), and the fact that it increases the detection rate very little when compared to the combined use of digital rectal examination and PSA testing.

MRI of the prostate allows for evaluation of the prostatic lesion as well as regional lymph nodes. The prostate has a homogenous appearance on T1-weighted images, while T2-weighted images can distinguish the zonal anatomy of the prostate. Prostatic cancer is usually associated with a decreased signal intensity on T2-weighted images. The sensitivity for detection of both capsular penetration and seminal vesicle invasion is similar for both transuretheral ultrasound and MRI. CT scanning plays little role in evaluation because of its inability to accurately identify or stage prostatic cancers.

Radionuclide bone scan is superior to conventional plain skeletal x-rays in detecting bony metastases. Most prostatic cancer metastases are multiple and are most commonly localized to the axial skeleton. Because of the high frequency of abnormal scans in patients in this age group, plain films are often useful in patients with indeterminate radionuclide findings. Intravenous urography and cystoscopy are not routinely used to evaluate patients with prostatic cancer.

Imaging can be tailored to the likelihood of advanced disease in newly diagnosed patients. Asymptomatic patients with well to moderately well differentiated cancers—thought to be localized to the prostate on digital rectal examination and transuretheral ultrasound and associated with normal or only modest elevations of PSA (ie, < 10 ng/mL)—need no further evaluation. The negative predictive value of bone scan approaches 99% in this group. Those with more advanced local lesions, symptoms of metastases (ie, bone pain), and elevations in PSA greater than 10 ng/mL should undergo radionuclide bone scan. Cross-sectional imaging of the prostate is usually indicated only in those patients in the latter group who have negative bone scans in an attempt to detect lymph node metastases. Patients found to have enlarged pelvic lymph nodes are candidates for fine-needle aspiration. Transrectal MRI and spectroscopy may provide superior imaging of the prostate compared to transuretheral ultrasound or digital rectal examination. Despite application of modern and sophisticated imaging, understaging of prostatic cancer is common.

Pathology & Staging

The majority of prostatic cancers are adenocarcinomas. Most arise in the periphery of the prostate (peripheral zone), though a small percentage arise in the central (5–10%) and transition zones (20%) of the gland. Most pathologists employ the Gleason grading system whereby a "primary" grade is applied to the architectural pattern of cancerous glands occupying the largest area of the specimen and a "secondary" pattern is assigned to the next largest area of cancerous growth. Grading is based on architectural (rather than histologic) criteria, and five possible "grades" are possible. Adding the score of the primary and secondary patterns gives a Gleason score. Grade correlates well with tumor volume, stage, and prognosis. The TNM classification of the American Joint Cancer Committee for prostatic cancer is shown in Table 21–6.

The patterns of prostatic cancer progression have been well defined. The likelihood of both local inva-

Table 21–6. TNM staging system for prostate cancer.

T: Primary tumor		
	Tx	Cannot be assessed
	T0	No evidence of primary tumor
	Tis	Carcinoma in situ (CIS)
	T1a	≤ Three foci of carcinoma in resection for benign disease; normal digital rectal examination
	T1b	≥ Three foci of carcinoma in resection for benign disease; normal digital rectal examination
	T1c	Detected from elevated PSA alone; normal digital rectal examination
	T2a	Tumor in less than half of one lobe
	T2b	Tumor in more than half of one lobe
	T2c	Tumor in both lobes
	T3a	Unilateral extracapsular extension
	T3b	Bilateral extracapsular extension
	T3c	Seminal vesicle involvement
	T4	Adjacent organ involvement
N: Regional lymph nodes		
	Nx	Cannot be assessed
	N0	No regional lymph node metastasis
	N1	Metastasis in a single lymph node 2 cm or less
	N2	Metastasis in a single lymph
	N3	node >2 cm and <5 cm or multiple nodes none >5cm
M: Distant metastasis		
	Mx	Cannot be assessed
	M0	No distant metastasis
	M1	Distant metastasis present

sion and metastases is greater in larger or less well differentiated cancers. Small and well-differentiated cancers (grades 1 and 2) are usually confined within the prostate, whereas large-volume (> 4 mL) or poorly differentiated (grades 4 and 5) cancers are more commonly locally extensive or metastatic to regional lymph nodes or bone. Penetration of the prostatic capsule by cancer is common and often occurs along perineural spaces. Seminal vesicle invasion is associated with a high likelihood of regional or distant disease. Lymphatic metastases are most often identified in the obturator lymph node chain. The axial skeleton, as mentioned previously, is the most common site of distant metastases.

Treatment

A. Localized Disease: What constitutes the optimal form of treatment for patients with clinically localized cancers remains controversial. Treatment decisions are at present made on the basis of tumor grade and stage and the age and health of the patient. Although selected patients may be candidates for surveillance based on age or health and the presence of small-volume or well-differentiated cancers, most patients with an anticipated survival in excess of 10 years should be considered for treatment with irradiation or surgery. Both radiation therapy and radical prostatectomy allow for acceptable levels of local control. Radical prostatectomy appears to be associated with a lower likelihood of local recurrence and a longer disease-free survival at 10 years. Although randomized trials are needed to determine what constitutes the best form of treatment for localized prostatic cancer, no such trials are ongoing at present. Patients need to be advised of all treatment options (including surveillance) along with their particular benefits, risks, and limitations.

B. Radical Prostatectomy: In radical prostatectomy, the seminal vesicles, prostate, and ampullae of the vas deferens are removed. Refinements in technique have allowed maintenance of urinary continence in almost all patients and erectile function in selected patients. However, the procedure should be used selectively. As capsular penetration is a common finding in patients with presumed localized prostatic cancer, preservation of the neurovascular bundle contiguous with a prostatic cancer may increase the likelihood of local tumor recurrence. Local recurrence is uncommon after radical prostatectomy, and its incidence is related to pathologic stage. Organ-confined cancers rarely recur (2% local, 1% distant). However, cancers found to be locally extensive (capsular penetration, seminal vesicle invasion) are associated with higher local (10–25%) and distant (20–25%) distant relapse rates.

Ideal candidates for the procedure include healthy patients with stages T1, T2, and selected T3 prostatic cancers. Patients with advanced local tumors (T3 and T4) and those with lymph node metastases are rarely candidates for this procedure. However, several recent reports suggest that selected patients with more advanced cancers may benefit from aggressive local treatment approaches. Some feel that outcome is positively influenced by tumor ploidy and the early application of androgen deprivation after surgery.

Patients with positive surgical margins are at an increased risk for local and distant tumor relapse. Such patients are often considered candidates for adjuvant therapy (radiation for positive margins or androgen deprivation for lymph node metastases). Although adjuvant radiation seems to be associated with fewer local recurrences (0–5% with radiation versus 15–30% without), it has little or no impact on distant failure rates (30–35% with radiation versus 30–45% without).

C. Radiation Therapy: Radiation can be delivered by a variety of techniques including use of external beam radiotherapy and transperineal implantation of radioisotopes. Morbidity is limited, and the survival of patients with localized cancers (T1, T2, and selected T3) approaches 65% at 10 years. As with surgery, the likelihood of local failure correlates with technique and tumor stage. The likelihood of a positive, prostatic biopsy more than 18 months after surgery varies between 20% and 60% in selected series. Patients with local recurrence are at an increased risk of cancer progression and cancer death compared with those who have negative biopsies. Ambiguous target definitions, inadequate radiation doses, and understaging of patients may be responsible for the failure noted in some series. Newer techniques of radiation (implantation, conformal therapy using three-dimensional reconstruction of CT-based tumor volumes, heavy particle, charged particle, and heavy charged particle) may improve local control rates.

D. Surveillance: A positive impact of localized prostatic cancer treatment with regard to survival has not been conclusively demonstrated. Surveillance alone may be an appropriate form of management for very selected patients with prostatic cancer. However, most patients in such series are older and have very small and well-differentiated cancers. Even in such a selected population, cancer death rates approach 10%. In addition, end points for intervention in patients on surveillance regimens have not been defined.

E. Locally and Regionally Advanced Disease: Prostatic cancers associated with minimal degrees of capsular penetration are candidates for standard irradiation or surgery. Those with locally extensive cancers, including those with seminal vesicle and bladder neck invasion, are at increased risk of both local and distant relapse despite conventional therapy. Currently, a variety of investigational regimens are being tested in an effort to improve local and distant relapse rates in such patients. Combination therapy (androgen deprivation combined with surgery or irradiation), cryosurgery, newer forms of

irradiation, and hormonal therapy alone are being tested in such patients. Similarly, patients with lymph node metastases may be benefited little by aggressive local therapy and are most often best treated with androgen deprivation due to the inevitability of distant relapse in the majority of such patients.

F. Metastatic Disease: Since death due to prostatic carcinoma is almost invariably a result of failure to control metastatic disease, research has emphasized efforts to improve control of distant disease. It is well known that most prostatic carcinomas are hormone-dependent, and approximately 70–80% of men with metastatic prostatic carcinoma will respond to various forms of androgen deprivation. Testosterone, the major circulating androgen, is produced by Leydig cells in the testes (95%), with a smaller amount being produced by peripheral conversion of other steroids. Although 98% of serum testosterone is protein-bound, free testosterone enters prostate cells and is converted to dihydrotestosterone, the major intracellular androgen. Dihydrotestosterone binds a cytoplasmic receptor protein, and the complex moves to the cell nucleus, where it modulates transcription. Androgen deprivation may be induced at several levels along the pituitary-gonadal axis using a variety of methods or agents (Table 21–7). Use of LHRH agonists (leuprolide, buserelin, nafarelin)—a new class of drugs delivered monthly by injection—has allowed induction of androgen deprivation without orchiectomy or administration of diethylstilbestrol. Presently, administration of LHRH agonists and orchiectomy are the most common forms of primary androgen blockade used. Because of its rapid onset of action, ketoconazole should be considered in patients with advanced prostatic cancer who present with spinal cord compression or disseminated intravascular coagulation. Although testosterone is the major circulating androgen, the adrenal gland secretes the androgens dehydroepiandrosterone, dehydroepiandrosterone sulfate, and androstenedione. Some investigators believe that suppressing both testicular and adrenal androgens will allow for a better initial and longer response than methods which inhibit production of only testicular androgens. Complete androgen blockade can be achieved by combining an antiandrogen with use of an LHRH agonist or orchiectomy. Flutamide is a nonsteroidal antiandrogen that appears to act by competitively binding the receptor for dihydrotestosterone, the intracellular androgen responsible for prostatic cell growth and development. When patients with metastatic prostatic cancer are stratified with regard to extent of disease and performance status, those patients with limited disease and a good performance status treated with combined androgen blockade (LHRH agonist and flutamide) seem to survive longer than those treated with an LHRH agonist alone. Additional trials examining the potential benefits of complete androgen deprivation are ongoing, and new antiandrogens are being tested.

Table 21–7. Androgen ablation for prostatic cancer.

Level	Agent	Sequelae	Dose
Pituitary, hypothalamus	Estrogens	Gynecomastia, hot flushes, thromboembolic disease, impotence	1–3 mg daily
	LHRH agonists	Impotence, hot flushes, gynecomastia, rarely anemia	Monthly injection
Adrenal	Ketoconazole	Adrenal insufficiency, nausea, gynecomastia, hepatic toxicity	400 mg 3 times daily
	Aminoglutethimide	Adrenal insufficiency, nausea, rash, ataxia	250 mg 4 times daily
	Glucocorticoids	Gastrointestinal bleeding, fluid retention	Prednisone: 20–40 mg daily
Testis	Orchiectomy	Gynecomastia, hot flushes, impotence	
Prostate cell	Antiandrogens	No impotence when used alone; nausea, diarrhea	Flutamide: 250 mg 3 times daily

Although androgen deprivation is effective, most patients with advanced disease so treated will experience disease relapse, usually within 3 years. Once relapse has been identified, survival is limited. Palliative care including adequate pain control and focal irradiation of symptomatic or unstable bone disease should be instituted in patients who have failed standard hormonal therapy. Secondary therapy with chemotherapeutic agents has had limited results but should be considered in patients with a reasonable performance status. Preliminary trials of suramin, a growth factor antagonist, suggest that it may have substantial activity in patients with hormone-refractory prostatic cancer.

Bagshaw MA, Cox RS, Ramback JE: Radiation therapy for localized prostate cancer. Urol Clin North Am 1990; 17:787.

Carroll PR, Narayan P: Treatment options for hormone-insensitive or independent prostatic carcinoma. Semin Urol 1988;6:322.

Catalona WJ et al: Measurement of prostate-specific antigen in serum as a screening test for prostate cancer. N Engl J Med 1991;324:1156.

Cooner WH et al: Prostate cancer detection in a clinical urological practice by ultrasonography, digital rectal examination and prostate specific antigen. J Urol 1990;143:1146.

Gittes R: Carcinoma of the prostate. N Engl J Med 1991; 324:236.

Johansson J-E et al: High 10-year survival rate in patients with early, untreated prostatic cancer. JAMA 1992; 267:2191.

BLADDER CANCER

Essentials of Diagnosis

- Irritative voiding symptoms.
- Gross or microscopic hematuria.
- Positive urinary cytology in most patients.
- Filling defect within bladder noted on imaging.

General Considerations

Bladder cancer is the second most common urologic cancer, occurs more commonly in men than women (2.7:1), and the mean age at diagnosis is 65 years. Cigarette smoking and exposure to industrial dyes or solvents are risk factors for the disease and account for approximately 60% and 15% of new cases, respectively.

Clinical Findings

A. Symptoms and Signs: Hematuria—gross or microscopic, chronic or intermittent—is the presenting symptom in 85–90% of patients with bladder cancer. Irritative voiding symptoms (urinary frequency and urgency) will occur in a small percentage of patients as a result of the location or size of the cancer. Most patients with bladder cancer will fail to have signs of the disease because of its superficial nature. Masses detected on bimanual examination may be present in patients with large-volume or deeply infiltrating cancers. Hepatomegaly or supraclavicular lymphadenopathy may be present in patients with metastatic disease, and lymphedema of the lower extremities may be present as a result of locally advanced cancers or metastases to pelvic lymph nodes.

B. Laboratory Findings: Urinalysis will reveal hematuria in the majority of cases. On occasion, it may be accompanied by pyuria. Azotemia may be present in a small number of cases associated with ureteral obstruction. Anemia may be due to chronic blood loss, which is unusual, or to replacement of the bone marrow with metastatic disease. Exfoliated cells from normal and abnormal urothelium can be readily detected in voided urine specimens. Cytology may be useful in detecting the disease at the time of initial presentation or to detect recurrence. Cytology is very sensitive in detecting cancers of higher grade and stage (80–90%) but less so in detecting superficial or well-differentiated lesions (50%). Sensitivity of detection using exfoliated cells may be enhanced by flow cytometry.

C. Imaging: Bladder cancers may be detected using intravenous urography, ultrasound, CT, or MRI where filling defects within the bladder are noted. However, the presence of cancer is confirmed by cystoscopy and biopsy, so imaging is useful primarily for evaluating the upper urinary tract and in staging the more advanced lesions.

D. Cystourethroscopy and Biopsy: The diagnosis and staging of bladder cancers is made by cystoscopy and transurethral resection. If cystoscopy—performed usually under local anesthesia—confirms the presence of bladder cancer, the patient is scheduled for transurethral resection under general or regional anesthesia. A careful bimanual examination is performed initially and at the end of the procedure, noting the size, position, and degree of fixation of a mass, if present. Any suspicious lesions are resected using electrocautery. Resection is carried down to the muscular elements of the bladder wall so as to allow complete staging. Random bladder and, on occasion, prostatic urethral biopsies are performed to detect occult disease elsewhere in the bladder and, therefore, identify patients at high risk of recurrence and progression.

Pathology & Selection of Treatment

Ninety-eight percent of primary bladder cancers are epithelial malignancies, with the majority being transitional cell carcinomas (90%). These latter cancers most often appear as papillary growths, but higher-grade lesions are often sessile and ulcerated. Grading is based on histologic architecture: size, pleomorphism, mitotic rate, and hyperchromatism. The frequency of recurrence and progression is strongly correlated with grade. Whereas progression may be noted in few grade I cancers (19–37%), it is common with poorly differentiated lesions (33–67%). Carcinoma in situ is recognizable as a flat, nonpapillary, anaplastic epithelium and may occur focally or diffusely, but it is most often found in association with papillary bladder cancers. Its presence identifies a patient at increased risk of recurrence and progression.

Adenocarcinomas and squamous cell cancers account for approximately 2% and 7% (respectively) of all bladder cancers detected in the USA. The latter is often associated with schistosomiasis, vesical calculi, or chronic catheter use.

Bladder cancer staging is based on the extent of bladder wall penetration and the presence of either regional or distant metastases. The TNM classification of the American Joint Cancer Committee for bladder cancer is shown in Table 21–8.

The natural history of bladder cancer is based on two separate but related processes: tumor recurrence and progression to higher stage disease. Both are related to tumor grade and stage. At initial presentation, approximately 50–80% of bladder cancers will be superficial: Ta, TIS, T1. Lymph node metastases and progression are uncommon in such patients when they are properly treated, and survival is excellent at 81%. Patients with superficial cancers (Ta, T1) are treated with complete transurethral resection and the

Table 21–8. TNM staging system for bladder cancer.

T: Primary tumor	
Tx	Cannot be assessed
T0	No evidence of primary tumor
Tis	Carcinoma in situ (CIS)
T1	Invasion into lamina propria
T2	Invasion into superficial layer of muscularis propria
T3a	Invasion into deep layer of muscularis propria
T3b	Invasion through serosa into perivesical fat
T4a	Invasion into adjacent organs
T4b	Invasion into pelvic sidewall
N: Regional lymph nodes	
Nx	Cannot be assessed
N0	No regional lymph node metastasis
N1	Metastasis in a single lymph node 2 cm or less
N2	Metastasis in a single lymph node >2 cm and <5 cm or multiple nodes none >5 cm
N3	Metastasis in lymph node >5 cm
M: Distant metastasis	
Mx	Cannot be assessed
M0	No distant metastasis
M1	Distant metastasis present

selective use of intravesical chemotherapy. The latter is used to prevent or delay recurrence. Patients who present with large, high-grade, recurrent Ta lesions, T1 cancers, and those with carcinoma in situ are good candidates for intravesical chemotherapy. Patients with more invasive (T2, T3) but still localized cancers are at risk of both nodal metastases and progression, and they require more aggressive surgery, irradiation, or the combination of chemotherapy and selective surgery or irradiation due to the much higher risk of progression compared to patients with lower-stage lesions. Patients with evidence of lymph node or distant metastases should undergo systemic chemotherapy initially.

Treatment

A. Intravesical Chemotherapy: Immuno- or chemotherapeutic agents can be delivered directly into the bladder by a urethral catheter. They can be used to eradicate existing disease or to reduce the likelihood of recurrence in those who have undergone complete transurethral resection. Such therapy is more effective in the latter situation. Most agents are administered weekly for 6–12 weeks. The use of maintenance therapy after the initial induction regimen may be beneficial. Efficacy may be increased by prolonging contact time to 2 hours. Common agents include thiotepa, mitomycin C, doxorubicin, and BCG, the latter being the most effective agent when compared with mitomycin C or doxorubicin. Side effects of intravesical chemotherapy include irritative voiding symptoms and hemorrhagic cystitis. Systemic effects are rare. Patients who develop symptoms from BCG may require antituberculous therapy.

B. Surgical Treatment: Although transurethral resection is the initial form of treatment for all bladder cancers as it is diagnostic, allows for proper staging, and will control superficial cancers, muscle infiltrating cancers will require more aggressive treatment. Partial cystectomy may be indicated in patients with solitary lesions and those with cancers in a bladder diverticulum. Radical cystectomy entails removal of the bladder, prostate, seminal vesicles, and surrounding fat and peritoneal attachments in men and in women also the uterus, cervix, urethra, anterior vaginal vault, and usually the ovaries. Bilateral pelvic lymph node dissection is performed simultaneously.

Urinary diversion can be performed using a conduit of small or large bowel. However, continent forms of diversion have been developed that avoid the necessity of an external appliance.

C. Radiotherapy: External beam radiotherapy delivered in fractions over a 6- to 8-week period is generally well tolerated, but approximately 10–15% of patients will develop bladder, bowel, or rectal complications. Unfortunately, local recurrence is common after radiotherapy (30–70%). Increasingly, radiotherapy is being combined with systemic chemotherapy in an effort to improve local and distant relapse rates.

D. Chemotherapy: Fifteen percent of patients with newly diagnosed bladder cancer will present with metastatic disease, and 40% of those thought to have localized disease at the time of cystectomy or definitive radiotherapy will develop metastases usually within 2 years after the start of treatment. Cisplatin-based combination chemotherapy will result in partial or complete responses in 15–35% and 15–45% of patients, respectively.

Combination chemotherapy has been integrated into trials of surgery and radiotherapy. It has been used before each in an attempt to preserve the bladder and decrease recurrence rates. Alternatively, it has been employed postoperatively in patients who have undergone cystectomy and have been found to be at high risk of recurrence. Both approaches seem to have merit and are the subject of ongoing clinical trials.

Carroll PR: Urothelial carcinoma: Cancers of the bladder, ureter and renal pelvis. In: *Smith's General Urology,* 13th ed. Tanagho EA, McAninch JW (editors). Appleton & Lange, 1992.
Droller M (editor): Advanced bladder cancer. Urol Clin North Am 1992;19:1.

CANCERS OF THE URETER & RENAL PELVIS

Cancers of the renal pelvis and ureter are rare and occur more commonly in smokers, in those with Balkan nephropathy, in those exposed to Thorotrast (a contrast agent in use until the 1960s), or those with a long history of analgesic abuse. The majority are transitional cell carcinomas. Gross or microscopic hematuria occurs in most patients, and flank pain secondary to bleeding and obstruction occurs less commonly. Like primary bladder cancers, urinary cytology is often positive. The most common signs identified at the time of intravenous pyelography include an intraluminal filling defect, unilateral nonvisualization of the collecting system, and hydronephrosis. Ureteral and renal pelvic tumors must be differentiated from calculi, blood clots, papillary necrosis, or inflammatory or infectious lesions. On occasion, such lesions are accessible to direct biopsy, fulguration, or resection using a ureteroscope. Treatment is based on the site, size, depth of penetration, and number of tumors present. Most such cancers are excised with nephroureterectomy (renal pelvic and upper ureteral lesions) or segmental excision of the ureter (distal ureteral lesions). Endoscopic resection may be indicated in patients with limited renal function and in the management of focal, low-grade, upper tract cancers.

PRIMARY TUMORS OF THE KIDNEY

1. RENAL CELL CARCINOMA

Essentials of Diagnosis

- Gross or microscopic hematuria.
- Flank pain or mass in some patients.
- Systemic symptoms such as fever, weight loss may be prominent.
- Solid renal mass on imaging.

General Considerations

Renal cell carcinoma accounts for 2.3% of all adult cancers. In the United States, approximately 27,000 cases will be diagnosed and 10,900 deaths will result from renal cell carcinoma in 1993. Renal cell carcinoma has a peak incidence in the sixth decade of life and a male-to-female ratio of 2:1.

The cause is unknown. Cigarette smoking is the only significant environmental risk factor that has been identified. Familial settings for renal cell carcinoma have been identified (von Hippel-Lindau syndrome) as well as an association with acquired cystic disease, but sporadic tumors are far more common.

Renal cell carcinoma originates from the proximal tubule cells. Various cell types (clear, granular, spindle) and histologic patterns (acinar, papillary, solid) are observed. However, cell type and histologic pattern do not affect treatment. The TNM classification of the American Joint Cancer Committee for kidney cancer is shown in Table 21–9.

Table 21–9. TNM staging system for kidney cancer.

T: Primary tumor

Tx	Cannot be assessed
T0	No evidence of primary tumor
T1	Tumor ≤ 2.5 cm limited to kidney
T2	Tumor > 2.5 cm limited to kidney
T3a	Tumor invades adrenal gland or perinephric tissue
T3b	Tumor extends into renal vein or vena cava
T4	Tumor invades outside of Gerota's fascia

N: Regional lymph nodes

Nx	Cannot be assessed
N0	No regional lymph node metastasis
N1	Metastasis in a single lymph node 2 cm or less
N2	Metastasis in a single lymph node >2 cm and <5 cm or multiple nodes none >5 cm
N3	Metastasis in lymph node >5 cm

M: Distant metastasis

Mx	Cannot be assessed
M0	No distant metastasis
M1	Distant metastasis present

Clinical Findings

A. Symptoms and Signs: Historically, 60% of patients presented with gross or microscopic hematuria. Flank pain or an abdominal mass was detected in approximately 30% of cases. The triad of flank pain, hematuria, and mass was found in only 10–15% of patients and is often a sign of advanced disease. Symptoms of metastatic disease (cough, bone pain) occur in 20–30% of patients at presentation. Because of the more widespread use of ultrasound and CT scanning for diverse indications, renal tumors are being detected incidentally in patients with no urologic symptoms.

B. Laboratory Findings: Hematuria is present in 60% of patients. Paraneoplastic syndromes are not uncommon in renal cell carcinoma. Erythrocytosis occurs in 5%, though anemia is far more common; hypercalcemia may be present in up to 10% of patients. Stauffer's syndrome is a reversible syndrome of hepatic dysfunction in the absence of metastatic disease.

C. Imaging: Renal masses are often first detected by intravenous urography; ultrasound determines whether they are cystic or solid. Further evaluation requires ultrasound to determine whether it is solid or cystic. CT scanning is the most valuable imaging test for renal cell carcinoma. It confirms the character of the mass and further stages the lesion with respect to regional lymph nodes, renal vein, or hepatic involvement. It also gives valuable information on the contralateral kidney (function, bilaterality of neoplasm). Chest radiographs exclude pulmonary metastases, and bone scans should be performed for large tumors and in patients with bone pain or elevated alkaline phosphatase levels. MRI is an excellent means of as-

sessing for the presence and extent of tumor thrombus within the renal vein or vena cava in selected patients.

Differential Diagnosis

Solid lesions of the kidney are renal cell carcinoma until proved otherwise. Other solid masses include angiomyolipomas (fat density usually visible by CT); transitional cell cancers of the renal pelvis (more centrally located, involvement of the collecting system, positive urinary cytology reports); adrenal tumors (supero-anterior to the kidney) and oncocytomas (indistinguishable from renal cell carcinoma preoperatively); and renal abscesses.

Treatment

Radical nephrectomy is the primary treatment for localized renal cell carcinoma. Tumors confined to the renal capsule (T1–T2) demonstrate 5-year disease-free survivals of 90–100%. Tumors extending beyond the renal capsule (T3 or T4) and node-positive tumors have 50–60% and 0–15% 5-year disease-free survivals, respectively.

No effective chemotherapy is available for metastatic renal cell carcinoma. Vinblastine is the single most effective agent, with short-term partial response rates of 15%. Biologic response modifiers have received much attention, including alpha interferon and interleukin-2. Partial response rates of 15–20% and 15–35%, respectively, have been reported. Responders tend to have lower tumor burdens, metastatic disease confined to the lung, and a high performance status. Multicenter trials with these agents are ongoing.

Prognosis

One subgroup of metastatic patients has demonstrated long-term survival, namely, those with solitary resectable metastases. In this setting, radical nephrectomy with resection of the metastasis has resulted in 5-year disease-free survival rates of 15–30%.

2. OTHER PRIMARY TUMORS OF THE KIDNEY

Oncocytomas account for 3–5% of renal tumors and are indistinguishable from renal cell carcinoma by all imaging modalities. The biologic potential of these lesions is not well defined. These tumors are seen in other organs, including the adrenals, the salivary glands, and the thyroid and parathyroid glands.

Angiomyolipomas are rare benign tumors composed of fat, smooth muscle, and blood vessels. They are most commonly seen in patients with tuberous sclerosis (often multiple and bilateral) or in young to middle-aged women. CT scanning may identify the fat component, which is diagnostic for angiomyolipoma. Asymptomatic lesions less than 5 cm in diameter usually do not require intervention.

Wilms' tumor is the most common solid renal tumor of childhood and accounts for 5% of all childhood cancers. The peak age at presentation is during the third year of life, and there is an equal sex distribution. As with renal cell carcinoma, Wilms' tumor occurs in familial and sporadic settings. The most common presentation is of an asymptomatic abdominal mass. Ultrasound can readily distinguish between a solid or cystic mass and is crucial to the assessment process, since hydronephrosis is a more common cause of flank mass in the pediatric age group. Treatment tends to be multimodal, including surgery, radiation therapy, and chemotherapy, depending upon the stage and histologic features.

Boring CC et al: Cancer statistics, 1993. CA 1993;43:7.
Dreicer R, Williams RD: Renal parenchymal neoplasms. In: *Campbell's Urology,* 6th ed. Walsh PC et al (editors). Saunders, 1992.
Sufrin G et al: Paraneoplastic and serologic syndromes of renal adenocarcinoma. Semin Urol 1989;7:158.

SECONDARY TUMORS OF THE KIDNEY

The kidney is not an infrequent site for metastatic disease. Of the solid tumors, the lung is the most common (20%), followed by breast (10%), stomach (10%), and the contralateral kidney (10%). Lymphoma, both Hodgkin's and non-Hodgkin's, may also involve the kidney, though it tends to be a diffusely infiltrative process resulting in renal enlargement rather than a discrete mass.

PRIMARY TUMORS OF THE TESTIS

Malignant tumors of the testis are rare, with approximately two to three new cases per 100,000 males being reported in the United States each year. Ninety to 95 percent of all primary testicular tumors are germ cell tumors (seminoma and nonseminoma), while the remainder are nongerminal neoplasms (Leydig cell, Sertoli cell, gonadoblastoma). The lifetime probability of developing testicular cancer is 0.2% for an American white male. For the purposes of this review, we will only consider germ cell tumors. Survival in testicular cancer has improved dramatically in recent years as a result of the development and application of effective combination chemotherapy.

Testicular cancer is slightly more common on the right than on the left, which parallels the increased incidence of cryptorchism on the right side. One to 2 percent of primary testicular tumors are bilateral, and up to 50% of these men have a history of unilateral or bilateral cryptorchism. Primary bilateral testicular tumors may occur synchronously or asynchronously but tend to be of the same histology. Seminoma is the most common histologic finding in bilateral *primary* testicular tumors, while malignant lymphoma is the most common bilateral testicular tumor.

While the cause of testicular cancer is unknown, both congenital and acquired factors have been associated with tumor development. Approximately 5% of testicular tumors develop in a patient with a history of cryptorchism, with seminoma being the most common. However, 5–10% of these tumors occur in the contralateral, normally descended testis. The relative risk of development of malignancy is highest for the intra-abdominal testis (1:20) and lower for the inguinal testis (1:80). Placement of the cryptorchid testis into the scrotum (orchiopexy) does not alter the malignant potential of the cryptorchid testis; however, it does facilitate examination and tumor detection.

Exogenous estrogen administration during pregnancy has been associated with an increased relative risk for testicular tumors ranging from 2.8 to 5.3. Other acquired factors such as trauma and infection-related testicular atrophy have been associated with testicular tumors; however, a causal relationship has not been established.

Histopathology & Clinical Staging

From a treatment standpoint, testicular carcinoma can be divided into two major categories: (1) nonseminomas, which include embryonal cell carcinomas (20%), teratomas (5%), choriocarcinomas (< 1%), and mixed cell types (40%); and (2) seminomas (35%). In the most commonly used staging system for germ cell tumors, a stage A lesion is confined to the testis; stage B demonstrates regional lymph node involvement in the retroperitoneum; and stage C indicates distant metastasis. For seminoma, the M.D. Anderson system is commonly used. In this system, a stage I lesion is confined to the testis, a stage II lesion has spread to the retroperitoneal lymph nodes, and a stage III lesion has supradiaphragmatic nodal or visceral involvement. The TNM classification of the American Joint Cancer Committee for testis cancer is shown in Table 21–10.

Clinical Findings

A. Symptoms and Signs: The most common symptom of testicular cancer is painless enlargement of the testis. Sensations of heaviness are not unusual. Patients are usually the first to recognize an abnormality, yet the typical delay in seeking medical attention ranges from 3 to 6 months. Acute testicular pain resulting from intratesticular hemorrhage occurs in approximately 10% of cases. Ten percent of patients are asymptomatic at presentation, and 10% manifest symptoms relating to metastatic disease such as back pain (retroperitoneal metastases), cough (pulmonary metastases), or lower extremity edema (vena cava obstruction).

Table 21–10. TNM staging system for testicular cancer.

T: Primary tumor

Tx	Cannot be assessed
T0	No evidence of primary tumor
Tis	Intratubular cancer (CIS)
T1	Limited to testis
T2	Invades beyond tunica albuginea or into epididymis
T3	Invades spermatic cord
T4	Invades scrotum

N: Regional lymph nodes

Nx	Cannot be assessed
N0	No regional lymph node metastasis
N1	Microscopic lymph node metastasis
N2A	Metastasis in $\leq$ 5 nodes, none >2 cm
N2B	Metastasis in >5 nodes, or any node >2 cm
N3	Extranodal invasion
N4	Unresectable retroperitoneal metastasis

M: Distant metastasis

Mx	Cannot be assessed
M0	No distant metastasis
M1	Distant metastasis present

A testicular mass or diffuse enlargement of the testis is found in the majority of cases on physical examination. Secondary hydroceles may be present in 5–10% of cases. In advanced disease, supraclavicular adenopathy may be detected, and abdominal examination may palpate a retroperitoneal mass. Gynecomastia is seen in 5% of germ cell tumors.

B. Laboratory Findings: Several biochemical markers are important in the diagnosis and treatment of testicular carcinoma, including human chorionic gonadotropin (hCG), alpha-fetoprotein, and LDH. Alpha-fetoprotein is never elevated in seminomas, and while hCG is occasionally elevated in seminomas, levels tend to be lower than those seen in nonseminomas. LDH may be elevated in either type of tumor. Liver function tests may be elevated in the presence of hepatic metastases, and anemia may be present in advanced disease. In patients with advanced disease who will receive chemotherapy, renal function is assessed with a 24-hour creatinine clearance urine collection.

C. Imaging: Scrotal ultrasound can readily determine whether the mass is intra- or extratesticular in origin. Once the diagnosis of testicular cancer has been established by inguinal orchiectomy, clinical staging of the disease is accomplished by chest radiograph and abdominal and pelvic CT scanning.

Differential Diagnosis

An incorrect diagnosis is made at the initial examination in up to 25% of patients with testicular tumors. The differential diagnosis of scrotal masses has been discussed previously in this chapter. Scrotal ultrasonography should be performed if any uncertainty exists with respect to the diagnosis. Although most intratesticular masses are malignant, one benign lesion, an epidermoid cyst, may rarely been seen. Epidermoids cysts are usually very small benign nodules located just underneath the tunica albuginea; on occasion, however, they can be large.

Treatment

Inguinal exploration with early vascular control of the spermatic cord structures is the initial intervention to exclude neoplasm. If cancer cannot be excluded by examination of the testis, radical orchiectomy is warranted. Scrotal approaches and open testicular biopsies should be avoided. Further therapy is dependent upon the histology of the tumor as well as the clinical stage.

The 5-year disease-free survival rates for stage I and IIa (retroperitoneal disease < 10 cm in diameter) seminomas treated by radical orchiectomy and retroperitoneal irradiation are 98% and 92–94%, respectively. High-stage seminomas of stage IIb (> 10 cm retroperitoneal involvement) and stage III receive primary chemotherapy (etoposide and cisplatin or cisplatin, etoposide, and bleomycin). Ninety-five percent of patients with stage III disease will attain a complete response following orchiectomy and chemotherapy. Surgical resection of residual retroperitoneal masses is warranted only if the mass is larger than 3 cm in diameter, under which circumstances 40% will harbor residual carcinoma.

Up to 75% of stage A nonseminomas are cured by orchiectomy alone. Currently, such patients may be treated by modified retroperitoneal lymph node dissections designed to preserve the sympathetic innervation for ejaculation. Selected patients who meet specific criteria may be offered surveillance. These criteria are as follows: (1) tumor is confined within the tunica albuginea (T1); (2) tumor does not demonstrate vascular invasion; (3) tumor markers normalize after orchiectomy; (4) radiographic imaging shows no evidence of disease (chest x-ray and CT); and (5) the patient is reliable. Surveillance should be considered an active process both by the physician and by the patient. Patients are followed monthly for the first 2 years and bimonthly in the third year. Tumor markers are obtained at each visit, and chest x-ray and CT scans are obtained every 3–4 months. Follow-up continues beyond the initial 3 years; however, the majority of relapses will occur within the first 8–10 months. With rare exceptions, patients who relapse can be cured by chemotherapy or surgery. The 5-year disease-free survival rate for patients with stage A disease ranges from 96% to 100%. For low-volume stage B disease, 90% 5-year disease-free survival is attainable.

Patients with bulky retroperitoneal disease (> 3 cm nodes) or metastatic nonseminomas are treated with primary cisplatin-based combination chemotherapy following orchiectomy (etoposide and cisplatin or cisplatin, etoposide, and bleomycin). If tumor markers normalize and a residual mass is apparent on imaging studies, resection of that mass is mandatory because 20% of the time it will harbor residual cancer and 40% of the time it will be teratoma. Even if patients have a complete response to chemotherapy, a recent study suggests that retroperitoneal lymphadenectomy is warranted in some patients as 10% of patients may harbor residual carcinoma and 10% may have teratoma in the retroperitoneum. If tumor markers fail to normalize following primary chemotherapy, salvage chemotherapy is required (cisplatin, etoposide, bleomycin, ifosfamide).

Prognosis

Patients with bulky retroperitoneal or disseminated disease treated with primary chemotherapy followed by surgery have a 5-year disease-free survival rate of 55–80%.

SECONDARY TUMORS OF THE TESTIS

Secondary tumors of the testis are rare. Lymphoma is the most common testis tumor in a patient over the age of 50 and is the most common secondary neoplasm of the testis, accounting for 5% of all testicular tumors. It may be seen in three clinical settings: (1) as a late manifestation of widespread lymphoma; (2) as the initial presentation of clinically occult disease; and (3) as primary extranodal disease. Radical orchiectomy is indicated to make the diagnosis. Prognosis is related to the stage of disease.

The testis is a common site of relapse for children with acute lymphocytic leukemia. Bilateral involvement may be present in half of cases. Testicular biopsy rather than orchiectomy is the diagnostic procedure of choice.

Metastasis to the testis is rare. The most common primary site is the prostate, followed by the lung, gastrointestinal tract, melanoma, and kidney.

Donohue JP et al: Nerve-sparing retroperitoneal lymphadenectomy with preservation of ejaculation. J Urol 1990;144:287.
Dunphy CH et al: Clinical stage I nonseminomatous and mixed germ cell tumors of the testis. A clinicopathologic study of 93 patients on a surveillance protocol after orchiectomy alone. Cancer 1988;62:1202.
Presti JC Jr, Herr HW: Genital tumors. In: *Smith's General Urology,* 13th ed. Tanagho EA, McAninch JW (editors). Appleton & Lange, 1992.
Toner GC et al: Adjunctive surgery after chemotherapy for nonseminomatous germ cell tumors: Recommendations for patient selection. J Clin Oncol 1990;8:1683.

MEDICAL RENAL DISEASE

Richard M. Freeman, MD

ACUTE RENAL FAILURE

Essentials of Diagnosis

- Sudden increase in serum urea nitrogen or creatinine.
- Often accompanied by oliguria.
- Oliguria is self-limiting over a few days to 4–6 weeks.

General Considerations

Acute renal failure occurs when elevations in the blood urea nitrogen and serum creatinine are noted within days after documented normal values. It is often accompanied by oliguria. In some clinical circumstances, the distinction between acute and chronic renal failure may not be readily apparent. Kidney size may be helpful in differentiation, since patients with acute renal failure often have kidneys of normal or slightly larger size and patients with chronic renal failure often have bilaterally small kidneys. Likewise, renal osteodystrophy suggests chronicity of disease.

Etiology & Clinical Findings

Causes of acute renal failure are listed in Table 21–11.

Before one can investigate the causes of acute renal failure, prerenal and postrenal causes of azotemia must be excluded (Table 21–12). The most common cause of prerenal azotemia is hypovolemia, but impaired cardiac function may also be responsible. In both circumstances, the BUN/creatinine ratio is often greater than 15:1. It is in distinguishing prerenal from

Table 21–11. Causes of acute renal failure.

Acute tubular necrosis
Postischemic
Nephrotoxic
Acute interstitial nephritis
Drug hypersensitivity
Immunologic disorders
Infections
Acute glomerulonephritis
Renal artery occlusion, bilateral
Thrombotic microangiopathy
Thrombotic thrombocytopenic purpura
Hemolytic uremic syndrome
Postpartum renal failure
Scleroderma
Malignant hypertension
Cortical necrosis
Gram-negative sepsis
Abruptio placentae
Placenta previa

Table 21–12. Causes of postrenal azotemia.[1]

Obstruction of ureters, bilateral
  Extraureteral
    Tumor: cervix, prostate, endometriosis
    Periureteral fibrosis
    Accidental ureteral ligation during pelvic operation
  Intraureteral
    Sulfonamide and uric acid crystals
    Blood clots
    Pyogenic debris
    Stones
    Edema
    Papillary necrosis
Bladder neck obstruction
  Prostatic hypertrophy
  Bladder carcinoma
  Functional: neuropathy or ganglionic blocking agents
Urethral obstruction

[1]Reproduced, with permission, from Anderson RJ, Conger JD: Acute renal failure including cortical necrosis. In: *Textbook of Nephrology*, vol 1, 2nd ed. Williams & Wilkins, 1989.

oliguric renal failure that urinary indices are of value (Table 21–13). Prerenal causes of oliguria are characterized by high urine osmolality, high urine/plasma urea nitrogen and urine/plasma creatinine ratios, and low urinary sodium excretion.

A. Renal Hypoperfusion: Hypoperfusion of the kidney is the most frequently recognized insult leading to acute renal failure in the setting of trauma, surgery, hemorrhage, or dehydration. Hypoperfusion is associated with a graded parenchymal injury that can range from none in prerenal azotemia to frank acute tubular necrosis.

B. Acute Tubular Necrosis: Acute tubular necrosis is often manifested by oliguric renal failure and in most patients is a reversible lesion. The duration of the oliguric phase is quite variable, ranging from a few days to 4–6 weeks. One to 2 days after diuresis ensues (usually defined as a urinary output > 1000 mL/d in adults), the blood urea nitrogen and serum creatinine will gradually decrease and will usually re-

Table 21–13. Summary of urinary indices in oliguric renal failure.[1]

	Prerenal	Oliguric Acute Renal Failure
Urine osmolality (mosm/kg)	>500	<350
Urine sodium (meq/L)	<20	>40
Urine/plasma urea nitrogen ratio	>8	<3
Urine/plasma creatinine ratio	>40	<20
Renal failure index	<1	>1
Fractional excretion of filtered sodium	<1	>1

[1]Reproduced, with permission, from Miller TR et al: Urinary diagnosis indices in acute renal failure: A prospective study. Ann Intern Med 1978;89:47.

turn to normal values in patients without previous evidence of renal dysfunction.

C. Drug Toxicity:

1. Nonsteroidal anti-inflammatory drugs– These commonly used agents, some of which (eg, ibuprofen—as Advil or Nupren) are available over the counter, may cause renal failure. This occurs typically in patients with previously impaired renal blood flow, as in congestive heart failure or acute volume depletion. Inhibition of prostaglandin-mediated compensatory renal vasodilation is responsible (see below).

2. Angiotensin-converting enzyme inhibitors– Also in wise use, these drugs reduce efferent arteriolar tone in the glomerulus. If the kidney had been dependent on this mechanism to maintain function (eg, in renal artery stenosis), hydrostatic pressure across the glomerulus falls, and renal dysfunction ensues. Hyperkalemia is often associated because of secondary hypoaldosteronism caused by reduction in angiotensin.

3. Aminoglycosides– In hospitalized patients, the aminoglycoside nephrotoxicity is encountered commonly. Neomycin, kanamycin, gentamicin, tobramycin, amikacin, and streptomycin have all been reported to cause renal damage. Damage has occurred even when plasma levels of these drugs appear to have been therapeutic. Aminoglycoside-induced acute renal failure is typically nonoliguric. As a rule, drug administration for 5–10 days is necessary for the nephrotoxic effect to be manifested; occasionally, the serum creatinine does not rise until the antibiotics have been discontinued.

4. Amphotericin B– Nephrotoxicity should be anticipated when the total dose of amphotericin B exceeds 2–3 g. Distal renal tubular acidosis may accompany the azotemia. Radiographic contrast material may be additively nephrotoxic.

5. Cyclosporine– Nephrotoxicity from cyclosporine is dose-dependent. Kidney biopsy may be necessary to distinguish transplant rejection from cyclosporine nephrotoxicity.

D. Myoglobinuria: Myoglobinuria as a consequence of rhabdomyolysis is a frequent cause of acute renal failure. The patient will often complain of muscle pain, and a high serum level of creatine kinase is expected. Red blood cells are not seen in the urine microscopically even though the urine is dipstick-positive for blood due to myoglobin. Rhabdomyolysis most often occurs in the settings of alcohol abuse, crush injury, muscle necrosis from prolonged unconsciousness, and seizures. Simultaneous presence of hypovolemia is necessary for myoglobin to produce nephrotoxicity.

E. Transfusion Reactions: Intravascular hemolysis secondary to transfusion reaction is a well-known but increasingly less common cause of acute renal failure.

Management of Acute Renal Failure

A. Dialysis: The universal availability of dialysis has had a major effect on how patients with acute renal failure are managed. In oliguric acute tubular necrosis, the oliguric stage can last from several days to 4–6 weeks. Once oliguric acute tubular necrosis has been established, dialysis should be initiated and performed on an intermittent basis until diuresis ensues. Mental status abnormalities, pericarditis, and hyperkalemia also constitute indications for dialysis. In nonoliguric acute renal failure, dialysis may also be necessary in order to minimize increases in urea nitrogen and creatinine, although hyperkalemia is generally not a problem.

B. Medical Treatment: Intravenous calcium gluconate or chloride, hypertonic sodium bicarbonate, and glucose with insulin all are effective initial methods of controlling hyperkalemia. Sodium polystyrene sulfonate orally or by rectum will remove potassium by exchanging it with sodium. Fluid overload is an additional indication for dialysis. The cautious use of loop diuretics in this situation is believed by some to convert oliguric to nonoliguric renal failure, an easier condition to manage.

Finn WF: Diagnosis and management of acute tubular necrosis. Med Clin North Am 1990;74:873.

Manske CL et al: Contrast nephropathy in azotemic diabetic patients undergoing coronary angiography. Am J Med 1990;89:615.

CHRONIC RENAL FAILURE

Essentials of Diagnosis

- Progressive azotemia over weeks and months.
- May be a consequence of many primary glomerular and tubular diseases.
- Urinary abnormalities are dependent upon the underlying disease, though isosthenuria is common when chronic renal failure is advanced.
- Hypertension develops in the majority of patients.

Clinical Findings

The symptoms of chronic renal failure are nonspecific. Nausea, vomiting, weakness, and lethargy are typical. Hiccup may be intractable, and some patients complain of itching. Decreased libido and menstrual irregularities are common, as is impaired concentration. Once symptoms begin, complications of uremia soon follow. These include pericarditis, platelet dysfunction, anemia, renal osteodystrophy, and peripheral neuropathy. The relationship of the development of symptoms to renal function studies is inconsistent, but chronic renal failure is considered to be present when glomerular filtration has been reduced by 75%. The rate of progression to end-stage renal failure requiring dialysis or transplant varies and depends on the underlying cause. Some patients, however, are free of symptoms at much higher levels.

Many of the signs and symptoms of chronic renal failure are listed in Table 21–14.

Complications & Treatment of Complications

A. Pericarditis: Pericarditis may develop during untreated renal failure but is also seen in patients who have been maintained with dialysis for months or years and who appear to be adequately dialyzed. Chest pain occurs in about two-thirds of cases. Fever is common also. A pericardial friction rub is almost always present but occasionally is intermittent. Disappearance of a friction rub may be a sign of accumulation of pericardial fluid. Electrocardiography may

Table 21–14. Clinical consequences of renal failure.

General: Nausea, vomiting, weakness, lethargy, hiccup
Cardiovascular
  Pericarditis with or without cardiac tamponade
  Congestive heart failure
  Hypertension
Hematopoietic
  Red blood cells: Anemia
    Decreased erythropoietin
    Low-grade hemolysis
    Iron deficiency (in hemodialysis patients)
  White blood cells
    Decreased phagocytosis and chemotaxis
    Decreased lymphocytes
  Platelets: Abnormal bleeding due to prolonged bleeding time (decreased platelet adhesiveness)
Neurologic
  Peripheral neuropathy
  Central nervous system: Seizures
    Hypertensive encephalopathy
    Disequilibrium syndrome (in dialysis patients)
    Dialysis encephalopathy
Musculoskeletal
  Renal osteodystrophy
    Subperiosteal resorption due to increased parathyroid hormone
    Osteomalacia
      Defective conversion of 25-hydroxycholecalciferol to 1,25-dihydroxycholecalciferol
      Aluminum excess
  Articular complications (dialysis patients)
Metabolic and endocrine disturbances
  Glucose intolerance
  Sexual dysfunction
  Lipid abnormalities
Gastrointestinal
  Gastrointestinal bleeding: Angiodysplasia
  Hepatitis (dialysis patients)
Electrolyte abnormalities
  Hyponatremia
  Hyperkalemia
  Metabolic acidosis
  Hypocalcemia or hypercalcemia
  Hyperphosphatemia
  Hypermagnesemia
Dermatologic
  Dry skin
  Itching

not disclose elevated ST segments, in contrast to other types of pericarditis; atrial fibrillation may occur. Echocardiography will demonstrate the absence or presence of pericardial effusion.

The most serious complication of pericarditis is **cardiac tamponade,** which may be manifested by shortness of breath and hypotension. Sudden onset of hypotension at the beginning of dialysis may be the first clinical sign. Emergent pericardiocentesis is required, but subsequent management is somewhat controversial. In some centers, a catheter is left in the pericardial sac after pericardiocentesis to remove fluid if it should continue to accumulate. In others, the preference is for pericardiectomy or placement of a pericardial window so that fluid will drain into the pleural space.

In most cases, the frequency or duration of dialysis should be increased after pericarditis develops. Pericarditis is an absolute indication for initiation of hemodialysis if the patient has not previously been dialyzed.

Though the value of indomethacin has not been substantiated by placebo-controlled studies, it is often used in patients with chest pain, especially if they have associated fever.

B. Congestive Heart Failure: Fluid overload occurs commonly in patients with renal failure, often in the absence of associated heart disease. If water and salt intakes are not controlled in the patient who is oliguric or anuric, plasma volume expansion and symptoms of congestive heart failure will ultimately ensue. Many patients with renal failure have underlying hypertensive cardiovascular disease that may contribute to the problem. As the dialysis patient population continues to age, more of the patients have coronary artery disease as well.

Diuretics may be of value in the patient with chronic renal failure. Thiazide diuretics are ineffective when the creatinine clearance is less than 10–15 mL/min and should therefore be avoided. Loop diuretics are commonly utilized, and higher doses will be necessary than in patients without renal failure. Digitalis should be used with caution, and the maintenance dose must be greatly reduced. Since digoxin is not dialyzed at the same rate as the serum potassium, cardiac arrhythmias typical of hypokalemia may occur in patients receiving hemodialysis.

C. Hypertension: Hypertension is both a cause and an effect of chronic renal failure. A variety of antihypertensive medications are available to control blood pressure. Rarely, an untreated patient will present with malignant or accelerated hypertension and require urgent therapy (see Chapter 11). With vigorous therapy, normal blood pressure can be achieved in the majority of dialysis patients. Most dialysis patients with hypertension are salt- and water-sensitive—ie, if one removes salt and water with the dialysis procedure and minimizes weight gain between dialyses with judicious dietary control of salt

and water intake, normal blood pressures can be achieved. About 25% of dialysis patients, however, are renin-sensitive. These patients characteristically have high predialysis blood pressure but exhibit an unpredictable response to that therapy. Though bilateral nephrectomy will often convert these patients to the more typically salt- and water-responsive type of hypertension, the availability of minoxidil and angiotensin-converting enzyme inhibitors has largely eliminated the use of bilateral nephrectomy in these patients. ACE inhibitors are better tolerated than minoxidil, though not all patients respond to the drugs.

D. Hematopoietic Abnormalities:

1. Anemia–As renal failure progresses, anemia develops. The anemia of renal failure is characteristically normochromic and normocytic; it is due mainly to decreased erythropoietin from the damaged kidneys, though low-grade hemolysis may play an additional role. In hemodialysis patients, iron is regularly given as a supplement because of the loss of red cells in the dialyzer. Supplements of water-soluble vitamins are also administered.

Erythropoietin (epoetin alfa) is generally used in patients whose hematocrit is less than 35%. The effective dose differs from patient to patient. The medication can be given either intravenously (most commonly in the hemodialysis patient) or subcutaneously (for patients receiving peritoneal dialysis or those who have not yet started dialysis therapy). Erythropoietin is very expensive, and iron stores must be adequate to ensure response to it. Simultaneous administration of an androgen (eg, nandrolone decanoate, 100 mg intramuscularly once weekly) will enhance the response to erythropoietin. Aluminum excess also prevents response to the drug; deferoxamine can be used to chelate aluminum in such patients. Finally, patients with chronic inflammatory processes may not respond to epoetin alfa.

Hypertension has recently been noted as a complication of erythropoietin therapy. It appears to develop more abruptly in patients with the lowest hematocrit values at the initiation of therapy. Patients receiving erythropoietin may therefore require adjustment of antihypertensive drugs or initiation of medication if they were previously not requiring any.

2. Coagulopathy–Purpura and petechiae are common manifestations of untreated uremia. Platelet counts in most patients are only moderately decreased or within normal limits. Even so, the bleeding time is prolonged, a defect that has been attributed to decreased platelet adhesiveness. This abnormality improves with dialysis, though it does not always completely normalize. Giving platelet transfusions to these patients is of limited value since the transfused platelets are quickly modified by the uremic environment. Cryoprecipitate has occasionally been used but has only a transient effect. Desmopressin is quite effective and is often used in preparation for surgery in order to minimize bleeding. Conjugated estrogens have recently been shown to have a beneficial effect and have the advantage of prolonged action (for several days or weeks).

E. Neurologic: Peripheral neuropathy was at one time a major complication of end-stage renal disease. Presumably as a result of the earlier initiation of dialysis, it is now seen less often. The response of peripheral neuropathy to dialysis is variable, however; some cases respond only to transplant.

Patients in whom the blood urea nitrogen is rapidly lowered sometimes develop headaches, nausea, muscular twitching, disorientation, and seizures. This symptom complex has been called the **dialysis disequilibrium syndrome.** The movement of urea from the blood through the dialysis membrane is more rapid than its transport from the cerebrospinal fluid to the bloodstream. This establishes an osmotic gradient by which water moves into the cerebrospinal fluid, producing the symptoms. The syndrome can largely be prevented by using lower blood flow rates or a shorter duration of hemodialysis when it is initiated.

Dialysis encephalopathy or **dialysis dementia** is an insidious syndrome characterized by speech disturbances, personality changes, progressive dementia, and seizures that occurs most commonly in patients who have received dialysis for several years. The symptoms appear to be a manifestation of aluminum intoxication. While the initial cases appeared to be related to the high aluminum content of the dialysate, the absorption of aluminum from aluminum hydroxide received by many patients with renal failure is also of importance. If the syndrome is identified early enough, it may respond to aluminum chelation with deferoxamine.

F. Skeletal: Renal osteodystrophy is a complex disorder with several pathogenetic factors. The most common component is osteitis fibrosa, manifested as subperiosteal resorption of bone. This is a consequence of decreased excretion as well as increased secretion of parathyroid hormone. In renal failure, small increments of serum phosphorus cause small decreases in serum calcium, stimulating the secretion of parathyroid hormone. Because of the phosphaturic effect of PTH, the serum phosphorus tends to be normalized but at the expense of a higher circulating PTH level; ultimately, progression of renal disease results in persistent hyperphosphatemia and hypocalcemia, leading to extremely high PTH concentrations. Aluminum hydroxide has been used to bind phosphorus in the gut in such patients. Because of concerns about aluminum toxicity, calcium carbonate is often used to minimize its intake. Newer preparations to bind phosphorus are now being tested.

Another important component of renal osteodystrophy is **osteomalacia.** Defective kidneys fail to convert 25-hydroxycholecalciferol to 1,25-dihydroxycholecalciferol. This leads to increased losses of calcium in the feces and defective mineralization in bone. Calcitriol or dihydrotachysterol can effectively overcome this problem. Standard vitamin D preparations should not be used in these patients, since hypercalcemia, if it occurs, may last for several weeks. In some patients with renal osteodystrophy, phosphate binders and vitamin D preparations are ineffective in reducing the parathyroid hormone level, and subtotal parathyroidectomy is required.

The least common type of renal osteodystrophy is **aluminum-induced osteomalacia.** In patients who have received aluminum for many years, the element may interfere with mineralization of bone. This diagnosis is confirmed by high serum aluminum levels and demonstration of aluminum in bone biopsy specimens. Chelation with deferoxamine may be effective.

G. Metabolic and Endocrine Disturbances: Glucose intolerance occurs with regularity in the nondiabetic patient once the serum creatinine exceeds 10–12 mg/dL. Its exact cause is controversial, but a dialyzable toxin is suspected since the abnormality seems to disappear after several weeks of adequate dialysis. Conversely, some patients with end-stage renal disease, usually of several years' duration, develop hypoglycemia. Reduced renal gluconeogenesis may play a role in pathogenesis.

Decreased libido and impotence occur in a high percentage of patients with chronic renal failure. Menstrual irregularities or amenorrhea is the rule, and successful pregnancy does not occur. There are many hormonal abnormalities that might play a role in these symptoms: decreased circulating testosterone in men, increased circulating prolactin in women. Sexual function appears to improve in patients whose hematocrits are normalized with erythropoietin.

H. Gastrointestinal: Gastrointestinal bleeding is a relatively common consequence of renal failure. Factors such as prolonged bleeding time and use of heparin during artificial kidney treatment may play a role. There appears to be increased frequency of angiodysplasia of the upper gastrointestinal tract. There is no increased incidence of peptic disease.

Both hepatitis B and hepatitis C are common in dialysis units. Both may result in chronic liver disease and cirrhosis. The use of hepatitis B vaccines has decreased the frequency of hepatitis in patients and staff. All patients and staff should receive this vaccine even though the antibody response to the vaccine in renal failure may be less than ideal. Although ascites may occur in association with chronic liver disease, dialysis patients also manifest on occasion an exudative ascites in the face of normal liver function. Its pathogenesis is unknown.

I. Electrolyte Abnormalities: Serum electrolyte abnormalities are universally found in patients with chronic renal failure. **Hyponatremia** may develop as a result of excessive water intake. **Hyperkalemia** is a clinical problem in chronic renal failure when it is accompanied by oliguria. However, hyporeninemic hypoaldosteronism may also cause hyperkalemia. Here, the serum potassium may be elevated when the serum creatinine is only moderately increased. Though typical of diabetic nephropathy, it occurs in all types of renal disease and may be worsened by the use of angiotensin-converting enzyme inhibitors.

Most **metabolic acidosis** in renal failure is due to inability of the damaged kidney to excrete hydrogen ion. Metabolic acidosis tends to be more severe in patients who have tubular rather than glomerular disease. Correction by sodium bicarbonate is seldom necessary in adequately dialyzed patients. Such patients tend to have mild metabolic acidosis immediately before and mild metabolic alkalosis at the end of the 3- to 4-hour procedure.

Hypermagnesemia occurs with regularity in the dialysis patient but generally is a clinical problem only in patients receiving magnesium-containing antacids, which are contraindicated in patients with renal failure. When serum magnesium exceeds 4–5 meq/L, orthostatic hypotension and constipation become prominent. Cardiac arrhythmias may occur with such levels, and coma may be induced if the serum magnesium level exceeds 7–8 meq/L.

Management of Chronic Renal Failure

A. Dietary Management: The dietary management of chronic renal failure is complex. A rationale exists for dietary restriction of protein, fat, carbohydrate, sodium, potassium, phosphorus, and water. It is therefore crucial to determine what the specific goals of therapy are in an individual patient and to discuss with the dietician how this can be practically achieved.

1. Protein restriction–There is some evidence that protein restriction may slow the deterioration of renal function in patients with a variety of renal diseases. The practicality of such an approach as well as its efficacy and nutritional value are uncertain. However, it is probably wise to restrict protein intake moderately to 1 g/kg daily.

2. Sodium restriction–Most patients with chronic renal failure can neither conserve nor excrete sodium effectively and thus lose a relatively fixed amount daily in the urine. In practical terms, this means that most patients should eat a diet with no added salt because of associated hypertension or edema. In patients who are neither hypertensive nor edematous, salt restriction may not be necessary. In rare cases (eg, the patient with medullary cystic disease), salt losing can be a prominent feature and supplemental sodium chloride is actually mandatory. In dialysis patients, sodium intake should be reduced in patients who gain excessive weight between dialyses.

3. Potassium restriction–Potassium restriction is usually not necessary until oliguria supervenes. Dialysis patients, however, should be educated with regard to what foods are high in potassium—nuts, dried fruits, bananas, etc—in order to avoid very high serum levels of potassium before each dialysis.

4. Water restriction–Like sodium, water is neither conserved nor excreted, and patients tend to have isosthenuria. Water restriction may be necessary if predialysis hyponatremia becomes prominent.

B. Dialysis: Although there is wide variability in the number, many patients with chronic renal failure start dialysis when the serum creatinine is around 10 mg/dL (or blood urea nitrogen around 100 mg/dL); patients with diabetic nephropathy often seem to require dialysis somewhat earlier. Whenever possible, an arteriovenous fistula should be placed on an outpatient basis several weeks before the anticipated initiation of hemodialysis. This allows maturation of the fistula and a higher blood flow through the dialyzer.

1. Hemodialysis–Several types of dialysis are now available. Hemodialysis can be performed either in a dialysis unit or in the home. Most patients will require hemodialysis three times weekly. The dialysis procedure itself lasts 3–6 hours depending on the type of membranes used, the size of the patient, and other criteria. Dialysis in a unit requires that the patient travel to and from the unit three times a week. Unless nighttime dialysis is available, the procedure may interfere with work.

Home hemodialysis has the advantage that it can be performed in the home at nighttime at the patient's convenience, though a regular schedule is still indicated. Patients receiving home hemodialysis must become much more knowledgeable about their treatment than patients treated in the center. Many believe that home dialysis patients do better for this reason, but selection bias obviously plays a role. A major disadvantage of home hemodialysis is that a helper must be available. Furthermore, training for home hemodialysis may take weeks to months.

2. Peritoneal dialysis–While the percentage of patients receiving home hemodialysis has declined over the past 10 years, the number of patients receiving continuous ambulatory peritoneal dialysis has greatly increased. Peritoneal dialysis is performed by the patient, and the continual nature of the dialysis leads to better clearance of poorly dialyzable compounds, especially phosphate. This in turn results in less dietary restriction for these patients. Similarly, continuous dialysis is not associated with symptom swings observed in hemodialysis.

When first introduced, it was hoped that the cost of continuous ambulatory peritoneal dialysis would be much less than the cost of hemodialysis. While the equipment costs are indeed less, the total cost of care of these patients is not much different. Peritonitis remains a major complication of peritoneal dialysis, and its treatment (which sometimes includes hospitalization) has been expensive. When vascular access for hemodialysis is hard to achieve, such as in small children and in some diabetic patients, continuous ambulatory peritoneal dialysis has been found to be a reasonable alternative. In patients who have been treated with both modalities, peritoneal dialysis is usually preferred.

C. Kidney Transplantation: In most patients who develop chronic renal failure, serious consideration should be given to the role of kidney transplantation. About two-thirds of the kidney transplants performed in the United States come from cadaveric donors and the remainder from living related donors. Posttransplant immunosuppression with corticosteroids, azathioprine, and cyclosporine—singly or in combination—are regularly required in cadaveric kidney transplants and generally in living related donor transplants as well, though the number of drugs and the duration of drug administration may be less depending upon the degrees of HLA matching.

The 2-year kidney graft survival rate for living related donor transplantations is 85%; the 2-year graft survival rate for cadaveric donor transplantations is 70%. There is some evidence that HLA mismatching has a greater effect on living related than it does on cadaveric donor kidney transplantation. Interestingly, pretransplant blood transfusion appears to improve graft survival, in contrast to its deleterious effect on marrow engraftment.

Delmez JA, Slatopolsky E: Hyperphosphatemia: Its consequences and treatment in patients with chronic renal disease. Am J Kidney Dis 1992;19:303.

Ersley AJ: Erythropoietin. N Engl J Med 1991;324:1339.

Felsenfeld AJ, Llach F: Parathyroid gland function in chronic renal failure. Kidney Int 1993;43:771.

Held PJ et al: Five-year survival for end-stage renal disease patients in the United States, Europe, and Japan, 1982 to 1987. Am J Kidney Dis 1990;15:451.

Humphries JE: Anemia of renal failure: Use of erythropoietin. Med Clin North Am 1992;76:711.

Mitch WE: Dietary protein restriction in patients with chronic renal failure. Kidney Int 1991;40:326. (Nephrology forum on dietary aspects of renal failure discussed by a leading expert.)

Nisserson AR, Fine RN: *Dialysis Therapy.* Mosby Year Book, 1992.

Rotellar C et al: Ten years' experience with continuous ambulatory peritoneal dialysis. Am J Kidney Dis 1991; 17:158.

NEPHROTIC SYNDROME

Essentials of Diagnosis

- Proteinuria (> 3.5 g/d).
- Hypoalbuminemia (< 3 g/dL).
- Hyperlipidemia with serum cholesterol > 300 mg/dL.
- Oval fat bodies and fatty casts in the urinary sediment.
- Edema.

General Considerations

Nephrotic syndrome is usually defined as the simultaneous presence of heavy proteinuria (usually > 3.5 g/1.73 m^2/24 h) together with hypoalbuminemia, lipiduria, hypercholesterolemia, and edema. It is a consequence of severe proteinuria, and patients often complain of foamy urine. Because a variety of disorders can produce nephrotic syndrome, symptoms and signs, except for the edema, otherwise are those of the causative diseases. It has been customary to order tests for antinuclear antibody, rheumatoid factor, cryoglobulins, complement, HBsAg, VDRL serology, and protein electrophoresis of the serum and urine in patients with heavy proteinuria. It is more appropriate to refine the selection of studies in light of the history and physical examination.

Histologic Classification

Nephrotic syndrome is invariably due to a glomerular lesion and is one of the most common indications for **renal biopsy,** particularly if the cause is unclear after initial evaluation. Nephrotic syndrome is a common sequela of certain systemic diseases. Diabetes mellitus is the commonest example, and it also occurs with systemic lupus erythematosus and amyloidosis. Histologic diagnoses of primary renal causes of nephrotic syndrome are discussed in the following paragraphs.

A. Minimal Change Disease (Lipoid Nephrosis, Nil Disease): Minimal change disease is so called because under light microscopy the glomeruli appear totally normal. Under electron microscopy, however, there is characteristic fusion of the epithelial foot processes. Immunofluorescence tests are usually negative.

Minimal change disease, though common in children, is seen occasionally in adults. The glomerular filtration rate is usually normal. This disorder responds very well to corticosteroids; in a few patients, however, it tends to recur after prednisone is decreased or discontinued. In such cases, the addition of cyclophosphamide or chlorambucil is often curative. In any case, progression to renal failure does not occur unless the biopsy shows glomerulosclerosis. The latter probably constitutes a separate entity, encountered most often in intravenous drug users.

B. Membranous Glomerulonephritis: Membranous glomerulonephritis is one of the most common biopsy findings in adults with nephrotic syndrome. Light microscopy reveals diffuse uniform thickening of the capillary wall which on silver staining may show some epimembranous projection of basement membrane material. Electron microscopy shows striking electron-dense deposits in the basement membrane. Immunofluorescence demonstrates a granular distribution of IgG.

Membranous glomerulonephritis may be idiopathic or associated with a variety of disorders (systemic lupus erythematosus, gold toxicity, penicillamine toxicity, hepatitis B, syphilis, solid tumors). The natural history of **idiopathic membranous glomerulonephritis** has been so variable that the influence of treatment is been difficult to assess. Most placebo-controlled studies have not demonstrated a major benefit from corticosteroids or immunosuppressant drugs, though many clinicians favor a trial of empiric prednisone for 6–8 weeks.

C. Mesangiocapillary Glomerulonephritis: Mesangiocapillary glomerulonephritis is characterized histologically by an increase in mesangial cells—producing, on light microscopy, a double contour of the capillary wall. There is often a lobular appearance to the glomeruli. Like membranous glomerulonephritis, mesangiocapillary glomerulonephritis can occur as a complication of a variety of diseases, such as systemic lupus erythematosus, or as a primary disease. On electron microscopy, deposits may be seen subendothelially or within the glomerular basement membrane. Patients are often hypocomplementemic.

Immunomodulation with steroids and antiplatelet agents are frequently attempted, with unimpressive results.

Treatment

A. Cholesterol Lowering: Hypercholesterolemia and hypertriglyceridemia are regular accompaniments of heavy proteinuria. The low-density lipoproteins are usually increased. The high-density lipoproteins may be normal or even increased early in the disease but generally are decreased because of losses in the urine. Increased hepatic production of lipids has been generally considered responsible for hyperlipidemia.

Dietary management appears to be of limited value in these patients if there has been no amelioration of hyperlipidemia with treatment of the causative diseases. The choice of which hypolipidemic agent to use is not clearly established, but in general that decision can be approached in the same fashion as hyperlipidemia without nephrotic syndrome (see Chapter 27). The accelerated atherosclerosis observed in many dialysis patients may be related in part to this hyperlipidemia but is observed in many renal failure patients without hyperlipidemia and nephrotic syndrome.

B. High-Protein Diet: High-protein diets are of debatable value. Indeed, in diabetics with nephrotic syndrome, urinary protein is often decreased after reduction in dietary protein intake. Since increased protein intake seems to have a theoretic adverse effect on renal function in some disease processes, moderation of protein intake in the nephrotic syndrome seems reasonable. An intake of 1 g/kg/d of protein should be adequate in most circumstances.

C. Sodium Restriction: In the presence of edema, sodium intake should be restricted. Patients who do not respond to corticosteroids may be managed with varying doses of diuretics.

D. Vitamin D: Some patients with nephrotic syndrome lose vitamin D metabolites in the urine. It is not clear whether vitamin D supplementation should be routinely used in these patients. Supplementation should be considered when nephrotic syndrome is chronic and unresponsive to other therapy.

Appel G: Lipid abnormalities in renal disease. Kidney Int 1991;39:169.

Austin HA et al: Membranous nephropathy. Ann Intern Med 1992;116:672. (Edited summary of NIH Conference on membranous nephropathy, including comments on pathology, immunosuppressive agents, and therapeutic studies.)

D'Amico G: Influence of clinical and histological features on actuarial renal survival in adult patients with idiopathic IgA nephropathy, membranous nephropathy, and membranoproliferative glomerulonephritis: Survey of the recent literature. Am J Kidney Dis 1992;20:315.

Howard AD et al: Routine serologic tests in the differential diagnosis of the adult nephrotic syndrome. Am J Kidney Dis 1990;15:24.

Pollack VE: Treatment of membranous glomerulonephritis. Am J Kidney Dis 1992;19:68. (Thoughtful editorial on the complexities in evaluating therapy in idiopathic membranous nephropathy.)

SPECIFIC DISEASES OF THE KIDNEY

1. POSTSTREPTOCOCCAL GLOMERULONEPHRITIS

Poststreptococcal glomerulonephritis is the result of infection with a nephritogenic strain of group A hemolytic streptococci. Subclinical cases are probably 4–5 times as common as those that come to the physician's attention. While in the United States the streptococci are usually isolated from patients with a sore throats, in tropical regions skin infection is a more important historical feature. The latent period between infection and onset of urinary symptoms is about 10 days.

Clinical Findings

Poststreptococcal glomerulonephritis is characterized by smoky or rust-colored urine, edema (especially of the face), increased blood pressure, and red blood cell urinary casts. Circulatory congestion is not unusual. While some proteinuria is present, it is typically not in the nephrotic range. Urinary sodium is low, with fractional excretion often less than 0.5%. While the ASO titer usually rises, this rise may be blunted by previous treatment with antibiotics. There is a decrease in the third component of complement in about 50% of cases.

Renal biopsy shows an exudative proliferative glomerulonephritis, and electron microscopy shows rather characteristic "humps" beneath the epithelial basement membrane.

Treatment

There is no specific treatment except for antihypertensives, salt restriction, and diuretics. Corticosteroids have not been of value. The disorder is generally considered self-limiting, but in some adults it may progress to chronic renal failure.

2. RAPIDLY PROGRESSIVE GLOMERULONEPHRITIS

Rapidly progressive glomerulonephritis can be defined as any glomerular disease in which extensive crescents are the principal finding on biopsy and in which there is a rapid loss of renal function over days and weeks rather than months and years. Many conditions are now known to produce this clinical syndrome (Table 21–15), though the symptoms of glomerulonephritis (hypertension, edema, dark urine, oliguria) are similar irrespective of the cause. If one biopsies such patients, about one-fifth of cases will be associated with anti-glomerular basement antibody. The remainder will be equally divided between those who show immunocomplexes and those who do not.

Treatment

Therapy for rapidly progressive glomerulonephritis has been difficult to assess because so many diverse conditions are associated with it. If one restricts the discussion to idiopathic rapidly progressive glomerulonephritis, however—ie, crescentic glomerulonephritis without either anti-GBM antibodies or im-

Table 21–15. Rapidly progressive glomerular nephritis.[1]

No immune deposit
  Vasculitis
    Polyarteritis
    Wegener's granulomatosis
  Idiopathic
Immune complex
  Postinfectious
    Poststreptococcal
    Visceral abscess
  Collagen vascular disease
    Lupus nephritis
    Henoch-Schönlein purpura
  Primary renal disease
    IgA nephropathy
    Membranoproliferative glomerulonephritis
Anti-GBM antibody
  With lung hemorrhage (Goodpasture's syndrome)
  Without lung hemorrhage

[1]Reproduced, with permission, from Couser WG: Rapidly progressive glomerulonephritis. Am J Kidney Dis 1988;11:449

mune complex deposition—there are noncontrolled studies suggesting a benefit from corticosteroid administration. Alternate-day high-dose intravenous methylprednisolone for 3 or 4 days followed by oral prednisone is perhaps the most common form of treatment. As many as 75% of such patients will show initial improvement, though some who improve will ultimately progress to end-stage renal disease. The evidence that plasmapheresis contributes to a favorable response is unconvincing.

Couser WG: Rapidly progressive glomerulonephritis: Classification, pathogenetic mechanisms, and therapy. Am J Kidney Dis 1988;11:449.
Pusey CD, Lockwood MC: Autoimmunity in rapidly progressive glomerulonephritis. Kidney Int 1989;35:929.

3. ANTI-GLOMERULAR BASEMENT MEMBRANE ANTIBODY DISEASE (Goodpasture's Syndrome)

Essentials of Diagnosis

- Progressive renal insufficiency in a patient with hemoptysis.
- Linear immunofluorescence of IgG deposits in glomerular basement membrane in kidney biopsy.
- Circulating anti-GBM antibodies in the serum.

General Considerations

An uncommon but rather distinctive renal lesion is characterized by the deposition of antibody on the glomerular basement membrane in a linear immunofluorescent pattern. Such a histologic picture is seen most often in young men, typically smokers, with hematuria, proteinuria, progressive renal failure, and bilateral pulmonary infiltrates. Hemoptysis is a consequence of pulmonary hemorrhage and frequently precedes clinical evidence of the renal lesion. Iron deficiency anemia often is present as well—in contrast to the usual normochromic normocytic anemia associated with renal failure—and is frequently out of proportion to the severity of azotemia and to the amount of hemoptysis. Early diagnosis is crucial for preservation of renal function.

On light microscopy, one observes a crescentic type of glomerular nephritis. On immunofluorescence, IgG is deposited in a linear fashion. Deposition of IgM or IgA occurs in less than 20% of cases. The serum complement level is normal. Two-thirds of patients with anti-GBM antibody disease have pulmonary involvement (Goodpasture's syndrome). There may be an inherited predisposition to this disease; both members of two sets of twins have been reported to be affected. HLA-DR2 occurs with increased frequency. Circulating serum antibodies to glomerular basement membrane are also diagnostic.

Treatment

This disorder is treated aggressively with corticosteroids as an anti-inflammatory agent and cyclophosphamide or azathioprine (or both) to suppress antibody production, and with daily plasma exchange for 2 weeks to remove circulating antibodies. This therapy is more effective in preserving renal function the earlier it is initiated. Dialysis-dependent patients seldom exhibit enough improvement to enable them to discontinue dialysis.

Kidney transplantation has been quite successful. Circulating serum antibodies to glomerular basement membrane, however, should be absent for several months before either cadaveric or living donor transplantation is undertaken.

Bruijn JA et al: Biology of disease: Pathogenesis of anti-basement membrane glomerulopathy and immune-complex glomerulonephritis: Dichotomy dissolved. Lab Invest 1989;61:480.

4. IgA NEPHROPATHY (BERGER'S DISEASE) & HENOCH-SCHÖNLEIN PURPURA

IgA nephropathy (Berger's disease) is a mesangial proliferative nephritis associated with IgA deposits in mesangial cells; small amounts of complement and IgG are sometimes also found. The disorder tends to present as an episode of macroscopic hematuria or is picked up incidentally after an abnormal urinalysis on an asymptomatic individual. In cases presenting with macroscopic hematuria, there is often a preceding episode of respiratory tract infection.

Occasionally, Berger's disease may present as hypertension. The serum IgA level is increased in 30–50% of patients; when increased, the IgA level is helpful diagnostically, though a normal value does not rule out the diagnosis. Despite evidence of complement deposition in some biopsy specimens, the serum complement level is uniformly normal. While Berger's disease has been generally considered to be a benign disorder, some patients do progress to renal failure. Kidney survival is over 90% at 10 years and about 80% at 20 years. Males are affected more often than females.

Mesangial deposition of IgA is also observed in the disorder known as anaphylactoid purpura (Henoch-Schönlein purpura). Although the renal lesion is identical, in anaphyalactoid purpura there is vascular involvement of the skin, joints, and gastrointestinal tract. Arthralgias and abdominal pain are common. Purpuric skin lesions are often located on the lower extremities, though the platelet count is normal. Like IgA nephropathy without purpuric lesions, there is no specific therapy. Further details about Henoch-Schönlein purpura appear in Chapter 19.

D'Amico G: Clinical features and natural history in adults with IgA nephropathy. Am J Kidney Dis 1988;12:353.
Leendert AV: Pathogenesis of IgA nephropathy. Kidney Int 1992;41:1720.

5. HEREDITARY NEPHRITIS

Hereditary nephritis accounts for 2–3% of patients receiving dialysis. When associated with anterior lenticonus or neurosensory deafness, it is often called Alport's syndrome. Inheritance of the disorder is still somewhat controversial. It is clear, however, that the disease affects men much more severely than women.

The patient usually presents with hematuria and nephrotic syndrome, with or without hypertension, between the ages of 15 and 25 years. The renal biopsy is relatively characteristic. On light microscopy, foamy tubular cells may be present, especially if the patient is nephrotic. On electron microscopy, the glomerular basement membrane is thickened and the lamina densa is split into strands. Immunofluorescence tests are negative.

Dialysis or kidney transplantation is generally necessary before age 30. The results in either case have been very good, presumably in part because of the young age of the patients and the absence of extrarenal major organ involvement.

Kashtan CE, Michael AF: Hereditary nephritis. Semin Nephrol 1989;9:135.

6. POLYCYSTIC KIDNEY DISEASE

Essentials of Diagnosis
- Presenting signs include hematuria, hypertension, and urinary tract infections.
- Autosomal dominant inheritance.
- Palpable abdominal masses may be present bilaterally.

Clinical Findings
A. Symptoms and Signs: The disease is inherited as an autosomal dominant and generally presents in the fifth or sixth decade of life unless the positive family history brings the patient to the physician, in which case asymptomatic involvement may be diagnosed with appropriate tests. Hematuria and hypertension are common presenting complaints. Cysts in the kidneys may become so large that the patient may complain of discomfort in the abdomen. Bilateral palpable masses in the abdomen are often noted on examination in such cases.

The cysts may not be restricted to the kidneys but may be found also in the liver, pancreas, and testis. In fact, cysts in the liver may occur in as many as 50% of cases. These cysts are largely asymptomatic and seldom produce functional abnormality of the liver.

On occasion, however, they may become huge, leading to palpable hepatomegaly and abdominal discomfort. Aneurysms of the cerebral vessels are commonly associated with polycystic kidneys.

Colonic diverticula are also noted in patients with polycystic kidney disease, and sudden abdominal pain in such a patient should lead one to consider a diagnosis of diverticular perforation. However, an infected cyst can also cause abdominal pain, as can hemorrhage into a cyst.

B. Laboratory Findings: Urinalysis is not a good screening test for polycystic kidney disease, since proteinuria tends to be minimal until advanced stages and cellular elements are not necessarily present. Pyuria suggests complicating infection.

Erythrocytosis is sometimes observed in patients with polycystic kidney disease and is presumably the consequence of increased erythropoietin production by the cysts. In a large dialysis population, patients with polycystic disease will have higher hematocrit levels than patients with other disorders.

C. Imaging Studies: Ultrasound and CT scanning of the abdomen have replaced intravenous urography and angiography in diagnosis. These studies readily delineate the size and extent of the cysts.

Treatment & Prognosis

Polycystic disease is slowly progressive. The serum creatinine may exceed 2 mg/dL for several years before kidney transplantation or dialysis is necessary—especially if one can control hypertension and kidney infections. Patients with polycystic kidney disease are generally good candidates for either long-term hemodialysis or kidney transplantation. Though often older than other transplant recipients, the absence of associated systemic disease and autoimmune phenomena makes these patients excellent candidates.

Genetic counseling should be offered to patients with polycystic disease, given its pattern of inheritance.

Fitzpatrick PM et al: Long-term outcome of renal transplantation in autosomal dominant polycystic kidney disease. Am J Kidney Dis 1990;15:535.
Gabow PA: Autosomal dominant polycystic kidney disease: More than a renal disease. Am J Kidney Dis 1990;16:403.
Milutinovic J: Clinical manifestations of autosomal dominant polycystic kidney disease in patients older than 50 years. Am J Kidney Dis 1990;15:237.

7. ACQUIRED CYSTIC DISEASE OF THE KIDNEYS

Acquired cystic disease of the kidneys is a recently recognized disorder in patients with renal failure, especially those receiving dialysis. It is best diagnosed by ultrasound or CT scanning. If one excludes patients with polycystic kidney disease, fewer than 10% of patients with renal failure have cysts in their kidneys at the initiation of dialysis. This percentage increases to around 50% at the end of 5 years and close to 90% after a decade of dialysis. Acquired cysts occur with equal frequency in men and women.

The disorder has attracted clinical interest because of a tendency toward malignant transformation in the cysts. Interestingly, although cyst development is of similar frequency in both sexes, cancer is much more common in men. In general, bilateral nephrectomy has been avoided in dialysis patients because of the severe anemia and need for blood transfusions in most anephric patients. The availability of erythropoietin may allow reconsideration of this view. In any event, the clinician should be alert to symptoms and signs of renal cell carcinoma in any dialysis patient.

Chandboke PS et al: Acquired cystic disease of kidney: Management dilemma. J Urol 1992;147:969. (Review of literature with guidelines for evaluation and therapy.)
Grantham JJ: Acquired cystic kidney disease. Kidney Int 1991;40:143. (Nephrology forum devoted to this increasingly important entity.)

8. ANALGESIC-ASSOCIATED NEPHROPATHY

Ingestion of analgesics in large doses over periods of years may lead to tubulointerstitial renal disease. This was observed more frequently when phenacetin was widely available in over-the-counter analgesic mixtures. The typical patient often had an ill-characterized chronic pain syndrome, eg, headache, which led to excessive self-medication. Symptoms include polyuria and occasionally renal colic secondary to papillary necrosis. Urinalysis reveals sterile hematuria and pyuria and isosthenuria but minimal proteinuria. This disorder has become uncommon in the United States with diminished use of phenacetin. More commonly observed is nephropathy associated with ingestion of nonsteroidal anti-inflammatory drugs. This is discussed above under drug-induced nephropathy.

Kincaid-Smith P: Analgesic nephropathy. Aust NZ J Med 1988;18:251.

MULTISYSTEM DISEASES WITH VARIABLE KIDNEY INVOLVEMENT

1. DIABETIC NEPHROPATHY

The nephropathy of diabetes mellitus is discussed in Chapter 26. By the time diabetic nephropathy develops, diabetic retinopathy is invariably present. Many patients will have additional evidence of vascular disease throughout the body. Hypertension should be treated aggressively early in the course of diabetes, since blood pressure control may slow the progress of the diabetes-associated renal lesion. Angiotensin-converting enzyme inhibitors are useful in many of these patients, but hyperkalemia should be looked for after such drugs are begun. Patients with insulin-dependent diabetes may become hypoglycemic as the nephropathy progresses unless the insulin dose is reduced, since a smaller percentage of the injected insulin is excreted in the kidney with progressive renal failure.

In general, patients with diabetic nephropathy appear to develop symptomatic uremia somewhat earlier than nondiabetic patients with renal failure (at least when one uses serum creatinine or creatinine clearance as an index of glomerular filtration rate). While one often looks to a serum creatinine level of 9–10 mg/dL as an indication for planning dialysis or kidney transplantation in the nondiabetic patient, a serum level of 5–6 mg/dL is often used in the diabetic. Because of increased vascular disease in the diabetic, placement of an arteriovenous fistula may be more difficult than in the nondiabetic, and it may take longer before it can be used for regular hemodialysis treatment.

The mortality rates of both dialysis and kidney transplantation in diabetics are twice as high as those observed in nondiabetic patients. Although patients have been maintained for several years with successful hemodialysis treatments, continuous ambulatory peritoneal dialysis has become quite popular. The use of peritoneal dialysis obviates the need for vascular access with hemodialysis. Salt and water removal with peritoneal dialysis can be achieved more slowly with peritoneal dialysis than with hemodialysis; this can be a major advantage with patients who have vascular instability related to coronary artery disease. Peritonitis, however, remains a major clinical problem with peritoneal dialysis in diabetics—as it does also in nondiabetics.

Kidney transplantation has been successful in patients with diabetes mellitus. Both living related and cadaveric donors have been utilized.

Bauer JH et al: A randomized double blind, placebo controlled trial to evaluate the effect of enalapril in patients with clinical diabetic nephropathy. Am J Kidney Dis 1992;20:443.

Breyer JA: Diabetic nephropathy in insulin-dependent patients. Am J Kidney Dis 1992;20:533.

Mauer SM et al: Symposium on the progress in diabetic nephropathy. Kidney Int 1992;41:717.

2. RENAL AMYLOIDOSIS

Amyloidosis is discussed in Chapter 18. Renal amyloidosis has a poor prognosis. In patients with nephrotic syndrome secondary to amyloid deposition in the glomerulus, the 3-year survival rate is less than 10%. One should always determine if the amyloidosis is secondary to a chronic inflammatory or infectious process (eg, osteomyelitis). If one can control this process, amyloid deposition in theory might be arrested. In patients treated with either dialysis or kidney transplantation, the prognosis is largely dependent on the sites and degree of amyloidosis in extrarenal organs, especially the heart and liver. Amyloidosis tends to recur in patients with kidney transplants.

3. MULTIPLE MYELOMA

Multiple myeloma is considered in detail in Chapter 13. It affects renal function in numerous ways. "Myeloma kidney" refers to light chains of immunoglobulins inspissated within tubules, causing renal failure associated on occasion with proximal renal tubular acidosis. Hypercalcemia results in polyuria, leading to dehydration. Hyperuricemia and uric acid stones may also be a problem, particularly after treatment is initiated. Rarely, the kidney itself is infiltrated by malignant plasma cells, and renal insufficiency may ensue. Finally, amyloidosis complicates myeloma in about 10% of cases, resulting in albuminuria and nephrotic syndrome. The amyloid protein consists of immunoglobulin light chain and is thus part of the primary expression of the plasma cell disorder.

Patients with renal failure due to multiple myeloma have been treated with both hemodialysis and peritoneal dialysis. Patients who have a good initial hematologic response to chemotherapy tend to do better than those who do not. In one study, survival after diagnosis in patients who responded to chemotherapy was about 48 months. Although continuous ambulatory peritoneal dialysis has been used in these patients with some success, the frequency of complicating peritonitis is high.

Iggo N, Parsons V: Renal disease in multiple myeloma: Current perspectives. Nephron 1990;56:229.

Korzets A et al: The role of continuous ambulatory peritoneal dialysis in end-stage renal failure due to multiple myeloma. Am J Kidney Dis 1990;16:216.

4. SYSTEMIC LUPUS ERYTHEMATOSUS

Lupus nephritis is a serious complication of systemic lupus erythematosus (see Chapter 19). A variety of renal histologic lesions have been observed in patients with SLE: focal, proliferative, membranoproliferative, diffuse proliferative, and membranous glomerulonephritis. Occasionally, interstitial nephritis is present as well. Although many of these lesions appear to respond to corticosteroid administration with or without other immunosuppressant drugs, some patients progress to renal failure. At the time dialysis is initiated in these patients, less than half will have extrarenal manifestations of SLE. Serologic evidence of activity—ie, increased levels of antinuclear antibodies and antibodies to double-stranded DNA—is still present in 80%, however. In patients receiving dialysis, the extrarenal manifestations of SLE become even less prominent with time. Serologic abnormalities also decrease.

Both dialysis and kidney transplantation have been quite successful in the management of patients with lupus nephritis. The 5-year survival rates of these patients approach 80%. Recurrence of lupus nephritis in grafted kidneys does not occur.

Cheigh JS, Stenzel KH: End-stage renal disease in systemic lupus erythematosus. Am J Kidney Dis 1993;21:2.

Levey AS et al: Progression and remission of renal disease in the lupus nephritis collaborative study. Ann Intern Med 1992;116:114. (Evaluation of prognostic factors in study of 86 patients.)

5. WEGENER'S GRANULOMATOSIS, POLYARTERITIS NODOSA, & ANTINEUTROPHIL CYTOPLASMIC AUTOANTIBODIES

Antineutrophil cytoplasmic autoantibodies have been described in some patients with necrotizing glomerulonephritis, with or without associated pulmonary hemorrhage, and in patients with active Wegener's granulomatosis. Wegener's granulomatosis is discussed in Chapter 19. Two types of antibodies have been described: one in which the staining is largely cytoplasmic and another in which staining is perinuclear. In addition to being potentially useful serologic tests for the diagnosis of these two disorders, the antibodies may be pathogenetically important in the development of some of the necrotizing lesions associated with the diseases.

Cees GM: Antineutrophil cytoplasmic antibodies: A still growing class of autoantibodies in inflammatory disorders. Am J Med 1992;93:675.

REFERENCES

Brenner BM, Rector FC Jr: *The Kidney,* 4th ed. Saunders, 1990.

Massry SG, Glassock RJ (editors): *Textbook of Nephrology,* 2nd ed. Williams & Wilkins 1989.

Schrier KW, Gottschalk CW: Disorders of the Kidney, 4th ed. Little, Brown, 1988.

Tanagho EA, McAninch JW (editors): *Smith's General Urology,* 13th ed. Appleton & Lange, 1992.

Walsh PC et al (editors): *Campbell's Urology,* 6th ed. Saunders, 1992.

Medical Genetics

22

Reed E. Pyeritz, MD, PhD

The rapid and in some cases spectacular advances in human genetics during the past decade have had important implications for clinical medicine. Familiarity with the fundamental principles of both basic and clinical genetics is now necessary if the physician is to provide a high standard of care. Within the professional lifetimes of most physicians practicing today, all 3 billion nucleotides of the human genome will have been sequenced. The great hope, of course, is that with this exponential growth in information will come new insights into the causes and pathogenetic mechanisms of human disease, more accurate diagnosis, and effective treatment for many disorders now considered beyond the practitioner's therapeutic reach. Along with this optimistic prospect, however, have come some urgent concerns about (1) the ethical, legal, and sociologic implications of what has been termed "genetic engineering" but is better and more broadly called "molecular medicine"; (2) the problem for medical educators of how best to transmit such an enormous body of information to their students and to physicians in practice; and (3) the seemingly esoteric nature of much of that information paired with the realization that any one of the obscure facts of medical genetics might achieve clinical relevance at any time.

This chapter is an attempt to introduce the medical reader to the field of knowledge encompassed by the term "medical genetics." The first section reviews basic genetic principles and emphasizes recent advances of clinical relevance. The second section focuses on the technology of medical genetics, the expanding scope of its clinical applications, and indications for use. The final section contains descriptions of some mendelian disorders. For more detailed treatment of these topics, the following contemporary texts are recommended.

Emery AEH, Rimoin DL (editors): *Principles of Medical Genetics,* 2nd ed. Churchill Livingstone, 1990. (Multiauthored compendium covering many chromosomal and mendelian conditions.)

Gelehrter TD, Collins FS: *Principles of Medical Genetics.* Williams & Wilkins, 1990. (Suitable for a medical school course in medical genetics.)

Holtzman NA: *Proceed With Caution.* Johns Hopkins Univ Press, 1989. (Social, legal, and ethical implications of contemporary issues in medical genetics.)

Pyeritz RE: A revolution in medicine like no other. FASEB J 1992;6:2761. (Current and future importance of genetics in clinical medicine.)

INTRODUCTION TO MEDICAL GENETICS

Physicians at one time concerned themselves only with what they could discover by bedside interrogation and inspection and laboratory investigation. In the parlance of genetics, the patient's signs and symptoms constitute his or her **phenotype.** Now the means are at hand for defining a person's **genotype,** the actual information content inscribed in the 2 meters of coiled DNA present in each cell of the body— or half that amount in every mature ovum or sperm. Virtually all phenotypic characteristics—and this includes diseases as well as human traits such as personality, height, and intelligence—are to some extent determined by the genes. The importance of the genetic contribution varies widely among human phenotypes, and methods are only now being developed to identify the gene involved in complex traits and most common diseases. Moreover, the importance of the environment and of interactions between environment and genotype in producing phenotypes cannot be overstated despite the obscurity of the actual mechanisms.

The billions of nucleotides in the nucleus of a cell are organized linearly along the DNA double helix in functional units called **genes,** and each of the 50,000–100,000 human genes is accompanied by various regulatory elements that control when it is active in producing **messenger RNA (mRNA)** by a process called **transcription.** In most situations, mRNA is transported from the nucleus to the cytoplasm, where its genetic information is **translated** into **proteins,** which perform the functions that ultimately determine phenotype. For example, proteins serve as enzymes that facilitate metabolism and cell synthesis; as DNA binding elements that regulate transcription of other genes; as structural elements of cells and the extracellular matrix; and as receptor molecules for intra- and intercellular communication.

Chromosomes are the vehicles in which the genes are carried from generation to generation. Each chromosome is a complex of protein and nucleic acid in which an unbroken double helix of DNA is coiled and supercoiled into a space many orders of magnitude less than the extended length of the DNA. Within the chromosome there occur highly complicated and integrated processes, including DNA replication, recombination, and transcription. Humans normally have 46 chromosomes, which are arranged in 23 pairs. One of these pairs, the **sex chromosomes** X and Y, determines the sex of the individual; females have the pair XX and males the pair XY. The remaining 22 pairs are called **autosomes** (Figure 22–1).

In all somatic cells, the 44 autosomes and one of the X chromosomes are transcriptionally active. In males, the active X is the only X; portions of the Y chromosome are also active. In females, the requirement for **dosage compensation** (to be equivalent to the situation in males) is satisfied by nearly complete inactivation of one of the X chromosomes early in the cell cycle. This process of X chromosomal inactiva-tion, while not understood biochemically, is known to be random, so that on average, in 50% of a female's cells, one of the X chromosomes will be active, and in the other 50% the **homologous** member of the pair will be active. The phenotype of the cell is determined by which genes on the chromosomes are active in producing mRNA at any given time.

GENES & CHROMOSOMES

In all genes, information is contained in parcels called **exons,** which are interspersed with stretches of DNA called **introns** that do not encode any information about the protein sequence. However, introns may contain genetic regulatory sequences, and some introns are so large that they encode an entirely distinct gene.

The exact location of a gene on a chromosome is its **locus,** and the array of loci constitutes the **human gene map.** Currently, the chromosomal site of more than 2400 genes is known, often to a high degree of resolution. A variation of this map, identifying selected loci known to be involved in human disease, is shown in Figure 22–2. The difference in resolution of

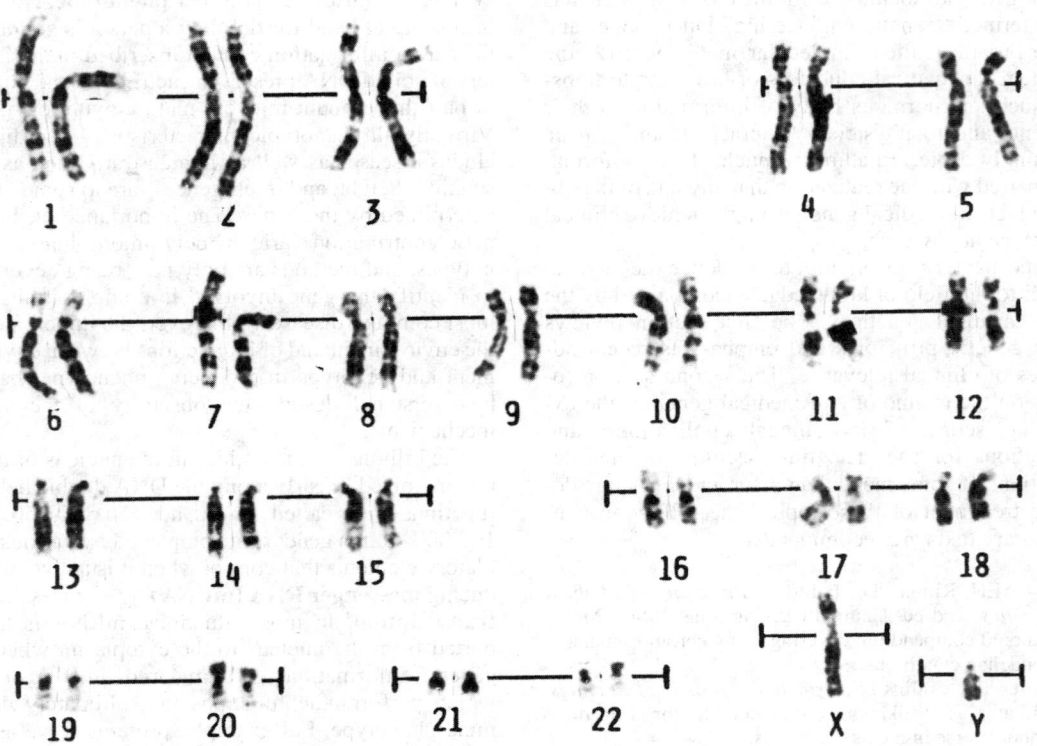

Figure 22–1. Normal karyotype of a human male. Prepared from cultured amniotic cells and stained with Giemsa's stain. About 400 bands are detectable per haploid set of chromosomes.

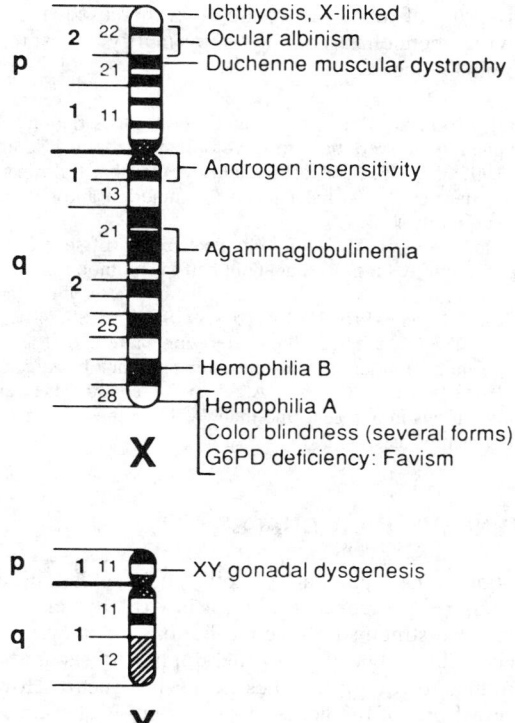

Figure 22–2. A partial "morbid map" of the human genome. Shown next to the ideogram of the human X and Y chromosomes are representative mendelian disorders caused by mutations at that locus. (Courtesy of McKusick and Strayer.)

the ordering of genes achievable by molecular techniques (such as linkage analysis) compared to cytogenetic techniques (such as visualization of small defects) is substantial, though the gap is narrowing. The chromosomes in the "standard" karyotype shown in Figure 22–1 have about 400 visible bands; under the best of cytologic and microscopic conditions, a total of about 1600 bands can be seen. But even in this extended configuration, each band contains dozens—sometimes hundreds—of individual genes. Thus, loss **(deletion)** of a small band, which is the smallest type of defect identifiable under the microscope, will involve loss of many coding sequences and will have diverse effects on the phenotype.

The number and arrangement of genes on homologous chromosomes are identical even though the actual coding sequences of homologous genes may not be. Homologous copies of a gene are termed **alleles.** In comparing alleles, it must be specified at what level of analysis the comparison is being made. When alleles are truly identical—in that their coding sequences are invariant—the individual is **homozygous** at that locus. At a coarser level, the alleles may

be functionally identical despite subtle variations in nucleotide sequence—with the result either that the proteins produced from the two alleles are identical or that whatever differences there may be in amino acid sequence will have no bearing on the function of the protein. If the individual is being analyzed at the level of the protein phenotype, allelic homozygosity would again be an apt descriptor. However, if the analysis were at the level of the DNA—as occurs in restriction enzyme examination or nucleotide sequencing—then, despite functional identity, the alleles would be viewed as different and the individual would be **heterozygous** for that locus. Heterozygosity based on differences in the protein products of alleles has been detectable for decades and was the first hard evidence concerning the high degree of human biologic variability. In the past decade, analysis of DNA sequences has shown this variability to be much more remarkable—differences in nucleotide sequence between individuals occur about once every 400 nucleotides.

McKusick VA: Current trends in mapping human genes. FASEB J 1991;5:12. (Methods of gene mapping and how the information is useful in clinical medicine.)

Watson JD et al: *Molecular Biology of the Gene,* 5th ed. Benjamin/Cummings, 1992.

MUTATION

Allelic heterozygosity most often results when different alleles are inherited from the egg and the sperm, but it also occurs as a consequence of spontaneous alteration in nucleotide sequence **(mutation).** Genetic change occurring during formation of an egg or a sperm is called a **germinal mutation.** When the change occurs after conception—from the earliest stages of embryogenesis to dividing cells in the body of the oldest adult—it is termed a **somatic mutation.** As is discussed below, the role of somatic mutation in the etiology of human disease is now increasingly recognized.

The coarsest type of mutation is alteration in the number or physical structure of chromosomes. For example, **nondisjunction** (failure of chromosome pairs to separate) during **meiosis**—the reduction division that leads to production of mature ova and sperms—causes the embryo to have too many or too few chromosomes, a situation called **aneuploidy.** Rearrangement of chromosome arms, such as occurs in **translocation** or **inversion,** is a mutation even if breakage and reunion does not disrupt any coding sequence. Thus, the phenotypic effect of gross chromosomal mutations can range from profound (as in aneuploidy) to nil.

A bit less coarse, but still detectable cytologically, are **deletions** of part of a chromosome. Such mutations almost always alter phenotype, because large numbers of genes are almost always lost; however, a deletion *may* involve only a single nucleotide, whereas about 1 million nucleotides (1 megabase) must be lost before the defect can be visualized by the most sensitive cytogenetic methods. Molecular biologic techniques are needed to detect smaller losses.

Mutations of one or a few nucleotides in exons have several potential consequences. Changes in one nucleotide can alter which amino acid is encoded; if the amino acid is in a critical region of the protein, function might in this way be severely deranged. On the other hand, some amino acid substitutions have no detectable effect on function, and the phenotype is therefore unaltered by the mutation. Similarly, because the genetic code is **degenerate** (2 or more different three-nucleotide sequences called **codons** encode some amino acids), nucleotide substitution does not necessarily alter the amino acid sequence of the protein. Three specific codons signal termination of translation; thus, a nucleotide substitution in an exon that generates one of the stop-codons usually causes a truncated protein, which is nearly always dysfunctional. Other nucleotide substitutions can disrupt the signals that direct splicing of the mRNA molecule and grossly alter the protein product. Finally, insertions and deletions of one or more nucleotides can have dramatic effects—any change that is not a multiple of three nucleotides disrupts the reading frame of the remainder of the exon—or potentially minimal effects (if the protein can tolerate the insertion or loss of an amino acid).

Mutations in introns may disrupt mRNA splicing signals or may be entirely silent with respect to the phenotype. A great deal of variation in nucleotide sequences among individuals (averaging one difference every few hundred nucleotides) resides within introns. Mutations in the DNA between adjacent genes may also be silent or may have a profound effect on phenotype if regulatory sequences are disrupted. A novel mechanism for mutation, which also helps explain clinical variation among relatives, has recently been discovered in myotonic dystrophy, spinal-bulbar muscular atrophy, and fragile X-mental retardation syndrome. A region of repeated sequences within a gene can be for unclear reasons unstable in some families; expansion of the number of repeated units within this segment is associated with a more severe phenotype.

Mutations may occur spontaneously or may be induced by such environmental factors as radiation, medication, or viral infections. Both advanced maternal and paternal age favor mutation, but of different types. In women, meiosis is completed only when an egg ovulates, and chromosomal nondisjunction is more common the older the egg. The risk that an aneuploid egg will result increases exponentially and becomes a major clinical worry for women older than their early 30s. In men, mutations of a subtler sort—affecting nucleotide sequences—increase with age.

Offspring of men over 40 are at an increased risk of having mendelian conditions, primarily autosomal dominant ones.

Harley HG et al: Expansion of an unstable DNA region and phenotypic variation in myotonic dystrophy. Nature 1992;355:545. (This article and the two that follow describe this "new" mechanism for mutation and clinical variability.)

Higuchi M et al: Molecular characterization of severe hemophilia A suggests that about half the mutations are not within the coding regions and splice junctions of the factor VIII gene. Proc Natl Acad Sci USA 1991;88:7405.

Sommer SS: Assessing the underlying pattern of human germline mutation: Lessons from the factor IX gene. FASEB J 1992;6:2767. (A review of all 604 different mutations in one gene and their effect on the protein and on hemostasis.)

GENES IN INDIVIDUALS

For some quantitative traits such as height or serum glucose concentration, it is virtually impossible to distinguish the contributions of individual genes; this is because in general, phenotypes are the products of multiple genes acting in concert. However, if one of the genes in the system is aberrant, a major departure from the "normal" or expected phenotype might arise. Whether the aberrant phenotype is serious (ie, a disease) or even recognized will depend on the nature of the defective gene product and how resilient the system is to disruption. The latter point emphasizes the importance of homeostasis in both physiology and development—many mutations go unrecognized because the system can cope, even though tolerances for further perturbation might be narrowed.

In other words, virtually all human characteristics are **polygenic,** while many of the disordered phenotypes thought of as "genetic" are **monogenic** but still influenced by other loci in a person's genome.

Phenotypes due to alterations at a single gene are also characterized as **mendelian,** after the monk and part-time biologist who studied the reproducibility and recurrence of variation in garden peas. Gregor Mendel showed that some traits were **dominant** to others, which he called **recessive.** The dominant traits required only one copy of a "factor" to be expressed, regardless of what the other copy was, whereas the recessive traits required two copies before expression occurred. In modern terms, the mendelian factors are genes, and the alternative copies of the gene are alleles. Let A be the common (normal) allele and let a be a mutant allele at a locus: If the same phenotype is present no matter whether the genotype is A/a or a/a, it is dominant, whereas if the phenotype is present only when the genotype is a/a, it is recessive.

In medicine, it is important to keep two considerations in mind: First, dominance and recessiveness are attributes of the phenotype, not the gene; and second, the concepts of dominance and recessiveness depend on how one defines the phenotype. To illustrate both points, consider sickle cell disease. This condition occurs when a person inherits two alleles for β^S globin, in which the normal glutamate at position 6 of the protein has been replaced by valine; the genotype for the β-globin locus is *HbS/HbS*, compared to the normal *HbA/HbA*. When the genotype is *HbS/HbA*, the individual does not have sickle cell disease, so this condition satisfies the criteria for being a recessive phenotype. But now consider the phenotype of sickled erythrocytes. Red cells with the genotype *HbS/HbS* clearly sickle—but, if the oxygen tension is reduced, so do cells with the genotype *HbS/HbA*. Therefore, sickling is a dominant trait.

A mendelian phenotype is characterized not only in terms of dominance and recessiveness but also according to whether the determining gene is on the X chromosome or on one of the 22 pairs of autosomes. Traits or diseases are therefore called autosomal dominant, autosomal recessive, X-linked recessive, and X-linked dominant.

Pyeritz RE: Formal genetics in humans: Mendelian and nonmendelian inheritance. In: *Genes, Brain and Behavior.* McHugh PR, McKusick VA (editors). Raven Press, 1991. (Behavior in families of phenotypes caused by autosomal, X-linked, and mitochondrial genes.)

GENES IN FAMILIES

Since the first decade of this century, the patterns of recurrence of specific human phenotypes have been explained in terms of principles first described by Mendel in the garden pea plant. Mendel's second principle—usually referred to as his first*—is called the **law of segregation** and states that a pair of factors (alleles) that determines some trait separates (segregates) during formation of gametes. In simple terms, a heterozygous (*A/a*) person will produce two types of gametes with respect to this locus—one containing only *A* and one containing only *a*, in equal proportions. Offspring of this person will have a 50–50 chance of inheriting the *A* allele and a similar chance of inheriting the *a* allele.

The concepts of genes in individuals and in fami-

---

*Mendel's first law stated that—from the perspective of the phenotype—it mattered not from which parent a particular allele was inherited. For years this principle was thought to be too obvious to be codified as anybody's "law" and was therefore ignored. In fact, however, recent evidence from studies of human disorders suggests that certain genes are "processed" (**imprinted**) as they move through the gonad and that processing in the testis is different from that in the ovary. Thus, not only is this first mendelian principle important, it was incorrect as originally formulated from observations in peas.

lies can be combined to specify how mendelian traits will be inherited.

Autosomal Dominant Inheritance

The characteristics of autosomal dominant inheritance in humans can be summarized as follows:

(1) There is a vertical pattern in the pedigree, with multiple generations affected (Figure 22–3).

(2) Heterozygotes for the mutant allele show an abnormal phenotype.

(3) Males and females are affected with equal frequency and severity.

(4) Only one parent must be affected for an offspring to be at risk for developing the phenotype.

(5) When an affected person mates with an unaffected one, each offspring has a 50% chance of inheriting the affected phenotype. This is true regardless of the sex of the affected parent—specifically, male-to-male transmission occurs.

(6) The frequency of sporadic cases is positively associated with the severity of the phenotype. More precisely, the greater the **reproductive fitness** of affected persons, the less likely it is that any given case resulted from a new mutation.

(7) The average age of fathers is advanced in the case of isolated (sporadic or new mutation) cases.

Autosomal dominant phenotypes are often age-dependent, less severe than autosomal recessive ones, and associated with malformations or other physical features. They are **pleiotropic** in that multiple, even seemingly unrelated clinical manifestations derive from the same mutation; and **variable** in that expression of the same mutation among people will differ.

Penetrance is a concept often associated with mendelian conditions—especially dominant ones—

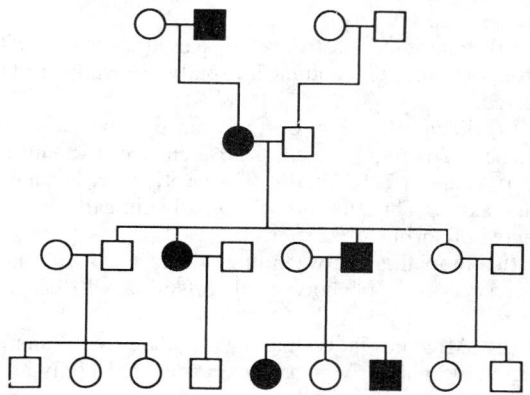

Figure 22–3. A pedigree illustrating autosomal dominant inheritance. Square symbols indicate males and circles females; open symbols indicate that the person is phenotypically unaffected, and filled symbols indicate that the phenotype is present to some extent.

and the term is often misused. It should be defined as an expression of the frequency of appearance of a phenotype (dominant or recessive) when one or more mutant alleles are present. For individuals, penetrance is an all-or-none phenomenon—the phenotype is either present (penetrant) or not (nonpenetrant). The term **variability**—not "incomplete penetrance"—should be used to denote differences in expression of an allele.

The most frequent cause of apparent nonpenetrance is insensitivity of the methods for detecting the phenotype. If an apparently normal parent of a child with a dominant condition were in fact heterozygous for the mutation, the parent would have a 50% chance at each subsequent conception of having another affected child. A common cause of nonpenetrance in adult-onset mendelian diseases is death of the affected person before the phenotype becomes evident but after transmission of the mutant allele to offspring. Thus, accurate genetic counseling demands careful attention to the family medical history and high-resolution scrutiny of both parents of a child with a condition known to be a mendelian dominant trait.

When both alleles are expressed in the heterozygote, as in blood group AB, in sickle trait (HbS/HbA), in the major histocompatibility antigens (eg, A2B5/A3B17), or in sickle-C disease (HbS/HbC), the phenotype is called **codominant.**

In human dominant phenotypes, the homozygous state for the mutant allele is almost always more severe than in heterozygotes.

Autosomal Recessive Inheritance

The characteristics of autosomal recessive inheritance in humans can be summarized as follows:

(1) There is a horizontal pattern in the pedigree, with a single generation affected (Figure 22–4).

(2) Males and females are affected with equal frequency and severity.

(3) Inheritance is from both parents, each a heterozygote (carrier) and each usually clinically unaffected.

(4) Each offspring of two carriers has a 25% chance of being affected, a 50% chance of being a carrier, and a 25% chance of inheriting neither mutant allele. Thus, two-thirds of all clinically unaffected offspring are carriers.

(5) In matings between individuals, each with the same recessive phenotype, all offspring will be affected.

(6) Affected individuals who mate with unaffected individuals who are not carriers have only unaffected offspring.

(7) The rarer the recessive phenotype, the more likely it is that the parents are **consanguineous** (related).

Autosomal recessive phenotypes are often associ-

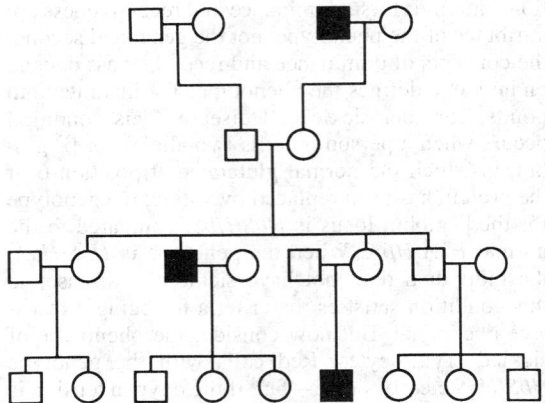

Figure 22–4. A pedigree illustrating autosomal recessive inheritance. (Symbols as in Figure 22–3.)

ated with deficient activity of enzymes and are thus termed **inborn errors of metabolism.** Such disorders include phenylketonuria, Tay-Sachs disease, and the various glycogen storage diseases and tend to be more severe, less variable, and less age-dependent than dominant conditions.

When an autosomal recessive condition is quite rare, the chance that the parents of affected offspring are consanguineous is increased. As a result, the prevalence of rare recessive conditions is high among inbred groups such as the Old Order Amish. On the other hand, when the autosomal recessive condition is common, the chance of consanguinity between parents of cases is no higher than in the general population (about 0.5%).

Two different *mutant* alleles at the same locus, as in HbS/HbC, form a **genetic compound.** The phenotype usually lies between those produced by either allele present in the homozygous state. Because of the large number of mutations possible in a given gene, many autosomal recessive phenotypes are probably due to genetic compounds. Sickle cell disease is an exception. Consanguinity is strong presumptive evidence for true homozygosity of mutant alleles and against a genetic compound.

X-Linked Inheritance

The general characteristics of X-linked inheritance in humans can be summarized as follows:

(1) There is no male-to-male transmission of the phenotype (Figure 22–5).

(2) Unaffected males do not transmit the phenotype.

(3) All of the daughters of an affected male are heterozygous carriers.

(4) Males are usually more severely affected than females.

(5) Whether a heterozygous female is counted as

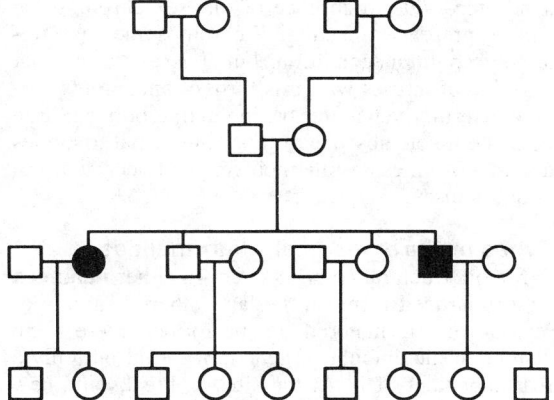

Figure 22–5. A pedigree illustrating X-linked recessive inheritance. (Symbols as in Figure 22–3.)

affected—and whether the phenotype is called "recessive" or "dominant"—depends often on the sensitivity of the assay or of the examination.

(6) Some mothers of affected males will not themselves be heterozygotes (ie, they will be homozygous normal) but will have a germinal mutation. The proportion of heterozygous (carrier) mothers is negatively associated with the severity of the condition.

(7) Heterozygous women transmit the mutant gene to one-half of sons, who are affected, and to one-half of daughters, who are heterozygotes.

(8) If an affected male mates with a heterozygous female, half of the male offspring will be affected, giving the false impression of male-to-male transmission. One-half of the female offspring of such matings will be affected as severely as the average hemizygous male; in small pedigrees, this pattern may simulate autosomal dominant inheritance.

The characteristics of X-linked inheritance depend on phenotypic severity. For some disorders, affected males do not survive to reproduce. In such cases, about two-thirds of affected males have a carrier mother; in the remaining third, the disorder arises by new germinal mutation in an X chromosome of the mother. When the disorder is nearly always manifest in heterozygous females (X-linked dominant inheritance), females tend to be affected about twice as often as males; and on average an affected female transmits the phenotype to half of her sons and half of her daughters.

X-linked phenotypes are often clinically variable—particularly in heterozygous females—and suspected of being autosomal dominant with nonpenetrance. For example, Fabry's disease (α-galactosidase A deficiency) may be clinically silent in carrier women or may cause stroke, renal failure, or myocardial infarction by middle age.

Germinal mosaicism occurs in mothers of boys with X-linked conditions. The chance of such a mother having a second affected son or a heterozygous daughter depends on the fraction of her oocytes that carries the mutation. Currently, this fraction is impossible to determine. However, the presence of germinal mosaicism can be detected in some conditions (eg, Duchenne's muscular dystrophy) in a family by analysis of DNA, and this knowledge becomes crucial for genetic counseling.

More than 5000 human genes have been identified through their phenotypes and inheritance patterns in families. This total represents 5–10% of all genes thought to be encoded by the 22 autosomes and 2 sex chromosomes. Victor McKusick coordinates an international effort to catalogue human mendelian variation (see first reference, below).

McKusick VA: *Mendelian Inheritance in Man,* 10th ed. Johns Hopkins Univ Press, 1992. (A catalogue consisting, for each phenotype, of a six-digit identification number—used extensively in the medical literature—a summary statement, and a list of pertinent references. Editions are published biennially, but the catalogue is updated continuously and is computer-accessible as Online Mendelian Inheritance in Man [OMIM]. For information, contact OMIM User Support, Welch Medical Library, 1830 East Monument Street, Third Floor, Baltimore, MD 21205; [410] 955–7058; FAX [410] 614–0434; Internet Help@Welch.JHU.edu.)

DISORDERS OF MULTIFACTORIAL CAUSATION

Many disorders cluster in families but are not associated with evident chromosomal aberrations or mendelian inheritance patterns. Examples include congenital malformations such as cleft lip, pyloric stenosis, and spina bifida; coronary artery disease; adult-onset diabetes mellitus; and various forms of neoplasia. They are often characterized by varying frequencies in different racial or ethnic groups, disparity in sexual predilection, and greater frequency (but less than full concordance) in monozygotic than in dizygotic twins. This inheritance pattern is called "multifactorial" to signify that multiple genes interact with various environmental agents to produce the phenotype. The familial clustering is assumed to be due to sharing of both alleles and environment.

For most multifactorial conditions, there is little understanding of which particular genes are involved, how they and their products interact, and in what way different nongenetic factors contribute to the phenotype. For some disorders, biochemical and genetic studies have identified mendelian conditions within the coarse phenotype: Defects of the low-density lipoprotein receptor account for a small fraction of cases of ischemic heart disease (a larger fraction if only patients under age 50 are considered); familial polyposis of the colon predisposes to adenocarcinoma; and some patients with emphysema have inherited deficiency of α_1-proteinase inhibitor. Despite these notable examples, this reductionistic preoccupation with mendelian phenotypes is unlikely to explain the great majority of human disease; but even so, in the last analysis, much of human pathology will prove to be associated with genetic factors in cause, pathogenesis, or both.

Our profound ignorance about fundamental genetic mechanisms has not completely restricted practical approaches to the genetics of multifactorial disorders. For example, recurrence risks are based on empiric data derived from observation of many families. The risk of recurrence of multifactorial disorders is increased in several instances, as follows: (1) to close relatives (sibs, offspring, and parents) of an affected individual; (2) when two or more members of a family have the same condition; (3) when the first case in a family is in the less commonly affected sex (eg, pyloric stenosis is five times more common in boys; an affected woman has a three- to fourfold greater risk of having a child with pyloric stenosis); and (4) in ethnic groups in which there is a high incidence of a particular condition (eg, spina bifida is 40 times more common in Caucasians—and even more frequent among the Irish—than in Asians).

For many apparently multifactorial disorders, enough families have not been examined to have established empiric risk data. A useful approximation of recurrence risk in close relatives is the square root of the incidence. For example, many common congenital malformations have an incidence of 1:2000 to 1:500 live births; the calculated recurrence risks are thus in the 2–5% range—values that correspond closely to experience.

King RA, Rotter JI, Motulsky AG (editors): *The Genetic Basis of Common Diseases.* Oxford Univ Press, 1992. (Standard reference work.)

Williams RR: Nature, nurture, and family predisposition. N Engl J Med 1988;318:769. (Prospects and pitfalls of understanding the causes and pathogenesis of disease.)

CHROMOSOMAL ABERRATIONS

Any deviation from the structure and number of chromosomes as displayed in Figure 22–1 is, technically, a chromosomal aberration. Not all aberrations cause problems in the affected individual, but some that do not may lead to problems in offspring. About 1:200 live-born infants have a chromosomal aberration that is detected because of some effect on phenotype. This frequency increases markedly the earlier in fetal life the chromosomes are examined. By the end of the first trimester of gestation, most fetuses with abnormal numbers of chromosomes have been lost through spontaneous abortion. For example, Turner's syndrome—due to absence of one sex chromosome and the presence of a single X chromosome—is a relatively common condition, but it is estimated that only 2% of fetuses with this form of aneuploidy survive to term. Even more striking in live-born children is the complete absence of most autosomal trisomies and monosomies despite their frequent occurrence in young fetuses.

Types of Chromosomal Abnormalities

Major structural changes occur in either **balanced** or **unbalanced** form. In the latter, there is a gain or loss of genetic material; in the former, there is no change in the amount of genetic material but only a rearrangement of it. At the sites of breaks and new attachments of chromosome fragments, there may be permanent structural or functional damage to one gene or to only a few genes. Despite no visible loss of material, the aberration may nonetheless be recognized as unbalanced through an abnormal phenotype and the chromosomal defect confirmed by molecular analysis of the DNA.

Aneuploidy results from nondisjunction—the failure of a chromatid pair to separate in a dividing cell. Nondisjunction in either the first or second division of meiosis results in gametes with abnormal chromosomal constitutions. In aneuploidy, more or fewer than 46 chromosomes are present (Table 22–1). The following are all forms of aneuploidy: (1) **monosomy,** in which only one member of a pair of chromosomes is present; (2) **trisomy,** in which three chromosomes are present instead of two; and (3) **polysomy,** in which one chromosome is represented four or more times.

If nondisjunction occurs in mitosis, **mosaic** patterns occur in somatic tissue, with some cells having one karyotype and other cells of the same organism another karyotype. Patients with a mosaic genetic constitution often have manifestations of each of the genetic syndromes associated with the various abnormal karyotypes.

Translocation results from an exchange of parts of two chromosomes.

Table 22–1. Clinical phenotypes resulting from aneuploidy.

Condition	Karotype	Incidence at Birth
Trisomy 13	47,XX or XY,+13	1:15,000
Trisomy 18	47,XX or XY,+18	1:11,000
Trisomy 21 (Down's syndrome)	47,XX or XY,+21	1:900
Klinefelter's syndrome	47,XXY	1:1000 males
XYY	47,XYY	1:1000 males
Turner's syndrome	45,X	1:7500 females
XXX syndrome	47,XXX	1:1000 females

Deletion is loss of chromosomal material.

Duplication is the presence of two or more copies of the same region of a given chromosome. The redundancy may occur in the same chromosome or in a nonhomologous chromosome. In the latter case, a translocation will also have occurred.

An **isochromosome** is one in which the arms on either side of the centromere have the same genetic material in the same order—ie, the chromosome has at some time divided in such a way that it has a double dose of one arm and absence of the other.

In an **inversion,** a chromosomal region becomes reoriented 180 degrees out of ordinary phase. The same genetic material is present, but in a different order.

Bickmore WA, Sumner AT: Mammalian chromosome banding: An expression of genome organization. Trends Genet 1989;5:144. (Association of chromosome bands and underlying genetic structure.)

Gardner RJ, Sutherland GR: *Chromosome Abnormalities and Genetic Counseling.* Oxford Univ Press, 1989. (Mechanisms, clinical presentations, and recurrence risks.)

Hall JG: Somatic mosaicism: Observations related to clinical genetics. Am J Hum Genet 1988;43:355. (Mechanisms of somatic mosaicism at the single gene or chromosome level and their relevance to clinical diagnosis and counseling.)

THE TECHNIQUES OF MEDICAL GENETICS

Without a doubt, the diagnosis and management of hereditary disorders involves in the first instance the skills and knowledge of a general physician. The disorders affect multiple organ systems and people of all ages. Many disorders are chronic ones, but often there are acute crises. The concerns of patients and families span a wide range of medical, psychologic, social, and economic issues. These characteristics emphasize the need for pediatricians, internists, obstetricians, and family practitioners to provide medical genetics services for their patients. Those physicians therefore need to know what laboratory and consultative services are available from clinical geneticists and the indications for their use. This section reviews these matters.

CYTOGENETICS

Cytogenetics is the study of chromosomes by light microscopy. The chromosomal constitution of a single cell or an entire individual is specified by a standardized notation. The total chromosome count is determined first, followed by the sex chromosome complement and then by any abnormalities. The autosomes are all designated by numbers from 1 to 22. A plus (+) or minus (–) sign indicates, respectively, a gain or loss of chromosomal material. For example, a normal male is 46,XY, while a girl with Down's syndrome caused by trisomy 21 is 47,XX,+21.

Chromosomal analyses are done by growing human cells in tissue culture, chemically inhibiting mitosis, and then staining, observing, photographing, sorting, and counting the chromosomes. The display of all of the chromosomes is termed the **karyotype** (Figure 22–1) and is the end result of the technical aspect of cytogenetics.

Specimens for cytogenetic analysis can be obtained for routine analysis from the peripheral blood, in which case T lymphocytes are examined; from amniotic fluid for culture of amniocytes; from trophoblastic cells from the chorionic villus; from bone marrow; and from cultured fibroblasts, usually obtained from a skin biopsy. Enough cells must be examined so that the chance of missing a cytogenetically distinct cell line (a situation of mosaicism) is statistically low. For most clinical indications, 20 mitoses are examined and counted under direct microscopic visualization, and two are photographed and karyotypes prepared. Observation of aberrations usually prompts more extended scrutiny and in many cases further analysis of the original culture.

A variety of methods can be used to reveal banding patterns—unique to each pair of chromosomes—in the analysis of aberrations. The number of bands that can be visualized is a function of how "extended" the chromosomes are, which in turn depends chiefly on how early in metaphase (or even in prophase for the most extensive banding) mitosis was arrested. The "standard" karyotype reveals about 400 bands per haploid set of chromosomes, whereas a prophase karyotype might reveal four times that number. As invaluable as extended karyotypes are in certain clinical circumstances, their interpretation is often difficult—in terms of the time and effort required and of ambiguity about what is abnormal, what is a normal variation, and what is a technical artifact. More recent techniques involve in situ hybridization of DNA probes for specific chromosomes. These probes can be labeled with radioactive isotopes or fluorescent dyes and can be used to identify chromosomes or fragments of chromosomes. Given proper technique, fluorescent in situ hybridization (FISH) yields sensitivities and specificities of virtually 100%. Some applications are being used routinely and marketed commercially.

Indications for Cytogenetic Analysis

The current indications are listed in Table 22–2. A wide array of clinical syndromes have been found to be associated with chromosomal aberrations, and analysis of the karyotype is useful any time a patient is discovered to have the manifestations of one of these syndromes. When a chromosomal aberration is revealed, not only does the patient's physician obtain valuable information about prognosis, but the parents gain insight into the cause of their child's problems and the family can be counseled accurately—and usually reassured—about the risks of recurrence.

Mental retardation is a frequent component of congenital malformation syndromes because of coincident defective development of the central nervous system. However, one of the most frequent causes of mental retardation is not associated with few systemic effects. The fragile-X syndrome—so called because of the gap, or **fragile site,** evident at the end of the long arm of the X chromosome—occurs in one of every 2000 males and is second only to Down's syndrome as a cause of retardation in males. This aberration is inherited from mothers who are heterozygous for the fragile-X site; many carrier women have apparently normal intellect, but some are retarded. Thus, any person with unexplained mental retardation should be studied by chromosomal analysis, with particular attention paid to this aberration. Since special techniques are required, the laboratory request must clearly indicate that a search for fragile sites is needed.

Abnormalities of sexual differentiation can only be understood once the patient's **genetic sex** is clarified. Hormonal therapy and plastic surgery can to some extent determine **phenotypic sex,** but genetic sex is dictated by the complement of sex chromosomes.

The best-known example of dichotomy between the genetic sex and phenotypic sex is the testicular feminization syndrome, in which the chromosomal constitution is 46,XY but, because of a defect in the testosterone receptor protein (specified by a gene on the Y chromosome), the external phenotype is completely female.

Failure or delay in developing secondary sexual characteristics occurs in Turner's syndrome (the most common cause being a form of aneuploidy, ie, monosomy for the X chromosome, 45,X), in Klinefelter's syndrome (the most common karyotype is 47,XXY), and in other much rarer chromosomal aberrations.

Tall stature is perhaps the only consistent phenotypic feature associated with having an extra Y chromosome (karyotype 47,XYY); most men with this chromosomal aberration lead normal lives, and thus tall stature in a male is itself no indication for chromosomal analysis. However, some evidence suggests that an increased prevalence of learning difficulties may be associated with this aberration. Furthermore, Klinefelter's syndrome often causes tall stature, albeit with a eunuchoid habitus, and learning and behavioral problems. Thus, the combination of learning or behavioral difficulties and unexpectedly increased height in a male should prompt consideration of cytogenetic analysis.

As discussed below, most tumors are associated with chromosomal aberrations, some of which are highly specific for certain malignancies. Cytogenetic analysis of tumor tissue may assist in diagnosis, prognosis, and management.

Whenever a person is shown to have a chromosome translocation—whether it be balanced and asymptomatic or unbalanced, causing a syndrome—the physician should consider the importance of identifying the source of the translocation. If the proband is a child and the parents are interested in having more children, both parents should be studied cytogenetically. How far the primary physician or consultant should go in tracking a translocation through a family is an unsettled question with legal and ethical as well as medical implications. Certainly the proband (if an adult) or the parents of the proband need to be counseled and the potential risks to relatives discussed. The physician should document, both in the medical record and by correspondence, that the burden of disclosing relevant data to the extended family has been assumed by specific named individuals.

Inability to produce offspring, either through failure to conceive or as a result of repeated miscarriages, is a frustrating and discouraging problem for affected couples and their physicians. Considerable progress in the urologic and gynecologic understanding of infertility has benefited many couples. However, chromosomal aberrations remain an important problem in reproductive medicine, and cytogenetic

---

Table 22–2. Indications for cytogenetic analysis.

1. Patients with malformations suggestive of one of the recognized syndromes associated with a specific chromosome aberration.
2. Patients of any age who are grossly retarded physically or mentally, especially if there are associated anomalies.
3. Any patient with ambiguous internal or external genitalia or suspected hermaphroditism.
4. Girls with primary amenorrhea and boys with delayed pubertal development. Up to 25% of patients with primary amenorrhea have a chromosomal abnormality.
5. Males with learning or behavioral disorders who are taller than expected (based on parental height).
6. Certain malignant and premalignant diseases (see Tables 22–8 and 22–9).
7. Parents of a patient with chromosome translocation.
8. Parents of a patient with a suspected chromosomal syndrome if there is a family history of similarly affected children.
9. Couples with a history of multiple spontaneous abortions of unknown cause.
10. Couples who are infertile after more common obstetric and urologic causes have been excluded.
11. Prenatal diagnosis (see Table 22–7).

analysis should be utilized at some stage in extended evaluation. Infertility can be caused by Klinefelter's and Turner's syndromes; the external phenotype may be subtle, particularly if the chromosomal aberration is mosaic. Any early spontaneous abortion may be due to fetal aneuploidy. Recurrence may be due to parental translocation predisposing to an unbalanced fetal karyotype.

Borgaonkar D: *Chromosomal Variation in Man: A Catalog of Chromosomal Variants and Anomalies,* 6th ed. Wiley, 1991. (The standard reference.)
Kuo W-L et al: Detection of aneuploidy involving chromosomes 13, 18, or 21 by fluorescence in situ hybridization (FISH) to interphase and metaphase amniocytes. Am J Hum Genet 1991;49:112. (Use of composite probes to detect numerical aberrations of chromosomes in fetal cells.)
Mitelman F: Catalog of Chromosome Aberrations in Cancer, 4th ed. Wiley, 1991. (Common and rare cytogenetic findings in tumors of all types.)

BIOCHEMICAL GENETICS

Biochemical genetics deals not only with enzymatic defects but also with proteins of all functions, including cytoskeletal and extracellular structure, regulation, and receptors. The principal functions of the biochemical genetics laboratory are to determine the presence or absence of proteins, to assess the qualitative characteristics of proteins, and to verify the effectiveness of proteins in vitro. The key elements from the referring physician's perspective are (1) to indicate what the suspected clinical diagnoses are and (2) to make certain that the proper specimen is obtained and transported to the laboratory in a timely manner.

Indications for Biochemical Investigations

Some inborn errors are relatively common in the general population, eg, hemochromatosis, defects of the low-density lipoprotein receptor, and cystic fibrosis (Table 22–3). Others, while rare across the entire population, are common in certain ethnic groups, such as Tay-Sachs disease in Ashkenazic Jews, sickle cell disease in African-Americans, and thalassemias in populations from around the Mediterranean basin. Many of these disorders are autosomal recessive, and the frequency of heterozygotes is many times that of the fully expressed disease. Screening for carrier status can be effective if certain requirements are satisfied (Table 22–4). For example, all of the United States and the District of Columbia require screening of newborns for one or more metabolic diseases. Such programs are cost-effective even for rare conditions such as phenylketonuria, which occurs in only one of every 11,000 births. Unfortunately, not all disorders that meet the requirements in Table 22–4 are screened for in every state. Furthermore, compliance is highly variable among programs, and follow-up diagnostic tests, management, and counseling are in some cases inadequate. Babies most likely to be missed are those born at home. In some states, parents can refuse to have their infants studied.

Use of the biochemical genetics laboratory for other than screening purposes must be justified by the need for data on which to base a diagnosis of specific disorders or classes of related disorders. The possibilities are limited only by the extent of knowledge, the enthusiasm of the primary physician or consultant, the willingness of the patient or family to pursue the diagnosis and specimens to be taken, and the availability of a laboratory to examine the specimens.

Though many inborn defects are so subtle they escape detection, there are a number of clinical situations in which an inborn error should be part of the differential diagnosis. The urgency with which the investigation is undertaken will vary depending on the severity of the disorder and the availability of treatment. Table 22–5 lists various clinical presentations.

The possibility of acute metabolic disease of the neonate is the most important indication, because

Table 22–3. Representative inborn errors of metabolism.

General Class of Defect	Example	Biochemical Defect	Inheritance
Aminoacidopathy	Phenylketonuria	Phenylalanine hydroxylase	AR
Connective tissue	Osteogenesis imperfecta type II	$\alpha_1(I)$ and $\alpha_2(I)$ procollagen	AD
Gangliosiodosis	Tay-Sachs disease	Hexosaminidase A	AR
Glycogen storage disease	Type I	Glucose-6-phosphatase	AR
Immune function	Chronic granulomatous disease	Cytochrome b, β chain	XL
Lipid metabolism	Familial hypercholesterolemia	LDL receptor	AD
Mucopolysaccharidosis	MPS II (Hunter's syndrome)	Iduronate sulfatase	XL
Porphyria	Acute intermittent	Porphobilinogen deaminase	AD
Transport	Cystic fibrosis	CF transmembrane conductance regulator	AR
Urea cycle	Citrullinemia	Arginosuccinate synthetase	AR

Table 22–4. Requirements for effective screening for inborn errors of metabolism.

1. The disease should be clinically severe or have potentially severe consequences.
2. The natural history of the disease should be understood.
3. Effective treatment should be generally available and depend on early diagnosis for optimal results.
4. The disease incidence should be high enough to warrant screening.
5. The screening test should have favorable specificity (low false-positive rate) and sensitivity (low false-negative rate).
6. The screening test should be available for and used by the entire population at risk.
7. An adequate system for follow-up of positive results should be provided.
8. The economic cost-benefit analysis should favor screening and treatment.

prompt diagnosis and treatment may often make the difference between life and death. The clinical features are nonspecific because the newborn has a limited repertoire of responses to severe metabolic insults. The physician must be both inclusive and systematic in evaluating such ill babies.

Brusilow SW, Valle DL, Arn P: Symptomatic inborn errors of metabolism. In: *Current Therapy in Neonatal-Perinatal Medicine.* Nelson NM (editor). BC Decker, 1990. (Approaches to mendelian conditions that cause serious disease in early life.)

Scriver CR et al (editors): *The Metabolic Basis of Inherited Diseases,* 6th ed. McGraw-Hill, 1989. (The standard reference work and source of information about most hereditary disorders.)

DNA ANALYSIS

Direct inspection of nucleic acids—often called "molecular genetics" or "DNA diagnosis"—is achieving an increasingly prominent role in a number of clinical areas, including oncology, infectious disease, forensic medicine, and the general study of pathophysiology. A major impact has been in the diagnosis of mendelian disorders. Once a particular gene is shown to be defective in a given condition, the nature of the mutation itself can be determined, often by sequencing the nucleotides and comparing the array with that of a normal allele. One of a variety of techniques can then be used to determine whether that same mutation is present in other patients with the same disorder. Genetic heterogeneity is so extensive that most mendelian conditions are associated with numerous mutations at one locus—or occasionally multiple loci—that produce the same phenotype. This fact complicates DNA diagnosis of patients and screening for carriers of defects in specific genes.

A few conditions are associated with relatively few mutations or with only one highly prevalent mutation. For example, all sickle cell disease is caused by exactly the same change of glutamate to valine at position 6 of β-globin, and that substitution in turn is due to a change of one nucleotide at the sixth codon in the β-globin gene. But such uniformity is the exception. In cystic fibrosis, about 70% of heterozygotes have an identical deletion of three nucleotides that causes loss of a phenylalanine residue from a chloride transport protein; however, the remaining 30% of mutations of that protein are diverse, so that no simple screening test will detect *all* carriers of cystic fibrosis.

Reviews of the current technical status of DNA analysis appear regularly in the medical literature. Polymerase chain reaction (PCR) studies have revolutionized many aspects of molecular biology, and DNA diagnosis has come to involve this technique in many instances. If the sequences of the 10–20 nucleotides at the ends of a region of DNA of interest (such as a portion of a gene) are known, then "primers" complementary to these sequences can be synthesized. When even a minute amount of DNA from a patient (eg, from a few leukocytes or hair bulbs) is combined with the primers in a reaction mixture that replicates DNA—and after several dozen cycles are then performed—the region of DNA between the primers will be amplified exponentially. For example, the presence of early HIV infection can be detected after PCR amplification of a portion of the viral genome.

Table 22–5. Manner of presentation of inborn errors of metabolism.

Presentation and Course	Examples
Acute metabolic disease of the neonate	Galactosemia, urea cycle disorders
Chronic disorders with little progression	Phenylketonuria, hypothyroidism
Chronic disorders with insidious, incessant progression	Tay-Sachs disease
Disorders causing abnormalities of structure	Skeletal dysplasias, Marfan's syndrome
Disorders of transport	Cystinuria, lactase deficiency
Disorders that determine susceptibilities	LDL receptor deficiency, agammaglobulinemia
Episodic disorders	Most porphyrias, G6PD deficiency
Disorders causing anemia	Pyruvate kinase deficiency, hereditary spherocytosis
Disorders interfering with hemostasis	Hemophilia A and B, von Willebrand disease
Congenital disorders with no possibility of reversal	Testicular feminization
Disorders with protean manifestations	Pseudohypoparathyroidism, hereditary amyloidoses
Inborn errors with no clinical effects	Pentosuria, histidinemia

Indications for DNA Diagnosis

The basic requirement for the use of nucleic acids in the diagnosis of hereditary conditions is that a **probe** be available for the gene in question. The probe may be a piece of the actual gene, a sequence close to the gene, or just a few nucleotides at the actual mutation. The closer the probe is to the actual mutation, the more accurate and the more useful will be the information derived. DNA diagnosis involves one of two general approaches: (1) direct detection of the mutation and (2) linkage analysis, whereby the presence of a mutation is inferred from the nature of a probe DNA sequence remote from the mutation. In the latter approach, as the probe moves farther from the mutation, the chances increase that recombination will have separated the two sequences and confused the interpretation of the data.

Some of the conditions for which direct detection is possible are listed in Table 22–6. Conditions that can be diagnosed only indirectly are also listed; while their number also is increasing, there is a gratifying shift to diagnosis by direct detection as the molecular nature of mutations is defined.

DNA diagnosis is finding frequent application in presymptomatic detection of individuals with age-dependent disorders such as Huntington's disease and adult polycystic kidney disease, screening for carriers of autosomal recessive conditions such as cystic fibrosis and thalassemias, screening for female heterozygotes of X-linked conditions such as Duchenne's muscular dystrophy and hemophilia A and B, and prenatal diagnosis (see below). The full range of indications is undefined at this time.

Logistics of DNA Diagnosis

Lymphocytes are a ready source of DNA; 10 mL of whole blood yields up to 0.5 mg of DNA, enough for dozens of analyses based on hybridization, each of which requires only 5 μg. If the analysis is quite narrowly focused on a specific mutation (such as in a family study, in which only one specific nucleotide change is addressed), PCR analysis can often be used and the amount of DNA needed is truly infinitesimal—a few hair bulbs or sperm are adequate. Once isolated, the DNA sample can be divided into aliquots and frozen. Alternatively, lymphocytes can be transformed with viruses into lymphoblasts; these cells are immortal, can be frozen, and—whenever DNA is required—can be thawed, propagated, and their DNA isolated. These stored specimens provide access to a person's genome long after the individual dies. This is such an important advantage that many clinical genetics centers and commercial laboratories "bank" DNA from patients and informative relatives even if the samples cannot be put to use immediately. The specimens may later prove invaluable to relatives or to other patients being evaluated. DNA in some instances has become more reliable than the medical record and even more readily retrievable!

Blood for DNA isolation should be drawn in EDTA anticoagulant (purple-top tubes); blood for lymphoblast culture should be drawn in heparin (green-top tubes). Neither should be frozen. Specimens for DNA isolation can be stored or shipped at room temperature over a period of a few days. Lymphoblast cultures should be established within 48 hours, so prompt shipment is essential.

Fetal DNA can be isolated from amniotic cells, from trophoblastic cells taken by chorionic villus sampling, or from either cell type grown in culture. Samples need to be processed promptly but can be shipped by overnight mail and *must not be frozen.*

Antonarakis S: Diagnosis of genetic disorders at the DNA level. N Engl J Med 1989;320:153. (Current techniques and copious references.)

Brandt J et al: Presymptomatic diagnosis of delayed-onset disease with linked DNA markers. JAMA 1989;

Table 22–6. Selected DNA probes with current diagnosis applications.

Gene Probe	Disorder	Diagnostic Application
β-Globin	Sickle cell disease	Prenatal
	Beta thalassemia	Prenatal
α-Globin	Alpha thalassemia	Prenatal
	Polycystic kidney disease	Presymptomatic, prenatal screening
Factor VIII	Hemophilia A	Prenatal, carrier detection
Dystrophin	Duchenne's muscular dystrophy	Presymptomatic, prenatal, carrier detection
α₁-AT	α₁-Antiprotease deficiency	Prenatal, screening
Phe hydroxylase	Phenylketonuria	Prenatal
CFTR	Cystic fibrosis	Prenatal, presymptomatic, carrier screening
G8, other chromosome 4 markers	Huntington's disease	Presymptomatic, prenatal
Growth hormone	Growth hormone deficiency	Prenatal, carrier detection, early diagnosis
HLA	Hemochromatosis Congenital adrenal hyperplasia	Presymptomatic, prenatal Prenatal

261:3108. (A model program for diagnosis and counseling.)

Kan YW: Development of DNA analysis for human disease. JAMA 1992;267:1532. (The discoverer of the first restriction fragment site polymorphism reviews the methods for and consequences of detecting the mutations causing hemoglobinopathies in his Lasker Award lecture.)

Kazazian HH Jr: Diagnosis by gene amplification. J Lab Clin Med 1989;114:95. (Utility of PCR in DNA diagnosis.)

PRENATAL DIAGNOSIS

It is possible to diagnose in utero, before the middle of the second trimester, several hundred mendelian disorders, all chromosome aberrations, and a number of congenital malformations that are not mendelian. The first step toward prenatal diagnosis is taken when the expecting couple, the primary physician, or the obstetrician thinks of the need for it. Recent surveys suggest that even for the most common indication for such service—advanced maternal age—well under half of all women 35 years and older are offered prenatal testing.

Techniques Used in Prenatal Diagnosis

Prenatal diagnosis depends on the ability to assay the fetus directly (fetal blood sampling, fetoscopy), indirectly (analysis of amniotic fluid, amniocytes or trophoblastic cells, ultrasound), or remotely (analysis of maternal serum). Some of these satisfy the requirements for screening (Table 22–4) and should be offered to all pregnant women; others carry considerable risk and should be reserved for specific circumstances.

Ultrasound scanning of the fetus is a safe, non-invasive procedure that can diagnose gross skeletal malformations as well as nonbony malformations known to be associated with specific diseases. Some obstetricians routinely perform fetal ultrasound at least once between 12 and 20 weeks of gestation, though this practice does not yet represent the standard of care.

Other prenatal diagnostic procedures—fetoscopy, fetography, and amniography—are more invasive and a definite risk to the mother and fetus. They are indicated only if the risk of the suspected abnormality is high and the information cannot be obtained by other means.

All of the cytogenetic, biochemical, and DNA analytic techniques discussed above can be applied to specimens from the fetus. Aside from screening for alpha-fetoprotein in maternal serum, analysis of fetal chromosomes is the most frequently performed test. Chromosomal analysis can be performed on amniotic cells and on trophoblastic cells grown in culture and directly on any trophoblastic cells that happen to be

undergoing mitosis. Amniotic fluid cells are derived chiefly from the fetal urinary system. Amniocentesis is best performed between gestational weeks 16 and 18 to permit unhurried sample analysis, transmission of results, and reproductive decisions. The time from obtaining the sample to a final reading of the karyotype has now been shortened to an average of 10–14 days, and automated methods may reduce the time a bit further. Sampling the chorionic villus for trophoblastic cells (derived embryologically from the same fertilized egg as the fetus) is usually done between gestational weeks 10 and 11. If the tissue can be analyzed directly, cytogenetic results can be obtained within a few hours; however, the quality of the karyotypes is inferior to that from cultured cells, and most laboratories routinely culture cells and reexamine any suspected abnormalities. The advantage of chorionic villus sampling is that the results are available early in pregnancy, so that if termination is elected the couple will have had less time to relate to the pregnancy and the obstetric complications of termination are fewer.

The risk of chorionic villus sampling is somewhat higher than that of amniocentesis, though both are relatively safe. Between 0.5% and 1% of pregnancies are lost as a complication of chorionic villus sampling, whereas less than one in 300 amniocenteses result in fetal loss. These figures are lower than but are in addition to the 2–3% spontaneous abortion rate after the first trimester ends.

Indications for Prenatal Diagnosis

The indications for prenatal diagnosis are listed in Table 22–7. A few deserve comment.

Most studies done for advanced maternal age will detect no chromosomal aberration, and the couple will be reassured by this news. However, it is always appropriate to emphasize that the average risk of producing a child with a defect evident at birth, such as a physical malformation or some inborn error of metabolism, is about 3%, and that the risk increases with the age of either parent. Simply examining the chromosomes reduces this risk minimally. On the other hand, unless one of the other indications is present, it is simply not possible to "screen" a pregnancy for most birth defects (neural tube defects being an exception).

Table 22–7. Indications for prenatal diagnosis.

Indications	Methods
Advanced maternal age, previous child with chromosome aberration, intrauterine growth delay	Cytogenetics (amniocentesis, chorionic villus sampling)
Biochemical disorder	Protein assay, DNA diagnosis
Congenital anomaly	Sonography, fetoscopy
Screening for neural tube defects and trisomy	Maternal serum α-fetoprotein

A history for cytogenetic aberrations emphasizes a chromosomal defect in a parent, a family history of a chromosomal defect, or a previous child or conceptus with a defined or undefined chromosomal defect. The factors that render some couples susceptible to repeated episodes of aneuploidy are unclear, and routine prenatal testing is warranted once a defect has occurred.

Cytogenetic analysis of the fetus will of course give information about the sex chromosomes. Some couples do not desire advance knowledge of the sex of their child, and the person transmitting the results to the couple should always address this issue first. On the other hand, some couples *only* want to know the sex of the fetus and plan to terminate the pregnancy if the undesired sex is detected. Virtually no centers in the United States consider sex selection to be an appropriate indication for prenatal diagnosis.

The level of α-fetoprotein in maternal serum changes with gestational age, with the mother's medical status, and with abnormalities of the fetus. If the first two factors can be well controlled, the assay can be used to provide information about the fetus. Levels are expressed as multiples of the median value for a particular gestational age. Higher than normal levels are associated with open neural tube defects (the conditions for which the test was developed), recent or impending fetal demise, gastroschisis, and fetal renal disease. Extremely high levels are highly specific for fetal anomalies—a level three times the median increases 20-fold the risk of meningomyelocele or anencephaly. Low α-fetoprotein levels in maternal serum are associated with fetal trisomy, especially Down's syndrome; the reason for this association remains unclear. The addition of two other compounds in maternal serum—human chorionic gonadotropin (hCG) and unconjugated estriol (uE3)—to the assay for α-fetoprotein (to produce the "triple screen") enhances by several times the ability to detect a fetus with trisomy 21 and trisomy 18. While the triple screen improves both the sensitivity and specificity of detection of trisomic pregnancies, all positive results need to be followed by amniocentesis for confirmation.

Ledbetter DH et al: Cytogenetic results of chorionic villus sampling: High success rate and diagnostic accuracy in the United States collaborative study. Am J Obstet Gynecol 1990;162:495. (Part of a multicenter collaborative study of chorionic villus sampling that proved its utility and documented its risks.)

Milunsky A (editor): *Genetic Disorders and the Fetus*, 3rd ed. Johns Hopkins Univ Press, 1992. (Multiauthored text that covers methods and specific fetal and maternal disorders.)

Staples AJ et al: A maternal serum screen for trisomy 18: An extension of maternal serum screening for Down syndrome. Am J Hum Genet 1991;49:1025. (βhCG and uE3 are the most powerful discriminators for screening maternal serum for trisomy in a pregnancy.)

NEOPLASIA: CHROMOSOMAL & DNA ANALYSIS

Studies of both chromosomes and nucleic acids support Boveri's 1914 hypothesis that cancer is caused by a change in genetic material at the cellular level. Two classes of genes have been discovered that function in neoplastic transformation.

Oncogenes arise from preexisting normal genes (proto-oncogenes) that have been altered by both viral and nonviral factors. As a result, the cells synthesize either normal proteins in inappropriate amounts or proteins that are aberrant in structure and function. Many of these proteins are cellular growth factors, controllers of messenger RNA, and initiators and regulators of RNA; others are receptors for growth factors. The net result of oncogene activation is unregulated cell division. Mutations that activate oncogenes virtually always arise in somatic cells and are not usually inherited. Although some oncogenes are more likely to be activated in certain tumors, in general the same mutations may be found in neoplasia arising in different cells and tissues.

Tumor suppressor genes can be viewed as the antithesis of oncogenes. Their normal function is to suppress transformation; mutation in both alleles is necessary to obliterate this important function. The first mutant allele at any tumor suppressor gene might arise spontaneously or might be inherited; mutation in the other allele (the "second hit") virtually always arises spontaneously, but by any of a number of molecular mechanisms. These genes show considerably more tumor specificity than do oncogenes; however, while some specific mutations are necessary for certain tumors to arise, no loss of single tumor suppressor function is sufficient. Clearly, a person who inherits one copy of a mutant tumor suppressor gene is at increased risk that in some susceptible cell, at some time during life, the function of that gene will be lost. This susceptibility is inherited as an autosomal dominant trait. For example, mutation in one allele of the p53 locus results in the Li-Fraumeni syndrome, in which susceptibility before age 45 years to sarcomas and other tumors occurs in males and females in successive generations. Inherited mutations in this locus also increase the risk that a second tumor will develop following radiation or chemotherapy for the first tumor, suggesting that the initial treatment may induce a "second hit" in a p53 locus in another tissue. However, inheriting a p53 mutation is not a guarantee that cancer will develop at an early age; much more needs to be learned about the pathogenesis of neoplasia before the genetic counseling of families with a molecular predisposition to cancer is clarified.

In selected cases, a patient's DNA can be analyzed for the presence of a mutated gene and thereby assess that individual's risk for developing a tumor. Examples are retinoblastoma and certain forms of Wilms' tumor. To illustrate how noninvasive and sensitive the methodology has become, it is possible to analyze stool for the presence of mutations in tumor suppressor genes that might indicate the presence of a clinically undetected adenocarcinoma of the colon. The analysis depends on the ability of the polymerase chain reaction to amplify minute quantities of the mutant DNA present in epithelial cells shed from the tumor.

This exciting work on the molecular nature of oncogenesis was preceded by years of study of the cytogenetics of tumors. Indeed, the retinoblastoma tumor suppression gene was ultimately isolated because a small number of patients with this tumor have a constitutive deletion of chromosome 13 where this gene maps. Other chromosomal aberrations have been found to be highly characteristic of—or even specific for—certain tumors (Table 22–8). Detection of one of these cytogenetic aberrations can thus aid in diagnosis.

Hematologic malignancies are especially amenable to study because of the relative ease of performing cytogenetic analysis. Such malignancies are associated with over 100 specific chromosomal rearrangements, chiefly translocations. Most of these rearrangements are restricted to a specific type of cancer (Table 22–9), and the remainder occur with many cancers.

In the leukemias, the chromosomal aberration is the basis of one of the subclassifications of the disease. When cytogenetic information is combined with the FAB classification, it is possible to define subsets of patients in which response to therapy, clinical course, and prognosis are predictable. If at the time of diagnosis there are no chromosomal changes in the bone marrow cells, the survival time is longer than if any or all of the bone marrow cells have abnormal cytogenetic characteristics. As secondary chromosomal changes occur, the leukemia becomes more aggressive, often associated with drug resistance and a reduced chance for complete or prolonged remission. The least ominous chromosomal change is numerical alteration without morphologic abnormality.

Table 22–8. Chromosome aberrations associated with representative solid tumors.

Tumor	Chromosome Aberration
Meningioma	del(22)(q11)[1]
Neuroblastoma	del(1)(p36)
Renal cell carcinoma	del(3)(p14.2-p25) or translocation of this region
Retinoblastoma, osteosarcoma	del(13)(q14.1) or translocation of this region
Small-cell lung carcinoma	del(3)(p14-p23)
Wilms' tumor	del(11)(p15)

[1]Nomenclature means, "a deletion at band q11 of chromosome 22."

Table 22–9. Chromosomal aberrations associated with representative hematologic malignancies.

Tumor	Chromosomal Aberration
Leukemias	
Acute myeloblastic	t(8;21)(q22;q11)[1]
Acute promyelocytic	t(15;17)(q22;q11-q12)
Acute monocytic	t(10;11)(p15-p11;q23)
Chronic myelogenous	t(9;22)(q34;q11)
Lymphomas	
Burkitt's	t(8;14)(q24.1;q32.3)
B cell	t(1;14)(q42;q43)
T cell	inv, del, and t of 1p13-p12
Premalignancy	
Polycythemia vera	del(20)(q11)

[1]Nomenclature means, "a translocation with the union at band q22 of chromosome 8 and q22 of chromosome 21."

Less cytogenetic information is available for lymphomas and premalignant hematologic disorders than for leukemia. In Hodgkin's disease, studies have been limited by the low yield of dividing cells and the low number of clear-cut aneuploid clones, so that complete chromosomal analyses with banding are available for far fewer patients with Hodgkin's disease than for any other type of lymphoma. In Hodgkin's disease, the modal chromosomal number tends to be triploid or tetraploid. About one-third of the samples have a 14q+ chromosome. In non-Hodgkin's lymphomas, high-resolution techniques of banding detect abnormalities in 95% of cases. Cytogenetic findings are now being correlated with the immunologic and histologic features and with prognosis.

In Burkitt's lymphoma, a solid tumor of B cell origin, 90% of patients have a translocation between the long arm of chromosome 8 and the long arm of chromosome 14, with chromosomal breakage sites being at or near immunoglobulin and oncogene loci.

Instability of chromosomes also predisposes to the development of some malignancies. In certain autosomal recessive diseases such as ataxia-telangiectasia, Bloom's syndrome, and Fanconi's anemia, the cells have a tendency to **genetic instability,** ie, to chromosomal breakage and rearrangement in vitro. These diseases are associated with a fairly high incidence of neoplasia, particularly leukemia and lymphoma.

Some chromosomal aberrations, better known for their effect on phenotype, also predispose to tumors. For example, patients with Down's syndrome (trisomy 21) have a 20-fold increase in the risk of leukemia; 47,XXY males (Klinefelter's syndrome) have a 30-fold increase in the risk of breast cancer; and XY phenotypic females have a heightened risk of developing ovarian cancer, primarily gonadoblastoma.

The indications for cytogenetic analysis of neoplasia continue to evolve. Not all tumors require study. However, in cases of tumors of unclear type (especially leukemias and lymphomas), with a strong family history of early neoplasia, or for certain tumors associated with potential generalized chromosomal defects (present in nonneoplastic cells), cytogenetic analysis should be strongly considered.

Fearon ER, Jones PA: Progressing toward a molecular description of colorectal cancer development. FASEB J 1992;6:2783. (Genes discovered thus far that are involved in the pathogenesis of adenocarcinoma of the colon.)

Frebourg T, Friend SH: Cancer risks from germline p53 mutations. J Clin Invest 1992;90:1637. (Convincing evidence that people who inherit a p53 mutation have a high risk of developing tumors of many types.)

Malkin D et al: Germline mutations of the p53 tumor-suppressor gene in children and young adults with second malignant neoplasms. N Engl J Med 1992;326:1309. (Heterozygosity for inherited mutations of p53 increase susceptibility to early-onset tumors.)

Shields PG, Harris: Molecular epidemiology and the genetics of environmental cancer. JAMA 1991;266:681. (How genes and exogenous factors interact in the genesis of neoplasia.)

Sidransky D et al: Identification of *ras* oncogene mutations in the stool of patients with curable colorectal tumors. Science 1992;256:102. (Makes finding a needle in a haystack seem mundane! Paves the way for screening high-risk patients, though sensitivity and specificity require further assessment.)

SELECTED GENETIC DISORDERS

MARFAN'S SYNDROME

Marfan's syndrome, a systemic connective tissue disease, is inherited as an autosomal dominant. Affected patients are typically tall, with particularly long arms, legs, and digits (arachnodactyly). Skeletal abnormalities are common, including frequent joint dislocations and pectus excavatum. Ectopia lentis may lead to severe myopia and retinal detachment. However, of most concern is disease of the ascending aorta—anuloaortic ectasia—which is associated with a dilated aortic root resulting in aortic regurgitation, and death in the fourth and fifth decades. Histology of the aorta shows diffuse medial abnormalities. Aortic and mitral valve leaflets are also abnormal, and mitral regurgitation may be present as well, often with elongated chordae tendineae, which on occasion may rupture.

Children with Marfan's syndrome require routine ophthalmologic and orthopedic surveillance to prevent or slow the development of amblyopia and scoliosis. Patients of all ages require regular echocardiography to monitor aortic diameter and mitral valve function;

chronic beta-adrenergic blockade and restriction of physical activity help slow aortic dilatation. Prophylactic replacement of the aortic root with a composite graft when the diameter reaches 55–60 mm prolongs life.

Dietz HC et al: Marfan phenotype variability in a family segregating a missense mutation in the EGF-like motif of the fibrillin gene. J Clin Invest 1992;89:1674. (The second mutation described in Marfan' syndrome illustrates that the clinical severity is not dependent solely on the fibrillin gene.)

Gott VL et al: Composite graft repair of Marfan aneurysm of the ascending aorta: Results in 100 patients. Ann Thorac Surg 1991;52:38. (Recent experience with aortic repair from the surgeon with the largest experience.)

Pyeritz RE: The Marfan syndrome. In: *Connective Tissue and Its Heritable Disorders: Molecular, Genetic and Medical Aspects.* Royce PM, Steinmann B (editors). Wiley-Liss, 1992. (Clinical, genetic, and biochemical aspects of this common connective tissue disorder.)

DOWN'S SYNDROME

Down's syndrome is usually diagnosed at birth on the basis of the typical facial features, hypotonia, and single palmar crease. Cytogenetic analysis should always be performed—even though most patients will have simple trisomy for chromosome 21—to detect unbalanced translocations; such patients will usually have a parent with a balanced translocation, and there will be a recurrence risk of Down's syndrome in future offspring. Some children have life-threatening problems (endocardial cushion defect, duodenal atresia, leukemia) that often can be successfully treated. Intelligence varies, but full independence in adulthood is uncommon. An Alzheimer-like dementia often occurs in the fourth and fifth decades and accounts for a reduced life expectancy.

Lott IT, McCoy EE (editors): *Down Syndrome: Advances in Medical Care.* Wiley, 1992. (Current perspectives on managing the diverse medical and social issues that arise in patients of all ages and their families.)

KLINEFELTER'S SYNDROME

Boys with an extra X chromosome are normal in appearance before puberty; thereafter, they have disproportionately long legs and arms, a female escutcheon, gynecomastia, and small testes. Infertility is due to azoospermia; the seminiferous tubules are hyalinized. The diagnosis is often not made until a couple is evaluated for inability to conceive. Although mental retardation is somewhat more common than in the general population, many men with Klinefelter's syndrome have learning problems. The risk of breast cancer is much higher in men with

Klinefelter's syndrome than in 46,XY men, as is the risk of diabetes mellitus. Treatment with testosterone after puberty is advisable but will not restore fertility.

Life expectancy is reduced, especially in untreated and pyridoxine-unresponsive patients; myocardial infarction, stroke, and pulmonary embolism are the most common causes of death. This condition is diagnosed by newborn screening for hypermethioninemia in some states; however, pyridoxine-responsive infants may not be detected.

HOMOCYSTINURIA

Homocystinuria in its classic form is caused by cystathionine β-synthase deficiency and exhibits an autosomal recessive pattern of inheritance. This results in extreme elevations of plasma and urinary homocystine levels, a basis for diagnosis of this disorder. Homocystinuria is similar in certain superficial aspects to Marfan's syndrome, since patients may show a similar body habitus and ectopia lentis is almost always present. However, mental retardation is often present, and the cardiovascular events are those of repeated venous and arterial thromboses whose precise cause remains obscure. Life expectancy is reduced, especially in untreated and pyridoxine-unresponsive patients; myocardial infarction, stroke, and pulmonary embolism are the most common causes of death. This condition is diagnosed by newborn screening for hypermethioninemia in some states; however, pyridoxine-responsive infants may not be detected. The diagnosis should be suspected in patients in the second and third decades of life who show evidence of arterial or venous thromboses and have no other risk factors.

About one-half of patients have a form of cystathionine β-synthase deficiency that improves biochemically and clinically through pharmacologic doses of pyridoxine and folate. For these patients, treatment from infancy can prevent retardation and the other clinical problems. Patients who are pyridoxine-nonresponders must be treated with dietary reduction in methionine and supplementation of cysteine, also from infancy. The vitamin betaine is also useful in reducing plasma methionine levels by facilitating a metabolic pathway that bypasses the defective enzyme. Patients who have suffered venous thrombosis should be anticoagulated, but there are no studies to support prophylactic use of warfarin or antiplatelet agents.

Pyeritz RE: Homocystinuria. In: *McKusick's Heritable Disorders of Connective Tissue,* 5th ed. Mosby, 1992. (Clinical, genetic, and biochemical aspects of an inborn error of metabolism with extensive effects on the extracellular matrix.)

GAUCHER'S DISEASE

Gaucher's disease is inherited as an autosomal recessive. A deficiency of β-glucocerebrosidase causes an accumulation of sphingolipid within phagocytic cells throughout the body. Anemia and thrombocytopenia are common and may be symptomatic; both are due primarily to hypersplenism, but marrow infiltration with Gaucher cells may contribute. Cortical erosions of bones, especially the vertebrae and femur, are due to local infarctions, but the mechanism is unclear. Episodes of bone pain (termed "crises") are reminiscent of those in sickle cell disease. A hip fracture in a patient with a palpable spleen—especially in a Jewish person of Eastern European origin—suggests the possibility of Gaucher's disease. Bone marrow aspirates reveal typical Gaucher cells, which have an eccentric nucleus and PAS-positive inclusions, along with wrinkled cytoplasm and inclusion bodies of a fibrillar type. In addition, the serum acid phosphatase is elevated. Definitive diagnosis requires the demonstration of deficient glucocerebrosidase activity in leukocytes.

Until recently, treatment has been supportive and has included splenectomy for thrombocytopenia secondary to platelet sequestration. The purification of sufficient quantities of alglucerase (glucocerebrosidase-β-glucosidase) to permit intravenous administration on a regular basis now permits a reduction in total body stores of glycolipid and improvement in orthopedic and hematologic manifestations. The major drawback is the exceptional cost of Alglucerase, which can exceed $350,000 per year, though recent studies suggest that more frequent administration of less enzyme (30 units/kg per month) is just as effective and reduces the cost to about $100,000 annually for an adult.

Figueroa ML et al: A less costly regimen of alglucerase to treat Gaucher's disease. N Engl J Med 1992;327:1632. (Establishes the standard treatment regimen.)

ACUTE INTERMITTENT PORPHYRIA

Though there are several different types of porphyrias, the one with serious consequences most commonly encountered in adulthood is acute intermittent porphyria, which is inherited as an autosomal dominant, though it remains clinically silent in the majority of patients who carry the trait. Those who develop clinical illness are usually women, with symptoms beginning in the teens or 20s. The disorder is caused by deficiency of porphobilinogen deaminase activity, leading to increased excretion of aminolevulinic acid and porphobilinogen in the urine. The diagnosis may be elusive if not specifically considered. Patients show intermittent abdominal pain of varying severity, and in some instances it may so simulate acute abdomen as to lead to exploratory laparotomy. Likewise, any part of the nervous system may be involved, with evidence for autonomic and peripheral neuropathy. Indeed, the abdominal pain may be due to abnormalities in autonomic innervation in the gut. Peripheral neuropathy may be symmetric or asymmetric and mild or profound; in the latter instance, it can even lead to quadriplegia with respiratory paralysis. Other central nervous system manifestations include seizures, psychosis, and abnormalities of the basal ganglia. In contrast to other forms of porphyria, cutaneous photosensitivity is absent in acute intermittent porphyria.

Attacks of acute intermittent porphyria are precipitated by numerous factors, especially drugs, with sulfonamides and barbiturates being the likely offending agents. Intercurrent infection and starvation diets also cause attacks.

Laboratory investigation often reveals profound hyponatremia, due in part to inappropriate release of antidiuretic hormone, though gastrointestinal loss of sodium in some patients may contribute. The diagnosis can be confirmed by demonstrating an increased amount of porphobilinogen in the urine during an acute attack. Freshly voided urine is of normal color but may turn dark upon standing in light and air.

Treatment with a high-carbohydrate diet diminishes the number of attacks in some patients and is a reasonable empiric gesture considering its benignity. Acute attacks may be life-threatening and require prompt diagnosis, withdrawal of the inciting agent (if possible), and treatment with analgesics and intravenous glucose and hematin.

Kappas A et al: The porphyrias. In: *The Metabolic Basis of Inherited Disease,* 6th ed. Criver CR et al (editors). Mc-Graw-Hill, 1989. (Review of all defects causing forms of porphyria, including the acute intermittent type.)

ALKAPTONURIA

Alkaptonuria is caused by a recessively inherited deficiency of the enzyme homogentisic acid oxidase. This acid derives from metabolism of both phenylalanine and tyrosine and is present in large amounts in the urine throughout the patient's life. An oxidation product accumulates slowly in cartilage throughout the body, leading to degenerative joint disease of the spine and peripheral joints. Indeed, examination of patients in the third and fourth decades shows a slight darkish blue color below the skin in areas overlying cartilage, such as in the ears, a phenomenon called "ochronosis." In some patients, a more severe hyperpigmentation can be seen in the sclera, conjunctiva, and cornea. Accumulation of metabolites in heart valves can lead to aortic or mitral stenosis. A predisposition to coronary artery disease also may be present. While the syndrome causes considerable morbidity, life expectancy is reduced only modestly. Symptoms are more often attributable to spondylitis with back pain, leading to a clinical picture difficult to distinguish from that of ankylosing spondylitis, though on radiographic assessment the sacroiliac joints are not fused in alkaptonuria.

The diagnosis is established by demonstrating homogentisic acid in the urine, which turns black spontaneously on exposure to the air; this reaction is particularly noteworthy if the urine is alkaline or when alkali is added to a specimen. Treatment of the arthritis is similar to that for other arthropathies. Though in theory rigid dietary restriction might reduce accumulation of the pigment, this has not proved to be of practical benefit.

La Du BN: Alcaptonuria. In: *The Metabolic Basis of Inherited Disease,* 6th ed. Criver CR et al (editors). McGraw-Hill, 1989. (Clinical and biochemical aspects of one of Garrod's original inborn errors of metabolism.)

Nervous System

Michael J. Aminoff, MD, FRCP

HEADACHE

Headache is such a common complaint and can occur for so many different reasons that its proper evaluation may be difficult. Although underlying structural lesions are not present in most patients presenting with headache, it is nevertheless important to bear this possibility in mind. About one-third of patients with brain tumors, for example, present with a primary complaint of headache.

The intensity, quality, and site of pain—and especially the duration of the headache and the presence of associated neurologic symptoms—may provide clues to the underlying cause. The onset of severe headache in a previously well patient is more likely than chronic headache to relate to an intracranial disorder such as subarachnoid hemorrhage or meningitis. Headaches that disturb sleep, exertional headaches, and late-onset paroxysmal headaches are also more suggestive of an underlying structural lesion, as are headaches accompanied by neurologic symptoms such as drowsiness, visual or limb problems, seizures, or altered mental status. Chronic headaches are commonly due to migraine, tension, or depression, but they may be related to intracranial lesions, head injury, cervical spondylosis, dental or ocular disease, temporomandibular joint dysfunction, sinusitis, hypertension, and a wide variety of general medical disorders. Depending on the initial clinical impression, the need for such investigations as CT scan or MRI of the head, electroencephalography, and lumbar puncture must be assessed on an individual basis. The diagnosis and treatment of primary neurologic disorders associated with headache are considered separately under these disorders.

Tension Headache

Patients frequently complain of poor concentration and other vague nonspecific symptoms, in addition to constant daily headaches that are often vise-like or tight in quality and may be exacerbated by emotional stress, fatigue, noise, or glare. The headaches are usually generalized, may be most intense about the neck or back of the head, and are not associated with focal neurologic symptoms.

When treatment with simple analgesics is not effective, a trial of antimigrainous agents (see Migraine, below) is worthwhile. Techniques to induce relaxation are also useful and include massage, hot baths, and biofeedback. Exploration of underlying causes of chronic anxiety is often rewarding.

Depression Headache

Depression headaches are frequently worse on arising in the morning and may be accompanied by other symptoms of depression. Headaches are occasionally the focus of a somatic delusional system. Tricyclic antidepressant drugs are often helpful, as may be psychiatric consultation.

Migraine

Classic migrainous headache is a lateralized throbbing headache that occurs episodically following its onset in adolescence or early adult life. In many cases, however, the headaches do not conform to this pattern, although their associated features and response to antimigrainous preparations nevertheless suggest that they have a similar basis. In this broader sense, migrainous headaches may be lateralized or generalized, may be dull or throbbing, and are sometimes associated with anorexia, nausea, vomiting, photophobia, and blurring of vision (so-called sick headaches). They usually build up gradually and may last for several hours or longer. They have been related to dilation and excessive pulsation of branches of the external carotid artery. Focal disturbances of neurologic function may precede or accompany the headaches and have been attributed to constriction of branches of the internal carotid artery. Visual disturbances occur quite commonly and may consist of field defects; of luminous visual hallucinations such as stars, sparks, unformed light flashes (photopsia), geometric patterns, or zigzags of light; or of some combination of field defects and luminous hallucinations (scintillating scotomas). Other focal disturbances such as aphasia or numbness, tingling, clumsiness, or weakness in a circumscribed distribution may also occur.

Patients often give a family history of migraine. Attacks may be triggered by emotional or physical stress, lack or excess of sleep, missed meals, specific foods (eg, chocolate), alcoholic beverages, menstruation, or use of oral contraceptives.

An uncommon variant is so-called **basilar artery**

migraine, in which blindness or visual disturbances throughout both visual fields are initially accompanied or followed by dysarthria, disequilibrium, tinnitus, and perioral and distal paresthesias and are sometimes followed by transient loss or impairment of consciousness or by a confusional state. This, in turn, is followed by a throbbing (usually occipital) headache, often with nausea and vomiting.

In **ophthalmoplegic migraine,** lateralized pain—often about the eye—is accompanied by nausea, vomiting, and diplopia due to transient external ophthalmoplegia. The ophthalmoplegia is due to third nerve palsy, sometimes with accompanying sixth nerve involvement, and may outlast the orbital pain by several days or even weeks. The ophthalmic division of the fifth nerve has also been affected in some patients. Ophthalmoplegic migraine is rare; more common causes of a painful ophthalmoplegia are internal carotid artery aneurysms and diabetes.

In rare instances, the neurologic or somatic disturbance accompanying typical migrainous headaches becomes the sole manifestation of an attack ("migraine equivalent"). Very rarely, the patient may be left with a permanent neurologic deficit following a migrainous attack, presumably because of irreversible cerebral ischemic damage.

The pathophysiology of migraine probably relates to the neurotransmitter serotonin. Headache may result from release of neuropeptides acting as neurotransmitters at trigeminal nerve branches, leading to an inflammatory process; another possible mechanism involves activation of the dorsal raphe nucleus.

Management of migraine consists of avoidance of any precipitating factors, together with prophylactic or symptomatic pharmacologic treatment if necessary.

During acute attacks, many patients find it helpful to rest in a quiet, darkened room until symptoms subside. A simple analgesic (eg, aspirin) taken right away often provides relief, but treatment with extracranial vasoconstrictors or other drugs is sometimes necessary. Cafergot, a combination of ergotamine tartrate (1 mg) and caffeine (100 mg), is often particularly helpful; one or two tablets are taken at the onset of headache or warning symptoms, followed by one tablet every 30 minutes, if necessary, up to six tablets per attack and ten tablets per week. Ergonovine maleate, up to five tablets (1 mg) taken at the onset of symptoms, may also provide relief. Because of impaired absorption or vomiting during acute attacks, oral medication sometimes fails to help. Cafergot given rectally as suppositories (one-half to one suppository containing 2 mg of ergotamine); ergotamine tartrate given by inhalation (0.36 mg per puff; up to six puffs per attack) or sublingually (2 mg tablets; not more than three tablets per 24 hours); or dihydroergotamine mesylate (0.5–1 mg intravenously or 1–2 mg subcutaneously or intramuscularly) may be useful in such cases. Ergotamine-containing preparations may affect the gravid uterus and thus should be avoided during pregnancy. Sumatriptan is a new, rapidly effective agent for aborting attacks when given subcutaneously by an autoinjection device. It has a high affinity for serotonin$_1$D receptors. It should probably be avoided in pregnancy.

Prophylactic treatment may be necessary if migrainous headaches occur more frequently than two or three times a month. Some of the more common drugs used for this purpose are listed in Table 23–1. Their mode of action is unclear and may involve both an effect on extracerebral vasculature and a cerebral effect, eg, by stabilizing serotonergic neurotransmission. Several drugs may have to be tried in turn before the headaches are brought under control. Once a drug has been found to help, it should be continued for several months. If the patient remains headache-free, the dose can then be tapered and the drug eventually withdrawn.

Calcium channel antagonist drugs may decrease the frequency of attacks after an interval of several weeks, but the severity and duration of attacks are not influenced.

Table 23–1. Prophylactic treatment of migraine.[1]

Drug	Usual Adult Daily Dose (mg)	Common Side Effects
Propranolol	80–240	Fatigue, lassitude, depression, insomnia, nausea, vomiting, constipation.
Amitriptyline	10–150	Sedation, dry mouth, constipation, weight gain, blurred vision, edema, hypotension, urinary retention.
Ergonovine maleate	0.6–2	Nausea, abdominal pain, diarrhea.
Cyproheptadine	12–20	Sedation, dry mouth, epigastric discomfort, gastrointestinal disturbances.
Clonidine	0.2–0.6	Dry mouth, drowsiness, sedation, headache, constipation.
Methysergide	4–8	Nausea, vomiting, diarrhea, abdominal pain, cramps, weight gain, insomnia, edema, peripheral vasoconstriction. Retroperitoneal and pleuropulmonary fibrosis and fibrous thickening of cardiac valves may occur; patients must be closely supervised.

[1]Reproduced with permission, from Aminoff MJ: Neurologic disorders. In: *Handbook of Medical Treatment,* 17th ed. Watts HD (editor). Jones, 1983.

Cluster Headache
(Migrainous Neuralgia)

Cluster headache affects predominantly middle-aged men. Its cause is unclear but may relate to a vascular headache disorder or a disturbance of serotonergic mechanisms. There is often no family history of headache or migraine. Episodes of severe unilateral periorbital pain occur daily for several weeks and are often accompanied by one or more of the following: ipsilateral nasal congestion, rhinorrhea, lacrimation, redness of the eye, and Horner's syndrome. Episodes usually occur at night, awaken the patient, and last for less than 2 hours. Spontaneous remission then occurs, and the patient remains well for weeks or months before another bout of closely spaced attacks occurs. During a bout, many patients report that alcohol triggers an attack; others report that stress, glare, or ingestion of specific foods occasionally precipitates attacks. In occasional patients, typical attacks of pain and associated symptoms recur at intervals without remission. This variant has been referred to as chronic cluster headache.

Examination reveals no abnormality apart from Horner's syndrome that either occurs transiently during an attack or, in long-standing cases, remains as a residual deficit between attacks.

Treatment of an individual attack with oral drugs is generally unsatisfactory, but use of ergotamine tartrate aerosol or inhalation of 100% oxygen (7 L/min for 15 minutes) may be effective. Butorphanol tartrate, a synthetic opioid agonist-antagonist, may also be helpful when administered by nasal spray. Ergotamine tartrate is an effective prophylactic and can be given as rectal suppositories (0.5–1 mg at night or twice daily), by mouth (2 mg daily), or by subcutaneous injection (0.25 mg three times daily for 5 days per week). Various prophylactic agents that have been found to be effective in individual patients are propranolol, amitriptyline, cyproheptadine, lithium carbonate (monitored by plasma lithium determination), prednisone (20–40 mg daily or on alternate days for 2 weeks, followed by gradual withdrawal), verapamil (240–480 mg daily), and methysergide (4–6 mg daily).

Giant Cell (Temporal or Cranial)
Arteritis

The superficial temporal, vertebral, ophthalmic, and posterior ciliary arteries are often the most severely affected pathologically. Most patients are elderly. The major symptom is headache, often associated with or preceded by myalgia, malaise, anorexia, weight loss, and other nonspecific complaints. Loss of vision is the most feared manifestation and occurs quite commonly. Clinical examination often reveals tenderness of the scalp and over the temporal arteries. Further details, including approaches to treatment, are given in Chapter 19.

Posttraumatic Headache

A variety of nonspecific symptoms may follow a closed head injury, regardless of whether consciousness is lost. Headache is often a conspicuous feature. Some authorities believe that psychologic factors may be important because there is no correlation of severity of the injury with neurologic signs.

The headache itself usually appears within a day or so following injury, may worsen over the ensuing weeks, and then gradually subsides. It is usually a constant dull ache, with superimposed throbbing that may be localized, lateralized, or generalized. It is sometimes accompanied by nausea, vomiting, or scintillating scotomas.

Disequilibrium, sometimes with a rotatory component, may also occur and is often enhanced by postural change or head movement. Impaired memory, poor concentration, emotional instability, and increased irritability are other common complaints and occasionally are the sole manifestations of the syndrome. The duration of symptoms relates in part to the severity of the original injury, but even trivial injuries are sometimes followed by symptoms that persist for months.

Special investigations are usually not helpful. The electroencephalogram may show minor nonspecific changes, while the electronystagmogram sometimes suggests either peripheral or central vestibulopathy. CT scans or MRI of the head usually show no abnormal findings.

Treatment is difficult, but optimistic encouragement and graduated rehabilitation, depending upon the occupational circumstances, are advised. Headaches often respond to simple analgesics, but severe headaches may necessitate treatment with amitriptyline, propranolol, or ergot derivatives.

Cough Headache

Severe head pain may be produced by coughing (and by straining, sneezing, and laughing) but, fortunately, usually lasts for only a few minutes or less. The pathophysiologic basis of the complaint is not known, and often there is no underlying structural lesion. However, intracranial lesions, usually in the posterior fossa (eg, Arnold-Chiari malformation, basilar impression), are present in about 10% of cases, and brain tumors or other space-occupying lesions may certainly present in this way. Accordingly, CT scanning or MRI should be undertaken in all patients and repeated annually for several years, since a small structural lesion may not show up initially.

The disorder is usually self-limited, although it may persist for several years. For unknown reasons, symptoms sometimes clear completely after lumbar puncture. Indomethacin (75–150 mg daily) may provide relief.

Headache Due to Other Neurologic Causes

Intracranial mass lesions of all types may cause headache owing to displacement of vascular structures. Posterior fossa tumors often cause occipital pain, and supratentorial lesions lead to bifrontal headache, but such findings are too inconsistent to be of value in attempts at localizing a pathologic process. The headaches are nonspecific in character and may vary in severity from mild to severe. They may be worsened by exertion or postural change and may be associated with nausea and vomiting, but this is true of migraine also. Headaches are also a feature of pseudotumor cerebri (see below). Signs of focal or diffuse cerebral dysfunction or of increased intracranial pressure will indicate the need for further investigation. Similarly, a progressive headache disorder or the new onset of headaches in middle or later life merits investigation if no cause is apparent.

Cerebrovascular disease may be associated with headache, but the mechanism is unclear. Headache may occur with internal carotid artery occlusion or carotid dissection and after carotid endarterectomy. Diagnosis is facilitated by the clinical accompaniments and the circumstances in which the headache developed.

Acute severe headache accompanies subarachnoid hemorrhage and meningeal infections, but the accompanying signs of meningeal irritation and the frequent impairment of consciousness then indicate the need for further investigations. A dramatically severe headache may also occur in association with paroxysmal hypertension in patients with pheochromocytoma.

Dull or throbbing headache is a frequent sequela of lumbar puncture and may last for several days. It is aggravated by the erect posture and alleviated by recumbency. The exact mechanism is unclear, but it is commonly attributed to leakage of cerebrospinal fluid through the dural puncture site. Its incidence may be reduced if a small-diameter needle is used for the spinal tap, and perhaps also if the patient lies prone or supine after the procedure.

Olesen J et al: Timing and topography of cerebral blood flow, aura, and headache during migraine attacks. Ann Neurol 1990;28:791.

Solomon S et al: Prophylactic therapy of cluster headaches. Clin Neuropharmacol 1991;14:116.

Subcutaneous Sumatriptan International Study Group: Treatment of migraine attacks with sumatriptan. N Engl J Med 1991;325:316.

FACIAL PAIN

Trigeminal Neuralgia

Trigeminal neuralgia ("tic douloureux") is most common in middle and later life. It affects women more frequently than men. The disorder is characterized by momentary episodes of sudden lancinating facial pain that commonly arises near one side of the mouth and then shoots toward the ear, eye, or nostril on that side. The pain may be triggered or precipitated by such factors as touch, movement, drafts, and eating. Indeed, in order to lessen the likelihood of triggering further attacks, many patients try to hold the face still while talking. Spontaneous remissions for several months or longer may occur. As the disorder progresses, however, the episodes of pain become more frequent, remissions become shorter and less common, and a dull ache may persist between the episodes of stabbing pain. Symptoms remain confined to the distribution of the trigeminal nerve (usually the second or third division) on one side only.

The characteristic features of the pain in trigeminal neuralgia usually distinguish it from other causes of facial pain. Neurologic examination shows no abnormality except in a few patients in whom trigeminal neuralgia is symptomatic of some underlying lesion, such as multiple sclerosis or a brain stem neoplasm, in which case the finding will depend on the nature and site of the lesion. Similarly, CT scans and radiologic contrast studies are normal in patients with classic trigeminal neuralgia.

In a young patient presenting with trigeminal neuralgia, multiple sclerosis must be suspected even if there are no other neurologic signs. In such circumstances, findings on evoked potential testing and examination of cerebrospinal fluid may be corroborative. When the facial pain is due to a posterior fossa tumor, CT scanning and MRI generally reveal the lesion.

The drug most helpful for treatment of trigeminal neuralgia is carbamazepine, given in a dose of up to 1200 mg/d, with monitoring by serial blood counts and liver function tests. If carbamazepine is ineffective or cannot be tolerated, phenytoin should be tried. (Doses and side effects of these drugs are shown in Table 23–2.) Baclofen (10–20 mg three or four times daily) may also be helpful, either alone or in combination with carbamazepine or phenytoin.

In the past, alcohol injection of the affected nerve, rhizotomy, or tractotomy were recommended if pharmacologic treatment was unsuccessful. More recently, however, posterior fossa exploration has frequently revealed some structural cause for the neuralgia (despite normal findings on CT scans, MRI, or arteriograms), such as an anomalous artery or vein impinging on the trigeminal nerve root. In such cases, simple decompression and separation of the anomalous vessel from the nerve root produce lasting relief of symptoms. In elderly patients with a limited life expectancy, radiofrequency rhizotomy is sometimes preferred because it is easy to perform, has few complications, and provides symptomatic relief for a period of time. Surgical exploration generally reveals

Table 23–2. Drug treatment for seizures.[1]

	Usual Adult Daily Dose (mg/kg)	Usual Adult Daily Dose (mg)	Minimum Number of Daily Doses	Time to Steady-State Drug Levels (days)	Optimal Blood Level (per mL)	Selected Side Effects and Idiosyncratic Reactions
Generalized tonic-clonic (grand mal) or partial (focal) seizures						
Phenytoin	4–8	200–400	1	5–10	10–20 µg	Nystagmus, ataxia, dysarthria, sedation, confusion, gingival hyperplasia, hirsutism, megaloblastic anemia, blood dyscrasias, skin rashes, fever, systemic lupus erythematosus, lymphadenopathy, peripheral neuropathy, dyskinesias.
Carbamazepine	5–25	600–1200	2	3–4	4–8 µg	Nystagmus, dysarthria, diplopia, ataxia, drowsiness, nausea, blood dyscrasias, hepatotoxicity.
Valproic acid	10–60	1500–2000	3	2–4	50–100 µg	Nausea, vomiting, diarrhea, drowsiness, alopecia, weight gain, hepatotoxicity, thrombocytopenia, tremor.
Phenobarbital	2–5	100–200	1	14–21	10–40 µg	Drowsiness, nystagmus, ataxia, skin rashes, learning difficulties, hyperactivity.
Primidone	5–20	750–1500	3	4–7	5–15 µg	Sedation, nystagmus, ataxia, vertigo, nausea, skin rashes, megaloblastic anemia, irritability.
Absence (petit mal) seizures						
Ethosuximide	20–35	100–1500	2	5–10	40–100 µg	Nausea, vomiting, anorexia, headache, lethargy, unsteadiness, blood dyscrasias, systemic lupus erythematosus, urticaria, pruritus.
Valproic acid	10–60	1500–2000	3	2–4	50–100 µg	See above.
Clonazepam	0.05–0.2		2	?	20–80 ng	Drowsiness, ataxia, irritability, behavioral changes, exacerbation of tonic-clonic seizures.
Myoclonic seizures						
Valproic acid	10–60	1500–2000	3	2–4	50–100 µg	See above.
Clonazepam	0.05–0.2		2	?	20–80 ng	See above.

[1]Modified and reproduced, with permission, from Aminoff MJ: Neurologic disorders. In: *Handbook of Medical Treatment*, 17th ed. Watts HD (editor). Jones, 1983.

no abnormality and is inappropriate in patients with trigeminal neuralgia due to multiple sclerosis.

Atypical Facial Pain

Facial pain without the typical features of trigeminal neuralgia is generally a constant, often burning pain that may have a restricted distribution at its onset but soon spreads to the rest of the face on the affected side and sometimes involves the other side, the neck, or the back of the head as well. The disorder is especially common in middle-aged women, many of them emotionally depressed, but it is not clear whether depression is the cause of or a reaction to the pain. Simple analgesics should be given a trial, as should tricyclic antidepressants, carbamazepine, and phenytoin; the response is often disappointing. Opiate analgesics should be avoided, since addiction is a very real danger in patients with this disorder. Attempts at surgical treatment are not indicated.

Glossopharyngeal Neuralgia

Glossopharyngeal neuralgia is an uncommon disorder in which pain similar in quality to that in trigeminal neuralgia occurs in the throat, about the tonsillar fossa, and sometimes deep in the ear and at the back of the tongue. The pain may be precipitated by swallowing, chewing, talking, or yawning and is sometimes accompanied by syncope. In most instances, no underlying structural abnormality is present. Carbamazepine is the treatment of choice and should be tried (in daily doses up to 1200 mg) before any surgical procedures are considered.

Postherpetic Neuralgia

Herpes zoster (shingles) is due to infection of the nervous system by varicella-zoster virus. About 10% of patients who develop shingles suffer from postherpetic neuralgia. This complication seems especially likely to occur in the elderly and when the first division of the trigeminal nerve is affected. A history of shingles and the presence of cutaneous scarring resulting from shingles aid in the diagnosis. Severe pain with shingles correlates with the intensity of postherpetic symptoms.

The incidence of postherpetic neuralgia may be reduced by the treatment of shingles with systemic corticosteroids (prednisone, 60 mg daily for 2 weeks, with rapid taper) but is not influenced by treatment with acyclovir. Management of the established complication is essentially medical. If simple analgesics fail to help, a trial of a tricyclic drug (eg, amitriptyline, up to 100–150 mg/d) in conjunction with a phenothiazine (eg, perphenazine, 2–8 mg/d) is often effective. Other patients respond to carbamazepine (up to 1200 mg/d) or phenytoin (300 mg/d).

Facial Pain Due to Other Causes

Facial pain may be caused by temporomandibular joint dysfunction in patients with malocclusion, abnormal bite, or faulty dentures. There may be tenderness of the masticatory muscles, and an association between pain onset and jaw movement is sometimes noted. Treatment consists of correction of the underlying problem.

A relationship of facial pain to chewing or temperature changes may suggest a dental disturbance. The cause is sometimes not obvious, and diagnosis requires careful dental examination and x-rays. Pain on mastication may also occur in giant cell arteritis. Sinusitis and ear infections causing facial pain are usually recognized by the history of respiratory tract infection, fever, and, in some instances, aural discharge. There may be localized tenderness. Radiologic evidence of sinus infection or mastoiditis is confirmatory.

Glaucoma is an important ocular cause of facial pain, usually localized to the periorbital region.

On occasion, pain in the jaw may be the principal manifestation of angina pectoris. Precipitation by exertion and radiation to more typical areas establish the cardiac origin.

EPILEPSY

Essentials of Diagnosis

- Recurrent seizures.
- Characteristic electroencephalographic changes accompany seizures.
- Mental status abnormalities or focal neurologic symptoms may persist for hours postictally.

General Considerations

The term epilepsy denotes any disorder characterized by recurrent seizures. A seizure is a transient disturbance of cerebral function due to an abnormal paroxysmal neuronal discharge in the brain. Epilepsy is common, affecting approximately 0.5% of the population in the USA.

Etiology

Epilepsy has several causes. Its most likely cause in individual patients relates to the age at onset.

A. Idiopathic or Constitutional Epilepsy: Seizures usually begin between 5 and 20 years of age but may start later in life. No specific cause can be identified, and there is no other neurologic abnormality.

B. Symptomatic Epilepsy: There are many causes for recurrent seizures.

1. Congenital abnormalities and perinatal injuries may result in seizures presenting in infancy or childhood.

2. Metabolic disorders such as hypocalcemia, hypoglycemia, pyridoxine deficiency, and phenylketonuria are major treatable causes of seizures in newborns or infants. In adults, withdrawal from alcohol or drugs is a common cause of recurrent seizures, and other metabolic disorders such as renal failure and diabetes may also be responsible.

3. Trauma is an important cause of seizures at any age, but especially in young adults. Posttraumatic epilepsy is more likely to develop if the dura mater was penetrated and generally becomes manifest within 2 years following the injury. However, seizures developing in the first week after head injury do not necessarily imply that future attacks will occur. There is suggestive evidence that prophylactic anticonvulsant drug treatment reduces the incidence of posttraumatic epilepsy.

4. Tumors and other space-occupying lesions may lead to seizures at any age, but they are an especially important cause of seizures in middle and later life, when the incidence of neoplastic disease increases. The seizures are commonly the initial symptoms of the tumor and often are partial (focal) in character. They are most likely to occur with structural lesions involving the frontal, parietal, or temporal regions. Tumors must be excluded by appropriate laboratory studies in all patients with onset of seizures after 30 years of age, focal seizures or signs, or a progressive seizure disorder.

5. Vascular diseases become increasingly frequent causes of seizures with advancing age and are the most common cause of seizures with onset at age 60 years or older.

6. Degenerative disorders such as Alzheimer's disease are a cause of seizures in later life.

7. Infectious diseases must be considered in all age groups as potentially reversible causes of seizures. Seizures may occur with an acute infective or inflammatory illness, such as bacterial meningitis or herpes encephalitis, or in patients with more longstanding or chronic disorders such as neurosyphilis or cerebral cysticercosis. In patients with AIDS, they may result from central nervous system toxoplasmosis, cryptococcal meningitis, secondary viral encephalitis, or other infective complications. Seizures are a common sequela of supratentorial brain abscess, developing most frequently in the first year after treatment.

Classification of Seizures

Seizures can be categorized in various ways, but the descriptive classification proposed by the International League Against Epilepsy is clinically the most useful. Seizures are divided into those that are generalized and those affecting only part of the brain (partial seizures).

A. Partial Seizures: The initial clinical and electroencephalographic manifestations of partial seizures indicate that only a restricted part of one cerebral hemisphere has been activated. The ictal manifestations depend upon the area of the brain involved. Partial seizures are subdivided into simple seizures, in which consciousness is preserved, and complex seizures, in which it is impaired. Partial seizures of either type sometimes become secondarily generalized, leading to a tonic, clonic, or tonic-clonic attack.

1. Simple partial seizures–Simple seizures may be manifested by focal motor symptoms (convulsive jerking) or somatosensory symptoms (eg, paresthesias or tingling) that spread (or "march") to different parts of the limb or body depending upon their cortical representation. In other instances, special sensory symptoms (eg, light flashes or buzzing) indicate involvement of visual, auditory, olfactory, or gustatory regions of the brain, or there may be autonomic symptoms or signs (eg, abnormal epigastric sensations, sweating, flushing, pupillary dilation). When psychic symptoms occur, they are usually accompanied by impairment of consciousness, but the sole manifestations of some seizures are phenomena such as dysphasia, dysmnesic symptoms (eg, déjà vu, jamais vu), affective disturbances, illusions, or structured hallucinations.

2. Complex partial seizures–Impaired consciousness may be preceded, accompanied, or followed by the psychic symptoms mentioned above, and automatisms may occur. Such seizures may also begin with some of the other simple symptoms mentioned above.

B. Generalized Seizures: There are several different varieties of generalized seizures, as outlined below. In some circumstances, seizures cannot be classified because of incomplete information or because they do not fit into any category.

1. Absence (petit mal) seizures–These are characterized by impairment of consciousness, sometimes with mild clonic, tonic, or atonic components (ie, reduction or loss of postural tone), autonomic components (eg, enuresis), or accompanying automatisms. Onset and termination of attacks are abrupt. If attacks occur during conversation, the patient may miss a few words or may break off in mid sentence for a few seconds. The impairment of external awareness is so brief that the patient is unaware of it. Absence seizures almost always begin in childhood and frequently cease by the age of 20 years, although occasionally they are then replaced by other forms of generalized seizure. Electroencephalographically, such attacks are associated with bursts of bilaterally synchronous and symmetric 3-Hz spike-and-wave activity. A normal background in the electroencephalogram and normal or above-normal intelligence imply a good prognosis for the ultimate cessation of these seizures.

2. Atypical absences–There may be more marked changes in tone, or attacks may have a more gradual onset and termination than in typical absences.

3. Myoclonic seizures–Myoclonic seizures consist of single or multiple myoclonic jerks.

4. Tonic-clonic (grand mal) seizures–In these seizures, which are characterized by sudden loss of consciousness, the patient becomes rigid and falls to the ground, and respiration is arrested. This tonic phase, which usually lasts for less than a minute, is followed by a clonic phase in which there is jerking of the body musculature that may last for 2 or 3 minutes and is then followed by a stage of flaccid coma. During the seizure, the tongue or lips may be bitten, urinary or fecal incontinence may occur, and the patient may be injured. Immediately after the seizure, the patient may either recover consciousness, drift into sleep, have a further convulsion without recovery of consciousness between the attacks (**status epilepticus**), or after recovering consciousness have a further convulsion (**serial seizures**). In other cases, patients will behave in an abnormal fashion in the immediate postictal period, without subsequent awareness or memory of events (**postepileptic automatism**). Headache, disorientation, confusion, drowsiness, nausea, soreness of the muscles, or some combination of these symptoms commonly occurs postictally.

5. Tonic, clonic, or atonic seizures–Loss of consciousness may occur with either the tonic or clonic accompaniments described above, especially in children. Atonic seizures (**epileptic drop attacks**) have also been described.

Clinical Findings

A. Symptoms and Signs: Nonspecific changes such as headache, mood alterations, lethargy, and myoclonic jerking alert some patients to an impending seizure hours before it occurs. These prodromal symptoms are distinct from the aura which may precede a generalized seizure by a few seconds or minutes and which is itself a part of the attack, arising locally from a restricted region of the brain.

In most patients, seizures occur unpredictably at any time and without any relationship to posture or ongoing activities. Occasionally, however, they occur at a particular time (eg, during sleep) or in relation to external precipitants such as lack of sleep, missed meals, emotional stress, menstruation, alcohol ingestion (or alcohol withdrawal; see below), or use of certain drugs. Fever and nonspecific infections may also precipitate seizures in known epileptics; in infants and young children, it may be hard to distinguish such attacks from febrile seizures. In a few patients, seizures are provoked by specific stimuli such as flashing lights or a flickering television set (**photosensitive epilepsy**), music, or reading.

Clinical examination between seizures shows no abnormality in patients with idiopathic epilepsy, but in the immediate postictal period, extensor plantar responses may be seen. The presence of lateralized or focal signs postictally suggests that seizures may have a focal origin. In patients with symptomatic epilepsy, the findings on examination will reflect the underlying cause.

B. Imaging: CT or MRI scan is indicated for patients with focal neurologic symptoms or signs, focal seizures, or electroencephalographic findings of a focal disturbance; some physicians routinely order imaging studies for all patients with new-onset seizure disorders. Such studies should certainly be performed in patients with clinical evidence of a progressive disorder and in those presenting with seizures after the age of 30 years, because of the possibility of an underlying neoplasm. A chest radiograph should also be obtained in such patients, since the lungs are a common site for primary or secondary neoplasms.

C. Laboratory and Other Studies: In patients older than 10 years, initial investigations should always include a full blood count, blood glucose determination, liver and renal function tests, and serologic tests for syphilis. The hematologic and biochemical screening tests are important both in excluding various causes of seizures and in providing a baseline for subsequent monitoring of long-term effects of treatment.

Electroencephalography may support the clinical diagnosis of epilepsy (by demonstrating paroxysmal abnormalities containing spikes or sharp waves), may provide a guide to prognosis, and may help classify the seizure disorder. Classification of the disorder is important for determining the most appropriate anticonvulsant drug with which to start treatment. For example, absence (petit mal) and complex partial seizures may be difficult to distinguish clinically, but the electroencephalographic findings and treatment of choice differ in these two conditions. Finally, by localizing the epileptogenic source, the electroencephalographic findings are important in evaluating candidates for surgical treatment.

Differential Diagnosis

The distinction between the various disorders likely to be confused with generalized seizures is usu-

ally made on the basis of the history. The importance of obtaining an eyewitness account of the attacks cannot be overemphasized.

A. Differential Diagnosis of Partial Seizures:

1. Transient ischemic attacks–These attacks are distinguished from seizures by their longer duration, lack of spread, and symptomatology. There is a loss of motor or sensory function (eg, weakness or numbness) with transient ischemic attacks, whereas positive symptomatology (eg, convulsive jerking or paresthesias) characterizes seizures.

2. Rage attacks–Rage attacks are usually situational and lead to goal-directed aggressive behavior.

3. Panic attacks–These may be hard to distinguish from simple or complex partial seizures unless there is evidence of psychopathologic disturbances between attacks and the attacks have a clear relationship to external circumstances.

B. Differential Diagnosis of Generalized Seizures:

1. Syncope–Syncopal episodes usually occur in relation to postural change, emotional stress, instrumentation, pain, or straining. They are typically preceded by pallor. sweating, nausea, and malaise and lead to loss of consciousness accompanied by flaccidity; recovery occurs rapidly with recumbency, and there is no postictal headache or confusion. Serum creatine kinase measured about 3 hours after the event is generally normal after syncopal episodes but markedly elevated after tonic-clonic seizures.

2. Cardiac dysrhythmias–Cerebral hypoperfusion due to a disturbance of cardiac rhythm should be suspected in patients with known cardiac or vascular disease or in elderly patients who present with episodic loss of consciousness. Prodromal symptoms are typically absent. A relationship of attacks to physical activity and the finding of a systolic murmur is suggestive of aortic stenosis. Repeated Holter monitoring may be necessary to establish the diagnosis; monitoring initiated by the patient ("event monitor") may be valuable if the disturbances of consciousness are rare.

3. Brain stem ischemia–Loss of consciousness is preceded or accompanied by other brain stem signs. Basilar artery migraine and vertebrobasilar vascular disease are discussed elsewhere in this chapter.

4. Pseudoseizures–The term pseudoseizures is used to denote both hysterical conversion reactions and attacks due to malingering when these simulate epileptic seizures. Many patients with pseudoseizures also have true seizures or a family history of epilepsy. Although pseudoseizures tend to occur at times of emotional stress, this may also be the case with true seizures.

Clinically, the attacks superficially resemble tonic-clonic seizures, but there may be obvious preparation before pseudoseizures occur. Moreover, there is usually no tonic phase; instead, there is an asynchronous thrashing of the limbs, which increases if restraints are imposed and which rarely leads to injury. Consciousness may be normal or "lost," but in the latter context the occurrence of goal-directed behavior or of shouting, swearing, etc, indicates that it is feigned. Postictally, there are no changes in behavior or neurologic findings.

Laboratory studies may aid in recognition of pseudoseizures. There are no electrocerebral changes, whereas the electroencephalogram changes during organic seizures accompanied by loss of consciousness. The serum level of prolactin has been found to increase dramatically between 15 and 30 minutes after a tonic-clonic convulsion in most patients, whereas it is unchanged after a pseudoseizure.

Treatment

A. General Measures: For patients with recurrent seizures, drug treatment is prescribed with the goal of preventing further attacks and is usually continued until there have been no seizures for at least 4 years. Epileptic patients should be advised to avoid situations that could be dangerous or life-threatening if further seizures should occur. State legislation may require physicians to report to the state department of motor vehicles any patients with seizures or other episodic disturbances of consciousness.

1. Choice of medication—The drug with which treatment is best initiated depends upon the type of seizures to be treated (Table 23–2). The dose of the selected drug is gradually increased until seizures are controlled, blood levels reach the upper limit of the optimal therapeutic range, or side effects prevent further increases. If seizures continue despite treatment at the maximal tolerated dose, a second drug is added and the dose increased until its blood levels are in the therapeutic range; the first drug is then gradually withdrawn. In treatment of partial and secondarily generalized tonic-clonic seizures, the success rate is higher with carbamazepine, phenytoin, or valproic acid than with phenobarbital or primidone. In most patients with seizures of a single type, satisfactory control can be achieved with a single anticonvulsant drug. Treatment with two drugs may further reduce seizure frequency or severity, but usually only at the cost of greater toxicity. Treatment with more than two drugs is almost always unhelpful unless the patient is having seizures of different types.

2. Monitoring—Monitoring plasma drug levels has led to major advances in the management of seizure disorders. The same daily dose of a particular drug leads to markedly different blood concentrations in different patients, and this will affect the therapeutic response. Steady-state drug levels in the blood should therefore be measured after treatment is initiated, dosage is changed, or another drug is added to the therapeutic regimen and when seizures are poorly controlled. Dose adjustments are then guided by the laboratory findings. The most common cause of a lower concentration of drug than expected for the prescribed dose is poor patient compliance. Compliance can be improved by limiting to a minimum the number of daily doses. Recurrent seizures or status epilepticus may result if drugs are taken erratically, and in some circumstances noncompliant patients may be better off without any medication.

All anticonvulsant drugs have side effects, and some of these are shown in Table 23–2. A complete blood count should be performed at least annually in all patients, because of the risk of anemia or blood dyscrasia. Treatment with certain drugs may require more frequent monitoring or use of additional screening tests. For example, periodic tests of hepatic function are necessary if valproic acid or carbamazepine is used, and serial blood counts are important with carbamazepine or ethosuximide.

3. Discontinuance of medication—Only when patients have been seizure-free for several (at least 4) years should withdrawal of medication be considered. Unfortunately, there is no way of predicting which patients can be managed successfully without treatment, although seizure recurrence is more likely in patients who initially failed to respond to therapy, those with seizures having focal features or of multiple types, and those with continuing electroencephalographic abnormalities. Dose reduction should be gradual over a period of weeks or months, and drugs should be withdrawn one at a time. If seizures recur, treatment is reinstituted with the same drugs used previously. Seizures are no more difficult to control after a recurrence than before.

B. Special Circumstances:

1. Solitary seizures—In patients who have had only one seizure, investigation should exclude an underlying cause requiring specific treatment. Prophylactic anticonvulsant drug treatment is generally not required unless further attacks occur or investigations reveal some underlying pathology that itself is untreatable. The risk of seizure recurrence varies in different series between about 30% and 70%. Epilepsy should not be diagnosed on the basis of a solitary seizure. If seizures occur in the context of a transient, nonrecurrent systemic disorders such as acute cerebral anoxia, the diagnosis of epilepsy is inaccurate, and long-term prophylactic anticonvulsant drug treatment is unnecessary.

2. Alcohol withdrawal seizures—One or more generalized tonic-clonic seizures may occur within 48 hours or so of withdrawal from alcohol after a period of high or chronic intake. If the seizures have consistently focal features, the possibility of an associated structural abnormality, often traumatic in origin, must be considered. Treatment with anticonvulsant drugs is generally not required for alcohol withdrawal seizures, since they are self-limited. Status epilepticus may rarely follow alcohol withdrawal and is managed along conventional lines (see below).

Further attacks will not occur if the patient abstains from alcohol.

3. Tonic-clonic status epilepticus—Poor compliance with the anticonvulsant drug regimen is the most common cause of tonic-clonic status epilepticus. Other causes include alcohol withdrawal, intracranial infection or neoplasms, metabolic disorders, and drug overdose. The mortality rate may be as high as 20%, and among survivors the incidence of neurologic and mental sequelae may be high. The prognosis relates to the length of time between onset of status epilepticus and the start of effective treatment.

Status epilepticus is a medical emergency. Initial management includes maintenance of the airway and 50% dextrose (25–50 mL) intravenously in case hypoglycemia is responsible. If seizures continue, 10 mg of diazepam is given intravenously over the course of 2 minutes, and the dose is repeated after 10 minutes if necessary. This is usually effective in halting seizures for a brief period but occasionally causes respiratory depression. Regardless of the response to diazepam, phenytoin (18–20 mg/kg) is given intravenously at a rate of 50 mg/min; this provides initiation of long-term seizure control. The drug is best injected directly but can also be given in saline; it precipitates, however, if injected into glucose-containing solutions. Because arrhythmias may develop during rapid administration of phenytoin, electrocardiographic monitoring is prudent. Hypotension may complicate phenytoin administration, especially if diazepam has also been given.

If seizures continue, phenobarbital is then given in a loading dose of 10–20 mg/kg intravenously by slow or intermittent injection. Respiratory depression and hypotension are common complications and should be anticipated; they may occur also with diazepam alone, though less commonly. If these measures fail, general anesthesia with ventilatory assistance and neuromuscular junction blockade may be required.

Other benzodiazepines than diazepam have been used in the immediate management of status epilepticus. Lorazepam given intravenously is effective but has no particular advantage over diazepam.

After status epilepticus is controlled, an oral drug program for the long-term management of seizures is started, and investigations into the cause of the disorder are pursued.

4. Nonconvulsive status epilepticus—Absence (petit mal) and complex partial status epilepticus are characterized by fluctuating abnormal mental status, confusion, impaired responsiveness, and automatism. Electroencephalography is helpful both in establishing the diagnosis and in distinguishing the two varieties. Initial treatment with intravenous diazepam is usually helpful regardless of the type of status epilepticus, but phenytoin, phenobarbital, carbamazepine, and other drugs may also be needed to obtain and maintain control in complex partial status epilepticus.

Bleck TP: Convulsive disorders: The use of anticonvulsant drugs. Clin Neuropharmacol 1990;13:198.

Lowenstein DH, Aminoff MJ, Simon RP: Barbiturate anesthesia in the treatment of status epilepticus: Clinical experience with 14 patients. Neurology 1988;38:395. (When standard pharmacologic maneuvers fail.)

Mattson RH et al: A comparison of valproate with carbamazepine for the treatment of complex partial seizures and secondarily generalized tonic-clonic seizures in adults. N Engl J Med 1992;327:765. (Comparative study showing valproic acid and carbamazepine equally effective for generalized tonic-clonic seizures, but valproic acid less effective and having greater side effects when given for complex partial seizures.)

Scheuer ML, Pedley TA: The evaluation and treatment of seizures. N Engl J Med 1990;323:1468.

Smith MC, Bleck TP: Convulsive disorders: Toxicity of anticonvulsants. Clin Neuropharmacol 1991;14:97.

NEUROLOGIC CAUSES OF SYNCOPE

The term syncope refers to transient loss of consciousness resulting from pancerebral hypoperfusion. The clinical features and certain general causes of syncope are discussed in detail in Chapter 10, and only the neurologic causes are considered here.

Syncope may occur because of orthostatic (postural) hypotension, which occurs in a variety of neurologic contexts when the baroreceptor reflex arc is interrupted. Spinal cord transection and other myelopathies (eg, due to tumor or syringomyelia) above the T6 level may lead to marked postural hypotension, as also do brain stem lesions such as syringobulbia and posterior fossa tumors. Postural hypotension is occasionally found in neurosyphilis (tabes dorsalis) and is a frequent and conspicuous complication of diabetic neuropathy. Other polyneuropathies associated with orthostatic hypotension include Guillain-Barré syndrome, primary amyloidosis, acute porphyric neuropathy, and that associated with carcinoma. An acute or subacute autonomic neuropathy may also develop on an autoimmune basis.

Primary degenerative disorders of the central nervous system may lead to dysautonomia occurring in isolation (primary autonomic failure) or in association with more widespread neurologic abnormalities (multisystem atrophy) that may include parkinsonian, pyramidal, lower motor neuron, and cerebellar deficits.

Manolis AS et al: Syncope: Current diagnostic evaluation and management. Ann Intern Med 1990;112:850.

SENSORY DISTURBANCES

Patients may complain of either lost or abnormal sensations. The term "numbness" is often used by patients to denote loss of feeling, but the word also has other meanings and the patient's intention must be clarified. Abnormal spontaneous sensations are generally called paresthesias, and unpleasant or painful sensations produced by a stimulus that is usually painless are called dysesthesias.

Sensory symptoms may be due to disease located anywhere along the peripheral or central sensory pathways. The character, site, mode of onset, spread, and temporal profile of sensory symptoms must be established and any precipitating or relieving factors identified. These features—and the presence of any associated symptoms—help identify the origin of sensory disturbances, as do the physical signs as well. Sensory symptoms or signs may conform to the territory of individual peripheral nerves or nerve roots. Involvement of one side of the body—or of one limb in its entirety—suggests a central lesion. Distal involvement of all four extremities suggests polyneuropathy, a cervical cord or brain stem lesion, or—when symptoms are transient—a metabolic disturbance such as hyperventilation syndrome. Short-lived sensory complaints may be indicative of sensory seizures or cerebral ischemic phenomena as well as metabolic disturbances. In patients with cord lesions, there may be a transverse sensory level. "Dissociated sensory loss" is characterized by loss of some sensory modalities with preservation of others. Such findings may be encountered in patients with either peripheral or central disease and must therefore be interpreted in the clinical context in which they are found.

The absence of sensory signs in patients with sensory symptoms does not mean that symptoms have a nonorganic basis. Symptoms are often troublesome before signs of sensory dysfunction have had time to develop.

WEAKNESS & PARALYSIS

Loss of muscle power may result from central disease involving the upper or lower motor neurons; from peripheral disease involving the roots, plexus, or peripheral nerves; from disorders of neuromuscular transmission; or from primary disorders of muscle. The clinical findings help to localize the lesion and thus reduce the number of diagnostic possibilities.

Weakness due to upper motor neuron lesions is characterized by selective involvement of certain muscle groups and is associated with spasticity, increased tendon reflexes, and extensor plantar responses. The site of upper motor neuron (pyramidal) involvement may be indicated by the presence of other clinical signs or by the distribution of the motor deficit. Lower motor neuron lesions lead to muscle wasting as well as weakness, with flaccidity and loss of tendon reflexes, but no change in the plantar responses unless the neurons subserving them are directly involved. Fasciculations may be evident over affected muscles. In distinguishing between a root, plexus, or peripheral nerve lesion, the distribution of the motor deficit and of any sensory changes is of particular importance. In patients with disturbances of neuromuscular transmission, weakness is patchy in distribution, often fluctuates over short periods of time, and is not associated with sensory changes. In myopathic disorders, weakness is usually most marked proximally in the limbs, is not associated with sensory loss or sphincter disturbance, and is not accompanied by muscle wasting or loss of tendon reflexes—at least not until an advanced stage.

TRANSIENT ISCHEMIC ATTACKS

Essentials of Diagnosis

- Risk factors for vascular disease often present.
- Focal neurologic deficit of acute onset.
- Clinical deficit resolves completely within 24 hours.

General Considerations

Transient ischemic attacks are characterized by focal ischemic cerebral neurologic deficits that last for less than 24 hours (usually less than 1–2 hours). About 30% of patients with stroke have a history of transient ischemic attacks, and proper treatment of the attacks is an important means of prevention. The incidence of stroke does not relate to either the number or the duration of individual attacks but is increased in patients with hypertension or diabetes.

Etiology

An important cause of transient cerebral ischemia is embolization. In many patients with these attacks, a source is readily apparent in the heart or a major extracranial artery to the head, and emboli sometimes are visible in the retinal arteries. Moreover, an embolic phenomenon explains why separate attacks may affect different parts of the territory supplied by the same major vessel. Cardiac causes of embolic ischemic attacks include rheumatic heart disease, mitral valve disease, cardiac arrhythmia, infective endocarditis, atrial myxoma, and mural thrombi complicating myocardial infarction. Atrial septal defects and patent foramen ovale may permit emboli from the veins to reach the brain ("paradoxical emboli"). An ulcerated plaque on a major artery to the brain may serve as a source of emboli. In the anterior circulation, atherosclerotic changes occur most commonly in the region of the carotid bifurcation extracranially, and these changes may cause a bruit. In some patients with transient ischemic attacks or strokes, an acute or recent hemorrhage is found to have occurred into this atherosclerotic plaque, and this finding may have pathologic significance. Patients with AIDS have an increased risk of developing transient ischemic deficits or strokes.

Other (less common) abnormalities of blood vessels that may cause transient ischemic attacks include fibromuscular dysplasia, which affects particularly the cervical internal carotid artery; inflammatory arterial disorders such as giant cell arteritis, systemic lupus erythematosus, polyarteritis, and granulomatous angiitis; and meningovascular syphilis. Hypotension may cause a reduction of cerebral blood flow if a major extracranial artery to the brain is markedly stenosed, but this is a rare cause of transient ischemic attack.

Hematologic causes of ischemic attacks include polycythemia, sickle cell disease, and hyperviscosity syndromes. Severe anemia may also lead to transient focal neurologic deficits in patients with preexisting cerebral arterial disease.

The **subclavian steal syndrome** may lead to transient vertebrobasilar ischemia. Symptoms develop when there is localized stenosis or occlusion of one subclavian artery proximal to the source of the vertebral artery, so that blood is "stolen" from this artery. A bruit in the supraclavicular fossa, unequal radial pulses, and a difference of 20 mm Hg or more between the systolic blood pressures in the arms should suggest the diagnosis in patients with vertebrobasilar transient ischemic attacks.

Clinical Findings

A. Symptoms and Signs: The symptoms of transient ischemic attacks vary markedly among patients; however, the symptoms in a given individual tend to be constant in type. Onset is abrupt and without warning, and recovery usually occurs rapidly, often within a few minutes.

If the ischemia is in the carotid territory, common symptoms are weakness and heaviness of the contralateral arm, leg, or face, singly or in any combination. Numbness or paresthesias may also occur either as the sole manifestation of the attack or in combination with the motor deficit. There may be slowness of movement, dysphasia, or monocular visual loss in the eye contralateral to affected limbs. During an attack, examination may reveal flaccid weakness with pyramidal distribution, sensory changes, hyperreflexia or an extensor plantar response on the affected side, dysphasia, or any combination of these findings. Subsequently, examination reveals no neurologic abnormality, but the presence of a carotid bruit or cardiac abnormality may provide a clue to the cause of symptoms.

Vertebrobasilar ischemic attacks may be characterized by vertigo, ataxia, diplopia, dysarthria, dimness or blurring of vision, perioral numbness and paresthesias, and weakness or sensory complaints on one, both, or alternating sides of the body. These symptoms may occur singly or in any combination. Drop attacks due to bilateral leg weakness, without headache or loss of consciousness, may occur, sometimes in relation to head movements.

The natural history of attacks is variable. Some patients will have a major stroke after only a few attacks, whereas others may have frequent attacks for weeks or months without having a stroke. Attacks may occur intermittently over a long period of time, or they may stop spontaneously. In general, carotid ischemic attacks are more liable than vertebrobasilar ischemic attacks to be followed by stroke.

B. Imaging: CT scan of the head will exclude the possibility of a small cerebral hemorrhage or a cerebral tumor masquerading as a transient ischemic attack. A number of noninvasive techniques, such as ultrasonography, have been developed for studying the cerebral circulation and imaging the major vessels to the head. Carotid duplex ultrasonography is useful for detecting significant stenosis of the internal carotid artery, but arteriography remains important for demonstrating the status of the cerebrovascular system. Accordingly, if findings on CT scan are normal, if there is no cardiac source of embolization, and if age and general condition indicate that the patient is a good operative risk, bilateral carotid arteriography should be considered in the further evaluation of carotid ischemic attacks, although the ultrasound findings may help in selecting patients for study.

C. Laboratory and Other Studies: Clinical and laboratory evaluation must include assessment for hypertension, heart disease, diabetes mellitus, hyperlipidemia, and peripheral vascular disease. It should include complete blood count, fasting blood glucose and serum cholesterol determinations, serologic tests for syphilis, and an ECG and chest x-ray. Echocardiography with bubble contrast is performed if a cardiac source is likely, and blood cultures are obtained if endocarditis is suspected. Holter monitoring is indicated if a transient, paroxysmal disturbance of cardiac rhythm is suspected.

Differential Diagnosis

Focal seizures usually cause abnormal motor or sensory phenomena such as clonic limb movements, paresthesias, or tingling, rather than weakness or loss of feeling. Symptoms generally spread ("march") up the limb and may lead to a generalized tonic-clonic seizure. The electroencephalogram may help in detecting the epileptogenic source.

Classic migraine is easily recognized by the visual premonitory symptoms, followed by nausea, headache, and photophobia, but less typical cases may be hard to distinguish. The patient's age and medical history (including family history) may be helpful in this regard. Patients with migraine commonly have a history of episodes since adolescence and report that other family members have a similar disorder.

Focal neurologic deficits may occur during periods of hypoglycemia in diabetic patients receiving insulin or oral hypoglycemic agent therapy, and the lack of general hypoglycemic symptoms does not exclude this possibility.

Treatment

When arteriography reveals a surgically accessible high-grade stenosis (70–99% in luminal diameter) on the side appropriate to carotid ischemic attacks and there is relatively little atherosclerosis elsewhere in the cerebrovascular system, operative treatment (carotid thromboendarterectomy) reduces the risk of ipsilateral carotid stroke, especially when transient ischemic attacks are of recent onset (< 2 months). When more extensive atherosclerotic disease is angiographically evident in the cerebral circulation, the benefits of surgery are less clear.

In patients with carotid ischemic attacks who are poor operative candidates (and thus have not undergone arteriography) or who are found to have extensive vascular disease, medical treatment should be instituted. Similarly, patients with vertebrobasilar ischemic attacks are treated medically and are not subjected to arteriography unless there is clinical evidence of stenosis or occlusion in the carotid or subclavian arteries.

Medical treatment is aimed at preventing further attacks and stroke. Cigarette smoking should be stopped, and cardiac sources of embolization, hypertension, diabetes, hyperlipidemia, arteritis, or hematologic disorders should be treated appropriately. If anticoagulants are indicated for the treatment of embolism from the heart, they should be started immediately, provided there is no contraindication to their use. There is no advantage in delay, and the common fear of causing hemorrhage into a previously infarcted area is misplaced, since there is a far greater risk of further embolism to the cerebral circulation if treatment is withheld. Treatment is initiated with intravenous heparin (in a loading dose of 5000–10,000 units, and maintenance infusion of 1000–2000 units per hour depending on the partial thromboplastin time) while warfarin sodium is introduced in a daily dose of 5–15 mg orally, depending on prothrombin time. Alternatively, aspirin (325 mg daily) may be used in patients with nonrheumatic atrial fibrillation to reduce the risk of stroke.

In patients with presumed or angiographically verified atherosclerotic changes in the extracranial or intracranial cerebrovascular circulation, antithrombotic medication is prescribed. The treatment selected will depend upon the patient's age, the likelihood of compliance in taking the drug, and the ready availability of medical and laboratory services. Some physicians use anticoagulant drugs (eg, warfarin, with temporary heparinization until the dose of warfarin is adequate) unless they are medically contraindicated, continuing them for 3–6 months before they are tapered and ulti-

mately replaced with aspirin, which is continued for another year. However, there is no convincing evidence that anticoagulant drugs are of value. Other physicians therefore prefer aspirin from the onset.

The evidence supporting a therapeutic role for aspirin to suppress platelet aggregation is convincing. Platelets adhere to and aggregate around an atherosclerotic plaque and release various substances including thromboxane A_2. One study found that treatment with aspirin significantly reduces the frequency of transient ischemic attacks and the incidence of stroke or myocardial infarcts in high-risk patients. A daily dose of 325 mg is adequate; higher doses may provide added benefit but are associated with a higher incidence of gastrointestinal side effects. Dipyridamole is not as effective, and when added to aspirin does not offer any advantage over aspirin alone for stroke prevention. In patients intolerant of aspirin, ticlopidine (another platelet aggregation inhibitor) may be used in a dose of 250 mg twice daily, but patients must be monitored closely for the development of neutropenia or agranulocytosis.

In recent years, many patients with transient ischemic attacks associated with stenotic lesions of the distal internal carotid or the proximal middle cerebral arteries have undergone surgical extracranial-intracranial arterial anastomosis. However, no benefit of surgical treatment could be demonstrated in a large controlled prospective study.

Cairns JA, Connolly SJ: Nonrheumatic atrial fibrillation: Risk of stroke and role of antithrombotic therapy. Circulation 1991;84:469.

Engstrom JW, Lowenstein DH, Bredesen DE: Cerebral infarctions and transient neurologic deficits associated with acquired immunodeficiency syndrome. Am J Med 1989;86:528.

European Carotid Surgery Trialists' Collaborative Group: MRC European carotid surgery trial. Lancet 1991; 337:1235. (Endarterectomy trial for symptomatic stenosis.)

NASCET Investigators: Clinical alert: Benefit of carotid endarterectomy for patients with high-grade stenosis of the internal carotid artery. Stroke 1991;22:816.

Sandercock P: Recent developments in the diagnosis and management of patients with transient ischaemic attacks and minor ischaemic strokes. Q J Med 1991;78:101.

Scheinberg P: Transient ischemic attacks: An update. J Neurol Sci 1991;101:133. (Pathogenesis, prognosis, and management.)

STROKE

Essentials of Diagnosis

- Sudden onset of characteristic neurologic deficit.
- Patient often has history of hypertension, diabetes mellitus, valvular heart disease, or atherosclerosis.
- Distinctive neurologic signs reflect the region of the brain involved.

General Considerations

In the USA, stroke remains the third leading cause of death, despite a general decline in the incidence of stroke in the last 30 years. The precise reasons for this decline are uncertain, but increased awareness of risk factors (hypertension, diabetes, hyperlipidemia, cigarette smoking, cardiac disease, AIDS, recreational drug abuse, heavy alcohol consumption, family history of stroke) and improved prophylactic measures and surveillance of those at increased risk have been contributory. A previous stroke makes individual patients more susceptible to further strokes.

For years, strokes have been subdivided pathologically into infarcts (thrombotic or embolic) and hemorrhages, and clinical criteria for distinguishing between these possibilities have been emphasized. However, it is often difficult to determine on clinical grounds the pathologic basis for stroke.

1. LACUNAR INFARCTION

Lacunar infarcts are among the most common cerebral vascular lesions. They are small infarcts (usually <5 mm in diameter) that occur in the distribution of short penetrating arterioles in the basal ganglia, pons, cerebellum, anterior limb of the internal capsule, and, less commonly, the deep cerebral white matter. Lacunar infarcts may be associated with poorly controlled hypertension or diabetes and have been found in conjunction with several clinical syndromes, including contralateral pure motor or pure sensory deficit, ipsilateral ataxia with crural paresis, and dysarthria with clumsiness of the hand. The neurologic deficit may progress over 24–36 hours before stabilizing.

Lacunar infarcts are sometimes visible on CT scans as small, punched-out, hypodense areas, but in other patients no abnormality is seen. In some instances, patients with a clinical syndrome suggestive of lacunar infarction are found on CT scanning to have a severe hemispheric infarct.

The prognosis for recovery from the deficit produced by a lacunar infarct is usually good, with partial or complete resolution occurring over the following 4–6 weeks in many instances.

2. CEREBRAL INFARCTION

Thrombotic or embolic occlusion of a major vessel leads to cerebral infarction. Causes include the disorders predisposing to transient ischemic attacks (see above) and atherosclerosis of cerebral arteries. The resulting deficit depends upon the particular vessel involved and the extent of any collateral circulation. Cerebral ischemia leads to release of excitatory and other neuropeptides that may augment calcium flux into neurons, thereby leading to cell death and increasing the neurologic deficit.

Clinical Findings

A. Symptoms and Signs: Onset is usually abrupt, and there may then be very little progression except that due to brain swelling. Clinical evaluation always includes examination of the heart and auscultation over the subclavian and carotid vessels to determine whether there are any bruits.

1. Obstruction of carotid circulation—Occlusion of the ophthalmic artery is probably symptomless in most cases because of the rich orbital collaterals, but its transient embolic obstruction leads to amaurosis fugax—sudden and brief loss of vision in one eye.

Occlusion of the anterior cerebral artery distal to its junction with the anterior communicating artery causes weakness and cortical sensory loss in the contralateral leg and sometimes mild weakness of the arm, especially proximally. There may be a contralateral grasp reflex, paratonic rigidity, and abulia (lack of initiative) or frank confusion. Urinary incontinence is not uncommon, particularly if behavioral disturbances are conspicuous. Bilateral anterior cerebral infarction is especially likely to cause marked behavioral changes and memory disturbances. Unilateral anterior cerebral artery occlusion proximal to the junction with the anterior communicating artery is generally well tolerated because of the collateral supply from the other side.

Middle cerebral artery occlusion leads to contralateral hemiplegia, hemisensory loss, and homonymous hemianopia (ie, bilaterally symmetric loss of vision in half of the visual fields), with the eyes deviated to the side of the lesion. If the dominant hemisphere is involved, global aphasia is also present. It may be impossible to distinguish this clinically from occlusion of the internal carotid artery. With occlusion of either of these arteries, there may also be considerable swelling of the hemisphere, leading to drowsiness, stupor, and coma in extreme cases. Occlusions of different branches of the middle cerebral artery cause more limited findings. For example, involvement of the anterior main division leads to a predominantly expressive dysphasia and to contralateral paralysis and loss of sensations in the arm, the face, and to a lesser extent, the leg. Posterior branch occlusion produces a receptive (Wernicke's) aphasia and a homonymous visual field defect. With involvement of the nondominant hemisphere, speech and comprehension are preserved, but there may be a confusional state, dressing apraxia, and constructional and spatial deficits.

2. Obstruction of vertebrobasilar circulation—Occlusion of the posterior cerebral artery may lead to a thalamic syndrome in which contralateral hemisensory disturbance occurs, followed by the development of spontaneous pain and hyperpathia.

There is often a macular-sparing homonymous hemianopia and sometimes a mild, usually temporary, hemiparesis. Depending on the site of the lesion and the collateral circulation, the severity of these deficits varies and other deficits may also occur, including involuntary movements and alexia. Occlusion of the main artery beyond the origin of its penetrating branches may lead solely to a macular-sparing hemianopia.

Vertebral artery occlusion distally, below the origin of the anterior spinal and posterior inferior cerebellar arteries, may be clinically silent because the circulation is maintained by the other vertebral artery. If the remaining vertebral artery is congenitally small or severely atherosclerotic, however, a deficit similar to that of basilar artery occlusion is seen unless there is good collateral circulation from the anterior circulation through the circle of Willis. When the small paramedian arteries arising from the vertebral artery are occluded, contralateral hemiplegia and sensory deficit occur in association with an ipsilateral cranial nerve palsy at the level of the lesion. An obstruction of the posterior inferior cerebellar artery or an obstruction of the vertebral artery just before it branches to this vessel leads ipsilaterally to spinothalamic sensory loss involving the face, ninth and tenth cranial nerve lesions, limb ataxia and numbness, and Horner's syndrome, combined with contralateral spinothalamic sensory loss involving the limbs.

Occlusion of both vertebral arteries or the basilar artery leads to coma with pinpoint pupils, flaccid quadriplegia and sensory loss, and variable cranial nerve abnormalities. With partial basilar artery occlusion, there may be diplopia, visual loss, vertigo, dysarthria, ataxia, weakness or sensory disturbances in some or all of the limbs, and discrete cranial nerve palsies. In patients with hemiplegia of pontine origin, the eyes are often deviated to the paralyzed side, whereas in patients with a hemispheric lesion, the eyes commonly deviate from the hemiplegic side.

Occlusion of any of the major cerebellar arteries produces vertigo, nausea, vomiting, nystagmus, ipsilateral limb ataxia, and contralateral spinothalamic sensory loss in the limbs. If the superior cerebellar artery is involved, the contralateral spinothalamic loss also involves the face; with occlusion of the anterior inferior cerebellar artery, there is ipsilateral spinothalamic sensory loss involving the face, usually in conjunction with ipsilateral facial weakness and deafness. Massive cerebellar infarction may lead to coma, tonsillar herniation, and death.

3. Coma–Infarction in either the carotid or vertebrobasilar territory may lead to loss of consciousness. For example, an infarct involving one cerebral hemisphere may lead to such swelling that the function of the other hemisphere or the rostral brain stem is disturbed and coma results. Similarly, coma occurs with bilateral brain stem infarction when this in-volves the reticular formation, and it occurs with brain stem compression after cerebellar infarction.

B. Imaging: Radiography of the chest may reveal cardiomegaly or valvular calcification; the presence of a neoplasm would suggest that the neurologic deficit is due to metastasis rather than stroke. A CT scan of the head (without contrast) is important in excluding cerebral hemorrhage, but it may not permit distinction between a cerebral infarct and tumor. CT scanning is preferable to MRI in the acute stage because it is quicker and because intracranial hemorrhage is not easily detected by MRI within the first 48 hours after a bleeding episode.

C. Laboratory and Other Studies: Investigations should include a complete blood count, sedimentation rate, blood glucose determination, and serologic tests for syphilis. Antiphospholipid antibodies (lupus anticoagulants and anticardiolipin antibodies) promote thrombosis and are associated with an increased incidence of stroke. Similarly, elevated serum cholesterol and lipids may indicate an increased risk of thrombotic stroke. Electrocardiography will help exclude a cardiac arrhythmia or recent myocardial infarction that might be serving as a source of embolization. Blood cultures should be performed if endocarditis is suspected, echocardiography if heart disease is suspected, and Holter monitoring if paroxysmal cardiac arrhythmia requires exclusion. Examination of the cerebrospinal fluid is not always necessary but may be helpful if there is diagnostic uncertainty; it should be delayed until after CT scanning.

Treatment

If the neurologic deficit progresses over the following minutes or hours, heparinization may be of value in limiting or arresting further deterioration. Since the signs of progressing stroke may be simulated by an intracerebral hematoma, the latter must be excluded by immediate CT scanning or angiography before the patient is heparinized.

Early management of a completed stroke consists of attention to general supportive measures. During the acute stage, there may be marked brain swelling and edema, with symptoms and signs of increasing intracranial pressure, an increasing neurologic deficit, or herniation syndrome. Corticosteroids have been prescribed in an attempt to reduce vasogenic cerebral edema. Prednisone (up to 100 mg/d) or dexamethasone (16 mg/d) has been used, but the evidence that corticosteroids are of any benefit is conflicting. Dehydrating hyperosmolar agents have also been prescribed in efforts to reduce brain swelling, but there is little evidence of any lasting benefit. Likewise, clinical benefit from treatment with vasodilators such as papaverine is minimal. Neither hypercapnia nor hypocapnia has been shown to have any benefit. Barbiturates are known to decrease neuronal metabolism and energy requirements and have been reported to improve functional recovery in experimental stroke models; their use in humans, however, is experimental. Attempts to lower the blood pressure of hypertensive patients during the acute phase of a stroke should be avoided, since there is loss of cerebral autoregulation and lowering the blood pressure may further compromise ischemic areas.

Anticoagulant drugs have no role in the management of patients with a completed stroke, except when there is a cardiac source of embolization. Treatment is then started with intravenous heparin while warfarin is introduced. If the CT scan shows no evidence of hemorrhage and the cerebrospinal fluid is clear, anticoagulant treatment may be started without delay. Some physicians, however, prefer to wait for 2 or 3 days (to reduce any risk of cerebral hemorrhage) before initiating anticoagulant treatment; the CT scan is then repeated and anticoagulant therapy is initiated if it again shows no evidence of hemorrhagic transformation.

Preliminary studies suggest that calcium channel blocking drugs such as nimodipine (30 mg orally every 6 hours for 4 weeks) may reduce the deficit produced by cerebral ischemia and the morbidity and mortality rates from stroke. Multicenter studies are now in progress to study further the effects of these agents in acute cerebral ischemia.

Blockage of glutamate, an excitatory neurotransmitter, reduces the sensitivity of central neurons to ischemia. The N-methyl-D-aspartate (NMDA) type of glutamate receptors are linked to calcium-permeable channels, and studies in animals have shown that specific NMDA-receptor antagonists reduce stroke size, deficits, and the percentage of severely ischemic neurons. The role of this therapeutic approach in humans is currently under study.

The role of tissue plasminogen activator as a means of providing thrombolytic therapy for acute stroke is also currently the subject of clinical trials.

Physical therapy has an important role in the management of patients with impaired motor function. Passive movements at an early stage will help prevent contractures. As cooperation increases and some recovery begins, active movements will improve strength and coordination. In all cases, early mobilization and active rehabilitation are important. Occupational therapy may improve morale and motor skills, while speech therapy may be beneficial in patients with expressive dysphasia or dysarthria. When there is a severe and persisting motor deficit, a device such as a leg brace, toe spring, frame, or cane may help the patient move about, and the provision of other aids to daily living may improve the quality of life.

Prognosis

The prognosis for survival after cerebral infarction is better than after cerebral or subarachnoid hemorrhage. Loss of consciousness after a cerebral infarct implies a poorer prognosis than otherwise. The extent of the infarct governs the potential for rehabilitation. Patients who have had a cerebral infarct are at risk for further strokes and for myocardial infarcts.

Bamford J et al: Classification and natural history of clinically identifiable subtypes of cerebral infarction. Lancet 1991;337:1521. (Site of infarction influences prognosis for recovery and risk of recurrence.)

Estol C, Caplan LR: Therapy of acute stroke. Clin Neuropharmacol 1990;13:91.

Levine SR et al: Cerebrovascular and neurologic disease associated with antiphospholipid antibodies: 48 cases. Neurology 1990;40:1181.

Rothrock JF, Hart RG: Antithrombotic therapy in cerebrovascular disease. Ann Intern Med 1991;115:885.

Scheinberg P: The biologic basis for the treatment of acute stroke. Neurology 1991;41:1867. (Experimental approaches to treatment.)

3. INTRACEREBRAL HEMORRHAGE

Spontaneous intracerebral hemorrhage in patients with no angiographic evidence of an associated vascular anomaly (eg, aneurysm or angioma) is usually due to hypertension. The pathologic basis for hemorrhage is probably the presence of microaneurysms that are now known to develop on perforating vessels of 100–300 μm in diameter in hypertensive patients. Hypertensive intracerebral hemorrhage occurs most frequently in the basal ganglia and less commonly in the pons, thalamus, cerebellum, and cerebral white matter. Hemorrhage may extend into the ventricular system or subarachnoid space, and signs of meningeal irritation are then found. Hemorrhages usually occur suddenly and without warning, often during activity.

In addition to its association with hypertension, nontraumatic intracerebral hemorrhage may occur with hematologic and bleeding disorders (eg, leukemia, thrombocytopenia, hemophilia, or disseminated intravascular coagulation), anticoagulant therapy, liver disease, cerebral amyloid angiopathy, and primary or secondary brain tumors. Bleeding is primarily into the subarachnoid space when it occurs from an intracranial aneurysm or arteriovenous malformation (see below), but it may be partly intraparenchymal as well. In some cases, no specific cause for cerebral hemorrhage can be identified.

Clinical Findings

A. Symptoms and Signs: With hemorrhage into the cerebral hemisphere, consciousness is initially lost or impaired in about one-half of patients. Vomiting occurs very frequently at the onset of bleeding, and headache is sometimes present. Focal symptoms and signs then develop, depending on the site of the hemorrhage. With hypertensive hemorrhage, there is generally a rapidly evolving neurologic deficit with hemiplegia or hemiparesis. A hemisensory disturbance is also present with more deeply placed lesions. With lesions of the putamen, loss of conjugate lateral gaze may be conspicuous. With thalamic hemorrhage, there may be a loss of upward gaze, downward or skew deviation of the eyes, lateral gaze palsies, and pupillary inequalities.

Cerebellar hemorrhage may present with sudden onset of nausea and vomiting, disequilibrium, headache, and loss of consciousness that may terminate fatally within 48 hours. Less commonly, the onset is gradual and the course episodic or slowly progressive—clinical features suggesting an expanding cerebellar lesion. In yet other cases, however, the onset and course are intermediate, and examination shows lateral conjugate gaze palsies to the side of the lesion; small reactive pupils; contralateral hemiplegia; peripheral facial weakness; ataxia of gait, limbs, or trunk; periodic respiration; or some combination of these findings.

B. Imaging: CT scanning (without contrast) is important not only in confirming that hemorrhage has occurred but also in determining the size and site of the hematoma. As indicated earlier, it is superior to MRI for detecting intracranial hemorrhage of less than 48 hours duration. If the patient's condition permits further intervention, cerebral angiography may be undertaken thereafter to determine if an aneurysm or arteriovenous malformation is present (see below).

C. Laboratory and Other Studies: A complete blood count, platelet count, bleeding time, prothrombin and partial thromboplastin times, and liver and renal function tests may reveal a predisposing cause for the hemorrhage. Lumbar puncture is contraindicated because it may precipitate a herniation syndrome in patients with a large hematoma, and CT scanning is superior in detecting intracerebral hemorrhage.

Treatment

Neurologic management is generally conservative and supportive, regardless of whether the patient has a profound deficit with associated brain stem compression, in which case the prognosis is grim, or a more localized deficit not causing increased intracranial pressure or brain stem involvement. Decompression is helpful, however, when a superficial hematoma in cerebral white matter is exerting a mass effect and causing incipient herniation. In patients with cerebellar hemorrhage, however, prompt surgical evacuation of the hematoma is appropriate, because spontaneous unpredictable deterioration may otherwise lead to a fatal outcome and because operative treatment may lead to complete resolution of the clinical deficit. The treatment of underlying structural lesions or bleeding disorders depends upon their nature.

4. SUBARACHNOID HEMORRHAGE

Between 5% and 10% of strokes are due to subarachnoid hemorrhage. Although hemorrhage is usually from rupture of an aneurysm or arteriovenous malformation, no specific cause can be found in 20% of cases.

Clinical Findings

A. Symptoms and Signs: Subarachnoid hemorrhage has a characteristic clinical picture. Its onset is with sudden headache of a severity never experienced previously by the patient. This may be followed by nausea and vomiting and by a loss or impairment of consciousness that can either be transient or progress inexorably to deepening coma and death. If consciousness is regained, the patient is often confused and irritable and may show other symptoms of an altered mental status. Neurologic examination generally reveals nuchal rigidity and other signs of meningeal irritation, except in deeply comatose patients. A focal neurologic deficit is occasionally present and may suggest the site of the underlying lesion.

B. Imaging: A CT scan should be performed immediately to confirm that hemorrhage has occurred and to search for clues regarding its source. It is preferable to MRI because it is faster and more sensitive in detecting hemorrhage in the first 24 hours. CT findings sometimes are normal in patients with suspected hemorrhage, and the cerebrospinal fluid must then be examined for the presence of blood or xanthochromia before the possibility of subarachnoid hemorrhage is discounted.

Cerebral arteriography may be undertaken to determine the source of bleeding; it is not performed unless or until the patient's condition has stabilized and is good enough so that operative treatment is feasible. In general, bilateral carotid and vertebral arteriography are necessary because aneurysms are often multiple, while arteriovenous malformations may be supplied from several sources.

Treatment

The medical management of patients is important. The measures outlined in the section on stupor and coma must be applied to comatose patients. Conscious patients are confined to bed, advised against any exertion or straining, treated symptomatically for headache and anxiety, and given laxatives or stool softeners to prevent straining. If there is severe hypertension, the blood pressure can be lowered gradually, but not below a diastolic level of 100 mm Hg. Phenytoin is generally prescribed routinely to prevent seizures. Further comment concerning the specific operative management of arteriovenous malformations and aneurysms follows.

5. INTRACRANIAL ANEURYSM

Saccular aneurysms ("berry" aneurysms) tend to occur at arterial bifurcations, are considerably more common in adults than in children, are frequently multiple (20% of cases), and are usually asymptomatic. They may be associated with polycystic kidney disease and coarctation of the aorta. Most aneurysms are located on the anterior part of the circle of Willis—particularly on the anterior or posterior communicating arteries, at the bifurcation of the middle cerebral artery, and at the bifurcation of the internal carotid artery.

Clinical Findings

A. Symptoms and Signs: Aneurysms may cause a focal neurologic deficit by compressing adjacent structures. However, most are asymptomatic or produce only nonspecific symptoms until they rupture, at which time subarachnoid hemorrhage results. There is often a paucity of focal neurologic signs in patients with subarachnoid hemorrhage, but when present, such signs may relate either to a focal hematoma or to ischemia in the territory of the vessel with the ruptured aneurysm. Hemiplegia or other focal deficit sometimes occurs after a delay of 4–14 days and is due to focal arterial spasm in the vicinity of the ruptured aneurysm. This spasm is of uncertain, probably multifactorial, cause, but it sometimes leads to significant cerebral ischemia or infarction, and it may further aggravate any existing increase in intracranial pressure. Subacute hydrocephalus due to interference with the flow of cerebrospinal fluid may occur after 2 or more weeks, and this leads to a delayed clinical deterioration that is relieved by shunting.

In some patients, "warning leaks" of a small amount of blood from the aneurysm precede the major hemorrhage by a few hours or days. They lead to headaches, sometimes accompanied by nausea and neck stiffness, but the true cause of these symptoms is often not appreciated until massive hemorrhage occurs.

B. Imaging: The CT scan generally confirms that subarachnoid hemorrhage has occurred, but occasionally it is normal. Angiography (bilateral carotid and vertebral studies) generally indicates the size and site of the lesion, sometimes reveals multiple aneurysms, and may show arterial spasm. If subarachnoid hemorrhage is confirmed by lumbar puncture or CT scanning but arteriograms show no abnormality, the examination should be repeated after 2 weeks, because vasospasm may have prevented detection of an aneurysm during the initial study.

C. Laboratory and Other Studies: The cerebrospinal fluid is bloodstained. The electroencephalogram sometimes indicates the side or site of hemorrhage but frequently shows only a diffuse abnormality. Electrocardiographic evidence of arrhythmias or myocardial ischemia has been well described

and probably relates to excessive sympathetic activity. Peripheral leukocytosis and transient glycosuria are also common findings.

Treatment

The major aim of treatment is to prevent further hemorrhages. Definitive treatment requires a surgical approach to the aneurysm and ideally consists of clipping of its base. If surgery is not feasible, medical management as outlined above for subarachnoid hemorrhage is continued for about 6 weeks and is followed by gradual mobilization.

The risk of further hemorrhage is greatest within a few days of the first hemorrhage; approximately 20% of patients will have further bleeding within 2 weeks and 40% within 6 months. Attempts have been made to reduce this risk pharmacologically. Since antifibrinolytic drugs prevent lysis of any blood clot that has formed near the site of rupture, aminocaproic acid (Amicar) is sometimes given for the first 2 weeks or so, or until surgery, to reduce the incidence of early recurrence of bleeding. The daily dose is 24–36 g (5 g initially, followed by 1–1.25 g hourly) given intravenously for the first week and then orally, while the streptokinase clot lysis time is monitored. Potential complications include venous thrombosis, pulmonary embolism, and ischemic focal neurologic deficits. Recent studies indicate that this approach may indeed lower the incidence of recurrent bleeding but that it is associated with such an increase in cerebral ischemic complications that the mortality rate and the degree of disability among survivors are unchanged. Thus, early operation (ie, within about 2 days of hemorrhage) is preferred for good operative candidates.

Calcium channel-blocking agents have helped to reduce or reverse experimental vasospasm, and nimodipine has been shown to reduce, in neurologically normal patients, the incidence of ischemic deficits from arterial spasm without producing any side effects. The dose of nimodipine is 60 mg every 4 hours for 21 days.

With regard to unruptured aneurysms, those that are symptomatic merit prompt surgical treatment, whereas small asymptomatic ones discovered incidentally are often followed arteriographically and corrected surgically only if they increase in size to over 5 mm. The natural history of unruptured aneurysms is not clearly defined.

Disney L, Weir B, Petruk K: Effect on management mortality of a deliberate policy of early operation on supratentorial aneurysms. Neurosurgery 1987;20:695.

Haley EC et al: The International Cooperative Study on the timing of aneurysmal surgery. Stroke 1992;23:205. (Surgery within 3 days after hemorrhage has the best outcome.)

Pickard JD et al: Effect of oral nimodipine on cerebral infarction and outcome following subarachnoid haemorrhage. Br Med J 1989;298:636.

6. ARTERIOVENOUS MALFORMATIONS

Arteriovenous malformations are congenital vascular malformations that result from a localized maldevelopment of part of the primitive vascular plexus and consist of abnormal arteriovenous communications without intervening capillaries. They vary in size, ranging from massive lesions that are fed by multiple vessels and involve a large part of the brain to lesions so small that they are hard to identify at arteriography, surgery, or autopsy. In approximately 10% of cases, there is an associated arterial aneurysm, while 1–2% of patients presenting with aneurysms have associated arteriovenous malformations. Clinical presentation may relate to hemorrhage from the malformation or an associated aneurysm or may relate to cerebral ischemia due to diversion of blood by the anomalous arteriovenous shunt or due to venous stagnation. Regional maldevelopment of the brain, compression or distortion of adjacent cerebral tissue by enlarged anomalous vessels, and progressive gliosis due to mechanical and ischemic factors may also be contributory. In addition, communicating or obstructive hydrocephalus may occur and lead to symptoms.

Clinical Findings
A. Symptoms and Signs:
1. Supratentorial lesions—Most cerebral arteriovenous malformations are supratentorial, usually lying in the territory of the middle cerebral artery. Initial symptoms consist of hemorrhage in 30–60% of cases, epilepsy in 20–40%, headache in 5–25%, and miscellaneous complaints (including focal deficits) in 10–15%. Up to 70% of arteriovenous malformations bleed at some point in their natural history, most commonly before the patient reaches the age of 40 years. This tendency to bleed is unrelated to the lesion site or to the patient's sex, but small arteriovenous malformations are more likely to bleed than large ones. Arteriovenous malformations that have bled once are more likely to bleed again. Hemorrhage is commonly intracerebral as well as into the subarachnoid space, and it has a fatal outcome in about 10% of cases. Focal or generalized seizures may accompany or follow hemorrhage, or they may be the initial presentation, especially with frontal or parietal arteriovenous malformations. Headaches are especially likely when the external carotid arteries are involved in the malformation. These sometimes simulate migraine but more commonly are nonspecific in character, with nothing about them to suggest an underlying structural lesion.

In patients presenting with subarachnoid hemorrhage, examination may reveal an abnormal mental status and signs of meningeal irritation. Additional findings may help to localize the lesion and sometimes indicate that intracranial pressure is increased. A cranial bruit always suggests the possibility of a cerebral arteriovenous malformation, but bruits may also be found with aneurysms, meningiomas, acquired arteriovenous fistulas, and arteriovenous malformations involving the scalp, calvarium, or orbit. Bruits are best heard over the ipsilateral eye or mastoid region and are of some help in lateralization but of no help in localization. Absence of a bruit in no way excludes the possibility of arteriovenous malformation.

2. Infratentorial lesions—Brain stem arteriovenous malformations are often clinically silent, but they may hemorrhage, cause obstructive hydrocephalus, or lead to progressive or relapsing brain stem deficits. Cerebellar arteriovenous malformations may also be clinically inconspicuous but sometimes lead to cerebellar hemorrhage.

B. Imaging: In patients presenting with suspected hemorrhage, CT scanning indicates whether subarachnoid or intracerebral bleeding has recently occurred, helps to localize its source, and may reveal the arteriovenous malformation. If the CT scan shows no evidence of bleeding but subarachnoid hemorrhage is diagnosed clinically, the cerebrospinal fluid should be examined.

When intracranial hemorrhage is confirmed but the source of hemorrhage is not evident on the CT scan, arteriography is necessary to exclude aneurysm or arteriovenous malformation. Even if the findings on CT scan suggest arteriovenous malformation, arteriography is required to establish the nature of the lesion with certainty and to determine its anatomic features so that treatment can be planned. The examination must generally include bilateral opacification of the internal and external carotid arteries and the vertebral arteries. Arteriovenous malformations typically appear as a tangled vascular mass with distended tortuous afferent and efferent vessels, a rapid circulation time, and arteriovenous shunting. Findings on plain radiographs of the skull are often normal unless an intracerebral hematoma is present, in which case there may be changes suggestive of raised intracranial pressure and displacement of a calcified pineal gland.

In patients presenting without hemorrhage, CT scan or MRI usually reveals the underlying abnormality, and MRI frequently also shows evidence of old or recent hemorrhage that may have been asymptomatic. The nature and detailed anatomy of any focal lesion identified by these means is delineated by angiography, especially if operative treatment is under consideration.

C. Laboratory and Other Studies: Electroencephalography is usually indicated in patients presenting with seizures and may show consistently focal or lateralized abnormalities resulting from the underlying cerebral arteriovenous malformation. This should be followed by CT scanning.

Treatment

Surgical treatment to prevent further hemorrhage is justified in patients with arteriovenous malformations that have bled, provided that the lesion is accessible and the patient has a reasonable life expectancy. Surgical treatment is also appropriate if intracranial pressure is increased or if there is cardiac decompensation, as occurs in children, and to prevent further progression of a focal neurologic deficit. In patients presenting solely with seizures, anticonvulsant drug treatment is usually sufficient, and operative treatment is unnecessary unless there are further developments.

Definitive operative treatment consists of excision of the arteriovenous malformation if it is surgically accessible. Arteriovenous malformations that are inoperable because of their location are sometimes treated solely by embolization; although the risk of hemorrhage is not reduced, neurologic deficits may be stabilized or even reversed by this procedure. Two other new techniques for the treatment of intracerebral arteriovenous malformations are injection of a vascular occlusive polymer through a flow-guided microcatheter and permanent occlusion of feeding vessels by positioning detachable balloon catheters in the desired sites and then inflating them with quickly solidifying contrast material. Proton beam therapy may also be useful in the management of inoperable cerebral arteriovenous malformations.

Aminoff MJ: Treatment of unruptured cerebral arteriovenous malformations. Neurology 1987;37:815. (Surgery is not necessary for unruptured malformations.)
Heros RC et al: Surgical excision of cerebral arteriovenous malformations: Late results. Neurosurgery 1990;26:570.
Steinberg GK et al: Stereotactic heavy-charged-particle Bragg-peak radiation for intracranial arteriovenous malformations. N Engl J Med 1990;323:96
Vinuela F et al: *Interventional Neuroradiology: Endovascular Therapy of the Central Nervous System.* Raven Press, 1992.

7. INTRACRANIAL VENOUS THROMBOSIS

Intracranial venous thrombosis may occur in association with intracranial or maxillofacial infections, hypercoagulable states, polycythemia, sickle cell disease, and cyanotic congenital heart disease and in pregnancy or during the puerperium. It is characterized by headache, focal or generalized convulsions, drowsiness, confusion, increased intracranial pressure, and focal neurologic deficits—and sometimes by evidence of meningeal irritation. The diagnosis is confirmed by CT scanning and MRI, MR venography, or angiography.

Treatment includes anticonvulsant drugs if sei-

zures have occurred and antiedema agents (eg, dexamethasone, 4 mg four times daily) to reduce intracranial pressure. Anticoagulation with dose-adjusted intravenous heparin reduces morbidity and mortality of venous sinus thrombosis.

Einhaupl KM et al: Heparin treatment in sinus venous thrombosis. Lancet 1991;338:597.

8. SPINAL CORD VASCULAR DISEASES

Infarction of the Spinal Cord

Infarction of the spinal cord is rare. It occurs only in the territory of the anterior spinal artery because this vessel, which supplies the anterior two-thirds of the cord, is itself supplied by only a limited number of feeders. Infarction usually results from interrupted flow in one or more of these feeders, eg, with aortic dissection, aortography, polyarteritis, or severe hypotension, or after surgical resection of the thoracic aorta. The paired posterior spinal arteries, by contrast, are supplied by numerous arteries at different levels of the cord.

Since the anterior spinal artery receives numerous feeders in the cervical region, infarcts almost always occur more caudally. Clinical presentation is characterized by acute onset of flaccid, areflexive paraplegia that evolves after a few days or weeks into a spastic paraplegia with extensor plantar responses. There is an accompanying dissociated sensory loss, with impairment of appreciation of pain and temperature but preservation of sensations of vibration and position. Treatment is symptomatic.

Epidural or Subdural Hemorrhage

Epidural or subdural hemorrhage may lead to sudden severe back pain followed by an acute compressive myelopathy necessitating urgent myelography and surgical evacuation. It may occur in patients with bleeding disorders or those who are taking anticoagulant drugs, sometimes following trauma or lumbar puncture. Epidural hemorrhage may also be related to a vascular malformation or tumor deposit.

Arteriovenous Malformation of the Spinal Cord

Arteriovenous malformations of the cord are congenital lesions that present with spinal subarachnoid hemorrhage or myeloradiculopathy. Since most of these malformations are located in the thoracolumbar region, they lead to motor and sensory disturbances in the legs and to sphincter disorders. Pain in the legs or back is often severe. Examination reveals an upper, lower, or mixed motor deficit in the legs; sensory deficits are also present and are usually extensive, although occasionally they are confined to radicular distribution. Cervical arteriovenous malformations lead also to symptoms and signs in the arms. Spinal MRI may not detect the arteriovenous malformation, and negative findings do not exclude the diagnosis. In general, the diagnosis is suggested at myelography (performed with the patient prone and supine) when serpiginous filling defects due to enlarged vessels are found. Selective spinal arteriography confirms the diagnosis. Most lesions are extramedullary, are posterior to the cord (lying either intra- or extradurally), and can easily be treated by ligation of feeding vessels and excision of the fistulous anomaly or by embolization procedures. Delay in treatment may lead to increased and irreversible disability or to death from recurrent subarachnoid hemorrhage.

INTRACRANIAL & SPINAL SPACE-OCCUPYING LESIONS

1. PRIMARY INTRACRANIAL TUMORS

Essentials of Diagnosis
- Generalized or focal disturbance of cerebral function, or both.
- Increased intracranial pressure in some patients.
- Neuroradiologic evidence of space-occupying lesion.

General Considerations
Approximately half of all primary intracranial neoplasms (Table 23–3) are gliomas, and the remainder are meningiomas, pituitary adenomas, neurofibromas, and other tumors. Certain tumors, especially neurofibromas, hemangioblastomas, and retinoblastomas, may have a familial basis, and congenital factors bear on the development of craniopharyngiomas. Tumors may occur at any age, but certain gliomas show particular age predilections (Table 23–3).

Clinical Findings
A. Symptoms and Signs: Intracranial tumors may lead to a generalized disturbance of cerebral function and to symptoms and signs of increased intracranial pressure. In consequence, there may be personality changes, intellectual decline, emotional lability, seizures, headaches, nausea, and malaise. If the pressure is increased in a particular cranial compartment, brain tissue may herniate into a compartment with lower pressure. The most familiar syndrome is herniation of the temporal lobe uncus through the tentorial hiatus, which causes compression of the third cranial nerve, midbrain, and posterior cerebral artery. The earliest sign of this is ipsilateral pupillary dilation, followed by stupor, coma, decerebrate posturing, and respiratory arrest.

Another important herniation syndrome consists of displacement of the cerebellar tonsils through the foramen magnum, which causes medullary compression leading to apnea, circulatory collapse, and death. Other herniation syndromes are less common and of less clear clinical importance.

Intracranial tumors also lead to focal deficits depending on their location.

1. Frontal lobe lesions–Tumors of the frontal lobe often lead to progressive intellectual decline, slowing of mental activity, personality changes, and contralateral grasp reflexes. They may lead to expressive aphasia if the posterior part of the left inferior frontal gyrus is involved. Anosmia may also occur as a consequence of pressure on the olfactory nerve. Precentral lesions may cause focal motor seizures or contralateral pyramidal deficits.

2. Temporal lobe lesions–These lesions may produce a variety of disturbances. Tumors of the uncinate region may be manifested by seizures with olfactory or gustatory hallucinations, motor phenomena such as licking or smacking of the lips, and some impairment of external awareness without actual loss of consciousness. Temporal lobe lesions also lead to depersonalization, emotional changes, behavioral disturbances, sensations of déjà vu or jamais vu, micropsia or macropsia, visual field defects (crossed upper quadrantanopia), and auditory illusions or hallucinations. Left-sided lesions may lead to dysnomia and receptive aphasia, while right-sided involvement sometimes disturbs the perception of musical notes and melodies.

3. Parietal lobe lesions–Tumors in this location characteristically cause contralateral disturbances of sensation and may cause sensory seizures, sensory loss or inattention, or some combination of these symptoms. The sensory loss is cortical in type and involves postural sensibility and tactile discrimination, so that the appreciation of shape, size, weight, and texture is impaired. Objects placed in the hand may not be recognized (astereognosis). Extensive parietal lobe lesions may produce contralateral hyperpathia and spontaneous pain (thalamic syndrome). Involvement of the optic radiation leads to a contralateral homonymous field defect that sometimes consists solely of lower quadrantanopia. Lesions of the left angular gyrus cause Gerstmann's syndrome (a combination of alexia, agraphia, acalculia, right-left confusion, and finger agnosia), whereas involvement of the left submarginal gyrus causes ideational apraxia. Anosognosia (the denial, neglect, or rejection of a paralyzed limb) is seen in patients with lesions of the nondominant (right) hemisphere. Constructional apraxia and dressing apraxia may also occur with right-sided lesions.

4. Occipital lobe lesions–Tumors of the occipital lobe characteristically produce crossed homonymous hemianopia or a partial field defect. With left-sided or bilateral lesions, there may be visual ag-

Table 23–3. Primary intracranial tumors.

Tumor	Clinical Features	Treatment and Prognosis
Glioblastoma multiforme	Presents commonly with nonspecific complaints and increased intracranial pressure. As it grows, focal deficits develop	Course is rapidly progressive, with poor prognosis. Total surgical removal is usually not possible, and response to radiation therapy is poor.
Astrocytoma	Presentation similar to glioblastoma multiforme but course more protracted, often over several years. Cerebellar astrocytoma, especially in children, may have a more benign course.	Prognosis is variable. By the time of diagnosis, total excision is usually impossible; tumor often is not radiosensitive. In cerebellar astrocytoma, total surgical removal is often possible.
Medulloblastoma	Seen most frequently in children. Generally arises from roof of fourth ventricle and leads to increased intracranial pressure accompanied by brain stem and cerebellar signs. May seed in subarachnoid space.	Treatment consists of surgery combined with radiation therapy and chemotherapy.
Ependymoma	Glioma arising from the ependyma of a ventricle, especially the fourth ventricle; leads early to signs of increased intracranial pressure. Arises also from central canal of cord.	Tumor is not radiosensitive and is best treated surgically if possible.
Oligodendroglioma	Slow-growing. Usually arises in cerebral hemisphere in adults. Calcification may be visible on skull x-ray.	Treatment is surgical, which is usually successful.
Brain stem glioma	Presents during childhood with cranial nerve palsies and then with long-tract signs in the limbs. Signs of increased intracranial pressure occur late.	Tumor is inoperable; treatment is by irradiation and shunt for increased intracranial pressure.
Cerebellar hemangioblastoma	Presents with disequilibrium, ataxia of trunk or limbs, and signs of increased intracranial pressure. Sometimes familial. May be associated with retinal and spinal vascular lesions, polycythemia, and hypernephromas.	Treatment is surgical.
Pineal tumor	Presents with increased intracranial pressure, sometimes associated with impaired upward gaze (Parinaud's syndrome) and other deficits indicative of midbrain lesion.	Ventricular decompression by shunting is followed by surgical approach to tumor; irradiation is indicated if tumor is malignant. Prognosis depends on histopathologic findings and extent of tumor.
Craniopharyngioma	Originates from remnants of Rathke's pouch above the sella, depressing the optic chiasm. May present at any age but usually in childhood, with endocrine dysfunction and bitemporal field defects.	Treatment is surgical, but total removal may not be possible.
Acoustic neurinoma	Ipsilateral hearing loss is most common initial symptom. Subsequent symptoms may include tinnitus, headache, vertigo, facial weakness or numbness, and long-tract signs. (May be familial and bilateral when related to neurofibromatosis.) Most sensitive screening tests are MRI and brain stem auditory evoked potential.	Treatment is excision by translabyrinthine surgery, craniectomy, or a combined approach. Outcome is usually good.
Meningioma	Originates from the dura mater or arachnoid; compresses rather than invades adjacent neural structures. Increasingly common with advancing age. Tumor size varies greatly. Symptoms vary with tumor site—eg, unilateral exophthalmos (sphenoidal ridge); anosmia and optic nerve compression (olfactory groove). Tumor is usually benign and readily detected by CT scanning; may lead to calcification and bone erosion visible on plain x-rays of skull.	Treatment is surgical. Tumor may recur if removal is incomplete.
Primary cerebral lymphoma	Associated with AIDS and other immunodeficient states. Presentation may be with focal deficits or with disturbances of cognition and consciousness. May be indistinguishable from cerebral toxoplasmosis.	Treatment is by whole-brain irradiation; chemotherapy may have an adjunctive role.

nosia both for objects and for colors, while irritative lesions on either side can cause unformed visual hallucinations. Bilateral occipital lobe involvement causes cortical blindness in which there is preservation of pupillary responses to light and lack of awareness of the defect by the patient. There may also be loss of color perception, prosopagnosia (inability to identify a familiar face), simultagnosia (inability to integrate and interpret a composite scene as opposed to its individual elements), and Balint's syndrome (failure to turn the eyes to a particular point in space, despite preservation of spontaneous and reflex eye movements). The denial of blindness or a field defect constitutes Anton's syndrome.

5. Brain stem and cerebellar lesions–Brain stem lesions lead to cranial nerve palsies, ataxia, incoordination, nystagmus, and pyramidal and sensory deficits in the limbs on one or both sides. Intrinsic brain stem tumors, such as gliomas, tend to produce an increase in intracranial pressure only late in their course. Cerebellar tumors produce marked ataxia of the trunk if the vermis cerebelli is involved and ipsilateral appendicular deficits (ataxia, incoordination and hypotonia of the limbs) if the cerebellar hemispheres are affected.

6. False localizing signs–Tumors may lead to neurologic signs other than by direct compression or infiltration, thereby leading to errors of clinical localization. These false localizing signs include third or sixth nerve palsy and bilateral extensor plantar responses produced by herniation syndromes, and an extensor plantar response occurring ipsilateral to a hemispheric tumor as a result of compression of the opposite cerebral peduncle against the tentorium.

B. Imaging: CT scanning or MRI may detect the lesion and may also define its location, shape, and size; the extent to which normal anatomy is distorted; and the degree of any associated cerebral edema or mass effect. CT scanning is less helpful with tumors in the posterior fossa, but MRI is of particular value there. The characteristic appearance of meningiomas on CT scanning is virtually diagnostic; ie, a lesion in a typical site (parasagittal and sylvian regions, olfactory groove, sphenoidal ridge, tuberculum sellae) that appears as a homogeneous area of increased density in noncontrast CT scans and enhances uniformly with contrast.

Arteriography may show stretching or displacement of normal cerebral vessels by the tumor and the presence of tumor vascularity. The presence of an avascular mass is a nonspecific finding that could be due to tumor, hematoma, abscess, or any space-occupying lesion. In patients with normal hormone levels and an intrasellar mass, angiography is necessary to distinguish with confidence between a pituitary adenoma and an arterial aneurysm.

C. Laboratory and Other Studies: The electroencephalogram provides supporting information concerning cerebral function and may show either a focal disturbance due to the neoplasm or a more diffuse change reflecting altered mental status. Lumbar puncture is rarely necessary; the findings are seldom diagnostic, and the procedure carries the risk of causing a herniation syndrome.

Treatment

Treatment depends on the type and site of the tumor (Table 23–3) and the condition of the patient. Complete surgical removal may be possible if the tumor is extra-axial (eg, meningioma, acoustic neuroma) or is not in a critical or inaccessible region of the brain (eg, cerebellar hemangioblastoma). Surgery also permits the diagnosis to be verified and may be beneficial in reducing intracranial pressure and relieving symptoms even if the neoplasm cannot be completely removed. Clinical deficits are sometimes due in part to obstructive hydrocephalus, in which case simple surgical shunting procedures often produce dramatic benefit. In patients with malignant gliomas, radiation therapy increases median survival rates regardless of any preceding surgery, and its combination with chemotherapy provides additional benefit. Indications for irradiation in the treatment of patients with other primary intracranial neoplasms depend upon tumor type and accessibility and the feasibility of complete surgical removal. Corticosteroids help reduce cerebral edema and are usually started before surgery. Herniation is treated with intravenous dexamethasone (10–20 mg as a bolus, followed by 4 mg every 6 hours) and intravenous mannitol (20% solution given in a dose of 1.5 g/kg over about 30 minutes). Anticonvulsants are also commonly administered in standard doses (Table 23–2).

Black P McL: Brain tumors. (Two parts.) N Engl J Med 1991;324:1471, 1555. (Epidemiology, pathogenesis, clinical features, and treatment.)

Rosenblum ML (editor): Role of surgery in brain tumor management. Neurosurg Clin North Am 1990;1:1. (Entire issue.)

2. METASTATIC INTRACRANIAL TUMORS

Cerebral Metastases

Metastatic brain tumors present in the same way as other cerebral neoplasms, ie, with increased intracranial pressure, with focal or diffuse disturbance of cerebral function, or with both of these manifestations. Indeed, in patients with a single cerebral lesion, the metastatic nature of the lesion may only become evident on histopathologic examination. In other patients, there is evidence of widespread metastatic disease, or an isolated cerebral metastasis develops during treatment of the primary neoplasm.

The most common source of intracranial metastasis is carcinoma of the lung; other primary sites are the breast, kidney, and gastrointestinal tract. Most cerebral metastases are located supratentorially. The laboratory and radiologic studies used to evaluate patients with metastases are similar to those described in the preceding section on primary neoplasms. They include MRI and CT scanning performed both with and without contrast material. Lumbar puncture is necessary only in patients with suspected carcinomatous meningitis (see below). In patients with verified cerebral metastasis from an unknown primary, investigation should be guided by symptoms and signs. In women, mammography is regularly indicated; in men, attention should be paid to a possible germ cell origin. Both have therapeutic implications.

In patients with only a single cerebral metastasis who are otherwise well, it may be possible to remove the lesion and then treat with irradiation. Alternatively, irradiation may be selected as the sole means of treatment. In patients with multiple metastases or widespread systemic disease, the long-term outlook is gloomy, and treatment by radiation therapy or chemotherapy is palliative.

Leptomeningeal Metastases (Carcinomatous Meningitis)

The neoplasms metastasizing most commonly to the leptomeninges are carcinoma of the breast, lymphomas, and leukemia. Leptomeningeal metastases lead to multifocal neurologic deficits, which may be associated with infiltration of cranial and spinal nerve roots, direct invasion of the brain or spinal cord, obstructive hydrocephalus, or some combination of these factors.

The diagnosis is confirmed by examination of the cerebrospinal fluid. Findings may include elevated cerebrospinal fluid pressure, pleocytosis, increased protein concentration, and decreased glucose concentration. Cytologic studies may indicate that malignant cells are present; if not, spinal tap should be repeated at least twice to obtain further samples for analysis.

CT scans showing contrast enhancement in the basal cisterns or showing hydrocephalus without any evidence of a mass lesion support the diagnosis. Gadolinium-enhanced MRI frequently shows enhancing foci in the leptomeninges. Myelography may show deposits on multiple nerve roots.

Treatment is by irradiation to symptomatic areas, combined with intrathecal methotrexate. The long-term prognosis is poor—only about 10% of patients survive for 1 year.

Rodesch G et al: Neuroradiologic findings in leptomeningeal carcinomatosis. Neuroradiology 1990;32:26. (Value of gadolinium-enhanced MRI for diagnosis.)

3. INTRACRANIAL MASS LESIONS IN AIDS PATIENTS

AIDS patients may present with **primary cerebral lymphoma.** This leads to disturbances in cognition or consciousness, focal motor or sensory deficits, aphasia, seizures, and cranial neuropathies. Similar clinical disturbances may result from **cerebral toxoplasmosis,** which is also a common complication in patients with AIDS. Neither CT nor MRI findings distinguish these two disorders, and serologic tests for toxoplasmosis are unreliable in AIDS patients. Accordingly, for neurologically stable patients, a trial of treatment with sulfadiazine (100 mg/kg/d up to 8 g/d in four divided doses) and pyrimethamine (75 mg/d for 3 days, then 25 mg/d) is recommended for 3 weeks; the imaging studies are then repeated, and if any lesion has improved, the antitoxoplasmosis regimen is continued indefinitely. If any lesion does not improve, cerebral biopsy is necessary. Primary cerebral lymphoma is treated with whole-brain irradiation.

Cryptococcal meningitis is also a commonly opportunistic infection in AIDS patients. Clinically, it may resemble cerebral toxoplasmosis or lymphoma, but cranial CT scans are usually normal. The diagnosis is made on the basis of cerebrospinal fluid studies, with positive India ink staining in 75–80% and cryptococcal antigen tests in 95% of cases. Treatment is with amphotericin B, sometimes accompanied by flucytosine, as set forth in Table 36–1.

4. PRIMARY & METASTATIC SPINAL TUMORS

Approximately 10% of spinal tumors are intramedullary. Ependymoma is the most common type of intramedullary tumor; the remainder are other types of glioma. Extramedullary tumors may be extradural or intradural in location. Among the primary extramedullary tumors, neurofibromas and meningiomas are relatively common, are benign, and may be intra- or extradural. Carcinomatous metastases, lymphomatous or leukemic deposits, and myeloma are usually extradural; in the case of metastases, the prostate, breast, lung, and kidney are common primary sites.

Tumors may lead to spinal cord dysfunction by direct compression, by ischemia secondary to arterial or venous obstruction, and, in the case of intramedullary lesions, by invasive infiltration.

Clinical Findings

A. Symptoms and Signs: Symptoms usually develop insidiously. Pain is often conspicuous with extradural lesions; is characteristically aggravated by coughing or straining; may be radicular, localized to the back, or felt diffusely in an extremity; and may be accompanied by motor deficits, paresthesias, or numbness, especially in the legs. When sphincter disturbances occur, they are usually particularly disabling. Pain, however, often precedes specific neurologic symptoms from epidural metastases.

Examination may reveal localized spinal tenderness. A segmental lower motor neuron deficit or dermatomal sensory changes (or both) are sometimes found at the level of the lesion, while an upper motor neuron deficit and sensory disturbance are found below it.

B. Imaging: Findings on plain radiography of the spine may be normal but are commonly abnormal when there are metastatic deposits. CT myelography or MRI may be necessary to identify and localize the site of cord compression. The combination of known tumor elsewhere in the body, back pain, and either abnormal plain films of the spine or neurologic signs of cord compression is an indication to perform these studies on an urgent basis. Some clinicians proceed to myelography based solely on new back pain in a cancer patient. If a complete block is present at lumbar myelography, a cisternal myelogram is performed to determine the upper level of the block and to investigate the possibility of block higher in the cord.

C. Laboratory Findings: The cerebrospinal fluid removed at myelography is often xanthochromic and contains a greatly increased protein concentration with normal cell content and glucose concentration.

Treatment

Intramedullary tumors are treated by decompression and surgical excision (when feasible) and by irradiation. The prognosis depends upon the cause and severity of cord compression before it is relieved.

Treatment of epidural spinal metastases consists of irradiation, irrespective of cell type. Dexamethasone is also given in a high dosage (eg, 25 mg four times daily for 3 days, followed by rapid tapering of the dosage, depending on response) to reduce cord swelling and relieve pain. Surgical decompression is reserved for patients with tumors that are unresponsive to irradiation or have previously been irradiated and for cases in which there is some uncertainty about the diagnosis. The long-term outlook is poor, but radiation treatment may at least delay the onset of major disability.

Sze G: Magnetic resonance imaging in the evaluation of spinal tumors. Cancer 1991;67:1229. (Role of CT scans and MRI.)

5. BRAIN ABSCESS

Infectious disorders are considered elsewhere in this book, but brief comment will be made here concerning cerebral abscess, which presents as an intracranial space-occupying lesion. Brain abscess may arise as a sequela of disease of the ear or nose, may be a metastatic complication of infection elsewhere in the body, or may result from infection introduced intracranially by trauma or surgical procedures. The most common infective organisms are streptococci, staphylococci, and anaerobes; mixed infections are not uncommon. Headache, drowsiness, inattention, confusion, and seizures are early symptoms, followed by signs of increasing intracranial pressure and then a focal neurologic deficit. There may be little or no evidence of systemic infection.

A CT scan of the head characteristically shows an area of contrast enhancement surrounding a low-density core. Similar abnormalities may, however, be found in patients with metastatic neoplasms. The MRI findings may also be abnormal and probably permit earlier recognition of focal cerebritis or an abscess. Arteriography indicates the presence of a space-occupying lesion, which appears as an avascular mass with displacement of normal cerebral vessels, but this procedure provides no clue to the nature of the lesion.

Treatment consists of intravenous antibiotics, combined with surgical drainage (aspiration or excision) if necessary to reduce the mass effect, or sometimes to establish the diagnosis. Abscesses smaller than 2 cm can often be cured medically. Broad-spectrum antibiotics are used if the infecting organism is unknown. In adults, a common regimen is penicillin G (2 million units every 2 hours intravenously) plus either chloramphenicol (1–2 g intravenously every 6 hours), metronidazole (750 mg intravenously every 6 hours), or both. Nafcillin is added if *Staphylococcus aureus* infection is suspected. Dexamethasone (4–25 mg four times daily, depending on severity, followed by tapering of dose, depending on response) may reduce any associated edema.

Tureen JH, Sande MA: Acute bacterial infections of the central nervous system. In: *Neurology and General Medicine.* Aminoff MJ (editor). Churchill Livingstone, 1989.

NONMETASTATIC NEUROLOGIC COMPLICATIONS OF MALIGNANT DISEASE

A variety of nonmetastatic neurologic complications of malignant disease can be recognized:

(1) Metabolic encephalopathy due to electrolyte abnormalities, infections, drug overdose, or the failure of some vital organ may be reflected by drowsiness, lethargy, restlessness, insomnia, agitation, confusion, stupor, or coma. The mental changes are usually associated with tremor, asterixis, and multifocal myoclonus. The electroencephalogram is generally diffusely slowed. Laboratory studies are necessary to detect the cause of the encephalopathy, which must then be treated appropriately.

(2) Immune suppression resulting from either the malignant disease or its treatment (eg, by chemotherapy) predisposes patients to brain abscess, progressive multifocal leukoencephalopathy, meningitis, herpes zoster infection, and other opportunistic infectious diseases. Moreover, an overt or occult cerebrospinal fluid fistula, as occurs with some tumors, may also increase the risk of infection. CT scanning aids in the early recognition of a brain abscess, but metastatic brain tumors may have a similar appearance. Examination of the cerebrospinal fluid is essential in the evaluation of patients with meningitis but is of no help in the diagnosis of brain abscess. Treatment should be specific for the infective organism.

(3) Cerebrovascular disorders that cause neurologic complications in patients with systemic cancer include nonbacterial thrombotic endocarditis and septic embolization. Cerebral, subarachnoid, or subdural hemorrhages may occur in patients with myelogenous leukemia and may be found in association with metastatic tumors, especially malignant melanoma. Spinal subdural hemorrhage sometimes occurs after lumbar puncture in patients with marked thrombocytopenia.

Disseminated intravascular coagulation occurs most commonly in patients with acute promyelocytic leukemia or with some adenocarcinomas and is characterized by a fluctuating encephalopathy, often with associated seizures, that frequently progresses to coma or death. There may be few accompanying neurologic signs.

Venous sinus thrombosis, which usually presents with convulsions and headaches, may also occur in patients with leukemia or lymphoma. Examination commonly reveals papilledema and focal or diffuse neurologic signs. Treatment is with anticonvulsants and drugs to lower the intracranial pressure. The role of anticoagulants is controversial.

(4) Paraneoplastic cerebellar degeneration occurs most commonly in association with carcinoma of the lung. Symptoms may precede those due to the neoplasm itself, which may be undetected for several months or even longer. Typically, there is a pancerebellar syndrome causing dysarthria, nystagmus, and ataxia of the trunk and limbs. The disorder probably has an autoimmune basis. Treatment is of the underlying malignant disease.

(5) Encephalopathy, characterized by impaired recent memory, disturbed affect, hallucinations, and seizures, occurs in some patients with carcinomas. The cerebrospinal fluid is often abnormal. EEGs may show diffuse slow-wave activity, especially over the temporal regions. Pathologic changes are most marked in the inferomedian portions of the temporal lobes. There is no specific treatment.

(6) Malignant disease may be associated with sensorimotor polyneuropathy and less commonly with pure sensory neuropathy (ie, dorsal root ganglionitis) or autonomic neuropathy. A subacute motor neuronopathy may be associated with lymphomas.

(7) Dermatomyositis or a myasthenic syndrome may be seen in patients with underlying carcinoma (see Chapter 19). The myasthenic syndrome has an autoimmune basis.

Posner JB: Paraneoplastic syndromes. Neurol Clin 1991; 9:919.

PSEUDOTUMOR CEREBRI
(Benign Intracranial Hypertension)

Symptoms of pseudotumor cerebri consist of headache, diplopia, and other visual disturbances due to papilledema and abducens nerve dysfunction. Examination reveals the papilledema and some enlargement of the blind spots, but patients otherwise look well. Investigations reveal no evidence of a space-occupying lesion, and the CT scan shows small or normal ventricles. Lumbar puncture confirms the presence of intracranial hypertension, but the cerebrospinal fluid is normal.

There are many causes of pseudotumor cerebri. Thrombosis of the transverse venous sinus as a noninfectious complication of otitis media or chronic mastoiditis is one cause, and sagittal sinus thrombosis may lead to a clinically similar picture. Other causes include chronic pulmonary disease, endocrine disturbances such as hypoparathyroidism or Addison's disease, vitamin A toxicity, and the use of tetracycline or oral contraceptives. Cases have also followed withdrawal of corticosteroids after long-term use. In many instances, however, no specific cause can be found, and the disorder remits spontaneously after several months.

Untreated pseudotumor cerebri leads to secondary optic atrophy and permanent visual loss. Repeated lumbar puncture to lower the intracranial pressure by removal of cerebrospinal fluid is effective, but pharmacologic approaches to treatment are now more satisfactory. Acetazolamide (250 mg orally three times daily) reduces formation of cerebrospinal fluid and can be used to start treatment. Oral corticosteroids (eg, prednisone, 60–80 mg daily) may also be necessary. Obese patients should be advised to lose weight. Treatment is monitored by checking visual acuity and visual fields, funduscopic appearance, and pressure of the cerebrospinal fluid.

If medical treatment fails to control the intracranial pressure, surgical placement of a lumboperitoneal or other shunt—or optic nerve sheath fenestration—should be undertaken to preserve vision.

In addition to the above measures, any specific cause of pseudotumor cerebri requires appropriate treatment. Thus, hormone therapy should be initiated if there is an underlying endocrine disturbance. Discontinuing the use of tetracycline, oral contraceptives, or vitamin A will allow for resolution of pseudotumor cerebri due to these agents. If corticosteroid withdrawal is responsible, the medication should be reintroduced and then tapered more gradually.

Giuseffi V et al: Symptoms and disease association in idiopathic intracranial hypotension. Neurology 1991;41:239.

Spoor TC et al: Treatment of pseudotumor cerebri by primary and secondary optic nerve sheath decompression. Am J Ophthalmol 1991;112:177.

SELECTED NEUROCUTANEOUS DISEASES

Tuberous Sclerosis

Tuberous sclerosis may occur sporadically or on a familial basis with autosomal dominant inheritance. Its pathogenesis is unknown. Neurologic presentation is with seizures and progressive psychomotor retardation beginning in early childhood. The cutaneous abnormality, adenoma sebaceum, becomes manifest usually between 5 and 10 years of age and typically consists of reddened nodules on the face (cheeks, nasolabial folds, sides of the nose, and chin) and sometimes on the forehead and neck. Other typical cutaneous lesions include subungual fibromas, shagreen patches (leathery plaques of subepidermal fibrosis, situated usually on the trunk), and leaf-shaped hypopigmented spots. Associated abnormalities include retinal lesions and tumors, benign rhabdomyomas of the heart, lung cysts, benign tumors in the viscera, and bone cysts.

The disease is slowly progressive and leads to increasing mental deterioration. There is no specific treatment, but anticonvulsant drugs may help in controlling seizures.

Neurofibromatosis

Neurofibromatosis may occur either sporadically or on a familial basis with autosomal dominant inheritance. Two distinct forms are recognized: Type 1 **(Recklinghausen's disease)** is characterized by multiple hyperpigmented macules and neurofibromas and type 2 by **eighth nerve tumors,** often accompanied by other intracranial or intraspinal tumors. Among familial cases, the gene for type 1 is located on chromosome 17 and that for type 2 on chromosome 22.

Neurologic presentation is usually with symptoms and signs of tumor. Multiple neurofibromas characteristically are present and may involve spinal or cranial nerves, especially the eighth nerve. Examination of the superficial cutaneous nerves usually reveals palpable mobile nodules. In some cases, there is an associated marked overgrowth of subcutaneous tissues (plexiform neuromas), sometimes with an underlying bony abnormality. Associated cutaneous lesions include axillary freckling and patches of cutaneous pigmentation (café au lait spots). Malignant degeneration of neurofibromas occasionally occurs and may lead to peripheral sarcomas. Meningiomas, gliomas (especially optic nerve gliomas), bone cysts, pheochromocytomas, scoliosis, and obstructive hydrocephalus may also occur.

It may be possible to correct disfigurement by plastic surgery. Intraspinal or intracranial tumors and tumors of peripheral nerves should be treated surgically if they are producing symptoms.

Mulvihill JJ et al: Neurofibromatosis 1 (Recklinghausen disease) and neurofibromatosis 2 (bilateral acoustic neurofibromatosis): An update. Ann Intern Med 1990; 113:39. (Clinical features, genetics, molecular biology, and management.)

Sturge-Weber Syndrome

Sturge-Weber syndrome consists of a congenital, usually unilateral, cutaneous capillary angioma involving the upper face, leptomeningeal angiomatosis, and, in many patients, choroidal angioma. It has no sex predilection and usually occurs sporadically. The cutaneous angioma sometimes has a more extensive distribution over the head and neck and is often quite disfiguring, especially if there is associated overgrowth of connective tissue. Focal or generalized seizures are the usual neurologic presentation and may commence at any age. There may be contralateral homonymous hemianopia, hemiparesis and hemisensory disturbance, ipsilateral glaucoma, and mental subnormality. Skull x-rays taken after the first 2 years of life usually reveal gyriform ("tramline") intracranial calcification, especially in the parieto-occipital region, due to mineral deposition in the cortex beneath the intracranial angioma.

Treatment is aimed at controlling seizures pharmacologically. Ophthalmologic advice should be sought concerning the management of choroidal angioma and of increased intraocular pressure.

MOVEMENT DISORDERS

1. BENIGN ESSENTIAL (FAMILIAL) TREMOR

The cause of benign essential tremor is uncertain, but it is sometimes inherited in an autosomal dominant manner. Tremor may begin at any age and is enhanced by emotional stress. The tremor usually involves one or both hands, the head, or the hands and head, while the legs tend to be spared. Examination reveals no other abnormalities. Ingestion of a small quantity of alcohol commonly provides remarkable but short-lived relief by an unknown mechanism.

Although the tremor may become more conspicuous with time, it generally leads to little disability, and treatment is often unnecessary. Occasionally, it interferes with manual skills and leads to impairment of handwriting. Speech may also be affected if the laryngeal muscles are involved. In such circumstances, propranolol may be helpful but will need to be continued indefinitely in daily doses of 60–240 mg. However, intermittent therapy is sometimes useful in patients whose tremor becomes exacerbated in specific predictable situations. It is not clear whether the response to propranolol depends on central or peripheral mechanisms. Primidone may be helpful when propranolol is ineffective, but patients with essential tremor are often very sensitive to it. They are therefore started on 50 mg daily, and the daily dose is increased by 50 mg every 2 weeks depending on the response; a maintenance dose of 125 mg three times daily is commonly effective.

2. PARKINSONISM

Essentials of Diagnosis

- Any combination of tremor, rigidity, bradykinesia, progressive postural instability.
- Seborrhea of skin quite common.
- Mild intellectual deterioration is often observed.

General Considerations

Parkinsonism is a relatively common disorder that occurs in all ethnic groups, with an approximately equal sex distribution. The most common variety, idiopathic Parkinson's disease (paralysis agitans), begins most often between 45 and 65 years of age.

Etiology

Postencephalitic parkinsonism is becoming increasingly rare. Exposure to certain toxins (eg, manganese dust, carbon disulfide) and severe carbon monoxide poisoning may lead to parkinsonism. Typical parkinsonism has occurred in individuals who have taken 1-methyl-4-phenyl-1,2,5,6-tetrahydropyridine (MPTP) for recreational purposes. This compound is converted in the body and selectively destroys dopaminergic neurons in the substantia nigra. Reversible parkinsonism may develop in patients receiving neuroleptic drugs (see Chapter 24) and has also been caused by reserpine and metoclopramide. Only rarely is hemiparkinsonism the presenting feature of a brain tumor or some other progressive space-occupying lesion.

In idiopathic parkinsonism, dopamine depletion due to degeneration of the dopaminergic nigrostriatal system leads to an imbalance of dopamine and acetylcholine, which are neurotransmitters normally present in the corpus striatum. Treatment is directed at redressing this imbalance by blocking the effect of acetylcholine with anticholinergic drugs or by the administration of levodopa, the precursor of dopamine.

Clinical Findings

Tremor, rigidity, bradykinesia, and postural instability are the cardinal features of parkinsonism and may be present in any combination. There may also be a mild decline in intellectual function. The tremor of about four to six cycles per second is most conspicuous at rest, is enhanced by emotional stress, and is often less severe during voluntary activity. Although it may ultimately be present in all limbs, the tremor is commonly confined to one limb or to the limbs on one side for months or years before it becomes more generalized. In some patients, tremor is absent.

Rigidity (an increase in resistance to passive movement) is responsible for the characteristically flexed posture seen in many patients, but the most disabling symptoms of parkinsonism are due to bradykinesia, manifested as a slowness of voluntary movement and a reduction in automatic movements such as swinging of the arms while walking. Curiously, however, effective voluntary activity may briefly be regained during an emergency (eg, the patient is able to leap aside to avoid an oncoming motor vehicle).

Clinical diagnosis of the well-developed syndrome is usually simple. The patient has a relatively immobile face with widened palpebral fissures, infrequent blinking, and a certain fixity of facial expression. Seborrhea of the scalp and face is common. There is often mild blepharoclonus, and a tremor may be present about the mouth and lips. Repetitive tapping (about twice per second) over the bridge of the nose produces a sustained blink response (Myerson's sign). Other findings may include saliva drooling from the mouth, perhaps due to impairment of swallowing; soft and poorly modulated voice; a variable rest tremor and rigidity in some or all of the limbs; slowness of voluntary movements; impairment of fine or rapidly alternating movements; and micrographia. There is typically no muscle weakness (provided that sufficient time is allowed for power to be developed) and no alteration in the tendon reflexes or plantar responses. It is difficult for the patient to arise from a sitting position and begin walking. The gait itself is characterized by small shuffling steps and a loss of the normal automatic arm swing; there may be unsteadiness on turning, difficulty in stopping, and a tendency to fall.

Differential Diagnosis

Diagnostic problems may occur in mild cases, especially if tremor is minimal or absent. For example, mild hypokinesia or slight tremor is commonly attributed to old age. Depression, with its associated expressionless face, poorly modulated voice, and reduction in voluntary activity, can be difficult to distinguish from mild parkinsonism, especially since the two disorders may coexist; in some cases, a trial of antidepressant drug therapy may be necessary. The family history, the character of the tremor, and lack of other neurologic signs should distinguish essential tremor from parkinsonism. Wilson's disease can be distinguished by its early age at onset, the presence of other abnormal movements, Kayser-Fleischer rings, and chronic hepatitis, and by increased concentrations of copper in the tissues. Huntington's disease presenting with rigidity and bradykinesia may be mistaken for parkinsonism unless the family history and accompanying dementia are recognized. In Shy-Drager syndrome, the clinical features of parkinsonism are accompanied by autonomic insufficiency (leading to postural hypotension, anhidrosis, disturbances of sphincter control, impotence, etc) and more widespread neurologic deficits (pyramidal, lower motor neuron, or cerebellar signs). In progressive supranuclear palsy, bradykinesia and rigidity are accompanied by a supranuclear disorder of eye movements, pseudobulbar palsy, and axial dystonia. Creutzfeldt-Jakob disease may be accompanied by features of parkinsonism, but dementia is usual, myoclonic jerking is common, ataxia and pyramidal signs may be conspicuous, and the electroencephalographic findings are usually characteristic. In patients with tremor, movement may produce an electrocardiographic artifact mimicking atrial flutter.

Treatment

A. Medical Measures: Drug treatment is not required early in the course of parkinsonism, but the nature of the disorder and the availability of medical treatment for use when necessary should be discussed with the patient.

1. Amantadine–Patients with mild symptoms but no disability may be helped by amantadine. This drug improves all of the clinical features of parkinsonism, but its mode of action is unclear. Side effects include restlessness, confusion, depression, skin rashes, edema, nausea, constipation, anorexia, postural hypotension, and disturbances of cardiac rhythm. However, these are relatively uncommon with the usual dose (100 mg twice daily).

2. Anticholinergic drugs–Anticholinergics are more helpful in alleviating tremor and rigidity than bradykinesia. Treatment is started with a small dose (Table 23–4) and gradually increased until benefit occurs or side effects limit further increments. If treatment is ineffective, the drug is gradually withdrawn and another preparation then tried.

Common side effects include dryness of the mouth, nausea, constipation, palpitations, cardiac arrhythmias, urinary retention, confusion, agitation, restlessness, drowsiness, mydriasis, increased intraocular pressure, and defective accommodation.

Anticholinergic drugs are contraindicated in patients with prostatic hypertrophy, narrow-angle glaucoma, or obstructive gastrointestinal disease and are often tolerated poorly by the elderly.

Table 23–4. Some anticholinergic antiparkinsonian drugs.[1]

Drug	Usual Daily Dose (mg)
Benztropine mesylate (Cogentin)	1–6
Biperiden (Akineton)	2–12
Chlorphenoxamine (Phenoxene)	150–400
Cycrimine (Pagitane)	5–20
Orphenadrine (Disipal, Norflex)	150–400
Procyclidine (Kemadrin)	7.5–30
Trihexyphenidyl (Artane)	6–20

[1]Modified, with permission, from Aminoff MJ: Pharmacologic management of parkinsonism and other movement disorders. In: *Basic & Clinical Pharmacology,* 5th ed. Katzung BG (editor). Appleton & Lange, 1992.

3. Levodopa–Levodopa, which is converted in the body to dopamine, improves all of the major features of parkinsonism, including bradykinesia, but does not stop progression of the disorder. The commonest early side effects of levodopa are nausea, vomiting, and hypotension, but cardiac arrhythmias may also occur. Dyskinesias, restlessness, confusion, and other behavioral changes tend to occur somewhat later and become more common with time. Levodopa-induced dyskinesias may take any conceivable form, including chorea, athetosis, dystonia, tremor, tics, and myoclonus. An even later complication is the "on-off phenomenon," in which abrupt but transient fluctuations in the severity of parkinsonism occur unpredictably but frequently during the day. The "off" period of marked bradykinesia has been shown to relate in some instances to falling plasma levels of levodopa. During the "on" phase, dyskinesias are often conspicuous but mobility is increased.

Carbidopa, which inhibits the enzyme responsible for the breakdown of levodopa to dopamine, does not cross the blood-brain barrier. When levodopa is given in combination with carbidopa, the extracerebral breakdown of levodopa is diminished. This reduces the amount of levodopa required daily for beneficial effects, and it lowers the incidence of nausea, vomiting, hypotension, and cardiac irregularities. Such a combination does not prevent the development of the "on-off phenomenon," and the incidence of other side effects (dyskinesias or psychiatric complications) may actually be increased.

Sinemet, a commercially available preparation that contains carbidopa and levodopa in a fixed ratio (1:10 or 1:4), is generally used. Treatment is started with a small dose—eg, one tablet of Sinemet 25/100 (containing 25 mg of carbidopa and 100 mg of levodopa) three times daily—and gradually increased depending on the response. Sinemet CR is a controlled-release formulation (containing 50 mg of carbidopa and 200 mg of levodopa). It is sometimes helpful in reducing fluctuations in clinical response to treatment and in reducing the frequency with which medication must be taken. Response fluctuations are also reduced by keeping the daily intake of protein at the recommended minimum and taking the main protein meal as the last meal of the day.

The dyskinesias and behavioral side effects of levodopa are dose-related, but reduction in dose may eliminate any therapeutic benefit. In such circumstances, a drug holiday may be helpful. Levodopa medication is gradually withdrawn over several days and not reinstated for 1–2 weeks. When it is reintroduced, up to two-thirds of patients show improved responsiveness and so derive benefit at a lower daily dose than previously required. The "on-off phenomenon" may also be improved by a drug holiday, but any benefit is usually so transient that a drug holiday is not recommended in this context. Complications of a drug holiday include depression, decubitus ulcers, aspiration pneumonia, and thromboembolism.

Levodopa therapy is contraindicated in patients with psychotic illness or narrow-angle glaucoma. It should not be given to patients taking monoamine oxidase A inhibitors or within 2 weeks of their withdrawal, because hypertensive crises may result. Levodopa should be avoided in patients with suspected malignant melanomas, which may be activated, and in patients with active peptic ulcers, which may bleed.

4. Bromocriptine–This ergot derivative acts directly on dopamine receptors, and its use in parkinsonism is associated with a lower incidence of the response fluctuations and dyskinesias that occur with long-term levodopa therapy. It was often reserved for patients who had either become refractory to levodopa or developed the "on-off phenomenon." However, it is now best given with a low dose of Sinemet-25/100 (carbidopa 25 mg and levodopa 100 mg), one tablet three times daily when dopaminergic therapy is first introduced; the dose of Sinemet is kept constant, while the dose of bromocriptine is gradually increased. The initial dosage of bromocriptine is 1.25 mg twice daily; this is increased by 2.5 mg at 2-week intervals until benefit occurs or side effects limit further increments. The usual daily maintenance dose in patients with parkinsonism is between 10 and 30 mg.

Side effects include anorexia, nausea, vomiting, constipation, postural hypotension, digital vasospasm, cardiac arrhythmias, various dyskinesias and mental disturbances, headache, nasal congestion, erythromelalgia, and pulmonary infiltrates.

Bromocriptine is contraindicated in patients with a history of mental illness or recent myocardial infarction and is probably best avoided in those with peripheral vascular disease or peptic ulcers (bleeding from peptic ulcers has been reported).

A number of other dopamine agonists have been used to treat parkinsonism. Only pergolide has been approved for use in the USA, and it seems to have no particular advantage over bromocriptine. It is started in a low dose (eg, 0.05 mg daily) and built up gradually depending on response and tolerance.

5. Selegiline–Selegiline is a monoamine oxidase B inhibitor that is sometimes used as adjunctive treatment for parkinsonism in patients receiving levodopa. By inhibiting the metabolic breakdown of dopamine, selegiline has been used to improve fluctuations or declining response to levodopa. In general, however, the response to treatment with it has been disappointing. The drug is taken in a standard dose of 5 mg with breakfast and 5 mg with lunch, and at this dose it does not have the hypertensive effect of the nonselective monoamine oxidase inhibitors. It may, however, increase any adverse effects of levodopa.

Treatment with selegiline may affect the natural history of Parkinson's disease by slowing down its progressive course. Studies have failed to establish this conclusively, but this remains an important consideration for patients who are young or have mild diseases.

B. General Measures: Physical therapy or speech therapy helps many patients. The quality of life can often be improved by the provision of simple aids to daily living, eg, rails or banisters placed strategically about the home, special table cutlery with large handles, nonslip rubber table mats, and devices to amplify the voice.

C. Surgical Measures: Thalamotomy is generally reserved for the patient who is relatively young, has predominantly unilateral tremor and rigidity that have failed to respond to medication, and has no evidence of diffuse vascular disease. Surgical implantation of adrenal medullary or fetal substantia nigra tissue into the caudate nucleus has recently been reported to benefit some patients, but other investigators have failed to substantiate such claims or have found only modest benefits, and the procedure is still being evaluated.

Ahlskog JE: Parkinson's disease: Update on pharmacologic options to slow progression and treat symptoms. Hosp Formul 1992;27:146.

Goetz GG et al: Neurosurgical horizons in Parkinson's disease. Neurology 1993;43:1.

Jenner P et al: New insights into the cause of Parkinson's disease. Neurology 1992;42:2241.

Parkinson Study Group: Effects of tocopherol and deprenyl on the progression of disability in early Parkinson's disease. N Engl J Med 1993;328:176. (Controlled clinical trial of treatment to slow disease progression.)

Standaert DG, Stern MB: Update on the management of Parkinson's disease. Med Clin North Am 1993:77:169.

3. HUNTINGTON'S DISEASE

Essentials of Diagnosis
- Gradual onset and progression of chorea and dementia.
- Family history of the disorder.

General Considerations

Huntington's disease is characterized by chorea and dementia. It is inherited in an autosomal dominant manner and occurs throughout the world, in all ethnic groups, with a prevalence rate of about 5 per 100,000. The gene responsible for the disease has been located on the short arm of chromosome No. 4. Symptoms do not usually develop until after 30 years of age, by which time the patient has usually had children, and so the disease continues from one generation to the next. The cause of Huntington's disease is unknown.

Clinical Findings

Clinical onset is usually between 30 and 50 years of age. The disease is progressive and usually leads to a fatal outcome within 15–20 years. The initial symptoms may consist of either abnormal movements or intellectual changes, but ultimately both occur. The earliest mental changes are often behavioral, with irritability, moodiness, antisocial behavior, or a psychiatric disturbance, but a more obvious dementia subsequently develops. The dyskinesia may initially be no more than an apparent fidgetiness or restlessness, but eventually choreiform movements and some dystonic posturing occur. Progressive rigidity and akinesia (rather than chorea) sometimes occur in association with dementia, especially in cases with childhood onset. CT scanning usually demonstrates cerebral atrophy and atrophy of the caudate nucleus in established cases. MRI and positron emission tomography (PET) have shown reduced glucose utilization in an anatomically normal caudate nucleus.

Chorea developing with no family history of choreoathetosis should not be attributed to Huntington's disease, at least not until other causes of chorea have been excluded clinically and by appropriate laboratory studies. In younger patients, self-limiting Sydenham's chorea develops after group A streptococcal infections on rare occasions. If a patient presents solely with progressive intellectual failure, it may not be possible to distinguish Huntington's disease from other causes of dementia unless there is a characteristic family history or a dyskinesia develops.

Treatment

There is no cure for Huntington's disease, progression cannot be halted, and treatment is purely symptomatic. The reported biochemical changes suggest a relative underactivity of neurons containing gamma-aminobutyric acid (GABA) and acetylcholine or a relative overactivity of dopaminergic neurons. Treatment with drugs blocking dopamine receptors, such as phenothiazines or haloperidol, may control the dyskinesia and any behavioral disturbances. Haloperidol treatment is usually begun with a dose of 1 mg once or twice daily, which is then increased every 3 or 4 days depending on the response. Tetrabenazine, a drug that depletes central monoamines, is widely used in Europe to treat dyskinesia but is not available in the USA. Reserpine is similar in its actions to tetrabenazine and may be helpful; the daily dose is built up gradually to between 2 and 5 mg, depending on the response. Behavioral disturbances may respond to clozapine. Attempts to compensate for the relative GABA deficiency by enhancing central GABA activity or to compensate for the relative cholinergic underactivity by giving choline chloride have not been therapeutically helpful. High levels of somatostatin (a neuropeptide) have recently been reported in certain areas of the brain in patients with Huntington's disease, and the therapeutic response to cysteamine (a selective depleter of somatostatin in the brain) is currently under study.

Offspring should be offered genetic counseling. Their probability of carrying the gene responsible for the disease can be estimated in many instances by identifying a specific DNA marker that is genetically linked to the gene, but this requires analysis of DNA samples from both affected and elderly unaffected family members.

Albin RL et al: Abnormalities of striatal projection neurons and N-methyl-D-aspartate receptors in presymptomatic Huntington's disease. N Engl J Med 1990;322:1293. (The findings bear on pathogenesis, suggesting that excitotoxins mediate cell death.)

4. IDIOPATHIC TORSION DYSTONIA

Essentials of Diagnosis
- Dystonic movements and postures.
- Normal birth and developmental history. No other neurologic signs.
- Investigations (including CT scan) reveal no cause of dystonia.

General Considerations

Idiopathic torsion dystonia may occur sporadically or on a hereditary basis, with autosomal dominant, autosomal recessive, and X-linked recessive modes of transmission. The responsible gene has been localized to the long arm of chromosome 9 in the dominantly inherited disorder and to the long arm of the X chromosome in the X-linked recessive form; the responsible gene in the autosomal recessive disorder is unknown. Symptoms may begin in childhood or later and persists throughout life.

Clinical Findings

The disorder is characterized by the onset of abnormal movements and postures in a patient with a normal birth and developmental history, no relevant past medical illness, and no other neurologic signs. Investigations (including CT scan) reveal no cause for the abnormal movements. Dystonic movements of the head and neck may take the form of torticollis, blepharospasm, facial grimacing, or forced opening or closing of the mouth. The limbs may also adopt abnormal but characteristic postures. The age at onset influences both the clinical findings and the prognosis. With onset in childhood, there is usually a family history of the disorder, symptoms commonly commence in the legs, and progression is likely until there is severe disability from generalized dystonia. In contrast, when onset is later, a positive family history is unlikely, initial symptoms are often in the arms or axial structures, and severe disability does not usually occur, although generalized dystonia may ultimately develop in some patients. If all cases are considered together, about one-third of patients eventually become so severely disabled that they are confined to chair or bed, while another one-third are affected only mildly.

Before a diagnosis of idiopathic torsion dystonia is made, it is imperative to exclude other causes of dystonia. For example, perinatal anoxia, birth trauma, and kernicterus are common causes of dystonia, but abnormal movements usually then develop before the age of 5, the early development of the patient is usually abnormal, and a history of seizures is not unusual. Moreover, examination may reveal signs of mental retardation or pyramidal deficit in addition to the movement disorder. Dystonic posturing may also occur in Wilson's disease, Huntington's disease, or parkinsonism; as a sequela of encephalitis lethargica or previous neuroleptic drug therapy; and in certain other disorders. In these cases, diagnosis is based on the history and accompanying clinical manifestations.

Treatment

Idiopathic torsion dystonia usually responds poorly to drugs. Levodopa, diazepam, baclofen, carbamazepine, amantadine, or anticholinergic medication (in high dosage) is occasionally helpful; if not, a trial of treatment with phenothiazines, haloperidol, or tetrabenazine (not available in the USA) may be worthwhile. In each case, the dose has to be individualized, depending on response and tolerance. However, the doses of these latter drugs that are required for benefit lead usually to mild parkinsonism. Stereotactic thalamotomy is sometimes helpful in patients with predominantly unilateral dystonia, especially when this involves the limbs.

Nygaard TG et al: Dopa-responsive dystonia. Neurology 1991;41:174. (Treatment response and prognosis.)

5. FOCAL TORSION DYSTONIA

A number of the dystonic manifestations that occur in idiopathic torsion dystonia may also occur as isolated phenomena. They are best regarded as focal dystonias that either occur as formes frustes of idiopathic torsion dystonia in patients with a positive family history or represent a focal manifestation of the adult-onset form of that disorder when there is no family history. Medical treatment is generally unsatisfactory. A trial of the drugs used in idiopathic torsion dystonia is worthwhile, however, since a few patients do show some response. In addition, with restricted dystonias such as blepharospasm or torticollis, local injection of botulinum A toxin into the overactive muscles may produce benefit for several weeks or months and can be repeated as needed.

Both blepharospasm and oromandibular dystonia may occur as an isolated focal dystonia. The former is characterized by spontaneous involuntary forced closure of the eyelids for a variable interval. Oromandibular dystonia is manifested by involuntary contraction of the muscles about the mouth causing, for example, involuntary opening or closing of the mouth, roving or protruding tongue movements, and retraction of the platysma.

Spasmodic torticollis, usually with onset between 25 and 50 years of age, is characterized by a tendency for the neck to twist to one side. This initially occurs episodically, but eventually the neck is held to the side. Spontaneous resolution may occur in the first year or so. The disorder is otherwise usually lifelong. Selective section of the spinal accessory nerve and the upper cervical nerve roots is sometimes helpful if medical treatment is unsuccessful. Local injection of botulinum A toxin may provide benefit in some cases.

Writer's cramp is characterized by dystonic posturing of the hand and forearm when the hand is used for writing and sometimes when it is used for other tasks, eg, playing the piano, using a screwdriver or eating utensils. Drug treatment is usually unrewarding, and patients are often best advised to learn to use the other hand for activities requiring manual dexterity.

Gelb DJ et al: Change in pattern of muscle activity following botulinum toxin injections for torticollis. Ann Neurol 1991;29:370.

Saint-Hilaire MH et al: Delayed-onset dystonia due to perinatal or early childhood asphyxia. Neurology 1991;41:216. (Postasphyxial and idiopathic dystonia may be clinically similar.)

Yoshimura DM et al: Botulinum toxin therapy for limb dystonias. Neurology 1992;42:627.

6. MYOCLONUS

Occasional myoclonic jerks may occur in anyone, especially when drifting into sleep. General or multifocal myoclonus is common in patients with idiopathic epilepsy and is especially prominent in certain hereditary disorders characterized by seizures and progressive intellectual decline, such as the lipid storage diseases. It is also a feature of various rare degenerative disorders, notably Ramsay Hunt syndrome, and is common in subacute sclerosing panencephalitis and Creutzfeldt-Jakob disease. Generalized myoclonic jerking may accompany uremic and other metabolic encephalopathies, result from levodopa therapy, occur in alcohol or drug withdrawal states, or follow anoxic brain damage. It also occurs on a hereditary or sporadic basis as an isolated phenomenon in otherwise healthy subjects.

Segmental myoclonus is a rare manifestation of a focal spinal cord lesion. It may also be the clinical expression of **epilepsia partialis continua,** a disorder in which a repetitive focal epileptic discharge arises in the contralateral sensorimotor cortex, sometimes from an underlying structural lesion. An electroencephalogram is often helpful in clarifying the epileptic nature of the disorder, and CT or MRI scan may reveal the causal lesion.

Myoclonus may respond to certain anticonvulsant drugs, especially valproic acid, or to one of the benzodiazepines, particularly clonazepam (Table 23–2). Myoclonus following anoxic brain damage is often responsive to oxitriptan (5-hydroxytryptophan), an investigational agent that is the precursor of serotonin, and sometimes to clonazepam. Oxitriptan is given in gradually increasing doses up to 1–1.5 mg daily. In patients with segmental myoclonus, a localized lesion should be searched for and treated appropriately.

Obeso J et al: The treatment of severe action myoclonus. Brain 1989;112:765. (Case reports and review.)

7. WILSON'S DISEASE

In this metabolic disorder, abnormal movements and postures of all sorts may occur with or without coexisting signs of liver involvement. It is discussed in detail in Chapter 15.

8. DRUG-INDUCED ABNORMAL MOVEMENTS

Phenothiazines and butyrophenones may produce a wide variety of abnormal movements, including parkinsonism, akathisia (ie, motor restlessness), acute dystonia, chorea, and tardive dyskinesia. These complications are discussed in Chapter 24. Chorea may also develop in patients receiving levodopa, bromocriptine, anticholinergic drugs, phenytoin, carbamazepine, lithium, amphetamines, or oral contraceptives, and it resolves with withdrawal of the offending substance. Similarly, dystonia may be produced by levodopa, bromocriptine, lithium, metoclopramide, or carbamazepine; and parkinsonism by reserpine, tetrabenazine, and metoclopramide. Postural tremor may occur with a variety of drugs, including epinephrine, isoproterenol, theophylline, caffeine, lithium, thyroid hormone, tricyclic antidepressants, and valproic acid.

9. GILLES DE LA TOURETTE'S SYNDROME

Essentials of Diagnosis
- Multiple motor and phonic tics.
- Symptoms begin before age 15 years.
- Chronic lifelong disorder with relapses and remissions.

Clinical Findings
Motor tics are the initial manifestation in 80% of cases and most commonly involve the face, whereas in the remaining 20%, the initial symptoms are phonic tics; all patients ultimately develop a combination of different motor and phonic tics. These are noted first in childhood, generally between the ages of 2 and 15. Motor tics occur especially about the face, head, and shoulders (eg, sniffing, blinking, frowning, shoulder shrugging, head thrusting, etc). Phonic tics commonly consist of grunts, barks, hisses, throat-clearing, coughs, etc, but sometimes also of verbal utterances including coprolalia (obscene speech). There may also be echolalia (repetition of the speech of others), echopraxia (imitation of others' movements), and palilalia (repetition of words or phrases). Some tics may be self-mutilating in nature, such as severe nail-biting, hair-pulling, or biting of the lips or tongue. The disorder is chronic, but the course may be punctuated by relapses and remissions.

Examination usually reveals no abnormalities other than the multiple tics. Psychiatric disturbances may occur, however, because of the associated cosmetic and social embarrassment. Investigations are unrevealing except that the EEG may show minor nonspecific abnormalities of no diagnostic relevance.

The diagnosis of the disorder is often delayed for years, the tics being interpreted as psychiatric illness or some other form of abnormal movement. Patients are thus often subjected to unnecessary and expensive treatments before the true nature of the disorder is recognized. The tic-like character of the abnormal movements and the absence of other neurologic signs should differentiate this disorder from other movement disorders presenting in childhood. Wilson's disease, however, can simulate the condition and should be excluded.

Treatment

Treatment is symptomatic and may need to be continued indefinitely. Haloperidol is generally regarded as the drug of choice. It is started in a low daily dose (0.25 mg) that is gradually increased (by 0.25 mg every 4 or 5 days) until there is maximum benefit with a minimum of side effects or until side effects limit further increments. A total daily dose of between 2 and 8 mg is usually optimal, but higher doses are sometimes necessary. Treatment with clonazepam (in a dose that depends on response and tolerance) or clonidine (2–5 μg/kg/d) may also be helpful, and it seems sensible to begin with one of these drugs in order to avoid some of the long-term extrapyramidal side effects of haloperidol. Phenothiazines, such as fluphenazine (2–15 mg daily), have been used, but patients unresponsive to haloperidol are usually unresponsive to these as well.

Pimozide, an oral dopamine-blocking drug related to haloperidol, may be helpful in patients who cannot tolerate or have not responded to haloperidol. Treatment is started with 1 mg daily and the daily dose increased by 1–2 mg every 10 days; the average dose is between 7 and 16 mg daily. The long-term safety of the drug is unclear.

There are a few anecdotal reports that calcium channel blockers may be helpful, but this requires further study.

Goetz CG et al: Adult tics in Gilles de la Tourette's syndrome: Description and risk factors. Neurology 1992;42:784. (Clinical features and prognostic factors in 58 cases.)

DEMENTIA

Dementia, the symptom complex of progressive global impairment of intellectual function, is a major medical, social, and economic problem that is worsening as the number of elderly people in the general population increases. It is discussed in Chapter 4, and the only point to be reiterated here is the importance of recognizing early any treatable or reversible causes of dementia, such as normal-pressure hydrocephalus, intracranial mass lesions, vascular disease, hypothyroidism, thiamin or vitamin B_{12} deficiency, Wilson's disease, hepatic or renal failure, neurosyphilis, and the chronic meningitides.

MULTIPLE SCLEROSIS

Essentials of Diagnosis

- Episodic symptoms that may include sensory abnormalities, blurred vision, sphincter disturbances, and weakness with or without spasticity.
- Patient usually under 55 years of age at onset.
- Single pathologic lesion cannot explain clinical findings.
- Multiple foci best demonstrated radiographically by MRI.

General Considerations

This common neurologic disorder of unknown cause has its greatest incidence in young adults. Epidemiologic studies indicate that multiple sclerosis is much more common in persons of western European lineage who live in temperate zones. No population with a high risk for multiple sclerosis exists between latitudes 40 °N and 40 °S. Genetic, dietary, and climatic factors cannot account for these differences. There may be a familial incidence of the disease, since affected relatives are sometimes reported. The strong association between multiple sclerosis and specific HLA antigens (HLA-DR2) provides support for a theory of genetic predisposition. Many believe that the disease has an immunologic basis. Pathologically, focal—often perivenular—areas of demyelination with reactive gliosis are found scattered in the white matter of brain and spinal cord and in the optic nerves.

Clinical Findings

A. Symptoms and Signs: The common initial presentation is weakness, numbness, tingling, or unsteadiness in a limb; spastic paraparesis; retrobulbar neuritis; diplopia; disequilibrium; or a sphincter disturbance such as urinary urgency or hesitancy. Symptoms may disappear after a few days or weeks, although examination often reveals a residual deficit.

In most patients, there is an interval of months or years after the initial episode before new symptoms develop or the original ones recur. Eventually, however, relapses and usually incomplete remissions lead to increasing disability, with weakness, spasticity, and ataxia of the limbs, impaired vision, and urinary incontinence. The findings on examination at this stage commonly include optic atrophy, nystagmus, dysarthria, and pyramidal, sensory, or cerebellar deficits in some or all of the limbs.

Less commonly, symptoms are steadily progressive from their onset, and disability develops at a relatively early stage. The diagnosis cannot be made with confidence unless the total clinical picture indicates involvement of different parts of the central nervous system at different times.

A number of factors (eg, infection, trauma) may precipitate or trigger exacerbations. Relapses are also more likely during the 2 or 3 months following pregnancy, possibly because of the increased demands and stresses that occur in the postpartum period.

B. Imaging: MRI of the brain or cervical cord is often helpful in demonstrating the presence of a multiplicity of lesions. CT scans are less helpful.

In patients presenting with myelopathy alone and in whom there is no clinical or laboratory evidence of more widespread disease, myelography or MRI may be necessary to exclude a congenital or acquired surgically treatable lesion. The foramen magnum region must be visualized to exclude the possibility of Arnold-Chiari malformation, in which part of the cerebellum and the lower brain stem are displaced into the cervical canal and produce mixed pyramidal and cerebellar deficits in the limbs.

C. Laboratory and Other Studies: A definitive diagnosis can never be based solely on the laboratory findings. If there is clinical evidence of only a single lesion in the central nervous system, multiple sclerosis cannot properly be diagnosed unless it can be shown that other regions are affected subclinically. The electrocerebral responses evoked in the clinical neurophysiology laboratory by monocular visual stimulation with a checkerboard pattern stimulus, by monaural click stimulation, and by electrical stimulation of a sensory or mixed peripheral nerve have been used to detect subclinical involvement of the visual, brain stem auditory, and somatosensory pathways, respectively. Other disorders may also be characterized by multifocal electrophysiologic abnormalities.

There may be mild lymphocytosis or a slightly increased protein concentration in the cerebrospinal fluid, especially soon after an acute relapse. Elevated IgG in cerebrospinal fluid and discrete bands of IgG, called oligoclonal bands, are present in many patients. The presence of such bands is not specific, however, since they have been found in a variety of inflammatory neurologic disorders and occasionally in patients with vascular or neoplastic disorders of the nervous system.

Treatment

At least partial recovery from acute exacerbations can reasonably be expected, but further relapses may occur without warning, and there is no means of preventing progression of the disorder. Some disability is likely to result eventually, but about half of all patients are without significant disability even 10 years after onset of symptoms.

Recovery from acute relapses may be hastened by treatment with corticosteroids, but the extent of recovery is unchanged. A high dose (eg, prednisone, 60 or 80 mg) is given daily for 1 week, after which medication is tapered over the following 2 or 3 weeks. Such a regimen is often preceded by methylprednisolone, 1 g intravenously for 3 days. Long-term treatment with steroids provides no benefit and does not prevent further relapses.

Several recent studies have suggested that intensive immunosuppressive therapy with cyclophosphamide or azathioprine may help to arrest the course of chronic progressive active multiple sclerosis. The evidence of benefit is incomplete, however, and further clinical trials are in progress. There is little evidence that plasmapheresis enhances any beneficial effects of immunosuppression in sclerosis, and its role in the management of the various clinical forms of multiple sclerosis is uncertain. The findings in a recent trial of systemic interferon therapy suggested some benefit in patients whose disease was characterized by relapses and remissions rather than by steady progression. Further studies to evaluate this form of treatment in selected patients are proceeding. Finally, preliminary studies suggest that Cop 1 (a random polymer-simulating myelin basic protein) may be beneficial in patients with the exacerbating-remitting form of multiple sclerosis, and further evaluation of this approach seems warranted.

Treatment for spasticity (see below) and for neurogenic bladder may be needed in advanced cases. Excessive fatigue must be avoided, and patients should rest during periods of acute relapse.

Beck RW et al: A randomized, controlled trial of corticosteroids in the treatment of acute optic neuritis. N Engl J Med 1992;326:581. (Intravenous methylprednisolone followed by oral prednisone speeds recovery after optic neuritis.)
Goodin DS: The use of immunosuppressive agents in the treatment of multiple sclerosis: A critical review. Neurology 1991;41:980.

VITAMIN E DEFICIENCY

Vitamin E deficiency may produce a disorder somewhat similar to Friedreich's ataxia (see below. There is spinocerebellar degeneration involving particularly the posterior columns of the spinal cord and leading to limb ataxia, sensory loss, absent tendon reflexes, slurring of speech, and, in some cases, pigmentary retinal degeneration. The disorder may occur as a consequence of malabsorption or on a hereditary basis. Treatment is with alpha-tocopheryl acetate (eg, Aquasol E capsules or drops), as discussed in Chapter 28.

Yokota T et al: Adult-onset spinocerebellar syndrome with idiopathic vitamin E deficiency. Ann Neurol 1987;22:84. (Case reports and review.)

SPASTICITY

The term "spasticity" is commonly used for an upper motor neuron deficit, but it properly refers to a velocity-dependent increase in resistance to passive movement that affects different muscles to a different extent, is not uniform in degree throughout the range of a particular movement, and is commonly associated with other features of pyramidal deficit. It is often a major complication of stroke, cerebral or spinal injury, static perinatal encephalopathy, and multiple sclerosis.

Physical therapy with appropriate stretching programs is important during rehabilitation after the development of an upper motor neuron lesion and in subsequent management of the patient. The aim is to prevent joint and muscle contractures and perhaps to modulate spasticity.

Drug management is important also, but treatment may increase functional disability when increased extensor tone is providing additional support for patients with weak legs. Dantrolene weakens muscle contraction by interfering with the role of calcium. It may be helpful in the treatment of spasticity but is best avoided in patients with poor respiratory function or severe myocardial disease. Treatment is begun with 25 mg once daily, and the daily dose is built up by 25 mg increments every 3 days, depending on tolerance, to a maximum of 100 mg four times daily. The drug should be withdrawn if no benefit has occurred after treatment with the maximum tolerated dose for about 2 weeks. Side effects include diarrhea, nausea, weakness, hepatic dysfunction (that may rarely be fatal, especially in women older than 35), drowsiness, light-headedness, and hallucinations.

Baclofen seems to be the most effective drug for treating spasticity of spinal origin. It is particularly helpful in relieving painful flexor (or extensor) spasms. The maximum recommended daily dose is 80 mg; treatment is started with a dose of 5 or 10 mg twice daily and then built up gradually. Side effects include gastrointestinal disturbances, lassitude, fatigue, sedation, unsteadiness, confusion, and hallucinations. Diazepam may modify spasticity by its action on spinal interneurons and perhaps also by influencing supraspinal centers, but effective doses often cause intolerable drowsiness and vary with different patients.

Motor-point blocks by intramuscular phenol have been used to reduce spasticity selectively in one or a few important muscles and may permit return of function in patients with incomplete myelopathies. Intrathecal injection of phenol or absolute alcohol may be helpful in more severe cases, but greater selectivity can be achieved by nerve root or peripheral nerve neurolysis. These procedures should not be undertaken until the spasticity syndrome is fully evolved, ie, only after about 1 year or so, and only if long-term drug treatment either has been unhelpful or carries a significant risk to the patient.

A number of surgical procedures, eg, adductor or heel cord tenotomy, may help in the management of spasticity. Neurectomy may also facilitate patient management. For example, obturator neurectomy is helpful in patients with marked adductor spasms that interfere with personal hygiene or cause gait disturbances. Posterior rhizotomy reduces spasticity, but its effect may be short-lived, whereas anterior rhizotomy produces permanent wasting and weakness in the muscles that are denervated.

Spasticity may be exacerbated by decubitus ulcers, urinary or other infections, and nociceptive stimuli.

Young RR: Treatment of spastic paraparesis. N Engl J Med 1989;320:1553.

MYELOPATHIES IN AIDS

Patients with AIDS may develop a subacute or chronic vacuolar myelopathy leading to paraparesis or quadriparesis, sphincter dysfunction, and sensory disturbances. There is no effective treatment. Myelitis or radiculomyelitis may occur also in AIDS patients as a result of opportunistic viral infections. When extradural lymphomatous deposits cause compressive myelopathy, pain and spinal tenderness are conspicuous, and MRI or myelography reveals the underlying lesion. Treatment is with corticosteroids, radiotherapy, and chemotherapy. Lymphomatous meningitis occurring in AIDS patients has the features described above.

Rosenblum M et al: Dissociation of AIDS-related vacuolar myelopathy and productive HIV-1 infection of the spinal cord. Neurology 1989;39:892. (Etiology of vacuolar myelopathy in AIDS.)

MYELOPATHY OF HUMAN T CELL LEUKEMIA VIRUS

Human T cell leukemia virus (HTLV-1), a human retrovirus, is transmitted by breast feeding, sexual contact, blood transfusion, and contaminated needles. Most patients are asymptomatic, but after a variable latent period (may be as long as several years) a myelopathy develops in some instances. The MRI, electrophysiologic, and cerebrospinal fluid findings are similar to those of multiple sclerosis, but HTLV-1 antibodies are present in serum and spinal fluid. There is no specific treatment.

Gessain A, Gout O: Chronic myelopathy associated with human T-lymphotropic virus type 1 (HTLV-1). Ann Intern Med 1992;117:933.

SUBACUTE COMBINED DEGENERATION OF THE SPINAL CORD

Subacute combined degeneration of the spinal cord is due to vitamin B_{12} deficiency, such as occurs in pernicious anemia. It is characterized by myelopathy with predominant pyramidal and posterior column deficits, sometimes in association with polyneuropathy, mental changes, or optic neuropathy. Megaloblastic anemia may also occur, but this does not parallel the neurologic disorder, and the former may be obscured if folic acid supplements have been taken. Treatment is with vitamin B$_{12}$. For pernicious anemia, a convenient therapeutic regimen is 100 mg cyanocobalamin intramuscularly daily for 1 week, then weekly for 1 month, and then monthly for the remainder of the patient's life.

Healton EB et al: Neurologic aspects of cobalamin deficiency. Medicine 1991;70:229. (Clinical features and response to treatment in a large series of patients.)

WERNICKE'S ENCEPHALOPATHY

Wernicke's encephalopathy is characterized by confusion, ataxia, and nystagmus leading to ophthalmoplegia (lateral rectus muscle weakness, conjugate gaze palsies); peripheral neuropathy may also be present. It is due to thiamin deficiency and in the USA occurs most commonly in alcoholics. It may also occur in patients with AIDS. In suspected cases, thiamin (50 mg) is given intravenously immediately and then intramuscularly on a daily basis until a satisfactory diet can be ensured. Intravenous glucose given before thiamin may precipitate the syndrome or worsen the symptoms. The diagnosis is confirmed by the response to treatment, which must not be delayed while laboratory confirmation is obtained.

Charness ME et al: Ethanol and the nervous system. N Engl J Med 1989;321:442.

STUPOR & COMA

The patient who is stuporous is unresponsive except when subjected to repeated vigorous stimuli, while the comatose patient is unarousable and unable to respond to external events or inner needs, although reflex movements and posturing may be present.

Coma is a major complication of serious central nervous system disorders. It can result from seizures, hypothermia, metabolic disturbances, or structural lesions causing bilateral cerebral hemispheric dysfunction or a disturbance of the brain stem reticular activating system. A mass lesion involving one cerebral hemisphere may cause coma by compression of the brain stem.

Assessment & Emergency Measures

The diagnostic workup of the comatose patient must proceed concomitantly with management. Supportive therapy for respiration or blood pressure is initiated if necessary. This is especially true in hypothermia, where all vital signs may be absent; all such patients should be rewarmed before the prognosis is assessed.

The patient can be positioned on one side with the neck partly extended, dentures removed, and secretions cleared by suction; if necessary, the patency of the airways is maintained with an oropharyngeal airway. Blood is drawn for serum glucose, electrolyte, and calcium levels; arterial blood gases; liver and renal function tests; and toxicologic studies if necessary. Dextrose 50% (25 g), naloxone (0.4–1.2 mg), and thiamin (50 mg) to counteract possible hypoglycemia, opiate overdosage, or thiamin deficiency should be given intravenously. The intravenous line is left in place to facilitate further access to the circulation.

After these initial measures, further details are obtained from attendants of the patient's medical history, the circumstances surrounding the onset of coma, and the time course of subsequent events. Abrupt onset of coma suggests subarachnoid hemorrhage, brain stem stroke, or intracerebral hemorrhage, whereas a slower onset and progression occur with other structural or mass lesions. A metabolic cause is likely with a preceding intoxicated state or agitated delirium. On examination, attention is paid to the behavioral response to painful stimuli, the pupils and their response to light, the position of the eyes and their movement in response to passive movement of the head and ice-water caloric stimulation, and the respiratory pattern.

A. Response to Painful Stimuli: Purposive limb withdrawal from painful stimuli implies that sensory pathways from and motor pathways to the stimulated limb are functionally intact, at least in part. Unilateral absence of responses despite application of stimuli to both sides of the body in turn implies a corticospinal lesion; bilateral absence of responsiveness suggests brain stem involvement, bilateral pyramidal tract lesions, or psychogenic unresponsiveness. Inappropriate responses may also occur. Decorticate posturing may occur with lesions of the internal capsule and rostral cerebral peduncle, decerebrate posturing with dysfunction or destruction of the midbrain and rostral pons, and decerebrate posturing in the arms accompanied by flaccidity or slight flexor responses in the legs in patients with extensive brain stem damage extending down to the pons at the trigeminal level.

B. Ocular Findings:

1. Pupils—Hypothalamic disease processes may lead to unilateral Horner's syndrome, while bilateral diencephalic involvement or destructive pontine lesions may lead to small but reactive pupils. Ipsilateral pupillary dilation with no direct or consensual response to light occurs with compression of the third cranial nerve, eg, with uncal herniation. The pupils are slightly smaller than normal but responsive to light in many metabolic encephalopathies; however, they may be fixed and dilated following overdosage with atropine, scopolamine, or glutethimide, and pinpoint (but responsive) with opiates. Pupillary dilation for several hours following cardiopulmonary arrest implies a poor prognosis.

2. Eye movements–Conjugate deviation of the eyes to the side suggests the presence of an ipsilateral hemispheric lesion or a contralateral pontine lesion. A mesencephalic lesion leads to downward conjugate deviation. Dysconjugate ocular deviation in coma implies a structural brain stem lesion unless there was preexisting strabismus.

The oculomotor responses to passive head turning and to caloric stimulation relate to each other and provide complementary information. In response to brisk rotation of the head from side to side and to flexion and extension of the head, normally conscious patients with open eyes do not exhibit contraversive conjugate eye deviation (doll's-head eye response) unless there is voluntary visual fixation or bilateral frontal pathology. With cortical depression in lightly comatose patients, a brisk doll's-head eye response is seen. With brain stem lesions, this oculocephalic reflex becomes impaired or lost, depending on the site of the lesion.

The oculovestibular reflex is tested by caloric stimulation using irrigation with ice water. In normal subjects, jerk nystagmus is elicited for about 2 or 3 minutes, with the slow component toward the irrigated ear. In unconscious patients with an intact brain stem, the fast component of the nystagmus disappears, so that the eyes tonically deviate toward the irrigated side for 2–3 minutes before returning to their original position. With impairment of brain stem function, the response becomes perverted and finally disappears. In metabolic coma, oculocephalic and oculovestibular reflex responses are preserved, at least initially.

C. Respiratory Patterns: Diseases causing coma may lead to respiratory abnormalities. Cheyne-Stokes respiration may occur with bihemispheric or diencephalic disease or in metabolic disorders. Central neurogenic hyperventilation occurs with lesions of the brain stem tegmentum; apneustic breathing (in which there are prominent end-inspiratory pauses) suggests damage at the pontine level (eg, due to basilar artery occlusion); and atactic breathing (a completely irregular pattern of breathing with deep and shallow breaths occurring randomly) is associated with lesions of the lower pontine tegmentum and medulla.

1. STUPOR & COMA DUE TO STRUCTURAL LESIONS

Supratentorial mass lesions tend to affect brain function in an orderly way. There may initially be signs of hemispheric dysfunction, such as hemiparesis. As coma develops and deepens, cerebral function

becomes progressively disturbed, producing a predictable progression of neurologic signs that suggest rostrocaudal deterioration.

Thus, as a supratentorial mass lesion begins to impair the diencephalon, the patient becomes drowsy, then stuporous, and finally comatose. There may be Cheyne-Stokes respiration; small but reactive pupils; doll's-head eye responses with side-to-side head movements but sometimes an impairment of reflex upward gaze with brisk flexion of the head; tonic ipsilateral deviation of the eyes in response to vestibular stimulation with cold water; and initially a positive response to pain but subsequently only decorticate posturing. With further progression, midbrain failure occurs. Motor dysfunction progresses from decorticate to bilateral decerebrate posturing in response to painful stimuli; Cheyne-Stokes respiration is gradually replaced by sustained central hyperventilation; the pupils become middle-sized and fixed; and the oculocephalic and oculovestibular reflex responses become impaired, perverted, or lost. As the pons and then the medulla fail, the pupils remain unresponsive; oculovestibular responses are unobtainable; respiration is rapid and shallow; and painful stimuli may lead only to flexor responses in the legs. Finally, respiration becomes irregular and stops, the pupils often then dilating widely.

In contrast, a subtentorial (ie, brain stem) lesion may lead to an early, sometimes abrupt disturbance of consciousness without any orderly rostrocaudal progression of neurologic signs. Compressive lesions of the brain stem, especially cerebellar hemorrhage, may be clinically indistinguishable from intraparenchymal processes.

A structural lesion is suspected if the findings suggest focality. In such circumstances, a CT scan should be performed before, or instead of, a lumbar puncture in order to avoid any risk of cerebral herniation. Further management is of the causal lesion and is considered separately under the individual disorders.

2. STUPOR & COMA DUE TO METABOLIC DISTURBANCES

Patients with a metabolic cause of coma generally have signs of patchy, diffuse, and symmetric neurologic involvement that cannot be explained by loss of function at any single level or in a sequential manner, although focal or lateralized deficits may occur in hypoglycemia. Moreover, pupillary reactivity is usually preserved, while other brain stem functions are often grossly impaired. Comatose patients with meningitis, encephalitis, or subarachnoid hemorrhage may also exhibit little in the way of focal neurologic signs, however, and clinical evidence of meningeal irritation is sometimes very subtle in comatose patients.

Examination of the cerebrospinal fluid in such patients is essential to establish the correct diagnosis.

In patients with coma due to cerebral ischemia and hypoxia, the absence of pupillary light reflexes at the time of initial examination indicates that there is little chance of regaining independence; by contrast, preserved pupillary light responses, the development of spontaneous eye movements (roving, conjugate, or better), and extensor, flexor, or withdrawal responses to pain at this early stage imply a relatively good prognosis.

Treatment of metabolic encephalopathy is of the underlying disturbance and is considered in other chapters. If the cause of the encephalopathy is obscure, all drugs except essential ones may have to be withdrawn in case they are responsible for the altered mental status.

Bates D: Defining prognosis in medical coma. J Neurol Neurosurg Psychiatry 1991;54:569. (Editorial review.)

3. BRAIN DEATH

The definition of brain death is controversial, and diagnostic criteria have been published by many different professional organizations. In order to establish brain death, the irreversibly comatose patient must be shown to have lost all brain stem reflex responses, including the pupillary, corneal, oculovestibular, oculocephalic, oropharyngeal, and respiratory reflexes, and should have been in this condition for at least 6 hours. Spinal reflex movements do not exclude the diagnosis, but ongoing seizure activity or decerebrate or decorticate posturing is not consistent with brain death. The apnea test (presence or absence of spontaneous respiratory activity at a $PaCO_2$ of at least 60 mm Hg) serves to determine whether the patient is capable of respiratory activity.

Reversible coma simulating brain death may be seen with hypothermia (temperature < 32 °C) and overdosage with central nervous system depressant drugs, and these conditions must be excluded. Certain ancillary tests may assist the determination of brain death but are not essential. An isoelectric electroencephalogram, when the recording is made according to the recommendations of the American Electroencephalographic Society, is especially helpful in confirming the diagnosis. Alternatively, the demonstration of an absent cerebral circulation by intravenous radioisotope cerebral angiography or by four-vessel contrast cerebral angiography can be confirmatory.

Chatrian GE: Electrophysiologic evaluation of brain death: A critical appraisal. In: *Electrodiagnosis in Clinical Neurology,* 3rd ed. Aminoff MJ (editor). Churchill Livingstone, 1992.

4. PERSISTENT VEGETATIVE STATE

Patients with severe bilateral hemispheric disease may show some improvement from an initially comatose state, so that, after a variable interval, they appear to be awake but lie motionless and without evidence of awareness or higher mental activity. This persistent vegetative state has been variously referred to as akinetic mutism, apallic state, or coma vigil. Most patients in this persistent vegetative state will die in months or years, but partial recovery has occasionally occurred and in rare instances has been sufficient to permit communication or even independent living.

5. LOCKED-IN SYNDROME (De-efferented State)

Acute destructive lesions (eg, infarction, hemorrhage, demyelination, encephalitis) involving the ventral pons and sparing the tegmentum may lead to a mute, quadriparetic but conscious state in which the patient is capable of blinking and of voluntary eye movement in the vertical plane, with preserved pupillary responses to light. Such a patient can mistakenly be regarded as comatose. Physicians should recognize that "locked-in" individuals are fully aware of their surroundings. Prognosis is variable, but recovery has occasionally been reported, in some cases including resumption of independent daily life, though this may take up to 2 or 3 years.

HEAD INJURY

Trauma is the most common cause of death in young people, and head injury accounts for almost half of these trauma-related deaths. The prognosis following head injury depends upon the site and severity of brain damage. Some guide to prognosis is provided by the mental status, since loss of consciousness for more than 1 or 2 minutes implies a worse prognosis than otherwise. Similarly, the degree of retrograde and posttraumatic amnesia provides an indication of the severity of injury and thus of the prognosis. Absence of skull fracture does not exclude the possibility of severe head injury. During the physical examination, special attention should be given to the level of consciousness and extent of any brain stem dysfunction.

Note: In general, patients who have lost consciousness for 2 minutes or more following head injury should be admitted to the hospital for observation, as should patients with focal neurologic deficits, lethargy, or skull fractures. If patients are not to be detained, responsible family members should be given clear instructions about the need for, and manner of, checking on them at regular (hourly) intervals and for obtaining additional medical help if necessary. Deterioration is an indication for further investigation.

Skull radiographs or CT scans may provide evidence of fractures. Because injury to the spine may have accompanied head trauma, cervical spine radiographs (especially in the lateral projection) should always be obtained in comatose patients and in patients with severe neck pain or a deficit possibly related to cord compression. CT scanning has an important role in demonstrating intracranial hemorrhage and may also provide evidence of cerebral edema and displacement of midline structures.

Cerebral Injuries

These are summarized in Table 23–5 along with comments about treatment.

Scalp Injuries & Skull Fractures

Scalp lacerations and depressed or compound depressed skull fractures should be treated surgically as appropriate. Simple skull fractures require no specific treatment.

The clinical signs of basilar skull fracture include bruising about the orbit (raccoon sign), blood in the external auditory meatus (Battle's sign), and leakage of cerebrospinal fluid (which can be identified by its glucose content) from the ear or nose. Cranial nerve palsies (involving especially the first, second, third, fourth, fifth, seventh, and eighth nerves in any combination) may also occur. If there is any leakage of cerebrospinal fluid, conservative treatment, with elevation of the head, restriction of fluids, and administration of acetazolamide (250 mg four times daily), is often helpful; but if the leak continues for more than a few days, lumbar subarachnoid drainage may be necessary. Antibiotics are given if infection occurs, based on culture and sensitivity studies. Only very occasional patients require intracranial repair of the dural defect because of persistence of the leak or recurrent meningitis.

Late Complications of Head Injury

The relationship of chronic subdural hemorrhage to head injury is not always clear. In many elderly persons there is no history of trauma, but in other cases a head injury, often trivial, precedes the onset of symptoms by several weeks. The clinical presentation is usually with mental changes such as slowness, drowsiness, headache, confusion, memory disturbances, personality change, or even dementia. Focal neurologic deficits such as hemiparesis or hemisensory disturbance may also occur but are less common. CT scan is an important means of detecting the hematoma, which is sometimes bilateral. Treatment is by surgical evacuation to prevent cerebral compression and tentorial herniation.

Normal-pressure hydrocephalus may follow head injury, subarachnoid hemorrhage, or meningoencephalitis.

Other late complications of head injury include posttraumatic seizure disorder and posttraumatic headache.

White RJ, Likavec MJ: The diagnosis and initial management of head injury. N Engl J Med 1992;327:1507.

SPINAL TRAUMA

While spinal cord damage may result from whiplash injury, severe injury usually relates to fracture-dislocation causing compression or angular deformity of the cord either cervically or in the lower thoracic and upper lumbar region. Extreme hypoten-

Table 23–5. Acute cerebral sequelae of head injury.

Sequelae	Clinical Features	Pathology
Concussion	Transient loss of consciousness with bradycardia, hypotension, and respiratory arrest for a few seconds followed by retrograde and posttraumatic amnesia. Occasionally followed by transient neurologic deficit.	Bruising on side of impact (coup injury) or contralaterally (contrecoup injury).
Cerebral contusion/laceration	Loss of consciousness longer than with concussion. May lead to death or severe residual neurologic deficit.	Cerebral contusion, edema, hemorrhage, and necrosis. May have subarachnoid bleeding.
Acute epidural hemorrhage	Headache, confusion, somnolence, seizures, and focal deficits occur several hours after injury and lead to coma, respiratory depression, and death unless treated by surgical evacuation.	Tear in meningeal artery, vein, or dural sinus, leading to hematoma visible on CT scan.
Acute subdural hemorrhage	Similar to epidural hemorrhage, but interval before onset of symptoms is longer. Treatment is by surgical evacuation.	Hematoma from tear in veins from cortex to superior sagittal sinus or from cerebral laceration, visible on CT scan.
Cerebral hemorrhage	Generally develops immediately after injury. Clinically resembles hypertensive hemorrhage. Surgical evacuation is sometimes helpful.	Hematoma, visible on CT scan.

sion following injury may also lead to cord infarction.

Total cord transection results in immediate flaccid paralysis and loss of sensation below the level of the lesion. Reflex activity is lost for a variable period, and there is urinary and fecal retention. As reflex function returns over the following days and weeks, spastic paraplegia or quadriplegia develops, with hyperreflexia and extensor plantar responses, but a flaccid atrophic (lower motor neuron) paralysis may be found depending on the segments of the cord that are affected. The bladder and bowels also regain some reflex function, permitting urine and feces to be expelled at intervals. As spasticity increases, flexor or extensor spasms (or both) of the legs become troublesome, especially if the patient develops bed sores or a urinary tract infection. Paraplegia with the legs in flexion or extension may eventually result.

With lesser degrees of injury, patients may be left with mild limb weakness, distal sensory disturbance, or both. Sphincter function may also be impaired, urinary urgency and urgency incontinence being especially common. More particularly, a unilateral cord lesion leads to an ipsilateral motor disturbance with accompanying impairment of proprioception and contralateral loss of pain and temperature appreciation below the lesion (Brown-Séquard's syndrome). A central cord syndrome may lead to a lower motor neuron deficit and loss of pain and temperature appreciation, with sparing of posterior column functions. A radicular deficit may occur at the level of the injury—or, if the cauda equina is involved, there may be evidence of disturbed function in several lumbosacral roots.

Treatment of the injury consists of immobilization and—if there is cord compression—decompressive laminectomy and fusion. Early treatment with high doses of corticosteroids (eg, methylprednisolone, 30 mg/kg by intravenous bolus, followed by 5.4 mg/kg/h for 23 hours) has been shown to improve neurologic recovery if commenced within 8 hours after injury. Treatment with GM1 ganglioside for 3 or 4 weeks is an experimental approach that has also been helpful. Anatomic realignment of the spinal cord by traction and other orthopedic procedures is also important. Subsequent care of the residual neurologic deficit—paraplegia or quadriplegia—requires treatment of spasticity and care of the skin, bladder, and bowels.

Walker MD: Acute spinal-cord injury. (Editorial.) N Engl J Med 1991;324:1885.

SYRINGOMYELIA

Destruction or degeneration of gray and white matter adjacent to the central canal of the cervical spinal cord leads to cavitation and accumulation of fluid within the spinal cord. The precise pathogenesis is unclear, but many cases are associated with Arnold-Chiari malformation, in which there is displacement of the cerebellar tonsils, medulla, and fourth ventricle into the spinal canal, sometimes with accompanying meningomyelocele. In such circumstances, the cord cavity connects with and may merely represent a dilated central canal. In other cases, the cause of cavitation is less clear. There is a characteristic clinical picture, with segmental atrophy and areflexia and loss of pain and temperature appreciation in a "cape" distribution owing to the destruction of fibers crossing in front of the central canal. Thoracic kyphoscoliosis is usually present. With progression, involvement of the long motor and sensory tracts occurs as well, so that a pyramidal and sensory deficit develops in the legs. Upward extension of the cavitation (syringobulbia) leads to dysfunction of the lower brain stem and thus to bulbar palsy, nystagmus, and sensory impairment over one or both sides of the face.

Syringomyelia, ie, cord cavitation, may also occur in association with an intramedullary tumor or following severe cord injury, and the cavity then does not communicate with the central canal.

In patients with Arnold-Chiari malformation, there are commonly skeletal abnormalities on plain x-rays of the skull and cervical spine. CT scans show caudal displacement of the fourth ventricle. MRI or positive contrast myelography may demonstrate the malformation itself. Focal cord enlargement is found at myelography or by MRI in patients with cavitation related to past injury or intramedullary neoplasms.

Treatment of Arnold-Chiari malformation with associated syringomyelia is by suboccipital craniectomy and upper cervical laminectomy, with the aim of decompressing the malformation at the foramen magnum. The cord cavity should be drained, and if necessary an outlet for the fourth ventricle can be made. In cavitation associated with intramedullary tumor, treatment is surgical, but radiation therapy may be necessary if complete removal is not possible. Posttraumatic syringomyelia is also treated surgically if it leads to increasing neurologic deficits or to intolerable pain.

Batzdorf U: Chiari I malformation with syringomyelia: Evaluation of surgical therapy by magnetic resonance imaging. J Neurosurg 1988;68:726.

MOTOR NEURON DISEASES

This group of disorders is characterized clinically by weakness and variable wasting of affected muscles, without accompanying sensory changes. Certain of these disorders, such as Werdnig-Hoffman disease and Kugelberg-Welander syndrome, occur in infants or children and are not considered further here.

Motor neuron disease in adults generally commences between 30 and 60 years of age. There is degeneration of the anterior horn cells in the spinal cord, the motor nuclei of the lower cranial nerves, and the corticospinal and corticobulbar pathways. The disorder is usually sporadic, but familial cases may occur.

Classification

Five varieties have been distinguished on clinical grounds.

A. Progressive Bulbar Palsy: Bulbar involvement predominates owing to disease processes affecting primarily the motor nuclei of the cranial nerves.

B. Pseudobulbar Palsy: Bulbar involvement predominates in this variety also, but it is due to bilateral corticobulbar disease and thus reflects upper motor neuron dysfunction.

C. Progressive Spinal Muscular Atrophy: This is characterized primarily by a lower motor neuron deficit in the limbs due to degeneration of the anterior horn cells in the spinal cord.

D. Primary Lateral Sclerosis: There is a purely upper motor neuron deficit in the limbs.

E. Amyotrophic Lateral Sclerosis: A mixed upper and lower motor neuron deficit is found in the limbs. This disorder is sometimes associated with dementia, parkinsonism, and other neurologic diseases.

Clinical Findings

A. Symptoms and Signs: Difficulty in swallowing, chewing, coughing, breathing, and talking (dysarthria) occur with bulbar involvement. In progressive bulbar palsy, there is drooping of the palate, a depressed gag reflex, pooling of saliva in the pharynx, a weak cough, and a wasted, fasciculating tongue. In pseudobulbar palsy, the tongue is contracted and spastic and cannot be moved rapidly from side to side. Limb involvement is characterized by motor disturbances (weakness, stiffness, wasting, fasciculations) reflecting lower or upper motor neuron dysfunction; there are no objective changes on sensory examination, though there may be vague sensory complaints. The sphincters are generally spared.

The disorder is progressive and usually fatal within 3–5 years; death usually results from pulmonary infections. Patients with bulbar involvement generally have the poorest prognosis.

B. Laboratory and Other Studies: Electromyography may show changes of chronic partial denervation, with abnormal spontaneous activity in the resting muscle and a reduction in the number of motor units under voluntary control. In patients with suspected spinal muscular atrophy or amyotrophic lateral sclerosis, the diagnosis should not be made with confidence unless such changes are found in at least three extremities. Motor conduction velocity is usually normal but may be slightly reduced, and sensory conduction studies are also normal. Biopsy of a wasted muscle shows the histologic changes of denervation. The serum creatine kinase may be slightly elevated but never reaches the extremely high values seen in some of the muscular dystrophies. The cerebrospinal fluid is normal.

There have been recent reports of juvenile spinal muscular atrophy due to hexosaminidase deficiency, with abnormal findings on rectal biopsy and reduced hexosaminidase A in serum and leukocytes. Pure motor syndromes resembling motor neuron disease may also occur in association with monoclonal gammopathy or multifocal motor neuropathies due to conduction block. A motor neuronopathy may also develop in Hodgkin's disease and has a relatively benign prognosis.

Treatment

There is no specific treatment except in patients with gammopathy, in whom plasmapheresis and immunosuppression may lead to improvement. Symptomatic and supportive measures may include prescription of anticholinergic drugs (such as trihexyphenidyl, amitriptyline, or atropine) if drooling is troublesome, braces or a walker to improve mobility, and physical therapy to prevent contractures. Spasticity may be helped by baclofen or diazepam. A semiliquid diet or nasogastric tube feeding may be needed if dysphagia is severe. Gastrostomy or cricopharyngomyotomy is sometimes resorted to in extreme cases of predominant bulbar involvement, and tracheostomy may be necessary if respiratory muscles are severely affected; however, in the terminal stages of these disorders, the aim of treatment should be to keep patients as comfortable as possible.

Rowland LP (editor): *Amyotrophic Lateral Sclerosis and Other Motor Neuron Diseases.* Raven Press, 1991.

PERIPHERAL NEUROPATHIES

Peripheral neuropathies can be categorized on the basis of the structure primarily affected. The predominant pathologic feature may be axonal degeneration (axonal or neuronal neuropathies) or paranodal or segmental demyelination. The distinction may be possible on the basis of neurophysiologic findings. Motor and sensory conduction velocity can be measured in accessible segments of peripheral nerves. In axonal neuropathies, conduction velocity is normal or reduced only mildly and needle electromyography provides evidence of denervation in affected muscles. In demyelinating neuropathies, conduction may be slowed considerably in affected fibers, and in more severe cases, conduction is blocked completely, without accompanying electromyographic signs of denervation.

Peripheral neuropathies may also occur as a result of disorders affecting the connective tissues of the nerves or the blood vessels supplying the nerves, but these are much less common than the preceding varieties.

Nerves may be injured or compressed by neighboring anatomic structures at any point along their course. Common **mononeuropathies** of this sort are considered below. They lead to a sensory, motor, or mixed deficit that is restricted to the territory of the affected nerve. A similar clinical disturbance is produced by peripheral nerve tumors, but these are rare except in patients with Recklinghausen's disease. Multiple mononeuropathies suggest a patchy multifocal disease process such as vasculopathy (eg, diabetes, arteritis), an infiltrative process (eg, leprosy, sarcoidosis), radiation damage, or an immunologic disorder (eg, brachial plexopathy). Diffuse **polyneuropathies** lead to a symmetric sensory, motor, or mixed deficit, often most marked distally. They include the hereditary, metabolic, and toxic disorders; idiopathic inflammatory polyneuropathy (Guillain-Barré syndrome); and the peripheral neuropathies that may occur as a nonmetastatic complication of malignant diseases. Involvement of motor fibers leads to flaccid weakness that is most marked distally; dysfunction of sensory fibers causes impaired sensory perception. Tendon reflexes are depressed or absent. Paresthesias, pain, and muscle tenderness may also occur.

1. POLYNEUROPATHIES & MONONEURITIS MULTIPLEX

The cause of polyneuropathy or mononeuritis multiplex is suggested by the history, mode of onset, and predominant clinical manifestations. Laboratory workup includes a complete blood count and sedimentation rate, serum protein electrophoresis, determination of plasma urea and electrolytes, liver and thyroid function tests, tests for rheumatoid factor and antinuclear antibody, HBsAg determination, a serologic test for syphilis, fasting blood glucose level, urinary heavy metal levels, cerebrospinal fluid examination, and chest radiography. These tests should be ordered selectively, as guided by symptoms and signs. Measurement of nerve conduction velocity is important in confirming the peripheral nerve origin of symptoms and providing a means of following clinical changes, as well as indicating the likely disease process (ie, axonal or demyelinating neuropathy). Cutaneous nerve biopsy may help establish a precise diagnosis (eg, polyarteritis, amyloidosis). In about half of cases, no specific cause can be established; of these, slightly less than half are subsequently found to be heredofamilial.

Treatment is of the underlying cause, when feasible, and is discussed below under the individual disorders. Physical therapy helps prevent contractures, and splints can maintain a weak extremity in a position of useful function. Anesthetic extremities must be protected from injury. To guard against burns, patients should check the temperature of water and hot surfaces with a portion of skin having normal sensation, measure water temperature with a thermometer, and use cold water for washing or lower the temperature setting of their hot-water heaters. Shoes should be examined frequently during the day for grit or foreign objects in order to prevent pressure lesions.

Patients with polyneuropathies or mononeuritis multiplex are subject to additional nerve injury at pressure points and should therefore avoid such behavior as leaning on elbows or sitting with crossed legs for lengthy periods.

Neuropathic pain is sometimes troublesome and may respond to simple analgesics such as aspirin. Narcotics or narcotic substitutes may be necessary for severe hyperpathia or pain induced by minimal stimuli, but their use should be avoided as far as possible. The use of a frame or cradle to reduce contact with bedclothes may be helpful. Many patients experience episodic stabbing pains, which may respond to phenytoin, carbamazepine, or tricyclic antidepressants.

Symptoms of autonomic dysfunction are occasionally troublesome. Postural hypotension is often helped by wearing waist-high elastic stockings and sleeping in a semierect position at night. Fludrocortisone reduces postural hypotension, but doses as high as 1 mg/d are sometimes necessary in diabetics and may lead to recumbent hypertension. Indomethacin (25 or 50 mg three times daily) is sometimes helpful. Impotence and diarrhea are difficult to treat; a flaccid neuropathic bladder may respond to parasympathomimetic drugs such as bethanechol chloride, 10–50 mg three or four times daily.

Inherited Neuropathies

A. Charcot-Marie-Tooth Disease: Several distinct varieties of Charcot-Marie-Tooth disease can be recognized. There is usually an autosomal dominant mode of inheritance, but occasional cases occur on a sporadic, recessive, or X-linked basis. The responsible gene is commonly located on the short arm of chromosome 17 and less often shows linkage to chromosome 1 or the X chromosome. Clinical presentation may be with foot deformities or gait disturbances in childhood or early adult life. Slow progression leads to the typical features of polyneuropathy, with distal weakness and wasting that begin in the legs, a variable amount of distal sensory loss, and depressed or absent tendon reflexes. Tremor is a conspicuous feature in some instances. Pathologic examination reveals segmental demyelination and remyelination of peripheral nerves, an increase in their transverse fascicular area, and hyperplasia of Schwann cells. Electrodiagnostic studies show a marked reduction in motor and sensory conduction velocity (hereditary motor and sensory neuropathy [HMSN] type I).

In other instances (HMSN type II), motor conduction velocity is normal or only slightly reduced, sensory nerve action potentials may be absent, and signs of chronic partial denervation are found in affected muscles electromyographically. The predominant pathologic change is axonal loss rather than segmental demyelination.

A similar disorder may occur in patients with progressive distal spinal muscular atrophy, but there is no sensory loss; electrophysiologic investigation reveals that motor conduction velocity is normal or only slightly reduced, and nerve action potentials are normal.

B. Dejerine-Sottas Disease (HMSN Type III): Most cases are sporadic or autosomal recessive. The recessive form has its onset in infancy or childhood and leads to a progressive motor and sensory polyneuropathy with weakness, ataxia, sensory loss, and depressed or absent tendon reflexes. The peripheral nerves may be palpably enlarged and are characterized pathologically by segmental demyelination, Schwann cell hyperplasia, and thin myelin sheaths. Electrophysiologically, there is slowing of conduction, and sensory action potentials may be unrecordable.

C. Friedreich's Ataxia: Patients generally present in childhood or early adult life with this autosomal recessive disorder. The gait becomes ataxic, the hands become clumsy, and other signs of cerebellar dysfunction develop accompanied by weakness of the legs and extensor plantar responses. Involvement of peripheral sensory fibers leads to sensory disturbances in the limbs and depressed tendon reflexes. There is bilateral pes cavus. Pathologically, there is a marked loss of cells in the posterior root ganglia and degeneration of peripheral sensory fibers. In the central nervous system, changes are conspicuous in the posterior and lateral columns of the cord. Electrophysiologically, conduction velocity in motor fibers is normal or only mildly reduced, but sensory action potentials are small or absent.

D. Refsum's Disease (HMSN Type IV): This autosomal recessive disorder is due to a disturbance in phytanic acid metabolism. Clinically, pigmentary retinal degeneration is accompanied by progressive sensorimotor polyneuropathy and cerebellar signs. Auditory dysfunction, cardiomyopathy, and cutaneous manifestations may also occur. Motor and sensory conduction velocity is reduced, often markedly, and there may be electromyographic evidence of denervation in affected muscles. Dietary restriction of phytanic acid and its precursors may be helpful therapeutically.

E. Porphyria: Peripheral nerve involvement may occur during acute attacks in both variegate porphyria and acute intermittent porphyria. Motor symptoms usually occur first, and weakness is often most marked proximally and in the upper limbs rather than the lower. Sensory symptoms and signs may be proximal or distal in distribution. Autonomic involvement

is sometimes pronounced. The electrophysiologic findings are in keeping with the results of neuropathologic studies suggesting that the neuropathy is axonal in type. Hematin (4 mg/kg intravenously over 15 minutes once or twice daily) may lead to rapid improvement. A high-carbohydrate diet and, in severe cases, intravenous glucose or levulose may also be helpful. Propranolol (up to 100 mg every 4 hours) may control tachycardia and hypertension in acute attacks. Porphyria is discussed further in Chapter 22.

Neuropathies Associated With Systemic & Metabolic Disorders

A. Diabetes Mellitus: In this disorder, involvement of the peripheral nervous system may lead to symmetric sensory or mixed polyneuropathy, asymmetric motor neuropathy (diabetic amyotrophy), thoracoabdominal radiculopathy, autonomic neuropathy, or isolated lesions of individual nerves. These may occur singly or in any combination.

Sensory polyneuropathy, the most common manifestation, may lead to no more than depressed tendon reflexes and impaired appreciation of vibration in the legs. When symptomatic, there may be pain, paresthesias, or numbness in the legs, but in severe cases distal sensory loss occurs in all limbs. Diabetic amyotrophy is characterized by asymmetric weakness and wasting involving predominantly the proximal muscles of the legs, accompanied by local pain. Thoracoabdominal radiculopathy leads to pain over the trunk. In patients with autonomic neuropathy, postural hypotension, impaired thermoregulatory sweating, postgustatory hyperhidrosis, constipation, flatulence, diarrhea, impotence, urinary retention, and incontinence may occur, and there may be abnormal pupillary responses. Isolated lesions of individual peripheral nerves are common and in the limbs tend to occur at sites of compression or entrapment. Treatment is symptomatic. Entrapment neuropathies may be helped by surgical decompression. Treatment of neuropathic pain is discussed above.

B. Uremia: Uremia may lead to a symmetric sensorimotor polyneuropathy that tends to affect the lower limbs more than the upper limbs and is more marked distally than proximally. The diagnosis can be confirmed electrophysiologically, for motor and sensory conduction velocity is moderately reduced. The neuropathy improves both clinically and electrophysiologically with renal transplantation and to a lesser extent with chronic dialysis.

C. Alcoholism and Nutritional Deficiency: Many alcoholics have an axonal distal sensorimotor polyneuropathy that is frequently accompanied by painful cramps, muscle tenderness, and painful paresthesias and is often more marked in the legs than in the arms. Symptoms of autonomic dysfunction may also be conspicuous. Motor and sensory conduction velocity may be slightly reduced, even in subclinical cases, but gross slowing of conduction is uncommon.

A similar distal sensorimotor polyneuropathy is a well-recognized feature of beriberi (thiamin deficiency). In vitamin B_{12} deficiency, distal sensory polyneuropathy may develop but is usually overshadowed by central nervous system manifestations (eg, myelopathy, optic neuropathy, or intellectual changes).

D. Paraproteinemias: A symmetric sensorimotor polyneuropathy that is gradual in onset, progressive in course, and often accompanied by pain and dysesthesias in the limbs may occur in patients (especially men) with multiple myeloma. The neuropathy is of the axonal type in classic lytic myeloma, but segmental demyelination (primary or secondary) and axonal loss may occur in sclerotic myeloma and lead to predominantly motor clinical manifestations. Both demyelinating and axonal neuropathies are also observed in patients with paraproteinemias without myeloma. A small fraction will develop myeloma if serially followed. The demyelinating neuropathy in these patients may be due to the monoclonal protein's reacting to a component of the nerve myelin. The neuropathy of classic multiple myeloma is poorly responsive to therapy. The polyneuropathy of benign monoclonal gammopathy may respond to immunosuppressant drugs and plasmapheresis.

Polyneuropathy may also occur in association with macroglobulinemia and cryoglobulinemia and sometimes responds to plasmapheresis. Entrapment neuropathy, such as carpal tunnel syndrome, is more common than polyneuropathy in patients with (nonhereditary) generalized amyloidosis. With polyneuropathy due to amyloidosis, sensory and autonomic symptoms are especially conspicuous, whereas distal wasting and weakness occur later; there is no specific treatment.

Neuropathies Associated With Infectious & Inflammatory Diseases

A. Leprosy: Leprosy is an important cause of peripheral neuropathy in certain parts of the world. Sensory disturbances are mainly due to involvement of intracutaneous nerves. In tuberculoid leprosy, they develop at the same time and in the same distribution as the skin lesion but may be more extensive if nerve trunks lying beneath the lesion are also involved. In lepromatous leprosy, there is more extensive sensory loss, and this develops earlier and to a greater extent in the coolest regions of the body, such as the dorsal surfaces of the hands and feet, where the bacilli proliferate most actively. Motor deficits result from involvement of superficial nerves where their temperature is lowest, eg, the ulnar nerve in the region proximal to the olecranon groove, the median nerve as it emerges from beneath the forearm flexor muscle to run toward the carpal tunnel, the peroneal nerve at the head of the fibula, and the posterior tibial nerve in the lower part of the leg; patchy facial muscular weakness may also occur owing to involvement of the superficial branches of the seventh cranial nerve.

Motor disturbances in leprosy are suggestive of multiple mononeuropathy, whereas sensory changes resemble those of distal polyneuropathy. Examination, however, relates the distribution of sensory deficits to the temperature of the tissues; in the legs, for example, sparing frequently occurs between the toes and in the popliteal fossae, where the temperature is higher. Treatment is with antileprotic agents (see Chapter 32).

B. AIDS: A variety of neuropathies occur in HIV-infected patients. Patients with AIDS may develop a chronic symmetric sensorimotor axonal **polyneuropathy** associated usually with no abnormal cerebrospinal fluid findings. Treatment is symptomatic. AIDS patients may also develop progressive **polyradiculopathy** or radiculomyelopathy that leads to leg weakness and urinary retention; sensory loss is less conspicuous than in polyneuropathy. The cerebrospinal fluid may show mononuclear pleocytosis and increased protein and low glucose concentrations. Cytomegalovirus is responsible in at least some cases. The prognosis is generally poor, but some patients respond to intravenous ganciclovir (2.5 mg/kg every 8 hours for 10 days, then 7.5 mg/kg daily 5 days per week).

An inflammatory **demyelinating polyradiculoneuropathy** sometimes occurs in HIV-seropositive patients without AIDS and may follow an acute, subacute, or chronic course. Weakness is usually more conspicuous distally than proximally and tends to overshadow sensory symptoms. Tendon reflexes are depressed or absent. The cerebrospinal fluid shows an increased cell count and protein concentration. Treatment with plasmapheresis has helped some patients. Spontaneous improvement may also occur. Seropositive patients without AIDS may also develop a **mononeuropathy multiplex** that sometimes responds to treatment with plasmapheresis.

C. Lyme Borreliosis: The neurologic manifestations of Lyme disease include meningitis, meningoencephalitis, polyradiculoneuropathy, mononeuropathy multiplex, and cranial neuropathy. Serologic tests establish the underlying disorder. Treatment is as described in Chapter 33.

D. Sarcoidosis: Cranial nerve palsies (especially facial palsy), multiple mononeuropathy, and, less commonly, symmetric polyneuropathy may all occur, the latter sometimes preferentially affecting either motor or sensory fibers. Improvement may occur with use of corticosteroids.

E. Polyarteritis: Involvement of the vasa nervorum by the vasculitic process may result in infarction of the nerve. Clinically, one encounters an asymmetric sensorimotor polyneuropathy (mononeuritis multiplex) that pursues a waxing and waning course. Steroids and cytotoxic agents—especially cyclophosphamide—may be of benefit in severe cases.

F. Rheumatoid Arthritis: Compressive or entrapment neuropathies, ischemic neuropathies, mild distal sensory polyneuropathy, and severe progressive sensorimotor polyneuropathy can occur in rheumatoid arthritis.

Toxic Neuropathies

Axonal polyneuropathy may follow exposure to industrial agents or pesticides such as acrylamide, organophosphorus compounds, hexacarbon solvents, methyl bromide, and carbon disulfide; metals such as arsenic, thallium, mercury, and lead; and drugs such as phenytoin, perhexiline, isoniazid, nitrofurantoin, vincristine, and pyridoxine in high doses. Detailed occupational, environmental, and medical histories and recognition of clusters of cases are important in suggesting the diagnosis. Treatment is by preventing further exposure to the causal agent. Isoniazid neuropathy is prevented by pyridoxine supplementation.

Diphtheritic neuropathy results from a neurotoxin released by the causative organism and is common in many areas. Palatal weakness may develop 2–4 weeks after infection of the throat, and infection of the skin may similarly be followed by focal weakness of neighboring muscles. Disturbances of accommodation may occur about 4–5 weeks after infection and distal sensorimotor demyelinating polyneuropathy after 1–3 months.

Neuropathies Associated With Malignant Diseases

Both a sensorimotor and a purely sensory polyneuropathy may occur as a nonmetastatic complication of malignant diseases. The sensorimotor polyneuropathy may be mild and occur in the course of known malignant disease; or it may have an acute or subacute onset, lead to severe disability, and occur before there is any clinical evidence of the cancer, occasionally following a remitting course.

Acute Idiopathic Polyneuropathy (Guillain-Barré Syndrome)

This acute or subacute polyradiculoneuropathy sometimes follows infective illness, inoculations, or surgical procedures. There is an association with preceding *Campylobacter jejuni* enteritis. The disorder probably has an immunologic basis, but the precise mechanism is unclear. The main complaint is of weakness that varies widely in severity in different patients and often has a proximal emphasis and symmetric distribution. It usually begins in the legs, spreading to a variable extent but frequently involving the arms and often one or both sides of the face. The muscles of respiration or deglutition may also be affected. Sensory symptoms are usually less conspicuous than motor ones, but distal paresthesias and dysesthesias are common, and neuropathic or radicular

pain is present in many patients. Autonomic disturbances are also common, may be severe, and are sometimes life-threatening; they include tachycardia, cardiac irregularities, hypotension or hypertension, facial flushing, abnormalities of sweating, pulmonary dysfunction, and impaired sphincter control.

The cerebrospinal fluid characteristically contains a high protein concentration with a normal cell content, but these changes may take 2 or 3 weeks to develop. Electrophysiologic studies may reveal marked abnormalities, which do not necessarily parallel the clinical disorder in their temporal course. Pathologic examination has shown that primary demyelination occurs in regions infiltrated with inflammatory cells, and it seems probable that myelin disruption has an autoimmune basis.

When the diagnosis is made, the history and appropriate laboratory studies should exclude the possibility of porphyric, diphtheritic, or toxic (heavy metal, hexacarbon, organophosphate) neuropathies. Poliomyelitis, botulism, and tick paralysis must also be considered. The presence of pyramidal signs, a markedly asymmetric motor deficit, a sharp sensory level, or early sphincter involvement should suggest a focal cord lesion.

Most patients eventually make a good recovery, but this may take many months, and 10–20% patients are left with persisting disability. Treatment with prednisone is ineffective and may actually affect the outcome adversely by prolonging recovery time. Plasmapheresis is of value; it is best performed within the first few days of illness and is best reserved for clinically severe or rapidly progressive cases or those with ventilatory impairment. Intravenous immunoglobulin (400 mg/kg/d for 5 days) is also helpful and imposes less stress on the cardiovascular system than plasmapheresis. Patients should be admitted to intensive care units if their forced vital capacity is declining, and intubation should be considered if the forced vital capacity reaches 15 mL/kg, dyspnea becomes evident, or the oxygen saturation declines. Respiratory toilet and chest physical therapy help prevent atelectasis. Marked hypotension may respond to volume replacement or pressor agents. Frequent turning of the patient helps prevent decubitus ulcers, and physical therapy helps prevent contractures. Low-dose heparin to prevent pulmonary embolism should be considered.

Approximately 3% of patients with acute idiopathic polyneuropathy have one or more clinically similar relapses, sometimes several years after the initial illness. Plasma exchange therapy may produce improvement in chronic and relapsing inflammatory polyneuropathy.

Chronic Inflammatory Polyneuropathy

Chronic inflammatory demyelinating polyneuropathy, an acquired immunologically mediated disorder, is clinically similar to Guillain-Barré syndrome except that it has a relapsing or steadily progressive course over months or years. In the relapsing form, partial recovery may occur after some relapses, but in other instances there is no recovery between exacerbations. Although remission may occur spontaneously with time, the disorder frequently follows a progressive downhill course leading to severe functional disability.

Electrodiagnostic studies show marked slowing of motor and sensory conduction, and focal conduction block. Signs of partial denervation may also be present owing to secondary axonal degeneration. Nerve biopsy may show chronic perivascular inflammatory infiltrates in the endoneurium and epineurium, without accompanying evidence of vasculitis. However, a normal nerve biopsy result or the presence of nonspecific abnormalities does not exclude the diagnosis.

Corticosteroids may be effective in arresting or reversing the downhill course. Treatment is usually begun with prednisone, 60 mg daily, continued for 2–3 months or until a definite response has occurred. If no response has occurred despite 3 months of treatment, a higher dose may be tried. In responsive cases, the dose is gradually tapered, but most patients become corticosteroid-dependent, often requiring prednisone, 20 mg daily on alternate days, on a long-term basis. Patients unresponsive to corticosteroids may benefit instead from treatment with a cytotoxic drug such as azathioprine. There are increasing anecdotal reports of short-term benefit with plasmapheresis; high-dose intravenous immunoglobulin treatment (eg, 400 mg/kg/d) may produce clinical improvement lasting for weeks to months.

Greene DA et al: Diabetic neuropathy. Annu Rev Med 1990;41:303.

Hallam PJ et al: Duplication of part of chromosome 17 is commonly associated with hereditary motor and sensory neuropathy type 1 (Charcot-Marie-Tooth disease type 1). Ann Neurol 1992;31:570.

Logigian EL et al: Chronic neurologic manifestations of Lyme disease. N Engl J Med 1990;323:1438. (Clinical features in 27 cases.)

Ropper AH: The Guillain-Barré syndrome. N Engl J Med 1992;326:1130.

Simpson DM, Olney RK: Peripheral neuropathies associated with human immunodeficiency virus infection. Neurol Clin 1992;10:685.

2. MONONEUROPATHIES

An individual nerve may be injured along its course or may be compressed, angulated, or stretched by neighboring anatomic structures, especially at a point where it passes through a narrow space (entrapment neuropathy). The relative contributions of mechanical factors and ischemia to the local damage are not clear. With involvement of a sensory or mixed nerve, pain is commonly felt distal to the lesion. Symptoms never develop with some entrapment neuropathies, resolve rapidly and spontaneously in others, and become progressively more disabling and distressing in yet other cases. The precise neurologic deficit depends on the nerve involved. Percussion of the nerve at the site of the lesion may lead to paresthesias in its distal distribution.

Entrapment neuropathy may be the sole manifestation of subclinical polyneuropathy, and this must be borne in mind and excluded by nerve conduction studies. Such studies are also indispensable for the accurate localization of the focal lesion.

In patients with acute compression neuropathy such as Saturday night palsy, no treatment is necessary. Complete recovery generally occurs, usually within 2 months, presumably because the underlying pathology is demyelination. However, axonal degeneration can occur in severe cases, and recovery then takes longer and may never be complete.

In chronic compressive or entrapment neuropathies, avoidance of aggravating factors and correction of any underlying systemic conditions is important. Local infiltration of the region about the nerve with corticosteroids may be of value; in addition, surgical decompression may help if there is a progressively increasing neurologic deficit or if electrodiagnostic studies show evidence of partial denervation in weak muscles.

Peripheral nerve tumors are uncommon, except in Recklinghausen's disease, but also give rise to mononeuropathy. This may be distinguishable from entrapment neuropathy only by noting the presence of a mass along the course of the nerve and by demonstrating the precise site of the lesion with appropriate electrophysiologic studies. Treatment of symptomatic lesions is by surgical removal if possible.

Carpal Tunnel Syndrome
See Chapter 19.

Pronator Teres or Anterior Interosseous Syndrome

The median nerve gives off its motor branch, the anterior interosseous nerve, below the elbow as it descends between the two heads of the pronator teres muscle. A lesion of either nerve may occur in this region, sometimes after trauma or owing to compression from, for example, a fibrous band. With anterior interosseous nerve involvement, there is no sensory loss, and weakness is confined to the pronator quadratus, flexor pollicis longus, and the flexor digitorum profundus to the second and third digits. Weakness is more widespread and sensory changes occur in an appropriate distribution when the median nerve itself is affected. The prognosis is variable. If improvement does not occur spontaneously, decompressive surgery may be helpful.

Ulnar Nerve Lesions

Ulnar nerve lesions are likely to occur in the elbow region as the nerve runs behind the medial epicondyle and descends into the cubital tunnel. In the condylar groove, the ulnar nerve is exposed to pressure or trauma. Moreover, any increase in the carrying angle of the elbow, whether congenital, degenerative, or traumatic, may cause excessive stretching of the nerve when the elbow is flexed. Ulnar nerve lesions may also result from thickening or distortion of the anatomic structures forming the cubital tunnel, and the resulting symptoms may also be aggravated by flexion of the elbow, because the tunnel is then narrowed by tightening of its roof or inward bulging of its floor. A severe lesion at either site causes sensory changes in the medial 1½ digits and along the medial border of the hand. There is weakness of the ulnar-innervated muscles in the forearm and hand. With a cubital tunnel lesion, however, there may be relative sparing of the flexor carpi ulnaris muscle. Electrophysiologic evaluation using nerve stimulation techniques allows more precise localization of the lesion.

If conservative measures are unsuccessful in relieving symptoms and preventing further progression, surgical treatment may be necessary. This consists of nerve transposition if the lesion is in the condylar groove, or a release procedure if it is in the cubital tunnel.

Ulnar nerve lesions may also develop at the wrist or in the palm of the hand, usually owing to repetitive trauma or to compression from ganglia or benign tumors. They can be subdivided depending upon their presumed site. Compressive lesions are treated surgically. If repetitive mechanical trauma is responsible, this is avoided by occupational adjustment or job retraining.

Radial Nerve Lesions

The radial nerve is particularly liable to compression or injury in the axilla (eg, by crutches or by pressure when the arm hangs over the back of a chair). This leads to weakness or paralysis of all the muscles supplied by the nerve, including the triceps. Sensory changes may also occur but are often surprisingly inconspicuous, being marked only in a small area on the back of the hand between the thumb and index finger. Injuries to the radial nerve in the spiral groove occur characteristically during deep sleep, as in intoxicated individuals (Saturday night palsy), and there is then sparing of the triceps muscle, which is supplied more proximally. The nerve may also be injured at or above the elbow; its purely motor posterior interosseous branch, supplying the extensors of the wrist and fingers, may be involved immediately below the elbow, but then there is sparing of the extensor carpi radialis longus, so that the wrist can still be extended. The superficial radial nerve may be compressed by handcuffs or a tight watch strap.

Femoral Neuropathy

The clinical features of femoral nerve palsy consist of weakness and wasting of the quadriceps muscle, with sensory impairment over the anteromedian aspect of the thigh and sometimes also of the leg to the medial malleolus, and a depressed or absent knee jerk. Isolated femoral neuropathy may occur in diabetics or from compression by retroperitoneal neoplasms or hematomas (eg, expanding aortic aneurysm). Femoral neuropathy may also result from pressure from the inguinal ligament when the thighs are markedly flexed and abducted, as in the lithotomy position.

Meralgia Paresthetica

The lateral femoral cutaneous nerve, a sensory nerve arising from the L2 and L3 roots, may be compressed or stretched in obese or diabetic patients and during pregnancy. The nerve usually runs under the outer portion of the inguinal ligament to reach the thigh, but the ligament sometimes splits to enclose it. Hyperextension of the hip or increased lumbar lordosis—such as occurs during pregnancy—leads to nerve compression by the posterior fascicle of the ligament. However, entrapment of the nerve at any point along its course may cause similar symptoms, and several other anatomic variations predispose the nerve to damage when it is stretched. Pain, paresthesia, or numbness occurs about the outer aspect of the thigh, usually unilaterally, and is sometimes relieved by sitting. Examination shows no abnormalities except in severe cases when cutaneous sensation is impaired in the affected area. Symptoms are usually mild and commonly settle spontaneously, so patients can be reassured about the benign nature of the disorder. Hydrocortisone injections about the nerve where it lies medial to the anterosuperior iliac spine often relieve symptoms temporarily, while nerve decompression by transposition may provide more lasting relief.

Sciatic & Common Peroneal Nerve Palsies

Misplaced deep intramuscular injections are probably still the most common cause of sciatic nerve palsy. Trauma to the buttock, hip, or thigh may also be responsible. The resulting clinical deficit depends on whether the whole nerve has been affected or only certain fibers. In general, the peroneal fibers of the sciatic nerve are more susceptible to damage than those destined for the tibial nerve. A sciatic nerve lesion may therefore be difficult to distinguish from peroneal neuropathy unless there is electromyographic evidence of involvement of the short head of the biceps femoris muscle. The common peroneal nerve itself may be compressed or injured in the region of the head and neck of the fibula, eg, by sitting with crossed legs or wearing high boots. There is weakness of dorsiflexion and eversion of the foot, accompanied by numbness or blunted sensation of the anterolateral aspect of the calf and dorsum of the foot.

Tarsal Tunnel Syndrome

The tibial nerve, the other branch of the sciatic, supplies several muscles in the lower extremity, gives origin to the sural nerve, and then continues as the posterior tibial nerve to supply the plantar flexors of the foot and toes. It passes through the tarsal tunnel behind and below the medial malleolus, giving off calcaneal branches and the medial and lateral plantar nerves that supply small muscles of the foot and the skin on the plantar aspect of the foot and toes. Compression of the posterior tibial nerve or its branches between the bony floor and ligamentous roof of the tarsal tunnel leads to pain, paresthesias, and numbness over the bottom of the foot, especially at night, with sparing of the heel. Muscle weakness may be hard to recognize clinically. Compressive lesions of the individual plantar nerves may also occur more distally, with similar clinical features to those of the tarsal tunnel syndrome. Treatment is surgical decompression.

Stewart J: *Focal Peripheral Neuropathies.* Elsevier Science, 1987.

Facial Neuropathy

An isolated facial palsy may occur in patients with HIV seropositivity, sarcoidosis, or Lyme disease (Chapter 33), but most often it is idiopathic (Bell's palsy).

3. BELL'S PALSY

Bell's palsy is an idiopathic facial paresis of lower motor neuron type that has been attributed to an inflammatory reaction involving the facial nerve near the stylomastoid foramen or in the bony facial canal. A relationship of Bell's palsy to reactivation of herpes simplex virus has recently been suggested, but there is little evidence to support this.

The clinical features of Bell's palsy are characteristic. The facial paresis generally comes on abruptly, but it may worsen over the following day or so. Pain about the ear precedes or accompanies the weakness in many cases but usually lasts for only a few days. The face itself feels stiff and pulled to one side. There may be ipsilateral restriction of eye closure and difficulty with eating and fine facial movements. A disturbance of taste is common, owing to involvement of chorda tympani fibers, and hyperacusis due to involvement of fibers to the stapedius occurs occasionally.

The management of Bell's palsy is controversial. Approximately 60% of cases recover completely without treatment, presumably because the lesion is so mild that it leads merely to conduction block. Considerable improvement occurs in most other cases, and only about 10% of all patients are seriously dissatisfied with the final outcome because of permanent disfigurement or other long-term sequelae. Treatment is unnecessary in most cases but is indicated for patients in whom an unsatisfactory outcome can be predicted. The best clinical guide to progress is the severity of the palsy during the first few days after presentation. Patients with clinically complete palsy when first seen are less likely to make a full recovery than those with an incomplete one. A poor prognosis for recovery is also associated with advanced age, hyperacusis, and severe initial pain. Electromyography and nerve excitability or conduction studies provide a guide to prognosis but not early enough to aid in the selection of patients for treatment.

The only medical treatment that may influence the outcome is administration of corticosteroids, but studies supporting this concept have been criticized. Many physicians nevertheless routinely prescribe corticosteroids for patients with Bell's palsy seen within 5 days of onset. The author prescribes them only when the palsy is clinically complete or there is severe pain. Treatment with prednisone, 60 or 80 mg daily in divided doses for 4 or 5 days, followed by tapering of the dose over the next 7–10 days, is a satisfactory regimen. It is helpful to protect the eye with lubricating drops (or lubricating ointment at night) and a patch if eye closure is not possible. There is no evidence that surgical procedures to decompress the facial nerve are of benefit.

DISCOGENIC NECK & BACK PAIN
(See also Chapter 19.)

1. LOW BACK PAIN

Spinal disease may lead to local pain, root pain, or both. It may also lead to pain that is referred to other parts of the involved dermatomes. Local pain may lead to protective reflex muscle spasm, which in turn causes further pain and may result in abnormal posture and limitation of movement. Radicular pain arises from compression, stretch, or irritation of nerve roots and usually radiates from the back to the territory of the affected root, being exacerbated by coughing, straining, or stretching of the nerve fibers, eg, by straight leg raising. Root disturbances may also lead to paresthesias and numbness in dermatomal (as opposed to peripheral nerve) distribution (Figure 23–1) and to weakness in segmental distribution; reflex changes may accompany involvement of motor or sensory fibers. Only pain due to disk disease is considered here; other causes have been considered in Chapter 19.

PERIPHERAL NERVE

NERVE ROOT

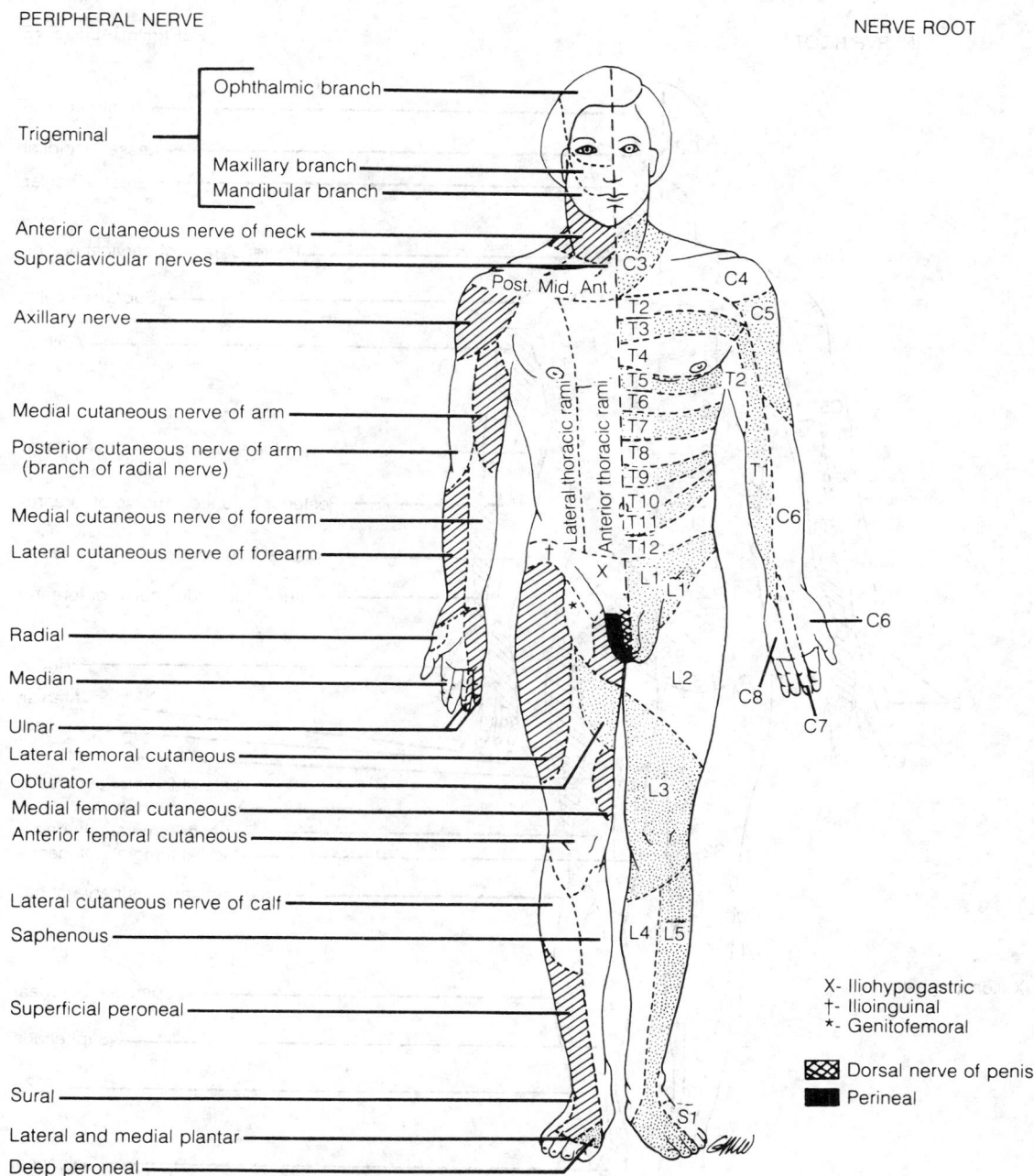

Trigeminal
- Ophthalmic branch
- Maxillary branch
- Mandibular branch

Anterior cutaneous nerve of neck

Supraclavicular nerves

Axillary nerve

Medial cutaneous nerve of arm

Posterior cutaneous nerve of arm
 (branch of radial nerve)

Medial cutaneous nerve of forearm

Lateral cutaneous nerve of forearm

Radial

Median

Ulnar

Lateral femoral cutaneous

Obturator

Medial femoral cutaneous

Anterior femoral cutaneous

Lateral cutaneous nerve of calf

Saphenous

Superficial peroneal

Sural

Lateral and medial plantar

Deep peroneal

Post. Mid. Ant.

Lateral thoracic rami

Anterior thoracic rami

C3 C4 C5
T2 T3 T4 T5 T6 T7 T8 T9 T10 T11 T12
T2 T1 C6 C7 C8
L1 L2 L3 L4 L5
X
S1

C6

X- Iliohypogastric
†- Ilioinguinal
*- Genitofemoral

Dorsal nerve of penis

Perineal

Figure 23–1. Cutaneous innervation (anterior view). The segmental or radicular (root) distribution is shown on the left side of the body and the peripheral nerve distribution on the right side. ***Above:*** anterior view; ***facing page:*** posterior view. (Reproduced, with permission, from Greenberg DA, Aminoff MJ, Simon RP: *Clinical Neurology,* 2nd ed. Appleton & Lange, 1993.)

NERVE ROOT

PERIPHERAL NERVE

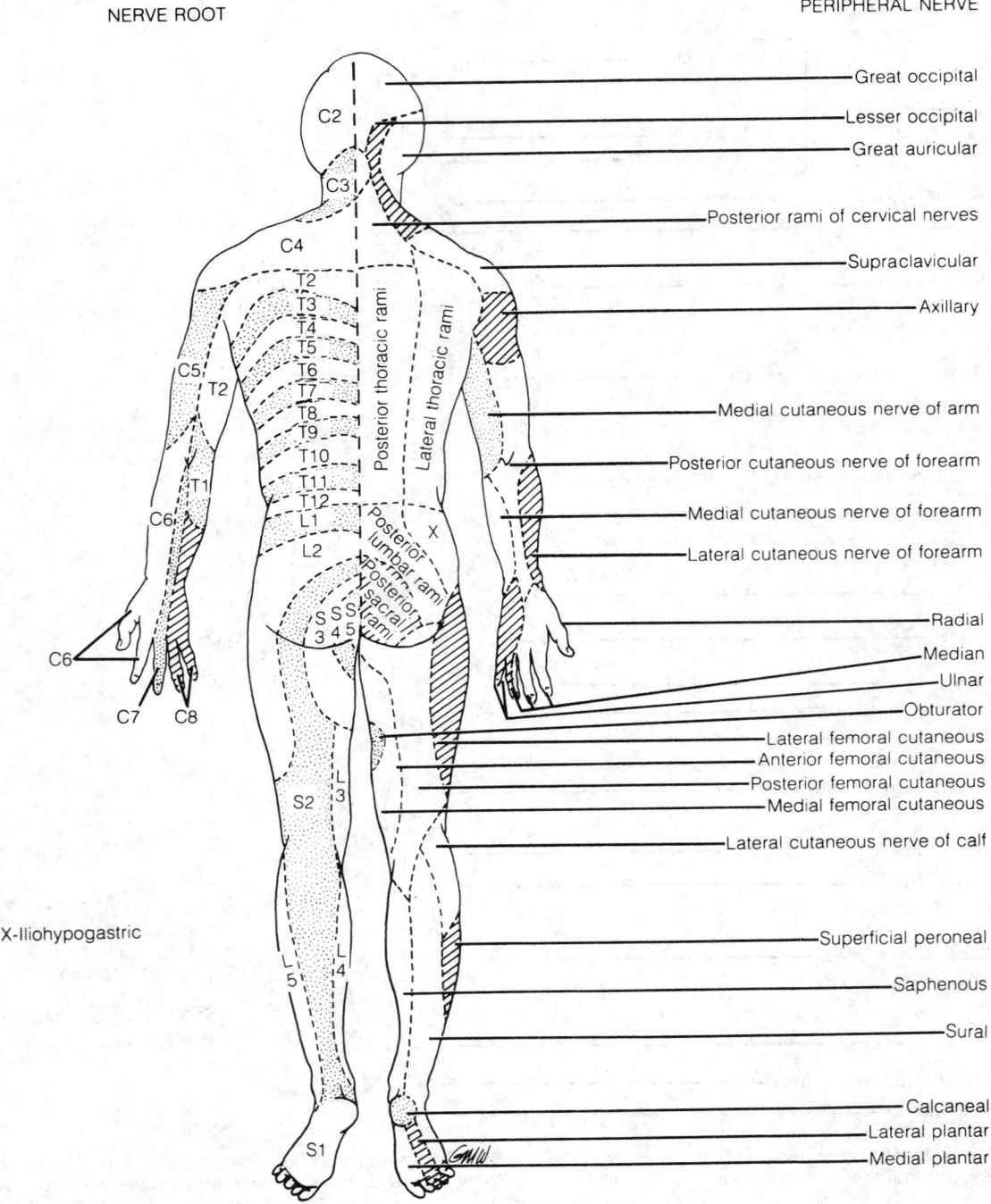

- Great occipital
- Lesser occipital
- Great auricular
- Posterior rami of cervical nerves
- Supraclavicular
- Axillary
- Medial cutaneous nerve of arm
- Posterior cutaneous nerve of forearm
- Medial cutaneous nerve of forearm
- Lateral cutaneous nerve of forearm
- Radial
- Median
- Ulnar
- Obturator
- Lateral femoral cutaneous
- Anterior femoral cutaneous
- Posterior femoral cutaneous
- Medial femoral cutaneous
- Lateral cutaneous nerve of calf
- Superficial peroneal
- Saphenous
- Sural
- Calcaneal
- Lateral plantar
- Medial plantar

X-Iliohypogastric

Figure 23–1. (continued)

Acute Lumbar Intervertebral Disk Prolapse

This cause of low back pain generally involves the L4–5 or the L5–S1 disk and leads to back and radicular (L5 or S1) pain. The L4 root is occasionally affected, but involvement of a higher lumbar root should arouse suspicion of other causes of root compression. There may be accompanying numbness and paresthesias in dermatomal distribution or segmental motor deficit. An L5 radiculopathy causes weakness of dorsiflexion of the foot and toes. With an S1 root lesion, there is weakness of eversion and plantar flexion of the foot and a depressed ankle jerk. A centrally prolapsed disk may lead to bilateral limb disturbances and sphincter involvement. Pelvic and rectal examination and plain x-rays of the spine help to exclude other disorders such as local primary cancers or metastatic deposits. Symptoms are often relieved with simple analgesics, diazepam, and bed rest on a firm mattress. Persisting pain, an increasing neurologic deficit, or any evidence of sphincter dysfunction calls for investigation by CT myelography—or, preferably, by MRI—followed by surgical treatment. The role of percutaneous discectomy is currently under study as an alternative to operative treatment.

Degenerative Lumbar Osteoarthropathy & Chronic Disk Degeneration

This process leads to local pain, stiffness, and restricted activity. The radiologic findings vary from minor degenerative abnormalities to marked osteophytic spurs, ridges, and other changes. Even minor changes may lead to root or cord dysfunction when there is also a congenitally narrowed spinal canal (spinal stenosis). Pain, sometimes accompanied by weakness or radicular sensory disturbances in the legs, then occurs with activity or with certain postures and is relieved by rest. This has been referred to as neurogenic claudication; surgical decompression may be helpful in selected cases.

Onik G et al: Automated percutaneous discectomy: A prospective multi-institutional study. Neurosurgery 1990; 26:228.

2. NECK PAIN

A variety of congenital abnormalities may involve the cervical spine and lead to neck pain; these include hemivertebrae, fused vertebrae, basilar impression, and instability of the atlantoaxial joint. Traumatic, degenerative, infective, and neoplastic disorders may also lead to pain in the neck. When rheumatoid arthritis involves the spine, it tends to affect especially the cervical region, leading to pain, stiffness, and reduced mobility; displacement of vertebrae or atlantoaxial subluxation may lead to cord compression that can be life-threatening if not treated by fixation. Further details are given in Chapter 19, and discussion here is restricted to disk disease.

Acute Cervical Disk Protrusion

Acute cervical disk protrusion leads to pain in the neck and radicular pain in the arm, exacerbated by head movement. With lateral herniation of the disk, motor, sensory, or reflex changes may be found in a radicular (usually C6 or C7) distribution on the affected side; with more centrally directed herniations, the spinal cord may also be involved, leading to spastic paraparesis and sensory disturbances in the legs, sometimes accompanied by impaired sphincter function. The diagnosis is confirmed by MRI or CT myelography. In mild cases, bed rest or intermittent neck traction may help, followed by immobilization of the neck in a collar for several weeks. If these measures are unsuccessful or the patient has a significant neurologic deficit, surgical removal of the protruding disk may be necessary.

Cervical Spondylosis

Cervical spondylosis results from chronic cervical disk degeneration, with herniation of disk material, secondary calcification, and associated osteophytic outgrowths. One or more of the cervical nerve roots may be compressed, stretched, or angulated; and myelopathy may also develop as a result of compression, vascular insufficiency, or recurrent minor trauma to the cord. Patients present with neck pain and restricted head movement, occipital headaches, radicular pain and other sensory disturbances in the arms, weakness of the arms or legs, or some combination of these symptoms. Examination generally reveals that lateral flexion and rotation of the neck are limited. A segmental pattern of weakness or dermatomal sensory loss (or both) may be found unilaterally or bilaterally in the upper limbs, and tendon reflexes mediated by the affected root or roots are depressed. The C5 and C6 nerve roots are most commonly involved, and examination frequently then reveals weakness of muscles supplied by these roots (eg, deltoids, supra- and infraspinatus, biceps, brachioradialis), pain or sensory loss about the shoulder and outer border of the arm and forearm, and depressed biceps and brachioradialis reflexes. Spastic paraparesis may also be present if there is an associated myelopathy, sometimes accompanied by posterior column or spinothalamic sensory deficits in the legs.

Plain radiographs of the cervical spine show osteophyte formation, narrowing of disk spaces, and encroachment on the intervertebral foramina, but such changes are common in middle-aged persons and may be unrelated to the presenting complaint. CT or MRI helps to confirm the diagnosis and exclude other structural causes of the myelopathy.

Restriction of neck movements by a cervical collar may relieve pain. Operative treatment may be necessary to prevent further progression if there is a significant neurologic deficit or if root pain is severe, persistent, and unresponsive to conservative measures.

BRACHIAL & LUMBAR PLEXUS LESIONS

Brachial Plexus Neuropathy

Brachial plexus neuropathy may be idiopathic, sometimes occurring in relationship to a number of different nonspecific illnesses or factors. In other instances, brachial plexus lesions follow trauma or result from congenital anomalies, neoplastic involvement, or injury by various physical agents. In rare instances, the disorder occurs on a familial basis.

Idiopathic brachial plexus neuropathy (neuralgic amyotrophy) characteristically begins with severe pain about the shoulder, followed within a few days by weakness, reflex changes, and sensory disturbances involving especially the C5 and C6 segments. Symptoms and signs are usually unilateral but may be bilateral. Wasting of affected muscles is sometimes profound. The disorder relates to disturbed function of cervical roots or part of the brachial plexus, but its precise cause is unknown. Recovery occurs over the ensuing months but may be incomplete. Treatment is purely symptomatic.

Cervical Rib Syndrome

Compression of the C8 and T1 roots or the lower trunk of the brachial plexus by a cervical rib or band arising from the seventh cervical vertebra leads to weakness and wasting of intrinsic hand muscles, especially those in the thenar eminence, accompanied by pain and numbness in the medial two fingers and the ulnar border of the hand and forearm. The subclavian artery may also be compressed, and this forms the basis of Adson's test for diagnosing the disorder; the radial pulse is diminished or obliterated on the affected side when the seated patient inhales deeply and turns the head to one side or the other. Electromyography, nerve conduction studies, and somatosensory evoked potential studies may help confirm the diagnosis. X-rays sometimes show the cervical rib or a large transverse process of the seventh cervical vertebra, but normal findings do not exclude the possibility of a cervical band. Treatment of the disorder is by surgical excision of the rib or band.

Lumbosacral Plexus Lesions

A lumbosacral plexus lesion may develop in association with diseases such as diabetes, cancer, or bleeding disorders or in relation to injury. It occasionally occurs as an isolated phenomenon similar to idiopathic brachial plexopathy, and pain and weakness then tend to be more conspicuous than sensory symptoms. The distribution of symptoms and signs depends on the level and pattern of neurologic involvement.

DISORDERS OF NEUROMUSCULAR TRANSMISSION

1. MYASTHENIA GRAVIS

Essentials of Diagnosis

- Fluctuating weakness of commonly used voluntary muscles, producing symptoms such as diplopia, ptosis, and difficulty in swallowing.
- Activity increases weakness of affected muscles.
- Short-acting anticholinesterases transiently improve the weakness.

General Considerations

Myasthenia gravis occurs at all ages, sometimes in association with a thymic tumor or thyrotoxicosis, as well as with rheumatoid arthritis and lupus erythematosus. It is commonest in young women with HLA-DR3; if thymoma is associated, older men are more commonly affected. Onset is usually insidious, but the disorder is sometimes unmasked by a coincidental infection that leads to exacerbation of symptoms. Exacerbations may also occur before the menstrual period or during or shortly after pregnancy. Symptoms are due to a variable degree of block of neuromuscular transmission. This probably has an immunologic basis, and autoantibodies binding to acetylcholine receptors are found in most patients with the disease. These antibodies have a primary role in reducing the number of functioning acetylcholine receptors. Additionally, cellular immune activity against the receptor is found. Clinically, this leads to weakness; initially powerful movements fatigue readily. The external ocular muscles and certain other cranial muscles, including the masticatory, facial, and pharyngeal muscles, are especially likely to be affected, and the respiratory and limb muscles may also be involved.

Clinical Findings

A. Symptoms and Signs: Patients present with ptosis, diplopia, difficulty in chewing or swallowing, respiratory difficulties, limb weakness, or some combination of these problems. Weakness may remain localized to a few muscle groups, especially the ocular muscles, or may become generalized. Symptoms often fluctuate in intensity during the day, and this diurnal variation is superimposed on a tendency to longer-term spontaneous relapses and remissions that may last for weeks. Nevertheless, the disorder follows a slowly progressive course and may have a fatal outcome owing to respiratory complications such as aspiration pneumonia.

Clinical examination confirms the weakness and fatigability of affected muscles. In most cases, the extraocular muscles are involved, and this leads to ocular palsies and ptosis, which are commonly asymmetric. Pupillary responses are normal. The bulbar and limb muscles are often weak, but the pattern of involvement is variable. Sustained activity of affected muscles increases the weakness, which improves after a brief rest. Sensation is normal, and there are usually no reflex changes.

The diagnosis can generally be confirmed by the response to a short-acting anticholinesterase. Edrophonium can be given intravenously in a dose of 10 mg (1 mL), 2 mg being given initially and the remaining 8 mg about 30 seconds later if the test dose is well tolerated; in myasthenic patients, there is an obvious improvement in strength of weak muscles lasting for about 5 minutes. Alternatively, 1.5 mg of neostigmine can be given intramuscularly, and the response then lasts for about 2 hours; atropine sulfate (0.6 mg) should be available to reverse muscarinic side effects.

B. Imaging: Lateral and anteroposterior x-rays of the chest and CT scans should be obtained to demonstrate a coexisting thymoma, but normal studies do not exclude this possibility.

C. Laboratory and Other Studies: Electrophysiologic demonstration of a decrementing muscle response to repetitive 2- or 3-Hz stimulation of motor nerves indicates a disturbance of neuromuscular transmission. Such an abnormality may even be detected in clinically strong muscles with certain provocative procedures. Needle electromyography of affected muscles shows a marked variation in configuration and size of individual motor unit potentials, and single-fiber electromyography reveals an increased jitter, or variability, in the time interval between two muscle fiber action potentials from the same motor unit.

Assay of serum for elevated levels of circulating acetylcholine receptor antibodies is another approach—increasingly used—to the laboratory diagnosis of myasthenia gravis and has a sensitivity of 80–90%.

Treatment

Medication such as aminoglycosides that may exacerbate myasthenia gravis should be avoided. Anticholinesterase drugs provide symptomatic benefit without influencing the course of the disease. Neostigmine, pyridostigmine, or both can be used, the dose being determined on an individual basis. The usual dose of neostigmine is 7.5–30 mg (average, 15 mg) taken four times daily; of pyridostigmine, 30–180 mg (average, 60 mg) four times daily. Overmedication may temporarily increase weakness, which is then unaffected or enhanced by intravenous edrophonium.

Thymectomy usually leads to symptomatic benefit or remission and should be considered in all patients younger than age 60, unless weakness is restricted to the extraocular muscles. If the disease is of recent onset and only slowly progressive, operation is sometimes delayed for a year or so, in the hope that spontaneous remission will occur.

Treatment with corticosteroids is indicated for patients who have responded poorly to anticholinesterase drugs and have already undergone thymectomy. It is introduced with the patient in the hospital, since weakness may initially be aggravated. Once weakness has stabilized after 2–3 weeks or any improvement is sustained, further management can be on an outpatient basis. Alternate-day treatment is usually well tolerated, but if weakness is enhanced on the nontreatment day it may be necessary for medication to be taken daily. The dose of corticosteroids is determined on an individual basis, but an initial high daily dose (eg, prednisone, 60–100 mg) can gradually be tapered to a relatively low maintenance level as improvement occurs; total withdrawal is difficult, however. Treatment with azathioprine may also be effective. The usual dose is 2–3 mg/kg orally daily after a lower initial dose.

In patients with major disability in whom conventional treatment is either unhelpful or contraindicated, plasmapheresis may be beneficial. It may also be useful for stabilizing patients before thymectomy and for managing acute crisis.

Levin KH, Richman DP: Myasthenia gravis. Clin Aspects Autoimm 1989;4:23.
Misulis KE, Fenichel GM: Genetic forms of myasthenia gravis. Pediatr Neurol 1989;5:205.

2. MYASTHENIC SYNDROME (Lambert-Eaton Syndrome)

Myasthenic syndrome may be associated with small-cell carcinoma, sometimes developing before the tumor is diagnosed, and occasionally occurs with certain autoimmune diseases. There is defective release of acetylcholine in response to a nerve impulse, and this leads to weakness especially of the proximal muscles of the limbs. As is not the case in myasthenia gravis, however, power steadily increases with sustained contraction. The diagnosis can be confirmed electrophysiologically, because the muscle response to stimulation of its motor nerve increases remarkably if the nerve is stimulated repetitively at high rates, even in muscles that are not clinically weak.

Treatment with plasmapheresis and immunosuppressive drug therapy (prednisone and azathioprine) may lead to clinical and electrophysiologic improvement, in addition to therapy aimed at tumor when present. Prednisone is usually initiated in a daily dose of 60–80 mg and azathioprine in a daily dose of 2 mg/kg. Guanidine hydrochloride (25–50 mg/kg/d in divided doses) is occasionally helpful in seriously disabled patients, but adverse effects of the drug include marrow suppression. The response to treatment with anticholinesterase drugs such as pyridostigmine or neostigmine, either alone or in combination with guanidine, is variable.

O'Neill JH et al: The Lambert-Eaton myasthenic syndrome. Brain 1988;111:577. (Review of 50 cases.)

3. BOTULISM

The toxin of *Clostridium botulinum* prevents the release of acetylcholine at neuromuscular junctions and autonomic synapses. Botulism occurs most commonly following the ingestion of contaminated home-canned food and should be suggested by the development of sudden, fluctuating, severe weakness in a previously healthy person. Symptoms begin within 72 hours following ingestion of the toxin and may progress for several days. Typically, there is diplopia, ptosis, facial weakness, dysphagia, and nasal speech, followed by respiratory difficulty and finally by weakness that appears last in the limbs. Blurring of vision (with unreactive dilated pupils) is characteristic, and there may be dryness of the mouth, constipation (paralytic ileus), and postural hypotension. Sensation is preserved, and the tendon reflexes are not affected unless the involved muscles are very weak. If the diagnosis is suspected, the local health authority should be notified and a sample of serum and contaminated food (if available) sent to be assayed for toxin. Support for the diagnosis may be obtained by electrophysiologic studies; with repetitive stimulation of motor nerves at fast rates, the muscle response increases in size progressively.

Patients should be hospitalized in case respiratory assistance becomes necessary. Treatment is with trivalent antitoxin, once it is established that the patient is not allergic to horse serum. Guanidine hydrochloride (25–50 mg/kg/d in divided doses) to facilitate release of acetylcholine from nerve endings sometimes helps to increase muscle strength. Anticholinesterase drugs are of no value. Respiratory assistance and other supportive measures should be provided as necessary. Further details are provided in Chapter 32.

Pickett JB: Botulism. Muscle Nerve 1988;11:1201. (Case report and review.)

4. DISORDERS ASSOCIATED WITH USE OF AMINOGLYCOSIDES

Aminoglycoside antibiotics, eg, gentamicin, may produce a clinical disturbance similar to botulism by preventing the release of acetylcholine from nerve endings, but symptoms subside rapidly as the responsible drug is eliminated from the body. These antibiotics are particularly dangerous in patients with preexisting disturbances of neuromuscular transmission and are therefore best avoided in patients with myasthenia gravis.

MYOPATHIC DISORDERS

Muscular Dystrophies

These inherited myopathic disorders are characterized by progressive muscle weakness and wasting. They are subdivided by mode of inheritance, age at onset, and clinical features, as shown in Table 23–6. In the Duchenne type, pseudohypertrophy of muscles frequently occurs at some stage; intellectual retardation is common; and there may be skeletal deformities, muscle contractures, and cardiac involvement. The serum creatine kinase level is increased, especially in the Duchenne and Becker varieties, and mildly increased also in limb-girdle dystrophy. Electromyography may help to confirm that weakness is myopathic rather than neurogenic. Similarly, histopathologic examination of a muscle biopsy specimen may help to confirm that weakness is due to a primary disorder of muscle and to distinguish between various muscle diseases.

A genetic defect on the short arm of the X chromosome has been identified in Duchenne dystrophy. The affected gene codes for the protein dystrophin, which is markedly reduced or absent from the muscle of patients with the disease. Dystrophin levels are generally normal in the Becker variety, but the protein is qualitatively altered.

Duchenne muscular dystrophy can now be recognized early in pregnancy in about 95% of women by genetic studies; in late pregnancy, DNA probes can be used on fetal tissue obtained for this purpose by amniocentesis. The gene causing facioscapulohumeral dystrophy has recently been localized to the long arm of chromosome 4. The genetic defect has been characterized, but the abnormal gene product is not yet known.

There is no specific treatment for the muscular dystrophies, but it is important to encourage patients to lead as normal lives as possible. Prolonged bed rest must be avoided, as inactivity often leads to worsening of the underlying muscle disease. Physical therapy and orthopedic procedures may help to counteract deformities or contractures.

Wijmenga C et al: Chromosome 4q DNA rearrangements associated with facioscapulohumeral muscular dystrophy. Nature Genet 1992;2:26.

Myotonic Dystrophy

Myotonic dystrophy, a slowly progressive, dominantly inherited disorder, usually manifests itself in the third or fourth decade but occasionally appears early in childhood. The genetic defect has been localized to the long arm of chromosome 19. Myotonia leads to complaints of muscle stiffness and is evidenced by the marked delay that occurs before affected muscles can relax after a contraction. This can often be demonstrated clinically by delayed relaxation of the hand after sustained grip or by percussion

Table 23–6. The muscular dystrophies.

Disorder	Inheritance	Age at Onset (years)	Distribution	Prognosis
Duchenne type	X-linked recessive	1–5	Pelvic, then shoulder girdle; later, limb and respiratory muscles.	Rapid progression. Death within about 15 years after onset.
Becker's	X-linked recessive	5–25	Pelvic, then shoulder girdle.	Slow progression. May have normal life span.
Limb-girdle (Erb's)	Autosomal recessive (may be sporadic or dominant)	10–30	Pelvic or shoulder girdle initially, with later spread to the other.	Variable severity and rate of progression. Possible severe disability in middle life.
Facioscapulo-humeral	Autosomal dominant	Any age	Face and shoulder girdle initially; later, pelvic girdle and legs.	Slow progression. Minor disability. Usually normal life span.
Distal	Autosomal dominant	40–60	Onset distally in extremities; proximal involvement later.	Slow progression.
Ocular	Autosomal dominant (may be recessive)	Any age (usually 5–30)	External ocular muscles. May also be mild weakness of face, neck, and arms.	
Oculopharyngeal	Autosomal dominant	Any age	As in the ocular form but with dysphagia.	

of the belly of a muscle. In addition, there is weakness and wasting of the facial, sternocleidomastoid, and distal limb muscles. Associated clinical features include cataracts, frontal baldness, testicular atrophy, diabetes mellitus, cardiac abnormalities, and intellectual changes. Electromyographic sampling of affected muscles reveals myotonic discharges in addition to changes suggestive of myopathy.

Myotonia can be treated with quinine sulfate (300–400 mg three times daily), procainamide (0.5–1 g four times daily), or phenytoin (100 mg three times daily). More recently, tocainide and mexiletine have been used. In myotonic dystrophy, phenytoin is preferred, since the other drugs may have undesirable effects on cardiac conduction. Neither the weakness nor the course of the disorder is influenced by treatment.

Ptacek LJ et al: Genetics and physiology of the myotonic muscle disorders. N Engl J Med 1993;328:482.

Shelbourne P et al: Direct diagnosis of myotonic dystrophy with a disease-specific DNA marker. N Engl J Med 1993;328:471. (Diagnosis is improved by a probe that detects the responsible mutation.)

Myotonia Congenita

Myotonia congenita is commonly inherited as a dominant trait. The locus of the responsible gene is on the long arm of chromosome 7. Generalized myotonia without weakness is usually present from birth, but symptoms may not appear until early childhood. Patients complain of muscle stiffness that is enhanced by cold and inactivity and relieved by exercise. Muscle hypertrophy, at times pronounced, is also a feature. A recessive form with later onset is associated with slight weakness and atrophy of distal

muscles. Treatment with quinine sulfate, procainamide, tocainide, mexiletine, or phenytoin may help the myotonia, as in myotonic dystrophy.

Polymyositis & Dermatomyositis

See Chapter 19.

Myopathies Associated With Other Disorders

Myopathy may occur in association with chronic hypokalemia, hyper- or hypothyroidism, hyper- or hypoparathyroidism, hyper- or hypoadrenalism, hypopituitarism, and acromegaly and in patients taking corticosteroids, chloroquine, colchicine, clofibrate, emetine, aminocaproic acid, lovastatin, bretylium tosylate, or drugs causing potassium depletion; weakness is mainly proximal, and serum creatine kinase is typically normal, except in certain cases of hypothyroidism and some of the toxic myopathies. Treatment is of the underlying cause. Myopathy also occurs with chronic alcoholism, whereas acute reversible muscle necrosis may occur shortly after acute alcohol intoxication. Inflammatory myopathy may occur in patients taking penicillamine; myotonia may be induced by diazocholesterol or clofibrate; and preexisting myotonia may be exacerbated or unmasked by depolarizing muscle relaxants (eg, suxamethonium), beta-blockers (eg, propranolol), fenoterol, ritodrine, and, possibly, certain diuretics.

EOSINOPHILIA-MYALGIA SYNDROME

This disorder is characterized by disabling myalgia and a variety of other neurologic disturbances, including weakness of the limb and bulbar muscles, distal sensory loss, and areflexia occurring in patients with peripheral blood eosinophil counts exceeding 1000/μL. Other symptoms include arthralgia, cough, fever, fatigue, and skin rashes. Electrophysiologic studies may show evidence of polyneuropathy, myopathy, or both. The disorder has been associated with the ingestion of supplementary L-tryptophan, and treatment involves the discontinuation of this amino acid and administration of analgesics, nonsteroidal anti-inflammatory drugs, and corticosteroids. Although occasional fatalities have been reported, most patients improve either partially or completely.

Medsger TA: Tryptophan-induced eosinophilia-myalgia syndrome. N Engl J Med, 1990;322:926. (Editorial and general review.)

PERIODIC PARALYSIS SYNDROME

Periodic paralysis may have a familial (dominant inheritance) basis. Episodes of flaccid weakness or paralysis occur, sometimes in association with abnormalities of the plasma potassium level. Strength is normal between attacks. The **hypokalemic** variety is characterized by attacks that tend to occur on awakening, after exercise, or after a heavy meal and may last for several days. Patients should avoid excessive exertion. A low-carbohydrate and low-salt diet may help prevent attacks, as may acetazolamide, 250–750 mg/d. An ongoing attack may be aborted by potassium chloride given orally or by intravenous drip, provided the ECG can be monitored and renal function is satisfactory. It is sometimes associated with hyperthyroidism, especially in young Asian men; treatment of the endocrine disorder may then prevent recurrences. In **hyperkalemic** periodic paralysis, attacks also tend to occur after exercise but usually last for less than an hour. They may be terminated by intravenous calcium gluconate (1–2 g) or by intravenous diuretics (furosemide, 20–40 mg), glucose, or glucose and insulin; daily acetazolamide or chlorothiazide may prevent recurrences. **Normokalemic** periodic paralysis is similar clinically to the hyperkalemic variety, but the plasma potassium level remains normal during attacks; treatment is with acetazolamide.

Ricker K et al: Adynamia episodica hereditaria: What causes the weakness? Muscle Nerve 1989;12:883. (Pathophysiology of hyperkalemic periodic paralysis.)

REFERENCES

Adams RD, Victor M: *Principles of Neurology*, 4th ed. McGraw-Hill, 1989.

Aminoff MJ (editor): *Electrodiagnosis in Clinical Neurology*, 3rd ed. Churchill Livingstone, 1992.

Aminoff MJ (editor): *Neurology and General Medicine: The Neurological Aspects of Medical Disorders*. Churchill Livingstone, 1989.

Asbury AK et al (editors): *Diseases of the Nervous System: Clinical Neurobiology*, 2nd ed. Saunders, 1992.

Dyck PJ et al (editors): *Peripheral Neuropathy*, 3rd ed. Saunders, 1993.

Rosenblum ML et al (editors): *AIDS and the Nervous System*. Raven Press, 1988.

Rowland LP (editor): *Merritt's Textbook of Neurology*, 8th ed. Lea & Febiger, 1989.

Walton JN (editor): *Disorders of Voluntary Muscle*, 5th ed. Churchill Livingstone, 1988.

Psychiatric Disorders

24

James J. Brophy, MD

Psychiatric disorders are functional impairments that may result from disturbance of one or more of the following interrelated factors: (1) biologic function, (2) psychodynamic adaptation, (3) learned behavior, and (4) social and environmental conditions. Although the clinical situation at a given time determines which area of dysfunction will be emphasized, proper patient care requires an approach that adequately evaluates all factors.

(1) Biologic function: Psychiatric disorders of biologic origin may be secondary to identifiable physical illness or caused by biochemical disturbances of the brain. A wide variety of psychiatric disorders (eg, psychosis, depression, delirium, anxiety), as well as nonspecific symptoms are caused by organic brain disease (particularly temporal lobe lesions) or by derangement of cerebral metabolism resulting from illness, biochemical aberrations (usually neurotransmitter dysfunction), nutritional deficiencies, or toxic agents.

Neurotransmitter functions have been correlated with the major psychiatric disorders. Cholinergic deficiency is present in some dementias, and adrenergic imbalance is important in some psychoses. Serotonergic mechanisms are significantly involved in affective disorders, aggression, autism, and the anxiety disorders, particularly obsessive-compulsive disorders.

Studies of the physiologic interactions that take place along the hypothalamic-pituitary-adrenocortical axis have resulted in a recognized association between depression and endocrine dysfunction.

Positron emission tomography (PET) promises to be a major advance in differentiating psychiatric disorders. For example, schizophrenics tend to have low metabolic levels in the frontal lobes and basal ganglia (which correlates with the role of the prefrontal cortex and organizational abilities).* The opposite occurs in obsessive-compulsive disorder, which is characterized by increased frontal lobe and caudate metabolism and clinical overorganization. The differences are more subtle, but in depressive disorders the

temporal lobes, striatal regions, and limbic systems are affected and are different on PET from tracings of schizophrenic patients. Patients with Alzheimer's disease show hypometabolism in the parietotemporal regions.

(2) Psychodynamic maladaptation involves intrapsychic aberrations and is usually treated by a psychotherapeutic approach. There are many forms of psychotherapy: supportive, interpretive, cognitive, persuasive, educative, or some combination of these. Depth, duration, intensity, and frequency of sessions may vary. Various theoretic frameworks may be employed—freudian, jungian, adlerian, sullivanian, kleinian, etc. The "dynamic" approaches have their roots in classic freudian psychoanalytic theory, whereas "experiential" psychotherapy is of more recent origin, including many tenuous offshoots of dubious long-term significance.

(3) Learned behavior is part of the pathogenetic mechanism in all psychiatric disorders. Although a biochemical abnormality may be the matrix of a schizophrenic process, the content of the psychotic material is to a great degree learned and socially relevant. Paranoid delusions reflect current concerns (eg, radar, electronic eavesdropping). In the case of anxiety disorders, many behavioral scientists feel that learned behavior is the major consideration. Appropriate parenting or training consists in great part of utilizing proper behavioral practices, rewarding correct behavior, and punishing delinquent behavior. Personality disorders are examples of failure to learn and incorporate patterns of behavior acceptable in societal surroundings.

(4) Social and environmental conditions have always been considered vital factors in the mental balance of the individual. Without the encounter with the environment, there can be no socially recognized illness: the exigencies of everyday life contribute both to the development of a stable personality and to the deviations from the norm. There is a constantly changing ethnic influence that determines which types of behavior will be tolerated or considered deviant as well as variations in the metabolism of drugs. Cultural attitudes and fears play key roles in the perception of illness and acceptance of treatment. Changes in the family unit have coincided with changes in work patterns of parents and in schooling

---

*Electroencephalographic evidence of weakened suppression of α_2 waves tends to support the hypofrontality hypothesis. Dopamine (D_2) receptor blockers such as haloperidol also increase frontal activity in PET scans.

and work patterns of young adults. The changes are complex and generally have lengthened the period of dependency and increased stresses in the family unit; this, in turn, affects the underlying social fabric.

Goodman A: Organic unity theory: The mind-body problem revisited. Am J Psychiatry 1991;148:553.

PSYCHIATRIC ASSESSMENT

Psychiatric diagnosis rests upon the established principles of a thorough history and examination. All of the forces contributing to the individual's life situation must be identified, and this can only be done if the examination includes the history; mental status; medical conditions (including drugs); and pertinent social, cultural, and environmental factors impinging on the individual.

Interview

The appearance and behavior of the interviewer influences the interviewee. The manner in which the history is taken is important not only because it affects success in eliciting pertinent data but also because it may be of therapeutic value in itself. The setting should be quiet, with an appropriate degree of professional decorum at all times, and patients should initially be allowed to talk about their problems in an unstructured way without interruption. The interviewer should minimize writing, unnecessary direct questioning, incoming phone calls, and interpretive comments. Long, rambling discussions may be controlled by subtly interjecting questions relevant to the topic, though the patient's digressions sometimes provide important clues to his or her mental status. The first few minutes are often the most important part of the interview.

The interviewer should be alert for key words or phrases that can be used to help the patient develop the theme of the main difficulty. For example, if the patient says, "Doctor, I hurt, and when we have marital problems, things just get worse"—the words "hurt" and "marital problems" are important clues that need amplification when the physician makes another comment. Nonverbal clues may be as important as words, and one should notice gestures, tones of voice, and facial expressions. Obvious omissions, shying away from painful subjects, and sudden shifts of subject matter give important clues to unconscious as well as conscious sources of difficulty.

Every psychiatric history should cover the following points: (1) complaint, from the patient's viewpoint; (2) the present illness, or the evolution of the complaints; (3) previous disorders and the nature and extent of treatment; (4) the family history—important for genetic aspects and family influences; (5) personal history—childhood development, adolescent adjustment, level of education, and adult coping patterns; (6) sexual history; (7) current life functioning, with attention to vocational, social, educational, and avocational areas; and (8) current medications, alcohol, or other drugs.

It is often essential to obtain additional information from the family. Observing interactions of significant other people with the patient in the context of a family interview may give significant diagnostic information and may even underscore the nature of the problem and suggest a therapeutic approach.

The Mental Status Examination

Observation of the patient and the content of the remarks made during the interview constitute the informal part of the mental status examination, ie, that which is obtained indirectly. The formal mental status examination is performed as noted below and should be particularly detailed when there is any evidence or high risk of cognitive dysfunction.

The mental status examination includes the following: (1) Appearance: Note unusual modes of dress, makeup, etc. (2) Activity and behavior: Gait, gestures, coordination of bodily movements, etc. (3) Affect: Outward manifestation of emotions such as depression, anger, elation, fear, resentment, or lack of emotional response. (4) Mood: Inward feelings, sum of statements, and observable emotional manifestations. (5) Speech: Coherence, spontaneity, articulation, hesitancy in answering, and duration of response. (6) Content of thought: Associations, preoccupations, obsessions, depersonalization, delusions, hallucinations, paranoid ideation, anger, fear, or unusual experiences. (7) Sensorium: (a) orientation to person, place, time, and circumstances; (b) remote and recent memory and recall; (c) calculations, digit retention (forward and backward), serial 7s or 3s; (d) general fund of knowledge (presidents, states, distances, events); (e) abstracting ability, often tested with common proverbs or with analogies and differences (eg, how are a lie and a mistake the same, and how are they different?); (f) ability to identify by naming, reading, and writing specified test names and objects; (g) ideomotor function, which combines understanding and the ability to perform a task (eg, "Show me how to throw a ball"); (h) ability to reproduce geometric constructions (eg, parallelogram, intersecting squares); and (i) right-left differentiation. (8) Judgment regarding commonsense problems such as what to do when one runs out of medicine. (9) Insight into the nature and extent of the current difficulty and its ramifications in the patient's daily life.

The mental status examination is important in establishing a diagnosis and must be *recorded carefully and clearly in the chart.*

Medical Examination

The examination of a psychiatric patient must include a complete medical history and physical examination (with emphasis on the neurologic examination) as well as all necessary laboratory and other special studies. Physical illness may frequently present as psychiatric disease, and vice versa. It is hazardous to assign a "functional" cause to symptoms simply because they arose during an emotional crisis.

Special Diagnostic Aids

Many tests and evaluation procedures are available that can be used to support and clarify initial diagnostic impressions.

A. Psychologic Testing: Psychologic testing by a trained psychologist may measure intelligence and cognitive functioning; provide information about personality, feelings, psychodynamics, and psychopathology; and differentiate psychic problems from organic ones. The place of such tests is similar to that of other tests in medicine—helpful in diagnostic problems but a useless expense when not needed.

1. Objective tests–These tests provide quantitative evaluation compared to standard norms.

a. Intelligence tests–The test most frequently used is the Wechsler Adult Intelligence Scale—Revised (WAIS-R). Intelligence tests often reveal more than IQ. The results, given expert interpretation, can lend objective support to the ultimate psychiatric diagnosis. They provide information regarding different aspects of cognitive functioning, eg, short-term memory, abstract reasoning skills, and judgment.

b. Minnesota Multiphasic Personality Inventory (MMPI)–The MMPI is an empirically based test of personality assessment. The patient's scores are interpreted in comparison with data about others with the same response pattern to assess psychopathologic changes.

c. Bender Gestalt Test–This test is used to elicit evidence of psychomotor dysfunction in persons with organic disorders.

d. Vocational aptitude and interest tests–Several are available and may be used as a source of advice regarding vocational plans.

e. Neuropsychologic assessment–Such an assessment is made when an organic deficit is present but information on anatomic location and extent of dysfunction is required.

f. Mini-mental status tests–These tests are short tests easily administered in the office by an assistant to screen for organic brain syndrome or to provide ongoing assessment of the progress of dementia. Unfortunately, they may not pick up on early changes.

2. Projective tests–These tests are unstructured, so that the subject is forced to respond in ways that reflect fantasies and individual modes of adaptation. Conscious and unconscious attitudes (particularly disordered thinking) may be deduced from the subject's responses.

a. Rorschach Psychodiagnostics–This test utilizes ten inkblots. It requires expert interpretation but can provide important information on psychodynamic themes and aberrations.

b. Thematic Apperception Test (TAT)–This test uses 20 pictures of people in different situations. Interpretation is based on psychoanalytic theory concerning defenses against feelings of anxiety and reflects areas of interpersonal conflicts.

c. Sentence completion tests, draw-a-person tests, etc–These tests are most useful in providing information about the patient's present concerns and conflicts.

3. Miscellaneous tests–Other tests designed for specific purposes include aphasia screening tests, inventories of depression, tests of different types of memory, and neurologic, behavior, and anxiety screening tests.

B. Neurologic Evaluation: Consultation is often necessary and may include specialized tests. Brain imaging is useful for detecting structural abnormalities in the patient who presents with a nondefinitive history and examination (eg, dissociative episodes, unusual psychotic episodes not explained by drug abuse). MRI studies (which, unlike CT, can image in all planes and produce a superb gray-white resolution) are particularly useful in delineating lesions, demyelinating disorders, and degenerative diseases (eg, Huntington's disease). Electroencephalography is particularly useful for general screening and diagnosis of seizure disorders. The significance of PET was noted above. Single photon emission computed tomography (SPECT) is a gamma imaging technology like PET, and both provide tomographic images of brain activity. SPECT is cheaper but has the disadvantages of lower image resolution and lower quantification of regional brain activity.

C. Amobarbital Interviews: The success of any of the sedative agents in eliciting clinically useful information is quite limited. The procedure can be helpful in differentiating psychosis from delirium; the former usually improves with amobarbital, whereas the latter worsens. Some cases of conversion disorders or dissociative disorders respond to this approach. Hypnosis can provide similar relief in selected subjects.

D. Biologic Markers: The dexamethasone suppression test (DST) and the thyrotropin-releasing hormone (TRH) test have been used as aids in the diagnosis, treatment, and follow-up of patients with depressive illness. Clinical usefulness of the tests is limited to difficult diagnostic problems (the DST may be measuring anxiety), but they represent progress in the search for reliable biologic markers.

Formulation of the Diagnosis

A psychiatric diagnosis must be based upon positive evidence accumulated by the above techniques. *It must not be based simply on the exclusion of organic findings.*

A thorough psychiatric evaluation has therapeutic as well as diagnostic value and should be expressed in ways best understood by the patient, family, and other physicians.

Gilman S: Advances in neurology. (Two parts.) N Engl J Med 1992;326:1608, 1671. (Imaging techniques and their value in common disorders.)

Thienhaus DJ: Emergency psychiatry: Rational physical evaluation in the emergency room. Hosp Community Psychiatry 1992;43:311. (Need for physical evaluation in psychiatric disorders.)

TREATMENT APPROACHES

The approaches to treatment of psychiatric patients are, in a broad sense, similar to those in other branches of medicine. For example, the internist treating a patient with heart disease uses not only **medical** measures such as digitalis and pacemakers but also **psychologic** techniques to change attitudes and behaviors, **social** and **environmental** manipulation to mitigate deleterious influences, and **behavioral** techniques to change behavior patterns.

Regardless of the methods employed, treatment must be directed toward an objective, ie, **goal-oriented.** This usually involves (1) obtaining active cooperation on the part of the patient; (2) establishing reasonable goals and modifying the goal downward if failure occurs; (3) emphasizing positive behavior (goals) instead of symptom behavior (problems); (4) delineating the method; and (5) setting a time frame (which can be modified later).

The physician must resist pressures for instantaneous results. In almost all cases, psychiatric treatment involves the *active participation* of the significant people in the patient's life. Time must be spent with the patient, but the frequency and duration of appointments are highly variable and should be adjusted to meet both the patient's psychologic needs and financial restrictions. Compliance (collaboration) is the end product of many factors, the most important being clear communication, attention to cost, and simple dosage regimens when drugs are prescribed. *The physician can unwittingly promote chronic illness by prescribing inappropriate medication.* The patient may come to believe that problems respond only to medication, and the more drugs prescribed, the stronger the misconception becomes.

Psychiatric Referrals

All physicians have always treated most psychiatric problems and are in an excellent position to meet their patients' emotional needs in an organized and competent way, referring to psychiatrists for consultation or treatment those patients who are considered beyond the expertise of the referring physician (just as in any other medical condition). The most pressing problems involve evaluation of suicidal or assaultive potential and diagnostic differentiation in mood disorders and psychoses. The psychiatric problems associated with unusual psychopharmacologic therapy and with medications used in other branches of medicine may require expert pharmacologic consultation. When a psychiatric referral is made, it should be conducted like any other referral: in an open manner, with full explanation of the problem to the patient and the referral appointment made while the patient is still in the office.

MEDICAL APPROACHES

1. ANTIPSYCHOTIC DRUGS (Neuroleptics, "Major Tranquilizers")

This group of drugs includes **phenothiazines** and **thioxanthenes** (both similar in structure), **butyrophenones, dihydroindolones,** and **dibenzoxazepines.** Table 24–1 lists the drugs in order of increasing milligram potency and decreasing side effects (with the exception of extrapyramidal symptoms). Thus, chlorpromazine has lower milligram potency and causes more severe side effects and fewer extrapyramidal complications than fluphenazine. All are efficacious in reducing symptoms.

The phenothiazines comprise the bulk of the currently used neuroleptic drugs. The only butyrophenone commonly used in psychiatry is haloperidol, which is totally different in structure but very similar in action and side effects to the piperazine phenothiazines such as fluphenazine, perphenazine, and trifluoperazine. These drugs and haloperidol (dopamine [D_2] receptor blockers) have high potency, a paucity of autonomic side effects and act to markedly lower arousal levels. Molindone and loxapine, while less potent, are similar in action, side effects, and safety to the piperazine phenothiazines. Clozapine, a dibenzoxazepine derivative, has high dopamine (D_4) receptor blocking activity as well as central serotonergic, histaminergic, and alpha-noradrenergic receptor blocking activity. It is about 30% effective in the treatment of psychoses resistant to other neuroleptic drugs.

None of the antipsychotics produce true physical dependency, and they have a wide safety margins between therapeutic and toxic effects. All decrease adrenergic response and are efficacious in ameliorating psychotic symptoms. Previous patient response, ex-

Table 24–1. Commonly used antipsychotics.

	Chlor- proma- zine Ratio	Usual Daily Oral Dose	Usual Daily Maximum Dose[1]
Phenothiazines			
Chlorpromazine (Thorazine and other trade names)	1:1	100–400 mg	1 g
Thioridazine (Mellaril)	1:1	100–400 mg	600 mg
Mesoridazine (Serentil)	1:2	50–200 mg	400 mg
Perphenazine (Trilafon)[2]	1:10	16–32 mg	64 mg
Trifluoperazine (Stelazine)[2]	1:20	5–15 mg	60 mg
Fluphenazine (Permitil, Prolixin)[2]	1:50	2–10 mg	60 mg
Thioxanthenes			
Chlorprothixene (Taractan)	1:1	100–400 mg	600 mg
Thiothixene[2] (Navane)	1:20	5–10 mg	80 mg
Butyrophenone			
Haloperidol (Haldol)	1:50	2–5 mg	80 mg
Dihydroindolone			
Molindone (Moban)	1:12	30–100 mg	225 mg
Dibenzoxazepine			
Clozapine (Clozaril)	1:1	300–450 mg	900 mg
Loxapine (Loxitane)	1:10	20–60 mg	200 mg

[1]Can be higher in some cases.
[2]Indicates piperazine structure.

perience with the drug, and its side effects dictate the choice of a drug.

Clinical Indications

The antipsychotics are used to treat all **psychoses,** including the **schizophrenias** and **psychotic ideation in organic brain psychoses, drug-induced psychoses, psychotic depression,** and **mania.** They are also effective in Tourette's disorder. They quickly lower the arousal (activity) level and, perhaps indirectly, gradually improve socialization and thinking. The improvement rate is about 80%. Patients whose behavioral symptoms worsen with use of antipsychotic drugs may have an undiagnosed organic condition.

Symptoms that are ameliorated by these drugs include hyperactivity, hostility, aggression, delusions, hallucinations, irritability, and poor sleep. Individuals with acute psychosis and good premorbid function respond quite well. Clozapine is helpful in reducing the negative symptoms (apathy, withdrawal,

anhedonia) in chronic schizophrenics. A full trial is 6–12 months. The most common cause of failure in the treatment of acute psychosis is inadequate dosage, and the most common cause of relapse is noncompliance.

Dosage Forms & Patterns

The dosage range is quite broad. For example, haloperidol, 1 mg orally at bedtime, may be sufficient for the elderly person with a mild organic brain syndrome, whereas 60 mg/d may be used in a young schizophrenic patient. A dosage of 10–20 mg/d is adequate initially for most patients. For quick response, one may start with haloperidol, 10 mg intramuscularly, which is absorbed rapidly and achieves an initial tenfold plasma level advantage over equal oral doses. Psychomotor agitation, racing thoughts, and general arousal are quickly reduced. The dose can be repeated every 3–4 hours; when the patient is less symptomatic, oral doses can replace parenteral administration in most cases.

Various factors play a role in the absorption of oral medications. Of particular importance are previous gastrointestinal surgery and concomitant administration of other drugs, eg, antacids (Table 24–2). There are racial differences in metabolizing the neuroleptic drugs—eg, many Asians require only about half the usual dosage. Bioavailability is influenced by other factors such as smoking or microsomal stimulation with alcohol or barbiturates and enzyme-altering drugs such as carbamazepine or methylphenidate. Plasma drug level determinations are not of major clinical assistance.

Divided daily doses are not necessary after a maintenance dose has been established, and most patients can then be maintained on a single daily dose, usually taken at bedtime. This is particularly appro-

Table 24–2. Antipsychotic drug interactions with other drugs.

Drug	Effects
Antacids	Decreased absorption of antipsychotic drugs.
All anticholinergics	Increased anticholinergic effects.
Barbiturates	Central nervous system depression and decreased antipsychotic drug levels.
Carbamazepine	Decreased neuroleptic levels.
Cimetidine	Increased chlorpromazine levels.
Tricyclic antidepressants	Increased antidepressant blood levels.
Guanadrel	Increased hypotensive effect.
Guanethidine	Decreased hypotensive effect.
Indomethacin	Severe drowsiness (with haloperidol).
Levodopa	Decreased antiparkinson effect.
Methyldopa	Decreased hypotensive effect.
Phenytoin	Increased phenytoin levels.
Propranolol	Increased thioridazine levels.
Thiazide diuretics	Increased hypotensive effect.
Trihexyphenidyl	Decreased antipsychotic levels.

priate in a case where the sedative effect of the drug is desired for nighttime sleep, and undesirable sedative effects can be avoided during the day. Costs of medication, nursing time, and patient unreliability are reduced when either a single daily dose or a large bedtime/smaller morning dose schedule is utilized. This requires adequate follow-up and decreases in dosage when possible. First-episode patients especially should be tapered off medications after about 6 months of stability and carefully monitored; their rate of relapse is lower than that of multiple-episode patients.

Psychiatric patients—particularly paranoid individuals—often neglect to take their medication. In these cases and in nonresponders to oral medication, the enanthate and decanoate (the latter is slightly longer lasting and has fewer extrapyramidal side effects) forms of fluphenazine or the decanoate form of haloperidol may be given by deep subcutaneous injection or intramuscularly to achieve an effect that will usually last 7–28 days. A patient who cannot be depended on to take oral medication (or who overdoses on minimal provocation) will generally agree to come to the physician's office for a "shot." The usual dose of the fluphenazine long-acting preparations is 25 mg every 2 weeks. Dosage and frequency of administration vary from about 100 mg weekly to 12.5 mg monthly. Use the smallest amount as infrequently as possible. A monthly injection of 25 mg of fluphenazine decanoate is equivalent to about 15–20 mg of oral fluphenazine daily. Concomitant use of a benzodiazepine (eg, lorazepam, 2 mg orally twice daily) may permit reduction of the required dosage of oral or parenteral antipsychotic drug.

Intravenous use of haloperidol (the only neuroleptic used in this manner) is reserved for special situations (eg, severely burned patients who have psychotic symptoms associated with delirium).

Side Effects

The side effects *decrease* as one goes from the sedating, lower milligram potency drugs such as chlorpromazine or thioridazine to those of higher milligram potency such as fluphenazine and haloperidol (Table 24–1). However, the extrapyramidal effects *increase* as one goes down the list (consider chlorprothixene as similar to chlorpromazine).

The most common anticholinergic side effects include dry mouth (which can lead to ingestion of caloric liquids and weight gain), blurred vision, urinary retention (particularly in elderly men with enlarged prostates), delayed gastric emptying, ileus, and precipitation of acute glaucoma in patients with narrow anterior chamber angles. Other autonomic effects include orthostatic hypotension and sexual dysfunction—problems in achieving erection, ejaculation (including retrograde ejaculation), and orgasm in males (approximately 50% of cases) and females (approximately 30%). Delay in achieving orgasm is often a factor in medication noncompliance. Electrocardiographic changes occur frequently, but clinically significant arrhythmias are much less common. Elderly patients and those with preexisting cardiac disease are at greater risk. The most frequently seen electrocardiographic changes include diminution of the T wave amplitude, appearance of prominent U waves, depression of the ST segment, and prolongation of the QT interval. These electrocardiographic findings do not alter treatment.

Metabolic and endocrine effects include weight gain, hyperglycemia, infrequent temperature irregularities (particularly in hot weather), and water intoxication that may be due to inappropriate antidiuretic hormone secretion. Lactation and menstrual irregularities are common (antipsychotic drugs should be avoided, if possible, in breast cancer patients because of potential trophic effects of elevated prolactin levels on the breast). Both antipsychotic and antidepressant drugs inhibit sperm motility. Bone marrow depression and cholestatic jaundice occur rarely; these are hypersensitivity reactions, and they usually appear in the first 2 months of treatment. They subside on discontinuance of the drug.

Clozapine is associated with a 1.6% risk of **agranulocytosis** (higher in persons of Jewish ancestry), and its use must be strictly monitored with weekly blood counts. It also lowers the seizure threshold and has many side effects, including sedation, hypotension, increased liver enzyme levels, hypersalivation, seizures, respiratory arrest, weight gain, and changes in both ECG and EEG. There is cross-sensitivity among all of the phenothiazines, and a drug from a different group must be used when allergic reactions occur.

Photosensitivity (including retinal effects) is commonly related to chlorpromazine use. Retinopathy and hyperpigmentation are associated with use of fairly high dosages of thioridazine and chlorpromazine. The appearance of particulate melanin deposits in the lens of the eye is related to the total dose given, and patients on long-term medication should have periodic eye examinations. Teratogenicity has not been causally related to these drugs, but prudence is indicated particularly in the first trimester of pregnancy. The seizure threshold is lowered, but it is safe to use these medications in epileptics controlled by anticonvulsants.

The **neuroleptic malignant syndrome (NMS)** is a catatonia-like state with extrapyramidal signs, blood pressure changes, altered consciousness, and hyperpyrexia; it is an uncommon but serious complication of neuroleptic treatment. Muscle rigidity, involuntary movements, confusion, dysarthria, and dysphagia are accompanied by pallor, cardiovascular instability, fever, pulmonary congestion, and diaphoresis and may result in stupor, coma, and death. The cause may be related to a number of factors, including poor dosage control of neuroleptic medication, affective illness, decreased serum iron, and increased sensitivity of dopamine receptor sites. Lithium in combination with a neuroleptic drug may increase vulnerability, which is already increased in patients with an affective disorder. In most cases, the symptoms develop within the first 2 weeks of antipsychotic drug treatment. The syndrome may occur with small doses of the drugs. Intramuscular administration is a risk factor. Elevated creatine kinase and leukocytosis with a shift to the left are present early in about half of cases. Treatment includes bringing down the temperature with cooling methods. Dopamine agonists such as bromocriptine, 2.5–10 mg orally three times a day, and amantadine, 100–200 mg orally twice a day, have also been useful. Dantrolene, 50 mg intravenously as needed, is used to alleviate rigidity (do not exceed 10 mg/kg/d). There is ongoing controversy about the efficacy of these three agents as well as the use of calcium channel blockers and benzodiazepines. Electroconvulsive therapy has been used effectively in resistant cases. Clozapine has been used with relative safety and fair success as an antipsychotic drug for patients who have had NMS. The syndrome must be differentiated from acute lethal catatonia, malignant hyperthermia, neurotoxic syndromes (including AIDS), and a variety of other conditions such as viral encephalitis, Wilson's disease, central anticholinergic syndrome, and hypertonic states (eg, tetany, strychnine poisoning).

Extrapyramidal symptoms. Akathisia is the most common (about 20%) so-called extrapyramidal symptom. It usually occurs early in treatment (but may persist after neuroleptics are discontinued) and is frequently mistaken for anxiety or exacerbation of psychosis. It is characterized by a subjective desire to be in constant motion followed by an inability to sit or stand still and consequent pacing. It may include feelings of fright, rage, terror, or sexual torment. Insomnia is often present. In all cases, reevaluate the dosage requirement or the type of neuroleptic drug. One should inquire also about cigarette smoking, which in women has been associated with an increased incidence of akathisia. Antiparkinsonism drugs such as trihexyphenidyl, 2–5 mg orally three times daily, or benztropine mesylate, 1–2 mg twice daily, may be helpful. High-potency neuroleptics often require concomitant antiparkinsonism drugs (see Table 23–4). In resistant cases, propranolol, 30–80 mg/d orally; diazepam, 5 mg three times daily; or amantadine, 100 mg orally three times daily, may alleviate the symptoms.

Acute dystonias usually occur early, though a late (tardive) occurrence is reported in patients (mostly males after several years of therapy) who previously had early severe dystonic reactions and a mood disorder (see below). Younger patients are at higher risk for acute dystonias. The most common signs are bizarre muscle spasms of the head, neck, and tongue. Frequently present are torticollis, oculogyric crises, swallowing or chewing difficulties, and masseter

spasms. Laryngospasm is particularly dangerous. Back, arm, or leg muscle spasms are occasionally reported. Diphenhydramine, 50 mg intramuscularly, is effective for the acute crisis; one should then give benztropine mesylate, 2 mg orally twice daily, for several weeks, and then discontinue gradually, since few of the extrapyramidal symptoms require long-term use of the antiparkinsonism drugs (all of which are about equally efficacious—though trihexyphenidyl tends to be mildly stimulating and benztropine mildly sedating).

Drug-induced parkinsonism is indistinguishable from idiopathic parkinsonism, but it is reversible, occurs later in treatment than the preceding extrapyramidal symptoms, and in some cases appears after neuroleptic withdrawal. The condition includes the typical signs of apathy and reduction of facial and arm movements (akinesia, which can mimic depression), festinating gait, rigidity, loss of postural reflexes, and the pill-rolling tremor. AIDS patients seem particularly vulnerable to extrapyramidal side effects. The neuroleptic should be reduced, and immediate relief can be achieved with antiparkinsonism drugs in the same dosages as above. After 4–6 weeks, these antiparkinsonism drugs can often be discontinued with no recurrent symptoms. In any of the extrapyramidal symptoms, amantadine, 100–400 mg daily, may be used instead of the antiparkinsonism drugs. Neuroleptic-induced catatonia is similar to catatonic stupor with rigidity, drooling, urinary incontinence, and cogwheeling. It usually responds slowly to withdrawal of the offending medication and use of antiparkinsonism agents.

Tardive dyskinesia is a syndrome of abnormal involuntary stereotyped movements of the face, mouth, tongue, trunk, and limbs that may occur after months or (usually) years of treatment with neuroleptic agents. The syndrome affects 20–35% of patients who have undergone long-term neuroleptic therapy. Predisposing factors include older age, many years of treatment, cigarette smoking, and diabetes mellitus. Pineal calcification is higher in this condition by a margin of 3:1. *There are no known differences among any of the antipsychotic drugs in the development of this syndrome.*

Early manifestations include fine wormlike movements of the tongue at rest, difficulty in sticking out the tongue, facial tics, increased blink frequency, or jaw movements of recent onset. Later manifestations may include bucco-linguo-masticatory movements, lip smacking, chewing motions, mouth opening and closing, disturbed gag reflex, puffing of the cheeks, disrupted speech, respiratory distress, or choreoathetoid movements of the extremities (the last being more prevalent in younger patients). The symptoms do not necessarily worsen and in rare cases may lessen even though neuroleptic drugs are continued. The dyskinesias do not occur during sleep and can be voluntarily suppressed for short periods. Stress and movements in other parts of the body will often aggravate the condition.

Early signs of dyskinesia must be differentiated from those reversible signs produced by ill-fitting dentures or nonneuroleptic drugs such as levodopa, tricyclic antidepressants (TCAs), antiparkinsonism agents, anticonvulsants, and antihistamines. Other neurologic conditions such as Huntington's chorea can be differentiated by history and examination.

The emphasis should be on prevention. Use the least amount of neuroleptic drug necessary to mute the psychotic symptoms. Detect early manifestations. When these occur, stop anticholinergic drugs and gradually discontinue neuroleptic drugs. If neuroleptic drugs are restarted (as they usually are), the use of adjunctive agents such as benzodiazepines or lithium may help directly or indirectly by allowing control of psychotic symptoms with a low dosage of neuroleptics. Weight loss and cachexia sometimes appear on withdrawal of neuroleptics. In an indeterminate number of cases, the dyskinesias will remit. Keep the patient off the drugs until reemergent psychotic symptoms dictate their resumption, at which point they are restarted in low doses and gradually increased until there is clinical improvement. If the dyskinesic syndrome recurs and it is necessary to continue neuroleptic drugs to control psychotic symptoms, informed consent should be obtained. Benzodiazepines, buspirone (in doses of 40–160 mg/d), phosphatidylcholine, clonidine, calcium channel blockers, vitamin E, and propranolol all have had limited usefulness in treating the dyskinetic side effects.

Reserpine has occasionally been successfully substituted for the neuroleptic drugs and does not cause dyskinesic syndrome. Depression and gastric symptoms are common with any of the rauwolfia derivatives.

Feltner DE, Hertzman M: Progress in the treatment of tardive dyskinesia: Theory and practice. Hosp Community Psychiatry 1993;44:25. (Literature review.)

Goff DC, Baldessarini RJ: Drug interactions with antipsychotic agents. J Clin Psychopharmacol 1993;13:57.

Kimberly A et al: Gender differences in pharmacokinetics and pharmacodynamics of psychotropic medication. Am J Psychiatry 1992;149:587.

2. LITHIUM

The use of lithium has dramatically affected both diagnosis and treatment in psychiatry. The discovery of lithium's effectiveness in bipolar mood disorders has shown that many of these patients were erroneously diagnosed as having a schizophrenic disorder.

Clinical Indications

As a prophylactic drug for bipolar affective disorder, lithium significantly decreases the frequency and severity of both manic and depressive attacks in about 70% of patients. A positive response is more predictable if the patient has a low frequency of episodes (no more than two per year with intervals free of psychopathology). A positive response occurs more frequently in individuals who have blood relatives with a diagnosis of manic or hypomanic attacks. Patients who swing rapidly back and forth between manic and depressive attacks (at least four cycles per year) usually respond poorly to lithium prophylaxis initially, but some improve with continued long-term treatment. Carbamazepine has been used with success in this group.

Acute manic or hypomanic symptoms will respond to lithium therapy, but it is common to use neuroleptic drugs to treat the excited or psychotic manic stage (as outlined in the treatment of the psychoses) and then make a decision with the patient and family about the feasibility of long-term prophylactic lithium therapy. The decision is usually based on the severity of the condition. Some schizoaffective disorders and some cases of so-called schizophrenia are probably atypical bipolar affective disorder, for which lithium treatment may be effective.

Lithium—either alone or combined with cyclic antidepressants in acute phases—is useful in the prophylaxis of some recurrent unipolar depressions (perhaps undiagnosed bipolar disorder). It is the most effective adjunctive drug with antidepressants in the treatment of resistant depression. Lithium may ameliorate nonspecific aggressive behaviors and dyscontrol syndromes. The dosages are the same as used in bipolar disorder. Most patients with bipolar disease can be managed with lithium alone, though some will require continued or intermittent use of a neuroleptic, antidepressant medication, or carbamazepine. An excellent resource for information pertaining to lithium is the Lithium Information Center, University of Wisconsin, Department of Psychiatry, 600 Highland Avenue, Madison, WI 53792.

Dosage Forms & Patterns

Lithium carbonate in generally prescribed in the 300 mg unit. In a small minority of patients, a slow release form or units of different dosage may be required. Lithium citrate is available as a syrup for patients in whom compliance is a problem. The dosage is that required to maintain blood levels in the therapeutic range. For acute attacks this ranges from 1 to 1.6 meq/L, whereas the prophylactic dose is usually 0.4–1 meq/L (though levels < 0.6 meq/L may lead to a higher frequency of relapses). Maintenance levels should be kept as low as clinically feasible. The dose required to meet this need will vary in individuals and should be determined by giving a test dose of 600 mg of lithium carbonate after the clinical workup, which should include a medical history and physical examination; complete blood count; T4, TSH, blood urea nitrogen, creatinine, and electrolyte determinations;

urinalysis; and ECG. Twenty-four hours after the administration of the test dose, a blood sample is drawn for lithium determination. (See Table 24–3 for dosage requirements based on a test dose.) Once-a-day dosage is acceptable, but most patients have less nausea when they take the drug in divided doses with meals.

Lithium is readily absorbed, with peak serum levels occurring within 1–3 hours and complete absorption in 8 hours. Half of the total body lithium is excreted in 18–24 hours (95% in the urine). *The blood for the lithium levels should be drawn 12 hours after the last dose.* Serum levels should be measured every 1–3 weeks in the early maintenance stage and thereafter when clinically indicated (at least every 3–4 months), particularly when there is any condition that causes volume depletion (eg, diarrhea; dehydration; use of diuretics). Patients receiving lithium should use diuretics with caution and only under close medical supervision. The thiazide diuretics cause increased lithium reabsorption from the proximal renal tubules, resulting in increased serum lithium levels (Table 24–4), and adjustment of lithium intake must be made to compensate for this. Reduce lithium dosage by 25–40% when the patient is receiving 50 mg of hydrochlorothiazide daily. Potassium-sparing diuretics (spironolactone, amiloride, triamterene) may also cause increased serum lithium levels and require careful monitoring of lithium levels. Loop diuretics (furosemide, ethacrynic acid, bumetanide) appear not to alter serum lithium levels. Concurrent use of lithium and ACE inhibitors requires a 50–75% reduction in lithium intake to achieve therapeutic lithium levels.

Side Effects

A. Early Side Effects: Mild gastrointestinal symptoms (take lithium with food), fine tremors (treat with propranolol, 20–60 mg/d orally, only if persistent), slight muscle weakness, and some degree of somnolence are early side effects that are usually transient. Moderate polyuria (reduced renal responsiveness to antidiuretic hormone) and polydipsia (as-

Table 24–3. Predicted lithium daily dosage necessary to produce therapeutic levels. (Based on 600-mg test dose).

24-h Lithium Level (meq/L)	Total Daily Dose (mg)
<0.05	3600
0.05–0.09	2700
0.10–0.14	1800
0.15–0.19	1200
0.20–0.23	900
0.24–0.30	600
>0.30	300

Table 24–4. Lithium interactions with other drugs.

Drug	Effects
ACE inhibitors	↑Lithium levels
Ibuprofen	↑Lithium levels
Indomethacin	↑Lithium levels
Methyldopa	Rigidity, mutism, fascicular twitching
Osmotic diuretics (urea, mannitol)	↑Lithium excretion
Phenylbutazone	↑Lithium levels
Potassium-sparing diuretics (spironolactone, amiloride, triamterene)	↑Lithium levels
Sodium bicarbonate	↑Lithium excretion
Succinylcholine	↑Duration of action of succinylcholine
Theophylline, aminophylline	↑Lithium excretion
Thiazide diuretics	↑Lithium levels
Valproic acid	↓Lithium levels

sociated with increased plasma renin concentration) are occasionally present. Potassium administration can blunt this effect. Weight gain (often a result of calories in fluids taken for polydipsia) and leukocytosis not due to infection are fairly common.

B. Other Side Effects: These include weight gain, goiter (3%; often euthyroid), occasionally hypothyroidism (10%; concomitant administration of lithium and iodide or lithium and carbamazepine enhances the hypothyroid and goitrogenic effect of either drug), changes in the glucose tolerance test toward a diabetes-like curve, nephrogenic diabetes insipidus (usually resolving about 8 weeks after cessation of lithium therapy), nephrotic syndrome, edema, folate deficiency, pseudotumor cerebri (do funduscopy if there are complaints of headache or blurred vision), and leukocytosis. A metallic taste, hair loss, and Raynaud's phenomena have been reported in a small number of cases. Thyroid and kidney function should be checked at 3- to 4-month intervals. Most of these side effects subside when lithium is discontinued; when residual side effects exist, they are usually not serious. Most clinicians treat lithium-induced hypothyroidism (more common in women) with thyroid hormone while continuing lithium therapy. Hypercalcemia and elevated parathyroid hormone levels occur in some patients. Electrocardiographic abnormalities (principally T wave flattening or inversion) may occur during lithium administration but are not of major clinical significance. Sinoatrial block may occur, particularly in the elderly. It is important that other drugs which prolong intraventricular conduction, such as TCAs, be used with caution in conjunction with lithium. Lithium impairs ventilatory function in patients with airway obstruction. Lithium alone does not have a significant effect on sexual function, but when combined with benzodiazepines (clonazepam in most of the symptomatic patients) it caused sexual dysfunction in about 50% of male patients. Lithium may precipitate or exacerbate psoriasis in some patients. Patients receiving long-term lithium therapy may have cogwheel rigidity and, occasionally, other extrapyramidal signs. Lithium potentiates the parkinsonian effects of haloperidol. A wide variety of neurologic sequelae have been reported; most remit quickly when lithium therapy is discontinued. (Taper slowly over 1 week.)

The long-term use of lithium has adverse effects on renal function (with interstitial fibrosis, tubular atrophy, and glomerulosclerosis) in some patients that are not always completely reversible. A rise in serum creatinine levels is an indication for in-depth evaluation of renal function. Incontinence has been reported in women, apparently related to changes in bladder cholinergic-adrenergic balance. Long-term lithium therapy has also been associated with a relative lowering of the level of memory and perceptual processing (affecting compliance in some cases). Some impairment of attention and emotional reactivity has also been noted. Lithium-induced delirium with therapeutic lithium levels is an infrequent complication and often persists for several days after serum levels have become negligible. Encephalopathy has occurred in patients on combined lithium/neuroleptic therapy and in those who have cerebrovascular disease, thus requiring careful evaluation of patients who develop neurotoxic signs at subtoxic blood levels.

Lithium exposure in early pregnancy increases the frequency of congenital anomalies, with a marked shift toward Ebstein's and other major cardiovascular anomalies. *It is advisable for women using lithium either to avoid pregnancy or to not use lithium at all during a planned pregnancy, particularly during the first trimester.* A recent prospective study does not support some previous beliefs about the risk (see reference below). Bottle-feeding should be considered in mothers using lithium, since concentration in breast milk is one-third to one-half that in serum.

C. Lithium Toxicity: Frank toxicity usually occurs at blood levels above 2 meq/L. This is often a result of sodium depletion or kidney disease, since sodium and lithium are reabsorbed at the same loci in the proximal renal tubules. Any sodium loss such as that which occurs with diarrhea, use of diuretics, or excessive perspiration results in increased lithium levels. Symptoms and signs include vomiting and diarrhea, the latter exacerbating the problem since more sodium is lost and more lithium is absorbed. Other signs and symptoms, some of which may not be reversible, include tremors, marked muscle weakness, confusion, dysarthria, vertigo, choreoathetosis, ataxia, hyperreflexia, rigidity, lack of coordination, myoclonus, seizures, opisthotonos, and coma. Toxicity is higher in the elderly, who should be maintained on slightly lower serum levels. Lithium overdosage may be accidental or intentional or may occur as a result of poor monitoring.

Compliance with lithium therapy is adversely affected by the loss of some hypomanic experiences valued by the patient. These include social extroversion and a sense of heightened enjoyment in many activities such as sex and business dealings, often with increased productivity in the latter. (Creativity has been positively correlated with bipolar disorder.)

Patients with massive ingestions of lithium or levels above 2.5 meq/L should be treated with induced emesis and gastric lavage. In normal renal function, osmotic and saline diuresis increases renal lithium clearance. Urinary alkalinization is also helpful, since sodium bicarbonate decreases lithium reabsorption in the proximal tubule, as does acetazolamide also. Aminophylline potentiates the diuretic effect by increasing the glomerular filtration rate of lithium. Drugs affecting the distal loop have no effect on lithium reabsorption. Levels above 2.5 meq/L (confirmed by cerebrospinal fluid lithium levels) should be considered an indication for hemodialysis or peritoneal dialysis.

Jacobson SJ et al: Prospective multicentre study of pregnancy outcome after lithium exposure during first trimester. Lancet 1992;339:530.

Kehoe RF et al: Lithium treatment: Prescribing and monitoring habits in hospital and general practice. Br Med J 1992;304:552. (Basic prescribing techniques in a general practice population.)

3. ANTIDEPRESSANT DRUGS

The term "antidepressant" is not completely descriptive, since the drugs in this class are also used in panic attacks, posttraumatic stress disorder, anxiety states, obsessive-compulsive disorder, aggressive conditions, pain syndromes, enuresis, bulimia, cocaine withdrawal, and affective symptoms in organic brain syndromes. The drugs may be conveniently classified into three groups: (1) the monoamine oxidase (MAO) inhibitors, (2) the tricyclic antidepressants (TCAs) and clinically similar drugs, and (3) the newer antidepressants.

Clinical Indications

A. Monoamine Oxidase Inhibitors: The MAO inhibitors have generally been used as second-line drugs (after a failure of tricyclics) because of the dietary and other restrictions (see below and Table 24–5). They should be considered as drugs of first choice in some anxious depressions, atypical depression, and panic disorders and for maintenance therapy of depression in the elderly.

B. Tricyclic Antidepressants (TCAs) and Clinically Similar Drugs: These drugs have been the mainstay of drug therapy for depression for many years. They have also been effective in panic disorders, pain syndromes, and anxiety states. Specific

Table 24–5. Principal dietary restrictions in MAO use.

1. Cheeses except cream and cottage cheese types and yogurt.
2. Fermented or aged meats such as bologna, salami.
3. Broad bean pods such as Chinese bean pods.
4. Liver of all types.
5. Meat and yeast extracts.
6. Red wine, sherry, vermouth, cognac, beer, ale.
7. Soy sauce, shrimp paste, sauerkraut.

Table 24–6. Commonly used antidepressants.

	Usual Daily Oral Dose (mg)	Usual Daily Maximum Dose (mg)
Monoamine oxidase inhibitors		
Isocarboxazid (Marplan)	10–30	60
Phenelzine (Nardil)	45–60	90
Tranylcypromine (Parnate)	20–30	50
Tricyclic and clinically similar compounds		
Amitriptyline (Elavil)	150–250	300
Amoxapine (Asendin)	150–200	400
Clomipramine (Anafranil)	100	250
Desipramine (Norpramin)	100–250	300
Doxepin (Sinequan)	150–200	300
Imipramine (Tofranil)	150–200	300
Maprotiline (Ludiomil)	100–200	300
Nortriptyline (Pamelor)	100–150	200
Protriptyline (Vivactil)	15–40	60
Trazodone (Desyrel)	100–300	400
Trimipramine (Surmontil)	75–200	200
Newer compounds		
Bupropion (Wellbutrin)	300	450[1]
Fluoxetine[2] (Prozac)	20	80
Paroxetine[2] (Paxil)	20–30	50
Sertraline[2] (Zoloft)	100	200

[1]No single dose should exceed 150 mg.
[2]Serotonin-selective reuptake inhibitors.

ones have been effective in obsessive-compulsive disorder (clomipramine), enuresis (imipramine), psychotic depression (amoxapine), and reduction of craving in cocaine withdrawal (desipramine).

C. Newer Antidepressants: This group includes the serotonin-selective reuptake inhibitors (SSRIs): fluoxetine, sertraline, and paroxetine. Also in the group is bupropion, which exerts its action through the dopamine neurotransmitter system. All are effective in the treatment of depression, both typical and atypical. The SSRI drugs have shown promise in the treatment of panic attacks, bulimia, and obsessive-compulsive disorders, while bupropion has been effective in the treatment of rapid-cycling bipolar disorder. They do not seem to be effective in pain syndromes.

Dosage Forms & Patterns

Caution: Depressed patients may have suicidal thoughts, and the amount of drug dispensed should be appropriately controlled. The older tricyclics have a narrow therapeutic index, and one advantage of the newer drugs is their wider margin of safety. In all cases of pharmacologic management of depressed states, caution is indicated until the risk of suicide is considered minimal.

A. MAO Inhibitors: MAO inhibitors are administered in gradual stepwise dosage and may be given in the morning or evening, depending upon the effect on sleep. They tend to take effect quickly in a fairly low dosage range (Table 24–6). Blood levels are not congruent with therapeutic response.

B. Tricyclic Antidepressants and Clinically Similar Drugs: These drugs are characterized more by their similarities to each other than by their differences. There is a lag in clinical response for up to several weeks, partly as a result of side effects that prevent rapid increase in dosage and partly because of their neurotransmitter effects. They tend to affect both serotonin and norepinephrine reuptake; some drugs act mainly on the former and others principally on the latter neurotransmitter system. Individuals receiving the same dosages vary markedly in therapeutic drug levels achieved (elderly patients require smaller doses), and determination of plasma drug levels is helpful when clinical response has been disappointing. Nortriptyline is usually effective when plasma levels are around 150 ng/mL; imipramine at plasma levels of 200–250 ng/mL; and desipramine at

plasma levels of about 125 ng/mL. High blood levels are not more effective than moderate levels and may be counterproductive (eg, delirium, seizures). Patients who have had gastric surgery frequently require higher doses to achieve satisfactory plasma levels. Most of the tricyclics can be given in a single dose at bedtime, starting at fairly low doses (eg, desipramine, 50 mg orally) and increasing by 50 mg every several days as tolerated until the therapeutic response is achieved (eg, desipramine, 150–200 mg) or to maximum dose if necessary (eg, desipramine, 300 mg). The most common cause of treatment failure is an inadequate trial. A full trial consists of giving maximum daily dosage for at least 2 weeks. To reach maximum dosage, the trial encompasses a total of about 4 weeks. Clomipramine is started at a low dose (25 mg/d orally) and increased slowly in divided doses up to 100 mg/d, held at that level for several days, and then gradually increased as necessary up to 250 mg/d. Any of the TCA-like drugs should be started at low doses and increased slowly in the treatment of panic disorder.

C. Newer Antidepressants: All of the drugs in this group tend to be activating and are given in the morning so as not to interfere with sleep. The SSRIs can be given in once-daily dosage except bupropion, which should be given in divided doses. There is a delay in response; fluoxetine, for example, requires 2–6 weeks to act in depression, 4–8 weeks to be effective in panic disorder, and 6–12 weeks in treatment of obsessive-compulsive disorder. The starting dose (20 mg) is the usual daily dose for depression, while obsessive-compulsive disorder may require up to 80 mg daily. The other SSRIs (sertraline, paroxetine) have shorter half-lives and a lesser effect on hepatic enzymes, which reduces their impact on the metabolism of other drugs (thus not increasing significantly the serum concentrations of tricyclic antidepressants or other drugs). The lesser side effects of these two newer drugs are an additional advantage.

D. Switching and Combination Therapy: If the therapeutic response has been poor, one should reassess the diagnosis after an adequate trial with the chosen drug. Assuming that the diagnosis is correct and the trial has been adequate, a trial with a drug from another group is appropriate. Combination therapy with antidepressant drugs is not usually feasible (Table 24–7), and in switching from one group to another an adequate "washout time" must be allowed. This is critical in certain situations—eg, in switching from an MAO inhibitor to a tricyclic, allow 2–3 weeks between stopping one drug and starting another; in switching from an SSRI to an MAO inhibitor, allow 4–5 weeks. In switching within groups —eg, from one tricyclic to another (amitriptyline to desipramine, etc)—no washout time is needed, and one can rapidly decrease the dosage of one drug while increasing the other.

However, in any of the three groups, one can augment the antidepressant drug if the therapeutic response has been less than satisfactory. Lithium is the most effective augmenting agent. It is added to the regimen and regulated in the usual fashion.

E. Maintenance and Tapering: When clinical relief of symptoms is obtained, medication is continued for 12 months in the effective maintenance dosage, which is usually about half the dosage required in the acute stage. After about 12 months of effective treatment, the dosage is slowly decreased and, if there is no resurgence of symptoms, discontinued.

Side Effects

A. MAO Inhibitors: The MAO inhibitors commonly cause symptoms of orthostatic hypotension (which may persist) and sympathomimetic effects of tachycardia, sweating, and tremor. Nausea, insomnia (often associated with intense afternoon drowsiness), and sexual dysfunction are common. Trazodone, 25–75 mg orally at bedtime, may ameliorate the MAO-induced insomnia. Central nervous system effects include agitation and toxic psychoses. Dietary limitations (Table 24–5) and abstinence from drug products containing phenylpropanolamine, phenylephrine, and pseudoephedrine are mandatory for MAO-A type inhibitors (those marketed for treatment of depression), since the reduction of available monoamine oxidase leaves the patient vulnerable to exogenous amines (eg, tyramine in foodstuffs).

Treatment for a resultant hypertensive crisis has been the same as for pheochromocytoma (see Chap-

Table 24–7. Antidepressant drug interactions with other drugs.

Drug	Effects
Tricyclic and other non-MAOI antidepressants	
Antacids	Decreased absorption of antidepressants.
Anticoagulants	Increased hypoprothrombinemic effect.
Cimetidine	Increased antidepressant blood levels and psychosis.
Clonidine	Decreased antihypertensive effect.
Digitalis	Increased incidence of heart block.
Disulfiram	Increased antidepressant blood levels.
Guanadrel	Decreased antihypertensive effect.
Guanethidine	Decreased antihypertensive effect.
Haloperidol	Increased clomipramine levels.
Insulin	Decreased blood sugar.
Lithium	Increased lithium levels with fluoxetine.
Methyldopa	Decreased antihypertensive effect.
Other anticholinergic drugs	Marked anticholinergic responses.
Phenytoin	Increased blood levels.
Procainamide	Decreased ventricular conduction.
Procarbazine	Hypertensive crisis.
Propranolol	Increased hypotension.
Quinidine	Decreased ventricular conduction.
Rauwolfia derivatives	Increased stimulation.
Sedatives	Increased sedation.
Sympathomimetic drugs	Increased pressor effect.
Monoamine oxidase inhibitors	
Antihistamines	Increased sedation.
Belladonna-like drugs	Increased blood pressure.
Dextromethorphan	Same as meperidine.
Guanadrel	Increased blood pressure.
Guanethidine	Decreased blood pressure.
Insulin	Decreased blood sugar.
Levodopa	Increased blood pressure.
Meperidine	Increased mood lability, agitation, seizures.
Methyldopa	Decreased blood pressure.
Reserpine	Increased blood pressure and temperature.
Succinylcholine	Increased neuromuscular blockage.
Sulfonylureas	Decreased blood sugar.
Sympathomimetic drugs	Increased blood pressure.

ter 25), but there have been reports of success with nifedipine, 10 mg sublingually, which normalized blood pressure in 1–5 minutes. The restrictions on the proscribed foodstuffs and sympathomimetic drugs are in effect during treatment and for 1 month after cessation of therapy. Termination of therapy with MAO inhibitors may be associated with anxiety, agitation, cognitive slowing, and headache. Very gradual withdrawal and short-term benzodiazepine therapy will ameliorate symptoms.

B. Tricyclic Antidepressants and Clinically Similar Drugs: These drugs have anticholinergic side effects (amitriptyline 100 mg is equivalent to atropine 5 mg) to varying degrees. One must be particularly wary of the effect in elderly men with prostatic hypertrophy. The anticholinergic effects also predispose to other medical problems such as heat stroke or dental problems such as xerostomia. Orthostatic hypotension is fairly common, may not remit with time, and is a major problem in elderly women with osteoporosis who may suffer a hip fracture after a fall. Cardiac effects of the TCAs are functions of the anticholinergic effect, direct myocardial depression (quinidine-like effect), and interference with adrenergic neurons. These factors produce altered rate, rhythm, and contractility, particularly in patients with preexisting cardiac disease, particularly bundle-branch or bifascicular block. Electrocardiographic changes range from benign ST segment and T wave changes and sinus tachycardia to a variety of complex and serious arrhythmias, the latter requiring a change in medication. The seizure threshold may be lowered and is of particular concern in patients with a propensity for seizures (eg, previous head injury, alcohol withdrawal). Loss of libido and erectile, ejaculatory, and orgasmic dysfunction are fairly common and seriously compromise compliance. Trazodone rarely causes priapism, which requires treatment (epinephrine 1:1000 injected into the corpus cavernosum) within 12 hours. Delirium, agitation, and mania are infrequent complications. Sudden discontinuation of some of these drugs can produce "cholinergic rebound," manifested by headaches and nausea with cramps. Overdoses of the tricyclic compounds are often serious because of the narrow therapeutic index.

C. Newer Antidepressants: The side effects common to all of these drugs are headache, nausea, tinnitus, insomnia, and nervousness. Akathisia and dyskinesia have been common with fluoxetine but less so with the other drugs. As with all the antidepressants, sexual side effects of impotence, retrograde ejaculation, and dysorgasmia are common. Cyproheptadine, 4 mg orally prior to sexual activity, may be helpful in countering drug-induced anorgasmia. Because of early research with bulimic patients, bupropion has been burdened with an unwarranted reputation for causing seizures. The SSRIs are strong serotonin uptake blockers and may in high dosage or in combination with other serotonin uptake blockers cause a "serotonin syndrome" manifested by rigidity, hyperthermia, autonomic instability, confusion, myoclonus, delirium, and coma. This syndrome can be a particularly troublesome problem in the elderly.

Kapur S, Mieczkowski T, Mann JJ: Antidepressant medication and the relative risk of suicide attempts and suicide. JAMA 1992;268:3441. (The newer antidepressant drugs are much safer than the older groups.)

Mann JJ, Kapur S: The emergence of suicidal ideation and behavior during antidepressant therapy. Am J Psychiatry 1991;148:1027. (Rather similar in the various antidepressant drugs.)

4. SEDATIVE-HYPNOTIC & OTHER ANTIANXIETY DRUGS (Anxiolytic Agents, "Minor Tranquilizers")

The sedatives are a heterogeneous group of drugs that differ in chemical structure but have quite similar pharmacologic and behavioral effects. Almost all of them produce the same behavioral profile as ethanol. They are often marketed as "minor tranquilizers" or "antianxiety agents," and all have hypnotic properties when given in adequate dosage. To varying degrees, all have the potential for dependency with tolerance and severe withdrawal symptoms. Short-acting drugs may present a greater risk of withdrawal reactions than longer-acting agents. Some have anticonvulsant and muscle relaxant properties, though muscle relaxation usually occurs in the ataxic dosage range.

The highly addicting drugs with a narrow margin of safety such as glutethimide, ethchlorvynol, methyprylon, meprobamate, and the barbiturates (with the exception of phenobarbital) should be avoided. Phenobarbital, in addition to its anticonvulsant properties, is a reasonably safe and very cheap sedative but has the disadvantage of enzyme stimulation (not the case with benzodiazepines), which markedly reduces its usefulness if any other medications are being used by the patient.

The benzodiazepines are most commonly used. Onset of action is a function of rate of absorption (related to lipophilic activity) and varies, with diazepam and clorazepate being the most rapidly absorbed. This characteristic, along with high lipid solubility, may explain the popularity of diazepam. The length of action of the benzodiazepines varies as a function of the active metabolites they produce. Short-acting benzodiazepines, which do not produce active metabolites, have half-lives of 5–20 hours, and ultra-short-acting ones have half-lives of less than 5 hours. The other benzodiazepines produce active metabolites and have half-lives of 1–8 days.

The antihistamines hydroxyzine and diphenhydramine are often prescribed for mild sedation because they are safe and produce no dependency.

Buspirone is the only marketed anxiolytic drug that is not a sedative. There is no evidence that it produces depressant effects or dependence. In fact, it is increasingly being used in the treatment of depression and compulsive behaviors. It differs from the sedatives in that motor skills are not impaired and it does not potentiate the effects of alcohol or cause a withdrawal syndrome, nor can it be used in benzodiazepine or alcohol withdrawal. There is a 2- to 3-week lag period before the drug takes effect.

Clinical Indications

The sedatives are used clinically for the treatment of anxiety, which may be the result of many factors, eg, transient situational problems, acute and chronic stresses of life, chronic medical problems, intractable pain exacerbated by apprehension and depression, and problems that people cannot or will not resolve (unhappy marriages, unsatisfactory jobs, etc). In higher doses these drugs act as hypnotics. Whether the indications are anxiety or insomnia, the drugs should be used judiciously. The longer-acting benzodiazepines are used for the treatment of alcohol withdrawal and anxiety symptoms; the shorter-acting drugs are useful as sedatives in sleep and medical procedures such as endoscopy.

Clonazepam, approved in the USA as an oral benzodiazepine antiseizure agent, has been found to be effective in a variety of other conditions. It has been shown to be effective as an antimanic drug (0.5–16 mg/d orally) and in the treatment of panic attacks (3–6 mg/d orally). Clonazepam is longer-acting than alprazolam and is an effective drug in panic disorders. It and lorazepam have been used as an adjunct to antipsychotic drugs in the treatment of agitation in the psychotic patient.

Dosage Forms & Patterns
(Table 24–8)

All of the sedatives may be given orally, and several are available in parenteral form. Short-acting benzodiazepines are absorbed rapidly when given intramuscularly. Disadvantages of intravenous use outweigh advantages in psychiatric disorders. Antacids significantly alter the absorption of clorazepate and prazepam; this is an important consideration, since many anxious individuals suffer from gastrointestinal disturbances and use both types of drugs concomitantly. Food also modifies the absorption of diazepam (and possibly the other benzodiazepines), initially slowing absorption but resulting in higher levels over many hours. In the average case of anxiety, diazepam, 5–10 mg orally every 6–8 hours as needed, is a reasonable starting regimen. Since people vary widely in their response and since the drugs are long-lasting, one must individualize the dosage. Once this is established, an adequate dose early in the course of symptom development will obviate the need for "pill-popping," which contributes to dependency problems. Flurazepam and temazepam are both longer-acting and should be avoided in elderly patients. The latter has a somewhat shorter duration of action but a delayed onset of action in the range of 1–3 hours. Triazolam has achieved popularity as a hypnotic drug because of its very short duration of action. There are problems in some patients with dependency, transient psychotic ideation, and anterograde amnesia.

Buspirone is given in dose of 30–40 mg/d. Higher doses tend to be counterproductive and produce gastrointestinal symptoms and dizziness. Sleep is sometimes negatively affected.

Table 24–8. Commonly used antianxiety and hypnotic agents.

	Usual Daily Oral Dose (mg)	Usual Daily Maximum Dose (mg)
Benzodiazepines (used for anxiety)		
Alprazolam (Xanax)	0.5	4
Chlordiazepoxide (Librium)	10–20	40
Clonazepam (Klonopin)	1–2	10
Clorazepate (Tranxene)	15–30	60
Diazepam (Valium)	5–15	30
Lorazepam (Ativan)[1]	2–4	10
Oxazepam (Serax)[1]	10–30	60
Prazepam (Centrax)	20–40	60
Benzodiazepines (used for sleep)		
Estazolam (Prosom)[1]	1	2
Flurazepam (Dalmane)	15	30
Quazepam (Doral)	7.5	15
Temazepam (Restoril)	15	30
Triazolam (Halcion)[2]	0.125	0.25
Miscellaneous (used for anxiety)		
Buspirone (Buspar)	10–30	60
Phenobarbital	15–30	90
Miscellaneous (used for sleep)		
Chloral hydrate (Noctec)[1]	500	1000
Hydroxyzine (Vistaril)	50	100

[1]Shorter-acting.
[2]Ultra-short-acting.

Side Effects

The side effects of all the sedatives are mainly behavioral and depend on patient reaction and dosage. As the dosage exceeds the levels necessary for sedation, the side effects include disinhibition, ataxia, dysarthria, nystagmus, and errors of commission. (Machinery should not be operated until the patient is well stabilized, and the patient should be so informed.) Agitation, anxiety, psychosis, confusion, mood lability, and anterograde amnesia have been reported, particularly with the shorter-acting benzodiazepines.

The sedatives produce **cumulative** clinical effects with repeated dosage (especially if the patient has not had time to metabolize the previous dose); **additive** effects when given with other classes of sedatives or alcohol (many "accidental" deaths are the result of concomitant use of sedatives and alcohol); and **residual** effects after termination of treatment (particularly in the case of drugs that undergo slow biotransformation).

Overdosage results in respiratory depression, hypotension, shock syndrome, coma, and death. Fortunately, flumazenil, a benzodiazepine antagonist, is now available. Treatment of overdoses (see Chapter 39) and withdrawal states are medical emergencies.

A serious side effect of chronic excessive dosage is drug dependency, which may involve tolerance, and physiologic dependency with withdrawal symptoms similar in morbidity and mortality to alcohol or barbiturate withdrawal (withdrawal effects must be distinguished from reemergent anxiety). Abrupt withdrawal of sedative drugs may cause serious and even fatal convulsive seizures. Psychosis, organic brain syndrome, and autonomic dysfunction have also been described. Both duration of action and duration of exposure are major factors. Common withdrawal symptoms after low to moderate daily use of benzodiazepines are classified as **somatic** (disturbed sleep, tremor, nausea, muscle aches), **psychologic** (anxiety, poor concentration, irritability, mild depression), or **perceptual** (poor coordination, mild paranoia, mild confusion). The presentation of symptoms will vary depending on the half-life of the drug. There are no significant side effects on organ systems other than the brain, and the drugs are safe in most medical conditions. Trazodone, 300 mg orally at bedtime, can mitigate the mild withdrawal effects and reduce craving if given regularly over a period of 3–6 months.

Benzodiazepine interactions with other drugs are listed in Table 24–9.

Rickels K et al: Long-term benzodiazepine users 3 years after participation in a discontinuation program. Am J Psychiatry 1991;148:757. (Continuation of drugs a function of both dependence and concurrent psychiatric disorders.)
Rifkin A: Benzodiazepines for anxiety disorders: Are the concerns justified? Postgrad Med 1990;87:209. (A pertinent question.)

5. OTHER DRUGS USED IN PSYCHIATRIC DISORDERS

Carbamazepine, an antiseizure drug that stabilizes the activity of cell membranes, has been used with increasing frequency in the treatment of bipolar patients who cannot be satisfactorily treated with lithium (nonresponsive or side effects). It has also been used in the treatment of resistant depressions, mania, rapid-cycling bipolar disorder, alcohol withdrawal, and hallucinations (in conjunction with neuroleptics) and in patients with behavioral dyscontrol or panic

Table 24–9. Benzodiazepine interactions with other drugs.

Drug	Effects
Antacids	Decreased absorption of benzodiazepines.
Cimetidine	Increased half-life of flurazepam, alprazolam.
Contraceptives	Increased levels of diazepam and triazolam.
Dicumarol	Decreased prothrombin time.
Digoxin	Alprazolam and diazepam raise digoxin level.
Disulfiram	Increased duration of action of sedatives.
Isoniazid	Increased plasma diazepam.
Levodopa	Inhibition of antiparkinsonism effect.
Propoxyphene	Impaired clearance of diazepam.
Rifampin	Decreased plasma diazepam.

attacks. It suppresses some phases of kindling (see Stimulants) and has been used to treat residual symptoms in previous stimulant abusers (eg, posttraumatic stress disorder with impulse control problems). Dose-related side effects include sedation and ataxia. Dosages start at 400–600 mg orally daily and are increased slowly to therapeutic levels. Skin rashes and a mild reduction in white count are common. SIADH occurs rarely. Congenital anomalies have been reported along with growth deficiency and developmental delay. Nonsteroidal anti-inflammatory drugs (except aspirin); the antibiotics erythromycin, troleandomycin, and isoniazid; the calcium channel blockers verapamil and diltiazem (but not nifedipine); fluoxetine, propoxyphene, and cimetidine all increase carbamazepine levels. Carbamazepine can be effective in conjunction with lithium, though there have been reports of reversible neurotoxicity with the combination. Carbamazepine stimulates liver enzymes and so tends to decrease levels of haloperidol and oral contraceptives. It also lowers T_4, free T_4, and T_3 levels. Cases of fetal malformation (particularly spina bifida) have been reported. Hepatic and hematologic status should be monitored in patients taking carbamazepine.

Valproic acid is an antiseizure drug whose activity is at least partially related to GABA neurotransmission. In psychiatric disorders, it is used as primary or adjunctive treatment of the same conditions for which carbamazepine is indicated. It has somewhat less neurotoxicity than carbamazepine when used in conjunction with lithium. Treatment is started at a dose of 750 mg/d orally, and dosage is then titrated to achieve therapeutic serum levels. Concomitant use of aspirin, carbamazepine, warfarin, or phenytoin may affect serum levels. Gastrointestinal symptoms are the main side effect. Hematologic and hepatic function should be monitored, and teratogenic problems are a concern.

Calcium channel blockers are increasingly being used in psychiatric conditions. This has come about with the realization that a number of drugs used in psychiatry (eg, lithium, antidepressants, neuroleptics, and carbamazepine) have calcium channel-blocking activity. Mania has been the principal disorder studied to date. There is also preliminary evidence that these drugs may be useful in the treatment of tardive dyskinesia and panic attacks.

Beta-blockers such as atenolol and propranolol have been used to mute the peripheral symptoms of anxiety without significantly affecting motor performance. They block symptoms mediated by sympathetic stimulation (eg, palpitations, tremulousness) but not noradrenergic symptoms (eg, diarrhea, muscle tension). Contrary to current belief, they do not generally cause depression as a side effect.

Amphetamines have some usefulness in geriatric patients for apathy and depression secondary to medical and surgical problems.

6. OTHER ORGANIC THERAPIES

Electroconvulsive therapy (ECT) causes a generalized central nervous system seizure (peripheral convulsion is not necessary) by means of electric current. The key objective is to exceed the seizure threshold, which can be accomplished by a variety of means. Electrical stimulation is more reliable and simpler than the use of chemical convulsants such as hexafluorodiethyl ether (flurothyl). The mechanism of action is not known, but it is thought to involve major neurotransmitter responses at the cell membrane. Current insufficient to cause a seizure produces no therapeutic benefit.

Electroconvulsive therapy is the most effective (about 70%) treatment of severe depression, particularly with delusions and agitation commonly seen with depression in the involutional period. It is indicated when medical conditions preclude the use of antidepressants or in cases of nonresponsiveness to these medications. Comparative controlled studies of electroconvulsive therapy in severe depression show that it is more effective than chemotherapy. It is also effective in the manic disorders and psychoses during pregnancy (when drugs may be contraindicated). It has not been shown to be helpful in chronic schizophrenic disorders, and it is generally not used in acute schizophrenic episodes unless drugs are not effective and it is urgent that the psychosis be controlled (eg, a catatonic stupor complicating an acute medical condition).

The most common side effects are memory disturbance and headache. Memory loss or confusion is usually related to number and frequency of electroconvulsive therapy treatments and proper oxygenation during treatment. Some memory loss is occasionally permanent, but most memory faculties return to full capacity within several weeks. There have been reports that lithium administration concurrent with electroconvulsive therapy resulted in greater memory loss. Before anesthesia was used, spinal compression fractures and severe anticipatory anxiety were common.

Increased intracranial pressure is a serious contraindication. Other problems such as cardiac disorders, aortic aneurysms, bronchopulmonary disease, and venous thrombosis are relative contraindications and must be evaluated in light of the severity of the medical problem versus the need for electroconvulsive therapy. Serious complications arising from electroconvulsive therapy occur in less than one in 1000 cases. Most of these problems are cardiovascular or respiratory in nature (eg, aspiration of gastric contents). Poor patient understanding and lack of acceptance of the technique by the public are the biggest obstacles to the use of electroconvulsive therapy.

Psychosurgery has a limited place in selected cases of severe, unremitting anxiety and depression, obsessional neuroses, and, to a lesser degree, some of the schizophrenias. The stereotactic techniques now being used, including modified bifrontal tractotomy, are great improvements over the crude methods of the past.

In the controversial area of **megavitamin treatment** for the schizophrenic patient, the overall therapeutic efficacy of nicotinic acid or nicotinamide as the sole or adjuvant medication is no better than that of an inactive placebo.

Acupuncture and **electrosleep** are of unproved usefulness for any psychiatric conditions.

Phototherapy is used in seasonal affective disorder (SAD). It consists of exposure (at a 3-foot distance) to a light source of 2500 lux for 2 hours daily in the morning. Light visors are an adaptation that provide greater mobility and an adjustable light intensity. The price of these full-spectrum light sources range between $300 and $400. The dosage varies, with some patients requiring morning and night exposure. One effect is alteration of biorhythm through melatonin mechanisms.

Garza-Trevino ES, Overall JE, Hollister MD: Verapamil versus lithium in acute mania. Am J Psychiatry 1992; 149:121.

Jenike MA et al: Cingulotomy for refractory obsessive-compulsive disorder. Arch Gen Psychiatry 1991;48:548. (The major role of psychosurgery.)

Lam RW et al: Ultraviolet versus non-ultraviolet light therapy for seasonal affective disorder. J Clin Psychiatry 1991;52:213.

7. HOSPITALIZATION

The need for hospital care may range from admission to a medical bed in a general hospital for an acute situational stress reaction to admission to a psychiatric ward when the patient is in acute psychosis. The trend over recent years has been to admit patients to general hospitals in the community, treat patients aggressively, and discharge them promptly to the next appropriate level of treatment—day hospital, halfway house, outpatient therapy, etc. Involuntary hospitalization should be objectively determined on the basis of patient and society welfare. Sixty percent of admissions are readmissions. The total "in residence" population (hospital plus residential) is about the same as the hospital total of 30 years ago. This does not include the homeless mentally ill, a population that would have been institutionalized in past years.

Hospital care may be indicated when patients are too sick to care for themselves or when they present serious threats to themselves or others; when observation and diagnostic procedures are necessary; or when specific kinds of treatment such as complex medication trials or hospital environment (milieu) are required. Symptoms correlating best with hospitalization are self-neglect, violent or bizarre behavior, paranoid ideation or delusions, marked intellectual impairment, and poor judgment.

The disadvantages of psychiatric hospitalization include decreased self-confidence as a result of needing hospitalization; the stigma of being a "psychiatric patient"; possible increased dependency and regression; and the expense. Generally, there is no advantage to prolonged hospital stays for most psychiatric disorders.

Dowart RA et al: A national study of psychiatric hospital care. Am J Psychiatry 1991;148:204.

PSYCHOLOGIC APPROACHES

Psychotherapy attempts to make sense of the chaotic aspects of a person's life and to change the patient's attitudes and behaviors. There are over 100 different types of psychotherapy, and all are reported to give similar results. Harm as well as good can be done by psychotherapy. Bad results can usually be shown to be due to the inexperience, poor judgment, or inflexibility of the therapist. The physician must at all times maintain an ethical relationship with the patient. Any sexual misconduct with a patient is increasingly being regarded as a criminal offense.

Dynamic psychotherapy. The basic concepts of dynamic psychotherapy rest in the role of the unconscious with libidinal drives and conflicts that remain out of awareness and in the importance of determinism, which emphasizes that each psychic event is determined by the ones that preceded it. The ideologic framework is not a critical factor. The variables that correlate highly with improvement are support by the therapist and identification with the therapist (both being functions of the patient-therapist relationship), improved self-esteem, and appropriate use of defense mechanisms.

The defense mechanisms of particular importance are **repression** (barring from consciousness), **reaction formation** (substituting a pleasant thought for a painful one), **isolation** (separating original memory from affective response), **denial** (refusing to deal with obvious reality issues), **projection** (attributing a wish or impulse to some other person), **rationalization** (substituting acceptable reason for unacceptable reason), and **undoing** (neutralizing objectionable thoughts).

The focus is rooted in the subjective past, and the mode of change is to make the unconscious conscious, ie, to achieve insight with an understanding of the early past and its connection with conflicts. To achieve reduction of the conflicts, the therapist in a dyadic relationship uses free associations, interpretations, and analysis of both resistance and transference of feelings (a repetition of the past that is inappropriate to the present) onto the therapist. The process is long-term—in classic psychoanalysis, with major psychic reorganization, daily sessions; in later modifications, weekly or twice weekly meetings with the focus on insight and change of behavior.

Experiential psychotherapy. This includes gestalt therapy, client-centered psychotherapy, cognitive therapy, existential analysis, and structural analysis. The focus of therapy is on the present. The mode of change is in the immediate experiencing of one's emotions. The past is not significant in the therapeutic process. The sharing is an important element in the encounter. The goals in this short-term process (weekly meetings for weeks or months) are self-determination; integration of new perceptions, thinking patterns, and self-awareness; rational thinking; creativity; and self-affirmation within a setting of adult, humanistic, peer-oriented relationships.

Cognitive therapy. Corrects faulty impressions (upon which the person acts) and counteracts learned behavior such as helplessness (eg, "Everybody must love me," or "If I make a mistake, I am no good"). The therapist challenges the patient's negative self-image, negative interpretations, and negative views of the future upon which previous behaviors were based. Daily logs often help the patient see the incongruity between established conceptions and reality and help substitute more reality-oriented and positive cognitions. A number of studies (particularly studies of depression and panic attack disorders) have substantiated the value of combined cognitive therapy and medications.

Supportive psychotherapy. It usually denotes a positive relationship with the patient, strengthening of existing defenses, assumption of responsibility by the patient, enhancing self-esteem (remoralization), and an emphasis on the here and now. The goals are primarily alleviation of symptoms and termination of therapy when this has been accomplished. There is little effort to make substantial changes in the personality structure. Termination should occur within the framework of therapist availability in the event of future needs.

Group therapy. The decision for group versus individual therapy is usually based on the patient's need to improve **interpersonal relationships,** and the group setting may provide the "laboratory" for improvisation and practice of new behaviors that can then be generalized to everyday activities. Personality disorders and posttraumatic stress disorders are conditions for which group psychotherapy may be preferred. Therapy groups are usually composed of individuals who have no outside connection with one another, but groups may be made up of couples or families.

The various schools of therapy often purport to be unique, more effective, or of more lasting value than others. In reality, they have many similarities and common derivations, with about the same results. The attitude of the patient, the cultural variations, and the skill of the therapist rather than the ideology are usually the major factors in producing change.

Council on Ethical and Judicial Affairs, American Medical Association: Sexual misconduct in the practice of medicine. JAMA 1991;266:2741.
Gabbard GO: Psychodynamic psychiatry in the "decade of the brain." Am J Psychiatry 1992;149:991.

SOCIAL APPROACHES

In contrast to psychologic techniques, which deal principally with intrapsychic phenomena and interpersonal problems, the social approaches to psychiatric treatment attempt to modify attitudes and behavior by altering the **environmental** factors contributing to the patient's maladaptation. The scope of the attempt may range from provision of a therapeutic milieu—eg, in a day hospital or residential community—to minor alterations in school procedures or daily family activities. The family, friends, and neighbors provide the major social support in the large majority of cases. Various psychologic and behavioral techniques are used within social approaches.

Part-Time Hospitalization

The patient either participates in the hospital milieu during the day (day hospitals—going home at night), or stays the night (night hospitals—going to work or school during the day), or spends several hours a day in the hospital for up to 5 or 6 days a week. This is a cost-effective alternative to full hospitalization.

Self-Help Communities & Substitute Homes

These are usually sponsored by nongovernmental agencies for the purpose of helping people with a particular type of difficulty. The individual lives-in full-time for varying periods and usually continues to be affiliated with the group after leaving. Examples of self-help communities include halfway houses, lodge societies (autonomous financial and social entities) across the USA, residences for people with alcohol or other drug problems, Salvation Army, and church-sponsored agencies. They are often a bridge between hospitalization and independent living. Substitute homes provide shelter and treatment-related programs for longer periods of time. An example is board-and-care homes, primarily for people who are disabled and unlikely to return to productive functioning.

Nonresidential Self-Help Organizations

The following are examples of organizations usually administered by people who have survived similar problems: Alcoholics Anonymous (and Al-Anon, to help families of alcoholics); Recovery Inc., organized and run by people who have had an emotional problem that required hospitalization; Schizophrenics Anonymous; Gamblers Anonymous; Overeaters Anonymous; colostomy clubs; mastectomy clubs; the Epilepsy Society; Body Positive, for AIDS patients; the Alzheimer's Disease and Related Disorders Association; the American Heart Association's Stroke Clubs of America; and burn recovery groups.

A national self-help clearinghouse at the City University of New York, 33 West 42nd St., New York, NY 10036, maintains up-to-date listings of mutual aid organizations in the USA.

Special Professional & Paraprofessional Organizations

Examples of special organizations of this type are Homemaker Service, made up of individuals who come into the home to help the partially disabled maintain the household; Visiting Nurse Associations, which usually provide more than medical assistance; adult protective services for the elderly; genetic counseling services; family service agencies, for marriage counseling and family problems; crisis centers, eg, "free clinics" and county-sponsored satellite clinics; and church-sponsored agencies. Religion (personal beliefs) and churches (organized groups) play major roles in psychosocial adjustment.

Stress Reduction

Social and environmental factors are major aids in lowering stress and should be part of the activities of daily living. Both active recreation (sports, physical exercise, participant hobbies) and passive pursuits (reading, music, painting) are necessary for a balanced life and alleviation of stress. Family structure and dynamics must be evaluated, and there will be occasions (eg, adult children living at home, presence of in-laws) when a social restructuring is in order.

BEHAVIORAL APPROACHES

Behavior therapy has its foundations in theories of the learning process. The role of the behavior therapist is that of a teacher who attempts to bring about change in the patient's maladaptation. The specific problem (target behavior) and the factors that play a role in precipitating or perpetuating the problem must first be identified. An attempt can then be made to alter those factors that perpetuate unwanted behavior.

The emphasis of behavior therapy is on "here and now" and *direct* change. The goal is to "unlearn" those destructive or unproductive types of behavior that result from faulty learning and to enhance the individual's repertoire of useful social and adaptive skills. Great emphasis is placed on identifying and then ablating whatever is maintaining the maladaptive behavior.

Whereas **conditioning** is understood by some to be synonymous with a specific type of learning (eg, Pavlov's dogs), behavior therapy is much broader. It includes the relationship with the therapist, utilizes some verbal techniques, though to a lesser degree than other therapies, and interprets "behavior" in a broad sense that includes thoughts and feelings. Behavior techniques are frequently blended with cognitive psychotherapy.

Many of the techniques of behavior therapy require a cooperative effort on the part of a number of people who must all understand and be consistent in their responses to specified behaviors. Thus, a cooperative social setting such as a milieu ward or the patient's own home and family is important in implementing many of the following techniques.

Techniques of Behavior Therapy

A. Modeling: Much learning occurs by imitation. From the earliest years of childhood, the individual's behavior is modeled after parents, teachers, peers, employers, public personalities, historical figures, etc ("significant others"). The therapist makes a conscious effort to serve as a model of particular kinds of behavior that are significant to and attainable by the patient. This device is particularly useful in treating patients with low self-esteem.

B. Operant Conditioning: Operant conditioning is the deliberate implementation of a system of rewards to encourage repetition of specific desired behaviors. A voluntary behavior is singled out for a specific reward every time the behavior is used. The objective is to develop a habit in the use of that behavior. Like modeling, operant conditioning is a common procedure in families, and the child soon learns that "good" behavior is rewarded.

C. Aversive Conditioning: Aversive conditioning is the opposite of operant conditioning but is a less potent shaper of behavior. Undesirable behavior (eg, alcohol ingestion) is paired with an unpleasant consequence (eg, vomiting induced by apomorphine, mild electric or sound shock), whereas satisfactory alternative responses are operantly encouraged. The most common conditions treated by this technique have been enuresis, smoking, alcoholism, and sexual arousal disorders.

D. Extinction: Extinction is the process of refusing to reinforce behavior on the theory that behavior cannot be sustained without some sort of reinforcement. Temper tantrums and noxious behavior, usually contrived to gain attention of any sort, are "extinguished" in this way.

E. Desensitization: Familiarity lessens anxiety and reduces the tendency to avoid exposure to the feared object, person, or situation. The subject is repeatedly exposed to the feared stimulus (eg, looking at a picture of an elevator when the fear has been ri-

ding in elevators) at such a low level of intensity that the fear response is minimal. Exposures are then gradually increased (eg, walking past a real elevator) until the subject is able to tolerate the real experience with markedly reduced fear. This technique has been most effective in the treatment of phobias and a variety of situations (such as frigidity or impotence) that engender fears of failure, disapproval, and embarrassment.

F. Emotive Imagery: Deliberate evocation of mental images that arouse certain feelings can be used as a way of warding off painful emotions resulting from stress-inducing circumstances. Noxious imagery can be used in aversive conditioning and "pleasant thoughts" in operant training. A graded exposure to the thoughts results in gradually lower anxiety levels.

G. Flooding: Flooding (implosion) consists of overwhelming the individual, in a safe setting, with anxiety-producing stimuli. The anxiety responses gradually lessen (law of diminishing returns) until extinction occurs. In some ways, flooding is a desensitization technique without the graded approach.

H. Role-Playing: In the role-playing technique, patients can practice various types of behaviors in anxiety-producing but "safe" situations. For example, the therapist may assume the role of an angry friend and the patient uses different ways of handling the situation. Role reversal—where the therapist and the patient change roles—then gives the patient a chance to experience the other's feelings and attitudes. Assertiveness training for inhibited individuals is a variant to help people learn to be more spontaneous.

I. Relaxation Techniques: These include muscle relaxation, self-hypnosis, and biofeedback procedures. The names are descriptive. Biofeedback requires some equipment to measure and signal physiologic change. It is particularly helpful in such somatic disorders as migraine headache and hyperactive bowel syndrome (see Somatoform Disorders). Relaxation, meditation, and hypnosis share some common features and are valuable ancillary modalities in effecting change and modifying symptoms.

COMMON PSYCHIATRIC DISORDERS

STRESS & ADJUSTMENT DISORDERS
(Situational Disorders)

Essentials of Diagnosis
- Anxiety or depression clearly secondary to an identifiable stress.
- Future symptoms of anxiety or depression commonly elicited by similar stress of lesser magnitude.
- Alcohol and other drugs are commonly used in self-treatment.

General Considerations
Stress exists when the adaptive capacity of the individual is overwhelmed by events. The event may be an insignificant one objectively considered, and even favorable changes (eg, promotion and transfer) requiring adaptive behavior can produce stress. For each individual, stress is subjectively defined, and the response to stress is a function of each person's personality and physiologic endowment.

Classification & Clinical Findings
Opinion differs about what events are most apt to produce stress reactions. The causes of stress are different at different ages—eg, in young adulthood, the sources of stress are found in the marriage or parent-child relationship, the employment relationship, and the struggle to achieve financial stability; in the middle years, the focus shifts to changing spousal relationships, problems with aging parents, and problems associated with having young adult offspring who themselves are encountering stressful situations; in old age, the principal concerns are apt to be retirement, loss of physical capacity, major personal losses, and thoughts of death.

An individual may react to stress by becoming anxious or depressed, by developing a physical symptom, by running away, by having a drink or starting an affair, or in limitless other ways. Common subjective responses are fear (of repetition of the stress-inducing event), rage (at frustration), guilt (over aggressive impulses), and shame (over helplessness). Acute and reactivated stress may be manifested by restlessness, irritability, fatigue, increased startle reaction, and a feeling of tension. Inability to concentrate, sleep disturbances (insomnia, bad dreams), and somatic preoccupations often lead to self-medication, most commonly with alcohol or other central nervous system depressants. Maladaptive behavior to stress is called adjustment disorder, with the major symptom specified (eg, "adjustment disorder with depressed mood").

Posttraumatic stress disorder (PTSD) is a syndrome with symptoms of reexperiencing the traumatic event (eg, rape, severe burns, military combat), along with decreased responsiveness to and avoidance of current events associated with the trauma, and physiologic hyperarousal, which includes startle reactions, intrusive thoughts, illusions, overgeneralized associations, sleep problems, nightmares, dreams about the precipitating event, impulsivity, difficulties in concentration, and hyperalertness. The symptoms may be precipitated or exacerbated by distant events that are a reminder of the original stress (less common with the anxiety disorders). Symptoms frequently arise after a long latency period (eg, child abuse can result in later posttraumatic stress syndrome). The sooner the symptoms arise after the initial trauma and the sooner therapy is initiated, the better the prognosis. The therapeutic approach is to facilitate the normal recovery that was blocked at the time of the trauma. Therapy at that time should be brief, simple (catharsis and working through of the traumatic experience), and expectant (of quick recovery and a rapid return to work).

Treatment initiated later, when symptoms have crystallized, includes programs for cessation of alcohol and other drug abuse, group psychotherapy, and social support systems.

Differential Diagnosis
Adjustment disorders must be distinguished from anxiety disorders, affective disorders, and personality disorders exacerbated by stress and from structural somatic disorders with psychic overlay.

Treatment
A. Behavioral: Stress reduction techniques include immediate symptom reduction (eg, rebreathing in a bag for hyperventilation) or early recognition and removal from a stress source before full-blown symptoms appear. It is often helpful for the patient to keep a daily log of stress precipitators, responses, and alleviators. Relaxation and exercise techniques are also helpful in reducing the reaction to stressful events. Specific behavioral techniques such as desensitization are indirectly helpful in anxiety reduction of stress reactions.

B. Social: The stress reactions of life crisis problems are—more than any other category—a function of psychosocial upheaval, and patients frequently present with somatic symptoms. While it is not easy for the patient to make necessary changes (or they would have been made long ago), it is important for the therapist to establish the framework of the problem, since the patient's denial system may obscure the issues. Clarifying the problem allows the patient to begin viewing it within the proper context and facilitates the sometimes difficult decisions the patient eventually must make (eg, change of job or relocation of adult dependent offspring).

C. Psychologic: Prolonged in-depth psychotherapy is seldom necessary in cases of isolated stress response or adjustment disorder. Supportive psychotherapy (see above) with an emphasis on the here and now and strengthening of existing defenses, is a helpful approach while time and the patient's own resiliency allow a restoration to the previous level of function. Posttraumatic stress syndromes respond to early catharsis and dynamic psychotherapy oriented toward acceptance of the event, with the expectation of quick recovery and return to the previous level of function. Marital problems are a major area of concern, and it is important that the physician have available a dependable referral source when marriage counseling is indicated. In posttraumatic stress disorder, group psychotherapy and individual counseling are both helpful.

D. Medical: Judicious use of sedatives (eg, lorazepam, 1–2 mg orally daily) for a limited time and as part of an overall treatment plan can provide relief from acute anxiety symptoms. Problems arise when the situation becomes chronic through inappropriate treatment or when the treatment approach supports the development of chronicity (see Sedative-Hypnotic Drugs, above).

In posttraumatic stress disorder, antidepressant drugs in full dosage are helpful in ameliorating depression, panic attacks, sleep disruption, and startle responses, though there is no way to predict which drug will be most useful. Beta-blockers are used to lessen the peripheral symptoms of anxiety (eg, tremors, palpitations). Antiseizure medications such as carbamazepine and valproic acid will often mitigate symptoms in patients with a history of alcohol and other drug abuse. Benzodiazepines such as clonazepam will reduce anxiety and panic attacks when used in adequate dosage, but dependency problems are a concern, particularly when the patient has had such problems in the past.

Prognosis

Return to satisfactory function after a short period is part of the clinical picture of this syndrome. Resolution may be delayed if others' responses to the patient's difficulties are thoughtlessly harmful or if the secondary gains outweigh the advantages of recovery. The longer the chronicity, the worse the prognosis.

Chrousos GP, Gold PW: The concepts of stress and stress system disorders: Overview of physical and behavioral homeostasis. JAMA 1992;267:1244.

Gersons BPR, Carlier IVE: Post-traumatic stress disorder: The history of a recent concept. Br J Psychiatry 1992;161:742.

Solomon SD, Gerrity ET, Muff AM: Efficacy of treatments for posttraumatic stress disorder: An empirical review. JAMA 1992;268:633. (Literature review.)

ANXIETY DISORDERS & DISSOCIATIVE DISORDERS (Neuroses)

Essentials of Diagnosis

- Overt anxiety or an overt manifestation of a defense mechanism (such as a phobia) or both.
- Not limited to an adjustment disorder.
- Somatic symptoms referable to the autonomic nervous system or to a specific organ system (eg, dyspnea, palpitations, paresthesias).
- Not a result of physical disorders, psychiatric conditions (eg, schizophrenia), or drug abuse (eg, cocaine).

General Considerations

Stress, fear, and anxiety all tend to be interactive. The principal components of anxiety are **psychologic** (tension, fears, difficulty in concentration, apprehension) and **somatic** (tachycardia, hyperventilation, palpitations, tremor, sweating). Other organ systems (eg, gastrointestinal) may be involved in multiple-system complaints. Fatigue and sleep disturbances are common. Sympathomimetic symptoms of anxiety are both a response to a central nervous system state and a reinforcement of further anxiety. Anxiety can become self-generating, since the symptoms reinforce the reaction, causing it to spiral. This is often the case when the anxiety is an epiphenomenon of other medical or psychiatric disorders.

Anxiety may be free-floating, resulting in acute anxiety attacks, occasionally becoming chronic. When one or several defense mechanisms (see above) are functioning, the consequences are well-known problems such as phobias, conversion reactions, dissociative states, obsessions, and compulsions. *Lack of structure is frequently a contributing factor,* as noted in those people who have "Sunday neuroses." They do well during the week with a planned work schedule but cannot tolerate the unstructured weekend. Planned-time activities tend to bind anxiety, and many people have increased difficulties when this is lost, as in retirement.

Some believe that various manifestations of anxiety are not a result of unconscious conflicts but are "habits"—persistent patterns of nonadaptive behavior acquired by learning. The "habits," being nonadaptive, are unsatisfactory ways of dealing with life problems—hence the resultant anxiety. Help is sought only when the anxiety becomes too painful. *Exogenous factors such as stimulants (eg, caffeine, cocaine) must be considered as a contributing factor.*

Clinical Findings

A. Generalized Anxiety Disorder: This is the most common of the clinically significant anxiety disorders. Initial manifestations appear at age 20–35 years, and there is a slight predominance in women.

The disabling anxiety symptoms of apprehension, worry, irritability, hypervigilance (preparation for threat), and somatic complaints are long-lasting and persist for at least 1 month. Manifestations include cardiac (eg, tachycardia, increased blood pressure), gastrointestinal (eg, increased acidity, epigastric pain), and neurologic (eg, headache, syncope) systems. Some of the origins or exacerbating causes of the anxiety may be identified in life situations.

B. Panic Disorder: This is characterized by short-lived, recurrent, unpredictable episodes of intense anxiety (with or without agoraphobia) accompanied by marked physiologic manifestations. Distressing signs and symptoms such as dyspnea, tachycardia, palpitations, headaches, dizziness, paresthesias, choking, smothering feelings, nausea, and bloating are associated with feelings of impending doom (alarm response). Recurrent sleep panic attacks (not nightmares) occur in about 30% of panic disorders. Anticipatory anxiety develops in all these patients and further constricts their daily lives. Panic disorder tends to be familial, with onset under age 25; it affects 3–5% of the population, is probably related to temporal lobe dysfunction, and there is a 2:1 prevalence in women. The premenstrual period is one of heightened vulnerability. Patients frequently undergo emergency medical evaluations (eg, for "heart attacks" or "hypoglycemia") before the correct diagnosis is made. Gastrointestinal symptoms are especially common, occurring in about one-third of cases. Myocardial infarction, pheochromocytoma, hyperthyroidism, and various recreational drug reactions can mimic panic disorder. Lactate infusion with reemergence of the symptoms is corroborative evidence of panic disorder. Cholecystokinin (sincalide) can also reproduce symptoms. PET scans are also diagnostic (there is intense activity in the frontal poles of the temporal lobes). *Mitral valve prolapse may be present but is not necessarily a significant factor.* Patients with recurrent panic disorder often become **demoralized, hypochondriacal, agoraphobic,** and **depressed.** Alcohol abuse (about 20%) results from self-treatment and is not infrequently combined with dependence on sedatives. Some patients have atypical panic attacks associated with seizure-like symptoms that often include psychosensory phenomena (a history of stimulant abuse often emerges). Suicide attempts are a significant complication. About 25% also have obsessive-compulsive disorder.

C. Obsessive-Compulsive Disorder: In the obsessive-compulsive reaction, the irrational idea or the impulse persistently intrudes into awareness. Obsessions (constantly recurring thoughts such as fears of exposure to germs) and compulsions (repetitive actions such as washing hands many times prior to peeling a potato) are recognized by the individual as absurd and are resisted, but anxiety is alleviated only by ritualistic performance or thought ritual. The primary underlying concern of the patient is to not lose control. Many patients do not mention the symptoms and must be asked about them. These patients are usually predictable, orderly, conscientious, and intelligent, traits that are seen in many compulsive behaviors such as bulimia and compulsive running. There is an overlapping of obsessive-compulsive disorder and tics, including trichotillomania (hair pulling), onychophagia (nail biting), hypochondriasis, Tourette's syndrome, and eating disorders (see Chapter 28). Major depression occurs in two-thirds of these patients during their lifetimes. The 2–3% incidence in the USA is a much higher incidence than was previously recognized. Male:female ratios are similar, with the highest rates occurring in the young, divorced, separated, and unemployed (all high stress periods). In these patients, neurologic abnormalities of fine motor coordination and involuntary movements are common. Under extreme stress, these patients sometimes exhibit paranoid and delusional behaviors, often associated with depression, and can mimic schizophrenia.

D. Phobic Disorder: Phobic ideation can be considered a mechanism of "displacement" in which the patients transfer feelings of anxiety from their true object to one that can be avoided. However, since phobias are ineffective defense mechanisms, there tends to be an increase in their scope, intensity, and number. Social phobias are global or specific; in the former, all social situations are poorly tolerated, while the latter group includes performance anxiety or well-delineated phobias. Agoraphobia (fear of open places and public areas) is frequently associated with severe panic attacks. Claustrophobia and acrophobia relate to agoraphobia, which term tends to be used in the broader sense. Patients often develop the syndrome in early adult life, making a normal lifestyle difficult.

E. Dissociative Disorder: Fugue, amnesia, somnambulism, and multiple personality are the usual dissociative states. The reaction is precipitated by emotional crisis, and although the primary gain is anxiety reduction, the secondary gain is a temporary solution of the crisis. Mechanisms include repression and isolation as well as particularly limited concentration such as seen in hypnotic states. This condition is similar in many ways to symptoms seen in patients with temporal lobe dysfunction.

Treatment

A. Medical: In all cases, underlying medical disorders must be ruled out (eg, cardiovascular, endocrine, respiratory, and neurologic disorders and substance-related syndromes, both intoxication and withdrawal states). These and other disorders can coexist with panic disorder. Benzodiazepines and buspirone are the anxiolytics of choice in most cases of generalized anxiety. Other classes of drugs, such as antipsychotics, and the older sedatives, such as the barbiturates, have no advantages over the benzodiazepines and numerous disadvantages. Beta-blockers such as propranolol may help reduce peripheral somatic symptoms. Ethanol is the most frequently self-administered drug and should be discontinued.

Panic attacks may be treated in several ways. A paper bag is used for rebreathing in hyperventilation episodes. Antidepressants are the initial drugs of choice (adequate blood levels will require dosages similar to those used in the treatment of depression. As in depression, lithium may be used to augment the antidepressant drugs. Fluoxetine is effective, particularly if obsessive-compulsive disorder is present with the panic disorder (25% of patients). Because of overresponsiveness to the tricyclics, *starting doses should be low and very gradually increased.* Clonazepam (1–8 mg/d orally) is effective as an alternative to antidepressants. Alprazolam (0.5–8 mg/d orally) is also effective but causes significant dependency problems. Because of chronicity of the disorders and the problem of dependency with benzodiazepine drugs, it is generally desirable to use antidepressant drugs as the principal pharmacologic approach. Nonresponse may indicate the presence of limbic overstimulation and warrant a trial of carbamazepine. Antidepressants have been used in conjunction with propranolol (40–160 mg/d orally) in resistant cases.

Phobic disorder may be part of the panic disorder and is treated within that framework. Global social phobias may be treated with MAO inhibitors in the same dosage as used for depression, while specific phobias such as performance anxiety may respond to moderate doses of β-blockers. A sustained effect is often not obtained with drugs alone; a combination of drugs, behavioral techniques, and cognitive psychotherapy is most effective. If there is any indication of seizure-like phenomena, carbamazepine or valproic acid should be considered.

Obsessive-compulsive disorders respond to serotonergic drugs in about 60% of cases. Clomipramine has proved effective in doses equivalent to those used for depression. Fluoxetine (an SSRI drug) has been widely used in this disorder but in doses higher than those used in depression (up to 60–80 mg/d). The other SSRI drugs such as sertraline and paroxetine are being used with early results comparable to those achieved with clomipramine and fluoxetine. Fluvoxamine, soon to be released, is effective also in obsessive-compulsive disorder. Buspirone in doses of up to 60 mg/d has shown promise. (It is also used to augment fluoxetine, but in lower doses, ie, 30 mg/d.) Tourette's syndrome has responded to fluoxetine, 20–40 mg/d orally.

B. Behavioral: Behavioral approaches are widely used in various anxiety disorders, often in conjunction with medication. Any of the behavioral techniques (see above) can be used beneficially in altering the contingencies (precipitating factors or rewards) supporting any anxiety-provoking behavior. Relaxation techniques can sometimes be helpful in reducing anxiety. Desensitization, by exposing the patient to graded doses of a phobic object or situation, is an effective technique and one that the patient can practice outside the therapy session. Emotive imagery, wherein the patient imagines the anxiety-provoking situation while at the same time learning to relax, helps to decrease the anxiety when the patient faces the real life situation. Physiologic symptoms in panic attacks respond well to relaxation training.

C. Psychologic: Cognitive approaches have been effective in treatment of panic disorders, phobias, and obsessive-compulsive disorder when erroneous beliefs need correction. The combination of medical and cognitive therapy is more effective than either alone. Other individual approaches such as reality therapy and transactional analysis are helpful when problems with interpersonal relationships are a major factor. Group therapy is the treatment of choice when the anxiety is clearly a function of the patient's difficulties in dealing with others, and if these other people are part of the family it is appropriate to include them and initiate family or couples therapy.

D. Social: Social modification may require measures such as family counseling to aid acceptance of the patient's symptoms and avoid counterproductive behavior in behavioral training. Any help in maintaining the social structure is anxiety-alleviating, and work, school, and social activities should be maintained. School and vocational counseling may be provided by professionals, who often need help from the physician in defining the patient's limitations.

Prognosis

Anxiety disorders are usually of long standing and may be quite difficult to treat. All can be relieved to varying degrees with medications and behavioral techniques. The prognosis is much better if one can break the commonly observed anxiety-panic-phobia-depression cycle with a combination of the therapeutic interventions discussed above.

Barr LC et al: The serotonin hypothesis of obsessive compulsive disorder: Implications of pharmacologic challenge studies. J Clin Psychiatry 1992;53(4 Suppl):17. (Role of serotonin.)

Friedman S et al: Suicidal ideation and suicide attempts among patients with panic disorder: A survey of two outpatient clinics. Am J Psychiatry 1992;149:680. (Suicide attempts are made by about 20% of patients with panic disorder.)

Gelernter CS et al: An examination of syndrome validity and diagnostic subtypes in social phobia and panic disorder. J Clin Psychiatry 1992;53. (Fair reliability.)

SOMATOFORM DISORDERS
(Psychophysiologic Disorders, Psychosomatic Disorders)

Essentials of Diagnosis

- Physical symptoms may involve one or more organ systems and are not intentional.
- Subjective complaints exceed objective findings.
- Correlations of symptom development and psychosocial stresses.
- Matrix of biogenetic and developmental patterns.

General Considerations

A major source of diagnostic confusion in medicine has been to assume cause-and-effect relationships when parallel events have been observed. This post hoc ergo propter hoc reasoning has been particularly vexing in many situations where the individual exhibits psychosocial distress that could well be secondary to a chronic illness but has been assumed to be primary and causative. An example is the person with a chronic bowel disease who becomes querulous and demanding. Is this a result of problems of coping with a chronic disease, or is it a personality pattern that causes the gastrointestinal problem?

Vulnerability in one or more organ systems and exposure to family members with somatization problems play a major role in the development of particular symptoms, and the "functional" versus "organic" dichotomy is a hindrance to good treatment.

In any patient presenting with a condition judged to be somatoform, depression must be considered in the diagnosis.

Clinical Findings

A. Conversion Disorder: "Conversion" (formerly "hysterical conversion") of psychic conflict into physical symptoms in parts of the body innervated by the sensorimotor system (eg, paralysis, aphonia) is a disorder that is more common in unsophisticated individuals and certain cultures. The defense mechanisms utilized in this condition are repression (a barring from consciousness) and isolation (a splitting of the affect from the idea). The somatic manifestation that takes the place of anxiety is typically paralysis, and in some instances the organ dysfunction may have symbolic meaning (eg, arm paralysis in marked anger). Hysterical seizures ("pseudoseizures") are usually difficult to differentiate from intoxication states or panic attacks. Retention of consciousness, random flailing with asynchronous movements of the right and left sides, and resistance to having the nose and mouth pinched closed *during the attack* all point toward a hysterical event. Electroencephalography during the attack is the most helpful diagnostic aid in excluding seizure states. Serum prolactin levels rise abruptly in the postictal state but not in pseudoseizures. There is usually a history of other conversion situations. La belle indifférence (a lack of affect) is not a significant characteristic as commonly believed. Important criteria in diagnosis include a history of conversion or somatization disorder, modeling, a serious precipitating emotional event, associated psychopathology (eg, schizophrenia, personality disorders), a temporal correlation between the precipitating event and the symptom, and a temporary "solving of the problem" by the conversion. *It is important to differentiate physical disorders with unusual presentations (eg, multiple sclerosis).*

B. Somatization Disorder (Briquet's Syndrome, Hysteria): This is characterized by multiple physical complaints referable to several organ systems. Anxiety, panic disorder, and depression are often present, and **major depression** is an important consideration in the differential diagnosis. There is a significant relationship (20%) to a lifetime history of panic-agoraphobia-depression. It usually occurs before age 30 and is more common in women. Polysurgery is often a feature of the history. Preoccupation with medical and surgical therapy becomes a life-style that excludes most other activities. The symptoms are a reflection of adaptive patterns, coping techniques, and reactivity of the particular organ system. There is often evidence of long-standing somatic symptoms (particularly dysmenorrhea, a lump in the throat, vomiting, shortness of breath, burning in the sex organs, painful extremities, and amnesia), often with a history of similar organ system involvement in other family members. Multiple symptoms that constantly change and inability of more than three doctors to make a diagnosis are strong clues to the problem.

C. Psychogenic Pain Disorder: This involves a long history of complaints of severe pain not consonant with anatomic and clinical signs. This diagnosis must not be one of exclusion and should be made only after extended evaluation has established a clear correlation of psychogenic factors with exacerbations and remissions of complaints.

D. Hypochondriasis: This is a fear of disease and preoccupation with the body, with perceptual amplification and heightened responsiveness. A process of social learning is usually involved, frequently with a role model who was a member of the family and may be a part of the underlying psychodynamic etiology. It is common in panic disorders.

E. Factitious Disorders: These disorders, in which symptom production is intentional, are not somatoform conditions. They are characterized by self-induced symptoms or false physical and laboratory findings for the purpose of deceiving physicians or other hospital personnel. The deceptions may involve self-mutilation, fever, hemorrhage, hypoglycemia, seizures, and an almost endless variety of manifestations—often presented in an exaggerated and dramatic fashion (Munchausen's syndrome). "Proxy Munchausen" is the term used when a parent creates an illness in a child so that treatment can be given to satisfy a somatization disorder in the parent. The duplicity may be either simple or extremely complex and difficult to recognize. The patients are frequently connected in some way with the health professions, they are often migratory, and their motivation in complex cases is usually unclear.

Complications

A poor doctor-patient relationship, with iatrogenic disorders and "doctor shopping," tends to exacerbate the problem. Sedative and analgesic dependency is the most common iatrogenic complication.

Treatment

A. Medical: Medical support with careful attention to building a therapeutic doctor-patient relationship is the mainstay of treatment. *It must be accepted that the patient's distress is real. Every problem not found to have an organic basis is not necessarily a mental disease.* Diligent attempts should be made to relate symptoms to adverse developments in the patient's life. It may be useful to have the patient keep a meticulous diary, paying particular attention to various pertinent factors evident in the history. Regular, frequent, short appointments may be helpful. Drugs (not infrequently abused) should not be prescribed to replace appointments. One doctor should be the primary physician, and consultants should be used mainly for evaluation. An emphatic, realistic, optimistic approach must be maintained in the face of the expected ups and downs. Ongoing re-evaluation is necessary, since somatization can coexist with a concurrent physical illness.

B. Psychologic: Psychologic approaches can be used by the primary physician when it is clear that the patient is ready to make some changes in life-style in order to achieve symptomatic relief. This is often best approached on a here-and-now basis and oriented toward pragmatic changes rather than an exploration of early experiences that the patient frequently fails to relate to current distress. Group therapy with other individuals who have similar problems is sometimes of value to improve coping, allow ventilation, and focus on interpersonal adjustment. Hypnosis or amobarbital interviews used early are helpful in resolving conversion disorders. If the primary physician has been working with the patient on psychologic problems related to the physical illness, the groundwork is often laid for successful psychiatric referral.

C. Behavioral: Behavioral therapy is probably best exemplified by biofeedback techniques. In biofeedback, the particular abnormality (eg, increased peristalsis) must be recognized and monitored by the patient and therapist (eg, by an electronic stethoscope to amplify the sounds). This is immediate feedback, and after learning to recognize it the patient can then learn to identify any change thus produced (eg, a decrease in bowel sounds) and so become a conscious

originator of the feedback instead of a passive recipient. Relief of the symptom operantly conditions the patient to utilize the maneuver that relieves symptoms (eg, relaxation causing a decrease in bowel sounds). With emphasis on this type of learning, the patient is able to identify symptoms early and initiate the countermaneuvers, thus decreasing the symptomatic problem. Migrainoid and tension headaches have been particularly responsive to biofeedback methods.

D. Social: Social endeavors include family, work, and other interpersonal activity. Family members should come for some appointments with the patient so that they can learn how best to live with the patient. This is particularly important in treatment of the somatization and psychogenic pain disorders. Ileostomy clubs and similar mutual aid groups provide a climate for encouraging the patient to accept and live with the problem. Ongoing communication with the employer may be necessary to encourage long-term continued interest in the employee. Employers can become just as discouraged as physicians in dealing with employees who have chronic problems.

Prognosis

The prognosis is much better if the primary physician is able to intervene early before the situation has deteriorated. After the problem has crystallized into chronicity, it is very difficult to effect change.

Creed F et al: Psychiatric referrals within the general hospital: Comparison with referrals to general practitioners. Br J Psychiatry 1993;162:204.
Katon W et al: Somatization: A spectrum of severity. Am J Psychiatry 1991;148:34.

CHRONIC PAIN DISORDERS

Essentials of Diagnosis

- Chronic complaints of pain.
- Symptoms frequently exceed signs.
- Minimal relief with standard treatment.
- History of many physicians.
- Frequent use of many nonspecific medications.

General Considerations

A problem in the management of pain is the lack of distinction between acute and chronic pain syndromes. Most physicians are adept at dealing with acute pain problems but have difficulty handling the patient with chronic pain. This type of patient frequently takes too many medications, stays in bed a great deal, has had many physicians, has lost skills, and experiences little joy in either work or play. All relationships suffer (including those with physicians), and life becomes a constant search for succor. The search results in complex physician-patient relationships that usually include many drug trials, particularly sedatives, with adverse consequences (eg, irritability, depressed mood) related to long-term use. Treatment failures provoke angry responses and depression from both the physician and the patient, and the pain syndrome is exacerbated. When frustration becomes too great, a new physician is found, and the cycle is repeated. The longer the existence of the pain, the more important the psychologic factors of anxiety and depression, which are often a consequence rather than a cause of chronic pain. As with all other conditions, it is counterproductive to speculate about whether the pain is "real." It is real to the patient, and acceptance of the problem underlines a mutual endeavor to alleviate the disturbance.

Clinical Findings

Components of the chronic pain syndrome consist of anatomic changes, chronic anxiety and depression, anger, and changed life-style. Usually, the anatomic problem is irreversible, since it has already been subjected to many interventions with increasingly unsatisfactory results.

Chronic anxiety and depression produce heightened irritability and overreaction to stimuli. A marked decrease in pain threshold is apparent. This pattern develops into a hypochondriacal preoccupation with the body and a constant need for reassurance. The pressure on the doctor becomes wearing and often leads to covert rejection devices, such as not being available or making referrals to other physicians. This is perceived by the patient, who then intensifies the effort to get help, and the typical cycle is under way. Anxiety and depression are seldom discussed, almost as if there is a tacit agreement not to deal with these issues.

Changes in life-style involve some of the so-called pain games. These usually take the form of a family script in which the patient accepts the role of being sick, and this role then becomes the focus of most family interactions and may become important in maintaining the family, so that neither the patient nor the family wants the patient's role to change. Demands for attention and efforts to control the behavior of others revolve around the central issue of control of other people (including physicians). Cultural factors frequently play a role in the behavior of the patient and how the significant people around the patient cope with the problem. Some cultures encourage demonstrative behavior, while others value the stoic role. The physician's recognition of this fact is important, since overt dramatization of the discomfort is sometimes helpful in alleviating the problem.

Another secondary gain that frequently maintains the patient in the sick role is financial compensation or other benefits ("green poultice"). Frequently, such systems are structured so that they reinforce the maintenance of sickness and discourage any attempts to give up the role. Physicians unwittingly reinforce this role because of the very nature of the practice of medicine, which is to respond to complaints of illness. Helpful suggestions are often met with responses like "Yes, but. . . ." Medications then become the principal approach, and drug dependency problems may develop.

Treatment

A. Behavioral: The cornerstone of a unified approach to chronic pain syndromes is a comprehensive behavioral program. This is necessary to identify and eliminate pain reinforcers, to decrease drug use, and to use effectively those positive reinforcers that shift the focus from the pain. *It is critical that the patient be made a partner in the effort to alleviate pain.* (Avoid the concept of cure.) The patient should agree to discuss the pain only with the physician and not with family members; this tends to stabilize the patient's personal life, since the family is usually tired of the subject. At the beginning of treatment, the patient should be assigned self-help tasks graded up to maximal activity, as a means of positive reinforcement. The tasks should not exceed capability. The patient can also be asked to keep a self-rating chart to log accomplishments, so that progress can be measured and remembered. Instruct the patient to record degrees of pain on a self-rating scale in relation to various situations and mental attitudes so that similar circumstances can be avoided or modified.

Avoid negative reinforcers such as sympathy and attention to pain. Emphasize a positive response to productive activities, which remove the focus of attention from the pain. Activity is also desensitizing, since the patient learns to tolerate increasing activity levels.

Biofeedback techniques (see Somatoform Disorders, above) and hypnosis have been successful in ameliorating some pain syndromes. Hypnosis tends to be most effective in those patients with a high level of denial, who are more responsive to suggestion. Hypnosis can be used to lessen anxiety, alter perception of the length of time that pain is experienced, and encourage relaxation.

B. Medical: A *single physician* in charge of the multiple treatment approach is the highest priority. Consultations as indicated and technical procedures done by others are appropriate, but the care of the patient should remain in the hands of the primary physician. Referrals should not be allowed to raise the patient's hopes unrealistically or to become a way for the physician to reject the case. The attitude of the doctor should be one of honesty, interest, and hopefulness—not for a cure but for control of pain and improved function. If the patient is heavily addicted to narcotics, detoxification may be an early treatment goal.

If analgesics or sedatives are prescribed, they should not be given on an "as-needed" schedule. A fixed schedule lessens the conditioning effects of these drugs. TCAs (eg, amitriptyline) in doses smaller than those used in depression may be helpful.

In addition to medications, a variety of alternative strategies may be offered, including physical therapy and acupuncture.

C. Social: *Involvement of family members and other significant persons in the patient's life should be an early priority.* The best efforts of both patient and therapists can be unwittingly sabotaged by other persons who may feel that they are "helping" the patient. They frequently tend to reinforce the negative aspects of the pain syndrome. The patient becomes more dependent and less active, and the pain syndrome becomes an immutable way of life. The more destructive "pain games" described by many experts in chronic pain syndromes are results of well-meaning but misguided efforts of family members. Ongoing therapy with the family can be helpful in the early identification and elimination of these behavior patterns.

D. Psychologic: In addition to group therapy with family members and others, groups of patients can be helpful if properly led. The major goal, whether of individual or group therapy, is to gain patient *involvement*. A group can be a powerful instrument for achieving this goal, with the development of group loyalties and cooperation. People will frequently make efforts with group encouragement that they would never make alone. Individual therapy should be directed toward strengthening existing defenses and improving self-esteem. The rapport between patient and physician, as in all psychotherapeutic efforts, is the major factor in therapeutic success.

Tyrer S: Psychiatric assessment of chronic pain. Br J Psychiatry 1992;160:733. (Contains an excellent flow chart of pain assessment.)

PSYCHOSEXUAL DISORDERS

The stages of sexual activity include **excitement** (arousal), **plateau, orgasm,** and **resolution.** The precipitating excitement or arousal is psychologically determined. Arousal response leading to plateau is a physiologic and psychologic phenomenon of vasocongestion, a parasympathetic reaction causing erection in the male and labial/clitoral congestion in the female. The orgasmic response includes emission in the male and clonic contractions of the analogous striated perineal muscles of both male and female. Resolution is a gradual return to normal physiologic status.

While the arousal stimuli—vasocongestive and orgasmic responses—constitute a single response in a well-adjusted person, they can be considered as separate stages that can produce different syndromes responding to different treatment procedures.

Clinical Findings

There are three major groups of sexual disorders.

A. Paraphilias (Sexual Arousal Disorders): In these conditions, formerly called "deviations" or "variations," the excitement stage of sexual activity is associated with sexual objects or orientations different from those usually associated with adult heterosexual stimulation. The stimulus may be a woman's shoe, a child, animals, instruments of torture, or incidents of aggression. The pattern of sexual stimulation is usually one that has early psychologic roots. Poor experiences with heterosexual activity frequently reinforce this pattern over time.

Exhibitionism is the impulsive behavior of exposing the genitalia in order to achieve sexual excitation. It is a childhood sexual behavior carried into adult life.

Transvestism is the wearing of clothes and the enactment of a role of the opposite sex for the purpose of sexual excitation. Such fetishistic cross-dressing can be part of masturbation foreplay. Transvestism in homosexuality and transsexualism is not done to cause sexual excitement but is a function of the homosexual preference or gender disorder.

Voyeurism involves the achievement of sexual arousal by secretly watching the activities of the opposite sex, usually in various stages of undress or sexual activity. In both exhibitionism and voyeurism, excitation leads to masturbation as a *replacement* for heterosexual activity.

Pedophilia is the use of a child of either sex to achieve sexual arousal and, in many cases, gratification. Contact is frequently oral, with either participant being dominant, but pedophilia includes intercourse of any type. Adults of both sexes engage in this behavior, but because of social and cultural factors it is more commonly identified with males. The pedophile has difficulty in adult sexual relationships, and males who perform this act are frequently impotent.

Incest involves a sexual relationship with a person in the immediate family, most frequently a child. In many ways it is similar to pedophilia (intrafamilial pedophilia). Incestuous feelings are fairly common, but cultural mores are usually sufficiently strong to act as a barrier to the expression of sexual feelings.

Bestiality is the attainment of sexual gratification by intercourse with an animal. The intercourse may involve penetration or simply contact with the human genitalia by the tongue of the animal. The practice is more common in rural or isolated areas and is frequently a substitute for human sexual contact rather than an expression of preference.

Sadism is the attainment of sexual arousal by inflicting pain upon the sexual object, and **masochism** is the attainment of sexual excitation by enduring pain. Much sexual activity has aggressive components (eg, biting, scratching). Forced sexual acquiescence (eg, rape) is considered to be primarily an act of aggression.

Bondage is the achievement of erotic pleasure by being humiliated, enslaved, physically bound, and restrained. It is life-threatening, since neck binding or partial asphyxiation usually forms part of the ritual. It is estimated that bondage is responsible for about 1000 accidental deaths a year in males (the practice is much less common in females).

Necrophilia is sexual intercourse with a dead body or the use of parts of a dead body for sexual excitation, often with masturbation.

B. Gender Identity Variations: *Core gender identity* reflects a biologic self-image—the conviction that "I am a male" or "I am a female." While this is a fixed self-image, *gender role identity* is a dynamic, changing self-representation. Variances of core gender identity are not common, while those of gender role identity are common. The major gender variation is transsexualism.

Transsexualism (a core gender identity problem) is an attempt to deny and reverse biologic sex by maintaining sexual identity with the opposite gender. Transsexuals do not alternate between gender roles; rather, they assume a fixed role of attitudes, feelings, fantasies, and choices consonant with those of the opposite sex, all of which clearly date back to early development. For example, male transsexuals in early childhood behave, talk, and fantasize as if they were girls. They do not grow out of feminine patterns, they do not work in professions traditionally considered to be masculine, and they have no interest in their own penises either as evidence of maleness or as organs for erotic behavior. The desire for sex change starts early and may culminate in assumption of a feminine life-style, hormonal treatment, and use of surgical procedures, eg, castration and vaginoplasty.

Homosexuality is no longer considered to be a classifiable sexual disorder. Problems arise in this group when the individual has difficulty accepting the sexual orientation or is under stress in a society that is intolerant.

C. Psychosexual Dysfunction: This category includes a large group of vasocongestive and orgasmic disorders. Often, they involve problems of sexual adaptation, education, and technique that are often initially discussed with, diagnosed by, and treated by the family physician.

There are two conditions common in the male: impotence and ejaculation disturbances.

Impotence (erectile dysfunction) is inability to achieve or maintain an erection firm enough for satisfactory intercourse; patients sometimes use the term to mean premature ejaculation. Careful questioning is necessary, since causes of this vasocongestive disorder can be psychologic, physiologic, or both. The majority are pathophysiologic and, to varying degrees, treatable. After onset of the problem, a history of occasional erections—especially nocturnal penile tu-

mescence, which may be evaluated by a simple monitoring device, or a sleep study in the sleep laboratory—is usually evidence that the dysfunction is psychologic in origin, with the caveat that decreased nocturnal penile tumescence occurs in some depressed patients. **Psychologic impotence** is caused by interpersonal or intrapsychic factors (eg, marital disharmony, depression). **Organic factors** (which usually develop gradually) include arteriosclerosis, hypertension, diabetes mellitus, drug abuse (alcohol, nicotine, narcotics, stimulants), pharmacologic agents (anticholinergic drugs, antihypertensive medication, antihistamines, disulfiram, all psychotherapeutic drugs, narcotics, estrogens), organ system failure (circulatory, cardiorespiratory, renal), surgical complications (prostatectomy, vascular and back surgery), trauma (disk and spinal cord injuries), endocrine disturbances (pituitary, thyroid, adrenal), zinc deficiency, nitric oxide deficiency, neurologic disorders (multiple sclerosis, tumors, peripheral neuropathies, injuries, pernicious anemia, syphilis), urologic problems (phimosis), and primary developmental abnormalities (Klinefelter's syndrome).

Ejaculation disturbances include premature ejaculation, inability to ejaculate, and retrograde ejaculation. (One may ejaculate even though impotent.) Ejaculation is usually connected with orgasm, and ejaculatory control is an acquired behavior that is minimal in adolescence and increases with experience. Pathogenic factors are those that interfere with learning control, most frequently sexual ignorance. Intrapsychic factors (anxiety, guilt, depression) and interpersonal maladaptation (marital problems, unresponsiveness of mate, power struggles) are also common. Organic causes include interference with sympathetic nerve distribution (often due to surgery or trauma) and the effects of pharmacologic agents on sympathetic tone.

In females, the two most common forms of sexual dysfunction are vaginismus and frigidity.

Vaginismus is a conditioned response in which a spasm of the perineal muscles occurs if there is any stimulation of the area. The desire is to avoid penetration. Sexual responsiveness and vasocongestion may be present, and orgasm can result from clitoral stimulation.

Frigidity is a complex condition in which there is a general lack of sexual responsiveness. The woman has difficulty in experiencing erotic sensation and does not have the vasocongestive response. Sexual activity varies from active avoidance of sex to an occasional orgasm. Orgasmic dysfunction—in which a woman has a vasocongestive response but varying degrees of difficulty in reaching orgasm—is sometimes differentiated from frigidity. Causes for the dysfunctions include poor sexual techniques, early traumatic sexual experiences, interpersonal disharmony (marital struggles, use of sex as a means of control), and intrapsychic problems (anxiety, fear, guilt). Organic causes include any conditions that might cause pain in intercourse, pelvic pathology, mechanical obstruction, and neurologic deficits.

Disorders of sexual desire refer to reduction or absence of sexual desire in either sex and may be a function of organic or psychologic difficulties (eg, anxiety, phobic avoidance). Any chronic illness can sap desire. Hormonal variations, including use of antiandrogen compounds such as cyproterone acetate, and chronic renal failure contribute to deterioration in sexual activity. Alcohol, sedatives, narcotics, marihuana, and some medications may affect sexual drive and performance.

Treatment

A. Paraphilias and Gender Identity Disorders:

1. Psychologic—Sexual arousal disorders involving variant sexual activity (paraphilia), particularly those of a more superficial nature (eg, voyeurism) and those of recent onset, are responsive to psychotherapy in a moderate percentage of cases. The prognosis is much better if the motivation comes from the individual rather than the legal system; unfortunately, however, court intervention is frequently the only stimulus to treatment, because the condition persists and is reinforced until conflict with the law occurs. Therapies frequently focus on barriers to normal arousal response; the expectation is that the variant behavior will decrease as normal behavior increases.

2. Behavioral—Aversive and operant conditioning techniques have been tried frequently in gender role disorders but have been only occasionally successful. In some cases, the sexual arousal disorders improve with modeling, role-playing, and conditioning procedures. Emotive imagery is occasionally helpful in lessening anxiety in fetish problems.

3. Social—Although they do not produce a change in sexual arousal patterns or gender role, self-help groups have facilitated adjustment to an often hostile society. Attention to the family is particularly important in helping persons in such groups to accept their situation and alleviate their guilt about the role they think they had in creating the problem.

4. Medical—Medroxyprogesterone acetate, a suppressor of libidinal drive, is used to mute disruptive sexual behavior in males of all ages. Onset of action is usually within 3 weeks, and the effects are generally reversible. Some preliminary results indicate that fluoxetine or other SSRI drugs may reduce some of the compulsive sexual behaviors. After careful evaluation, some transsexuals are treated with hormones and genital surgery, though more careful selection markedly reduces this approach.

B. Psychosexual Dysfunction:

1. Medical—Identification of a contributory reversible cause is most important. Even if the condition is not reversible, identification of the specific

cause helps the patient to accept the condition. Marital disharmony, with its exacerbating effects, may thus be avoided. Of all the sexual dysfunctions, impotence is the condition most likely to have an organic basis. As part of the evaluation, vascular factors can be assessed in the office by injections of papaverine and phentolamine to produce an erection (apparently raising nitric oxide levels or relaxing smooth muscle through other pathways). Ultrasound examination is helpful in detecting arterial abnormalities. Yohimbine, 18 mg orally daily, has had modest effectiveness in both organic and psychogenic impotence. When the condition is irreversible, penile implants may be considered. Revascularization surgery has been done in patients with impotence due to circulatory problems. Evaluation of the problem and use of the above drugs are usually best handled by a urologic specialist in sexual disorders.

2. Behavioral—Syndromes resulting from conditioned responses have been treated by conditioning techniques, with excellent results. Vaginismus responds well to desensitization with graduated Hegar dilators along with relaxation techniques. Masters and Johnson have used behavioral approaches in all of the sexual dysfunctions, with concomitant supportive psychotherapy and with improvement of the communication patterns of the couple.

3. Psychologic—The use of psychotherapy by itself is best suited for those cases in which interpersonal difficulties or intrapsychic problems predominate. Anxiety and guilt about parental injunctions against sex constitute the most frequent psychopathology contributing to sexual dysfunction. Even in these cases, however, a combined behavioral-psychologic approach usually produces results most quickly.

4. Social—The proximity of other people (eg, a mother-in-law) in a household is frequently an inhibiting factor in sexual relationships. In such cases, some social engineering may alleviate the problem.

Bailey JM, Pillard RC: A genetic study of male sexual orientation. Arch Gen Psychiatry 1991;48:1089.

Gregoire A: New treatments for erectile impotence. Br J Psychiatry 1992;160:315.

PERSONALITY DISORDERS

Essentials of Diagnosis

- Long history dating back to childhood.
- Recurrent maladaptive behavior.
- Low self-esteem and lack of confidence.
- Minimal introspective ability.
- Major difficulties with interpersonal relationships or society.
- Depression with anxiety when maladaptive behavior fails.

General Considerations

Personality—a hypothetical construct—is the result of a genetic substrate and the prolonged interaction of an individual with personal drives and with outside influences (parent-child interactions, peer influences, random events), the sum being the enduring and unique patterns of behavior which are adopted in order to cope with the environment and which characterize one as an individual. The personality structure, or character, is an integral part of self-image and is important to one's sense of identity.

The classification of subtypes depends upon the predominant symptoms and their severity. The most severe disorders—those that bring the patient into greatest conflict with society—tend to be classified as antisocial (psychopathic) or borderline.

Personality disorders can be considered a matrix for some of the more severe psychiatric problems (eg, schizotypal, relating to schizophrenia; avoidance types, relating to some anxiety disorders).

Classification & Clinical Findings

Paranoid: Defensive, oversensitive, secretive, suspicious, hyperalert, with limited emotional response.

Schizoid: Shy, introverted, withdrawn, avoids close relationships.

Compulsive: Perfectionist, egocentric, indecisive, with rigid thought patterns and need for control.

Histrionic (hysterical): Dependent, immature, seductive, histrionic, egocentric, vain, emotionally labile (a mnemonic device describing these traits is *dishevel*).

Schizotypal: Superstitious, socially isolated, suspicious, with limited interpersonal ability and odd speech.

Narcissistic: Exhibitionist, grandiose, preoccupied with power, lacks interest in others, with excessive demands for attention.

Avoidant: Fears rejection, hyperreacts to rejection and failure, with poor social endeavors and low self-esteem.

Dependent: Passive, overaccepting, unable to make decisions, lacks confidence, with poor self-esteem.

Passive-aggressive: Stubborn, procrastinating, argumentative, sulking, helpless, clinging, negative to authority figures.

Antisocial: Selfish, callous, promiscuous, impulsive, unable to learn from experience, has legal problems.

Borderline: Impulsive; has unstable and intense interpersonal relationships; is suffused with anger, fear, and guilt; lacks self-control and self-fulfillment; has identity problems and affective instability; is suicidal (a serious problem—up to 80% of hospitalized borderline patients make an attempt at some time during treatment, and the incidence of completed suicide is as high as 5%);

aggressive behavior, feelings of emptiness, and occasional psychotic decompensation. This group has a high drug abuse rate, which plays a role in symptomatology. There is extensive overlap with other diagnostic categories, particularly mood disorders and posttraumatic stress disorder.

Differential Diagnosis

Patients with personality disorders tend to show anxiety and depression when pathologic techniques fail, and their symptoms can be similar to those occurring with anxiety disorders. Occasionally, the more severe cases may decompensate into psychosis under stress and mimic other psychotic disorders.

Treatment

A. Social: Social and therapeutic environments such as day hospitals, halfway houses, and self-help communities utilize peer pressures to modify the self-destructive behavior. The patient with a personality disorder often has failed to profit from experience, and difficulties with authority impair the learning experience. The use of peer relationships and the repetition possible in a structured setting of a helpful community enhances the behavioral treatment opportunities and increases learning. When problems are detected early, both the school and the home can serve as foci of intensified social pressure to change the behavior, particularly with the use of behavioral techniques.

B. Behavioral: The behavioral techniques used are principally operant and aversive conditioning. The former simply emphasizes the recognition of acceptable behavior and reinforcement of this with praise or other tangible rewards. Aversive responses usually mean punishment, though this can range from a mild rebuke to some specific punitive responses such as verbal abuse or deprivation of privileges. Extinction plays a role in that an attempt is made not to respond to inappropriate behavior, and the lack of response eventually causes the person to abandon that type of behavior. Pouting and tantrums, for example, diminish quickly when such behavior elicits no reaction.

C. Psychologic: Psychologic intervention is most usefully accomplished in group settings. Group therapy is helpful when specific interpersonal behavior needs to be improved (eg, schizoid and inadequate types, in which involvement with people is markedly impaired). This mode of treatment also has a place with so-called acting-out patients, ie, those who frequently act in an impulsive and inappropriate way. The peer pressure in the group tends to impose restraints on rash behavior. The group also quickly identifies the patient's types of behavior and helps to improve the validity of the patient's self-assessment, so that the antecedents of the unacceptable behavior can be effectively handled, thus decreasing its frequency. Individual therapy should initially be supportive, ie, helping the patient to restabilize and mobilize defenses. If the individual has the ability to observe his or her own behavior, a longer-term and more introspective therapy may be warranted. The therapist must be able to handle countertransference feelings (which are frequently negative), maintain appropriate boundaries in the relationship (no physical contacts, however well-meaning), and refrain from premature confrontations and interpretations.

D. Medical: Hospitalization is rarely indicated except in the case of serious suicidal danger. In most cases, treatment can be accomplished in the day treatment center or self-help community. Antipsychotics may be required for short periods in conditions that have temporarily decompensated into transient psychoses (eg, haloperidol, 2–5 mg orally every 3–4 hours until the patient has quieted down and is regaining contact with reality). In most cases, these drugs are required only for several days and can be discontinued after the patient has regained a previously established level of adjustment. Carbamazepine, 800 mg orally daily in divided doses, decreases the severity of behavioral dyscontrol. Antidepressants have improved anxiety, depression, and sensitivity to rejection in some borderline patients.

Prognosis

Antisocial and borderline categories generally have a guarded prognosis. Those patients with poor outcomes are more likely to have a history of parental abuse and a family history of mood disorder, whereas persons with mild schizoid or passive-aggressive tendencies have a good prognosis with appropriate treatment.

Gunderson JG, Sabo AN: The phenomenological and conceptual interface between borderline personality and PTSD. Am J Psychiatry 1993;150:19. (Preexisting problems in many patients.)

Perry JC: Problems and considerations in the valid assessment of personality disorders. Am J Psychiatry 1992;149:1645. (Diagnosis of these disorders is much too casual.)

Searight HR: Borderline personality disorder: Diagnosis and management in primary care. J Fam Pract 1992;34:605. (Psychiatric referral is recommended.)

SCHIZOPHRENIC & OTHER PSYCHOTIC DISORDERS

Essentials of Diagnosis (Schizophrenia)

- Social withdrawal, usually slowly progressive, often with deterioration in personal care.
- Loss of ego boundaries, with inability to perceive oneself as a separate entity.
- Loose thought associations, often with slowed thinking or overinclusive and rapid shifting from topic to topic.
- Autistic absorption in inner thoughts and frequent sexual or religious preoccupations.
- Auditory hallucinations, often of a derogatory nature.
- Delusions, frequently of a grandiose or persecutory nature.
- Symptoms of at least 6 months' duration.

Frequent additional signs:
- Flat affect and rapidly alternating mood shifts irrespective of circumstances.
- Hypersensitivity to environmental stimuli, with a feeling of enhanced sensory awareness.
- Variability or changeable behavior incongruent with the external environment.
- Concrete thinking with inability to abstract; inappropriate symbolism.
- Impaired concentration worsened by hallucinations and delusions.
- Depersonalization, wherein one behaves like a detached observer of one's own actions.

General Considerations

The schizophrenic disorders are a group of syndromes manifested by massive disruption of thinking, mood, and overall behavior, as well as poor filtering of stimuli. The characterization and nomenclature of the disorders are quite arbitrary and are influenced by sociocultural factors and schools of psychiatric thought.

It is currently believed that the schizophrenic disorders are of multifactorial cause, with genetic, environmental, neuroendocrine, and pathophysiologic components. At present, there is no laboratory method to confirm the diagnosis of schizophrenia. There may or may not be a history of a major disruption in the individual's life (failures, losses, physical illness) before gross psychotic deterioration is evident.

"Other psychotic disorders" are conditions that are similar to schizophrenic illness in their acute symptoms but have a less pervasive influence over the long term. The individual usually attains higher levels of functioning. The acute psychotic episodes tend to be less disruptive of the person's life-style, with a fairly quick return to previous levels of functioning.

Classification

A. Schizophrenic Disorders: Schizophrenic disorders are subdivided on the basis of certain prominent phenomena that are frequently present. **Disorganized (hebephrenic) schizophrenia** is characterized by marked incoherence and an incongruous or silly affect. **Catatonic schizophrenia** is distinguished by a marked psychomotor disturbance of either excitement (purposeless and stereotyped) or rigidity with mutism. Infrequently, there may be rapid alternation between excitement and stupor (see under catatonic syndrome, below). **Paranoid schizophrenia** includes marked persecutory or grandiose delusions often consonant with hallucinations of similar content. **Undifferentiated schizophrenia** denotes a category in which symptoms are not specific enough to warrant inclusion of the illness in the other subtypes. **Residual schizophrenia** is a classification that includes persons who have clearly had an episode warranting a diagnosis of schizophrenia but who at present have no overt psychotic symptoms, though they show milder signs such as social withdrawal, flat affect, and eccentric behaviors.

B. Paranoid (Delusional) Disorders: Paranoid disorders are psychoses in which the predominant symptoms are persistent persecutory delusions, with minimal impairment in daily function (the schizophrenic disorders show significant impairment). Intellectual and occupational activities are little affected, whereas social and marital functioning tend to be markedly involved. Hallucinations are not usually present. Many of these patients are misdiagnosed as paranoid schizophrenics.

C. Schizoaffective Disorders: Schizoaffective disorders are those cases that fail to fit comfortably either in the schizophrenic or in the affective categories. They are usually cases with affective symptoms that precede or develop concurrently with psychotic manifestations.

D. Schizophreniform Disorders: Schizophreniform disorders are similar in their symptoms to schizophrenic disorders except that the duration is less than 6 months but more than 1 week.

E. Brief Reactive Psychotic Disorders: These disorders last less than 1 week. They are the result of psychologic stress. The shorter duration is significant and correlates with a more acute onset and resolution as well as a much better prognosis.

F. Late Life Psychosis: Brain abnormalities occur in 40% of patients who develop psychotic symptoms after age 60. The psychotic symptoms are typical, and there are other findings such as low IQ scores and diminished cognitive function.

G. Atypical Psychoses: This group includes a wide range of conditions with psychotic symptomatology. The cause is often not clear, but later events (eg, new symptoms) may clarify the diagnosis. The most common example is chronic psychosis developing either during periods of heavy abuse of drugs or at some time after the drug use has ceased. Other conditions include temporal lobe dysfunction, HIV infection, and a number of the conditions noted in the differential diagnosis (see below). They often have a good premorbid history, a precipitous onset, and an episodic course with symptom-free intervals.

Clinical Findings (Schizophrenia)

The signs and symptoms vary markedly among individuals as well as in the same person at different times. **Appearance** may be bizarre, though the usual finding is a mild to moderate unkempt blandness. **Motor activity** is generally reduced, though extremes ranging from catatonic stupor to frenzied excitement occur. **Social behavior** is characterized by marked withdrawal, coupled with disturbed interpersonal relationships and a reduced ability to experience pleasure. Dependency and a poor self-image are common. **Verbal utterances** are variable, the language being concrete yet symbolic, with unassociated rambling statements (at times interspersed with mutism) during an acute episode. Neologisms (made-up words or phrases), echolalia (repetition of words spoken by others), and verbigeration (repetition of senseless words or phrases) are occasionally present. **Affect** is usually flattened and shallow, with occasional inappropriateness. **Depression** is ubiquitous but may be less apparent during the acute psychotic episode and become more obvious during recovery. Depression is sometimes confused with akinetic side effects of antipsychotic drugs. It is also related to **boredom,** which increases symptoms and decreases the response to treatment. Work is generally unavailable and time hangs heavy, providing opportunities for counterproductive activities such as drug abuse, withdrawal, and increased psychotic symptoms.

Thought content may vary from a paucity of ideas to a rich complex of delusional fantasy with archaic thinking. One frequently notes after a period of conversation that little if any information has actually been conveyed. Incoming stimuli produce varied responses. In some cases a simple question may trigger explosive outbursts, whereas at other times there may be no overt response whatsoever (catatonia). When paranoid ideation is present, the patient is often irritable and less cooperative. **Delusions** (false beliefs) are characteristic of paranoid thinking, and they usually take the form of a preoccupation with the supposedly threatening behavior exhibited by other individuals. This ideation may cause the patient to adopt active countermeasures such as locking doors and windows, taking up weapons, covering the ceiling with aluminum foil to counteract radar waves, and other bizarre efforts. Somatic delusions revolve around issues of bodily decay or infestation. **Perceptual distortions** usually include auditory hallucinations—visual hallucinations are more commonly associated with organic mental states—and may include illusions (distortions of reality) such as figures changing in size or lights varying in intensity. Cenesthetic hallucinations (eg, burning sensation in the brain, feeling blood flowing in blood vessels) occasionally occur. Lack of humor, feelings of dread, depersonalization (a feeling of being apart from the self), and fears of annihilation may be present. Any of the above symptoms generate higher anxiety levels, with heightened arousal and occasional panic and suicidal ideation, as the individual fails to cope.

Ventricular enlargement and cortical atrophy, as

seen on the CT scan, has been correlated with a chronic course, severe cognitive impairment, and nonresponsiveness to neuroleptic medications.

The development of the acute episode in schizophrenia frequently is the end product of a gradual decompensation. Frustration and anxiety appear early, followed by depression and alienation, along with decreased effectiveness in day-to-day coping. This often leads to feelings of panic and increasing disorganization, with loss of the ability to test and evaluate the reality of perceptions. The stage of so-called psychotic resolution includes delusions, autistic preoccupations, and psychotic insight, with acceptance of the decompensated state. The process is frequently complicated by the use of caffeine, alcohol, and other recreational drugs. Life expectancy of schizophrenics is as much as 20% shorter than that of cohorts in the general population (usually because of a higher mortality rate in younger people).

Polydipsia and polyuria with secondary hyponatremia may produce water intoxication—characterized by symptoms of confusion, lethargy, psychosis, seizures, and occasionally death—in any psychiatric disorder, but most commonly schizophrenia. These problems exacerbate the schizophrenic symptoms. Possible pathogenetic factors include a hypothalamic defect, inappropriate ADH secretion (exclude medical causes of SIADH), neuroleptic medications (anticholinergic effects, stimulation of hypothalamic thirst center, effect on ADH), smoking (nicotine and SIADH), psychotic thought processes (delusional beliefs), and other medications (eg, diuretics, antidepressants, lithium, alcohol). Other causes must be ruled out (eg, diabetes mellitus, diabetes insipidus, renal disease).

Differential Diagnosis

One should not hesitate to reconsider the diagnosis of schizophrenia in any person who has received that diagnosis in the past, particularly when the clinical course has been atypical. A number of these patients have been found to actually have atypical episodic affective disorders that have responded well to lithium. Manic episodes often mimic schizophrenia. Also, many individuals have been diagnosed as schizophrenic because of inadequacies in psychiatric nomenclature. Thus, persons with brief reactive psychoses, obsessive-compulsive disorder, paranoid disorders, and schizophreniform disorders were often inappropriately diagnosed as having schizophrenia.

Psychotic depressions, psychotic organic mental states, and any illness with psychotic ideation tend to be confused with schizophrenia, partly because of the regrettable tendency to use the terms interchangeably. Adolescent phases of growth and counterculture behaviors constitute another area of diagnostic confusion. It is particularly important to avoid a misdiagnosis in these groups, because of the long-term

implications arising from having such a serious diagnosis made in a formative stage of life.

Medical disorders such as thyroid dysfunction, adrenal and pituitary disorders, reactions to toxic materials (eg, mercury, PCBs), and practically all of the organic mental states in the early stages must be ruled out. Postpartum psychosis is discussed under mood disorders. **Complex partial seizures,** especially when psychosensory phenomena are present, are an important differential consideration. Toxic drug states arising from prescription, over-the-counter, and street drugs may mimic all of the psychotic disorders. *The chronic use of amphetamines, cocaine, and other stimulants frequently produces a psychosis that is almost identical to the acute paranoid schizophrenic episode.* The presence of formication and stereotypy suggests the possibility of stimulant abuse. Phencyclidine (see below) has become a very common street drug, and in many cases a reaction to it is difficult to distinguish from other psychotic disorders. Cerebellar signs, excessive salivation, dilated pupils, and increased deep tendon reflexes should alert the physician to the possibility of a toxic psychosis. Industrial chemical toxicity (both organic and metallic), degenerative disorders, and metabolic deficiencies must be considered in the differential diagnosis.

Catatonic syndrome, frequently assumed to exist solely as a component of schizophrenic disorders, is actually the end product of a number of illnesses, including various organic conditions. Neoplasms, viral and bacterial encephalopathies, central nervous system hemorrhage, metabolic derangements such as diabetic ketoacidosis, sedative withdrawal, and hepatic and renal malfunction have all been implicated. It is particularly important to realize that drug toxicity (eg, overdoses of antipsychotic medications such as fluphenazine or haloperidol) can cause catatonic syndrome, which may be misdiagnosed as a catatonic schizophrenic disorder and inappropriately treated with more antipsychotic medication.

Treatment

A. Medical: Hospitalization is often necessary, particularly when the patient's behavior shows gross disorganization. The presence of competent family members lessens the need for hospitalization, and each case should be judged individually. The major considerations are to prevent self-inflicted harm or harm to others and to provide the patient's basic needs. A full medical evaluation and CT scanning or MRI should be considered in first episodes of schizophreniform disorder and other psychotic episodes of unknown cause.

Antipsychotic medications (see Antipsychotic Drugs) are the treatment of choice. They block the response to stimulation. The relapse rate can be reduced by 50% with proper maintenance neuroleptic therapy. Long-acting neuroleptics are used in noncompliant patients or nonresponders to oral medication. So-called **positive symptoms** such as hallucinations and delusions respond best, while **negative symptoms** such as withdrawal, psychomotor retardation, and poor interpersonal relationships may show little improvement. Clozapine may reduce these symptoms. Antidepressant drugs may be used in conjunction with neuroleptics if significant depression is present. Resistant cases may require concomitant use of lithium, carbamazepine, or valproic acid. The addition of a benzodiazepine drug to the neuroleptic regimen may prove helpful in treating the agitated or catatonic psychotic patient who has not responded to neuroleptics alone—lorazepam, 1–2 mg orally, can produce a rapid resolution of catatonic symptoms; the benzodiazepine may make possible maintenance with a lower neuroleptic dose. ECT has also been effective in treating catatonia. Clozapine may be helpful in schizophrenics with negative symptoms who have not responded to other antipsychotic drugs.

B. Social: Environmental considerations are most important in the individual with a chronic illness, who usually has a history of repeated hospitalizations, a continued low level of functioning, and symptoms that never completely remit. Family rejection and work failure are common. In these cases, board and care homes experienced in caring for psychiatric patients are most important. There is frequently an inverse relationship between stability of the living situation and the amounts of required antipsychotic drugs, since the most salutary environment is one that reduces stimuli.

Nonresidential self-help groups such as Recovery, Inc. should be utilized whenever possible. They provide a setting for sharing, learning, and mutual support and are frequently the only social involvement with which this type of patient is comfortable. Work agencies (eg, Goodwill Industries, Inc.) and vocational rehabilitation departments provide assessment, training, and job opportunities at a level commensurate with the person's clinical condition.

C. Psychologic: The need for psychotherapy varies markedly depending on the patient's current status and history. In a person with a single psychotic episode and a previously good level of adjustment, supportive psychotherapy may be helpful in assisting the patient to reintegrate the experience, gain some insight into antecedent problems, and become a more self-observant individual who can recognize early signs of stress. Insight-oriented psychotherapy is often counterproductive in this type of disorder. More importantly, family therapy should be given concomitantly to help alleviate the patient's stress and to assist relatives in coping with the patient.

D. Behavioral: Behavioral techniques (see above) are most frequently used in therapeutic settings such as day treatment centers, but there is no reason why they cannot be incorporated into family situations or any therapeutic setting. Many behavioral techniques are used unwittingly (eg, positive reinforcement—whether it be a word of praise or an approving nod—after some positive behavior), and with some careful thought, this approach can be a most powerful instrument for helping a person learn behaviors that will facilitate social acceptance. Music from portable cassette players with earphones is one of many ways to divert the patient's attention away from auditory hallucinations.

Prognosis

In any psychosis, the prognosis for alleviation of positive symptoms with medication is excellent in the large majority of patients. Negative symptoms are much more difficult to treat and are the principal reason schizophrenic patients do not achieve optimal function. Unavailability of structured work situations and lack of family therapy are two other reasons why the prognosis is so guarded in such a large percentage of schizophrenic patients. Psychosis connected with a history of serious drug abuse has a guarded prognosis because of the central nervous system damage, usually from the drugs themselves and associated medical illnesses.

Böker W, Brenner HD: Onset and course of schizophrenic disorders: Dynamic interactions between relevant factors. Br J Psychiatry 1992;(Suppl 18):161. (Genesis, progress, and treatment of a complex disorder.)

McGlashan TH, Fenton WS: The positive-negative distinction in schizophrenics: Review of natural history validators. Arch Gen Psychiatry 1992;49:63. (The distinction has validity and is a factor in treatment selection.)

Rifkin A et al: Dosage of haloperidol for schizophrenics. Arch Gen Psychiatry 1991;48:166.

MOOD DISORDERS
(Depression & Mania)

Essentials of Diagnosis

Present in most depressions:

- Lowered mood, varying from mild sadness to intense feelings of guilt, worthlessness, and hopelessness.
- Difficulty in thinking, including inability to concentrate, ruminations, and lack of decisiveness.
- Loss of interest, with diminished involvement in work and recreation.
- Somatic complaints such as headache; disrupted, lessened, or excessive sleep; loss of energy; change in appetite; decreased sexual drive.
- Anxiety.

Present in some severe depressions:

- Psychomotor retardation or agitation.
- Delusions of a hypochondriacal or persecutory nature.
- Withdrawal from activities.
- Physical symptoms of major severity, eg, anorexia,

insomnia, reduced sexual drive, weight loss, and various somatic complaints.

- Suicidal ideation.

Present in mania:

- Sleep disruption.
- Hyperactivity.
- Racing thoughts.
- Grandiosity.
- Variable psychotic symptoms.

General Considerations

Depression, like anxiety (with which it is associated), is ubiquitous and is a reality of everyday life. It may be the final expression of (1) genetic factors (neurotransmitter dysfunction), (2) developmental problems (personality defects, childhood events), or (3) psychosocial stresses (divorce, job loss). It frequently presents in the form of somatic complaints with negative medical workup. It can be a normal reaction to a wide variety of events and must be evaluated as such. When the depression is appropriate to a life event and is not of major magnitude, specific treatment is not necessary. The whole issue of depression is further confused by the fact that the word is used as an expression of a mood, a symptom, a syndrome, or a disease.

Mania is often combined with depression and may occur alone or cycle with depression.

Clinical Findings

In general, there are three major groups of depressions, with similar symptoms in each group.

A. Reactive to Psychosocial Factors: Depression may occur in reaction to some outside (exogenous) adverse life situation, usually loss of a person by death (grief reaction), divorce, etc; financial reversal (crisis); or loss of an established role, such as being needed. Anger is frequently associated with the loss, and this in turn often produces a feeling of guilt. Adjectives such as reactive and neurotic (implying anxiety, which is often present in these depressions) are often used in this group of depressions. They are properly classified as adjustment disorders with depressed mood. The symptoms range from mild sadness, anxiety, irritability, worry, lack of concentration, discouragement, and somatic complaints to the more severe symptoms of the next group.

B. Depressive Disorders: The subclassifications include major depressive episodes and dysthymia.

1. A major depressive episode (eg, endogenous unipolar disorder, involutional melancholia) is a period of serious mood depression that occurs at any time of life relatively independently of the patient's life situations or events. Many consider a physiologic or metabolic aberration to be causative. Complaints vary widely but most frequently include a loss of interest and pleasure (anhedonia), withdrawal from activities, and feelings of guilt. Also included are

inability to concentrate, some cognitive dysfunction, anxiety, chronic fatigue, feelings of worthlessness, somatic complaints (unidentifiable somatic complaints frequently indicate depression), and loss of sexual drive. Diurnal variation with improvement as the day progresses is common. Vegetative signs that frequently occur are insomnia, anorexia with weight loss, and constipation. Occasionally, severe agitation and psychotic ideation (paranoid thinking, somatic delusions) are present. These symptoms are more common in postmenopausal depression (involutional melancholia). Paranoid symptoms may range from general suspiciousness to ideas of reference with delusions. The somatic delusions frequently revolve around feelings of impending annihilation or hypochondriacal beliefs (eg, that the body is rotting away with cancer). Hallucinations are uncommon.

Atypical depression is a subtype that is characterized by hypersomnia, overeating, lethargy, and rejection sensitivity. These patients should be carefully evaluated for bipolar disorder. **Seasonal affective depression (SAD)** is a dysfunction of circadian rhythms that occurs more commonly in the winter and is believed to be due to decreased exposure to full-spectrum light. Common symptoms include carbohydrate craving, lethargy, hyperphagia, and hypersomnia.

Prenatal and postpartum depressive disorders occur in approximately 20% of pregnancies, usually in the postpartum period. The symptoms are those usually seen in serious depression, with an increased emphasis on concerns related to the baby (obsessive thoughts about harming it or inability to care for it). When psychotic symptoms occur, there is frequently associated sleep deprivation, volatility of behavior, and manic-like symptoms. Biologic vulnerability with hormonal changes and psychosocial stresses all play a role. The chances of a second episode are about 25%.

2. Dysthymia is a chronic depressive disturbance. Sadness, loss of interest, and withdrawal from activities over a period of 2 or more years with a relatively persistent course is necessary for this diagnosis. Generally, the symptoms are milder but longer-lasting than those in a major depressive episode.

C. Bipolar Disorders: Bipolar disorders (manic and depressive episodes) and individual manic episodes usually occur earlier (late teens or early adult life) than major depressive episodes.

1. A manic episode is a mood change characterized by elation with hyperactivity, overinvolvement in life activities, low irritability threshold, flight of ideas, easy distractibility, and little need for sleep. The overenthusiastic quality of the mood and the expansive behavior initially attract others, but the irritability, mood lability, aggressive behavior, and grandiosity usually lead to marked interpersonal difficulties. Activities may occur that are later regretted, eg, excessive spending, resignation from a job, a hasty marriage, sexual acting out, and exhibitionistic behavior, with alienation of friends and family. Atypical manic episodes can include gross delusions, paranoid ideation of severe proportions, and auditory hallucinations usually related to some grandiose perception. The episodes begin abruptly (sometimes precipitated by life stresses) and may last from several days to months. Spring and summer tend to be the peak periods. Generally, the manic episodes are of shorter duration than the depressive episodes. In almost all cases, the manic episode is part of a broader bipolar (manic-depressive) disorder. Patients with more than four complete cycles without remission in 1 year are called "rapid cyclers." (Substance abuse, particularly cocaine, can mimic rapid cycling.) These patients have a higher incidence of hypothyroidism. Manic patients differ from schizophrenics in that the former use more effective interpersonal maneuvers, are more sensitive to the social maneuvers of others, and are more able to utilize weakness and vulnerability in others to their own advantage. Creativity has been positively correlated with mood disorders, but the best work done is between episodes of mania and depression.

2. Cyclothymic disorders are chronic mood disturbances with episodes of depression and hypomania. The symptoms must have at least a 2-year duration and are milder than those in a depressive or manic episode. Occasionally, the symptoms will escalate into a full-blown manic or depressive episode, in which case it would be classified as a bipolar disorder.

D. Mood Disorders Secondary to Illness and Drugs: (All are classified as organic mood disorders.) Any illness, severe or mild, can cause significant depression. Conditions such as rheumatoid arthritis, multiple sclerosis, and chronic heart disease are particularly likely to be associated with depression, as are all other chronic illnesses. Hormonal variations clearly play a role in some depressions. Varying degrees of depression occur at various times in schizophrenic disorders, central nervous system disease (including cerebral dysrhythmias), and organic mental states. **Alcohol dependency** frequently coexists with serious depression.

The classic model of drug-induced depression occurs with the use of reserpine, both in a clinical and a neurochemical sense. Corticosteroids and oral contraceptives are commonly associated with affective changes. Antihypertensive medications such as methyldopa, guanethidine, and clonidine have been associated with the development of depressive syndromes, as have digitalis and antiparkinsonism drugs. Infrequently, disulfiram and anticholinesterase drugs may be associated with symptoms of depression. All stimulant use results in a depressive syndrome when the drug is withdrawn. Alcohol, sedatives, opiates, and most of the psychedelic drugs are depressants

and, paradoxically, are often used in self-treatment of depression.

Differential Diagnosis

Since depression may be a part of any illness—either reactively or as a secondary symptom—careful attention must be given to personal life adjustment problems, the role of medications (eg, reserpine, steroids, levodopa). Schizophrenia, partial complex seizures, brain syndromes, panic disorders, and anxiety disorders must be differentiated. Subtle thyroid dysfunction must be ruled out.

Complications

The longer the depression continues, the more crystallized it becomes—particularly when there is an element of secondary reinforcement. The most important complication is **suicide,** which always includes some elements of aggression. Suicide rates vary from 9 per 100,000 in Spain to 20 per 100,000 in the USA to 58 per 100,000 in Hungary. Males tend toward successful suicide, particularly in older age groups, whereas women make more attempts with lower mortality rates. An increased suicide rate is being observed in the younger population, ages 15–35. Patients with cancer, respiratory illnesses, AIDS, and those being maintained on hemodialysis have higher suicide rates. Alcohol is a significant factor in many suicide attempts.

There are four major groups of people who make suicide attempts:

(1) Those who are overwhelmed by problems in living (the despair of ordinary people). By far the greatest number fall into this category. There is often great ambivalence; they don't really want to die, but they don't want to go on as before either. These may be impulsive or aggressive acts not associated with significant depression.

(2) Those who are clearly attempting to control others. This is the blatant attempt in the presence of a significant other person in order to hurt or control that person.

(3) Those with severe depressions *(high-risk group).* This group includes both exogenous (eg, AIDS, which has a suicide rate many times that of the general population) and endogenous conditions (eg, panic disorders). It also includes those who may not be diagnosed as having depression but who are overwhelmed by a serious stressful situation (eg, the man charged with child molestation who hangs himself in his cell). Anxiety, panic, and fear are major findings in suicidal behavior. A patient may seem to make a dramatic improvement, but the lifting of depression may be due to the patient's decision to commit suicide.

(4) Those with psychotic illness *(high-risk group).* These individuals tend not to verbalize their concerns, are unpredictable, and are often successful but comprise a small percentage of the total. (Suicide is ten times more prevalent in schizophrenics than in the general population, and jumping from bridges is more common. In one study of 100 jumpers, 47% were schizophrenic.) Borderline personality disorders are included in this group.

The immediate goal of psychiatric evaluation is to assess the current suicidal risk and the need for hospitalization versus outpatient management. The intent is less likely to be truly suicidal, for example, if small amounts of poison or drugs were ingested or scratching of wrists was superficial; if the act was performed in the presence of others or with early notification of others; or if the attempt was arranged so that early detection would be anticipated. Alcohol, hopelessness, delusional thoughts, and complete or nearly complete loss of interest in life or ability to experience pleasure are all positively correlated with suicide attempts. Other risk factors are previous attempts, a family history of suicide, medical or psychiatric illness (eg, anxiety, depression, psychosis), male sex, older age, contemplation of violent methods, and drug use (including long-term sedative or alcohol use), which contributes to impulsiveness or mood swings. Successful treatment cannot be achieved if the patient continues to abuse drugs.

The patient's current mood status is best evaluated by direct evaluation of plans and concerns about the future, personal reactions to the attempt, and thoughts about the reactions of others. The patient's immediate resources should be assessed—people who can be significantly involved (most important), family support, job situation, financial resources, etc.

If hospitalization is not indicated (eg, gestures, impulsive attempts; see above), the physician must formulate and institute a treatment plan or make an adequate referral. Medication should be dispensed in small amounts to at-risk patients. The risk of suicide *attempts* does not differ among the antidepressants, but overdoses with the older tricyclic antidepressant drugs results in a higher death rate. *Guns and drugs should be removed from the patient's household.* Driving should be interdicted until the patient improves. The problem is often worsened by the long-term complications of the suicidal attempt, eg, brain damage due to hypoxia; peripheral neuropathies caused by staying for long periods in one position, causing nerve compressions; and medical or surgical problems such as esophageal strictures and tendon dysfunctions.

The reasons for self-mutilation, most commonly wrist cutting (but also autocastration, autoamputation, and autoenucleation, which are associated with psychoses), may be very different from the reasons for a suicide attempt. The initial treatment plan, however, should presume suicidal ideation, and conservative treatment should be initiated as for attempted suicide.

Sleep disturbances in the depressions are discussed below.

Treatment

A. Medical:

1. Depression–Depression associated with reactive disorders usually does not call for drug therapy and can be managed by psychotherapy and the passage of time. In severe cases—particularly when vegetative signs are present or impending—antidepressant drug therapy (see Antidepressant Drugs) is often effective. Drug selection depends on previous response if that information is available. If no background information is available, a safe and economical drug such as desipramine can be selected and a *full trial* instituted. If the response is inadequate, the serum level is measured and the diagnosis of depression reassessed. If the diagnosis is supportive by review and drug levels are adequate, a drug from a different group (eg, an MAO inhibitor) is given a trial. If the second drug fails, then a drug from the third group (eg, fluoxetine) may be given a trial. It is important to take note of washout times (see above). With any of the antidepressants, it is permissible to use lithium as an adjunctive drug in patients who do not respond to the antidepressant alone. Dysthymia is also treated in this way.

Psychotic depression can be treated with amoxapine, and if that drug is not adequate, a combination of an antipsychotic such as perphenazine (used initially) and an antidepressant such as desipramine is usually effective.

Atypical depression (including SAD) can be treated with an MAO inhibitor or a newer drug such as fluoxetine with good results. Light therapy is preferentially used in SAD.

Stimulants have little if any place in the treatment of depression but are helpful in the treatment of apathy in geriatric cases and medical convalescent problems.

Electroconvulsive therapy is effective in all types of depression (particularly involutional melancholia) and will also rapidly resolve a manic episode. It is also very effective for postpartum depression.

Hospitalization is necessary if suicide is a major consideration or if complex treatment modalities are required.

2. Mania–Manic episodes are treated with haloperidol, 5–10 mg orally or intramuscularly every 2–3 hours until symptoms subside. A decision must then be made about the need for long-term lithium maintenance in the bipolar patient. The dosage of haloperidol is gradually reduced after lithium is started (see Lithium, above).

If lithium is contraindicated or if problems develop with lithium (eg, kidney dysfunction), clonazepam alone (0.5–16 mg/d orally) may be effective in acute episodes but is questionable for long-term prophylaxis. Carbamazepine, 800–1600 mg/d orally, is also an effective substitute. Carbamazepine or bupropion, 400–500 mg/d orally, is effective in rapid-cycling bipolar patients. Valproic acid in initial studies has been shown to be comparable in effectiveness to carbamazepine for mania but is not effective in depression. Both carbamazepine and valproic acid should be brought to therapeutic serum levels. Calcium channel blockers are increasingly being used in the treatment of mania in patients for whom lithium or carbamazepine is either ineffective or contraindicated (eg, verapamil is safer than lithium or carbamazepine during pregnancy, though it decreases uterine contractility and must be discontinued before delivery).

B. Psychologic: It is seldom possible to engage an individual in penetrating psychotherapeutic endeavors during the acute stage of a severe depression. While medications may be taking effect, a supportive approach to strengthen existing defenses and appropriate consideration of the patient's continuing need to function at work, to engage in recreational activities, etc, are necessary as the severity of the depression lessens. If the patient is not seriously depressed, it is often quite appropriate to initiate intensive psychotherapeutic efforts, since flux periods are a good time to effect change. A catharsis of repressed anger and guilt may be beneficial. Therapy during or just after the acute stage may focus on coping techniques, with some practice of alternative choices. When lack of self-confidence and identity problems are factors in the depression, individual psychotherapy can be oriented to ways of improving self-esteem, increasing assertiveness, and lessening dependency. As previously noted, numerous studies have shown that the combination of drug therapy plus cognitive psychotherapy is more effective than either modality alone. It is usually helpful to involve the spouse or other significant family members early in treatment.

C. Social: Flexible use of appropriate social services can be of major importance in the treatment of depression. Since alcohol is often associated with depression, early involvement in alcohol treatment programs such as Alcoholics Anonymous can be important to future success (see Alcohol Dependency and Abuse, below). The *structuring* of daily activities during severe depression is often quite difficult for the patient, and loneliness is often a major factor. The help of family, employer, or friends is often necessary to mobilize the patient who experiences no joy in daily activities and tends to remain uninvolved and to deteriorate. Insistence on sharing activities will help involve the patient in simple but important daily functions. In some severe cases, the use of day treatment centers or support groups of a specific type (eg, mastectomy groups) is indicated. It is not unusual for a patient to have multiple legal, financial, and vocational problems requiring legal and vocational assistance.

D. Behavioral: When depression is a function of self-defeating coping techniques such as passivity, the role-playing approach can be useful. Behavioral techniques, including desensitization, may be used in problems such as phobias where depression is a by-product. When depression is a regularly used interpersonal style, behavioral counseling to family members or others can help in extinguishing the behavior in the patient.

Prognosis

Reactive depressions are usually time-limited, and the prognosis with treatment is good if a pathologic pattern of adjustment does not intervene. Major affective disorders frequently respond well to a full trial of drug treatment. Mania and bipolar disorder have a good prognosis with adequate treatment.

Eisenberg L: Treating depression and anxiety in primary care. N Engl J Med 1992;326:1080.

Klerman GL, Weissman MM: The course, morbidity and costs of depression. Arch Gen Psychiatry 1992;49:831. (All three are grossly underestimated.)

Winokur G, Black DW: Suicide: What can be done? (Editorial.) N Engl J Med 1992;327:490.

SLEEP DISORDERS

Sleep consists of two distinct states as shown by electroencephalographic studies: REM (rapid eye movement) sleep, also called dream sleep, D state sleep, paradoxic sleep; and NREM (non-REM) sleep, also called S stage sleep, which is divided into stages 1, 2, 3, and 4 recognizable by different electroencephalographic patterns. Stages 3 and 4 are "delta" sleep. Dreaming occurs mostly in REM and to a lesser extent in NREM sleep.

Sleep is a cyclic phenomenon, with four or five REM periods during the night accounting for about one-fourth of the total night's sleep (1½–2 hours). The first REM period occurs about 80–120 minutes after onset of sleep and lasts about 10 minutes. Later REM periods are longer (15–40 minutes) and occur mostly in the last several hours of sleep. Most stage 4 (deepest) sleep occurs in the first several hours.

Age-related changes in normal sleep include an unchanging percentage of REM sleep and a marked decrease in stage 3 and stage 4 sleep, with an increase in wakeful periods during the night. These normal changes, early bedtimes, and daytime naps play a role in the increased complaints of insomnia in older people. Variations in sleep patterns may be due to circumstances (eg, "jet lag") or to idiosyncratic patterns ("night owls") in persons who perhaps because of different "biologic rhythms" habitually go to bed late and sleep late in the morning. Creative facilities and rapidity of response to unfamiliar situations are impaired by loss of sleep. There are also rare individuals who have chronic difficulty in adapting to a 24-hour sleep-wake cycle (desynchronization sleep disorder), which can be resynchronized by altering exposure to light.

The three major sleep disorders are discussed below.

Dyssomnias (Insomnia)

Patients may complain of difficulty getting to sleep or staying asleep, intermittent wakefulness during the night, early morning awakening, or combinations of any of these. Transient episodes are usually of little significance. Stress, caffeine, physical discomfort, daytime napping, and early bedtimes are common factors.

A. Clinical Conditions: Psychiatric disorders are often associated with persistent insomnia. **Depression** is usually associated with fragmented sleep, decreased total sleep time, earlier onset of REM sleep, a shift of REM activity to the first half of the night, and a loss of slow wave sleep—all of which are nonspecific findings. In **manic disorders,** sleeplessness is a cardinal feature and an important early sign of impending mania in bipolar cases. Total sleep time is decreased, with shortened REM latency and increased REM activity. Sleep-related panic attacks occur in the transition from stage 2 to stage 3 sleep in some patients with a longer REM latency in the sleep pattern preceding the attacks.

Abuse of alcohol may cause or be secondary to the sleep disturbance. There is a tendency to use alcohol as a means of getting to sleep without realizing that it disrupts the normal sleep cycle. Acute alcohol intake produces a decreased sleep latency with reduced REM sleep during the first half of the night. REM sleep is increased in the second half of the night, with an increase in total amount of slow wave sleep (stages 3 and 4). Vivid dreams and frequent awakenings are common. Chronic alcohol abuse increases stage 1 and decreases REM sleep (most drugs delay or block REM sleep), with symptoms persisting for many months after the individual has stopped drinking. Acute alcohol or other sedative withdrawal causes delayed onset of sleep and REM rebound with intermittent awakening during the night.

Heavy smoking (more than a pack a day) causes difficulty falling asleep—apparently independently of the often associated increase in coffee drinking. Excess intake near bedtime of caffeine, cocaine, and other stimulants (eg, over-the-counter cold remedies) causes decreased total sleep time—mostly NREM sleep—with some increased sleep latency.

Sedative-hypnotics—specifically, the benzodiazepines, which are the prescription drugs of choice to promote sleep—tend to increase total sleep time, decrease sleep latency, and decrease nocturnal awakening, with variable effects on NREM sleep. Withdrawal causes just the opposite effects and results in continued use of the drug for the purpose of preventing withdrawal symptoms. Antidepressants decrease REM sleep (with marked rebound on withdrawal in the form of nightmares) and have varying effects on NREM sleep. The effect on REM sleep correlates with reports that REM sleep deprivation parallels improvement in some depressions.

Persistent insomnias are also related to a wide variety of medical conditions, particularly delirium, pain, respiratory distress syndromes, uremia, asthma, and hypothyroidism. Adequate analgesia and proper treatment of medical disorders will reduce symptoms and decrease the need for sedatives.

B. Treatment: In transient insomnias, deemphasis and reassurance are sufficient treatment. The patient should be given commonsense advice about consistent bedtimes, room temperature (cool is best), late snacks (a small amount of food or liquid), daily exercise, avoidance of noxious habits (too much coffee, alcohol, cigarettes), and avoidance of daytime naps (including dozing at the TV set). To be avoided are clock-watching, restless bed partners (easier said than done), and lying in bed trying to force sleep to come. A relaxed attitude toward the problem should be emphasized. Medications should be avoided if possible. Patients in acute distress may require a short course of benzodiazepine (eg, temazepam, 15 mg at bedtime). Antihistamines such as diphenhydramine or hydroxyzine are acceptable milder substitutes for benzodiazepines. Antidepressive and antipsychotic drugs with sedative effects (eg, trazodone, thioridazine) may be selected when dyssomnia is a symptom of the underlying condition requiring these types of medication.

Hypersomnias (Disorders of Excessive Sleepiness)

The hypersomnias are a more severe problem than insomnia.

A. Clinical Conditions:

1. Sleep apnea–This disorder is characterized by cessation of breathing for at least 30 episodes (each lasting 10 seconds) during the night. There are two types: obstructive and central. The obstructive type is discussed in Chapter 9. Central sleep apnea is due to failure during sleep of the respiratory drive mechanism. Obese middle-aged and older men with hypertension and associated congestive heart failure) are most often affected. Both types may occur simultaneously. Symptoms include snoring, restless sleep, and excessive daytime sleepiness, which may be associated with headaches, memory impairment, and *depression.* Cardiac arrhythmias (particularly bradycardia) and blood gas irregularities occur during episodes. The patients tend to have poor judgment and a history of work-related problems. Definitive diagnostic evaluation may include thyroid evaluation and otolaryngologic examination; polysomnography in the hospital to record sleep, heart rate, and respiratory movement; and oxygen saturation studies. Moderate alcohol intake at bedtime has produced sleep apnea episodes (10–12 nightly) in healthy men.

2. Narcolepsy–Narcolepsy consists of a tetrad

of symptoms: (1) Sudden, brief (about 15 minutes) sleep attacks that may occur during any type of activity; (2) cataplexy—sudden loss of muscle tone involving specific small muscle groups or generalized muscle weakness that may cause the person to slump to the floor, unable to move, often associated with emotional reactions and sometimes confused with seizure disorder; (3) sleep paralysis—a generalized flaccidity of muscles with full consciousness in the transition zone between sleep and waking; and (4) hypnagogic hallucinations, visual or auditory, which may precede sleep or occur during the sleep attack. The attacks are characterized by an abrupt transition into REM sleep—a necessary criterion for diagnosis. The disorder begins in early adult life, affects both sexes equally, and usually levels off in severity at about 30 years of age.

REM sleep behavior disorder, characterized by motor dyscontrol and often violent dreams during REM sleep, may be related to narcolepsy.

3. Kleine-Levin syndrome–This syndrome, which occurs mostly in young males, is characterized by hypersomnic attacks three or four times a year lasting up to 2 days, with hyperphagia, hypersexuality, irritability, and confusion on awakening. It has often been associated with antecedent neurologic insults. It usually remits after age 40.

4. Nocturnal myoclonus–Periodic lower leg movements occur during sleep with subsequent daytime sleepiness, anxiety, depression, and cognitive impairment.

B. Treatment: Treatment of sleep apnea may include medical measures such as weight reduction and administration during sleep of air under fairly high pressure through the nasopharynx. Surgical treatment is discussed in Chapter 9. Diaphragmatic pacing has also been helpful for central sleep apnea. Trials with protriptyline have improved daytime somnolence and nocturnal oxygenation, with no significant change, however, in the number of apneic episodes. Acetazolamide has shown some promise, probably by creating a metabolic acidosis and the resultant hypercapnic ventilatory response.

Narcolepsy is managed by daily administration of a stimulant such as amphetamine sulfate, 10 mg in the morning, with increased dosage as necessary. Imipramine, 75–100 mg daily, has been effective in treatment of cataplexy but not narcolepsy.

Nocturnal myoclonus and REM sleep behavior disorder can be is treated with clonazepam with variable results. There is no treatment for Kleine-Levin syndrome.

Parasomnias (Abnormal Behaviors During Sleep)

These disorders are fairly common in children and less so in adults.

A. Clinical Presentations: Sleep terror (pavor nocturnus) is an abrupt, terrifying arousal from sleep, usually in preadolescent boys though it may occur in adults as well. It is distinct from sleep panic attacks. Symptoms are fear, sweating, tachycardia, and confusion for several minutes, with amnesia for the event. **Nightmares** occur during REM sleep; sleep terrors in stage 3 or stage 4 sleep. **Sleepwalking (somnambulism)** includes ambulation or other intricate behaviors while still asleep, with amnesia for the event. It affects mostly children aged 6–12 years, and episodes occur during stage 3 or stage 4 sleep in the first third of the night and in REM sleep in the later sleep hours. Sleepwalking in elderly people is a feature of organic brain syndrome. Idiosyncratic reactions to drugs (eg, marihuana, alcohol) and medical conditions (eg, partial complex seizures) may be causative factors in adults.

Enuresis is involuntary micturition during sleep in a person who usually has voluntary control. Like other parasomnias, it is more common in children, usually in the 3–4 hours after bedtime, but is not limited to a specific stage of sleep. Confusion during the episode and amnesia for the event are common.

B. Treatment: Treatment for sleep terrors is with benzodiazepines (eg, diazepam, 5–20 mg at bedtime), since it will suppress stage 3 and stage 4 sleep. Somnambulism responds to the same treatment for the same reason, but simple safety measures should not be neglected. Enuresis may respond to imipramine, 50–100 mg at bedtime, though desmopressin nasal spray (an antidiuretic hormone preparation) has increasingly become the treatment of choice for nocturnal enuresis. Behavioral approaches (eg, bells that ring when the pad gets wet) have also been successful.

Becker PM, Jamieson AO: Insomnia: Use of a decision tree to assess and treat. Postgrad Med 1993;93:66. (Concise overview.)

Schenck CH: Motor dyscontrol in narcolepsy: Rapid-eye movement (REM) sleep without atonia and REM sleep behavior disorder. Ann Neurol 1992;32:3. (There are probably a number of REM sleep problems as yet undifferentiated from narcolepsy.)

DISORDERS OF AGGRESSION

Acts performed with the deliberate intent of causing physical harm to persons or property have a wide variety of causative factors. Aggression and violence are symptoms rather than diseases, and most frequently they are *not* associated with an underlying medical condition. Clinicians are unable to predict dangerous behavior with greater than chance accuracy. In terms of demographic characteristics, the perpetrator of an act of aggression is often a male under age 25, a member of a minority group, a person in socially and economically deprived circumstances, and a resident of an inner-city area. Depression, schizophrenia, personality disorders, mania, paranoia, temporal lobe dysfunction, and organic mental states may be associated. Violence and suicide are correlated.

In the USA, a significant proportion of all violent deaths are alcohol-related. The ingestion of even small amounts of alcohol can result in pathologic intoxication that resembles an acute organic mental condition. Amphetamines, crack cocaine, and other stimulants are frequently associated with aggressive behavior. Phencyclidine is a drug commonly associated with violent behavior that is occasionally of a bizarre nature, partly due to lowering of the pain threshold. Impulse control disorders are characterized by physical abuse, usually of wife or children, pathologic intoxication, impulsive sexual activities, and automobile misuse.

Wife beating and rape are much more widespread than heretofore recognized. Awareness of the problem is to some degree due to increasing recognition of the rights of women and the understanding by women that they do not have to accept abuse. Acceptance of this kind of aggression inevitably leads to more, with the ultimate aggression being murder— 20–50% of murders in the USA occur within the family. Police are called in more domestic disputes than *all other criminal incidents combined.* Children who are a part of such relationships inevitably become victims. The majority of abused children come from this type of household.

Features of individuals who have been subjected to chronic physical or sexual abuse are as follows: trouble expressing anger, staying angry longer, general passivity in relationships, feeling "marked for life" with accompanying feeling of deserving to be victimized, lack of trust, and dissociation of affect from experiences. They may also have symptoms related to posttraumatic stress, as discussed above. The physician should be suspicious about the origin of any injuries not fully explained, particularly if such incidents recur.

Treatment

A. Psychologic: Management of any violent individual includes appropriate psychologic maneuvers. Move slowly, talk slowly with clarity and reassurance, and evaluate the situation. Strive to create a setting that is minimally disturbing and eliminate people or things threatening to the violent individual. Do not threaten or abuse and do not touch or crowd the person. Allow no weapons in the area (an increasing problem in hospital emergency rooms). Proximity to a door is comforting to both the patient and the examiner. Use a negotiator whom the violent person can relate to comfortably. Food and drink are helpful in defusing the situation (as are cigarettes for those who smoke). Honesty is important. Make no false promises, bolster the patient's self-esteem, and continue to engage the subject verbally until the situation is under control. This type of individual does better with strong external controls to replace the lack of inner controls over the long term. Close probationary supervision and court-mandated restrictions can be most helpful. There should be a major effort to help the individual avoid drug use (eg, Alcoholics Anonymous). Victims of abuse are essentially treated as any victim of trauma and, not infrequently, have evidence of posttraumatic stress disorder.

B. Pharmacologic: Pharmacologic means are often necessary whether or not psychologic approaches have been successful. This is particularly true in the agitated or psychotic patient. The drug of choice in psychotic aggressive states is haloperidol, 10 mg intramuscularly every hour until symptoms are alleviated. Benzodiazepine sedatives (eg, diazepam, 5 mg orally or intravenously every several hours) can be used for mild to moderate agitation, but an antipsychotic drug is preferred for management of the seriously violent and psychotic patient. Chronic aggressive states, particularly in retardation and brain damage (rule out causative organic conditions and medications such as anticholinergic drugs in amounts sufficient to cause confusion) have been ameliorated with propranolol, 40–240 mg/d orally, or pindolol, 5 mg twice daily orally (pindolol causes less bradycardia and hypotension). Carbamazepine and valproic acid are effective in the treatment of aggression and explosive disorders, particularly when associated with known or suspected brain lesions. Lithium and potent serotonin reuptake blockers (eg, trazodone) are also effective for intermittent explosive outbursts. Buspirone (10–40 mg/d orally) is helpful for aggression, particularly in mentally retarded patients.

C. Physical: Physical management is necessary if psychologic and pharmacologic means are not sufficient. It requires the active and visible presence of an adequate number of personnel (five or six) to reinforce the idea that the situation is under control despite the patient's lack of inner controls. Such an approach often precludes the need for actual physical restraint. When adequate personnel are not available, however, two people shielded by a mattress (single-bed size) can usually corner and subdue the patient without injury to anyone. Seclusion rooms and restraints should be used only when necessary (ambulatory restraints are an alternative), and the patient must then be observed at frequent intervals. Design of corridors and seclusion rooms is important. Narrow corridors, small spaces, and crowded areas exacerbate the potential for violence in an anxious patient.

D. Other: The treatment of victims (eg, beaten

wives) is a frustrating experience, chiefly because of the woman's reluctance to leave the situation. Reasons for staying vary, but common themes include the fear of more violence because of leaving; the hope that the situation may ameliorate (in spite of steady worsening); and the financial aspects of the situation, which are seldom to the woman's advantage. Concerns for the children often finally compel the woman to seek help. An early step is to get the woman into a therapeutic situation that provides the support of others in similar straits. Al-Anon is frequently a valuable asset and quite appropriate when alcohol is one of the factors in the abuse of the woman. The group can support the victim while she gathers strength to consider alternatives without being paralyzed by fear. Many cities now offer temporary emergency centers and counseling. Use the available resources, attend to any medical or psychiatric problems, and maintain a compassionate interest.

Bownes IT, O'Gorman EC, Sayers A: Assault characteristics and posttraumatic stress disorder in rape victims. Acta Psychiatr Scand 1991;83:27.
Council on Scientific Affairs, American Medical Association: Violence against women: Relevance for medical practitioners. JAMA 1992;267:3184.
Marzuk PM, Tardiff K, Hirsch CS: The epidemiology of murder-suicide. JAMA 1992;267:3179.

SUBSTANCE USE DISORDERS (Drug Dependency, Drug Abuse)

The term "drug dependency" is used in a broad sense here to include both addictions and habituations. It involves the triad of compulsive drug use referred to as drug addiction, which includes (1) a **psychologic craving** or dependence and the behavior included in the procurement of the drug ("hustle"); (2) **physiologic dependence,** with withdrawal symptoms on discontinuance of the drug; and (3) **tolerance,** ie, the need to increase the dose to obtain the desired effects. Drug dependency is a function of the amount of drug used and the duration of usage. The amount needed to produce dependency varies with the nature of the drug and the idiosyncratic nature of the user. The frequency of use is usually daily, and the duration is inevitably greater than 2–3 weeks. Polydrug abuse is very common. Transgenerational continuity of drug abuse is also common. A large percentage of drug abusers present themselves for something other than treatment (eg, avoiding legal consequences, obtaining more drugs).

There is accumulating evidence that an impairment syndrome exists in many former (and current) drug users. It is believed that drug use has damaged neurotransmitter receptor sites and that the consequent imbalance produces symptoms that may mimic other psychiatric illnesses. **"Kindling"**—repeated stimulation of the brain—renders the individual more susceptible to focal brain activity with minimal stimulation. Stimulants and depressants can produce kindling, leading to relatively spontaneous effects no longer dependent on the original stimulus. These effects may be manifested as mood swings, panic, psychosis, and occasionally overt seizure activity. The imbalance also results in an individual who simply does not produce: poor job retention, marriage problems, poor planning, and generally erratic behavior. Patients with posttraumatic stress disorder frequently have been self-treated with a variety of drugs. Chronic abusers of a wide variety of drugs exhibit cerebral atrophy on CT scans, a finding that may relate to the above symptoms. Early recognition is important, mainly to establish realistic treatment programs that are chiefly symptom-directed.

The physician faces three problems with substance abuse: (1) the prescribing of substances such as sedatives, stimulants, or narcotics that might produce dependency; (2) the treatment of individuals who have already abused drugs, most commonly alcohol; and (3) the detection of illicit drug use in patients presenting with psychiatric symptoms. The usefulness of urinalysis for detection of drugs varies markedly with different drugs and under different circumstances (pharmacokinetics is a major factor). Water-soluble drugs (eg, alcohol, stimulants, opioids) are eliminated in a day or so. Lipophilic substances (eg, barbiturates, tetrahydrocannabinol) appear in the urine over longer periods of time: several days in most cases, 1–2 months in chronic marihuana users. Sedative drug determinations are quite variable, amount of drug and duration of use being important determinants. False-positives can be a problem related to ingestion of some legitimate drugs or foods (eg, phenytoin for barbiturates, phenylpropanolamine for amphetamines, chlorpromazine for opiates) and some foods (eg, poppy seeds for opiates, coca leaf tea for cocaine). Manipulations can alter the legitimacy of the testing. Dilution, either in vivo or in vitro, can be detected by checking urine specific gravity. Addition of ammonia, vinegar, or salt may invalidate the test, but odor and pH determinations are simple. Hair analysis can determine drug use over longer periods, particularly sequential drug-taking patterns. The sensitivity and reliability of such tests are considered good, and the method may be complementary to urinalysis.

Cottler LB et al: Posttraumatic stress disorder among substance users from the general population. Am J Psychiatry 1992;149:664. (It is difficult to sort out traumas in any population, but it is clear that a large number of

PTSD patients use a large number of drugs for a long period of time.)

Regier DA et al: Comorbidity of mental disorders with alcohol and other drug abuse. JAMA 1991;264:2511.

ALCOHOL DEPENDENCY & ABUSE (Alcoholism)

Essentials of Diagnosis

Major criteria:

- Physiologic dependence as manifested by evidence of withdrawal when intake is interrupted.
- Laboratory tests (see below).
- Tolerance to the effects of alcohol.
- Evidence of alcohol-associated illnesses, such as alcoholic liver disease, cerebellar degeneration.
- Continued drinking despite strong medical and social contraindications and life disruptions.
- Impairment in social and occupational functioning. Depression.
- Blackouts.

Other signs:

- Alcohol stigmas: Alcohol odor on breath, alcoholic facies, flushed face, scleral injection, tremor, ecchymoses, peripheral neuropathy.
- Surreptitious drinking.
- Unexplained work absences.
- Frequent accidents, falls, or injuries of vague origin; in smokers, cigarette burns on hands or chest.

General Considerations

Alcoholism is a syndrome consisting of two phases: problem drinking and alcohol addiction. Problem drinking is the repetitive use of alcohol, often to alleviate anxiety or solve other emotional problems. Alcohol addiction is a true addiction similar to that which occurs following the repeated use of other sedative-hypnotics. There is a high incidence among homeless individuals. Alcohol and other drug abuse patients have a much higher prevalence of lifetime psychiatric disorders. While male-to-female ratios in alcoholic treatment agencies remain at 4:1, there is evidence that the rates are converging. Women delay seeking help, and when they do they tend to seek it in medical or mental health settings. Adoption and twin studies indicate some genetic influence. Ethnic distinctions are important—eg, 40% of Japanese have aldehyde dehydrogenase deficiency and are more susceptible to the effects of alcohol. *Depression is often present and should be evaluated carefully.* The majority of suicides and intrafamily homicides involve alcohol, and it is a major factor in rapes and other assaults.

Clinical Findings

A. Acute Intoxication: The signs of alcoholic intoxication are the same as those of overdosage with any other central nervous system depressant: drowsiness, errors of commission, psychomotor dysfunction, disinhibition, dysarthria, ataxia, and nystagmus. For a 70-kg person, an ounce of whiskey, a glass of wine, or a 12-oz bottle of beer raises the level of alcohol in the blood by 25 mg/dL. Blood levels below 50 mg/dL rarely cause significant motor dysfunction. Intoxication as manifested by ataxia, dysarthria, and nausea and vomiting indicates a blood level above 150 mg/dL, and lethal blood levels range from 350 to 900 mg/dL. In severe cases, overdosage is marked by respiratory depression, stupor, seizures, shock syndrome, coma, and death. Serious overdoses are frequently due to a combination of alcohol with other sedatives.

B. Withdrawal: There is a wide spectrum of manifestations of alcoholic withdrawal, ranging from anxiety, decreased cognition, and tremulousness through increasing irritability and hyperreactivity to full-blown **delirium tremens.** The latter is an acute organic psychosis that is usually manifest within 24–72 hours after the last drink (but may occur up to 7–10 days later). It is characterized by mental confusion, tremor, sensory hyperacuity, visual hallucinations (often of snakes, bugs, etc), autonomic hyperactivity, diaphoresis, dehydration, electrolyte disturbances (hypokalemia, hypomagnesemia), seizures, and cardiovascular abnormalities. The acute withdrawal syndrome is often completely unexpected and occurs when the patient has been hospitalized for some unrelated problem and presents as a diagnostic problem. *Suspect alcohol withdrawal in every unexplained delirium.* Seizures occur early (the first 24 hours) and are more prevalent in persons who have a history of withdrawal syndromes. The mortality rate from delirium tremens has steadily decreased with early diagnosis and improved treatment.

In addition to the immediate withdrawal symptoms, there is evidence of persistent longer-term ones, including sleep disturbances, anxiety, depression, excitability, fatigue, and emotional volatility. These symptoms may persist for 3–12 months, and in some cases they become chronic.

C. Alcoholic (Organic) Hallucinosis: This syndrome occurs either during heavy drinking or on withdrawal and is characterized by a paranoid psychosis without the tremulousness, confusion, and clouded sensorium seen in withdrawal syndromes. The patient appears normal except for the auditory hallucinations, which are frequently persecutory and may cause the patient to behave aggressively and in a paranoid fashion.

D. Chronic Alcoholic Brain Syndromes: These encephalopathies are characterized by increasing erratic behavior, memory and recall problems, and emotional instability—the usual signs of organic brain syndrome due to any cause. Early recognition and treatment of the alcoholic with intravenous thiamine and B complex vitamins can minimize damage.

Differential Diagnosis

The differential diagnosis of problem drinking is essentially between primary alcoholism (when no other major psychiatric diagnosis exists) and secondary alcoholism, when alcohol is used as self-medication for major underlying psychiatric problems such as schizophrenia or affective disorder. The differentiation is important, since the latter group requires treatment for the specific psychiatric problem.

The differential diagnosis of alcoholic withdrawal includes other sedative abuse. Acute alcoholic hallucinosis must be differentiated from other acute paranoid states such as amphetamine psychosis or acute paranoid schizophrenia. An accurate history is the most important differentiating factor. The history and laboratory test results are the most important features in differentiating chronic organic brain syndromes due to alcohol from those due to other causes. The form of the brain syndrome is of little help—eg, chronic brain syndromes from lupus erythematosus may be associated with confabulation similar to that resulting from long-standing alcoholism.

Complications

The medical, economic, and psychosocial problems of alcoholism are staggering. The central and peripheral nervous system complications include chronic brain syndromes, cerebellar degeneration, cardiovascular disorders, and peripheral neuropathies. Direct effects on the liver include cirrhosis, esophageal varicosities, and eventual hepatic failure. Indirect effects include protein abnormalities, coagulation defects, hormone deficiencies, and an increased incidence of liver neoplasms.

Fetal alcohol syndrome includes one or more of the following developmental defects in the offspring of alcoholic women: (1) low birth weight and small size with failure to catch up in size or weight; (2) mental retardation, with an average IQ in the 60s; and (3) a variety of birth defects, with a large percentage of facial and cardiac abnormalities. The fetuses are very quiet in utero, and there is an increased frequency of breech presentations. There is a higher incidence of delayed postnatal growth and behavior development. The risk factors are appreciably higher the more alcohol ingested by the mother each day. Cigarette and marihuana smoking can produce similar effects on the fetus.

Treatment of Problem Drinking

A. Psychologic: The most important consideration for the physician is to suspect the problem early and take a nonjudgmental attitude, though this does not mean a passive one. The problem of **denial** must be met, preferably with significant family members at the first meeting. This means dealing from the beginning with any enabling behavior of the spouse or other significant people. This is particularly true when the problem has become a "chronic rescue operation."

There must be an emphasis on the things that can be done. This approach emphasizes the fact that the physician cares and strikes a positive and hopeful note early in treatment. Valuable time should not be wasted trying to find out why the patient drinks; come to grips early with the immediate problem of how to stop the drinking. Total abstinence (not "controlled drinking") should be the primary goal.

B. Social: Get the patient into Alcoholics Anonymous (AA) and the spouse into Al-Anon. Success is usually proportionate to the utilization of AA, religious counseling, and other resources. The patient should be seen frequently for short periods and charged an appropriate fee.

Do not underestimate the importance of religion, particularly since the alcoholic is often a dependent person who needs a great deal of support. Early enlistment of the help of a concerned religious adviser can often provide the turning point for a personal conversion to sobriety.

One of the most important considerations is the job; it is usually lost or in jeopardy. The business community has become painfully aware of the problem, with the result that about 70% of the Fortune 500 companies offer programs to their employees to help with the problem of alcoholism. In the latter case, some specific recommendations to employers can be offered: (1) Avoid placement in jobs where the alcoholic must be alone, eg, traveling buyer or sales executive. (2) Use supervision but not surveillance. (3) Keep competition with others to a minimum. (4) Avoid positions that require quick decision making on important matters (high stress situations).

C. Medical: Hospitalization is not usually necessary at this stage, which is not an acute one. It is sometimes used to dramatize a situation and force the patient to face the problem of alcoholism, but generally it should be used on medical indications.

Because of the many medical complications of alcoholism, a complete physical examination with appropriate laboratory tests is mandatory, with special attention to the liver and nervous system. Two tests that may provide clues to an alcohol problem are γ-glutamyl transferase measurement (levels above 30 mU/mL are suggestive of heavy drinking) and mean corpuscular volume (> 95 fL in males and > 100 fL in females). If both are elevated, there is a probability of a serious drinking problem. Use of other recreational drugs with alcohol skews and negates the significance of these tests. HDL cholesterol elevations combined with elevated γ-glutamyl transferase concentrations also can help to identify heavy drinkers. *Use of sedatives as a replacement for alcohol is not desirable.* The usual result is concomitant use of sedatives and alcohol and worsening of the problem. Lithium is not helpful in the treatment of primary alcoholism.

Disulfiram has been used for many years as an

aversive drug to discourage alcohol use. The results have generally been disappointing.

In preliminary studies, naltrexone (an opiate antagonist) has been helpful in lowering relapse rates over the 3–6 months after cessation of drinking, apparently by lessening the pleasurable effects of alcohol.

D. Behavioral: Conditioning approaches have been used in some settings in the treatment of alcoholism, most commonly as a type of aversion therapy. For example, the patient is given a drink of whiskey and then a shot of apomorphine, and proceeds to vomit. In this way a strong association is built up between the vomiting and the drinking. Although this kind of treatment has been successful in some cases, many people do not retain the learned aversive response.

Treatment of Withdrawal & Hallucinosis

A. Medical:

1. Alcoholic hallucinosis–Alcoholic hallucinosis, which can occur either during or on cessation of a prolonged drinking period, is not a typical withdrawal syndrome and is handled differently. Since the symptoms are primarily those of a psychosis in the presence of a clear sensorium, they are handled like any other psychosis: hospitalization (when indicated) and adequate amounts of antipsychotic drugs. Haloperidol, 5 mg orally twice a day for the first day or so, usually ameliorates symptoms quickly, and the drug can be decreased and discontinued over several days as the patient improves. It then becomes necessary to deal with the chronic alcohol abuse, which has been discussed.

2. Withdrawal symptoms–Withdrawal symptoms, ranging from a mild syndrome to the severe state usually called delirium tremens, are a medical problem with a significant morbidity and mortality rate. They usually occur when an intake of at least 7–8 pints of beer or 1 pint of spirits daily for several months has been stopped (onset 12 hours, peak intensity 48–72 hours after cessation of alcohol intake). The patient should be hospitalized and given adequate central nervous system depressants (eg, benzodiazepines, phenobarbital) to counteract the excitability resulting from the sudden cessation of alcohol. Monitoring of vital signs and fluids and electrolyte levels is essential for the severely ill patient. Antipsychotic drugs such as chlorpromazine should *not* be used. The choice of the specific sedative is less important than using *adequate* doses to bring the patient to a level of moderate sedation, and this will vary from person to person. Mild to moderate dependency requires "drying out"—a short course of oral benzodiazepines on an outpatient basis with *no alcohol intake*. In severe withdrawal, hospitalize and use diazepam orally in a dosage of 5–10 mg every 1–4 hours depending on the clinical need. In severe withdrawal, intravenous administration is nec-

essary. After stabilization, the amount of diazepam required to maintain a sedated state may be given orally every 8–12 hours. If restlessness, tremulousness, and other signs of withdrawal persist, the dosage is increased until moderate sedation occurs. The dosage is then gradually reduced by 20% every 24 hours until withdrawal is complete. This usually requires a week or so of treatment. Clonidine, 5 µg/kg orally every 2 hours, or patches of appropriate dosage strength, suppresses cardiovascular signs of withdrawal and also has some anxiolytic effect. Carbamazepine, 400–800 mg daily orally, compares favorably with benzodiazepines for alcohol withdrawal.

Meticulous examination for other medical problems is necessary. Alcoholic hypoglycemia can occur with low blood alcohol levels (see Chapter 26). Alcoholics commonly have liver disease and associated clotting problems and are also prone to injury—and the combination all too frequently leads to undiagnosed subdural hematoma.

Anticonvulsant drugs are not needed unless there is a history of seizures. In these situations, phenytoin can be given in a loading dose—500 mg orally and, several hours later, another 500 mg orally (ie, 1 g over 4–6 hours). This drug is then continued in a dosage of 300 mg daily, which is checked by serum drug level.

A general diet should be given, and vitamins in high doses: thiamine, 50 mg intravenously initially, then intramuscularly on a daily basis; pyridoxine, 100 mg/d; folic acid, 5 mg three times a day; and ascorbic acid, 100 mg twice a day. Intravenous glucose solutions should not be given prior to the vitamins for fear of precipitation of Wernicke's syndrome. Concurrent administration is satisfactory, and hydration should be meticulously assessed on an ongoing basis.

Chronic brain syndromes secondary to a long history of alcohol intake are not responsive to any specific measures. Attention to the social and environmental care of this type of patient is paramount.

B. Psychologic and Behavioral: The comments in the section on problem drinking apply here also; these methods of treatment become the primary consideration after the successful treatment of withdrawal or alcoholic hallucinosis. Psychologic and social measures should be initiated in the hospital shortly before discharge. This increases the possibility of continued posthospitalization treatment.

Delbanco TL: Patients who drink too much: Where are their doctors? JAMA 1992;267:702.

Morse RM et al: The definition of alcoholism. JAMA 1992;268:1012. (An attempt to define the disorder by a committee of experts.)

OTHER DRUG & SUBSTANCE DEPENDENCIES

Opiates

The terms "opiates" and "narcotics" are used interchangeably and include a group of drugs with actions that mimic those of morphine. The group includes natural derivatives of opium, synthetic surrogates, and a number of polypeptides, some of which have been discovered to be natural neurotransmitters. The principal narcotic of abuse is heroin (metabolized to morphine), which is not used as a legitimate medication. A large percentage of heroin addicts are infected with HIV because of nonsterile needles. The other common narcotics are prescription drugs and differ in milligram potency, duration of action, and agonist and antagonist capabilities (see Chapter 1). All of the narcotic analgesics can be reversed by the narcotic antagonist naloxone.

The clinical signs of mild narcotic intoxication include needle tracks; changes in mood, with feelings of euphoria; drowsiness; nausea with occasional emesis; and miosis. The incidence of snorting and inhaling heroin ("smoking") is increasing, particularly among cocaine users. This coincides with a decrease in the availability of methaqualone (no longer on the market) and other sedatives used to temper the cocaine "high." Overdosage causes respiratory depression, peripheral vasodilatation, pinpoint pupils, pulmonary edema, coma, and death.

Dependency is a major concern when continued use of narcotics occurs, though withdrawal causes only moderate morbidity (about the severity of a bout with the "flu"). Addicts sometimes consider themselves more addicted than they really are and may not require a withdrawal program. Grades of withdrawal are categorized from 0–4: grade 0 includes craving and anxiety; grade 1, yawning, lacrimation, rhinorrhea, and perspiration; grade 2, previous symptoms plus mydriasis, piloerection, anorexia, tremors, and hot and cold flashes with generalized aching; grades 3 and 4, increased intensity of previous symptoms and signs, with increased temperature, blood pressure, pulse, and respiratory rate and depth. In withdrawal from the most severe addiction, vomiting, diarrhea, weight loss, hemoconcentration, and spontaneous ejaculation or orgasm commonly occur.

Treatment for overdosage (or suspected overdosage) is naloxone (Narcan), 2 mg intravenously. If an overdose has been taken, the results are dramatic and occur within 2 minutes. Since the length of action of naloxone is much shorter than that of the narcotics, the patient must be under close observation. Hospitalization, supportive care, repeated naloxone administration, and observation for withdrawal from other drugs should be maintained for as long as necessary. Complications of heroin administration include infections (eg, pneumonia, septic emboli, hepatitis), traumatic insults (eg, arterial spasm due to drug injection, gangrene), and pulmonary edema.

Treatment for withdrawal begins if grade 2 signs develop. If a withdrawal program is necessary, use methadone, 10 mg orally (use parenteral administration if the patient is vomiting), and observe. If signs (piloerection, mydriasis, cardiovascular changes) persist for more than 4–6 hours, give another 10 mg; continue to administer methadone at 4- to 6-hour intervals until signs are not present (rarely more than 40 mg of methadone in 24 hours). Divide the total amount of drug required over the first 24-hour period by 2 and give this dose every 12 hours. Each day, reduce the total 24-hour dose by 5–10 mg. Thus, a moderately addicted patient initially requiring 30–40 mg of methadone could be withdrawn over a 4- to 8-day period. Clonidine, 0.1 mg in several divided doses over a 10- to 14-day period, is an alternative adjunct to methadone detoxification; it is not necessary to taper the dose. Clonidine is helpful in alleviating cardiovascular symptoms but does not significantly relieve anxiety, insomnia, or generalized aching. There is a protracted abstinence syndrome of metabolic, respiratory, and blood pressure changes over a period of 3–6 months.

Methadone maintenance programs are of some value in chronic recidivism. Under carefully controlled supervision, the narcotic addict is maintained on fairly high doses of methadone (40–120 mg/d) that satisfy craving and block the effects of heroin to a great degree. Methadyl acetate is longer lasting and is replacing methadone in some programs. Abrupt withdrawal from methadyl acetate does not result in more severe withdrawal problems than gradual withdrawal.

Narcotic antagonists (eg, naltrexone) can also be used successfully for treatment of the patient who has been free of opioids for 7–10 days. Naltrexone blocks the narcotic "high" of heroin when 50 mg is given orally every 24 hours initially for several days and then 100 mg is given every 48–72 hours. Liver disorders are a major contraindication. Compliance tends to be poor, partly because of the dysphoria that can persist long after opioid discontinuance.

Sedatives (Anxiolytics)

See Sedative-Hypnotic and Other Antianxiety Drugs.

Psychedelics

About 6000 species of plants have psychoactive properties. All of the common psychedelics (LSD, mescaline, psilocybin, dimethyltryptamine, and other derivatives of phenylalanine and tryptophan) can produce similar behavioral and physiologic effects. An initial feeling of tension is followed by emotional release such as crying or laughing (1–2 hours). Later, perceptual distortions occur, with visual illusions and hallucinations, and occasionally there is fear of ego disintegration (2–3 hours). Major changes in time sense and mood lability then occur (3–4 hours). A feeling of detachment and a sense of destiny and control occur (4–6 hours). Of course, reactions vary among individuals, and some of the drugs produce markedly different time frames. Occasionally, the acute episode is terrifying (a "bad trip") which may include panic, depression, confusion, or psychotic symptoms. Preexisting emotional problems, the attitude of the user, and the setting where the drug is used affect the experience.

Treatment of the acute episode primarily involves protection of the individual from erratic behavior that may lead to injury or death. A structured environment is usually sufficient until the drug is metabolized. In severe cases, antipsychotic drugs with minimal side effects (eg, haloperidol, 5 mg intramuscularly) may be given every several hours until the individual has regained control. In cases where "flashbacks" occur (mental imagery from a "bad trip" that is later triggered by mild stimuli such as marihuana, alcohol, or psychic trauma), a short course of an antipsychotic drug (eg, trifluoperazine, 5 mg orally) for several days is usually sufficient. An occasional patient may have "flashbacks" for much longer periods and require small doses of neuroleptic drugs over the longer term.

Phencyclidine

Phencyclidine (PCP, angel dust, peace pill, hog), developed as an anesthetic agent, first appeared as a street drug deceptively sold as tetrahydrocannabinol (THC). Because it is simple to produce and mimics to some degree the traditional psychedelic drugs, it has become a common deceptive substitute for LSD, THC, and mescaline. It is available in crystals, capsules, and tablets to be inhaled, injected, swallowed, or smoked (it is commonly sprinkled on marihuana).

Absorption after smoking is rapid, with onset of symptoms in several minutes and peak symptoms in 15–30 minutes. Mild intoxication produces a euphoria accompanied by a feeling of numbness. Moderate intoxication (5–10 mg) results in disorientation, detachment from surroundings, distortion of body image, combativeness, unusual feats of strength (partly due to its anesthetic activity), and loss of ability to integrate sensory input, especially touch and proprioception. Physical symptoms include dizziness, ataxia, dysarthria, nystagmus, retracted upper eyelid with blank stare, hyperreflexia, and tachycardia. There are increases in blood pressure, respiration, muscle tone, and urine production. Usage in the first trimester of pregnancy is associated with an increase in spontaneous abortion and congenital defects. Severe intoxication (20 mg or more) produces an increase in degree of moderate symptoms, with the addition of seizures, deepening coma, hypertensive crisis, and severe psychotic ideation. The drug is particularly long lasting (several days to several weeks)

owing to high lipid solubility, gastroenteric recycling, and the production of active metabolites. Overdosage may be directly fatal, with the major causes of death being hypertensive crisis, respiratory arrest, and convulsions. Acute rhabdomyolysis has been reported and can result in myoglobinuric renal failure.

Differential diagnosis involves the whole spectrum of street drugs, since in some ways phencyclidine mimics sedatives, psychedelics, and marihuana in its effects. Blood and urine testing can detect the acute problem.

Treatment is discussed in Chapter 39.

Marihuana

Cannabis sativa, a hemp plant, is the source of marihuana. The parts of the plant vary in potency. The resinous exudate of the flowering tops of the female plant (hashish, charas) is the most potent, followed by the dried leaves and flowering shoots of the female plant (bhang) and the resinous mass from small leaves of inflorescence (ganja). The least potent parts are the lower branches and the leaves of the female plant and all parts of the male plant. Mercury may be a contaminant in marihuana grown in volcanic soil. The drug is usually inhaled by smoking. Effects occur in 10–20 minutes and last 2–3 hours. "Joints" of good quality contain about 500 mg of marihuana (which contains approximately 5–15 mg of tetrahydrocannabinol with a half-life of 7 days). Marihuana soaked in formaldehyde and dried ("AMP") has produced unusual effects, including autonomic discharge and severe, transient cognitive impairment.

With moderate dosage, marihuana produces two phases: mild euphoria followed by sleepiness. In the acute state, the user has an altered time perception, less inhibited emotions, psychomotor problems, impaired immediate memory, and conjunctival injection. High doses produce transient psychotomimetic effects. No specific treatment is necessary except in the case of the occasional "bad trip," in which case the person is treated in the same way as for psychedelic usage. Marihuana frequently aggravates existing mental illness, adversely affects motor performance, and slows the learning process in children.

Studies of long-term effects have conclusively shown abnormalities in the pulmonary tree. Laryngitis and rhinitis are related to prolonged use, along with chronic obstructive pulmonary disease. Electrocardiographic abnormalities are common, but no long-term cardiac disease has been linked to marihuana use. Chronic usage has resulted in depression of plasma testosterone levels and reduced sperm counts. Abnormal menstruation and failure to ovulate have occurred in some female users. Cognitive impairments are probable, though studies are not conclusive. Sudden withdrawal produces insomnia, nausea, myalgia, and irritability. Psychologic effects of chronic marihuana usage are still unclear. Urine testing is reliable if samples are carefully collected and tested. Detection periods span 4–6 days in acute users and 20–50 days in chronic users.

Stimulants

Stimulant abuse is quite common, either alone or in combination with abuse of other drugs. The **amphetamines,** including methedrine ("speed")—the latest variant is a "smokable" form called "ice," which gives an intense and fairly long-lasting high—methylphenidate, and phenmetrazine, are under prescription control, but street availability remains high. Moderate usage of any of the stimulants produces hyperactivity, a sense of enhanced physical and mental capacity, and sympathomimetic effects. The clinical picture of acute stimulant intoxication includes sweating, tachycardia, elevated blood pressure, mydriasis, hyperactivity, and an acute brain syndrome with confusion and disorientation. Tolerance develops quickly and, as the dosage is increased, hypervigilance, paranoid ideation (with delusions of parasitosis), stereotypy, bruxism, and full-blown psychoses occur, often with aggressive responses. Stimulant withdrawal is characterized by depression with symptoms of hyperphagia and hypersomnia.

People who have used stimulants chronically (eg, anorexigenics) occasionally become sensitized (**"kindling"**) to future use of stimulants. In these individuals, even small amounts of mild stimulants such as caffeine can cause symptoms of paranoia and auditory hallucinations.

Cocaine is a stimulant, not a narcotic. It is a product of the coca plant. The derivatives include seeds, leaves, coca paste, cocaine hydrochloride, and the free base of cocaine. Coca paste is a crude extract that contains 40–80% cocaine sulfate and other impurities. Cocaine hydrochloride is the salt and the most commonly used form. Free base, a purer (and stronger) derivative called "crack" is prepared by simple extraction from cocaine hydrochloride.

There are various modes of use. Coca leaf chewing involves toasting the leaves and chewing with alkaline material (eg, the ash of other burned leaves) to enhance buccal absorption. One achieves a mild high, with onset in 5–10 minutes and lasting for about an hour. Intranasal use is simply snorting cocaine through a straw. Absorption is slowed somewhat by vasoconstriction (which may eventually cause tissue necrosis and septal perforation); the onset of action is in 2–3 minutes, with a moderate high (euphoria, excitement, increased energy) lasting about 30 minutes. The purity of the cocaine is a major determinant of the high. Intravenous use of cocaine hydrochloride or free-base cocaine is effective in 30 seconds and produces a short-lasting, fairly intense high of about 15 minutes' duration. The combined use of cocaine and ethanol results in the metabolic production of cocaethylene by the liver. This substance produces more intense and long-lasting cocaine-like effects. Smoking free-base cocaine (volatilized cocaine because of the lower boiling point) acts in seconds and results in an intense high lasting several minutes. The intensity of the reaction is related to the marked lipid solubility of the free-base form and produces by far the most severe medical and psychiatric symptoms.

Cardiovascular collapse, arrhythmias, myocardial infarction, and transient ischemic attacks have been reported. Seizures, strokes, migraine symptoms, hyperthermia, and lung damage may occur, and there are several obstetric complications, including spontaneous abortion, abruptio placentae, teratogenic effects, delayed fetal growth, and prematurity. Cocaine can cause anxiety, mood swings and delirium, and chronic use can cause the same problems as other stimulants (see above).

Physicians should be alert to cocaine use in patients presenting with unexplained nasal bleeding, headaches, fatigue, insomnia, anxiety, depression, and chronic hoarseness. Sudden withdrawal of the drug is not life-threatening but usually produces craving, sleep disturbances, hyperphagia, lassitude, and severe depression (sometimes with suicidal ideation) lasting days to weeks.

Treatment is imprecise and difficult. Since the high is related to blockage of dopamine reuptake, the dopamine agonist bromocriptine, 1.5 mg orally three times a day, alleviates some of the symptoms of craving associated with acute cocaine withdrawal. Other dopamine agonists such as apomorphine, levodopa, and amantadine are under study for this purpose. There is preliminary evidence that carbamazepine in the usual doses reduces craving in withdrawal (probably owing to its effect on kindling), and desipramine in moderate doses has been useful in helping maintain abstinence in the early stages of treatment. Treatment of psychosis is the same as that of any psychosis: antipsychotic drugs in dosages sufficient to alleviate the symptoms. Any medical symptoms (eg, hyperthermia, seizures, hypertension) are treated specifically. These approaches should be used in conjunction with a structured program, most often based on the AA model. Hospitalization may be required if the self-harm or violence toward others is a perceived threat (usually indicated by paranoid delusions).

Caffeine

Caffeine, along with nicotine and alcohol, is one of the most commonly used drugs worldwide. About 10 billion pounds of coffee (the richest source of caffeine) are consumed yearly throughout the world. Tea, cocoa, and cola drinks also contribute to an intake of caffeine that is often astoundingly high in a large number of people. Low and moderate doses (30–200 mg/d) tend to improve some aspects of performance (eg, vigilance). The approximate content of caffeine in a (180 mL) cup of beverage is as follows: brewed coffee, 80–140 mg; instant coffee, 60–100 mg; decaffeinated coffee, 1–6 mg; black leaf tea, 30–80 mg; tea bags, 25–75 mg; instant tea, 30–60 mg;

cocoa, 10–50 mg; and 12-oz cola drinks, 30–65 mg. A 2-oz chocolate candy bar has about 20 mg. Some herbal teas (eg, "morning thunder") contain caffeine. Caffeine-containing analgesics usually contain approximately 30 mg per unit. Symptoms of caffeinism (usually associated with ingestion of over 500 mg/d) include anxiety, agitation, restlessness, insomnia, a feeling of being "wired," and somatic symptoms referable to the heart and gastrointestinal tract. *It is common for a case of caffeinism to present as an anxiety disorder.* It is also common for caffeine and other stimulants to precipitate severe symptoms in compensated schizophrenic and manic-depressive patients. Chronically depressed patients often use caffeine drinks as self-medication. This diagnostic clue may help distinguish some major affective disorders. Withdrawal from caffeine (> 250 mg/d) can produce headaches, irritability, lethargy, and occasional nausea.

Nicotine

Nicotine is generally taken via snuff, chewing, or smoking tobacco products. While the percentage of people in the USA who smoke tobacco has decreased to about one-third of the population, the use of snuff or chewing tobacco has increased, and tobacco smoking in the rest of the world remains highly prevalent. Nicotine enhances alertness, with later muscular relaxation. It is highly addicting, with abstinence symptoms that include irritability, anxiety, craving, sleep problems, headache, tremor, and lethargy. Withdrawal symptoms may continue for 4–6 weeks, and craving may continue for many months.

Treatment involves some medical approaches such as substitution therapy with nicotine-containing chewing gum (nicotine polacrilex; Nicorette), one piece for each cigarette habitually smoked in a 24-hour period, gradually reduced. Nicotine skin patches are also available for gradually reducing the physiologic dependency (see Chapter 1). Patches produce 6-month abstinence rates of 22–44% versus placebo patch rates of 5–28%. Clonidine, 0.1–0.4 mg/d orally, reduces symptoms such as tremor and tachycardia. Many treatment programs combine the above medications with a behavioral approach.

Miscellaneous Drugs & Solvents

The principal over-the-counter drugs (OTC) of concern are phenylpropanolamine (PPA) and an assortment of antihistaminic agents. Frequently, these drugs are sold in combination with a mild analgesic as cold remedies (eg, Dristan, Triaminic). Most appetite suppressant drugs are combinations of phenylpropanolamine and caffeine (fenfluramine is an exception); these drugs are also heavily marketed as "stay-awake" drugs. Practically all of the so-called sleep aids are now antihistamines. Scopolamine and bromides have generally been removed from the over-the-counter market.

The major problem in the use of all these drugs relates to phenylpropanolamine, which has all the side effects of any stimulant, including precipitation of anxiety states, increased pressor effect, auditory and visual hallucinations, paranoid ideation, and, occasionally, delirium. Aggressiveness and some loss of impulse control have been reported. Sleep disturbances are common even with reasonably small doses.

Antihistamines usually produce some central nervous system depression—thus their use as over-the-counter sedatives. Drowsiness may be a problem. The mixture of antihistamines with alcohol usually exacerbates the central nervous system effects.

The abuse of laxatives sometimes can lead to electrolyte disturbances that may contribute to the manifestations of an organic brain syndrome. The greatest use of laxatives tends to be in the elderly, who are most vulnerable to physiologic changes.

Anabolic steroids are being abused by people who wish to increase muscle mass for cosmetic reasons or for greater strength. In addition to the medical problems, the practice is associated with significant mood swings, aggressiveness, and paranoid delusions. Alcohol and stimulant use is higher in these individuals. Withdrawal symptoms of steroid dependency include fatigue, depressed mood, restlessness, and insomnia.

Amyl nitrite, a drug useful in angina pectoris, has been used in recent years as an "orgasm expander." The changes in time perception, "rush," and mild euphoria caused by the drug prompted its nonmedical use, and popular lore concerning the effects of inhalation just prior to orgasm has led to increased use. Subjective effects last from 5 seconds to 15 minutes. Tolerance develops readily, but there are no known withdrawal symptoms. Abstinence for several days reestablishes the previous level of responsiveness. Long-term effects may include damage to the immune system and respiratory difficulties.

Sniffing of solvents and inhaling of gases (including aerosols) produce a form of inebriation similar to that of the volatile anesthetics. Agents include gasoline, toluene, petroleum ether, lighter fluids, cleaning fluids, paint thinners, solvents are present in many household products (eg, nail polish, typewriter correction fluid). Typical intoxication states include euphoria, slurred speech, hallucinations, and confusion, and with high doses, acute manifestations are unconsciousness and cardiorespiratory depression or failure; chronic exposure produces a variety of symptoms related to the liver, kidney, or bone marrow. Lead encephalopathy can be associated with sniffing leaded gasoline. In addition, studies of workers chronically exposed to jet fuel showed significant increases in neurasthenic symptoms, including fatigue, anxiety, mood changes, memory difficulties, and somatic complaints. These same problems have been noted in long-term solvent abuse.

The so-called designer drugs are synthetic substitutes for commonly used recreational drugs and are produced in small, clandestine laboratories. The most common designer drugs have been methyl analogues of fentanyl and have been used as heroin substitutes. MDMA, an amphetamine derivative sometimes called "ecstasy," is also a designer drug with high abuse potential and neurotoxicity. Manufacture and use of these substances are a vexing problem for law enforcement, since the newest drugs have not yet reached an illegal status and there are no tests developed for detection. Furthermore, they present problems for physicians faced with symptoms from a totally unknown cause.

D'Aunno T, Vaughn TE: Variations in methadone treatment practices: Results from a national study. JAMA 1992;267:253.

Fiore MC et al: Tobacco dependence and the nicotine patch: Clinical guidelines for effective use. JAMA 1992; 268:2687.

Mirin SM et al: Psychopathology in drug abusers and their families. Compr Psychiatry 1991;32:36.

Rounsaville BJ et al: Psychiatric diagnoses of treatment-seeking cocaine abusers. Arch Gen Psychiatry 1991; 48:43.

Silverman K et al: Withdrawal syndrome after the double-blind cessation of caffeine consumption. N Engl J Med 1992;327:1109. (Lower than previously thought.)

ORGANIC MENTAL SYNDROMES (Organic Brain Syndrome [OBS])

Essentials of Diagnosis

- Transient or permanent brain dysfunction.
- Cognitive impairment to varying degrees: may include impaired recall and recent memory, inability to focus attention, random psychomotor activity such as stereotypy, and problems in perceptual processing, often with psychotic ideation.
- Emotional disorders frequently present: depression, anxiety, irritability.
- Behavioral disturbances may include problems of impulse control, sexual acting out, attention, aggression, exhibitionism.

General Considerations

The organic problem may be a primary brain disease or a secondary manifestation of some general disorder. All of the brain syndromes show some degree of cognitive impairment depending on the site of involvement, the rate of onset and progression, and the duration of the underlying brain lesion. Emo-

tional disturbances (eg, depression) are often inversely proportionate to the severity of the cognitive disorder. The behavioral disturbances tend to be more common with chronicity, more directly related to the underlying personality or central nervous system vulnerability to drug side effects, and not necessarily correlated with cognitive dysfunction.

Etiology

A. Intoxication: Alcohol, sedatives, bromides, anticholinergic drugs, antidepressants, analgesics (eg, pentazocine), psychedelic drugs, stimulants, salicylates (chronic use), a wide variety of over-the-counter and prescribed drugs, and household solvents.

B. Drug Withdrawal: Withdrawal from alcohol, sedative-hypnotics, corticosteroids.

C. Long-Term Effects of Alcohol: Wernicke-Korsakoff syndrome.

D. Infections: Septicemia; meningitis and encephalitis due to bacterial, viral, fungal, parasitic or tuberculous organisms or to central nervous system syphilis; acute and chronic infections due to the entire range of microbiologic pathogens.

E. Endocrine Disorders: Thyrotoxicosis, hypothyroidism, adrenocortical dysfunction (including Addison's disease and Cushing's syndrome), pheochromocytoma, insulinoma, hypoglycemia, hyperparathyroidism, hypoparathyroidism, panhypopituitarism, diabetic ketoacidosis.

F. Respiratory Disorders: Hypoxia, hypercapnia.

G. Metabolic Disturbances: Fluid and electrolyte disturbances (especially hyponatremia, hypomagnesemia, and hypercalcemia), acid-base disorders, hepatic disease (hepatic encephalopathy), renal failure, porphyria.

H. Nutritional Deficiencies: Deficiency of vitamin B_1 (beriberi), vitamin B_{12} (pernicious anemia), folic acid, nicotinic acid (pellagra); protein-calorie malnutrition.

I. Trauma: Subdural hematoma, subarachnoid hemorrhage, intracerebral bleeding, concussion syndrome.

J. Cardiovascular Disorders: Cardiac infarctions, arrhythmias, cerebrovascular spasms, hypertensive encephalopathy, hemorrhages, embolisms, and occlusions indirectly cause decreased cognitive function.

K. Neoplasms: Primary or metastatic lesions of the central nervous system, cancer-induced hypercalcemia.

L. Seizure Disorders: Ictal and interictal dysfunction.

M. Collagen and Immunologic Disorders: Autoimmune disorders, including systemic lupus erythematosus, Sjögren's syndrome, and AIDS.

N. Degenerative Diseases: Alzheimer's disease, Pick's disease, multiple sclerosis, parkinsonism, Huntington's chorea, normal pressure hydrocephalus.

Clinical Findings

The manifestations are many and varied and include problems with orientation, short or fluctuating attention span, loss of recent memory and recall, impaired judgment, emotional lability, lack of initiative, impaired impulse control, inability to reason through problems, depression (worse in mild to moderate types), confabulation (not limited to alcohol organic brain syndrome), constriction of intellectual functions, visual and auditory hallucinations, and delusions. Physical findings will naturally vary according to the cause. The EEG is often abnormal.

A. Delirium: Delirium (acute confusional state) is a transient global disorder of attention, with clouding of consciousness, usually a result of systemic problems (eg, drugs, hypoxemia). Onset is usually rapid. The mental status fluctuates (impairment is usually least in the morning), with varying inability to concentrate, maintain attention, and sustain purposeful behavior. ("Sundowning"—mild to moderate delirium at night—is more common in patients with preexisting dementia and may be precipitated by drugs and sensory deprivation.) There is a marked deficit of short-term memory and recall. Anxiety and irritability are common. Amnesia is retrograde (impaired recall of past memories) and anterograde (inability to recall events after the onset of the delirium). Orientation problems follow the inability to retain information. Perceptual disturbances (often visual hallucinations) and psychomotor restlessness with insomnia are common. Autonomic changes include tachycardia, dilated pupils, and sweating. The average duration is about 1 week, with full recovery in most cases. Delirium can coexist with dementia.

B. Dementia: (See also Chapter 4.) Dementia is characterized by chronicity and deterioration of selective mental functions. Onset is insidious in most cases. Dementia is usually progressive, more common in the elderly, and rarely reversible even if underlying disease can be corrected. Dementia can be classified as cortical or subcortical.

There are three types of cortical dementia: (1) primary degenerative dementia, accounting for about 50–60% of cases; (2) atherosclerotic (multi-infarct) dementia, 15–20% of cases (this figure is probably low because of the tendency to overuse the diagnosis of Alzheimer's dementia); and (3) mixtures of the first two types or dementia due to miscellaneous causes, 15–20% of cases (see also Chapter 4). Examples of primary degenerative dementia are Alzheimer's dementia (most common) and Pick, Parkinson, Creutzfeldt-Jakob, and Huntington dementias (less common).

Dementia of the Alzheimer type (DAT) has in many cases a genetic link and is characterized by initial short-term memory loss (both anterograde and retrograde), gradual loss of expressive and comprehensive language (aphasia of a word finding type occurs early), constructional apraxia, visuoperceptual defects, a decreased sense of smell, problem-solving difficulties, and personality changes, including thought disorder (usually paranoid) and increased irritability. There is enormous diversity in symptoms and momentum of the disease. Sudden onset, seizures, gait disturbance, or focal neurologic signs tend to rule out the diagnosis.

Subcortical forms include degeneration of subcortical structures (eg, parkinsonism, Huntington's disease) and are less likely to be associated with aphasia, agnosia, or loss of higher associative functions but more likely to produce movement disorders and major problems in retrieval of information (very poor on recall but much better at recognition of items), major attention deficits, early arithmetic difficulties, speech disorders, some constructional apraxia, and personality changes in which depression—which imposes an increased suicidal risk— is a major feature (this adversely affects neuropsychologic testing). Localization of the lesion plays a significant role in producing depression.

In all types, loss of impulse control (sexual and language) is common. The tenuous level of functioning makes the individual most susceptible to minor physical and psychologic stresses. The course depends on the underlying cause, and the general trend is steady deterioration.

HIV infection can produce primary neurogenic disorder (partially due to neuronal loss) and secondary effects due to opportunistic infections, neoplasias, or the effects of drug therapy. At present there has been a reduction in dementia symptoms in both early and late stages, perhaps due to earlier use of AZT. The general trend is variable, and patients require ongoing monitoring of neuropsychiatric status.

Pseudodementia is a term applied to depressed patients who appear to be demented. It is occasionally used to include other reversible conditions that mimic dementia (eg, mass lesions, effects of medication). Neurologic findings are absent.

C. Amnestic Syndrome: This is a memory disturbance without delirium or dementia. It is usually associated with thiamine deficiency and chronic alcohol use (eg, Korsakoff's syndrome). It impairs selective areas of cognitive functioning. The onset is usually sudden, but the course is usually chronic.

D. Organic Hallucinosis: This condition is characterized by persistent or recurrent hallucinations (usually auditory) without the other symptoms usually found in delirium or dementia. Alcohol or hallucinogens are often the cause. There does not have to be any other mental disorder, and there may be complete spontaneous resolution.

E. Organic Personality Syndrome: This syndrome is characterized by emotional lability and loss of impulse control along with a general change in personality. Cognitive functions are preserved. Social inappropriateness is common. Loss of interest and lack of concern with the consequences of one's actions are often present. The course depends on the underlying cause (eg, frontal lobe contusion may resolve completely).

Differential Diagnosis

The differential diagnosis consists mainly of schizophrenia and the other psychoses, which are sometimes confused with organic brain syndrome, which itself often has psychotic symptoms.

Complications

Chronicity may result from delayed correction of the defect, eg, subdural hematoma, low-pressure hydrocephalus. Accidents secondary to impulsive behavior and poor judgment are a major consideration. Secondary depression and impulsive behavior not infrequently lead to suicide attempts. Drugs, particularly sedatives, may worsen thinking abilities and contribute to the overall problems.

Treatment
(See also Chapter 4.)

A. Medical: Provide a pleasant, comfortable, nonthreatening, and physically safe environment with adequate nursing or attendant services. *Establish the diagnosis and correct underlying medical problems* (electrolyte abnormalities, abnormal thyroid function, etc). Discontinue drugs that may be contributing to the problem (eg, alcohol, cimetidine, lidocaine, *anticholinergic drugs,* analgesics, central nervous system depressants). Do not overlook any possibility of reversible organic disease. CT, MRI, PET, and SPECT evaluations are helpful in diagnosis. Give antipsychotics in small doses at first (eg, haloperidol, 2 mg orally at bedtime) and increase according to the need to reduce psychotic ideation or excessive irritability. Aggressiveness and rage states in central nervous system lesions can be reduced with lipophilic beta-blockers (eg, propranolol, metoprolol) in moderate doses. Since the serotonergic system has been implicated in arousal conditions, drugs that affect serotonin have been studied and found to be of some benefit in aggression and agitation. Included in this group are lithium, trazodone, buspirone, and clonazepam. Dopamine blockers (eg, the neuroleptic drugs such as haloperidol) have been used for many years to attenuate aggression. There are recent reports of reduced agitation in Alzheimer's disease from carbamazepine, 100–400 mg/d orally (with slow increase as needed). Emotional lability in some cases responds to small doses of imipramine, 25 mg three times daily, or fluoxetine, 20 mg/d orally; and depression, which often occurs early in the course of Alzheimer type dementia, responds to the usual doses of antidepressant drugs, preferably those with the least anticholinergic side effects eg, MAO inhibitors and SSRIs).

Cerebral vasodilators were originally used on the assumption that cerebral arteriosclerosis and ischemia were the principal causes of the dementias. Although there is a slight reduction of blood flow in primary degenerative dementia (probably as a result of the basic disorder), there is no evidence that this is a major factor in this group of disorders or that vasodilators are of value. Ergotoxine alkaloids (ergoline mesylates; Hydergine, others) have been studied, with mixed results; improvement in ambulatory self-care and depressed mood has been noted, but there has been no improvement of cognitive functioning on any standardized tests. Hyperbaric oxygen treatment has not produced significant improvement. Stimulant drugs (eg, methylphenidate) do not change cognitive function but can improve affect and mood, which helps the caretakers cope with the problem. Since there is a cholinergic deficiency in Alzheimer's disease, recent research has focussed on drugs to increase cholinergic activity (eg, tacrine, phosphatidyl choline). Tacrine (tetrahydroaminoacridine, THA) has produced some positive results, but there is disagreement among researchers regarding its efficacy.

Failing sensory functions should be supported as necessary, with hearing aids, cataract surgery, etc.

B. Social: Substitute home care, board care, or convalescent home care may be most useful when the family is unable to care for the patient. The setting should include familiar people and objects, lights at night, and a simple schedule. Family counseling may help the family to cope with problems that may occur and may help keep the patient at home as long as possible. Information about local Information about local groups can be obtained from the Alzheimer's Disease and Related Disorders Association, 70 East Lake Street, Suite 600, Chicago, IL 60601. Volunteer services, including homemakers, visiting nurses, and adult protective services may be helpful in maintaining the patient at home.

C. Behavioral: Behavioral techniques include operant responses that can be used to induce positive behaviors, eg, paying attention to the patient who is trying to communicate appropriately, and extinction by ignoring inappropriate responses. Alzheimer's patients can learn skills and retain them but do not recall the circumstances in which they were learned.

D. Psychologic: Formal psychologic therapies are not usually helpful and may make things worse by taxing the patient's limited cognitive resources.

Prognosis

The prognosis is good in acute (reversible) cases, fair in moderate cases, and poor in deteriorated states.

Engel PA, Gelber J: Does computed tomographic brain imaging have a place in the diagnosis of dementia? Arch Intern Med 1992;152:1437. (Yes.)

Levkoff SE et al: Delirium: The occurrence and persistence of symptoms among elderly hospitalized patients. Arch Intern Med 1992;152:334. (It is common and prolongs the hospital stay.)

Skoog I et al: A population-based study of dementia in 85-year-olds. N Engl J Med 1993;328:153. (A surprising percentage of vascular dementias with treatment implications.)

Small GW: Tacrine for treating Alzheimer's disease. JAMA 1992;268:2564.

GERIATRIC PSYCHIATRIC DISORDERS
(See also Chapter 4.)

There are three basic factors in the process of aging: biologic, sociologic, and psychologic.

The complex **biologic** changes depend on inherited characteristics (the best guarantee of long life is to have long-lived parents), nutrition, declining sensory functions such as hearing or vision, disease, trauma, and life-style. A definite correlation between hearing loss and paranoid ideation exists in the elderly. (See Organic Brain Syndrome, above.) As a person ages, relatively minor disorders or combinations of disorders may cause deficits in cognition and affective response. Hypochondriasis is frequently a mechanism of compensating for decreased function (eg, preoccupation with bowel function).

The **sociologic** factors derive from stresses connected with occupation, family, and community. Any or all of these areas may be disrupted in a general phenomenon of "disengagement" and lack of intimacy that older people experience as friends die, the children move away, and the surroundings become less familiar. Retirement commonly precipitates a major disruption in a well-established life structure. This is particularly stressful in the person whose compulsive devotion to a job has precluded other interests, so that sudden loss of this outlet leaves a void that is not easily filled.

The **psychologic** withdrawal of the elderly person is frequently related to a loss of self-esteem, which is based on the economic insecurity of older age with its congruent loss of independence, the realization of decreasing physical and mental ability, loneliness, and the fear of approaching death. The process of aging is often poorly accepted, and the real or imagined loss of physical attractiveness may have a traumatic impact that the plastic surgeon can only soften for a time. In a culture that stresses physical and sexual attractiveness, it is difficult for most people to accept the change.

Clinical Findings & Complications

The most common psychiatric syndrome in the elderly is organic brain syndrome of varying degree. Psychotic ideation (usually paranoid) may coexist with the organic brain syndrome. Frequently, in milder cases, the individual is aware of the deficiency in sensorium and becomes *depressed* about actual or threatened loss of function. Unless the examination is done with great care, organic brain syndrome is missed, and the patient is treated for the secondary symptom of depression without evaluation of the organic problem.

Overt depression, often presenting as a somatic complaint, is often related to life exigencies (80% of people over age 65 have some kind of medical problem). Alcoholism is present in approximately 15% of older patients presenting with psychiatric symptoms. The incidence of suicide is higher in elderly people—loneliness, age, and medical problems being directly related. Deprivation of full-spectrum light may be a factor in some patients (eg, nursing home residents). Anxiety, often associated with organic illness, heightens preexisting confusion in the patient with organic brain syndrome.

Abuse of the elderly—both physical neglect (passive) and physical injury (active)—demands early recognition. Bruises, welts, fractures, and debilitation should alert the physician. The battered elderly are probably just as numerous as battered children, but less reported, and require the same diligence in physician recognition.

Polypharmacy (with both prescription and over-the-counter drugs) is a major cause of accidents (often with resultant hip fracture) and illness in the elderly. Cognitive impairment increases as the number of drugs used increases; sedatives and anticholinergic drugs are the major culprits (eg, overuse in sleep problems). The increased and varied complaints are often an attempt to compensate and divert attention from decreased mental function.

Treatment

A. Social: Socialization, a structured schedule of activities, familiar surroundings, continued achievement, and avoidance of loneliness (probably the most important factor) are some of the major considerations in prevention and amelioration of the psychiatric problems of older age. The patient can be supported in the primary environment by various agencies that can help avoid a premature change of habits. For patients with disabilities that make it difficult to cope with the problems of living alone, homemaker services can assist in continuing the day-to-day activities of the household; visiting nurses can administer medications and monitor the physical condition of the patient; and geriatric social groups can help maintain socialization and human contacts. In the hospital or nursing home, attention to the kinds of people placed in the same room is most important (mix active and inactive patients).

B. Medical: Treatment of any reversible components of an organic brain syndrome is obviously the major medical consideration. One commonly overlooked factor is self-medication, frequently with over-the-counter drugs that further impair the patient's already precarious functioning. Common culprits are antihistamines and anticholinergic drugs, sometimes mixed with ethanol abuse.

Any signs of psychosis, such as paranoid ideation, agitation, and delusions, respond very well to *small amounts* of antipsychotics. Trifluoperazine, 2–5 mg orally once a day, or fluphenazine, 1–2 mg orally daily, will usually decrease psychotic ideation markedly.

Do not use drugs that cause significant orthostatic hypotension (resulting in dizziness, falls, fractures).

Antidepressants (in one-half to one-third the doses given to young adults) are used when indicated for depression. Occasionally, a stimulant in small doses (eg, methylphenidate, 5–10 mg orally daily) can be used to treat apathy. The stimulant may help increase the patient's energy for social involvement and help the patient to maintain life activities.

The appropriate use of wine and beer for mild sedative effects is quite rewarding in the hospital and other care facilities as well as at home.

C. Behavioral: The impaired cognitive abilities of the geriatric patient necessitate simple behavioral techniques. Positive responses to appropriate behavior encourage the patient to repeat desirable kinds of behavior, and frequent repetition offsets to some degree the defects in recent memory and recall. It also results in participation—a most important element, since there is a tendency in the older population to withdraw, thus increasing isolation and functional decline.

One must be careful not to reinforce and encourage obstreperous behavior by responding to it; in this way, extinction or at least gradual reduction of inappropriate behavior will occur. At the same time, the obstreperous behavior often represents a nondirective response to frustration and inability to function, and a structured program of activity is necessary.

D. Psychologic: Patients may require help in adjusting to changing roles and commitments and in finding new goals and viewpoints. The older person steadily loses an important commodity—the future—and may attempt to compensate for this by preoccupation with the past. Involvement with the present and psychotherapy on a here-and-now basis can help make the adjustment easier.

Becker PM, Jamieson AO: Common sleep disorders in the elderly: Diagnosis and treatment. Geriatrics 1992;47:41. (Probably the most common complaint from elderly patients.)

Ray WA: Psychotropic drugs and injuries among the elderly: A review. J Clin Psychopharmacol 1992;12:386. (Hip fractures are a major worry.)

DEATH & DYING

As Thomas Browne said, "The long habit of living indisposeth us for dying." It is only when death comes close to us that we really begin to respond to the possibility of our own death.

Death means different things to different people. For some it may represent an escape from unbearable suffering or other difficulties; for others, entrance into a new transcendental life. Death may come as a narcissistic attempt to find lasting fame or importance in martyrdom or heroic adventure, or it may be an atonement for real or imagined guilt or a means of extorting from others posthumously the affection that was not forthcoming during life.

How each individual responds to imminent death is a function not only of what death means to that person but also of the mechanisms used to deal with problems—and these are usually the same as those used throughout life. Patients usually worry more about *how* they will die than about death itself. Responses frequently seen in the dying patient include denial, anger, bargaining, depression, and acceptance—stages that are seen in many people as they go through any significant flux or loss. Seldom are these stages seen in isolation, and the complexity of the process contributes to the juxtaposition of the stages and the noted lability of mood and attitude in the dying patient.

An ill person may at first deny any concern with dying and then later admit to a fear of going to sleep because of the possibility of not waking up. This is often demonstrated by a need to keep the light on and to call frequently during the night with minor complaints. Some find it necessary to deny impending death to the end. Their families and doctors will often join in the conspiracy of denial, either out of sympathy or for their own reasons. It is important not to force the patient to realize the truth but to allow the opportunity, *when the patient is ready,* to discuss and deal with the problem of impending death. Frank discussion can mitigate the terror some patients feel. For many it is a comfort to be actively involved in the process of dying, sharing in the anticipation of death, and making whatever plans may be important. Alleviation of pain and unnecessary prolongation of life are primary concerns of many patients. The physician should not be concerned about addiction to narcotics when treating a dying patient.

The reactions of the family are often a combination of pain, anger, sadness, and depression. They react to each other and to the personnel caring for the patient. The problem to be resolved with the survivors is the guilt feelings they may have—that they continue to exist while the other person has died. Also to be reconciled are the vague sense of being responsible for the death and the subconscious refusal to believe that the person is really dead. The staff must be careful to achieve a proper balance between empathic caring and emotional overinvestment.

Conwell Y, Caine ED: Rational suicide and the right to die: Reality and myth. N Engl J Med 1991;325:1100.
Kjellstrand CM: Who should decide about your death? JAMA 1991;267:103. (Editorial on the role of the physician.)

PSYCHIATRIC PROBLEMS ASSOCIATED WITH HOSPITALIZATION & MEDICAL & SURGICAL DISORDERS

Diagnostic Categories
A. Acute Problems:
1. Psychotic organic brain syndrome secondary to the medical or surgical problem, or compounded by effect of treatment.

2. Acute anxiety, often related to ignorance and fear of the immediate problem as well as uncertainty about the future.

3. Anxiety as an intrinsic aspect of the medical problem (eg, hyperthyroidism).

4. Denial of illness, which may present during acute or intermediate phases of illness.

B. Intermediate Problems:
1. Depression as a function of the illness or acceptance of the illness, often associated with realistic or fantasied hopelessness about the future.

2. Behavioral problems, often related to denial of illness and, in extreme cases, causing the patient to leave the hospital against medical advice.

C. Recuperative Problems:
1. Decreasing cooperation as the patient sees improvement and is not compelled to follow orders closely.

2. Readjustment problems with family, job, and society.

General Considerations
A. Acute Problems:
1. **"Intensive care unit psychosis"** is a type of delirium. It is an expression of organic (frequently including a preexisting organic brain syndrome), psychologic, and environmental factors. Some factors include sleep deprivation, sedative and analgesic medications, alcohol withdrawal, metabolic fluctuations (particularly hypoxemia and hyponatremia), fear, and overstimulation. It is important to consider and recognize the problem early when it is more easily treated. (See Organic Mental Disorders, above.)

2. **Pre- and postsurgical anxiety** states are common—and commonly ignored. Presurgical anxiety is ubiquitous and is principally a fear of death (note the high number of surgical patients who make out their wills). Patients may be fearful of anesthesia (improved by the preoperative anesthesia interview), the mysterious operating room, and the disease processes that might be uncovered by the surgeon. Such fears frequently cause people to delay examinations that might result in earlier surgery and a greater incidence of cure.

The opposite of this is **surgery proneness,** the quest for surgery to escape from overwhelming life stresses. Polysurgery patients are not easily categorized. Dynamic motivations include narcissism, societal pressures (eg, breast implants), unconscious guilt, a masochistic need to suffer, an attempt to deal with another family member's illness, and psychogenic pain. More apparent reasons may include an attempt to get relief from pain and a life-style that has become almost exclusively medically oriented, with all of the risks entailed in such an endeavor.

Postsurgical anxiety states are usually related to pain, procedures, and loss of body image. Acute pain problems are quite different from chronic pain disorders (see Chronic Pain Disorders, above); the former are readily handled with *adequate* analgesic medication. The alteration in body image is particularly difficult for mastectomy patients. Any procedure that results in a stoma has the attendant concern about relationships with others.

3. **Iatrogenic problems** usually pertain to medications, complications of diagnostic and treatment procedures, and impersonal and unsympathetic staff behavior. Polypharmacy is often a factor. Patients with unsolved diagnostic problems are at higher risk. They are desirous of relief, and the quest engenders more diagnostic procedures with a higher incidence of complications. The upset patient and family may be very demanding. Excessive demands usually result from anxiety. Such behavior is best handled with calm and measured responses.

B. Intermediate Problems:
1. **Prolonged hospitalization** presents unique problems in certain hospital services, eg, burn units, orthopedic services, and tuberculosis wards. The acute problems of the severely burned patient are discussed in Chapter 38. The problems often are behavioral difficulties related to length of hospitalization and necessary procedures. For example, in burn units, pain is a major problem in addition to anxiety about procedures. Disputes with staff are common and often concern pain medication or ward privileges.

Some patients regress to infantile behavior and dependency. Staff members must agree about their approach to the patient in order to ensure the smooth functioning of the unit.

Denial of illness may present in the patient with acute myocardial infarction. Intervention by an authority figure (eg, immediate work supervisor) may help the patient accept treatment and eventually abandon the defense of denial.

2. Depression frequently intervenes during this period. Therapeutic drugs (eg, corticosteroids) may be a factor. It can contribute to irritability and overt anger. Severe depression can lead to anorexia, which further complicates healing and metabolic balance. It is during this period that the issue of disfigurement arises—relief at survival gives way to concern about future function and appearance.

C. Recuperative Problems:

1. Anxiety about return to the posthospital environment can cause regression to a dependent position. Complications increase, and staff forbearance again is tested. Anxiety at this stage usually is handled more easily than previous behavior problems.

2. Posthospital adjustment is related to the severity of the deficits and the use of outpatient facilities (eg, physical therapy, rehabilitation programs, psychiatric outpatient treatment). Some patients may experience posttraumatic stress symptoms (eg, trauma victims). Lack of appropriate follow-up can contribute to depression in the patient, who may feel that he or she is making poor progress and may have thoughts of "giving up." Reintegration into work, educational, and social endeavors may be slow. Life is simply much more difficult when one is disfigured, disabled, or disfranchised.

Clinical Findings

The symptoms that occur in these patients are similar to those discussed in previous sections of this chapter, eg, organic brain syndrome, stress and adjustment disorders, anxiety, and depression. Behavior problems may include lack of cooperation, increased complaints, demands for medication, sexual approaches to nurses, threats to leave the hospital, and actual signing out against medical recommendations. The underlying personality structure of the individual is a major factor in coping styles (eg, compulsive increases indecision, hysterical increases dramatic behavior).

Differential Diagnosis

Organic brain syndrome (including cases associated with HIV infection and drug abuse) must always be ruled out, since it often presents with symptoms resembling anxiety, depression, or psychosis. Personality disorders existing prior to hospitalization often underlie the various behavior problems, but particularly the management problems.

Complications

Prolongation of hospitalization causes increased expense, deterioration of patient-staff relationships, and increased probabilities of iatrogenic and legal problems. The possibility of increasing posthospital treatment problems is enhanced.

Treatment

A. Medical: The most important consideration by far is to have *one* physician in charge, a physician whom the patient trusts and who is able to oversee multiple treatment approaches (see Somatoform Disorders, above). In the acute problems, attention must be paid to metabolic imbalance, alcohol withdrawal, and previous drug use—prescribed, recreational, or over-the-counter. Adequate sleep and analgesia are important in the prevention of delirium.

Most physicians are attuned to the early detection of the surgery-prone patient. Plastic and orthopedic surgeons are at particular risk. Appropriate consultations may help detect some problems and mitigate future ones.

Postsurgical anxiety states can be alleviated by personal attention from the surgeon. Anxiety is not so effectively lessened by ancillary medical personnel, whom the patient perceives as lesser authorities, until after the physician has reassured the patient. Inappropriate use of "as needed" analgesia places an unfair burden on the nurse. "Patient-controlled analgesia" can improve pain control, decrease anxiety, and minimize side effects (see Chapter 1).

Depression should be recognized early. If severe, it may be treated by antidepressant medications (see Antidepressant Drugs, above). High levels of anxiety can be lowered with *judicious* use of anxiolytic agents. Unnecessary medications tend to reinforce the patient's impression that there must be a serious illness or medication would not be required.

B. Psychologic: Prepare the patient and family for what is to come. This includes the types of units where the patient will be quartered, the procedures that will be performed, and any disfigurements that will result from surgery. Repetition improves understanding. The nursing staff can be helpful, since patients frequently confide a lack of understanding to a nurse but are reluctant to do so to the physician.

Denial of illness is frequently a block to acceptance of treatment. This, too, should be handled with family members present (to help the patient face the reality of the situation) in a series of short interviews (for reinforcement). Dependency problems resulting from long hospitalization are best handled by focusing on the changes to come as the patient makes the transition to the outside world. Key figures are teachers, vocational counselors, and physical therapists. Challenges should be realistic and practical and handled in small steps.

Depression is usually related to the loss of familiar hospital supports, and the outpatient therapists and counselors help to lessen the impact of the loss. Some of the impact can be alleviated by anticipating, with the patient and family, the signal features of the common depression to help prevent the patient from assuming a permanent sick role (invalidism).

Suicide is always a concern when a patient is faced with despair. An honest, compassionate, and supportive approach will help sustain the patient during this trying period.

C. Behavioral: Prior desensitization can significantly allay anxiety about medical procedures. A "dry run" can be done to reinforce the oral description. Cooperation during acute problem periods can be enhanced by the use of appropriate reinforcers such as a favorite nurse or *helpful* family member. People who are positive reinforcers are even more helpful during the intermediate phases when the patient becomes resistant to the seemingly endless procedures (eg, debridement of burned areas).

Specific situations (eg, psychologic dependency on the respirator) can be corrected by weaning with appropriate reinforcers (eg, a loved one allowed in the room only when the patient is disconnected from the respirator). Behavioral approaches should be done in a positive and optimistic way for maximal reinforcement.

Relaxation techniques and attentional distraction can be used to block side effects of a necessary treatment (eg, nausea in cancer chemotherapy).

D. Social: A change in environment requires adaptation. Because of the illness, admission and hospitalization may be more easily handled than discharge. Reintegration into society can be difficult. In some cases, the family is a negative influence. A pre-discharge evaluation must be made to determine whether the family will be able to cope with the physical or mental changes in the patient. Working with the family while the patient is in the acute stage may presage a successful transition later on.

A positive work situation is critical to the restoration of self-esteem. In many cases, the previous form of employment is no longer available. Vocational counseling should be started in the hospital as early as possible and may include the occupational therapists.

Development of a new social life can be facilitated by various self-help organizations (eg, the stoma club). Sharing problems with others in similar circumstances eases the return to a social life which may be quite different from that prior to the illness.

Prognosis

The prognosis is good in all patients who have reversible medical and surgical conditions. It is guarded when there is serious functional loss that impairs vocational, educational, or societal possibilities—especially in the case of progressive and ultimately life-threatening illness.

Federoff J et al: Depression in patients with acute traumatic brain injury. Am J Psychiatry 1992;149:918. (Thirty percent incidence—same as stroke.)
Soderstrom CA et al: Psychoactive substance dependence among trauma center patients. JAMA 1992;267:2756. (Seventy-five percent used alcohol or other drugs.)

REFERENCES

Colt GH: *The Enigma of Suicide.* Summit Books, 1991.
Foy DW: *Treating PTSD: Cognitive-Behavioral Strategies.* Guilford, 1992.
Goldman HH (editor): *Review of General Psychiatry,* 3rd ed. Appleton & Lange, 1992.
Lowinson JH, Ruiz P, Millman RB (editors): *Substance Abuse: A Comprehensive Textbook,* 2nd ed. Williams & Wilkins, 1992.
Shorter E: *From Paralysis to Fatigue: A History of Psychosomatic Illness in the Modern Era.* The Free Press, 1992.
Weiner MF (editor): *The Dementias.* American Psychiatric Press, 1991.
Wolf N: *The Beauty Myth.* Morrow, 1991.

25

Endocrine Disorders

Paul A. Fitzgerald, MD

Hormones exert their effects by interacting with receptors on the cell surface (catecholamines and polypeptide hormones) or inside the cell (thyroid and steroid hormones). Endocrine disorders result from an excess or deficiency of hormonal effects.

Baniahmad A, Tsa MJ: Mechanisms of transcriptional activation by steroid hormone receptors. J Cellular Biochem 1993;51:151.
DeGroot LJ: Mechanism of thyroid hormone action. Adv Exp Med Biol 1991;299:1.

COMMON PRESENTATIONS IN ENDOCRINOLOGY

Short Stature

There is tremendous normal genetic variation in growth, which makes the definition of short stature relatively imprecise. There is also a certain sex bias in that boys are referred for evaluation twice as frequently as girls. The criteria for short stature can be stated as follows: (1) height below the fifth percentile plotted on a growth chart that is appropriate for gender and race, or (2) growth velocity below the fifth percentile plotted on an incremental growth chart that is appropriate for gender and race.

All children with short stature require careful evaluation. The most thorough testing is given to those children whose height or growth velocity falls below the fifth percentile for age or whose clinical evaluation suggests a medical problem.

Various cause of short stature are set forth in Table 25–1.

Lippe BM, Nakamoto JM: Conventional and nonconventional uses of growth hormone. Recent Prog Horm Res 1993;48:179.
Moore WV et al: Long term treatment with growth hormone of children with short stature and normal growth hormone secretion. J Pediatr 1992;120:702.
Underwood LE: Growth hormone therapy for short stature: Yes or No? Hosp Pract [Off] 1992;27(4):192.

Excessive Growth

Excessive growth may be a familial or ethnic characteristic or a physiologic event (eg, the growth spurt of puberty) as well as a sign of endocrine disease. Precocious puberty tends to produce tall children whose ultimate adult height is less than expected because of premature closure of the epiphyses. Pituitary tumors secreting excess growth hormone cause gigantism if present before puberty and acromegaly if growth hormone excess occurs after closure of the epiphysial plates of long bones. A few cases of nonpituitary "cerebral gigantism" have been described. Marfan's syndrome and Klinefelter's syndrome and its variants can also be associated with tall stature. Individuals with XYY genotype are often tall and may exhibit mental retardation and antisocial behavior. Purely hypogonadal individuals tend to be tall, with eunuchoid proportions (span exceeds height; excessive length of floor-to-pubis segment of body).

Underwood LE, Van Wyk JJ: Normal and aberrant growth. In: *Williams' Textbook of Endocrinology,* 8th ed. Wilson JD, Foster DW (editors). Saunders, 1992.

Obesity

Although obesity is a common presenting "endocrine" complaint, the overwhelming majority of cases are due to excessive food intake or physical inactivity, or both. Some obese individuals may have lower rates of thermogenesis. Studies of twins separated soon after birth have emphasized the importance of genetic factors in obesity.

A rapid onset of massive obesity associated with lethargy or polyuria suggests a hypothalamic lesion. Some cases of obesity are associated with delayed puberty. Hypothyroidism is usually *not* associated with marked obesity. In Cushing's syndrome, there is roundness of the face with characteristic supraclavicular fat pads, "buffalo hump," and truncal obesity with thin extremities. Striae are common with any type of obesity. They are wider (> 10 mm) and more violaceous in Cushing's syndrome. Amenorrhea, hypertension, and glucose intolerance are commonly associated with obesity and often improve after adequate weight loss. Insulin-secreting adenomas are often associated with weight gain, but these tumors are quite rare.

Table 25–1. Causes of short stature.[1]

Variations of normal	Syndromes of short stature
Constitutional (delayed bone age)	Turner's syndrome (syndrome of gonadal dysgenesis)
Genetic (short familial heights)	Noonan's syndrome (pseudo-Turner's syndrome)
	Prader-Willi syndrome
Endocrine disorders	Laurence-Moon-Biedl syndrome
GH deficiency	Autosomal abnormalities
Congenital	Dysmorphic syndromes
Isolated GH deficiency	Pseudohypoparathyroidism
With other pituitary hormone deficiencies	
With midline defects	**Chronic disease**
Pituitary agenesis	Cardiac disorders
Acquired	Left-to-right shunt
Hypothalamic/pituitary tumors	Congestive heart failure
Histiocytosis X	Pulmonary disorders
CNS infections and granulomas	Cystic fibrosis
Head trauma (birth and later)	Asthma
Hypothalamic/pituitary radiation	Gastrointestinal disorders
CNS vascular accidents	Malabsorption (eg, celiac disease)
Hydrocephalus	Disorders of swallowing
Psychosocial dwarfism (functional GH deficiency)	Hepatic disorders
Amphetamine treatment for hyperactivity	Hematologic disorders
Biologically inactive GH	Sickle cell anemia
Laron's dwarfism (increased GH and decreased IGF-I)	Thalassemia
Pygmies (normal GH and IGF-II but decreased IGF-1 at	Renal disorders
puberty)	Renal tubular acidosis
Hypothyroidism	Chronic uremia
Glucocorticoid excess	Immunologic disorders
Endogenous	Connective tissue disease
Exogenous	Juvenile rheumatoid arthritis
Diabetes mellitus under poor control	Chronic infection
Diabetes insipidus (untreated)	Hereditary fructose intolerance
Virilizing congenital adrenal hyperplasia (tall child, short	
adult); P450c21, P450c11 deficiencies	**Malnutrition**
	Inadequate food availability
Skeletal dysplasias	Iron deficiency
Osteogenesis imperfecta	Zinc deficiency
Osteochondroplasias	Anorexia due to chemotherapy of neoplasms
	Malabsorption
Lysosomal storage diseases	
Mucopolysaccharidoses	
Mucolipidoses	

[1]Reproduced, with permission, from Fitzgerald PA: *Handbook of Clinical Endocrinology.* Appleton & Lange, 1992.

Women with polycystic ovary syndrome are often obese. Patients who quit smoking usually gain weight.

Patients with *morbid* obesity may be considered for surgical treatment if concerted attempts at restrictive diets have failed. Gastric procedures are now favored over jejunoileal bypass. In one series, isolated gastric bypass had a higher success rate than vertical gastric bypass or vertical banded gastroplasty. However, such procedures appear to have variable success rates and morbidity in other hands.

Bray GA, York B, Delany J: A survey of the opinions of obesity experts on the causes and treatment of obesity. Am J Clin Nutr 1992;55:1515.

Maclean LD et al: Results of the surgical treatment of obesity. Am J Surg 1993;165:155.

Weight Loss

Weight loss from uncontrolled diabetes mellitus may be associated with polyphagia, polydipsia, and polyuria. Anorexia and nausea may be seen with diabetic ketoacidosis and with adrenal insufficiency (due either to pituitary ACTH deficiency or to Addison's disease). Patients with severe diabetes insipidus may also lose weight. Patients with hyperthyroidism typically lose weight despite increased appetite; some patients with hypothyroidism lose weight because of diminished appetite.

A great variety of nonendocrine conditions enter into the differential diagnosis of unintended weight loss. These include brain lesions or any cause of decreased alertness. Malignancies typically produce diminished appetite and cachexia. Tuberculosis may cause weight loss even when occult. Chronic respiratory insufficiency is often associated with weight loss. Psychiatric illnesses producing diminished appetite include depressed or agitated affective disorder, catatonia, and anorexia nervosa. Anorexia is frequently a side effect of medications or radiation therapy and is also seen with azotemia, AIDS, and many gastrointestinal conditions.

Abnormal Skin Pigmentation or Color

Increased skin pigmentation is often present in conditions associated with ACTH excess such as Addison's disease. It may be very marked after bilateral adrenalectomy for Cushing's disease (Nelson's syndrome). Pregnancy and, less frequently, the ingestion of oral contraceptives may be associated with spotty brown pigmentation, especially over the face (chloasma). Nonendocrine conditions such as sprue, chronic iron deposition, chronic ingestion of chlorpromazine, arsenic poisoning, severe malnutrition, etc, may also be associated with hyperpigmentation.

Vitiligo is common in Addison's disease and is often associated with autoimmune endocrinopathies.

Gynecomastia

Gynecomastia is a glandular enlargement of the male breast that may be tender and is often asymmetric or unilateral. It must be distinguished from tumors and from the fatty breast enlargement of obesity.

Pubertal gynecomastia is common and is characterized by tender discoid enlargement of breast tissue 2–3 cm in diameter beneath the areola; the swelling usually subsides spontaneously within a year. Gynecomastia is also common among elderly men, particularly when there is associated weight gain. Gynecomastia can be the first sign of a serious disorder such as a testicular tumor, and medical evaluation is always indicated when breast enlargement occurs.

The causes of gynecomastia are multiple and diverse (Table 25–2).

The history and physical examination will often clarify the cause of gynecomastia. An adolescent with slight gynecomastia or a patient with prostatic carcinoma taking diethylstilbestrol needs no further study. Careful examination of the testes is mandatory to look for a testicular tumor. The small, firm testes of Klinefelter's syndrome are characteristic. Eunuchoid features, signs of liver disease, or the enlarged thyroid of Graves' disease are also helpful.

Laboratory investigation of unclear cases should include the following:

(1) A chest x-ray to search for metastatic or primary lung tumors.

(2) Measurements of plasma levels of the beta subunit of human chorionic gonadotropin (β-hCG). High levels implicate a choriocarcinoma or other hCG-secreting tumors.

(3) Measurements of plasma testosterone and luteinizing hormone (LH) are valuable in the diagnosis of primary or secondary hypogonadism. A low testosterone and high LH are seen in primary hypogonadism. High testosterone levels *plus* high LH levels characterize partial androgen resistance.

(4) Serum estradiol is usually normal. Many estro-

Table 25–2. Causes of gynecomastia.

Idiopathic	Drugs
Physiologic uses	Alcohol
Neonatal period	Alkylating agents
Puberty	Amiodorone
Aging	Amphetamines
Obesity	Androgens
	Busulfan
Endocrine diseases	Butyrophenones
Androgen resistance	Chorionic gonadotropin
syndromes	Cimetidine
Hyperprolactinemia	Clomiphene
Hyperthyroidism	Cyclophosphamide
Klinefelter's syndrome	Diazepam
Male hypogonadism	Diethylstilbestrol
	Digitalis
Systemic diseases	Domeperidone
Chronic liver disease	Estrogens
Refeeding after	Ethionamide
starvation	Flutamide
	Hydroxyzine
Neoplasms	Isoniazid
Adrenal tumors	Ketoconazole
Bronchogenic carcinoma	Marihuana
Carcinoma of the breast	Meprobamate
Hepatoma (rare)	Methadone
Testicular tumors	Methyldopa
	Metoclopramide
	Narcotics
	Omeprazole
	Penicillamine
	Phenothiazines
	Progestins
	Reserpine
	Spironolactone
	Testosterone
	Tricyclic antidepressants

gens and substances with estrogen activity are *not* detected by estradiol radioimmunoassay. Other laboratory tests such as serum prolactin, serum thyroxine and TSH, and chromosomal analysis (for Klinefelter's syndrome) can be helpful also.

The treatment of gynecomastia is that of the underlying condition. Idiopathic and pubertal gynecomastia usually resolve spontaneously within 1–2 years. Painful gynecomastia may be treated with tamoxifen (an antiestrogen), 10 mg orally twice daily; discomfort improves, but breast size reduction occurs in only 50% and is usually minor. Surgical correction is reserved for persistent or severe gynecomastia, since results are often disappointing. Subcutaneous liposuction mastectomy by a surgeon experienced in the technique may produce acceptable results.

Braunstein GD: Gynecomastia. N Engl J Med 1993;328: 490.

Thompson DF, Carter JR: Drug-induced gynecomastia. Pharmacotherapy 1993;13:37.

Galactorrhea

Lactation that occurs in the absence of nursing is

termed galactorrhea. A small amount of breast milk can be expressed from the nipple in many parous women and is not cause for concern. Galactorrhea requires evaluation when it occurs in significant amounts or in nulliparous women or when it is associated with amenorrhea, headache, visual field abnormalities, or other symptoms implying systemic illness.

Evaluation begins with serum prolactin measurement; a persistently elevated level should prompt further investigation to determine its cause (Table 25–3). Treatment is directed at correcting the cause of the elevated prolactin. Galactorrhea may occur in the absence of elevated serum prolactin levels (idiopathic). Whatever the cause, galactorrhea can be reduced with bromocriptine administration.

Precocious Puberty (in Both Sexes)

In the USA, puberty is considered precocious if it occurs before age 8 in girls or age 9 in boys. Distinction is made between "true" puberty (LH- and FSH-dependent) and "pseudoprecocious" puberty (LH- and FSH-independent—ie, caused by tumor hCG secretion or primary gonadal secretion of sex hormones due to hyperplasia or tumor). True precocious puberty is often a familial trait. Many cases are idiopathic, especially in girls presenting between the ages of 6 and 8 years. However, all children require evaluation.

The history should screen for androgen or estrogen intake (eg, mother's oral contraceptives). A dietary history should exclude the ingestion of chicken necks or beef from a single source, which might rarely have excessive concentrations of estrogens. The abdomen is examined for adrenal or ovarian tumor. Genitalia are checked for ambiguity, which is frequently present in congenital adrenal hyperplasia. Serum sodium and potassium are obtained to screen for the salt-losing form of 21-hydroxylase deficiency; patients with the rarer 11β-hydroxylase deficiency have hypokalemia and hypertension. Boys require examination of the testes in search of hypertrophy or Leydig cell tumor.

Laboratory evaluation should include a serum free thyroxine and TSH to screen for hypothyroidism. Boys should have measurements of serum hCG, which is secreted by some central nervous system tumors (eg, germinoma, teratoma, chorioepithelioma) and non-central nervous system neoplasms (eg, teratoma, seminoma, hepatoma, choriocarcinoma). They should also have determinations of serum testosterone, FSH, and LH. Girls may have elevated serum estradiol, FSH, and LH. Children with suppressed levels of LH and FSH may require adrenal CT scan or pelvic ultrasound to search for tumors.

If no obvious cause for precocious puberty is found outside the central nervous system, a brain MRI scan is required. A variety of central nervous system conditions can cause true precocious puberty, including trauma; hypothalamic tumors, cysts, or granulomas; infection, and hydrocephalus.

Treatment usually consists of first treating the cause. However, some central nervous system lesions (eg, hamartomas of the tuber cinereum) are indolent and situated in such a way that careful observation may be preferable to immediate aggressive surgical or radiation therapy.

Children with true precocious puberty may be treated with a gonadotropin inhibitor, GnRHa. Available preparations of GnRHa include leuprolide acetate (300 µg/kg by depot intramuscular injection every 4 weeks) and nafarelin acetate (800–1600 µg by intranasal administration daily).

Boys with premature Leydig cell maturation (familial testotoxicosis) usually respond favorably to carefully administered ketoconazole; medroxyprogesterone acetate may also be helpful.

Girls may develop gonadotropin-independent sexual precocity from ovarian cysts. Treatment with testolactone is frequently effective; medroxyprogesterone acetate may also be used.

Table 25–3. Causes of hyperprolactinemia.

Physiologic Causes	Pharmacologic Causes	Pathologic Causes
Exercise	Amoxepin	Acromegaly
Idiopathic	Amphetamines	Chronic chest wall stimulation
Pregnancy	Anesthetic agents	(postthoracotomy, postmastectomy,
Puerperium	Butyrophenones	herpes zoster, breast problems, etc)
Sleep (REM phase)	Cimetidine	Cirrhosis
Stress (trauma, surgery)	Estrogens	Hypothalamic disease
Suckling	Hydroxyzine	Hypothyroidism
	Methyldopa	Pituitary stalk section
	Metoclopramide	Prolactin-secreting tumors
	Narcotics	Pseudocyesis
	Nicotine	Renal failure
	Phenothiazines	Spinal cord lesions
	Progestins	
	Reserpine	
	Tricyclic antidepressants	
	Verapamil	

Kaplan SL, Grumbach MM: Pathophysiology and treatment of sexual precocity. J Clin Endocrinol Metab 1990; 71:785.

Impotence & Lack of Libido in Males

Erectile impotence is a frequent problem. Psychogenic factors as well as endocrine, vascular, or neurologic abnormalities may be important. Hypogonadism of whatever origin (Table 25–17) is associated with lack of libido and consequent erectile dysfunction. These can also be the first clinical manifestations of a hyperprolactinemic disorder (Table 25–3). Other endocrine causes include hyperthyroidism, Addison's disease, and acromegaly. Impotence in diabetes may be related to inadequate penile blood flow or autonomic neuropathy. Vascular disease is a frequent factor in impotence in elderly men.

Many pharmacologic agents are known to cause impotence through a variety of mechanisms; some interfere directly with the neural erectile reflex, and a few induce hyperprolactinemia or interfere with testosterone action (Table 25–4). All drugs that are associated with impotence are variable in effect, with some patients developing severe impotence with a given dose and others retaining normal erectile function. If the cause is in doubt, the suspected offending agent should be discontinued and the patient's response evaluated.

Evaluation and treatment of erectile dysfunction are covered in Chapter 21.

Althof SE et al: Through the eyes of women: The sexual and psychological responses of women to their partner's treatment with self-injection or external vacuum therapy. J Urol 1992;147:1024.
Morley JE, Kaiser FE: Impotence: The internist's approach to diagnosis and treatment. Adv Intern Med 1993;38: 151.

Cryptorchism

One or both testes may be absent from the scrotum at birth in about 20% of premature males and in 3–6% at full term. Cryptorchism is found in 1–2% of males after 1 year of age. Examination in a warm room with the patient in a cross-legged position is necessary to see if the testis can be milked down from an inguinal location; such retractile testes require no treatment. True cryptorchism should be corrected before age 18–24 months in an attempt to reduce the risk of infertility, which occurs in up to 75% of men with bilateral cryptorchism and in 50% with unilateral cryptorchism. Many patients have underlying hypogonadism.

Medical therapy may be used to stimulate gonadal testosterone secretion, which in turn may prompt descent of a cryptorchid testis. Human chorionic gonadotropin (hCG) may be given twice weekly for 5 weeks in doses of 250 units intramuscularly for boys under age 2 years, 500 units for boys ages 2–6 years, and 1000 units for boys over age 6 years. If neither testis descends, a serum testosterone measurement is obtained during hCG treatment; failure to see a rise in testosterone indicates bilateral anorchia.

Surgical orchiopexy is used for boys with an inguinal hernia or ectopic testis and in cases where endocrine therapy has been unsuccessful. It is not clear whether early orchiopexy improves ultimate fertility. Orchiectomy after puberty is an option for intra-abdominal testes. Boys with other causes of infertility or with severe mental retardation are not usually candidates for orchiopexy that does not decrease the risk of neoplasia when performed after age 10. Orchiopexy does not enhance the detection rate or contribute to the treatment of neoplasia, so adults are usually not treated.

The incidence of testicular neoplasia is about 0.002% in normal males, 0.06% in cryptorchid males, and up to 5% in patients with intra-abdominal testes.

Benson RC Jr et al: Malignant potential of the cryptorchid testis. Mayo Clin Proc 1991;66:372.
Palmer TM: The undescended testicle. Endocrinol Metab Clin North Am 1991;20:231.

Bone Pain & Pathologic Fractures

Onset of pathologic fractures at an early age is seen in osteogenesis imperfecta (blue scleras may be present). Painful bowing of the bones and pseudofractures suggest rickets or osteomalacia. Hyperparathyroidism or malignancy is suspected in patients with bone pain and hypercalcemia. Back pain or pathologic fractures in hypogonadal men and women implicate osteoporosis. In cases of osteopenia of unknown cause, hyperthyroidism and Cushing's syndrome should also be considered. Bone pain may occur also as a result of metastatic tumors, multiple myeloma, and Paget's disease. Treatment is that of the underlying disorder.

Muscle Cramps & Tetany

Muscle cramps are usually caused by sports or occupational muscle injury. Nocturnal leg cramps are commonly idiopathic but are seen in diabetes mellitus. They may also occur with Parkinson's disease,

Table 25–4. Drugs causing impotence.

Alcohol	Leuprolide
Amphetamines	Marihuana
Antihistamines	Methadone
Barbiturates	Methyldopa
Beta-blockers	Monoamine oxidase
Butyrophenones	inhibitors
Cimetidine	Narcotics
Clonidine	Phenothiazines
Cocaine	Spironolactone
Guanethidine	Thiazides
Ketoconazole	Tricyclic antidepressants

central nervous system lesions, and a variety of neuromuscular conditions. Muscle cramping is also frequently seen in patients undergoing hemodialysis and in those receiving cisplatin or vincristine chemotherapy. Alkalosis due to any cause (eg, severe vomiting or hyperventilation during an anxiety attack) may cause muscle cramping and paresthesias.

Diffuse, recurrent, or severe muscle cramping requires evaluation for hypocalcemia (Table 20–9). Severe hypocalcemia will also produce convulsions. Treatment of hypocalcemia is discussed elsewhere in Chapter 20. Magnesium deficiency must be considered in tetany unresponsive to calcium. Nocturnal leg cramping may be treated with quinine sulfate, 200-500 mg in the evening.

Connolly PS et al: Treatment of nocturnal leg cramps: A crossover trial of quinine vs vitamin E. Arch Intern Med 1992;152:1877.

Lees AJ et al: Treatment of cervical dystonia, hand spasms, and laryngeal dystonia with botulinum toxin. J Neurol 1992;239:1.

Simchak AC, Pascuzzi RM: Muscle cramps. Semin Neurol 1991;11:281.

Walton T, Kolb KW: Treatment of nocturnal leg cramps and restless leg syndrome. Clin Pharm 1991;10:427.

Mental Changes

Disturbances of mentation may be important indications of underlying endocrine disorders. Nervousness and excitability are characteristic of the menopause, hyperthyroidism, and anxiety states. Prolonged hypothyroidism in infancy is associated with severe mental deficits. In adults, hypothyroidism is accompanied by mental slowness, depression, and lethargy. Occasionally it may be manifested by delusional psychosis ("myxedema madness"). Prolonged hypocalcemia from untreated hypoparathyroidism may be associated with intellectual deterioration. Hypoglycemia of any origin may cause confusion, abnormal speech, and behavioral or personality changes as well as sudden loss of consciousness, somnolence and prolonged lethargy, or coma. Frank psychosis can occur but is rare. Hypercalcemia leads to somnolence and lethargy, with marked weakness. Confusion may occur in hypopituitarism or Addison's disease. Confusion, lethargy, and nausea may be the presenting symptoms of hyponatremia. Insomnia, mood changes, anxiety, and psychosis can be associated with Cushing's syndrome. Rapid changes in glucocorticoid status (either a sudden increase or a sudden decrease) may be associated with acute psychosis.

DISEASES OF THE HYPOTHALAMUS & PITUITARY GLAND

Anterior pituitary gland function is controlled by regulating hormones produced by the hypothalamus and by direct feedback inhibition. The **posterior pituitary** receives antidiuretic hormone and oxytocin from the hypothalamus, secreting them under central nervous system control (Table 25–5). Hypothalamic hormones generally stimulate the pituitary except for dopamine, which inhibits the pituitary from spontaneously secreting prolactin.

Hypothalamic injury thus produces variable degrees of anterior pituitary hormone deficiencies plus hyperprolactinemia; it may also cause ADH deficiency, manifest as diabetes insipidus. Hypothalamic damage may also be associated with neurologic damage (somnolence, hyperphagia and obesity, hypothermia, organic brain syndrome). Visual field defects may be caused by compression of the optic nerves.

Pituitary tumors may present with symptoms of pituitary excess or deficiency or with local symptoms (headache, visual field defects, or cranial nerve III palsy). Patients with a pituitary tumor or any problem apparently related to pituitary hormonal excess or deficiency need complete endocrine evaluation to detect deficiencies (see below) or excesses that may not be obvious. Patients require evaluation for acromegaly and Cushing's disease and serum prolactin, TSH, LH, and FSH measurements. Serum hCG is measured in women of childbearing age to rule out pregnancy, which can cause pituitary enlargement, amenorrhea, and hyperprolactinemia.

Katznelson L et al: Clinically nonfunctioning pituitary adenomas. J Clin Endocrinol Metab 1993;76:1089.

Lechan RM: Neuroendocrinology of pituitary hormone regulation. Endocrinol Metab Clin North Am 1987;16:475.

Molitch ME (editor): Pituitary tumors. (Symposium.) Endocrinol Metab Clin North Am 1987;16:475.

HYPOPITUITARISM

Essentials of Diagnosis

- Sexual dysfunction; weakness; easy fatigability; lack of resistance to stress, cold, and fasting; axillary and pubic hair loss.
- Low blood pressure; may have visual field defects.
- Low or normal free thyroxine index; deficient cortisol response to cosyntropin.
- Low or normal serum testosterone (men); amenorrhea; serum prolactin may be elevated; FSH and LH are low or low normal.
- CT scan or MRI may reveal a pituitary or hypothalamic lesion.

Table 25–5. Pituitary hormones.[1]

	Structure	Serum Half-Life (Approximate)
Anterior pituitary		
Growth hormone (GH)[2]	Polypeptide, 191 amino acids	35 min
Prolactin (PRL)	Polypeptide, 198 amino acids	35 min
Adrenocorticotropic hormone (ACTH)	Polypeptide, 39 amino acids	10 min
Thyroid-stimulating hormone (TSH)	Glycopeptide, α subunit, 89 amino acids; β subunit, 112 amino acids	50 min
Luteinizing hormone (LH)[3]	Glycopeptide, α subunit, 89 amino acids; β subunit, 115 amino acids	50 min
Follicle-stimulating hormone (FSH)	Glycopeptide, α subunit, 89 amino acids; β subunit, 115 amino acids	50 min
Posterior pituitary		
Arginine vasopressin (AVP)[4]	Ringed polypeptide, 9 amino acids	4 min
Oxytocin (OT)	Ringed polypeptide, 9 amino acids	4 min

[1]Reproduced with permission from Fitzgerald PA: *Handbook of Clinical Endocrinology.* Appleton & Lange, 1992.
[2]GH closely resembles human placental lactogen (hPL).
[3]LH closely resembles human chorionic gonadotropin (hCG).
[4]AVP is identical with antidiuretic hormone (ADH).

General Considerations

Patients with hypopituitarism may have single or multiple hormonal deficiencies. When one hormonal deficiency is discovered, others must be sought.

Causes include mass lesions such as pituitary adenomas, brain tumors or aneurysms, apoplexy, metastatic carcinoma, granulomas, multifocal Langerhans cell granulomatosis, and pituitary abscess. Autoimmune hypophysitis and postpartum pituitary necrosis (Sheehan's syndrome) are rare causes. Causes of hypopituitarism without mass lesions include trauma, radiation or surgery, encephalitis, hemochromatosis, and stroke.

A pituitary tumor may be part of the syndrome of multiple endocrine adenomatosis (type I), with concomitant tumors of the parathyroid glands and pancreatic islets.

Clinical Findings

These vary with the degree of pituitary destruction and are related to lack of hormones from the "target" endocrine glands.

A. Symptoms and Signs: Fatigue and weakness, diminished libido, and sexual dysfunction (lack of development of secondary sex characteristics, or regression of function) are the most common symptoms. In expanding lesions of the sella, compression of the optic chiasm may produce temporal hemianopia or other visual field defects. Short stature is the rule if onset is during the growth period. Amenorrhea and galactorrhea may be the first indications of a pituitary tumor. In men, decreased libido or impotence is usually an early complaint.

In long-standing hypopituitarism, there is sparseness of axillary and pubic hair. Men may note diminished beard growth.

The skin is often dry, with lack of sweating, and the patient appears pale. The face has fine wrinkles and a "sleepy" appearance.

The heart is usually small and the blood pressure low. Orthostatic hypotension is often present. Hypopituitarism (GH deficiency) has been reported to stabilize diabetic retinopathy and nephropathy; insulin requirements are greatly reduced.

B. Laboratory Findings: The fasting blood glucose may be low. Hyponatremia is often present. Hyperkalemia usually does not occur, since aldosterone production is not affected.

Children and adolescents with delayed growth may require assessment for hypothyroidism, Cushing's syndrome, or growth hormone deficiency. Adults are not assessed or treated for GH deficiency.

The T_4 level is low, and TSH is not elevated. Cosyntropin (synthetic ACTH) stimulation testing may show a subnormal cortisol response. Serum ACTH is normal or low. Plasma levels of sex steroids (testosterone and estradiol) are low or low normal, and so are the serum gonadotropins. Elevated prolactin levels are found in patients with prolactinomas, acromegaly, and hypothalamic disease.

The demonstration of a low level of a hormone secreted by a target gland in the presence of a low level of a trophic hormone is strongly suggestive of hypothalamic or pituitary disease (low plasma cortisol *and* ACTH, T_4 *and* TSH, estradiol or testosterone *and* LH).

C. Imaging: MRI provides the best visualization of parasellar lesions. The posterior pituitary normally has a high-intensity signal on sagittal MRI that is lacking in central diabetes insipidus.

Differential Diagnosis

Anorexia nervosa may occasionally simulate hypopituitarism. In fact, severe malnutrition may give rise to functional hypopituitarism. Cachexia is rare in hypopituitarism. Loss of axillary and pubic hair is unusual in anorexia nervosa. Plasma cortisol is normal or high and may respond rapidly to cosyntropin stimulation; the gonadotropins are usually present at low levels. Thyroid function tests are not abnormal in anorexia nervosa except for low T_3. Pituitary growth hormone assays show high levels in anorexia nervosa and very low levels in hypopituitarism.

Primary adrenal or thyroid insufficiency is easily differentiated from pituitary insufficiency, since serum ACTH or TSH is invariably elevated in the former conditions.

Complications

In addition to those of the primary lesion (eg, tumor), complications may develop at any time as a result of the patient's inability to cope with stressful illness. This may lead to high fever, shock, coma, and death. Sensitivity to thyroid may rarely precipitate adrenal crisis if thyroid hormone is administered without glucocorticoid treatment. Rarely, acute hemorrhage may occur in large pituitary tumors, manifested by rapid loss of vision, headache, and evidence of acute pituitary failure (pituitary apoplexy) requiring emergency decompression of the sella.

Treatment

The pituitary lesion, if a tumor, is treated by surgical removal, x-ray irradiation, or both. Removal is usually via a transsphenoidal approach, which in expert hands is an effective and safe surgical procedure. Craniotomy is rarely necessary. Endocrine substitution therapy must be used before, during, and often permanently after such procedures.

The mainstay of substitution therapy for pituitary insufficiency remains the lifetime replacement of the end-organ deficiencies (adrenal, thyroid, and gonad).

A. Corticosteroids: Give hydrocortisone tablets, 15–25 mg/d orally in divided doses. Most patients do well with 15 mg in the morning and 5–10 mg in the late afternoon. Some patients feel better taking prednisone, 5–7.5 mg/d, or dexamethasone, 0.25 mg/d. A mineralocorticoid is rarely needed. Additional hydrocortisone must be given during states of stress, eg, during infection, trauma, or surgical procedures.

B. Thyroid: Thyroid should rarely, if ever, be used in panhypopituitarism unless the patient is receiving corticosteroids. Because of lack of adrenal function, patients may be exceedingly sensitive to these drugs. Levothyroxine is the drug of choice. The usual maintenance dose is 0.125 mg daily (range, 0.1–0.2 mg daily).

C. Sex Hormones:

1. Androgen replacement is usually administered as testosterone enanthate (or testosterone cypionate); the average requirement is about 300 mg every 3 weeks intramuscularly.

2. Estrogen replacement is discussed below in the section on Turner's syndrome.

3. For fertility induction in males, chorionic gonadotropin is given at a dosage of 2000–5000 units intramuscularly three times weekly. For males who have never entered puberty, menotropins (hMG) may

be added. Leuprolide (GnRH analogue) by intermittent subcutaneous infusion may also help.

4. For fertility induction in females, ovulation may be induced with clomiphene, 50 mg daily for 5 days every 2 months. Menotropins and chorionic gonadotropin can induce multiple births and should be used only by those experienced with their administration. (See Chapter 17.)

D. Human Growth Hormone: This 191-amino-acid polypeptide hormone is now synthesized by recombinant DNA techniques. hGH (somatrem, somatropin) is administered by injection daily to children with demonstrated GH deficiency by clinicians expert in its use. Adults with growth hormone deficiency have been noted to have an improved sense of well-being and work capacity when administered GH in doses of 0.04–0.1 U/kg body weight/day; muscle mass increases, fat is lost and bone density improves. However, GH deficiency is not usually treated due to the very high cost of therapy.

E. Other Drugs: Bromocriptine may reverse the hypogonadism seen in hyperprolactinomas. (See Disorders of Prolactin Secretion.)

Prognosis

The prognosis depends on the primary cause. Hypopituitarism resulting from a pituitary tumor may be reversible with careful selective resection of the tumor. Functional hypopituitarism due to starvation, suppression by hypercortisolism, or hyperthyroidism is also correctable.

Hypopituitarism is usually permanent. However, with appropriate therapy, a patient with hypopituitarism can expect a normal life span.

Blondell RD: Hypopituitarism. Am Fam Physician 1991; 43:2029.

Frasier SD, Lippe BM: The rational use of growth hormone during childhood. J Clin Endocrinol Metab 1990;71:269.

Libber SM et al: Long-term follow-up of hypopituitary patients treated with human growth hormone. Medicine 1990;69:46.

Plumb M et al: Hypopituitarism stabilizes the renal and retinal complications of diabetes. Am J Nephrology 1992;12:265.

DIABETES INSIPIDUS

Essentials of Diagnosis

- Polyuria (2–40 L/d); polydipsia.
- Urine specific gravity usually < 1.006 during ad libitum fluid intake.
- Vasopressin reduces urine output (except in nephrogenic diabetes insipidus).

General Considerations

Diabetes insipidus is an uncommon disease characterized by an increase in thirst and the passage of large quantities of urine of low specific gravity. The urine is otherwise normal. It is caused by a deficiency of or resistance to vasopressin.

The causes may be classified as follows:

A. Due to Deficiency of Vasopressin:

1. Primary diabetes insipidus (without an identifiable organic lesion noted on MRI of the pituitary and hypothalamus) may be familial, occurring as a dominant trait, or sporadic ("idiopathic").

2. Secondary diabetes insipidus is due to damage to the hypothalamus or pituitary stalk by anoxic encephalopathy, surgical or accidental trauma, infection (eg, encephalitis, tuberculosis, syphilis), sarcoidosis, primary tumor, metastatic carcinoma, or multifocal Langerhans cell (eosinophilic) granulomatosis ("histiocytosis X").

3. Vasopressinase-induced diabetes insipidus may be seen in the last trimester of pregnancy and in the puerperium; it is often associated with preeclampsia or hepatic dysfunction. The condition usually responds to desmopressin therapy (see below) and subsides spontaneously.

B. "Nephrogenic" Diabetes Insipidus: This disorder is due to a defect in the kidney tubules that interferes with water reabsorption. The polyuria is unresponsive to vasopressin. In fact, these patients have normal secretion of vasopressin. It occurs as a familial X-linked trait; adults often have hyperuricemia as well. Acquired forms of vasopressin-resistant diabetes insipidus are seen in some patients with pyelonephritis, renal amyloidosis, myeloma, potassium depletion, Sjögren's syndrome, sickle cell anemia, or chronic hypercalcemia. The disorder may occur also as a glucocorticoid effect or as an acute side effect of diuretics. Certain drugs (eg, demeclocycline, lithium, foscarnet, or methicillin) may induce nephrogenic diabetes insipidus.

Clinical Findings

A. Symptoms and Signs: The symptoms of the disease are intense thirst, especially with a craving for ice water, and polyuria, the volume of ingested fluid varying from 4 L to 20 L daily, with correspondingly large urine volumes. Patients with impaired thirst mechanisms may present with lethargy due to hypernatremia. Partial diabetes insipidus presents with less intense symptoms and should be suspected in patients with unremitting enuresis. Restriction of fluids causes marked weight loss and muscular pains. Signs include tachycardia, dehydration, and orthostatic hypotension.

B. Laboratory Findings: Evaluation for diabetes insipidus should include a 24-hour urine collection for volume, glucose, and creatinine. Blood is assayed for glucose, urea nitrogen, calcium, potassium, and sodium.

The diagnosis of diabetes insipidus as a cause of polyuria or hypernatremia requires mostly clinical judgment. There is no single diagnostic laboratory test. If the clinical situation implicates central diabetes insipidus (and no other causes for polyuria are present; see Differential Diagnosis, below), a supervised "vasopressin challenge test" may be given: Desmopressin acetate is given in an initial dose of 0.05 mL intranasally (or 1 μg subcutaneously or intravenously), with measurement of prior and subsequent urine volumes. Serum sodium is measured every 12 hours and "stat" in the event of fatigue or other symptoms of hyponatremia. The dosage of desmopressin is doubled if the response is marginal. Patients with true central diabetes insipidus will notice a distinct reduction in their thirst and polyuria; serum sodium usually stays normal except in some salt-losing conditions (Table 25–6).

A vasopressin challenge test is ideally done in the hospital.

Patients who have nephrogenic diabetes insipidus will not respond to desmopressin. When nephrogenic diabetes insipidus is a diagnostic consideration, measurement of serum vasopressin is done during modest fluid restriction; typically, the vasopressin level is high.

In true nonfamilial central diabetes insipidus, MRI of the pituitary and hypothalamus and of the skull is done to look for mass lesions in the hypothalamus, a lesion in the pituitary stalk, or a bone lesion indicative of eosinophilic granuloma. Absence of a posterior pituitary "bright spot" on T1-weighted MRI is also suggestive of central diabetes insipidus.

Differential Diagnosis of Polyuria

Central diabetes insipidus must be distinguished from polyuria caused by excessive fluid intake seen in psychogenic polydipsia, central nervous system sarcoidosis, and intravenous fluid administration.

Central diabetes insipidus is easily distinguished from diabetes mellitus by checking the urine for glucose. It must be distinguished also from nephrogenic diabetes insipidus (see above).

Complications

If water is not readily available, the excessive output of urine will lead to severe dehydration. Patients with an impaired thirst mechanism are very prone to hypernatremia. All the complications of the primary disease may eventually become evident. In patients who are receiving antidiuretic therapy, there is a danger of induced water intoxication. In untreated subjects, the passage of large volumes of urine for many years may be associated with dilation of the ureters and bladder.

Treatment

A. Desmopressin: Desmopressin acetate (DDAVP) is the treatment of choice for central diabetes insipidus. It is also useful in pregnancy- or puerperium-associated diabetes insipidus, since desmo-

Table 25–6. Differential diagnosis of hyponatremia.[1,2]

Artifactual: hyperglycemia, hypertriglyceridemia
Syndrome of inappropriate ADH release or action (SIADH)
  Central nervous system lesions; reset osmostat
  Pulmonary lesions
  Other: acute intermittent porphyria, positive-pressure
    breathing
  Ectopic ADH production: especially small-cell carcinoma
    of the lung
  Drug-induced SIADH

Chlorpropamide	Vincristine
Amitriptyline	Vinblastine
Clofibrate	Cyclophosphamide
Carbamazepine	Vasopressin
Phenothiazines	Oxytocin
Barbiturates	Melphalan
Morphine	Ifosfamide
Thiothixene	Trimethoprim-sulfamethoxazole
	(intravenously)

Hyponatremia with hypervolemia
  Decreased water excretion; natriuresis for atriopeptin
    Congestive heart failure
    Cirrhosis
    Renal failure
  Excessive water intake
    Restriction of dietary salt without water restriction
    Compulsive water drinking
    Intravenous water
Hyponatremia due to sodium depletion
  Renal losses
    Diuretics
    Addison's disease; congenital adrenal hyperplasia; se-
      lective hypoaldosteronism
    Renal diseases: tubulointerstitial disease, renal tubular
      acidosis
    Central nervous system-induced natriuresis (associated
      with central nervous sytem injury, especially sub-
      arachnoid hemorrhage; also pituitary surgery)
    Nonsteroidal anti-inflammatory agents
  Gastrointestinal losses
    Vomiting
    Diarrhea
    Fistulas
  Third space losses
    Burns
    Pancreatitis
    Crush injuries
    Major surgery
Hypothyroidism
Severe illness

[1]Reproduced with permission, from Fitzgerald PA: *Handbook of Clinical Endocrinology.* Appleton & Lange, 1992.
[2]Two or more conditions may coexist.

pressin is resistant to degradation by the circulating vasopressinase. It is usually given intranasally every 12–24 hours as needed for thirst and polyuria. The nasal solution contains 100 μg per mL. It may be administered via metered-dose inhaler containing 0.1 mL/spray. The drug also is available in vials with a teat from which the solution is squeezed into a narrow calibrated plastic tube (rhinyle). Patients are started with 0.05–0.1 mL, and the dose is then individualized according to response.

Desmopressin is also available as a parenteral preparation containing 4 μg/mL. For central diabetes insipidus, it is given intravenously, intramuscularly,

or subcutaneously in doses of 1–4 μg every 12–24 hours as needed to treat thirst or hypernatremia.

Patients having an adverse reaction to desmopressin (eg, agitation or erythromelalgia) may receive lypressin nasal spray (1–4 sprays in each nostril every 6–8 hours). Aqueous vasopressin is an alternative parenteral agent given as 0.05–0.1 unit/kg subcutaneously every 4–8 hours as needed.

B. Other Measures: Mild cases require no treatment other than adequate fluid intake. Reduction of aggravating factors (eg, glucocorticoids) will improve polyuria. Both central and nephrogenic diabetes insipidus respond partially to hydrochlorothiazide, 50–100 mg/d (with potassium supplement or amiloride). Chlorpropamide is sometimes effective for central diabetes insipidus and can improve thirst sensation in patients with recurrent hypernatremia; however, chlorpropamide is usually reserved for special cases due to the danger of hypoglycemia. Nephrogenic diabetes insipidus may respond to combined treatments of indomethacin-hydrochlorothiazide and indomethacin-desmopressin.

Psychotherapy is required for most patients with compulsive water drinking. Thioridazine and lithium are best avoided if drug therapy is needed, since they cause polyuria.

Prognosis

Central diabetes insipidus appearing after pituitary surgery usually remits after days to weeks but may be permanent if the superior pituitary stalk is cut.

Central diabetes insipidus is made transiently worse by glucocorticoids in high doses frequently given perioperatively.

Chronic diabetes insipidus is more an inconvenience than a dire medical condition. Treatment with desmopressin allows normal sleep and activity. Hypernatremia can occur, especially when the thirst center is damaged, but diabetes insipidus itself does not reduce life expectancy, and the prognosis is that of the underlying disorder.

Blevins LS Jr, Wand GS: Diabetes insipidus. Crit Care Med 1992;20:69.

Narins RG, Riley LJ Jr: Polyuria: Simple and mixed disorders. Am J Kidney Dis 1991;17:237.

Robinson AG, Amico JA: "Non-sweet" diabetes of pregnancy. N Engl J Med 1991;324:556.

Stasoir DS et al: Nephrogenic diabetes insipidus responsive to indomethacin plus DDAVP. N Engl J Med 1991; 324:850.

ACROMEGALY & GIGANTISM

Essentials of Diagnosis

- Excessive growth of hands (increased glove and ring size), feet (increased shoe width), jaw (protru-

sion of lower jaw), and internal organs; or gigantism before closure of epiphyses.
- Coarsening facial features; deeper voice.
- Amenorrhea, headaches, visual field loss, sweating, weakness.
- Increased heel pad thickness.
- Soft, doughy, sweaty handshake.
- Serum GH not suppressed following oral glucose.
- Elevated insulin-like growth factor I (IGF-I).
- Imaging: Terminal phalangeal "tufting" on radiographs. CT or MRI demonstration of pituitary tumor in 90%.

General Considerations

Growth hormone seems to exert its growth-promoting effects through the release of IGF-I produced in the liver and other tissues.

An excessive amount of growth hormone is most often produced by a benign pituitary adenoma. Many growth hormone-secreting tumors have a genetic mutation in the "G" peptide associated with the growth hormone-releasing hormone (GHRH) receptor. Acromegaly is usually sporadic in distribution but may rarely be familial. The disease may be associated with adenomas elsewhere, such as in the parathyroids or pancreas (multiple endocrine neoplasia type I). Acromegaly may also be seen in McCune-Albright syndrome and as part of Carney's complex (atrial myxoma, acoustic neuroma, and spotty skin pigmentation). Acromegaly is rarely caused by ectopic GHRH or GH secreted by hypothalamic or bronchial carcinoid or pancreatic tumors. If the onset precedes closure of the epiphyses, gigantism will result. If the epiphyses have already closed at onset, only overgrowth of soft tissues and terminal skeletal structures (acromegaly) results. Rarely, the disease is transient and followed by partial pituitary insufficiency.

Clinical Findings

A. Symptoms and Signs: Concurrent secretion of prolactin and crowding of other hormone-producing cells causes hypogonadism. Production of excessive growth hormone causes doughy enlargement of the hands, with spade-like fingers; large feet, face, tongue, and internal organs; wide spacing of the teeth; and an oily, tough, "furrowed" skin and scalp. There is frequently enlargement of the jaw, with prognathism and malocclusion. Hoarseness is common. Sleep apnea may occur. Acanthosis nigricans may be present. Pituitary tumor enlargement may cause headache, bitemporal hemianopia, and diplopia. Other hormonal changes may include diabetes mellitus, goiter, and abnormal lactation. Less commonly, these may be the presenting picture in acromegaly. Excessive sweating may be the most reliable clinical sign of activity of the disease. Carpal tunnel syndrome and spinal stenosis may cause neurologic symptoms.

B. Laboratory Findings: After an overnight fast, a fasting serum specimen is obtained and assayed for prolactin (cosecreted by many GH-secreting tumors); IGF-I (increased in most acromegalics); glucose (diabetes is common in acromegaly); liver function tests and BUN; serum inorganic phosphorus (frequently elevated); serum T_4 index; and TSH (secondary hypothyroidism is common in acromegaly; primary hypothyroidism may increase prolactin).

Glucose syrup (100 g) is then administered orally, and serum GH is measured 60 minutes afterward. A GH level higher than 2 ng/mL (males) or 5 ng/mL (females) is evidence of acromegaly. High serum GH levels can be caused by exercise or eating just prior to the test, acute illness or agitation, hepatic or renal failure, malnourishment, diabetes mellitus or concurrent treatment with estrogens, beta-blockers, or clonidine. Some patients with acromegaly have normal serum GH concentrations.

C. Imaging: MRI shows a pituitary tumor in 90% of acromegalics. MRI is generally superior to CT scanning, especially in the postoperative setting. X-rays of the skull may show an enlarged sella and thickened skull. X-rays may also show tufting of the terminal phalanges of the fingers and toes. A lateral view of the feet shows increased thickness of the heel pad.

Differential Diagnosis

Gigantism from a GH-secreting pituitary tumor must be distinguished from other causes of tall stature: genetic or constitutional (bone age advanced), sexual precocity, thyrotoxicosis, Beckwith-Wiedemann syndrome (omphalocele, neonatal hypoglycemia, macroglossia, etc), Marfan's syndrome, Kleinfelter's syndrome, XYY syndromes, and cerebral gigantism (Sotos syndrome, infant rapid growth, hypertelorism, prominent forehead, sharp chin).

Active acromegaly must be distinguished from familial coarse features, large hands and feet, and isolated prognathism. It must also be distinguished from inactive ("burned-out") acromegaly in which there has been a spontaneous remission due to infarction of the pituitary adenoma. Acromegaly is distinguished from these conditions by testing (see above) and by ongoing enlargement in ring or shoe size and by progressive coarsening of facial features, which can be seen in serial photographs.

Complications

Complications include hypopituitarism, hypertension, glucose intolerance or frank diabetes mellitus, cardiac enlargement, and cardiac failure. The carpal tunnel syndrome, due to compression of the median nerve at the wrist, may cause disability of the hand. Arthritis of hips, knees, and spine can be troublesome. Cord compression may be seen. Visual field defects may be severe and progressive. Acute loss of vision or cranial nerve palsy may occur if the tumor undergoes spontaneous hemorrhage and necrosis (pituitary apoplexy).

Treatment

Transsphenoidal pituitary microsurgery removes the adenoma while preserving anterior pituitary function in most patients. Growth hormone levels fall immediately, but IGF-I levels fall gradually over days to weeks. Diaphoresis and carpal tunnel syndrome often improve within a day after surgery. Patients in remission tend to gain some weight. Pituitary irradiation is useful if operative therapy fails. Periodic reassessment of pituitary function after these procedures is advisable. Large doses of bromocriptine (eg, 20 mg/d) may control GH secretion in some patients, especially those with concomitant prolactin secretion.

Octreotide, a somatostatin analogue, can be useful in treating acromegaly. It may be used as first therapy in locales where transsphenoidal surgery is not available. Octreotide must be administered by injection at doses averaging 100 μg subcutaneously three times daily. Most patients experience at least a partial response. Headache often improves, but tumor shrinkage is usually marginal. Octreotide may also be effective in ectopic acromegaly. Side effects are experienced by about 36% of patients and include injection site pain, loose acholic stools, and abdominal discomfort. Combined therapy with bromocriptine and octreotide may have an additive effect.

Prognosis

Patients with untreated acromegaly tend to have premature cardiovascular disease and progressive acromegalic symptoms. Transsphenoidal pituitary surgery is successful in 90% of patients with tumors less than 2 cm diameter and GH levels less than 50 ng/mL. Postoperatively, normal pituitary function is usually preserved. Conventional radiation therapy (alone) produces a remission in about 38% by 2 years and 73% by 5 years after treatment. Heavy particle pituitary radiation produces a remission in about 70% by 2 years and 80% by 5 years but is not generally available. Radiation therapy eventually produces some degree of hypopituitarism in most patients. Bromocriptine has an adequate effect in up to 50% of patients and is usually used as an interim measure.

Barkan AL: Acromegaly: Diagnosis and therapy. Endocrinol Metab Clin North Am 1989;18:277.

Goffman TE et al: Persistent or recurrent acromegaly: Long-term endocrinologic efficacy and neurologic safety of postsurgical radiation therapy. Cancer 1992;69:271.

Landis CA et al: GTPase inhibiting mutations activate the alpha chain of Gs and stimulate adenylyl cyclase in human pituitary tumours. Nature 1989;340:692.

Melmed S: Extrapituitary acromegaly. Endocrinol Metab Clin North Am 1991;20:507.

Melmed S et al: Acromegaly. N Engl J Med 1990;322:966.

Sano T et al: Growth hormone-releasing hormone-produc-

ing tumors: Clinical, biochemical and morphological manifestations. Endocr Rev 1988;9:357.

Vance ML, Harris AG: Long term treatment of 189 acromegalic patients with the somatostatin analog octreotide: Results of the International Multicenter Acromegaly Study Group. Arch Intern Med 1991;151:1573.

Yen RS et al: The syndrome of right atrial myxoma, spotty skin pigmentation, and acromegaly. Am Heart J 1992;123:243.

HYPERPROLACTINEMIA

Essentials of Diagnosis

- Women: Menstrual cycle disturbances (oligomenorrhea, amenorrhea); galactorrhea; infertility.
- Men: Hypogonadism; decreased libido and erectile dysfunction; infertility.
- Elevated serum prolactin.
- CT scan or MRI often demonstrates pituitary adenoma.

Normal Physiology

Prolactin is a 198-amino-acid polypeptide hormone which is secreted by the pituitary. In mammalian species, its main role is to induce lactation. Serum prolactin levels increase during pregnancy from a normal (follicular phase) level of less than 20 ng/mL to as high as 600 ng/mL by the time of delivery. Under the combined effect of prolactin, increased estrogen, and progesterone, breast development takes place, with eventual formation of milk in the acini. Estrogens inhibit the actual secretion of milk. After parturition, the sudden withdrawal of estrogen caused by expulsion of the placenta results in the onset of lactation. During the puerperal period, suckling constitutes a powerful stimulus for the continued production of prolactin. Lactation will cease if prolactin secretion is interrupted by prolactin-lowering drugs or by pituitary destruction. Prolactin is an unusual hormone in terms of control of secretion in that it is under mainly inhibitory control. Thus, section of the pituitary stalk will result in marked increases in prolactin secretion. Prolactin inhibitory factor (PIF) is dopamine.

Elevated serum prolactin can be caused by numerous conditions (Table 25–3).

Clinical Consequences of Prolactin Excess

In women, prolactin excess produces disturbances of pituitary ovarian function with anovulatory cycles, oligomenorrhea, or (frequently) amenorrhea and (less commonly) galactorrhea. In men, excess prolactin is associated with erectile dysfunction and decreased libido (very common), hypogonadism (common), and gynecomastia (unusual).

Of all women with nongestational secondary amenorrhea, about 30% have hyperprolactinemia. Of women with nonpuerperal secondary amenorrhea and galactorrhea, about 70% have elevated serum prolactin levels. In men, increased prolactin concentrations are usually not associated with galactorrhea because the male breast tissue has not been primed by estrogens and progesterone.

Most women with hyperprolactinemia have amenorrhea, oligomenorrhea, or infertility. The combination of amenorrhea and galactorrhea is characteristic of hyperprolactinemic syndromes, but amenorrhea is more common than galactorrhea. Hyperprolactinemic women tend to have decreased bone density and are therefore ultimately at increased risk to develop clinical osteoporosis if left untreated.

The most important cause of high serum prolactin is a pituitary tumor. As many as 65% of all pituitary tumors may be associated with hyperprolactinemia. The tumors may be small (microadenomas) or may produce clear-cut enlargement of the sella (macroadenomas). A number of hormone stimulation tests have been devised to distinguish a prolactin-secreting tumor from other causes of hyperprolactinemia. All of them are unreliable. The actual level of serum prolactin is useful, however. In the absence of renal failure or late pregnancy, levels greater than 250 ng/mL are almost diagnostic of prolactinoma. Macroadenomas tend to cause higher levels of serum prolactin than microadenomas and are more frequently associated with decreased secretion of gonadotropins (LH and FSH). MRI or CT scan of the pituitary often demonstrates small prolactinomas. Differentiation from normal variants, however, is not always possible.

All possible causes of nontumorous hyperprolactinemia (Table 25–3) must be considered; tests for hypothyroidism and unsuspected pregnancy are usually indicated.

Treatment

The treatment of hyperprolactinemia depends upon the cause. Medications known to increase prolactin are stopped, if possible. If hyperprolactinemia is due to hypothyroidism, administration of thyroxine will rapidly correct it. Patients with hyperprolactinemia not induced by drugs, hypothyroidism, or pregnancy should be examined by pituitary MRI. Patients with persistent hyperprolactinemia who have amenorrhea or other significant symptoms are usually treated with dopamine agonists (eg, bromocriptine, pergolide). these drugs bind to the pituitary dopamine receptor and thus inhibit prolactin secretion from the gland.

Bromocriptine and pergolide are about equally effective in improving symptoms and reducing serum prolactin levels when given at therapeutically comparable doses, ie, bromocriptine, 2.5–20 mg/d, or pergolide, 25–200 mg/d.

Therapy should be started with a small dose (eg, bromocriptine, 1.25 mg/d) given at bedtime to mini-

mize side effects of nausea, dizziness, and orthostatic hypotension. Fatigue commonly occurs, as do a variety of psychiatric side effects; these are not dose-related and may take many weeks to resolve once the dopamine agonist is discontinued. A patient who has been unable to tolerate one dopamine agonist may sometimes be able to tolerate another. *Note:* Most adverse symptoms may be reduced in women by *intravaginal administration* of the bromocriptine tablet. The dose is then gradually increased as necessary to bring prolactin levels down to normal.

Bromocriptine can normalize serum prolactin in 67% of patients, with 90% having a fall in prolactin to 10% or less of basal levels. Shrinkage of a pituitary adenoma occurs early, but maximum effect may take up to 6 months. Nearly half shrink more than 50%. Discontinuing therapy even after many years usually results in reappearance of hyperprolactinemia and galactorrhea-amenorrhea. Since fertility is usually promptly restored with bromocriptine, many pregnancies have resulted—with no clear evidence that the drug is teratogenic. Patients with microadenomas may have bromocriptine safely withdrawn during pregnancy. Macroadenomas may enlarge significantly during pregnancy; if bromocriptine is withdrawn, patients should be followed most carefully clinically and with computer-assisted visual field perimetry.

Transsphenoidal surgery may be urgently required for large tumors causing visual compromise or apoplexy. It is also used electively for patients who do not tolerate or respond to bromocriptine.

Blackwell RE: Hyperprolactinemia: Evaluation and management. Endocrinol Metab Clin North Am 1992; 21:105.

Ginsberg J et al: Vaginal bromocriptine: Clinical and biochemical effects. Gynecol Endocrinol 1992;6:119.

Klibanski A, Zervas NT: Diagnosis and management of hormone-secreting pituitary adenomas. N Engl J Med 1991;324:822.

Molitch ME: Pathologic hyperprolactinemia. Endocrinol Metab Clin North Am 1992;21:877.

DISEASES OF THE THYROID GLAND

An adult's thyroid gland normally weighs about 15–20 g. Its two lobes, flanking the trachea, are joined by an isthmus. A pyramidal lobe arises superiorly from the isthmus in about 30% of cases, being derived embryologically from the thyroglossal duct. Embryologic defects may result in a rare lingual thyroid, retrosternal thyroid, or agenesis of one or both lobes.

Thyroid examination involves inspection of the neck during swallowing. The normal thyroid is commonly visualized in thin necks; thyroid nodules and goiter are often quite noticeable. Palpation of the thyroid is best performed with the examiner behind the seated patient. The three middle fingers of each hand are placed on either side of the lower trachea while the patient swallows water. The thyroid moves upward with swallowing, making it easier to appreciate its size, shape, consistency, and nodularity. Any abnormality may be traced on the skin and measured. Patients with goiter may also have their neck circumference (average of several measurements) recorded for future comparison.

Thyroid-stimulating hormone (TSH, thyrotropin) is secreted by the pituitary and stimulates several steps of thyroid hormone production: trapping of iodine, peroxidase linking of iodine to tyrosine, coupling of monoiodotyrosine or diiodotyrosine to form T_3 (triiodothyronine) or T_4 (thyroxine), and release of T_3 and T_4. The thyroid secretes mostly T_4 and very little T_3. About 90% of circulating T_3, the most active thyroid hormone, is derived from peripheral deiodination of T_4. Circulating thyroid hormones have a direct feedback inhibition effect upon the pituitary thyrotroph cells, desensitizing them from the stimulatory effect of hypothalamic thyrotropin-releasing hormone (TRH).

Over 99% of circulating thyroid hormones are bound to serum proteins, mostly thyroid-binding globulin (TBG). Only free hormone enters cells, binding to its nuclear hormone receptor, which regulates DNA control of oxidative processes throughout the body.

The thyroid tests discussed in the following section are ordinarily very helpful in the evaluation of thyroid disorders. However, many conditions and drugs alter serum thyroxine levels without affecting clinical status (Table 25–7). Furthermore, a serum thyroxine determination is not sufficiently sensitive to detect mild degrees of hypo- or hyperthyroidism. Therefore, other tests have been developed, but all are imperfect.

TESTS OF THYROID FUNCTION (Table 25–8)

The tests most widely used in clinical practice are T_4 and "free" T_4 immunoassays. When the latter is not available, the resin uptake of T_3 (with determination of free thyroxine index) is useful. The TSH assay has been of great help in diagnosis.

1. SERUM THYROID TESTS

Free Thyroxine Immunoassay (FT₄)

Adult normal range: 0.9–1.7 ng/dL. (Varies with assay. Higher in newborns and in children.)

FT_4 is a direct measurement of the serum concentration of free (unbound) thyroxine. FT_4 represents only about 0.025% of the serum concentration of the

Table 25–7. Factors altering serum thyroxine measurements without affecting clinical status.[1,2]

Factors Increasing T_4	Factors Decreasing T_4
Acute illness (eg, viral hepatitis, chronic active hepatitis; primary biliary cirrhosis; acute intermittent porphyria; AIDS)	Severe illness (eg, chronic renal failure, major surgery, caloric deprivation)
High-estrogen states (may also increase T_3)	Acute psychiatric problems
Oral estrogen-containing contraceptives	Cirrhosis
Pregnancy	Nephrotic syndrome
Estrogen replacement therapy	Hereditary TBG deficiency
Neonatal period	Drugs
Acute psychiatric problems	Phenobarbital
Hyperemesis gravidarum and morning sickness (may also increase T_3)	Phenytoin (T_4 may be as low as 2 µg/dL)
Familial dysalbuminemic hyperthyroxinemia	Carbamazepine
Familial X-linked TBG excess (may also increase T_3)	Triiodothyronine (T_3) therapy
Generalized resistance to thyroid hormone (Refetoff's syndrome)	Androgens
Drugs	Fluorouracil
Levothyroxine (T_4) replacement therapy	Halofenate (lowers triglycerides and uric acid; not marketed in USA)
Amiodarone	Mitotane
Heparin, intravenously	Phenylbutazone
Amphetamines	Fenclofenac (nonsteroidal anti-inflammatory agent; not marketed in USA)
Methadone (may also increase T_3)	Salicylates (large doses)
Heroin	Chloral hydrate
Perphenazine	Asparaginase
Clofibrate	

[1]Reproduced, with permission from Fitzgerald PA: *Handbook of Clinical Endocrinology.* Appleton & Lange, 1992.
[2]Symptomatic hyperthyroidism or hypothyroidism may also be present incidentally.

Table 25–8. Appropriate use of thyroid tests.

Purpose	Test	Comment
Screening	Free T$_4$	Excellent test
	T$_4$ (RIA)	Varies with TBG
	T$_3$ resin uptake	Varies with TBG
	Free thyroxine index	Useful combination
For hypothyroidism	Serum TSH	Primary versus secondary hypothyroidism. "Feedback" T$_4$ and T$_3$.
	Antithyroglobulin and anti-microsomal antibodies	Elevated in Hashimoto's thyroiditis
For hyperthyroidism	Serum TSH (sensitive assay)	Usually suppressed
	T$_3$ (RIA)	Elevated
	^{123}I uptake and scan	Increased diffuse versus "hot" areas
	Antithyroglobulin and anti-microsomal	Elevated in Graves' disease
	Thyroid-stimulating immunoglobulin (TSI)	Usually positive in Graves' disease
For nodules	Fine-needle aspiration	Best diagnostic method for thyroid cancer
	^{123}I uptake and scan	"Warm" versus "cold"
	^{99m}Tc scan	Vascular versus avascular
	Echo scan	Solid versus cystic. Pure cysts are usually not malignant.
	Thyroglobulin (TG)	High in metastatic, papillary, or follicular carcinomas and thyroiditis
	Calcitonin	High in medullary thyroid and other carcinomas

total T$_4$. It is the only metabolically active fraction of T$_4$ that freely enters cells to produce its effects.

When performed properly, this assay is superior to the total T$_4$ assay and free thyroxine index, since it is not affected by variations in protein binding. It is the procedure of choice for following the thyroid's changing secretion of T$_4$ during treatment for hyperthyroidism. Unfortunately, even the FT$_4$ assay has some shortcomings; serum FT$_4$ levels may be suppressed in patients with severe nonthyroid illness. FT$_4$ levels (in vitro) can be misleadingly low in euthyroid patients receiving heparin even in the small doses from a heparin lock. Serum FT$_4$ levels may rise transiently in acute nonthyroidal illness, when TBP frequently falls.

T$_4$ Immunoassay

Adult normal range: 5–11 μg/dL. (Varies with assay. Higher in newborns and in children.)

This test measures the total serum concentration of thyroxine (bound and free). An increased serum T$_4$ confirms a clinical diagnosis of hyperthyroidism, while a decreased serum T$_4$ confirms a clinical diagnosis of hypothyroidism. It is affected by altered states of thyroxine binding (see Table 25–7). Therefore, this test is usually run with a resin T$_3$ uptake to provide a free thyroxine index (see below).

Resin T$_3$ (or T$_4$) Uptake

Normal range: 25–35%. (Varies with assay.)

This is an indirect inverse test of serum thyroid-binding proteins (TBP)—ie, it is high when thyroid-binding proteins are low. It is used because direct measurement of the various thyroid-binding proteins is rather difficult. The assay involves adding labeled T$_3$ or T$_4$ to a sample of the patient's serum; it is allowed to compete and equilibrate with the patient's thyroxine for binding to TBP. An aliquot of this mixture is then added to a thyroid hormone-binding resin. The resin is then assayed for its uptake of the label. A high resin uptake indicates that the patient's serum contains relatively low amounts of TBP or high levels of thyroxine.

This test is used as a "fudge factor" to correct a total serum thyroxine measurement for the effect of increased or decreased binding, creating a free thyroxine index (see below). A low resin uptake (high TBP) is seen with estrogen therapy, pregnancy, acute hepatitis, genetic TBP increase, and hypothyroidism. A low resin uptake with low TBP may be seen in severe illness. A high resin uptake (low TBP) is seen with chronic liver disease, nephrotic syndrome, anabolic steroid administration, high-dose glucocorticoid administration, and hyperthyroidism.

Free Thyroxine Index (FTI)

The normal range varies in different laboratories. It is higher in newborns and children than in adults.

The product of T_4 and resin T_3 uptake ($T_4 \times T_3$ uptake) helps correct for abnormalities of thyroxine binding. If a good free T_4 assay is available, this calculation is unnecessary.

The FTI, when calculated using the RT_3U, may be elevated in euthyroid patients with familial dysalbuminemic hyperthyroxinemia. This is a benign autosomal dominant trait in which an abnormal albumin molecule binds T_4 with much greater affinity than T_3. The RT_3U is not decreased (failing to compensate for the increased binding, as it would for TBG excess), because the T_3 used in the RT_3U assay is not significantly affected. Serum levels of free thyroxine and TSH are normal.

T_3

Adult normal: 95–190 ng/mL. (Higher in newborns and children.)

This test is of value in the diagnosis of thyrotoxicosis with normal T_4 values (T_3 thyrotoxicosis). It is not useful for the diagnosis of hypothyroidism.

2. THYROID RADIOACTIVE IODINE UPTAKE & SCAN

Radioiodine (^{123}I) Uptake of Thyroid Gland

Normal in the USA: 5–15% at 5 hours and 10–30% at 24 hours. The normal range has been markedly lowered in the USA because of an increased of dietary intake of iodine.

A. Elevated: Graves' disease, dietary iodine deficiency, toxic nodular goiter, pregnancy, early Hashimoto's thyroiditis, some thyroid enzyme deficiencies, nephrotic syndrome, recovery from subacute thyroiditis, recovery from thyroid hormone suppression.

B. Low: Administration of iodides or iodine in any form (drugs, radiology contrast dyes, etc), antithyroid drugs, subacute thyroiditis, thyroid hormone administration, thyroid gland damage (from thyroiditis, surgery, or radioiodine), hypopituitarism, ectopic functioning thyroid tissue, thyroid aplasia, azotemia, severe (high-turnover) Graves' disease, heart failure, and some thyroid enzyme abnormalities.

A rectilinear scan over the thyroid may be obtained after ^{123}I administration, thereby obtaining a life-sized picture of thyroid uptake. A technetium 99m Tc camera scan may also be obtained for better resolution in some cases.

3. OTHER THYROID TESTS

Thyroid-Stimulating Hormone (TSH) Immunoassay

Adult normal range: 0.4–4.8 µU/mL. (Varies with assay. Higher in newborns and children.)

Immunoassays for TSH have become increasingly more sensitive. First-generation assays are able to detect TSH down to 1 µU/mL, second-generation assays down to 0.1 µU/mL, and third-generation assays down to 0.01 µU/mL. Laboratory technique also affects the assay's sensitivity. The clinician must know the sensitivity of the TSH assay used by a particular laboratory in order to know its diagnostic limitations.

TSH levels are elevated with any of the above assays in primary hypothyroidism, either clinical or subclinical. TSH may also be elevated or inappropriately normal in the very rare cases of hyperthyroidism due to pituitary neoplastic inappropriate secretion of thyrotropin or nonneoplastic inappropriate secretion of thyrotropin. TSH may be transiently elevated during recovery for nonthyroidal illness and in about 14% of patients with acute psychiatric admissions; the TSH returns to normal in the great majority of these patients. TSH may be mildly elevated as a normal variant in some individuals, especially the elderly (over 2% incidence). Such euthyroid patients with normal T_4 levels must be followed carefully, since about 18% later become hypothyroid.

TSH levels are decreased (in sensitive assays) in patients with primary hyperthyroidism (eg, Graves' disease, toxic multinodular goiter, toxic nodule, subacute thyroiditis, hashitoxicosis). TSH levels may also be suppressed in some clinically euthyroid individuals with autonomous thyroid secretion (eg, euthyroid Graves' ophthalmopathy). TSH can also be suppressed by thyroid hormone administration in either excessive or adequate replacement amounts. TSH is also frequently low during severe nonthyroidal illness; distinction from hypopituitarism can usually be made clinically and by using a good third-generation ultrasensitive assay: TSH levels are usually above 0.05 µU/mL in nonthyroidal illness. TSH levels are low or inappropriately normal in hypothyroidism due to pituitary insufficiency.

Dopamine can cause suppression of TSH and may cause true secondary hypothyroidism during prolonged administration. Other conditions associated with decreased TSH include pregnancy (especially with morning sickness), hCG-secreting trophoblastic tumors, acute psychiatric illness (1% incidence), and acute administration of glucocorticoids. Certain drugs cause mild suppression of TSH without clinical hypothyroidism; these include nonsteroidal anti-inflammatory agents, narcotics, and certain calcium channel blockers (especially nifedipine; also vera-pamil, but not diltiazem). TSH may be low as a normal variant, especially in the elderly (5% incidence, with an even higher incidence among men over age 70).

Effect of Nonthyroidal Illness & Drugs Upon Thyroid Function Tests

Many factors affect thyroid function tests, causing misleading laboratory evidence of hypothyroidism or hyperthyroidism in patients who are clinically euthyroid. See Table 25–8.

Patients with severe illness, caloric deprivation, or major surgery have a shift in the peripheral conversion of serum T_4 to more inactive reverse T_3 (rT_3) and less active T_3. In most patients who are critically ill, there is a circulating inhibitor of thyroid hormone binding to serum thyroid binding proteins. This causes the resin uptake of thyroid hormone (rT_3U) to be misleadingly low, causing the computed free thyroxine index to be very low. The presence of a very low serum T_4 in severe nonthyroidal illness indicates a poor prognosis. In one series of such patients with serum T_4 levels under 3 µg/dL, there was a mortality rate of 84%.

Direct assays of free thyroxine often show low levels of FT_4 in severe illness. Since studies of giving replacement thyroxine to such patients have shown no improvement in survival, they are considered "euthyroid." Serum TSH tends to be suppressed in severe nonthyroidal illness, making the diagnosis of primary hypothyroidism quite difficult, although the presence of a goiter suggests the diagnosis.

The clinician must decide whether such severely ill patients (with a low serum T_4 but nonelevated TSH) might have hypothyridism due to pituitary insufficiency. The distinction can usually be made by considering the clinical setting. Patients without symptoms of prior brain lesion or hypopituitarism are very unlikely to suddenly develop hypopituitarism during an unrelated illness. In adults, loss of beard, axillary, or pubic hair is a sign of chronic hypopituitarism. Although the serum TSH may be low in nonthyroidal illness, it is generally above 0.05 µU/mL in sensitive third-generation assays, helping distinguish it from hypopituitarism, in which the sensitive TSH levels is usually lower. Patients with diabetes insipidus, hypopituitarism or other signs of a central nervous system lesion may have thyroxine given empirically. Patients receiving prolonged dopamine infusions in the intensive care unit may develop true secondary hypothyroidism due to direct dopamine suppression of TSH-secreting cells; it is thus reasonable to give short courses of thyroxine to such patients.

Thyroid Antibodies

Antibodies against several thyroid constituents (antithyroglobulin and antimicrosomal) are most commonly found in Hashimoto's thyroiditis but are also found in most patients with Graves' disease. Antithyroid antibodies are found in about 5–10% of normal subjects. There is an increasing incidence with age. About 20% of hospitalized patients have detectable antithyroid antibodies. In the latter, the titers tend to be low, and they increase with age. Thyroid-stimulating immunoglobulin (TSI) titers are elevated in approximately 80% of patients with Graves' disease. These titers—and those of antithyroglobulin and antimicrosomal antibodies—often decrease during pregnancy and during treatment of Graves' disease with antithyroid drugs. TSI titers have been used with variable results to predict the rate of relapse of Graves' disease after chronic thiourea therapy and to predict neonatal hyperthyroidism.

Serum Thyroglobulin

The level of serum thyroglobulin rises in autoimmune thyroid disease, thyroid injury or inflammation, and thyroid cancer. Levels are of little value in diagnosing or distinguishing among these conditions, but they provide a useful marker in thyroid cancer to indicate recurrence of disease and the need for further studies and therapy. Do not confuse serum thyroglobulin with serum thyroid binding globulin (see above).

Ultrasound

This simple technique has been used to determine if thyroid lesions are solid or cystic. Cysts are less likely to be malignant, since thyroid carcinomas rarely undergo cystic degeneration. One should remember, however, that most solid lesions are also benign.

Fine-Needle Thyroid Biopsy

Aspiration of thyroid tissue with a fine needle (25-gauge) is helpful in the diagnosis of thyroid disorders, especially nodular lesions. This technique has become the preferred approach to the diagnosis of thyroid masses.

Calcitonin Assay

This test is elevated in newborns and in medullary thyroid carcinoma, azotemia, hypercalcemia, pernicious anemia, thyroiditis, and pregnancy. High levels are also seen in many malignancies other than medullary thyroid carcinoma.

Gharib H, Goellner JR: Fine-needle aspiration biopsy of the thyroid: An appraisal. Ann Intern Med 1993;118:282.

Lewis GF et al: Low serum free thyroxine index in ambulatory elderly is due to a resetting of the threshold for thyrotropin feedback suppression. J Clin Endocrinol Metab 1991;73:843.

Nicoloff JT, Spencer CA: The use and misuse of sensitive thyrotropin assays. J Clin Endocrinol Metab 1990; 71;553.

Parle JV et al: Prevalence and follow-up of abnormal thyrotrophin (TSH) concentrations in the elderly in the United Kingdom. Clin Endocrinol 1991;34:77.

ENDEMIC GOITER

Essentials of Diagnosis
- Common in regions of the world with low-iodine diets.
- High rate of congenital hypothyroidism and cretinism.
- Goiters may become multinodular and grow to great size.
- Most adults with endemic goiter are found to be euthyroid; however, some are hypothyroid or hyperthyroid.

General Considerations
Approximately 5% of the world's population have goiters. Of these, about 75% are in persons dwelling in geologic regions characterized by past or current unsupplemented iodine deficiency. Such areas include Central Africa, New Guinea, the Andes, and the Himalayas. In certain endemic areas, up to 50% of the population may have goiters. Up to 0.5% of such populations may have full-blown cretinism, with less severe manifestations of congenital hypothyroidism being even more common (eg, isolated deafness, short stature, or impaired mentation). Although iodine deficiency is the most common cause of endemic goiter, other goitrogenic substances exist in certain foods or water supplies that can themselves cause goiter or aggravate a goiter proclivity caused by iodine deficiency. Some individuals are particularly susceptible to goiter owing to congenital partial defects in thyroid enzyme activity.

Clinical Findings
A. Symptoms and Signs: Endemic goiters may become multinodular and very large, causing compressive symptoms. Endemic iodine-deficient goiters may enlarge during pregnancy, when a woman's iodine requirement increases. Although cretinism is more common with early childhood endemic goiter, most individuals with such goiters are euthyroid. Some may become hypothyroid. Others may become thyrotoxic as the goiter grows and becomes more autonomous. Such hyperthyroidism occurs especially if large amounts of iodine are suddenly added to the diet.

B. Laboratory Findings: The serum thyroxine is usually normal. Serum TSH is generally normal or slightly elevated. TSH falls in the presence of hyperthyroidism if a multinodular goiter has become autonomous in the presence of sufficient amounts of iodine for thyroid hormone synthesis. Thyroid radioactive iodine uptake is usually elevated, but it may be normal if the iodine intake has improved. Serum levels of antithyroid antibodies are usually either undetectable or in low titers.

Differential Diagnosis
Endemic goiter must be distinguished from all other forms of goiter that may coexist in an endemic region.

Prevention
Before the days of dietary iodine supplementation, the Great Lakes region of the USA was known as a "goiter belt." In certain cantons of Switzerland, nearly all schoolchildren had goiters and 30% of young men were declared unfit for military service because of their large goiters. Iodine supplementation was started in Switzerland in 1922, initially by adding 3.75 mg of iodide per kilogram of salt, with later increases to the current level of 15 mg/kg salt. This practice has virtually eliminated endemic iodine-deficient goiter and cretinism. The minimum dietary requirement for iodine is about 50 μg daily, with optimal iodine intake being 150–300 μg daily.

Treatment
Dietary supplementation with iodine successfully prevents iodine-deficient goiter and cretinism but is less successful in shrinking established goiter in such regions. Attempts to shrink such goiters with thyroxine are generally unsuccessful. Furthermore, unless the individual is hypothyroid, thyroxine supplementation may cause thyrotoxicosis, since nodular goiters tend to become autonomous over time. Adults with large multinodular goiter may require thyroidectomy for cosmesis, compressive symptoms, or thyrotoxicosis; but following partial thyroidectomy in iodine-deficient geographic areas, there is a high goiter recurrence rate.

Greenspan FS: The problem of the multinodular goiter. Med Clin North Am 1991;75:195.
Woeber KA: Iodine and thyroid disease. Med Clin North Am 1991;75:169.

HYPOTHYROIDISM

Thyroid hormone deficiency may affect virtually all body functions. The degree of severity ranges from mild and unrecognized hypothyroid states to striking myxedema.

Hypothyroidism may be due to primary disease of the thyroid gland itself or lack of pituitary TSH or hypothalamic TRH. A true end-organ insensitivity to normal amounts of circulating hormone has been rarely observed. Although gross forms of hypothyroidism, ie, myxedema and cretinism, are readily recognized on clinical grounds alone, the far more common mild forms often escape detection without adequate laboratory testing.

1. CRETINISM & JUVENILE HYPOTHYROIDISM

Congenital hypothyroidism occurs in the USA in about one in 4000 births. Untreated, it results in a syndrome called cretinism. Acquired hypothyroidism is fairly common in children. (See also above.)

The causes of cretinism and juvenile hypothyroidism are as follows:

A. Congenital (Cretinism):

1. Thyroid gland absent or rudimentary (embryogenic defect; most cases of sporadic cretinism).

2. Thyroid gland present but defective in hormone secretion. Due to deficient iodine or goitrogenic substances (in most cases of endemic cretinism); or due to familial enzymatic defects in thyroid hormone synthesis. Deficiency in pituitary TSH occurs occasionally.

B. Acquired (Juvenile Hypothyroidism): Atrophy of the gland or defective function may be due to unknown causes, thyroiditis, or operative removal (lingual thyroid or toxic goiter) or secondary to pituitary deficiency.

Clinical Findings

A. Symptoms and Signs: Delayed growth and skeletal maturation; apathy; physical and mental torpor; dry skin with coarse, dry, brittle hair; constipation; slow teething; poor appetite; large tongue; "pot belly" with umbilical hernia; deep voice; cold extremities and cold sensitivity; and true myxedema of subcutaneous and other tissues. A yellow skin due to carotenemia is not infrequent. The thyroid gland is usually not palpable, but a large goiter may be present that may be diffusely enlarged or nodular. Sexual development is usually retarded, but maturation eventually occurs. Conversely, some children with severe hypothyroidism have precocious puberty. Deafness is occasionally associated with congenital goiter (Pendred's syndrome).

Critical thyroid-dependent brain development occurs during the first 18 months of life. A delay of only 3 months in treatment of neonatal hypothyroidism causes significant irreversible mental retardation.

Acquired juvenile hypothyroidism occurring after 18 months is associated with reversible mental slowness. Such patients are often considered quiet, "good" children and may actually do well in school. Growth is usually delayed. Hypothyroidism diagnosed in early childhood (ages 1–5 years) is usually due to maldeveloped or ectopic thyroid tissue. Goiter in such cases is usually absent, but lingual thyroid tissue at the base of the tongue is sometimes seen.

B. Laboratory Findings: Screening tests for hypothyroidism are suggested for all newborns; a TSH over 30 μU/mL or a T_4 under 6 μg/dL is suggestive of neonatal hypothyroidism. Note that TSH levels in newborns are normally higher than adult levels; TSH values then normally decline during the neonatal period. Serum T_4 levels also fluctuate in the newborn; levels of 4.6–13 μg/dL are seen in cord blood and increase to 11.8–23.2 μg/dL at 1–3 days, declining gradually thereafter.

C. Imaging: Delayed skeletal maturation is a constant finding, often with "stippling" of the epiphyses (especially of the femoral head), with flattening; widening of the cortices of the long bones, absence of the cranial sinuses, and delayed dentition may also be noted.

Differential Diagnosis

It is important to measure serum TSH to differentiate primary hypothyroidism (high) from pituitary failure (low). Cretinism is sometimes confused with Down's syndrome, although retarded skeletal development is rare in mongoloid infants. In children and adolescents, any unexplained decrease in the rate of growth should alert the physician to the possibility of early hypothyroidism.

Treatment

See Myxedema, below.

Prognosis

The progress and outcome of the disease depend largely upon the duration of thyroid deficiency and the adequacy and persistence of treatment. Since mental development is at stake, it is of utmost importance to start treatment early.

The prognosis for full mental and physical maturation is much better if the onset of disease occurs later in life. Congenital cretins often have variable degrees of permanent intellectual impairment. With implementation of large-scale thyroid screening programs at birth, appropriate therapy is being instituted much earlier than before, and patients so treated have reasonably normal mental development.

By and large, the response to thyroid therapy is gratifying, but thyroxine replacement therapy usually must be continued throughout life.

Larsen PR: Maternal thyroxine and congenital hypothyroidism. N Engl J Med 1989;321:44.

Rallison ML et al: Natural history of thyroid abnormalities: Prevalence, incidence, and regression of thyroid disease in adolescents and young adults. Am J Med 1991;91:363.

Willi SM, Neoshang T Jr: Diagnostic dilemmas: Results of screening tests for hypothyroidism. Pediatr Clin North Am 1991;38:555.

2. ADULT HYPOTHYROIDISM & MYXEDEMA

Essentials of Diagnosis

- Weakness, fatigue, cold intolerance, constipation, weight change, depression, menorrhagia, hoarseness.

- Dry, cold, yellow, puffy skin; scant eyebrows; thick tongue; bradycardia; delayed return of deep tendon reflexes.
- Anemia, hyponatremia.
- T_4 and radioiodine uptake usually low.
- TSH elevated in primary myxedema.

General Considerations

Goiter is frequently noted when hypothyroidism is due to Hashimoto's thyroiditis, iodide deficiency, genetic thyroid enzyme defects, drug goitrogens (lithium, iodide, propylthiouracil or methimazole, phenylbutazone, sulfonamides, amiodarone), food goitrogens in iodide-deficient areas (eg, turnips, cassavas), or, rarely, peripheral resistance to thyroid hormone or infiltrating diseases (eg, cancer, sarcoidosis).

Goiter is usually absent when hypothyroidism is due to: deficient pituitary TSH secretion, thyroid dysgenesis, or destruction of the gland by surgery, external radiation, or ^{131}I. Primary hypothyroidism may also be idiopathic.

Amiodarone, because of its high iodine content, causes clinically significant hypothyroidism in about 8% of patients. The T_4 level is normal or low, and the TSH is elevated, usually over 20 ng/dL. Another 17% of patients develop milder elevations of TSH and are asymptomatic. Cardiac patients with amiodarone-induced symptomatic hypothyroidism are treated with just enough thyroxine to relieve symptoms.

Clinical Findings

These may vary from the rather rare full-blown myxedema to mild states of hypothyroidism, which are far more common and may escape detection unless looked for.

A. Symptoms and Signs:

1. Early–The principal symptoms are weakness, fatigue, arthralgias or myalgias, muscle cramps, cold intolerance, constipation, lethargy, dryness of skin, headache, and menorrhagia. Physical findings may be few or absent. Outstanding features are thin, brittle nails; thinning of hair, which may be coarse; and pallor, with poor turgor of the mucosa. Delayed return of deep tendon reflexes is often noted.

2. Late–The principal symptoms are slow speech, absence of sweating, constipation, peripheral edema, pallor, hoarseness, decreased sense of taste and smell, muscle cramps, aches and pains, dyspnea, weight changes (usually gain, but weight loss is not rare), and deafness. Some women have amenorrhea; others have menorrhagia. Galactorrhea may also be present. Physical findings include puffiness of the face and eyelids, typical carotenemic skin color, thinning of the outer halves of the eyebrows, thickening of the tongue, hard pitting edema, and effusions into the pleural, peritoneal, and pericardial cavities, as well as into joints. Cardiac enlargement ("myxedema heart") is often due to pericardial effusion. The heart rate is slow; the blood pressure is more often normal than low, and even diastolic hypertension reversible with treatment may be found. Hypothermia may be present. Pituitary enlargement due to hyperplasia of TSH-secreting cells, which is reversible following thyroid therapy, may be seen in long-standing hypothyroidism. True obesity is relatively unusual in hypothyroidism.

B. Laboratory Findings: The T_4 is usually under 5.0 µg/dL; the free T_4 is less than 0.9 ng/dL. TSH is increased in patients with primary hypothyroidism. Serum T_4 levels may be low or low-normal. Other laboratory abnormalities may often be seen: increased serum cholesterol, liver enzymes, and creatine kinase; increased serum prolactin; hyponatremia, hypoglycemia, and anemia (with normal or increased corpuscular volume). Antithyroid antibody titers (antimicrosomal and antithyroglobulin) are high in patients with Hashimoto's thyroiditis. Serum T_3 is not a good test for hypothyroidism.

A number of factors can lower serum T_4 levels without causing true hypothyroidism (Table 25–7). Euthyroid patients with severe nonthyroidal illness often have decreased serum free T_4 and free thyroxine indices. TSH levels are usually not elevated, helping make the distinction from true primary hypothyroidism. Patients with severe illness (with low serum T_4 and without elevated TSH) can usually be assumed not to have hypopituitarism (TSH deficiency) in the absence of pituitary or hypothalamic disease or other pituitary hormone deficiencies. The hypothyroxinemia of severe illness is not thought to be clinically significant, since treatment of such patients with thyroxine does not improve survival.

Differential Diagnosis

Hypothyroidism must be considered in many states of neurasthenia, unexplained menstrual disorders, myalgias, constipation, weight change, hyperlipidemia, and anemia. Myxedema enters into the differential diagnosis of unexplained heart failure that does not respond to digitalis or diuretics, and unexplained ascites. The protein content of myxedematous effusions is high. The thick tongue may be confused with that seen in primary amyloidosis. Pernicious anemia may be suggested by the pallor and the macrocytic anemia sometimes seen in myxedema; the two disorders may even coexist. Some cases of depression, primary psychosis and structural diseases of the brain have been confused with myxedema. The pituitary is often quite enlarged in primary hypothyroidism due to reversible hyperplasia of TSH-secreting cells; the concomitant hyperprolactinemia seen in hypothyroidism can lead to the mistaken diagnosis of a pituitary adenoma.

Complications

Complications are mostly cardiac in nature, occurring as a result of advanced coronary artery disease and congestive failure, which may be precipitated by too vigorous thyroid therapy. There is an increased susceptibility to infection. Megacolon has been described in long-standing hypothyroidism. Organic psychoses with paranoid delusions may occur ("myxedema madness"). Rarely, adrenal crisis may be precipitated by thyroid therapy of pituitary or primary myxedema. Hypothyroidism is a rare cause of infertility, which may respond to thyroid medication. Pregnancy in a woman with untreated hypothyroidism often results in miscarriage. On the other hand, if the hypothyroidism is due to autoimmune disease, it may improve during pregnancy. Sellar enlargement and even well-defined TSH-secreting tumors may develop in untreated cases. These tumors decrease in size after replacement therapy is instituted.

A rare complication of severe hypothyroidism is deep stupor, at times progressing to **myxedema coma,** with severe hypothermia, hypoventilation, hypoxia, hypercapnia, and hypotension. Water intoxication and severe hyponatremia are common. Convulsions and abnormal central nervous system signs may occur. Myxedema coma is often induced by an underlying infection; cardiac, respiratory, or central nervous system illness; cold exposure; or drug use. It is most often seen in elderly women. The mortality rate is high. Myxedematous patients are unusually sensitive to opiates and may die from average doses.

Refractory hyponatremia is often seen in severe myxedema. Inappropriate secretion of antidiuretic hormone has been observed in some patients, but a defect in distal tubular reabsorption of sodium and water has been demonstrated in many others.

Treatment

A. Specific Therapy: Levothyroxine is the drug of choice. Other thyroid preparations are still available (Table 25–9), but their use is discouraged. Levothyroxine is readily available, inexpensive, and well standardized. Levothyroxine is converted in the body to T_3, the most active thyroid hormone, in an enzymatically regulated manner that best meets the metabolic needs of the patient.

1. When treating patients with severe myxedema or myxedema heart disease—or elderly patients with hypothyroidism who have other associated heart disease—begin with small doses of levothyroxine, 25–

50 µg daily for 1 week, and increase the dose every 1–2 weeks by 25 µg daily up to a total of 100–150 µg daily. This dosage should be continued as long as signs of hypothyroidism have vanished and the TSH normalizes.

2. Patients with early hypothyroidism may be started with larger doses, 50–100 µg daily, increasing by 25 µg every 1–2 weeks until the TSH normalizes.

3. Maintenance–Each patient's dose must be adjusted to obtain the optimal effect. The proper dose should be decided mainly by careful clinical assessment. A serum TSH can be helpful, since persistently elevated levels usually indicate underreplacement with thyroxine. Once a patient is feeling completely well, the dose is kept constant, and repeat determinations of serum thyroxine or TSH are unnecessary and can be misleading. Serum thyroxine is usually high-normal or high in patients receiving adequate doses of a purely T_4 compound. Serum thyroxine levels in euthyroid patients may be quite high in patients also taking estrogen preparations. Serum TSH should be normal or slightly low. Most patients require 100–200 µg daily for maintenance.

4. Myxedema coma is a medical emergency with a high mortality rate. Levothyroxine sodium is given intravenously and repeated daily in a dose of 100 µg. Hydrocortisone, 100 mg as an initial bolus, followed by 25–50 mg every 8 hours, may be lifesaving. The patient must not be warmed except by blanket. Infection is often present and must be aggressively treated. Assisted mechanical ventilation is almost always necessary to correct the hypercapnia.

5. There are special situations where the daily maintenance dose of thyroxine may have to be altered: Slightly higher doses may be necessary during pregnancy or in patients taking phenobarbital or bile acid binding resins. Conversely, lower doses are often required in aging patients.

B. Needless Use of Thyroid: Thyroid medication should not be used as nonspecific stimulating therapy. The doses usually employed merely suppress the activity of the patient's own gland. Larger doses given to euthyroid individuals to induce weight loss may induce cardiac arrhythmias, osteoporosis, muscle weakness, and anxiety.

The use of thyroid in cases of amenorrhea or infertility is indicated only if the patient is proved to be hypothyroid.

Prognosis

The patient may rarely die from the complications of myxedema coma. With early treatment, striking transformations take place both in appearance and mental function. Return to a normal state is usually the rule, but relapses will occur if treatment is interrupted. On the whole, response to thyroid treatment is most satisfactory. Chronic maintenance therapy with unduly large doses of thyroid hormone may lead to

Table 25–9. Approximate equivalency of thyroid preparations.

Levothyroxine Sodium (Levothroid, Synthroid, etc)	Liothyronine Sodium (T3, Cytomel)	Liotrix (Euthroid, Thyrolar)
0.05 mg	12.5 µg	Code: ½
0.1 mg	25 µg	1
0.2 mg	50 µg	2
0.3 mg	75 µg	3

subtle but important side effects (eg, bone demineralization) and is to be avoided.

Camargo CA: Hypothyroidism and goiter during pregnancy. In: *Endocrine Disorders in Pregnancy.* Brody SA, Ueland K (editors). Appleton & Lange, 1989.

Gavin LA: Thyroid crises. Med Clin North Am 1991; 75:179.

Myers L, Hays J: Myxedema coma. Crit Care Clin 1991; 7:43.

Nademanee K et al: Amiodarone and thyroid function. Prog Cardiovasc Dis 1989;31:427.

Utiger RD: Therapy of hypothyroidism: When are changes needed? N Engl J Med 1990;323:126.

Wolf PG, Meek JC: Practical approach to the treatment of hypothyroidism. Am Fam Physician 1992;45:722.

HYPERTHYROIDISM
(Thyrotoxicosis)

Essentials of Diagnosis

- Sweating, weight change, nervousness, loose stools, heat intolerance, irritability, fatigue, weakness, menstrual irregularity.
- Tachycardia; warm, thin, soft, moist skin; stare; tremor.
- In Graves' disease: goiter (often with bruit); ophthalmopathy.
- Suppressed TSH in primary hyperthyroidism; increased T_4, free T_4, and free T_4 index.

General Considerations

The term "thyrotoxicosis" denotes a series of clinical disorders associated with increased circulating levels of free thyroxine or triiodothyronine.

The various causes include the following:

(1) Graves' disease: By far the most common form of thyrotoxicosis is that associated with diffuse enlargement of the thyroid, hyperactivity of the gland, and the presence of antibodies against different fractions of the thyroid gland. This autoimmune thyroid disorder is called **Graves' disease** (Basedow's disease). It is much more common in women than in men (8:1), and its onset is usually between the ages of 20 and 40. It may be accompanied by infiltrative ophthalmopathy (Graves' exophthalmos) and, less commonly, by infiltrative dermopathy (pretibial myxedema). It may also be associated with other systemic autoimmune disorders such as pernicious anemia, myasthenia gravis, diabetes mellitus, etc. It has a familial tendency, and histocompatibility studies have shown an association with group HLA-B8 and HLA-DR3. The pathogenesis of the hyperthyroidism of Graves' disease involves the formation of autoantibodies that bind to the TSH receptor in thyroid cell membranes and stimulate the gland to hyperfunction. These thyroid-stimulating immunoglobulins (TSI) are demonstrable in the plasma of about 80% patients with Graves' disease. Other antibodies are generated in Graves' disease, with antimicrosomal or antithyroglobulin antibodies being increased in most patients.

(2) Autonomous toxic adenomas of the thyroid may be single (Plummer's disease) or multiple (toxic multinodular goiter). This is not accompanied by infiltrative ophthalmopathy or dermopathy. Antithyroid antibodies are usually not present in the plasma, and tests for TSI are negative.

(3) Subacute thyroiditis (thought to be due to viral infection) is characterized by a moderately enlarged, tender thyroid. Radioactive iodine uptake is low. If the gland is nontender, the disorder is called "silent thyroiditis." Interleukin-2 therapy can cause a similar problem; hyperthyroidism is followed by hypothyroidism. During thyrotoxicosis, thyroid RAIU is low. Treatment is with propranolol and analgesics until the condition subsides, usually over several months.

(4) Jodbasedow disease, or iodine-induced hyperthyroidism, may occur in patients with multinodular goiters after intake of large amounts of iodine in the form of radiographic contrast materials or drugs, especially amiodarone.

(5) Thyrotoxicosis factitia is due to ingestion of excessive amounts of exogenous thyroid hormone. An unusual variant has been reported, with epidemics of thyrotoxicosis due to consumption of ground beef contaminated with bovine thyroid gland.

(6) Struma ovarii: Thyroid tissue is contained in about 3% of ovarian dermoid tumors and teratomas. This thyroid tissue may autonomously secrete thyroid hormone due to a toxic nodule or in concert with the woman's thyroid gland in Graves' disease or toxic multinodular goiter.

(7) TSH-secreting tumor of the pituitary gland is a rare cause of hyperthyroidism. Serum TSH is normal or elevated (ie, not suppressed as determined by a sensitive TSH assay) in the presence of thyrotoxicosis. No ophthalmopathy is present. Antithyroid antibodies and TSI are usually normal. It may be caused by a pituitary adenoma, in which case it is known as neoplastic inappropriate secretion of thyrotropin. The tumor may present as a mass lesion following treatment of hyperthyroidism (mistaken for Graves' disease) with radioactive iodide or surgery. The adenoma can usually be seen on MRI of the pituitary. Treatment usually consists of transsphenoidal selective resection of the adenoma when possible. Large tumors may require radiation therapy. Tumors may sometimes also respond to bromocriptine or octreotide. Hyperthyroidism is treated symptomatically with propranolol.

This condition may also be due to pituitary hyperplasia, in which case it is known as "nontumorous inappropriate secretion of thyrotropin)." Pituitary hyperplasia may be detected on MRI scan as pituitary enlargement without a discrete adenoma being visible. This condition appears to be due to a diminished feedback effect of T_4 upon the pituitary. It may be familial, but it can also be caused by prolonged untreated hypothyroidism, especially in youth. Hyperthyroid symptoms are treated with propranolol. Definitive treatment is with radioactive iodine or thyroid surgery.

(8) Hashimoto's thyroiditis may cause with transient hyperthyroidism during the initial destructive phase. It may occur transiently postpartum.

(9) hCG-secreting trophoblastic tumors of the testis or ovary secrete huge amounts of hCG, which resemble TSH enough that thyroid TSH receptors are stimulated to produce hyperthyroidism.

(10) Metastatic functioning thyroid carcinoma is a rare cause of thyrotoxicosis.

(11) Amiodarone causes symptomatic hyperthyroidism in about 2.5% of patients. Since high levels of T_4 and free T_4 are normally seen in patients taking amiodarone, suppressed TSH (sensitive assay) must be present along with a greatly elevated T_4 (> 20 μg/dL) or T_3 (> 200 ng/dL). Treatment involves withdrawing the drug. Other options include thiourea drugs and radioactive iodine if the radioiodine uptake is adequate for treatment.

Clinical Findings

A. Symptoms and Signs: Thyrotoxicosis due to any cause produces many different manifestations of variable intensity among different individuals. Patients may complain of nervousness, restlessness, heat intolerance, increased sweating, fatigue, weakness, muscle cramps, frequent bowel movements, or weight change (usually loss). There may be palpitations or angina pectoris. Women frequently report menstrual irregularities. Hypokalemic periodic paralysis may occur, especially in Asian or Native American men.

Signs of thyrotoxicosis may include stare and lid lag, tachycardia or atrial fibrillation, fine resting finger tremors, moist warm skin, hyperreflexia, fine hair, onycholysis, and (rarely) heart failure. Chronic thyrotoxicosis may cause osteoporosis. At times there may be clubbing and swelling of the fingers (acropachy). Graves' disease usually presents with additional findings of goiter (often with a bruit). Ophthalmopathy occurs in most patients with Graves' disease, but only 5–10% manifest severe eye changes; chemosis and conjunctivitis are frequent. Lymphocytic infiltration of the eye muscles produces exophthalmos and sometimes diplopia due to extraocular muscle entrapment. The optic nerve may be compressed in severe cases. Corneal drying may occur with inadequate lid closure. Eye changes may sometimes be asymmetric or unilateral. The severity of the eye disease is not closely correlated with the severity of the thyrotoxicosis. In some cases of ophthalmopathy, the patient may be clinically euthyroid. Skin changes include occasional vitiligo and "myxedema"; the latter occurs in about 3% of Graves' dis-

ease patients and usually in the pretibial region. Its texture resembles the skin of an orange.

Thyroid "storm," rarely seen today, is an extreme form of thyrotoxicosis that may occur with stressful illness, thyroid surgery, or radioactive iodine administration and is manifested by marked delirium, severe tachycardia, vomiting, diarrhea, dehydration, and, in many cases, very high fever. The mortality rate is high.

B. Laboratory Diagnosis: Serum T_3, T_4, thyroid resin uptake, and free thyroxine index are usually all increased. Sometimes the T_4 level may be normal but the serum T_3 elevated. A reliable TSH assay is the most sensitive test for thyrotoxicosis; it is suppressed except in the very rare cases of pituitary inappropriate secretion of thyrotropin. Other laboratory abnormalities may include hypercalcemia, increased alkaline phosphatase, anemia, and decreased granulocytes.

Patients with Graves' disease usually also have increased serum antimicrosomal or antithyroglobulin antibodies. TSI levels also are usually high (80%), but TSI measurement is not ordinarily required for diagnosis. Antithyroglobulin or antimicrosomal antibodies are usually elevated in Graves' disease; serum ANA and anti-double-stranded DNA antibodies are also usually elevated without any evidence of lupus erythematosus or other collagen vascular disease.

Patients with subacute thyroiditis often have an increased erythrocyte sedimentation rate.

Thyroid radioactive iodine uptake and scan is usually performed on patients with an established diagnosis of thyrotoxicosis. A high radioactive iodine uptake is seen in Graves' disease and toxic nodular goiter but can be seen in other conditions as well. A low radioactive iodine uptake is characteristic of subacute thyroiditis but can also be seen in other conditions. (For conditions affecting radioactive iodine uptake, see section tests of thyroid function.)

C. Imaging: MRI of the orbits is the imaging method of choice to visualize Graves' ophthalmopathy affecting the extraocular muscles. CT scanning and ultrasound can also be used. Imaging is required only in severe cases or in euthyroid exophthalmos that must be distinguished from orbital tumors or other disorders.

Differential Diagnosis

True thyrotoxicosis must be distinguished from those condition elevating serum thyroxine without affecting clinical status (Table 25–7).

Hyperthyroidism may be confused with anxiety neurosis or mania, but in the latter the thyroid is not enlarged and thyroid function tests are usually normal. Problems of diagnosis occur in patients with acute psychiatric disorders, about 30% of whom have hyperthyroxinemia without thyrotoxicosis. The TSH is not suppressed, distinguishing psychiatric disorder from true hyperthyroidism. Levels return to normal gradually.

Exogenous thyroid administration will present the same laboratory features as thyroiditis. A rare pituitary tumor may produce the picture of thyrotoxicosis with high levels of TSH.

Some states of hypermetabolism without thyrotoxicosis—notably severe anemia, leukemia, polycythemia, and cancer—rarely cause confusion. Pheochromocytoma is often associated with hypermetabolism, tachycardia, weight loss, and profuse sweating. Acromegaly may also produce tachycardia, sweating, and thyroid enlargement. Appropriate laboratory tests will easily distinguish these entities.

Cardiac disease (eg, atrial fibrillation, cardiac failure) refractory to treatment with digitalis, quinidine, or diuretics suggests the possibility of underlying ("apathetic") hyperthyroidism. Other causes of ophthalmoplegia (eg, myasthenia gravis) and exophthalmos (eg, orbital tumor) must be considered. Graves' ophthalmopathy closely resembles pseudotumor of the orbit. Thyrotoxicosis must also be considered in the differential diagnosis of muscle weakness and osteoporosis. Hypercalciuria and bone demineralization may resemble hyperparathyroidism. Diabetes mellitus and Addison's disease may coexist with thyrotoxicosis.

Complications

Cardiac complications of thyrotoxicosis include atrial fibrillation with a ventricular response that is difficult to control. Episodes of periodic paralysis induced by exercise or heavy carbohydrate ingestion and accompanied by hypokalemia may complicate thyrotoxicosis in Oriental men. Hypercalcemia and nephrocalcinosis may occur. Decreased libido, impotence, decreased sperm count, and gynecomastia may be noted in men with hyperthyroidism.

Treatment

The methods used to treat thyrotoxicosis will vary according to several considerations, including the cause and severity of the hyperthyroidism, the patient's age, the clinical situation, and the desires of the patient.

A. Graves' Disease: The treatment of Graves' disease involves a choice of methods rather than a method of choice:

1. Propranolol–Propranolol is generally used for symptomatic relief until the hyperthyroidism is resolved. It effectively relieves the tachycardia, tremor, diaphoresis, and anxiety that occur with hyperthyroidism due to any cause. It is the initial treatment of choice for thyroid storm. The periodic paralysis seen in association with thyrotoxicosis, especially among Oriental men, is also effectively treated with beta blockade. It has no effect on thyroid hormone secretion. Treatment is usually begun with 10 mg orally and increased progressively until an ad-

equate response is achieved. The ultimate dosage required is usually 20 mg four times daily, but doses as high as 80 mg four times daily are occasionally required.

2. Thiourea drugs–Methimazole or propylthiouracil is generally used for children, young adults, or pregnant women and for patients with mild thyrotoxicosis, small goiters, or fear of isotopes. These drugs are also useful for preparing hyperthyroid patients for surgery and elderly patients for radioactive iodide treatment. They drugs do not permanently damage the thyroid and are associated with a lower chance of posttreatment hypothyroidism (compared with radioactive iodide or surgery). Unfortunately, there is a high rate of recurrent hyperthyroidism (over 50%) after a year or more of therapy. A greater likelihood of long-term remission is seen in patients with small goiters or mild hyperthyroidism. Patients whose microsomal and thyroglobulin antibodies remain high after 2 years of therapy have been reported to have only a 10% rate of relapse.

a. Methimazole–Methimazole is the thiourea drug most commonly used in Japan and Europe and is now also being used more frequently in the USA. It has the advantage of requiring less frequent dosing and fewer pills than propylthiouracil, making treatment more convenient. It apparently also is associated with a lower incidence of acute hepatic necrosis. Rare complications peculiar to methimazole include serum sickness, cholestatic jaundice, loss of taste, alopecia, nephrotic syndrome, and hypoglycemia. Methimazole (available as 10 mg tablets) is given orally in initial doses of 30–60 mg once daily. The dosage is usually reduced as manifestations of hyperthyroidism resolve and as the free thyroxine level becomes normal.

b. Propylthiouracil–Propylthiouracil has been considered the drug of choice during pregnancy, being less likely to cause aplasia cutis in the newborn. It blocks the peripheral conversion of T_4 to T_3 and is of some theoretic advantage over methimazole in thyroid storm, but this effect has not been demonstrated to be clinically significant. Rare complications which appear to be more common with propylthiouracil include hepatitis, arthritis, lupus erythematosus, aplastic anemia, thrombocytopenia, and hypoprothrombinemia; rash is fairly common. Propylthiouracil (available as 50 mg tablets) is given orally in initial doses of 300–600 mg daily in four divided doses. The dosage and frequency of administration is generally reduced as symptoms of hyperthyroidism resolve and the free thyroxine level becomes normal. During pregnancy, the dose is kept below 200 mg/d in order to avoid goitrous hypothyroidism in the infant.

Some authorities add thyroxine in doses of about 0.1 mg daily may be added to either thiourea drug regimen—once the patient has become euthyroid.

c. Complications of thioureas–Agranulocytosis is an uncommon but serious complication of thiourea therapy, being reported in about 0.1% of patients taking methimazole and about 0.4% of patients taking propylthiouracil. A pretreatment white blood count is usually obtained, since mild leukopenia is common with thyrotoxicosis. Patients are warned that if they develop a sore throat or febrile illness, they should stop the drug while a white blood count is rechecked. The agranulocytosis is generally reversible when discovered early. Periodic surveillance of the white blood count during treatment has been advocated by some clinicians, but onset is generally abrupt.

Other side effects common to thiourea drugs include pruritus, allergic dermatitis, nausea, and dyspepsia. Antihistamines may control mild pruritus without discontinuation of the drug. Since the two thiourea drugs are similar, patients who have had a major side effect from one should not be given another.

Another complication seen with thiourea therapy is primary hypothyroidism. The patient may become clinically hypothyroid for 2 weeks or more before TSH levels rise, having been suppressed by the preceding hyperthyroidism. Therefore, the patient's changing thyroid status is best followed clinically and with serum levels of free thyroxine. Rapid growth of the goiter usually occurs if the patient is allowed to develop prolonged hypothyroidism; the goiter may sometimes become massive but usually regresses rapidly with thyroid hormone replacement.

3. Radioactive iodine (^{131}I)–The administration of radioiodine has proved to be an excellent method of destruction of overfunctioning thyroid tissue (either diffuse or toxic nodular goiter). The rationale of treatment is that the radioiodine, being concentrated in the thyroid, will destroy the cells that concentrate it. Objections to radioiodine therapy include the possibility of carcinogenesis and of damage to the individual's genetic pool, but studies to date have failed to show evidence of these effects. Nevertheless, the use of radioiodine is generally limited to older patients (age 25 or above); the age restriction is not absolute, however, and some children may be best treated with radioiodine. Since fetal radiation is harmful, *radioactive iodine should not be given to pregnant women.*

Most patients may receive radioiodine while being symptomatically treated with just propranolol, which is then reduced in dosage as hyperthyroxinemia resolves. However, some patients (those with coronary diseases, elderly people, or those with severe hyperthyroidism) are usually rendered euthyroid with a thiouracil drug (see above) while the dosage of propranolol is reduced; once the patient is euthyroid, the thiourea is discontinued 3–5 days before ^{131}I treatment is given. There is a high incidence of hypothyroidism several years after this form of treatment even when small doses are given. However, hypothyroidism also occurs quite frequently years after surgical or medical treatment of Graves' disease, and eventual hypothyroidism may be part of the natural history of this condition. Prolonged follow-up, preferably with T_4 and TSH measurements, is therefore mandatory.

4. Thyroid surgery–Thyroid surgery for Graves' disease and toxic nodular goiter has been performed less frequently as radioiodine treatment has become more widely accepted. Surgery is usually preferred for children, for pregnant women whose thyrotoxicosis is not controlled with low doses of thioureas, for patients with particularly large goiters, and whenever there is a significant chance of malignancy.

Thyrotoxic patients must have adequate preparation for thyroid surgery. Patients must be rendered euthyroid with a thiourea drug or with ipodate preoperatively. Propranolol is given until the T_3 is normal preoperatively. Iodine is given (eg, Lugol's solution, 2–3 drops orally daily) for about 10 days preoperatively to reduce thyroid vascularity.

Morbidity includes possible damage to the recurrent laryngeal nerve that causes vocal cord paralysis. Hypoparathyroidism also occurs, which means that calcium levels must be checked postoperatively. These complications are unusual (< 1%) when the surgery is performed by a competent, experienced neck surgeon.

5. Iodinated contrast agents–Iopanoic acid and ipodate sodium are radiologic contrast agents now seldom used in radiology. (Procurement is sometimes a problem.) They are given orally (ipodate, 500 mg once daily) and quickly block hepatic conversion of T_4 to T_3 as well as T_4 release. Within 24 hours, serum T_3 levels fall an average of 62%. Treatment periods of 8 months or more are possible, but the effect tends to wane with time. These agents provide an important therapeutic option for patients in thyroid storm (see below), patients intolerant to thioureas, and newborns with thyrotoxicosis (due to maternal Graves' disease). Thyroid radioiodine uptake may be suppressed during treatment but returns to pretreatment uptake by 7 days after discontinuing the drug, allowing ^{131}I treatment.

B. Toxic Solitary Thyroid Nodules: Hyperthyroidism caused by a single hyperfunctioning thyroid nodule may be treated symptomatically with propranolol as in Graves' disease. Definitive treatment is with surgery or radioactive iodine. For patients under age 40, surgery is usually recommended; patients are made euthyroid with a thiourea preoperatively and given 10 days of iodine therapy before surgery as in Graves' disease (see above). Transient postoperative hypothyroidism resolves spontaneously. Permanent hypothyroidism occurs in about 14% of patients by 6 years after surgery. Patients over age 40 with a toxic solitary nodule are offered radioactive iodine. Permanent hypothyroidism occurs in about one-third of patients by 8 years after radioactive iodine. The nodule remains palpable in half and may grow in 10% of patients after radioactive iodine.

C. Toxic Multinodular Goiter: Hyperthyroidism caused by a toxic multinodular goiter may also be treated symptomatically with propranolol as in Graves' disease. This disorder usually affects older individuals, so radioactive iodine is ordinarily selected over surgery as definitive treatment. Thioureas do reverse hyperthyroidism, but there is a 95% recurrence rate after they are stopped. Older patients who are quite thyrotoxic are rendered nearly euthyroid with a thiourea, which is stopped about 3 days before radioactive iodine treatment. Meanwhile, the patient follows a low-iodine diet; this is done to enhance the thyroid gland's uptake of radioactive iodine, which may be relatively low in this condition (compared to Graves' disease). Relatively high doses of radioactive iodine are usually required; recurrent thyrotoxicosis and hypothyroidism are common, so patients must be followed closely. Surgery is generally reserved for pressure symptoms or cosmetic indications. Patients are prepared for surgery as in Graves' disease (see above).

D. Subacute Thyroiditis: Patients with subacute thyroiditis are best treated symptomatically with propranolol. The condition subsides spontaneously within weeks to months. Thioureas are ineffective, since thyroid hormone production is actually low in this condition. Radioactive iodine is ineffective, since the thyroid's iodine uptake is low. Since periods of hypothyroidism may occur following the initial inflammatory episode, patients should have close clinical follow-up, with serum free thyroxine measurement when necessary. Prompt treatment of the transient hypothyroidism may reduce the incidence of recurrent thyroiditis. Pain can usually be managed with aspirin or other nonsteroidal anti-inflammatory agents.

E. Hashitoxicosis: Some rare patients develop hyperthyroidism as a result of release of stored thyroid hormone during severe Hashimoto's thyroiditis. The microsomal or thyroglobulin antibodies are usually high, but radioiodine uptake is low, thus distinguishing it from Graves' disease. This is especially common in postpartum women, in whom it may be transient. Treatment is with propranolol. Patients are followed carefully for the development of hypothyroidism and treated according to their thyroid status.

F. Treatment of Complications:
1. Graves' ophthalmopathy–Graves' ophthalmopathy is due to lymphocytic infiltration of the extraocular muscles. Clinically detectable ophthalmopathy occurs in 20–40%, with 85% of cases occurring within 18 months of the hyperthyroidism. Only about 10% of these cases are severe. Treatment is usually not required in mild cases. For progressive exophthalmos, prednisone is given in doses of 40–60 mg/d, with dosage reduction over several weeks.

Higher initial prednisone doses of 80–120 mg/d are used when there is optic nerve compression. Hypothyroidism and hyperthyroidism must be treated, but no treatment modality has proved superior with regard to ophthalmopathy, which seems to run an independent course. Other treatment options include low-dose radiation therapy to the extraocular muscles, avoiding the cornea and lens. For severe cases, orbital decompression surgery may save vision, though diplopia often persists postoperatively. General eye protective measures include wearing glasses to protect the protruding eye and taping the lids shut during sleep if corneal drying is a problem. Methylcellulose drops and gels ("artificial tears") may also help. Tarsorrhaphy or canthoplasty can frequently help protect the cornea and provide improved appearance.

2. Cardiac complications–
a. Some degree of tachycardia is almost always found if normal rhythm is present in thyrotoxicosis. This requires only the treatment of the thyrotoxicosis. Severe tachycardia responds promptly to propranolol therapy.

b. Congestive failure tends to occur in longstanding thyrotoxicosis, especially in older people. Treatment is as for congestive failure due to any cause.

c. Atrial fibrillation may occur in association with thyrotoxicosis. Ventricular response rates remain rapid despite digitalis. Many cases revert to normal rhythm soon after toxicity is removed. However, if fibrillation persists after euthyroidism is achieved, electrical conversion is necessary after appropriate anticoagulation therapy to prevent embolism.

d. Apathetic hyperthyroidism may present with angina pectoris. Treatment is directed at reversing the hyperthyroidism as well as providing standard antianginal therapy. Coronary angioplasty or bypass grafting can often be avoided by prompt diagnosis and treatment.

3. Thyroid crisis or "storm"–A thiourea drug is given (eg, propylthiouracil, 150–250 mg every 6 hours; or methimazole, 15–25 mg every 6 hours). Iodide is given 1 hour later as Lugol's solution (10 drops three times daily orally) or as sodium iodide (1 g intravenously slowly). Ipodate sodium (500 mg/d orally) can be helpful if begun after the thiourea. Propranolol is given in a dosage of 0.5–2 mg intravenously every 4 hours or 20–120 mg orally every 6 hours. Glucocorticoids are usually given in doses of 50 mg every 6 hours, with rapid dosage reduction as the clinical situation improves. Aspirin is avoided. Definitive treatment with ^{131}I or surgery is delayed until the patient is euthyroid.

4. Hyperthyroidism and pregnancy–Diagnosis may be difficult, since normal pregnancy may be accompanied by tachycardia, warm skin, heat intolerance, increased sweating, and a palpable thyroid. Laboratory tests are helpful: Although the T_4 is elevated in all pregnant women, values over 20 mg/dL are encountered only in hyperthyroidism. TSH is suppressed. The T_3 resin uptake, which is low in normal pregnancy because of high TBG concentration, is normal in thyrotoxic subjects. The free T_4 is clearly elevated. Pregnancy often has a beneficial effect upon the thyrotoxicosis of Graves' disease, with decreasing antibody titers and decreasing free T_4 levels as the pregnancy advances. Pregnant women with hyperthyroidism are best treated with propylthiouracil in the smallest dose possible, permitting mild hyperthyroidism to occur since it is usually well tolerated. The drug does cross the placenta and rarely may induce TSH hypersecretion and thyroid enlargement in the fetus. Thyroid hormone administration to the mother does not prevent hypothyroidism in the fetus, since T_4 and T_3 do not freely cross the placenta. Fetal hypothyroidism is rare, however, since the mother's hyperthyroidism is often controlled with small daily doses of propylthiouracil (50–150 mg/d). If hyperthyroidism is severe, surgery may be necessary—best done during the second trimester.

Rarely, the child may be born with transient thyrotoxicosis due to placental passage of maternal thyroid stimulators. This neonatal thyrotoxicosis resolves spontaneously in 3–12 weeks. On occasion, hyperthyroidism may persist because of the presence of active Graves' disease in the infant.

A question often arises about whether a mother taking thioureas should breast feed her baby. Only minimal amounts of propylthiouracil are transferred to the maternal milk, so breast feeding is apt to be safe. Apparently this is less true for methimazole, which appears in higher concentrations in the milk.

5. Dermopathy–An uncommon complication of Graves' disease, dermopathy is an abnormal thickening of the skin due to deposition of glycosaminoglycans. It is known as "pretibial myxedema" since it usually occurs in the anterior lower leg, sometimes also including the dorsum of the foot. Treatment involves application of a topical glucocorticoid (eg, fluocinolone) with nocturnal plastic occlusive dressings.

Prognosis

Graves' disease may subside spontaneously and may even result in spontaneous hypothyroidism. More commonly, however, it progresses. The ocular, cardiac, and psychologic complications often are more serious than the chronic wasting of tissues and may become irreversible even after treatment. Permanent hypoparathyroidism and vocal cord palsy are risks of surgical thyroidectomy. Recurrences are common following thiourea therapy but also occur after low-dose ^{131}I therapy or subtotal thyroidectomy. With adequate treatment and long-term follow-up, the results are good. Posttreatment hypothyroidism is common. It may occur within a few months or up to several years after radioactive iodine therapy or sub-

total thyroidectomy. Use of ^{131}I to treat Graves' disease has not resulted in any demonstrable increase of thyroid cancer, leukemia, or other cancers. Malignant exophthalmos has a poor prognosis unless treated aggressively.

Barrie WE: Graves' ophthalmopathy. West J Med 1993; 158:591.
Gavin LA: Thyroid crises. Med Clin North Am 1991; 75:179.
McDougall IR: Graves' disease: Current concepts. Med Clin North Am 1991;75:79.
Schimke RN: Hyperthyroidism: The clinical spectrum. Postgrad Med 1992;91:229.
Singer PA: Thyroiditis: Acute, subacute, and chronic. Med Clin North Am 1991;75:61.
Woeber KA: Thyrotoxicosis and the heart. N Engl J Med 1992;327:94.

THYROID CANCER

Essentials of Diagnosis

- Painless swelling in region of thyroid.
- Thyroid function tests usually normal.
- Past history of irradiation to head and neck region may be present.
- Positive thyroid needle aspiration.

General Considerations (Table 25–10)

Although carcinoma of the thyroid is rarely associated with functional abnormalities, it enters into the differential diagnosis of all types of thyroid lesions. It is common in all age groups but especially in patients who have received radiation therapy in childhood or infancy to the face, neck, or upper chest.

Papillary carcinoma is the most common and least aggressive thyroid malignancy. Pure papillary or mixed papillary-follicular carcinoma represents about 70% of all thyroid cancers. Follicular carcinoma represents about 15% of thyroid malignancies but is more likely to have distant metastases. Papillary and follicular thyroid carcinomas are classified as differentiated thyroid carcinoma. Medullary thyroid carcinoma represents less than 5% of thyroid cancers. Of all cases of medullary thyroid cancer, about one-third are sporadic, one-third are isolated familial occurrences, and another third are associated with multiple endocrine neoplasia type II. Anaplastic thyroid carcinoma represents only about 1% of thyroid malignancies. Other malignancies involving the thyroid include lymphomas and metastases (especially melanoma, breast, renal, and bronchogenic carcinomas).

Clinical Findings

A. Symptoms and Signs: The principal signs of thyroid cancer are a painless nodule, a hard nodule in an enlarged thyroid gland, so-called lateral aber-

Table 25–10. Some characteristics of thyroid cancer.

	Papillary	Follicular	Medullary	Anaplastic
Incidence[1] (%)	61	18	6	15
Average age[1]	42	50	50	57
Females[1] (%)	70	72	56	56
Deaths due to thyroid cancer[1,2] (%)	6	24	33	98
Invasion: Juxtanodal	+++++	+	++++++	+++
Blood vessels	+	+++	+++	+++++
Distant sites	+	+++	++	++++
Resemblance to normal thyroid	+	+++	+	±
[123]I uptake	+	++++	0	0
Degree of malignancy	+	++ to +++	+++	+++++++

[1]Data based upon 885 cases analyzed by Woolner et al; figures have been rounded to the nearest digit. (After Woolner.)

[2]Some patients have been followed up to 32 years after diagnosis.

rant thyroid tissue, or palpable lymph nodes with thyroid enlargement. Metastatic functioning differentiated thyroid carcinoma can sometimes secrete enough thyroid hormone to produce thyrotoxicosis. Signs of pressure or invasion of surrounding tissues are present in anaplastic or long-standing tumors with recurrent laryngeal nerve palsy, fixation of nodule to neighboring structures, etc.

B. Fine-Needle Aspiration Biopsy: This is the best way to assess a nodule for malignancy. A 25-gauge needle is used to biopsy suspicious nodules. The needle is attached to a syringe and special syringe holder. The biopsy is done without local anesthesia. Care must be taken to avoid bloody dilution of the specimens. Material obtained is placed on a slide; a thin smear is obtained by laying a second slide over the material and then drawing the slides apart. One slide is air-dried while the other is preserved in 95% alcohol. Two or more biopsies may be obtained. Reading by an experienced cytopathologist is mandatory.

In one review of thyroid biopsies, about 70% were benign, 10% suspicious, 5% malignant and 15% nondiagnostic. About 30% of patients with suspicious cytology harbor a malignancy. Patients with suspicious cytology usually undergo immediate thyroid surgery; however, those electing not to have surgery appear to have a benign course for at least several years (Cerosimo, 1993).

C. Laboratory Findings: With very few exceptions, all thyroid function tests are normal unless the disease is associated with thyroiditis. The scintiscan usually shows a "cold" nodule. Serum thyroid autoantibodies are sometimes found. Thyroglobulin levels are high in metastatic papillary and follicular tumors. In medullary carcinoma, the calcitonin levels are elevated, especially after stimulation by a pentagastrin or calcium infusion. Calcitonin assay is a reliable clue to silent medullary carcinoma in the familial syndrome; a pentagastrin stimulation test is

used to detect early medullary carcinoma in these kindreds.

D. Imaging: [123]I or ^{99m}Tc scanning usually shows malignancies as hypofunctioning ("cold") relative to the rest of the gland. Functioning ("hot") nodules are generally benign. Exceptions occur frequently enough to make this assessment method unreliable. Fine-needle aspiration biopsy has largely supplanted it.

Extensive bone and soft tissue metastases (some of which may take up radioiodine) may be demonstrable on radiographs or radioisotope scans. Calcified areas may be seen in medullary carcinoma (primary tumor or metastases).

Differential Diagnosis (Table 25–11)

Nonmalignant enlargements of the thyroid gland are far more common than carcinoma. The incidence of malignancy is much greater in single than in multinodular lesions, and far greater in nonfunctioning than in functioning nodules. The differentiation from chronic thyroiditis is at times most difficult, and the two lesions may occur together. Any thyroid nodule that increases rapidly in size must be considered carcinoma until proved otherwise. Thyroid suppression therapy was traditionally used to differentiate benign from malignant nodules, the benign ones being expected to decrease in size. This has unfortunately proved unreliable. Percutaneous needle aspiration biopsy has been extremely useful in diagnosis and is the diagnostic procedure of choice to distinguish benign from malignant lesions prior to surgery. If there is a history of neck radiation in childhood or adolescence, excision of the thyroid nodule is usually required.

Complications

The complications vary with the type of carcinoma. Papillary tumors invade local structures, such as lymph nodes; follicular tumors metastasize

Table 25–11. Differential diagnosis of thyroid nodules.[1]

Clinical Evidence	Low Index of Suspicion	High Index of Suspicion
History	Family history of goiter; residence in area of endemic goiter	Previous therapeutic irradiation of head, neck, or chest; hoarseness
Physical characteristics	Older women; soft nodule; multinodular goiter	Children, young adults, men; solitary, firm nodule; vocal cord paralysis; enlarged lymph nodes; distant metastatic lesions
Serum factors	High titer of antithyroid antibody; hypothyroidism; hyperthyroidism	Elevated serum calcitonin; high serum thyroglobulin
Scanning techniques Uptake of ^{123}I Echo scan Roentgenogram	"Hot" nodule Cystic lesion Shell-like calcification	"Cold" nodule Solid lesion Punctate calcification
Thyroxine therapy	Regression after 0.2 mg/d for 6 months or more	Increase in size

[1]Adapted from Greenspan FS: Thyroid nodules and thyroid cancer. West J Med 1974;121:359.

through the bloodstream; anaplastic carcinomas are highly aggressive, both locally and systemically. One-third of medullary carcinomas may secrete serotonin and prostaglandins, producing flushing and diarrhea and may be complicated by the coexistence of pheochromocytomas or hyperparathyroidism. The complications of radical neck surgery often include permanent hypoparathyroidism and, less commonly, vocal cord palsy; permanent hypothyroidism is expected and should always be treated adequately.

Treatment

Surgical removal is the treatment of choice for thyroid carcinomas. Highly skilled surgeons can perform near-total thyroidectomies with a less than 1% rate of serious complications (hypoparathyroidism or recurrent laryngeal nerve damage). Other series have reported up to an 11% incidence of permanent hypoparathyroidism after total thyroidectomy. The incidence of hypoparathyroidism may be reduced if accidentally resected parathyroids are immediately autotransplanted into the neck muscles. The advantage of near-total thyroidectomy for differentiated thyroid carcinoma is that multicentric foci of carcinoma are more apt to be resected and there is then less normal thyroid tissue to compete with cancer for ^{131}I administered later for scans or treatment. Other surgeons prefer to do more conservative procedures. Neck muscle dissections are avoided for differentiated thyroid carcinoma. Thyroxine is prescribed in doses of 0.1–0.15 mg/d postoperatively. Serum TSH should be kept suppressed during long-term follow-up of differentiated thyroid carcinoma.

About 2–4 months after surgery, a whole-body ^{131}I scan is performed: Iodide uptake is enhanced by stopping thyroxine for 4–6 weeks prior to the scan, thereby causing hypothyroidism; TSH then rises and stimulates iodide uptake. Iodine-containing foods and contrast media are avoided. Patients with significant ^{131}I uptake are given ablative doses of ^{131}I. For patients with significant normal thyroid uptake or minimal uptake, doses of ^{131}I of 30–50 mCi are given

on an outpatient basis. Patients with extrathyroidal uptake from metastatic disease may be given larger doses of 100–150 mCi in the hospital.

False-positive ^{131}I scans are common with normal residual thyroid tissue and have been reported with Zenker's diverticulum, ovary, pleuropericardial cyst, gastric pull-up, and ^{131}I-contaminated bodily secretions. False-negative ^{131}I scans are common in early metastatic differentiated thyroid carcinoma but occur also in more advanced disease, including 14% of bone metastases.

Patients with differentiated thyroid carcinoma are followed clinically with neck palpation, physical examination, and chest x-ray and observed for thyrotoxicosis that might indicate functioning metastases. About 6–12 months after their postoperative scan, patients usually receive another ^{131}I whole body scan and serum thyroglobulin measurement while hypothyroid; these have a combined sensitivity of 95% for metastases. Serum thyroglobulin in a patient receiving thyroxine has a lower sensitivity of 62%.

Thallium-201 (^{201}Tl) scans may be more sensitive for detecting metastatic differentiated thyroid carcinoma and have the advantage over ^{131}I of lower radiation exposure, immediate postinjection imaging, and no requirement for withdrawal from thyroxine replacement. Whether it can substitute for ^{131}I scanning remains to be determined.

Patients with papillary carcinoma should have at least two consecutively negative scans before they are considered in remission. Further scans may be required for patients with more aggressive follicular carcinomas, prior metastases, rising serum thyroglobulin, or other evidence of metastases. Patients with anaplastic thyroid carcinoma are treated with local resection and radiation for palliation only. Thyroid lymphomas are best treated with external radiation therapy.

Patients with medullary thyroid carcinoma are treated surgically; medullary carcinoma does not take up ^{131}I but may be scanned with thallium 201, especially when serum calcitonin levels exceed 1000 ng/L.

Prognosis

The prognosis is directly related to the cell type. The anaplastic carcinomas advance rapidly in spite of early diagnosis and treatment. Papillary carcinomas, when treated, are not associated with a significant mortality rate, and life expectancy is nearly normal. Follicular carcinomas are generally more aggressive but still have a good prognosis. Patients with papillary and follicular carcinoma may be followed with serum thyroglobulin levels, which serve as a tumor marker after thyroidectomy. Hürthle cell carcinoma, perhaps a variant of follicular carcinoma, is more aggressive than papillary or follicular carcinoma. Early detection (followed by removal) of medullary carcinomas by finding elevated calcitonin levels may lead to a better prognosis. In general, the prognosis is less favorable in elderly patients. Anaplastic carcinoma is locally aggressive; the 1-year survival rate is about 10%, and the 5-year rate is about 5%. Medullary thyroid carcinoma has a variable prognosis. Patients with sporadic disease usually have lymph node involvement at the time of diagnosis, whereas distal metastases may not be noted for years; the 10-year survival rate is 46%. Familial cases or those associated with MEN IIa tend to be less aggressive; the 10-year survival rate is higher, in part due to earlier detection. Women with medullary thyroid carcinoma who are under age 40 also have a better prognosis.

Medullary thyroid carcinoma carries a worse prognosis if tumor tissue stains heavily for calcitonin or myelomonocytic antigen Leu-M1.

Serum calcitonin levels may be used as a tumor marker for medullary thyroid carcinoma. Serum CEA is also elevated in 70% of cases. Since these levels may remain elevated in patients with apparent complete resections and long-term remissions, it is a rising level of these markers (rather than the absolute level) that best indicates progression of the malignancy.

Brennan MD et al: Follicular thyroid cancer treated at the Mayo Clinic, 1946 through 1979: Initial manifestations, pathologic findings, therapy, and outcome. Mayo Clin Proc 1991;61:11.

Cerosimo E et al: "Suspicious" thyroid cytologic findings: Outcomes in patients without immediate surgical treatment. Mayo Clin Proc 1993;68:343.

Galloway JW et al: Changing trends in thyroid surgery: 38 years experience, Am Surg 1991;57:18.

Gharib H, Goellner JR: Fine needle aspiration biopsy of the thyroid: An appraisal. Ann Intern Med 1993;118:282.

Ramanna L et al: Thallium-201 scintigraphy in differentiated thyroid cancer: Comparison with radioiodine scintigraphy and serum thyroglobulin determinations. J Nucl Med 1991;32:441.

Robbins J et al: Thyroid cancer: A lethal endocrine neoplasm. Ann Intern Med 1991;115:133.

Samaan NA et al: The results of various modalities of treatment of well differentiated thyroid carcinomas: A retrospective review of 1599 patients. J Clin Endocrinol Metab 1992;75:714.

THYROIDITIS

Essentials of Diagnosis

- Swelling of thyroid gland, often causing pressure symptoms in acute and subacute forms; painless enlargement in chronic form.
- Thyroid function tests variable; discrepancy in T_4 and radioiodine uptake common.
- Serum antithyroid antibody tests often positive.

General Considerations

Thyroiditis may be classified as follows: (1) chronic lymphocytic ("Hashimoto's") thyroiditis due to autoimmunity, (2) subacute thyroiditis, (3) suppurative thyroiditis, and (4) Riedel's thyroiditis.

Clinical Findings

A. Symptoms and Signs:

1. Hashimoto's thyroiditis–Hashimoto's thyroiditis—also called struma lymphomatosa, lymphadenoid goiter, and chronic lymphocytic thyroiditis—is the most common form of thyroiditis and probably the most common thyroid disorder. Onset of enlargement of the thyroid gland is insidious, with few pressure symptoms. The gland is firm, symmetrically enlarged, lobulated, and nontender to palpation. Thyroid antibody titers (antithyroglobulin and antimicrosomal) are usually high. The condition is more frequent in women and has a familial clustering. It occurs at all ages. Signs of thyroid dysfunction are common. The disease is frequently subclinical and not detected. Thyroid antibodies are found in up to 15% of hospitalized patients, most of whom have no thyroid dysfunction. Many patients do gradually develop hypothyroidism, usually associated with goiter. Acute Hashimoto's thyroiditis can rarely cause transient hyperthyroidism from cell damage (hashitoxicosis). Hashimoto's thyroiditis and high antithyroid antibody levels are usually present to some degree in most cases of Graves' disease. The presence of an antibody to the TSH receptor in Graves' disease causes gland hyperfunction, distinguishing it from Hashimoto's thyroiditis. Postpartum thyroiditis is a form of autoimmune thyroiditis occurring soon after parturition and accompanied by transient hyperthyroidism followed by hypothyroidism. Recovery of normal function occurs in most cases.

2. Subacute thyroiditis–This fairly common disorder—also called de Quervain's thyroiditis, granulomatous thyroiditis, giant cell thyroiditis—is an acute, usually painful enlargement of the thyroid gland, with dysphagia. The pain may radiate to the ears. If there is no pain, it is called "silent thyroiditis." The manifestations may persist for weeks or months and may be associated with signs of thyrotoxicosis and malaise. Young and middle-aged women are most commonly affected. Viral infection has been suggested as the cause. The erythrocyte sedimentation rate is markedly elevated, and antithyroid antibodies are low, which helps differentiate this form of thyroiditis from others. Radioactive iodine, uptake is low, distinguishing this disorder from Graves' disease. Aspiration biopsy is usually not required but shows characteristic giant multinucleated cells.

3. Suppurative thyroiditis–Suppurative thyroiditis is a rare disorder causing severe pain, tenderness, redness, and fluctuation in the region of the thyroid gland. It is caused by pyogenic organisms, usually in the course of systemic infection.

4. Riedel's thyroiditis–Riedel's thyroiditis is also called chronic fibrous thyroiditis, Riedel's struma, woody thyroiditis, ligneous thyroiditis, and invasive thyroiditis. It usually causes hypothyroidism and may cause hypoparathyroidism as well. It is the rarest form of thyroiditis and is found most frequently in middle-aged women. Enlargement is often asymmetric; the gland is stony hard and adherent to the neck structures, causing signs of compression and invasion, including dysphagia, dyspnea, and hoarseness. It is usually a manifestation of a multifocal systemic fibrosis syndrome with retroperitoneal, mediastinal, and biliary tract sclerosis.

B. Laboratory Findings: The T_4 and T_3 resin uptake are usually markedly elevated in acute and subacute thyroiditis and normal or low in the chronic forms. Radioiodine uptake is characteristically very low in the initial, hyperthyroid phase of subacute thyroiditis; it may be high with an uneven scan in chronic thyroiditis, with enlargement of the gland, and low in Riedel's struma. Thyroid autoantibodies are most commonly demonstrable in Hashimoto's thyroiditis but are also found in the other types. The serum TSH level is elevated if thyroid hormone is not elaborated in adequate amounts by the thyroid gland.

Complications

In the suppurative forms of thyroiditis, any of the complications of infection may occur; the subacute and chronic forms of the disease are complicated by the effects of pressure on the neck structures: dyspnea and, in Riedel's struma, vocal cord palsy. Hashimoto's thyroiditis may lead to hypothyroidism. Carcinoma or lymphoma may be associated with chronic thyroiditis and must be considered in the diagnosis of uneven painless enlargements that continue in spite of treatment. Hashimoto's thyroiditis may be associated with Addison's disease, hypoparathyroidism, diabetes, pernicious anemia, biliary cirrhosis, vitiligo, and other autoimmune conditions.

Differential Diagnosis

Thyroiditis must be considered in the differential diagnosis of all types of goiters, especially if enlargement is rapid. The very low radioiodine uptake in subacute thyroiditis with elevated T_4 and T_3 are helpful. Chronic thyroiditis, especially if the enlargement is uneven and if there is pressure on surrounding structures, may resemble carcinoma, and both disorders may be present in the same gland. The subacute and suppurative forms of thyroiditis may resemble any infectious process in or near the neck structures. Thyroid autoantibody tests have been of help in the diagnosis of chronic lymphocytic (Hashimoto's) thyroiditis, but the tests are not specific and may also be positive in patients with goiters, carcinoma, and thyrotoxicosis—though the titers are often higher in Hashimoto's thyroiditis. Biopsy may be required for diagnosis.

Treatment

A. Suppurative Thyroiditis: Treatment is with antibiotics and with surgical drainage when fluctuation is marked.

B. Subacute Thyroiditis: All treatment is empiric and must be continued for several weeks. Recurrence is common. The drug of choice is aspirin, which relieves pain and inflammation. Thyrotoxic symptoms are treated with propranolol, 10–40 mg every 6 hours. Transient hypothyroidism is treated with thyroxine (0.05–0.1 mg/d) if symptomatic.

C. Hashimoto's Thyroiditis: Levothyroxine should be given in the usual doses (0.1–0.15 mg daily) if hypothyroidism or large goiter is present. If the thyroid gland is only minimally enlarged and the patient is euthyroid (with normal TSH levels), regular observation is in order, since hypothyroidism may develop subsequently—often years later.

D. Riedel's Struma: Partial thyroidectomy is often required to relieve pressure; adhesions to surrounding structures make this a difficult operation.

Prognosis

The course of this group of diseases is quite variable. Spontaneous remissions and exacerbations are common in the subacute form, and therapy is nonspecific. The disease process may smolder for months. Hashimoto's thyroiditis may be associated with other autoimmune disorders (diabetes mellitus, Addison's disease, pernicious anemia, etc), with all the complications of those diseases. In general, however, patients with Hashimoto's thyroiditis have an excellent prognosis, since the condition either remains stable for years or progresses slowly to hypothyroidism, which is easily treated.

Utiger RD: The pathogenesis of autoimmune thyroid disease. N Engl J Med 1991;325:278.

THE PARATHYROIDS

Parathyroid hormone (PTH) is a polypeptide hormone composed of 84 amino acids. Together with 1,25-dihydroxycholecalciferol, the active form of vitamin D, parathyroid hormone is responsible for maintenance of calcium, phosphate, and magnesium balance and for the integrity and normal mineralization of bone.

The main physiologic effects of PTH are as follows: (1) It increases the osteoclastic activity in bone, with increased delivery of calcium and phosphorus to the extracellular compartment and the circulation; (2) it increases the renal tubular reabsorption of calcium in the glomerular filtrate; (3) it inhibits the net absorption of phosphate and bicarbonate by the renal tubule; and (4) it stimulates the synthesis of 1,25-dihydroxycholecalciferol by the kidney. All of these steps result in a net increase in the amount of ionized calcium circulating in plasma.

Vitamin D is a hormone with a complex set of actions and mechanism of synthesis. Cholecalciferol (vitamin D_3) is synthesized in the skin, under the influence of ultraviolet radiation, from 7-dehydrocholesterol. Two sequential hydroxylations, are necessary for full biologic activity: The first one takes place in the liver—to 25-hydroxycholecalciferol—and the second one in the kidney, resulting in the formation of the most potent biologic metabolite of vitamin D, 1,25-dihydroxycholecalciferol (1,25[OH]$_2$ D_3). The main action of vitamin D is the acceleration of calcium and phosphate absorption in the intestine. Deficiency or excess of vitamin D results in profound disturbances of calcium homeostasis.

HYPOPARATHYROIDISM & PSEUDOHYPOPARATHYROIDISM

Essentials of Diagnosis
- Tetany, carpopedal spasms, tingling of lips and hands, muscle and abdominal cramps, psychologic changes.
- Positive Chvostek's sign and Trousseau's phenomenon; defective nails and teeth; cataracts.
- Serum calcium low; serum phosphate high; alkaline phosphatase normal; urine calcium excretion reduced.
- Basal ganglia calcification on x-ray or CT scan of the head.

General Considerations
Hypoparathyroidism is most commonly seen following thyroidectomy or surgery for primary hyperparathyroidism. Rarely, it follows x-ray irradia-

tion to the neck. Transient hypoparathyroidism occurs in a significant number of patients after thyroidectomy. After surgical removal of parathyroid adenoma for primary hyperparathyroidism, hypocalcemia may occur as a result of suppression of the remaining normal parathyroids and accelerated remineralization of the skeleton (hungry bone syndrome).

Hypoparathyroidism may be autoimmune and occur sporadically or as part of polyglandular autoimmune syndrome (PGA type I). This is also known as autoimmune polyendocrinopathy-candidiasis-ectodermal dystrophy (APECED). Type I PGA includes at least two of the following: candidiasis (beginning about age 3–6 years), hypoparathyroidism (age 5–8 years), and Addison's disease (age 8–11 years). Such patients may also have cataracts, uveitis, and alopecia. They may later develop vitiligo or thyroid immune disease.

Parathyroid deficiency can also occur from dysembryogenesis (DiGeorge's syndrome) or as a result of damage from heavy metals (Wilson's disease, transfusion hemosiderosis, hemochromatosis), granulomas, metastatic tumors, or infection.

Functional hypoparathyroidism may also occur as a result of magnesium deficiency (malabsorption, chronic alcoholism), which prevents the secretion of PTH. Correction of hypomagnesemia results in rapid disappearance of the condition.

Pseudohypoparathyroidism is a genetic defect associated with short stature, round face, obesity, bone abnormalities including short metacarpals and metatarsals, and ectopic bone formation. There may be mild mental retardation. The disorder can be inherited as an X-linked dominant trait known as Albright's hereditary osteodystrophy. The parathyroids are present and often hyperplastic, but there is resistance to the hormone action. It appears to be a heterogeneous group of disorders, with several different subgroups having been identified. The classic cases present with clinical and chemical evidence of hypoparathyroidism and elevated serum PTH. Most patients with the phenotypic abnormalities just described have tissue resistance to PTH and to other hormones that act by stimulating cAMP (glucagon, vasopressin, TSH). Patients without hypocalcemia but sharing the phenotypic abnormalities are said to have **pseudopseudohypoparathyroidism.**

Clinical Findings
A. Symptoms and Signs: Acute hypoparathyroidism causes tetany, with muscle cramps, irritability, carpopedal spasm, and convulsions; tingling of the circumoral area, hands, and feet is almost always present. Symptoms of the chronic disease are lethargy, personality changes, anxiety state, blurring of vision due to cataracts, and mental retardation.

Chvostek's sign (facial muscle contraction on tapping the facial nerve in front of the tragus) is positive, and Trousseau's phenomenon (carpal spasm after application of a cuff) is present. Cataracts may occur; the nails may be thin and brittle; the skin is dry and scaly, at times with fungus infection (candidiasis), and there may be loss of hair (eyebrows); deep tendon reflexes may be hyperactive. Papilledema and elevated cerebrospinal fluid pressure are occasionally seen. Teeth may be defective if the onset of the disease occurs in childhood. Branchial anomalies (eg, cleft palate) may be found. In pseudohypoparathyroidism, the fingers and toes are short, especially the fourth finger, where a dimple instead of a knuckle is seen on making a fist, due to a short fourth metacarpal bone.

B. Laboratory Findings: Serum calcium is largely bound to albumin. Therefore, the serum calcium level should be corrected for serum albumin level as follows:

"Corrected" serum calcium = Serum calcium mg/dL + [0.8 ×(4.0 – Albumin g/dL)]

Serum calcium is low, serum phosphate high, urinary phosphate low, urinary calcium low, and alkaline phosphatase normal. Alkaline phosphatase may be elevated in pseudohypoparathyroidism. Parathyroid hormone levels are low or absent in hypoparathyroidism but normal or markedly elevated in pseudohypoparathyroidism.

C. Imaging: Radiographs or CT scans of the skull may show basal ganglia calcifications; the bones may be denser than normal. In pseudohypoparathyroidism, short metacarpals and ectopic bone may be seen and bones may be demineralized.

D. Other Examinations: Slit-lamp examination may show early posterior lenticular cataract formation. The ECG shows prolonged QT intervals and T wave abnormalities.

Complications

Acute tetany with stridor, especially if associated with vocal cord palsy, may lead to respiratory obstruction requiring tracheostomy. The complications of chronic hypoparathyroidism depend largely upon the duration of the disease and the age at onset. If it starts early in childhood, there may be stunting of growth, malformation of the teeth, and retardation of mental development. There may be associated sprue syndrome, pernicious anemia, and Addison's disease. In pseudohypoparathyroidism, tissue resistance to the action of other hormones (TSH, glucagon, vasopressin) may be present. In long-standing cases, cataract formation and calcification of the basal ganglia are seen. Occasionally, parkinsonian symptoms develop. Ossification of the paravertebral ligaments may occur with nerve root compression; surgical decompression may be required. Seizures are common in untreated patients. Overtreatment with vitamin D and calcium may produce impairment of renal function and nephrocalcinosis.

Differential Diagnosis

The symptoms of hypocalcemic tetany may be confused with paresthesias, muscle cramps, or tetany due to respiratory alkalosis, in which the serum calcium is normal. In fact, hyperventilation tends to accentuate hypocalcemic symptoms.

Hypocalcemia may also be due to malabsorption of calcium, magnesium, or vitamin D; patients do not always have diarrhea. It may also be caused by certain drugs such as loop diuretics, plicamycin (mithramycin), and phenytoin. In addition, hypocalcemia may be seen in cases of rapid intravascular volume expansion or due to chelation from transfusions of large volumes of citrated blood. Transient hypocalcemia is also frequently seen following parathyroidectomy for hyperparathyroidism. It is also observed in patients with acute pancreatitis. Some patients with certain metastatic carcinomas (especially breast, prostate) may develop hypocalcemia instead of the expected hypercalcemia. Hypocalcemia with hyperphosphatemia (simulating hypoparathyroidism) may be caused by large doses of intravenous, oral, or rectal phosphate preparations and by chemotherapy of responsive lymphomas or leukemias.

Neonatal hypocalcemia is seen in infants whose mothers had hypercalcemia during gestation. Infants fed cow's milk or high-phosphate formula may also develop hypocalcemia.

At times hypoparathyroidism is misdiagnosed as idiopathic epilepsy, choreoathetosis, or brain tumor (on the basis of brain calcifications, convulsions, choked disks) or, more rarely, as "asthma" (on the basis of stridor and dyspnea).

Treatment

A. Emergency Treatment for Acute Attack (Hypoparathyroid Tetany): This usually occurs after surgery and requires immediate treatment.

1. Be sure an adequate airway is present.

2. Calcium gluconate, 10–20 mL of 10% solution intravenously, may be given *slowly* until tetany ceases. Ten to 50 mL of 10% calcium gluconate may be added to 1 L of 5% glucose in water or saline and administered by slow intravenous drip. The rate should be so adjusted that the serum calcium is raised above 7 mg/dL and maintained between 8 and 9 mg/dL.

3. Oral calcium–Calcium salts should be given orally as soon as possible to supply 1–2 g of calcium daily. Calcium carbonate (40% calcium) is effective and is the calcium salt of choice. Tablets containing 250 mg of calcium are well tolerated; the dosage is four to eight tablets per day. Other calcium preparations, such as calcium lactate, gluconate, or citrate have lower calcium content and are more expensive.

They can be used by patients with gastrointestinal intolerance to calcium carbonate.

4. Vitamin D preparations–(Table 25–12.) Therapy should be started as soon as oral calcium is begun. The treatment of choice for chronic hypoparathyroidism is vitamin D_2 (ergocalciferol), which has been used successfully for many years. The usual daily dose ranges from 25,000 to 150,000 units/d. It is a slow-acting preparation, and if toxicity develops, hypercalcemia—treatable with hydration and prednisone—may persist for weeks after the drug is discontinued. Ergocalciferol gives a more stable serum calcium level than do the shorter-acting preparations.

Dihydrotachysterol is faster in onset of action and is three times more potent than ergocalciferol. The usual daily maintenance dose is 0.125–1 mg/d. It is more expensive than vitamin D_2.

The active metabolite of vitamin D, 1,25-dihydroxycholecalciferol (calcitriol), has a very rapid onset of action, and if toxicity develops it is not long-lasting. Because of its very high cost, it has been used primarily in the treatment of acute hypocalcemia in doses ranging from 1–4 μg/d rather than for chronic therapy.

Calcifediol (25-hydroxyvitamin D_3) is another option for treatment which has an intermediate onset and duration of action; the usual starting dose is 20 μg/d orally.

5. Magnesium–If hypomagnesemia is present (chronic alcoholism, malnutrition, renal loss, drugs such as cisplatin, etc), it must be corrected in order to treat the resulting hypocalcemia. Acutely, $MgSO_4$ is given intravenously, 1–2 g every 6 hours. Chronic magnesium replacement may be given as magnesium oxide tablets (600 mg), one or two per day, or as a combined magnesium and calcium preparation (Dolomite, others).

B. Maintenance Treatment: The goal should be to maintain the serum calcium in a slightly low but asymptomatic range (8–8.6 mg/dL). This will minimize the hypercalciuria that would otherwise occur and provides a margin of safety against overdosage and hypercalcemia, which may produce permanent damage to renal function. Calcium supplementation (1–2 g/d) is continued, and a vitamin D preparation (see above) is given. Monitoring of serum calcium at regular intervals (at least every 3 months) is mandatory. One should also monitor urine calcium with "spot" urine determinations and keep the level below 30 mg/dL if possible.

Caution: Phenothiazine drugs should be administered with caution to hypocalcemic patients, since they may precipitate extrapyramidal symptoms. Furosemide should be avoided, since it may enhance hypocalcemia.

Prognosis

The outlook is good if the diagnosis is made promptly and treatment instituted. Some changes (eg, in the electroencephalogram) are reversible by appropriate treatment, but the dental changes, cataracts, and brain calcifications are permanent. Periodic blood chemical evaluation is required, since changes in calcium levels may call for modification of the treatment schedule. Hypercalcemia that develops in patients with seemingly stable, treated hypoparathyroidism (especially in children with PGA type I) may be a presenting sign of Addison's disease.

Ahonen P et al: Clinical variation of autoimmune polyendocrinopathy-candidiasis-ectodermal dystrophy (APECED) in a series of 68 patients. N Engl J Med 1990;322:1829.
Faull CM et al: Pseudohypoparathyroidism: Its phenotypic variability and associated disorders in a large family. Q J Med 1991;78:251.

HYPERPARATHYROIDISM

Essentials of Diagnosis

- Patients frequently asymptomatic, detected by screening.
- Renal stones, nephrocalcinosis, polyuria, polydip-

Table 25–12. Vitamin D preparations used in the treatment of hypoparathyroidism.[1]

	Potency[2]	How Supplied	Daily Dose (Range)	Time Required for Toxic Effects to Subside
Ergocalciferol (ergosterol, vitamin D_2)	40,000 USP units/mg.	Capsules of 25,000 and 50,000 units; solution, 500,000 units/mL.	25,000–200,000 units	6–18 weeks.
Dihydrotachysterol (Hytakerol)	120,000 USP units/mg.	Tablets of 0.125, 0.2, and 0.4 mg.	0.2–1 mg.	1–3 weeks.
Calcifediol (Calderol)	...	Capsules of 20 and 50 μg.	20–200 μg	3–6 weeks.
Calcitriol (Rocaltrol)	...	Capsules of 0.25 and 0.5 μg.	0.25–5 μg.	½–2 weeks.

[1]Reproduced, with permission, from Greenspan FS (editor): *Basic & Clinical Endocrinology*, 3rd ed. Appleton & Lange, 1990.
[2]Number of units of vitamin D provided by 1 mg of the preparation.

sia, hypertension, uremia, intractable peptic ulcer, pancreatitis, constipation, mental changes.
- Bone pain, cystic lesions, and, rarely, pathologic fractures.
- Serum and urine calcium elevated; urine phosphate high with low to normal serum phosphate; alkaline phosphatase normal to elevated.
- Elevated parathyroid hormone.

General Considerations

Primary hyperparathyroidism is an increasingly recognized disorder. Surveys suggest that hyperfunction of the parathyroids, often as asymptomatic hypercalcemia, may be present in 0.1% of patients examined. It should always be suspected in obscure bone and renal disease, especially if nephrocalcinosis or calculi are present. At least 5% of renal stones are associated with this disease. It is more frequent in persons over the age of 50 and more common in women than in men. It is hereditary in about 5% of cases.

The disease is due to hypersecretion of parathyroid hormone either by hyperplastic glands or by a parathyroid adenoma or carcinoma (< 2% of all cases). The pathologic classification of parathyroid adenoma versus hyperplasia is difficult when examining an isolated gland.

Multiple neoplasms, often familial, of the pancreas, pituitary, thyroid, and adrenal glands may be associated with primary hyperparathyroidism due to adenoma or, more commonly, due to hyperplasia of the parathyroids (multiple endocrine adenomatosis types I, IIa, and IIb; see Table 25–19).

Hyperparathyroidism causes excessive excretion of calcium and phosphate by the kidneys; this can result in either calculus formation within the urinary tract or, less commonly, diffuse parenchymal calcification (nephrocalcinosis). Chronic bone resorption induced by excessive PTH in the circulation may produce diffuse demineralization, pathologic fractures, or cystic bone lesions throughout the skeleton ("osteitis fibrosa cystica").

In chronic renal failure, hyperphosphatemia and decreased renal production of $1,25(OH)_2D_3$ initially produce a decrease in ionized calcium The parathyroid glands are stimulated (secondary hyperparathyroidism) and may enlarge, becoming autonomous (tertiary hyperparathyroidism). The bone disease seen in this setting is known as "renal osteodystrophy." Diabetics seem somewhat less prone to develop this syndrome. Hypercalcemia often occurs after renal transplant but usually subsides spontaneously.

Clinical Findings

A. Symptoms and Signs: In most patients, the disease is discovered when they are entirely asymptomatic as the result of a blood "multipanel" screening test that reveals unsuspected hypercalcemia. Parathyroid adenomas are usually so small and deeply located in the neck that they are almost never palpable; when a mass is palpated, it usually turns out to be an incidental thyroid nodule.

Patients are said to have problems with "bones, stones, abdominal groans, psychic moans, with fatigue overtones." The manifestations are more formally categorized as follows:

1. Skeletal manifestations–These may vary from simple back pain, joint pains, painful shins, and similar complaints, to actual pathologic fractures of the spine, ribs, or long bones, with loss of height and progressive kyphosis. At times an epulis of the jaw (actually a "brown tumor") may be the telltale sign of osteitis fibrosa.

2. Urinary tract manifestations–Polyuria and polydipsia may be present and are due to hypercalcemia. Stones containing calcium oxalate or phosphate may be passed. Nephrocalcinosis and renal failure may eventually occur.

3. Manifestations of hypercalcemia–Mild hypercalcemia is often asymptomatic. In more severe cases, thirst, anorexia, and nausea and vomiting are outstanding symptoms. Often one finds a history of peptic ulcer, with obstruction or even hemorrhage. There may be stubborn constipation, asthenia, anemia, and weight loss. Hypertension is commonly found. Some patients present primarily with neuromuscular disorders such as muscle weakness, easy fatigability, or paresthesias. Depression and psychosis may occur. Intense pruritus may accompany severe hypercalcemia. Calcium may precipitate in the corneas ("band keratopathy"). In secondary (renal) hyperparathyroidism, calcium also precipitates in the soft tissues, especially around the joints. Recurrent pancreatitis occurs in some patients.

B. Laboratory Findings: The hallmark of primary hyperparathyroidism is hypercalcemia (serum calcium > 10.5 mg/dL when corrected for serum albumin). In hyperproteinemic states, the total serum calcium may be elevated but the ionized fraction is normal, whereas in primary hyperparathyroidism the ionized calcium is almost always elevated. The serum phosphate is often low (< 2.5 mg/dL). The urine calcium excretion may be high or normal, but it is usually low for the degree of hypercalcemia. There is an excessive loss of phosphate in the urine in the presence of low to low normal serum phosphate (low tubular reabsorption of phosphate [below 80–90%]). The alkaline phosphatase is elevated only if bone disease is present. The plasma chloride and uric acid levels may be elevated. (In secondary hyperparathyroidism due to renal failure, the serum phosphate is high.) Elevated levels of parathyroid hormone confirm the diagnosis. Multiple radioimmunoassays are available. The best recognizes the intact molecule at two different sites—the N-terminal and the C-terminal ends—with two different antibodies. This assay, known as *immunoradiometric assay* (IRMA), is specific, sensitive, and makes it easy to differentiate primary hyperparathyroidism from other causes of hypercalcemia.

The localization of parathyroid tumors by determinations of PTH in multiple serum samples taken during selective venous catheterization is rarely done—only after an unsuccessful prior neck exploration.

C. Imaging: Since the gland or glands affected are rarely larger than 1.5 cm in diameter (and usually *much* smaller), preoperative imaging techniques are often unsuccessful. Imaging techniques include ultrasonsography, CT, MRI, and thallium/technetium subtraction studies. MRI sensitivity may be enhanced using the flat suppression short-tau inversion recovery (STIR) sequence. The accuracy of a given technique depends upon the available equipment and technical personnel. Angiography and selective venous sampling for PTH are rarely required. Unsuspected small intrathyroidal nodules are discovered incidentally in nearly half of patients with hyperparathyroidism who have imaging with ultrasound or MRI.

Bone x-rays may show diffuse demineralization, subperiosteal resorption of bone (especially in the radial aspects of the fingers), and often loss of the lamina dura of the teeth. There may be cysts throughout the skeleton, mottling of the skull ("salt-and-pepper appearance"), or pathologic fractures. Articular cartilage calcification (chondrocalcinosis) is sometimes found. One may find calculi in the urinary tract or diffuse stippled calcifications in the region of the kidneys (nephrocalcinosis). Patients with renal osteodystrophy may have ectopic calcifications around joints or in soft tissue. Such patients may exhibit x-ray changes of osteopenia, osteitis fibrosa, or osteosclerosis, alone or in combination. Osteosclerosis of the vertebral bodies is known as "rugger jersey spine."

Complications

Pathologic fractures are more common, especially in women. Urinary tract infection due to stone and obstruction may lead to renal failure and uremia. If the serum calcium level rises rapidly, clouding of sensorium, renal failure, and rapid precipitation of calcium throughout the soft tissues may occur. Peptic ulcer and pancreatitis may be intractable before surgery. Insulinomas or gastrinomas may be associated, as well as pituitary tumors (multiple endocrine neoplasia type I). Pseudogout may complicate hyperparathyroidism both before and after surgical removal of tumors. Subcutaneous, soft tissue, and extensive vascular calcification—as well as dermal necrosis—may occur in secondary hyperparathyroidism due to renal insufficiency.

Differential Diagnosis

(1) Artifact: A report of hypercalcemia may be due to laboratory error or excess tourniquet time and should always be repeated. Hypercalcemia may be due to high serum protein concentrations; serum calcium should be corrected for albumin (see above). It may also be seen with dehydration.

(2) Hypercalcemia of malignancy: Many malignant tumors (breast, lung, pancreas, uterus, hypernephroma, etc) can produce hypercalcemia. In some cases (breast carcinoma especially), bony metastases are present. In others, no metastases to bone can be demonstrated. Most of these tumors secrete a polypeptide substance that has effects on bone resorption similar to those of parathyroid hormone. This peptide amino acid sequence has homology with PTH in amino acids 1–13 only but has tertiary structural homologies with PTH. It has been named parathyroid hormone-related peptide (PTH-RP), and its gene locus has been identified in the short arm of chromosome 12 (the PTH gene is in the short arm of chromosome 11). A radioimmunoassay is now commercially available and has proved useful to separate the humoral hypercalcemia of malignancy from other forms of hypercalcemia. The clinical features of the hypercalcemia of cancer can closely simulate hyperparathyroidism. Serum phosphate is often low, but the plasma level of PTH by IRMA is *low*.

Multiple myeloma is a common cause of hypercalcemia in the older population. Many other hematologic cancers such as monocytic leukemia, T cell leukemia and lymphoma, Burkitt's lymphoma, etc, have also been associated with hypercalcemia. Multiple myeloma causes renal dysfunction; resultant increased levels of C-terminal PTH may cause it to be confused with hyperparathyroidism if a C-terminal PTH assay is used. Serum protein and urine electrophoresis and bone marrow biopsy establish the diagnosis.

(3) Sarcoidosis and other granulomatous disorders: Macrophages and perhaps other cells present in granulomatous tissue have the ability to synthesize 1,25-dihydroxycholecalciferol. Hypercalcemia has been reported in patients with tuberculosis, berylliosis, histoplasmosis, coccidioidomycosis, leprosy, and even foreign-body granuloma. Increased intestinal calcium absorption and hypercalciuria are more common than hypercalcemia. Serum levels of 1,25-dihydroxycholecalciferol are elevated.

(4) Calcium or vitamin D ingestion: The history of peptic ulcer and prolonged therapy with milk or antacids such as sodium bicarbonate or calcium carbonate is of paramount importance. Hypercalcemia is rapidly reversible following discontinuance of such therapy. If it persists, the possibility of associated hyperparathyroidism should be strongly considered.

In vitamin D intoxication, patients may take large amounts of vitamin D for unclear reasons, and a check of all medications is important. Serum levels of 25-hydroxycholecalciferol are helpful to confirm the diagnosis. A brief course of glucocorticoid therapy may be necessary if hypercalcemia is severe.

(5) Familial hypocalciuric hypercalcemia: This benign condition can be easily mistaken for mild hyperparathyroidism. It is an autosomal dominant inherited disorder characterized by hypocalciuria (usually < 50 mg/24 h), variable hypermagnesemia, and normal or minimally elevated levels of PTH. These patients do not normalize their hypercalcemia after subtotal parathyroid removal and should not be subjected to surgery. The condition has an excellent prognosis and is easily diagnosed with family history and urinary calcium clearance determination.

(6) Adrenal insufficiency: Hypercalcemia is common in untreated Addison's disease. The mechanism is unclear, but a partial explanation relates to the hyperproteinemia often found in a dehydrated, hemoconcentrated addisonian patient, so that it is the total rather than the ionized calcium that is elevated.

(7) Hyperthyroidism: Increased calcium turnover is a feature of thyrotoxicosis. Mild hypercalcemia may also be present.

(8) Other causes: Other causes of hypercalcemia include bone fractures, acute renal failure, and vitamin A intoxication. Modest hypercalcemia is also occasionally seen in patients taking thiazide diuretics. Prolonged immobilization at bed rest may also cause hypercalcemia, especially in children, adolescents, and patients with extensive Paget's disease of bone. Mild hypercalcemia is also commonly seen in acutely ill patients being treated in intensive care units.

Treatment

A. Surgical Measures: Not every patient with hyperparathyroidism requires surgical treatment. Patients with mild hypercalcemia (< 11 mg/dL) may be followed medically unless they show evidence of deterioration of renal function, bone demineralization, significant hypertension, etc. (See Table 25–13.) The mainstay of therapy for primary hyperparathyroidism is surgical removal of the excess parathyroid tissue. Removal of a parathyroid adenoma usually results in surgical cure. Multiple tumors occur so frequently that bilateral neck exploration is usually advisable. Parathyroid glands are not uncommonly supernumerary (five or more) or ectopic (eg, intrathyroidal, carotid sheath, mediastinum).

Parathyroid hyperplasia, commonly seen with chronic renal failure, is best treated with subtotal parathyroidectomy. Alternatively, one may perform total parathyroidectomy with autotransplantation to the forearm. Recurrent hyperparathyroidism due to graft hyperplasia may be treated by excision of grafted tissue. After surgery, the patient may develop tetany (usually transient) as a result of rapid fall of blood calcium even though the calcium level may fall only to the normal range. Therefore, frequent postoperative monitoring of serum calcium and albumin (once or twice daily) is recommended. Postoperative serum PTH levels are not as useful and may be mis-

Table 25–13. Categories of treatment for patients with primary hyperparathyroidism.[1]

Criteria	Preferred Treatment
1. One or more of the following: Serum calcium > 11 mg/dL. Osteitis fibrosa cystica. Progressive osteopenia. Metabolically active nephrolithiasis. Intractable peptic ulcer. Pancreatitis. Serious psychiatric disease. Severe hypertension.	Surgical removal of parathyroid lesion.
2. Unsuccessful surgery, or recurrence with manifestations noted in category 1.	Surgical removal of parathyroid lesion; preoperative localization may be indicated.
3. Serum calcium < 11 mg/dL. Abnormal serum iPTH. Absence of manifestations noted in category 1.	Surgical removal of parathyroid lesion or medical management (see text).
4. Surgery contraindicated.	Medical management for hypercalcemia and prevention of nephrolithiasis (see text).

[1]Reproduced, with permission, from Greenspan FS (editor): *Basic & Clinical Endocrinology*, 3rd ed. Appleton & Lange, 1990.

leading. Transient thyrotoxicosis may also occur postoperatively.

Caution: Postoperative hypocalcemia may require large amounts of calcium and short-acting vitamin D. Additional magnesium salts may be required postoperatively.

B. Fluids: A large fluid intake ensures a diluted urine to minimize the formation of calcium-containing renal stones.

C. Treatment of Hypercalcemia: If symptomatic and severe, hypercalcemia requires hospitalization and intensive hydration with intravenous saline. Loop diuretics such as furosemide are helpful for inducing calcium excretion and lowering the serum calcium. If used initially, however, furosemide may further dehydrate the patient and worsen the hypercalcemia. It should be used, therefore, only *after* circulatory volume has been restored by saline administration. Thiazide diuretics should not be used, since they decrease calcium excretion and worsen the hypercalcemia. In subjects in renal failure, hemodialysis may be necessary.

Pamidronate disodium is a potent inhibitor of bone resorption. It may be used for treatment of hypercalcemia due to hyperparathyroidism as well as that due to malignancy. It has also been used successfully to relieve bone pain in patients with metastatic prostate and breast carcinoma. Pamidronate, 30 mg, is mixed in 500 mL of normal saline solution and administered intravenously over 4 hours. Side effects may include mild transient leukopenia and mild fever (temperature rise of < 2 °C). Pamidronate causes a gradual decline in serum calcium over several days that tends to last for weeks to months.

Glucocorticoid therapy is very useful in cases of hypercalcemia from vitamin D intoxication, sarcoidosis, and other granulomatous disorders. The patient with hypercalcemia is very sensitive to the toxic effects of digitalis. Propranolol may be useful in preventing the adverse cardiac effects of hypercalcemia.

D. Medical Treatment of Hyperparathyroidism: Since this disorder is more frequently recognized by routine chemical screening procedures, a number of patients with relatively mild hypercalcemia (< 11 mg/dL) and few symptoms are encountered. They are best managed by forcing fluids; avoiding immobilization and thiazides; adding phosphate preparations if renal function is good; and giving estrogenic hormones if the patient is postmenopausal. If the patient cannot be followed periodically or becomes symptomatic—eg, passes a stone or shows progressive bone disease—neck exploration must be considered. Pamidronate (see above) may be used for patients unable to have surgery or to prepare patients for surgery.

Renal osteodystrophy may be prevented by avoiding the hyperphosphatemia that usually accompanies renal failure. Oral phosphate binders are usually used, most commonly calcium carbonate or calcium acetate. Aluminum hydroxide antacids are also good phosphate binders but are used less now to avoid aluminum-induced osteomalacia, an adynamic osteodystrophy. Diabetics are particularly prone to the latter condition. Calcitriol, given orally or intravenously after dialysis, also suppresses parathyroid hyperplasia and reduces the risk of renal osteodystrophy.

Prognosis

The disease is usually a chronic progressive one unless treated successfully by surgical removal of the abnormal parathyroid glands. There are at times unexplained exacerbations and partial remissions. Completely asymptomatic patients with mild hypercalcemia may be followed by means of serial calcium determinations and treated medically as outlined above.

Spontaneous cure due to necrosis of the tumor has been reported but is exceedingly rare. The prognosis is directly related to the degree of renal impairment. The bones, in spite of severe cyst formation, deformity, and fracture, will heal if a tumor is successfully removed. Significant renal damage, however, may progress even after removal of an adenoma. Parathyroid carcinoma tends to invade local structures and may sometimes metastasize; repeat surgical resections can prolong life. The presence of pancreatitis increases the mortality rate.

Bessel JR et al: Parathyroidectomy in the treatment of patients with chronic renal failure: A 10-year review. Br J Surg 1993;80:40.

Bilezikian JP: Management of acute hypercalcemia. N Engl J Med 1992;326:1196.

Carter WB et al: Cause and current management of reoperative hyperparathyroidism. Am Surg 1993;59:120.

Deftos LF et al: Management of primary hyperparathyroidism. Annu Rev Med 1993;44:19.

Kaplan EL et al: Primary hyperparathyroidism in the 1990's: Choice of surgical procedures for this disease. Ann Surg 1992;215:300.

Kelly TR: Primary hyperparathyroidism during pregnancy. Surgery 1991;110:1028.

Kohri K et al: Comparison of imaging methods for localization of parathyroid tumors. Am J Surg 1992;164:140.

Kinney TB, Deluca SA: Parathyroid hyperplasia as a cause of recurrent hyperparathyroidism. Am Fam Physician 1991;44:1253.

Marons R: Laboratory diagnosis of hyperparathyroidism. Endocrinol Metab Clin North Am 1989;18:647.

Nottingham JM et al: Bilateral neck exploration for primary hyperparathyroidism. Am Surg 1993;59:115.

Walfish PG et al: Postparathyroidectomy: Transient thyrotoxicosis. J Clin Endocrinol Metab 1992;75:224.

Winzelberg GG: Parathyroid imaging. Ann Intern Med 1989;107:64.

Wright AA et al: Fat-suppression magnetic resonance imaging in the preoperative localization of parathyroid adenomas. Clin Radiol 1992;46:324.

METABOLIC BONE DISEASE

The term "metabolic bone disease" denotes those conditions producing diffusely decreased bone density (osteopenia) and diminished bone strength. It is categorized by histologic appearance: osteoporosis (common; bone matrix and mineral both decreased) and osteomalacia (unusual; bone matrix intact, mineral decreased).

OSTEOPOROSIS

Essentials of Diagnosis

- Asymptomatic to severe backache.
- Spontaneous fractures and collapse of vertebrae often discovered accidentally on radiography; loss of height.
- Fracture of hip, ribs, or other bones with minimal or no trauma.
- Serum parathyroid hormone, 25(OH)D$_2$, calcium, phosphorus, and alkaline phosphatase usually normal.
- Demineralization, especially of spine and pelvis.

General Considerations

Osteoporosis is the most common metabolic bone disease in the USA and the cause of hundreds of thousands of fractures every year. The morbidity and indirect mortality rates are very high. Since the usual form of the disease is clinically evident in middle life and beyond and since women are more frequently affected than men, it may be referred to as "senile" or "postmenopausal" osteoporosis. It is characterized by a decrease in the amount of bone present to a level below which it is capable of maintaining the structural integrity of the skeleton. The rate of bone formation is often normal, whereas the rate of bone resorption is increased. There is a greater loss of trabecular bone than compact bone, accounting for the primary features of the disease, ie, crush fractures of vertebrae, fractures of the neck of the femur, and fractures of the distal end of the radius. Whatever bone is present is normally mineralized.

Osteogenesis imperfecta (see Chapter 19) is caused by a major mutation in the gene encoding for type I collagen, the major collagen constituent of bone. This causes severe osteoporosis. Spontaneous fractures occur in utero or during childhood. Less severe mutations in the type I collagen gene are common, resulting in collagen disarray and predisposing to hypogonadal (eg, menopausal), senile, or idiopathic osteoporosis.

Etiology

The causes of osteoporosis are listed in Table 25–14.

Clinical Findings

A. Symptoms and Signs: Osteoporosis may first be discovered on x-ray examination. It may pre-sent as backache of varying degrees of severity or as a spontaneous fracture or collapse of a vertebra. Loss of height is common.

B. Laboratory Findings: Serum calcium, phosphate, and alkaline phosphatase are normal. Serum PTH is normal. The alkaline phosphatase may be slightly elevated.

C. Imaging: The principal areas of demineralization are the spine and pelvis, especially in the femoral neck and head; demineralization is less marked in the skull and extremities. Compression of vertebrae is common. Bone densitometry (dual photon or CT) makes screening for premature bone loss feasible in high-risk individuals and allows assessment of response to therapy.

Differential Diagnosis

It is important not to confuse osteoporosis with other metabolic bone diseases, especially osteomalacia, osteogenesis imperfecta, hypophosphatasia, and hyperparathyroidism; or with the diffuse demineralization sometimes seen in myeloma and metastatic bone disease. Bone scintiscans and biopsy may be required, since these conditions may coexist.

Treatment

A. Specific Measures: Specific treatment varies with the cause; hormone therapy is most often used, though its effectiveness is greater in preventing bone loss than in increasing bone mass.

1. Sex hormones–Estrogens appear to decrease bone resorption. Before beginning estrogen therapy in a postmenopausal woman, pelvic examination should be performed to rule out neoplasm. A breast examination and mammograms are also recommended.

Estrogen preparations include conjugated estrogens in doses of 0.625–1.25 mg/d, ethinyl estradiol in doses of 0.02–0.05 mg/d, and estradiol, 1–2 mg/d.

Women with an intact uterus must take estrogen with a progestin (medroxyprogesterone acetate) in order to reduce the risk of endometrial carcinoma. This may be done on a cycled regimen: estrogen on days 1–25 every month with medroxyprogesterone acetate, 5–10 mg, added on days 16–25. Alternatively, estrogen may be given daily along with medroxyprogesterone acetate, 2.5–5 mg. The latter regimen usually produces intermittent bleeding during the first few months but is usually well tolerated ultimately, with amenorrhea and little breakthrough bleeding.

Women who have had a hysterectomy may take estrogen daily. If breast tenderness becomes a problem during daily estrogen therapy, the dose may be reduced or the estrogen may be cycled—ie, taken on days 1–25 each month or on 5 out of 7 days per week. (See below and Chapter 17.)

Men with osteoporosis and hypogonadism should be treated with parenteral **testosterone** after assess-

Table 25–14. Etiologic classification of osteoporosis.[1]

Senile	**Genetic disorders**
Hormone deficiency	Type I collagen mutations
Estrogen (women)	Osteogenesis imperfecta
Androgen (men)	Adult osteoporosis
	Ehlers-Danlos syndrome
Hormone excess	Marfan's syndrome
Cushing's syndrome or	Menke's syndrome
glucocorticoid adminis-	Homocystinuria
tration	
Thyrotoxicosis	**Miscellaneous**
Hyperparathyroidism	Diabetes mellitus
Excessive vitamin D ad-	Protein-calorie malnutrition
ministration	Liver disease
	Rheumatoid arthritis
Immobilization	Heparin therapy
	Vitamin C deficiency
Malignancy, especially mul-	Copper deficiency
tiple myeloma	Juvenile osteoporosis
	Systemic mastocytosis
	Alcoholism-induced

[1]Modified, with permission, from Fitzgerald PA: *Handbook of Clinical Endocrinology.* Appleton & Lange, 1992.

ing for prostate disease (rectal examination and serum prostate-specific antigen).

2. Calcitonin has been approved by the FDA for the treatment of osteoporosis in doses of 100 IU/d. It must be used parenterally and has limited efficacy. It is sometimes used (in patients having acute pain from an osteoporosis-induced vertebral compression fracture) for its reputed analgesic effect.

3. Diphosphonates–These agents inhibit osteoclast-induced bone resorption. Etidronate (200 mg tablets) is given in a dose of 400 mg daily for 2 weeks every 3 months.

Pamidronate is available as a parenteral preparation (30 mg/vial, lyophilized). It is a potent inhibitor of bone resorption. It has been formally approved for the treatment of hypercalcemia of malignancy but has also been demonstrated to inhibit glucocorticoid-induced osteoporosis. It is currently unclear whether the pamidronate's short-term salutary effect on bone density will be maintained with long-term glucocorticoid use. Pamidronate and other investigational diphosphonates are expected to reduce glucocorticoid-induced pathologic fractures, but their actual effect on fracture rates is still unknown. Intravenous infusions of pamidronate (eg, 30 mg in 500 L of normal saline solution over 4 hours) have been given prophylactically at approximately 3-month intervals; it may benefit certain selected patients at high risk for the development of osteoporosis. Such individuals include those expected to require high-dose long-term glucocorticoids.

B. General Measures: The diet should be adequate in protein, calcium, and vitamin D. Increased calcium intake by use of supplementary calcium salts (eg, calcium carbonate), up to 1 g calcium per day, is advisable. Additional vitamin D (2000–5000 units/d) may be needed if there is associated malabsorption or osteomalacia. Thiazides may be useful if hypercalciuria is present. Regular weight-bearing exercise is recommended. Patients should be kept active; bedridden patients should be given active or passive exercises. The spine may be adequately supported (eg, with a brace or corset), but rigid or excessive immobilization must be avoided. Patients must be protected from falling. Alcohol should be avoided.

Prognosis

The prognosis is good for postmenopausal osteoporosis if estrogen therapy is started early and maintained for years. There may be improvement in osteoporosis (especially glucocorticoid-induced) once treatment is begun and the offending agent is stopped. Periodic records of the patient's height will indicate whether the disease has stabilized. Periodic measurements of bone mass in a given individual may alert the physician to a progressive bone loss before clinical or x-ray evidence of osteoporosis occurs. Measures to prevent progressive loss of bone mass

are more effective than treatment of the clinical disease.

Avioli LV: Osteoporosis syndromes: Patient selection for calcitonin therapy. Geriatrics 1992;47:58.

Christiansen C: Prevention and treatment of osteoporosis: A review of current modalities. Bone 1992;13(Suppl 1):S35.

Lukert BP, Raisz LG: Glucocorticoid induced osteoporosis: Diagnosis and management. Ann Intern Med 1990;112:352.

Riggs BL: A new option for treating osteoporosis. N Engl J Med 1990;323:124. (Editorial on diphosphonates.)

Riggs BL et al: The prevention and treatment of osteoporosis. N Engl J Med 1992;327:620.

Stevenson JC: Pathogenesis, prevention, and treatment of osteoporosis. Obstet Gynecol 1990;75(No. 4 Suppl):36S.

Watts NB et al: Intermittent cyclical etidronate treatment of postmenopausal osteoporosis. N Engl J Med 1990; 323:73.

RICKETS & OSTEOMALACIA

Essentials of Diagnosis

- Bone deformities (rickets) in growing children.
- Bone tenderness common.
- Decreased bone density from diminished mineralization of osteoid.
- Depending on cause, laboratory abnormalities are common (versus osteoporosis) and may include increases in alkaline phosphatase, decreased 25-hydroxyvitamin D or 1,25-dihydroxyvitamin D, $25(OH)D_2$ or $1,25(OH)_2D_3$ hypocalcemia, hypocalciuria, hypophosphatemia, secondary hyperparathyroidism.
- Classic radiologic features.

General Considerations

Defective mineralization of the growing skeleton in childhood causes rickets. The same defects occurring in adults cause osteomalacia.

Etiology
(Table 25–15)

Rickets and osteomalacia can be caused by any condition that results in inadequate calcium or phosphate mineralization of bone osteoid.

A. Calcium Deficiency: Calcium deficiency can be caused by inadequate vitamin D from insufficient sun exposure, malnutrition, or malabsorption (pancreatic insufficiency, gluten-sensitive enteropathy, etc). The minimal vitamin D requirement is 2.5 μg (100 IU) daily; the recommended daily allowance is at least 10 μg (400 IU) daily. In the USA, with the exception perhaps of Alaska, the latitude is adequate to allow sufficient sun exposure of infants and children so that ultraviolet radiation can convert 7-dehydrocholesterol to cholecalciferol (vitamin D_3) in the skin, thus providing vitamin D necessary for

Table 25–15. Causes of rickets and osteomalacia.[1]

Vitamin disorders
  Decreased availability of vitamin D
    Insufficient sunlight exposure
    Nutritional deficiency of vitamin D
    Malabsorption
    Nephrotic syndrome
  Abnormal response to vitamin D
  Vitamin D-dependent rickets type I
  X-linked hypophosphatemic rickets
  Tumoral hypophosphatemic osteomalacia
  Liver disease
  Chronic renal failure
  Phenytoin or barbiturate therapy

Calcium deficiency

Phosphate deficiency
  Decreased intestinal absorption
    Nutritional deficiency of phosphorus
    Malabsorption
    Phosphate-binding antacid therapy

Increased renal loss
  Vitamin D-resistant rickets
  Tumoral hypohposphatemic osteomalacia
  Association with other disorders, including
    paraproteinemias, glycogen storage diseases,
    galactosemia, tyroisinemia, cystinosis,
    neurofibromatosis, Wilson's disease,
    Fanconi's syndrome

Disorders of bone matrix
  Hypophosphatasia
  Fibrogenesis imperfecta
  Axial osteomalacia

Inhibitors of mineralization
  Aluminum
  Diphosphonates

[1]Reproduced, with permission, from Fitzgerald PA: *Handbook of Clinical Endocrinology.* Appleton & Lange, 1992.

calcium absorption. However, human milk is a poor source of vitamin D; infants who are otherwise thriving on pure breast feeding may develop mild rickets during the winter months unless they receive vitamin D supplements or adequate ultraviolet exposure.

Children and adults in the USA generally receive nutritional supplements of plant vitamin D (ergocalciferol, vitamin D_2) in milk or other processed foods, so that serious vitamin D deficiency is now quite rare. Nutritional vitamin D deficiency is common in less developed areas of the world.

Patients may have other defects of vitamin D synthesis or resistance. Renal disease causes deficient 1-hydroxylation of 25-hydroxyvitamin D.

Rickets and osteomalacia may also be caused by anticonvulsant medication, especially phenytoin and phenobarbital, probably by causing resistance to 1,25-hydroxyvitamin D. Familial 1,25-hydroxyvitamin D resistance syndromes have also been described.

B. Phosphate Deficiency: Phosphate deficiency is caused most commonly by a familial X-linked renal tubular defect of phosphate resorption vitamin D-resistant rickets). It can also be caused by

malabsorption due to gut-binding by aluminum hydroxide antacids. Hypophosphatemia can also be caused by benign soft tissue tumors that secrete a substance which causes phosphaturia and total body phosphate depletion.

C. Hypophosphatasia: Diminished activity of bone alkaline phosphatase is an inherited disorder of bone mineralization. Manifestations are quite variable, ranging from death in utero to dental dysplasia or fractures that may present in childhood or adulthood. Serum alkaline phosphatase is usually low. Urinary phosphoethanolamine excretion is usually increased. Treatment is entirely symptomatic.

Clinical Findings

The clinical manifestations of defective bone mineralization depend on the age at onset and the severity. Bones growing fastest are affected the most. Infants develop cranial defects with "frontal bossing"; the infant's posterior skull may become flattened (craniotabes). The costochondral junctions become enlarged (rachitic rosary), and thoracic deformities are common. Growing children's legs tend to bow (genu varum) or become knock-kneed (genu valgus) and are shorter than normal. Children are usually very weak and may suffer convulsions or tetany if severely hypocalcemic.

Diagnostic Tests

Serum is obtained for calcium, albumin, phosphate, alkaline phosphatase, parathyroid hormone. and 25-hydroxyvitamin D 25(OH)D_2 determinations. Serum 1,25-hydroxyvitamin D 1,25(OH)$_2D_3$ measurements may sometimes be helpful. Urine is obtained for calcium and phosphate excretion rates. Bone densitometry helps document the degree of osteopenia. X-rays may show diagnostic features of rickets (see above). Pseudofractures may sometimes be seen, as well as other radiologic features characteristic of osteomalacia or rickets. Bone biopsy can be helpful when this is a consideration, since unmineralized osteoid will be apparent. Laboratory features of hypophosphatasia include a low serum alkaline phosphatase, low urinary hydroxyproline, and high serum and urinary concentrations of phosphorylethanolamine and pyrophosphate.

Differential Diagnosis

Rickets and osteomalacia usually can be distinguished from osteoporosis by the relative absence of biochemical abnormalities in the latter.

Treatment

Treatment of rickets and osteomalacia depends upon the cause. Nutritional vitamin D deficiency is treated with ergocalciferol. Large doses are sometimes required in malabsorption syndromes.

Vitamin D resistance syndromes may be reversed

with 25-OH vitamin D (cacifediol) or 1,25-$(OH)_2$ vitamin D (calcitriol).

Phosphate deficiency from renal phosphate wasting (vitamin D-resistant rickets) responds to lifetime phosphate supplementation; vitamin D must be given also to improve the impaired calcium absorption caused by the phosphate.

Hypophosphatasia has been treated with oral phosphates, but responses are often disappointing.

Campbell GA: Osteomalacia: Diagnosis and Management. Br J Hosp Med 1990;44:332.

Feldman KW et al: Nutritional rickets. Am Fam Phys 1990;42:1311.

Goodman WG, Coburn JW: the use of 1,25-dihydroxy vitamin D_3 in early renal failure. Ann Rev Med 1992;43:227.

Hutchinson FN, Bell NH: Osteomalacia and rickets. Semin Nephrol 1992;12:127.

Mankin HJ: Rickets, osteomalacia, and renal osteodystrophy: An update. Orthop Clin North Am 1990;21:81.

Tzamalovkas AH: Diagnosis and management of bone disorder in chronic renal failure and dialyzed patients. Med Clin North Am 1990;74:961.

NONMETABOLIC BONE DISEASE

POLYOSTOTIC FIBROUS DYSPLASIA

Polyostotic fibrous dysplasia is the bone manifestation of a rare disorder known as **McCune-Albright syndrome.** It presents in childhood with bone lesions, patchy skin pigmentation, precocious puberty, and a variety of other endocrine problems. These seemingly unrelated disorders are caused by a mosaic distribution of a mutated "G protein."

Peptide hormones (from the hypothalamus and pituitary; catecholamines) direct their messages to "target" tissues by binding to unique cell surface receptors. The hormone-receptor complex causes a conformational change in an adjacent common transmembrane G protein. The altered G protein regulates (usually enhances) the activity of adenylyl cyclase, an enzyme bound to the cytoplasmic side of the cell membrane. Adenylyl cyclase catalyzes ATP to form cAMP; this stimulates protein kinases to alter the activity of important enzymes, thus producing the hormonal effect.

Levine MA: The McCune-Albright syndrome: The whys and wherefores of abnormal signal transduction. (Editorial.) N Engl J Med 1991;325:1738.

PAGET'S DISEASE
(Osteitis Deformans)

Essentials of Diagnosis
- Often asymptomatic.
- Bone pain may be the first symptom.
- Kyphosis, bowed tibias, large head, waddling gait, and frequent fractures that vary with location of process.
- Serum calcium and phosphate normal; alkaline phosphatase elevated; urinary hydroxyproline elevated.
- Dense, expanded bones on x-ray.

General Considerations
Paget's disease is a nonmetabolic bone disease of unknown cause, though virus infection has been suggested. It causes excessive bone destruction and repair—with associated deformities, since the repair takes place in an unorganized fashion. Up to 3% of persons over age 50 have isolated lesions, but clinically important disease is much less common. There is a strong familial incidence of Paget's disease. A rare form occurs in young people.

Clinical Findings
A. Symptoms and Signs: Paget's disease is often mild or asymptomatic. Deep "bone pain" is usually the first symptom. The bones become soft, leading to bowed tibias, kyphosis, and frequent fractures with slight trauma. If the skull is involved, the patient may report headaches and an increased hat size. Increased vascularity over the involved bones causes increased warmth.

B. Laboratory Findings: Serum calcium and phosphorus are normal, but serum alkaline phosphatase is markedly elevated. Urinary hydroxyproline is also elevated in active disease. Serum calcium may be elevated, particularly if the patient is at bed rest.

C. Imaging: On radiographs the involved bones are expanded and denser than normal. Multiple fissure fractures may be seen in the long bones. The initial lesion may be destructive and radiolucent, especially in the skull ("osteoporosis circumscripta"). Technetium pyrophosphate bone scans are helpful in delineating activity of bone lesions even before any radiologic changes are apparent.

Differential Diagnosis
Paget's disease must be differentiated from primary bone lesions such as osteogenic sarcoma, multiple myeloma, and fibrous dysplasia and from secondary bone lesions such as metastatic carcinoma and osteitis fibrosa cystica. Fibrogenesis imperfecta ossium is a rare symmetric disorder that can mimic the features of Paget's disease; alkaline phosphate is likewise elevated. If serum calcium is elevated, hyperparathyroidism may be present in some patients as well.

Complications

Fractures are frequent and occur with minimal trauma. If immobilization takes place and there is an excessive calcium intake, hypercalcemia and kidney stones may develop. Vertebral collapse may lead to spinal cord compression. Osteosarcoma may develop in long-standing lesions. Sarcomatous change is suggested by marked increase in bone pain, sudden rise in alkaline phosphatase, and appearance of a new lytic lesion. The increased vascularity may give rise to high-output cardiac failure. Arthritis frequently develops in joints adjacent to involved bone.

Extensive skull involvement may cause cranial nerve palsies from impingement of the neural foramina. Ischemic neurologic events may occur as a result of a vascular "steal" phenomenon. Involvement of the auditory region frequently causes hearing loss (mixed sensorineural and conductive) and occasionally tinnitus or vertigo.

Treatment

Asymptomatic patients require no treatment.

The calcitonins (porcine, human, and salmon) act by reducing osteoclastic activity. **Synthetic salmon calcitonin** is given in doses of 50–100 IU subcutaneously daily or three times weekly for months to years. Aside from local sensitivity reactions, systemic side effects—eg, flushing, nausea—are common but usually quite mild. Calcimar is the drug of choice for painful pagetic lesions. It is expensive, and antibody formation occurs in about 20% of patients, reducing its effectiveness; such patients may respond to human calcitonin. Nasal calcitonin is due to become available in 1994 or 1995. It is given in doses of 400 IU nasally twice weekly (along with oral calcium and a thiazide) with efficacy similar to that achieved by the parenteral route.

The **diphosphonates** inhibit osteoclast-mediated bone resorption. Etidronate disodium is available in 200 mg and 400 mg tablets. The safest dose is 5 mg/kg daily for 90–180 days. In severe disease, 10 mg/kg/d may be used for 90 days, with rest periods before another course is given. Etidronate disodium is effective orally with minor side effects (eg, diarrhea), but it must never be used for periods longer than 6 months because it may have adverse effects on bone mineralization. Etidronate can aggravate bone pain.

Pamidronate is effective in treating Paget's disease. The dosage is 30 mg diluted in 500 mL normal saline solution and given intravenously over 4 hours. Improvement may last several months.

Plicamycin (mithramycin) rapidly suppresses osteoclastic activity and has been effective in severe cases. Because of renal, hepatic, and bone marrow toxicity, however, this drug should be used only in the most serious cases.

Patients may respond to one agent after they have escaped from the beneficial effects of another.

Prognosis

The prognosis in general is good, but sarcomatous changes (in 1–3%) or renal complications secondary to hypercalciuria alter the prognosis unfavorably. In general, the prognosis is worse the earlier in life the disease starts. Fractures usually heal well. In the severe forms, marked deformity, intractable pain, and cardiac failure are found.

Merkow RL, Lane JM: Paget's disease of bone. Endocrinol Metab Clin North Am 1990;19:177.

Posen S: Paget's disease: Current concepts. Aust N Z J Surg 1992;62:17.

DISEASES OF THE ADRENAL CORTEX

ADRENAL CORTEX PHYSIOLOGY

Aldosterone is the major mineralocorticoid secreted by the zona glomerulosa, the outer layer of the adrenal cortex. It stimulates the renal tubule to reabsorb sodium and excrete potassium, thereby protecting against hypovolemia and hyperkalemia.

Aldosterone secretion is stimulated by hypovolemia in an indirect way: Hypovolemia causes the renal juxtaglomerular cells to secrete renin; renin stimulates the peripheral conversion of angiotensin I to angiotensin II; angiotensin II then causes aldosterone secretion. Hypokalemia directly stimulates aldosterone secretion. Secretion is inhibited by atrial natriuretic factor and by dopamine.

Cortisol is the major glucocorticoid secreted by the middle zona fasciculata and the inner zona reticularis of the adrenal cortex. It exerts complex effects via cytoplasmic receptors found in nucleated cells throughout the body.

Cortisol is secreted in a diurnal pattern, being highest upon awakening and lowest at bedtime. It is required for production of angiotensin II, thereby helping maintain adequate vascular tone.

Cortisol counters insulin effects, tending to cause hyperglycemia by inhibiting insulin secretion and by increasing hepatic gluconeogenesis, substrate being provided by the increased amino acids made available by cortisol's inhibition of protein synthesis in muscles.

Cortisol production normally increases during exercise, making more glucose and fatty acids available for energy. Cortisol is also secreted in response to acute trauma, infection, and other stresses; it dampens defense mechanisms, helping prevent their dangerous overactivity. It inhibits the production or action of many mediators of inflammation and immunity such as lymphokines, prostaglandins, and histamine.

Glucocorticoids also increase renal free water clearance. They lower serum calcium by inhibiting calcium uptake by the renal tubule and gut and by redistributing calcium intracellularly.

Androgens are produced in the adrenal cortex, mostly by the inner zona fasciculata. This zone is prominent during fetal life, producing vast amounts of dehydroepiandrosterone sulfate (DHEAS), which is acted upon by the sulfatases in the placenta (and other tissues) to become DHEA, the precursor to maternal estrogen. The adrenal cortex's fetal zone atrophies after birth, but the adrenal continues to make large amount of DHEAS and DHEA, which have no known significance during adult life, having minimal androgenic activity; but they continue to be the adrenals' most abundantly secreted steroids. DHEAS secretion declines steadily with age. There are individual differences in secretion, and—for unknown reasons—there is a direct positive correlation between DHEAS levels and longevity.

Testosterone and androstenedione are the major functional androgens secreted by the adrenal. Their secretion causes adrenarche, which precedes gonadal androgen secretion and stimulates the first sexual hair of puberty.

All hormones secreted by the adrenal cortex are steroids. They are lipid-soluble, entering cells readily, where they bind to specific intracellular receptors. Those hormone-receptor complexes then bind to specific DNA sequences considered to be hormone-dependent transcription enhancers. These regulate gene expression, producing and amplifying the hormonal effect.

ADRENOCORTICAL HYPOFUNCTION (Adrenocortical Insufficiency)

1. ACUTE ADRENAL INSUFFICIENCY (Adrenal Crisis)

Essentials of Diagnosis

- Weakness, abdominal pain, fever, confusion, nausea and vomiting.
- Low blood pressure, dehydration; skin pigmentation may be increased.
- Serum potassium high, sodium low, blood urea nitrogen high.
- Cosyntropin (ACTH$_{1-24}$) unable to stimulate a normal increase in serum cortisol.

General Considerations

Acute adrenal insufficiency is an emergency caused by insufficient cortisol. Crisis may occur in the course of chronic insufficiency in a known addisonian patient, or it may be the presenting manifes-

tation of adrenal insufficiency. Acute adrenal crisis is more commonly seen in primary adrenal insufficiency (Addison's disease) than in disorders of the pituitary gland causing secondary adrenocortical hypofunction.

Adrenal crisis may occur in the following situations: (1) Following stress, eg, trauma, surgery, infection, or prolonged fasting in a patient with latent insufficiency. (2) Following sudden withdrawal of adrenocortical hormone in a patient with chronic insufficiency or in a patient with temporary insufficiency due to suppression by exogenous glucocorticoids. (3) Following bilateral adrenalectomy or removal of a functioning adrenal tumor that had suppressed the other adrenal. (4) Following sudden destruction of the pituitary gland (pituitary necrosis), or when thyroid is given to a patient with hypoadrenalism. (5) Following injury to both adrenals by trauma, hemorrhage, anticoagulant therapy, thrombosis, infection, or, rarely, metastatic carcinoma. In overwhelming sepsis, massive bilateral adrenal hemorrhage may occur (Waterhouse-Friderichsen syndrome).

Clinical Findings

A. Symptoms and Signs: The patient complains of headache, lassitude, nausea and vomiting, abdominal pain, and often diarrhea. Confusion or coma may be present. Fever may be 40.6 °C (105 °F) or more. The blood pressure is low. Other signs may include cyanosis, petechiae (especially with meningococcemia), dehydration, skin hyperpigmentation, and sparse axillary hair (if hypogonadism is also present).

B. Laboratory Findings: The eosinophil count may be high. Hyponatremia or hyperkalemia (or both) are usually present. Hypoglycemia is frequent. Hypercalcemia may be present. Blood, sputum, or urine culture may be positive if bacterial infection is the precipitating cause.

The diagnosis is made by the cosyntropin stimulation test, which is performed as follows: (1) Serum is obtained for a baseline cortisol and ACTH determination at least 12 hours after any prior administration of hydrocortisone. (2) Synthetic ACTH$_{1-24}$ (cosyntropin), 0.25 mg, is then given parenterally. (3) Serum is obtained for cortisol 60 minutes after cosyntropin is administered. Normally, serum cortisol rises at least 8 μg/dL above baseline to a peak of over 16 μg/dL. Both criteria are important, since some patients with adrenal insufficiency have serum cortisol levels in the "normal range" but insufficient cortisol reserve to deal with a stressful illness.

Plasma ACTH is markedly elevated if the patient has primary adrenal disease (generally > 200 pg/mL).

Differential Diagnosis

This condition must be differentiated from other causes of coma and confusion, such as diabetic coma, cerebrovascular accident, and acute poisoning, and from other causes of high fever. The high serum potassium is not specific, but it should alert the physician to the possibility of adrenal insufficiency. The blood glucose is usually low, but the condition may coexist with diabetes mellitus, in which case the blood sugar is high, which may be misleading. Eosinophilia and lymphocytosis, which are usually absent in other emergencies, are characteristic.

Treatment

A. Acute Phase: If the diagnosis is suspected, draw a blood sample for cortisol determination and treat with hydrocortisone, 100–300 mg intravenously, and saline *immediately*, without waiting for the results. Thereafter, give hydrocortisone phosphate or hydrocortisone sodium succinate, 100 mg intravenously immediately, and continue intravenous infusions of 50–100 mg every 6 hours for the first day. Give the same amount every 8 hours on the second day and then adjust the dosage in view of the clinical picture.

Since bacterial infection is frequently the precipitating factor of acute adrenal crisis, it is wise to administer broad-spectrum antibiotics empirically while waiting for the results of initial cultures. Hypoglycemia should be vigorously treated while serum electrolytes, blood urea nitrogen, and creatinine are monitored.

B. Convalescent Phase: When the patient is able to take food by mouth, give oral hydrocortisone, 10–20 mg every 6 hours, and reduce dosage to maintenance levels as needed. Most patients ultimately require hydrocortisone twice daily (AM, 10–20 mg; PM, 5–10 mg). Mineralocorticoid therapy is not needed when large amounts of hydrocortisone are being given, but as the dose is reduced it is usually necessary to add fludrocortisone acetate, 0.05–0.2 mg daily. Some patients never require fludrocortisone and become edematous when it is taken.

Prognosis

Before the era of glucocorticoid replacement therapy and antibiotics, acute adrenal crisis was usually rapidly fatal. Even today, if aggressive treatment is not provided early, death may occur. Once the crisis has passed, the patient must be investigated to assess the degree of permanent adrenal insufficiency and to establish the cause if possible.

Claussen MS et al: Acute adrenal insufficiency presenting as shock after trauma and surgery: Three cases and review of the literature. Trauma 1992;32:94.

Frederick R et al: Addisonian crisis: Emergency presentation of primary adrenal insufficiency. Ann Emerg Med 1991;20:802.

2. CHRONIC ADRENOCORTICAL INSUFFICIENCY (Addison's Disease)

Essentials of Diagnosis

- Weakness, easy fatigability, anorexia, weight loss; nausea and vomiting, diarrhea; abdominal pain, muscle and joint pains; amenorrhea.
- Sparse axillary hair; increased skin pigmentation, especially of creases, pressure areas, and nipples.
- Hypotension, small heart.
- Serum sodium may be low; potassium, calcium, and urea nitrogen may be elevated; neutropenia, mild anemia, eosinophilia, and relative lymphocytosis may be present.
- Plasma cortisol levels are low or fail to rise after administration of corticotropin.
- Plasma ACTH level elevated.

General Considerations

Addison's disease is an uncommon disorder caused by destruction of the adrenal cortices. It is characterized by chronic deficiency of cortisol, aldosterone, and adrenal androgens and causes skin pigmentation that can be strikingly dark or subtle. Volume and sodium depletion and potassium excess eventually occur in primary adrenal failure. In contrast, if chronic adrenal insufficiency is secondary to pituitary failure (atrophy, necrosis, tumor), mineralocorticoid production (controlled by the renin-angiotensin system) persists and hyperkalemia is not present. Furthermore, if ACTH is not elevated, skin pigmentary changes are not encountered.

The term "Addison's disease" should be reserved for adrenal insufficiency due to adrenocortical disease. Autoimmune destruction of the adrenals is the most common cause of Addison's disease in the USA (accounting for about 80% of spontaneous cases). It may be isolated or may occur as part of a polyglandular autoimmune syndrome (PGA). **Type I PGA** begins in early childhood with chronic mucocutaneous candidiasis followed by hypoparathyroidism and Addison's disease by age 10–12 years. **Type II PGA** consists of Addison's disease, thyroid disease (hyperthyroidism 5%; hypothyroidism 10%) or insulin-dependent diabetes (10%). This syndrome is also known as "autoimmune polyendocrinopathy-candidiasis-ectodermal dysplasia (APECED)." The combination of Addison's disease and hypothyroidism is known as Schmidt's syndrome.

Other problems seen with autoimmune Addison's disease include vitiligo, premature primary ovarian failure (40% of women before age 50), testicular failure (5%), and pernicious anemia (4%).

Tuberculosis was formerly a leading cause of Addison's disease. The association is now relatively rare in the USA but common where tuberculosis is more prevalent.

Rare causes include metastatic carcinoma, coccidioidomycosis, histoplasmosis, cytomegalovirus infection (more frequent in patients with AIDS), syphilitic gummas, scleroderma, amyloid disease, and hemochromatosis. Bilateral adrenal hemorrhage may occur in patients taking anticoagulants, during open heart surgery, and during birth or other major trauma. Some cases are associated with antiphospholipid antibody syndrome.

Clinical Findings

A. Symptoms and Signs: The symptoms may include weakness and fatigability, weight loss, anorexia, nausea and vomiting, and, less frequently, diarrhea and nervous and mental irritability. Pigmentary changes consist of diffuse tanning over non-exposed as well as exposed parts or multiple freckles; hyperpigmentation is especially prominent over the knuckles, elbows, knees, and posterior neck and in palmar creases and nail beds. Nipples and areolas tend to darken. The skin in pressure areas such as the belt or brassiere lines and the buttocks also darkens. New scars are pigmented. Some patients have associated vitiligo. Arthralgias, myalgias, and muscle stiffness may occur. Emotional changes are common. Hypoglycemia, when present, may worsen the patient's weakness and mental functioning, rarely leading to coma. Manifestations of other autoimmune disease (see above) may be present. Other findings include hypotension with small heart, hyperplasia of lymphoid tissues, stiffness and calcification of the cartilages of the ear, and scant axillary and pubic hair (especially in women).

B. Laboratory Findings: The white count shows moderate neutropenia (about 5000/µL), lymphocytosis (35–50%), and a total eosinophil count over 300/µL. Serum potassium and urea nitrogen are elevated; serum sodium may be low. Fasting blood glucose may be low. Hypercalcemia may be present.

Low plasma cortisol (< 5 mg/dL) at 8 AM is diagnostic, especially if accompanied by simultaneous elevation of the plasma ACTH level (usually > 200 pg/mL). The cosyntropin stimulation test is performed as described above. Antiadrenal antibodies are found in the serum in about 50% of cases of autoimmune Addison's disease. Antibodies to thyroid (45%) and other tissues may be present.

C. Imaging: When Addison's disease is not clearly autoimmune, a chest x-ray is obtained to look for tuberculosis, fungal infection, or cancer as possible causes. CT scan of the abdomen will show small noncalcified adrenals in autoimmune Addison's disease. The adrenals are enlarged in about 85% of cases due to metastatic or granulomatous disease. Calcification is noted in about 50% of cases of tuberculous Addison's disease but is also seen with hemorrhage, fungal infection, pheochromocytoma, and melanoma.

Differential Diagnosis

Addison's disease should be considered in any patient with hypotension and hyperkalemia. Unexplained weight loss, weakness, and anorexia may be mistaken for occult cancer. Nausea, vomiting, diarrhea, and abdominal pain may be misdiagnosed as intrinsic gastrointestinal disease. The hyperpigmentation may be confused with that due to ethnic or racial factors. Weight loss may simulate anorexia nervosa. Hemochromatosis also enters the differential diagnosis of skin hyperpigmentation, but it should be remembered that it may truly be a cause of Addison's disease as well as diabetes mellitus and hypoparathyroidism. Serum ferritin is increased in most cases of hemochromatosis and is a useful screening test.

Complications

Any of the complications of the underlying disease (eg, tuberculosis) are more likely to occur, and the patient is susceptible to intercurrent infections that may precipitate crisis. Diabetes mellitus and, rarely, thyrotoxicosis, as well as Hashimoto's thyroiditis, hypoparathyroidism, pernicious anemia, and ovarian failure of autoimmune origin may be associated with idiopathic adrenal failure.

Treatment

A. Specific Therapy: Replacement therapy should include a combination of glucocorticoids and mineralocorticoids. In mild cases, hydrocortisone alone may be adequate.

1. Hydrocortisone is the drug of choice. Most addisonian patients are well maintained on 15–25 mg of hydrocortisone orally daily in two divided doses, two-thirds in the morning and one-third in the late afternoon or early evening. Some patients respond better to prednisone in a dosage of about 3 mg in the morning and 2 mg in the evening. Many patients, however, do not obtain sufficient salt-retaining effect and require fludrocortisone supplementation or extra dietary salt.

2. Fludrocortisone acetate has a potent sodium-retaining effect. The dosage is 0.05–0.3 mg orally daily or every other day. If postural hypotension, hyperkalemia, or weight loss occurs, raise the dose. If edema, hypokalemia, or hypertension ensues, lower the dose.

B. General Measures: If replacement therapy is adequate, most patients need no special diets or precautions. Treat all infections immediately and vigorously, and raise the dose of hydrocortisone appropriately. The dose of glucocorticoid should also be raised in case of trauma, surgery, stressful diagnostic procedures, or other forms of stress. Patients are advised to wear a medical alert bracelet or medal reading, "Adrenal insufficiency—takes hydrocortisone."

Prognosis

With adequate replacement therapy, the life expectancy of patients with Addison's disease is markedly prolonged. Active tuberculosis responds to specific treatment. Withdrawal of treatment or increased demands due to infection, trauma, surgery, or other types of stress may precipitate crisis with a sudden fatal outcome unless large doses of parenteral corticosteroids are employed. Pregnancy may be followed by exacerbation of the disease. With appropriate therapy, however, a fully active life is possible for most patients.

Johnson TL: Tuberculous Addison's disease. Postgrad Med 1991;90:139.
Kasperlik-Zaluska AA et al: Association of Addison's disease with autoimmune disorders: A long-term observation of 180 patients. Postgrad Med J 1991;76;984.
Muir A, Maclaren NK: Autoimmune diseases of the adrenal glands, parathyroid glands, gonads, and hypothalamic-pituitary axis. Endocrinol Metab Clin North Am 1991;20:619.
Norbiato G et al: Cortisol resistance in acquired immunodeficiency syndrome. J Clin Endocrinol Metab 1992; 74:608.

CUSHING'S SYNDROME (Hypercortisolism)

Essentials of Diagnosis

- Central obesity, muscle wasting, thin skin, easy bruisability, psychologic changes, hirsutism, purple striae.
- Osteoporosis, hypertension, poor wound healing.
- Hyperglycemia, glycosuria, leukocytosis, lymphocytopenia, hypokalemia.
- Elevated serum cortisol and urinary free cortisol. Lack of normal suppression by dexamethasone.

General Considerations

The term Cushing's "syndrome" refers to the manifestations of hypercortisolism due to any cause. ACTH hypersecretion by the pituitary is the most common cause of the disorder and is referred to as Cushing's "disease" (about 90% due to a pituitary adenoma, the rest due to hyperplasia). It accounts for about 70–80% of cases of spontaneous hypercortisolism in adults. Hypercortisolism may also be due to an autonomous adrenal tumor (adenoma or carcinoma, 10–15%), ectopic secretion of ACTH by a nonpituitary neoplasm (5–15%), or bilateral nodular hyperplasia without ACTH (< 1%). In Cushing's syndrome in children, adrenal neoplasms are relatively more common while ectopic ACTH is uncommon.

Chronic administration of corticotropin causes adrenal hyperplasia; administration of supraphysiologic doses of glucocorticoid causes adrenal atrophy associated with features of Cushing's syndrome. These effects are partially reversible when medication is withdrawn.

Adrenal carcinoma may sometimes not be hormonally active or may produce Cushing's syndrome with severe virilization.

Certain extra-adrenal malignant tumors (eg, small-cell carcinoma of the lung) may secrete ACTH or, more rarely, corticotropin-releasing factor and produce severe Cushing's syndrome with bilateral adrenal hyperplasia. Severe hypokalemia and hyperpigmentation are commonly found in this group.

Clinical Findings

A. Symptoms and Signs: Patients with Cushing's syndrome usually have central obesity with a plethoric "moon face," "buffalo hump," supraclavicular fat pads, protuberant abdomen, and thin extremities; oligomenorrhea or amenorrhea (or impotence in the male); weakness, backache, headache; hypertension; and acne and superficial skin infections. Patients may have thirst and polyuria (with or without glycosuria), renal calculi, glaucoma, purple striae (especially around the thighs, breasts, and abdomen), and easy bruisability. Wound healing is impaired. Mental symptoms may range from increased lability of mood to frank psychosis. Patients are subject to infections.

B. Laboratory Findings: Glucose tolerance is impaired as a result of insulin resistance. Polyuria is present as a result of increased free water clearance; diabetes mellitus with glycosuria may worsen it. Patients with Cushing's syndrome often have leukocytosis with relative granulocytosis and lymphopenia. Hypokalemia may be present, particularly in cases of ectopic ACTH secretion.

Tests for Hypercortisolism

The easiest screening test for hypercortisolism involves giving dexamethasone, 1 mg, at 11 PM and collecting serum for cortisol determination at about 8 AM the next morning; a cortisol level under 5μg/dL excludes Cushing's syndrome with 98% certainty. Other patients require further investigation, which includes a 24-hour urine collection for cortisol and creatinine; free cortisol excretion of over 100 μg/d—or over 95 mg per milligram of creatinine—helps confirm hypercortisolism.

A suppression test can also be done by giving dexamethasone, 0.5 mg orally every 6 hours for 48 hours; urine is collected on the second day. Urine free cortisol over 20 μg/d or urine 17-hydroxycorticosteroid over 4.5 mg/d also helps confirm hypercortisolism.

Samples for serum cortisol determinations may be obtained at 8 AM and 11 PM; an 11 PM cortisol over 50% of the 8 AM level indicates lack of diurnal variation that is characteristic of Cushing's syndrome in adults. Conditions that cause false-positive testing (see below) should be considered.

Finding the Cause of Hypercortisolism

Once hypercortisolism is confirmed, a baseline plasma ACTH is obtained. It must be collected properly on ice and processed quickly by a laboratory with a reliable, sensitive assay. A level of ACTH below the normal range (20 pg/mL) indicates a probable adrenal tumor, whereas higher levels are produced by pituitary or ectopic tumors.

Localizing Techniques

In ACTH-dependent Cushing's syndrome, MRI of the pituitary can demonstrate a pituitary adenoma in about 50% of cases. When the pituitary MRI is not helpful, selective inferior petrosal venous sampling for ACTH is performed (often during CRH stimulation) to confirm a pituitary ACTH source, distinguishing it from an occult nonpituitary tumor secreting ACTH.

In non-ACTH-dependent Cushing's syndrome, a CT scan of the adrenals can localize the adrenal tumor in most cases.

Differential Diagnosis

Alcoholic patients can have hypercortisolism and many clinical manifestations of Cushing's syndrome. Depressed patients also have hypercortisolism that can be nearly impossible to distinguish biochemically from Cushing's syndrome. Patients with severe obesity frequently have an abnormal dexamethasone suppression test, but the urine free cortisol is usually normal, as is diurnal variation of serum cortisol. Patients with familial cortisol resistance have hyperandrogenism and hypertension along with hypercortisolism that does not produce actual Cushing's syndrome. Certain drugs such as phenytoin, phenobarbital, and primidone accelerate the metabolism of dexamethasone, thereby causing a "false-positive" dexamethasone suppression test. Estrogens—during pregnancy or as medication—also frequently cause lack of dexamethasone suppressibility. In pregnancy, urine free cortisol is increased, while 17-hydroxycorticosteroids remain normal and diurnal variability of serum cortisol is normal.

Complications

Cushing's syndrome, if untreated, produces serious morbidity and even death. The patient may suffer from any of the complications of hypertension or of diabetes. Susceptibility to infections is increased. Compression fractures of the osteoporotic spine and aseptic necrosis of the femoral head may cause marked disability. Nephrolithiasis and psychosis may occur. Following bilateral adrenalectomy for Cushing's disease, a pituitary adenoma may enlarge progressively, causing local destruction (eg, visual field impairment) and hyperpigmentation; this complication is known as Nelson's syndrome.

Treatment

Cushing's disease is best treated by selective transsphenoidal resection of the pituitary adenoma. After selective resection of a pituitary adenoma causing Cushing's disease, the rest of the pituitary usually returns to normal function; however, the normal corticotrophs are suppressed and require 6–36 months to recover normal function. Hydrocortisone replacement therapy is necessary in the meantime. Patients who fail to have a remission should undergo bilateral adrenalectomy. Patients may also receive pituitary irradiation, but only about 23% of patients are cured, and remissions require up to 6 months. Patients who are not surgical candidates may be given a trial of ketoconazole in doses of about 200 mg every 6 hours; liver enzymes must be monitored for progressive elevation.

Adrenal neoplasms secreting cortisol are treated with surgical resection via a flank approach. The contralateral adrenal is suppressed, so postoperative hydrocortisone replacement is required until recovery occurs. Metastatic adrenal carcinomas may be treated with mitotane; ketoconazole or metyrapone can help suppress hypercortisolism in unresectable adrenal carcinoma.

Ectopic ACTH-secreting tumors should be surgically resected. If that cannot be done, medical treatment with ketoconazole or metyrapone (or both) may at least suppress the hypercortisolism, whereas metyrapone may exacerbate female virilization.

Prognosis

The best prognosis for total recovery is for patients in whom a benign adrenal adenoma has been removed and who have survived the postadrenalectomy state of adrenal insufficiency. Patients with Cushing's disease can be cured by transsphenoidal surgery, but there is a failure rate of about 10–20%. Those patients who have a complete remission after transsphenoidal surgery have about a 15–20% chance of recurrence over the next 10 years. Even patients who undergo bilateral adrenalectomy may have a recurrence of hypercortisolism due to growth of an adrenal remnant, stimulated by the high levels of ACTH found after adrenalectomy. The prognosis for ectopic ACTH-producing tumors is dependent upon the aggressiveness and metastatic status of the particular tumor type.

Findling JW: Cushing's syndromes: An enlarged clinical spectrum. N Engl J Med 1989;321:1677.
Kaye TB, Crapo L: The Cushing's syndrome: An update on diagnostic tests. Ann Intern Med 1990;112:434.
Schteingart D: Cushing's syndrome. Endocrinol Metab Clin North Am 1989;18:311.

3. HIRSUTISM & VIRILIZATION

Essentials of Diagnosis

- Menstrual disorders, hirsutism, acne.
- Virilization may occur: increased muscularity,

balding, deepening of the voice, enlargement of the clitoris.

- Occasionally a palpable pelvic tumor.
- Urinary 17-ketosteroids and serum DHEAS and androstenedione elevated in adrenal disorders, variable in others.
- Serum testosterone often elevated.

General Considerations

Important androgens include testosterone, androstenedione, and dehydroepiandrosterone sulfate (DHEAS). In women, circulating testosterone is derived from direct ovarian secretion (60%) and from peripheral conversion from androstenedione (40%). Androstenedione is secreted in about equal amounts by the adrenals and ovaries. DHEAS is secreted exclusively by the adrenals.

Testosterone is the most potent androgen, but 98% circulates in a bound state: About 65% is strongly bound to sex hormone-binding globulin (SHBG), while 33% is weakly bound to albumin. Only free testosterone and a portion of the weakly bound testosterone can enter target cells to exert androgenic effect. Assays have therefore been devised to measure "total," "free," or "free and weakly bound" testosterone.

Testosterone is converted in the skin to dihydrotestosterone (DHT), which actually stimulates the hair follicle. DHT is metabolized to androstanediol glucuronide, which can be measured and is elevated in most cases of hirsutism.

Etiology

Hirsutism may be caused by the following disorders:

(1) Polycystic ovary syndrome (hyperthecosis, Stein-Leventhal syndrome): This is a common functional disorder of the ovaries. Patients frequently have amenorrhea or oligomenorrhea with anovulation and obesity. The serum LH:FSH ratio is often greater than 2.0. Both adrenal and ovarian androgen hypersecretion are commonly present.

(2) Ovarian tumors are very uncommon causes of hirsutism and include arrhenoblastomas, Sertoli-Leydig cell tumors, dysgerminomas, and hilar cell tumors.

(3) Cushing's syndrome due to ACTH secretion by the pituitary or an ectopic source is an uncommon cause of hirsutism.

(4) Adrenal carcinoma is a rare cause of hyperandrogenism that can be quite virilizing.

(5) Adrenal enzyme defects: "Classic" 21-hydroxylase deficiency accounts for over 90% of congenital adrenal enzyme defects (adrenal hyperplasia) noted at birth. Female infants frequently have ambiguous genitalia and may become virilized unless treated with corticosteroid replacement; about half of such patients have clinically evident mineralocorticoid deficiency (salt-wasting) as well.

About 1–6% of patients with adult-onset hirsutism have been found to have a partial defect in adrenal 21-hydroxylase, whose phenotypic expression is delayed until adolescence or adulthood; such patients do not have salt wasting.

Some rare patients with hyperandrogenism and hypertension are found to have an 11-hydroxylase deficiency. This can be distinguished from the likewise rare cortisol resistance syndrome by high cortisol levels in the latter and by high 11-deoxycortisol levels in the former.

(6) Other cause of hirsutism are acromegaly, ovarian luteoma of pregnancy, and central nervous system lesions. Pharmacologic causes include minoxidil, cyclosporine, phenytoin, anabolic steroids, diazoxide, and certain progestins.

(7) Idiopathic or familial: Many patients with hirsutism have no detectable hyperandrogenism. Patients often have a strong familial predisposition to hirsutism that may be considered normal in the context of their genetic background. Such patients may have elevated serum levels of androstanediol glucuronide, a metabolite of dihydrotestosterone that is produced by skin in cosmetically unacceptable amounts.

Clinical Findings

A. Symptoms and Signs: Modest androgen excess from any source increases sexual hair (chin, upper lip, abdomen, and chest) and increases sebaceous gland activity, producing acne. Menstrual irregularities, anovulation, and amenorrhea are common. If androgen excess is pronounced, defeminization (decrease in breast size, loss of feminine adipose tissue) and virilization (frontal balding, muscularity, clitoromegaly, and deepening of the voice) occurs. Virilization implicates the presence of an androgen-producing neoplasm.

Hypertension may be seen in patients with Cushing's syndrome, adrenal 11-hydroxylase deficiency, or cortisol resistance syndrome.

A pelvic examination may disclose clitoromegaly or ovarian enlargement that may be cystic or neoplastic.

B. Laboratory Testing and Imaging: Serum androgen testing is mainly useful to screen for rare occult adrenal or ovarian neoplasms. Some general guidelines are presented here, though exceptions are common:

A serum testosterone level greater than 200 ng/dL or free testosterone greater than 40 ng/dL indicates the need for pelvic examination and ultrasound. If that is negative, an adrenal CT scan is performed.

A serum androstenedione greater than 1000 ng/dL also implicates an ovarian or adrenal neoplasm.

Patients with milder elevations of serum testosterone or androstenedione usually are treated with an oral contraceptive. If androgens are not reduced significantly or if hirsutism progresses, ovarian ultrasound or adrenal CT may be performed, but such studies are usually negative.

Patients with very elevated serum DHEAS (> 700 µg/dL) have an adrenal source of androgen. This usually is due to hyperplasia and rarely to adrenal carcinoma. An adrenal CT scan may be performed directly or in selected cases not suppressible to normal with dexamethasone (0.5 mg orally every 6 hours for 5 days).

No firm guidelines exist as to which patients (if any) with hyperandrogenism should be screened for "late-onset" 21-hydroxylase deficiency. The evaluation requires levels of serum 17-hydroxyprogesterone to be drawn at baseline and at 30–60 minutes after the intramuscular injection of 0.25 mg of cosyntropin ($ACTH_{1-24}$). Patients with congenital adrenal hyperplasia will usually have a baseline 17-hydroxyprogesterone over 300 ng/dL or a stimulated level over 1000 ng dL. The diagnosis, once made, is interesting academically but not helpful to the patient since glucocorticoid treatment is not particularly more effective in this condition than are other treatment modalities (see below).

Patients with any clinical signs of Cushing's syndrome should receive a screening test: (1) dexamethasone 1 mg is given at 11 PM, and an 8 AM serum cortisol is drawn (normal: < 5 µg/dL), or (2) 24-hour urine collection for free cortisol and creatinine. The latter test is preferable for very obese patients. (See Cushing's syndrome.)

Serum levels of FSH and LH are elevated if amenorrhea is due to ovarian failure. An LH:FSH ratio greater than 2.0 is common in patients with polycystic ovaries.

Treatment

Any underlying cause of hyperandrogenism must be detected and treated if possible. Cushing's syndrome or acromegaly must be corrected. An ovarian or adrenal neoplasm is resected. Any drugs causing hirsutism may be stopped. In cases of mild hyperandrogenism that is idiopathic or thought due to polycystic ovaries, an oral contraceptive is usually prescribed to ameliorate the hirsutism and normalize menses. An antiandrogen such as spironolactone or cyproterone acetate is usually also required for adequate treatment, especially in severe cases of hirsutism. Patients without demonstrably elevated serum androgens often respond well to these same measures.

Patients with "late-onset" 21-hydroxylase deficiency also usually respond better to estrogens or antiandrogens than to glucocorticoids.

(1) Oral contraceptives containing estrogen suppress ovarian androgen production and decrease free testosterone levels by increasing SHBG. Oral contraceptives are becoming available with new progestins (desogestrel, gestodene) that have a salutary effect on hirsutism; they may lower blood pressure and improve serum lipids. Side effects may include weight gain, headache, nausea, or mood change.

(2) Spironolactone may be taken in doses of 50–100 mg twice daily on days 5–25 of the menstrual cycle or daily if used concomitantly with an oral contraceptive. Hyperkalemia or hyponatremia may occur, but not commonly.

(3) Cyproterone acetate is a potent antiandrogen with progestational activity. It is available in some countries compounded with estrogen as an oral contraceptive. It is not available in the USA. It is available elsewhere as the progestin element in an oral contraceptive (Diane-35: ethinyl estradiol 35 µg with cyproterone acetate 2 mg). The dose of 2 mg appears to be about as effective as the much larger doses previously prescribed. An oral contraceptive is usually prescribed also. Side effects may include fatigue, nausea, or depression.

(4) Dexamethasone in doses of 0.125–0.25 mg at bedtime may be effective in some patients not responsive or intolerant to other measures noted above. Some rare patients with hyperandrogenism due to cortisol resistance have high basal levels of cortisol without Cushing's syndrome; such patients respond to higher doses of dexamethasone. Most patients are best not treated with this drug or at least must be followed very closely for the development of cushingoid features. Patients treated long-term may develop osteoporosis; periodic bone densitometry measurements are recommended to screen for this.

(5) Ketoconazole in doses of about 400 mg orally every 12 hours inhibits androgen production and can be very effective in some cases. Increases in liver enzymes may occur and must be followed for any progressive increase. Since liver toxicity is the main concern, patients are cautioned against excess alcohol consumption. Absorption of ketoconazole is decreased by H_2-blocking drugs. Drug interactions may also occur with: oral hypoglycemics, phenytoin, cyclosporine, warfarin, rifampin, and isoniazid.

(6) Local treatment by shaving or depilatories, waxing, electrolysis, or bleaching should be encouraged.

(7) GnRH analogues inhibit pituitary FSH and LH, thereby decreasing ovarian androgen and estrogen secretion. Leuprolide is given by monthly depot injections and has been approved for treatment of prostate cancer. Nafarelin is given as a nasal spray twice daily. It has been approved for treatment of endometriosis. Oral contraceptives are required to treat the hypogonadism thus produced. GnRH analogues are very expensive.

(8) Other antiandrogens: Finasteride is a newly released inhibitor of 5α-reductase, the enzyme that converts testosterone to dihydrotestosterone. Taken orally once daily, it has been approved for the treatment of benign prostatic hypertrophy, but it may be useful for cases of severe hirsutism and male pattern baldness as well. Flutamide inhibits androgen receptor uptake or nuclear binding (or both). Taken three times daily, it has been approved for use with leuprolide in the treatment of prostate cancer, but it may be useful for some cases of severe hirsutism. Doses of 250 mg/d are used.

Note: Antiandrogen treatments must be given only to nonpregnant women. Women must be counseled to take oral contraceptives, when indicated, and avoid pregnancy. Use during pregnancy causes malformations and pseudohermaphroditism in male infants.

Barnes R, Rosenfield RL: The polycystic ovary syndrome: Pathogenesis and treatment. Ann Intern Med 1989; 110:386.

Jurzyk RS et al: Antiandrogens for the treatment of acne and hirsutism. Am Fam Physician 1992;45:1803.

Schriock EA, Schriock ED: Treatment of hirsutism. Clin Obstet Gynecol 1991;34;852.

PRIMARY HYPERALDOSTERONISM

Essentials of Diagnosis

- Hypertension, polyuria, polydipsia, muscular weakness.
- Hypokalemia, alkalosis.
- Elevated plasma and urine aldosterone levels and low plasma renin level.

General Considerations

Primary hyperaldosteronism is a relatively rare disorder caused by aldosterone excess. It accounts for about 0.5% of cases of hypertension. It is more common in females. The two main types of primary hyperaldosteronism are those due to unilateral adrenocortical adenoma (Conn's syndrome) and those due to bilateral cortical hyperplasia. Hyperaldosteronism due to bilateral adrenal hyperplasia is sometimes glucocorticoid-suppressible. The latter is due to an autosomal-dominant genetic defect wherein the expression of the gene for P450 aldosterone synthetase is abnormally linked to the expression of the gene for 11β-hydroxylase which is regulated by ACTH. This genetic defect can now be detected by Southern blot analysis of DNA from the blood of suspected patients and their relatives.

Clinical Findings

A. Symptoms and Signs: Hypertension, muscular weakness (at times with paralysis simulating periodic paralysis), paresthesias with frank tetanic manifestations, headache, polyuria, and polydipsia are the outstanding complaints. Edema is rarely present. Some patients have only diastolic hypertension, without other signs or symptoms. Hypertension is typically moderate. Malignant hypertension is rare. Edema is rarely seen in primary hyperaldosteronism.

B. Laboratory Findings: The patient must have a high sodium intake (> 120 meq/d) during the entire

evaluation period; serum potassium is low. Cushing's syndrome should be eliminated clinically or with a 24-hour urine collection for free cortisol determination (see p 894); the urine is assayed for aldosterone. A low plasma renin activity (<5 μg/dL) with 24-hour urine aldosterone over 20 μg indicates hyperaldosteronism. A urine aldosterone of less than 20 μg/24 h is seen with rare adrenal or gonadal enzyme defects in the activity of 17α-hydroxylase (associated with ambiguous genitalia or primary amenorrhea) or 11β-hydroxylase (associated with virilization).

Once hyperaldosteronism is diagnosed, plasma is assayed for 18-hydroxycorticosterone; a level over 85 μg/dL is seen with adrenal neoplasms, whereas levels under 85 μg/dL are seen with idiopathic hyperplasia. Additionally, plasma can be assayed for aldosterone at 8 AM while the patient is supine after overnight recumbency and again after 4 hours upright. Patients with an adrenal adenoma usually have a baseline plasma aldosterone greater than 20 μg/dL which does not rise. Patients with hyperplasia typically have a baseline plasma aldosterone less than 20 μg/dL which rises during upright posture.

If an adrenal adenoma is diagnosed by the above testing, a CT scan of the adrenals can lateralize it with 80% success. If not visualized by CT, the adenoma may be localized by adrenal vein catheterization for aldosterone or by a dexamethasone-suppressed iodocholesterol adrenal scan.

Differential Diagnosis

This important reversible cause of hypertension must be considered in the differential diagnosis in any patient who shows muscular weakness and tetanic manifestations; and in the differential diagnosis of periodic paralysis, potassium- and sodium-losing nephritis, nephrogenic diabetes insipidus, and hypokalemia. (Be certain the patient has not been receiving diuretic agents.) Excessive ingestion of real licorice may simulate hyperaldosteronism, as may diuretics and laxative abuse. The oral contraceptives may raise aldosterone secretion in some patients. Unilateral renal vascular disease producing secondary hyperaldosteronism with severe hypertension must be ruled out. Plasma renin activity is low in primary hyperaldosteronism and elevated in renal vascular disease. Excessive secretion of deoxycorticosterone and corticosterone may produce a similar clinical picture. Low renin levels are found in about 25% of cases of essential hypertension. Their response to diuretics and their prognosis are better than those of patients with hypertension associated with high renin levels. Excess of an as yet unidentified mineralocorticoid is thought by some to be responsible. Aldosteronism due to a malignant ovarian tumor has been reported.

Complications

All of the complications of chronic hypertension

are encountered in primary hyperaldosteronism. Progressive renal damage is less reversible than hypertension.

Treatment

Conn's syndrome (unilateral adrenal adenoma secreting aldosterone) is treated by surgical removal of the lesion, though lifelong spironolactone therapy is an option. Bilateral adrenal hyperplasia is best treated with spironolactone. Bilateral adrenalectomy corrects the hypokalemia but not the hypertension and should *not* be performed. Antihypertensive agents may also be necessary. A rare type of hyperplasia responds well to dexamethasone suppression.

Prognosis

The hypertension is reversible in about two-thirds of cases but persists or returns in spite of surgery in the remainder.

The prognosis is much improved by early diagnosis and treatment.

Case records of the Massachusetts General Hospital Weekly Clinicopathological Exercises: Case 24–1992. A 52-year-old man with hypertension, hypokalemia, and an adrenal mass. N Engl J Med 1992;326:1617.

Lifton RP et al: A chimeric 11β-hydroxylase/aldosterone synthetase gene causes glucocorticoid-remediable aldosteronism and human hypertension. Nature 1992; 355:262.

Radin DR et al: Diagnosis of primary hyperaldosteronism: Importance of correlating CT findings with endocrinologic studies. AJR Am J Roentgenol 1992;158:553.

Rich GM et al: Glucocorticoid-remediable aldosteronism in a large kindred: Clinical spectrum and diagnosis using a characteristic biochemical phenotype. Ann Intern Med 1992;116:813.

Young WF Jr et al: Primary aldosteronism: Diagnosis and treatment. Mayo Clin Proc 1990;65:96.

DISEASES OF THE ADRENAL MEDULLA

PHEOCHROMOCYTOMA

Essentials of Diagnosis

- "Attacks" of headache, perspiration, palpitations.
- Hypertension, frequently sustained but often paroxysmal, especially during surgery or delivery.
- Attacks of nausea, thoracic or abdominal pain, weakness, dyspnea, visual disturbance.
- Hypermetabolism with anxiety, tremor, weight loss, or heat intolerance.
- Normal T_4 and TSH. Elevated urinary catecholamines or their metabolites.

General Considerations

Pheochromocytoma is a rare disease characterized by paroxysmal or sustained hypertension due to a tumor located in either or both adrenals or anywhere along the sympathetic nervous chain, and rarely in such aberrant locations as the thorax, bladder, or brain. Primary extra-adrenal pheochromocytomas are known as "paragangliomas." Pheochromocytomas are characterized by a rough "rule of ten": About 10% of cases are not associated with hypertension; in about 10%, the tumor involves both adrenal glands; 10% are extra-adrenal, and of those about 10% are extra-abdominal; 10% occur in children; most tumors are sporadic with only 10–15% familial (bilateral adrenal tumors tend to occur more frequently in familial cases); and about 10% of tumors are malignant.

Familial pheochromocytoma may occur without other abnormalities or associated with the following: islet cell tumors of the pancreas, calcitonin-secreting medullary carcinoma of the thyroid and hyperparathyroidism (multiple endocrine neoplasia type II), medullary carcinoma of the thyroid and the syndrome of multiple mucosal neuromas, without hyperparathyroidism (multiple endocrine neoplasia type IIb), neurofibromatosis (Recklinghausen's disease), or von Hippel-Lindau disease (hemangioblastomas of retina, cerebellum, and other parts of the nervous system).

Clinical Findings

A. Symptoms and Signs: Pheochromocytoma is manifested by attacks of severe headache, palpitations, tachycardia, profuse sweating, vasomotor changes (including facial pallor), precordial or abdominal pain, increasing nervousness and irritability, increased appetite, and loss of weight. Anginal attacks may occur. Physical findings may include hypertension, either in attacks or sustained, with cardiac enlargement; postural tachycardia (change of more than 20 beats/min) and postural hypotension; and mild elevation of basal body temperature. Retinal hemorrhage or papilledema occurs occasionally.

The manifestations of pheochromocytoma can be quite varied. Besides the above symptoms, some patients can present with psychosis or confusion, seizures, hyperglycemia, bradycardia, hypotension, paresthesias, or Raynaud's phenomenon. Other patients may have pulmonary edema and heart failure due to cardiomyopathy. Still other patients may be entirely asymptomatic or may have abdominal discomfort due to a pheochromocytoma presenting as a large abdominal mass.

B. Laboratory Findings: Hypermetabolism is present; thyroid function tests are normal, including serum T_4, free T_4, T_3, and TSH; and glycosuria or hyperglycemia (or both) may be present.

C. Special Tests: Pharmacologic provocative and suppressive tests that evaluate the rise or fall in blood pressure are usually not required or recommended.

1. Assay of urinary catecholamines (total and fractionated), metanephrines, vanilmandelic acid (VMA), and creatinine detects most pheochromocytomas, especially when samples are obtained during or immediately following an episodic attack. A 24-hour urine specimen is usually obtained, although a shorter collection may be used for screening; patients with pheochromocytomas generally have more that 2.2 µg of metanephrine per milligram of creatinine and more than 5.5 µg of VMA per milligram creatinine.

Many drugs and chemicals and some foods can affect the tests for pheochromocytoma (Table 25–16).

2. Direct assay of epinephrine and norepinephrine in blood and urine during or following an attack is the most sensitive test for pheochromocytoma associated with paroxysmal hypertension.

High epinephrine levels favor tumor localization within the adrenal gland. Proper, quiet collection of specimens is essential.

3. Imaging–CT scan and MRI have been very helpful in the confirmation and localization of pheochromocytoma. They should not ordinarily replace urinary catecholamine assays since incidental adrenal adenomas are not uncommon (over 2%) and may cause misdiagnosis. [123]I MIBG scan helps localize tumors.

Differential Diagnosis

Pheochromocytoma should always be suspected in any patient with labile hypertension, especially if some of the other features such as hypermetabolism or hyperglycemia are present in a young person. Because of such symptoms as tachycardia, tremor, palpitation, and hypermetabolism, pheochromocytoma may be confused with thyrotoxicosis. It should be

Table 25–16. Drugs, foods, and conditions affecting chemical tests for pheochromocytoma.[1]

Test	Increase	Decrease
Universally affecting catecholamines, metanephrines, and vanilmandelic acid (VMA)	Sympathomimetics (amphetamines, ephedrine, nasal decongestants, bronchodilators) Levodopa Rapid clonidine withdrawal Excess ingestion of bananas Vasodilators (nitroprusside, nitroglycerin) Methylxanthines (theophylline, aminophylline) Severe stress (emotion, exercise, pain, myocardial infarction) Diseases: intracranial lesions, acute psychosis, Guillain-Barré syndrome, lead poisoning, eclampsia, hypoglycemia, carcinoid, acute porphyria, acrodynia, quadriplegia, amyotrophic lateral sclerosis Fluorescent substances (fluorimetric method[2]): quinidine, chloral hydrate, tetracyclines, methenamine, methocarbamol, nicotinic acid, erythromycin, quinine, riboflavin, bretylium, sulfobromophthalein, phenolsulfonphthalein	Large doses of ganglionic blockers: guanethidine, reserpine (with chronic administration; acute administration causes initial increases) Fenfluramine (anorectic) Renal insufficiency Diseases: malnutrition, dysautonomia, quadriplegia (quiescent)
Catecholamines	Ethanol, isoproterenol, methyldopa, monoamine oxidase inhibitors, phenothiazines, α-methyl-*p*-tyrosine, methenamine, urine bilirubin, labetalol	
Metanephrines	Ethanol, methyldopa, monoamine oxidase inhibitors, benzodiazepines, phenothiazines	Radiopaque media (methylglucamine): Renografin, Hypaque-M,[3] Renovist, Cardiografin, Urografin, Conray
Vanilmandelic acid (VMA)	Lithium, nalidixic acid, methocarbamol, glycerol guaiacolate, *p*-aminosalicylic acid, salicylates, mephenesin, sulfonamides, excess ingestion of (fluorimetric method[2]) chocolate, citrus, tea, vanilla, coffee	Ethanol, monoamine oxidase inhibitors, disulfiram, clofibrate, mandelamine, salicylates (Pisano method)

[1]Reproduced, with permission, from Fitzgerald PA: *Handbook of Clinical Endocrinology.* Appleton &Lange, 1992.
[2]Fluorimetric assay methods are subject to most types of interference. The most specific assays use chromatographic and spectrophotometric methods. Drugs should be stopped for 1 week before testing.
[3]Hypaque as diatrizoate sodium is alright.

considered in patients with unexplained acute anginal attacks. Pheochromocytoma may also be misdiagnosed as essential hypertension, myocarditis, glomerulonephritis or other renal lesions, toxemia of pregnancy, eclampsia, and psychoneurosis (anxiety attack). It can sometimes be mistaken for an acute abdomen.

Other conditions that have manifestations similar to those of pheochromocytoma include acute intermittent porphyria, hypogonadal vascular instability (hot flushes), cocaine or amphetamine use, clonidine withdrawal, hypertensive crisis caused by foods containing tyramine (eg, cheeses) in patients taking MAO inhibitor antidepressants, labile hypertension, and unstable angina.

Complications

All of the complications of severe hypertension may be encountered. Hypertensive crises with sudden blindness or cerebrovascular accidents are not uncommon. These may be precipitated by sudden movement, by manipulation during or after pregnancy, by emotional stress or trauma, or during surgical removal of the tumor. Cardiomyopathy may develop. Occasionally, the initial manifestation of pheochromocytoma may be hypotension or even shock.

After removal of the tumor, a state of severe hypotension and shock (resistant to epinephrine and norepinephrine) may ensue with precipitation of renal failure or myocardial infarction. These complications can be avoided by judicious preoperative and operative use of catecholamine-blocking agents such as phenoxybenzamine and labetalol by the use of blood or plasma to restore blood volume. Hypotension and shock may occur from spontaneous infarction or hemorrhage of the tumor; emergency surgical removal of the tumor is necessary in these cases.

On rare occasions, a patient dies as a result of the complications of diagnostic tests or during surgery. No patient with suspected pheochromocytoma should be subjected either to an invasive diagnostic procedure or to surgery unless there has been adequate alpha blockade with phenoxybenzamine.

Treatment

Surgical removal of the tumor or tumors is the treatment of choice. Administration of α-adrenergic blocking drugs preoperatively has made pheochromocytoma surgery a great deal safer in recent years. Give phenoxybenzamine, 10 mg orally every 12 hours, and increase the dose gradually—about every 3 days—until hypertension is controlled. The usual maintenance dose is 40–120 mg daily. Do not increase the dose further when postural hypotension and nasal stuffiness become manifest.

After appropriate α-adrenergic receptor blockade with phenoxybenzamine, the beta-blocker propranolol or the combined alpha- and beta-blocker labetalol can be employed to control tachycardia and other arrhythmias. Maintain adrenergic blockade for a minimum of 10 days or until optimal cardiac status is established. Monitor the ECG until it becomes stable. (It may take a week or even months to correct electrocardiographic changes in patients with catecholamine myocarditis, and it is prudent to defer surgery until then in such cases.) Patients must be very closely monitored during surgery in order to promptly detect and control sudden changes in blood pressure or cardiac arrhythmias.

Since there may be multiple tumors, it is essential to recheck urinary catecholamine levels postoperatively (1–2 weeks after surgery).

Oral phenoxybenzamine has been successfully used as chronic treatment in inoperable carcinoma.

Metyrosine is a competitive blocker in the synthesis of catecholamines. It is useful in the medical management of malignant or inoperable tumors. The initial dosage is 250 mg four times daily, increased daily by increments of 250–500 mg to a maximum of 4 g/d.

Metastatic or unresectable pheochromocytomas may be treated with combination chemotherapy or with high doses of ^{131}I MIBG, which is available at some medical centers.

Prognosis

The prognosis depends upon how early the diagnosis is made. The malignancy of a pheochromocytoma cannot be determined by histologic examination. A tumor is considered malignant if metastases are present; this may take many years to become clinically evident. If the tumor is successfully removed before irreparable damage to the cardiovascular system has occurred, a complete cure is usually achieved. Complete cure (or improvement) may follow removal of a tumor that has been present for many years. In some cases, hypertension persists or returns in spite of successful surgery. Although this may be essential hypertension, biochemical reevaluation is then required, looking for a second or metastatic pheochromocytoma.

Before the advent of blocking agents, the surgical mortality rate was as high as 30%, but this has rapidly decreased. The importance of a team approach—endocrinologist, anesthesiologist, and surgeon—cannot be overemphasized. With optimal management, the surgical mortality rate is less than 3%.

Patients with symptomatic pheochromocytoma have a median survival of about 4.5 years; however, prolonged survivals do occur.

Benowitz NL: Pheochromocytoma. Adv Intern Med 1990; 35:195.

Bravo EL: Diagnosis of pheochromocytoma: Reflections on a controversy. Hypertension 1991;17:744.

Breslow MJ, Legier B: Hyperadrenergic states. Crit Care Med 1991;19:1566.

Cryer PE: Pheochromocytoma. West J Med 1992;156:399.

Grossman E et al: Glucagon and clonidine testing in the diagnosis of pheochromocytoma. Hypertension 1991; 17:733.

Hanson MW et al: Iodine 131-I-labeled metaiodobenzylguanidine scintigraphy and biochemical analysis in suspected pheochromocytoma. Arch Intern Med 1991; 151:397.

Krakoff LR, Garbowit D: Adreno-medullary hypertension: A review of syndromes, pathophysiology, diagnosis, and treatment. Clin Chem 1991;37:1849.

Schwartz RW et al: Diagnosis and treatment of primary adrenal tumors. Curr Opin Oncol 1991;3:121.

Sheps SG: Pheo or not a pheo, that is the question. (Editorial.) West J Med 1992;156:433.

Stein PP, Black HR: A simplified diagnostic approach to pheochromocytoma: A review of the literature and report of one institution's experience. Medicine 1991;70:46.

Whalen RK et al: Extra-adrenal pheochromocytoma. J Urol 1992;147:1.

DISEASES OF THE PANCREATIC ISLET CELLS*

ISLET CELL FUNCTIONING PANCREATIC TUMORS

The pancreatic islets are composed of several types of cells, each with distinct chemical and microscopic features: the A cells (20%) secrete glucagon, the B cells (70%) secrete insulin, and the D cells (5%) secrete somatostatin or gastrin. F cells secrete "pancreatic polypeptide." Each type of cell may give rise to benign or malignant neoplasms that may be multiple and usually present with a clinical syndrome related to hypersecretion of a native or ectopic hormonal product. The diagnosis of a particular pancreatic islet neoplasm depends upon first suspecting it from its clinical manifestations. The serum concentration of that particular hormone may then be assayed.

Insulinomas are usually (about 85%) benign and secrete excessive amounts of insulin (as well as proinsulin and C-peptide), which causes hypoglycemia. The tumors may be multiple, especially in familial cases of MEN type I or in cases of nesidioblastosis. The latter is seen mostly in children and is characterized by excessive insulin secretion from histologically normal-appearing B cells.

Gastrinomas are generally benign and secrete excessive gastrin (as well as "big" gastrin), which stimulates the stomach to hypersecrete acid, thereby causing peptic ulceration (Zollinger-Ellison syndrome).

Glucagonomas secrete excessive glucagon and may cause a peculiar dermatitis called **necrolytic migratory erythema.** Such patients also usually have diabetes mellitus, weight loss, and liver metastases by the time of diagnosis.

Somatostatinomas are very rare and are associated with weight loss, diabetes mellitus, malabsorption, and hypochlorhydria.

Other rare tumors secrete excessive amounts of **vasoactive intestinal polypeptide (VIP),** a substance that causes profuse watery diarrhea (Verner-Morrison syndrome). Treatment with octreotide improves the symptoms but does not halt tumor growth. Symptomatic improvement with calcitonin treatment has also been reported.

In addition to the native hormones, aberrant or ectopic hormones are often secreted by islet cell tumors, including ACTH, melanocyte-stimulating hormone, serotonin, and chorionic gonadotropin, with a variety of clinical syndromes. Islet cell tumors may be part of the syndrome of multiple endocrine adenomatosis type I (with pituitary and parathyroid adenomas).

Direct resection of the tumor (or tumors), which often spreads locally, is the primary form of therapy for all types of islet cell neoplasm except Zollinger-Ellison syndrome, where treatment choices include blockade of acid secretion by the gastric mucosa with H_2 blocking agents or removal of the end organ (total gastrectomy). A new class of "acid pump" inhibitors (omeprazole) may become the therapy of choice for Zollinger-Ellison syndrome. Palliation of functioning malignant disease often requires both antihormonal and anticancer chemotherapy. The use of streptozocin, doxorubicin, and asparaginase, especially for malignant insulinoma, has produced some encouraging results, though these drugs are quite toxic. Octreotide, a somatostatin analogue, is now used in the therapy of islet cell tumor. The hypoglycemia of insulinoma may be counteracted by verapamil or diazoxide.

The prognosis in these neoplasms is variable. Long-term survival in spite of widespread metastases has been reported. Earlier diagnosis by hormonal assay may lead to earlier detection and a higher cure rate.

Antonelli A et al: Calcitonin, as SMS 201–995, ameliorates the VIPoma syndrome. J Endocrinol Invest 1993;16:57.

Cherner JA, Sawyers JL: Benefit of resection of metastatic gastrinoma in multiple endocrine neoplasia type I. Gastroenterology 1992;102:1049.

Doppman JL: Pancreatic endocrine tumors: The search goes on. N Engl J Med 1992;326:1770.

Jaffe BM: Current issues in the management of Zollinger-Ellison syndrome. Surgery 1992;111:241.

Kasper CS: Necrolytic migratory erythema: Unresolved problems in diagnosis and pathogenesis: A case report and literature review. Cutis 1992;49:120.

Pasieka JL: Surgical approach to insulinomas: Assessing

---

*Diabetes mellitus and the hypoglycemic states are discussed in Chapter 26.

the need for preoperative localization. Arch Surg 1992;127:442.

Rothmund M et al: Endocrine pancreatic carcinoma. Eur J Surg Oncol 1991;17:191.

Solcia E et al: The gastroenteropancreatic endocrine system and related tumors. Gastroenterol Clin North Am 1989; 18:671.

van Hecke E et al: Glucagonoma syndrome. Curr Probl Dermatol 1991;20:24.

Willberg B, Muller E: Surgery for nesidioblastosis: Indications, treatment, and results. Prog Pediatr Surg 1991; 26:76.

Winocour PH et al: Difficulties in localization and treatment of insulinomas in type I multiple endocrine adenomatosis (MEA). Postgrad Med J 1992;68:196.

DISEASES OF THE TESTES

Table 25–17. Causes of male hypogonadism.

Hypogonadotropic (Low or Normal LH)	Hypergonadotropic (High LH)
Constitutinal delay	Klinefelter's syndrome
Chronic illness	Bilateral anorchia
Malnourishment	Sertoli cell only syndrome
Kallmann's syndrome	Noonan's syndrome
Prader-Willi syndrome	Bilateral anorchia
Laurence-Moon-Biedl syndrome	Testicular trauma
Alström's syndrome	Orchitis
Cushing's syndrome	Mumps
Hypothyroidism	Leprosy
Hypopituitarism	Tuberculosis
Pituitary tumors	Lymphoma
Hypothalamic lesions	Myotonic dystrophy
Hemochromatosis	Antitumor chemotherapy
Drugs	Radiation therapy
Alcohol	Male climacteric
Marihuana	Idiopathic
Spironolactone	
Ketoconazole	
Idiopathic isolated gondotropin deficiency	

MALE HYPOGONADISM

Male hypogonadism may be classified according to time of onset, ie, prepubertal or postpubertal. It may also be classified as to whether the lesion is in the testes (hypergonadotropic) or in the hypothalamic-pituitary area (hypogonadotropic).

The etiology of hypogonadism is determined by careful history, physical examination, and laboratory tests (Table 25–17).

1. DELAYED PUBERTY IN BOYS

In the USA, boys who have no sign of sexual development by age 14 are considered to have delayed puberty. Arrested pubertal development also requires evaluation. Such boys require a careful family and personal history as well as physical examination and laboratory testing, which includes serum levels of LH, FSH, and testosterone.

Evaluation

A. Hypogonadotropic Hypogonadism: Boys without elevations in serum FSH and LH but with a low testosterone may have either temporary (constitutional delay in growth and adolescence) or permanent hypogonadotropic hypogonadism. They may need further endocrine evaluation for hypothyroidism (free thyroxine and TSH). They may also require further evaluation for Cushing's syndrome or adrenal insufficiency, depending upon the clinical picture. The sense of smell should always be tested.

Boys with constitutional growth delay are usually thin, short, have a delayed bone age, and frequently have a family history of delayed puberty. Other causes of temporarily delayed puberty include chronic illness, dieting, and malnourishment. Vigorous physical training does not cause delayed puberty in boys as it does in girls.

Patients with permanent hypogonadotropic hypogonadism may have signs of other pituitary hormone deficiencies. They may have syndromes associated with hypogonadotropic hypogonadism: Prader-Willi syndrome (obesity, mental retardation, hypotonia, microphallus, small hands and feet), Laurence-Moon-Biedl syndrome (obesity, polydactyly, retinitis pigmentosa), or Alström's syndrome (obesity, nerve deafness, retinitis pigmentosa).

Patients with an impaired sense of smell are usually found to have **Kallmann's syndrome,** caused by a congenitally defective neural migration factor. This keeps the GnRH-secreting neurons, which originate in the olfactory placode, from migrating to the hypothalamus. Aplasia or hypoplasia of the olfactory bulbs and tracts may be seen by MRI. Patients with Kallmann's syndrome are usually otherwise normal, though they may have other developmental neurologic abnormalities, eg, mental retardation, spatial attention abnormalities, cerebellar dysfunction, pes cavus, spastic paraplegia, color vision disturbance, or hearing loss. Other associated developmental defects may be associated, such as facial dysraphism (cleft palate or lip), unilateral renal agenesis, or horseshoe kidney. It is genetically heterogeneous, being inherited as either an autosomal dominant or recessive trait.

Boys who do not have a clear etiology for delayed puberty or who have symptoms of a possible brain tumor (eg, headaches) or other pituitary hormone deficiencies should have an MRI of the pituitary and hypothalamus to look for a destructive lesion.

B. Hypergonadotropic Hypogonadism: Boys with elevated serum FSH and LH concentrations but low testosterone levels are considered to have primary testicular failure. The most common cause is Klinefelter's syndrome (see below).

Boys without palpable testes may have bilateral anorchia. This can be distinguished from cryptorchid testes by administering chorionic gonadotropin, 2000 units subcutaneously every 3 days for 2 weeks. Plasma testosterone rises to over 100 ng/dL with cryptorchid or retractile testes.

Other conditions that can lead to early testicular failure include viral infection, irradiation or antitumor chemotherapy, XY gonadal dysgenesis, and autoimmunity.

Patients with androgen-insensitivity syndromes may have increases in LH and testosterone but variable degrees of gynecomastia, hypospadias, cryptorchism, and hypogonadism (Reifenstein's syndrome).

Treatment

Whatever the cause, boys with delayed puberty should be treated with gradually increasing doses of testosterone every 3–4 weeks. Begin with testosterone enanthate, 50 mg intramuscularly, and increase by 50 mg at each dose up to about 300 mg. In patients with apparent constitutional delay, this treatment is usually continued for 1–2 years and then stopped to see if natural puberty has started. Patients with permanent hypogonadism require lifelong testosterone replacement.

Phenotypic males with androgen insensitivity may require larger doses of testosterone.

Management of Infertility

Men with permanent hypogonadotropic hypogonadism are usually infertile. Exceptions do occur in rare cases of isolated LH deficiency (fertile eunuch syndrome). A semen analysis must be obtained. Fertility may be induced (without cryptorchism) in men with hypothalamic hypogonadotropism by means of intermittent infusion of pulsatile leuprolide (GnRH analogue) every 2 hours subcutaneously, delivered by an externally worn pump. Alternatively, chorionic gonadotropin (hCG) may be injected three times weekly for a year, with menotropins (hMG) then added to the regimen. Such treatments for infertility are expensive and may be unsuccessful.

Bagatell CJ et al: Physiologic testosterone levels in normal men suppress high-density lipoprotein cholesterol levels. Ann Intern Med 1992;116:967.

Schopohl J et al: Comparison of gonadotropin-releasing hormone and gonadotropin therapy in male patients with idiopathic hypogonadotropic hypogonadism. Fertil Steril 1991;56:1143.

Winters SJ: Expanding the differential diagnosis of male hypogonadism. N Engl J Med 1991;326:193.

2. KLINEFELTER'S SYNDROME

Klinefelter's syndrome (seminiferous tubule dysgenesis) is the expression of an abnormal karyotype, classically 47,XXY. Other forms are common, eg, 46,XY/47,XXY mosaicism, 48,XXYY, 48,XXXY, or 46,XX males.

The manifestations of Klinefelter's syndrome are variable. Testes feel normal during childhood, but during adolescence they usually become firm, fibrotic, small, and nontender to palpation. This is due to fibrosis of the sperm-producing seminiferous tubules, which ordinarily comprise about 85% of the testicular mass. The Leydig cells that produce testosterone are variably affected. Therefore, although puberty occurs at the normal time, the degree of virilization is variable. There is usually diminished pubic, axillary, and body hair. Other men have virtually normal virilization but may have infertility or gynecomastia. About 85% have gynecomastia of variable severity at puberty.

Other common findings include tall stature and abnormal body proportions (height greater than arm span; crown-pubis length greater than pubis-floor). This is the *opposite* of the eunuchoid proportions typically seen in other forms of prepubertal hypogonadism. Some rare patients may be short (46,XX males). Patients with multiple X or Y chromosomes are more apt to have mental deficiency and other abnormalities such as clinodactyly or synostosis. They may also exhibit problems with coordination and social skills. Certain other problems seen more commonly in adult men with Klinefelter's syndrome include a higher incidence of breast cancer, chronic pulmonary disease, varicosities of the legs, and diabetes mellitus (8%); impaired glucose tolerance occurs in an additional 19%.

Most men (about 95%) have azoospermia. Exceptions occur, however, especially in men with 46,XY/47,XXY mosaicism, who may have oligospermia or may even be fertile. Thus, Klinefelter's syndrome also enters the differential diagnosis of postpubertal primary hypogonadism or new-onset infertility in men who have fathered children.

The serum testosterone is low, and FSH and LH are elevated. Sometimes the serum testosterone is in the normal range despite signs of hypogonadism; serum free testosterone measurements may better document decreased available testosterone in such cases.

All causes of gynecomastia (Table 25–2) must be differentiated from Klinefelter's syndrome. Testicular size, plasma LH, FSH, and prolactin and, if necessary, chromosomal analysis will settle the diagnosis.

Testosterone replacement should be given if secondary sexual characteristics have failed to appear or if impotence and low blood testosterone develop later in life. There is no treatment for the infertility. If gynecomastia is disfiguring, plastic surgical removal is indicated.

Castro-Magana M et al: Genetic forms of male hypogonadism. Urology 1990;35:195.

Schwartz ID, Rout AW: The Klinefelter syndrome of testicular dysgenesis. Endocrinol Metab Clin North Am 1991;20:153.

3. POSTPUBERTAL (ACQUIRED) MALE HYPOGONADISM

Clinical Findings

A. Symptoms and Signs: Men with acquired hypogonadism have variable manifestations. Most men experience decreased libido. Others complain of erectile dysfunction, hot sweats, asthenia, or depression. Their presenting complaint may also be infertility, gynecomastia, headache, fracture, or other symptoms related to the cause or result of the hypogonadism. The patient's history often gives a clue to the cause (Table 25–17).

Physical signs associated with hypogonadism may include decreased body, axillary, beard, or pubic hair; such diminished sexual hair growth is not reliably present except after years of severe hypogonadism. Examination should include measurements of arm span and height. Testicular size should be assessed with an orchidometer (normal volume is about 10–25 mL; normal maximal diameter is usually over 6 cm). Testicular size usually remains normal in men with postpubertal hypogonadotropic hypogonadism, but it may be diminished with testicular injury or Klinefelter's syndrome. The testes must also be carefully palpated for masses, since Leydig cell tumors may secrete estrogen and present with hypogonadism.

B. Laboratory Findings: The hemoglobin and hematocrit may be slightly below the male range due to hypogonadism. Laboratory evaluation for male hypogonadism should always include measurement of serum testosterone. There are different sorts of testosterone assays. An assay for serum free testosterone is more sensitive than that for total testosterone. Testosterone levels fluctuate, generally being higher in the morning, so that more than one assay may be necessary for careful evaluation. In patients with low or borderline-low serum testosterone levels, serum LH and FSH should be measured. LH and FSH tend to be high in patients with primary hypogonadism but low or inappropriately normal in men with hypogonadotropic hypogonadism. Bone densitometry may be reduced in long-standing male hypogonadism.

1. Acquired hypogonadotropic hypogonadism–Men with hypogonadotropic hypogonadism have low serum testosterone levels without a compensatory increase in gonadotropins. Such men require careful evaluation for other manifestations of hypopituitarism, Cushing's syndrome, hemochromatosis, pituitary tumor, or brain tumor. Olfactory testing is performed even though Kallmann's syndrome ordinarily presents with delayed puberty. A serum prolactin determination is obtained but may be elevated for many reasons (Table 25–3). The serum estradiol level may be elevated in patients with cirrhosis and in rare cases of estrogen-secreting tumors (testicular Leydig cell tumor or adrenal carcinoma). Men with no discernible definite cause for hypogonadotropic hypogonadism should have an MRI of the pituitary and hypothalamic region to look for a tumor or other lesion.

2. Acquired hypergonadotropic hypogonadism–Men with hypergonadotropic hypogonadism have low serum testosterone levels with a compensatory increase in gonadotropins. It is most commonly seen in elderly men, in whom the cause is usually idiopathic (male climacteric). Younger men require a particularly careful evaluation. Patients should be examined for features of Klinefelter's syndrome. Patients must be assessed for uremia. Uremic patients may have suppressed serum testosterone with an elevated LH level but may also have a suppressed LH level due to hyperprolactinemia. Patients with myotonic dystrophy also tend to have primary hypogonadism. The testicles must be carefully examined for evidence of trauma, infiltrative lesions (eg, lymphoma), or ongoing infection (eg, leprosy, tuberculosis). Testicular biopsy is usually reserved for younger patients in whom the reason for primary hypogonadism is unclear.

Treatment

Hypogonadism is usually treated with parenteral testosterone (enanthate or cypionate). The usual dose is about 300 mg intramuscularly every 3 weeks. The preparation is oil-based and is usually given in the gluteal area. The dose is adjusted according to the patient's response. Side effects include acne and suppressed HDL cholesterol. Transdermal testosterone preparations are becoming available; these are usually applied to the scrotum. Oral androgen preparations are available and include methyltestosterone and fluoxymesterone. These oral preparations have occasionally caused liver tumors or peliosis hepatis with long-term use. Furthermore, the oral androgens are not as effective as parenteral testosterone.

Management of Infertility

Men with male infertility usually (50–60%) have idiopathic seminiferous tubular failure. Another 20% have varicocele with oligospermia. About 10% have obstruction, and another 10% have ejaculatory dysfunction. Only about 10% of male infertility cases are associated with an endocrine problem. Operations for varicocele have produced a pregnancy rate of 42% versus 45% for a nonoperated group. Men with primary testicular failure usually have infertility due to azoospermia. Some patients with oligospermia may successfully father children via sperm concentration or in vitro fertilization techniques. Men with acquired hypogonadotropic hypogonadism may have fertility restored by use of chorionic gonadotropin (hCG). Doses of about 2000 units injected subcutaneously three times weekly will ordinarily restore serum testosterone levels to normal; sperm counts usually rise to normal over the course of several months to a year. The addition of menotropins (hMG) or the use of pulsatile leuprolide (GnRH analogue) infusions (as in prepubertal hypogonadotropic hypogonadism; see above) is not as frequently required in this group of men.

Prognosis of Hypogonadism

If hypogonadism is due to a pituitary lesion, the prognosis is that of the primary disease (eg, tumor, necrosis). The prognosis for restoration of virility is good if testosterone is given. The sooner administration is started, the fewer stigmas of eunuchoidism remain (unless therapy is discontinued).

Fisch, Lipshultz LI: Diagnosing male factors of infertility. Arch Pathol Lab Med 1992;116:398.
Foster MB: Aberrant puberty. Obstet Gynecol Clin North Am 1992;19:59.
Meikle AW et al: Enhanced transdermal delivery of testosterone across nonscrotal skin produces physiological concentrations of testosterone and its metabolites in hypogonadal men. J Clin Endocrinol Metab 1992; 74:623.
Puberty and its disorders. (Review.) Endocrinol Metab Clin North Am 1991;20:1.
Rageth JC et al: Long-term results of varicocelectomy. Urol Int 1992;48:327.
Styne DM, Grumbach MM: Puberty in the male and female: Its physiology and disorders. In: *Reproductive Endocrinology.* Yen SSC, Jaffe RD (editors). Saunders, 1991.
Wise P: Male infertility update. West J Med 1991;155:635.

TESTICULAR TUMORS IN ADULTS
(See also Chapter 21.)

Testicular tumors generally present as a testicular lump; about 30% are painful. They must be distinguished from more common scrotal masses (spermatocele, epididymitis, hydrocele). When the diagnosis is in doubt, excisional biopsy is usually prudent.

About 95% of testicular tumors are germ cell tumors (seminomas or nonseminomas). They may produce (as serum markers) hCG and alpha-fetoprotein. Seminomas do not produce alpha-fetoprotein, but about 5–10% produce some hCG; nonseminomas, on the other hand, produce increased serum levels of one or both of these markers in about 90% of cases.

About 5% of testicular tumors are Leydig or Sertoli cell tumors. Leydig cell tumors tend to produce estrogen (75%) and cause gynecomastia and impotence on that basis; they may sometimes produce androgens that can cause pseudoprecocious puberty in boys. Sertoli cell tumors may also produce estrogen (30%) with feminization; gynecomastia may be due to hCG secretion (25%).

Some testicular tumors may be small and nonpalpable yet may secrete sufficient amounts of hCG or estrogen to cause gynecomastia or impotence. Therefore, in any man with gynecomastia without obvious cause, serum levels of hCG and estradiol should be determined to screen for such hidden tumors. Testicular ultrasound may help reveal small tumors.

Treatment & Prognosis

Testicular tumors are generally resected by inguinal orchiectomy. Patients with seminomas generally have radiation to retroperitoneal nodes; radiation therapy is extended to the mediastinum for metastatic disease. Seminomas with distant metastases are treated effectively with chemotherapy (cisplatin, bleomycin, and vinblastine), which achieves nearly 100% remission rates. Malignant nonseminomas are treated with lymph node dissection and chemotherapy (same as above); remissions occur in about 90%.

Benign Leydig and Sertoli cell tumors can be simply resected. Malignant tumors have a poor prognosis.

Brown ER et al: Long-term outcome of patients with relapsed and refractory germ cell tumors treated with high-dose chemotherapy and autologous bone marrow rescue. Ann Intern Med 1992;117:124.
Foster RS, Donohue JP: Surgical treatment of clinical stage A nonseminomatous testis cancer. Semin Oncol 1992; 19:166.
Williams SD, Roth BJ: Chemotherapy of testis cancer: A review. Int J Radiat Oncol Biol Phys 1992;22:213.

DISEASES OF THE OVARIES
(See also Chapter 17.)

FEMALE HYPOGONADISM

The outstanding symptom of female hypogonadism is amenorrhea (see below). Partial deficiencies—principally corpus luteum failure—may occur; these do not always cause amenorrhea but more often produce anovulatory periods, oligomenorrhea, or metrorrhagia.

Primary pituitary disorders are much less common causes of hypogonadism in the female than primary ovarian disorders and are often associated with other signs of pituitary failure.

Ovarian failure starting in early life will lead to delayed closure of the epiphyses and retarded bone age, often resulting in tall stature with long extremities. On the other hand, in gonadal dysgenesis due to chromosomal disorder, short stature is the rule (see below). In adult-onset ovarian failure, changes are more subtle, with some regression of secondary sex characteristics, including breast atrophy, diminished vaginal secretions, changes in vaginal epithelium, etc. Vasomotor instability with "hot flushes" is a typical sign of estrogen secretory failure. In estrogenic deficiency of long standing in any age group, osteoporosis, especially of the spine, is usually found, since estrogen protects bone against excessive resorption.

Ovarian failure can also be caused by Cushing's syndrome and by hyperandrogenism due to any cause (eg, congenital adrenal hyperplasia, ovarian or adrenal tumors).

1. AMENORRHEA

Since regular menstruation depends upon normal function of the entire physiologic axis extending from the hypothalamus and pituitary to the ovary and the uterine lining, it is not surprising that menstrual disorders are among the most common presenting complaints of endocrine disease in women. Correct diagnosis depends upon proper evaluation of each component of the axis, and nonendocrine factors must also be considered.

If menstruation is defined as shedding of endometrium which has been stimulated by estrogen or by estrogen and progesterone which are subsequently withdrawn, it is obvious that amenorrhea can occur either when hormones are deficient or lacking (the hypohormonal or ahormonal type) or when these hormones, though present in adequate amounts, are never withdrawn (the continuous hormonal type).

In primary amenorrhea, menses have never been established. This diagnosis is not usually made before the age of about 16. In secondary amenorrhea, menses once established have ceased (temporarily or permanently).

The most common type of hypohormonal amenorrhea is the **menopause**, or physiologic failure of ovarian function. The most common example of continuous hormonal amenorrhea is that due to **pregnancy**, when cyclic withdrawal is prevented by the placental secretions. These two conditions should always be considered before extensive diagnostic studies are undertaken in a patient who presents with a complaint of amenorrhea.

The principal diagnostic aids used in the study of amenorrhea are as follows: (1) vaginal smear for estrogen effect; (2) endometrial biopsy; (3) "medical D&C" (see below); (4) basal body temperature determination; (5) serum FSH, LH, and prolactin; (6) serum testosterone; and (7) MRI of the hypothalamic and pituitary areas in cases of hypogonadotropic hypogonadism.

Primary Amenorrhea

Because of the frequency with which "delayed puberty" is found in otherwise normal females, the diagnosis of primary amenorrhea usually is not made until the patient is clearly beyond the age at which normal menarche occurs. In the USA, the mean age at menarche is 12½ years. If menses have not started by age 16, primary amenorrhea is definitely present, and the cause should be investigated.

Patients with primary amenorrhea require careful assessment for systemic illness, short stature, signs of Turner's syndrome, and physical examination to verify the presence of the uterus and hymenal patency. Endocrine evaluation may include serum determinations of FSH, LH, PRL, and hCG (pregnancy test). A serum testosterone is drawn to screen for androgen insensitivity syndrome (testicular feminization).

Girls with low or normal FSH and LH—especially those with high PRL—may have a hypothalamic or pituitary lesion; such patients are evaluated with MRI or CT scan of the hypothalamus and pituitary.

Patients with an elevated serum FSH are likely to have ovarian dysgenesis.

The chromosomal sex pattern must be determined in many cases. Laparoscopy or pelvic exploration may be required to establish the diagnosis. In large series, the most common cause has always been Turner's syndrome (gonadal dysgenesis).

The causes are as follows:

(1) Hypothalamic causes: Constitutional delay in onset, severe malnutrition, serious organic illness, lack of LHRH (GnRH).

(2) Pituitary causes (with low or absent FSH): Pituitary tumors, nonsecreting or secreting prolactin, growth hormone, or ACTH (Cushing's disease); other destructive tumors (eg, craniopharyngiomas). Conditions without a mass lesion can cause lack of pituitary gonadotropins, either isolated or as part of panhypopituitarism: head trauma, encephalitis, midline defects, optic dysplasia, or damage from neonatal kernicterus.

(3) Ovarian causes (with high FSH): Ovarian dysgenesis with XO karyotype (Turner's syndrome), mosaic variants, mixed gonadal dysgenesis (XO,XY karyotype), pure gonadal dysgenesis, etc. Rarely, "resistant ovaries" syndrome. Rare congenital steroid enzyme defects that can cause hypogonadism include side chain cleavage enzyme deficiency (associated with adrenal insufficiency) and 17α-hydroxylase deficiency (associated with hypertension and hypokalemia).

(4) Uterine causes: Malformations, congenital müllerian dysgenesis, imperforate hymen, hermaphroditism, unresponsive or atrophic endometrium.

(5) Miscellaneous causes: All forms of male

pseudohermaphroditism (enzymatic defects in testosterone synthesis, androgen resistance syndromes), androgen excess syndromes (adrenal or ovarian tumors, adrenal enzymatic defects with excess androgen formation, such as 21- or 11β-hydroxylase deficiencies, polycystic ovaries).

Since primary amenorrhea is only a manifestation of multiple and often complex underlying defects, treatment must be individualized according to the specific cause.

Secondary Amenorrhea

Temporary cessation of menses is extremely common and usually does not usually require extensive endocrine investigation. In women of childbearing age, pregnancy must be ruled out. In women beyond the childbearing age, menopause should be considered first. States of emotional stress, malnutrition, anemia, and similar disorders may be associated with temporary amenorrhea, and correction of the primary disorder will usually also reestablish menses. Some women fail to menstruate regularly for prolonged intervals after stopping oral contraceptive pills. Lactation may be associated with amenorrhea, either physiologically or for abnormally prolonged periods after delivery. An increasing number of small prolactin-secreting pituitary tumors causing secondary amenorrhea and often lactation have been discovered by means of prolactin assays and pituitary imaging studies.

Young women with secondary amenorrhea should therefore be assessed for pregnancy with a β-hCG determination. FSH and LH may be determined; FSH is especially elevated in primary ovarian failure (eg, Turner's syndrome or menopause). An LH:FSH ratio greater than 2.0 is seen in polycystic ovary syndrome. Serum prolactin may be determined to screen for prolactin-secreting pituitary tumor or a hypothalamic lesion. Normal or low levels of serum LH and FSH are seen with anorexia nervosa, drug use, frequent flying ("jet lag"), severe illness or psychic stress, pituitary or hypothalamic disease, or uterine problems (eg, uterine synechiae [Asherman's syndrome]). Patients must be assessed for hyper- or hypothyroidism with a sensitive serum TSH. Routine tests for renal and hepatic function are performed. Serum electrolytes help screen for Addison's disease. Screening tests for Cushing's syndrome are performed when indicated clinically. Serum testosterone and other androgens may be elevated in androgen resistance syndromes and in hyperandrogen states (such as congenital adrenal hyperplasia, polycystic ovary syndrome, or tumors of the adrenal or ovary).

Estrogen Replacement Therapy

The aim of therapy is not only to reestablish menses (though this may be valuable for psychologic reasons) but also to attempt to establish the cause (eg, pituitary tumor) of the amenorrhea and to restore reproductive function.

Treatment depends upon the underlying disease. It is not necessary to treat all cases, especially temporary amenorrhea or irregular menses. Patients who have normal menses after a short course of medroxyprogesterone acetate (see above) may have menses induced every 1–3 months in this manner.

Women who have had a hysterectomy are given conjugated estrogens, 0.625–1.25 mg, either daily or cycled on days 1–25 of the calendar month.

Women with an intact uterus may be treated with estrogen (as above) but must also receive a progestin in order to decrease the risk of estrogen-induced endometrial carcinoma. The progestin of choice is medroxyprogesterone acetate. It may be given as 5 mg daily with the estrogen; this tends to cause irregular spotting for about 4 months, but bleeding then usually stops by 1 year, and women are not bothered by menstruation. Continued abnormal bleeding necessitates a pelvic examination; endometrial biopsy may be done using a Vibra aspiration technique. Alternatively, medroxyprogesterone acetate (5–10 mg) is given on days 16–25 of the calendar month; conjugated estrogens, 0.625–1.25 mg, is given daily on days 1–25 of the month. These regimens can be tailored to the individual's requirements and response.

Patients with an elevation in serum FSH are assumed to have inadequate ovarian estrogen secretion. Patients (nonpregnant) without such FSH elevation can be assessed for adequacy of estrogenization with a progestin withdrawal test: medroxyprogesterone acetate, 10 mg, is given daily for 10 days. Patients with adequate estrogenization usually have withdrawal menstruation. Women without withdrawal bleeding usually have more serious estrogen deficiency, which is likely to cause osteoporosis; such women are considered for estrogen replacement therapy.

The effect of estrogen upon the risk of breast cancer is controversial. A review of 24 articles, three meta-analyses, and five studies attempting to minimalize detection bias concluded that the risk was not increased (Henrich, 1992). Nevertheless, women should have regular breast examinations and mammography.

In patients who are unresponsive to progesterone and whose urinary gonadotropin levels are low, treatment of a pituitary lesion may restore menstruation. In patients with the galactorrhea-amenorrhea syndromes associated with elevated prolactin levels, restoration of ovulatory menses has been achieved with bromocriptine. Transsphenoidal resection of small prolactin-producing pituitary adenomas likewise has resulted in restoration of fertility. Hydrocortisone may restore menstruation in patients with congenital adrenal hyperplasia or Addison's disease.

General measures include dietary management as required to correct overweight or underweight; psychotherapy in cases due to emotional disturbance; and correction of anemia and any other metabolic abnormality that may be present (eg, mild hypothyroidism).

Barrett-Connor E: Risks and benefits of replacement estrogen. Annu Rev Med 1992;43:239.

Foster MB: Aberrant puberty. Obstet Gynecol Clin North Am 1992;19:59.

Henrich JB: The postmenopausal estrogen/breast cancer controversy. JAMA 1992;268:1900.

Ott SM: Estrogen therapy for osteoporosis—even in the elderly. Ann Intern Med 1992;117:85.

Puberty and its disorders. (Review.) Endocrinol Metab Clin North Am 1991;20:1.

Rubin SM, Cummings SR: Results of bone densitometry affect women's decisions about taking measures to prevent fractures. Ann Intern Med 1992;116:990.

Styne DM, Grumbach MM: Puberty in the male and female: Its physiology and disorders. In: *Reproductive Endocrinology.* Yen SSC, Jaffe RD (editors). Saunders, 1991.

2. TURNER'S SYNDROME (Gonadal Dysgenesis)

Turner's syndrome is a chromosomal disorder associated with primary hypogonadism, short stature, and other phenotypic anomalies. It is a common cause of primary amenorrhea. Patients with the classic syndrome lack one of the two X chromosomes and have a 45,XO karyotype.

Typical Turner's Syndrome (45,XO Gonadal Dysgenesis)

Typical features of Turner's syndrome are noted in Table 25–18. 45,XO zygotes account for about 0.8% of all conceptuses, making this the most common major chromosomal abnormality in humans. Less than 3% of these zygotes survive to term, with the incidence of Turner's syndrome being about 1:10,000 female newborns.

Girls with Turner's syndrome may be diagnosed at birth, since they tend to be small and may exhibit severe lymphedema. Evaluation for childhood short stature often leads to the diagnosis. Patients tend to be very short, falling below the third percentile for age, and do not have a pubertal growth spurt. Growth hormone and somatomedin levels are normal. Hypogonadism presents as "delayed adolescence"; FSH and LH are high, making a diagnosis of primary hypogonadism. A blood karyotype showing 46,XO establishes the diagnosis.

Treatment of girls with Turner's syndrome is largely supportive. Short stature does not respond significantly enough to injections of growth hormone to warrant this expensive and arduous treatment. At the usual time of puberty, these girls will not mature sexually. Replacement of cycled estrogens should not be delayed, since such delay has not produced im-

Table 25–18. Manifestations of Turner's syndrome.

Distinctive facial features:
  Ptosis
  Micrognathia
  Low-set ears
  Epicanthal folds
Short stature
Sexual infantilism due to gonadal dysgenesis
Webbed neck (40%)
Low hairline
High-arched palate
Cubitus valgus
Short fourth metacarpals (50%)
Lymphedema of hands and feet (Bonnevie-Ulrich syndrome) (30%)
Hypoplastic widely spaced nipples
Hyperconvex nails
Pigmented nevi
Keloid formation
Recurrent ear infections
Renal abnormalities (60%)
  Horseshoe kidney
  Hydronephrosis
Hypertension (idiopathic or due to coarctation or renal disease)
Gastrointestinal bleeding from intestinal telangiectases (rare)
Impaired space-form recognition, direction sense, and mathematical reasoning
Cardiovascular anomalies
  Coarctation of the aorta (10–20%)
  Aortic stenosis
  Bicuspid aortic valve
  Aortic dissection due to coarctation and cystic medial necrosis of aorta (rare)
  Associated conditions
  Obesity
  Diabetes mellitus
  Hashimoto's thyroiditis
  Achlorhydria
  Cataracts: lenticular or corneal
  Rheumatoid arthritis
  Inflammatory bowel disease

proved adult height. Replacement estrogen is begun at age 12 or 13 years with low doses of conjugated estrogens (0.3 mg) or ethinyl estradiol (5μg) given on days 1–25 per month; the dose is gradually increased over 2–3 years to 0.625–1.25 mg of conjugated estrogens or 10–20 μg of ethinyl estradiol. Medroxyprogesterone acetate, 5 mg, is added on days 16–25 of the month to induce menses.

Turner's Syndrome Variants

A. 46,X (Abnormal X) Karyotype: An abnormality or deletion of certain genes on the short arm of the X chromosome causes short stature and other signs of Turner's syndrome; some gonadal function and even fertility is possible. Abnormalities or deletions of other genes located on both the long and short arms of the X chromosome can produce gonadal dysgenesis with few of the usual somatic features of Turner's syndrome.

B. 45,XO/46,XX Mosaicism: This karyotype results in a modified form of Turner's syndrome. Such girls tend to be taller and may have more gonadal function and fewer other manifestations of Turner's syndrome.

C. Other Variants: 45,XO/46,XY mosaicism can produce some manifestations of Turner's syndrome. Patients typically have ambiguous genitalia.

D. Noonan's Syndrome: This disorder is manifested by short stature and many of the features of Turner's syndrome. However, these patients tend to have pectus excavatum and right-sided heart disease (pulmonary stenosis in 50%; atrial or ventricular septal defects). They have a normal karyotype. Renal anomalies are uncommon. Male patients may have cryptorchism, hypogonadism, and a small penis. Females may have delayed puberty but eventually have normal ovarian function. Patients tend to have more severe mental retardation than those with Turner's syndrome.

Mora S et al: Effect of estrogen replacement therapy on bone mineral content in girls with Turner syndrome. Obstet Gynecol 1992;79:747.

Takano K et al: Treatment of 46 patients with Turner's syndrome with recombinant human growth hormone (YM-17798) for 3 years: A multicenter study. Acta Endocrinol (Copenh) 1992;126:296.

Verschraegen-Spae MR et al: Familial Turner syndrome. Clin Genet 1992;41:218.

MULTIPLE ENDOCRINE NEOPLASIA

Several familial syndromes with multiple gland involvement have been described. The most common one is multiple endocrine neoplasia (or adenomatosis) type I (MEN I or MEA I; see Table 25–19), which is inherited as an autosomal dominant trait.

MEN I
(Wermer's Syndrome)

In MEN I, hyperparathyroidism occurs in over 80% of patients; it presents with hypercalcemia and usually involves hyperplasia or adenomas of several parathyroid glands. Pancreatic islet cell tumors occur in about 75% of patients; gastrinomas are the most common tumor and can result in gastric hyperacidity (Zollinger-Ellison syndrome) with peptic ulcer disease or diarrhea. Islet cell tumors may also secrete insulin, somatostatin, or glucagon. Pituitary adenomas occur in about 60% and may secrete prolactin, growth hormone, or ACTH but are usually nonfunctional; such tumors may produce local pressure effects and hypopituitarism. About 37% of these patients have adrenal cortical adenomas or hyperplasia—bilateral in about half. they are generally benign and nonfunctional. In one series, one out of 12 such patients developed a feminizing adrenal carcinoma. These adrenal lesions are pituitary-independent and are a secondary phenomenon in MEN I.

In this condition, tumors of the pituitary gland, the parathyroid gland, and the pancreatic islets occur in the same patient, though not necessarily at the same time. Some individuals in the same family express the abnormality as children, whereas in others the clinical manifestations may not appear until late in adult life. The clinical manifestations of MEN I are extremely variable, since the glandular tumors may secrete a variety of different hormones.

The kindreds expressing MEN I have been shown to harbor a gene mutation on the long arm of chromosome 11. Genetic linkage analysis can be used to determine which other family members will express this syndrome, permitting informed genetic counseling and avoiding unnecessary testing for unaffected individuals.

Table 25–19. Multiple endocrine neoplasia (MEN) syndromes.[1]

	MEN I	MEN IIa	MEN IIb
Synonym	Wermer's syndrome	Sipple's syndrome	
Genetic transmission	Autosomal dominant	Autosomal dominant	(?) Autosomal dominant
Tumor types (incidence)			
Parathyroid	>80%	50%	Rare
Pancreatic	75%		
Pituitary	60%		
Medullary thyroid carcinoma		>90%	80%
Pheochromocytoma		20%	60%
Mucosal and gastrointestinal ganglioneuromas		Rare	>90%
Lipoma	Occasional		
Adrenocortical adenoma	Occasional		
Carcinoid	Occasional		
Thyroid adenoma	Occasional		

[1]From Fitzgerald PA (editor): *Handbook of Clinical Endocrinology.* Appleton & Lange, 1992.

MEN IIa
(Sipple's Syndrome)

A separate disorder of familial hypersecretion of hormones is the so-called multiple endocrine neoplasia type II (MEN II or MEA II), or Sipple's syndrome. It too is inherited as an autosomal dominant trait. In MEN II, patients may have medullary thyroid carcinoma (> 90%); hyperparathyroidism (20–50%), due to hyperplasia or multiple adenomas in over 70% of cases; or pheochromocytomas (20–35%), which are often bilateral. The medullary thyroid carcinoma generally occurs in the third or fourth decade and is of mild to moderate aggressiveness. Patients may have periodic serum calcitonin measurements after pentagastrin stimulation to screen for early medullary thyroid carcinoma: pentagastrin, 0.5 µg/kg, is given intravenously over 15 seconds; serum samples for calcitonin are obtained at 1½-, 5-, and 10-minute intervals; a peak level over 190 pg/mL in males or over 80 pg/mL in females implicates an occult medullary thyroid carcinoma.

MEN IIb

Patients with MEN IIb (III) have a syndrome characterized by mucosal neuromas (> 90% with bumpy lips, enlarged tongue, Marfan-like habitus), pheochromocytomas (60%), and medullary thyroid carcinoma (80%), which can be quite aggressive. Patients also have intestinal abnormalities (75%), skeletal abnormalities (87%), and delayed puberty (43%). The medullary thyroid carcinoma tends to present in the third to fourth decades. Prophylactic thyroidectomy is reasonable treatment for such patients with mucosal neuromas and family members with the syndrome.

Nanes MS, Catherwood BD: The genetics of multiple endocrine neoplasia syndromes. Annu Rev Med 1992;43:253.

Ponder BA: Genetic screening for multiple endocrine neoplasia type 2. Exp Clin Endocrinol 1993;101:53.

Rave F, Zink A: Clinical features of multiple endocrine neoplasia type I and type 2. Horm Res 1992;38(Suppl 2):31.

Skogseid B et al: Clinical and genetic features of adrenocortical lesions in multiple endocrine neoplasia type I. J Clin Endocrinol Metab 1992;75:76.

Vasen HF et al: The natural course of multiple endocrine neoplasia type IIb: A study of 18 cases. Arch Intern Med 1992;152:1250.

CLINICAL USE OF CORTICO-STEROIDS & CORTICOTROPIN (ACTH)

Both pituitary adrenocorticotropin (ACTH), acting by adrenal stimulation, and the adrenal corticosteroids have been shown to have profound modifying effects on many pathologic processes, especially those associated with immunologic problems and inflammation.

These agents do not "cure." Their action is primarily anti-inflammatory and appears to be related to multiple effects upon blood vessels, leukocytes, macrophages, fibroblasts, cell membrane permeability, etc, rather than to one discrete, all-encompassing effect. They suppress the immune process but do not deal with the underlying cause of the disease. When they are discontinued, the disease often recurs.

There is no reason to use ACTH, given its parenteral route of administration and the unpredictability of its corticosteroid response. Both ACTH and the corticosteroids cause varying degrees of pituitary suppression. Secondary hypoadrenalism is present if either are stopped. They should not be stopped suddenly, and during periods of stress (eg, surgery, trauma), additional amounts of rapidly acting corticosteroids must be provided.

The systemic and topical efficacies of the corticosteroids are compared in Table 25–20.

It is recommended that an organized program be instituted for each patient receiving corticosteroids in order to recognize or prevent complications. Such a program is outlined in Table 25–21.

Table 25–20. Systemic versus topical activity of corticosteroids.
(Hydrocortisone = 1 in potency.)

	Systemic Activity	Topical Activity
Prednisolone	4–5	1–2
Fluprednisolone	8–10	10
Triamcinolone	5	1
Triamcinolone acetonide	5	40
Dexamethasone	30–120	10
Betamethasone	30	5–10
Betamethasone valerate		50–150
Methylprednisolone	5	5
Fluocinolone acetonide		40–100
Flurandrenolone acetonide		20–50
Fluorometholone	1–2	40

Table 25–21. Management of patients receiving glucocorticoids.[1]

1. Do not administer glucocorticoids unless absolutely indicated and more conservative measures have failed.
2. Keep dosage and length of administration to the minimum required for adequate treatment. Consider alternate-day or local therapy for certain conditions. Asthmatics who are prednisone-dependent may be able to reduce their systemic dosage of glucocorticoids if inhaled beclomethasone is added to the regimen; systemic absorption and oral candidiasis caused by beclomethasone may be reduced by using a spacer device to catch large droplets prior to inhalation.
3. Obtain a pretreatment chest x-ray, and apply a PPD (purified protein derivative) preparation. Treat any latent tuberculosis as indicated to avoid reactivation. Repeat the chest x-ray periodically.
4. Screen for diabetes mellitus before treatment and at each physician visit. Train the patient to test urine weekly with Tes-Tape, Diastix, Chemstrip uGK strips, or Clinistix.
5. Screen for hypertension before treatment and at each physician visit.
6. Screen for glaucoma and cataracts before treatment, 3 months after treatment, and then at least yearly.
7. Prepare the patient and family for possible adverse effects on mood, memory, and cognitive function. Inform them about other possible side effects.
8. Institute a vigorous physical exercise and isometric regimen tailored to each patient's disabilities.
9. Avoid prolonged bed rest that will accelerate muscle weakness and bone mineral loss. Ambulate early after fractures.
10. Treat hypogonadism in women or men.
11. Administer calcium (1 g elemental calcium) orally daily. Check spot morning urines, and alter dosage to keep urine calcium concentration below 30 mg/dL. If the patient is receiving thiazide diuretics, check for hypercalcemia, and administer only 500 mg elemental calcium daily. Consider pamidronate (ADP) therapy for prophylaxis against osteoporosis in selected patients (see text).
12. Avoid elective surgery, if possible. Vitamin A in a daily dose of 20,000 units orally for a week may improve wound healing.
13. Avoid activities that could cause falls or other trauma.
14. Watch for fungal or yeast infections of skin, nails, mouth, vagina, and rectum, and treat appropriately. Nail mycoses may be prevented or treated with twice-daily applications of ciclopirox olamine cream (Loprox 1%).
15. Ulcer prophylaxis: Administer oral glucocorticoids with meals. Consider prophylaxis with sucralfate, 1 g, an hour before meals or at bedtime. Ranitidine may also be used. Avoid large doses of antacids containing aluminum hydroxide (many popular brands) unless the patient is azotemic; aluminum hydroxide binds phosphate and may cause a hypophosphatemic osteomalacia that can compound glucocorticoid osteoporosis. If calcium carbonate is used (eg, Tums, Titralac), the total calcium dose must be monitored and screening done for hypercalciuria and hypercalcemia.
16. Treat any infections aggressively. Consider unusual pathogens.
17. Weigh daily. Use dietary measures to avoid obesity and optimize nutrition.
18. Measure height frequently. In children, this serves to document the degree of growth retardation. In adults, it serves to document the degree of axial spine demineralization and compression.
19. Treat edema as indicated.
20. Monitor plasma potassium for hypokalemia. Treat as indicated.
21. With dosage reduction, watch for signs of adrenal insufficiency or glucocorticoid withdrawal syndrome.

[1]Reproduced, with permission, from Fitzgerald PA: *Handbook of Clinical Endocrinology.* Appleton & Lange, 1992.

Horber FF et al: Evidence that prednisone-induced myopathy is reversed by physical training. J Clin Endocrinol Metab 1985;61:83.

Reid IR et al: Two-year follow-up of bisphosphonate (APD) treatment in steroid osteoporosis. Lancet 1988;2:1144.

Walkema R et al: Maintained improvement in calcium balance and bone mineral content in patients with osteoporosis treated with the bisphosphonate (APD). Bone Miner 1989;5:183.

REFERENCES

Bardin CW (editor): *Current Therapy in Endocrinology and Metabolism,* 4th ed. BC Decker, 1991.

Baulieu EE, Kelly PA (editors): *Hormones. From Molecules to Disease.* Chapman & Hall, 1990.

Becker KL et al (editors): *Principles and Practice of Endocrinology and Metabolism.* Lippincott, 1990.

Braverman LE, Utiger RD (editors): *Werner and Ingbar's The Thyroid: A Fundamental and Clinical Text,* 7th ed. Lippincott, 1992.

Fitzgerald PA (editor): *Handbook of Clinical Endocrinology,* 2nd ed. Appleton & Lange, 1992.

Greenspan FS (editor): *Basic and Clinical Endocrinology,* 3rd ed. Appleton & Lange, 1991.

Hadley ME: *Endocrinology,* 3rd ed. Prentice-Hall, 1992.

Wilson JD, Foster DW (editors): *Williams' Textbook of Endocrinology,* 8th ed. Saunders, 1992.

Yen SSC, Jaffe RB (editors): *Reproductive Endocrinology,* 3rd ed. Saunders, 1991.

Diabetes Mellitus & Hypoglycemia 26

John H. Karam, MD

DIABETES MELLITUS

Essentials of Diagnosis

Type I diabetes, or insulin-dependent diabetes mellitus (IDDM):

- Polyuria, polydipsia, and rapid weight loss associated with unequivocal hyperglycemia.
- Plasma glucose of 140 mg/dL or higher after an overnight fast, documented on more than one occasion.
- Ketonemia, ketonuria, or both.

Type II diabetes, or non-insulin-dependent diabetes mellitus (NIDDM):

- Most patients are over 40 years of age and obese.
- Polyuria and polydipsia. Ketonuria and weight loss generally are uncommon at time of diagnosis. Candidal vaginitis in women may be an initial manifestation. Many patients have few or no symptoms.
- Plasma glucose of 140 mg/dL or higher after an overnight fast on more than one occasion. After 75 g oral glucose, diagnostic values are 200 mg/dL or more 2 hours after the oral glucose and at least once between 0 and 2 hours.
- Hypertension, hyperlipidemia, and atherosclerosis are often associated.

Classification & Pathogenesis

Diabetes mellitus represents a syndrome with disordered metabolism and inappropriate hyperglycemia due to either an absolute deficiency of insulin secretion or a reduction in its biologic effectiveness or both. It is classified into two major types in which age at onset is not a criterion (Table 26–1).

A. Type I: Insulin-Dependent Diabetes Mellitus (IDDM): This severe form is associated with ketosis in the untreated state. It occurs most commonly in juveniles but occasionally in adults, especially the nonobese and those who are elderly when hyperglycemia first appears. It is a catabolic disorder in which circulating insulin is virtually absent, plasma glucagon is elevated, and the pancreatic B cells fail to respond to all insulinogenic stimuli. Exogenous insulin is there-

fore required to reverse the catabolic state, prevent ketosis, reduce the hyperglucagonemia, and bring the elevated blood glucose level down.

The highest prevalence of type I diabetes is in Scandinavia, where it comprises as many as 20% of the total number of patients with diabetes. This decreases in prevalence to 13% in southern Europe and 8% in the USA, while in Japan and China less than 1% of patients with diabetes have type I diabetes.

Certain human leukocyte antigens (HLA) are strongly associated with the development of type I diabetes. About 95% of type I patients possess either HLA-DR3 or HLA-DR4, compared to 45–50% of Caucasian controls. HLA-DQ genes are even more specific markers of type I susceptibility, since a particular variety (HLA-DQw3.2) is generally found in the DR4 patients with type I, while a "protective" gene (HLA-DQw3.1) is often present in the DR4 controls. In addition, circulating islet cell antibodies have been detected in as many as 85% of patients tested in the first few weeks of their diabetes, and when sensitive immunoassays are used, the majority of these patients also have detectable anti-insulin antibodies prior to receiving insulin therapy. It has recently been documented that most islet cell antibodies are directed against glutamic acid decarboxylase (GAD), a 64,000-MW enzyme localized within pancreatic B cells. Immunoassay kits for this sensitive antibody marker of type I diabetes are presently undergoing clinical trials in Denmark. These kits will facilitate screening of siblings of affected children as well as adults with atypical features of type II for the presence of an autoimmune cause for their diabetes.

Because of these immune characteristics, type I diabetes is felt to result from an infectious or toxic environmental insult to pancreatic B cells of persons whose immune system is genetically predisposed to develop a vigorous autoimmune response either against altered pancreatic B cell antigens or against molecules of the B cell resembling the viral protein (molecular mimicry). Extrinsic factors that affect B cell function include damage caused by viruses such as mumps or coxsackie B4 virus, by toxic chemical agents, or by destructive cytotoxins and antibodies released from sensitized immunocytes. Specific HLA genes may increase susceptibility to a diabetogenic

Table 26–1. Clinical classification of idiopathic diabetes mellitus syndromes.

Type	Ketosis	Islet Cell Antibodies	HLA Association	Treatment
(I) Insulin-dependent (IDDM)	Present	Present at onset	Positive	Insulin (mixtures of rapid- and intermediate-acting, at least twice daily) and diet
(II) Non-insulin-dependent (NIDDM) (a) Nonobese	Absent	Absent	Negative	(1) Eucaloric diet alone (2) Diet plus insulin or sulfonylureas
(b) Obese				(1) Weight reduction (2) Hypocaloric diet, plus sulfonylureas or insulin for symptomatic control only

virus or be linked to certain immune response genes that predispose patients to a destructive autoimmune response against their own islet cells (autoaggression). Amelioration of hyperglycemia in patients given cyclosporine shortly after onset of type I diabetes lends further support to the pathogenetic role of autoimmunity.

B. Type II: Non-Insulin-Dependent Diabetes Mellitus (NIDDM): This represents a heterogeneous group comprising milder forms of diabetes that occur predominantly in adults but occasionally in juveniles. More than 90% of all diabetics in the USA are included under this classification. Circulating endogenous insulin is sufficient to prevent ketoacidosis but is inadequate in the face of increased needs owing to tissue insensitivity. Type II diabetes is defined in essentially negative terms: It is a *non*ketotic form of diabetes that is *not* linked to HLA markers on the sixth chromosome; it has *no* islet cell antibodies or any other immune component; and it is *not* dependent on exogenous insulin therapy to sustain life, thereby being termed "*non*-insulin-dependent diabetes mellitus" (NIDDM). In most cases of this type of diabetes, the cause is unknown.

An element of tissue insensitivity to insulin has been noted in most type II patients irrespective of weight and has been attributed to several interrelated factors. These include a primary (and as yet undefined) genetic factor, which is aggravated in time by additional enhancers of insulin resistance such as aging and abdominal-visceral obesity. In addition, there is an accompanying deficiency in the response of pancreatic B cells to glucose. Both the tissue resistance to insulin and the impaired B cell response to glucose appear to be further aggravated by increased hyperglycemia, and both defects are ameliorated by treatment that reduces the hyperglycemia toward normal. Attempts to identify a genetic marker for type II have as yet been unsuccessful. However, most epidemiologic data indicate strong genetic influences, since in monozygotic twins over 40 years of age, concordance is uniform within a year whenever one twin develops type II.

Two subgroups of patients with type II diabetes are currently distinguished by the absence or presence of obesity. The degree and prevalence of obesity varies among different racial groups. While obesity occurs in less than 30% of Chinese and Japanese patients with type II, it is found in 75–80% of North Americans, Europeans, or Africans with type II and approaches 100% of patients with type II among Pima Indians or Pacific Islanders from Nauru or Samoa.

1. Nonobese type II patients–These patients generally show an absent or blunted early phase of insulin release in response to glucose; however, it may often be elicited in response to other insulinogenic stimuli such as acute intravenous administration of sulfonylureas, glucagon, or secretin. Among this heterogeneous subgroup may be certain unrecognized patients with a milder expression of type I diabetes who initially retain enough B cell function to avoid ketosis but later develop increasing dependency on insulin therapy. Also included within this subgroup are those with diabetes characterized as "maturity-onset diabetes of the young" (MODY), whose strongly positive family history of a mild form of diabetes shows autosomal dominant transmission. In France, 18 families have been found to have mutations of the glucokinase gene of chromosome 7, resulting in impaired beta cell function. Another large MODY kindred in Michigan has had its as yet unidentified genetic defect traced to the large arm of chromosome 20.

The hyperglycemia in this subgroup of patients often responds to oral hypoglycemic agents or, at times, to dietary therapy alone. Occasionally, insulin therapy is required to achieve satisfactory glycemic control even though it is not needed to prevent ketoacidosis.

Although residual insulin resistance may persist after therapeutic correction of the hyperglycemia in some cases, it does not seem to be clinically relevant to the treatment of nonobese type II patients, who generally respond to appropriate therapeutic supplements of insulin in the absence of rare associated conditions such as lipoatrophy or acanthosis nigricans.

2. Obese type II patients–This form of diabetes is secondary to extrapancreatic factors that produce insensitivity to endogenous insulin. It is characterized by nonketotic mild diabetes, mainly in adults but occasionally also in children. The primary problem is a "target organ" disorder resulting in ineffective insulin action (Table 26–2) that can secondarily influence pancreatic B cell function. Hyperplasia of pancreatic B cells is often present and probably accounts for the fasting hyperinsulinism and exaggerated insulin and proinsulin responses to glucose and other stimuli seen in the milder forms of this disorder. In more severe cases, secondary (but potentially reversible) failure of B cell secretion may result after exposure to prolonged fasting hyperglycemia. This phenomenon has been called "desensitization" of the pancreatic B cell. It is selective for glucose, and the B cell recovers sensitivity to glucose stimulation once the sustained hyperglycemia is corrected by any form of therapy, including diet, sulfonylureas, and insulin. Obesity is common in this type of diabetes and is generally associated with abdominal distribution of fat, producing an abnormally high waist-to-hip ratio. Refined radiographic techniques of assessing abdominal fat distribution with CT scans have documented that a "visceral" obesity, due to accumulation of fat in the omental and mesenteric regions, correlates with insulin resistance, whereas fat predominantly in subcutaneous tissues of the abdomen has little if any association with insulin insensitivity. Lipolysis of visceral fat directly into the portal circulation alters liver metabolism and increases hepatic glucose output much more than when peripheral fat is mobilized into systemic veins. In obese patients, insulin insensitivity is positively correlated with the presence of distended adipocytes, but liver and muscle cells also resist the deposition of additional glycogen and triglycerides in their storage depots.

A major cause of the observed resistance to insulin in target tissues of obese patients is believed to be a postreceptor defect in insulin action. This is associated with overdistended storage depots, and there is a reduced ability to clear nutrients from the circulation after meals. A resulting hyperinsulinism can further enhance insulin resistance by down-regulation of insulin receptors. Moreover, when hyperglycemia develops, a specific glucose transporter protein within insulin target tissue also becomes down-regulated

Table 26–2. Factors reducing response to insulin.

Prereceptor inhibitors: Anti-insulin antibodies
Receptor inhibitors:
  Insulin receptor antibodies
  "Down regulation" of receptors by hyperinsulinism:
    Primary hyperinsulinism (B cell adenoma)
    Hyperinsulinism secondary to a postreceptor defect
      (obesity, Cushing's syndrome, acromegaly, pregnancy) or prolonged glycemia (diabetes mellitus, postglucose tolerance test)
Postreceptor influences:
  Poor responsiveness of principal target organs; obesity; hepatic disease; muscle inactivity; sustained hyperglycemia
  Hormonal excess: glucocorticoids, growth hormone, oral contraceptive agents, progesterone, human chorionic somatomammotropin, catecholamines, thyroxine

---

after continuous activation. This contributes to further defects in postreceptor insulin action, thereby aggravating the hyperglycemia.

When overfeeding is corrected so that storage depots become less saturated, the cycle is interrupted. There is improvement in insulin sensitivity, which is further restored toward normal by a reduction of both the hyperinsulinism and the hyperglycemia.

Epidemiologic Considerations

An estimated 8 million people in the USA are known to have diabetes, of which 680,000 have the insulin-dependent type. Use of the current "therapeutic" classification has been widely accepted throughout the world, but its deficiencies are apparent in many individual cases. For example, a 23-year-old nonobese woman whose mild diabetes is presently responding adequately to diet alone and who shows a low-normal C-peptide response to stimuli had presented with severe diabetes with ketosis and required insulin for several weeks following diagnosis. In addition, she has an associated autoimmune disorder, myasthenia gravis. From an etiologic standpoint, she probably has type I diabetes, but her present clinical status is "non-insulin-dependent." Similarly, many diabetics classified as "non-insulin-dependent" require insulin therapy. With the soon-to-be-available sensitive immunoassay kits to detect islet cell antibodies to the 64,000-MW B cell antigen GAD (see above), a new classification will be forthcoming relating to cause and independent of therapy. To retain the acronyms, type I could aptly be termed "immune-dependent diabetes mellitus" (IDDM), and type II "non-immune-dependent diabetes mellitus" (NIDDM).

Insulin resistance syndrome (syndrome X, CHAOS). investigators have speculated that the well-known association of **hyperglycemia, hyperinsulinemia, hyperlipidemia,** and **hypertension,** which lead to coronary artery disease and stroke, may result from a genetic defect producing insulin resistance, particularly when obesity aggravates the degree of insulin resistance. They suggest that insulin resistance predisposes to hyperglycemia, which results in hyperinsulinemia, which may or may not be of sufficient magnitude to correct the hyperglycemia; and that this excessive insulin level then contributes to increased VLDL production in the liver, leading to hyperlipidemia and to increased sodium retention by renal tubules, thus inducing hypertension. Moreover, they propose that high insulin levels can stimulate endothelial proliferation—by virtue of insulin's action on growth factor receptors—to initiate atherosclerosis. Australian epidemiologists have called this association of disorders "CHAOS" (acronym for *c*oronary artery disease, *h*ypertension, *a*therosclerosis, *o*besity, and *s*troke). While these associations have been well known, the mechanism for their interrelationship remains speculative and an invitation to experimental investigation. Some investigators question the etiologic role of hyperinsulinism on hypertension, since these two manifestations, which often coexist in Caucasians, are not highly associated in blacks or Pima Indians. Moreover, patients with hyperinsulinism due to insulinoma are generally not hypertensive, and there is no fall in blood pressure after surgical removal of the insulinoma restores normal insulin levels. The main value of grouping these disorders as a syndrome, however, is to remind physicians that the therapeutic goals are not only to correct hyperglycemia but also to manage the elevated blood pressure and hyperlipidemia that result in increased cerebrovascular and cardiac morbidity and mortality in these patients. Physicians aware of this syndrome are less likely to prescribe therapies that correct hypertension but raise lipids (diuretics, beta-blockers) or that correct hyperlipidemia but increase insulin resistance, with aggravation of diabetes (niacin). Finally, the use of long-acting insulins and sulfonylureas that promote sustained hyperinsulinism may have to be moderated and other drugs considered if the hypothesis behind the insulin-resistance syndrome is ever substantiated.

Clinical Findings

The principal clinical features of the two major types of diabetes mellitus are listed for comparison in Table 26–3.

Patients with type I diabetes (IDDM) present with a characteristic symptom complex, as outlined below. An absolute deficiency of insulin results in excessive accumulation of circulating glucose and fatty acids, with consequent hyperosmolality and hyperketonemia. The severity of the insulin deficiency and the acuteness with which the catabolic state develops determine the intensity of the osmotic and ketotic excess.

Patients with type II diabetes (NIDDM) may or may not present with characteristic signs and symptoms. The presence of obesity or a strongly positive family history for mild diabetes suggests a high risk for the development of type II diabetes.

Table 26–3. Clinical features of diabetes at diagnosis.

	Diabetes Type I (IDDM)	Diabetes Type II (NIDDM)
Polyuria and thirst	++	+
Weakness or fatigue	++	+
Polyphagia with weight loss	++	−
Recurrent blurred vision	+	++
Vulvovaginitis or pruritus	+	++
Peripheral neuropathy	+	++
Nocturnal enuresis	++	−
Often asymptomatic	−	++

A. Symptoms and Signs:

1. Type I diabetes (IDDM)–Increased urination is a consequence of osmotic diuresis secondary to sustained hyperglycemia. This results in a loss of glucose as well as free water and electrolytes in the urine. Enuresis may signal the onset of diabetes in very young children. Thirst is a consequence of the hyperosmolar state, as is blurred vision, which often develops as the lenses and retinas are exposed to hyperosmolar fluids.

Weight loss despite normal or increased appetite is a common feature of type I when it develops subacutely over a period of weeks. The weight loss is initially due to depletion of water, glycogen, and triglyceride stores; thereafter, reduced muscle mass occurs as amino acids are diverted to form glucose and ketone bodies.

Lowered plasma volume produces dizziness and weakness due to postural hypotension when sitting or standing. Total body potassium loss and the general catabolism of muscle protein contribute to the weakness.

Paresthesias may be present at the time of diagnosis of type I diabetes, particularly when the onset is subacute. They reflect a temporary dysfunction of peripheral sensory nerves, which clears as insulin replacement restores glycemic levels closer to normal, suggesting neurotoxicity from sustained hyperglycemia.

When insulin deficiency is absolute and of acute onset, the above symptoms progress in an accelerated manner. Ketoacidosis exacerbates the dehydration and hyperosmolality by producing anorexia and nausea and vomiting, thus interfering with oral fluid replacement.

The patient's level of consciousness can vary depending on the degree of hyperosmolality. When insulin deficiency develops relatively slowly and sufficient water intake is maintained, patients remain relatively alert and physical findings may be minimal. When vomiting occurs in response to worsening ketoacidosis, dehydration progresses and compensatory mechanisms become inadequate to keep serum osmolality below 320–330 mosm/L. Under these circumstances, stupor or even coma may occur. The fruity breath odor of acetone further suggests the diagnosis of diabetic ketoacidosis.

Hypotension in the recumbent position is a serious prognostic sign. Loss of subcutaneous fat and muscle wasting are features of more slowly developing insulin deficiency. In occasional patients with slow, insidious onset of insulin deficiency, subcutaneous fat may be considerably depleted. An enlarged liver, eruptive xanthomas on the flexor surface of the limbs and on the buttocks, and lipemia retinalis indicate that chronic insulin deficiency has resulted in chylomicronemia, with circulating triglycerides elevated usually to over 2000 mg/dL.

2. Type II diabetes (NIDDM)–Most patients

with type II diabetes have an insidious onset of hyperglycemia and may be relatively asymptomatic initially. This is particularly true in obese patients, whose diabetes may be detected only after glycosuria or hyperglycemia is noted during routine laboratory studies. Occasionally, type II patients may present with evidence of neuropathic or cardiovascular complications because of underlying occult disease present for some time prior to diagnosis. Chronic skin infections are common. Generalized pruritus and symptoms of vaginitis are frequently the initial complaints of women with type II. Diabetes should be suspected in women with chronic candidal vulvovaginitis as well as in those who have delivered large babies (> 9 lb, or 4.1 kg) or have had polyhydramnios, preeclampsia, or unexplained fetal losses.

Obese diabetics may have any variety of fat distribution; however, diabetes seems to be more often associated in both men and women with localization of fat deposits on the upper segment of the body (particularly the abdomen, chest, neck, and face) and relatively less fat on the appendages, which may be quite muscular. Standardized tables of waist-to-hip ratio indicate that ratios of "greater than 0.9" in men and "greater than 0.8" in women are associated with an increased risk of diabetes in obese subjects. Mild hypertension is often present in obese diabetics.

B. Laboratory Findings:

1. Urinalysis–

a. Glucosuria–A specific and convenient method to detect glucosuria is the paper strip impregnated with glucose oxidase and a chromogen system (Clinistix, Diastix, TesTape), which is sensitive to as little as 0.1% glucose in urine. Diastix can be directly applied to the urinary stream, and differing color responses of the indicator strip reflect glucose concentration.

Certain common therapeutic agents interfere with this determination. When taken in large doses, ascorbic acid, salicylates, methyldopa, and levodopa can give false-negative results, since these powerful reducing agents interfere with the color reaction and thus prevent accurate estimation of glucose in the urine of diabetics. A normal renal threshold for glucose as well as reliable bladder emptying is essential for interpretation.

b. Ketonuria–Qualitative detection of ketone bodies can be accomplished by nitroprusside tests (Acetest or Ketostix). Although these tests do not detect β-hydroxybutyric acid, which lacks a ketone group, the semiquantitative estimation of ketonuria thus obtained is nonetheless usually adequate for clinical purposes.

2. Blood testing procedures–

a. Glucose tolerance test–

(1) Methodology and normal fasting glucose: Plasma or serum from venous blood samples may be used and has the advantage over whole blood of providing values for glucose that are independent of hematocrit and that reflect the glucose concentration to which body tissues are exposed. For these reasons, and because plasma and serum are more readily measured on automated equipment, plasma and serum glucose measurements are rapidly replacing the whole blood glucose determinations used heretofore in most laboratories. Fluoride anticoagulant in the collecting tube prevents enzymatic glycolysis by blood corpuscles and prevents pseudohypoglycemia, seen in states of extreme leukocytosis. If serum is used, samples should be refrigerated and separated within 1 hour after collection.

(2) Criteria for laboratory confirmation of diabetes mellitus: If the fasting plasma glucose level is over 140 mg/dL on more than one occasion, further evaluation of the patient with a glucose challenge is unnecessary. However, when fasting plasma glucose is less than 140 mg/dL in suspected cases, a standardized oral glucose tolerance test may be done (see Table 26–4).

For proper evaluation of the test, the subjects should be normally active and free from acute illness. Medications that may impair glucose tolerance include diuretics, contraceptive drugs, glucocorticoids, nicotinic acid, and phenytoin.

Because of difficulties in interpreting oral glucose tolerance tests and the lack of standards related to aging, these tests are generally being replaced by documentation of fasting hyperglycemia as a means of diagnosing diabetes mellitus.

Since fasting plasma glucose is known to increase with aging, physicians should be more tolerant of slight abnormalities of fasting glucose values in elderly people (over 70 years of age) and not deprive patients of occasional sugar-containing snacks when symptoms are not evident. However, an occasional elderly patient may benefit from the diagnosis of mild diabetes in that macular edema may be detected

Table 26–4. National Diabetes Data Group criteria for evaluating standard oral glucose tolerance test.[1]

	Normal Glucose Tolerance	Impaired Glucose Tolerance	Diabetes Mellitus[2]
Fasting plasma glucose (mg/dL)	< 115	116–139	> 140
Points between 0 and 120 minutes (mg/dL)	< 200	< 200	200 at least once
Two hours post glucose load (mg/dL)	< 140	> 140 but < 200	> 200

[1]Give 75 g of glucose dissolved in 300 mL of water for adults (1.75 g/kg ideal body weight for children) after an overnight fast in subjects who have been receiving at least 150–200 g of carbohydrate daily for 3 days before the test.

[2]A fasting plasma glucose greater than 140 mg/dL is diagnostic of diabetes. However, if the plasma glucose is less than 140 mg/dL, both of the lower columns must be fulfilled to make the diagnosis of diabetes mellitus.

earlier and laser treatment initiated before vision deteriorates permanently.

b. Glycosylated hemoglobin (hemoglobin A₁) measurements–Glycosylated hemoglobin is abnormally high in diabetics with chronic hyperglycemia and reflects their metabolic control. It is produced by nonenzymatic condensation of glucose molecules with free amino groups on the globin component of hemoglobin. The higher the prevailing ambient levels of blood glucose, the higher will be the level of glycosylated hemoglobin. The major form of glycohemoglobin is termed hemoglobin A_{1c}, which normally comprises only 4–6% of the total hemoglobin. The remaining glycohemoglobins (2–4% of the total) consist of phosphorylated glucose or fructose and are termed hemoglobin A_{1a} and hemoglobin A_{1b}. Most laboratories measure the sum of these three glycohemoglobins and report it as hemoglobin A_1.

Since glycohemoglobins circulate within red blood cells whose life span lasts up to 120 days, they generally reflect the state of glycemia over the preceding 8–12 weeks, thereby providing an improved method of assessing diabetic control. When glycohemoglobins are measured in a reliable laboratory, they are extremely useful in monitoring the progress of patients. Measurements should be made in patients with either type of diabetes mellitus at 3- to 4-month intervals. In patients monitoring their own blood glucose levels, glycohemoglobin values provide a valuable check on the accuracy of monitoring. In patients who do not monitor their own blood glucose levels, glycohemoglobin values are essential for adjusting therapy. Attempts to use glycohemoglobin methods for diabetes screening have been controversial. Sensitivity in detecting known diabetes cases by hemoglobin A_{1c} measurements is only 85%, indicating that diabetes cannot be excluded by a normal value. On the other hand, elevated hemoglobin A_{1c} assays are quite specific (91%) in identifying the presence of diabetes mellitus.

Occasionally, fluctuations in hemoglobin A_1 are due to an acutely generated, reversible, intermediary (aldimine-linked) product that can falsely elevate glycohemoglobins when measured with "short-cut" chromatographic methods. This can be eliminated by using more intricate methods or by dialysis of the hemolysate before chromatography. When hemoglobin variants are present, such as negatively charged hemoglobin F, acetylated hemoglobin from high-dose aspirin therapy, or carbamoylated hemoglobin produced by the complexing of urea with hemoglobin in uremia, falsely *high* "hemoglobin A_1" values are obtained with commonly used chromatographic methods. In the presence of positively charged hemoglobin variants such as hemoglobin S or C, or when the life span of red blood cells is reduced by increased hemolysis or hemorrhage, falsely *low* values for "hemoglobin A_1" result.

Serum fructosamine is formed by nonenzymatic glycosylation of serum proteins (predominantly albumin). Since serum albumin has a much shorter half-life than hemoglobin, serum fructosamine generally reflects the state of glycemic control for only the preceding 2 weeks. When abnormal hemoglobins or hemolytic states affect the interpretation of glycohemoglobin or when a narrower time frame is required, such as for ascertaining glycemic control at the time of conception in a diabetic woman who has recently become pregnant, serum fructosamine assays offer some advantage. Normal values are 1.5–2.4 mmol/L when serum albumin levels are 5 g/dL.

c. Self-monitoring of blood glucose–Capillary blood glucose measurements performed by patients themselves, as outpatients, are extremely useful, particularly in type I patients in whom "tight" metabolic control is attempted. A portable battery-operated Glucometer II (Ames Co.) or Glucoscan II (Lifescan, Inc.) provides a digital readout of the intensity of color developed when glucose oxidase paper strips are exposed to a drop of capillary blood for up to 60 seconds. Similar diagnostic strips made by Bio-Dynamics Corp. (Chemstrip-bG) have two chromogen indicators that permit *visual* estimation of the glucose concentration when compared to a series of color standards. The Chemstrip-bG can also be read by a reflectance meter (Accu-chek II). Second-generation glucometers—One Touch II (Lifescan, Inc) or ExacTech (Baxter Corp)—automatically time the reaction as soon as a drop of blood is applied to the previously inserted test strip. This relieves patients of the need to wipe off the strip after an exact interval of time and eliminates technical errors from improper blotting or timing. Glucose meters are relatively inexpensive, ranging from $50.00 to $100.00 dollars each. However, test strips remain a major expense, costing 50–75 cents apiece. In self-monitoring of blood glucose, patients must prick their finger with a small lancet (Monolet, Ames Co.), which can be facilitated by a small plastic trigger device such as an Autolet (Ames Co.), Autoclix (Bio-Dynamics), or Penlet (Lifescan, Inc.). When used for multiple patients, as in a clinic, physician's office, or hospital ward, *disposable* finger-rest platforms are required to avoid inadvertent transmission of blood-borne viral diseases.

The accuracy of data obtained by glucose monitoring requires careful education and training of the patient in sampling and measuring procedures as well as in proper calibration of the instruments. Bedside glucose monitoring in a hospital setting requires rigorous quality control programs and certification of personnel to avoid serious errors. When this is not feasible, glucose testing at the bedside is best done by technicians from the central laboratory.

3. Capillary morphometry (biopsy of the quadriceps muscle)–The basement membrane of capillaries from skeletal muscle tissue of the quadriceps area is abnormally thickened in cases of overt spontaneous diabetes in adults with fasting hyperglycemia of 140 mg/dL or more. Capillary morphometry appears to be less useful in diabetic children, being normal in as many as 60% of those below age 18.

Whether basement membrane thickening in diabetics can result from hyperglycemia alone with no genetic component appears to have been resolved by documented observation of thickened capillary basement membranes in the muscle of patients with acquired chronic hyperglycemia after ingestion of a diabetogenic toxin (Vacor rodenticide) during attempted suicide. While this finding establishes that glucose toxicity can produce abnormally thick membranes, it is still possible that the degree of abnormal thickening may depend on varying genetic susceptibility among diabetic patients. Moreover, it remains unclear whether a thickened capillary basement membrane of skeletal muscle has clinical significance, since it has not been possible to demonstrate a correlation between this marker and clinically evident renal dysfunction or renal mesangial changes associated with progressive diabetic nephropathy.

Differential Diagnosis

A. Hyperglycemia Secondary to Other Causes: (Table 26–5.) Secondary hyperglycemia has been associated with various disorders of insulin target tissues (liver, muscle, and adipose tissue).

Other secondary causes of carbohydrate intolerance include endocrine disorders—often specific endocrine tumors—associated with excess production of growth hormone, glucocorticoids, catecholamines, glucagon, or somatostatin. In the first four situations, peripheral responsiveness to insulin is impaired. With excess of glucocorticoids, catecholamines, or glucagon, increased hepatic output of glucose is a contributory factor; in the case of catecholamines, decreased insulin release is an additional factor in producing carbohydrate intolerance, and with excess somatostatin production it is the major factor.

A rare syndrome of extreme insulin resistance as-

Table 26–5. Secondary causes of hyperglycemia.

Hyperglycemia due to tissue insensitivity to insulin
  Hormonal tumors (acromegaly, Cushing's syndrome, glucagonoma, pheochromocytoma)
  Pharmacologic agents (glucocorticoids, sympathomimetic drugs, nicotinic acid)
  Liver disease (cirrhosis, hemochromatosis)
  Muscle disorders (myotonic dystrophy)
  Adipose tissue disorders (lipoatrophy, lipodystrophy, truncal obesity)
  Insulin receptor disorders (acanthosis nigricans syndromes, leprechaunism)
Hyperglycemia due to reduced insulin secretion
  Hormonal tumors (somatostatinoma, pheochromocytoma)
  Pancreatic disorders (pancreatitis, hemosiderosis from excess transfusions, idiopathic hemochromatosis)
  Pharmacologic agents (thiazide diuretics, phenytoin, pentamidine, Vacor rodenticide)

---

sociated with acanthosis nigricans afflicts either young women with androgenic features as well as insulin receptor mutations or older people, mostly women, in whom a circulating immunoglobulin binds to insulin receptors and reduces their affinity to insulin.

Medications such as thiazide diuretics, phenytoin, and high-dose glucocorticoids can produce hyperglycemia that is reversible once the drugs are discontinued. Chronic pancreatitis reduces the number of functioning B cells and can result in a metabolic derangement very similar to that of genetic diabetes mellitus except that a concomitant reduction in pancreatic A cells may reduce glucagon secretion so that relatively lower doses of insulin replacement are needed. Insulin-dependent diabetes is occasionally associated with Addison's disease and autoimmune thyroiditis (Schmidt's syndrome). This occurs particularly in women and probably represents an autoimmune disorder in which there are circulating antibodies to adrenocortical and thyroid tissue, thyroglobulin, and gastric parietal cells.

B. Nondiabetic Glycosuria: Nondiabetic glycosuria (renal glycosuria) is a benign, asymptomatic condition wherein glucose appears in the urine despite a normal amount of glucose in the blood, either basally or during a glucose tolerance test. Its cause may vary from an autosomally transmitted genetic disorder to one associated with dysfunction of the proximal renal tubule (Fanconi's syndrome, chronic renal failure), or it may merely be a consequence of the increased load of glucose presented to the tubules by the elevated glomerular filtration rate during pregnancy. As many as 50% of pregnant women normally have demonstrable sugar in the urine, especially during the third and fourth months. This sugar is practically always glucose except during the late weeks of pregnancy, when lactose may be present.

Treatment

A. Goals of Treatment of Diabetes: Diabetes mellitus is a chronic disease that requires ongoing medical care as well as patient and family education both to prevent acute illness and to reduce the risk of long-term complications. Therapy directed toward these goals should not be too restrictive to the patient's quality of life. The recent dramatic results of the diabetes control and complications trial (see below) indicate that the therapeutic objective is to restore known metabolic derangements toward normal in order to prevent and delay progression of diabetic complications. This objective should be approached while making every effort to avoid severe hypoglycemia.

B. Treatment Regimens:

1. Diet—A well-balanced, nutritious diet remains a fundamental element of therapy. However, in more than half of cases, diabetic patients fail to follow their diet. Consultation with a registered dietician is recommended. In prescribing a diet, it is important to relate dietary objectives to the type of diabetes. In obese patients with mild hyperglycemia, the major goal of diet therapy is weight reduction by caloric restriction. Thus, there is less need for exchange lists, emphasis on timing of meals, or periodic snacks, all of which are so essential in the treatment of insulin-requiring nonobese diabetics. This type of patient represents the most frequent challenge for the physician. Weight reduction is an elusive goal that can only be achieved by close supervision and education of the obese patient. See Chapter 28 for dietary management of obesity.

a. ADA diet–Exchange lists for meal planning can be obtained from the American Diabetes Association and its affiliate associations or from the American Dietetic Association, 430 North Michigan Avenue, Chicago 60611. The ADA diet stresses the major goal of caloric restriction as a means of achieving or maintaining ideal weight. A prudent diet is recommended, which includes restriction of fat intake to 35% or less of the total calories and suggests that saturated fat be reduced to only one-third of this by substituting poultry, veal, and fish for red meats as a major protein source. At the same time, cholesterol is restricted to less than 300 mg daily. Carbohydrates may be consumed liberally (as much as 50–60% of total calories) as long as refined and simple sugars are avoided as snacks. In obese type II patients, however, who tend to have elevated triglycerides with low HDL cholesterol on high-carbohydrate diets, it seems prudent to replace some of the dietary carbohydrate with noncholesterologenic monounsaturated oils (olive oil, canola oil). This maneuver is also indicated in type I patients on intensive insulin regimens in whom near-normoglycemic control is less achievable with carbohydrate content of the diet exceeding 50%. Unrefined carbohydrates with a fiber content sufficient to provide 15–20 g of fiber daily are recommended for both type I and type II diabetic patients.

b. Dietary fiber–Plant components such as cellulose, gum, and pectin are indigestible by humans and are termed dietary "fiber." Insoluble fibers such as cellulose or hemicellulose, as found in bran, tend to increase intestinal transit and may have beneficial effects on colonic function. In contrast, soluble fibers such as gums and pectins, as found in beans, oatmeal, or apple skin, tend to retard nutrient absorption rates so that glucose absorption is slower and hyperglycemia is diminished. Although the ADA diet does not include insoluble fiber supplements such as added bran, it recommends food such as oatmeal, cereals, and beans with relatively high soluble fiber content as staple components of the diet in diabetics. High soluble fiber content in the diet may also have a favorable effect on blood cholesterol levels.

c. Artificial sweeteners–Aspartame (Nutra-Sweet) has proved to be a popular sweetener for diabetic patients. It consists of two amino acids (aspartic acid and phenylalanine) that combine to produce a nutritive sweetener 180 times as sweet as sucrose. A major limitation is that it cannot be used in baking or cooking because of its lability to heat.

The nonnutritive sweetener saccharin continues to be available in certain foods and beverages despite recent warnings by the FDA about its potential long-term carcinogenicity to the bladder. A restriction on the use of saccharin in children and pregnant women is recommended; however, in patients with diabetes or obesity, physicians should determine on an individual basis its comparative benefit versus risk.

Nutritive sweeteners such as sorbitol and fructose have recently increased in popularity. Except for acute diarrhea induced by ingestion of large amounts of sorbitol-containing foods, their relative risk has yet to be established. Fructose represents a "natural" sugar substance that is a highly effective sweetener which induces only slight increases in plasma glucose levels.

2. Oral hypoglycemic drugs–Only the sulfonylureas remain in use as oral hypoglycemic drugs in the USA. Some discussion of the biguanides is included here because these drugs are still used in other countries.

a. Sulfonylureas–(Table 26–6.) Slight modifications of the basic structure produce agents that have similar qualitative actions but differ widely in potency. The mechanism of action of the sulfonylureas when they are acutely administered is due to their insulinotropic effect on pancreatic B cells. Sulfonylureas apparently specifically bind to an ATP-sensitive potassium channel of the pancreatic B cell and close it, thereby depolarizing the cell membrane. This results in an influx of extracellular calcium through voltage-gated calcium channels, which causes insulin granules to move toward the cell surface, facilitating exocytosis. However, it remains unclear whether this well-documented *acute* action requires additional extrapancreatic effects such as enhanced peripheral glucose utilization, hepatic glucose output suppression, and increased binding of insulin receptors to better explain the hypoglycemic effect of sulfonylureas during chronic administration.

Sulfonylureas are presently not indicated in the juvenile type ketosis-prone insulin-dependent diabetic, since these drugs seem to depend on functioning pancreatic B cells. There is little, if any, potentiation of insulin effectiveness on long-term glycemic control when sulfonylureas are added in type I patients.

The sulfonylureas seem most appropriate for use in the nonobese insulinopenic mild maturity-onset diabetic in whom acute administration improves the early phase of insulin release that is refractory to acute glucose stimulation. In obese mild diabetics and others with peripheral insensitivity to levels of circulating insulin, primary emphasis should be on weight reduction. When hyperglycemia in obese diabetics has been more severe, with consequent impair-

Table 26–6. Sulfonylureas.

Drug	Tablet Size (mg)	Daily Dose	Duration of Action (hours)
Tolbutamide (Orinase)[1]	250,500	0.25–2 g in 2 or 3 divided doses	6–12
Tolazamide (Tolinase)[1]	100,250,500	0.1–1 g as single dose or in 2 divided doses	Up to 24
Acetohexamide (Dymelor)[1,2]	250,500	0.25–1.5 g as single dose or in 2 divided doses	8–24
Chlorpropamide (Diabinese)[1,2]	100,250	0.1–0.5 g as single dose	24–72
Glyburide (Diaβeta, Micronase)	1.25,2.5,5	1.25–20 mg as single dose or in 2 divided doses	Up to 24
Glipizide (Glucotrol)	5,10	2.5–30 mg as single dose or in 2 or 3 divided doses on an empty stomach	6–12

[1]Generic available.

[2]There has been a decline in use of these formulations. In the case of chlorpropamide, the decline is due to its numerous side effects (see text).

ment of pancreatic B cell function, sulfonylureas may improve glycemic control until concurrent measures such as diet, exercise, and weight reduction can sustain the improvement without the need for oral drugs. Sulfonylureas are generally contraindicated in patients with hepatic or renal impairment.

(1) Tolbutamide is supplied in tablets of 250 and 500 mg. It is rapidly oxidized in the liver to inactive metabolites, and its approximate duration of effect is relatively short (6–10 hours). Tolbutamide is probably best administered in divided doses (eg, 500 mg before each meal and at bedtime); however, some patients require only one or two tablets daily. Because of its short duration of action, which is independent of renal function, tolbutamide is probably the safest sulfonylurea to use in elderly patients, in whom hypoglycemia would be a particularly serious risk. Prolonged hypoglycemia has been reported rarely, mostly in patients receiving certain antibacterial sulfonamides (sulfisoxazole), or phenylbutazone for arthralgias. These drugs apparently compete with sulfonylureas for plasma protein binding sites and for oxidative enzyme systems in the liver, resulting in maintenance of high levels of unmetabolized, active sulfonylureas in the circulation.

(2) Chlorpropamide is supplied in tablets of 100 and 250 mg. This drug, with a half-life of 32 hours, is slowly metabolized, with approximately 20–30% excreted unchanged in the urine. Since the metabolites retain hypoglycemic activity, elimination of the biologic effect is almost completely dependent on renal excretion. Its use is therefore contraindicated in patients with renal insufficiency because of its increased duration of action and prolonged half-life. The average maintenance dose is 250 mg daily, given as a single dose in the morning. Chlorpropamide is a potent agent, and prolonged hypoglycemic reactions are more common than with tolbutamide, particularly

in elderly patients, in whom chlorpropamide therapy should be monitored with special care. Doses in excess of 500 mg daily increase the risk of cholestatic jaundice. A flush may occur when alcohol is ingested by patients taking chlorpropamide, appearing within 8 minutes of ingesting the alcohol and lasting for 10–12 minutes; it is believed to be dose-related and similar to a disulfiram reaction, though much milder.

Hyponatremia is a complication of chlorpropamide therapy in some patients, especially those taking diuretics. Chlorpropamide both stimulates vasopressin secretion and potentiates its action at the renal tubule, resulting in dilutional hyponatremia. The antidiuretic effect of chlorpropamide is relatively unique, since four other sulfonylureas (acetohexamide, tolazamide, and glyburide) facilitate water excretion in humans. Since other sulfonylureas have now become available with comparable potency but without the disadvantage of causing water retention or alcohol-induced flushing, there is less need to prescribe chlorpropamide in managing patients with type II.

(3) Tolazamide is supplied in tablets of 100, 250, and 500 mg. It is comparable to chlorpropamide in potency but has a shorter duration of action and does not cause water retention. Tolazamide is more slowly absorbed than the other sulfonylureas, with effects on blood glucose not appearing for several hours. Its duration of action may last up to 20 hours, with maximal hypoglycemic effect occurring between the fourth and 14th hours. Tolazamide is metabolized to several compounds that retain hypoglycemic effects. If more than 500 mg/d is required, the dose should be divided and given twice daily. Doses larger than 1000 mg daily do not improve the degree of glycemic control.

(4) Acetohexamide is supplied in tablets of 250 and 500 mg. Its duration of action is about 10–16 hours, being intermediate in action between tolbutamide and chlorpropamide. A dose of 0.25–1.5 g is given daily in one or two doses. Liver metabolism is rapid, but the metabolite produced remains active.

(5) Second-generation sulfonylureas (glyburide and glipizide): Glyburide and glipizide are 100-fold more potent than tolbutamide. These drugs should be used with caution in patients with cardiovascular disease or in elderly patients, in whom prolonged hypoglycemia would be especially dangerous.

Diabetic patients who have not responded to tolbutamide or even tolazamide may respond to the more potent first-generation sulfonylurea chlorpropamide or to either of the second-generation sulfonylureas. Unfortunately, substantial glycemic benefit has not always resulted when a maximum therapeutic dose of chlorpropamide has been replaced with that of a second-generation drug in type II patients whose glucose control has been unsatisfactory.

(a) Glyburide–Glyburide is available in 1.25, 2.5, and 5 mg tablets. The usual starting dose is 2.5 mg/d, and the average maintenance dose is 5–10 mg/d given as a single morning dose; maintenance doses higher than 20 mg/d are not recommended. Glyburide is metabolized in the liver into products with such low hypoglycemic activity that they are considered clinically unimportant. Although assays specific for the unmetabolized compound suggest a plasma half-life of only 1–2 hours, the biologic effects of glyburide are clearly persistent 24 hours after a single morning dose in diabetic patients. Glyburide is unique among sulfonylureas in that it not only binds to a pancreatic B cell membrane receptor but also becomes sequestered within the B cell. This may explain its prolonged biologic effect despite its relatively short circulating half-life. A recently marketed "Press Tab" formulation of "micronized" glyburide—easy to divide in half with slight pressure if necessary—is currently available in tablet sizes of 1.5 mg and 3 mg. However, there is some question about its bioequivalency as compared to nonmicronized formulations, so that the FDA recommends careful monitoring to retitrate dosage when switching from standard glyburide doses or from other sulfonylurea drugs.

Glyburide has few adverse effects other than its potential for causing hypoglycemia. Flushing has rarely been reported after ethanol ingestion. It does not cause water retention, as chlorpropamide does, but rather slightly enhances free water clearance. Glyburide is absolutely contraindicated in the presence of hepatic impairment and probably should not be used in patients with renal insufficiency, in elderly patients, or in those who would be put at serious risk from an episode of hypoglycemia.

(b) Glipizide–Glipizide is available in 5 and 10 mg tablets. For maximum effect in reducing postprandial hyperglycemia, this agent should be ingested 30 minutes before meals, since rapid absorption is delayed when the drug is taken with food. The recommended starting dose is 5 mg/d with up to 15 mg/d given as a single daily dose before breakfast. When higher daily doses are required, they should be divided and given before meals. The maximum recommended dose is 40 mg/d.

At least 90% of glipizide is metabolized in the liver to inactive products, and 10% is excreted unchanged in the urine. Glipizide therapy is therefore contraindicated in patients with hepatic or renal impairment, who would therefore be at high risk for hypoglycemia, but because of its lower potency and shorter duration of action it is preferable to glyburide in elderly patients.

b. Biguanides–These compounds were introduced in the 1950s for the management of non-insulin-dependent diabetes mellitus. Phenformin was available in the USA until 1977, when it was discontinued because of its association with lactic acidosis. While it is still prescribed in some other countries to a limited extent, it has generally been replaced by other biguanides such as buformin and particularly metformin. Only metformin is discussed here.

Metformin (1,1-dimethylbiguanide hydrochloride) was introduced in France in 1957 as an oral agent for therapy of type II diabetes, either alone or in conjunction with sulfonylureas. It is awaiting FDA approval in the USA pending the outcome of multicenter clinical trials. It is marketed in many parts of the world under the brand name Glucophage and is also known as Diabefagos and Haurymellin.

(1) Clinical pharmacology: The exact mechanism of action of metformin remains unclear. It reduces both the fasting level of blood glucose and the degree of postprandial hyperglycemia in patients with type II diabetes but has no effect on fasting blood glucose in normal subjects. Metformin does not stimulate insulin action, yet is particularly effective in reducing hepatic gluconeogenesis. Other proposed mechanisms include a slowing down of gastrointestinal absorption of glucose and increased glucose uptake by skeletal muscle, which have been reported in some but not all clinical studies.

Metformin has a half-life of $1\frac{1}{2}$–3 hours, is not bound to plasma proteins, and is not metabolized in humans, being excreted unchanged by the kidneys.

(2) Indications and dosage: Metformin may be used as an adjunct to diet for the control of hyperglycemia and its associated symptomatology in patients with type II diabetes, particularly those who are obese or are not responding optimally to maximal doses of sulfonylureas. A side benefit of metformin therapy is its tendency to improve hyperglycemia and hypertriglyceridemia in obese diabetics without the weight gain associated with insulin or sulfonylurea therapy. Metformin is not indicated for patients with type I diabetes and is contraindicated in diabetics with renal or hepatic insufficiency, alcoholism, or a propensity to develop hypoxia (eg, disease associated with cardiorespiratory insufficiency).

Metformin is dispensed as 500 mg or 850 mg tablets, and the dosage range is from 500 mg to a maximum of 2.5 g daily, with the lowest possible effective dose being recommended. It is important that metformin be taken in divided doses—and with meals—to reduce minor gastrointestinal upsets. A common schedule would be one 500 mg tablet four times a day with meals or one 850 mg tablet twice daily at breakfast and dinner.

(3) Adverse reactions: The most frequent side effects of metformin are gastrointestinal symptoms (anorexia, nausea, vomiting, abdominal discomfort, diarrhea), which occur in up to 20% of patients. These effects are dose-related, tend to occur at onset of therapy, and often are transient. However, in 3–5% of patients, therapy may have to be discontinued because of persistent diarrheal discomfort.

Hypoglycemia does not occur with therapeutic doses of metformin, which permits its description as a "euglycemic" or "antihyperglycemic" drug rather than an oral hypoglycemic agent. Dermatologic or hematologic toxicity is rare.

Lactic acidosis (see below) has been reported as a side effect but is uncommon with metformin in contrast to phenformin, and almost all reported cases have involved subjects with associated risk factors that should have contraindicated its use (renal, hepatic, or cardiorespiratory insufficiency, alcoholism, advanced age).

c. Safety of the oral hypoglycemic agents– The University Group Diabetes Program (UGDP) reported that the number of deaths due to cardiovascular disease in diabetic patients treated with tolbutamide or the no longer used phenformin was excessive compared to either insulin-treated patients or those receiving placebos. Controversy persists about the validity of the conclusions reached by the UGDP because of concerns about the heterogeneity of the population studied, with its preponderance of obese subjects, and because of certain features of the experimental design such as the use of a fixed dose of oral drug. At present, a warning label is inserted in each package of sulfonylureas, but there is no restriction to recommending their use by the American Diabetes Association.

Idiosyncratic reactions to sulfonylureas are rare, with skin rashes or hematologic toxicity (transient leukopenia, thrombocytopenia) occurring in less than 0.1% of patients.

3. Insulin–Insulin is indicated for type I (IDDM) diabetics as well as for nonobese type II diabetics with insulinopenia whose hyperglycemia does not respond to diet therapy either alone or combined with oral hypoglycemic drugs.

With the development of highly purified human insulin preparations, immunogenicity has been markedly reduced, thereby decreasing the incidence of therapeutic complications such as insulin allergy, immune insulin resistance, and localized lipoatrophy at the injection site. However, the problem of achieving optimal insulin delivery remains unsolved with the present state of technology. It has not been possible to reproduce the physiologic patterns of intraportal insulin secretion with subcutaneous injections of soluble or longer-acting insulin suspensions. Even so, with the help of appropriate modifications of diet and exercise and careful monitoring of capillary blood glucose levels at home, it has often been possible to achieve acceptable control of blood glucose by using various mixtures of short- and longer-acting insulins injected at least twice daily or portable insulin infusion pumps.

a. Characteristics of available insulin preparations–Commercial insulin preparations differ with respect to the animal species from which they are obtained, their purity and solubility, and the time of onset and duration of their biologic action. More than 40 different formulations of insulin are available in the USA.

(1) Species of insulin: Human insulin is now produced by recombinant DNA techniques (biosynthetic human insulin). It has been introduced for clinical use as Humulin (Eli Lilly) and as Novolin (Novo Nordisk) and dispensed as either Regular (R), NPH (N), Lente (L), or Ultralente (U) formulations (see Table 26–7). In addition to human insulin, insulin from pork and beef sources continues to be widely used throughout the world.

Because the supply of pork insulin has been too limited to satisfy the insulin requirements of all diabetic patients, most commercial insulins contain the slightly more antigenic beef insulin, which differs by three amino acids from human insulin (in contrast to the single amino acid distinguishing pork and human insulins). Standard preparations of Iletin I (Eli Lilly) are mixtures containing 70% beef and 30% pork insulin. However, a limited supply of monospecies pork or beef insulin (Iletin II) has been available for use in certain patients with insulin allergy or immune insulin resistance. The production of highly purified insulins by Danish manufacturers has resulted in a substantial increase in the availability of porcine insulin. The cost of human insulin is approximately 1¼ times the cost of standard beef or pork insulin but slightly less than the cost of purified pork or beef insulin.

(2) Purity of insulin: Recent improvements in purification techniques for insulins extracted from animal pancreas have reduced or eliminated contaminating insulin precursors which were capable of inducing anti-insulin antibodies. The degree of purification in which proinsulin contamination is greater than 10 but less than 25 ppm characterizes the main form of insulin produced commercially in the USA by Eli Lilly as Iletin I. When proinsulin content is reduced to less than 10 ppm, manufacturers are entitled by FDA regulations to label the insulin as "purified." Such highly purified insulins are presently marketed in the USA by Eli Lilly and Novo Nordisk.

Table 26–7. Insulin preparations available in the USA.[1]

Preparation	Special Source	Concentration
SHORT-ACTING INSULINS		
Standard[2]		
Regular (Novo Nordisk)	Pork	U100
Regular Iletin I (Lilly)	Beef and pork	U100
Semilente (Novo Nordisk)	Beef	U100
Semilente Iletin I (Lilly)	Beef and pork	U100
"Purified"[3]		
Regular (Novo Nordisk)[4]	Pork or human	U100
Regular Humulin (Lilly)	Human	U100
Regular Iletin II (Lilly)	Pork or beef	U100, U500[5]
Semilente (Novo Nordisk)	Pork	U100
Velosulin (Novo Nordisk)	Pork or human	U100
Humulin BR (Lilly)[6]	Human	U100
INTERMEDIATE-ACTING INSULINS		
Standard[2]		
Isophane NPH (Novo Nordisk)	Beef	U100
Lente (Novo Nordisk)	Beef	U100
Lente Iletin I (Lilly)	Beef and pork	U100
NPH Iletin I (Lilly)	Beef and pork	U100
"Purified"[3]		
Insulatard NPH (Novo Nordisk)[4]	Pork or human	U100
Lente Humulin (Lilly)	Human	U100
Lente Iletin II (Lilly)	Pork or beef	U100
Lente (Novo Nordisk)[4]	Pork or human	U100
NPH Humulin (Lilly)	Human	U100
NPH Iletin II (Lilly)	Pork or beef	U100
NPH (Novo Nordisk)	Pork or human	U100
PREMIXED INSULINS **(70% NPH, 30% REGULAR)**		
Mixtard (Novo Nordisk)	Pork	U100
Novolin 70/30 (Novo Nordisk)	Human	U100
Humulin 70/30 (Lilly)	Human	U100
LONG-ACTING INSULINS		
Standard[2]		
Ultralente (Novo Nordisk)	Beef	U100
Ultralente Iletin I (Lilly)	Beef and pork	U100
"Purified"[3]		
Ultralente (Novo Nordisk)	Beef	U100
Ultralente Humulin (Lilly)	Human	U100

[1]These agents are all available without prescription. Wholesale prices for all preparations are similar.
[2]Greater than 10 but less than 25 ppm proinsulin.
[3]Less than 10 ppm proinsulin.
[4]Novo Nordisk human insulins are termed Novolin R, L, and N.
[5]U500 available only as pork insulin.
[6]Humulin BR (Buffered Regular) is recommended for use only in pumps. Its phosphate buffer precludes its being mixed with lente insulin.

The Eli Lilly product is called Iletin II to identify this highly purified insulin, and it presently is available only as a monospecies pork or beef insulin. All human insulins are also highly purified.

Purified insulins seem to preserve their potency quite well, so that refrigeration is recommended but not crucial. During travel, reserve supplies of insulin can thus be readily transported for weeks without losing potency if protected from extremes of heat or cold.

(3) Concentration of insulin: At present, most insulins are available in a concentration of 100 units/mL (U100), and all are dispensed in 10 mL vials. With the popularity of "low-dose" (0.5 or 0.3 mL) disposable insulin syringes, U100 can be measured with acceptable accuracy in doses as low as 1–2 units, and the manufacture of all U40 concentrations has therefore been discontinued in the United States. For use in rare cases of severe insulin resistance in which large quantities of insulin are required, a limited supply of U500 regular porcine insulin (Iletin II) is available from Eli Lilly.

b. Insulin preparations–(Table 26–7.) Three principal types of insulins are available: (1) short-acting, with rapid onset of action; (2) intermediate-acting; and (3) long-acting, with slow onset of action (Figure 26–1). Short-acting insulin (unmodified insulin) is a crystalline zinc insulin provided in soluble form and thus is dispensed as a clear solution. It is the only type of insulin that can be administered intravenously. All other commercial insulins have been specially modified to retain more prolonged action and are dispensed as turbid suspensions at neutral pH with either protamine in phosphate buffer (NPH) or varying concentrations of zinc in acetate buffer (ultralente and semilente). These preparations are designed for subcutaneous use. The use of semilente preparations is currently decreasing, and almost no

indications for its use remain. A long-acting protamine zinc insulin formulation (PZI) is no longer available in the United States.

(1) Regular insulin is a short-acting soluble crystalline zinc insulin whose effect appears within 15 minutes after subcutaneous injection and lasts 5–7 hours when usual quantities are administered. Intravenous infusions of regular insulin are particularly useful in the treatment of diabetic ketoacidosis and during the perioperative management of insulin-requiring diabetics. Regular insulin is also preferred when the insulin requirement is changing rapidly, such as after surgery or during acute infections.

Two preparations of regular insulin are used for insulin infusion pumps since they contain a phosphate buffer that prevents aggregation in the tubing. These are Velosulin (Novo Nordisk) and a specially prepared Humulin BR (Eli Lilly) which is only recommended for pump use.

(2) Lente insulin is a mixture of 30% semilente (an amorphous precipitate of insulin with zinc ions) with 70% ultralente insulin (an insoluble crystal of zinc and insulin). Its onset of action is delayed for up to 2 hours (Figure 26–1), and because its duration of action often is less than 24 hours (with a range of 18–24 hours), most patients require at least two injections daily to maintain a sustained insulin effect. Lente insulin has its peak effect in most patients between 8 and 12 hours, but individual variations in peak response time must be considered when interpreting unusual or unexpected patterns of glycemic responses in individual patients. While lente insulin is the most widely used of the lente series, particularly in conjunction with regular insulin, there has recently been a resurgence of the use of ultralente in combination with multiple injections of regular insulin as a means of attempting optimal control in type I patients. Ultralente has a very slow onset of action

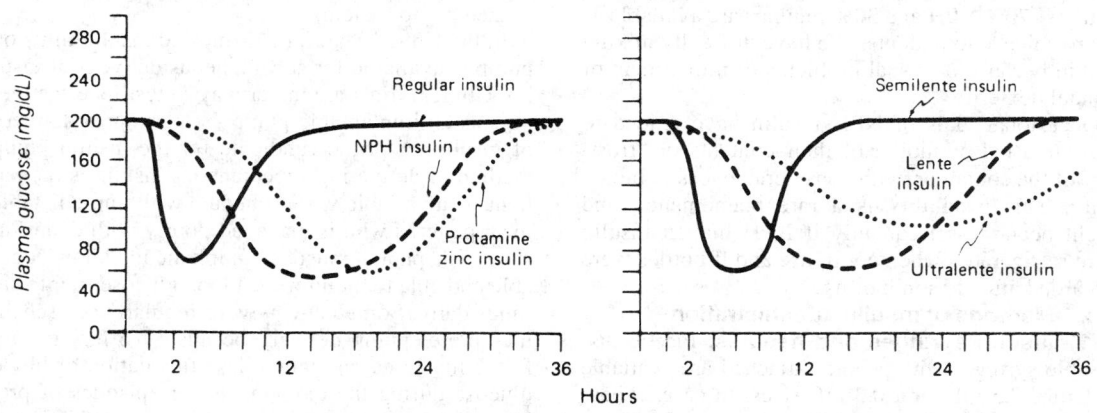

Figure 26–1. Extent and duration of action of various types of insulin (in a fasting diabetic). Duration of action is extended considerably when the dose of a given insulin formulation increases above the average therapeutic doses depicted here.

with a prolonged duration (Figure 26–1), and its administration once or twice daily has been advocated to provide a basal level of insulin comparable to that achieved by basal endogenous secretion or the overnight infusion rate programmed into insulin pumps.

(3) NPH (neutral protamine Hagedorn or isophane) insulin is an intermediate-acting insulin whose onset of action is delayed by combining two parts soluble crystalline zinc with 1 part protamine zinc insulin. This produces equivalent amounts of insulin and protamine, so that neither is present in an uncomplexed form ("isophane").

The onset and duration of action of NPH insulin are comparable to those of lente insulin (Figure 26–1); it is usually mixed with regular insulin and given at least twice daily for insulin replacement in type I patients.

(4) Mixtures of insulin: Since intermediate insulins require several hours to reach adequate therapeutic levels, their use in type I patients requires supplements of regular insulin preprandially. Recent reports caution that insulin mixtures containing increased proportions of lente to regular insulins may retard the rapid action of admixed regular insulin. The excess zinc in lente insulin may bind the soluble insulin and partially blunt its action, particularly when a relatively small proportion of regular insulin is mixed with lente (eg, 1 part regular to 1½ or more parts lente). NPH preparations that do not contain excess protamine do not delay absorption of admixed regular insulin. They are therefore preferable to lente when mixtures of intermediate and regular insulins are prescribed. For convenience, regular or NPH insulin may be mixed together in the same syringe and injected subcutaneously in split dosage before breakfast and supper. It is recommended that the regular insulin be withdrawn first, then the NPH insulin. No attempt should be made to mix the insulins in the syringe, and the injection is preferably given immediately after loading the syringe. Stable premixed insulins (70% NPH and 30% regular) are available as a convenience to patients who have difficulty mixing insulin because of visual problems or impairment of manual dexterity.

Occasional vials of NPH insulin have tended to show unusual clumping of their contents or "frosting" of the container, with considerable loss of bioactivity. This instability is a rare phenomenon and might occur less frequently if NPH human insulin were refrigerated when not in use and if bottles were discarded after 1 month of use.

c. Methods of insulin administration–

(1) Insulin syringes and needles: Plastic disposable syringes with needles attached are available in 1 mL, 0.5 mL, and 0.3 mL sizes. In cases where very low insulin doses are prescribed, as in young children, the specially calibrated 0.5 mL and 0.3 mL disposable syringes facilitate accurate measurement of U100 insulin in doses up to 50 or 30 units, respec-

tively. The "low-dose" syringes have become increasingly popular, because diabetics generally should not take more than 30–50 units of insulin in a single injection, except in rare instances of extreme insulin resistance. Several recent reports have indicated that "disposable" syringes may be reused until blunting of the needle occurs (usually after three to five injections). Sterility adequate to avoid infection with reuse appears to be maintained by refrigerating syringes between uses. One concern, however, arises from a recent report that flecks of silicone may become suspended in insulin bottles in which disposable syringes have repeatedly been reused; the silicone flecks seem to reduce the activity of the insulin.

(2) Site of injection: Any part of the body covered by loose skin can be used, such as the abdomen, thighs, upper arms, flanks, and upper buttocks. Rotation of sites continues to be recommended to avoid delayed absorption when fibrosis or lipohypertrophy occurs from repeated use of a single site. However, considerable variability of absorption rates from different sites, particularly with exercise, may contribute to the instability of glycemic control in certain type I patients if injection sites are rotated too frequently in different areas of the body. Consequently, it is best to limit injection sites to a single region of the body and rotate sites within that region. The abdomen is recommended for subcutaneous injections, since regular insulin has been shown to absorb more rapidly from that site than from other subcutaneous sites.

(3) Insulin delivery systems: Efforts to administer soluble insulin by "closed-loop" systems (glucose-controlled insulin infusion system) have been successful for acute situations such as diabetic ketoacidosis or for administering insulin to diabetics during surgery. However, chronic use is prevented by the need for continually aspirating blood to reach an external glucose sensor and the large size of the computerized pump system.

In the United States, the MiniMed insulin infusion pump is available for subcutaneous delivery of insulin. Clinical trials are under way to test its effectiveness as an implantable pump for peritoneal delivery of insulin. A prime candidate for the insulin pump method of delivering subcutaneous insulin is the patient on a variable work schedule with unpredictable meal patterns who is managed poorly with depot insulin. The patient must be compliant and knowledgeable and able to monitor the blood glucose four to six times daily. Some patients with regular work schedules prefer pump delivery because it offers greater flexibility in eating habits, less fluctuation of blood glucose during the day, and fewer episodes of prebreakfast hyperglycemia. The high cost of infusion pumps and the time demanded of physicians and staff in initiating therapy has limited their use in type I diabetes despite the potential advantages. Conventional methods of insulin administration with multiple subcutaneous injections of soluble, rapid-acting insulin and a single injection of either long-acting insulin or intermediate-acting insulin at bedtime are therefore widely used for intensive insulin therapy. These regimens usually provide acceptable glycemic control if frequent self-monitoring of blood glucose is practiced.

To facilitate these multiple injection regimens, portable pen-sized injectors have been introduced which contain cartridges of U100 regular human insulin and retractable needles (NovoPen, NovolinPen, Insuject). These injectors eliminate the need for patients to carry an insulin bottle and syringes during the day while adhering to a regimen of multiple injections of regular insulin supplementing a single injection of long-acting insulin.

C. General Considerations in Treatment of Diabetes: Patients with diabetes can have a full and satisfying life. However, "free" diets and unrestricted activity are still not advised for insulin-requiring diabetics. Until new methods of insulin replacement are developed that provide more normal patterns of insulin delivery in response to metabolic demands, multiple feedings will continue to be recommended, and certain occupations potentially hazardous to the patient or others will continue to be prohibited because of risks due to hypoglycemia.

Exercise increases the effectiveness of insulin, and moderate exercise is an excellent means of improving utilization of fat and carbohydrate in diabetic patients. A judicious balance of the size and frequency of meals with moderate regular exercise can often stabilize the insulin dosage in diabetics who tend to slip out of control easily. Strenuous exercise could precipitate hypoglycemia in an unprepared patient, and diabetics must therefore be taught to reduce their insulin dosage in anticipation of strenuous activity or to take supplemental carbohydrate. Injection of insulin into a site farthest away from the muscles most involved in exercise may help ameliorate exercise-induced hypoglycemia, since insulin injected in the proximity of exercising muscle may be more rapidly mobilized.

All diabetic patients must receive adequate instruction on personal hygiene, especially with regard to care of the feet (see below), skin, and teeth. All infections—but especially pyogenic infections with fever and toxemia—provoke the release of high levels of insulin antagonists such as catecholamines or glucagon and thus bring about a marked increase in insulin requirements. Supplemental regular insulin is often required to correct hyperglycemia during infection.

Psychologic factors are of great importance in the control of diabetes, particularly when the disease is difficult to stabilize. One reason the diabetic may be particularly sensitive to emotional upset is that pancreatic A cells of diabetics are hyperresponsive to physiologic levels of epinephrine, producing excessive levels of glucagon with consequent hyperglycemia.

Counseling should be directed at avoiding extremes of compulsive rigidity or self-destructive neglect and is especially important for adolescents.

D. The Diabetes Control and Complications Trial (DCCT): In June 1993, a long-term randomized prospective study involving 1441 type I patients in 29 medical centers reported that "near" normalization of blood glucose resulted in a delay in the onset and a major slowing of the progression of established microvascular and neuropathic complications of diabetes during an up to 10-year follow-up.

Multiple insulin injections (66%) or insulin pumps (34%) were used in the intensively treated group who were trained to modify their therapy depending on frequent glucose monitoring. The conventionally treated groups used no more than two insulin injections, and clinical well-being was the goal with no attempt to modify management based on HbA_{1c} or their glucose results.

In one-half of the subjects, a mean hemoglobin A_{1c} of 7.2% (normal: < 6%) and a blood glucose of 155 mg/dL was achieved using intensive therapy, while in the conventionally treated group, HbA_{1c} averaged 8.9% with an average blood glucose of 225 mg/dL. Over the study period, which averaged 7 years, there was an approximately 60% reduction in risk between the two groups in regard to diabetic retinopathy, nephropathy, and neuropathy.

Intensively treated patients had a threefold greater risk of serious hypoglycemia as well as a greater tendency toward weight gain. However, there were no deaths from hypoglycemia in any subjects in the DCCT study, and no evidence of posthypoglycemic neurologic damage was detected.

The general consensus of the American Diabetes Association is that intensive insulin therapy associated with comprehensive self-management training should become standard therapy in type I patients after the age of puberty. Exceptions include those with advanced renal disease and the elderly, since, in these groups, the detrimental risks of hypoglycemia outweigh the benefits of tight glycemic control—particularly since diabetic complications do not seem to occur until some years after the onset of puberty.

While patients with type II were not studied in the DCCT, there is no reason to believe that the effects of better control of blood glucose levels would not also apply to type II. The eye, kidney, and nerve abnormalities are quite similar in both types of diabetes, and it is likely that similar underlying mechanisms apply. However, because weight gain may be greater in obese type II patients receiving intensive insulin therapy and because of an increased prevalence of macrovascular disease in older patients with type II—in whom hypoglycemia may be more hazardous—the American Diabetes Association feels that

INSTRUCTIONS IN THE CARE OF THE FEET
FOR PERSONS WITH DIABETES MELLITUS OR VASCULAR DISTURBANCES

Hygiene of the Feet

(1) Wash feet daily with mild soap and luke-warm water. Dry thoroughly between the toes by pressure. Do not rub vigorously, as this is apt to break the delicate skin.

(2) When feet are thoroughly dry, rub well with vegetable oil to keep them soft, prevent excess friction, remove scales, and prevent dryness. Care must be taken to prevent foot tenderness.

(3) If the feet become too soft and tender, rub them with alcohol about once a week.

(4) When rubbing the feet, always rub upward from the tips of the toes. If varicose veins are present, massage the feet very gently; never massage the legs.

(5) If the toenails are brittle and dry, soften them by soaking for one-half hour each night in lukewarm water containing 1 tbsp of powdered sodium borate (borax) per quart. Follow this by rubbing around the nails with vegetable oil. Clean around the nails with an orangewood stick. If the nails become too long, file them with an emery board. File them straight across and no shorter than the underlying soft tissues of the toe. Never cut the corners of the nails. (The podiatrist should be informed if a patient has diabetes.)

(6) Wear low-heeled shoes of soft leather that fit the shape of the feet correctly. The shoes should have wide toes that will cause no pressure, fit close in the arch, and grip the heels snugly. Wear new shoes one-half hour only on the first day and increase by 1 hour each day following. Wear thick, warm, loose stockings.

Treatment of Corns & Calluses

(1) Corns and calluses are due to friction and pressure, most often from improperly fitted shoes and stockings. Wear shoes that fit properly and cause no friction or pressure.

(2) To remove excess calluses or corns, soak the feet in lukewarm (not hot) water, using a mild soap, for about 10 minutes and then rub off the excess tissue with a towel or file. Do not tear it off. Under no circumstances must the skin become irritated.

(3) Do not cut corns or calluses. If they need attention it is safer to see a podiatrist.

(4) Prevent callus formation under the ball of the foot (a) by exercise, such as curling and stretching the toes several times a day; (b) by finishing each step on the toes and not on the ball of the foot; and (c) by wearing shoes that are not too short and that do not have high heels.

Aids in Treatment
of Impaired Circulation
(Cold Feet)

(1) Never use tobacco in any form. Tobacco contracts blood vessels and so reduces circulation.

(2) Keep warm. Wear warm stockings and other clothing. Cold contracts blood vessels and reduces circulation.

(3) Do not wear circular garters, which compress blood vessels and reduce blood flow.

(4) Do not sit with the legs crossed. This may compress the leg arteries and shut off the blood supply to the feet.

(5) If the weight of the bedclothes is uncomfortable, place a pillow under the covers at the foot of the bed.

(6) Do not apply any medication to the feet without directions from a physician. Some medicines are too strong for feet with poor circulation.

(7) Do not apply heat in the form of hot water, hot water bottles, or heating pads without a physician's consent. Even moderate heat can injure the skin if circulation is poor.

(8) If the feet are moist or the patient has a tendency to develop athlete's foot, a prophylactic dusting powder should be used on the feet and in shoes and stockings daily. Change shoes and stockings at least daily or oftener.

Treatment of Abrasions
of the Skin

(1) Proper first-aid treatment is of the utmost importance even in apparently minor injuries. Consult a physician immediately for any redness, blistering, pain, or swelling. Any break in the skin may become ulcerous or gangrenous unless properly treated by a physician.

(2) Dermatophytosis (athlete's foot), which begins with peeling and itching between the toes or discoloration or thickening of the toenails, should be treated immediately by a physician or podiatrist.

(3) Avoid strong irritating antiseptics such as tincture of iodine.

(4) As soon as possible after any injury, cover the area with sterile gauze, which may be purchased at drugstores. Only fine paper tape or cellulose tape (Scotch Tape) should be used on the skin if adhesive retention of the gauze is required.

(5) Elevate and, as much as possible until recovery, avoid using the foot.

common sense and clinical judgment on an individual basis should determine whether tight glycemic control is appropriate in type II.

Steps in the Management of the Diabetic Patient

A. Diagnostic Examination: Any features of the clinical picture that suggest end-organ insensitivity to insulin, such as obesity, must be identified. The family history should document not only the incidence of diabetes in other members of the family but also the age at onset, whether it was associated with obesity, and whether insulin was required. Other factors that increase cardiac risk, such as smoking history, presence of hypertension or hyperlipidemia, or oral contraceptive pill use, should be recorded.

Laboratory diagnosis should document fasting plasma glucose levels above 140 mg/dL or postprandial values consistently above 200 mg/dL and whether ketonuria accompanies the glycosuria. A glycohemoglobin measurement is useful for assessing the effectiveness of future therapy. Some flexibility of clinical judgment is appropriate when diagnosing diabetes mellitus in the elderly patient with borderline hyperglycemia.

Baseline values include fasting plasma triglycerides, total cholesterol and HDL cholesterol, electrocardiography, renal function studies, peripheral pulses, and neurologic, podiatric, and ophthalmologic examinations to help guide future assessments.

B. Patient Education: Since diabetes is a lifelong disorder, education of the patient and the family is probably the most important obligation of the physician who provides initial care. The best persons to manage a disease that is affected so markedly by daily fluctuations in environmental stress, exercise, diet, and infections are the patients themselves and their families. The "teaching curriculum" should include explanations by the physician or nurse of the nature of diabetes and its potential acute and chronic hazards and how they can be recognized early and prevented or treated. The importance of regular tests for glucose on either capillary blood or double-voided urine specimens should be stressed and instructions on proper testing and recording of data provided. Moreover, patients should be provided with algorithms they can use to adjust the timing and quantity of their insulin dose, food, and exercise in response to recorded blood glucose values for optimal blood glucose control. The targets for blood glucose control should be elevated appropriately in elderly patients since they have the greatest risk if subjected to hypoglycemia and the least long-term benefit from more rigid glycemic control. Advice on personal hygiene, including detailed instructions on foot care, as well as individual instruction on diet and specific hypoglycemic therapy, should be provided. Patients should be told about community agencies, such as Diabetes Association chapters, that can serve as a continuing source of instruction. Finally, vigorous efforts should be made to persuade new diabetics who smoke to give up the habit, since large vessel peripheral vascular disease and debilitating retinopathy are less common in nonsmoking diabetic patients.

C. Self-Monitoring of Blood Glucose: Monitoring of blood glucose by patients has allowed greater flexibility in management while achieving improved glycemic control.

Self-monitoring of blood glucose is particularly useful in brittle diabetics, those attempting "ideal" glycemic control such as during pregnancy, patients who have little or no early warning of hypoglycemic attacks, and those with dysfunctional bladders from diabetic neuropathy or altered renal thresholds for glucose. Self-monitoring of blood glucose is recommended for all insulin-treated diabetic patients. The expert consensus on self-monitoring is that its proper use is to develop a data base as an aid in making day-to-day informal decisions about therapy as well as to determine when emergency situations arise. It is particularly valuable as an educational and training tool to enhance understanding of diabetes by patients and their families. The usefulness of self-monitoring depends on the accuracy of the results obtained. Patients must be taught proper techniques, cautioned to calibrate instruments each day despite the expense of strips, to keep proper records, and, particularly, how to respond to unacceptably high or low blood glucose levels with appropriate therapeutic maneuvers. Self-monitoring has proved to be an effective and safe clinical tool that can improve glycemic control in compliant patients.

D. Initial Therapy: Treatment must be individualized on the basis of the type of diabetes and specific needs of each patient. However, certain general principles of management can be outlined for hyperglycemic states of different types.

1. The obese type II patient–The most common type of diabetic patient is obese, is non-insulin-dependent, and has hyperglycemia because of insensitivity to normal or elevated circulating levels of insulin.

a. Weight reduction–Treatment is directed toward achieving weight reduction, and prescribing a diet is only one means to this end. Behavior modification to achieve adherence to the diet, as well as increased physical activity to expend energy, is also required. Cure can be achieved by reducing adipose stores, with consequent restoration of tissue sensitivity to insulin. The presence of diabetes with its added risk factors may motivate the obese diabetic to greater efforts to lose weight. (See also Chapter 28.)

b. Hypoglycemic agents–Neither insulin nor sulfonylureas are indicated for long-term use in the obese patient with mild diabetes. The weight reduction program can be upset by real or imagined hypoglycemic reactions when insulin therapy is used and weight gain is a frequent complication. It is also possible that administration of insulin to an obese patient who already has excessive circulating levels may have the ill effects of maintaining insulin insensitivity of receptor sites as well as interfering with catabolic mechanisms during caloric deprivation. The obese diabetic who has been previously treated with conventional beef-pork insulin—often in interrupted fashion—and who requires high doses both to offset excess caloric intake and to overcome tissue insensitivity may develop immune insulin resistance. This not only increases the requirements for exogenous insulin but also impairs the effectiveness of endogenous insulin and may even precipitate ketosis.

Oral sulfonylureas have a role in the management of obese patients with moderately severe diabetes causing nocturia, blurred vision, or candidal vulvovaginitis. Insulin injections may be required if a trial of sulfonylurea therapy does not ameliorate symptoms. In such cases, short-term therapy (weeks or months) with either sulfonylureas or insulin may be indicated to abate symptoms until simultaneous caloric restriction leading to weight reduction can occur.

Combining sulfonylureas with insulin replacement has not been effective in reducing insulin requirements or improving glycemic control in type I patients who have no residual pancreatic B cell function. On the other hand, type II patients do show modest glycemic improvement with a combined sulfonylurea-insulin regimen, but one that generally can be achieved with insulin therapy alone. At present, there is no overall consensus for using combined sulfonylurea therapy with insulin in type II. One regimen has been proposed that adds a bedtime intermediate-acting insulin to reduce excessive nocturnal hepatic glucose output in type II patients doing poorly on maximal doses of sulfonylureas, but until more data are available to validate this approach, most diabetologists recommend stopping the sulfonylureas in these circumstances and changing over to insulin therapy alone. It is only in the case of type II patients requiring excessive amounts of insulin—exceeding 100 units/d—that it is considered a reasonable option to add sulfonylureas to improve glycemic control rather than prescribing higher insulin doses.

2. The nonobese patient–In the nonobese diabetic, mild to severe hyperglycemia is usually due to refractoriness of B cells to glucose stimulation. Treatment depends on whether insulinopenia is mild (type II or mild type I in partial remission) or severe, with ketoacidosis (IDDM).

a. Diet therapy–If hyperglycemia is mild, normal metabolic control can occasionally be restored by means of multiple feedings of a diet limited in simple sugars and with a caloric content sufficient to maintain ideal weight. Restriction of saturated fats and cholesterol is also strongly advised.

b. Oral hypoglycemic agents–When diet therapy is not sufficient to correct hyperglycemia, a trial of sulfonylureas is often successful in reducing the

glycohemoglobin concentration below 9.5%. Once the dosage of one of the more potent sulfonylureas reaches the upper recommended limit in a compliant patient without maintaining blood glucose below 200 mg/dL during the day, insulin therapy is recommended by the American Diabetes Association.

c. Treatment of type I with insulin–(Table 26–8.) The patient requiring insulin therapy should be initially regulated under conditions of optimal diet and normal daily activities. In patients with type I, information and counseling should be provided about the advantages of taking multiple injections of insulin in conjunction with self blood glucose monitoring. If tight control is attempted, urine glucose measurements are not sufficient, and at least three measurements of capillary blood glucose are required daily to avoid frequent hypoglycemic reactions. A single injection of long-acting insulin is not recommended in patients with type I for the reasons given in Table 26–8, which describes the advantages and disadvantages of various insulin regimens in this type of diabetes.

(1) Conventional split-dose insulin mixtures: A typical initial dose schedule in a 70-kg patient taking 2200 kcal divided into six or seven feedings might be 10 units of regular and 15 units of NPH insulin in the morning and 5 units of regular and 5 units of NPH insulin in the evening. The morning capillary blood glucose gives a measure of the effectiveness of NPH insulin administered the previous evening; the noon blood glucose reflects the effects of the morning regular insulin; and the 5:00 PM and 9:00 PM sugars represent the effects of the morning NPH and evening regular insulins, respectively. A properly educated patient should be taught to adjust insulin dosage by observing the pattern of glycemia and correlating it with the approximate duration of action and the time of peak effect after injection of the various insulin preparations (Figure 26–1). Adjustments to correct patterns of hyperglycemia should include the following options, either alone or in combination: modification of diet and exercise programs and changes in the insulin dose or its preprandial timing.

(2) Intensive insulin therapy: In cases where conventional split doses of insulin mixtures cannot maintain near normalization of blood glucose without hypoglycemia, particularly at night, multiple injections of insulin may be required. An increasingly popular regimen consists of reducing or omitting the evening dose of intermediate insulin and adding a portion of it at bedtime. For example, 10 units of regular insulin mixed with 10 units of NPH insulin in the morning, 8–10 units of regular insulin before the evening meal, and 6 units of NPH insulin at bedtime is often more efficacious than the conventional split-dose regimen mentioned above.

In cases where hypoglycemia occurs unexpectedly and at inconsistent times day or night, variable or delayed insulin absorption from large subcutaneous de-

Table 26–8. Advantages and disadvantages of various insulin regimens in treatment of type I diabetes.

Single Injection of NPH or Lente	Conventional Split Dose of Mixture (Regular and NPH Twice Daily)	Three Injections (Mixture of Regular and NPH in AM; Regular at Dinner; NPH at Bedtime)	Four Injections (Regular Before Meals and NPH, Lente, or Ultralente at Bedtime) or Subcutaneous Infusion of Regular Insulin With Pump
Advantages			
Convenience only.	Relatively convenient. Controls postprandial glycemia at breakfast and dinner.	Controls postprandial glycemia at breakfast and dinner. Can prevent prebreakfast hyperglycemia with less risk of nocturnal hypoglycemia. Less variability of absorption of NPH, since lower doses are injected to last overnight.	Controls postprandial glycemia. Allows flexibility of meal schedules and quantity. Less variability of absorption of small doses of insulins given more frequently. Tight glycemic control is possible with least risk of hypoglycemia.
Disadvantages			
Poor glycemic control or nocturnal hypoglycemia. Requires frequent feedings to avoid hypoglycemia if acceptable control attempted. Inflexible feeding schedules. Variability of absorption of large doses predisposes to hypoglycemia, which is common. Because of these disadvantages, this regimen is not recommended.	Prebreakfast hyperglycemia is common. Increased risk of nocturnal hypoglycemia in attempt to control prebreakfast hyperglycemia. Variability of absorption due to relatively large NPH doses to last overnight.	Less convenient. Lunch schedule is relatively inflexible as to time and quantity to avoid hypoglycemia from morning NPH. Dinner schedule cannot be delayed without extra feedings.	Relatively inconvenient. Pumps are expensive and are generally less convenient than multiple injections and add risk of skin infections and pump failures.

pots containing regular and NPH insulin may be a contributing factor. Reducing the size and changing the character of the depots by administering small doses of regular insulin more frequently (eg, four times a day), with one injection of a long-acting insulin (eg, ultralente insulin) at bedtime has often been most helpful in reducing the frequency and severity of hypoglycemia in patients attempting near normalization of blood glucose. This regimen has become more convenient with the advent of pen-injectors and gives greater flexibility regarding meal patterns and diet than conventional therapy with split-dose insulin mixtures. Certain patients do not accept multiple injections of regular insulin but often prefer continuous subcutaneous infusions with portable open-loop insulin pumps, which require subcutaneous needle insertion only every 48 hours.

(3) Management of early morning hyperglycemia in type I: (Table 26–9.) One of the more difficult therapeutic problems in managing patients with type I is determining the proper adjustment of insulin dose when the prebreakfast blood glucose level is high.

(a) Somogyi effect: Patients with type I may develop nocturnal hypoglycemia, which may in turn stimulate a surge of counterregulatory hormones (Somogyi effect) to produce high blood glucose levels by 7:00 AM.

Clinicians have often observed that by reducing inappropriately high doses of administered insulin, hyperglycemia on the following morning may improve substantially. This "Somogyi effect" remains a factor to be considered as contributing to early morning hyperglycemia in patients treated with relatively high doses of insulin. Prescribing a lower dose of intermediate-acting insulin before dinner or at bedtime is a reasonable therapeutic option, particularly when nocturnal hypoglycemia is suspected.

(b) Dawn phenomenon: The dawn phenomenon is present in as many as 75% of type I patients and occurs in most type II and normal subjects as well. It is characterized by reduced tissue sensitivity to insulin developing between 5:00 AM and 8:00 AM. Recent evidence suggests that this phenomenon is evoked by spikes of growth hormone released hours before, at the onset of sleep. When the dawn phenomenon occurs alone, it may produce only mild hyperglycemia in the early morning, but when it is associated with the Somogyi effect or the waning phenomenon (or both), the hyperglycemia may be more severe.

(c) Waning of circulating insulin levels: The most common cause of prebreakfast hyperglycemia is probably the waning of circulating insulin levels.

Table 26–9. Prebreakfast hyperglycemia: Classification by blood glucose and insulin levels.

	Blood Glucose (mg/dL)			Free Immunoreactive Insulin (μU/mL)		
	10:00 PM	3:00 AM	7:00 AM	10:00 PM	3:00 AM	7:00 AM
Somogyi effect	90	40	200	High	Slightly high	Normal
Dawn phenomenon	110	110	150	Normal	Normal	Normal
Waning of insulin dose plus dawn phenomenon	110	190	220	Normal	Low	Low
Waning of insulin dose plus dawn phenomenon plus Somogyi effect	110	40	380	High	Normal	Low

This would suggest that *more* rather than less intermediate-acting insulin should be given in the evening.

The Somogyi effect, the dawn phenomenon, and the waning of insulin levels are not mutually exclusive; if they occur together, more severe hyperglycemia develops.

Table 26–9 shows that diagnosis of the cause of prebreakfast hyperglycemia can be facilitated by self-monitoring of blood glucose at 3:00 AM in addition to the usual bedtime and 7:00 AM measurements. This is required for only a few nights until the diagnosis is established and appropriate adjustment of bedtime insulin dose or nighttime feeding is achieved.

(d) Therapy of prebreakfast hyperglycemia: When a particular pattern emerges from monitoring blood glucose levels overnight, appropriate therapeutic measures can be taken. The Somogyi effect can be treated by reducing the dose of intermediate insulin at dinnertime, giving a portion of it at bedtime, or supplying more food at bedtime. When the dawn phenomenon alone is present, the dosage of intermediate insulin can be divided between dinnertime and bedtime, or when insulin pumps are used, the basal infusion rate can be increased (eg, from 0.8 unit/h to 1 unit/h from 6:00 AM until breakfast). With waning insulin levels, either increasing the evening dose or shifting it from dinnertime to bedtime, or both, can be effective.

d. Treatment of type II with insulin–When sulfonylureas fail and type II patients require insulin to control their hyperglycemia, various insulin regimens may be effective. Although a single morning injection of insulin is not recommended in type I diabetes (see Table 26–8), in some patients with type II diabetes enough residual insulin secretion persists to allow a single morning injection of 25–30 units of NPH or lente insulin to replace their deficient insulin secretion. If prebreakfast hyperglycemia persists on this regimen, a number of alternatives are available. A convenient regimen includes split doses of a fixed 70:30 mixture of NPH:regular insulin, which can be started as 20 units before breakfast and 15 units before dinner and increased appropriately depending on target blood glucoses at 7:00 AM and 5:00 PM. When more than 50 units a day are required without achieving proper control, these patients may benefit from three or four injection regimens as described for type I in Table 26–8.

e. Acceptable levels of glycemic control: See above for a discussion of the Diabetes Control and Complications Trial and its implications for type II therapy. Limited data are available concerning the level of glucose control needed to avoid diabetic complications. Postprandial blood glucose levels below 200 mg/dL have been advocated by retrospective analysis of two populations of type II patients. A reasonable aim of therapy is to approach normal glycemic excursions without provoking severe or frequent hypoglycemia. What has been considered "acceptable" control includes blood glucose levels of 80–130 mg/dL before meals and after an overnight fast and levels no higher than 180 mg/dL 1 hour after meals and 150 mg/dL 2 hours after meals. Glycohemoglobin levels should be no higher than 1% or 2% above the upper limit of the normal range for any particular laboratory. In elderly patients, criteria for optimal control should be adjusted upward, with glycohemoglobins 2–3% above the upper limits of normal and preprandial blood glucose levels below 200 mg/dL being acceptable.

Indications for Purified Insulins

Human insulin or purified pork insulins are indicated when insulin of conventional purity and containing beef species has been associated with allergy, immune resistance, or lipoatrophy. Also, they are preferable in any patient undergoing insulin therapy for the first time, since they reduce or eliminate the risk of occurrence of these rare immune complications. Moreover, absent or very low levels of anti-insulin antibodies enhance recovery from insulin-induced hypoglycemia and facilitate the measurement of therapeutic levels of circulating insulin as a guide for optimal management. In patients with type II whose therapy with insulin is to be for a limited time (eg, in gestational diabetes or during acute infections or surgery), human insulin or purified insulin reduces the risks of immunologic sensitization to future exposures to insulin.

Complications of Insulin Therapy

A. Hypoglycemia: Hypoglycemic reactions, the most common complication of insulin therapy, may result from delay in taking a meal or unusual physical exertion. With more type I patients attempting "tight" control, this complication has become even more frequent. In older diabetics, in those taking only longer-acting insulins, and often in those attempting to maintain euglycemia on infusion pumps, autonomic counterregulatory responses are less readily elicited, and the manifestations are mainly from impaired function of the central nervous system, ie, mental confusion, bizarre behavior, and ultimately coma. Even focal neurologic deficits mimicking stroke may be observed. More rapid development of hypoglycemia from the effects of regular insulin causes signs of autonomic hyperactivity, both sympathetic (tachycardia, palpitations, sweating, tremulousness) and parasympathetic (nausea, hunger), that may progress to coma and convulsions. Except for sweating, most of the sympathetic symptoms of hypoglycemia are blunted in patients receiving beta-blocking agents for angina or hypertension. Though not absolutely contraindicated, these drugs must be used with great caution in insulin-requiring diabetics, and, whenever possible, beta-selective blocking agents should be used.

1. Altered awareness of hypoglycemia– Since autonomic responses correlate strongly with "awareness" of hypoglycemia, many poorly controlled diabetics—whose nervous systems have adapted to chronic hyperglycemia—may trigger adrenergic alarms at levels of blood glucose above the usual hypoglycemic range. Conversely, type I patients overtreated with insulin may be unaware of critically low levels of blood glucose because of an adaptive blunting of their alarm systems owing to repeated episodes of hypoglycemia. This is potentially reversible if higher average blood glucose levels are maintained in these patients to avoid recurrent hypoglycemia.

Controversy exists over whether there is a link between switching from animal insulin to human insulin and development of reduced awareness for hypoglycemia. However, in the absence of large-scale prospective studies, the consensus of most diabetologists is that the data questioning the safety of human insulin are insufficient to justify a restriction of its use at this time. They feel that loss of awareness can be induced by repeated episodes of hypoglycemia. The latter may occur in as many as half of patients switched from animal to human insulin if the switch is made at equivalent or nearly equivalent dosages, without taking the precaution of beginning with a 20–25% lower human insulin dose to compensate for the reduced neutralization of the injected insulin by preexisting anti-beef or anti-pork insulin antibodies. Another cause of frequent hypoglycemia could be the inclination of patients and their physicians to attempt tighter glycemic control at the time of switching from animal to human insulin as part of a general upgrading of their diabetes care. As evi-

denced by preliminary results of the Diabetes Control and Complications Trial, the risk of frequent hypoglycemic episodes is greatly increased when "normalization" of the blood glucose is attempted with presently available methods of insulin delivery, and this is independent of the species of insulin used.

2. Lack of glucagon response in type I–For unexplained reasons, patients with type I lose their glucagon responses to hypoglycemia (but not to amino acids in protein-containing meals) within a year or so after developing diabetes. These patients then rely predominantly on the sympathetic nervous system to counterregulate hypoglycemia and are at special risk in later years when aging or autonomic neuropathy blunts their sympathetic responses.

3. Prevention and treatment of hypoglycemia–Because of the potential danger of insulin reactions, the diabetic patient should carry packets of table sugar or a candy roll at all times for use at the onset of hypoglycemic symptoms. *Tablets containing 3 g of glucose are available* (dextrosol). The educated patient soon learns to take the amount of glucose needed and avoids the excess that may occur with eating candy or drinking orange juice, causing very high hyperglycemia. An ampule of glucagon (1 mg) should be provided to every diabetic receiving insulin therapy, and family or friends should be instructed how to inject it intramuscularly in the event that the patient is unconscious or refuses food. *An identification Medic Alert bracelet, necklace, or card in the wallet or purse should be carried by every diabetic receiving hypoglycemic drug therapy.* The telephone number for the Medic Alert Foundation International in Turlock, California, is 1-800-ID-ALERT.

All of the manifestations of hypoglycemia are rapidly relieved by glucose administration. If more severe hypoglycemia has produced unconsciousness or stupor, the treatment is 50 mL of 50% glucose solution by rapid intravenous infusion. If intravenous therapy is not available, 1 mg of glucagon injected intramuscularly will usually restore the patient to consciousness within 15 minutes to permit ingestion of sugar. If the patient is stuporous and glucagon is not available, small amounts of honey or syrup can be inserted within the buccal pouch, but, in general, oral feeding is contraindicated in unconscious patients. Rectal administration of syrup or honey (30 mL per 500 mL of warm water) has been effective.

B. Immunopathology of Insulin Therapy: At least five molecular classes of insulin antibodies are produced during the course of insulin therapy in diabetes, including IgA, IgD, IgE, IgG, and IgM. With the increased therapeutic use of purified pork and human insulin in Western countries, the various immunopathologic syndromes such as insulin allergy, immune insulin resistance, and lipoatrophy have become quite rare. However, wherever less purified forms of beef insulin are still used, these disorders remain a clinical concern among insulin-treated patients.

1. Insulin allergy–Insulin allergy, or immediate-type hypersensitivity, is a rare condition in which local or systemic urticaria is due to histamine release from tissue mast cells sensitized by adherence of anti-insulin IgE antibodies. In severe cases, anaphylaxis results. A subcutaneous nodule appearing several hours later at the site of insulin injection and lasting for up to 24 hours has been attributed to an IgG-mediated complement-binding Arthus reaction. When only human insulin has been used from the onset of insulin therapy, insulin allergy is exceedingly rare. When allergy to beef or, more rarely, pork insulin is present, a species change (eg, to human insulin) may correct the problem, although in many cases cross-reaction between human and animal insulins results in persistent allergic responses. Antihistamines, corticosteroids, and even desensitization may be required, especially for systemic hypersensitivity.

2. Immune insulin resistance–All insulin-treated patients develop a low titer of circulating IgG anti-insulin antibodies that neutralize to a small extent the action of insulin. In some diabetic patients, principally those with some degree of tissue insensitivity to insulin (such as in the obese) and with a history of interrupted exposure to therapy with beef insulin, a high titer of circulating IgG anti-insulin antibodies develops. This results in extremely high insulin requirements—often more than 200 units daily. This is often a self-limited condition and may clear spontaneously after several months. However, in cases where the circulating antibody is specifically more reactive with beef insulin—a more potent immunogen in humans than pork insulin—changing the patient to a less antigenic insulin (pork or human) may make possible a dramatic reduction in insulin dosage or at least may shorten the duration of immune resistance. In some adults, the foreign insulin can be completely discontinued and the patient maintained on diet along with oral sulfonylureas. This is possible only when the circulating antibodies do not effectively neutralize endogenous (human) insulin. Owing to the usual effectiveness of human insulin in treating this syndrome, immunosuppressive therapy with high doses of glucocorticoids is no longer required.

C. Lipodystrophy at Injection Sites: Atrophy of subcutaneous fatty tissue leading to disfiguring excavations and depressed areas may rarely occur at the site of injection. This complication results from an immune reaction, and it has become rarer with the development of pure insulin preparations. Injection of these preparations directly into the atrophic area often results in restoration of normal contours. Lipohypertrophy, on the other hand, is a consequence of the pharmacologic effects of insulin being deposited in the same location repeatedly. It can occur with purified insulins and is best treated with localized liposuction of the hypertrophic areas by an experienced plastic surgeon. Rotation of injection sites will prevent lipohypertrophy.

Chronic Complications of Diabetes

Late clinical manifestations of diabetes mellitus include a number of pathologic changes that involve small and large blood vessels, cranial and peripheral nerves, the skin, and the lens of the eye. These lesions lead to hypertension, renal failure, blindness, autonomic and peripheral neuropathy, amputations of the lower extremities, myocardial infarction, and cerebrovascular accidents. The cause of these late manifestations is not well understood, but they correlate with the duration of the diabetic state. In type I diabetes, up to 40% of patients develop end-stage renal disease, compared to only about 20% of patients with type II diabetes. However, because of the much greater numbers who have type II diabetes, this group comprises the bulk of patients with end-stage renal disease. As regards proliferative retinopathy, it ultimately develops to a similar degree (prevalence of 25%) in both types of diabetes. In patients with type I diabetes, complications from end-stage renal disease are a major cause of death, whereas patients with type II diabetes are more likely to have macrovascular diseases leading to myocardial infarction and stroke as the main causes of death.

A. Ocular Complications:

1. Diabetic cataracts–Premature cataracts occur in diabetic patients. These opacities resemble those found in elderly patients with "senile" cataracts but occur at a younger age and seem to correlate with both the duration of diabetes and the severity of chronic hyperglycemia. Nonenzymatic glycosylation of lens protein is twice as high in diabetic patients as in age-matched nondiabetic persons and may contribute to the premature occurrence of cataracts.

2. Diabetic retinopathy–Three main categories exist: background, or "simple," retinopathy, consisting of microaneurysms, hemorrhages, exudates, and retinal edema; proliferative retinopathy with arteriolar ischemia manifested as cotton-wool spots (small infarcted areas of retina); and proliferative, or "malignant," retinopathy, consisting of newly formed vessels. Proliferative retinopathy is a leading cause of blindness in the USA, particularly since it increases the risk of retinal detachment. After 10 years of diabetes, half of all patients have retinopathy, and this proportion increases to more than 80% after 15 years of diabetes. Annual consultation with an ophthalmologist should be arranged for patients who have had type I diabetes for more than 5 years and for *all* patients with type II diabetes, because they were probably diabetic for an extensive period of time before diagnosis. Extensive "scatter" xenon or argon photocoagulation and focal treatment of new vessels reduce severe visual loss in those cases in which proliferative retinopathy is associated with *recent* vitreous hemorrhages or in which extensive new vessels are located on or near the optic disk. Macular edema, which is more common than proliferative retinopathy in patients with type II diabetes (about 6% prevalence), has also responded to this therapy with improvement in visual acuity. Avoiding tobacco use and correction of associated hypertension are important therapeutic measures in the management of diabetic retinopathy.

3. Glaucoma–Glaucoma occurs in approximately 6% persons with diabetes. It is generally responsive to the usual therapy for open-angle disease. Neovascularization of the iris in diabetics can predispose to closed-angle glaucoma, but this is relatively uncommon except after cataract extraction, when growth of new vessels has been known to progress rapidly, involving the angle of the iris and obstructing outflow.

B. Diabetic Nephropathy: (See also Chapter 21.) As many as 4000 cases of end-stage renal disease occur each year among diabetic people in the United States. This is about one-fourth of all patients being treated for end-stage renal disease and represents a considerable national health expense.

Patients developing diabetes before the age of 20 years have a 50% chance of having diabetic nephropathy after 20 years—in contrast to those with diabetes occurring after the age of 40 years, who have only a 4% incidence of diabetic renal disease after 20 years.

Diabetic nephropathy is initially manifested by proteinuria; subsequently, as kidney function declines, urea and creatinine accumulate in the blood.

1. Microalbuminuria–New methods of detecting small amounts of urinary albumin have permitted detection of microgram concentrations—in contrast to the less sensitive dipstick strips, whose minimal detection limit is 0.3–0.5%. Conventional 24-hour urine collections, in addition to being inconvenient for patients, also show wide variability of albumin excretion, since several factors such as sustained erect posture, dietary protein, and exercise tend to increase albumin excretion rates. For these reasons, most laboratories prefer to screen patients with a timed overnight urine collection beginning at bedtime, when the urine is discarded and the time noted. Normal subjects excrete less than 15 μg/min during overnight urine collections; values of 20 μg/min or higher are considered to represent abnormal microalbuminuria.

Subsequent renal failure can be predicted by urinary albumin excretion rates exceeding 30 μg/min. Increased microalbuminuria correlates with increased levels of blood pressure, and this may explain why increased proteinuria in diabetic patients is associated with an increase in cardiovascular deaths even in the absence of renal failure. Careful glycemic control as well as a low-protein diet (0.6 g/kg/d) may reduce both the hyperfiltration and the elevated microalbuminuria in patients in the early stages of diabetes and those with incipient diabetic nephropathy. Antihypertensive therapy also decreases microalbuminuria, and clinical trials with inhibitors of angiotensin I converting enzyme (eg, enalapril, 20 mg/d) show a documented reduction of microalbuminuria in diabetic patients even in the absence of hypertension.

2. Progressive diabetic nephropathy–Progressive diabetic nephropathy consists of proteinuria of varying severity occasionally leading to nephrotic syndrome with hypoalbuminemia, edema, and an increase in circulating betalipoproteins as well as progressive azotemia. In contrast to all other renal disorders, the proteinuria associated with diabetic nephropathy does not diminish with progressive renal failure (patients continue to excrete 10–11 g daily as creatinine clearance diminishes). As renal failure progresses, there is an elevation in the renal threshold at which glycosuria appears.

Hypertension develops with progressive renal involvement, and coronary and cerebral atherosclerosis seems to be accelerated. Approximately two-thirds of adult patients with diabetes have hypertension. Once diabetic nephropathy has progressed to the stage of hypertension, proteinuria, or early renal failure, glycemic control is not beneficial in influencing its course. In this circumstance, antihypertensive medications, including ACE inhibitors, and restriction of dietary protein to 0.6 g/kg body weight per day are recommended.

When the serum creatinine reaches 3 mg/dL, consultation with a nephrologist or a diabetologist experienced in the treatment of diabetic nephropathy is recommended. When the serum creatinine reaches 5 mg/dL, consultation with personnel at a center where renal transplantation is performed is indicated.

Dialysis has been of limited value in the treatment of renal failure due to diabetic nephropathy. At present, experience in renal transplantation—especially from related donors—is more promising and is the treatment of choice in cases where there are no contraindications such as severe cardiovascular disease.

C. Gangrene of the Feet: The incidence of gangrene of the feet in diabetics is 20 times the incidence in matched controls. The factors responsible for its development are ischemia, peripheral neuropathy, and secondary infection. Occlusive vascular disease involves both microangiopathy and atherosclerosis of large and medium-sized arteries. Cigarette smoking should be avoided, and prevention of foot disease should be emphasized, since treatment is difficult once ulceration and gangrene have developed (see above). Patients should be instructed to inspect their feet daily for reddened areas, blisters, abrasions, or lacerations, particularly when the foot is insensitive. Physicians should inspect the feet of diabetic patients at each visit and instruct patients as necessary on filing calluses with an emery board, cutting toenails straight across, not walking barefoot, and avoiding tight shoes. When an uncomplicated neuropathic ulcer is present and blood flow is not impaired, consultation with a podiatrist or orthopedist is recommended. If blood supply is diminished or absent, patients with foot ulcers should be referred to an appropriate specialist (vascular or orthopedic surgeon). Special custom-built shoes are usually required to redistribute weight evenly over an insensitive foot, particularly when it has been deformed by surgery or asymptomatic fractures (Charcot's joint). Amputation of the lower extremities is sometimes required.

Nonselective beta-blockers are relatively contraindicated in patients with ischemic foot ulcers, because these drugs reduce peripheral blood flow.

D. Diabetic Neuropathy: Peripheral and autonomic neuropathy, the two most common chronic complications of diabetes, are poorly understood. Peripheral neuropathy is generally bilateral, symmetric, and associated with dulled perception of vibration, pain, and temperature, particularly in the lower extremities. At times, discomfort of the lower extremities can be incapacitating. Both motor and sensory nerve conduction are delayed in peripheral nerves, and ankle jerks may be absent.

Contrasting with this axonal neuropathic process is ischemic neuropathy resulting from small vessel disease of the vasa nervorum. Femoral and cranial nerves are commonly involved, and motor abnormalities predominate. These can result in sudden onset of diplopia due to ophthalmoplegia or in acute pain and weakness of thigh muscles (diabetic amyotrophy). Spontaneous resolution of these ischemic neuropathies generally occurs in 6–12 weeks. In more severe cases with extensive atrophy of limb musculature, this disorder has been termed "malignant cachexia" and mimics the end stages of advanced neoplasia, particularly when depression produces anorexia and weight loss. With this more severe manifestation of diabetic amyotrophy, recovery of muscle function may only be partial.

Amitriptyline, 25–75 mg at bedtime, has been recommended for pain associated with diabetic neuropathy. Dramatic relief has often resulted within 48–72 hours. This rapid response is in contrast to the 2 or 3 weeks required for an antidepressive effect. Patients often attribute benefit to their having a full night's sleep after amitriptyline compared to many previously sleepless nights occasioned by neuropathic pain. Mild to moderate morning drowsiness is a side effect that generally improves with time or can be lessened by giving the medication several hours before bedtime. This drug should not be continued if improvement has not occurred after 5 days of therapy. Desipramine in doses of 25–150 mg/d seems to have the same efficacy as amitriptyline. Other drugs used include carbamazepine and phenytoin, both of questionable benefit for leg pain. There has also been interest in use of the antiarrhythmic drug mexiletine for this purpose in doses of up to 10 mg/kg/d.Capsaicin,

a topical irritant, has recently been advocated for local nerve pain; it is dispensed as a cream (Zostrix 0.025%, Zostrix-HP 0.075%) to be rubbed into the skin over the painful region two to four times daily. A multicenter 8-week double-blind study (see Capsaicin Study Group reference) has recently reported that topical 0.075% capsaicin is effective in reducing pain among a population of 277 diabetic patients with painful diabetic neuropathy.

With autonomic neuropathy, there is evidence of postural hypotension, decreased cardiovascular response to Valsalva's maneuver, gastroparesis, alternating bouts of diarrhea (particularly nocturnal) and constipation, inability to empty the bladder, and impotence. Gastroparesis should be considered in insulin-dependent diabetic patients who develop unexpected fluctuations and variability in their blood glucose levels after meals. Impotence due to neuropathy differs from psychogenic impotence in that the latter may be intermittent (erections occur under special circumstances), whereas diabetic impotence is usually persistent; aortoiliac occlusive disease may contribute to this problem.

Local injection of papaverine into the corpus cavernosum produces a penile erection if blood supply is competent. This helps differentiate erectile disabilities due to neuropathic causes from those that do not respond to papaverine because of vasculopathy. Impotence is usually permanent, and a penile prosthesis should be considered as a therapeutic option in appropriate cases. External vacuum therapy (Erec-Aid System) is a nonsurgical treatment consisting of a suction chamber operated by a hand pump that creates a vacuum around the penis. This draws blood into the penis to produce an erection which is maintained by a specially designed tension ring inserted around the base of the penis and which can be kept in place for up to 20–30 minutes. This approach has met with acceptance by a majority of patients with impotence, while others have opted for surgical implant of a penile prosthesis.

There is no consistently effective treatment for diabetic autonomic neuropathy. Metoclopramide has been of some help in treating diabetic gastroparesis over the short term, but its effectiveness seems to diminish over time. It is a dopamine antagonist that has central antiemetic effects as well as a cholinergic action to facilitate gastric emptying. It can be given intravenously (10 mg three or four times a day, 30 minutes before meals and at bedtime) or orally (20 mg of liquid metoclopramide) before breakfast and dinner. Drowsiness, restlessness, fatigue, and lassitude are common adverse effects. Tardive dyskinesia and extrapyramidal effects also occur. Diarrhea associated with autonomic neuropathy has occasionally responded to broad-spectrum antibiotic therapy, though it often undergoes spontaneous remission. Refractory diabetic diarrhea is often associated with impaired sphincter control and fecal incontinence. Therapy with loperamide, 4–8 mg daily, or diphenoxylate with atropine, two tablets up to four times a day, may provide relief. In more severe cases, tincture of paregoric or codeine (60 mg tablets) may be required to reduce the frequency of diarrhea and improve the consistency of the stools. Clonidine has been reported to lessen diabetic diarrhea, but its tendency to lower blood pressure in these patients who already have autonomic neuropathy and some orthostatic hypotension often limits its usefulness. Bethanechol in doses of 10–50 mg three times a day has occasionally improved emptying of the atonic urinary bladder. Catheter decompression of the distended bladder has been reported to improve its function, and considerable benefit has been reported after surgical severing of the internal vesicle sphincter. Mineralocorticoid therapy with fludrocortisone, 0.2–0.3 mg/d, and elastics stockings or pressure suits have reportedly been of some help in patients with orthostatic hypotension occurring as a result of loss of postural reflexes.

E. Skin and Mucous Membrane Complications: Chronic pyogenic infections of the skin may occur, especially in poorly controlled diabetic patients. Eruptive xanthomas can result from hypertriglyceridemia, associated with poor glycemic control. An unusual lesion termed **necrobiosis lipoidica diabeticorum** is usually located over the anterior surfaces of the legs or the dorsal surfaces of the ankles. They are oval or irregularly shaped plaques with demarcated borders and a glistering yellow surface and occur in women two to four times more frequently than in men.

"Shin spots" are not uncommon in adult diabetics. They are brownish, rounded, painless atrophic lesions of the skin in the pretibial area. Candidal infection can produce erythema and edema of intertriginous areas below the breasts, in the axillas, and between the fingers. It causes vulvovaginitis in most chronically uncontrolled diabetic women with persistent glucosuria and is a frequent cause of pruritus.

While antifungal creams containing nystatin offer immediate relief of vulvovaginitis, recurrence is frequent unless glucosuria is reduced.

F. Special Situations:

1. Insulin replacement during surgery–During major surgery and in the immediate recovery period in patients with insulin-requiring diabetes, 5% dextrose in physiologic saline should be infused intravenously at a rate of 100–200 mL/h with regular human insulin (25 units/250 mL normal saline) infused into the intravenous tubing at a rate of 1–3 units/h. The patient's blood glucose should be monitored every hour initially and the rates of insulin or dextrose adjusted to maintain blood glucose values between 120 and 190 mg/dL.

Most patients with type II, whether or not they are receiving insulin therapy for their diabetes, should be treated with insulin during major surgery. In these patients, 10 units of regular insulin added to 1000 mL of a 5% dextrose/water solution containing 20 meq of potassium chloride and infused at a rate of 100 mL/h (1 unit/h) is generally adequate to regulate glycemia during surgery. The patient's glucose should be monitored hourly to prevent extremes of hyper-or hypoglycemia. If blood glucose values remain above 250 mg/dL at 1–2 hours, an infusion concentration of 15 units/L can be substituted.

2. Pregnancy and the diabetic patient–Several features distinguish the management of diabetics during pregnancy from the general therapy of diabetes. These include the following: (1) Oral hypoglycemic agents are contraindicated. (2) Weight reduction is not advised, since fetal nutrition can be adversely affected. (3) Intensive insulin therapy with frequent self-monitoring of blood glucose is generally recommended to improve the likelihood of having healthy normal babies. Every effort should be made, utilizing multiple injections of insulin or a continuous infusion of insulin by pump, to maintain near-normalization of fasting and preprandial blood glucose values while avoiding hypoglycemia. Glycohemoglobin should be maintained in the normal range.

Since many diabetic pregnancies persist beyond the expected term—or because the infants are usually large and hydramnios may be present—it has been suggested that pregnancy be terminated early (at 37–38 weeks), especially if glycemic control during pregnancy has been inadequate (eg, glycohemoglobin > 10%). There is a present trend away from elective cesarean section and toward induction of labor.

See Chapter 17 for further details.

Prognosis

Despite the present inadequacy of subcutaneous insulin delivery systems for physiologic insulin replacement, over 60% of patients with type I do reasonably well over the long term. The remainder develop severe disability leading to blindness, end-stage renal failure, and early demise.

The period between 10 and 20 years after onset of type I diabetes seems to be a critical one. If the patient survives this period without fulminating complications, there is a strong likelihood that reasonably good health will continue. In addition to poorly understood genetic factors relating to differences in individual susceptibility to development of long-term complications of hyperglycemia, it is clear that in both types of diabetes, the diabetic patient's intelligence, motivation, and awareness of the potential complications of the disease contribute significantly to the ultimate outcome.

Classification, Pathophysiology, & Diagnosis of Diabetes Mellitus

Bjorntorp P: Metabolic implications of body fat distribution. Diabetes Care 1991;14:1132. (Visceral fat contributes most to metabolic abnormalities of plasma glucose, triglycerides, and insulin resistance.)

DeFronzo RA, Bonadonna RC, Ferrannini E: Pathogenesis of NIDDM: A balanced overview. Diabetes Care 1992;15:318. (Defects both in insulin action and insulin secretion are necessary in causing type II.)

Karam JH: Type II diabetes and syndrome X: Pathogenesis and glycemic management. Endocrinol Metab Clin North Am 1992;21:329. (The controversy over whether insulin resistance is responsible for most of the other components of syndrome X or merely an associated manifestation.)

Leahy JL, Bonner-Weir S, Weir GC: Beta cell dysfunction induced by chronic hyperglycemia: Current ideas on mechanism of impaired glucose-induced insulin secretion. Diabetes Care 1992;15:442. (Mechanisms by which defects of insulin secretion in type II may be an acquired consequence of hyperglycemia.)

Muir A, Schatz DA, Maclaren NK: The pathogenesis, prediction, and prevention of insulin-dependent diabetes mellitus. Endocrinol Metab Clin North Am 1992;21:199. (The autoimmune etiology of type I and the current status of immunosuppression clinical trials in its prevention.)

Therapy of Diabetes Mellitus

American Diabetes Association Committee on Professional Practice: Standards of medical care for patients with diabetes mellitus. Diabetes Care 1989;12:365. (Standards for appropriate care of diabetic patients.)

DCCT Research Group: Epidemiology of severe hypoglycemia in the Diabetes Control and Complications Trial. Am J Med 1991;90:450. (Severe hypoglycemia is a major risk factor in type I patients attempting tight glycemic control.)

Dunn FL: Management of hyperlipidemia in diabetes mellitus. Endocrinol Metab Clin North Am 1992; 21:395.

Gavin LA: Perioperative management of the diabetic patient. Endocrinol Metab Clin North Am 1992;21:457.

Genuth S: Management of the adult onset diabetic with sulfonylurea failure. Endocrinol Metab Clin North Am 1992;21:351. ("Pseudo" failure due to poor compliance versus "true" failure to respond to sulfonylureas.)

Lebovitz HE (editor): Therapy for diabetes mellitus and related disorders. Alexandria, Virginia, American Diabetes Association 1991.

Nathan DM: The rationale for glucose control in diabetes mellitus. Endocrinol Metab Clin North Am 1992; 21:221.

Nolte MS: Insulin therapy in insulin-dependent (type I) diabetes mellitus. Endocrinol Metab Clin North Am 1992;21:281.

Selam J-L, Charles MA: Devices for insulin administration. Diabetes Care 1990;13:955. (Jet injectors, insulin pens, conventional subcutaneous insulin pumps, and programmable implantable insulin pumps—specific advantages and risks.)

Tamborlane WV, Amiel SA: Hypoglycemia in the treated diabetic patient: A risk of intensive insulin therapy. Endocrinol Metab Clin North Am 1992; 21:313.

Vinik AI, Wing RR: The good, the bad, the ugly in diabetic diets. Endocrinol Metab Clin North Am 1992; 21:237.

Wu MS et al: Effect of metformin on carbohydrate and lipoprotein metabolism in NIDDM patients. Diabetes Care 1990;13:1. (Improved glycemic control as well as lipoprotein metabolism during a 4-month trial in 12 patients.)

Chronic Complications of Diabetes Mellitus

Capsaicin Study Group: Effect of treatment with capsaicin on daily activities of patients with painful diabetic neuropathy. Diabetes Care 1992;15:159. (This derivative of chili pepper is an irritant that desensitizes nerve endings and reduces pain sensation in painful diabetic neuropathy.)

Davis MD: Diabetic retinopathy. Diabetes Care 1992; 15:1884.

Microalbuminuria Collaborative Study Group: Microalbuminuria in type I diabetic patients: Prevalence and clinical characteristics. Diabetes Care 1992;15:495.

Ogbonnaya KI, Arem R: Diabetic diarrhea. Arch Intern Med 1990;150:262.

Pecoraro RE, Reiber GE, Burgess EM: Pathways to diabetic limb amputation: Basis for prevention. Diabetes Care 1990;13:513.

Vinik AI et al: Diabetic neuropathies. Diabetes Care 1992;15:1926.

Watkins PJ: Diabetic autonomic neuropathy. N Engl J Med 1990;322:1078.

DIABETIC COMA

Coma may be due to a variety of causes not directly related to diabetes. Certain causes directly related to diabetes require differentiation: (1) Hypoglycemic coma resulting from excessive doses of insulin or oral hypoglycemic agents. (2) Hyperglycemic coma associated with either severe insulin deficiency (diabetic ketoacidosis) or mild to moderate insulin deficiency (hyperglycemic nonketotic hyperosmolar coma). (3) Lactic acidosis associated with diabetes, particularly in diabetics stricken with severe infections or with cardiovascular collapse.

DIABETIC KETOACIDOSIS

Essentials of Diagnosis

- Hyperglycemia > 300 mg/dL.
- Acidosis with blood pH < 7.3.
- Serum bicarbonate < 15 meq/L.
- Serum positive for ketones.

General Considerations

Diabetic ketoacidosis may be the initial manifestation of type I diabetes or may result from increased insulin requirements in type I diabetes patients during the course of infection, trauma, myocardial infarction, or surgery. Type II diabetics may develop ketoacidosis under severe stress such as sepsis. Recently, diabetic ketoacidosis has been found to be one of the more common serious complications of insulin pump therapy, occurring in approximately one per 80 patient-months of treatment. Many patients who monitor capillary blood glucose regularly ignore urine ketone measurements, which would signal the possibility of insulin leakage or pump failure before serious illness develops. Poor compliance is one of the most common causes of diabetic ketoacidosis, particularly when episodes are recurrent.

Clinical Findings

A. Symptoms and Signs: The appearance of diabetic ketoacidotic coma is usually preceded by a day or more of polyuria and polydipsia associated with marked fatigue, nausea and vomiting, and, finally, mental stupor that can progress to coma. On physical examination, evidence of dehydration in a stuporous patient with rapid deep breathing and a "fruity" breath odor of acetone would strongly suggest the diagnosis. Hypotension with tachycardia indicates profound fluid and electrolyte depletion, and mild hypothermia is usually present. Abdominal pain and even tenderness may be present in the absence of abdominal disease. Conversely, cholecystitis or pancreatitis may occur with minimal symptoms and signs.

B. Laboratory Findings: (Table 26–10.) Glycosuria of 4+ and strong ketonuria with hyperglycemia, ketonemia, low arterial blood pH, and low plasma bicarbonate are typical of diabetic ketoacidosis. Serum potassium is often elevated despite total body potassium depletion resulting from protracted

polyuria or vomiting. Elevation of serum amylase is common but often represents salivary as well as pancreatic amylase. Thus, in this setting, serum amylase is not a good marker for acute pancreatitis. Multichannel chemical analysis of serum creatinine (SMA-6) is falsely elevated by nonspecific chromogenicity of keto acids and glucose. Most laboratories can correct for these interfering substances on request, and newer analyzers are being introduced that routinely eliminate this interference. Leukocytosis as high as 25,000/μL with a left shift may occur with or without associated infection. The presence of an elevated temperature would suggest the presence of an infection, since patients with diabetic ketoacidosis are generally hypothermic if uninfected.

Complications

The two major metabolic aberrations of diabetic ketoacidosis are hyperglycemia and ketoacidemia, both due to insulin lack associated with hyperglucagonemia.

A. Hyperglycemia: Hyperglycemia results from increased hepatic production of glucose as well as diminished glucose uptake by peripheral tissues. Hepatic glucose output is a consequence of increased gluconeogenesis resulting from insulinopenia as well as from an associated hyperglucagonemia. When serum hyperosmolality exceeds 320–330 mosm/L, central nervous system depression or coma may ensue. Coma in a diabetic patient with a lower osmolality should prompt a search for cause of coma other than hyperosmolality.

B. Ketoacidemia: Ketoacidemia represents the effect of insulin lack at multiple enzyme loci. Insulin lack associated with elevated levels of growth hormone and glucagon contributes to an increase in lipolysis from adipose tissue and in hepatic ketogenesis. In addition, there is evidence that reduced ketolysis by insulin-deficient peripheral tissues contributes to the ketoacidemia. The only true

Table 26–10. Laboratory diagnosis of coma in diabetic patients.

	Urine		Plasma		
	Glucose	Acetone	Glucose	Bicarbonate	Acetone
Related to diabetes					
Hypoglycemia	0[1]	0 or +	Low	Normal	0
Diabetic ketoacidosis	++++	++++	High	Low	++++
Nonketotic hyperglycemic coma	++++	0	High	Normal or slightly low	0
Lactic acidosis	0 or +	0 or +	Normal or low or high	Low	0 or +
Unrelated to diabetes					
Alcohol or other toxic drugs	0 or +	0 or +	May be low	Normal or low[2]	0 or +
Cerebrovascular accident or head trauma	+ or 0	0	Often high	Normal	0
Uremia	0 or +	0	High or normal	Low	0 or +

[1]Leftover urine in bladder might still contain glucose from earlier hyperglycemia.
[2]Alcohol can elevate plasma lactate as well as keto acids to reduce pH.

"keto" acid present is acetoacetic acid, which, along with its by-product acetone, is measured by nitroprusside reagents (Acetest and Ketostix). The sensitivity for acetone, however, is poor, requiring over 10 mmol, which is seldom reached in the plasma of ketoacidotic subjects—although this detectable concentration is readily achieved in urine. Thus, in the plasma of ketotic patients, only acetoacetate is measured by these reagents. The more prevalent β-hydroxybutyric acid has no ketone group and is therefore not detected by conventional nitroprusside tests. This takes on special importance in the presence of circulatory collapse during diabetic ketoacidosis, wherein an increase in lactic acid can shift the redox state to increase β-hydroxybutyric acid at the expense of the readily detectable acetoacetic acid. Bedside diagnostic reagents would then be unreliable, suggesting no ketonemia in cases where β-hydroxybutyric acid is a major factor in producing the acidosis.

Treatment

A. Prevention: Education of diabetic patients to recognize the early symptoms and signs of ketoacidosis has done a great deal to prevent severe acidosis. Urine ketones should be measured in patients with signs of infection or in insulin pump-treated patients when capillary blood glucose is unexpectedly and persistently high. When heavy ketonuria and glycosuria persist on several successive examinations, supplemental regular insulin should be administered and liquid foods such as lightly salted tomato juice and broth should be ingested to replenish fluids and electrolytes. The patient should be instructed to contact the physician if ketonuria persists, and especially if vomiting develops or if appropriate adjustment of the infusion rate on an insulin pump does not correct the hyperglycemia and ketonuria. In juvenile-onset diabetics, particularly in the teen years, recurrent episodes of severe ketoacidosis often indicate poor compliance with the insulin regimen, and these patients will require intensive family counseling.

B. Emergency Measures: If ketosis is severe, the patient should be placed in the hospital for correction of the hyperosmolality as well as the ketoacidemia.

1. Therapeutic flow sheet—One of the most important steps in initiating therapy is to start a flow sheet listing vital signs and the time sequence of diagnostic laboratory values in relation to therapeutic maneuvers. Indices of the metabolic defects include urine glucose and ketones as well as arterial pH, plasma glucose, acetone, bicarbonate, serum urea nitrogen, and electrolytes. Serum osmolality should be estimated and tabulated during the course of therapy. A convenient method of estimating *effective* serum osmolality is as follows (normal values in humans are 280–300 mosm/L:

$$\text{mosm/L} = 2[\text{Na}^+ + \text{K}^+] = \frac{\text{Glucose (mg/dL)}}{18}$$

These calculated estimates are usually 10–20 mosm/L lower than values recorded by standard cryoscopic techniques in patients with diabetic coma. One physician should be responsible for maintaining this therapeutic flow sheet and prescribing therapy. An indwelling catheter is required in all comatose patients but should be avoided if possible in a fully cooperative diabetic because of the risk of introducing bladder infection. Fluid intake and output should be recorded. Gastric intubation is recommended in the comatose patient to correct the commonly associated gastric dilatation that may lead to vomiting and aspiration. The patient should not receive sedatives or narcotics.

2. Insulin replacement—Only regular insulin should be used initially in all cases of severe ketoacidosis, and it should be given immediately after the diagnosis is established. Regular insulin can be given in a loading dose of 0.3 unit/kg as an intravenous bolus followed by 0.1 unit/kg/h, continuously infused or given hourly as an intramuscular injection; this is sufficient to replace the insulin deficit in most patients. Replacement of insulin deficiency helps correct the acidosis by reducing the flux of fatty acids to the liver, reducing ketone production by the liver, and also improving removal of ketones from the blood. Insulin treatment reduces the hyperosmolality by reducing the hyperglycemia. It accomplishes this by increasing removal of glucose through peripheral utilization as well as by decreasing production of glucose by the liver. This latter effect is accomplished by direct inhibition of gluconeogenesis and glycogenolysis, as well as by lowered amino acid flux from muscle to liver and reduced hyperglucagonemia.

The insulin dose should be "piggy-backed" into the fluid line so the rate of fluid replacement can be changed without altering the insulin delivery rate. For optimal effects, continuous low-dose insulin infusions should always be preceded by a rapid intravenous loading dose of regular insulin, 0.3 unit/kg, to prime the tissue insulin receptors. If the plasma glucose level fails to fall at least 10% in the first hour, a repeat loading dose is recommended. The availability of bedside glucometers and of laboratory instruments for rapid and accurate glucose analysis (Beckman or Yellow Springs glucose analyzer) has contributed much to achieving optimal insulin replacement. Rarely, a patient with immune insulin resistance is encountered, and this requires doubling the insulin dose every 2–4 hours if hyperglycemia does not improve after the first two doses of insulin.

3. Fluid and electrolyte replacement—In most patients, the fluid deficit is 4–5 L. Initially, normal saline solution is the solution of choice to help reexpand the contracted vascular volume. The use of sodium bicarbonate has been questioned because of the following potentially harmful consequences: (1) Hypokalemia from rapid potassium shifts into cells. (2) Tissue anoxia from reduced dissociation of oxygen from hemoglobin when acidosis is rapidly reversed. (3) Cerebral acidosis resulting from a reduction of cerebrospinal fluid pH. However, these considerations are relatively less important in certain clinical settings, and 1–2 ampules of sodium bicarbonate (44 meq per 50 mL ampule) added to a bottle of *hypotonic* saline solution may be administered whenever the blood pH is 7.0 or less or blood bicarbonate is below 9 meq/L. Once the pH reaches 7.2, no further bicarbonate should be given, since it aggravates rebound metabolic alkalosis as ketones are metabolized. Alkalosis causes potassium shifts that increase the risk of cardiac arrhythmias. In the first hour, at least 1 L of normal saline should be infused, and fluid should be given thereafter at a rate of 300–500 mL/h with careful monitoring of serum potassium. If the blood glucose is above 500 mg/dL, 0.45% saline solution may be used after the first hour, since the water deficit exceeds the sodium loss in uncontrolled diabetes with osmotic diuresis. When blood glucose falls to 250 mg/dL or less, 5% glucose solutions should be used to maintain blood glucose between 200 and 300 mg/dL while insulin therapy is continued in order to clear the ketonemia. Glucose administration has the dual advantage of preventing hypoglycemia and furthermore of reducing the likelihood of cerebral edema, which could result from too rapid a decline in hyperglycemia.

During therapy, hyperchloremic acidosis develops because of the considerable loss of keto acids in the urine during the initial phase of treatment. A portion of the bicarbonate deficit is replaced with chloride ions infused in large amounts as saline to correct the dehydration. Thus, in most patients, as the ketoacidosis clears during insulin replacement, they show a hyperchloremic, low bicarbonate pattern with a normal anion gap. This is a relatively benign condition that reverses itself over the subsequent 12–24 hours once intravenous saline is no longer being administered.

4. Potassium and phosphate replacement– Total body potassium loss from polyuria as well as from vomiting may be as high as several hundred milliequivalents. However, because of shifts from cells due to the acidosis, serum potassium is usually normal or high until after the first few hours of treatment, when acidosis improves and serum potassium returns into cells. Potassium in doses of 20–30 meq/h should be infused within 2–3 hours after beginning therapy, or sooner if initial serum potassium is inappropriately low. Potassium replacement should be deferred if serum potassium remains above 5.8 meq/L, as in cases of renal insufficiency. An ECG can be of help in monitoring the patient and reflecting the state of potassium balance at the time, but it should not replace accurate laboratory measurements.

Foods high in potassium content can be prescribed when the patient has recovered sufficiently to take food orally. (Tomato juice and grapefruit juice contain 14 meq of potassium per 240 mL and a medium-sized banana 10 meq.) See Chapter 20 for potassium content of foods.

If severe hypophosphatemia of less than 0.35 mmol/L (< 1 mg/dL) develops during insulin therapy of diabetic ketoacidosis, a small amount of phosphate can be replaced as the potassium salt. Hypophosphatemia of this severity is detrimental to membranes of skeletal muscle and may lyse red blood cells. The potassium need is several times that of phosphate and should be replaced separately, since replacing phosphorus ions too rapidly (while meeting potassium requirements) can precipitate a drop in serum calcium in the tissues and induce tetany.

A significant therapeutic benefit of routine phosphate replacement has not been documented in several randomized trials. However, certain potential advantages have been suggested. Treatment of hypophosphatemia helps to restore the buffering capacity of the plasma, thereby facilitating renal excretion of hydrogen; and it corrects the impaired oxygen dissociation from hemoglobin by regenerating 2,3-diphosphoglycerate. To minimize the risk of inducing tetany from an overload of phosphate replacement, an average deficit of 40–50 mmol phosphate in adults with diabetic ketoacidosis should be replaced by intravenous infusion *at a rate not to exceed 3 mmol/h.*

A stock solution available from Abbott Laboratories provides a mixture of 1.12 g KH_2PO_4 and 1.18 g K_2HPO_4 in a 5 mL single-dose vial representing 22 meq potassium and 15 mmol phosphate (27 meq). Five milliliters of this stock solution in 2 L of either 0.45% saline or 5% dextrose in water, infused at 400 mL/h, will replace the phosphate at the optimal rate of 3 mmol/h and will provide 4.4 meq of potassium per hour. If serum phosphate remains below 0.8 mmol/L (2.5 mg/dL), a repeat 5-hour infusion of potassium phosphate at a rate of 3 mmol/h would be reasonable.

5. Treatment of associated infection–Antibiotics are prescribed as indicated. Cholecystitis and pyelonephritis may be particularly severe in these patients.

Prognosis

The frequency of deaths due to diabetic ketoacidosis has been dramatically reduced by improved therapy of young diabetics, but this complication remains a significant risk in the aged and in patients in profound coma in whom treatment has been delayed. Acute myocardial infarction and infarction of the bowel following prolonged hypotension worsen the outlook. A serious prognostic sign is renal failure, and prior kidney dysfunction worsens the prognosis considerably because the kidney plays a key role in compensating for massive pH and electrolyte abnormalities. Cerebral edema has been reported to occur rarely as metabolic deficits return to normal. This is best prevented by avoiding sudden reversal of marked hyperglycemia. Maintaining glycemic levels of 200–300 mg/dL for the initial 24 hours after correction of severe hyperglycemia reduces this risk.

NONKETOTIC HYPERGLYCEMIC COMA

Essentials of Diagnosis

- Hyperglycemia > 600 mg/dL.
- Serum osmolality > 310 mosm/kg.
- No acidosis; blood pH above 7.3.
- Serum bicarbonate > 15 meq/L.
- Normal anion gap (< 14 meq/L).

General Considerations

This second most common form of hyperglycemic coma is characterized by severe hyperglycemia in the absence of significant ketosis, with hyperosmolality and dehydration. It occurs in patients with mild or occult diabetes, and most patients are at least middle-aged to elderly. Lethargy and confusion develop as serum osmolality exceeds 310 mosm/kg, and coma can occur if osmolality exceeds 320–330 mosm/kg. Underlying renal insufficiency or congestive heart failure is common, and the presence of either worsens the prognosis. A precipitating event such as infection, myocardial infarction, stroke, or recent operation is often present. Certain drugs such as phenytoin, diazoxide, glucocorticoids, and diuretics have been implicated in its pathogenesis, as have procedures associated with glucose loading such as peritoneal dialysis.

Pathogenesis

A partial or relative insulin deficiency may initiate the syndrome by reducing glucose utilization of muscle, fat, and liver while inducing hyperglucagonemia and increasing hepatic glucose output. With massive glycosuria, obligatory water loss ensues. If a patient is unable to maintain adequate fluid intake because of an associated acute or chronic illness or has suffered excessive fluid loss, marked dehydration results. As plasma volume contracts, renal insufficiency develops, and the resultant limitation of renal glucose loss leads to increasingly higher blood glucose concentrations. Severe hyperosmolality develops that causes mental confusion and finally coma. It is not clear why ketosis is virtually absent under these conditions of insulin insufficiency, although reduced levels of growth hormone may be associated along with portal vein insulin concentrations sufficient to restrain ketogenesis.

Clinical Findings

A. Symptoms and Signs: Onset may be insidious over a period of days or weeks, with weakness, polyuria, and polydipsia. The lack of features of ketoacidosis may retard recognition of the syndrome and delay therapy until dehydration becomes more profound than in ketoacidosis. Reduced intake of fluid is not an uncommon historical feature, due to either inappropriate lack of thirst, nausea, or inaccessibility of fluids to elderly, bedridden patients. Lethargy and confusion develop, progressing to convulsions and deep coma. Physical examination confirms the presence of profound dehydration in a lethargic or comatose patient without Kussmaul respirations.

B. Laboratory Findings: Severe hyperglycemia is present, with blood glucose values ranging from 600 to 2400 mg/dL. In mild cases, where dehydration is less severe, dilutional hyponatremia as well as urinary sodium losses may reduce serum sodium to 120–125 meq/L, which protects to some extent against extreme hyperosmolality. However, as dehydration progresses, serum sodium can exceed 140 meq/L, producing serum osmolality readings of 330–440 mosm/kg. Ketosis and acidosis are usually absent or mild. Prerenal azotemia is the rule, with serum urea nitrogen elevations over 100 mg/dL being typical.

Treatment

A. Saline: Fluid replacement is of paramount importance in treating nonketotic hyperglycemic coma. The onset of hyperosmolarity is more insidious in elderly people without ketosis than in younger individuals with high serum ketone levels. Consequently, diagnosis and treatment are often delayed until fluid deficit has reached levels of 6–10 L.

If hypovolemia is present, fluid therapy should be initiated with isotonic saline. In all other cases, hypotonic (0.45%) saline appears to be preferable as the initial replacement solution because the body fluids of these patients are markedly hyperosmolar. As much as 4–6 L of fluid may be required in the first 8–10 hours. Careful monitoring of the patient is required for proper sodium and water replacement. Once blood glucose reaches 250 mg/dL, fluid replacement should include 5% dextrose in either water, 0.45% saline solution, or 0.9% saline solution. The rate of dextrose infusion should be adjusted to maintain glycemic levels of 250–300 mg/dL in order to reduce the risk of cerebral edema. An important end point of fluid therapy is to restore urine output to 50 mL/h or more.

B. Potassium: With the absence of acidosis, there may be no initial hyperkalemia unless associated renal failure is present. This results in less severe total potassium depletion than in diabetic ketoacidosis, and less potassium replacement is therefore needed. However, because initial serum potassium is usually not elevated and because it declines rapidly as a result of insulin's effect on driving potassium intracellularly, it has been recommended that potassium replacement be initiated earlier than in ketotic patients, assuming that no renal insufficiency or oliguria is present. Potassium chloride (10 meq/L) can be added to the initial bottle of fluids administered if the patient's serum potassium is not elevated.

C. Phosphate: When hypophosphatemia develops during insulin therapy, phosphate replacement can be given as described for ketoacidotic patients (at 3 mmol/h).

D. Insulin: Less insulin may be required to reduce the hyperglycemia in nonketotic patients as compared to those with diabetic ketoacidotic coma. In fact, fluid replacement alone can reduce hyperglycemia considerably by correcting the hypovolemia, which then increases both glomerular filtration and renal excretion of glucose. An initial dose of only 15 units intravenously and 15 units subcutaneously of regular insulin is usually quite effective, and in most cases subsequent doses need not be greater than 10–25 units subcutaneously every 4 hours.

Prognosis

The overall mortality rate of hyperglycemic, hyperosmolar, nonketotic coma is more than ten times that of diabetic ketoacidosis, chiefly because of its higher incidence in older patients, who may have compromised cardiovascular systems or associated major illnesses and whose dehydration is often excessive because of delays in recognition and treatment. (When patients are matched for age, the prognoses of these two hyperglycemic emergencies are reasonably comparable.) When prompt therapy is instituted, the mortality rate can be reduced from nearly 50% to that related to the severity of coexistent disorders.

LACTIC ACIDOSIS
(See also Biguanides.)

Essentials of Diagnosis

- Severe acidosis with hyperventilation.
- Blood pH below 7.30.
- Serum bicarbonate < 15 meq/L.
- Anion gap > 15 meq/L.
- Absent serum ketones.
- Serum lactate > 7 mmol/L.

General Considerations

Lactic acidosis is characterized by accumulation of excess lactic acid in the blood. Normally, the principal sources of this acid are the erythrocytes (which lack enzymes for aerobic oxidation), skeletal muscle, skin, and brain. Conversion to glucose and oxidation principally by the liver but also by the kidneys represent the chief pathways for its removal. Overproduction of lactic acid (tissue hypoxia), deficient removal (hepatic failure), or both (circulatory collapse) can

cause accumulation. Lactic acidosis is not uncommon in any severely ill patient suffering from cardiac decompensation, respiratory or hepatic failure, septicemia, or infarction of bowel or extremities. With the discontinuance of phenformin therapy in the USA, lactic acidosis in patients with diabetes mellitus has become uncommon, but it still must be considered in the acidotic diabetic, especially if the patient is seriously ill.

Clinical Findings

A. Symptoms and Signs: The main clinical features of lactic acidosis are marked hyperventilation. When lactic acidosis is secondary to tissue hypoxia or vascular collapse, the clinical presentation is variable, being that of the prevailing catastrophic illness. However, in the idiopathic, or spontaneous, variety, the onset is rapid (usually over a few hours), blood pressure is normal, peripheral circulation is good, and there is no cyanosis.

B. Laboratory Findings: Plasma bicarbonate and blood pH are quite low, indicating the presence of severe metabolic acidosis. Ketones are usually absent from plasma and urine or at least not prominent. The first clue may be a high anion gap (serum sodium minus the sum of chloride and bicarbonate anions [in meq/L] should be no greater than 15). A higher value indicates the existence of an abnormal compartment of anions. If this cannot be clinically explained by an excess of keto acids (diabetes), inorganic acids (uremia), or anions from drug overdosage (salicylates, methyl alcohol, ethylene glycol), then lactic acidosis is probably the correct diagnosis. (See Chapter 20 also.) In the absence of azotemia, hyperphosphatemia may be a clue to the presence of lactic acidosis. The diagnosis is confirmed by demonstrating, in a sample of blood that is promptly chilled and separated, a plasma lactic acid concentration of 7 mmol/L or higher (values as high as 30 mmol/L have been reported). Normal plasma values average 1 mmol/L, with a normal lactate/pyruvate ratio of 10:1. This ratio is greatly exceeded in lactic acidosis.*

Treatment

Aggressive treatment of the precipitating cause of lactic acidosis is the main component of therapy. Empiric antibiotic coverage should be given after culture samples are obtained in any patient in whom the cause of the lactic acidosis is not apparent.

Alkalinization with intravenous sodium bicarbonate to keep the pH above 7.2 has been recommended in the emergency treatment of severe lactic acidosis. Massive doses may be required (as much as 2000

---

*In collecting samples, it is essential to rapidly chill and separate the blood in order to remove red cells, whose continued glycolysis at room temperature is a common source of error in reports of high plasma lactate. Frozen plasma remains stable for subsequent assay.

meq in 24 hours has been used); however, there is no evidence that the mortality rate is favorably affected by administering bicarbonate, and the matter is at present controversial. Hemodialysis may be useful in cases where large sodium loads are poorly tolerated. Dichloroacetate, an anion that facilitates pyruvate removal by activating pyruvate dehydrogenase, reverses certain types of lactic acidosis in animals is of no clinical utility in humans. In a recent prospective controlled clinical trial involving 252 cases of lactic acidosis, dichloroacetate failed to alter either hemodynamics or survival.

Prognosis

The mortality rate of spontaneous lactic acidosis approaches 80%. The prognosis in most cases is that of the primary disorder that produced the lactic acidosis.

Cefalu WT: Diabetic ketoacidosis. Crit Care Clin 1991; 7:89.

Cooper DJ et al: Bicarbonate does not improve hemodynamics in critically ill patients who have lactic acidosis. Ann Intern Med 1990;112:492.

Henderson G. The psychosocial treatment of recurrent diabetic ketoacidosis: An interdisciplinary team approach. Diabetes Educat 1991;17:119. (An often neglected approach.)

Morris LR, Murphy MB, Kitabachi AE: Bicarbonate therapy in severe ketoacidosis. Ann Intern Med 1986; 105:836.

Narins RG, Cohen JJ: Bicarbonate therapy for organic acidosis: The case for its continued use. Ann Intern Med 1987;106:615.

Rosenbloom AL: Intracerebral crises during treatment of diabetic ketoacidosis. Diabetes Care 1990;13:22.

Rumbak MJ, Kitabachi AE: Diabetic ketoacidosis: Etiology, pathophysiology, and treatment. Compr Ther 1991;17:46.

Siperstein MD: Diabetic ketoacidosis and hyperosmolar coma. Endocrinol Metab Clin North Am 1992;21:415.

Stacpoole PW et al: A controlled clinical trial of dichloroacetate for treatment of lactic acidosis in adults. N Engl J Med 1992;327:1564. (A placebo-controlled randomized clinical trial of intravenous dichloroacetate in 252 patients with lactic acidosis. This therapy failed to alter either hemodynamics or survival.)

Wrenn KD et al: The syndrome of alcoholic ketoacidosis. Am J Med 1991;91:119.

THE HYPOGLYCEMIC STATES

Spontaneous hypoglycemia in adults is of two principal types: fasting and postprandial. Fasting hypoglycemia is often subacute or chronic and usually presents with neuroglycopenia as its principal manifestation; postprandial hypoglycemia is relatively acute and is often heralded by symptoms of adrenergic discharge (sweating, palpitations, anxiety, tremulousness).

Differential Diagnosis (Table 26–11)

Fasting hypoglycemia may occur in certain endocrine disorders, such as hypopituitarism, Addison's disease, or myxedema; in disorders related to liver malfunction, such as acute alcoholism or liver failure; and in instances of renal failure, particularly in patients requiring dialysis. These conditions are usually obvious, with hypoglycemia being only a secondary feature. When fasting hypoglycemia is a primary manifestation developing in adults without apparent endocrine disorders or inborn metabolic diseases from childhood, the principal diagnostic possibilities include (1) hyperinsulinism, due to either pancreatic B cell tumors or surreptitious administration of insulin (or sulfonylureas); and (2) hypoglycemia due to non-insulin-producing extrapancreatic tumors.

Postprandial (reactive) hypoglycemia may be classified as early (within 2–3 hours after a meal) or late (3–5 hours after eating). Early, or alimentary, hypoglycemia occurs when there is a rapid discharge of ingested carbohydrate into the small bowel followed by rapid glucose absorption and hyperinsulinism. It may be seen after gastrointestinal surgery and is particularly associated with the dumping syndrome after gastrectomy. In some cases, it is functional and may represent overactivity of the parasympathetic nervous system mediated via the vagus nerve. Rarely, it results from defective counterregulatory responses such as deficiencies of growth hormone, glucagon, cortisol, or autonomic responses.

Alcohol hypoglycemia is due to hepatic glycogen

Table 26–11. Common causes of hypoglycemia.[1]

Fasting hypoglycemia
  Hyperinsulinism
    Pancreatic B cell tumor
    Surreptitious administration of insulin or sulfonylureas
  Extrapancreatic tumors
Postprandial (reactive) hypoglycemia
  Early hypoglycemia (alimentary)
    Postgastrectomy
    Functional (increased vagal tone)
  Late hypoglycemia (occult diabetes)
    Delayed insulin release due to B cell dysfunction
  Counterregulatory deficiency
  Idiopathic
Alcohol hypoglycemia
Immunopathologic hypoglycemia
  Idiopathic anti-insulin antibodies (which release their bound insulin)
  Antibodies to insulin receptors (which act as agonists)
Pentamidine-induced hypoglycemia

[1]In the absence of clinically obvious endocrine or hepatic disorders and exclusive of diabetes treated with hypoglycemic drugs.

depletion combined with alcohol-mediated inhibition of gluconeogenesis. At presentation, blood ethanol may be below levels usually associated with legal standards relating to being "under the influence."

Immunopathologic hypoglycemia is an extremely rare condition in which anti-insulin antibodies or antibodies to insulin receptors develop spontaneously. In the former case, the mechanism is unclear, but it may relate to increasing dissociation of insulin from circulating pools of bound insulin. When antibodies to insulin receptors are found, most patients do not have hypoglycemia but rather severe insulin-resistant diabetes and acanthosis nigricans. However, during the course of the disease in these patients, certain anti-insulin receptor antibodies with agonist activity mimicking insulin action predominate, producing severe hypoglycemia.

Factitious hypoglycemia is self-induced hypoglycemia due to surreptitious administration of insulin or sulfonylureas.

HYPOGLYCEMIA DUE TO PANCREATIC B CELL TUMORS

Fasting hypoglycemia in an otherwise healthy, well-nourished adult is rare, and is most commonly due to an adenoma of the islets of Langerhans. Ninety percent of such tumors are single and benign, but multiple adenomas can occur as well as malignant tumors with functional metastases. B cell hyperplasia as a cause of fasting hypoglycemia is rare and not well documented in adults. Adenomas may be familial, and multiple adenomas have been found in conjunction with tumors of the parathyroids and pituitary (Werner's syndrome; multiple endocrine neoplasia type I).

Clinical Findings

A. Symptoms and Signs: The signs and symptoms are those of subacute or chronic hypoglycemia, which may progress to permanent and irreversible brain damage. Delayed diagnosis has often resulted in prolonged psychiatric care or treatment for psychomotor epilepsy before the true diagnosis was established. In long-standing cases, obesity can result as a consequence of overeating to relieve symptoms.

Whipple's triad is characteristic of hypoglycemia regardless of the cause. It consists of (1) a history of hypoglycemic symptoms, (2) an associated fasting blood glucose of 40 mg/dL or less,* and (3) immediate recovery upon administration of glucose. The hypoglycemic symptoms in insulinoma often develop in the early morning or after missing a meal. Occasionally, they occur after exercise. They typically begin

*Plasma glucose values are generally 10–15% higher than blood glucose values.

with evidence of central nervous system glucose lack and can include blurred vision or diplopia, headache, feelings of detachment, slurred speech, and weakness. Personality and mental changes vary from anxiety to psychotic behavior, and neurologic deterioration can result in convulsions or coma. Sweating and palpitations may not occur.

B. Laboratory Findings: B cell adenomas do not reduce secretion in the presence of hypoglycemia, and the critical diagnostic test is to demonstrate inappropriately elevated serum insulin levels at a time when hypoglycemia is present. A reliable serum insulin level of 8 μU/mL or more in the presence of blood glucose values below 40 mg/dL is diagnostic of inappropriate hyperinsulinism. Other causes of hyperinsulinemic hypoglycemia must be considered, including factitious administration of insulin or sulfonylureas. An elevated circulating proinsulin level is characteristic of most B cell adenomas and does not occur in factitious hyperinsulinism.

C. Diagnostic Tests:

1. Prolonged fasting under hospital supervision until hypoglycemia is documented is probably the most dependable means of establishing the diagnosis, especially in men. In patients with insulinoma, the blood glucose levels often drop below 40 mg/dL after an overnight fast. In normal male subjects, the blood glucose does not fall below 55–60 mg/dL during a 3-day fast. In contrast, in premenopausal women who have fasted for only 24 hours, the plasma glucose may fall normally to such an extent that it can reach values as low as 35 mg/dL. After 36 hours of fasting, premenopausal normal women occasionally achieve such low levels of glucose that clinical evaluation of this test for insulinoma becomes quite difficult. In these cases, however, the women are not symptomatic, presumably owing to the development of sufficient ketonemia to supply energy needs to the brain. Insulinoma patients, on the other hand, become symptomatic when plasma glucose drops to subnormal levels, since inappropriate insulin secretion restricts ketone formation. Moreover, the demonstration of a nonsuppressed insulin level (≥ 8 units/mL) in the presence of hypoglycemia and of an *increasing* ratio of insulin to glucose (ie, glucose falls more rapidly than does insulin) suggests the diagnosis of insulinoma, since normal females show a falling insulin-to-glucose ratio during a fast. If hypoglycemia does not develop in a male patient after fasting for up to 72 hours—and particularly when this prolonged fast is terminated with a period of moderate exercise—insulinoma must be considered an unlikely diagnosis. Studies have not yet been done on postmenopausal women's ability to maintain euglycemia during fasting and whether or not estrogen replacement affect this.

2. Proinsulin determinations—In contrast to normal subjects, whose proinsulin concentration is less than 20% of the total immunoreactive insulin, patients with insulinoma have elevated levels of proinsulin representing 30–90% of total immunoreactive insulin. New assays for human proinsulin incorporating specific monoclonal antibodies offer considerable potential for the evaluation of patients with suspected insulinoma.

3. Stimulation tests with pancreatic B cell secretagogues such as tolbutamide, glucagon, or leucine are generally not needed in most cases if basal insulin is found to be nonsuppressible and therefore inappropriately elevated during fasting hypoglycemia. However, in occasional patients with a relatively fixed level of circulating insulin that is only barely inappropriate, stimulation may be helpful, bearing in mind that false-negative results can occur if the tumor is poorly differentiated and agranular.

Intravenous glucagon (1 mg over 1 minute) can be useful in patients with "borderline" fasting inappropriate hyperinsulinism. A rise above baseline of 200 μU/mL or more at 5 and 10 minutes strongly suggests insulinoma, although poorly differentiated tumors may not respond. Glucagon has the advantage over tolbutamide of correcting rather than provoking hypoglycemia during stimulation testing and is diagnostic in 60–70% of patients with insulinoma.

D. Preoperative Localization of B Cell Tumors: Pancreatic arteriography has been disappointing, with an accuracy rate of only 20% and a false-positive rate of about 5%. A promising modification correlates imaging from selective arteriography of segments of the pancreas with simultaneous hepatic vein sampling for insulin during a bolus of intra-arterial calcium delivered selectively to these same pancreatic segments. Calcium has been found to be a secretagogue only for insulinomas and not for normal islet tissue, so that a rise in hepatic insulin concentration indicates segmental localization of the insulinomas. CT scan and MRI are not helpful in the preoperative localization of insulinoma because they do not distinguish small tumors within the pancreas. However, intraoperative ultrasound is proving to be a valuable means of localizing small tumors within the pancreas not palpable at laparotomy.

Percutaneous transhepatic pancreatic vein catheterization with insulin assay is also useful for localizing small insulinomas; it is particularly helpful when multiple insulinomas are suspected, as in patients with coexisting pituitary or parathyroid adenomas. However, this technique is not widely available and is associated with considerable discomfort.

Treatment

A. Surgical Measures: Resection is the treatment of choice, preferably by a surgeon with previous experience in removing islet cell tumors. Diazoxide, 300–400 mg/d orally, inhibits insulin release from tumors and is useful in the interval prior to surgery for prevention of hypoglycemic episodes. Hydrochlorothiazide, 25–50 mg daily, should also be prescribed to counteract the edema and hyperkalemia secondary to diazoxide therapy as well as to potentiate its hyperglycemic effect. However, because effective doses are tolerated poorly over the long term, diazoxide and hydrochlorothiazide are not considered desirable alternatives to surgical excision. Blood glucose should be monitored throughout surgery, and 10% dextrose in water should be infused at a rate of 100 mL/h or faster. In cases where the diagnosis has been established but no adenoma is located after careful palpation and use of intraoperative ultrasound, subtotal pancreatectomy is usually indicated, including the entire body and tail of the pancreas. Total pancreatectomy is seldom required now in view of the efficacy of long-term medical therapy with diazoxide in most patients with insulinomas.

B. Diet and Medical Therapy: In patients with inoperable functioning islet cell carcinoma or in patients in whom subtotal removal of the pancreas has failed to produce cure, reliance on frequent feedings is necessary. Since most tumors are not responsive to glucose, carbohydrate feedings every 2–3 hours are usually effective in preventing hypoglycemia, although obesity may become a problem. Glucagon should be available for emergency use as indicated in the discussion of treatment of diabetes. Diazoxide, 300–600 mg daily orally, has been useful with concomitant thiazide diuretic therapy to control concomitant sodium retention. When patients are unable to tolerate diazoxide because of gastrointestinal upset, hirsutism, or edema, the calcium channel blocker verapamil may be beneficial in view of its inhibitory effect on insulin release from insulinoma cells. Recently, a potent long-acting synthetic octapeptide analogue of somatostatin (octreotide, Sandoz) has been used to inhibit release of hormones from a number of endocrine tumors, including inoperable insulinomas. When hypoglycemia persists after attempted surgical removal of the insulinoma and if diazoxide or verapamil is poorly tolerated or ineffective, a trial of 50 μg of octreotide acetate injected subcutaneously twice daily may control the hypoglycemic episodes in conjunction with multiple small feedings. Streptozocin is useful in decreasing insulin secretion in islet cell carcinomas, and effective doses have been achieved without the undue renal toxicity that characterized early experience.

Prognosis

When insulinoma is diagnosed early and cured surgically, complete recovery is likely, although brain damage following severe hypoglycemia is not reversible. A significant increase in survival rate has been shown in streptozocin-treated patients with islet cell carcinoma, with reduction in tumor mass as well as decreased hyperinsulinism.

HYPOGLYCEMIA DUE TO EXTRAPANCREATIC TUMORS

These rare causes of hypoglycemia include mesenchymal tumors such as retroperitoneal sarcomas, hepatomas, hepatocellular carcinomas, adrenocortical carcinomas, and miscellaneous epithelial type tumors. The tumors are frequently large and readily palpated or visualized on urograms.

Laboratory diagnosis depends upon fasting hypoglycemia associated with serum insulin levels that are generally below 8 μU/mL. The mechanism of these tumors' hypoglycemic effect remains obscure. Although they do not release immunoreactive insulin, it has been suggested that they may produce certain insulin-like substances similar to the somatomedins or growth factors that may bind to the insulin receptor. A high-molecular-weight form of IGF-II has recently been implicated as a cause of hypoglycemia in patients with hepatocellular tumors.

The prognosis for these tumors is generally poor, and surgical removal should be attempted when feasible. Dietary management of the hypoglycemia is the mainstay of medical treatment, since diazoxide is usually ineffective.

POSTPRANDIAL HYPOGLYCEMIA (Reactive Hypoglycemia)

Postgastrectomy Alimentary Hypoglycemia

Reactive hypoglycemia following gastrectomy is a consequence of hyperinsulinism resulting from rapid gastric emptying of ingested food. Symptoms result from adrenergic hyperactivity in response to the hypoglycemia. Treatment consists of more frequent feedings with smaller portions of less rapidly assimilated carbohydrate and more slowly absorbed fat and protein.

Functional Alimentary Hypoglycemia

This syndrome is classified as functional when no postsurgical explanation exists for the presence of early alimentary type reactive hypoglycemia. It is most often associated with chronic fatigue, anxiety, irritability, weakness, poor concentration, decreased libido, headaches, hunger after meals, and tremulousness. However, most patients with these symptoms do not have hypoglycemia. (See Chronic Fatigue Syndrome in Chapter 1.)

Indiscriminate use and overinterpretation of glucose tolerance tests have led to an unfortunate tendency to overdiagnose functional hypoglycemia. *As many as one-third or more of* normal *subjects have hypoglycemia reaching nadirs as low as 40–50 mg/dL with or without symptoms during a 4-hour glucose tolerance test.* Accordingly, to increase diagnostic reliability, hypoglycemia should preferably be documented during a spontaneous symptomatic episode accompanying routine daily activity, with clinical improvement following feeding.

In patients with documented postprandial hypoglycemia on a functional basis, there is no harm and occasional benefit in reducing the proportion of carbohydrate in the diet while increasing the frequency and reducing the size of meals. Support and mild sedation should be the mainstays of therapy, with dietary manipulation only an adjunct.

Late Hypoglycemia (Occult Diabetes)

This condition is characterized by a delay in early insulin release from pancreatic B cells, resulting in initial exaggeration of hyperglycemia during a glucose tolerance test. In response to this hyperglycemia, an exaggerated insulin release produces a late hypoglycemia 4–5 hours after ingestion of glucose. These patients are usually quite different from those with early hypoglycemia, often being obese and frequently having a family history of diabetes mellitus.

In obese patients, treatment is directed at weight reduction to achieve ideal weight. Like all patients with postprandial hypoglycemia, regardless of cause, these patients often respond to reduced carbohydrate intake with multiple, spaced, small feedings high in protein. They should be considered potential diabetics and advised to have periodic medical evaluations.

ALCOHOL HYPOGLYCEMIA

Fasting Hypoglycemia After Ethanol

During the postabsorptive state, normal plasma glucose is maintained by hepatic glucose output derived from both glycogenolysis and gluconeogenesis. With prolonged starvation, glycogen reserves become depleted within 18–24 hours and hepatic glucose output becomes totally dependent on gluconeogenesis. Under these circumstances, a blood concentration of ethanol as low as 45 mg/dL (considerably below the California legal "under the influence" level for drivers of 80 mg/dL) can induce profound hypoglycemia by blocking gluconeogenesis. Neuroglycopenia in a patient whose breath smells of alcohol may be mistaken for alcoholic stupor. Prevention consists of adequate food intake during ethanol ingestion. Therapy consists of glucose administration to replenish glycogen stores until gluconeogenesis resumes.

Postethanol Reactive Hypoglycemia

When sugar-containing soft drinks are used as mixers to dilute alcohol in beverages (gin and tonic, rum and cola), there seems to be a greater insulin release than when the soft drink alone is ingested and a tendency for more of a late hypoglycemic overswing to occur 3–4 hours later. Prevention would consist of avoiding sugar mixers while ingesting alcohol or ensuring supplementary food intake to provide sustained absorption.

FACTITIOUS HYPOGLYCEMIA

Factitious hypoglycemia may be difficult to document. A suspicion of self-induced hypoglycemia is supported when the patient is associated with the health professions or has access to insulin or sulfonylurea drugs taken by a diabetic member of the family. The triad of hypoglycemia, high immunoreactive insulin, and suppressed plasma C peptide immunoreactivity is pathognomonic of exogenous insulin administration. Demonstration of circulating antibodies supports this diagnosis in suspected cases. When sulfonylureas are suspected as a cause of factitious hypoglycemia, a chemical test of the plasma to detect the presence of these drugs may be required to distinguish laboratory findings from those of insulinoma.

IMMUNOPATHOLOGIC HYPOGLYCEMIA

This rare cause of hypoglycemia, documented in isolated case reports, may occur as two distinct disorders: one associated with spontaneous development of circulating anti-insulin antibodies and another associated with antibodies to insulin receptors, in which the antibodies apparently have agonist capabilities.

PENTAMIDINE-INDUCED HYPOGLYCEMIA
(See also Chapter 27.)

With the increased prevalence of pulmonary infection by *Pneumocystis carinii* in patients with ac-

quired immune deficiency syndrome, pentamidine given intravenously or by aerosol is being used more frequently and in 10–20% of patients produce symptomatic hypoglycemia. This apparently is due to lytic destruction of pancreatic B cells, causing acute hyperinsulinemia and hypoglycemia, followed later by insulinopenia and hyperglycemia which occasionally is persistent. Intravenous glucose should be administered during pentamidine administration and for the period immediately following to prevent or ameliorate hypoglycemic symptoms. Following a complete course of therapy with pentamidine, fasting blood glucose or a subsequent glycohemoglobin should be monitored to assess the extent of pancreatic B cell recovery or residual damage.

Doherty GM et al: Results of a prospective strategy to diagnose, localize and resect insulinomas. Surgery 1991; 110:989.

Grunberger G et al: Factitious hypoglycemia due to surreptitious administration of insulin: Diagnosis, treatment, and long-term follow-up. Ann Intern Med 1988;108:252.

Marks V, Teale JD: Tumors producing hypoglycemia. Diabetes Metab Rev 1991;7:79. (Pathogenesis and therapy of hypoglycemia produced by pancreatic and extrapancreatic neoplasms.)

Palardy J et al: Blood glucose measurements during symptomatic episodes in patients with suspected postprandial hypoglycemia. N Engl J Med 1989;321:1421.

Polansky KS: A practical approach to fasting hypoglycemia. N Engl J Med 1992;326:1020.

Service FJ: Hypoglycemias. West J Med 1991;154:442.

Service FJ et al: Functioning insulinoma: Incidence, recurrence, and long-term survival of patients—a 60-year study. Mayo Clin Proc 1991;66:711.

Waskin H et al: Risk factors for hypoglycemia associated with pentamidine therapy for *Pneumocystis* pneumonia. JAMA 1988;260:345.

Lipid Abnormalities

27

Warren S. Browner, MD, MPH

Serum lipoproteins are of importance to the clinician mainly because of their relation to atherosclerotic vascular disease, especially coronary heart disease. Several clinical trials showing that lowering high blood cholesterol reduces the incidence of coronary heart disease have given impetus to nationwide campaigns to reduce serum cholesterol levels. A major problem for clinicians is that current therapies for high blood cholesterol do not reduce total mortality, in part because their use has been associated with an unexplained increase in deaths from noncardiovascular causes. Another problem is that most of the clinical trials have been conducted in middle-aged men; the effects of cholesterol-lowering in women, in young men, and in the elderly are not known.

LIPIDS & LIPOPROTEINS

The two main lipids in blood are cholesterol and triglyceride. They are carried in lipoproteins, which are globular packages that also contain proteins known as apoproteins. Cholesterol is an essential element of all animal cell membranes and forms the backbone of steroid hormones and bile acids; triglycerides are important in transferring energy from food into cells. Why lipids are deposited into the walls of large and medium-sized arteries—an event with potentially lethal consequences—is not known.

Lipoproteins are usually classified on the basis of how dense they are. Density is determined by the amounts of triglyceride (which makes them less dense) and apoproteins (which have the opposite effect). The least dense particles, known as chylomicrons, are normally found in the blood only after fat-containing foods have been eaten. Chylomicrons rise as a creamy layer when nonfasting serum is allowed to stand. The other lipoproteins are suspended in serum and must be separated using a centrifuge. The densest (and smallest) family of particles consists mainly of apoproteins and cholesterol and are called high-density lipoproteins (HDLs). Somewhat less dense are the low-density lipoproteins (LDLs). Least dense are the large, very low density lipoproteins (VLDLs), consisting mainly of triglyceride. In fasting serum, most of the cholesterol is carried on LDL particles and is therefore referred to as LDL cholesterol; most of the triglyceride is found in VLDL particles. Specific apoproteins are associated with each lipoprotein class.

A less common way to classify lipoproteins takes advantage of their different electrical charges and weights by using electrophoresis to separate them. This results in an alternative nomenclature, based on the alpha (HDL), beta (LDL), and prebeta (VLDL) bands that form.

Chylomicrons are made in the gut and travel via the portal vein into the liver and via the thoracic duct into the circulation. They are normally completely metabolized, transferring energy from food into muscle and fat cells. The liver manufactures VLDL particles from its own stores of fat and carbohydrate. VLDL particles transfer triglyceride to cells; after losing enough, they eventually become LDL particles, which provide cholesterol for cellular needs. (Along the way, there is also a class of transient molecules that are between VLDLs and LDLs in density, known as intermediate-density lipoproteins.) Excess LDL particles are taken up by the liver, and the cholesterol they contain is then excreted into the bile. HDL particles are made in the liver and intestine and appear to facilitate the transfer of apoproteins among lipoproteins. They also participate in reverse cholesterol transport, either by transferring cholesterol into other lipoproteins or directly into the liver.

LIPOPROTEINS & ATHEROGENESIS

The plaques found in the arterial walls of patients with atherosclerosis contain large amounts of cholesterol, providing an early clue that serum cholesterol might be an important factor in their development. Epidemiologic studies have clearly established that the higher the level of LDL cholesterol, the greater the risk of atherosclerotic heart disease; conversely, the higher the level of HDL cholesterol, the lower the risk of coronary heart disease. This is true in men and women, in different racial and ethnic groups, and at all adult ages. Because most cholesterol in serum is LDL cholesterol, high total cholesterol levels are also

1014 / CHAPTER 27

associated with an increased risk of coronary heart disease. Middle-aged men whose serum cholesterol levels are in the highest quintile for age (above about 230 mg/dL) have a risk of coronary death before age 65 of about 11%; men in the lowest quintile (below about 170 mg/dL) have a 3% risk. Death from coronary heart disease before age 65 is less common in women, so the equivalent risks would be about one-third those of men. As a general approximation in men, each 10 mg/dL increase in cholesterol (or LDL cholesterol) increases the risk of coronary heart disease by about 10%; each 5 mg/dL increase in HDL reduces the risk by about 10%. The effect of HDL cholesterol is greater in women, whereas the effects of total and LDL cholesterol are smaller. All of these relationships tend to diminish with age.

The exact mechanism by which LDL particles result in the formation of atherosclerotic plaques—or the means whereby HDL particles protect against their formation—is not known. The simple model of LDL carrying cholesterol into the walls of arteries, with HDL removing it, is more useful as a mnemonic than as a representation of what is known. Recent work suggests that LDL particles which have become oxidized (a process that occurs naturally) may be particularly atherogenic. There are receptors on the surface of macrophages within atherosclerotic plaques that bind and accumulate oxidized LDLs. The formation of antibodies to oxidized LDLs may also be important in plaque formation. Thus, there is growing interest in the role of antioxidants, such as vitamins C and E and perhaps estrogens, in the prevention of atherosclerosis. Another recent discovery has been that high levels of a variant type of LDL, the lipoprotein antigen, or Lp(a), are associated with an increased risk of coronary heart disease. Finally, the size of the LDL molecule itself may influence its atherogenesis; at the same LDL concentrations, those persons with large numbers of smaller particles appear to be at high risk for coronary heart disease.

The relationship of VLDL cholesterol to atherogenesis is less certain. Perhaps the number or size of VLDL particles—rather than the total amount in serum—is important. In addition, HDL and VLDL levels are inversely related, so that the patient with a high VLDL level is likely to have a low HDL level and thus be at increased risk for coronary heart disease for that reason alone.

There are several genetic disorders that provide insight into the pathogenesis of lipid-related diseases. Most important—but fortunately rare in the homozygous state (about one per million)—is a condition in which the cell-surface receptors for the LDL molecule are absent or defective. This disorder is also known as familial hypercholesterolemia. These patients have reduced ability to metabolize LDL particles, resulting in high LDL levels and premature atherosclerosis. Patients with two abnormal genes (homozygotes) have extremely high LDL levels—up

to eight times normal—and may present with atherosclerotic disease in childhood. Homozygotes may require liver transplantation to correct their severe lipid abnormalities. Those with one defective gene (heterozygotes) have LDL concentrations that are approximately twice normal; persons men with this condition often present with coronary heart disease in their 30s or 40s.

Another rare condition is characterized by an abnormality of lipoprotein lipase, the enzyme that enables peripheral tissues (muscle and adipose cells, for example) to take up triglyceride from chylomicrons and VLDL particles. Patients with this condition (which is one of the causes of familial hyperchylomicronemia) have a marked increase in triglyceride concentrations and usually present with recurrent pancreatitis and hepatosplenomegaly in childhood.

There are several other genetic abnormalities of lipid metabolism, usually named for the abnormality that appears when serum is electrophoresed (eg, dysbetaliproteinemia) or from the particular combinations of lipid abnormalities that appear in families (eg, familial combined hyperlipidemia). These entities are important to the clinician because they emphasize the need to screen family members of patients with severe lipid disorders. Some of these patients have abnormalities in the production of various apoproteins, such as increased levels of apoprotein B and its affiliated lipoproteins, LDL and VLDL, or reduced production of apoprotein AII and its affiliated particle, HDL.

Lipids may also be related to the risk of coronary heart disease through effects other than the formation of atherosclerotic plaques. In particular, there may be an association between certain types of lipids and thrombogenesis. This may explain the lower rates of coronary disease in persons who consume diets that have certain types of fats, such as those found in marine fish. These fats in the n-3 (or omega-3) family have a double bond after the third carbon atom in the fatty acid chain of the fat molecule and appear to reduce platelet aggregation. Recent studies have also suggested that there are important differences in whether fatty acids are in the *trans* or *cis* configuration; partially hydrogenated vegetable oils, used to make margarine and shortening, for example, have artificial *trans* isomers and have been associated with increased risk of coronary heart disease.

Antibodies to oxidized LDL in atherosclerosis. Lancet 1992;339:899. (The importance of oxidized LDLs in atherogenesis.)

Martin MJ et al: Serum cholesterol, blood pressure and mortality: Implications from a cohort of 361,662 men. Lancet 1986;2:933. (The higher the cholesterol, the greater the coronary risk.)

NCEP Adult Treatment Panel: Report of the National Cholesterol Education Program Expert Panel on detection, evaluation, and treatment of high blood cholesterol in adults. Arch Intern Med 1988;148:36.

Simon J: Vitamin C and cardiovascular disease: A review. J Am Coll Nutr 1992;11:107.

Toronto Working Group: Asymptomatic hypercholesterolemia: A clinical policy review. J Clin Epidemiol 1990; 43:1029. (A less aggressive approach than that of the NCEP.)

Willett WC et al: Intake of *trans* fatty acids and risk of coronary heart disease among women. Lancet 1993; 341:581. (Women in the highest quintile of consumption of *trans* isomers [from margarine and shortening in baked goods] had a 50% higher risk of coronary heart disease. By contrast, consumption of butter and red meat were not associated with coronary heart disease.)

LIPID FRACTIONS & THE RISK OF CORONARY HEART DISEASE

In fasting serum, cholesterol is carried on three different lipoproteins—the VLDL, LDL, and HDL molecules. Total cholesterol equals the sum of these three components:

Total cholesterol = HDL cholesterol + VLDL cholesterol + LDL cholesterol

Most clinical laboratories measure the total cholesterol and the total triglyceride as well as the amount of cholesterol found in the HDL fraction, which is easily precipitated from serum. The vast majority of triglyceride is found in VLDL particles, which contain about five times as much triglyceride by weight as cholesterol. Thus, the amount of cholesterol found in the VLDL fraction can be estimated by dividing the triglyceride by 5:

$$\text{VLDL cholesterol} = \frac{\text{Triglycerides}}{5}$$

Because the triglyceride level is used as a proxy for the amount of VLDL, this formula only works in fasting samples. (Chylomicrons, which contain almost no cholesterol, elevate the triglyceride level in nonfasting samples.) Furthermore, it only works when the triglyceride level is less than 500–600 mg/dL. At higher triglyceride levels (as is the case when serum appears lipemic, or cloudy), LDL and VLDL cholesterol levels can be determined after centrifugation.

The total cholesterol is reasonably stable over time; however, measurements of HDL and especially triglyceride may vary considerably because of error in the laboratory and because of real day-to-day variation in a patient's triglyceride level. Thus, the LDL should always be estimated as the mean of at least two determinations; if those two estimates differ by more than 10%, a third lipid profile should be obtained. It is estimated as follows:

$$\text{LDL cholesterol} = \text{Total cholesterol} - \text{HDL cholesterol} - \frac{\text{Triglycerides}}{5}$$

Note that when using SI units (which measure lipids by moles rather than weight), the equivalent formula becomes:

$$\text{LDL cholesterol} = \text{Total cholesterol (mmol/L)} - \text{HDL cholesterol (mmol/L)} - \frac{\text{Triglycerides (mmol/L)}}{2.2}$$

Understanding the relationships of the different types of lipoproteins leads to a more sophisticated understanding of a patient's lipid-related coronary risk than simply knowing the total cholesterol level. Two persons with the same total cholesterol of 275 mg/dL may have very different lipid profiles. One may have an HDL of 110 mg/dL with a triglyceride of 150 mg/dL, with an estimated LDL cholesterol of 135 mg/dL; the other may have an HDL of 25 mg/dL with a triglyceride of 200 mg/dL and an LDL cholesterol of 210 mg/dL. All other risk factors being equal, the second patient would have more than a tenfold higher coronary heart disease risk than the first. Because high HDL cholesterol levels are common in women, many women with apparently high total cholesterol levels actually have favorable lipid profiles.

Some authorities use the ratio of the total cholesterol to HDL cholesterol as an indicator of lipid-related coronary risk: the lower this ratio is, the better. (In the example from the previous paragraph, the first person would have a ratio of 275 ÷ 110 = 2.5, while the second would have a much less favorable ratio of 275 ÷ 25 = 11.) While intuitively convenient as a summary measure, the ratio may obscure potentially important information (a total cholesterol of 300 mg/dL and an HDL of 60 mg/dL results in the same ratio of 5 as a total cholesterol of 150 mg/dL with an HDL of 30 mg/dL). Moreover, errors in the measurement of HDL cholesterol are common in many laboratories, and the total cholesterol-to-HDL cholesterol ratio magnifies their importance.

There is no "normal" range for serum lipids. In Western populations, cholesterol values are about 20% higher than in Asian populations and exceed 300 mg/dL in nearly 5% of adults. About 10% of adults have LDL cholesterol levels above 200 mg/dL. In general, total and LDL cholesterol levels rise with age.

Declines in cholesterol levels are seen when a patient is acutely ill. Thus, it is rarely appropriate to measure lipid levels in an ill or hospitalized patient, with the notable exception of the serum triglyceride level in a patient with pancreatitis. Cholesterol levels (even when expressed as an age-matched percentile rank, such as the highest 20%) do not remain constant over time, especially from childhood through adolescence and young adulthood. Thus, children and young adults with relatively high cholesterol levels may have lower levels later in life, whereas those with low cholesterol levels may later have higher levels.

Garber AM, Sox HC Jr, Littenberg B: Screening asymptomatic adults for cardiac risk factors: The serum cholesterol level. Ann Intern Med 1989;110:622.

Hulley SB et al: Should we be measuring blood cholesterol levels in young adults? JAMA 1993;269:1416. (Recommends against screening in men and women at least until middle age.)

Newman TB, Browner WS, Hulley SB: The case against childhood cholesterol screening. JAMA 1990; 264:3039.

THERAPEUTIC EFFECTS OF LOWERING CHOLESTEROL

Most studies of the effect of cholesterol lowering have distinguished between primary prevention (treating high blood cholesterol in persons free of coronary heart disease) and secondary prevention (treating persons with manifest coronary heart disease). The important distinction is that primary prevention trials enroll healthy subjects who have relatively low rates of coronary disease but in whom other causes of morbidity and mortality are relatively common. Secondary prevention trials, on the other hand, follow patients who have a high rate of subsequent coronary disease; other causes of mortality are relatively less important.

Several clinical trials have established that reducing cholesterol levels in healthy middle-aged men without coronary heart disease reduces their risk and that the reduction in risk is proportionate to the reduction in LDL cholesterol and the increase in HDL cholesterol. Patients in the treatment groups have had statistically significant and clinically important reductions in the rates of myocardial infarctions, new cases of angina, and need for coronary artery bypass procedures. As with most primary prevention interventions, however, large numbers of healthy patients need to be treated to prevent a single event; for cholesterol lowering, it may be necessary to treatment more than 600 patients for several years to prevent a single coronary death or five or six nonfatal coronary events.

Beneficial effects on the risk of coronary heart disease have been seen with the bile acid binding resins and with gemfibrozil; the evidence for benefit from dietary reduction of cholesterol is less clear. However, none of these studies have shown a reduction in total mortality. On the contrary, pooling the results of the primary prevention trials indicates that the use of cholesterol-lowering therapies has been associated with statistically significant increases in deaths from cancer (by 43%) and from injuries and violence (by 76%). These adverse effects remain unexplained, but they should not be ignored.

In patients—again, mainly middle-aged men—who already have coronary heart disease, the net benefits of cholesterol lowering are clearer, with reductions in the progression of coronary atherosclerosis, fewer subsequent coronary events, less mortality from coronary heart disease, and perhaps a reduction in mortality from all causes. The important exceptions among currently available therapies are the fibric acid derivatives (clofibrate and gemfibrozil), which have not shown benefits in the secondary prevention of coronary heart disease, and probucol, which has not been studies with clinical end points. Several studies have also shown that cholesterol lowering actually causes regression of atherosclerotic plaques in some patients, including women. This effects appears to occur throughout the range of LDL cholesterol levels; the lower the LDL, the greater the regression. The important exceptions among currently available therapies are the fibric acid derivatives (clofibrate and gemfibrozil), which have not shown benefits in the secondary prevention of coronary heart disease, and probucol, which has not been studied with clinical end points.

These apparent disparities highlight several important points. The benefits and adverse effects of cholesterol lowering appear to be specific to each type of drug; the clinician cannot assume that the effects will generalize to other classes of medication. Second, the net benefits from cholesterol lowering depend upon the underlying risk of coronary heart disease and of other disease. In patients with manifest atherosclerosis, morbidity and mortality rates associated with coronary heart disease are high, and measures that reduce coronary heart disease are more likely to be beneficial even if they have no effect—or even slightly harmful effects—on other diseases. Third, we do not know the effect of cholesterol lowering in women and among older and younger men. At this time, our intentions are better than our results with the available interventions.

Cashin-Hemphill L et al: Beneficial effects of colestipol-niacin on coronary atherosclerosis: A 4-year follow-up. JAMA 1990;264:3013. (Among middle-aged men who had previously undergone coronary artery bypass grafting, regression and nonprogression of lesions occurred more frequently in the treated group.)

Kane JP et al: Regression of coronary atherosclerosis during treatment of familial hypercholesterolemia with combined drug regimens. JAMA 1990;264:3007. (Of the 40 treatment subjects [mean LDL cholesterol 283 mg/dL] who completed the trial, 13 had definite regression of coronary lesions, compared with 4 of 32 in the control group. Results were generally similar in men and women.)

Lipid Research Clinical Investigators: The Lipid Research Clinic Coronary Primary Prevention Trials. Results of 6 years of post-trial follow-up. Arch Intern Med 1992;

152:1399. (Follow-up after the trial found no significant differences between the treatment and placebo group in most important outcomes, such as total mortality, coronary heart disease incidence, or cancer incidence.)

Muldoon M, Manuck S, Matthews K: Lowering cholesterol concentrations and mortality: A quantitative review of primary prevention trials. Br Med J 1990;310:309. (Pooling the results shows harmful effects of cholesterol-lowering on deaths from injuries and cancer.)

Peto R, Yusuf S, Collins R: Cholesterol-lowering trial results in their epidemiologic context. J Am Coll Cardiol 1991;17:III-451. (Adverse effects may be due to chance.)

Silberberg JS, Henry DA: The benefits of reducing cholesterol levels: The need to distinguish primary from secondary prevention. I. A meta-analysis of cholesterol-lowering trials. Med J Aust 1991;155:665. (Estimates that in secondary prevention, about 38 persons need to be treated with cholesterol-lower therapies for several years to prevent one coronary death, compared with 675 persons in primary prevention.)

LOW CHOLESTEROL & OTHER DISEASES

While high cholesterol levels are clearly associated with an increased risk of coronary heart disease, low cholesterol levels (especially < 160 mg/dL) are associated with an increased risk of mortality from other causes, including cancer, respiratory disease, injuries and accidents, and liver disease. The biologic explanation for this excess mortality is not known. Some studies have suggested that low cholesterol represents a preclinical manifestation of the underlying disease, eg, an undiagnosed malignancy. More recent analyses have found that the increase in risk persists for at least several years. Thus, the net effect is that the overall relationship between cholesterol and mortality is somewhat bowl-shaped, with mortality rates being highest in those with either low or high cholesterol levels.

Jacobs D et al: Conference on Low Blood Cholesterol Levels: Mortality associations. Circulation 1992;86:1046. (See also accompanying editorial by Hulley, Newman, and Walsh.)

SECONDARY CONDITIONS THAT AFFECT LIPID METABOLISM

Several factors, including drugs, can influence serum lipids (Table 27–1). These are of importance for two reasons: abnormal lipid levels (or changes in lipid levels) may be the presenting sign of some of these conditions, and correction of the underlying condition may obviate the need to treat an apparent lipid disorder. Diabetes and alcohol use, in particular, are commonly associated with high triglyceride levels that decline with improvements in glycemic control or reduction in alcohol use, respectively. While it

Table 27–1. Secondary causes of lipid abnormalities.

Cause	Associated Lipid Abnormality
Obesity	Increased triglyceride, decreased HDL cholesterol
Sedentary lifestyle	Decreased HDL cholesterol
Diabetes	Increased triglyceride, increased total cholesterol
Alcohol use	Increased triglyceride, increased HDL cholesterol
Hypothyroidism	Increased total cholesterol
Hyperthyroidism	Decreased total cholesterol
Nephrotic syndrome	Increased total cholesterol
Chronic renal insufficiency	Increased total cholesterol, increased triglyceride
Hepatic disease (cirrhosis)	Decreased total cholesterol
Obstructive liver disease	Increased total cholesterol
Malignancy	Decreased total cholesterol
Cushing's disease (or steroid use)	Increased total cholesterol
Oral contraceptives	Increased triglyceride, increased total cholesterol
Diuretics	Increased total cholesterol, increased triglyceride
Beta-blockers[1]	Increased total cholesterol, decreased HDL

[1]Beta-blockers with intrinsic sympathomimetic activity, such as pindolol and acebutolol, do not affect lipid levels.

is not necessary to rule out each of these secondary causes, the clinician should consider each possibility.

CLINICAL PRESENTATIONS

Most patients with high cholesterol levels have no specific signs or symptoms. The vast majority of patients with lipid abnormalities are detected by the laboratory, either as part of the workup of a patient with vascular disease, as part of a preventive screening strategy, or on a "routine" chemistry panel. Extremely high levels of chylomicrons or VLDL particles (triglyceride level above 1000 mg/dL) result in the formation of eruptive xanthomas (red-yellow papules, especially on the buttocks). High LDL levels result in xanthomas on certain tendons (Achilles, patella, back of the hand). Such xanthomas usually indicate one of the underlying genetic hyperlipidemias. Lipemia retinalis (cream-colored blood vessels in the fundus) is seen with extremely high triglyceride levels (above 2000 mg/dL).

SCREENING FOR HIGH BLOOD CHOLESTEROL

All patients with cardiovascular disease—whether manifest (eg, angina, claudication) or asymptomatic (inferior Q waves, femoral bruit)—should be screened for elevated lipids (Figure 27–1); the only exceptions would be patients in whom lipid-lowering is not indicated or desirable for other reasons (such as end-stage pulmonary disease or dementia). Patients who already have evidence of atherosclerosis are the group at highest risk of suffering additional manifestations in the near term and thus have the most to gain. Additional risk reduction measures for atherosclerosis are discussed in Chapter 10; lipid lowering should be just one aspect of a program to reduce the progression and effects of the disease.

Given the high prevalence of underlying lipid abnormalities in patients with cardiovascular disease, a complete lipid profile (total cholesterol, HDL cholesterol, and triglyceride levels) should be obtained as a screening test. Those whose estimated LDL cholesterol level is high should have at least one repeat measurement. Specific treatments for high LDL cholesterol levels are discussed below. The goal of therapy should be to reduce the LDL cholesterol as far as possible, even to below about 100 mg/dL. If this goal cannot be reached, the clinician should recognize that any reduction in LDL is better than no reduction. Moreover, the benefits of LDL reduction are greatest (in terms of coronary events prevented) at the high end; further reductions carry progressively less benefit. In patients with coronary heart disease in whom

dietary therapy is unlikely to reduce the LDL cholesterol sufficiently (such as a patient with a confirmed LDL cholesterol of 200 mg/dL who is already following a reasonably low-fat diet), drug therapy can be considered immediately.

The best strategy for the remainder of the adult population who do not have atherosclerotic cardiovascular disease is not clear. Whatever strategy is chosen, its purpose should be clear: to reduce the risk of coronary heart disease in persons with elevated levels of cholesterol by treating them with safe and effective therapies. This requires that the clinician determine, almost on a case-by-case basis, what constitutes an elevated cholesterol, and then to balance the potential benefits, risks, and costs of treatment (Figure 27–2). Coronary heart disease is a multifactorial disease; thus, a cholesterol level of 250 mg/dL in a 45-year-old woman with no coronary risk factors is associated with much less coronary risk than the same cholesterol level in a 45-year-old male smoker with hypertension and diabetes. Known risk factors for coronary heart disease include age and sex (coronary disease is rare in men before age 40 and in women before age 50), a family history of premature coronary heart disease (myocardial infarction or sudden cardiac death before age 55 in a first-degree relative), hypertension (whether treated or not), cigarette smoking (especially > 10 cigarettes a day), diabetes mellitus (whether treated or not), obesity (above 130% of ideal weight), and a low HDL cholesterol (< 35 mg/dL). Given that a high HDL level is protective against coronary heart disease, clinicians may "subtract" one risk factor in persons with an HDL

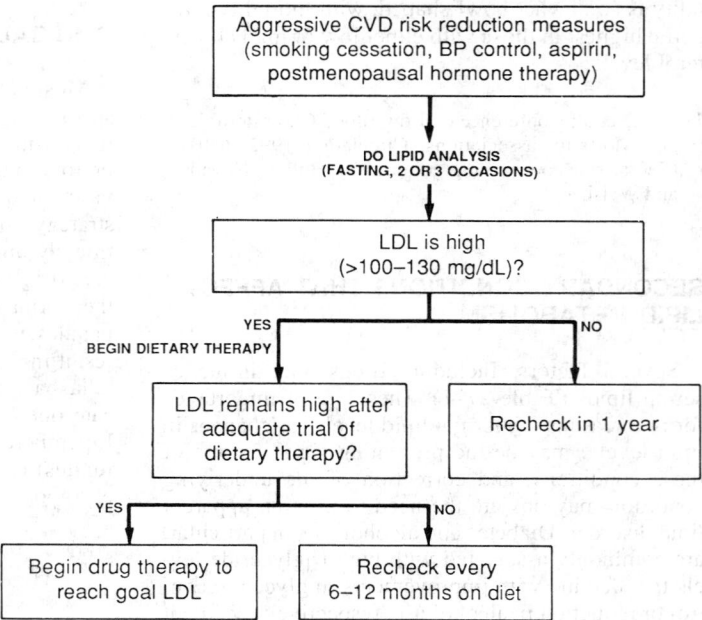

Figure 27–1. Suggested algorithm for screening and management of patients with known cardiovascular disease. Treatment cutpoints and goals discussed in text.

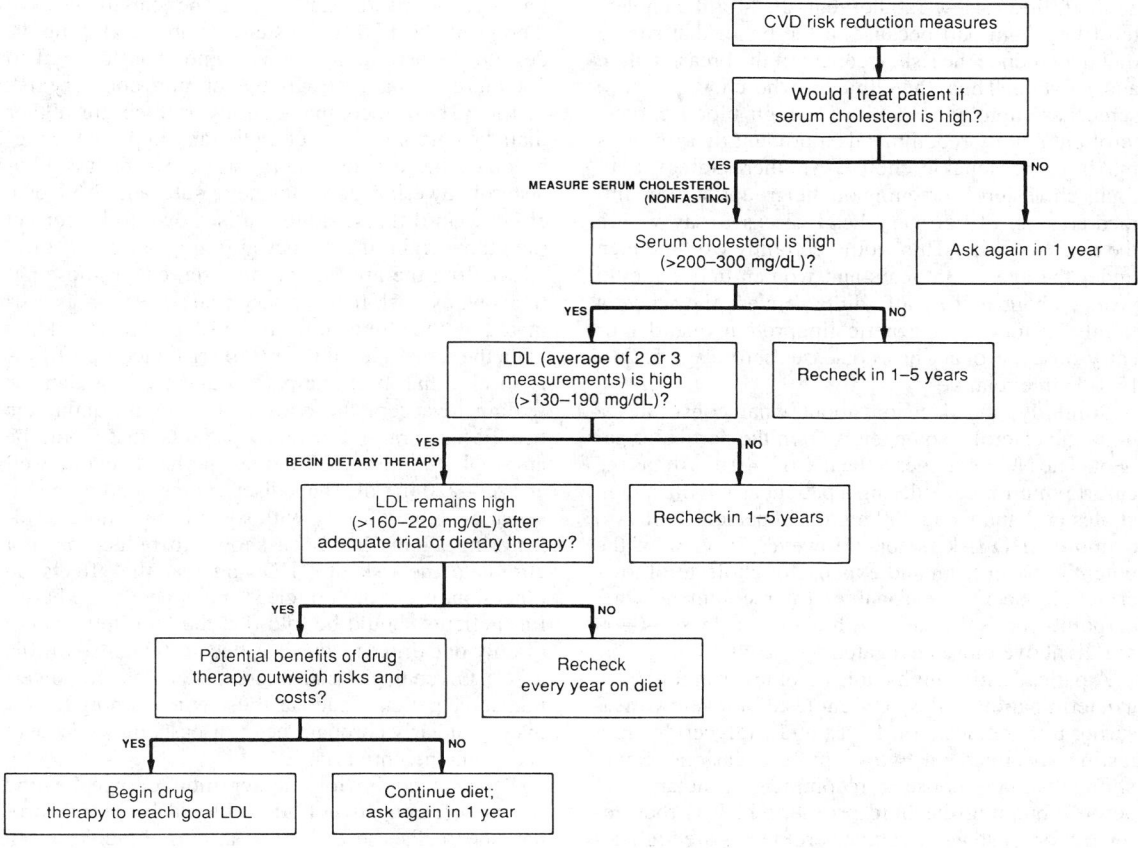

Figure 27–2. Suggested algorithm for screening and management of patients free of cardiovascular disease. Treatment cutpoints and goals discussed in text.

cholesterol above about 50 mg/dL and two risk factors in those with an HDL cholesterol above 70 mg/dL.

Each risk factor about doubles the risk of coronary heart disease. Thus, at the same serum cholesterol level, someone with five risk factors (a 45-year-old man with diabetes and hypertension who smokes and has a low HDL concentration) would be at more than a 30-fold (ie, $2 \times 2 \times 2 \times 2 \times 2$) increase in risk for coronary heart disease compared with a woman of about that age with no risk factors. Since the potential benefits of cholesterol lowering are roughly proportionate to the underlying risk of coronary heart disease, they would be more than 30 times greater in the high-risk man than in the low-risk woman. The costs and potential harm from therapy, however, would be comparable in the two patients.

While there are substantial epidemiologic data supporting the hypothesis that patients with several risk factors should derive more benefit from treatment, the clinician should be aware that the two major studies of intervention programs designed to reduce multiple risk factors simultaneously (the Multiple Risk Factor Intervention Trial, or MRFIT, in high-risk middle-aged men in the USA, and a Finnish study in high-risk middle-aged male executives) both failed to demonstrate a benefit from such an intervention strategy among healthy men. In fact, in the Finnish study, the intervention group had significantly more deaths (including more deaths from coronary heart disease) in long-term follow-up. Satisfactory explanations for the results of these studies are lacking.

Some clinicians may prefer to screen all adults, believing that all are eventually at risk of atherosclerosis. This is the strategy recommended by the National Cholesterol Education Program (NCEP) and by many experts in the field of lipid metabolism. The clinician who chooses this option should recognize that many patients will have persistently high cholesterol levels despite nonpharmacologic therapies. The clinician will then face the dilemma whether to use drugs of uncertain efficacy or safety in a healthy patient. Moreover, most authorities recommend (and many adults follow) a low-fat diet regardless of the cholesterol level—in part because of the belief that such a diet may reduce the risk of cancer of the breast, colon, and prostate. Thus, the clinician who chooses not to screen asymptomatic adults for high blood cholesterol but simply recommends a prudent diet for all is making a reasonable choice. Another strategy is to focus cholesterol screening on the groups at more immediate risk of coronary heart disease—say within the next 10 years. This would certainly exclude men under the age of 35 years and women under age 45 years—about half of all adults—unless they have a family history of a genetic lipoprotein disorder or early-onset coronary heart disease (before age 55 in a first-degree relative).

Similarly, the decision about what constitutes a high cholesterol also depends upon the particular patient. The NCEP suggests the use of 240 mg/dL as the cutoff point for considering a patient as having a high cholesterol and using 200 mg/dL in persons with two or more CHD risk factors. However, in view of the potential harm from and expense of cholesterol lowering, it seems reasonable to recommend that cutpoints be substantially higher—at least 40–60 mg/dL above those advocated by the NCEP.

A patient with a high cholesterol level should have a determination of the LDL cholesterol level by measuring total cholesterol, HDL, and triglycerides in a fasting specimen on two or more occasions. Some clinicians may choose to recommend a dietary trial before obtaining the lipid profile, which is then reserved for those whose cholesterol levels are high despite a cholesterol-lowering diet. Others may choose to estimate the LDL cholesterol before making such a recommendation.

Patients with a high LDL cholesterol should be counseled about nonpharmacologic methods to lower their LDL. Many clinicians may wish to refer such patients to a dietician or to provide patients with a book on cholesterol-lowering diets.* Again, the determination of what is a high LDL cholesterol should be made in light of the patient's other coronary risk factors. The NCEP Expert Panel suggests that values above 160 mg/dL are high; the cutpoint for non-pharmacologic therapy is lowered to 130 mg/dL in patients with two or more coronary risk factors.

The patient should be allowed 6–12 months to make the recommended dietary changes. In many patients, the LDL cholesterol remains high despite an adequate trial of diet therapy, and the question will then arise whether treatment with cholesterol-lowering drugs is indicated. The decision to start a healthy patient on a drug that may cost more than $100 a month and that may increase noncardiovascular mortality should be made cautiously. The NCEP Expert Panel recommends that patients be started on drug therapy if the LDL cholesterol is above 190 mg/dL despite dietary therapy; this cutpoint is lowered to 160 mg/dL in patients with two or more coronary risk factors. These recommendations—which are higher than the cutpoints for dietary therapy in partial recognition of the costs of drug therapy—assume that cholesterol lowering does not have substantial adverse effects. Until that assumption is shown to be correct (and the weight of evidence currently suggests otherwise), drug therapy should be reserved for those patients whose risk for coronary heart disease—as estimated by the clinician from the LDL cholesterol and from the remainder of their CHD risk factor profile—is so high that both the patient and the clinician are willing to accept the current uncertainty about the benefit/harm ratio. For many patients, that would be an LDL cholesterol above—perhaps even well above—220 mg/dL. This discussion should point out to patients that therapy with some of the cholesterol-lowering agents has been shown to reduce but not eliminate the risk of CHD and that the effects on other conditions are not clear and appear to be harmful. Patients should be told that the long-term safety of only one drug (niacin) has been established (Table 27–2). Given the intense interest in cholesterol lowering, some patients, such as those with a strong family history of early coronary heart disease, may decide to accept the potential risks.

There is no obvious upper limit of age beyond which screening is not advisable. The risk of coronary heart disease is highest among the elderly: an 80-year-old has more than a 1000-fold higher risk than a 20-year-old. The results of cholesterol lowering in persons with manifest coronary heart disease suggest that from the standpoint of the degree of atherosclerosis, it is never too late to lower an elevated cholesterol concentration. However, elderly persons may be more set in their dietary habits, may have more problems with drug side effects and interactions, and may have less to gain in terms of averted morbidity or life expectancy. Balancing these factors suggests that there are clearly patients in whom screening and treatment would be inappropriate because of very advanced age or other medical conditions.

Krahn M et al: Comparison of an aggressive (U.S.) and a less aggressive (Canadian) policy for cholesterol screening and treatment. Ann Intern Med 1991;115:248.

Rossouw J, Lewis B, Rifkind B: The value of lowering cholesterol after myocardial infarction. N Engl J Med 1990;323:1112. (Cholesterol remains a risk factor even after coronary heart disease has become manifest, and treatment is indicated.)

Siegel D et al: Risk factor modification after myocardial infarction. Ann Intern Med 1988;109:213. (Multifactorial approach.)

Sox HC Jr: Screening for lipid disorders under health care systems reform. N Engl J Med 1993;328:1269. (In

---

*A useful selection is Goor R, Goor N: *Eater's Choice: A Food Lover's Guide to Lower Cholesterol.* Houghton-Mifflin, 1987.

Table 27–2. Effects of selected cholesterol-lowering drugs.

Drug	Effect on CHD	Long-Term Safety	Effects on LDL	Effects on HDL	Effects on Triglyceride	Monthly Cost (Dose)[1]
Niacin	Reduce	Yes	↓	↑	↓	$6.00 (3 g)
Cholestyramine	Reduce	?	↓	+ / –	↑	$90.00 (16 g)[2]
Colestipol	Reduce	?	↓	+ / –	↑	$80.00 (20 g)[2]
Lovastatin	?	?	↓↓	↑	Å	$58.00 (20 mg)
Simvastatin	?	?	↓↓	↑	Å	$52.00 (10 mg)
Pravastatin	?	?	↓↓	↑	Å	$50.00 (20 mg)
Gemfibrozil	Reduce	Probably not[3]	Slight ↓	↑	ÅÅ	$60.00 (1200 mg)

[1]Wholesale price of average daily dose, 1993. Costs to patients, or for higher doses, will be higher.
[2]Cost for individual packets or bars is higher.
[3]See text for discussion of fibric acid derivatives and cancer.

healthy people, the evidence does not clearly support routine cholesterol testing.)

Strandberg TE et al: Long-term mortality after 5-year multifactorial primary prevention of cardiovascular disease in middle-aged men. JAMA 1991;266:1225. (A Finnish study showing increased CHD and total mortality in the intervention group.)

TREATMENT OF HIGH LDL CHOLESTEROL

Reduction of LDL cholesterol is just one part of a program to reduce the risk of cardiovascular disease. Other measures—including smoking cessation and hypertension control—are also of central importance. Less well studied but potentially of great value is raising the HDL cholesterol level. Several "healthy habits" have more than one benefit. Quitting smoking, for example, reduces the effect of other cardiovascular risk factors (such as a high cholesterol level); it may also increase the HDL cholesterol level. Exercise (and weight loss) may reduce the LDL cholesterol level and increase the HDL cholesterol level. Modest alcohol use (1–2 ounces a day) also raises HDL levels and appears to have a salutary effect on coronary heart disease rates. While the clinician may not wish to recommend alcohol use to patients, its safe use in moderation need not be discouraged.

Diet

Dietary modifications are assigned the central role in most algorithms for treatment of elevated lipid levels. The assumption is that the beneficial effects on coronary heart disease rates with drugs that lower cholesterol will generalize to lipid-lowering diets—and the reasonable hope is that the harmful effects will not. The primary recommendation is to reduce the consumption of total dietary fat to less than 30% of total calories, which should be set at the level required to achieve and then maintain ideal body weight. Most Americans currently eat 35–40% of calories as fat. In someone eating 2000 kcal a day, 30% of calories as fat would correspond to about 67 g of fat (one pat of butter or margarine contains 15 g). Many clinicians without special expertise and interest in dietary therapy find it advantageous to refer patients to a dietitian. This may be especially helpful if stringent diets (20% calories as fat, with < 7% as saturated fat) are prescribed.

In particular, saturated fats (mainly found in animal products, including meats and dairy products) should be reduced to at most 10% of calories. Dietary cholesterol should be reduced to less than 300 mg/d (slightly more than the amount in a single egg yolk). Previous advice to substitute polyunsaturated fats (such as those found in many vegetable oils) or *trans* monounsaturated fats (such as found in margarine) has been changed; instead, foods rich in *cis* monounsaturated fats, such as olive oil, are now recommended. The average effect of cholesterol-lowering diets varies considerably, suggesting that genetic or other factors influence an individual's diet responsiveness. Overall, most studies of free-living patients have shown that low-fat diets result in only modest changes in serum cholesterol levels, with reductions in both the LDL and HDL fractions of a few mg/dL. One recent study comparing a low-fat diet (26% of calories) with a high-fat diet (41% of calories) found a reduction of about 10 mg/dL in LDL cholesterol and a reduction of about 4 mg/dL in patients eating the low-fat diet. It is not known whether the dietary-induced changes in LDL and HDL cholesterol will affect the coronary risk.

Soluble fiber, such as that found in oat bran or psyllium, may reduce LDL cholesterol levels by about 5%. Insoluble fiber (found in wheat bran, for example) does not affect lipid levels.

Browner WS, Westenhouse J, Tice J: What if Americans ate less fat? A quantitative estimate of the effect on mortality. JAMA 1991;265:3285. (Perhaps 40,000 deaths would be delayed each year, with an average increase in life expectancy of 3–4 months.)

Grover SA et al: The benefits of treating hyperlipidemia to prevent coronary heart disease. JAMA 1992;267:816. (Similar conclusions.)

Hunninghake DB et al: The efficacy of intensive dietary therapy alone or combined with lovastatin in outpatients with hypercholesterolemia. N Engl J Med 1993; 328:1213. (A diet containing 28% of calories as fat was relatively ineffective, lowering LDL cholesterol by 5% but also lower HDL cholesterol by 6%.)

Manson JE et al: The primary prevention of myocardial infarction. N Engl J Med 1992;326:1406. (Major risk factors.)

Ramsay LE, Yeo WW, Jackson PR: Dietary reduction of serum cholesterol concentration: Time to think again. Br Med J 1991;303:953. (Effects of a diet containing 30% calories as fat diet, when studied in populations, are not as great as one would hope: decline of only 0–4% in cholesterol levels.)

Pharmacologic Agents

All patients whose risk from coronary heart disease is considered high enough to warrant pharmacologic therapy of an elevated LDL cholesterol should be given aspirin prophylaxis at a dose of about 325 mg every other day unless there are contraindications such as aspirin sensitivity, bleeding diatheses, or active peptic ulcer disease. Current data suggest that the effect of aspirin in reducing the risk of coronary heart disease is equal to or even greater than that of cholesterol lowering.

Treatment of postmenopausal women with oral estrogen replacement therapy is associated with a reduction in LDL levels and an increase in HDL levels. These lipid effects appear to be responsible for about half of the possible benefit of postmenopausal estrogens on reducing CHD. The addition of a progesterone to the hormone regimen may diminish the beneficial effect on lipids.

If the decision to treat a patient with an LDL-lowering drug is made, the clinician must select an appropriate agent based on the safety, efficacy, cost, and effects on other lipid levels (Table 27–2) and set a goal for treatment. Current recommendations do not include therapy to use drugs to treat low HDL levels in patients who do not also have high LDL levels. As with all therapies for chronic conditions, the therapeutic goal is best approached slowly and steadily, watching carefully for side effects and encouraging continued compliance with nonpharmacologic measures. Combinations of drugs may be necessary. Once the goal is reached, the lipid profile should be monitored periodically (every 6–12 months), with consideration given to periodic reductions in drug dose or even drug holidays. With the exception of niacin (available generically for a few dollars per month), all of these drugs are expensive and may cost more than $100 per month. Moreover, they may need to be given for decades. Thus, their cost-effectiveness is generally low. Therapy with lovastatin, for example, has been estimated to cost more than $1 million per year of life saved if it is used to treat a 35-year-woman with a cholesterol level of 300 mg/dL who has no other coronary risk factors (and this estimate assumes that there are no adverse effects of therapy).

A. Niacin (Nicotinic Acid): Niacin is the only lipid-lowering agent which has been associated with a reduction in total mortality. Long-term follow-up of a secondary prevention trial of middle-aged men with previous myocardial infarction disclosed that about 52% of those who had been previously treated with niacin had died, compared with 58% in the placebo group. This favorable effect on mortality was not seen during the trial itself, though there was a reduction in the incidence of coronary heart disease.

Niacin reduces the production of VLDL particles, with secondary reduction in LDL and increases in HDL cholesterol levels. The average effect of niacin is to reduce LDL levels by about 10–15% and triglyceride levels by up to half and to increase HDL levels by 10%. It is best to begin at a low dose (at 50 mg/d, using the "vitamin" preparations of niacin), slowly increasing to the therapeutic range, usually 0.5–2 g three times a day with meals. Niacin causes a prostaglandin-mediated flushing; some patients may complain of hot flashes or pruritus. This problem can usually be ameliorated by pretreatment with aspirin (325 mg 30 minutes before each dose) or other nonsteroidal anti-inflammatory agents. Niacin may exacerbate gout and peptic ulcer disease and may provoke hyperglycemia in patients with diabetes. Hepatitis is an important side effect, perhaps especially among patients treated with a sustained-release preparation, which is also more expensive. Whether routine monitoring of liver function tests helps to avoid this side effect is not known.

B. Bile Acid-Binding Resins (Cholestyramine, Colestipol): Treatment with these agents has been shown to reduce the incidence of coronary events (such as myocardial infarction) in middle-aged men by about 20%, with no significant effect on total mortality. The resins work by binding bile acids in the intestine. The resultant reduction in the enterohepatic circulation causes the liver to increase its production of bile acids, using hepatic cholesterol to do so. Thus, hepatic LDL receptor activity increases, with a decline in plasma LDL levels. The triglyceride level tends to increase slightly in some patients treated with bile acid-binding resins; they should be used with caution in those with elevated triglycerides and probably not at all in patients who have triglyceride levels above about 500 mg/dL. The clinician can anticipate a reduction of 20–30% in LDL cholesterol level, with minor changes in the HDL level.

The usual dose of cholestyramine is 12–36 g of resin per day in divided doses with meals, mixed in water or, more palatably, juice. The prepackaged 4 g doses are more expensive than the bulk form; the "candy bars" are even more expensive. Doses of colestipol are 20% higher (the packets each contain 5 g of resin).

These agents often cause gastrointestinal symptoms, such as constipation and gas. They may interfere with the absorption of fat-soluble vitamins (thereby complicating the management of patients receiving warfarin) and may bind other drugs in the intestine. Concurrent use of psyllium may ameliorate the gastrointestinal side effects.

C. HMG-CO Reductase Inhibitors (Lovastatin, Pravastatin, Simvastatin): The effects of these agents in preventing coronary heart disease—and their long-term safety—are not known. They appear to be effective in reducing progression of atherosclerosis among patients with manifest cardiovascular disease. They work by inhibiting the rate-limiting enzyme in the formation of cholesterol. Cholesterol synthesis in the liver is reduced, with a compensatory increase in hepatic LDL receptors (presumably so that the liver can take more of the cholesterol that it needs from the blood), and a reduction in the circulating LDL cholesterol level by up to 35%. There are also modest increases in HDL levels and decreases in triglyceride levels.

Several agents are available in the USA. Doses of lovastatin are 20–80 mg/d; pravastatin and simvastatin doses are 10–40 mg/d. These agents are usually given once a day in the evening (most cholesterol synthesis takes place overnight); at the high end of the dose ranges, twice-a-day dosing may be used. Side effects include myositis, whose incidence may be higher in patients concurrently taking fibrates or niacin. Manufacturers recommend monitoring liver and muscle enzymes. Several agents (notably erythromycin and cyclosporine) reduce the metabolism of these agents.

D. Fibric Acid Derivatives (Gemfibrozil, Clofibrate): In the largest clinical trial that used clofibrate, there were significantly more deaths—especially due to cancer—in the treatment group than in the control. Although still available, clofibrate is rarely used given the availability of its equally effective (but only possibly safer) relative, gemfibrozil. Gemfibrozil reduced coronary heart disease rates in hypercholesterolemic middle-aged men free of coronary disease in the Helsinki Heart Study, perhaps only among those who also had high triglyceride levels. Among men with previous myocardial infarction, however, gemfibrozil increased overall mortality as well as that due to coronary heart disease. Clinicians should also be aware of the trend toward increased

numbers of cancer deaths among subjects treated with gemfibrozil in the Helsinki Heart Study.

The fibrates reduce the synthesis and increase the breakdown of VLDL particles, with secondary effects on LDL and HDL levels. They reduce LDL levels by about 10% and triglyceride levels by about 40% and raise HDL levels by about 20% The usual dose of gemfibrozil is 600 mg once or twice a day. Side effects include cholelithiasis, hepatitis, and myositis. The incidence of the latter two conditions may be higher among patients also taking other lipid-lowering agents. Given that clofibrate caused a statistically significant increase in cancer mortality, it should not be used.

E. Probucol: The effects of probucol on coronary heart disease—and its long-term safety—are not known. It does reduce the deposition of LDL into xanthomas in humans (and into atherosclerotic plaques in rabbits). The mechanism of action of probucol is not clear. It apparently reduces the amount of oxidized LDL (it was originally used as an industrial antioxidant). Probucol reduces LDL levels by 10–15% but has the potentially important adverse effect of lowering HDL levels by up to 10%. It also may be cardiotoxic. Probucol, if used at all, should be reserved for patients with a clear genetic disorder who have failed other therapies.

Davey Smith G, Pekkanen J: Should there be a moratorium on the use of cholesterol lowering drugs? Br Med J 1992;304:431. (An appraisal of the unexplained risks of cholesterol-lowering drugs.)

Stampfer MJ et al: Postmenopausal estrogen therapy and cardiovascular disease. Ten-year follow-up from the Nurses' Health Study. N Engl J Med 1991;325:756. (A reminder about the importance of estrogens.)

Goldman L et al: Cost-effectiveness of HMG-CO reductase inhibition for primary and secondary prevention of CHD. JAMA 1991;265:1145. (Among otherwise low-risk middle-aged persons with cholesterol levels > 300 mg/dL, cost-effectiveness varies from $10,000 to more than $1,000,000 per year of life saved, depending upon the underlying coronary risk.)

Choice of cholesterol-lowering drugs. Med Lett Drugs Ther 1991;33:1. (Surprisingly, does not discuss effects on overall mortality risk.)

HIGH BLOOD TRIGLYCERIDES

Patients with very high levels of serum triglycerides are at risk of pancreatitis. The pathophysiology is not certain, since there are some patients with very high triglyceride levels who never develop pancreatitis. Most patients with congenital abnormalities in triglyceride metabolism present in childhood; hypertriglyceridemia-induced pancreatitis that first presents in adults is more commonly due to an acquired problem in lipid metabolism.

Although there are no clear triglyceride levels that

always result in pancreatitis, most clinicians are uncomfortable with levels above 1000 mg/dL. The risk of pancreatitis may be more related to the triglyceride level following consumption of a fatty meal. Because postcibal increases in triglyceride are inevitable if fat-containing foods are eaten, fasting triglyceride levels in persons prone to pancreatitis should be kept well below that level.

The primary therapy for high triglyceride levels is dietary, avoiding alcohol and fatty foods. Control of secondary causes of high triglyceride levels (see Table 27–1) may also be helpful. In patients with persistent elevations in the pancreatitis range despite adequate dietary compliance—and certainly in those with a previous episode of pancreatitis—therapy with a triglyceride-lowering drug (eg, niacin, in doses as described above) is indicated.

Whether patients with elevated triglycerides (> 250 mg/dL) and no other lipoprotein abnormalities are at increased risk of atherosclerotic disease is not known. Some of these patients may belong to families with a genetic disorder known as familial combined hyperlipidemia. This disorder is characterized by a variety of lipid abnormalities in different family members: Some have high cholesterol levels, some high triglyceride levels, and some both. It now appears that the common link is an abnormality in one of the LDL-associated apoproteins (B-100), and that this may be a coronary risk factor. However, the effect on coronary heart disease risk of treating an isolated high triglyceride level in these patients is not known. Some authorities recommend treating an isolated high triglyceride level in patients with known coronary heart disease, reasoning that such patients are likely to have some abnormality in lipid metabolism. Treatment is primarily nonpharmacologic, with an emphasis on weight loss, a low-fat diet, avoidance of excess alcohol, and exercise.

Criqui MH et al: Plasma triglyceride level and mortality from coronary heart disease. N Engl J Med 1993; 328:1220. (There was no evidence that an elevated triglyceride level was an independent predictor of death from coronary disease.)

Nutrition

28

Robert B. Baron, MD, MS

NUTRITIONAL REQUIREMENTS

Approximately 40 nutrients are required by the human body. Nutrients are considered essential if they cannot be synthesized by the body and if a deficiency causes recognizable abnormalities that disappear when the deficit is corrected. Required nutrients include the essential amino acids, water-soluble vitamins, fat-soluble vitamins, minerals, and the essential fatty acids. The body also requires an adequate energy substrate, a small amount of metabolizable carbohydrate, indigestible carbohydrate (fiber), additional nitrogen, and water.

Most of the required nutrients are harmful when consumed in excessive amounts. Thus, a range of acceptable intake levels can be established for most of them.

Nutritional requirements are most commonly expressed as the average daily amounts of nutrients a population group should consume. In the USA, the most widely used estimates of nutritional requirements are the Recommended Dietary Allowances (RDAs) developed by a subcommittee of the Food and Nutrition Board of the National Academy of Sciences. RDAs have been established for energy and protein; the water-soluble vitamins thiamin, riboflavin, niacin, vitamin B_6, folic acid, vitamin B_{12}, and vitamin C; the fat-soluble vitamins A, D, and K; and the minerals calcium, phosphorus, magnesium, iron, zinc, iodine, and selenium (Table 28–1).

The RDAs exceed the actual requirements of most individuals in the population because they are stated as 2 SD above the estimated mean requirement. Therefore, a dietary intake of less than the RDA of a specific nutrient is not necessarily inadequate for a given individual—it increases the *risk* of an inadequate intake. For most clinical situations, two-thirds of the RDA is considered an adequate nutritional intake.

The RDAs for energy are treated in a different manner. Because energy needs vary so greatly among individuals, the RDA Committee sets forth estimates of the average needs of the population rather than recommended intakes for individuals. About half of the population will require more energy than the RDA and half will require less.

Nutritional requirements vary not only from one individual to the next but from one day to the next in any given subject. They differ also with age, sex, and body size and during pregnancy and lactation. Different RDAs have been developed for different age and sex groups. Requirements vary also with such clinical circumstances as premature birth, aging, metabolic disorders, infections, chronic illness, medications, extremes of climate and physical activity, and the route of ingestion. The RDAs do not cover such situations—they are intended only for healthy populations.

ENERGY

The human body requires energy to support normal functions and physical activity, growth, and repair of damaged tissues. Energy is provided by oxidation of dietary protein, fat, carbohydrate, and alcohol. Oxidation of 1 g of each provides 4 kcal of energy from protein and carbohydrate, 9 kcal from fat, and 7 kcal from alcohol.

In healthy adults, energy expenditure is primarily determined by three factors: basal energy expenditure (BEE), thermic effect of food (TEF), and physical activity.

The BEE is the amount of energy required to maintain basic physiologic functions. It is measured while the subject is resting in a warm room, not having eaten for 12 hours. In healthy persons, the BEE (in kcal/24 h) can be estimated by the Harris-Benedict equation, which will correctly predict measured BEE in 90% + 10% of healthy subjects (see Nutritional Requirement, below). In clinical practice, patients rarely meet the strict criteria for basal measurement. Energy expenditure measured in individuals at rest without food for 2 hours is the resting metabolic expenditure (RME) and is about 10% greater than BEE.

TEF is the amount of energy expended during and following the ingestion of food. TEF averages approximately 10% of the BEE.

Physical activity has a major impact on energy ex-

Table 28–1. Recommended daily dietary allowances for adults (revised 1989).[1]

Category	Age (years) or Condition	Weight (kg)	Weight (lb)	Height (cm)	Height (in)	Protein (g)	Fat-Soluble Vitamins Vitamin A (mg RE)	Vitamin D (mg)	Vitamin E (mg α-TE)	Vitamin K (mg)	Water-Soluble Vitamins Vitamin C (mg)	Thiamine (mg)	Riboflavin (mg)	Niacin (mg NE)	Vitamin B6 (mg)	Folate (μg)	Vitamin B12 (μg)	Minerals Calcium (mg)	Phosphorus (mg)	Magnesium (mg)	Iron (mg)	Zinc (mg)	Iodine (μg)	Selenium (μg)
Males	15–18	66	145	176	69	59	1,000	10	10	65	60	1.5	1.8	20	2.0	200	2.0	1,200	1,200	400	12	15	150	50
	19–24	72	160	177	70	58	1,000	10	10	70	60	1.5	1.7	19	2.0	200	2.0	1,200	1,200	350	10	15	150	70
	25–50	79	174	176	70	63	1,000	5	10	80	60	1.5	1.7	19	2.0	200	2.0	800	800	350	10	15	150	70
	51+	77	170	173	68	63	1,000	5	10	80	60	1.2	1.4	15	2.0	200	2.0	800	800	350	10	15	150	70
Females	15–18	55	120	163	64	44	800	10	8	55	60	1.1	1.3	15	1.5	180	2.0	1,200	1,200	300	15	12	150	50
	19–24	58	128	164	65	46	800	10	8	60	60	1.1	1.3	15	1.6	180	2.0	1,200	1,200	280	15	12	150	55
	25–50	63	138	163	64	50	800	5	8	65	60	1.1	1.3	15	1.6	180	2.0	800	800	280	15	12	150	55
	51+	65	143	160	63	50	800	5	8	65	60	1.0	1.2	13	1.6	180	2.0	800	800	280	10	12	150	55
Pregnant						60	800	10	10	65	70	1.5	1.6	17	2.2	400	2.2	1,200	1,200	320	30	15	175	65
Lactating	1st 6 months					65	1,300	10	12	65	95	1.6	1.8	20	2.1	280	2.6	1,200	1,200	355	15	19	200	75
	2nd 6 months					62	1,200	10	11	65	90	1.6	1.7	20	2.1	260	2.6	1,200	1,200	340	15	16	200	75

[1] From: National Research Council: *Recommended Dietary Allowances*, 10th ed. National Academy of Sciences, 1989.

penditure. The average energy expenditure per hour by adults engaged in typical activities is shown in Table 28–2.

Daily recommended energy intakes for healthy individuals are shown in Table 28–3.

PROTEIN

Protein is required for growth and for maintenance of body structure and function. Although the nutritional requirement is commonly stated in grams of protein, the true requirement is for nine **essential amino acids** plus additional nitrogen for protein synthesis. The essential amino acids are leucine, isoleucine, lysine, methionine, phenylalanine, threonine, tryptophan, valine, and histidine.

Adequate protein must be consumed each day to replace essential amino acids lost through protein turnover. On a protein-free diet, the average male loses 3.8 g of nitrogen per day—equivalent to 24 g of protein. Allowing for differences in protein quality and utilization and for individual variability, the RDA for protein is 56 g/d for men and 45 g/d for women.

Protein and energy requirements are closely related. Diets that provide insufficient energy will require additional protein to maintain nitrogen equilibrium.

CARBOHYDRATE

As long as adequate energy and protein are provided in the diet, there is no specific requirement for dietary carbohydrate. A small amount of carbohydrate—approximately 100 g/d—is necessary to prevent ketosis. In practice, however, most dietary energy should be provided by carbohydrate. In the USA, the average diet contains 45% of calories as carbohydrate. Current recommendations are to increase carbohydrate intakes to 55–60% of total calories in the diet.

Dietary carbohydrates include simple sugars, complex carbohydrates (starches), and indigestible carbohydrates (dietary fiber). Although simple sugars and complex carbohydrates provide equal amounts of calories, the bulk of dietary carbohydrates should be derived from starches. Sugars—particularly sucrose—are concentrated sources of calories without other sources of essential nutrients. Sucrose consumption is also thought to be an important factor in the development of tooth decay. Complex carbohydrates, when unrefined, provide carbohydrate calories and vitamins, minerals, and dietary fiber.

Dietary fiber is that portion of plant foods that cannot be digested by the human intestine. Fiber increases the bulk of the stool and facilitates excretion. Epidemiologic evidence suggests that diets high in dietary fiber are associated with a lower incidence of digestive and cardiovascular diseases. The more insoluble fibers, such as those found in wheat bran, have the greatest impact on colonic function. Soluble fibers such as those found in legumes, oats, and fruit result in lower blood sugar levels in diabetics and lower blood cholesterol.

FAT

Dietary fat is the most concentrated source of food energy. Like energy from dietary carbohydrate, energy derived from fat can support protein synthesis. Dietary fat also provides the essential fatty acid linoleic acid. Other than the need for adequate quantities of linoleic acid, there is no specific requirement for dietary fat as long as the diet provides adequate nutrients oxidizable for energy. Although the average American diet contains 40% of calories as fat, current recommendations are to limit dietary fat to 30% or less of total calories. Diets containing as little as 5–10% of total calories as fat appear to be safe and well tolerated.

Dietary fats are composed chiefly of fatty acids and dietary cholesterol. Fatty acids contain either no double bonds (saturated), one double bond (mono-

Table 28–2. Average energy calories expended per hour by adults at selected weights engaged in various activities.[1]

Activity	54 kg (120 lb)	64 kg (140 lb)	73 kg (160 lb)	82 kg (180 lb)	91 kg (200 lb)	100 kg (220 lb)
Sleeping: Reclining	50	58	69	78	86	99
Very light: Sitting	73	83	103	115	127	150
Light: Walking on level, shopping, light housekeeping	143	166	200	225	250	290
Moderate: Cycling, dancing, skiing, tennis	226	262	307	345	382	430
Heavy: Walking uphill, shoveling, swimming, playing basketball or football	440	512	598	670	746	840

Note: Range of rate of expenditure of calories per minute of activity (for a 70-kg man or a 58-kg woman): Sleeping, 0.9–1.2: very light, 1.5–2.5; light, 2–4.9; moderate, 5–7.4; heavy, 6–12.

[1]Data from: *Recommended Dietary Allowances*, 9th ed. National Academy of Sciences—National Research Council, 1980. Adapted from McArdle WD, Katch FI, Katch VL: *Exercise Physiology: Energy, Nutrition and Human Performance.* Lea & Febiger, 1981.

Table 28–3. Median heights and weights and recommended energy intake (REE) for nonpregnant adults.[1]

Category	Age (years)	Weight (kg)	Weight (lb)	Height (cm)	Height (in)	REE (Kcal/d)	Average Energy Allowance[2] (kcal) Multiples of REE	Per kg	Per day[3]
Males	19–24	72	160	177	70	1780	1.67	40	2900
	25–50	79	174	176	70	1800	1.60	37	2900
	51+	77	170	173	68	1530	1.50	30	2300
Females	19–24	58	128	164	65	1350	1.60	38	2200
	25–50	63	138	163	64	1380	1.55	36	2200
	51+	65	143	160	63	1280	1.50	30	1900

[1]Modified form: National Research Council: *Recommended Dietary Allowances,* 19th ed. National Academy of Sciences, 1989.
[2]In the range of light to moderate activity, the coefficient of variation is ± 20%.
[3]Figure is rounded.

unsaturated), or more than one double bond (polyunsaturated). Current dietary recommendations are to decrease total fat and replace saturated fats with mono- and polyunsaturated fatty acids. Saturated fatty acids are associated with increased serum cholesterol, while polyunsaturated and monounsaturated fatty acids lower serum cholesterol. Saturated fats are solid at room temperature and in general are derived from animal foods; unsaturated fats are liquid at room temperature and in general are derived from plant foods.

The polyunsaturated fatty acid **linoleic acid** is an essential nutrient, required by the body for the synthesis of arachidonic acid, the major precursor of prostaglandins. Deficiencies of linoleic acid result in dermatitis, hair loss, and impaired wound healing. For individuals with average energy requirements, approximately 5 g of linoleic acid per day—1–2% of total calories—is required to prevent essential fatty acid deficiency.

Cholesterol is a major constituent of cell membranes. It is synthesized easily by the body and is not an essential nutrient. Diets that contain large amounts of cholesterol partially inhibit endogenous cholesterol synthesis but result in a net increase in serum cholesterol concentrations because of suppression of synthesis of low-density lipoprotein receptors. Average American diets contain approximately 450 mg/d of cholesterol. Current recommendations are to limit dietary cholesterol to 300 mg or less per day.

VITAMINS

Vitamins are a heterogeneous group of organic molecules required by the body for a variety of essential metabolic functions. They are grouped as **water-soluble vitamins:** thiamin, riboflavin, niacin, vitamin B_6 (pyridoxine), vitamin B_{12} (cobalamin), folate, pantothenic acid, biotin, and vitamin C (ascorbic acid); and **fat-soluble vitamins:** A, D, E, and K. Disorders of vitamin metabolism are discussed below.

MINERALS

The body also requires a number of inorganic minerals, commonly grouped as the **major minerals** calcium, magnesium, and phosphorus; the **electrolytes** sodium, potassium, and chloride; and the **trace elements** iron, zinc, copper, manganese, molybdenum, fluoride, iodine, cobalt, chromium, and selenium. Important characteristics of major minerals and electrolytes are summarized in Table 28–4.

DRUG-NUTRIENT INTERACTIONS

Many commonly used medications can have important effects on nutritional requirements. Chronic therapy with a variety of drugs can induce nutrient deficiencies by appetite suppression, intestinal malabsorption, and alterations in nutrient metabolism or excretion. The effects of selected drugs on nutrient absorption and metabolism are summarized in Table 28–5.

DIETARY RECOMMENDATIONS

Prior to 1977, the emphasis in nutrition education and diet planning was to ensure that the RDAs were met by diets that contained a wide variety of foods. The most important dietary education tool used for this purpose was *The Four Food Groups,* published by the United States Department of Agriculture (USDA). According to this model, two servings per day from both the milk group and the meat group and four servings per day from both the fruit and vegetable group and the cereal group would meet the minimal nutritional requirements for most individuals.

Although this model ensured that the RDAs were met by a variety of foods, it did not guarantee that selected foods were of high quality. The effects of food processing on the nutrient density of food, the balance of macronutrients (percentages of fat, carbo-

Table 28–4. Essential macrominerals: Summary of major characteristics.[1]

Elements	Functions	Deficiency Disease or Symptoms	Toxicity Disease or Symptoms[2]
Calcium	Constituent of bones, teeth; regulation of nerve, muscle function.	Children: rickets. Adults: osteomalacia. May contribute to osteoporosis.	Occurs with excess absorption due to hypervitaminosis D or hypercalcemia due to hyperparathyroidism, or other causes of hypercalcemia.
Phosphorus	Constituent of bones, teeth, ATP, phosphorylated metabolic intermediates. Nucleic acids.	Children: rickets. Adults: osteomalacia.	Low serum $Ca^{2+}:P_i$ ratio stimulates secondary hyperparathyroidism; may lead to bone loss.
Sodium	Principal cation in extracellular fluid. Regulates plasma volume, acid-base balance, nerve and muscle function, Na^+/K^+-ATPase.	Unknown on normal diet; secondary to injury or illness.	Hypertension (in susceptible individuals).
Potassium	Principal cation in intracellular fluid; nerve and muscle function, Na^+/K^+-ATPase.	Occurs secondary to illness, injury, or diuretic therapy; muscular weakness, paralysis, mental confusion.	Cardiac arrest, small bowel ulcers.
Chloride	Fluid and electrolyte balance; gastric fluid.	Infants fed salt-free formula. Secondary to vomiting, diuretic therapy, renal disease.	Cardiac arrest, small bowel ulcers.
Magnesium	Constituent of bones, teeth; enzyme cofactor (kinases, etc).	Secondary to malabsorption or diarrhea, alcoholism.	Depressed deep tendon reflexes and respiration.

[1]Reproduced, with permission, from Murray RK et al: *Harper's Biochemistry,* 21st ed. Appleton & Lange, 1988.
[2]Excess mineral intake produces toxic symptoms. Unless otherwise specified, symptoms include nonspecific nausea, diarrhea, and irritability.

hydrate, and protein), and the character of macronutrients (simple versus complex carbohydrate; saturated versus unsaturated fat) are omitted.

Since 1977, literally dozens of governmental, professional, and public health agencies and associations have published dietary recommendations that attempt to deal with these issues. Although attention has been directed to the differences between these reports, most agree on the basic principles of eating a wide variety of foods; increasing the consumption of foods containing complex carbohydrates; restricting the intake of sugar, fat (particularly saturated fat), cholesterol, salt, and alcohol; and maintaining an ideal body weight.

A new nutrition education guide, the "Food Guide Pyramid" (Figure 28–1), has been recently published by the USDA, replacing the "Four Food Groups." The Pyramid places greatest emphasis on consumption of bread, cereal, rice, and pasta (six to eleven servings), vegetables (three to five servings), and fruit (two to four servings), lesser emphasis on milk, yogurt, and cheese (two or three servings), and meat, poultry, fish, dry beans, eggs, and nuts (two or three servings); and recommends that fats, oils, and sweets be used sparingly.

National Research Council: *Diet and Health: Implications for Reducing Chronic Disease Risk.* National Academy Press, 1989.
National Research Council: *Recommended Dietary Allowances,* 10th ed. National Academy Press, 1989.
Trovato A, Nuhlicek DN, Midtling JE: Drug-nutrient interactions. Am Fam Physician 1991;44:1651. (Commonly prescribed drugs associated with drug-nutrient interactions.)
US Department of Health and Human Services: *The Surgeon General's Report on Nutrition and Health.* DHHS (PHS) Publication No. 88–50210. US Government Printing Office, 1988.

ASSESSMENT OF NUTRITIONAL STATUS

The prevention and treatment of nutritional problems require the identification of patients at risk for the development of malnutrition and the identification of patients who already show symptoms and signs of malnutrition. Unfortunately, no single biochemical test or clinical technique is sufficiently accurate to serve as a reliable test for malnutrition. Current techniques of nutritional assessment utilize a combination of methods, including evaluation of dietary intake, anthropometric measurements, clinical examination, and laboratory tests. Some patients require serial measurements and close observation to confirm the diagnosis of malnutrition.

DIETARY HISTORY

Virtually all patients undergoing a complete history and physical examination should be asked screening dietary questions to help identify those high-risk patients who require further evaluation. Of

Table 28–5. Effect of drugs on nutrient absorption and metabolism.

Drug	Effect
Analgesics and anti-inflammatories	
Salicylates	Decreases serum ascorbic acid; increases urinary loss of ascorbic acid, potassium, and amino acids.
Sulfasalazine	Impairs folate absorption and antagonizes folate supplementation.
Antacids	
Aluminum antacids	Decrease absorption of phosphate and vitamin A.
H_2 blockers	Decrease iron and vitamin B_{12} absorption.
Octreotide acetate	Hypo- and hyperglycemia; decrease fat and carotide absorption.
Anticonvulsants	
Phenobarbital	Decreases serum folate; increases vitamin D and vitamin K turnover and may cause deficiency.
Phenytoin	Decreases serum folate; increases vitamin D and vitamin K turnover and may cause deficiency.
Primidone	Decreases serum folate and vitamins B_6, B_{12}, decreases calcium absorption; increases vitamin D and vitamin K turnover and may cause deficiency.
Antimicrobials	
Neomycin	Binds bile acids and decreases absorption of fat, carotene; vitamins A, D, K, B_{12}; potassium, sodium, calcium, nitrogen.
Amphotericin B	Decreases serum magnesium and potassium.
Aminosalicyclic acid	Increases absorption of folate, vitamin B_{12}, iron, cholesterol, fat.
Chloramphenicol	Increases need for vitamins B_2, B_6, B_{12}; increases serum iron.
Penicillin	Hypokalemia; renal potassium wasting.
Tetracycline	Calcium, iron, magnesium inhibit drug absorption; decreases vitamin K synthesis.
Cycloserine	May decrease absorption of calcium, magnesium; may decrease serum folate and vitamins B_6, B_{12}; decreases protein synthesis.
Isoniazid	Vitamin B_6 antagonist; may cause deficiency.
Sulfonamides	Decrease absorption of folate; decrease serum folate, iron.
Nitrofurantoin	Decreases serum folate.
Pyrimethamine	Decreases serum B_{12} and folate.
Antimitotics	
Methotrexate	Decreases activation of folate.
Colchicine	Decreases absorption of vitamin B_{12}, carotene, fat, sodium, potassium, cholesterol, lactose, nitrogen.
Cathartics	
Phenolphthalein	Malabsorption, hypokalemia; deficiency of vitamin D, calcium
Mineral oil	Malabsorption; decreased absorption of vitamins A, D, K.
Diuretics	Some cause hypokalemia, hypomagnesemia; may increase urinary excretion of vitamins B_1, B_6; calcium, magnesium, potassium.
Hypocholesterolemics	
Cholestyramine	Binds bile acids; decreases absorption of fat, carotene; vitamins A, D, K, B_{12}; folate, iron.
Clofibrate	Decreases absorption of carotene, vitamin B_{12}, iron, glucose.
Hypotensives	
Hydralazine	Vitamin B_6 deficiency.
Captopril	May cause hyponatremia, hyperkalemia; decreased taste acuity.
Oral contraceptives	Vitamin B_6, folate deficiency; may increase the need for other nutrients.

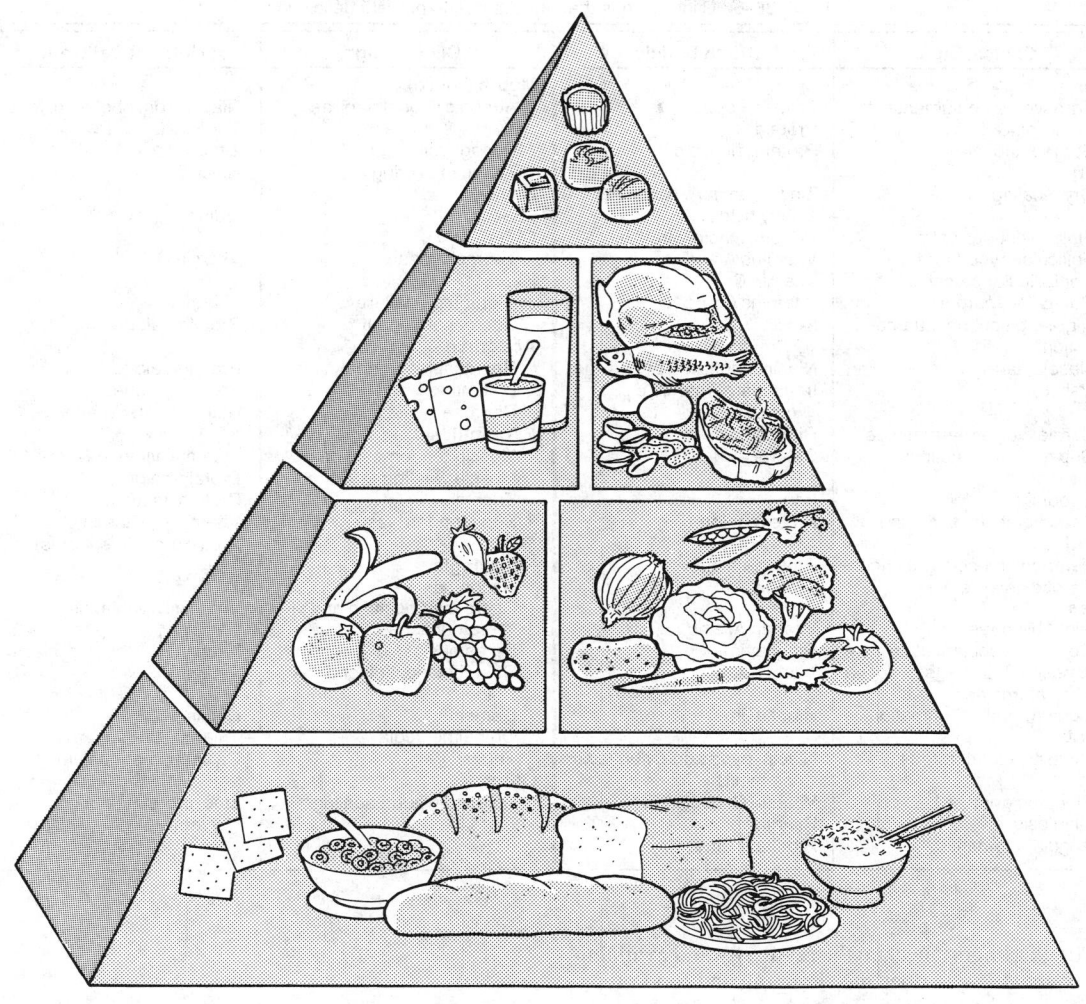

MAJOR FOOD GROUP	RECOMMENDED DAILY AMOUNTS	FATS and SUGARS (relative amounts)
Fats, oils, and sweets	Use sparingly	▼▼▼▼▼▼▼▼▼▼▼▼▼ ▼▼▼▼▼▼▼▼▼▼▼▼▼ ●●●●●●●●●●
Milk, yogurt, and cheese	2–3 servings	▼▼▼▼ ●●●●●●●●
Meat, poultry, fish, dry beans, eggs, and nuts	2–3 servings	●●●●●●●●●●
Fruits	2–4 servings	▼▼▼▼▼
Vegetables	3–5 servings	●●●●●
Bread, cereal, rice, and pasta	6–11 servings	▼▼▼▼▼▼▼▼ ●●●●●●●●

▼ Sugars (added)

● Fat (naturally occurring and added)

Figure 28–1. The Food Guide Pyramid. A guide to daily food choices.

Table 28–6. Clinical signs that may be due to nutrient deficiency.

Clinical Sign	Nutrient Deficiency	Clinical Sign	Nutrient Deficiency
Hair		**Mouth** (cont'd)	
Transverse depigmentation	Protein, copper	Atrophic lingual papillae	Niacin, iron, riboflavin, folate, vitamin B_{12}
Easily pluckable	Protein	Hypogeusia	Zinc, vitamin A
Sparse and thin	Protein, zinc, biotin	Tongue fissuring	Niacin
Skin		**Neck**	
Dry, scaling	Zinc, vitamin A, essential fatty acids	Goiter	Iodine
		Chest	
Flaky paint dermatitis	Protein, niacin, riboflavin	Thoracic rosary	Vitamin D
Follicular hyperkeratosis	Vitamins A and C	**Heart**	
Perifollicular petechiae	Vitamin C	High-output failure	Thiamin
Petechiae, purpura	Vitamins C and K	Decreased output	Protein-calorie
Pigmentation, desquamation	Niacin	**Abdomen**	
		Hepatosplenomegaly	Protein-calorie
Nasolabial seborrhea	Niacin, riboflavin, pyridoxine	Distention	Protein-calorie
Pallor	Iron, folate, vitamin B_{12}, copper	Diarrhea	Niacin, folate, vitamin B_{12}
Scrotal/vulvar dermatoses	Riboflavin	**Extremities**	
Subcutaneous fat loss	Calorie	Muscle tenderness, pain	Thiamin, vitamin C
Nails		Muscle wasting	Protein-calorie
Spooning	Iron	Edema	Protein, thiamin
Transverse lines, ridging	Protein-calorie	Bone tenderness	Vitamin D, vitamin C, calcium, phosphorus
Head			
Temporal muscle wasting	Protein-calorie	**Neurologic**	
Parotid enlargement	Protein	Hyporeflexia	Thiamin
Eyes		Decreased position and vibratory sense	Vitamin B_{12}, thiamin
Night blindness	Vitamin A, zinc		
Corneal vascularization	Riboflavin	Paresthesias	Vitamin B_{12}, thiamin, niacin
Xerosis, Bitot spots, keratomalacia	Vitamin A	Confabulation, disorientation	Thiamin
Conjunctival inflammation	Riboflavin	Dementia	Niacin
Mouth		Opthalmoplegia	Thiamin, phosphorus
Glossitis (scarlet, raw)	Niacin, pyridoxine, riboflavin, vitamin B_{12}, folate	Tetany	Calcium, magnesium
		Other	
Bleeding gums	Vitamin C, riboflavin	Delayed wound healing	Zinc, protein-calorie, vitamin C
Cheilosis	Riboflavin		
Angular stomatitis	Riboflavin, iron		

particular importance are the regularity and availability of meals; who does the shopping and food preparation; recent changes in appetite, intake, or body weight; use of special diets or dietary supplements; use of alcohol, drugs, or medications; food preferences and food allergies; and the presence of illnesses that affect nutritional intakes, losses, or requirements. Elderly and adolescent patients, pregnant or lactating women, and the poor and socially isolated are at particular risk for nutritional problems.

Further quantification of dietary intake can be performed using a variety of techniques. **Twenty-four-hour diet recalls** can be performed quickly and easily and provide rough estimates of nutrient intakes. Patients are asked to describe their dietary intake over the preceding 24 hours, including snacks, beverages, and alcohol. Problems with this technique include inaccurate reporting by patients, difficulties in estimating serving sizes, and the usual problems of generalizing from inadequate data: in this case, a single day's intake. More accurate quantitative information can be obtained by asking patients to complete a **3- to 5-day diet record.** Nutrient composition can then be analyzed with the aid of standard handbooks

Table 28–7. Acceptable weights (in pounds) for men and women.[1,2]

	Age	
Height	**19–34 Years**	**35 years and Older**
5'0"	97–128	108–138
5'1"	101–132	111–143
5'2"	104–137	115–148
5'3"	107–141	119–152
5'4"	111–146	122–157
5'5"	114–150	126–162
5'6"	118–156	130–167
5'7"	121–160	134–172
5'8"	125–164	138–178
5'9"	129–169	142–183
5'10"	132–174	146–188
5'11"	136–179	151–194
6'0"	140–184	155–199
6'1"	144–189	159–205
6'2"	148–195	164–210

[1]Weights based on weighing in without shoes or clothes.
[2]Source: United States Department of Agriculture and United States Department of Health and Human Resources, 1990.

or computer software. Although this technique is prospective and less likely to be invalidated by memory lapses, omissions are still common as well as the usual difficulties in estimating serving sizes.

CLINICAL EXAMINATION

A nutritionally focused physical examination should be performed on each patient at risk for nutritional problems. The examination emphasizes muscle wasting, fat stores, volume status, and signs of micronutrient deficiencies (Table 28–6).

Evaluation of body weight is particularly useful. Body weight in relationship to height should be checked against reference tables of desirable weight (Table 28–7) and expressed as **relative weight:** (current weight/desirable weight × 100). A recent change in body weight is a better index of undernutrition than a low relative weight. Changes in body weight are best expressed as a percentage of usual weight lost per unit of time. A loss of 10% or more of usual weight within a period of 1–2 months is generally considered to be predictive of a poor clinical outcome.

Evaluation of body composition—particularly fat stores and skeletal muscle—can be performed by visual inspection or, more quantitatively, by using **anthropometric measurements.** The most commonly used are the triceps skin fold, and mid arm muscle circumference. Because of significant individual variations and technical variations in measurement, however, anthropometry has limited clinical utility.

A number of more sophisticated techniques are available for more precise assessment of body composition. Most, however, have little role in patient care. These include bioimpedance analysis, total body electrical conductivity, dual energy x-ray absorptiometry, underwater weighing, total body water and potassium, neutron activation analysis, and MRI.

LABORATORY TESTS

Serum albumin is the most important test for the diagnosis of protein-calorie undernutrition. Most patients with severe protein depletion will have abnormally low serum albumin levels. Unfortunately, many nonnutritional conditions can also cause low levels of serum albumin—particularly liver disease and severe illness in general. Other serum proteins with shorter half-lives (transferrin, prealbumin, etc) may more accurately reflect short-term changes in nutritional status but suffer from similar shortcomings.

Qualitative and quantitative tests of cellular immunity are also abnormal in many patients with protein-calorie undernutrition. Measurements of the **total lymphocyte count** and **delayed hypersensitivity reactions** to common skin test antigens are commonly used but are also nonspecific; ie, abnormalities may be due to nonnutritional factors.

Despite their uncertain diagnostic utility, these tests are useful prognostic indicators. Patients with abnormal nutritional assessment parameters have a markedly increased risk of poor clinical outcomes.

Despite the use of a nutritionally focused history and physical examination and judicious use of laboratory tests, it is often difficult to confirm a diagnosis of malnutrition. Continued close observation is often necessary. Monitoring dietary intakes during hospitalization can be quite helpful. **Calorie counts** by registered dietitians can be used to estimate energy and protein intakes for comparison with estimated requirements. Serial measurements of body weight and serial clinical assessments should also be performed.

Dwyer JT, Gallo JJ, Reichel W: Assessing nutritional status in elderly patients. Am Fam Physician 1993;47:613. (Special considerations in nutritional assessment of the elderly.)

Smith LC, Mullen JL: Nutritional assessment and indications for nutritional support. Surg Clin North Am 1991;71:449. (Multifactorial approach to nutritional assessment.)

NUTRITIONAL DISORDERS

PROTEIN-CALORIE UNDERNUTRITION

Essentials of Diagnosis

- Manifestations range from weight loss and growth failure to distinct syndromes, kwashiorkor, and marasmus.
- In severe cases, virtually all organ systems affected.
- History of decreased intake of calories or protein, increased nutrient losses, or increased nutrient requirements.

General Considerations

Protein-calorie undernutrition occurs as a result of a relative or absolute deficiency of calories and protein. It may be primary, due to inadequate food intake, or secondary, as a result of other illness. For most developing nations, primary protein-calorie undernutrition remains the most important nutritional problem and among the most significant of all health problems. Classically, primary protein-calorie undernutrition has been described as two distinct syndromes. **Kwashiorkor,** caused by a deficiency of protein in the presence of adequate calories, is typically seen in weaning infants at the birth of a sibling in areas where foods containing protein are insufficiently abundant. **Marasmus,** caused by combined protein and calorie deficiency, is most commonly seen where adequate quantities of food are not available.

In industrialized societies, protein-calorie undernutrition is most often secondary to other diseases. As many as 20% of all patients admitted to the hospital have significant protein-calorie undernutrition. In these patients, protein-calorie undernutrition is caused either by decreased intake of calories and protein, increased nutrient losses, or increased nutrient requirements dictated by the underlying illness. For example, diminished oral intake may result from poor dentition or various gastrointestinal disorders. Loss of nutrients results from malabsorption and diarrhea as well as from glycosuria. Requirements are increased by fever, surgery, neoplasia, and burns. Few patients are sick enough to require acute hospitalization without manifesting some of these risk factors.

Pathophysiology

Protein-calorie undernutrition results in important pathophysiologic changes that can affect virtually every organ system. The most obvious results are loss of body weight, adipose stores, and skeletal muscle mass. Weight losses of 5–10% are usually tolerated without significant loss of physiologic function; losses of 35–40% of body weight usually result in death. Loss of protein from skeletal muscle and internal organs is usually proportionate to weight loss. Protein mass is lost from the liver, gastrointestinal tract, kidneys, and heart.

As protein-calorie undernutrition progresses, organ dysfunction may develop. Hepatic synthesis of serum proteins decreases, and depressed levels of circulating proteins may be observed. Cardiac output and contractility are decreased, and the ECG may show decreased voltage and a rightward axis shift. Autopsies of patients who die with severe undernutrition show myofibrillar atrophy and interstitial edema of the heart.

The lungs are affected primarily by weakness and atrophy of the muscles of respiration. Vital capacity and tidal volume are depressed, and mucociliary clearance is abnormal. The gastrointestinal tract is most importantly affected by mucosal atrophy and loss of villi of small intestine, resulting in a decrease in absorptive capacity. Intestinal disaccharidase deficiency and mild pancreatic insufficiency can also develop and result in malabsorption.

Changes in immunologic function are among the most important changes seen in protein-calorie undernutrition. The total lymphocyte count is commonly decreased, primarily because of a reduction in circulating T cells. T cell function is also depressed. Changes in B cell function are more variable. Other aspects of immunologic function are also affected, including total complement activity, granulocyte function, and anatomic barriers to infection. Virtually every phase of wound healing is also affected.

Clinical Findings

The clinical manifestations of protein-calorie undernutrition are diverse, ranging from mild growth failure and weight loss to a number of distinct clinical syndromes. Children in the developing world, for example, may manifest the classic syndromes of marasmus and kwashiorkor. In secondary protein-calorie undernutrition as seen in industrialized nations, clinical manifestations are affected by the degree of protein and calorie deficiency, the underlying illness that resulted in the deficiency, and the patient's nutritional status prior to illness.

In mild cases of secondary protein-calorie undernutrition, weight loss may be the only manifestation. In more severe cases, manifestations include depletion of fat stores in the face and extremities and loss of skeletal muscle, best seen in the interosseous and temporal muscles. The skin is often dry and the hair thin. If serum albumin is decreased, dependent edema or anasarca may be present.

The clinical manifestations of protein-calorie malnutrition may be obscured in two other circumstances. Patients with significant obesity often appear to be overnourished because of their excess adipose stores. Rapid weight loss, however—particularly when due to illness—commonly results in depletion of skeletal and visceral protein and can lead to the pathophysiologic abnormalities described above despite the external appearance of obesity. In such patients, significant weight loss and depletion of serum proteins may be the only clues to protein depletion. Acutely ill patients—particularly those who are "hypermetabolic" and unable to eat—may develop visceral protein depletion rapidly without manifesting significant weight loss or other signs of undernutrition. In these patients, signs of hypermetabolism and decreased levels of serum protein may be the only clues to the diagnosis of undernutrition.

Treatment

The treatment of severe protein-calorie undernutrition is a slow process requiring great care. Initial efforts should be directed at correcting fluid and electrolyte abnormalities and any significant acute infections. Of particular concern is depletion of potassium, magnesium, and calcium and acid-base abnormalities. The second phase of treatment is directed at repletion of protein, energy, and micronutrients. Treatment should be started with modest quantities of protein and calories calculated according to the patient's actual body weight. Adult patients can initially be given 0.8 g of protein and 30 kcal per kilogram. Concomitant administration of vitamins and minerals is necessary. Either the enteral or parenteral route can be used, although the former is preferable.

Enteral fat and lactose are usually withheld initially. Patients with less severe protein-calorie undernutrition can be given calories and protein simultaneously with the correction of fluid and electrolyte abnormalities. Similar quantities of protein and calories are recommended for initial treatment.

All patients initially treated for protein-calorie undernutrition require close follow-up. Both calories and protein can be advanced as tolerated. Adult patients can be advanced to 1.5 g/kg/d of protein and 40 kcal/kg/d of calories.

Patients who are refed too rapidly can develop a number of untoward clinical sequelae. During refeeding, circulating potassium, magnesium, phosphorus, and glucose move intracellularly and can result in low serum levels of each. The administration of water and sodium in combination with carbohydrate refeeding can overload hearts with depressed cardiac function and result in congestive heart failure. Enteral refeeding can result in malabsorption and diarrhea due to abnormalities in the gastrointestinal tract.

Refeeding edema is a benign condition that must be differentiated from congestive heart failure. Changes in renal sodium reabsorption and poor skin and blood vessel integrity result in the development of edema in dependent areas without other signs of congestive heart failure. Treatment is with reassurance, elevation of the dependent area, and modest sodium restriction. Diuretics are usually ineffective in this situation, may aggravate electrolyte deficiencies, and should not be used.

The prevention and early detection of protein-calorie malnutrition in hospitalized patients require constant awareness of that possibility by the physicians and others responsible for their care. Each patient admitted to the hospital should be screened for risk factors. Patients at risk require formal assessment of nutritional status and close observation of dietary intake, body weight, and nutritional requirements during the hospital stay.

Baron RB: Protein-energy malnutrition. In: *Cecil Textbook of Medicine,* 19th ed. Wyngaarden JB, Smith LH, Bennett JC (editors). Saunders, 1991.

McMahon MM, Bistrian BR: The physiology of nutrition assessment and therapy in protein-calorie malnutrition. Dis Mon (July) 1990;36:373. (Emphasis on hormonal responses to simple starvation and to injury; the effects of malnutrition on immune response; and the response to refeeding.)

OBESITY

Essentials of Diagnosis

- Excess adipose tissue, resulting in body weight 20% or more in excess of expected ("desirable") weight.
- Upper body obesity (abdomen and flank) of greater health consequence than lower body obesity (buttocks and thighs).
- Associated with multiple metabolic and structural disorders.

General Considerations

Obesity is one of the most common disorders in medical practice and among the most frustrating and difficult to manage. Little progress has been made in obesity treatment in the last 25 years, yet major changes have occurred in our understanding of its causes and its implications for health.

Definition & Measurement

Obesity is defined as an excess of adipose tissue. The exact criterion for how much is too much is controversial. Accurate quantification of body fat requires sophisticated techniques not usually available in clinical practice. In most situations, physical examination is sufficient to detect excess body fat. Two methods commonly used for more quantitative evaluation are relative weight (RW) and body mass index (BMI).

Relative weight (RW) is the measured body weight divided by the "desirable weight" × 100. Desirable weight is defined as the midpoint value recommended for a "medium-frame" person in the recently revised weight tables published by the United States government (Table 28–7). RW does not differentiate between patients with excess fat or "excess" muscle.

The **body mass index (BMI),** more accurately reflects the presence of excess adipose tissue. BMI is calculated by dividing measured body weight in kilograms by the height in meters squared. The "normal" BMI is 20–25 kg/m^2.

The National Institutes of Health currently define obesity as a relative weight over 120% (BMI > 27.5 kg/m^2): Mild obesity is a relative weight of 120–140% (BMI 27.5–30 kg/m^2); moderate obesity is a relative weight of 140–200% (BMI 30–40 kg/m^2); and severe or "morbid" obesity is a relative weight over 200% (BMI > 40 kg/m^2). Other factors besides total weight, however, are also important. Recent data suggest that upper body obesity (excess fat around the waist and flank) is a greater health hazard than lower body obesity (fat in the thighs and buttocks). Obese patients with high waist-hip ratios (> 1.0 in men; > 0.8 in women) have a significantly greater risk of diabetes mellitus, stroke, coronary artery disease, and early death than equally obese patients with lower ratios. Further differentiation of the location of excess fat suggests that visceral fat within the abdominal cavity is more hazardous to health than subcutaneous fat around the abdomen.

Age is also an important factor. As age increases, moderate increases in body weight are not associated with increased mortality rates. Current weight tables published by the Departments of Agriculture and of

Health and Human Services account for the effect of age.

About 25% of people in the USA have relative weights in excess of 120%. Blacks—particularly black women—are more apt to be obese than whites, and the poor are more obese than the rich regardless of race.

Health Consequences of Obesity

Obesity is associated with significant increases in both morbidity and mortality. A great many disorders occur with greater frequency in obese people. The most important and common of these are hypertension, type II diabetes mellitus, hyperlipidemia, coronary artery disease, degenerative joint disease, and psychosocial disability; but certain cancers (colon, rectum, and prostate in men; uterus, biliary tract, breast, and ovary in women), thromboembolic disorders, digestive tract diseases (gallstones, reflux esophagitis), and skin disorders are also more prevalent in the obese. Surgical and obstetric risks are greater as well. Obese patients also have a greater risk of pulmonary functional impairment, endocrine abnormalities, proteinuria, and increased hemoglobin concentration.

The death rate increases in proportion to the degree of obesity: Relative weights of 130% are associated with an excess mortality rate of 35% and relative weights of 150% a greater than two-fold excess death rate. Patients with "morbid" obesity (relative weight > 200%) have as much as a ten-fold increase in death rate.

Etiology

Until recently, obesity was considered to be the direct result of a sedentary life-style plus chronic ingestion of excess calories. Obese people were *blamed* for being obese—by their friends and families, their employers, their physicians, and even by themselves. Although these factors are undoubtedly the principal cause of obesity in some cases, there is now evidence for strong genetic influences on the development of obesity. A recent study of 540 adopted children demonstrated a close relationship between their body mass index and that of their biologic parents. No such relationship was found between the children and their adoptive parents. Twin studies have also demonstrated substantial genetic influences on body mass index and little influence from the childhood environment. Although studies vary, as much as 50–75% of obesity can be explained by genetic influences.

The exact mechanisms by which genetic influences affect body weight are unknown; however, most evidence suggests that genetically determined differences in appetite control and in energy expenditure are particularly important.

Further research will probably permit classification of obese patients into subgroups according to different etiologic features. Given our imperfect understanding of the causes of obesity, it is essential not to hold the patients personally responsible for their condition.

Medical Evaluation of the Obese Patient

The history and physical examination are the most important parts of the evaluation of obese patients. Historical information should be obtained about age at onset, recent weight changes, family history of obesity, occupational history, eating and exercise behavior, cigarette and alcohol use, previous weight loss experience, and psychosocial factors. Particular attention should be directed at use of laxatives, diuretics, hormones, nutritional supplements, and over-the-counter medications.

Physical examination should assess the degree and distribution of body fat, overall nutritional status, and signs of secondary causes of obesity.

Less than 1% of obese patients have an identifiable secondary cause of obesity. Hypothyroidism and Cushing's syndrome are important examples that can usually be diagnosed by physical examination in patients with unexplained recent weight gain. Such patients with physical findings suggesting hypothyroidism or Cushing's syndrome may require further endocrinologic evaluation, including serum TSH determination and dexamethasone suppression testing (see Chapter 25).

All obese patients should be evaluated for medical consequences of their obesity. Fasting levels of glucose, cholesterol, and triglycerides should be measured.

Treatment

There is no single effective method of treatment for obesity. Using conventional techniques, only 20% of patients will lose 20 lb and maintain the loss for over 2 years; 5% will maintain a 40-lb loss. Continued close provider-patient contact appears to be more important for success of treatment than the specific features of any given treatment regimen. Careful patient selection will improve success rates and lessen frustration of both patients and therapists. Only sufficiently motivated patients should enter treatment programs. Specific attempts to identify motivated patients—eg, requesting a 3-day diet record—are often useful.

Most successful programs employ a multidisciplinary approach to weight loss, with hypocaloric diets, behavior modification or other strategies to change eating behavior, aerobic exercise, and social support. Emphasis must be on *maintenance* of weight loss.

Dietary instructions should incorporate the same principles that apply to healthy people who are not obese, ie, a low-fat, high-complex carbohydrate, high-fiber diet. This is achieved by emphasizing intake of a wide variety of predominantly "unprocessed" foods. Special attention is usually paid to limiting foods that provide large amounts of calories without other nutrients, ie, fat, sucrose, and alcohol. There is no special advantage to diets that restrict carbohydrates, advocate large amounts of protein or fats, or recommend ingestion of foods one at a time.

Long-term changes in eating behavior are required to maintain weight loss. Although formal **behavior modification** programs are available to which patients can be referred, the clinician caring for obese patients can teach a number of useful behavioral techniques. The most important technique is to emphasize planning and record keeping. Patients can be taught to plan menus and exercise sessions and to record their actual behavior. Record keeping not only aids in behavioral change; the availability of records also helps the health care provider to make specific suggestions for problem solving. Patients can be taught to recognize "eating cues" (emotional, situational, etc) and how to avoid or control them. Reward systems and refundable financial contracts are also useful for many patients.

Exercise offers a number of advantages to patients trying to lose weight and keep it off. Aerobic exercise directly increases the daily energy expenditure and is particularly useful for long-term weight maintenance. Exercise will also preserve lean body mass and partially prevent the decrease in basal energy expenditure seen with semistarvation.

Social support is essential for a successful weight loss program. Continued close contact with the therapist, family and peer group involvement, etc, are useful techniques for reinforcing behavioral change and preventing social isolation.

Patients with severe obesity may require more aggressive treatment regimens. **Very low calorie diets** (400–500 kcal/d) result in rapid weight loss and marked improvement in obesity-related metabolic complications. Side effects such as fatigue, orthostatic hypotension, cold intolerance, and fluid and electrolyte disorders are common and require regular supervision by a physician. Other less common complications include gout, gallbladder disease, and cardiac arrhythmias. Patients are commonly maintained on such programs for 4–6 months and lose an average of 2–4 lb a week. Long-term weight maintenance is less predictable and requires concurrent behavior modification and exercise.

Medications for obesity are widely available over the counter and with prescription. The most commonly used medications are phenylpropanolamine, phentermine, mazindol, fenfluramine, diethylpropion, phenmetrazine, phendimitrazine, and the antidepressant fluoxetine. Controversy exists concerning the efficacy of these agents and specific indications for their use. Although many studies show a short-term benefit, there is little evidence of long-term weight loss.

Although it is generally considered to be the last resort for the treatment of obesity, more than 100,000 obese patients have had **surgical therapy.** Few controlled trials exist, and the development of rational indications for surgery has been difficult. Most surgeons require relative weights greater than 200% before they will proceed. Gastric operations, such as the vertical-banded gastroplasty and gastric bypass procedures, are now the operations of choice. Although both types of procedures result in significant weight loss, direct comparisons tend to favor gastric bypass. The perioperative mortality rate averages less than 1% but ranges from nil to 4% at different centers. When reversals, revisions, and patients lost to follow-up are considered, failure rates approach 50%. Jejunoileal bypass operations have been abandoned by most surgeons owing to unacceptable long-term complications.

A recent concern has been the possible deleterious health effects of fluctuations of body weight produced by repeated cycles of weight loss and gain ("yo-yo dieting"). Six studies have evaluated the effect of weight fluctuations on coronary heart disease and all-cause mortality. To date, four studies have shown a positive relationship; two have not. These concerns reinforce the common-sense approach to avoiding casual or short-lived attempts to lose weight. On the other hand, motivated individuals at risk for obesity-related illness should still be encouraged to lose weight, with particular emphasis on long-term weight maintenance.

Bray GA: Barriers to the treatment of obesity. Ann Intern Med 1991;115:152. (A call for further evaluation of pharmacologic management of obesity.)

Lee IM, Paffenberger RS: Change in body weight and longevity. JAMA 1992;268:2045. (Additional evidence that weight changes may increase the risk of coronary heart disease.)

Stunkard AJ et al: The body mass index of twins who have been reared apart. N Engl J Med 1990;322:1483.

Wadden TA, Van Itallie TB, Blackburn GL: Responsible and irresponsible use of very-low-calorie diets in the treatment of obesity. JAMA 1990;263:83.

Wilber JF: Neuropeptides, appetite regulation, and human obesity. JAMA 1991;266:257.

EATING DISORDERS

ANOREXIA NERVOSA

Essentials of Diagnosis

- Disturbance of body image and intense fear of becoming fat.
- Weight loss leading to body weight 25% below expected.

- Absence of at least three consecutive menstrual cycles.

General Considerations

Anorexia nervosa characteristically begins in the years between adolescence and young adulthood. Approximately 90% of patients are females, most commonly from the middle and upper socioeconomic strata. The diagnosis is based on weight loss leading to body weight 25% below expected, a distorted body image, and fear of weight gain or of loss of control over food intake. Other medical or psychiatric illnesses that can account for anorexia and weight loss must be excluded.

Recent studies suggest that the prevalence of anorexia nervosa is greater than previously suggested. In Rochester, Minnesota, for example, the prevalence of anorexia nervosa per 100,000 population is estimated to be about 270 for females and 22 for males. In Caucasian adolescent girls from middle and upper class families, anorexia nervosa is an even more common illness. Many other adolescent girls have features of the disorder without the severe weight loss.

The cause of anorexia nervosa is not known. Although multiple endocrinologic abnormalities exist in these patients, most authorities believe they are secondary to malnutrition and not primary disorders. Most authors favor a primary psychiatric origin, but no single psychiatric hypothesis satisfactorily explains all cases. The patient characteristically comes from a family whose members are highly goal- and achievement-oriented. Interpersonal relationships may be inadequate or destructive. The parents are usually overly directive and concerned with slimness and physical fitness, and much of the family conversation centers around dietary matters. One theory holds that the patient's refusal to eat is an attempt to regain control of her body in defiance of parental control. The patient's unwillingness to inhabit an "adult body" may also represent a rejection of adult responsibilities and the implications of adult interpersonal relationships. Patients are commonly perfectionistic in behavior and exhibit obsessional personality characteristics. Marked depression or anxiety may be present.

Clinical Findings

A. Symptoms and Signs: Clinically, patients with anorexia nervosa may exhibit severe emaciation and may complain of cold intolerance or constipation. Amenorrhea is almost always present. Bradycardia, hypotension, and hypothermia may be present in severe cases. Examination demonstrates loss of body fat, dry and scaly skin, and increased lanugo body hair. Parotid enlargement and edema may also be present.

B. Laboratory Findings: Laboratory findings are variable but may include anemia, leukopenia, electrolyte abnormalities, and elevations of BUN and serum creatinine. Serum cholesterol levels are often increased. Endocrine abnormalities included depressed levels of luteinizing and follicle-stimulating hormones and impaired response of LH to luteinizing hormone-releasing hormone.

Diagnosis & Differential Diagnosis

The diagnosis of anorexia nervosa can be difficult, since many common social and cultural factors promote and maintain anorexic behavior. Diagnosis depends upon identification of the common behavioral features and exclusion of medical disorders that would account for weight loss.

Behavioral features required for the diagnosis include intense fear of becoming obese, disturbance of body image, weight loss of at least 25%, and refusal to maintain body weight over a minimal normal weight.

The differential diagnosis includes endocrine and metabolic disorders such as panhypopituitarism, Addison's disease, hyperthyroidism, and diabetes mellitus; gastrointestinal disorders such as Crohn's disease and celiac sprue; chronic infections and cancers such as tuberculosis and lymphoma; and rare central nervous system disorders such as hypothalamic tumors.

Treatment

The goal of treatment is restoration of normal body weight and resolution of psychologic difficulties. Hospitalization is usually necessary for frank anorexia nervosa. Treatment programs conducted by experienced teams are successful in about two-thirds of cases, restoring normal weight and menstruation. One-half continue to experience difficulties with eating behavior and psychiatric problems. Occasional patients with anorexia develop obesity after treatment. Two to 6% of patients die from the complications of the disorder or commit suicide.

Various treatment methods have been used without clear evidence of superiority of one over another. Supportive care by physicians and nurses is probably the most important feature of therapy. Structured behavioral therapy, intensive psychotherapy, and family therapy may be tried. A variety of medications including polycyclic antidepressants and lithium carbonate are effective in some cases. Patients with severe malnutrition must be hemodynamically stabilized and may require enteral or parenteral feeding. Forced feedings should be reserved for life-threatening situations, since the goal of treatment is to reestablish normal eating behavior.

Buckner ET: Do you have patients with anorexia nervosa or bulimia? Understanding is the first step in helping. Postgrad Med 1991;89:209. (Detection and treatment.)

Comerci GD: Medical complications of anorexia nervosa and bulimia nervosa. Med Clin North Am 1990;74:1293.

Lucas AR et al: 50-year trends in the incidence of anorexia nervosa in Rochester, Minn: A population-based study. Am J Psychiatry 1991;148:917. (Prevalence greater than previously estimated and still increasing.)

BULIMIA NERVOSA

Essentials of Diagnosis

- Uncontrolled episodes of binge eating followed by self-induced purging.
- Overconcern with weight and body shape.

General Considerations

Bulimia nervosa is the episodic uncontrolled ingestion of large quantities of food followed by purging by self-induced vomiting, diuretics or cathartics, or strict dieting or vigorous exercise.

Like anorexia nervosa, bulimia nervosa is predominantly disorders of young, white middle- and upper-class women. It is more difficult to detect than anorexia, and some studies have estimated the prevalence to be as high as 19% in college-age women.

Patients with bulimia nervosa typically consume large quantities of easily ingested high-calorie foods, usually in secrecy. Some patients may have several such episodes a day for a few days; others report regular and persistent patterns of binge eating. Binging is usually followed by vomiting, cathartics, or diuretics and is usually accompanied by feelings of guilt or depression. Periods of binging may be followed by intervals of self-imposed starvation. Body weights may fluctuate but generally are within 20% of desirable weights.

Some patients with bulimia nervosa also have a cryptic form of anorexia nervosa with significant weight losses and amenorrhea. Family and psychologic issues are generally similar to those encountered among patients with anorexia nervosa. Bulimics, however, have a higher incidence of premorbid obesity, greater use of cathartics and diuretics, and more impulsive or antisocial behaviors. Weights are closer to normal, and menstruation is usually preserved.

Depending on the type and severity of abnormal behavior, a variety of medical complications can occur. Gastric dilatation and pancreatitis have been reported after binges. Vomiting can result in poor dentition, pharyngitis, esophagitis, aspiration, and electrolyte abnormalities. Cathartic and diuretic abuse also commonly result in electrolyte abnormalities or dehydration. Constipation and hemorrhoids are common.

Treatment of bulimia and bulimarexia requires supportive care and psychotherapy. Individual, group, family, and behavioral therapy have all been utilized with modest success. Antidepressants may be helpful in some patients. The best published results to date have been with fluoxetine hydrochloride. Although death from bulimia is rare, the long-term psychiatric prognosis in severe bulimia is worse than the prognosis in anorexia nervosa, which suggests that the underlying psychiatric disorder may be more severe.

Carlat DJ, Camargo CA Jr: Review of bulimia nervosa in males. Am J Psychiatry 1991;148:831. (As with anorexia, men account for about 10% of bulimics.)

Devlin MJ et al: Metabolic abnormalities in bulimia nervosa. Arch Gen Psychiatry 1990;47:1448.

Fitzgerald BA, Wright JH, Atala KD: Bulimia nervosa: Uncovering a secret disorder. Postgrad Med (Aug) 1988; 84:119. (Early recognition results in improved outcome.)

See also references under Anorexia Nervosa, above.

DISORDERS OF VITAMIN METABOLISM

Deficiencies of single vitamins are rarely encountered in current clinical practice, even in developing countries. Deficiencies of multiple vitamins are more commonly seen along with protein-calorie undernutrition. Although any cause of protein-calorie undernutrition can result in concurrent vitamin deficiency, most such instances are associated with malabsorption, alcoholism, medications, hemodialysis, total parenteral nutrition, food faddism, or inborn errors of metabolism.

Vitamin deficiency syndromes develop gradually. Symptoms are commonly nonspecific, and the physical examination is rarely helpful in early diagnosis. Most characteristic physical findings, such as the perifollicular hemorrhages associated with vitamin C deficiency, are seen late in the course of the syndrome. Other characteristic physical findings, such as glossitis and cheilosis, are seen with deficiencies of many B vitamins. Such abnormalities strongly suggest the presence of a nutritional deficiency but do not indicate which nutrient is deficient.

Despite the relative ease of meeting the recommended daily allowances with a mixed diet, many adults in the USA take vitamin supplements. In fact, syndromes of vitamin excess may be more common than deficiency syndromes, particularly those due to excess of vitamins A, D, and B_6. Most claims for significant health benefits of such supplements, particularly those taken in megadoses, remain unsubstantiated.

Some vitamins can be used efficaciously as drugs. Derivatives of vitamin A are used to treat cystic acne and, more recently, skin wrinkles. Niacin is an effective medication for hyperlipidemia. Vitamin-responsive inborn errors of metabolism also commonly require pharmacologic doses of vitamins.

Coodley G, Girard DE: Vitamins and minerals in HIV infections. J Gen Intern Med 1991;6:472.

Council on Scientific Affairs: Vitamin preparations as dietary supplements and as therapeutic agents. JAMA 1987;257:1929.

Suter PM, Russell RM: Vitamin requirements of the elderly. Am J Clin Nutr 1987;45:501.

WATER-SOLUBLE VITAMINS

1. THIAMIN (B₁)

The primary role of thiamin is as precursor of thiamin pyrophosphate, a coenzyme required for several important biochemical reactions necessary for carbohydrate oxidation. Thiamin is also thought to have an independent role in nerve conduction in peripheral nerves. The recommended daily allowances of thiamin are listed in Table 28–1.

Thiamin Deficiency

A. Clinical Findings: Most thiamin deficiency in the USA is due to alcoholism. Chronic alcoholics may have poor dietary intakes of thiamin and impaired thiamin absorption, metabolism, and storage. Thiamin deficiency is also associated with malabsorption, dialysis, and other causes of chronic protein-calorie undernutrition. Thiamin deficiency can be precipitated in patients with marginal thiamin status with intravenous dextrose solutions.

Early manifestations of thiamin deficiency include anorexia, muscle cramps, paresthesias, and irritability. Advanced deficiency affects chiefly the cardiovascular system ("wet beriberi") or the nervous system ("dry beriberi"). Wet beriberi occurs if severe physical exertion and high carbohydrate intakes accompany thiamin deficiency, whereas dry beriberi is seen with inactivity and low-calorie intake.

Beriberi heart disease is characterized by marked peripheral vasodilation resulting in classic high-output heart failure with dyspnea, tachycardia, cardiomegaly, and pulmonary and peripheral edema, with warm extremities mimicking cellulitis.

Involvement of the nervous system can include both the peripheral and the central nervous systems. Peripheral nerve involvement is typically a symmetric motor and sensory neuropathy with pain, paresthesias, and loss of reflexes. The legs are usually affected more than the arms. Central nervous system involvement results in Wernicke-Korsakoff syndrome. Wernicke's encephalopathy consists of nystagmus progressing to ophthalmoplegia, truncal ataxia, and confusion. Korsakoff's syndrome is characterized by amnesia, confabulation, and impaired learning.

B. Diagnosis: A variety of biochemical tests are available to assess thiamin deficiency. In most instances, however, the clinical response to empirical thiamine therapy is used to support a diagnosis of thiamin deficiency. The most commonly used and widely available biochemical tests are measurement of erythrocyte transketolase activity and urinary thiamin excretion. A transketolase activity coefficient greater than 15–20% suggests thiamin deficiency.

C. Treatment: Suspected thiamin deficiency should be treated promptly with large parenteral doses of thiamine. Fifty to 100 mg/d are typically administered for the first few days, followed by daily oral doses of 5–10 mg/d. All patients should simultaneously receive therapeutic doses of other water-soluble vitamins. Although treatment results in complete resolution in one-half of patients (one-fourth immediately and another one-fourth over days), the other half obtain only partial resolution or no benefit.

Thiamine Toxicity

Although extremely large doses of thiamine can be administered either orally or parenterally without significant toxicity, prolonged injections of large doses can result in an anaphylactoid reaction.

Seligmann H et al: Thiamine deficiency in patients with congestive heart failure receiving long-term furosemide therapy: A pilot study. Am J Med 1991;91:151. (Patients with congestive heart failure treated with furosemide demonstrated thiamin deficiency. Repletion of thiamin resulted in improved cardiac function in most of the small subset of patients that were treated.)

2. RIBOFLAVIN (B₂)

Riboflavin—as the coenzymes flavin mononucleotide and flavin adenine dinucleotide—participates in a variety of important oxidation-reduction reactions and is an essential component of a number of other enzymes. The recommended daily allowances of riboflavin are listed in Table 28–1.

Riboflavin Deficiency

A. Clinical Findings: Riboflavin deficiency almost always occurs in combination with deficiencies of other vitamins. Dietary inadequacy, interactions with a variety of medications, alcoholism, and other causes of protein-calorie undernutrition are the most common causes of riboflavin deficiency.

Manifestations of riboflavin deficiency include mouth soreness, cheilosis, angular stomatitis, glossitis, seborrheic dermatitis, weakness, corneal vascularization, and anemia.

B. Diagnosis: Riboflavin deficiency is usually treated empirically when the diagnosis is clinically suspected. Deficiency can be confirmed by measuring the riboflavin-dependent enzyme erythrocyte glutathione reductase. Activity coefficients greater than 1.2–1.3 are suggestive of riboflavin deficiency. Urinary riboflavin excretion and serum levels of plasma and red cell flavins can also be measured.

C. Treatment: Riboflavin deficiency is easily treated with riboflavin-containing foods such as meat, fish, and dairy products or with oral preparations of the vitamin. Administration of 5–15 mg/d until clinical findings are resolved is usually adequate. Riboflavin can also be given parenterally, but it is poorly soluble in aqueous solutions.

Riboflavin Toxicity

There is no known toxicity of riboflavin.

Campbell TC et al: Human requirements for riboflavin. Am J Clin Nutr 1990;51:436.

3. NIACIN

Niacin is a generic term for nicotinic acid and other derivatives with similar nutritional activity. Unlike most other vitamins, niacin can be synthesized by the human body from the essential amino acid tryptophan. Niacin is an essential component of the coenzymes nicotinamide adenine dinucleotide (NAD) and nicotinamide adenine dinucleotide phosphate (NADP), which are involved in many oxidation-reduction reactions. The recommended daily allowances of niacin are listed in Table 28–1; major food sources are protein foods containing tryptophan and numerous cereals, vegetables, and dairy products.

Niacin can also be used therapeutically for the treatment of hypercholesterolemia and hypertriglyceridemia. Daily doses of 3–6 g can result in significant reductions in levels of low-density lipoproteins (LDL) and very low density lipoproteins (VLDL) and in elevation of high-density lipoproteins (HDL). Niacinamide does not exhibit the lipid-lowering effects of nicotinic acid.

Niacin Deficiency

A. Clinical Findings: Historically, niacin deficiency occurred when corn, which is relatively deficient in both tryptophan and niacin, was the major source of calories. Currently, niacin deficiency is more commonly due to alcoholism and nutrient-drug interactions. Niacin deficiency can also occur in inborn errors of metabolism.

As with other B vitamins, the early manifestations of niacin deficiency are nonspecific. Common complaints include anorexia, weakness, irritability, mouth soreness, glossitis, stomatitis, and weight loss. More advanced deficiency results in the classic triad of pellagra: dermatitis, diarrhea, and dementia. The characteristic dermatitis is symmetric, involving sun-exposed areas. Skin lesions are dark, dry, and scaling. The dementia begins with insomnia, irritability, and apathy and progresses to confusion, memory loss, hallucinations, and psychosis. The diarrhea can be severe and may result in malabsorption due to atrophy of the intestinal villi. Advanced pellagra can result in death.

B. Diagnosis: In advanced cases, the diagnosis of pellagra can be made on clinical grounds. In early cases, diagnosis requires a high index of suspicion and attempts at confirmation of niacin deficiency. Niacin metabolites, particularly N-methylnicotinamide, can be measured in the urine. Low levels suggest niacin deficiency but may also be found in patients with generalized undernutrition. Serum and red cell levels of NAD and NADP are also low but are similarly nonspecific.

C. Treatment: Pellagra can be effectively treated with oral niacin, usually given as nicotinamide. Doses ranging from 10 to 150 mg/d have been used without difficulty.

Niacin Toxicity

At the high doses of niacin used to treat hyperlipidemia, side effects are common. These include cutaneous flushing (partially prevented by pretreatment with aspirin, 325 mg/d) and gastric irritation. Elevation of liver enzymes, hyperglycemia, and gout are less common untoward effects.

Etchason JA et al: Niacin-induced hepatitis: A potential side effect with low dose time-release niacin. Mayo Clin Proc 1991;66:23.

4. VITAMIN B₆ (Pyridoxine)

Vitamin B_6 ("pyridoxine") is actually a group of closely related substances involved in intermediary metabolism. These include pyridoxine itself, pyridoxal, pyridoxamine, and their 5-phosphate esters. As the major coenzyme involved in the metabolism of amino acids, pyridoxal 5-phosphate is the most important. Pyridoxal phosphate is also required for the synthesis of heme. The recommended daily allowances of vitamin B_6 are listed in Table 28–1.

Vitamin B₆ Deficiency

A. Clinical Findings: Vitamin B_6 deficiency most commonly occurs as a result of interactions with medications—especially isoniazid, cycloserine, penicillamine, and oral contraceptives—or of alcoholism. A number of inborn errors of metabolism and other pyridoxine-responsive syndromes, particularly pyridoxine-responsive anemia, are not clearly due to vitamin deficiency but commonly respond to high doses of the vitamin.

Manifestations of vitamin B_6 deficiency result in a

clinical syndrome similar to that seen with deficiencies of other B vitamins, including mouth soreness, glossitis, cheilosis, weakness, and irritability. Severe deficiency can result in peripheral neuropathy, anemia, and seizures.

B. Diagnosis: The diagnosis of vitamin B_6 deficiency can be confirmed by measurement of pyridoxal phosphate in blood. Normal levels are greater than 50 ng/mL.

C. Treatment: Vitamin B_6 deficiency can be effectively treated with oral vitamin B_6 supplements. Doses of 10–20 mg/d are usually adequate, though some patients taking medications that interfere with pyridoxine metabolism may need doses as high as 100 mg/d. Inborn errors of metabolism and the pyridoxine-responsive syndromes often require up to 600 mg/d.

Vitamin B_6 should be routinely prescribed for patients receiving medications (such as isoniazid) that interfere with pyridoxine metabolism to prevent vitamin B_6 deficiency. This is particularly true for elderly patients, the urban poor, and alcoholics, who are more likely to have diets marginally adequate in vitamin B_6.

Large doses of vitamin B_6 have also been advocated for treatment of premenstrual syndrome and carpal tunnel syndrome. No significant clinical benefits have been consistently demonstrated.

Vitamin B_6 Toxicity

A sensory neuropathy, at times irreversible, occurs in patients receiving large doses of vitamin B_6. Although most patients have taken 2 g or more per day, some patients have taken only 200 mg/d.

Leklem JE: Vitamin B-6: A status report. J Nutr 1990; 120(Suppl 11):1503.

5. VITAMIN B_{12} & FOLATE

Vitamin B_{12} (cobalamin) and folate are discussed in Chapter 13. The recommended daily allowances of vitamin B_{12} and folate are listed in Table 28–1. Vitamin B_{12} is abundant in meat and dairy products; fresh fruits and vegetables supply ample folic acid.

6. VITAMIN C (Ascorbic Acid)

Vitamin C is a potent antioxidant involved in many oxidation-reduction reactions and is also required for the synthesis of collagen. It increases the absorption of nonheme iron and is involved in tyrosine metabolism, wound healing, and drug metabolism. With the exception of collagen synthesis, the exact mechanism of action for most of these functions is poorly understood. The recommended daily allowances of vitamin

C are listed in Table 28–1; major food sources are fresh fruits and vegetables.

Vitamin C Deficiency

A. Clinical Findings: Most cases of vitamin C deficiency seen in the USA are due to dietary inadequacy, most commonly in the urban poor, the elderly, and chronic alcoholics. Patients with chronic illnesses such as cancer and chronic renal failure and individuals who smoke cigarettes are also at risk for vitamin C deficiency. Infants 6–12 months of age whose diets are not supplemented with vitamin C or vitamin C-containing foods are also at high risk.

Early manifestations of vitamin C deficiency are nonspecific and include malaise and weakness. In more advanced stages, the typical features of scurvy develop. Manifestations may include perifollicular hemorrhages, perifollicular hyperkeratotic papules, petechiae and purpura, splinter hemorrhages, bleeding gums, joint hemorrhages, and subperiosteal hemorrhages. Anemia is common, and wound healing is impaired. The late stages of scurvy are characterized by edema, oliguria, neuropathy, intracerebral hemorrhage, and death.

B. Diagnosis: The diagnosis of advanced scurvy can be made clinically on the basis of the characteristic skin lesions and other manifestations. The diagnosis can be confirmed with decreased plasma ascorbic acid levels, typically below 0.1 mg/dL. Platelet levels can also be measured.

C. Treatment: Adult scurvy can be treated with 300–1000 mg of ascorbic acid per day. Improvement typically occurs, even in advanced cases, within days. Numerous epidemiologic studies have suggested that high intakes of vitamin C are associated with a decreased risk of cancer. Vitamin C may also protect against coronary heart disease by modifying blood cholesterol levels and preventing LDL-cholesterol from oxidation. A recent large study showed a significant decrease in all-cause and coronary heart disease mortality in individuals with high intakes (approximately 300–400 mg/d).

Vitamin C Toxicity

Although generally extremely safe, very large doses of vitamin C can have side effects. Most common are gastric irritation, flatulence, or diarrhea. Oxalate kidney stones are of theoretic concern because ascorbic acid is metabolized to oxalate, but stone formation has not been frequently reported. Vitamin C can also confuse common diagnostic tests by causing false-negative tests for fecal occult blood and both false-negative and false-positive tests for urine glucose.

Block G: Vitamin C and cancer prevention: The epidemiologic evidence. Am J Clin Nutr 1991;53(Suppl):270S.
Block G, Henson DE, Levine M: Vitamin C: A new look. Ann Intern Med 1991;114:909. (Recommending fre-

quent measurements of fasting ascorbic acid levels in patient at high risk for deficiency.)

FAT-SOLUBLE VITAMINS

1. VITAMIN A

Vitamin A (retinol) is a high-molecular-weight alcohol either ingested preformed or synthesized from plant carotenoids, particularly β-carotene. Isomers and derivatives of retinol are commonly called retinoids. Vitamin A is essential for normal retinal function and plays an important but still not fully understood role in cell growth and differentiation, particularly of epithelial cells. Vitamin A is also necessary for normal wound healing. The recommended daily allowances of vitamin A are listed in Table 28–1; the principal food sources are highly pigmented vegetables.

Because of its role in cell differentiation, vitamin A has been postulated to have a role in cancer prevention. The role of retinoids for chemoprevention of cancer is under intense investigation. The provitamin β-carotene may play an even more important role in prevention of cancer and heart disease by virtue of its antioxidant activity.

Vitamin A Deficiency
A. Clinical Findings: Vitamin A deficiency is one of the most common vitamin deficiency syndromes, particularly in developing countries. In many such regions, vitamin A deficiency is the most common cause of blindness. In the USA, vitamin A deficiency is usually due to fat malabsorption syndromes, alcoholism, or laxative abuse with mineral oil and occurs most commonly in the elderly and the urban poor.

Night blindness is the earliest symptom of vitamin A deficiency. Dryness of the conjunctiva (xerosis) and the development of small white patches on the sclera (Bitot's spots) are early signs. Ulceration and necrosis of the cornea (keratomalacia), perforation, endophthalmitis, and blindness are late manifestations. Xerosis and hyperkeratinization of the skin and loss of taste may also occur.

B. Diagnosis: Abnormalities of dark adaptation are strongly suggestive of vitamin A deficiency. Serum levels below the normal range of 30–65 mg/dL are commonly seen in advanced deficiency.

C. Treatment: Night blindness, poor wound healing, and other signs of early deficiency can be effectively treated with 30,000 IU of vitamin A daily for 1 week. Advanced deficiency with corneal damage calls for administration of 20,000 IU/kg for at least 5 days. The potential antioxidant effects of β-carotene can be achieved with supplements of 25,000–50,000 IU of β-carotene.

Vitamin A Toxicity
Excess intake of β-carotenes (hypercarotenosis) results in a benign staining of the skin a yellow-orange color but is otherwise benign. Skin changes are most marked on the palms and soles, while the scleras remain white, clearly distinguishing hypercarotenosis from jaundice. Large doses of β-carotene are otherwise safe.

Excessive vitamin A (hypervitaminosis A), on the other hand, can be quite toxic. Chronic toxicity usually occurs after ingestion of daily doses of over 50,000 IU/d for more than 3 months. Early manifestations include dry, scaly skin, hair loss, mouth sores, painful hyperostoses, anorexia, and vomiting. More serious findings include increased intracranial pressure, with papilledema, headaches, and decreased cognition; and hepatomegaly, occasionally progressing to cirrhosis. Acute toxicity can result from ingestion of massive doses of vitamin A, such as in drug overdoses or consumption of polar bear liver. Manifestations include nausea, vomiting, abdominal pain, headache, papilledema, and lethargy.

The diagnosis can be confirmed by elevations of serum vitamin A levels. The only treatment is withdrawal of vitamin A from the diet. Most symptoms and signs improve rapidly.

Byers T, Perry G: Dietary carotenes, vitamin C and vitamin E as protective antioxidants in human cancers. Annu Rev Nutr 1992;12:139. (Beta-carotene but not vitamin A has been associated with decreased risk of cancer.)

Lippman SM et al: Comparison of low-dose isotretinoin with β-carotene to prevent oral carcinogenesis. N Engl J Med 1993;328:15. (Low-dose vitamin A was more effective than beta-carotene in preventing the progression of leukoplakia to oral cancer.)

2. VITAMIN D

Vitamin D is discussed in Chapter 25. The recommended daily allowances of vitamin D are listed in Table 28–1; a major food source is fortified milk, but sunlight on the skin is a prime resource as well.

3. VITAMIN E

Vitamin E activity is derived from at least eight naturally occurring tocopherols, the most potent of which is α-tocopherol. Although the exact function and mechanism of action of vitamin E in humans are unclear, it is commonly thought to function as an antioxidant, protecting membranes and other cellular structures from attack by free radicals. Dietary selenium and other antioxidants work in conjunction with vitamin E and may partially spare its requirement and reverse signs of vitamin E deficiency in animals. The recommended daily allowances of vitamin E are listed in Table 28–1; the major food source is vegetable seed oil.

Vitamin E, like β-carotene and vitamin C, may also play a role in protection against cancer, coronary heart disease, and cataracts through its antioxidant function.

Vitamin E Deficiency

A. Clinical Findings: Clinical deficiency of vitamin E is most commonly due to severe malabsorption, the genetic disorder abetalipoproteinemia, or, in children with chronic cholestatic liver disease, biliary atresia or cystic fibrosis. Manifestations of deficiency include areflexia, disturbances of gait, decreased proprioception and vibration, and ophthalmoplegia.

B. Diagnosis: Plasma vitamin E levels can be measured; normal levels are 0.5–0.7 mg/dL or higher. Since vitamin E is normally transported in lipoproteins, the serum level should be interpreted in relation to circulating lipids.

C. Treatment: The optimum therapeutic dose of vitamin E has not been clearly defined. Large doses, often administered parenterally, can be used to improve the neurologic complications seen in abetalipoproteinemia and cholestatic liver disease. The potential antioxidant effects of vitamin E can be achieved with supplements of 100–400 IU/d.

Vitamin E Toxicity

Vitamin E is the least toxic of the fat-soluble vitamins. Large doses, 20–80 times the recommended daily requirement, have been taken for extended periods of time without apparent harm, although nausea, flatulence, and diarrhea have been reported. Large doses of vitamin E can increase the vitamin K requirement and can result in bleeding in patients taking oral anticoagulants.

Comstock GW, Bush TL, Helzlsouer K: Serum retinol, beta-carotene, vitamin E, and selenium as related to subsequent cancer of specific sites. Am J Epidemiol 1992;135:115. (Higher blood levels of vitamin E are associated with a slight decrease in cancer risk.)

Packer L: Protective role of vitamin E in biological systems. Am J Clin Nutr 1991;53(Suppl):1050S. (Increasing evidence that vitamin E plays an important role in minimizing damage from free radicals associated with cancer and other illnesses.)

4. VITAMIN K

Vitamin K is discussed in Chapter 13. The recommended daily allowances of vitamin K are listed in Table 28–1; it is synthesized by intestinal bacteria.

DIET THERAPY

Specific therapeutic diets can be designed to facilitate the medical management of most common illnesses. In most cases, consultation with a registered dietitian is necessary in order to design and implement major dietary changes. Physicians should be familiar with the indications for special diets and their basic composition to facilitate patient referrals and to maximize patient compliance.

Diet therapy is a difficult process, and not all patients are able to cooperate fully. Before starting specific dietary changes, one should assess the patient's motivation for change in eating habits. Patients who are not adequately motivated or who for other reasons are unable to change their diets should not be started on diet therapy, since embarking on a course that can only fail will interfere with other aspects of the therapeutic relationship between doctor and patient. Requesting the patient to record dietary intake for 3–5 days may provide useful insight into the patient's motivation.

Prescribed diets should take into account personal food preferences, cultural habits, and eating behavior. Changes should be introduced gradually. Close follow-up and a close patient-therapist relationship are necessary for sustained dietary change.

Therapeutic diets can be divided into three groups: (1) diets that alter the consistency of food; (2) diets that restrict or otherwise modify dietary components; and (3) diets that supplement dietary components.

DIETS THAT ALTER CONSISTENCY

Clear Liquid Diet

This diet provides adequate water, 500–1000 kcal as simple sugar, and some electrolytes. It is fiber-free and requires minimal digestion or intestinal motility.

A clear liquid diet is useful for patients with resolving postoperative ileus, acute gastroenteritis, partial intestinal obstruction, and as preparation for diagnostic gastrointestinal procedures. It is commonly used as the first diet for patients who have been taking nothing by mouth for long periods. Because of the low calorie and minimal protein content of the clear liquid diet, it should be used only for short periods.

Full Liquid Diet

The full liquid diet provides adequate water and can be designed to provide adequate calories and protein. Vitamins and minerals—especially folic acid, iron, and vitamin B_6—may be inadequate and should be provided in the form of supplements. Dairy products, soups, eggs, and soft cereals are used to supplement clear liquids. Commercial oral supplements can also be incorporated into the diet or used alone.

This diet is low in residue and can be used in many instances instead of the clear liquid diet described above—especially in patients with difficulty in chewing or swallowing, with partial obstructions, or in preparation for some diagnostic procedures. Full liquid diets are commonly used following clear liquid diets to "advance" diets in patients who have been taking nothing by mouth for long periods.

Soft Diets

Soft diets are designed for patients unable to chew or swallow hard or coarse food. Tender foods are used, and most raw fruits and vegetables and coarse breads and cereals are eliminated. Soft diets are commonly used to assist in progression from full liquid diets to regular diets in postoperative patients and patients who are too weak or those whose dentition is too poor to handle a general diet.

Mechanical soft diets include chopped, ground, and pureed foods as well as any foods patients are able to masticate. These diets are used for head and neck surgical patients, those with dental problems and esophageal strictures, and other patients who have difficulty with chewing or swallowing.

The soft diet can be designed to meet all nutritional requirements.

DIETS THAT RESTRICT NUTRIENTS

Diets can be designed to restrict (or eliminate) virtually any nutrient or food component. The most commonly used restricted diets are those that limit sodium, fat, and protein. Other restrictive diets include gluten restriction in sprue, potassium and phosphate reduction in renal insufficiency, and various elimination diets for food allergies.

Sodium-Restricted Diets

Low-sodium diets are useful in the management of hypertension and in conditions in which sodium retention and edema are prominent features, particularly congestive heart failure, chronic liver disease, and chronic renal failure. Sodium restriction is beneficial with or without diuretic therapy. When used in conjunction with diuretics, sodium restriction allows lower dosage of the diuretic medication and may prevent side effects. Potassium excretion, in particular, is directly related to distal renal tubule sodium delivery, and sodium restriction will decrease diuretic-related potassium losses.

Typical American diets contain about 4–6 g (175–260 meq) of sodium per day. A no-added-salt diet contains approximately 3 g of sodium (132 meq) per day. Further restriction can be achieved with sodium diets 2 g or 1 g per day. Diets with more severe re-

striction are poorly accepted by patients and are rarely used.

Dietary sodium includes sodium naturally occurring in foods, sodium added during food processing, and sodium added by the consumer during cooking and at the table. About a third of current dietary intake is derived from each. Diets that allow 2000 mg of sodium daily are easiest to design and implement. Such diets generally eliminate added salt, most processed foods, and selected foods with particularly high sodium content. Patients who follow such diets for 2–3 months lose their craving for salty foods and can often continue to restrict their sodium intake indefinitely. Many patients with mild hypertension will achieve significant reductions in blood pressure (approximately 5 mm Hg diastolic) with this degree of sodium restriction. Other patients require more severe sodium restriction (approximately 1000 mg of sodium per day) for reduction in blood pressure, and others may actually have increased blood pressure with sodium restriction.

Diets allowing 1000 mg and 500 mg of sodium require further restriction of commonly eaten foods. Special "low-sodium" products are now available to facilitate such diets. These diets are difficult for most people to follow and are generally reserved for hospitalized patients and highly motivated outpatients—most commonly those with severe liver disease and ascites.

Fat-Restricted Diets

Traditional fat-restricted diets are useful in the treatment of fat malabsorption syndromes. Such diets will improve the symptoms of diarrhea with steatorrhea independently of the primary physiologic abnormality by limiting the quantity of fatty acids that reach the colon. The degree of fat restriction necessary to control symptoms must be individualized. Patients with severe malabsorption can be limited to 40–60 g of fat per day. Diets containing 60–80 g of fat per day can be designed for patients with less severe abnormalities.

In general, fat-restricted diets require broiling, baking, or boiling meat and fish; discarding the skin of poultry and fish and using those foods as the main protein source; using nonfat dairy products; and avoiding desserts, sauces, and gravies.

Low-Cholesterol, Low-Saturated Fat Diets

Fat-restricted diets that specifically restrict saturated fats and dietary cholesterol are the mainstay of dietary treatment of hyperlipidemia (see Chapter 27). Similar diets are recommended also for diabetes (Chapter 26) and for the prevention of coronary artery disease (Chapter 10). Current recommendations for the prevention of cancer by dietary modification also include fat restriction.

The aim of these diets is to restrict total fat to 30%

of calories and to achieve a normal body weight by caloric restriction. Saturated fat and dietary cholesterol are further restricted. In the first phase of treatment ("step 1"), saturated fat is restricted to 10% of total calories and dietary cholesterol to 300 mg/d. "Step 2" consists of further reduction of saturated fat to 7% of total calories and dietary cholesterol to 200 mg/d. In both cases, up to 10% of calories is derived from polyunsaturated fats and 10–15% is monounsaturated. In both diets also, 50–60% of calories is from carbohydrates, particularly complex carbohydrates high in dietary fiber. Ideally, the "step 1" diet can lead to a decrease in serum cholesterol of 15–20% and the "step 2" diet a further 5% reduction.

Protein-Restricted Diets

Protein-restricted diets are most commonly used in patients with hepatic encephalopathy due to chronic liver disease and in patients with renal failure to ameliorate the progression of early disease and to decrease symptoms of uremia in more severe disease. Patients with selected inborn errors of amino acid metabolism and other abnormalities resulting in hyperammonemia also require restriction of protein or of specific amino acids.

Protein restriction is intended to limit the production of nitrogenous waste products. Energy intake must be adequate to facilitate the efficient use of dietary protein. Proteins must be of high biologic value and be provided in sufficient quantity to meet minimal requirements. For most patients, the diet should contain at least 0.6 g/kg/d of protein. Patients with encephalopathy who fail to respond to this degree of restriction are unlikely to respond to more severe restriction.

DIETS THAT SUPPLEMENT NUTRIENTS

High-Fiber Diet

Dietary fiber is a diverse group of plant constituents that are resistant to digestion by the human digestive tract. Typical American diets contain about 5–10 g of dietary fiber per day. Epidemiologic evidence has suggested that populations consuming greater quantities of fiber have a lower incidence of certain gastrointestinal disorders, including diverticulitis and colon cancer. Most authorities currently recommend higher intakes of dietary fiber for health maintenance.

Diets high in dietary fiber (20–35 g/d) are also commonly used in management of a variety of gastrointestinal disorders, particularly the irritable bowel syndrome and recurrent diverticulitis. Diets high in fiber may also be useful to reduce blood sugar in patients with diabetes and to reduce cholesterol levels in patients with hypercholesterolemia. Such diets include greater intakes of fresh fruits and vegetables, whole grains, legumes and seeds, and bran products. For some patients, the addition of psyllium seed (2 tsp per day) or natural bran ($\frac{1}{2}$ cup per day) may be preferable.

High-Potassium Diets

Potassium-supplemented diets are used most commonly to compensate for potassium losses caused by diuretics. Although potassium losses can be partially prevented by using lower doses of diuretics, concurrent sodium restriction, and potassium-sparing diuretics, some patients require additional potassium to prevent hypokalemia. Epidemiologic and experimental evidence suggests that high-potassium diets may also have a direct antihypertensive effect. Typical American diets contain about 3 g (80 meq) of potassium per day. High-potassium diets commonly contain 4.5–7 g (120–180 meq) of potassium per day.

Most fruits, vegetables, and their juices contain high concentrations of potassium (see Chapter 20). Supplemental potassium can also be provided with potassium-containing salt substitutes (up to 20 meq in $\frac{1}{4}$ tsp) or as potassium chloride in solution or capsules, but this is rarely necessary if the above measures are followed to prevent potassium losses and supplement dietary potassium.

High-Calcium Diets

Additional intakes of dietary calcium have recently been recommended for the prevention of postmenopausal osteoporosis, the prevention and treatment of hypertension, and the prevention of colon cancer. Although the evidence in each case is preliminary, most authorities currently recommend intakes of 1 g of calcium per day for most adults and 1.5 g/d for postmenopausal women. Current USA intakes are approximately 700 mg/d.

Low-fat and nonfat dairy products are the mainstay of supplemental calcium intakes. Patients with lactose intolerance who cannot tolerate liquid dairy products may be able to tolerate nonliquid products such as cheese and yogurt. Leafy green vegetables and canned fish with bones also contain high concentrations of calcium, although the latter is also very high in sodium.

American Dietetic Association: Health implications of dietary fiber. J Am Diet Assoc 1988;88:216.

Baron RB: Management of hypercholesterolemia: A primary care perspective. West J Med 1989;150:562. (Practical suggestions for implementing diet therapy.)

Cappuccio FP, MacGregor GA: Does potassium supplementation lower blood pressure? A meta-analysis of published trials. J Hypertens 1991;9;465. (A meta-analysis of 19 published trials showing a modest decrease in blood pressure with potassium supplementation.)

Macgregor GA et al: Double-blind study of three sodium intakes and long-term effects of sodium restriction in essential hypertension. Lancet 1989;2:1244. (Reduction of blood pressure was achieved and maintained for 1 year by moderate sodium restriction.)

NUTRITIONAL SUPPORT

Nutritional support is the provision of nutrients to patients who cannot meet their nutritional requirements by eating standard diets. Nutrients may be delivered enterally, using oral nutritional supplements, nasogastric and nasoduodenal feeding tubes, and tube enterostomies; or parenterally, using lines or catheters placed in peripheral or central veins, respectively. Current nutritional support techniques permit adequate nutrient delivery to virtually any patient. Nutrition support should only be utilized, however, if it is likely to improve the patient's clinical outcome. The financial costs and risks of side effects must be balanced against the potential advantages of improved nutritional status in each clinical situation.

INDICATIONS FOR NUTRITIONAL SUPPORT

The precise indications for nutritional support remain controversial. Most authorities agree that nutritional support is indicated for at least four groups of adult patients: (1) those with inadequate bowel syndromes; (2) those with severe prolonged hypercatabolic states (eg, due to extensive burns, multiple trauma, mechanical ventilation); (3) those requiring prolonged therapeutic bowel rest; and (4) those with severe protein-calorie undernutrition with a treatable

disease who have sustained a loss of over 25% of body weight.

It has been difficult to prove the efficacy of nutritional support in the treatment of most other conditions. Over 100 randomized controlled clinical trials have been conducted in an attempt to address this question. In most cases it has not been possible to show a clear advantage of treatment by means of nutritional support over treatment without such support. Unfortunately, most of these studies have design flaws and do not disprove the effectiveness of nutritional support.

The American Society for Parenteral and Enteral Nutrition (ASPEN) has published recommendations for the rational use of nutritional support. The recommendations emphasize the need to individualize the decision to begin nutritional support, carefully weighing the risks and costs against the benefit to each patient. They also demonstrate the need to identify high-risk malnourished patients by nutritional assessment.

NUTRITIONAL SUPPORT METHODS

Selection of the most appropriate nutritional support method involves consideration of gastrointestinal function, the anticipated duration of nutritional support, and the ability of each method to meet the patient's nutritional requirements. The method chosen should meet the patient's nutritional needs with the lowest risk and lowest cost possible. For most patients, enteral feeding is safer and cheaper and offers significant physiologic advantages. An algorithm for selection of the most appropriate nutritional support method is presented in Figure 28–2.

Prior to initiating specialized enteral nutritional support, efforts should be made to supplement food

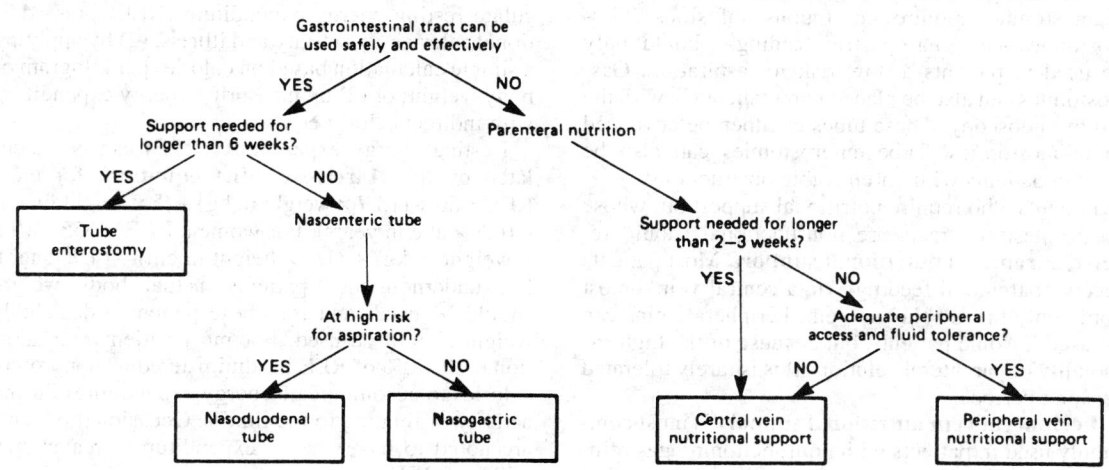

Figure 28–2. Nutritional support method decision tree.

intake. Careful attention to patient preferences, timing of meals, diagnostic procedures and use of medications, and the use of foods brought to the hospital by family and friends can often significantly increase oral intake. Patients unable to eat enough at regular mealtimes to meet their nutritional requirements can be given **oral supplements** as snacks or to replace low-calorie beverages. Supplements of differing nutritional composition are available for the purpose of individualizing the diet in accordance with specific clinical requirements. Fiber and lactose content, caloric density, protein level, and amino acid profiles can all be modified as necessary.

Patients unable to take adequate oral nutrients who have functioning gastrointestinal tracts and who meet the criteria for nutritional support are candidates for **tube feedings.** Small-bore feeding tubes are placed via the nose into the stomach or duodenum. Patients able to sit up in bed who can protect their airways can be fed into the stomach. Because of the increased risk of aspiration, patients who cannot adequately protect their airways should be fed nasoduodenally. Feeding tubes can be passed into the duodenum by leaving an extra length of tubing and placing the patient in the right decubitus position. Metoclopramide, 10 mg intravenously, can be given 20 minutes prior to insertion and continued every 6 hours thereafter to facilitate passage through the pylorus. Occasionally patients will require fluoroscopy or endoscopic guidance to insert the tube distal to the pylorus. Placement of nasogastric and, particularly, nasoduodenal tubes should be confirmed radiographically before delivery of feeding solutions.

Feeding tubes can also be placed directly into the gastrointestinal tract using **tube enterostomies.** Most tube enterostomies are placed in patients who require long-term enteral nutritional support. The most common application is the surgical placement of gastrostomies and jejunostomies. Gastrostomies have the advantage of allowing bolus feedings, while jejunostomies require continuous infusions. Gastrostomies—like nasogastric feeding—should only be used in patients at low risk for aspiration. Gastrostomies can also be placed percutaneously with the aid of endoscopy. These tubes can then be advanced to jejunostomies. Tube enterostomies can also be used in patients with unrelievable obstructions.

Patients who require nutritional support but whose gastrointestinal tracts are nonfunctional should receive **parenteral nutritional support.** Most patients receive parenteral feedings via a central vein—most commonly the subclavian vein. Peripheral veins can be used in some patients, but because of the high osmolality of parenteral solutions this is rarely tolerated for long periods.

Peripheral vein nutritional support is most commonly used in patients with nonfunctioning gastrointestinal tracts who require immediate support but whose clinical status is expected to improve within 1–2 weeks, allowing enteral feeding. Peripheral vein nutritional support is administered via standard intravenous lines. Solutions should always include lipid and dextrose in combination with amino acids to provide adequate nonprotein calories. Serious side effects are infrequent, but there is a high incidence of phlebitis and infiltration of intravenous lines.

Central vein nutritional support is most commonly delivered via intravenous catheters placed percutaneously using aseptic technique. Proper placement in the superior vena cava is documented radiographically before the solution is allowed to start running. Catheters must be carefully maintained by experienced nursing personnel and not used for anything other than nutritional support.

NUTRITIONAL REQUIREMENTS

Each patient's nutritional requirements should be determined independently of the method chosen. In most situations, solutions of equal nutrient value can be designed for delivery via enteral and parenteral routes, but differences in absorption must be considered. A complete nutritional support solution must contain water, energy, amino acids, electrolytes, vitamins, minerals, and essential fatty acids.

Water

For most patients, water requirements can be calculated by allowing 1500 mL for the first 20 kg of body weight plus 20 mL for every kilogram over 20. Additional losses should be replaced as they occur. For average-sized adult patients, fluid needs are about 30–35 mL/kg, or approximately 1 mL/kcal of energy required (see below).

Energy

Energy requirements can be estimated by one of three methods: (1) by using standard equations to calculate resting energy expenditure (REE) plus additional calories for activity and illness; (2) by applying a simple calculation based on calories per kilogram of body weight; or (3) by measuring energy expenditure with indirect calorimetry.

Resting energy expenditure (REE) can be calculated by the **Harris-Benedict equation:** for men, REE = 66 + (13.7 × weight in kg) + (5 × height in cm) − (6.8 × age in years). For women, REE = 655 + (9.5 × weight in kg) + (1.7 × height in cm) − (4.7 × age). For undernourished patients, actual body weight should be used; and for obese patients, ideal body weight should be used. For most patients, an additional 20–50% of REE is administered as nonprotein calories to accommodate energy expenditures during activity or relating to the illness. Occasional patients are noted to have energy expenditures greater than 150% of REE.

Energy requirements can be estimated also by multiplying actual body weight in kilograms (for obese patients, ideal body weight) by 30–35 kcal.

Both of these methods provide imprecise estimates of actual energy expenditures, especially for the markedly underweight, overweight, and critically ill patient. Studies using indirect calorimetry have demonstrated that as many as 30–40% of patients will have measured expenditures 10% above or below estimated values. For accurate determination of energy expenditure, indirect calorimetry should be used.

Protein

Protein and energy requirements are closely related. If adequate calories are provided, most patients can be given 0.8–1.2 g of protein per kilogram per day. Patients undergoing moderate to severe stress should receive up to 1.5 g/kg/d. As in the case of energy requirements, actual weights should be used for normal and underweight patients and ideal weights for patients with significant obesity.

Patients who are receiving protein without adequate calories will catabolize protein for energy rather than utilizing it for protein synthesis. Thus, when energy intake is low, excess protein is needed for nitrogen balance. If both energy and protein intakes are low, extra energy will have a more significant positive effect on nitrogen balance than extra protein.

Electrolytes & Minerals

Requirements for sodium, potassium, and chloride vary widely. Most patients require 45–145 meq/d of each. The actual requirement in individual patients will depend on the patient's cardiovascular, renal, endocrine, and gastrointestinal status as well as measurements of serum concentration.

Patients receiving enteral nutritional support should receive adequate vitamins and minerals according to the recommended daily allowances (Table 28–1). Most premixed enteral solutions provide adequate vitamins and minerals as long as adequate calories are administered.

Patients receiving parenteral nutritional support require smaller amounts of minerals: calcium, 10–15 meq/d; phosphorus, 15–20 meq per 1000 nonprotein calories; and magnesium, 16–24 meq/d. Most patients receiving nutritional support do not require supplemental iron because body stores are adequate. Iron nutrition should be monitored closely by following the hemoglobin concentration, MCV, and iron studies. Parenteral administration of iron is associated with a number of adverse effects and should be reserved for iron-deficient patients unable to take oral iron.

Patients receiving parenteral nutritional support should be given the trace elements zinc (about 5 mg/d) and copper (about 2 mg/d). Patients with diarrhea will require additional zinc to replace fecal losses. Additional trace elements—especially chro-

mium, manganese, and selenium—are provided to patients receiving long-term parenteral nutrition.

Parenteral vitamins are provided daily. Standardized multivitamin solutions are currently available to provide adequate quantities of vitamins A, B_{12}, C, D, E, thiamin, riboflavin, niacin, pantothenic acid, pyridoxine, folic acid, and biotin. Vitamin K is not given routinely but administered when the prothrombin time becomes abnormal.

Essential Fatty Acids

Patients receiving nutritional support should be given 2–4% of their total calories as linoleic acid to prevent essential fatty acid deficiency. Most prepared enteral solutions contain adequate linoleic acid. Patients receiving parenteral nutrition should be given at least 250 mL of a 20% intravenous fat (emulsified soybean or safflower oil) about two or three times a week. Intravenous fat can also be used as an energy source in place of dextrose.

Table 28–8. Enteral solutions.

Complete
   Blenderized (eg, Compleat Regular, Compleat Modified,[1] Vitaneed[1])
   Whole protein, lactose-containing (eg, Meritene, Sustacal)
   Whole protein, lactose-free, low-residue:
      1 kcal/mL (eg, Ensure, Entralife,[1] Newtrition, Isocal,[1] Osmolite[1])
      1.5 kcal/mL (eg, Ensure Plus, Sustacal HC, Comply)
      2 kcal/mL (eg, Isocal HCN, Magnacal, TwoCal HN)
      High-Nitorgen: >15% total calories from protein (eg, Ensure HN, Attain,[1] Isocal HN, Newtrition HN,[1] Osmolite HN,[1] Replete)
   Whole protein, lactose-free, high-residue
      1 kcal/mL (eg, Enrich, Jevity,[1] Profiber[1])
   Chemically defined peptide or amino acid based
      (Accupep HPF, Criticare HN, Isotein HN,[1] Peptamen,[1] Reablin, Vital HN, Vivonex HN)
   "Disease-specific" formulas:
      Renal failure: with essential amino acids (eg, Amin-Acid, Travasorb Renal, Replena)
      Malabsorption: with medium-chain triglycerides (eg, Portagen,[1] Travasorb MCT)
      Respiratory failure: with >50% calories from fat (eg, Pulmocare, Traumacal)
      Hepatic encephalopathy: with high amounts of branched-chain amino acids (eg, Hepatic-Acid II, Travasorb Hepatic)

Incomplete (modular)
   Protein (eg, Nutrisource Protein, Promed, Propac)
   Carbohydrate (eg, Nutrisource Carbohydrate, Polycose, Sumacal)
   Fat (eg, MCT Oil, Microlipid, Nutrisource Lipid)
   Vitamins (eg, Nutrisource Vitamins)
   Minerals (eg, Nutrisource Minerals)

[1]Isotonic.

ENTERAL NUTRITIONAL SUPPORT SOLUTIONS

Most patients who require enteral nutritional support can be given commercially prepared enteral solutions (Table 28–8). Nutritionally complete solutions have been designed to provide adequate proportions of water, energy, protein, and micronutrients. Nutritionally incomplete solutions are also available to provide specific macronutrients (eg, protein, carbohydrate, and fat) to supplement complete solutions for patients with unusual requirements or to design solutions that are not available commercially.

Nutritionally complete solutions are characterized as follows: (1) by osmolality (isotonic or hypertonic), (2) by lactose content (present or absent), (3) by the molecular form of the protein component (intact proteins; peptides or amino acids), (4) by the quantity of protein and calories provided, and (5) by fiber content (present or absent). For most patients, isotonic solutions containing no lactose or fiber are preferable. Such solutions generally contain relatively higher quantities of fat and intact protein. Most commercial isotonic solutions contain 1000 kcal and about 37–45 g of protein per liter.

Solutions containing hydrolyzed proteins or crystalline amino acids and with no significant fat content are called elemental solutions, since macronutrients are provided in their most "elemental" form. These solutions have been designed for patients with malabsorption, particularly pancreatic insufficiency and limited fat absorption. Elemental diets are extremely hypertonic and often result in more severe diarrhea. Their use should be limited to patients who cannot tolerate isotonic solutions.

Although formulas have been designed for specific clinical situations—solutions containing primarily essential amino acids (for renal failure), medium-chain triglycerides (for fat malabsorption), more fat (for respiratory failure and CO_2 retention), and more branched-chain amino acids (for hepatic encephalopathy and severe trauma)—they have not been shown to be superior to standard formulas for most patients.

Enteral solutions should be administered via continuous infusion, preferably with an infusion pump. Isotonic feedings should be started at full strength at about 25–33% of the estimated final infusion rate. Feedings can be advanced by similar amounts every 12 hours as tolerated. Hypertonic feedings should be started at half strength. The strength and the rate can then be advanced every 6 hours as tolerated.

COMPLICATIONS OF ENTERAL NUTRITIONAL SUPPORT

Minor complications of tube feedings occur in 10–15% of patients. Gastrointestinal complications include diarrhea (most common), inadequate gastric emptying, emesis, esophagitis, and occasionally gastrointestinal bleeding. Diarrhea associated with tube feeding may be due to intolerance to the osmotic load or to one of the macronutrients (eg, fat, lactose) in the solution. Patients being fed in this way may also have diarrhea from other causes (as side effect of antibiotics or other drugs; associated with infection, etc), and these possibilities should always be investigated in appropriate circumstances.

Mechanical complications of tube feedings are potentially the most serious. Of particular importance is aspiration. All patients receiving nasogastric tube feedings are at risk for this life-threatening complication. Limiting nasogastric feedings to those patients who can adequately protect their airway and careful monitoring of patients being fed by tube should limit these serious complications to 1–2% of cases. Minor mechanical complications are common and include tube obstruction and dislodgment.

Metabolic complications during enteral nutritional support are common but in most cases easily managed. The most important problem is hypernatremic dehydration, most commonly seen in elderly patients given excessive protein intake who are unable to respond to thirst. Abnormalities of potassium, glucose, and acid-base balance may also occur.

PARENTERAL NUTRITIONAL SUPPORT SOLUTIONS

Parenteral nutritional support solutions can be designed to deliver adequate nutrients to virtually any patient. The basic parenteral solution is composed of dextrose, amino acids, and water. Electrolytes, minerals, trace elements, vitamins, and medications can also be added. Most commercial solutions contain the monohydrate form of dextrose that provides 3.4

Table 28–9. Typical TPN solution (for stable patients without organ failure).

Dextrose (3.4 kcal/g)	25%
Amino acids (4 kcal/g)	6%
Na^+	50 meq/L
K^+	40 meq/L
Ca^{2+}	5 meq/L
Mg^{2+}	8 meq/L
Cl^-	60 meq/L
P	12 mmol/L
Acetate	Balance
MVI-12 (vitamins)	10 mL/d
MTE (trace elements)	5 mL/d
Fat emulsion 20%	250 mL five times a week
Typical rate	Day 1: 30 mL/h Day 2: 60 mL/h
By day 2, solution provides	Calories 1925 kcal total Protein 86 g Fat 19% of total kcal Fluid 1690 mL

kcal/g. Crystalline amino acids are available in a variety of concentrations, so that a broad range of solutions can be made up that will contain specific amounts of dextrose and amino acids as required.

Typical solutions for central vein nutritional support contain 25–35% dextrose and 2.75–6% amino acids depending upon the patient's estimated nutrient and water requirements. These solutions typically have osmolalities in excess of 1800 mosm/L and require infusion into a central vein. A typical formula for patients without organ failure is shown in Table 28–9.

Solutions with lower osmolalities can also be designed for infusion into peripheral veins. Typical solutions for peripheral infusion contain 5–10% dextrose and 2.75–4.25% amino acids. These solutions have osmolalities between 800 and 1200 mosm/L and result in a high incidence of thrombophlebitis and line infiltration. These solutions will provide adequate protein for most patients but inadequate energy. Additional energy must be provided in the form of emulsified soybean or safflower oil. Such intravenous fat solutions are currently available in 10% and 25% solutions providing 1.1 and 2.2 kcal/mL, respectively. Intravenous fat solutions are isosmotic and well tolerated by peripheral veins. Typical patients are given 200–500 mL of a 20% solution each day. As much as 60% of total calories can be administered in this manner.

Intravenous fat can also be provided to patients receiving central vein nutritional support. In this instance, dextrose concentrations should be decreased to provide a fixed concentration of energy. Intravenous fat has been shown to be equivalent to intravenous dextrose in providing energy to "spare protein." Intravenous fat is associated with less glucose intolerance, less production of carbon dioxide, and less fatty infiltration of the liver and has been increasingly utilized in patients with hyperglycemia, respiratory failure, and liver disease. Intravenous fat has also been increasingly used in patients with large estimated energy requirements. Recent studies suggest that the maximum glucose utilization rate is approximately 5–7 mg/min/kg. Patients who require additional calories can be given them as fat to prevent excess administration of dextrose. Intravenous fat can also be used to prevent essential fatty acid deficiency. The optimal ratio of carbohydrate and fat in parenteral nutritional support has not been determined.

Infusion of parenteral solutions should be started slowly to prevent hyperglycemia and other metabolic complications. Typical solutions are given initially at a rate of 50 mL/h and advanced by about the same amount every 24 hours.

COMPLICATIONS OF PARENTERAL NUTRITIONAL SUPPORT

Complications of central vein nutritional support occur in up to 50% of patients. Although most are minor and easily managed, about 5% of patients will develop significant complications. Complications of central vein nutritional support can be divided into catheter-related complications and metabolic complications.

Catheter-related complications can occur during insertion or while the catheter is in place. Pneumothorax, hemothorax, arterial laceration, air emboli, and brachial plexus injury can occur during catheter placement. The incidence of these complications is inversely related to the experience of the physician performing the procedure but will occur in at least 1–2% of cases even in major medical centers. Each catheter placement should be documented by chest radiograph prior to initiation of nutritional support.

Catheter thrombosis and catheter-related sepsis are the most important complications of indwelling catheters. Patients with indwelling central vein catheters who develop signs of sepsis without an apparent source should have their lines removed immediately, the tip cultured, and antibiotics begun empirically. Patients with less significant fevers without an appar-

Table 28–10. Metabolic complications of parenteral nutritional support.

Complication	Common Causes	Possible Solutions
Hyperglycemia	Too rapid infusion of dextrose, "stress," glucocorticoids.	Decrease glucose infusion. Insulin. Replacement of dextrose with fat.
Hyperosmolar non-ketotic dehydration	Severe, undetected hyperglycemia.	Insulin, hydration, potassium.
Hyperchloremic metabolic acidosis	High chloride administration.	Decrease chloride.
Azotemia	Excessive protein administration.	Decrease amino acid concentration.
Hyperphosphatemia. hypokalemia, hypomagnesemia	Extracellular to intracellular shifting with refeeding.	Increase solution concentration.
Liver enzyme abnormalities	Lipid trapping in hepatocytes, fatty liver.	Decrease dextrose.
Acalculous cholecystitis	Biliary stasis.	Oral fat.
Zinc deficiency	Diarrhea, small bowel fistulas.	Increase concentration.
Copper deficiency	Biliary fistulas.	Increase concentration.

ent source should have their lines removed and be observed without antibiotics. Catheter-related sepsis occurs in 2–3% of patients even if maximal efforts are made to prevent infection.

Metabolic complications of central vein nutritional support occur in over 50% of patients (Table 28–10). Most are minor and easily managed, and termination of support is seldom necessary.

PATIENT MONITORING DURING NUTRITIONAL SUPPORT

Every patient receiving enteral or parenteral nutritional support should be followed closely. Formal nutritional support teams composed of a physician, a nurse, a dietitian, and a pharmacist have been shown to decrease the rate of complications.

Patients should be monitored both for the adequacy of treatment and to prevent complications or detect them early when they occur. Because estimates of nutritional requirements are imprecise, frequent reassessment is necessary. Daily intakes should be recorded and compared with estimated requirements. Body weight, hydration status, and overall clinical status should be followed. Patients who do not appear to be responding as anticipated can be evaluated for nitrogen balance by means of the following equation:

$$\frac{\text{Nitrogen}}{\text{balance}} = \frac{\text{24-hour protein intake (g)}}{6.25} - \left(\frac{\text{24-hour urinary}}{\text{nitrogen (g)}} + 4\right)$$

Patients with positive nitrogen balances can be continued on their current regimens; patients with negative balances should receive moderate increases in calorie and protein intake and then be reassessed.

Feeding tubes and catheters should be examined often to avoid mechanical and infectious complications.

Monitoring for metabolic complications should include urine glucose determination every 6 hours and daily measurements of electrolytes; serum glucose, phosphorus, magnesium, calcium, and creatinine; and BUN until the patient is stabilized. Once the patient is stabilized, electrolytes, phosphorus, calcium, magnesium, and glucose should be checked at least twice weekly. Red blood cell folate, zinc, and copper should be checked at least once a month.

Meguid MM, Muscaritoli M: Current uses of total parenteral nutrition. Am Fam Physician 1993;47:383.Pillar B, Perry S (editors): Evaluating total parenteral nutrition: Core statement of the technology assessment and practice guidelines forum. Nutrition 1990;6:475.

Task Force on Nutrition Support in AIDS: Guidelines for nutrition support in AIDS. Nutrition 1989;5:39.

Veterans Affairs Total Parenteral Nutrition Cooperative Study Group: Perioperative total parenteral nutrition in surgical patients. N Engl J Med 1991;325:525. (Preoperative TPN is only effective in severely malnourished patients.)

REFERENCES

Brown ML (editor): *Present Knowledge in Nutrition,* 6th ed. International Life Sciences Institute, Nutrition Foundation, 1990.

National Research Council: *Recommended Dietary Allowances,* 10th ed. National Academy of Science, 1989.

Kinney JM et al: *Nutrition and Metabolism in Patient Care.* Saunders, 1988.

Rombeau JL, Caldwell MD: *Enteral Nutrition,* 2nd ed. Saunders, 1990.

Shils ME, Young VR: *Modern Nutrition in Health and Disease,* 7th ed. Lea & Febiger, 1988.

Wyngaarden JB, Smith LH, Bennett JC: Nutritional diseases. Part XV of: *Cecil Textbook of Medicine,* 19th ed. Wyngaarden JB, Smith LH, Bennett JC (editors). Saunders, 1992.

General Problems in Infectious Diseases

29

Richard A Jacobs, MD, PhD

Most infections are confined to specific organ systems. In a book such as this—arranged principally by organ system—many of the important infectious disease entities are discussed in chapters dealing with specific anatomic areas. In this chapter are discussed some important general problems related to infectious diseases that are not covered elsewhere.

FEVER OF UNKNOWN ORIGIN (FUO)

To fulfill the criteria of FUO, a patient must have an illness of at least 3 weeks' duration, fever over 38.3 °C (101 °F), and must remain undiagnosed after 1 week of study in the hospital. The intervals specified are arbitrary ones intended to exclude patients with protracted but self-limited viral illnesses and to allow time for the usual radiographic, serologic, and cultural studies to be performed. Because of concerns over costs of hospitalization and the availability of most screening tests on an outpatient basis, the criterion requiring 1 week of hospitalization is often ignored.

Etiologic Considerations

Certain general principles about FUO should be kept in mind in the diagnostic approach to these patients.

A. Common Causes: Most cases represent unusual manifestations of common diseases and not rare or exotic diseases—ie, tuberculosis, endocarditis, and gallbladder disease are more common causes of FUO than Whipple's disease or familial Mediterranean fever.

B. Age of Patient: In adults, infections (30–40% of cases) and cancer (20–35% of cases) account for the majority of FUOs. In children, infections are the most common cause of FUO (30–50% of cases) and cancer a rare cause (5–10% of cases). Autoimmune disorders occur with equal frequency in adults and children (10–20% of cases), but the diseases differ. Juvenile rheumatoid arthritis is particularly common in children, whereas systemic lupus erythematosus,

Wegener's granulomatosis, and polyarteritis nodosa are more common in adults.

C. Duration of Fever: The cause of FUO changes dramatically in patients who have been febrile for a prolonged period of time—ie, 6 months or longer. Infection, cancer, and autoimmune disorders combined account for only 20% of FUOs in these patients. Instead, other entities such as granulomatous diseases (granulomatous hepatitis, Crohn's disease, ulcerative colitis) and factitious fever become important causes. Up to 27% of patients who say they have been febrile for 6 months or longer actually have no true fever or underlying disease. Instead, the usual normal circadian variation in temperature (temperature 1–2 °F higher in the afternoon than in the morning) is interpreted as abnormal.

D. Immunologic Status: In the neutropenic patient, fungal infections and occult bacterial infection are important and common causes of FUO. In the patient taking immunosuppressive medications (particularly organ transplant patients), cytomegalovirus infections are a frequent cause of fever, as are fungal infections.

E. Classification of Causes of FUO: Most patients with FUO will fit into one of five categories.

1. Infection–Both systemic and localized infections can cause FUO. Tuberculosis and endocarditis are the most common systemic infections, but mycoses, viral diseases (particularly infection with Epstein-Barr virus and cytomegalovirus), toxoplasmosis, brucellosis, salmonellosis, malaria, and many other less common infections have been implicated. Primary infection with human immunodeficiency virus (HIV) or opportunistic infections associated with the acquired immunodeficiency syndrome (AIDS)—particularly mycobacterial infections—can also present as FUO. The most common form of localized infection causing FUO is an occult abscess. Liver, spleen, kidney, brain, and bone are organs in which abscess may be difficult to find. A collection of pus may form in the peritoneal cavity or in the subdiaphragmatic, subhepatic, paracolic, or other areas. Cholangitis, osteomyelitis, urinary tract infection, dental abscess, or a collection of pus in a paranasal sinus may cause prolonged fever.

2. Neoplasms–Many cancers can present as FUO. The most common are lymphoma and leukemia. Primary and metastatic tumors of the liver also are frequently associated with fever, as are renal cell carcinomas. Chronic lymphocytic leukemia and multiple myeloma are rarely associated with fever, and the presence of fever in patients with these diseases should prompt a careful search for infection.

3. Autoimmune disorders–Still's disease, systemic lupus erythematosus, and polyarteritis nodosa are the most common autoimmune causes of FUO.

4. Miscellaneous causes–Many other diseases have been associated with FUO but less commonly than the foregoing types of illness. Examples include temporal arteritis, sarcoidosis, Whipple's disease, familial Mediterranean fever, recurrent pulmonary emboli, alcoholic hepatitis, drug fever, factitious fever, and others.

5. Undiagnosed FUO–Despite extensive evaluation, in 10–15% of patients the diagnosis remains elusive. In about three-fourths of these patients, the fever abates spontaneously and the clinician never knows the cause; in the remainder, more classic manifestations of the underlying disease appear over time, and the diagnosis then becomes obvious.

Approach to Diagnosis of FUO

Because the evaluation of a patient with FUO is so costly and time-consuming, it is imperative to document the presence of fever. This is done most reliably by observing the patient while the temperature is being taken to make certain that fever is not factitious (self-induced). Associated findings that usually accompany fever include tachycardia, chills, and piloerection. A thorough history—including family, occupational, social (sexual preference, use of intravenous drugs), and travel histories—may give clues to the underlying diagnosis. Detailed and repeated physical examination may reveal subtle, evanescent clinical findings that are the key to diagnosis.

In addition to "routine" laboratory studies, blood cultures should always be obtained, preferably when the patient is off antibiotics. Serologic studies may be diagnostic for certain immunologic diseases but are less useful in diagnosing infectious causes of FUO. A single elevated titer rarely allows one to make a diagnosis of infection; instead, one must demonstrate a fourfold rise or fall in titer to confirm a specific infectious cause.

Almost all patients with FUO should have a chest radiograph, sinus films, upper gastrointestinal series with small bowel follow-through, barium enema, proctosigmoidoscopy, and evaluation of gallbladder function. CT scan of the abdomen and pelvis is also frequently performed and can be quite useful in evaluating patients with FUO. When positive, the findings on CT scan are usually confirmed and often lead to a specific diagnosis. It is important to realize that a negative CT scan is not quite as useful; even with a negative CT scan, more invasive procedures such as exploratory laparotomy may lead to the diagnosis. The role of MRI in the investigation of FUO has not been evaluated. The usefulness of radionuclide studies has not been extensively studied in FUO. Theoretically, a gallium scan would be more helpful than an indium-labeled white blood cell scan, because gallium is useful for detecting infection and neoplasm whereas the indium scan is useful only for detecting infection. Both studies are limited by a high rate of false positivity. Indium-labeled immunoglobulin is another radionuclide study that may prove to be useful in detecting infection and neoplasm and is presently under investigation.

Invasive procedures are often required for diagnosis. Any abnormal finding should be aggressively evaluated: headache calls for lumbar puncture to rule out meningitis; skin from an area of rash should be biopsied to look for cutaneous manifestations of collagen vascular disease or infection; and enlarged lymph nodes should be aspirated or biopsied and examined for cytologic features to rule out neoplasm and sent for culture. Bone marrow aspiration with biopsy is a relatively low-yield procedure, but the risk is low and the procedure should be done if other less invasive tests have not yielded a diagnosis. Liver biopsy will yield a specific diagnosis in 10–15% of patients with FUO. One should consider this procedure in any patient with abnormal liver function tests even if the liver is normal in size on physical examination. The role of exploratory laparotomy is debatable. Studies on the usefulness of laparatomy in the diagnosis of FUO have not been done since the advent of CT scanning and MRI. One should consider laparotomy in the deteriorating patient if the diagnosis is elusive despite extensive evaluation.

Therapeutic Trials

Therapeutic trials are indicated if a diagnosis is strongly suspected—eg, it is reasonable to give antituberculous drugs if one suspects tuberculosis, or tetracycline if brucellosis is suspected. However, if there is no clinical response in several weeks, it is imperative to stop therapy and reevaluate the situation.

Empiric use of steroids should be discouraged; these agents can suppress fever if given in high enough doses, but they can also exacerbate many infections, and infection remains a leading cause of FUO. Suppression of fever with low doses of nonsteroidal anti-inflammatory agents (eg, naproxen, 250 mg twice daily) has been reported to be specific for fever associated with malignancy, but published data are limited.

Chang JC: Neoplastic fever: A proposal for diagnosis. Arch Intern Med 1989;149:1728. (Reviews clinical aspects of neoplastic fever and proposes approach to diagnosis.)
Dinarello CA, Cannon JG, Wolff SM: New concepts on the

pathogenesis of fever. Rev Infect Dis 1988;10:168. (Extensive review of molecular basis of fever.)

Knockaert DC et al: Fever of unknown origin in the 1980's: An update of the diagnostic spectrum. Ann Intern Med 1992;152:51. (Documents change in etiology of FUO.)

Quinn MJ et al: Computed tomography of the abdomen in evaluation of patients with fever of unknown origin. Radiology 1980;136:407. (Only large study addressing role of CT in diagnosis of FUO.)

INFECTIONS IN THE IMMUNOCOMPROMISED PATIENT

A description of the cellular basis of immune response, the role of various host responses in maintaining health, and the methods used for detection of deficiencies in the immune system can be found in Chapter 18.

"Compromised hosts" are individuals who have one or more defects in their natural defense mechanisms that put them at an increased risk of developing infections. Not only is the risk of infection greater in these individuals, but once infection develops it is often severe, rapidly progressive, and can be life-threatening. In addition, microorganisms that are not usually pathogens in the noncompromised patient may cause serious disease in the compromised patient. Individuals are most commonly compromised because of dysfunction of their immune system (granulocytopenia, T and B cell deficiency, hypogammaglobulinemia), but the presence of coexisting illness can also predispose to infection.

Granulocytopenia is common following bone marrow transplantation—as a result of myelosuppressive chemotherapy—and in acute leukemias. The risk of infection begins to increase when the absolute granulocyte count falls below 500/µL, with a dramatic increase in frequency and severity when the granulocyte count falls below 100/µL. The granulocytopenic patient is particularly susceptible to infections with gram-negative enteric organisms, *Pseudomonas,* gram-positive cocci (particularly *Staphylococcus aureus* and *Staphylococcus epidermidis*), *Candida,* and *Aspergillus.*

Defects in humoral immunity are often congenital, though hypogammaglobulinemia can occur in multiple myeloma and chronic lymphocytic leukemia. Patients with defects in humoral immunity lack opsonizing antibodies and are at particular risk of infection with encapsulated organisms such as *Haemophilus influenzae* and *Streptococcus pneumoniae.*

Patients with cellular immune deficiency encompass a large and rather heterogeneous group that includes patients with AIDS (see Chapter 30), those with lymphoreticular malignancies such as Hodgkin's disease (which is associated with dysfunction of cellular immunity), and patients receiving immunosuppressive medications such as corticosteroids, cyclosporine, azathioprine, and other cytotoxic drugs. This latter group—immunosuppressed as a result of medications—includes transplant patients, many solid tumor patients receiving therapy, and patients receiving prolonged high-dose steroid treatment (for asthma, temporal arthritis, systemic herpes, etc). Patients with cellular immune dysfunction are susceptible to infections by a large number of organisms particularly ones that replicate intracellularly. Examples include bacteria such as *Listeria, Legionella, Salmonella,* and *Mycobacterium;* viruses such as herpes simplex, varicella, and cytomegalovirus; fungi such as *Cryptococcus, Coccidioides,* and *Histoplasma;* and protozoa such as *Pneumocystis* and *Toxoplasma.*

Patients who are functionally or anatomically asplenic fail to clear organisms from the bloodstream and are at an increased risk of overwhelming bacteremia with encapsulated bacteria (primarily *Streptococcus pneumoniae* but also *H influenzae* and *Neisseria meningitides*).

Finally, a large group of patients who are not classically immunodeficient are at increased risk of infection because of debilitating injury (eg, burns or severe trauma), invasive procedures (eg, hyperalimentation lines, Foley catheters, dialysis catheters), central nervous system dysfunction (which predisposes to aspiration pneumonia and decubitus ulcers), the presence of obstructing lesions (eg, pneumonia due to an obstructed bronchus, pyelonephritis due to nephrolithiasis, cholangitis secondary to cholelithiasis), and use of broad-spectrum antibiotics.

Despite the generalizations made above about the relationship between type of immunosuppression and likely pathogen, it is important to remember that any pathogen can occur in any immunosuppressed patient at any time. Thus, a systematic evaluation to identify a specific organism is required.

Organisms not usually considered pathogens in the noncompromised patient may cause serious life-threatening infection in the compromised patient (eg, *S epidermidis, Corynebacterium jeikeium, Propionobacterium acnes, Bacillus* spp). Therefore, one must interpret culture results with caution and not disregard isolates as mere "contaminants." A contaminating organism in the competent patient may be a pathogen in the compromised one.

Approach to Diagnosis

Because infection can be rapidly progressive in the compromised patient evaluation must be prompt and thorough.

(1) Routine evaluation includes complete blood count with differential, chest x-ray, and blood cultures; urine and sputum cultures should be obtained if indicated clinically or radiographically. Any focal complaints (localized pain, headache, rash) should prompt a thorough evaluation and cultures appropriate to the site.

(2) If an infection is identified, one should attempt to obtain specimens that could lead to specific diagnosis.

(3) Patients who remain febrile for no obvious reason should be evaluated for viral infection (cytomegalovirus blood cultures), abscesses (which usually occur near previous operative sites), or systemic candidiasis or aspergillosis that involves the liver or spleen. Serologic evaluation may be helpful if toxoplasmosis is a possible pathogen.

(4) Consider special diagnostic procedures. The cause of pulmonary infiltrates can be easily determined with simple techniques in some situations— eg, induced sputum yields a diagnosis of *P carinii* pneumonia in 50–80% of AIDS patients with this infection. In other situations, more invasive procedures may be required (bronchoalveolar lavage, transbronchial biopsy, or even open lung biopsy). Other procedures such as skin, liver, or bone marrow biopsy may be helpful in establishing a diagnosis.

It is important to remember that not all fevers are due to infection. Transplant rejection, organ ischemia and necrosis, thrombophlebitis, and lymphoma may all present as fever and must be considered in the differential diagnosis.

Because infections in the immunocompromised patient can be rapidly progressive and life-threatening, diagnostic procedures must be done promptly, and empiric therapy is often instituted before a specific diagnostic agent has been isolated.

Prevention of Infection

There is great interest in preventing infection with prophylactic antimicrobial regimens, but there is no uniformity of opinion about what the optimal drug or dosage regimen should be.

Trimethoprim-sulfamethoxazole is frequently used to prevent *P carinii* infections. It may also decrease the incidence of bacterial pneumonia, urinary tract infections, and nocardial infections. Acyclovir has been shown to be effective in preventing herpes simplex and cytomegalovirus infections in renal and bone marrow transplant patients. Ganciclovir has recently been shown to prevent cytomegalovirus infections (particularly pneumonia) in bone marrow transplant recipients, but whether it is more effective than acyclovir is not known. In the neutropenic patient, handwashing is the simplest and most effective means of decreasing the incidence of infection. Oral nonabsorbable antibiotics and quinolones have been used as "gastrointestinal decontamination" in neutropenic patients in an attempt to decrease bacteremia from this site. The role of prophylactic antifungal agents is presently under investigation.

It is important in the control of nosocomial infections to limit the use of peripheral and central venous lines and Foley catheters. The need for these devices should be continually assessed and their use discontinued at the earliest possible time.

Handwashing is the simplest and most effective means of decreasing nosocomial infections in *all* patients, especially the compromised host. Invasive devices such as central and peripheral lines and Foley catheters are a potential source of infection. The need for these devices should be continually assessed and their use discontinued at the earliest possible time.

Approach to Treatment

In addition to providing antimicrobial therapy, it is important to improve host defenses whenever possible, correct electrolyte imbalances, and maintain adequate nutrition. Because immunosuppression is often the reason for infection, it is important to decrease immunosuppressive medications even in organ transplant patients. Reduction or discontinuation of immunosuppressive medication may jeopardize the viability of the transplanted organ, but in life-threatening infections it is necessary as an adjunct to effective antimicrobial therapy.

Antimicrobial drug therapy should be rationally based on culture results (see Chapter 37). Therapy should be specific for isolated pathogens, and bactericidal agents should be used. Combinations of antimicrobials are often required to provide synergy, to prevent resistance, or to serve as broad-spectrum coverage of multiple pathogens (since infections in these patients are often polymicrobial).

Empiric therapy is often instituted at the earliest sign of infection in the immunosuppressed patient because prompt therapy favorably affects outcome. The antibiotic or combination of antibiotics used depends on the type of immunocompromise and the site of infection. For example, in the febrile neutropenic patient, one is concerned primarily about bacterial and fungal infections. A number of different antibiotics have been used to treat this patient population. (See discussion in Chapter 37.) If the patient fails to respond in 3 days, amphotericin B is usually added. In the organ transplant patient with interstitial infiltrates, one is concerned mainly about *P carinii* or *Legionella* spp, so that empiric treatment with intravenous erythromycin and trimethoprim-sulfamethoxazole would be reasonable. If the patient fails to respond to empiric treatment, one must often decide between empiric addition of more antimicrobial agents or undertaking invasive procedures (see above) to make a specific diagnosis. By making a specific diagnosis, therapy can be specific and "polypharmacy" with multiple potentially toxic agents avoided.

Ho M et al: Infections in solid organ transplant recipients. In: *Principles and Practice of Infectious Diseases*, 3rd ed. Mandell GL, Douglas RG, Bennett JE (editors). Churchill Livingstone, 1990. (Comprehensive review of etiology and timing of infections after organ transplants.)

Hughes WT et al: Guidelines for the use of antimicrobial agents in neutropenic patients with unexplained fever. J Infect Dis 1990;161:381. (A consensus statement about empiric therapy and duration of treatment.)

Myers JD: Infections in marrow transplant recipients. In: *Principles and Practice of Infectious Diseases,* 3rd ed. Mandell GL, Douglas RG, Bennett JE (editors). Churchill Livingstone, 1990. (General discussion of etiology and timing of infections in bone marrow transplant recipients.)

NOSOCOMIAL INFECTIONS

Nosocomial infections are by definition those acquired in the course of hospitalization. At present in the USA, 3–7% of patients who enter the hospital free from infection acquire a nosocomial infection. Generally, patients acquire hospital infections with common organisms because of their own increased susceptibility to infection or because of procedures performed in the hospital.

Nosocomial infections can be attributed principally to the following aspects of contemporary medical care:

(1) Many hospitalized patients (especially in tertiary care hospitals, which have the highest nosocomial infection rate) are compromised because of deficiencies in their immunologic responses or impaired host defenses (skin ulcers, aspiration tendencies, etc). These may be congenital but commonly are acquired as a result of the administration of drugs for the treatment of cancer, for the maintenance of transplants, or for the suppression of autoimmune processes. The very young and the elderly are particularly susceptible to infection.

(2) Many aspects of medical care now require the use of invasive techniques for diagnosis, monitoring, and therapy. Examples are the indwelling urinary catheter; intravascular lines used for measurements, infusions of fluids or drugs, or parenteral alimentation; drainage tubes; and shunts.

(3) Materials administered in the intensive care unit may themselves be vectors of infection. Common examples are contaminated intravenous solutions or their containers; respirators and humidifiers that may introduce microorganisms into particularly susceptible lungs; and plastic tubing that may carry infectious agents into the body.

(4) The widespread use of antimicrobial drugs contributes to the selection of drug-resistant microorganisms both in the individual patient and in the hospital environment. Thus, nosocomial infections are often attributable to members of the endogenous human microflora or free-living microorganisms that happen to be particularly resistant to antimicrobial drugs, presenting difficult management problems. Such organisms often are not established human pathogens but can be classed as opportunists.

The principal anatomic sites of hospital-acquired infection are the urinary tract, surgical wounds, the respiratory tract, and skin sites where indwelling needles or tubes penetrate. Most notorious among nosocomial infections are those due to gram-negative enteric bacteria, staphylococci, or mycotic organisms that develop in patients with granulocyte counts below 500/µL as a result of cancer chemotherapy or organ transplant. In such patients, bloodstream invasion often occurs without a well-defined portal of entry. Patients with markedly depressed cell-mediated immunity may also develop viral infections in the hospital, eg, varicella-zoster, cytomegalovirus, and hepatitis. They are likewise open to opportunists such as *Legionella, Nocardia,* and other bacteria and protozoa, eg, *P carinii.*

In general, organisms that cause nosocomial infections tend to be multidrug-resistant and are often not sensitive to antibiotics used to treat community-acquired infections. For example, *Staphylococcus aureus* strains that cause hospital infections may be resistant to nafcillin and cephalosporins; *S epidermidis*—a frequent pathogen in patients with foreign bodies (shunts, hyperalimentation catheters, prosthetic heart valves, etc)—similarly may be resistant to nafcillin and sensitive only to vancomycin; and gram-negative organisms that cause nosocomial infections may be unusual (*Enterobacter* spp, *Acinetobacter* spp, *Pseudomonas*) and sensitive only to aminoglycosides. For these reasons, it is often necessary to institute empiric therapy with drugs such as vancomycin and tobramycin (or amikacin) until a specific agent is isolated and sensitivities are known, at which time the least toxic and least costly active drug can be used. The bacteriology and sensitivity patterns of nosocomial infections are quite variable, and one must be aware of local patterns to best treat these patients.

Prevention is of paramount importance in controlling nosocomial infections. Foley catheters, intravenous lines, hemodynamic monitoring devices, hyperalimentation lines, and similar such "invasive" devices should only be used when critical to patient care and, when used, should be discontinued at the earliest possible time. Peripheral intravenous lines should be replaced every 3 days and arterial lines every 4 days. Lines in the central venous circulation (including those placed peripherally) can be left in indefinitely and are changed or removed when they are clinically suspected of being infected, when they are nonfunctional, or when they are no longer needed. Selective decontamination of the digestive tract with nonabsorbable antibiotics to prevent nosocomial pneumonia is widely used in Europe, but the therapeutic efficacy of this expensive intervention is controversial. Attentive nursing care (positioning to prevent decubitus ulcers, wound care, elevating the head during tube feedings to prevent aspiration) is critical in preventing nosocomial infections. In addition, careful monitoring of high-risk areas (intensive care units, neonatal units, surgical floors, hemodialysis and transplant units, etc) by skilled personnel—hospital epidemiologists—to detect increases in infection rates early is a key factor in prevention of these types of infections.

Gastinne H et al: A controlled trial in intensive care units of selective decontamination of the digestive tract with non-absorbable antibiotics. N Engl J Med 1992;326:594. (Evaluates efficacy of nonabsorbable antibiotic in preventing nosocomial pneumonia and death.)

Proceedings of the Third Decennial International Conference of Nosocomial Infections. Am J Med 1991;91(3B). (Entire issue. Reviews recent trends of several aspects of nosocomial infections.)

INFECTIONS OF THE CENTRAL NERVOUS SYSTEM

Infections of the central nervous system can be caused by almost any infectious agent but most commonly are due to bacteria, mycobacteria, fungi, spirochetes, and viruses. Certain symptoms and signs are common to all types of central nervous system infection: headache, fever, sensorial disturbances, neck and back stiffness, positive Kernig and Brudzinski signs, and cerebrospinal fluid abnormalities. Although it is rare for all of these manifestations to be present in any one individual, the presence of even one of them should suggest the possibility of a central nervous system infection.

Central nervous system infection constitutes a *medical emergency.* Immediate diagnostic steps must be instituted to establish the specific cause. Normally, these include the history, physical examination, blood count, blood culture, lumbar puncture followed by careful study and culture of the cerebrospinal fluid, and a chest film. The fluid must be examined for cell count, glucose, and protein, and a smear must be stained for bacteria (and acid-fast organisms when appropriate) and cultured for pyogenic organisms and for mycobacteria and fungi when indicated. Counterimmunoelectrophoresis and latex agglutination tests can detect antigens of encapsulated organisms. These tests are particularly helpful when the patient has already received antibiotics, so that cultures are likely to be negative. In bacterial meningitis, prompt therapy is essential to prevent death and minimize serious sequelae.

Since performing a lumbar puncture in the presence of a space-occupying lesion (brain abscess, subdural hematoma, subdural abscess) can result in brain stem herniation and death, a CT scan is often performed prior to lumbar puncture. If delays are encountered in obtaining a CT scan and bacterial meningitis is suspected, antibiotics should be administered even before cerebrospinal fluid is obtained for culture to avoid unnecessary delays in treatment (Table 29–1). Animal studies suggest that antibiotics given within 4 hours of obtaining culture cerebrospinal fluid will not affect culture results.

Etiologic Classification

Central nervous system infections can be divided into several categories that usually can be readily distinguished from each other by cerebrospinal fluid examination as the first step toward etiologic diagnosis (Table 29–2).

A. Purulent Meningitis: Patients with bacterial meningitis usually present acutely within hours or 1–2 days after onset of symptoms. The organisms responsible depend primarily on the age of the patient as summarized in Table 29–1. The diagnosis is usually based on the gram-stained smear (positive in 60–80%) or culture (positive in over 90%).

B. Chronic Meningitis: Patients with chronic meningitis present less acutely with a history of symptoms lasting weeks to months. The most common pathogens are *Mycobacterium tuberculosis,* atypical mycobacteria, fungi (*Cryptococcus, Coccidioides, Histoplasma*), and *Treponema pallidum* (meningovascular syphilis). The diagnosis is made

Table 29–1. Initial antimicrobial therapy for purulent meningitis of unknown cause.

Age Group	Common Microorganisms	Standard Therapy
3 months to 18 years	H influenzae, N meningitidis, S pneumoniae	Third-generation cephalosporin[1] or ampicillin[2] + chloramphenicol[3]
18–60 years	S pneumoniae, N meningitidis	Penicillin G[4] or ampicillin
Over 60 years	S pneumoniae, N meningitidis, L monocytogenes, gram-negative bacilli	Ampicillin + third-generation cephalosporin
Postsurgical or posttraumatic	S aureus, S pneumoniae, gram-negative bacilli	Third-generation cephalosporin with or without nafcillin[5]

[1]Third-generation cephalosporins are cefotaxime, ceftizoxime, and ceftriaxone. In infants > 1 month of age (including adults), 50 mg/kg IV every 6 hours. The dosage of ceftriaxone (including adults) is 50 mg/kg IV every 12 hours.
[2]For infants > 7 days of age, children, and adults, 50–100 mg/kg IV every 6 hours.
[3]Chloramphenicol dosage is 100 mg/kg/d IV in divided doses in children, 50 mg/kg/d IV in divided doses in adults.
[4]Penicillin G dosage is 3–4 million units IV every 4 hours.
[5]Nafcillin dosage is 2 g IV every 4 hours.

Table 29–2. Typical cerebrospinal fluid findings in various central nervous system diseases.

Diagnosis	Cells/μL	Glucose (mg/dL)	Protein (mg/dL)	Opening Pressure
Normal	0–5 lymphocytes	45–85[1]	15–45	70–180 mm H$_2$0
Purulent meningitis (bacterial)[2] (community-acquired)	200–20,000 polymorphonuclear neutrophils	Low (< 45)	High (> 50)	++++
Granulomatous meningitis (mycobacterial, fungal)[2,3]	100–1000, mostly lymphocytes	Low (< 45)	High (> 50)	+++
Aseptic meningitis, viral or meningoencephalitis[4]	100–1000, mostly lymphocytes[3]	Normal	Moderately high (> 50)	Normal to +
Spirochetal meningitis	25–2000, mostly lymphocytes[3]	Normal or low	High (> 50)	+
"Neighborhood" reaction[5]	Variably increased	Normal	Normal or high	Variable

[1]Cerebrospinal fluid glucose must be considered in relation to blood glucose level. Normally, cerebrospinal fluid glucose is 20–30 mg/dL lower than blood glucose, or 50–70% of the normal value of blood glucose.
[2]Organisms in smear or culture of cerebrospinal fluid; counterimmunoelectrophoresis or latex agglutination may be diagnostic.
[3]Polymorphonuclear neutrophils may predominate early.
[4]Viral isolation from cerebrospinal fluid early; antibody titer rise in paired specimens of serum.
[5]May occur in mastoiditis, brain abscess, epidural abscess, sinusitis, septic thrombus, brain tumor. Cerebrospinal fluid culture results usually negative.

by culture or in some cases by serologic tests (cryptococcosis, coccidioidomycosis, syphilis).

C. Aseptic Meningitis: Aseptic meningitis—a much more benign and self-limited syndrome—is caused principally by viruses, especially mumps virus, the enterovirus group (including coxsackieviruses and echoviruses), and herpesviruses. Infectious mononucleosis may be accompanied by aseptic meningitis. Leptospiral infection is usually placed in the aseptic group because of the lymphocytic cellular response and its relatively benign course. This type of meningitis also occurs during secondary syphilis and stage 2 Lyme disease.

D. Encephalitis: Encephalitis (due to herpesviruses, arboviruses, and many other viruses) produces disturbances of the sensorium, seizures, and many other manifestations. Cerebrospinal fluid may be entirely normal or may show some lymphocytes.

E. Partially Treated Bacterial Meningitis: Previous effective antibiotic therapy given for 12–24 hours will decrease the rate of positive Gram stain results by 20% and culture by 30–40% but will have little effect on cell count, protein, or glucose. Occasionally, previous antibiotic therapy will change a predominantly polymorphonuclear response to a lymphocytic pleocytosis, and some of the cerebrospinal fluid findings may be similar to those seen in aseptic meningitis.

F. "Neighborhood" Reaction: As noted in Table 29–2, this term denotes a purulent infectious process in close proximity to the central nervous system that spills some of the products of the inflammatory process—white blood cells or protein—into the cerebrospinal fluid. Such an infection might be a brain abscess, osteomyelitis of the vertebrae, epidural abscess, subdural empyema, or bacterial sinusitis.

G. Noninfectious Meningeal Irritation: Meningismus, presenting with the classic signs of

meningeal irritation with totally normal cerebrospinal fluid findings, may occur in the presence of other infections such as pneumonia and shigellosis. Carcinomatous meningitis, sarcoidosis, systemic lupus erythematosus, and chemical meningitis can also produce signs and symptoms of meningeal irritation with associated cerebrospinal fluid pleocytosis, increased protein, and low or normal glucose.

H. Brain Abscess: Brain abscess presents as a space-occupying lesion; symptoms may include vomiting, fever, change of mental status, or focal neurologic manifestations. If brain abscess is suspected, a CT scan should precede lumbar puncture.

I. Amebic Meningoencephalitis: These infections are caused by free-living amebas and present as two distinct syndromes. The diagnosis is confirmed by culture or identification of the organism in cerebrospinal fluid or on biopsy specimens. No effective therapy is available.

1. Primary amebic meningoencephalitis is caused by *Naegleria fowleri* and is an acute fulminant disease characterized by signs of meningeal irritation that rapidly progresses to encephalitis and death. Anecdotal reports of cure of primary amebic meningoencephalitis have been reported with intravenous and intraventricular administration of amphotericin B.

2. Granulomatous amebic encephalitis is caused by *Acanthamoeba* species. It is an indolent disease characterized by headache, nausea, vomiting, cranial neuropathies, seizures, and hemiparesis.

Treatment

Treatment consists of supporting circulation, ventilation, the airway, and other vital functions that may be compromised by infection and resulting disturbance of the central nervous system. Increased intracranial pressure due to brain edema often requires therapeutic attention. Hyperventilation, mannitol

(24–50 g as a bolus intravenous infusion), and even drainage of cerebrospinal fluid through placement of ventricular catheters have been employed to control cerebral edema and increased intracranial pressure. Dexamethasone (4 mg every 4–6 hours) may also decrease cerebral edema. In the case of purulent meningitis, proper antimicrobial treatment is imperative. Since the identity of the causative microorganism may remain unknown or doubtful for a few days, initial antibiotic treatment as set forth in Table 29–1 should be directed against the microorganisms most common for each age group.

The usual duration of therapy for most bacterial meningitides is 10–14 days. Meningitis caused by gram-negative bacilli should be treated longer (ie, for 3 weeks). Dexamethasone therapy (0.15 mg/kg every 6 hours for 4 days) for bacterial meningitis in infants and children is beneficial in preventing hearing loss and decreasing the incidence of neurologic sequelae (ataxia and seizures) but has no effect on the mortality rate. Its role in the therapy of acute bacterial meningitis in adults is under study.

Therapy of other types of meningitis is discussed elsewhere in this book (fungal meningitis, Chapter 36; syphilis and Lyme borreliosis, Chapter 33; tuberculous meningitis, Chapter 32).

Odio CA et al: The beneficial effects of early dexamethasone administration in infants and children with bacterial meningitis. N Engl J Med 1991;324:1525. (Compares outcome of meningitis in patients treated with dexamethasone and placebo.)

Tunkel AR, Wispelway B, Schald M: Bacterial meningitis: Recent advances in pathophysiology and treatment. Ann Intern Med 1990;112:610. (Superb review of pathophysiology, diagnosis, and therapy.)

Whitley RJ: Viral encephalitis. N Engl J Med 1990; 323:242. (Thorough review of etiology, diagnosis, and therapy.)

ANIMAL & HUMAN BITE WOUNDS

About 1% of emergency room visits in urban areas are for treatment of animal and human bites. Dog bites occur most commonly in the summer months, and most occur in children. Biting animals are usually known by their victims, and most biting incidents are provoked (ie, bites occur while playing with the animal or after surprising the animal or waking it abruptly from sleep). Failure to elicit a history of provocation is important, because an unprovoked attack raises the possibility that the animal is rabid. Human bites are usually inflicted by children while playing or fighting; in adults, bites are associated with alcohol use and closed-fist injuries that occur during fights.

The animal inflicting the bite, the location of the bite, and the type of injury inflicted are all important determinants of whether these injuries become in-fected. Cat bites are more likely to become infected than human bites—between 30% and 50% of all cat bites subsequently become infected. Infections following human bites are variable: Those inflicted by children rarely become infected, because they are superficial; and bites by adults become infected in 15–20% of cases, with a particularly high rate of infection in closed-fist injuries. Dog bites, for unclear reasons, become infected only 5% of the time. Bites of the head, face, and neck are less likely to become infected than bites on the extremities. Puncture wounds become infected more frequently than lacerations, probably because the latter are easier to irrigate and debride.

The bacteriology of bite infections depends upon the biting animal and when the infection occurs after the biting incident. Early infections (within 24 hours after the bite) following dog and cat bites are most frequently caused by *Pasteurella multocida.* These infections are characterized by rapid onset and progression, fevers, chills, cellulitis, and local adenopathy. Early infections following human bites are usually caused by mixed aerobic and anaerobic mouth flora and can produce a rapidly progressive necrotizing infection. Late infections (longer than 24 hours after the bite) are caused mainly by staphylococci and streptococci, but innumerable organisms have been implicated in these infections. *Capnocytophaga canimorsus* (formerly called a DF2 organism), a gram-negative organism that is part of canine oral flora; *Eikenella corrodens,* another gram-negative organism that can be part of human mouth flora; *Haemophilus* spp, *Pseudomonas* spp, and other gram-negative organisms—all have been implicated in bite infections.

The possibility of AIDS transmission from a bite by an HIV-infected person is exceedingly remote. There have been no documented cases of HIV transmission by this route.

Treatment

A. Local Care: Vigorous cleansing and irrigation of the wound as well as debridement of necrotic material are the most important factors in decreasing the incidence of infections. X-rays should be obtained to look for fractures and the presence of foreign bodies. Careful examination to assess the extent of the injury (tendon laceration, joint space penetration) is critical to appropriate care.

B. Suturing: If wounds require closure for cosmetic or mechanical reasons, suturing can be done. However, one should never suture a wound that is already infected, and wounds of the hand should generally not be sutured since a closed-space infection of the hand can result in loss of function.

C. Prophylactic Antibiotics: Prophylaxis is indicated in high-risk bites, eg, cat bites in any location (dicloxacillin, 0.5 g orally four times a day for 3–5 days) and hand bites by any animal or by humans (penicillin V, 0.5 g orally four times a day for 3–5 days). Although dicloxacillin and penicillin have been most extensively studied for prophylaxis, there is concern about their use because of their narrow spectrum of activity. Based on the microbiology of bite wounds noted above, other agents that have not been adequately studied but that have broader spectrums of activity may be even more effective as prophylactic agents. Examples include cefuroxime and amoxicillin-clavulanic acid. Immunocompromised patients and especially individuals without functional spleens are at risk for developing overwhelming bacteremia and sepsis following animal bites and thus should also receive prophylaxis.

D. Antibiotics: For wounds that are infected, antibiotics are clearly indicated. How they are given (orally or intravenously) and the need for hospitalization are individualized clinical decisions. In general, *P multocida* is best treated with penicillin or a tetracycline. Response to therapy is slow, and therapy should be continued for at least 2–3 weeks. Human bites frequently require admission to the hospital and intravenous therapy with either penicillin or clindamycin. Because the bacteriology of these infections is so variable, one should always culture infected wounds and adjust therapy appropriately, especially if the patient is not responding to initial empiric treatment.

E. Tetanus and Rabies: All patients must be evaluated for the need for tetanus (see Chapter 32) and rabies (see Chapter 31) prophylaxis.

Callaham ML: When an animal bites. Emerg Med June 15,1988:119.
Goldstein EJC: Bite wounds and infection. Clin Infect Dis 1992;14:633.
Weber DJ, Hansen AR: Infections resulting from animal bites. Infect Dis Clin North Am 1991;5:663. (Etiology, epidemiology, and therapy.)

SEXUALLY TRANSMITTED DISEASES

Some infectious diseases are transmitted most commonly—or most efficiently—by sexual contact. The frequency of some of these infections (eg, gonorrhea) has increased markedly in recent years as a result of changing patterns of sexual behavior. Others (eg, herpetic and chlamydial genital infections) are only now beginning to be appreciated as important systemic infections with a primarily sexual mode of transmission. Rectal and pharyngeal infections caused by these microorganisms are common as a result of varied sexual practices.

Most of the infectious agents that cause sexually transmitted diseases are fairly easily inactivated when exposed to a harsh environment. They are thus particularly suited to transmission by contact with mucous membranes. They may be bacteria (eg, gono-

cocci), spirochetes (syphilis), chlamydiae (nongonococcal urethritis, cervicitis), viruses (eg, herpes simplex, hepatitis B virus, cytomegalovirus, AIDS virus), or protozoa (eg, *Trichomonas*). In most infections caused by these agents, early lesions occur on genitalia or other sexually exposed mucous membranes; however, wide dissemination may occur, and involvement of nongenital tissues and organs may mimic many noninfectious disorders. All sexually transmitted diseases have subclinical or latent phases that may play an important role in long-term persistence of the infection or in its transmission from infected (but largely asymptomatic) persons to other contacts. Laboratory examinations are of particular importance in the diagnosis of such asymptomatic patients. Simultaneous infection by several different agents is common, and any person with a sexually transmitted disease should be tested for syphilis. If the test is negative, a repeat study should be done in 3 months, since seroconversion can be delayed.

For each patient, there are one or more sexual contacts who require diagnosis and treatment. As a rule, sexual partners should be treated simultaneously to avoid prompt reinfection. Finding a sexually transmitted disease in a child strongly suggests sexual abuse, and such cases must be reported to the authorities. The commonest sexually transmitted diseases are gonorrhea,* syphilis,* condyloma acuminatum, chlamydial genital infections, herpesvirus genital infections, *Trichomonas* vaginitis, chancroid,* granuloma inguinale,* scabies, and louse infestation. However, shigellosis,* hepatitis,* amebiasis,* giardiasis, cryptosporidiasis, salmonellosis,* and campylobacteriosis may also be transmitted by sexual (oral-anal) contact, especially in homosexual males. Homosexual contact is the most prevalent method of transmission of HIV and AIDS,* though bidirectional heterosexual transmission can also occur (see Chapter 30).

The risk of developing a sexually transmitted disease following a sexual assault has not been extensively studied. Victims of assault have a high baseline rate of infection (*Neisseria gonorrhoeae* 6%, *Chlamydia trachomatis* 10%, *Trichomonas vaginalis* 15%, and bacterial vaginosis 34%), and the risk of acquiring infection as a result of the assault is significant but is lower than the preexisting rate (*N gonorrhoeae* 4%, *C trachomatis* 2%, *T vaginalis* 12% and bacterial vaginosis 19%). Victims should be evaluated within 24 hours after the assault, and cultures for *N gonorrhoeae*, *C trachomatis* and herpes simplex virus should be obtained and vaginal secretions examined for *Trichomonas* and bacterial vaginosis. In addition, a blood sample should be obtained for serologic testing for syphilis. (An additional sample should be stored for future testing for

*Reportable to public health authorities.

HIV and hepatitis B if needed.) Follow-up serologic testing for syphilis should be performed in 3 months. If infection is found, it should be treated. Use of presumptive therapy is controversial, some workers feeling that all patients should receive it and others that it should be limited to those in whom follow-up cannot be ensured or that it should be given only to those who request it. If therapy is given, a reasonable regimen would be one dose of ceftriaxone, 250 mg intramuscularly, followed by doxycycline, 100 mg orally twice daily, and metronidazole, 500 mg orally twice daily, for 7 days.

Holmes KK et al: *Sexually Transmitted Diseases,* 2nd ed. McGraw-Hill, 1990.
Jenny C et al: Sexually transmitted diseases in victims of rape. N Engl J Med 1990;322:713. (Over 200 victims.)
Sexually transmitted diseases: Treatment guidelines. MMWR Morb Mortal Wkly Rep 1989;38:38.

INFECTIONS IN DRUG ADDICTS

The abuse of parenterally administered narcotic drugs has increased enormously in recent years. There are now an estimated 300,000 or more narcotic addicts in the USA, mostly in or near large urban centers. Consequently, physicians and hospitals serving such urban and suburban populations must deal with many problems—including infections—related to drug abuse.

Common Infections That Occur With Greater Frequency in Drug Users

(1) Skin infections are associated with poor hygiene and multiple needle punctures, commonly due to *S aureus.*

(2) Hepatitis is nearly universal among habitual drug users and is transmissible both by the parenteral and by the fecal-oral route. Many addicts experience hepatitis more than once.

(3) Aspiration pneumonia and its complications (lung abscess, empyema, brain abscess) result from altered consciousness associated with drug abuse. Mixed aerobic and anaerobic mouth flora are usually involved.

(4) Pulmonary septic emboli may originate from venous thrombi or right-sided endocarditis.

(5) Sexually transmitted diseases are not directly related to drug abuse but, for social reasons, occur with greater frequency in population groups that are also involved in drug abuse.

(6) AIDS has a high incidence among intravenous drug abusers and their sexual contacts and the offspring of infected women (see Chapter 30).

(7) Infective endocarditis (see below).

Infections Rare in USA Except in Drug Users

(1) Tetanus: Drug users now form a majority of cases of tetanus in the USA, especially in unimmunized female addicts who inject drugs subcutaneously ("skin-popping").

(2) Malaria: Needle transmission occurs from addicts who acquired the infection in malaria-endemic areas outside the USA.

(3) Melioidosis: This chronic pulmonary infection caused by *Pseudomonas pseudomallei* is occasionally seen in debilitated drug users.

Osteomyelitis & Septic Arthritis

Osteomyelitis involving vertebral bodies, sternoclavicular joints, and other sites usually results from hematogenous distribution of injected organisms or septic venous thrombi. Pain and fever precede radiographic changes by several weeks. While staphylococci—often methicillin-resistant—are common organisms, *Serratia, Pseudomonas,* and other pathogens rarely encountered in "spontaneous" bone or joint disease are found in addicts who use drugs intravenously.

Infective Endocarditis

The organisms that cause infective endocarditis in those who use drugs intravenously are most commonly *S aureus, Candida* (especially *Candida parapsilosis*), *Streptococcus faecalis,* other streptococci, and gram-negative bacteria (especially *Pseudomonas* and *Serratia marcescens*).

Involvement of the right side of the heart is somewhat more frequent than involvement of the left side, and infection of more than one valve is not infrequent. Right-sided involvement, especially in the absence of murmurs, is often suggested by manifest pulmonary emboli. The diagnosis must be established by blood culture. Therapy, including empiric treatment, is discussed below.

Dobkin JF: Infections in parenteral drug abusers. In: *Principles and Practice of Infectious Diseases.* Mandell GL, Douglas RG, Bennett JE (editors). Churchill Livingstone, 1990.
Scheidegger C, Zimmerli W: Infectious complications in drug addicts: Seven-year review of 269 hospitalized narcotics abusers in Switzerland. Rev Infect Dis 1989; 11:486. (Retrospective review from 1980–1986 of infections seen in past and current drug abusers.)

INFECTIVE ENDOCARDITIS

Discussions of the pathogenesis, clinical findings, complications, and prevention of infective endocarditis can be found in Chapter 10. Antimicrobial therapy of bacterial endocarditis is discussed in this section.

Approximately 90% of cases of native valve endocarditis are due to viridans streptococci (60%), *S aureus* (20%), and enterococci (5–10%). Gram-negative organisms and fungi account for a small percentage.

The microbiology of native valve endocarditis in intravenous drug users differs from that of other patients. *S aureus* accounts for 60% or more of all cases and for 80–90% of cases in which the tricuspid valve is infected. Enterococci and streptococci comprise the balance in about equal proportions. Gram-negative aerobic bacilli, fungi, and unusual organisms that rarely infect others may cause endocarditis in intravenous drug users.

The microbiology of prosthetic valve endocarditis also is distinctive. Early infections (ie, those occurring within 2 months after valve implantation) are commonly caused by staphylococci—both coagulase-positive and coagulase-negative—gram-negative organisms, and fungi. Late prosthetic valve endocarditis resembles native valve endocarditis, with the majority of infections caused by streptococci, though coagulase-negative staphylococci still cause a significant proportion of cases.

Diagnosis

Blood culture is the single most important procedure for diagnosis of endocarditis. The incidence of positive cultures depends primarily upon the etiologic agent and whether prior antibiotics have been administered. In streptococcal endocarditis, the first blood culture is positive in 96% of cases, and one of two cultures is positive in 98% of cases. If antibiotics have been administered within 2 weeks prior to obtaining cultures, only 65–90% of cultures will be positive. In nonstreptococcal endocarditis, the first blood culture is positive in 85% of cases; and if two cultures are taken, 100% are positive.

The current recommendation for maximizing the yield of blood cultures is to obtain three sets of blood cultures over a 24-hour period before starting antibiotics unless the patient is acutely ill. Even when this is done, a small but significant number of infected patients (5% of cases) will be culture-negative. These cases my be due to a fungus (50% of patients with fungal endocarditis have negative blood cultures), organisms that require special media for growth (eg, *Legionella* spp, nutritionally deficient streptococci), organisms that do not grow on artificial media (agents of Q fever, psittacosis), or organisms that are slow-growing and may require several weeks to grow (eg, *Brucella,* anaerobes, certain *Haemophilus* spp, *Actinobacillus actinomycetemcomitans, Cardiobacterium hominis, Eikenella corrodens,* and *Kingella* spp).

Echocardiography may provide adjunctive information useful for identifying the specific valve or valves that are infected. The sensitivity of echocardiography is between 30% and 75%; therefore, it cannot reliably rule out endocarditis but may confirm a clinical suspicion. Transesophageal echocardiography is useful in identification of valve ring abscess and is more sensitive than two-dimensional and M-mode echocardiography.

Prevention

Antimicrobial prophylaxis is described in Chapter 37 (Table 37–9).

Treatment

Empiric regimens for endocarditis while culture results are pending should include agents active against staphylococci, streptococci, and enterococci. Nafcillin or oxacillin, 1.5 g every 4 hours, plus penicillin, 4 million units every 4 hours (or ampicillin, 1.4 g every 4 hours), plus gentamicin, 1 mg/kg every 8 hours, is such a regimen. Vancomycin, 1 g every 12 hours, may be used instead of the penicillins in the penicillin-allergic patient.

A. Streptococci: For penicillin-susceptible viridans group streptococcal endocarditis (ie, MIC ≤ 0.1 μg/mL), penicillin G, 3 million units (400,000 units/kg for children) intravenously every 4 hours for 4 weeks, is recommended. The duration of therapy can be shortened to 2 weeks if streptomycin, 7.5 mg/kg (not to exceed 500 mg) intramuscularly every 12 hours, or gentamicin, 1 mg/kg every 8 hours, is added to the regimen. For infections due to nutritionally deficient streptococci and organisms that are relatively resistant to penicillin (ie, MIC > 0.1 μg/mL but < 0.5 μg/mL), total duration of therapy should be 4 weeks, with addition of gentamicin for the first 2 weeks.

For the penicillin-allergic patient, either cefazolin, 1 g every 8 hours for 4 weeks, or vancomycin, 1 g every 12 hours for 4 weeks, may be used. Two-week regimens including aminoglycosides have not been proved to be effective except with penicillin. Recent data from clinical trials suggest that 2 g of ceftriaxone given once daily intravenously or intramuscularly for 4 weeks is also effective therapy for endocarditis due to penicillin-sensitive strains (MIC ≤ 0.1 μg/mL).

For viridans streptococci with a penicillin MIC greater than 0.5 μg/mL, both penicillin and either gentamicin or streptomycin should be used for 4 weeks. This regimen is recommended also for prosthetic valve infection.

B. Enterococci: For enterococcal endocarditis, the relapse rate is unacceptably high when penicillin is used alone; either streptomycin or gentamicin must be included in the regimen. Because aminoglycoside resistance occurs in enterococci, susceptibility to it should be documented. Gentamicin is probably the aminoglycoside of choice, because streptomycin resistance is more common than gentamicin resistance and the nephrotoxicity of gentamicin is generally more easily managed than the vestibular toxicity of streptomycin. Penicillin, 4 million units every 4 hours (or vancomycin, 1 g every 12 hours in penicillin-allergic patients), plus gentamicin, 1 mg/kg every 8 hours for at least 4 weeks, is recommended. Patients who have had symptoms of endocarditis for 3 months or longer may be more prone to relapse and should be treated for 6 weeks with the combination.

C. Staphylococci: For methicillin-susceptible *S aureus,* nafcillin or oxacillin, 1.5 g every 4 hours for 4 weeks, is the preferred therapy. For penicillin-allergic patients, cephalothin, 2 g every 4 hours, cefazolin, 1 g every 6 hours, or vancomycin, 1 g every 12 hours, may be used. For methicillin-resistant strains, vancomycin is the only agent of proved effectiveness.

The role of aminoglycoside combination regimens for *S aureus* endocarditis remains unclear, but they may be useful in shortening the duration of bacteremia. In selected patients (such as intravenous drug users) with tricuspid valve endocarditis (with or without pulmonary involvement) who do not have serious extrapulmonary sites of infection, the total duration of therapy can be shortened from 4 weeks to 2 weeks.

Because coagulase-negative staphylococci—a common cause of prosthetic valve endocarditis—are routinely resistant to methicillin, β-lactam antibiotics should not be used for this infection until the isolate is known to be susceptible. A combination of vancomycin for 6 weeks, rifampin, 300 mg twice daily for 6 weeks, and gentamicin, 1 mg/kg every 8 hours for the first 2 weeks, is the regimen of choice.

Response to Therapy

Most patients respond rapidly to institution of appropriate antibiotics, with 50% becoming afebrile in 3 days, 72% in 1 week, and 84% by 2 weeks, but this is organism-dependent. If infection is caused by viridans streptococci, enterococci, or coagulase-negative staphylococci, defervescence occurs in 3–4 days on average, whereas if infection is caused by *Staphylococcus aureus* or *Pseudomonas aeruginosa,* patients may remain febrile for 9–12 days. If fevers persist, blood cultures should be obtained to ensure adequacy of therapy. Other causes of persistent fever are myocardial or metastatic abscess, sterile embolization, and drug reaction. Careful posttreatment monitoring is critical. Most relapses occur within 2 months after completion of therapy. Obtaining one or two blood cultures during this period allows for early detection of recurrent infection.

Bisno AL et al: Antimicrobial treatment of infective endocarditis due to viridans streptococci, enterococci, and staphylococci. JAMA 1989;261:1471. (Consensus statement.)

Chambers HF, Miller RT, Newman MG: Right-sided *S aureus* endocarditis in intravenous drug abusers: Two-week combination therapy. Ann Intern Med 1988; 109:619. (Nafcillin plus tobramycin for 2 weeks.)

"FOOD POISONING" & ACUTE GASTROENTERITIS

Food poisoning is a nonspecific term often applied to the syndrome of acute anorexia, nausea, vomiting, or diarrhea that is attributed to food intake, particularly if it afflicts groups of people and is not accompanied by fever. The actual cause of such acute gastrointestinal upsets might be emotional stress, viral or bacterial infections, food intolerance, inorganic (eg, sodium nitrite) or organic (eg, mushroom, shellfish) poisons, or drugs (eg, antimicrobials). More specifically, the term "food poisoning" denotes disorders caused by toxins produced by bacteria growing in food (staphylococci, clostridia, *Bacillus cereus*), or acute food infections with short incubation periods and a mild course (*Salmonella enterocolitis* [see above]), or infection with enterotoxigenic *Escherichia coli,* shigellae, or vibrios (*Vibrio cholerae,* El Tor vibrios, marine vibrios including *Vibrio parahaemolyticus, Vibrio vulnificus*). *Campylobacter jejuni* and *Yersinia enterocolitica* may produce similar clinical enterocolitis and can be identified only by special stool culture methods. *E coli* O157:H7 is an infrequent cause of hemorrhagic colitis. Adenoviruses, rotaviruses, astroviruses, and Norwalk-type viruses may produce a similar syndrome. Various protozoa (*Entamoeba histolytica, Giardia,* and others) can also cause acute or chronic diarrhea. (See Chapter 34.) Some prominent features of some of these "food poisonings" are listed in Table 29–3. In general, the diagnosis must be suspected when groups of people who have shared a meal develop acute vomiting or diarrhea. Food and stools must be obtained for bacteriologic and toxicologic examination. In febrile patients, blood cultures are indicated.

Treatment usually consists of replacement of fluids and electrolytes and, very rarely, management of hypovolemic shock and respiratory embarrassment. If botulism is suspected, polyvalent antitoxin must be administered. Historically, antimicrobial drugs have not been recommended unless a specific microbial agent producing progressive systemic involvement can be identified. Preliminary data now suggest that ciprofloxacin, 500 mg every 12 hours for 5 days, may shorten the duration of diarrhea and lead to a more rapid resolution of symptoms. Antimotility drugs may relieve cramping and decrease diarrhea in mild cases. Their use should be limited to patients without fever and without dysentery (bloody stools), and they should be used in low doses.

Blackow NR, Greenberg NB: Viral gastroenteritis. N Engl J Med 1991;325:252. (A review.)

Goodman LJ et al: Empiric antimicrobial therapy of domestically acquired acute diarrhea in urban adults. Arch Intern Med 1990;150:541. (Empiric ciprofloxacin shortens course.)

Table 29–3. Acute bacterial diarrheas and "food poisoning."

Organism	Incubation Period (Hours)	Vomiting	Diarrhea	Fever	Epidemiology	Pathogenesis	Clinical Features
Staphylococcus	1–8, rarely up to 18	+++	+	–	Staphylococci grow in meats, dairy, bakery products and produce enterotoxin.	Enterotoxin acts on receptors on gut that transmit impulse to medullary centers.	Abrupt onset, intense vomiting for up to 24 hours, regular recovery in 24–48 hours. Occurs in persons eating the same food. No treatment usually necessary except to restore fluids and electrolytes.
Bacillus cereus	1–8, rarely up to 18	+++	+	–	Reheated fried rice causes vomiting or diarrhea.	Enterotoxins formed in food or in gut from growth of *B cereus*.	After 1–6 hours, mainly vomiting. After 8–16 hours, mainly diarrhea. Both self-limited to less than 1 day.
Clostridium perfringens	8–16	±	+++	–	Clostridia grow in rewarmed meat dishes and produce enterotoxin.	Enterotoxin produced in food and in gut causes hypersecretion in small intestine.	Abrupt onset of profuse diarrhea; vomiting occasionally. Recovery usual without treatment in 1–4 days. Many clostridia in cultures of food and feces of patients.
Clostridium botulinum	24–96	±	Rare	–	Clostridia grow in anaerobic foods and produce toxin.	Toxin absorbed from gut blocks acetylcholine at neuromuscular junction.	Diplopia, dysphagia, dysphonia, respiratory embarrassment. Treatment requires clear airway, ventilation, and intravenous polyvalent antitoxin (see text). Toxin present in food and serum. Mortality rate high.
Clostridium difficile	?	–	+++	+	Associated with antimicrobial drugs, eg, clindamycin.	Enterotoxin causes epithelial necrosis in colon; pseudomembranous colitis.	Especially after abdominal surgery, abrupt bloody diarrhea, and fever. Toxin in stool. Oral vancomycin useful in therapy.
Escherichia coli (some strains)	24–72	±	+	–	Organisms grow in gut and produce toxin. May also invade superficial epithelium.	Enterotoxin causes hypersecretion in small intestine.	Usually abrupt onset of diarrhea; vomiting rare. A serious infection in neonates. In adults, "traveler's diarrhea" is usually self-limited in 1–3 days. Use diphenoxylate with atropine but no antimicrobials.

(continued)

Table 29-3. Acute bacterial diarrheas and "food poisoning." (continued)

Organism	Incubation Period (Hours)	Vomiting	Diarrhea	Fever	Epidemiology	Pathogenesis	Clinical Features
Vibrio parahaemolyticus	6–96	+	+	±	Organisms grow in seafood and in gut and produce toxin, or invade.	Hypersecretion in small intestine; stools may be bloody.	Abrupt onset of diarrhea in groups consuming the same food, especially crabs and other seafood. Recovery is usually complete in 1–3 days. Food and stool cultures are positive.
Vibrio cholerae (mild cases)	24–72	+	+++	–	Organisms grow in gut and produce toxin.	Enterotoxin causes hypersecretion in small intestine. Infective dose: 10^7–10^9 organisms.	Abrupt onset of liquid diarrhea in endemic area. Needs prompt replacement of fluids and electrolytes IV or orally. Tetracyclines shorten excretion of vibrios. Stool cultures positive.
Campylobacter jejuni	2–10 days	–	+++	+	Organism grows in jejunum and ileum.	Invasion and enterotoxin production uncertain.	Fever, diarrhea; PMNs and fresh blood in stool, especially in children. Usually self-limited. Special media needed for culture at 43 °C. Erythromycin in severe cases with invasion. Usual recovery in 5–8 days.
Shigella spp (mild cases)	24–72	±	+	+	Organisms grow in superficial gut epithelium and gut lumen and produce toxin.	Organisms invade epithelial cells; blood, mucus, and PMNs in stools. Infective dose: 10^2–10^3 organisms.	Abrupt onset of diarrhea, often with blood and pus in stools, cramps, tenesmus, and lethargy. Stool cultures are positive. In severe cases, give trimethoprim-sulfamethoxazole, ampicillin, or chloramphenicol. Do not give opiates. Restore fluids. Often mild and self-limited.
Salmonella spp	8–48	±	+	+	Organisms grow in gut. Do not produce toxin.	Superficial infection of gut, little invasion. Infective dose: 10^5 organisms.	Gradual or abrupt onset of diarrhea and low-grade fever. No antimicrobials unless systemic dissemination is suspected. Stool cultures are positive. Prolonged carriage is frequent.
Yersinia enterocolitica	?	±	+	+	Fecal-oral transmission (occasionally). Foodborne. In pets.	Gastroenteritis or mesenteric adenitis. Occasional bacteremia. Enterotoxin produced.	Severe abdominal pain, diarrhea, fever; PMNs and blood in stool; polyarthritis, erythema nodosum in children. If severe, give tetracycline or gentamicin. Keep stool at 4 °C before culture.

Guerrant RL, Bobak DA: Bacterial and protozoal gastroenteritis. N Engl J Med 1991;325:327. (A review.)

TRAVELER'S DIARRHEA

Whenever a person travels from one country to another—particularly if the change involves a marked difference in climate, social conditions, or sanitation standards and facilities—diarrhea is likely to develop within 2–10 days. There may be up to ten or even more loose stools per day, often accompanied by abdominal cramps, nausea, occasionally vomiting, and rarely fever. The stools do not usually contain mucus or blood, and aside from weakness, dehydration, and occasionally acidosis, there are no systemic manifestations of infection. The illness usually subsides spontaneously within 1–5 days; rarely, it lasts 2–3 weeks.

Stool cultures rarely reveal salmonellae or shigellae. Contributory causes may at times include unusual food and drink, change in living habits, occasional viral infections adenoviruses or rotaviruses), and change in bowel flora. A significant number of cases of traveler's diarrhea are caused by acquisition of strains of *Escherichia coli* that produce an enterotoxin.

Other less common pathogens are *Salmonella, Shigella, Campylobacter,* and *Entamoeba.* In patients with fever and bloody diarrhea, stool culture may be indicated, though the illness usually has resolved by the time the patient seeks medical attention. Chronic watery diarrhea may be due to amebiasis or giardiasis or, rarely, tropical sprue.

For most individuals, the affliction is short-lived, and symptomatic therapy with opiates or diphenoxylate with atropine is all that is required provided the patient is not systemically ill (fever ≥ 39 °C [102.2 °F]) and does not have dysentery (bloody stools). Avoidance of fresh foods and water sources that are likely to be contaminated is recommended for travelers to developing countries, where infectious diarrheal illnesses are endemic. For prophylaxis, bismuth subsalicylate is effective. Numerous antimicrobial regimens for prophylaxis also are effective, such as norfloxacin, 400 mg, ciprofloxacin, 500 mg, or trimethoprim-sulfamethoxazole, 160/800 mg, once daily. Tetracyclines also are effective, but photosensitization with these drugs makes them less desirable. Because not all travelers will have diarrhea and because most episodes are brief and self-limited, an alternative approach that is currently recommended is to provide the traveler with a 3- to 5-day supply of antimicrobials to be taken if significant diarrhea occurs during the trip. Commonly used regimens include ciprofloxacin, 500 mg twice daily, and trimethoprim-sulfamethoxazole, 160/800 mg twice daily. Aztreonam, a poorly absorbed monobactam with activity against most bacterial enteropathogens,

also is efficacious when given orally in a dose of 100 mg three times daily for 5 days.

Ericsson CD et al: Treatment of traveler's diarrhea with sulfamethoxazole and trimethoprim and loperamide. JAMA 1990;263:257.

Gorbach SL (editor): Infectious diarrhea. Infect Dis Clin North Am 1988;2:1. (Specific agents, diagnosis, and therapy.)

Wolfe MD: Acute diarrhea associated with travel. Am J Med 1990;88(Suppl 6A):34S. (Etiology, prophylaxis, and therapy.)

ACTIVE IMMUNIZATION AGAINST INFECTIOUS DISEASES

RECOMMENDED IMMUNIZATION OF CHILDREN

Every individual—child or adult—should maintain an adequate defense against infectious disease by immunization. The recommended schedules and dosages change often, so that one should always consult the manufacturer's package inserts.

The schedule for active immunizations in children is presented in Table 29–4.

RECOMMENDED IMMUNIZATION OF ADULTS

Several vaccines are recommended for adults depending upon the individual's previous vaccination status and the risks of exposure to certain diseases.

Tetanus-Diphtheria Toxoid

Everyone should receive a primary series of immunizations against tetanus and diphtheria once (Table 29–4). Thereafter, routine booster doses of tetanus-diphtheria toxoid for adults (Td) should be given every 10 years. Adults who have not previously been immunized should receive two doses of Td 1–2 months apart, followed by a booster dose 6–12 months later. Adults partially immunized in childhood with DTP need only a total of three doses of tetanus and diphtheria toxoid (ie, if one dose was given in childhood, give two doses of Td; if two doses were given, only one dose of Td is needed to complete primary immunization). If booster doses are given too frequently, an Arthus reaction as well as severe local pain and swelling can occur. Pertussis vaccine, which is combined with tetanus-diphtheria toxoid for use in children (DTP), should not be used in adults because of the frequency of adverse reactions

Table 29–4. Recommended schedule of active immunization of children.

Age	Product Administered[1]
Birth to just before hospital discharge	HBV[2]
2 months	DTP-1,[3] OPV-1,[4] HbCV,[5] HBV
4 months	DTP-2, OPV-2, HbCV
6 months	DTP-3, HBV
12 months	HbCV
15 months[6]	MMR-1,[7] DTP-4, OPV-3
4–6 years	DTP-5, OPV-4, MMR-2
14–16 years and every 10 years thereafter	Td[8]

(Adapted from: General recommendations on immunization: Guidelines from the Immunization Practices Advisory Committee. Ann Intern Med 1989;111:133.)

[1] Package insert should be consulted for doses, storage, and handling. Preparations from different manufacturers may vary, and individual manufacturers may change their products from time to time.

[2] HBV = hepatitis B vaccine. Two regimens are available. In addition to the one listed in the table, an alternative option is three doses, the first given at 1–2 months, the second at 4 months, and the third at 6–18 months. This vaccine can be administered simultaneously with DTP, HbCV, MMR, and OPV.

[3] DTP = diphtheria and tetanus toxoids and pertussis vaccine, absorbed. DTP can be used up to the seventh birthday.

[4] OPV = live oral poliovirus vaccine, trivalent (contains poliovirus types 1, 2, and 3).

[5] HbCV = *Haemophilus influenzae* type b polysaccharide antigen conjugated to a protein carrier. The conjugated vaccine is preferred over the polysaccharide vaccine. If the conjugate is not available, the polysaccharide vaccine can be given at 24 months or later. Children less than 5 years of age who have been previously vaccinated with polysaccharide vaccine between ages 18 and 23 months should be revaccinated with the conjugated vaccine.

[6] At least 6 months should have elapsed since DTP-3; or, if fewer than three doses of DTP have been given, at least 6 weeks should have elapsed since the last DTP or OPV. MMR should not be delayed to allow for MMR, DTP-4, and OPV-3 to be given simultaneously. Giving MMR at 15 months and DTP-4 and OPV-3 at 18 months is acceptable.

[7] MMR = measles, mumps, rubella virus vaccine, live. In high-risk areas (five or more cases of measles in preschool children in each of the last 5 years, or a county with a recent outbreak among unvaccinated children of preschool age), initial vaccination with MMR should be at 12 months of age.

[8] Td = tetanus and diphtheria toxoids, absorbed. For use in persons older than 7 years. Contains the same amount of tetanus as DTP but less diphtheria toxoid.

to the whole-cell pertussis component. The recently released acellular pertussis vaccine (DTaP) appears to be immunogenic and well-tolerated in adults but is not yet recommended for adult immunization.

Measles

Adults born before 1957 are considered immune to measles. Adults born in 1957 or later who were not immunized after age 1 year and who do not have a physician-documented history or laboratory evidence of previous infection should receive at lest one dose of vaccine. Persons born between 1963 and 1967—a period when inactivated measles vaccine was the only product available—should also receive one dose of live attenuated vaccine at least 1 month apart. Persons vaccinated before their first birthday should also be revaccinated. Because outbreaks of measles have occurred in young adults who have received a single dose of measles vaccine, revaccination is recommended, particularly before going to college, entering a health care profession, or embarking on foreign travel to areas where measles is endemic. Entrants to colleges and universities and employees of health care institutions who have not previously been vaccinated should receive two doses of vaccine at least 1 month apart. Revaccination of an immune person is

not associated with adverse effects—if the vaccination status is unknown and an indication for vaccination exists, it can be safely done. Vaccination of susceptible adults within 72 hours after exposure to an active case of measles is protective.

About 5–15% of unimmunized individuals will develop fever and about 5% a mild rash 5–12 days after vaccination. Fever and rash are self-limiting, lasting only 2–3 days. Local swelling and induration are particularly common in individuals previously vaccinated with inactivated vaccine. Pregnant women, immunosuppressed persons (with the exception of HIV-infected individuals, who should be vaccinated if susceptible), and persons with a history of anaphylaxis to eggs or egg products should not be vaccinated. Milder allergic reactions to eggs are not a contraindication to vaccination.

Rubella

The major purpose of rubella vaccination is to prevent transmission to the fetus. Immunization is recommended for all adults but particularly for women of childbearing age who have not previously been immunized. In addition, both male and female hospital workers who may be exposed to patients with rubella or who might have contact with pregnant patients should be immunized. A single immunization is given. Because of the expense of routine serologic testing to identify susceptible individuals and because revaccination of immune individuals is not associated with adverse effects, serologic testing is not required prior to vaccination.

Adverse effects are usually mild. Up to 40% of unvaccinated adults (usually women) experience joint pain. Joint symptoms begin 1–3 weeks after vaccination and are self-limited, lasting 3–10 days. Frank arthritis is rare. Although vaccination of pregnant women is *not* recommended, available data suggest that with the RA27/3 vaccine strain (the one presently available), the congenital rubella syndrome does not occur in the offspring of those inadvertently vaccinated during pregnancy or within 3 months before conception. Persons immunosuppressed by virtue of disease or medication should not receive vaccine. HIV infection is an exception—vaccine should be given to asymptomatic individuals and may be considered in symptomatic patients. Since the vaccine contains trace amounts of neomycin, a history of anaphylaxis to this agent is a contraindication to vaccine use.

Mumps

Mumps vaccine is recommended for all adults thought to be susceptible. Persons born before 1957 are considered to be naturally immune and do not require vaccination. Those born in 1957 or later should be considered susceptible unless they can document infection, prove vaccination, or have laboratory evidence of immunity. Vaccination in those already immune is not associated with an increased incidence of adverse effects

Mumps vaccine is generally safe. It should not be given to those who are immunosuppressed (except HIV-infected individuals) or who have a history of anaphylaxis to eggs or neomycin.

Influenza

Influenza vaccination is recommended yearly. Those at greatest risk for severe complications of influenza should have priority in vaccination programs: (1) Adults and children with chronic cardiopulmonary disease, including children with asthma. (2) Residents of nursing homes and other chronic care facilities. (3) Healthy adults 65 years of age or older. (4) Adults and children who have required either regular medical follow-up or hospitalization in the last year for chronic metabolic disorders (including diabetes) or renal disease, those with hemoglobinopathies, and those receiving immunosuppressive drugs. (5) Children and teenagers who are on long-term aspirin therapy and would be at increased risk for developing Reye's syndrome following influenza. Certain high-risk groups of patients (the elderly, persons with AIDS, transplant patients) may have a poor antibody response to vaccine, but there is no reason not to

vaccinate them. In an attempt to prevent disease in high-risk patients, vaccination of household members and health care providers who have contact with these high-risk patients should also be vaccinated. Vaccination is recommended also for otherwise healthy adults who provide essential community services.

Local reactions (erythema and tenderness) at the site of injection are common, but fevers, chills, and malaise (which lasts in any case only 2–3 days) are rare. Like measles, mumps, and yellow fever vaccines, influenza vaccine is prepared using embryonated chicken eggs, and persons with a history of anaphylaxis to eggs should not be vaccinated. Influenza vaccination may be associated with multiple false-positive serologic tests to HIV, HTLV-1, and hepatitis C. Seropositivity is self-limited, lasting 2–5 months.

Pneumococcal Pneumonia

Pneumococcal vaccine contains purified polysaccharide from 23 of the most common strains of *Streptococcus pneumoniae,* which cause 90% of bacteremic episodes in the USA. Antibody response following vaccination is dependent upon the patient's immune status and the presence of concomitant disease. Healthy adults have an excellent antibody response, as do patients who are postsplenectomy and those with sickle cell disease. Elderly individuals and those with chronic diseases (diabetes mellitus, alcoholic cirrhosis, chronic obstructive pulmonary disease) have increased antibody levels following vaccination but to a lesser extent than young healthy adults. Patients with Hodgkin's disease respond to vaccination if it is given before splenectomy, radiation, or chemotherapy, whereas patients with leukemia, lymphoma, and HIV infection respond poorly.

Although the efficacy of pneumococcal vaccine has been questioned, most postlicensure studies indicate that vaccination is about 60% effective in preventing bacteremic disease in immunocompetent persons. It is less effective in immunocompromised patients (only 10% effective) largely because of inability to mount an antibody response in this population of patients. It is presently recommended for patients at increased risk for developing severe pneumococcal disease, especially asplenic patients and those with sickle cell disease. It is also recommended for adults who are at increased risk of developing pneumococcal disease, including those with chronic illnesses (eg, cardiopulmonary disease, alcoholism, cirrhosis, cerebrospinal fluid leaks), those who are immunocompromised (eg, patients with Hodgkin's disease, lymphoma, chronic renal failure, nephrotic syndrome, and asymptomatic or symptomatic HIV infection), and those taking immunosuppressive medications. In addition, it is recommended for all individuals over 65 years of age. A single dose of vaccine usually confers lifelong immunity. Revaccination every 5–6 years should be considered only in those at highest risk of fatal pneumococcal infection (eg, asplenic patients) and those known to have a rapid decline in antibody titers (eg, those with nephrotic syndrome or renal failure, transplant recipients). Revaccination should also be considered for high-risk individuals previously immunized with the older 14-valent vaccine. Since immunocompetent patients respond best to the vaccine, it should be given 1 month before splenectomy or before starting chemotherapy if that can be anticipated.

Mild reactions (erythema and tenderness) occur in up to 50% of recipients, but systemic reactions are uncommon. The incidence of adverse reactions with revaccination is unknown but is probably related to the interval between vaccinations. Early reports suggested frequent adverse reactions when revaccination occurred within 1–2 years. Subsequent reports have indicated few adverse reactions when revaccination occurs 5 or more years later.

Hepatitis B

Recombinant hepatitis B vaccine is given on three separate occasions—the first two doses 1 month apart and the last dose 5 months after the second one. It is recommended for all individuals at increased risk of developing hepatitis B for social reasons (intravenous drug users, male homosexuals), family reasons (household and sexual contacts of hepatitis B carriers), or occupational reasons (those with frequent exposure to blood and blood products, hemodialysis patients and staff, house officers, medical students, morticians). Although most often used for preexposure prophylaxis, the vaccine is also given as postexposure prophylaxis along with hepatitis B immunoglobulin following needle stick injury or mucous membrane exposure to blood from an individual who is HBsAg-positive. It is also given along with hepatitis B immunoglobulin to infants of mothers who are HBsAg-positive. Immunity wanes with time, but recommendations for revaccination have not been established. Adverse reactions are minor and limited to local soreness.

RECOMMENDED IMMUNIZATIONS FOR TRAVELERS

Individuals traveling to other countries frequently require immunizations in addition to those listed above and may benefit from chemoprophylaxis against various diseases. Every traveler must fulfill the immunization requirements of the health authorities of different countries. These are listed in *Health Information for International Travel,* published by the Centers for Disease Control. An updated version is published yearly and is available from the Superintendent of Documents, United States Government Printing Office, Washington, DC 20402.

When individuals request information and vaccinations for travel from a physician, their entire immunization history should be reviewed and updated, including those immunizations listed above that are not specifically required for travel.

Various vaccines can be given simultaneously at different sites. Some, such as cholera, plague, and typhoid vaccine, which cause significant discomfort, are best given at different times. In general, live attenuated vaccines (measles, mumps, rubella, yellow fever, and oral poliovaccine) should not be given to immunosuppressed individuals or household members of immunosuppressed people or to pregnant women. Immunoglobulin should not be given for 3 months before or at least 2 weeks after live virus vaccines, because it may attenuate the antibody response.

Chemoprophylaxis of malaria is discussed in Chapter 34.

Cholera

Because the incidence of cholera among travelers is very low and because the vaccine is only marginally effective, the World Health Organization does not routinely require immunization even for persons traveling to and from endemic areas. Certain countries, however, still require vaccination for travel (Middle Eastern countries, Asian countries, occasionally others).

Cholera vaccine contains a suspension of killed vibrios, including prevalent antigenic types. Two injections are given intramuscularly 2–6 weeks apart, followed by booster injections every 6 months during periods of possible exposure. Protection depends largely on booster doses. An inactivated oral vaccine appears to be more effective than the parenteral vaccine but is not available in the USA. A live attenuated oral vaccine is being investigated. The WHO certificate is valid for 6 months only.

Hepatitis A

No active immunization is available for hepatitis A. Temporary passive immunity may be induced by the intramuscular injection of immune globulin, 0.02 mL/kg every 2–3 months or 0.1 mL/kg every 6 months. Protection with immune globulin is recommended for persons traveling to all parts of the world where sanitation is poor and the risk of exposure to hepatitis A is high because of contaminated food and water supplies and contact with infected persons. Preparation of immunoglobulin from plasma involves steps that inactivate the HIV virus, thus making immunoglobulin preparations incapable of transmitting HIV infection.

Hepatitis B

Persons traveling to and spending more than 6 months in endemic areas of HBV infection who will have close contact with the local population should be considered for vaccination. Short-term travelers to areas of moderate or high endemic infection (Southeast Asia and sub-Saharan Africa) who will be in contact with potentially infected body secretions of residents should be vaccinated. Vaccination should begin at least 6 months before travel to allow for completion of the series.

Meningococcal Meningitis

If travel is contemplated to an area where meningococcal meningitis is epidemic (Nepal, sub-Saharan Africa, New Delhi) or highly endemic, polysaccharide vaccines from types A, C, W-135, and Y may be indicated. Follow the manufacturer's dosage recommendations. The vaccine is also recommended for persons with anatomic or functional asplenia and those with terminal complement deficiencies.

Plague

Plague vaccine is a suspension of killed plague bacilli that is given intramuscularly. Three injections are given—the second, 4 months after the initial injection; and the third, 5 months after the second. Vaccination is generally recommended only for travelers who will have exposure to rodents or rabbits in rural areas where plague is endemic. (Some areas in South America, southeast Asia, occasionally others.) For continuing exposures, booster doses at intervals of 1–2 years are recommended.

Poliomyelitis

Adult travelers to tropical or developing countries who have not previously been immunized against poliomyelitis should receive a primary series of three doses of inactivated enhanced-potency poliovaccine (IPV), as follows: two doses of 0.5 mL subcutaneously 4–8 weeks apart and then a third dose at least 4 weeks and preferably 6–12 months after the second dose. Because of the risk of vaccine-associated paralytic poliomyelitis, live attenuated oral poliovaccine (OPV) should not be routinely used to vaccinate adults. It may be used if protection is needed within 4 weeks of travel, in which case a single dose of OPV or IPV is given and primary immunization is then completed with either IPV or OPV. (Primary immunization with OPV includes two doses given 6–8 weeks apart and a third dose given at least 6 weeks and preferably 8–12 months after the second dose.) Travelers who have previously been fully immunized with OPV or IPV should receive a one-time booster dose with either OPV or IPV.

Rabies

For travelers to areas where rabies is common in domestic animals (eg, India, Asia, Mexico), preexposure prophylaxis with human diploid cell vaccine or rabies vaccine adsorbed should be considered. It usually consists of two intramuscular (deltoid area) injections of 1 mL of human diploid cell vaccine or ra-

bies vaccine adsorbed given 1 week apart with a booster dose 2–3 weeks later. Alternatively, two intradermal injections of 0.1 mL of human diploid cell vaccine are given 1 week apart, with a booster dose given 2–3 weeks later. Chloroquine can blunt the immunologic response to rabies vaccine. If malaria prophylaxis with this agent is required, vaccination should be given intramuscularly (*not* intradermally) to ensure adequate antibody response. There are no data on the interaction between mefloquine and rabies vaccine. It would seem reasonable to administer rabies vaccine intramuscularly if mefloquine is to be given until further studies are done.

Typhoid

Typhoid vaccination is recommended for travelers to developing countries (especially Latin America, Africa, and Asia) who will have prolonged exposure to contaminated food and water. Two preparations of approximately equal efficacy (51–77% effective) are available. An oral live-attenuated Ty21a vaccine supplied as enteric-coated capsules is given as one capsule every other day for four doses; or two doses of a suspension of killed *Salmonella typhi* are given subcutaneously 4 weeks apart. A booster dose of the parenteral vaccine is recommended every 3 years if continued exposure is a probability. The optimal booster dose for the oral preparation has not been firmly established. The manufacturer currently recommends repeating the entire four-dose series every 5 years.

Yellow Fever

The live attenuated yellow fever virus vaccine is administered once subcutaneously. The WHO certificate requires registration of the manufacturer and the batch number of the vaccine. Vaccination is available in the USA only at approved centers. (Contact the local health department for available resources.) Vaccination must be repeated at intervals of 10 years or less. (Africa, South America.)

Because it is a live attenuated vaccine prepared in embryonated eggs, the yellow fever vaccine should not be given to immunosuppressed individuals or those with a history of anaphylaxis to eggs. Pregnancy is a relative contraindication to vaccination.

Japanese B Encephalitis

This is a mosquito-borne viral encephalitis that affects primarily children and older adults (65 years and older) and occurs primarily from June to September. It is prevalent in India and Asia. The vaccine is an inactivated viral preparation given three times at weekly intervals. Vaccination is recommended for those traveling to endemic areas in the summer months who will be exposed for 3 weeks or more.

Guide for Adult Immunization, 2nd ed. American College of Physicians, 1990. (Comprehensive review in textbook format.)

Update on adult immunization. Recommendations of the Immunization Practices Advisory Committee (ACIP). MMWR Morb Mortal Wkly Rep 1991;40(RR-12):1. (Official policy statement.)

HYPERSENSITIVITY TESTS & DESENSITIZATION

One should test for hypersensitivity before injecting antitoxin, materials derived from animal sources, or drugs (eg, penicillin) to which a patient has had a severe reaction in the past. If the test described below is negative, desensitization is not necessary, and a full dose of the material may be given. If the test is positive, alternative drugs should be strongly considered. If that is not feasible, desensitization is necessary.

Intradermal Test for Hypersensitivity

Penicillin is the drug that most frequently serves as an indication for sensitivity testing and desensitization. Skin testing requires two preparations: PPL (penicilloyl-polylysine) and a minor determinant mixture. Several points should be emphasized in performing and interpreting these tests. Whenever possible, both PPL and a minor determinant should be used, since 85% of skin test reactors are positive to PPL but 15% react only to the minor determinant mixture. In addition, if penicillin G is used instead of the minor determinant mixture, some allergic patients will be missed. About 25% of individuals who react to minor determinant mixture may not react to penicillin G, and such patients may still have an anaphylactic or accelerated reaction to penicillin. A "pinprick" test is performed with each solution at different sites by placing a small drop of solution on the skin and making small indentations of the skin with a needle. If there is no reaction within 10 minutes, 0.01–0.02 mL is injected intradermally, raising a small bleb. Development of a wheal greater than 5 mm in diameter is considered a positive test and an indication for desensitization. If the test is negative, the drug can be administered with the precautions listed below. Even if the test is negative, about 1% of patients will have an immediate or accelerated reaction. Thus, the drug can be administered with relative safety, but the precautions below should be followed.

Desensitization

A. Precautions:

1. The desensitization procedure is not innocuous—deaths from anaphylaxis have been reported. If extreme hypersensitivity is suspected, it is advisable to use an alternative structurally unrelated drug and to reserve desensitization for situations when treatment cannot be withheld and no alternative drug is available.

2. An antihistaminic drug (25–50 mg of hydroxyzine or diphenhydramine intramuscularly or orally) should be administered before desensitization is begun in order to lessen any reaction that occurs. An airway device must be available.

3. Epinephrine, 1 mL of 1:1000 solution, must be ready for immediate administration.

B. Desensitization Method: Several methods of desensitization have been described for penicillin, including use of both oral and intravenous preparations. All methods start with very small doses of drug and gradually increase the dose until therapeutic doses are achieved. For penicillin, 1 unit of drug is given intravenously and the patient observed for 15–30 minutes. If there is no reaction, some recommend doubling the dose while others recommend increasing it tenfold every 15–30 minutes until a dosage of 2 million units is reached; then give the remainder of the desired dose.

For recommendations on skin testing and desensitization for other preparations (botulism antitoxin, diphtheria antitoxin, etc), one should consult the manufacturer's package inserts.

Treatment of Reactions

A. Mild Reactions: If a mild reaction occurs, drop back to the next lower dose and continue with desensitization. If a severe reaction occurs, administer epinephrine (see below) and discontinue the drug unless treatment is urgently needed. If desensitization is imperative, continue slowly, increasing the dosage of the drug more gradually.

B. Severe Reactions: If bronchospasm occurs, epinephrine, 0.3–0.5 mL of 1:1000 dilution, should be given subcutaneously every 10–20 minutes. The following can also be given if symptoms persist: inhaled metaproterenol (0.3 mL of a 5% solution in 2.5 mL of saline), intravenous aminophylline (0.3–0.9 mL/kg/h maintenance after a 6 mg/kg loading dose over 30 minutes), or corticosteroids (250 mg of hydrocortisone or 50 mg of methylprednisolone intravenously every 6 hours for two to four doses). Hypotension should be treated with intravenous fluids (saline or colloid), epinephrine (1 mL of 1:1000 dilution in 500 mL of D_5W intravenously at a rate of 0.5–5 µg/min), and antihistamines (25–50 mg of hydroxyzine or diphenhydramine intramuscularly or orally every 6–8 hours as needed). Cutaneous reactions, manifested as urticaria or angioedema, respond to epinephrine subcutaneously and antihistamines in the doses set forth above.

Bochner BS, Lichtenstein LM: Anaphylaxis. N Engl J Med 1991;324:1785. (Review of pathophysiology and therapy.)

Borish L, Tamir R, Rosenwasser L: Intravenous desensitization to beta-lactam antibiotics. J Allergy Clin Immunol 1987;30:314. (Experience with 15 desensitizations in 12 patients.)

Penicillin allergy. Med Lett Drugs Ther 1988;30:79. (Summary of current recommendations.)

REFERENCES

Feigin RD, Cherry JD: *Textbook of Pediatric Infectious Diseases,* 3rd ed. Saunders, 1992.

Brooks GF, Butel JS, Ornston LN: *Jawetz, Melnick, & Adelberg's Medical Microbiology,* 19th ed. Appleton & Lange, 1991.

Mandell GL, Douglas RG Jr, Bennett JE: *Principles and Practice of Infectious Disease,* 3rd ed. Churchill Livingstone, 1990.

30

HIV Infection

Harry Hollander, MD, & Mitchell H. Katz, MD

Essentials of Diagnosis

- Risk factors: sexual contact with an infected person, parenteral exposure to infected blood by transfusion or needle sharing, perinatal exposure.
- Prominent systemic complaints such as sweats, diarrhea, weight loss, and wasting.
- Opportunistic infections due to diminished cellular immunity—often life-threatening.
- Aggressive cancers, particularly Kaposi's sarcoma and extranodal lymphoma.
- Neurologic manifestations, including dementia, aseptic meningitis, and neuropathy.

General Considerations

When AIDS was first recognized in the USA in 1981, cases were identified by finding severe opportunistic infections such as *Pneumocystis carinii* pneumonia that indicated profound defects in cellular immunity in the absence of other causes of immunodeficiency. When the syndrome was found to be caused by the human immunodeficiency virus (HIV), it became obvious that severe opportunistic infections and unusual neoplasms were at one end of a spectrum of disease, while healthy seropositive individuals were at the other end.

In 1993, the Centers for Disease Control and Prevention expanded the AIDS definition (Table 30–1). The 1993 definition includes all 23 opportunistic infections (eg, *P carinii* pneumonia) and neoplasms (eg, Kaposi's sarcoma) that were included in the 1987 definition. As with the 1987 definition, it also includes as AIDS cases persons with documented weight loss, diarrhea, or dementia and a positive HIV serology. There remain criteria for both definitive and presumptive diagnoses. The expansion is that persons with a positive HIV serology and a "lowest accurate" CD4 lymphocyte count below 200 cells/μL or a CD4 lymphocyte percentage below 14% will be considered to have AIDS. Inclusion of persons with low CD4 counts as AIDS cases reflects the recognition that immunodeficiency is the defining characteristic of AIDS. The choice of a cutoff point at 200 cells/μL is supported by several cohort studies showing that over 80% of persons with counts below this level will develop AIDS within 3 years. The 1993 definition was also expanded to include persons with positive HIV serology and pulmonary tuberculosis, recurrent pneumonia, and invasive cervical cancer. It is thought that the expanded definition will result in HIV-infected persons being diagnosed with AIDS an average of 1.6 years earlier in the course of the disease. The definition will double to triple the number of new cases of AIDS in 1993. However, the impact of the new definition on the number of new cases will be less in future years.

The goal of the new definition is to enhance efforts at surveillance of HIV disease. It probably will not affect eligibility for most social services benefits, since the Social Security Administration has decided not to use the CDC definition as presumptive eligibility of disability. Instead, SSA has developed a functional assessment for determining eligibility for benefits for HIV-infected persons. In general, the term "AIDS-related complex" (ARC) was used to denote those HIV-infected patients who were symptomatic but did not fit the CDC definition of AIDS. This group of patients is heterogeneous, with varying clinical problems and prognoses. Therefore, the use of the term "ARC" should be avoided. Because the CDC's definition is for surveillance purposes and does not stratify patients by severity of illness, other classification systems have been developed. The Walter Reed System stratifies individuals based on clinical manifestations, skin testing, and CD4 counts.

Epidemiology

The modes of transmission of HIV are similar to those of hepatitis B, in particular with respect to sexual, parenteral, and vertical transmission. The risk of sexual transmission varies with particular sexual practices; anal intercourse is the riskiest. The risk of sustaining HIV infection from a needle stick with infected blood is approximately 1:250, which is significantly less than the risk of contracting hepatitis B from a contaminated needle stick. Between 30% and 50% of children born to HIV-infected mothers contract HIV-infection. The HIV virus has not been shown to be transmitted by respiratory droplet spread, by vectors such as mosquitoes, or by casual nonsexual contact.

Current estimates are that about 1 million Americans are infected with HIV. Estimates of the number of people who will develop AIDS in the 1990s have been scaled down from prior estimates, based on re-

Table 30–1. CDC AIDS case definition for surveillance of adults and adolescents.

Definitive AIDS diagnoses (with or without laboratory evidence of HIV infection)
1. Candidiasis of the esophagus, trachea, bronchi, or lungs.
2. Cryptococcosis, extrapulmonary.
3. Cryptosporidiosis with diarrhea persisting > 1 month.
4. Cytomegalovirus disease of an organ other than liver, spleen, or lymph nodes.
5. Herpes simplex virus infection causing a mucocutaneous ulcer that persists longer than 1 month; or bronchitis, pneumonitis, or esophagitis of any duration.
6. Kaposi's sarcoma in a patient < 60 years of age.
7. Lymphoma of the brain (primary) in a patient < 60 years of age.
8. *Mycobacterium avium* complex or *Mycobacterium kansasii* disease, disseminated (at a site other than or in addition to lungs, skin, or cervical or hilar lymph nodes).
9. *Pneumocystis carinii* pneumonia.
10. Progressive multifocal leukoencephalopathy.
11. Toxoplasmosis of the brain.

Definitive AIDS diagnoses (with laboratory evidence of HIV infection)
1. Coccidioidomycosis, disseminated (at a site other than or in addition to lungs or cervical or hilar lymph nodes).
2. HIV encephalopathy.
3. Histoplasmosis, disseminated (at a site other than or in addition to lungs or cervical or hilar lymph nodes).
4. Isosporiasis with diarrhea persisting > 1 month.
5. Kaposi's sarcoma at any age.
6. Lymphoma of the brain (primary) at any age.
7. Other non-Hodgkin's lymphoma of B cell or unknown immunologic phenotype.
8. Any mycobacterial disease caused by mycobacteria other than *Mycobacterium tuberculosis*, disseminated (at a site other than or in addition to lungs, skin, or cervical or hilar lymph nodes).
9. Disease caused by extrapulmonary *M tuberculosis*.
10. *Salmonella* (nontyphoid) septicemia, recurrent.
11. HIV wasting syndrome.
12. CD4 lymphocyte count below 200 cells/μL or a CD4 lymphocyte percentage below 14%.
13. Pulmonary tuberculosis.
14. Recurrent pneumonia.
15. Invasive cervical cancer.

Presumptive AIDS diagnoses (with laboratory evidence of HIV infection)
1. Candidiasis of esophagus: (a) recent onset of retrosternal pain on swallowing; and (b) oral candidiasis.
2. Cytomegalovirus retinitis. A characteristic appearance on serial ophthalmoscopic examinations.
3. Mycobacteriosis. Specimen from stool or normally sterile body fluids or tissue from a site other than lungs, skin, or cervical or hilar lymph nodes, showing acid-fast bacilli of a species not identified by culture.
4. Kaposi's sarcoma. Erythematous or violaceous plaque-like lesion on skin or mucous membrane.
5. *Pneumocystis carinii* pneumonia: (a) a history of dyspnea on exertion or nonproductive cough of recent onset (within the past 3 months); and (b) chest x-ray evidence of diffuse bilateral interstitial infiltrates or gallium scan evidence of diffuse bilateral pulmonary disease; and (c) arterial blood gas analysis showing an arterial oxygen partial pressure of < 70 mm Hg or a low respiratory diffusing capacity of < 80% of predicted values or an increase in the alveolar-arterial oxygen tension gradient; and (d) no evidence of a bacterial pneumonia.
6. Toxoplasmosis of the brain: (a) recent onset of a focal neurologic abnormality consistent with intracranial disease or a reduced level of consciousness; and (b) brain imaging evidence of a lesion having a mass effect or the radiographic appearance of which is enhanced by injection of contrast medium; and (c) serum antibody to toxoplasmosis or successful response to therapy for toxoplasmosis.
7. Recurrent pneumonia: (a) more than one episode in a 1-year period; and (b) acute (new symptoms, signs, or radiologic evidence not present earlier) pneumonia diagnosed on clinical or radiologic grounds by the patient's physician.
8. Pulmonay tuberculosis: (a) apical or miliary infiltrates and (b) radiographic and clinical response to antituberculosis therapy.

cent AIDS incidence data. It is estimated that in 1994 there will between 134,000 and 228,000 people alive with AIDS (based on the 1987 definition), with between more 43,000 and 93,000 new cases per year. In the USA, 63% of AIDS cases are reported in gay or bisexual men, and 23% are intravenous drug users, the majority of whom live in major metropolitan areas. The remainder of cases occur in infants of infected mothers, heterosexual contacts of infected individuals, and recipients of contaminated blood or blood products. Among risk groups, the most rapid percentage increases are anticipated among women and inner city intravenous drug users, especially blacks and Latinos.

The rapid increase of AIDS cases among women is of great concern. Whereas women represented only 7% of cases prior to 1985, they represented 13% of AIDS cases in 1992. It is projected that there will be between 7000 and 16,000 new cases of AIDS among women (based on the 1987 definition) in 1994. Intravenous drug use and heterosexual contact with an infected partner are the two major risk factors for women. With the rapid increase of HIV infection among women, there has been a corresponding rise in the number of perinatally infected children.

It is not known whether the natural history of HIV infection is different in women than in men; several cohort studies have been initiated in an attempt to answer this question. It appears that HIV-infected women tend to present later for medical care than gay and bisexual men, and this may explain why some cross-sectional studies have found that women progress more rapidly to AIDS than men. Women are at risk for gynecologic complications of HIV infection, including recurrent candidal vaginitis, pelvic inflammatory disease, and cervical dysplasia.

HIV infection will continue to spread outward from major metropolitan areas to suburban and rural parts of the country. Because blood donor screening using the HIV-enzyme-linked immunosorbent assay (ELISA) is universally practiced in the USA, the number of new AIDS cases due to transfusion has already peaked and is expected to decline further. The current risk of contracting HIV from a screened unit of blood is 1:100,000. Since 1983, transmission of HIV to at-risk gay men in San Francisco has dramatically fallen to about 1% per year. Recent surveys have indicated a relapse from "safe sex" practices among certain populations of gay men, raising concern that there will be an increase in the number of new seroconverters. This finding underlines the need for continued counseling and education of at-risk individuals.

There are an estimated 10 million persons infected worldwide. In Central and East Africa in some urban areas, as many as a third of sexually active adults are infected. HIV infection began to spread in Asia in the late 1980s, and it is expected that new infections in Asia will exceed new infections in Africa by the mid to late 1990s. The most common mode of transmission is bidirectional heterosexual spread. The reason for the greater risk for transmission with heterosexual intercourse in Africa and Asia than in the United States may relate to cofactors such as general health status, the presence of genital ulcers, and the number of sexual partners.

Etiology

The syndromes described below are due to infection with human retroviruses known as human immunodeficiency viruses (HIV or HIV-1, formerly HTLV-III or LAV). Retroviruses depend upon a unique enzyme, reverse transcriptase (RNA-directed DNA-polymerase), to replicate within host cells. The other major pathogenic human retrovirus, HTLV-I, is associated with lymphoma, while HIV is not directly oncogenic. The genome of HIV viruses contains genes for three basic structural proteins and at least five other regulatory proteins; *gag* codes for group antigen proteins, *pol* codes for polymerase, and *env* codes for the external envelope protein. The greatest variability in strains of HIV occurs in the viral envelope. Since neutralizing activity is found in antibodies directed against the envelope, this variability presents problems for vaccine development.

In addition to the classic AIDS virus (HIV-1), a group of related viruses, HIV-2, have been isolated in West African patients. HIV-2 has the same genetic organization as HIV-1, but there are significant differences in the envelope glycoproteins. Some infected individuals exhibit AIDS-like illnesses, but most West Africans infected with HIV-2 are currently asymptomatic. HIV-2 has been found in several people in the USA. Thus, this variant may be less pathogenic or have a longer period of latency preceding disease.

Pathogenesis

The hallmark of symptomatic HIV infection is immunodeficiency. The virus can infect all cells expressing the T4 (CD4) antigen, which serves as a receptor for HIV. Once it enters a cell, HIV can replicate and cause cell fusion or death by unknown mechanisms. In many cases, a latent state is established, with integration of the HIV genome into the cell's genome. The cell principally infected is the CD4 (helper-inducer) lymphocyte, which directs many other cells in the immune network. With increasing duration of infection, the number of CD4 lymphocytes falls. Some of the immunologic defects, however, are explained not by *quantitative* abnormalities of lymphocyte subsets but by *qualitative* defects in CD4 responsiveness induced by HIV.

Other cells in the immune network that are infected by HIV include B lymphocytes and macrophages. The defect in B cells is partly due to disordered CD4 lymphocyte function. However, HIV can also alter B cell function directly. These direct and indirect effects can lead to generalized hypergammaglobulinemia and can also depress B cell responses to new antigen challenges. Because of these defects, the immunodeficiency of HIV is mixed. Elements of humoral and cellular immunodeficiency are present, especially in children.

The role of macrophage-monocyte infection in immunodeficiency is not as clear. It is possible that macrophage dysfunction plays a role in some of the clinical manifestations of the disease, such as *P carinii* pneumonia. Macrophages also act as a reservoir for HIV and serve to disseminate it to other organ systems (eg, the central nervous system).

Apart from the immunologic effects of HIV, the virus can also directly cause a variety of neurologic effects. Rare glial cells and oligodendrocytes express CD4 antigen and thus may be permissive of infection by HIV. However, these cells are rarely infected, whereas multinucleated giant cells of macrophage origin are more commonly seen in brain specimens of infected individuals. The envelope of HIV is homologous with neuroleukins; the neuropathologic features may be partly dependent upon inhibition of neurologic growth factors by the virus. Other factors such as coexistent CMV infection may also be important. Perturbations of excitatory neurotransmitters and calcium flux may contribute to neurologic dysfunction.

Pathology

Most histopathologic changes in HIV infection are caused by secondary opportunistic infections or neoplasms rather than direct effects of HIV infection. Several pathologic findings, however, are unique to HIV. The lymph nodes may demonstrate different pathologic changes at different stages of clinical disease. Early, a pattern of benign but florid follicular hyperplasia is seen. Immunologic staining reveals a profound decrease in CD4 lymphocytes in the paracortical areas of the lymph nodes, consistent with the depressed CD4 lymphocyte count in peripheral blood. Later, as immunodeficiency progresses, involution and atrophy of formerly hyperplastic lymph nodes often take place. Pulmonary involvement by HIV may result in a lymphocytic interstitial pneumonitis seen in lung biopsies. Whether this pathologic pattern represents direct HIV infection or is an autoimmune response to infection is unclear. This pathologic pattern is common in childhood HIV infection and is being recognized more commonly in adults. It has a variable clinical course.

Pathologic involvement of the nervous system is frequent in infected individuals. Over 90% of patients dying of AIDS have abnormal brain histopathologic findings, with diffuse involvement of the cerebrum and cerebellum. Findings include focal subcortical demyelination and, less commonly, the presence of multinucleated giant cells. A vacuolar myelopathy resembling that due to vitamin B_{12} deficiency may also be seen.

Finally, a variety of pathologic changes have been observed in peripheral nerves, ranging from demyelinating neuropathy, which resembles Guillain-Barré syndrome, to an axonal sensory neuropathy with little surrounding inflammatory response. Thus, HIV does leave some pathologic footprints in several organ systems. Far more common, however, is secondary disease due to immunodeficiency.

Pathophysiology

Clinically, the syndromes caused by HIV infection are usually explicable by one of three known mechanisms. Some HIV-associated manifestations, however, are not explained by any of these proposed mechanisms.

A. Immunodeficiency: Immunodeficiency is a direct result of the effects of HIV upon immune cells. A spectrum of infections and neoplasms is seen, as in other congenital or acquired immunodeficiency states. Two remarkable features of HIV immunodeficiency are the low incidence of certain infections such as listeriosis and aspergillosis and the frequent occurrence of certain neoplasms such as lymphoma or Kaposi's sarcoma. This latter complication has been seen primarily in gay or bisexual men, and its incidence has steadily declined through the first 10 years of the epidemic. This epidemiologic fact and other basic science advances suggest that Kaposi's sarcoma is not a true neoplasm but a multicentric hyperplasia of endothelial elements stimulated by an unidentified sexually transmitted or behaviorally related cofactor.

B. Autoimmunity: Autoimmunity can occur as a result of disordered cellular immune function or B lymphocyte dysfunction. Examples of both lymphocytic infiltration of organs (eg, lymphocytic interstitial pneumonitis) and autoantibody production (eg, immunologic thrombocytopenia) occur. These phenomena may be the only clinically apparent disease or may coexist with obvious immunodeficiency.

C. Neurologic Dysfunction: Little is known about the mechanisms of neurologic dysfunction, since relatively few neural cells are infected and the inflammatory response is minimal. Possibilities include homology with and blockade of neurologic growth factors, other toxic effects of viral products, or release of neurotoxic compounds from infected macrophages.

Clinical Findings

Primary care physicians, in consultation with specialists, are playing an increasing role in the care of HIV-infected individuals. With 1 million HIV-infected Americans, it would be impossible for all care to be delivered by infectious disease and oncology specialists. Moreover, with early antiviral therapy and prophylaxis for opportunistic infections, HIV disease shares features of other multisystem chronic diseases characterized by acute exacerbations and end-stage manifestations.

While the majority of general internists, family physicians, and general practitioners do treat HIV-infected patients, many feel uncomfortable doing so. The discomfort stems from attitudes toward gay men and intravenous drug users, lack of sufficient knowledge to treat the disease, and inadequate reimbursement for the time-consuming care required by AIDS patients. Resources are available to help clinicians care for HIV-infected persons. Clinicians should call their state medical associations for a list of local resources.

Primary care physicians should provide risk factor assessment of their patients and, when appropriate, screening for HIV infection with pre- and posttest counseling. Pretest counseling should include review of risk factors for HIV infection, discussion of safe sex (see Prevention), and the meaning of a positive test. Posttest counseling should include a review of the importance of safe sex practices. For persons who test positive, information on available medical and mental health services should be provided as well as guidance for contacting sexual or needle-sharing partners.

For HIV-infected patients, primary care providers should perform periodic physical examinations, monitor prognostic markers (eg, CD4 lymphocyte counts), prescribe initial antiviral and prophylactic therapy, initiate diagnostic evaluation and therapy for HIV-related complications, provide supportive counseling, and offer assistance with terminal care (eg, pain control and durable power of attorney for health care). Specialists should be consulted for patients intolerant of standard antiviral drugs, those in need of systemic chemotherapy, and those with complicated opportunistic infections, particularly when invasive procedures or experimental therapies are needed. In many cases, a single consultation with follow-up to the primary care physician will provide the needed expertise while ensuring continuity in care.

A. Symptoms and Signs: Many individuals with HIV infection remain asymptomatic for years, with a mean time of approximately 10 years between exposure and development of AIDS. When symptoms occur, they may be remarkably protean and nonspecific. Systemic complaints such as weight loss, fevers, and night sweats are common. Ear, nose, and throat complaints include sinus fullness and drainage, painful swallowing, mouth lesions (candidal plaques, hairy leukoplakia), and gingival and periodontal inflammation and ulceration. Cough or shortness of breath raises a suspicion of HIV-related pulmonary disease. Gastrointestinal complaints include changes in bowel function, especially diarrhea. Central nervous system symptoms include depression, changes in personality, difficulty in concentrating, and frank confusion. Tingling, numbness, and weakness suggest peripheral neuropathy. Cutaneous complaints are common and include dry skin, new rashes, and nail changes. Since virtually all of these findings may be seen with other diseases, a combination of complaints is more suggestive of HIV infection than any one symptom.

Physical examination may be entirely normal. Abnormal findings range from completely nonspecific to highly specific for HIV infection. Those that are predictive of HIV infection include hairy leukoplakia of the tongue and disseminated Kaposi's sarcoma. Hairy leukoplakia is commonly seen as a white lesion on the lateral aspect of the tongue. It may be flat or slightly raised, is usually corrugated, and has vertical parallel lines with fine or thick ("hairy") projections. Kaposi's lesions may appear anywhere; careful examination of the eyelids, conjunctiva, pinnae, palate, and toe webs is mandatory to locate potentially occult lesions. In light-skinned individuals, Kaposi's lesions usually appear as purplish, nonblanching lesions that can be papular or nodular. In dark-skinned individuals, the lesions may appear more brown. In the mouth, lesions are most often palatal papules, though exophytic lesions of the tongue and gingivae may also be seen. Kaposi's lesions may be confused with other vascular lesions such as angiomas and pyogenic granulomas. A funduscopic finding of cytomegalovirus retinitis (perivascular hemorrhages and fluffy exudates) and the presence of oral candidiasis are both suggestive if no other cause of these conditions is found. Other less specific findings include evidence of recent weight loss, folliculitis, seborrheic dermatitis, onycholysis, retinal cotton-wool spots, oral aphthous ulcerations, angular cheilitis, and generalized lymphadenopathy. Neuropsychiatric findings may include depression, emotional lability, psychomotor slowing, abnormalities of pursuit eye movements, focal deficits, decreased vibratory sensation, and depressed or accentuated reflexes.

B. Laboratory Findings: Specific tests for HIV include antibody and antigen detection (Table 30–2). Screening serology is done by enzyme-linked immunosorbent assay (ELISA). Positive specimens are then confirmed by a different method (eg, Western blot). False-positive screening tests may occur as normal biologic variants or in association with other disease states, such as connective tissue disease. These are usually detected by negative confirmatory tests. The specificity of positive results by two different methods approaches 100%, even in low-risk populations. Similarly, the sensitivity of screening serologic tests is now over 99.5%. Newer molecular biology techniques (polymerase chain reaction) show a small incidence of individuals (< 1%) who are infected with HIV for up to 36 months without generating an antibody response. However, the vast majority will develop antibodies detectable by screening serologic tests within several months of infection. Core protein antigen (p24) may be detectable before a serologic response occurs, and antigenemia may also reappear in the course of the disease as immunosuppression progresses.

Nonspecific laboratory findings with HIV infection may include anemia, leukopenia (particularly lymphopenia) and thrombocytopenia in any combination, polyclonal hypergammaglobulinemia, and hypocholesterolemia. Cutaneous anergy is frequent early in the course and becomes universal as the disease progresses.

Several laboratory markers are available to provide prognostic information and guide therapy decisions. The most widely used marker is the absolute CD4 lymphocyte count. As counts decrease, the risk of opportunistic infection increases.

With the increased use of the CD4 count, the limitations of the test have become more apparent. There is substantial diurnal variation (counts are generally lower in the morning), and counts may be depressed by any intercurrent illness. Therefore, the trend in counts is more important than any single value. Because of laboratory variation, serial counts should be performed in the same laboratory. The frequency of performance of counts depends on the patient's health status. Patients whose CD4 counts are substantially above the threshold for initiation of antiviral therapy (500 cells/μL), should have counts performed every 6 months. Those who have counts near 500 cells/μL should have counts performed every 3 months. All persons with CD4 counts below 350

Table 30–2. Laboratory findings with HIV infection.

Test	Significance
HIV enzyme-linked immunosorbent assay (ELISA)	Screening test for HIV infection. Sensitivity > 99.5%; to avoid false-positive results, repeatedly reactive results must be confirmed with Western blot.
Western blot	Confirmatory test for HIV. Specificity when combined with ELISA > 99.9%. Indeterminate results with early HIV infection, HIV-2 infection, false-positive results.
CBC	Anemia, neutropenia, and thrombocytopenia common with advanced HIV infection.
Absolute CD4 lymphocyte count	Most widely used predictor of HIV progression. Risk of progression to AIDS high with CD4 < 200 cells/µL.
CD4 lymphocyte percentage	Percentage may be more reliable than the CD4 count. Risk of progression to AIDS high with percentage < 14%.
β_2-Microglobulin	Cell surface protein indicative of macrophage-monocyte stimulation. Levels > 3.5 mg/dL associated with rapid progression of disease. Not useful with intravenous drug users.
p24 antigen	Indicates active HIV replication. Tends to be positive prior to seroconversion and with advanced disease.

cells/µL should also have counts performed every 3 months. This is necessary for evaluating the efficacy of antiviral therapy and for initiating *P carinii* prophylactic therapy when the CD4 count drops below 200 cells/µL). Some studies suggest that the percentage of CD4 lymphocytes is a more reliable indicator of prognosis than the absolute counts because the percentage does not depend on calculating a manual differential.

Tests that determine evidence of macrophage-monocyte stimulation may provide additional useful prognostic information in infected individuals. Beta$_2$-microglobulin, for example, is a cell surface protein that tends to rise in a high percentage of cases over the course of HIV disease. Asymptomatic individuals with elevated serum β_2-microglobulin concentrations may have a twofold to threefold increased incidence of disease progression. However, this test must be interpreted cautiously, since autoimmune processes, malignant tumors, and other infections are also associated with elevated values. Because many intravenous drug users have chronically elevated β_2-microglobulin levels, this test is not generally helpful for patients in this group.

The presence of detectable p24 antigen in serum indicates a higher risk of progression of disease even after adjusting for the level of CD4 lymphocyte count. A new immune-complex-dissociated p24 assay is more sensitive and appears useful for demonstrating antiviral activity of drugs. Newer techniques for viral quantitation include measurements of plasma viremia and viral RNA as well as assays for viral DNA in infected mononuclear cells. Viral burden as measured by any of these techniques correlates with stage of disease. The appropriate use of these expensive new tests in clinical practice has not yet been defined.

Differential Diagnosis

HIV infection may mimic a variety of other medical illnesses. Specific differential diagnosis depends upon the mode of presentation. In patients presenting with constitutional symptoms such as weight loss and fevers, differential considerations include cancer, chronic infections such as tuberculosis and endocarditis, and endocrinologic diseases such as hyperthyroidism. When pulmonary processes dominate the presentation, acute and chronic lung infections must be considered as well as other causes of diffuse interstitial pulmonary infiltrates. When neurologic disease is the mode of presentation, conditions that cause mental status changes or neuropathy—eg, alcoholism, liver disease, renal dysfunction, thyroid disease, and vitamin deficiency—should be considered. If a patient presents with headache and a cerebrospinal fluid pleocytosis, other causes of chronic meningitis enter the differential. When diarrhea is a prominent complaint, infectious enterocolitis, antibiotic-associated colitis, inflammatory bowel disease, and malabsorptive symptoms must be considered.

Complications & Sequelae

The complications of HIV-related infections and neoplasms affect virtually every organ. The general approach to the HIV-infected person with symptoms is to evaluate the organ systems involved, aiming to diagnose treatable conditions rapidly.

A. Systemic Complaints: Fever, night sweats, and weight loss are common symptoms in HIV-infected patients and may occur without a complicating opportunistic infection. Patients with persistent fever and no localizing symptoms should nonetheless be carefully examined, and evaluated with a chest radiograph (*P carinii* pneumonia can present without respiratory symptoms), bacterial blood cultures if the fever is greater than 38.5 °C (101.3 °F), serum cryptococcal antigen, and mycobacterial cultures of the blood. Sinus radiographs or sinus CT scans should be considered to evaluate occult sinusitis. If these studies are normal, patients should be observed closely. Antipyretics are useful because HIV-infected patients have a propensity for high fevers and subsequent dehydration. Generally, nonsteroidal anti-inflammatory agents are more effective than aspirin or acetaminophen in the relief of fever.

Weight loss is a particularly distressing complication of long-standing HIV infection. The mechanism of HIV-related cachexia is not well understood. Frequent episodes of anorexia, nausea, vomiting, and diarrhea all contribute to weight loss among AIDS patients. Depression and adrenal insufficiency are two potentially treatable causes of weight loss.

For some patients with poor appetite, the progestational agent megestrol acetate (80 mg four times a day) can increase appetite and lead to subsequent weight gain. Side effects from megestrol acetate are rare. Thromboembolic phenomena, edema, nausea, vomiting, and rash have been reported.

Nausea leading to weight loss is sometimes due to esophageal candidiasis. Patients with oral candidiasis and nausea should be empirically treated with an oral antifungal agent (Table 30–3). Patients with weight loss due to nausea of unclear origin may benefit from use of antiemetics prior to meals (prochlorperazine, 10 mg three times daily, or metoclopramide, 10 mg three times daily). Effective fever control decreases the metabolic rate and may slow the pace of weight loss. Dronabinol (5 mg three times daily) can also be used to increase appetite.

Many patients will benefit from the use of high-caloric food supplementation. Selected patients with otherwise good functional status and weight loss due to unrelenting nausea, vomiting, or diarrhea may benefit from total parenteral nutrition.

B. Sinopulmonary Disease: The lungs are a frequently involved site of disease. *P carinii* pneumonia is the most common opportunistic infection, affecting 75% of patients. *P carinii* pneumonia may be difficult to diagnose because the symptoms—fever, cough, and shortness of breath—are nonspecific. Furthermore, the severity of symptoms ranges from fever and no respiratory symptoms through mild cough or dyspnea to frank respiratory distress.

The cornerstone of diagnosis is the chest radiograph. Diffuse or perihilar infiltrates are most characteristic, but only two-thirds of patients with *P carinii* pneumonia have this finding. Normal chest radiographs are seen in 5–10% of patients with *P carinii* pneumonia, while the remainder have atypical infiltrates. Apical infiltrates are commonly seen among patients with *P carinii* pneumonia who have been receiving aerosolized pentamidine prophylaxis, presumably because the drug is not well distributed in the upper zones. Isolated elevations of serum lactate dehydrogenase concentrations are consistent with a diagnosis of *P carinii* pneumonia, as well as lymphoma, disseminated histoplasmosis, and long-term treatment with zidovudine.

Definitive diagnosis can be obtained by Wright-Giemsa stain of induced sputum in 50–80% of cases at centers with experience performing this test. Sputum induction is performed by having patients inhale an aerosolized solution of 3% saline produced by an ultrasonic nebulizer. Patients should not eat for at least 8 hours (to avoid vomiting) and should not use toothpaste or mouthwash prior to the procedure to avoid substances that can interfere with test interpretation. A negative sputum induction does not, however, rule out the disease. Therefore, the next step for patients suspected of having *P carinii* pneumonia should be bronchoalveolar lavage. This technique establishes the diagnosis in over 95% of cases. The use of fluorescent antibodies for staining sputum samples may increase the sensitivity of sputum examination, decreasing the need for bronchoscopy.

In patients with symptoms suggestive of *P carinii* pneumonia but with negative or atypical chest radiographs and negative sputum examinations, other diagnostic tests may provide additional information in deciding whether to proceed to bronchoalveolar lavage. Patients with serum lactate dehydrogenase levels of 220 IU/L or less and erythrocyte sedimentation rates less than 50 mm/h are unlikely to have *P carinii* pneumonia and may be clinically followed. Patients with elevated levels of either test may require additional monitoring such as pulmonary function tests with carbon monoxide diffusing capacity, lung gallium scanning, and exercise oximetry. In addition, a CD4 count above 250 cells/μL within 2 months prior to evaluation of respiratory symptoms makes a diagnosis of *P carinii* pneumonia unlikely.

Pneumothoraces are common in HIV-infected patients with a history of *P carinii* pneumonia, especially if they have received aerosolized pentamidine treatment. Because patients may have a pneumothorax as their presenting symptom of *P carinii* pneumonia, such patients who have not had therapy for *P carinii* pneumonia in the preceding 3 months may need bronchoscopic evaluation. Pneumothoraces in HIV-infected individuals should be treated initially in the same fashion as in other patients. Unfortunately, they frequently recur with clamping or removal of the chest tube. Sclerosis with bleomycin or talc is the treatment of choice for recurrent pneumothoraces, but it is not uniformly successful even when multiple treatments are performed. If sclerosis fails, thoracoscopic stapling or thoracotomy may be required.

Other infectious causes of pulmonary disease in AIDS patients include bacterial, mycobacterial, and viral pneumonias. An increased incidence of pneumococcal pneumonia with septicemia and *Haemophilus influenzae* pneumonia has been reported. The incidence of infection with *Mycobacterium tuberculosis* has markedly increased in metropolitan areas because of HIV infection as well as homelessness. Tuberculosis occurs in an estimated 4% of persons who have AIDS. It is thought to result mainly from reactivation of prior infection; atypical infiltrates and disseminated disease occur more commonly than among immunocompetent hosts. Multidrug-resistant

Table 30–3. Treatment of AIDS-related opportunistic infections and malignancies.[1]

Infection	Treatment	Complications
P carinii infection[2]	Trimethoprim-sulfamethoxazole, 15 mg/kg/d (based on TMP component) orally or IV	Nausea, neutropenia, anemia, hepatitis, drug rash, Stevens-Johnson syndrome
	Pentamidine, 3–4 mg/kg/d for IV 14–21 days	Hypotension, hypoglycemia, anemia, neutropenia, pancreatitis, hepaitis
	Trimethoprim, 15 mg/kg/d orally, with dapsone, 100 mg/d orally, for 14–21 days	Nausea, rash, hemolytic anemia in G6PD-deficient patients. Methemoglobinemia (weekly levels should be < 10% of total hemoglobin).
	Primaquine, 15–30 mg/d orally, and clindamycin, 600 mg every 8 hours orally, for 14–21 days	Hemolytic anemia in G6PD-deficient patients. Methemoglobinemia, neutropenia, colitis.
	Atovaquone,[3] 750 mg orally 3 times daily	Rash, elevated aminotransferases, anemia, neutropenia.
	Aerosolized pentamidine	Bronchospasm
	Trimetrexate,[3] 45 mg/m^2 IV for 21 days (given with leucovorin calcium)	Leukopenia, rash, mucositis

M avium-intracellulare infection	Clarithromycin, 750–1000 mg orally twice daily,[3] plus at least 2 of the following:
	  Clofazimine, 100 mg orally daily, plus–
	  Ethambutol, 15 mg/kg/d orally (maximum, 1 g)
	  Rifampin, 10 mg/kg/d orally (maximum, 600 mg daily)
	  Ciprofloxacin, 750 mg orally twice daily
	  Amikacin, 7.5 mg/kg every 12–24 hours IV for 2–4 weeks (consider in addition to above treatments)
		Hepatitis, nausea, diarrhea
		
		Abdominal pain, discoloration of skin
		Hepatitis, optic neuritis
		
		Rash, hepatitis
		
		Anaphylaxis, nausea, rash
		Nephrotoxicity, ototoxicity

Toxoplasmosis	Pyrimethamine, 100–200 mg orally as loading dose, followed by 50–75 mg/d, combined with sulfadiazine, 4–6 g orally daily in 4 divided doses, and folinic acid, 10 mg daily for 4–8 weeks; then pyrimethamine, 25–50 mg/d, with sulfadiazine, 2 g/d, and folinic acid, 5 mg/d	Leukopenia, rash
	Pyrimethamine, 100–200 mg orally as loading dose, followed by 50–75 mg/d, combined with clindamycin, 600 mg orally every 6 hours for 4–8 weeks, and folinic acid, 10 mg orally daily; then pyrimethamine, 25–50 mg/d, with clindamycin, 300–600 mg, every 6 hours, and folinic acid, 5 mg daily	Abdominal pain, nausea, rash
Lymphoma	Combination chemotherapy (eg, modified CHOP, M-BACOD,[4] with or without G-CSF or GM-CSF).[5] Central nervous system disease: radiation treatment with dexamethasone for edema.	Nausea, vomiting, anemia, leukopenia, cardiotoxicity (with doxorubicin)
Cryptococcal meningitis	Amphotericin B, 0.6 mg/kg/d IV, to a total dose of about 1.5 g.	Fever, anemia, hypokalemia, and azotemia
	Fluconazole, 400 mg orally daily for 6 weeks, then 200 mg orally daily	Hepatitis
Cytomegalovirus infection	Ganciclovir, 10 mg/kg/d IV in 2 divided doses for 10 days, followed by 6 mg/kg 5 days a week indefinitely. (Decrease dose for renal impairment.)	Neutropenia
	Foscarnet, 60 mg/kg IV 3 times daily for 10–14 days(induction), followed by 90 mg/kg once daily. (Adjust for changes in renal function.)	Nausea, hypokalemia, hypocalcemia, hyperphosphatemia
Esophageal candidiasis or recurrent vaginal candidiasis	Ketoconazole, 200 mg orally twice daily for 2–4 weeks	Hepatitis, adrenal insufficiency; ventricular tachycardia when given with terfenadine or astemizole
	Fluconazole, 100–200 mg daily for 2–4 weeks	Hepatitis, development of imidazole resistance

(continued)

Table 30–3. Treatment of AIDS-related opportunistic infections and malignancies. (continued)

Infection	Treatment	Complications
Herpes simplex infection	Acyclovir, 200 mg 5 times daily for 7–10 days; or acyclovir, 5 mg/kg IV every 8 hours for severe cases.	Resistant herpes simplex with chronic therapy
	Foscarnet, 40 mg/kg IV every 8 hours, for acyclovir-resistant cases. (Adjust for changes in renal function.)	See above.
Herpes zoster	Acyclovir, 800 mg orally 4–5 times daily for 7–10 days. Intravenous therapy at 10 mg/kg every 8 hours for ocular involvement, disseminated disease.	See above.
	Foscarnet, 40 mg/kg IV every 8 hours for acyclovir-resistant cases. (Adjust for changes in renal function.)	See above.
Kaposi's sarcoma Limited cutaneous disease	Observation, intralesional vinblastine	Inflammation, pain at site of injection
Extensive or aggressive cutaneous disease	Systemic chemotherapy (eg, alternating weekly vinca alkaloids). Alpha interferon (for patients with CD4 > 200 cells/μL and no constitutional symptoms). Radiation (amelioration of edema).	Bone marrow suppression, peripheral neuritis, flu-like syndrome
Visceral disease (eg, pulmonary)	Combination chemotherapy (eg, daunorubicin, bleomycin, vinblastine)	Bone marrow suppression, cardiac toxicity, fever

[1]For treatment of *Mycobacterium tuberculosis* infection, see Chapter 9.
[2]For moderate to severe *P carinii* infection (oxygen saturation < 90%), corticosteroids should be given with specific treatment. Dosage recommendations in text.
[3]Experimental drugs or unapproved indications.
[4]CHOP = cyclophosphamide, doxorubicin, vincristine, and prednisone. Modified M-BACOD = methotrexate, bleomycin, doxorubicin, cyclophosphamide, vincristine, and dexamethasone.
[5]G-CSF = granulocyte colony stimulating factor; GM-CSF = granulocyte macrophage colony stimulating factor.

tuberculosis has emerged as a major problem in several metropolitan areas. Noncompliance with prescribed antituberculous drugs is a major risk factor. Several of the reported outbreaks appear to implicate nosocomial spread. Affected individuals have generally not defervesced or shown improvement within several weeks of starting aggressive antituberculous therapy. The most effective therapy has not been defined, and the mortality rate is greater than 50%. Atypical mycobacteria can cause pulmonary disease in AIDS patients with or without preexisting lung disease and responds variably to treatment. Isolation of cytomegalovirus from bronchoalveolar lavage fluid occurs commonly in AIDS patients but does not establish a definitive diagnosis. Diagnosis of cytomegalovirus pneumonia requires biopsy; response to treatment is poor.

Noninfectious causes of lung disease include Kaposi's sarcoma, non-Hodgkin's lymphoma, and interstitial pneumonitis. In patients with known Kaposi's sarcoma, pulmonary involvement complicates the course in approximately one-third of cases. Non-Hodgkin's lymphoma may involve the lung as the sole site of disease but more commonly involves other organs as well, especially the brain, liver, and gastrointestinal tract. Both of these processes may show nodular or diffuse parenchymal involvement, pleural effusions, and mediastinal adenopathy on chest radiographs.

Nonspecific interstitial pneumonitis may mimic *P carinii* pneumonia. Typically, these patients present with several months of mild cough and dyspnea; chest radiographs show interstitial infiltrates. Many patients with this entity undergo transbronchial biopsies in an attempt to diagnose *P carinii* pneumonia. Instead, the tissue shows interstitial inflammation ranging from an intense lymphocytic infiltration (consistent with lymphoid interstitial pneumonitis) to a mild mononuclear inflammation. Corticosteroids may be helpful in some cases.

Chronic sinusitis can be a frustrating problem for HIV-infected patients. Symptoms include sinus congestion and discharge, headache, and fever. Some patients may have radiographic evidence on sinus x-ray or sinus CT scan of sinus disease in the absence of significant symptoms. Patients with purulent discharge should be treated with amoxicillin (for smokers) or amoxicillin-potassium clavulanate (for nonsmokers), 250 mg orally three times a day in either case. Guaifenesin, 600 mg orally twice daily, may be helpful in relieving sinus congestion. Some patients may require referral to an otolaryngologist for sinus drainage.

C. Central Nervous System Disease: Central nervous system disease in HIV-infected patients can be divided into intracerebral space-occupying lesions, encephalopathy, meningitis, and spinal cord processes.

Toxoplasmosis is the most common space-occupying lesion in HIV-infected patients. Patients may present with headache, focal neurologic deficits, seizures, or altered mental status. The diagnosis is usually made presumptively based on the characteristic appearance of cerebral imaging studies. Typically, toxoplasmosis appears as multiple lesions, contrast-enhancing on CT scan, with a predilection for the basal ganglia.

Single lesions are atypical of toxoplasmosis. When a single lesion has been detected by CT scanning, MRI scanning—because of its greater sensitivity—may reveal multiple lesions. If a patient has a single lesion on MRI and is neurologically stable, clinicians may either pursue an immediate tissue diagnosis or a 2-week empiric trial of toxoplasmosis therapy. A repeat scan should be performed at 2 weeks. If the lesion has not diminished in size, biopsy of the lesion should be performed. Since many HIV-infected patients will have detectable titers, a positive *Toxoplasma* serologic test does not confirm the diagnosis. Conversely, as many as 15% of patients with toxoplasmosis have negative titers by enzyme immunoassay or immunofluorescence assays.

Non-Hodgkin's lymphoma is the second most common space-occupying lesion in HIV-infected patients. Symptoms are similar to those with toxoplasmosis. While imaging techniques cannot distinguish these two diseases with certainty, lymphoma more often is solitary. Other less common lesions should be suspected if there is preceding bacteremia, positive tuberculin test, fungemia, or intravenous drug use. These include bacterial abscesses, cryptococcomas, tuberculomas, and *Nocardia* lesions.

Because techniques for stereotactic brain biopsy have improved, this procedure plays an increasing role in diagnosing cerebral lesions. Biopsy should be strongly considered if lesions are solitary or do not respond to toxoplasmosis treatment, especially if they are easily accessible. Diagnosis of lymphoma is important because patients who have not had a prior opportunistic infection are likely to benefit from treatment (radiation therapy).

AIDS dementia complex (HIV-associated cognitive/motor complex) is the most common cause of mental status changes in HIV-infected patients. The diagnosis is one of exclusion based on a brain imaging study and spinal fluid analysis which exclude other pathogens. Neuropsychiatric testing is helpful in distinguishing patients with dementia from those with depression. Patients with AIDS dementia complex typically have difficulty with cognitive tasks and exhibit diminished motor speed. Patients may first notice a deterioration in their handwriting. The manifestations of dementia may wax and wane, with persons exhibiting periods of lucidity and confusion over the course of a day. Although the mechanism by which HIV causes neurologic dysfunction is not completely understood, many patients improve with zidovudine. The calcium channel blocker nimodipine is also being studied as a potential therapeutic intervention. Metabolic abnormalities may also cause changes in mental status: hypoglycemia, hyponatremia, hypoxia, and drug overdose are important considerations in this population. Other less common infectious causes of encephalopathy include progressive multifocal leukoencephalopathy, cytomegalovirus, syphilis, and herpes simplex encephalitis.

Cryptococcal meningitis typically presents with fever and headache. Less than 20% of patients have meningismus. Diagnosis is based on a positive latex agglutination test or positive culture of spinal fluid for *Cryptococcus*. Seventy to ninety percent of patients with cryptococcal meningitis have a positive serum agglutination test for *Cryptococcus* (CRAG). Thus, a negative serum CRAG test makes a diagnosis of cryptococcal meningitis unlikely and can be useful in the initial evaluation of a patient with headache, fever, and normal mental status. HIV meningitis, characterized by lymphocytic pleocytosis of the spinal fluid with negative culture, is common early in HIV infection and may mimic cryptococcal meningitis in its clinical presentation.

Spinal cord function may also be impaired in HIV-infected individuals. HIV myelopathy presents with leg weakness and incontinence. Spastic paraparesis and sensory ataxia are seen on neurologic examination. Myelopathy is usually a late manifestation of HIV disease, and most patients will have concomitant HIV encephalopathy. Pathologic evaluation of the spinal cord reveals vacuolation of white matter. Because HIV myelopathy is a diagnosis of exclusion, symptoms suggestive of myelopathy should be evaluated by lumbar puncture to rule out cytomegalovirus polyradiculopathy (described below) and an MRI or CT scan to exclude epidural lymphoma.

D. Peripheral Nervous System: Peripheral nervous system syndromes include inflammatory polyneuropathies, sensory neuropathies, and mononeuropathies.

An inflammatory demyelinating polyneuropathy similar to Guillain-Barré syndrome occurs in HIV-infected patients, usually prior to frank immunodeficiency. The syndrome in many cases improves with plasmapheresis, supporting an autoimmune basis of the disease. Cytomegalovirus can cause an ascending polyradiculopathy characterized by lower extremity weakness and a neutrophilic pleocytosis on spinal fluid analysis with a negative bacterial culture. Transverse myelitis can be seen with herpes zoster or cytomegalovirus.

About 30% of patients with advanced HIV disease develop sensory neuropathies. Affected patients typically complain of numbness, tingling, and pain in their lower extremities. Symptoms are disproportionate to findings on gross sensory and motor evaluation. In contrast to inflammatory demyelinating polyneuropathy, sensory neuropathies occur late in

HIV-disease progression and are due to axonal loss. Evaluation should rule out other causes of sensory neuropathy such as alcoholism, thyroid disease, vitamin B_{12} deficiency, and syphilis. Severe sensory neuropathy is a contraindication to initiation of three newer antiretroviral drugs, the dideoxynucleosides didanosine zalcitabine, and d4T. Occasionally, sensory neuropathies improve with zidovudine therapy, but more commonly treatment is symptomatic with amitriptyline.

E. Rheumatologic Manifestations: Arthritis, involving single or multiple joints, with or without effusion, has been commonly noted in HIV-infected patients. While the cause of HIV-related arthritis is unknown, most patients will respond to nonsteroidal anti-inflammatory agents. Patients with a sizable effusion, especially if the joint is warm or erythematous, should have the joint tapped, followed by culture of the fluid to rule out suppurative arthritis as well as fungal and mycobacterial disease.

Several rheumatologic syndromes, including Reiter's syndrome, psoriatic arthritis, sicca syndrome, and systemic lupus erythematosus, have been reported in HIV-infected patients (Chapter 17). However, it is unclear if the prevalence is greater than in the general population.

F. Myopathy: Myopathies are increasingly noted in HIV-infected patients. Proximal muscle weakness is typical, and patients may have varying degrees of muscle tenderness. The most important clinical distinction is between myopathy due to the primary effect of HIV and that due to zidovudine. Patients with symptomatic myopathy, especially with creatine kinase levels greater than 1000 IU/L, should have their dose of zidovudine decreased or stopped and be considered for alternative antiviral therapy (didanosine or zalcitabine). A muscle biopsy can distinguish HIV myopathy from zidovudine myopathy and should be considered in patients for whom continuation of zidovudine is essential.

G. Retinitis: Complaints of visual changes must be evaluated immediately in HIV-infected patients. Cytomegalovirus retinitis is the most common retinal infection in AIDS patients and can be rapidly progressive. In contrast, cotton wool spots, which are also common in HIV-infected people, are benign, remit spontaneously, and appear as small indistinct white spots without exudation or hemorrhage. This distinction may be difficult at times for the nonspecialist, and patients with visual changes should be seen by an ophthalmologist. Other rare retinal processes include other herpesvirus infections or toxoplasmosis.

H. Oral Lesions: The findings of oral candidiasis and hairy leukoplakia are significant for several reasons. First, these lesions are almost pathognomonic for HIV infection. Second, several studies have indicated that patients with these lesions have a high rate of progression to AIDS, though it is not known whether this increased risk is independent of other parameters of immune function, such as the CD4 count.

Hairy leukoplakia is caused by the Epstein-Barr virus. The lesion is not usually troubling to patients and sometimes regresses spontaneously. Patients who are bothered by hairy leukoplakia can be treated with acyclovir, 800 mg orally four times a day. Oral candidiasis can be bothersome to patients, many of whom report an unpleasant taste or mouth dryness. There are two types of oral candidiasis: pseudomembranous (removable white plaques) and erythematous (red friable plaques). Treatment is with topical agents such as clotrimazole troches (one four or five times a day). Patients with candidiasis that does not respond to topical antifungals can be treated with oral ketoconazole (200 mg once a day). Ketoconazole is better absorbed from the gastrointestinal tract when taken with cranberry or other acidic fruit juice. Patients taking ketoconazole should avoid taking terfenadine or astemizole because of the possibility of malignant ventricular arrhythmias. Candidiasis that does not improve with ketoconazole therapy can be treated with fluconazole (50–100 mg orally once a day). Chronic suppression of oral candidiasis with fluconazole has been associated with development of candidiasis resistant to all available azoles (including ketoconazole). Chronic suppression with this agent should be avoided except in frequently recurring cases.

Angular cheilitis—fissures at the sides of the mouth—is usually due to *Candida* as well and can be treated topically with ketoconazole cream (2%) twice a day.

Gingival disease is common in HIV-infected patients and is thought to be due to an overgrowth of microorganisms. It usually responds to professional dental cleaning and chlorhexidine rinses. Some HIV-infected patients will develop a particularly aggressive gingivitis or periodontitis; these patients should be started on antibiotics that cover anaerobic oral flora (eg, metronidazole, 250 mg four times a day for 4 or 5 days) and referred to oral surgeons with experience with these entities.

Aphthous ulcers are painful and may interfere with eating. They can be treated with fluocinonide (0.05% ointment mixed 1:1 with plain Orabase and applied six times a day to the ulcer). For lesions that are difficult to reach, patients should use dexamethasone swishes (0.5 mg in 5 mL elixir three times a day). The pain of the ulcers can be relieved with use of an anesthetic spray (10% lidocaine). Other lesions seen in the mouths of HIV-infected patients include Kaposi's sarcoma (usually on the hard palate), and warts.

I. Gastrointestinal Manifestations: Esophageal candidiasis is a common AIDS infection. Typically, patients complain of substernal pain or burning, worse with swallowing. Nausea may also occur. In a patient with these characteristic symptoms and oral candidiasis, empiric antifungal treatment is begun. Patients who can take oral medications should be started on ketoconazole (200 mg twice a day). Patients who do not improve with ketoconazole may be given fluconazole (200 mg daily). Further evaluation to identify other causes of esophagitis (herpes simplex, cytomegalovirus) is reserved for patients who do not improve with treatment or those without visible oral candidiasis.

Autopsy studies have demonstrated that the liver is a frequent site of infections and neoplasms in HIV-infected patients. However, many of these infections are not clinically symptomatic. Clinicians may note elevations of alkaline phosphatase and aminotransferases on routine chemistry panels. Mycobacterial disease, cytomegalovirus, hepatitis B virus, and lymphoma cause liver disease and can present with varying degrees of nausea, vomiting, and right upper quadrant abdominal pain. Sulfonamide drugs and ketoconazole have also been associated with hepatitis. HIV-infected patients with chronic active hepatitis tend to have less severe bouts of hepatitis because of the concomitant immunodeficiency. Percutaneous liver biopsy may be helpful in diagnosing liver disease, but frequently the cause can be determined by other tests (eg, blood culture, biopsy of a more accessible site). Moreover, because the majority of hepatic infections do not respond well to treatment (eg, *M avium* complex), liver biopsy should be reserved for people with persistent symptoms and laboratory abnormalities in whom no other cause for illness can be determined.

Biliary disease is common in AIDS patients. Cholecystitis presents with similar manifestations as seen in immunocompetent hosts but is more likely to be acalculous. Sclerosing cholangitis and papillary stenosis have also been increasingly reported in HIV-infected patients. Typically, the syndrome presents with severe nausea, vomiting, and right upper quadrant pain. Liver function tests generally show alkaline phosphatase elevations disproportionate to elevation of the aminotransferases. Although dilated ducts can be seen on ultrasound, the diagnosis is made by endoscopic retrograde cholangiopancreatography, which reveals intraluminal irregularities of the proximal intrahepatic ducts with "pruning" of the terminal ductal branches. Stenosis of the distal common bile duct at the papilla is commonly seen with this syndrome. Cytomegalovirus and *Cryptosporidium* are thought to play inciting roles in this syndrome. Initial reports of symptomatic improvement with performance of sphincterotomies were encouraging, but enthusiasm for the procedure has waned because many patients had recurrence of symptoms.

Enterocolitis is a common problem in HIV-infected individuals. Organisms known to cause enterocolitis include bacteria *(Campylobacter, Salmonella, Shigella)*, viruses (cytomegalovirus, adeno-virus), and protozoans *(Cryptosporidium, E histolytica, Giardia)*. HIV itself may cause enterocolitis. Several of the organisms causing enterocolitis in HIV-infected individuals also cause diarrhea in immunocompetent hosts. However, HIV-infected patients tend to have more severe symptoms, including high fevers and severe abdominal pain that can mimic acute abdominal catastrophes. Bacteremia and concomitant biliary involvement are also more common with enterocolitis in HIV-infected patients. Relapses of enterocolitis following adequate therapy have been reported with both *Salmonella* and *Shigella* infections.

Because of the wide range of agents known to cause enterocolitis, a stool culture and multiple stool examinations for ova and parasites (including modified acid-fast staining for *Cryptosporidium*) should be performed. Those patients who have *Cryptosporidium* on one stool with improvement in symptoms in less than 1 month should not be considered to have AIDS, as *Cryptosporidium* is a cause of self-limited diarrhea in HIV-negative hosts. More commonly, HIV-infected patients with *Cryptosporidium* have persistent enterocolitis with profuse watery diarrhea.

To date, no consistently effective treatments have been developed for *Cryptosporidium* infection. There are anecdotal reports of good responses to paromomycin, 25 mg/kg/d orally. Immune bovine colostrum is being evaluated as oral therapy. Patients should be given diphenoxylate with atropine (one or two tablets orally three or four times a day). Those who do not respond may be given paregoric with bismuth (5–10 mL orally three or four times a day). Subcutaneous octreotide has been found to ameliorate symptoms in approximately 40% of patients with cryptosporidial or idiopathic HIV-associated diarrhea. This agent is used in escalating doses (starting at 0.05 mg subcutaneously every 8 hours for 48 hours).

Patients with a negative stool examination and persistent symptoms should be evaluated with colonoscopy and biopsy. Patients whose symptoms last longer than 1 month with no identified cause of diarrhea are considered to have a presumptive diagnosis of AIDS enteropathy. A primary effect of the HIV virus on the colonic epithelium may be the cause. Upper endoscopy with small bowel biopsy is not recommended as a routine part of the evaluation. Many patients who undergo upper endoscopy have nonspecific abnormalities, but these rarely reflect treatable diseases.

Two other important gastrointestinal abnormalities in HIV-infected patients are gastropathy and malabsorption. It has been documented that some HIV-infected patients do not produce normal levels of stomach acid and therefore are unable to absorb drugs such as ketoconazole that require an acid medium. This decreased acid production may explain, in part, the susceptibility of HIV-infected patients to

Campylobacter, Salmonella, and *Shigella,* all of which are sensitive to acid concentration.

A malabsorption syndrome occurs commonly in HIV-infected patients. It can be due to infection of the small bowel with *M avium* complex or *Cryptosporidium.* In other cases, biopsy of the small bowel reveals no pathogens but histologic changes consistent with Whipple's disease.

J. Endocrine: The adrenal gland is the most commonly afflicted endocrine gland in patients with AIDS. Abnormalities demonstrated on autopsy include infection (especially with cytomegalovirus and *M avium-intracellulare*), infiltration with Kaposi's sarcoma, and injury from hemorrhage and presumed autoimmunity. The prevalence of clinically significant adrenal insufficiency is unknown. Patients with suggestive symptoms should undergo a cosyntropin stimulation test. Those who do not achieve a cortisol level of 20 µg/dL (552 nmol/L) with cosyntropin administration should undergo a 3-day ACTH stimulation test.

While frank deficiency of cortisol is rare, an isolated defect in mineralocorticoid metabolism may lead to salt wasting and hyperkalemia. Such patients should be treated with fludrocortisone (0.1–0.2 mg daily).

AIDS patients appear to have abnormalities of thyroid function different from patients with other chronic diseases. AIDS patients have been shown to have high levels of triiodothyroninine (T_3), thyroxine (T_4), and thyroid-binding globulin and low levels of reverse triiodothyronine (rT_3). The causes and clinical significance of these abnormalities are unknown.

K. Skin: HIV-infected patients commonly develop skin manifestations that can be grouped into viral, bacterial, fungal, neoplastic, and nonspecific dermatitides.

Herpes simplex infections occur more frequently, tend to be more severe, and are more likely to disseminate in AIDS patients than in immunocompetent hosts. Because of the risk of progressive local disease, all herpes simplex attacks should be treated with acyclovir, 200 mg orally five times a day. To avoid the complications of attacks, many clinicians recommend chronic acyclovir administration (400 mg orally twice a day) for HIV-infected patients with a history of recurrent herpes. However, the finding of acyclovir resistance among some herpes strains cultured from HIV-infected patients raises concern about this practice.

Herpes zoster is a common manifestation of HIV-infection. As with herpes simplex infections, patients with zoster should be treated with acyclovir to prevent dissemination (800 mg orally four or five times per day). Vesicular lesions should be cultured if there is any question about their origin, since herpes simplex responds to much lower doses of acyclovir. Disseminated zoster and cases with ocular involvement

should be treated with intravenous (10 mg/kg every 8 hours) rather than oral acyclovir.

Molluscum contagiosum is seen in HIV-infected patients, as in other immunocompromised patients. Lesions have a propensity for spreading widely over the patient's skin and should be treated with topical liquid nitrogen.

Staphylococcus is the most common bacterial cause of skin disease in HIV-infected patients; it usually presents as folliculitis, superficial abscesses (furuncles), or bullous impetigo. Because dissemination with sepsis has been reported, attempts should be made to treat these lesions aggressively. Folliculitis is initially treated with topical clindamycin, and patients may benefit from regular washing with an antibacterial soap such as chlorhexidine (Hibiclens). Intranasal mupirocin has been used successfully for staphylococcal decolonization in other settings. In HIV-infected patients with recurrent staphylococcal infections, weekly intranasal mupirocin should be considered in addition to topical care and systemic antibiotics. Abscesses often require incision and drainage. Patients may need antistaphylococcal antibiotics such as dicloxacillin, 250–500 mg orally four times daily, or erythromycin, 250 mg orally four times daily, for severe folliculitis.

Bacillary angiomatosis is a newly recognized entity in HIV-infected patients. It is caused by a recently identified organism (*Rochalimaea henselae*), which is related to the organism of cat scratch disease (*Afipia felis*). The epidemiology suggests zoonotic transmission. The most common manifestation is raised, reddish, highly vascular skin lesions that can mimic the lesions of Kaposi's sarcoma. Fever is a common manifestation of this infection; involvement of bone, lymph nodes, and liver has also been reported. Responses to ciprofloxacin, 500 mg orally twice daily, and erythromycin, 250 mg orally four times daily, have been reported.

The majority of fungal rashes afflicting AIDS patients are due to dermatophytes and *Candida.* These are particularly common in the inguinal region but may occur anywhere on the body. Fungal rashes generally respond well to topical clotrimazole (1% twice a day) or ketoconazole (2% twice a day).

Kaposi's sarcoma lesions are red or purple, flat or raised papules that generally do not blanch. Cutaneous lesions can be treated with radiation or with intralesional injection of vinblastine, 0.01–0.02 mg in 0.1 mL of saline. Other dermatologic malignancies seen disproportionately among HIV-infected persons include basal cell and squamous cell carcinomas.

Seborrheic dermatitis is more common in HIV-infected patients. Scrapings of seborrhea have revealed *Pityrosporum ovale,* implying that the seborrhea is caused by this fungus. Consistent with the isolation of this fungus is the clinical finding that seborrhea responds well to topical clotrimazole (1% cream) as well as hydrocortisone (1% cream).

Xerosis presents in HIV-infected patients with severe pruritus. The patient may have no rash, or nonspecific excoriations from scratching. Treatment is with emollients (eg, absorption base cream) and antipruritic lotions (eg, camphor 9.5% and menthol 0.5%).

Psoriasis can be very severe in HIV-infected patients. Phototherapy and etretinate (0.25–9.75 mg/kg/d orally in divided doses) may be used for recalcitrant cases in consultation with a dermatologist. Because of the underlying immunodeficiency, methotrexate should be avoided.

L. HIV-related Malignancies: Four cancers are currently included in the CDC classification of AIDS: Kaposi's sarcoma, non-Hodgkin's lymphoma, primary lymphoma of the brain, and invasive cervical carcinoma. Epidemiologic studies have shown that between 1973 and 1987 among single men in San Francisco, the risk of Kaposi's sarcoma increased more than 5000-fold and the risk of non-Hodgkin's lymphoma more than tenfold. The increase in incidence of malignancies is probably a function of impaired cell-mediated immunity. As the epidemic progresses, other cancers may be noted to be occurring with increased frequency also. For example, there is evidence of an increased incidence of Hodgkin's disease in HIV-infected men.

Kaposi's sarcoma is still the most common HIV-related malignancy. About 40% of patients with dermatologic Kaposi's sarcoma will develop visceral disease (eg, gastrointestinal, pulmonary). Rapidly progressive dermatologic or visceral disease is best treated with systemic chemotherapy. Commonly used regimens include alternating weekly vincristine and vinblastine or combination doxorubicin, bleomycin, and vincristine. Alpha interferon has activity against Kaposi's sarcoma and may result in remission of lesions in minimally symptomatic patients with high CD4 counts and no history of opportunistic infection. However, even in this subgroup, subjective symptoms (eg, malaise, anorexia) limit the utility of this therapy. Bulky lesions of the lower extremities accompanied by lymphedema are a common presentation of Kaposi's sarcoma. Radiation and conservative measures (eg, leg elevation, elastic stockings) may be helpful.

Non-Hodgkin's lymphoma in HIV-infected persons tends to be very aggressive. The malignancies are usually of B cell origin and characterized as diffuse large-cell tumors. Over 90% of the malignancies are extranodal, with the central nervous system being a common site.

Patients with central nervous system disease are treated with radiation therapy. Systemic disease is treated with chemotherapy. Common regimens are CHOP (cyclophosphamide, doxorubicin, vincristine, and prednisone) and modified M-BACOD (methotrexate, bleomycin, doxorubicin, cyclophosphamide, vincristine, and dexamethasone). Granulo-

cyte colony-stimulating factor (G-CSF; filgrastim) is used to maintain white blood counts with this latter regimen.

Although Hodgkin's disease is not included as part of the CDC definition of AIDS, studies have found that HIV-infection is associated with a fivefold increase in the incidence of Hodgkin's disease. HIV-infected persons with Hodgkin's disease are more likely to have mixed cellularity and lymphocyte depletion subtypes of Hodgkin's disease and to present at an advanced stage of disease.

Anal dysplasia and squamous cell carcinoma have been noted in HIV-infected homosexual men. These lesions have been strongly correlated with previous infection by human papillomavirus (HPV). While many of the infected men report a history of anal warts or have visible warts, a significant percentage have silent papillomavirus infection. Cytologic (using Papanicolaou smears) and papillomavirus DNA studies can easily be performed on specimens obtained by anal swab. Although many questions remain unanswered, the growing frequency of these problems and the risk of progression from dysplasia to cancer in immunocompromised patients suggest that annual anal swabs for cytologic examination should be done in all HIV-infected persons who have engaged in anal intercourse.

HPV also appears to play a causative role in cervical dysplasia and neoplasia. The incidence and clinical course of cervical disease in HIV-infected women are discussed below.

M. Gynecologic Manifestations: Vaginal candidiasis, cervical dysplasia and neoplasia, and pelvic inflammatory disease are more common in HIV-infected women than in uninfected women. These manifestations also tend to be more severe when they occur in association with HIV infection. Therefore, HIV-infected women need frequent gynecologic care. Vaginal candidiasis may be treated with topical agents (see Chapter 36). However, HIV-infected women with recurrent or severe vaginal candidiasis may need systemic therapy (Table 30–3).

The incidence of cervical dysplasia in HIV-infected women is 40%. Because of this finding, HIV-infected women should have Papanicolaou smears every 6 months. Some clinicians recommend routine colposcopy or cervicography because cervical intraepithelial neoplasia has occurred in women with negative Papanicolaou smears. Cone biopsy is indicated in cases of serious cervical dysplasia.

Cervical neoplasia appears to be more aggressive among HIV-infected women. Most HIV-infected women with cervical cancer die of that disease rather than of AIDS. Because of its frequency and severity, cervical neoplasia was added to the CDC definition of AIDS in 1993.

While pelvic inflammatory disease appears to be more common in HIV-infected women, the bacteriology of this condition appears to be the same as among

HIV-uninfected women. At present, HIV-infected women with pelvic inflammatory disease should be treated the same regimens as uninfected women (see Chapter 17). However, inpatient therapy is generally recommended.

Treatment

Treatment for HIV infection can be divided into four categories: therapy for opportunistic infections and malignancies, antiretroviral treatment, hematopoietic stimulating factors, and prophylaxis of opportunistic infections.

Experimental treatment regimens for HIV infection are constantly changing. Clinicians may obtain up-to-date information on experimental treatments by calling the AIDS Clinical Trials Information Service (ACTIS), 1-800-TRIALS-A (English and Spanish); the National AIDS Hot Line, 1-800-342-AIDS (English), and 1-800-344-SIDA (Spanish), and 1-800-AIDS-TTY (hearing impaired).

A. Therapy for Opportunistic Infections and Malignancies:

Treatment of common HIV infections and malignancies is detailed in Table 30–3. In general, AIDS patients require protracted therapy, including lifelong therapy for toxoplasmosis, cryptococcosis, and cytomegalovirus retinitis. The emergence of resistance is more common for some infections of HIV-infected people (eg, acyclovir-resistant herpes simplex) than among immunocompetent individuals. In addition, HIV-infected patients have an increased incidence of side effects to standard drugs such as trimethoprim-sulfamethoxazole.

Treating patients with repeated episodes of the same opportunistic infection can pose difficult therapeutic challenges. For example, patients with second or third episodes of *P carinii* pneumonia may have developed allergic reactions to standard treatments with a prior episode. Fortunately, there are several alternatives available for the treatment of *P carinii* infection. Trimethoprim with dapsone—and prima-

quine and clindamycin—are two combinations that often are tolerated in patients with a prior allergic reaction to trimethoprim-sulfamethoxazole and intravenous pentamidine. On the positive side, patients who develop second episodes of *P carinii* pneumonia while taking prophylaxis tend to have milder courses.

Well-established alternative regimens now also exist for most AIDS-related opportunistic infections: amphotericin B or fluconazole for cryptococcal meningitis; ganciclovir or foscarnet for cytomegalovirus infection; and sulfadiazine or clindamycin with pyrimethamine for toxoplasmosis.

Although conceptually it would seem that corticosteroid therapy should be avoided in HIV-infected patients, steroid use has been shown to improve the course of patients with moderate to severe pneumocystosis (oxygen saturation < 90%) when administered within 72 hours after diagnosis. The dose of prednisone is 40 mg twice daily for 5 days, then 40 mg daily for 5 days, and then 20 mg daily until therapy is complete. The mechanism of action is presumed to be a decrease in alveolar inflammation.

B. Antiretroviral Treatment:
The development of drugs that suppress the HIV infection itself rather than its complications has been an important development (Table 30–4). Zidovudine (azidothymidine; AZT) was the first approved antiviral drug for HIV infection. It has been proved to decrease symptoms and prolong the life of patients with AIDS or severe symptomatic disease. Zidovudine has also been shown to slow the progression to severe disease among patients with mild symptoms as well as asymptomatic patients with CD4 counts below 500 cells/µL. Results from a Veterans Administration cooperative trial confirmed delay of disease progression in persons who started zidovudine with a CD4 count of 200–500 cells/µL. However, this study showed no ultimate survival benefit. The study was done before the availability of other retroviral agents, and its conclusions must be interpreted cautiously.

Subgroup analysis of this Veterans Administration

Table 30–4. Antiretroviral therapy.

Drug	Indication	Dose	Common Side Effects	Monitoring
Zidovudine (AZT)	CD4 ≤500 cells/µL	500–600 mg orally daily in 3 divided doses	Anemia, neutropenia, nausea, malaise, headache, insomnia	Complete blood count and differential (every 3 months once stable)
Didanosine (ddI)	CD4 ≤500 cells/µL and intolerant to AZT or with progression of disease on AZT	125–300 mg orally twice a day (for pill formulation)	Peripheral neuropathy, pancreatitis, dry mouth, hepatitis	CBC and differential, aminotransferases, K+, amylase, triglycerides, monthly neurologic examination
Dideoxycytidine (ddC)		0.375–0.75 mg orally 3 times a day	Peripheral neuropathy, aphthous ulcers, hepatitis	Monthly neurologic examination, aminotransferases
Stavudine (d4T) (experimental)	CD4 ≤300 cells/µL and intolerant to ddI, ddC, and AZT	Per protocol	Peripheral neuropathy, hepatitis, ?pancreatitis	Monthly neurologic examination, aminotransferases, amylase

cooperative trial initially suggested that zidovudine was less effective in blacks and Latinos. More recent reviews of this issue, however, have not verified any significant difference in response rates to zidovudine.

While the dosing of zidovudine had been controversial, a total daily dose of 500 mg for an individual of average weight (50–74 kg) is now standard based upon studies in both early and late disease. While some antiviral effect is preserved at a total daily dose of 300 mg, a recent study has suggested that this is a suboptimal dose. Conversely, the only setting in which a higher dose might be considered would be in the patient who develops dementia despite receiving the standard dose. One study suggested dose-related amelioration of neurologic symptoms.

Although all of the major trials of zidovudine have used every 4 hour dosing, clinicians are increasingly using three times a day dosing to improve patient compliance. The rationale for less frequent dosing is the long half-life of zidovudine once phosphorylated inside of infected cells (in contrast to the short half-life of zidovudine in the serum). The cost of zidovudine (at a dose of 500 mg/d) is approximately $200 a month.

Side effects seen with zidovudine are listed in Table 30–4. Approximately 40% of patients will experience subjective side effects that generally remit within 6 weeks. The common dose-limiting side effects of zidovudine are anemia and neutropenia. Although the anemia is usually macrocytic, it does not respond to vitamin B_{12} or folic acid supplementation. Both the anemia and the neutropenia generally respond to dose reductions and interruptions. Erythropoietin (epoetin alfa) and G-CSF (filgastrim) may also be used to ameliorate these side effects if the use of other antiretroviral agents is not possible.

In monitoring patients receiving zidovudine, complete blood counts—with platelet and differential counts—should be done monthly for the first 2 months of therapy and then every 1–3 months depending on the clinical situation. Liver function tests and creatine phosphokinase levels should be checked every 3 months. Zidovudine can be taken concomitantly with other medicines except probenecid, which prolongs the serum half-life of zidovudine. In the initial zidovudine trial, acetaminophen use was associated with an increased incidence of neutropenia. However, this association has been disproved. Therefore, acetaminophen can be used in patients with contraindications to aspirin or nonsteroidal anti-inflammatory agents. Because of the synergistic bone marrow toxicity with some antibiotics, it may be prudent to withhold zidovudine while treating patients for serious opportunistic infections such as *P carinii* pneumonia. Long-term administration of zidovudine with ganciclovir can pose a difficult problem. Only 15% of patients tolerate this combination without significant hematologic toxicity. One approach to neutropenia is to add G-CSF (filgastrim) to the regimen;

another is to substitute didanosine for zidovudine. Finally, foscarnet has been shown to be well tolerated with concomitant zidovudine therapy. Since longer survival has been demonstrated in patients given foscarnet than in those given ganciclovir—perhaps because they were better able to tolerate simultaneous zidovudine—foscarnet probably represents the optimal approach at present.

The demonstration of in vitro resistance to zidovudine in patients who had been treated for longer than 6 months, has raised new questions about zidovudine, especially its use in early infection. This finding must be interpreted cautiously, since the resistance was quantitative, and patients in whom resistance was demonstrated were doing well clinically. To date, it has been impossible to correlate the development of zidovudine resistance definitively with clinical deterioration. Nonetheless, development of resistance is consistent with experience with other antimicrobial agents and with the clinical observation that in many AIDS patients, the benefits of zidovudine do not last beyond 18 months. It appears that resistance is much slower to emerge in individuals who are started on zidovudine therapy earlier in the course of disease and with higher CD4 counts. Thus, in determining when to initiate zidovudine therapy, clinicians must weigh all of the factors discussed above. However, most clinicians still recommend zidovudine for individuals who present with CD4 counts of less than 500 cells/µL.

Concern about zidovudine resistance is also tempered by the finding that resistant isolates were not resistant to other related dideoxynucleosides (eg, didanosine, zalcitabine). Another observation is the return of zidovudine sensitivity once this agent has been withdrawn for several months and didanosine has been substituted. This suggests that alternating drug regimens may delay emergence of resistance. Both didanosine (dideoxyinosine; ddI) and zalcitabine (dideoxycytidine; ddC) have been approved by the FDA. Didanosine and zalcitabine are recommended for patients who are intolerant to zidovudine or have progressive HIV disease (eg, a significant drop of the CD4 lymphocyte count despite zidovudine treatment). Both drugs have been shown to increase CD4 lymphocyte counts and lower p24 antigen levels in a manner similar to zidovudine.

Didanosine alone has been shown to be superior to zidovudine alone in some patients who have taken zidovudine for at least 8–16 weeks. Because this finding has not yet been replicated by other studies, most clinicians do not automatically switch patients who are doing well on zidovudine to didanosine after 16 weeks of zidovudine therapy. Instead, most clinicians wait until patients show signs of clinical or laboratory progression of disease despite receiving zidovudine.

Administration of didanosine is inconvenient. Because the drug is degraded by stomach acid, patients must take the medication on an empty stomach (1 hour before or 2–3 hours after meals). It is supplied in two forms: pills and packets of powder. To receive adequate buffering agent, the pills should be taken two at a time and thoroughly chewed or dissolved in water. Because the tablets are hard to chew, the powder, which is dissolved in water before ingestion, may be preferred by some patients. Diarrhea (due to the buffering agent used) is more common with the powder.

Dosing of these two formulations is by weight. For adults weighing 35–49 kg, dosing is 125 mg (tablets) or 167 mg (powder) twice a day; for adults weighing 50–74 kg, 200 mg (tablets) or 250 mg (powder) twice a day; and for adults weighing over 75 kg, 300 mg (tablets) or 375 mg (powder) twice a day. Unlike zidovudine, didanosine does not cause anemia but may cause neutropenia. It has also been associated with pancreatitis. The incidence of pancreatitis with didanosine is 5–10%—of fatal pancreatitis, less than 0.4%. Patients with a history of pancreatitis, as well as those taking other medications associated with pancreatitis (including trimethoprim-sulfamethoxazole and intravenous pentamidine) are at higher risk of this complication. Patients should be warned not to use alcohol while taking didanosine. Clinicians should also teach patients to watch for the symptoms of pancreatitis and to stop treatment if they develop abdominal pain, nausea, or vomiting while taking didanosine until it can be determined if they have pancreatitis. Other common side effects with didanosine include a dose-related, reversible, painful peripheral neuropathy which occurs in about a third of patients, and dry mouth. Fulminant hepatic failure and electrolyte abnormalities, including hypokalemia, hypocalcemia, and hypomagnesemia, have been reported in patients taking didanosine.

Zalcitabine has several advantages as a potential antiviral agent. It is inexpensive, easy to administer, and has no known hematologic side effects. The usual dosage of zalcitabine is approximately 0.005–0.01 mg/kg orally every 8 hours. This drug is formulated in 0.375 mg and 0.75 mg tablets. A comparative trial of zidovudine and zalcitabine as single antiretroviral agents in patients without prior therapy showed superiority of zidovudine. However, zalcitabine has shown promise in combination with zidovudine (see below) and appears to be as efficacious as didanosine when used as monotherapy in persons who have previously received zidovudine.

Zalcitabine, like didanosine, may cause peripheral neuropathy. It is also associated with aphthous ulcers, rash, and rare cases of pancreatitis.

Stavudine (d4T) has shown promise as an antiretroviral drug. It has been found to increase CD4 counts and decrease p24 antigenemia. It is currently available as an investigational new drug for patients with CD4 counts below 300 cells/μL who are intolerant to didanosine and zidovudine or who have shown

progression of disease. Side effects noted are peripheral neuropathy and hepatitis. Pancreatitis has been reported in patients taking stavudine, but it is unclear if the drug was the cause of the pancreatitis. Doses being used in clinical trials are 20-80 mg daily. Physicians can inquire about enrolling patients for stavudine by calling 1–800–842–8036.

The recommended use of antiretroviral agents is evolving as more agents and clinical data become available. Most clinicians advocate starting zidovudine alone for persons with CD4 counts between 200 and 500 cells/μL. Didanosine is utilized as an alternative single agent if zidovudine cannot be tolerated.

The weight of evidence favoring combination antiretroviral therapy is increasing, especially for patients who have progression of disease while receiving zidovudine alone. Two studies show encouraging trends toward increased CD4 counts in patients treated with zidovudine plus zalcitabine compared with those treated with zidovudine alone. These studies have found increased antiretroviral activity with simultaneous regimens as well as alternating regimens (eg, alternating monthly between zidovudine and zalcitabine). Several studies of combination zidovudine and didanosine therapy are in progress. Until further data are available, it seems prudent to individualize therapeutic decisions based upon degree of illness, contraindications to available agents, and patient preferences. For example, combination therapy has theoretic advantages compared with zidovudine alone for patients who present with low CD4 counts (< 200 cells/μL). However, this strategy has not yet been proved superior to single-agent therapy. Clinicians must also keep in mind that combination antiretroviral regimens are not necessarily better. d4T appears to be antagonistic to zidovudine in vitro, and the drugs should not be used together. Because didanosine and zalcitabine have overlapping toxicities, these two drugs should not be given together. An approach to currently available antiretroviral therapy is outlined in Table 30–5.

Combination antiretroviral therapy will become increasingly important with the development of additional classes of drugs that act upon different parts of the HIV replication cycle. Alpha-interferon has synergistic antiretroviral activity when administered with the nucleoside drugs. However, it has not been widely utilized in clinical practice because of its cost, need for parenteral administration, and toxicities. A recent report regarding in vitro combination of zidovudine, didanosine, and nevirapine, a new non-nucleoside reverse transcriptase inhibitor, suggests an enhanced antiretroviral effect of a three-drug combination. Clinical trials have started to look at this question. Trials have also begun with two novel classes of agents that have in vitro synergy with nucleoside analogues. These are inhibitors of HIV protease and peptides that block the action of the *tat* gene product of HIV.

Table 30–5. Approach to antiretroviral therapy.

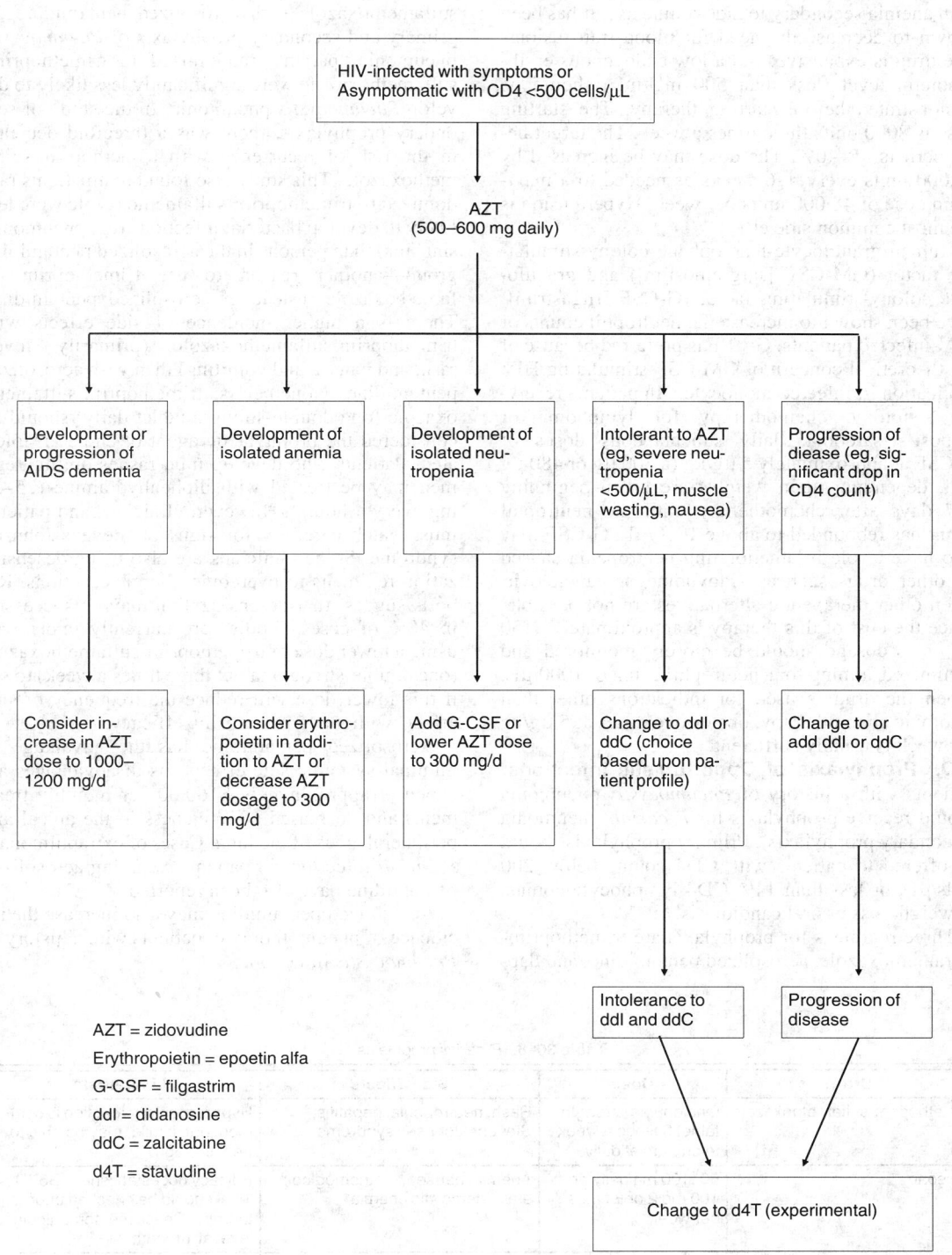

HIV-infected with symptoms or
Asymptomatic with CD4 <500 cells/µL

↓

AZT
(500–600 mg daily)

Development or progression of AIDS dementia	Development of isolated anemia	Development of isolated neutropenia	Intolerant to AZT (eg, severe neutropenia <500/µL, muscle wasting, nausea)	Progression of diease (eg, significant drop in CD4 count)
Consider increase in AZT dose to 1000–1200 mg/d	Consider erythropoietin in addition to AZT or decrease AZT dosage to 300 mg/d	Add G-CSF or lower AZT dose to 300 mg/d	Change to ddl or ddC (choice based upon patient profile)	Change to or add ddl or ddC

Intolerance to ddl and ddC

Progression of disease

↓

Change to d4T (experimental)

AZT = zidovudine
Erythropoietin = epoetin alfa
G-CSF = filgastrim
ddl = didanosine
ddC = zalcitabine
d4T = stavudine

C. Hematopoietic Stimulating Factors: Erythropoietin (epoetin alfa) has been approved for use in HIV-infected patients with anemia, including those with anemia secondary to zidovudine use. It has been shown to decrease the need for blood transfusions. The drug is expensive, and a low endogenous erythropoietin level (less than 500 mU/mL) should be demonstrated before starting therapy. The starting dose is 8000 units three times a week. The target hematocrit is 35–40%. The dose may be increased by 12,000 units every 4–6 weeks as needed to a maximum dose of 48,000 units per week. Hypertension is the most common side effect.

Human granulocyte-macrophage colony-stimulating factor (GM-CSF [sargramostim]) and granulocyte colony-stimulating factor (G-CSF [filgastrim]) have been shown to increase the neutrophil counts of HIV-infected patients. G-CSF is preferred because of the theoretical concern of GM-CSF-stimulating HIV replication in infected monocytes. In patients receiving cytotoxic chemotherapy for lymphoma or Kaposi's sarcoma, daily subcutaneous doses of G-CSF at approximately 5 µg/kg (a 300 µg or 480 µg vial, depending upon weight) are given beginning 5–7 days after chemotherapy until the neutrophil count has rebounded to above 1000/µL. G-CSF may also have a role in ameliorating neutropenia caused by other drugs such as zidovudine or ganciclovir, when other therapeutic alternatives are not possible. Since the cost of this therapy is approximately $150 per vial, dosage should be closely monitored and minimized, aiming for a neutrophil count of 1000/µL. When the drug is used for indications other than cytotoxic chemotherapy, one or two doses at 5 µg/kg per week is usually sufficient.

D. Prophylaxis of Opportunistic Infections: Patients with a history of *Pneumocystis* pneumonia should receive prophylaxis for *P carinii* pneumonia (secondary prophylaxis). Primary prophylaxis should be offered to patients with CD4 counts below 200 cells/µL, or less than 14% CD4 lymphocyte counts, or weight loss or oral candidiasis.

Three regimens for prophylaxis are trimethoprim-sulfamethoxazole, aerosolized pentamidine, and dapsone (see Table 30–6). Trimethoprim-sulfamethoxazole is inexpensive and widely available. In two recent studies comparing once-daily trimethoprim-sulfamethoxazole with aerosolized pentamidine for primary and secondary prophylaxis of *Pneumocystis* pneumonia, patients randomized to trimethoprim-sulfamethoxazole were significantly less likely to develop *Pneumocystis* pneumonia. In the study of secondary prophylaxis, there was a threefold decrease in the risk of recurrence with trimethoprim-sulfamethoxazole. This study also found that patients randomized to trimethoprim-sulfamethoxazole were less likely to develop bacterial infections (eg, pneumonia, sinusitis) than persons in the aerosolized pentamidine group—another reason to use trimethoprim-sulfamethoxazole instead of aerosolized pentamidine. There is a higher incidence of side effects with trimethoprim-sulfamethoxazole (primarily fever, rash, and nausea and vomiting) than with aerosolized pentamidine. Nonetheless, trimethoprim-sulfamethoxazole (one double-strength tablet daily) should be considered the prophylactic agent of choice if tolerated. Patients who develop mild rashes on this regimen may be treated with diphenhydramine (25–50 mg every 4 hours). However, clinicians and patients must watch carefully for signs of Stevens-Johnson syndrome. Some clinicians are also using desensitization regimens to overcome allergic reactions. Reports suggest that desensitization may be successful in 40% of cases. Studies are currently under way using a lower dose of trimethoprim-sulfamethoxazole (one double-strength tablet three times a week) to see if this lower dose will reduce the frequency of side effects without compromising efficacy.

Aerosolized pentamidine has the advantage of minimal systemic side effects. Its disadvantages are expense (approximately $160.00 per monthly treatment) and decreased effectiveness in the apical and peripheral areas of the lung. Cases of extrapulmonary *P carinii* infections in patients receiving aerosolized pentamidine have also been reported.

Aerosolized pentamidine may also increase the incidence of pneumothorax in patients with a history of *Pneumocystis* infection.

Table 30–6. *P carinii* prophlaxis.

Drug	Dose	Side Effects	Limitations
Trimethoprim-sulfamethoxazole	One double-strength tablet 3 times a week to one tablet daily	Rash, neutropenia, hepatitis, Stevens-Johnson syndrome	Hypersensitivity reaction is common, but, if mild, may be able to treat through.
Dapsone	50–100 mg daily or 100 mg 2 or 3 times per week	Anemia, nausea, methemoglobinemia, hemolytic anemia	Efficacy not established. G6PD level should be checked prior to therapy. Check methemoglobin level at 1 month.
Aerolized pentamidine	300 mg monthly	Bronchospasm (pretreat with bronchodilators); rare reports of pancreatitis	Apical *P carinii* pneumonia, extrapulmonary *P carinii* infections, pneumothorax.

Although dapsone has not been widely studied, it appears to be an effective prophylactic agent with minimal side effects. As with trimethoprim-sulfamethoxazole, it is inexpensive and widely available and may be used in patients with an allergic reaction to trimethoprim-sulfamethoxazole. Before prescribing dapsone, clinicians should document that the patient is not G6PD-deficient. Such patients are at high risk of developing hemolytic anemia with dapsone therapy. Patients taking dapsone concomitantly with didanosine should take the dapsone at least 2 hours prior to the didanosine. Dapsone is not absorbed well in the neutral pH stomach environment created by the didanosine buffering agent.

Patients who develop *P carinii* infection on a particular prophylactic regimen should be switched to a different one or should receive a combination regimen (eg, aerosolized pentamidine plus trimethoprim-sulfamethoxazole).

Prophylaxis for *M tuberculosis*—isoniazid, 300 mg daily for 9 months to a year—should be given to all HIV-infected patients with positive PPD reactions (defined for HIV-infected patients as > 5mm of induration). The use of prophylaxis for other AIDS infections, including toxoplasmosis, *M avium-intracellulare* infection, cytomegalovirus infection, cryptococcal infection, and histoplasmosis, is under study. Rational use of prophylactic regimens will require identification of patients at high risk for infection and efficacious oral regimens with acceptable side effect profiles.

Toxoplasmosis prophylaxis would be desirable in patients with positive IgG *Toxoplasma* serology. Pyrimethamine and clindamycin have been studied, but both were found to be unacceptable because of a high incidence of cutaneous reactions. Trimethoprim-sulfamethoxazole offers some protection against toxoplasmosis. *M avium-intracellulare* infection occurs commonly in patients with CD4 counts of fewer than 50 cells/μL; thus, prophylaxis for this infection would also be desirable. Rifabutin, 300 mg/d orally, delays the onset of disseminated *M avium intracellulare* in persons with fewer than 200 CD4 cells/μL. However, the paucity of agents with activity against this organism and the rapid development of antibiotic resistance make single-agent prophylaxis of this infection unlikely. Cytomegalovirus infection is also common in late HIV disease. Studies of an orally bioavailable preparation of ganciclovir are going forward; acyclovir, 2–4 g/d orally, has been shown to decrease the incidence of cytomegalovirus infection in other immunocompromised populations, but its efficacy is not of proved value in the setting of HIV disease. Cryptococcosis and endemic fungal diseases are also candidates for prophylaxis. Since cryptococcal meningitis is seen in a smaller percentage of patients than the above opportunistic infections, it is difficult to recommend routine use of fluconazole for prophylaxis without further clinical trials. In areas of the world where histoplasmosis and coccidioidomycosis are endemic and are frequent complications of HIV infection, prophylactic use of fluconazole or, eventually, itraconazole may prove to be useful prophylactic strategies.

Since individuals with advanced HIV infection are susceptible to a number of opportunistic pathogens, the use of agents with activity against more than one pathogen is envisioned. It has been shown, for example, that trimethoprim-sulfamethoxazole confers some protection against toxoplasmosis in individuals receiving this drug for *P carinii* prophylaxis. The newer macrolide antibiotics such as clarithromycin offer promise in this regard, since they have activity against bacterial, mycobacterial, and parasitic pathogens.

Prevention

A. Primary Prevention: In the past several years, primate model data have suggested that development of a protective vaccine may be possible. Clinical trials in humans are under way using recombinant gp120 or its precursor, gp160. It seems likely that information about the immunogenicity of vaccine prototypes will emerge over the next few years. However, proof of vaccine efficacy will take far longer.

A second aspect of vaccine development focuses on boosting the immunologic responses of individuals who are already HIV-infected. One study suggests the possibility of eliciting new humoral and cellular immune responses in seropositive individuals with CD4 counts of over 500 cells/μL. Furthermore, there is preliminary evidence that these vaccine responders may experience at least a short-term stabilization of the CD4 count.

Until vaccination is a reality, prevention of HIV infection will depend upon effective precautions regarding sexual practices and intravenous drug use, screening of blood products, and infection control practices in the health care setting. It is the duty of physicians to counsel HIV-negative patients on how to avoid exposure to the HIV virus. Patients should be counseled not to exchange bodily fluids unless they are in a long-term mutually monogamous relationship with someone who has tested HIV antibody-negative and has not engaged in unsafe sex for at least 6 months prior to or at any time since the negative test.

Only latex condoms should be used, along with a water-soluble lubricant. Although nonoxynol-9, a spermicide, kills HIV, it can not be enthusiastically recommended as an ingredient in lubricants because of the possibility that it may cause genital ulcers which could facilitate HIV transmission. Patients should be counseled that condoms are not 100% effective. They should be made familiar with the use of condoms, including, specifically, the advice that condoms must be used every time; that space should be left at the tip of the condom as a receptacle for semen; that intercourse with a condom should not be attempted if the penis is only partially erect; that men should hold on to base of the condom when withdrawing the penis to prevent slippage; and that condoms should not be reused. Although anal intercourse remains the sexual practice at highest risk of transmitting HIV, seroconversions have been documented with vaginal and oral intercourse as well. Therefore, condoms should be used when engaging in these activities. Women as well as men should understand how to use condoms so as to be sure that their partners are using them correctly.

Persons using intravenous drugs should be cautioned never to exchange needles or other drug paraphernalia. When sterile needles are not available, bleach does appear to inactivate HIV and should be used to clean needles.

Current efforts to screen blood and blood products have lowered the risk of HIV transmission with transfusion to 1:100,000.

In the hospital, concerns about nosocomial infection have led to the recommendation for universal body fluid precautions. This involves the rigorous use of gloves when handling any body fluid and the addition of gown, mask, and goggles for procedures that may result in splash or droplet spread. Reports of transmission of drug-resistant tuberculosis in health care settings also have had infection control implications. All patients with cough in outpatient settings should be encouraged to wear masks. Hospitalized HIV-infected patients with cough should be placed in respiratory isolation until tuberculosis can be excluded by chest x-ray and sputum smear examination.

B. Secondary Prevention: The percentage of HIV-infected persons who will ultimately progress to AIDS is not known. However, cohort studies of individuals with documented dates of seroconversion demonstrate that approximately 50% of untreated seropositive persons develop AIDS within 10 years. The risk of developing AIDS is inversely correlated with the CD4 count; over 80% of patients with a CD4 count below 200 cells/μL develop AIDS within 3 years. A CD4 count of less than 50 cells/μL is also an important natural history landmark, since most deaths occur once the count has fallen below this level.

However, there is increasing evidence that medical intervention can slow the progression of disease among healthy HIV-infected people. Epidemiologic studies indicate that the progression from HIV seroconversion to AIDS has been slowed by the use of antiviral and prophylactic treatments. Recommended interventions for health care maintenance of HIV-infected individuals are listed in Table 30–7.

Because of the increased occurrence of tuberculosis among HIV-infected patients, all such individuals should undergo PPD testing. Although anergy is common among AIDS patients, the likelihood of a false-negative result is much lower when the test is done early in infection. Those with positive tests (defined for HIV-infected patients as > 5 mm of induration) need a chest x-ray. Patients with an infiltrate in any location, especially if accompanied by mediastinal adenopathy, should have sputum sent for acid-fast staining. Those patients with a positive PPD but negative evaluations for active disease should receive isoniazid (300 mg daily) for 9 months to a year regardless of their age. Recent analysis suggests also that HIV-infected individuals at high risk for tuberculosis should receive a course of isoniazid prophylaxis regardless of PPD status. This would include homeless individuals and injection drug users.

HIV-infected patients are at increased risk of reactivation of syphilis and progression to tertiary syphilis despite standard treatment. Because the only widely available tests for syphilis are serologic and because HIV-infected individuals are known to have disordered antibody production, there is concern about the interpretation of these titers. This concern has been fueled by a report of an HIV-infected patient with secondary syphilis and negative syphilis serologic testing. Furthermore, HIV-infected individuals may lose FTA-ABS reactivity after treatment for syphilis, particularly if they have low CD4 counts. Thus, in this population, a nonreactive treponemal test does not rule out a past history of syphilis. In addition, persistence of treponemes in the spinal fluid after one dose of benzathine penicillin has been demonstrated in HIV-infected patients with primary and secondary syphilis. Therefore, the CDC has recommended an aggressive diagnostic approach to HIV-infected patients with reactive RPR or VDRL tests of greater than 1 year or unknown duration. All such patients should have a lumbar puncture with cerebrospinal fluid cell count and CSF-VDRL. Those with a

Table 30–7. Health care maintenance of HIV-infected individuals.

For all HIV-infected individuals
CD4 counts every 3–6 months
PPD with anergy controls
INH for those with positive PPD and normal chest x-ray
RPR or VDRL
Toxoplasma IgG serology
Pneumococcal vaccine
Influenza vaccine in season
Hepatitis vaccine for those who are HBsAb-negative
Haemophilus influenzae b vaccination
Papanicolaou smears every 6 months for women

For HIV-infected individuals with CD4 <500 cells/μL
Zidovudine (AZT) or other antiretroviral drug as indicated (see Table 30–5)

For HIV-infected individuals with CD4 <200 cells/μL
P carinii prophylaxis

For HIV-infected individuals with CD4 <100 cells/μL
M avium-intracellulare prophylaxis

normal cerebrospinal fluid evaluation are treated as having late latent syphilis (benzathine penicillin G, 2.4 million units intramuscularly weekly for 3 weeks) with follow-up titers. Those with a pleocytosis or a positive CSF-VDRL test are treated as having neurosyphilis (aqueous penicillin G, 2–4 million units intravenously every 4 hours; or procaine penicillin G, 2.4 million units intramuscularly daily, with probenecid, 500 mg four times daily, for 10 days.) Some clinicians take a less aggressive approach to patients who have low titers (less than 1:8), a history of having been treated for syphilis, and a normal neurologic examination. Close follow-up of titers is mandatory if such a course is taken.

The efficacy of pneumococcal, *Haemophilus influenzae* b, and influenza vaccines is debated, but since they are safe, HIV-infected individuals should receive them. Patients without evidence of hepatitis B surface antibody should receive hepatitis B vaccination. Live vaccines, such as yellow fever vaccine, should be avoided. Measles vaccination, while a live virus vaccine, appears relatively safe when administered to HIV-infected individuals and should be given if the patient has never had measles or been adequately vaccinated.

HIV-infected individuals should be counseled with regard to safe sex. Because of the risk of transmission, they should be warned to use condoms with sexual intercourse, including oral intercourse. HIV-infected women should use latex barriers such as dental dams (available at dental supply stores) to prevent their partners from having direct oral contact with vaginal secretions. Substance abuse treatment should be recommended for persons who are using recreational drugs. They should be warned to avoid consuming raw meat or eggs to avoid infections with *Toxoplasma, Campylobacter,* and *Salmonella.* Because of the emotional impact of HIV infection and subsequent illness, many patients will benefit from supportive counseling.

C. HIV Risk for Health Care Professionals: Epidemiologic studies show that needle sticks occur commonly among health care professionals, especially among surgeons performing invasive proce-

dures and inexperienced hospital house staff. Efforts to reduce needle sticks should focus on avoiding recapping needles and, whenever possible, doing invasive procedures under controlled circumstances. The risk of HIV transmission from a needle stick with blood from an HIV-infected patient is about 1:250. The risk from mucous membrane contact is too low to quantitate.

Health care professionals who sustain needle sticks should be counseled and offered HIV testing as soon as possible. HIV testing is done to establish a negative baseline for worker's compensation claims in case there is a subsequent conversion. Follow-up testing is usually performed at 6 weeks, 3 months, and 6 months.

There is no definitive evidence that postexposure administration of zidovudine reduces the risk of seroconversion. Because of the low rate of seroconversion following needle sticks and the difficulties in randomizing health care providers, it is unlikely that there will ever be a definitive answer concerning the efficacy of zidovudine in preventing HIV infection. However, data from animal models suggest potential efficacy of zidovudine when given within 8 hours after exposure. Therefore, providers should be offered the option of zidovudine therapy (1200 mg daily for 6 weeks). Unfortunately, there have been documented cases of seroconversion following parenteral exposure to HIV despite prompt use of zidovudine prophylaxis. Counseling of the provider should include "safe sex" guidelines.

Course & Prognosis

The rate of progression to symptomatic disease is reviewed above. Once clinical findings develop, outcome varies. With improvements in therapy, some cohorts of patients are living longer after the diagnosis of AIDS. In San Francisco, mean survival after a first bout of *Pneumocystis* pneumonia is 18–24 months. This is increased from approximately 12 months at the start of the epidemic. However, survival after diagnosis of HIV-related lymphomas still averages less than 8 months.

REFERENCES

Epidemiology
1993 revised classification system for HIV infection and expanded surveillance case definition for AIDS among adolescents and adults. MMWR Morb Mortal Wkly Rep 1992;41(RR-17):1. (Explains the 1993 AIDS case definition.)
Markovitz DM: Infection with the human immunodeficiency virus type 2. Ann Intern Med 1993;118:211. (This strain can cause AIDS, but the rate of development of disease is much slower than with HIV-1.)

Projections of the number of persons diagnosed with AIDS and the number of immunosuppressed HIV-infected persons—United States, 1992–94. MMWR Morb Mortal Wkly Rep 1992;41(RR17):1. (Projections of the AIDS epidemic including the number of persons with CD4 counts below 200 cells/μL.)

Opportunistic Infections and Malignancies
Armitage K et al: Treatment of cryptosporidiosis with

paromomycin. Arch Intern Med 1992;152:2497. (Five cases with apparent response to this agent.)

Dannemann B et al: Treatment of toxoplasmic encephalitis in patients with AIDS. Ann Intern Med 1992; 116:33. (Multicenter study suggesting the equivalence of clindamycin and sulfadiazine in addition to pyrimethamine therapy.)

Fischl MA et al: An outbreak of tuberculosis caused by multiple-drug-resistant tubercle bacilli among patients with HIV infection. Ann Intern Med 1992; 117:177. (Classic description of the disease profile and documentation of nosocomial spread.)

Gourevich MN et al: Effects of HIV infection on the serologic manifestations and response to treatment of syphilis in intravenous drug users. Ann Intern Med 1993;118:350. (HIV infection did not affect the presentation or treatment outcome of syphilis in this cohort.)

Greenson JK et al: AIDS enteropathy: Occult enteric infections and duodenal mucosal alterations in chronic diarrhea. Ann Intern Med 1991;114:366. (A high incidence of poorly treatable opportunistic infections and nonspecific histologic abnormalities.)

Katz MH et al: Risk stratification of ambulatory patients suspected of *Pneumocystis* pneumonia. Arch Intern Med 1991;51:105. (Diagnostic algorithm for respiratory symptoms based on 302 patients at risk for HIV.)

Kerlikowske K et al: *Mycobacterium avium* complex and *Mycobacterium tuberculosis* in patients infected with the human immunodeficiency virus. West J Med 1992;157:144. (Reviews epidemiology, clinical aspects, and principles of treatment of these important infections.)

Masur H: Drug therapy: Prevention and treatment of *Pneumocystis* pneumonia. N Engl J Med 1992; 327:1853. (Summary of available treatments for prophylaxis and treatment.)

The NIH-University of California Expert Panel: Consensus statement on the use of corticosteroids as adjunctive therapy for *Pneumocystis* pneumonia in the acquired immunodeficiency syndrome. N Engl J Med 1990;323:1500. (Concise review of available studies that suggest benefit of early corticosteroid administration in moderate to severe disease.)

Pappas PG et al: Blastomycosis in patients with the acquired immunodeficiency syndrome. Ann Intern Med 1992;116:847. (Rapid disease progression like histoplasmosis and coccidioidomycosis.)

Powderly WG et al: A controlled trial of fluconazole or amphotericin-B to prevent relapse of cryptococcal meningitis in patients with the acquired immunodeficiency syndrome. N Engl J Med 1992;326:793. (Fluconazole was clearly superior and less toxic.)

Rabkin CS, Biggar RJ, Horm JW: Increasing incidence of cancers associated with the human immunodeficiency virus epidemic. Int J Cancer 1991;47:692. (Marked increase in incidence of Kaposi's sarcoma and non-Hodgkin's lymphoma between 1973 and 1987.)

Ruskin J: Low-dose co-trimoxazole for prevention of *Pneumocystis carinii* in human immunodeficiency virus disease. Lancet 1991;337:468. (A retrospective study showing apparent prevention of P carinii pneumonia with low dose therapy. Acceptable toxicity profile.)

Saag MS et al: Comparison of amphotericin B with fluconazole in the treatment of acute AIDS-associated cryptococcal meningitis. N Engl J Med 1992;326:83. (Fluconazole and amphotericin B are equivalent in neurologically intact patients with cryptococcal meningitis.)

Safrin S et al: Foscarnet therapy in five patients with AIDS and acyclovir-resistant varicella-zoster virus infection. Ann Intern Med 1991;115:19. (Four of five patients with resistant virus had good clinical outcomes with foscarnet.)

Sepkowitz KA et al: Pneumothorax in AIDS. Ann Intern Med 1991;114:455. (Twenty patients, 19 of whom had active *Pneumocystis* pneumonia. Strong associations with prior *Pneumocystis* pneumonia and inhaled pentamidine usage.)

Small PM et al: Treatment of tuberculosis in patients with advanced human immunodeficiency virus infection. N Engl J Med 1991;324:289. (Majority presented before developing other AIDS-related infections and had a favorable response to therapy if compliant. Extrapulmonary disease present in 62% of cases.)

Studies of Ocular Complications of AIDS Research Group: Mortality in patients with the acquired immunodeficiency syndrome treated with either foscarnet or ganciclovir for cytomegalovirus retinitis. N Engl J Med 1992;326:213. (Foscarnet-treated patients had a survival advantage, but the ganciclovir-treated group received less antiretroviral therapy.)

Tompkins DC et al: *Rochalimaea*'s role in cat scratch disease and bacillary angiomatosis. Ann Intern Med 1993;118:388. (Current state of knowledge about these newly identified organisms.)

White MV et al: Desensitization to trimethoprim sulfamethoxazole in patients with acquired immune deficiency syndrome and *Pneumocystis carinii* pneumonia. Ann Allergy 1989;62:177. (Outlines one regimen for desensitization.)

Antiretroviral Treatment

Hamilton JD et al: A controlled trial of early versus late treatment with zidovudine in symptomatic human immunodeficiency virus infection. N Engl J Med 1992;326:43. (Rekindles controversy about timing of zidovudine therapy.)

Kahn J et al: A controlled trial comparing continued zidovudine with didanosine in human immunodeficiency virus infection. N Engl J Med 1992;327:581. (Patients switched from zidovudine to didanosine had a lower rate of disease progression than those maintained on zidovudine.)

Meng T et al: Combination therapy with zidovudine and dideoxycytidine in patients with advanced human immunodeficiency virus infection. Ann Intern Med 1992;116:13. (Phase I study showing superiority of zalcitabine plus zidovudine compared with zidovudine alone on CD4 response.)

Shih C et al: Post-exposure prophylaxis with zidovudine suppresses human immunodeficiency virus type I infection in SCID-hu mice in a time-dependent manner. J Infect Dis 1991;163:625. (In contrast to other animal models, using other retroviruses, zidovudine had significant protective effect up to 8 hours postexposure.)

Skowron G et al: Alternating and intermittent regimen of

zidovudine and dideoxycytidine in patients with AIDS or AIDS-related complex. Ann Intern Med 1993;118:321. (Explores the sequential strategy of antiretroviral drug use and finds some sparing of toxicity.)

Prevention

Holmberg SD et al: Biologic factors in the sexual transmission of human immunodeficiency virus. J Infect Dis 1989;160:116. (Review of factors affecting transmission of HIV.)

Jewett JF, Hecht FM: Preventive health care for adults with HIV infection. JAMA 1993;269:1144. (Review of evidence supporting preventive medical interventions for HIV-infected persons.)

Koop CE: Talking to patients about AIDS. J Fam Pract 1991;32:367. (Advice from the former Surgeon General about what to say to patients to lower their risk of exposure.)

Makadon HJ: Assessing HIV infection in primary care practice. J Gen Intern Med 1991;6(Suppl):S2. (Review of risk assessment, counseling and testing, and medical evaluation in primary care practice.)

Minkoff HL et al: Care of women infected with the human immunodeficiency virus. JAMA 1991;266:2253. (Review of gynecologic and obstetric care for HIV-infected women.)

Steinhoff MC et al: Antibody responses to *Haemophilus influenzae* type b vaccines in men with human immunodeficiency virus infection. N Engl J Med 1991;325:1837. (As with pneumococcal vaccine, response correlates with CD4 count.)

31

Infectious Diseases: Viral & Rickettsial

Wayne Shandera, MD, & Eva Patricia Gill, MD

I. VIRAL DISEASES

DIAGNOSIS OF VIRAL INFECTIONS

Although some viral illnesses present with clear clinical syndrome (measles, mumps, chickenpox), in many instances the clinical picture is suggestive of viral infection but the causative agent could be any one of a number of viruses. For example, aseptic meningitis can be caused by mumps virus, lymphocytic choriomeningitis virus, or any of several enteroviruses, and specific diagnosis requires laboratory assistance, which may be costly and not always relevant. Symptoms of respiratory disease associated with many viruses are similar: epithelial involvement, erythema, nasal secretions, minimal purulent response, and interstitial disease when pneumonia is present. In most cases, specific identification of a virus is required only for confirmation of atypical cases or for differential diagnosis of confusing syndromes. The frequency with which certain pathogens cause certain diseases allows for educated guesses, eg, respiratory syncytial virus (RSV) for bronchiolitis or parainfluenza virus for croup. However, in certain instances, rapid diagnosis may aid in patient management.

Laboratory Considerations

Three basic laboratory techniques are used for diagnosis of viral infections:

A. Isolation and Identification Of Virus: Prompt transport (in viral transport medium, on wet ice) to the laboratory and inoculation of appropriate specimens into appropriate cell culture, live animals, or embryonated eggs are required. Identification may be as simple as a stain (eg, the nonspecific Tzanck smear for herpes) or may involve laborious procedures (eg, identification of coxsackieviruses requires growth on cell cultures or in suckling mice). Isolation of virus from a normally sterile site (cerebrospinal fluid, lung) or from a lesion (vesicles) is diagnosti-

cally significant. From nonsterile sites (nasopharynx, stool), finding virus may denote only carriage, and seroconversion or pathologic change is needed for diagnosis. In the future, the shell vial centrifugation technique will be increasingly used to diagnose viral infection.

B. Microscopic Methods: Microscopic techniques are used to examine cells, body fluids, biopsy material, or aspirates in search of virus or cytologic changes specific for one or a group of viruses (eg, multinucleated giant cells at the base of herpes lesions, rotavirus structures on electron micrographs of diarrheal stools).

Immunofluorescent methods, often with monoclonal antibodies, can rapidly identify some antigens (rabies, varicella, herpes simplex, respiratory syncytial virus) in desquamated or scraped cells.

C. Immunologic Studies of Sera: Specific antibodies to viruses rise during the course of illness, though timing of a rise in titer and persistence of titer depend on the virus. A fourfold rise in titer during illness is usually considered evidence of disease.

Single titers are seldom helpful, and many laboratories require paired sera (2–3 weeks apart). Serologic panels against many viruses are not practical in individual patients, since serologic studies require suspicion of the involved virus. Antigenic detection is used for certain viruses (HBsAg, HIV) and detects viral persistence without comment regarding duration of disease or host response to infection.

HERPESVIRUSES OF HUMANS

These viruses share features important in human disease. Six identified human herpesviruses include herpes simplex virus (HSV) type 1, HSV type 2, varicella-zoster virus (type 3), Epstein-Barr (EB)-infectious mononucleosis virus (type 4), and cytomegalovirus (CMV) (type 5). A sixth agent (HHV-6) has been identified as the cause of roseola (exanthem subitum), and a seventh is in search of a disease.

Subclinical primary infection with the herpesviruses is more common than clinically manifest illness. Each persists in a latent state for the remainder of the host's life. Reactivation producing clinical recurrence of disease may follow known or unknown triggering mechanisms. With HSV and VZV, virus is latent in sensory ganglia, and upon reactivation lesions appear in the distal sensory nerve distribution. As a result of disease-, drug-, or radiation-induced immunosuppression, virus reactivation may lead to widespread lesions in affected organs such as the central nervous system. Severe or fatal illness may occur in infants and the immunodeficient.

Hall CB: Herpes and the rash of roses: A new virus, HHV-6, as a cause of an old childhood disease, roseola. Pediatr Ann 1990;19:517.

Oren I, Sobel JD: Human herpesvirus type 6: Review. Clin Infect Dis 1992;14:741.

1. HERPESVIRUSES 1 & 2

Herpesviruses can infect the fetus and induce congenital malformations. The viruses have also been linked to cervical carcinoma and Burkitt's lymphoma, but the relationship is uncertain. When epithelial surfaces are involved, prolonged shedding of herpesviruses and spread to contacts may occur.

Herpes simplex encephalitis presents with symptoms and signs of encephalitis (see below). A distinguishing feature is a propensity to temporal lobe disease ("mass-like" lesions on scans, temporal lobe seizure foci on EEGs). Encephalitis is definitively diagnosed by brain biopsy with immunofluorescent stain and viral culture. Perfusion scintigraphy using single-photon emission computed tomography (SPECT) can reportedly distinguish HSV and non-HSV encephalitis. If diagnosed and treated early, before coma ensues, encephalitis is not associated with as high a mortality rate. Many survivors are not neurologically normal.

Herpes simplex type 1 mucocutaneous lesions largely involve the mouth and oral cavity ("herpes labialis") but also cause whitlows, keratitis, and a minority of urogenital infections. Herpes simplex type 2 lesions largely involve the genital tract; latency in presacral ganglia with reactivation under unknown influences is responsible for recurrent disease. A manifestation of primary infection in many women is aseptic meningitis requiring treatment (see below). Asymptomatic shedding for weeks follows primary type 2 infection in almost 20% and appears to be responsible for transmission.

Drugs that inhibit replication of herpesviruses 1 and 2 include idoxuridine and trifluridine (for keratitis) and acyclovir and vidarabine (for encephalitis or disseminated disease). Because of a need for rapid treatment and the difficulties of brain biopsy, patients with suspected encephalitis are typically given intravenous acyclovir (10 mg/kg every 8 hours for 10 days, adjusting for renal function) prior to biopsy.

Acyclovir orally is beneficial in symptomatic primary genital infections, especially in women. Given in a dosage of 200 mg five times a day, oral acyclovir can reduce the frequency and severity of recurrent herpetic lesions. Acyclovir is given intravenously for disseminated (simplex and varicella) lesions of neonates or immunosuppressed patients (administered as 5 mg/kg intravenously every 8 hours for 5 days). Topical acyclovir is also available. Applied as a 5% solution six times per day, it can reduce viral shedding and local pain and shorten healing time, but it has little effect on recurrent lesions or on recurrence rate; it can aid in treating mucocutaneous lesions in immunocompromised patients. Acyclovir-resistant isolates have been described with mucocutaneous infections, especially in the HIV-positive population. The agent of choice for resistant HSV infections is foscarnet (phosphonoformic acid), 40–60 mg/kg intravenously every 8 hours, adjusting for renal dysfunction. As a consequence of a recent nosocomial outbreak, mucosal surface barrier precautions are probably needed to prevent spread from respiratory HSV-1 cases.

The basic properties of acyclovir and other antiviral agents are summarized in Table 31–1.

Gibson JJ et al: A cross-sectional study of herpes simplex types 1 and 2 in college students: Occurrence and determinants of infection. J Infect Dis 1990;162:306.

Koelle DM et al: Asymptomatic reactivation of herpes simplex virus in women after the first episode of genital herpes. Ann Intern Med 1992;116:433.

Mertz GJ et al: Long-term acyclovir suppression of frequently recurring genital herpes simplex virus infection. JAMA 1988;260:201.

Mertz GJ et al: Risk factors for the sexual transmission of genital herpes. Ann Intern Med 1992;116:197.

Perl TM et al: Transmission of HSV type 1 in an intensive care unit. Ann Intern Med 1992;117:584.

Safrin S et al: Foscarnet therapy for acyclovir-resistant mucocutaneous HSV infection in 26 AIDS patients. J Infect Dis 1990;161:1078.

Straus SE et al: Acyclovir suppression of frequently recurring genital herpes. JAMA 1988;260:2227.

Whitley RJ, Gnann JW Jr: Acyclovir: A decade later. (Drug Therapy.) N Engl J Med 1992;327:782.

2. VARICELLA (Chickenpox) & HERPES ZOSTER (Shingles)

Essentials of Diagnosis

- Fever and malaise just before or with eruption.
- Rash: pruritic, centripetal, papular, changing to vesicular ("dewdrops on a rose petal"), pustular, and finally crusting.
- Exposure 14–20 days previously.

General Considerations

Varicella-zoster virus is human herpesvirus 3. Dis-

Table 31–1. Agents for systemic viral infections.

Drug	Dosing	Renal Clearance?/ Hemodialysis?	CSF Penetration	Toxicities	Spectrum
Acyclovir	200–800 mg orally 5 times daily; 250–500 mg/m² IV every 8 hours for 7 days	Yes/Yes	Yes	Neurotoxic reactions, reversible renal dysfunction, local reactions	Herpesviruses
Amantadine	200 mg/d orally (100 mg in elderly)	Yes/No	Yes	Confusion, gastrointestinal symptoms	Influenza A
Didanosine (ddI)	125–300 mg orally twice daily based on weight	Yes (moderate)/–	Yes	Pancreatitis, neuropathy; magnesium toxicity in renal failure	HIV-1, HIV-2
Foscarnet	20 mg/kg IV bolus, then 60 mg/kg IV every 8 hours for 2 weeks; maintain with 60 mg/kg/d IV for 5 days each week	Yes/Yes	Yes	Nephrotoxicity, genital ulcerations, calcium disturbances	Cytomegalovirus, HSV resistant to acyclovir, V2V, HIV-1
Ganciclovir	5 mg/kg IV bolus every 12 hours for 14–21 days; maintain with 5–7 mg/kg/d IV for 5 days each week	Yes/Yes	Yes	Neutropenia, thrombocytopenia, CNS side effects	Cytomegalovirus
Idoxuridine	Topical, 0.1% every 1–2 hours for 3–5 days	–	–	Local reactions	HSV keratitis
Interferon alfa-2b	3–5 million IU SC 3 times weekly to daily. Intralesionally: 1 million IU per 0.1 mL in up to 5 warts 3 times weekly for 3 weeks.	Yes/Yes	–	Influenza-like syndrome, myelosuppression, neurotoxicity	HBV, HCV, papillomavirus
Ribavirin	Aerosol: 1.1 g/d as 20 mg/mL dilution over 12–18 hours. See text for Lassa fever doses.	Yes/No	Yes	Wheezing	Respiratory syncytial virus, severe influenza A or B, Lassa fever
Trifluridine	Topical, 1% drops every 2 hours to 9 drops/d	–	–	Local reactions	HSV keratitis
Vidarabine	15 mg/kg/d IV for 10 days	Yes/Yes	Yes	Teratogenic, megaloblastosis, neurotoxicity	HSV, VZV
Zalcitabine (ddC)	0.75 mg twice daily	Yes/–	Yes	Rash, fevers, aphthous stomatitis, neurotoxicity; rarely, pancreatitis and myelosuppression	HIV-1, HIV-2
Zidovudine (AZT)	100 mg every 4–6 hours to 200 mg orally every 8 hours (total daily dose: 400–600 mg)	Yes (moderate)/ Yes(moderate)	Yes	Bone marrow suppression, neurotoxicity	HIV-1, HIV-2

ease manifestations are either chickenpox or shingles (herpes zoster, a reactivation of varicella). Chickenpox is highly contagious and is generally a disease of childhood, with spread by inhalation of infective droplets or contact with lesions after 10–20 days (average, 14–15 days).

Clinical Findings

A. Varicella:

1. Symptoms and signs–(Table 31–2.) Fever and malaise are usually mild in children and more severe in adults. Vesicular lesions, quickly rupturing to form small ulcers, may appear first in the oropharynx. The pruritic rash is centripetal and most prominent on the face, scalp, and trunk, but to a lesser extent it commonly involves the extremities. Maculopapules change in a few hours to vesicles that become pustular and eventually form crusts. New lesions may erupt for 1–5 days, so that all stages of the eruption are generally present simultaneously. The crusts usually slough in 7–14 days. The vesicles and pustules are superficial and elliptic, with slightly serrated borders. Many infections are subclinical.

The generalized nondermatomal distribution and the evolution of lesions (all stages simultaneous) distinguish primary varicella from herpes zoster.

2. Laboratory findings–Leukopenia is common. Multinucleated giant cells are evident on Tzanck smear of scrapings of vesicle bases. Virus is isolable from vesicles using human diploid fibroblasts, though diagnosis by detection of antigens in vesicle fluid using immunofluorescent antibodies is easier. Diagnosis is usually made on the basis of clinical findings.

B. Herpes Zoster: Pain is often severe and may precede the appearance of rash. Lesions follow nerve root distributions, with thoracic and lumbar roots most common, but cervical or trigeminal involvement is possible. In most cases a single unilateral dermatome is involved.

Skin lesions resemble those of chickenpox, developing as maculopapules and evolving into vesicles and pustules. Lesions on the tip of the nose indicate ophthalmic division disease, while facial palsy, lesions of the external ear with or without tympanic membrane involvement, vertigo and tinnitus, and deafness signify geniculate ganglion involvement (Ramsay Hunt syndrome). In either of these cases, treatment is mandatory (see below).

Complications

A. Varicella: Secondary bacterial infections of lesions, whose range includes cellulitis, erysipelas, and scarlet fever, are common, and pitted scars are frequent sequelae. Interstitial pneumonia is more common in adults and may result in ARDS or death. Encephalitis is infrequent (1:1000), is characterized by ataxia and nystagmus, and usually results in complete recovery.

Reye's syndrome (hepatic encephalopathy) is a severe sequela of varicella (and other viruses, especially influenza B) and has been associated with aspirin therapy (see below).

Varicella in immunosuppressed patients (eg, those receiving antitumor chemotherapy, transplant patients) is often severe and may be fatal.

When contracted during the first or second trimesters of pregnancy, varicella carries a risk of congenital malformations whose constellation includes cicatricial lesions of an extremity, growth retardation, microphthalmia, cataracts, chorioretinitis, deafness, and cerebrocortical atrophy. If a mother develops varicella within 5 days after delivery, the newborn is at great risk of severe disease and should receive varicella-zoster immune globulin (VZIG). (See below for dosage.)

B. Herpes Zoster: In immunosuppressed patients, herpes zoster may disseminate, producing skin lesions beyond the dermatome, visceral lesions, and encephalitis. This is a serious, sometimes fatal complication.

Postherpetic neuralgias occur in 50% of zoster patients over age 60.

Prevention

A. Varicella: Varicella-zoster immune globulin (VZIG) is effective in preventing chickenpox in exposed susceptible immunosuppressed individuals. It is given by deep intramuscular injection in a dosage of 12.5 units/kg up to a maximum of 625 units, with a repeat dose in 3 weeks if a high-risk patient remains exposed. VZIG has no place in therapy, however. VZIG may be obtained by calling the nearest regional Red Cross Blood Center or the Centers for Disease Control and Prevention, Atlanta; day phone (404) 639–1870.

A live attenuated vaccine for immunocompromised susceptible children appears to be safe and effective, with a few recipients developing a mild rash. Attack rates are significantly reduced. However, the vaccine is not available as of 1993.

B. Zoster: There are no known means of effectively preventing zoster eruptions.

Treatment

A. General Measures: Isolate the patient until primary crusts have disappeared, and keep at bed rest until afebrile. Hospital patients with varicella-zoster should be placed in isolation rooms, and personnel entering the room should wear gowns, gloves, and masks. Keep the skin clean by means of frequent tub baths or showers when afebrile. Oral antihistamines, topical calamine lotion, and colloidal oatmeal baths may relieve pruritus. If antipyretics are necessary, acetaminophen rather than aspirin should be given to avoid risk of Reye's syndrome.

B. Treatment of Complications: Secondary bacterial infections of lesions are managed with baci-

Table 31–2. Diagnostic features of some acute exanthems.

Disease	Prodromal Signs and Symptoms	Nature of Eruption	Other Diagnostic Features	Laboratory Tests
Measles (rubeola)	3–4 days of fever, coryza, conjunctivitis, and cough.	Maculopapular, brick-red; begins on head and neck; spreads downward. In 5–6 days rash brownish, desquamating. See atypical measles.	Koplik's spots on buccal mucosa.	White blood count low. Virus isolation in cell culture. Antibody tests by hemagglutination inhibition or neutralization.
Atypical measles	Same as measles.	Maculopapular centripetal rash, becoming confluent.	History of measles vaccination.	Measles antibody present in past, with titer rise during illness.
Rubella	Little or no prodrome.	Maculopapular, pink; begins on head and neck, spreads downward, fades in 3 days. No desquamation.	Lymphadenopathy, postauricular or occipital.	White blood count normal or low. Serologic tests for immunity and definitive diagnosis (hemagglutination inhibition).
Varicella (chickenpox)	0–1 day of fever, anorexia, headache.	Rapid evolution of macules to papules, vesicles, crusts; all stages simultaneously present; lesions superficial, distribution centripetal.	Lesions on scalp and mucous membranes.	Specialized complement fixation and virus neutralization in cell culture. Fluorescent antibody test of smear of lesions.
Scarlet fever	½–2 days of malaise, sore throat, fever, vomiting.	Generalized, punctate, red; prominent on neck, in axilla, groin, skinfolds; circumoral pallor; fine desquamation involves hands and feet.	Strawberry tongue, exudative tonsillitis.	Group A hemolytic streptococci cultures from throat; antistreptolysin O titer rise.
Exanthem subitum (Roseola)	3–4 days of high fever.	As fever falls by crisis, pink maculopapules appear on chest and trunk; fade in 1–3 days.		White blood count low.
Erythema infectiosum	None. Usually in epidemics.	Red, flushed cheeks; circumoral pallor; maculopapules on extremities.	"Slapped face" appearance.	White blood count normal.
Meningococcemia	Hours of fever, vomiting.	Maculopapules, petechiae, purpura.	Meningeal signs, toxicity, shock.	Cultures of blood, cerebrospinal fluid. High white blood count.
Rocky Mt. spotted fever	3–4 days of fever, chills, severe headaches.	Maculopapules, petechiae, initial distribution centripetal (extremities to trunk).	History of tick bite.	Agglutination (OX19, OX2), complement fixation.
Typhus	3–4 days of fever, chills, severe headaches.	Maculopapules, petechiae, initial distribution centrifugal (trunk to extremities).	Endemic area, lice.	Agglutination (OX19), complement fixation.
Infectious mononucleosis	Fever, adenopathy, sore throat.	Maculopapular rash resembling rubella, rarely papulovesicular.	Splenomegaly, tonsillar exudate.	Atypical lymphocytes in blood smears; heterophil agglutination. Monospot test.
Enterovirus infections	1–2 days of fever, malaise.	Maculopapular rash resembling rubella, rarely papulovesicular or petechial.	Aseptic meningitis.	Virus isolation from stool or cerebrospinal fluid; complement fixation titer rise.
Drug eruptions	Occasionally fever.	Maculopapular rash resembling rubella, rarely papulovesicular.		Eosinophilia.
Eczema herpeticum	None.	Vesiculopustular lesions in area of eczema.		Herpes simplex virus isolated in cell culture. Multinucleate giant cells in smear of lesion.
Kawasaki disease	Fever, adenopathy, conjunctivitis.	Cracked lips, strawberry tongue, maculopapular polymorphous rash, peeling skin on fingers and toes.	Edema of extremities. Angiitis of coronary arteries.	Thrombocytosis, electrocardiographic changes.

tracin-neomycin, mupirocin (2% ointment), or anti-staphylococcal oral antibiotics if lesions are extensive (eg, dicloxacillin, 250 mg four times daily for 10 days). In immunocompromised patients, antiviral therapy with high-dose acyclovir (30 mg/kg/d in three divided doses intravenously for at least 7 days) should be started as soon as possible. It should also be instituted for severe disease (pneumonitis, corneal or trigeminal ganglion involvement) in immunocompetent persons (see Chapter 37).

The mainstay of antiviral therapy for varicella infections is acyclovir, which is effective in reducing the severity and shortening the duration of chickenpox and shingles both in adults and in children. However, acyclovir has little effect on postherpetic pain. Corticosteroids have been used to reduce the incidence of postherpetic neuralgia in the elderly but the drugs are usually ineffective; a short course will probably not have deleterious effects. Acyclovir-resistant varicella has been observed in AIDS patients receiving chronic acyclovir therapy.

Eye involvement in zoster demands ophthalmologic referral and use of mydriatics, topical steroids, and perhaps antivirals (vidarabine).

Prognosis

The total duration of varicella from onset of symptoms to disappearance of crusts rarely exceeds 2 weeks. Fatalities are rare except in immunosuppressed patients. Zoster resolves in 2–6 weeks. Antibodies persist longer and at higher levels than with primary varicella.

Benoldi D et al: Prevention of post-herpetic neuralgia: Evaluation of treatment with oral prednisone, oral acyclovir, and radiotherapy. Int J Dermatol 1991;30:288.

Gershon AA et al: Varicella vaccine: The American experience. J Infect Dis 1992;166(Suppl 1):S63.

Haake DA et al: Early treatment with acyclovir for varicella pneumonia in otherwise healthy adults: Retrospective controlled study and review. Rev Infect Dis 1990; 12:788.

Jacobson MA et al: Acyclovir-resistant varicella zoster virus infection after chronic oral acyclovir therapy in patients with AIDS. Ann Intern Med 1990;112:187.

Weller TH: Varicella and herpes zoster: A perspective and overview. J Infect Dis 1992;166(Suppl 1):S1.

Whitley RJ: Therapeutic approaches to varicella-zoster virus infections. J Infect Dis 1992;166(Suppl 1):S51.

3. INFECTIOUS MONONUCLEOSIS

Essentials of Diagnosis

- Fever, sore throat, malaise, lymphadenopathy.
- Splenomegaly and occasionally a maculopapular rash.
- Positive heterophil agglutination test (Monospot).
- "Atypical" large lymphocytes in blood smear; lymphocytosis.

- Hepatitis; occasionally myocarditis, neuritis, encephalitis.

General Considerations

Infectious mononucleosis is an acute infectious disease due to the Epstein-Barr (EB) virus (human herpesvirus 4). It is universal in distribution and may occur at any age but usually occurs between the ages of 10 and 35, either in an epidemic form or as sporadic cases. Rare cases have been reported in the elderly, usually without the full complex of symptoms. Its mode of transmission is probably by saliva. The incubation period is probably 5–15 days or longer.

Clinical Findings

A. Symptoms and Signs: Symptoms are varied but typically include fever; discrete, nonsuppurative, slightly painful, enlarged lymph nodes, especially those of the posterior cervical chain; and, in approximately half of cases, splenomegaly. Sore throat is often present, and toxic symptoms (malaise, anorexia, and myalgia) occur frequently in the early phase of the illness. A maculopapular or occasionally petechial rash occurs in fewer than 15% of cases unless ampicillin has been given (when rash may be seen in > 90%). Exudative pharyngitis, tonsillitis, or gingivitis may occur.

Other manifestations of infectious mononucleosis are hepatitis, nausea, anorexia, and jaundice; central nervous system involvement with headache, neck stiffness, photophobia, painful neuritis, and occasionally even Guillain-Barré syndrome; pulmonary involvement with chest pain, dyspnea, and cough; and myocardial involvement with tachycardia and arrhythmias.

The varying symptoms of infectious mononucleosis—especially sore throat, hepatitis, rash, and lymphadenopathy—raise difficult problems in differential diagnosis.

B. Laboratory Findings: Initially, there is a granulocytopenia followed within 1 week by a lymphocytic leukocytosis. Many lymphocytes are atypical, ie, are larger than normal mature lymphocytes, stain more darkly, and frequently show vacuolated, foamy cytoplasm and dark chromatin in the nucleus. Hemolytic anemia secondary to anti-i antibodies (cold agglutinin disease) is occasionally encountered, as is thrombocytopenia (at times severe).

Heterophil (sheep cell agglutination) antibody tests and the correlated mononucleosis spot (Monospot) test usually become positive in infectious mononucleosis before the fourth week after onset of illness. Heterophil-negative tests are not uncommon in children. Titer rises in antibodies directed at several EB virus antigens can be detected by immunofluorescence. During acute illness there is a rise in IgM antibody to EB virus capsid antigen (VCA), while antibodies to EB virus nuclear antigen (EBNA) appear at 3–4 weeks after onset. A false-positive VDRL or RPR test occurs in 10% of cases.

In central nervous system involvement, the cerebrospinal fluid may show increase of pressure, abnormal lymphocytes, and protein.

With myocardial involvement, the electrocardiographic studies may show abnormal T waves and prolonged PR intervals.

Hepatic serum aminotransferases and bilirubin are commonly elevated.

Differential Diagnosis

Causes of pharyngitis with exudate include diphtheria and adenovirus, herpes simplex, gonococcal, and streptococcal infections. Cytomegalovirus infection, toxoplasmosis, and rubella may be indistinguishable from infectious mononucleosis due to EB virus, but the heterophil antibody and Monospot tests are negative. Mycoplasmal infection may also present primarily with pharyngitis, though lower respiratory symptoms usually predominate.

Complications

These usually consist of secondary throat infections, often streptococcal, and (rarely) rupture of the spleen or hypersplenism (usually during the second or third weeks of illness). Rarely, there may be a variety of neurologic involvements, eg, transverse myelitis.

Treatment

A. General Measures: No specific treatment is available, and acyclic antiviral compounds (acyclovir, ganciclovir) are not helpful. The patient requires support and reassurance because of the frequent feeling of lassitude and the duration of symptoms. Symptomatic relief can be afforded by the administration of aspirin or another nonsteroidal antiinflammatory agent, and hot saline throat irrigations or gargles three or four times daily. In severely ill patients, when enlarged lymphoid tissue threatens to obstruct the airway, a 5-day course of corticosteroids (eg, prednisolone, 50 mg/d for 3 days, with tapering) may be beneficial; severe thrombocytopenia and autoimmune hemolytic anemia also may respond to corticosteroids; pericarditis and impending splenic rupture are not clear-cut indications for corticosteroid therapy.

B. Treatment of Complications: Hepatitis, myocarditis, and encephalitis are treated symptomatically. Rupture of the spleen requires emergency splenectomy. In order to avoid this complication, it is best to avoid frequent deep palpation of the spleen or vigorous activity.

Prognosis

In uncomplicated cases, fever disappears in 10 days and lymphadenopathy and splenomegaly in 4

weeks. The debility sometimes lingers for 2–3 months.

Death is uncommon; when it does occur it is usually due to splenic rupture or hypersplenic phenomena (severe hemolytic anemia, thrombocytopenic purpura) or to encephalitis.

Cheeseman SH: Infectious mononucleosis. Semin Hematol 1988;25:261.
See also references at end of next section.

4. OTHER EBV SYNDROMES

EB virus infections rarely are associated with B cell lymphomas. A special case, Burkitt's lymphoma of the jaw in African children, regularly shows the presence of EB viral antigens. The etiologic role of EB virus in this neoplasm is not established. While Burkitt's lymphoma in Africa responds to radiation therapy or anticancer chemotherapy, the effect of antiviral drugs is unknown. The rare cases of Burkitt's lymphoma in the USA are much more invasive, respond poorly to therapy, and are not regularly associated with EB virus. EB virus has also been associated with nasopharyngeal carcinoma in some populations, but again, the role of the virus is unclear.

An inability to eliminate EBV has a well-established association with the X-linked lymphoproliferative syndrome, affecting young males. Lymphoproliferative disease due to EBV is also seen in congenital and acquired immunodeficiencies, including up to 3% of renal transplants, wherein the presentation is typically a solid tumor often invading the allograft and frequently involving the small intestine or central nervous system. There is no credible evidence that chronic fatigue syndrome is caused by chronic EBV infection; instead, this syndrome is associated with elevated antibody titers to many viruses; further, few markers of lymphocyte activation are present, as is seen in EBV infections. Oral hairy leukoplakia is discussed in Chapter 8.

Radiation and anticancer chemotherapy are the treatment of choice for Burkitt's lymphoma. For EBV-induced lymphoproliferative syndrome, the mainstay of therapy is decreasing the dose of immunosuppressive agents plus resection of bulky lesions.

Andersson JP: Clinical aspects on Epstein-Barr infection. Scand J Infect Dis Suppl 1991;80:94.
Cohen JI: Epstein-Barr virus lymphoproliferative disease associated with acquired immunodeficiency. Medicine 1991;70:137.

5. CYTOMEGALOVIRUS DISEASE

Most cytomegalovirus infections in healthy individuals are asymptomatic, with the virus remaining latent (exact cells of latency are not known). However, the virus is isolable from up to 25% of salivary glands, 10% of uterine cervices, and 1% of neonatal urine samples. Seroprevalence increases with age and with the number of sexual partners; detectable antibody is present in the serum of most homosexual men. Transmission is sexual, congenital, through blood products or transplantation, and person-to-person (eg, day care centers). Severe disease occurs primarily in the immunocompromised, especially those with AIDS and transplant patients.

Clinical Findings

A. Classification: There are three recognizable clinical syndromes.

1. Perinatal disease and cytomegalovirus inclusion disease–Intrauterine infection of infants whose mothers had a primary infection during pregnancy results in a neonatal syndrome of jaundice, hepatosplenomegaly, thrombocytopenia, periventricular central nervous system calcifications, mental retardation, motor disability, and purpura. Diagnosis is confirmed by viruria within the first week after birth or serum IgM antibodies to cytomegalovirus. Hearing deficits occur in over 15% and mental retardation in up to 30%. Neonatally acquired disease may resemble mononucleosis; while it is often asymptomatic, neurologic deficits may ensue later in life.

2. Acute acquired cytomegalovirus infection–This syndrome, akin to EBV-associated infectious mononucleosis, is characterized by fever, malaise, myalgias and arthralgias (but not pharyngitis or respiratory symptoms), atypical lymphocytes, and abnormal liver function tests. Unlike EBV-associated infectious mononucleosis, the heterophil antibody is not found. Transmission can be by sexual contact, by milk, by respiratory droplets (probably) among nursery or day care center attendants, and by (usually massive) transfusions of blood.

3. Disease in immunocompromised hosts–Tissue (kidney, heart, lung, liver) and bone marrow transplant recipients are at a definite increased risk for cytomegalovirus infection, with pneumonia particularly occurring among bone marrow transplant recipients; pathology is due to the immune response and is seen up to 100 days after allograft transplantation. The immunosuppression of AIDS can result in cytomegalovirus disease with the most common manifestation being retinitis. Patients can be screened by asking for visual symptoms, although diagnosis requires documenting neovascular, proliferative lesions ("pizza-pie" retinopathy). Cytomegalovirus in AIDS affects many parts of the gastrointestinal and hepatobiliary tract. Esophagitis presents with pain on swallowing; pancreatitis, when not due to ddI, ddC, or pentamidine, is often due to cytomegalovirus; and hepatobiliary involvement often includes other pathogens including *Cryptosporidium*. Polyradiculopathy, encephalitis, and pneumonia can be due to cytomegalovirus but are uncommon in AIDS. Cytomegalovirus itself is immunosuppressive and may worsen manifestations of HIV infection including *Pneumocystis carinii* pneumonia.

B. Laboratory Findings: Cytomegalovirus is isolable from urine, cervical secretions, semen, saliva, blood, and other tissues, but virus isolation is most useful when combined with pathologic findings, including large cells with intranuclear and intracytoplasmic inclusions that resemble owl's eyes; cultures alone are of little use in diagnosing AIDS-related cytomegalovirus infections. Retinitis among AIDS patients is diagnosed clinically. The acute mononucleosis syndrome is associated with a lymphocytosis, often 2 weeks after the fever. Serologic tests (indirect fluorescent antibody [IFA], anti-complement immunofluorescent antibody [ACIF]) are useful primarily in seroepidemiologic studies. In AIDS patients, titers may be depressed, and seroconversions are seldom documented, with most seroconversions having occurred in the past. Antigen detection by virus technology (including the polymerase chain reaction technique) must be interpreted in the context of clinical and pathologic findings.

Prevention

Cytomegalovirus hyperimmune globulin given to seronegative bone marrow or renal transplant recipients may be prophylactic. Limiting transfusions, using products filtered to remove leukocytes, and selecting cytomegalovirus-seronegative donors are all important in reducing the rate of cytomegalovirus transmission. Acyclovir and ganciclovir also reduce the incidence of cytomegalovirus disease after transplant.

Treatment

Two antiviral agents with efficacy against cytomegalovirus are ganciclovir (an acyclovir analogue, also called DHPG), given in a dosage of 5 mg/kg intravenously every 12 hours for 14–21 days (maintenance: 5–7 mg/kg/d for 5 days each week, with dose reduction for renal impairment); and foscarnet, given as a loading dose of 20 mg/kg intravenously and then 60 mg/kg every 8 hours over 2 weeks (maintenance: 60 mg/kg/d). The induction phase is essential for AIDS patients with cytomegalovirus disease involving critical parts of the retina; for less critical areas, maintenance therapy can be used from the outset. Both agents are effective in preventing progression of retinitis, and ganciclovir is useful in cytomegalovirus colitis; treatment is usually lifelong in patients with AIDS. Complications include neutropenia with ganciclovir (preventing concomitant zidovudine therapy) and renal impairment with foscarnet (often manageable with hydration) (Table 31–1).

Drew WL: Clinical use of ganciclovir for CMV infection and the development of drug resistance. J Acquir Immune Defic Syndr 1991;4:S42.

Jabs DA, Enger C, Bartlett JG: Cytomegalovirus retinitis and acquired immunodeficiency syndrome. Arch Ophthalmol 1989;107:75.

Levinson ML, Jacobson PA: Treatment and prophylaxis of cytomegalovirus disease. Pharmacotherapy 1992;12:300.

Merigan TC, Resta S: Cytomegalovirus: Where have we been and where are we going? Rev Infect Dis 1990;12:S693.

Meyers JD: Chemoprophylaxis of viral infection in immunocompromised patients. Eur J Cancer Clin Oncol 1989;25:1369.

Sayers MHJ et al: Reducing the risk for transfusion-related CMV infection. Ann Intern Med 1992;116:55.

MAJOR VACCINE-PREVENTABLE VIRAL INFECTIONS

1. MEASLES

Essentials of Diagnosis

- Prodrome of fever, coryza, cough, conjunctivitis, photophobia, Koplik's spots.
- Rash: brick-red, irregular, maculopapular; onset 3–4 days after onset of prodrome; face to trunk to extremities.
- Leukopenia.
- Exposure 10–14 days previously in an unvaccinated patient.

General Considerations

Measles is an acute systemic viral (paramyxovirus) infection transmitted by inhalation of infective droplets. It is the cause of death for 1 million children worldwide yearly. Its highest incidence is in young children. Illness confers permanent immunity. Communicability is greatest during the preeruptive stage but continues as long as the rash remains. Sporadic recent outbreaks of the disease in adults, adolescents, and unvaccinated preschool children in dense urban areas have led to changes in recommendations concerning prevention (see below).

Clinical Findings

A. Symptoms and Signs: (Table 31–2.) Fever is often as high as 40–40.6 °C (104–105 °F). It persists through the prodrome and early rash (about 5–7 days). Malaise may be marked. Coryza (nasal obstruction, sneezing, and sore throat) resembles that seen with upper respiratory infections. Cough is persistent and nonproductive. There is conjunctivitis, with redness, swelling, photophobia, and discharge.

Koplik's spots are pathognomonic of measles. They appear about 2 days before the rash and last 1–4 days as tiny "table salt crystals" on the dull red mucous membranes of the cheeks and often on inner conjunctival folds and vaginal mucous membranes. Other findings include pharyngeal erythema, a yellowish exudate on the tonsils, coating of the tongue in the center with a red tip and margins, moderate generalized lymphadenopathy, and occasionally splenomegaly.

The rash usually appears first on the face and behind the ears 4 days after the onset of symptoms. The initial lesions are pinhead-sized papules which coalesce to form a brick-red, irregular, blotchy maculopapular rash; in severe cases, the rash may coalesce to form a nearly uniform erythema on some body areas. The rash next appears on the trunk, followed by the extremities, including the palms and soles. It fades in order of appearance. Hyperpigmentation remains in fair-skinned individuals and severe cases. Slight desquamation may follow.

Atypical measles is a syndrome occurring in adolescents or adults who have received inactivated measles vaccine (available 1963–1967) or who received live measles vaccine before age 12 months and as a result have developed hypersensitivity rather than protective immunity. When they are infected with wild measles virus, such individuals may develop a severe illness with high fever, unusual rashes (papular, hemorrhagic) without Koplik's spots, headache, arthralgias, hepatitis, and interstitial infiltrates, occasionally with pleural effusions. It can be fatal.

B. Laboratory Findings: Leukopenia is usually present unless secondary bacterial complications exist. Proteinuria is often present. Although technically difficult, virus can be cultured from nasopharyngeal washings and from blood. A fourfold rise in serum hemagglutination inhibition antibody supports the diagnosis.

Complications

A. Central Nervous System Complications: Encephalitis occurs in approximately 1:2000–1:1000 cases. Its onset is usually 3–7 days after the rash. Vomiting, convulsions, coma, and a variety of severe neurologic signs and symptoms develop. Treatment is symptomatic and supportive. Virus is usually not found in the central nervous system, though demyelination is prominent. There is an appreciable mortality rate (10–20%), and many patients are left with permanent sequelae.

Subacute sclerosing panencephalitis (SSPE) is a very late central nervous system complication, the measles virus acting as a "slow virus" to produce degenerative central nervous system disease years after the initial infection. SSPE is rare (1:100,000 cases of measles) and occurs more often when measles develops early in life, among males, and among rural cases.

An acute progressive encephalitis, characterized by seizures, neurologic deficits, and often progressive stupor and death, can occur among immunosuppressed patients; measles virus is found as an opportunistic invader in the central nervous system.

B. Respiratory Tract Disease: Early in the course of the disease, bronchopneumonia or bronchiolitis due to the measles virus may occur in 1–7% and result in serious difficulties with ventilation. Pneumonia occurring with or without an evanescent rash is seen in atypical measles.

C. Secondary Bacterial Infections: Immediately following measles, secondary bacterial infection—particularly cervical adenitis, otitis media, and pneumonia—occurs in about 15% of patients.

D. Tuberculosis: Measles produces temporary anergy to the tuberculin skin test; there may be exacerbations in tuberculosis patients.

Prevention

In the United States, most children receive their first vaccine dose at 15 months and a second at age 4–6 years prior to entry into school (see Table 29–4). In high-risk areas and in counties with large inner city populations—or if there have been recent cases among unvaccinated preschool children—the first dose may be administered at 12 months. Students beyond high school and medical staff starting employment must have the above vaccination schedule documented—or must have serologic evidence of immunity—if they were born after 1956. For individuals born before 1957, herd immunity can be assumed; health care workers should probably be screened and vaccinated if necessary regardless of date of birth.

Outbreak control is similar. If outbreaks are occurring in preschool children under 1 year of age, initial vaccination may be given at 6 months, with repeat at 15 months. When outbreaks take place in day care centers, K–12 institutions, or colleges and universities, revaccination is probably indicated for all, in particular for students and their siblings born after 1956 who do not have documentation of immunity as defined above. Susceptible personnel who have been exposed should be isolated from patient contact from the fifth to the 21st day after exposure irrespective of whether they have been vaccinated or have received immune globulin; if they should develop measles, they should be isolated from patient contact until 7 days after the rash develops.

When susceptible individuals are exposed to measles, the live virus vaccine can prevent disease if given within 5 days of exposure. This is rarely feasible in a household. Later, gamma globulin (0.25 mL/kg [0.11 mL/lb] body weight) can be injected for prevention of clinical illness. This must be followed by active immunization with live measles vaccine 3 months later.

Vaccination of all immunocompetent persons born after 1956 who travel to the developing world is essential.

Pregnant women and the immunosuppressed in general should not receive this or other live virus vaccines, though measles vaccination is recommended for all HIV-infected children and may be associated with improved survival following severe measles. Immune globulin should be considered for postexposure prophylaxis to any HIV-infected person exposed to measles.

Treatment

A. General Measures: Isolate the patient for the week following onset of rash and keep at bed rest until afebrile. Treat symptomatically as necessary. Vitamin A, 400,000 IU/d orally, has been shown to reduce pediatric morbidity and mortality rates in hospitalized measles patients.

B. Treatment of Complications: Secondary bacterial infections are treated with appropriate antimicrobial drugs. Postmeasles encephalitis, including SSPE, can only be treated symptomatically.

Prognosis

The mortality rate of measles in children in the USA is 0.2%, but it may be as high as 10% in children in developing nations. Deaths in the USA are due principally to encephalitis (15% mortality rate) and bacterial pneumonia and are more common for successive generations of a given outbreak. Deaths in the developing world are mainly related to diarrhea and protein-losing enteropathy.

Hersh BS et al: The geographic distribution of measles in the United States, 1980 through 1989. JAMA 1992; 267:1936.

Hussey GD, Klein M: A randomized, controlled trial of vitamin A in children with severe measles. N Engl J Med 1990;323:160.

Isaacs D, Menser M: Measles, mumps, rubella, and varicella. Lancet 1990;335:1384.

Kaplan LJ et al: Severe measles in immunocompromised patients. JAMA 1992;267:1237.

Lepow ML: Measles vaccine and measles control. Pediatr Ann 1990;19:542, 548.

Mast EE et al: Risk factors for measles in a previously vaccinated population and cost-effectiveness of revaccination strategies. JAMA 1990;264:2529.

The National Vaccine Advisory Committee: The measles epidemic: The problems, barriers, and recommendations. JAMA 1991;266:1547.

Peter G: Childhood immunizations. (Current Concepts.) N Engl J Med 1992;327:1794.

Schwarcz S, McCaw B, Fukushima P: Prevalence of measles susceptibility in hospital staff. Arch Intern Med 1992;152:481.

2. MUMPS

Essentials of Diagnosis

- Painful, swollen salivary glands, usually parotid.
- Exposure 14–21 days previously.
- Frequent involvement of other tissues, including

testes, pancreas, and meninges, in unvaccinated individuals.

General Considerations

Mumps is a viral (paramyxovirus) disease spread by respiratory droplets that usually produces inflammation of the salivary glands and, less commonly, orchitis, aseptic meningitis, pancreatitis, and oophoritis. Most patients are children. The incubation period is 14–21 days (average, 18 days). Infectivity precedes the symptoms by about 1 day, is maximal for 3 days but may last a week.

Clinical Findings

A. Symptoms and Signs: Fever and malaise are variable but are often minimal in young children. High fever usually accompanies orchitis or meningitis. Pain and swelling of one or both (75%) of the parotid or other salivary glands occur, usually in succession 1–3 days apart. Occasionally, one gland subsides completely (usually in 7 days or less) before others become involved. Orchitis occurs in 25% of postpubertal men. Headache and lethargy suggest meningitis. Upper abdominal pain and nausea and vomiting suggest pancreatitis. Lower abdominal pain suggesting oophoritis occurs in 25% of postpubertal women.

Tender parotid swelling and overlying facial edema are the commonest physical finding. Swelling and tenderness of the submaxillary and sublingual glands are variable. The orifice of Stensen's duct may be reddened and swollen. Salivary gland involvement must be differentiated from lymph node involvement in the anterior cervical space. Neck stiffness and other signs of meningeal irritation suggest meningitis. Testicular swelling and tenderness (unilateral in 75%) denote orchitis. Epigastric tenderness suggests pancreatitis. Lower abdominal tenderness and ovarian enlargement may be noted in mumps oophoritis, but the diagnosis is often difficult.

B. Laboratory Findings: Relative lymphocytosis may be present. Serum amylase is commonly elevated with or without pancreatitis. Lymphocytic pleocytosis (and normal to low glucose) of the cerebrospinal fluid is present in meningitis, which may be asymptomatic. The diagnosis is confirmed by isolating mumps virus from saliva or cerebrospinal fluid or demonstrating a fourfold rise in complement-fixing antibodies in paired sera.

Differential Diagnosis

Swelling of the parotid gland may be due to calculi in the parotid ducts or to a reaction to iodides. Other causes include starch ingestion, sarcoidosis, cirrhosis, diabetes, and bulimia. Parotitis may also be produced by pyogenic organisms (eg, *S aureus*), particularly in debilitated individuals, drug reaction (phenylbutazone, phenothiazines, propylthiouracil), and other viruses (influenza A, parainfluenza, EBV infection, coxsackieviruses). Swelling of the parotid gland must be differentiated from inflammation of the lymph nodes that are located more posteriorly and inferiorly than the parotid gland.

Complications

The "complications" of mumps are simply other manifestations of the disease less common than inflammation of the salivary glands. These usually follow the parotitis but may precede it or occur without salivary gland involvement: meningitis (30%), orchitis (occurs mainly after puberty in 25% of infected men, and on rare occasion leads to priapism or testicular infarction), pancreatitis, oophoritis, thyroiditis, neuritis, myocarditis, thrombocytopenic purpura, migratory arthralgias, and nephritis.

Aseptic meningitis is common during the course of mumps and may occur without salivary gland involvement. This is a very benign self-limited illness. Rare neurologic complications include encephalitis, Guillain-Barré syndrome, and transverse myelitis. Encephalitis is associated with cerebral edema, serious neurologic manifestations, and sometimes death. Deafness may develop (rarely) as a result of eighth nerve neuritis.

Prevention

Mumps live virus vaccine is safe and highly effective. It is recommended for routine immunization for children over age 1 year, either alone or in combination with other virus vaccines (eg, with measles and rubella—in MMR vaccine). It should not be given to immunocompromised individuals or to pregnant women. Its use has markedly decreased the incidence of mumps in the USA. The mumps skin test is less reliable in determining immunity than are serum neutralization titers.

Treatment

A. General Measures: Isolate the patient until swelling subsides and keep at bed rest during the febrile period. Treat symptomatically as needed.

B. Management of Complications:

1. Meningitis–The treatment of aseptic meningitis is purely symptomatic. The management of encephalitis requires attention to cerebral edema, the airway, and vital functions.

2. Orchitis–Suspend the scrotum in a suspensory or toweling "bridge" and apply ice bags. Incision of the tunica may be necessary in severe cases. Give codeine or morphine as necessary for pain. Pain can also be relieved by injection of the spermatic cord at the external inguinal ring with 10–20 mL of 1% procaine solution. Hydrocortisone sodium succinate (100 mg intravenously, followed by 20 mg orally every 6 hours for 2 or 3 days) to reduce the inflammatory reaction, is of questionable benefit.

3. Pancreatitis–Provide symptomatic treatment only and parenteral fluids if necessary.

4. Oophoritis–Give symptomatic treatment only.

Prognosis

The entire course of mumps rarely exceeds 2 weeks. Fatalities (from encephalitis) are rare.

Orchitis often makes the patient very uncomfortable but very rarely results in sterility. Mumps is not known to be associated with stillbirths or teratogenicity.

Cochi SL, Preblud SR, Orenstein WA: Perspectives on the relative resurgence of mumps in the United States. Am J Dis Child 1988;142:499.

Mumps prevention. MMWR Morb Mortal Wkly Rep 1989;38(22):388, 397.

Mumps: United States, 1985–1988. MMWR Morb Mortal Wkly Rep 1989;38(7):101.

3. POLIOMYELITIS

Essentials of Diagnosis

- Muscle weakness, headache, stiff neck, fever, nausea and vomiting, sore throat.
- Lower motor neuron lesion (flaccid paralysis) with decreased deep tendon reflexes and muscle wasting.
- Cerebrospinal fluid shows excess leukocytes. Lymphocytes predominate; rarely more than 500/μL.

General Considerations

Poliomyelitis virus, an enterovirus, is present in throat washings and stools. Infection is most commonly acquired by the fecal-oral route. Since the introduction of effective vaccine, poliomyelitis has become a rare disease in developed areas of the world. Among 86 cases in the United States over the last decade, 5 were imported and 80 were vaccine-associated, either in recipients (30), contacts (36), or the immunocompromised (14). Poliomyelitis is nearly eradicated from the Western Hemisphere.

Three antigenically distinct types of poliomyelitis virus (I, II, and III) are recognized, with no cross-immunity between them.

The incubation period is 5–35 days (usually 7–14 days). Infectivity is maximal during the first week, but virus is excreted in stools for several weeks.

Clinical Findings

A. Symptoms and Signs: At least 95% of infections are asymptomatic, but in those who become ill the following manifestations are seen.

1. Minor illness (abortive poliomyelitis)–The symptoms are fever, headache, vomiting, diarrhea, constipation, and sore throat.

2. Nonparalytic poliomyelitis–In addition to the above symptoms, signs of meningeal irritation and muscle spasm occur.

3. Paralytic poliomyelitis–Paralytic poliomyelitis represents 0.1% of all poliomyelitis cases. Paralysis may occur at any time during the febrile period. Tremors, muscle weakness, constipation, and ileus may appear. Paralytic poliomyelitis may be divided into two forms, which may coexist: (1) spinal poliomyelitis, with weakness of the muscles supplied by the spinal nerves; and (2) bulbar poliomyelitis, with weakness of the muscles supplied by the cranial nerves, involvement of the respiratory and vasomotor centers, and variable "encephalitis" symptoms.

In spinal poliomyelitis, paralysis of the shoulder girdle often precedes intercostal and diaphragmatic paralysis, which leads to diminished chest expansion and decreased vital capacity. Cyanosis (due to hypoxia) and stridor may appear later. Paralysis may quickly become maximal or may progress over a period of several days until the temperature becomes normal. Deep tendon reflexes are diminished or lost, often asymmetrically, in involved areas.

In bulbar poliomyelitis, symptoms include diplopia (uncommonly), facial weakness, dysphagia, dysphonia, nasal voice, weakness of the sternocleidomastoid and trapezius muscles, difficulty in chewing, inability to swallow or expel saliva, and regurgitation of fluids through the nose. In bulbar poliomyelitis there may be loss of gag reflex, loss of movement of palate and pharyngeal muscles, pooling of secretions in the oropharynx, deviation of tongue, and loss of movement of the vocal cords. The most life-threatening aspect of bulbar poliomyelitis is respiratory paralysis.

Lethargy or coma may be due to encephalitis or hypoxia, most often from hypoventilation. Hypertension, hypotension, and tachycardia may occur. Convulsions are rare.

B. Laboratory Findings: The peripheral white blood cell count may be normal or mildly elevated. Cerebrospinal fluid pressure and protein are normal or slightly increased; glucose is not decreased; cells usually number fewer than 500/μL (predominantly lymphocytes; polymorphonuclear cells may be elevated at first). Cerebrospinal fluid is normal in 5% of patients. The virus may be recovered from throat washings (early) and stools (early and late). Neutralizing and complement-fixing antibodies appear during the first or second week of illness.

Differential Diagnosis

Nonparalytic poliomyelitis is very difficult to distinguish from other forms of aseptic meningitis due to other enteroviruses. The distinction is made by laboratory means. Acute infectious polyneuritis (Guillain-Barré) and tick bite paralysis (see Chapter 6) may initially resemble poliomyelitis. In Guillain-Barré syndrome (see Chapter 23), the weakness is more symmetric and ascending, and the cerebrospinal fluid usually has a high protein content but normal cell count.

Complications

Urinary tract infection, atelectasis, pneumonia, myocarditis, and pulmonary edema may occur. Respiratory failure may be a result of paralysis of respiratory muscles, airway obstruction from involvement of cranial nerve nuclei, or lesions of the respiratory center.

Prevention

Oral live trivalent virus vaccine (Sabin) is easily administered, safe, and very effective in providing local gastrointestinal immunity as well as a good level of circulating antibody. It is essential for primary immunization of all immunocompetent infants, among whom the third (6-month) dose is not needed in the developed world, although doses at 2 and 4 months and at 4 and 6 years are required. Routine immunization of adults in the USA is not recommended because of the low incidence of the disease. However, adults who are exposed to poliomyelitis or plan to travel to endemic areas and who have not received polio immunization within the past decade should be given inactivated poliomyelitis vaccine (Salk). This vaccine should also be given when immunization of immunodeficient or immunosuppressed individuals and members of their households is required.

In the developing world, the interval between OPV doses should probably be longer than 1 month (because of interference from enteric pathogens). Universally, it is being considered that the enhanced inactivated poliovirus vaccine be used for the first one or two doses in a combination regimen with OPV to prevent vaccine-associated poliomyelitis.

Treatment

Strict bed rest in the first few days of illness reduces the rate of paralysis. Cranial nerve involvement must be detected promptly. Maintain comfortable but changing positions in a "polio bed": firm mattress, foot board, sponge rubber pads or rolls, sandbags, and light splints. Fecal impaction and urinary retention (especially with paraplegia) must be managed. In cases of respiratory paralysis or weakness, intensive care is needed.

Prognosis

During the febrile period, paralysis may develop or progress. Mild weakness of small muscles is more likely to regress than severe weakness of large muscles. Bulbar poliomyelitis carries the highest mortality rate (up to 50%). New muscle weakness may develop and progress slowly years after recovery from acute paralytic poliomyelitis. This entity, referred to as postpoliomyelitis syndrome, presents with signs of chronic and new denervation, is not infectious in origin, and is associated with increasing dysfunction of surviving motor neurons.

Agre JC et al: Late effects of polio: Critical review of the literature on neuromuscular function. Arch Phys Med Rehabil 1991;72:923.

Patriarca PA, Wright PF, John TJ: Factors affecting the immunogenicity of oral poliovirus vaccine in developing countries: Review. Rev Infect Dis 1991;13:926.

Peters G: Childhood immunizations. N Engl J Med 1992;327:1794.

Strebel PM et al: Epidemiology of poliomyelitis in the United States after the last reported case of indigenous wild virus-associated disease. J Infect Dis 1992;14:568.

4. RUBELLA

Essentials of Diagnosis

- No prodrome in children (mild in adults); mild symptoms (fever, malaise, coryza) coinciding with eruption.
- Posterior cervical and postauricular lymphadenopathy 5–10 days before rash.
- Fine maculopapular rash of 3 days' duration; face to trunk to extremities.
- Leukopenia, thrombocytopenia.
- Exposure 14–21 days previously.
- Arthralgia, particularly in young women.

General Considerations

Rubella is a systemic disease caused by a togavirus transmitted by inhalation of infective droplets. It is only moderately communicable. One attack usually confers permanent immunity. The incubation period is 14–21 days (average, 16 days). The disease is transmissible from 1 week before the rash appears until 15 days afterward.

The clinical picture of rubella is difficult to distinguish from other viral illnesses such as infectious mononucleosis, echovirus infections, and coxsackievirus infections. Definitive diagnosis can only be made by isolating the virus or by serologic means.

The principal importance of rubella lies in the devastating effect this virus has on the fetus in utero, producing teratogenic effects and a continuing congenital infection. Congenital rubella syndrome is not eliminated in the United States, and a Southern California cluster of 21 affected infants occurred in 1990–91.

Clinical Findings

A. Symptoms and Signs: (Table 31–2.) Fever and malaise, usually mild, accompanied by tender suboccipital adenitis, may precede the eruption by 1 week. Mild coryza may be present. Joint pain (polyarthritis) occurs in about 25% of adult cases. These symptoms usually subside within 7 days but may persist for weeks.

Posterior cervical and postauricular lymphadenopathy is very common. Erythema of the palate and throat, sometimes patchy, may be noted. A fine, pink maculopapular rash appears on the face, trunk, and extremities in rapid progression (2–3 days) and fades quickly, usually lasting 1 day in each area. Rubella without rash may be at least as common as the exanthematous disease. Diagnosis can be suspected when there is epidemiologic evidence of the disease in the community but requires laboratory confirmation.

B. Laboratory Findings: Leukopenia may be present early and may be followed by an increase in plasma cells. Virus isolation and serologic tests of immunity (rubella virus hemagglutination inhibition and fluorescent antibody tests) are available. Definitive diagnosis is based on a fourfold rise in the antibody titer.

Complications

A. Exposure During Pregnancy: It is important to know whether rubella antibodies are present at the beginning of pregnancy, since fetal infection during the first trimester may lead to congenital rubella in at least 80% of fetuses.

If a pregnant woman is exposed to a possible case of rubella, an immediate hemagglutination-inhibiting rubella antibody level should be obtained. If antibodies are found, there is no reason for concern. If no antibodies are found, careful clinical and serologic follow-up is essential. If the occurrence of rubella in the expectant mother can be confirmed, therapeutic abortion may be considered. Judgment in this regard is tempered by personal, religious, legal, and other considerations. The risk to the fetus is highest in the first trimester but continues into the second.

B. Congenital Rubella: An infant acquiring the infection in utero may be normal at birth but more likely will have a wide variety of manifestations, including growth retardation, maculopapular rash, thrombocytopenia, cataracts, deafness, congenital heart defects, organomegaly, and others. Viral excretion in the throat and urine persists for many months despite high antibody levels. The diagnosis is confirmed by isolation of the virus. A specific test for IgM rubella antibody is useful for making this diagnosis in the newborn. Treatment is directed to the many anomalies.

C. Postinfectious Encephalopathy: In 1:6000 cases, postinfectious encephalopathy develops 1–6 days after the rash; the virus is not always isolable. The mortality rate is 20%, but residual deficits are rare among those who recover. The mechanism is not established.

Prevention

Live attenuated rubella virus vaccine should be given to all infants and to susceptible girls before the menarche. When women are immunized, they must not be pregnant, and the absence of antibodies should be established. (In the USA, about 80% of 20-year-old women are immune to rubella.) Birth control must be practiced for at least 3 months after the use of this live vaccine. Arthritis following rubella vaccination (more common in women) may relate to hormonal and genetic influences of the immune response to rubella proteins. It is often more severe than that which occurs with the disease.

There are no reports of congenital rubella syndrome after rubella immunization, and inadvertent immunization of a pregnant woman is not considered an indication for therapeutic abortion.

Treatment

Give acetaminophen as required for symptomatic relief. Encephalitis and thrombocytopenia can only be treated symptomatically.

Prognosis

Rubella (other than the congenital form) is a mild illness and rarely lasts more than 3–4 days. Congenital rubella, on the other hand, has a high mortality rate, and the associated congenital defects are largely permanent. The association between chronic arthritis and rubella vaccination is currently under study.

Howson CP, Katz ML: Chronic arthritis after rubella vaccination. Clin Infect Dis 1992;15:307.

Mitchell LA, Zhang T, Tingle AJ: Differential antibody responses to rubella virus infections in males and females. J Infect Dis 1992;166:1258.

Lee SH et al: Resurgence of congenital rubella syndrome in the 1990s. JAMA 1992;267:2616.

Rubella prevention. Recommendations of the Immunization Practices Advisory Committee (ACIP). MMWR Morb Mortal Wkly Rep 1990;39(RR-15):1.

OTHER NEUROTROPIC VIRUSES

1. RABIES

Essentials of Diagnosis

- Paresthesia, hydrophobia, rage alternating with calm.
- Convulsions, paralysis, thick tenacious saliva.
- History of animal bite.

General Considerations

Rabies is a viral (rhabdovirus) encephalitis transmitted by infected saliva that gains entry into the body by a bite or an open wound. Bats, skunks, foxes, and raccoons are widely infected. Dogs and cats are infected in developing countries. Rodents and lagomorphs (eg, rabbits) are unlikely to have rabies. The virus gains entry into the salivary glands of dogs 5–7 days before their death from rabies, thus limiting their period of infectivity. The incubation period may range from 10 days to many years but is usually 3–7 weeks. The interval is dependent in part on distance of the wound from the central nervous system. The virus travels in the nerves to the brain, multiplies there, and then migrates along the efferent nerves to the salivary glands.

Rabies is almost uniformly fatal. Rare cases may be due to rabies-related viruses. The most common clinical problem confronting the physician is the management of a patient bitten by an animal (see Prevention).

Clinical Findings

A. Symptoms and Signs: There is usually a history of animal bite. Pain appears at the site of the bite, followed by paresthesias. The skin is quite sensitive to changes of temperature, especially air currents. Attempts at drinking cause extremely painful laryngeal spasm, so that the patient refuses to drink (hydrophobia). The patient is restless and behaves in a peculiar manner. Muscle spasm, laryngospasm, extreme excitability, convulsions, and paralysis occur. Convulsions occur. Large amounts of thick tenacious saliva are present.

B. Laboratory Findings: Biting animals who are apparently well should be kept under observation for 7–10 days. Sick or dead animals should be examined for rabies. A wild animal, if captured, should be sacrificed and the head shipped on ice to the nearest laboratory qualified to examine the brain for rabies. When the animal cannot be examined, skunks, bats, coyotes, foxes, and raccoons should be presumed to be rabid. The diagnosis of rabies in the brain of a rabid animal may be made rapidly by the fluorescent antibody technique.

Fluorescent antibody testing of skin biopsy material from the posterior neck or a corneal impression may be positive early in the disease; the test may become negative after antibodies develop.

Prevention

Since the disease is almost always fatal, prevention is the only available approach. Immunization of household dogs and cats and active immunization of persons with significant animal exposure (eg, veterinarians) are important. However, the most important common decisions concern animal bites.

A. Local Treatment of Animal Bites and Scratches: Thorough cleaning, debridement, and repeated flushing and cleansing of wounds with soap and water are important. If rabies immune globulin or antiserum is to be used, a portion should be infiltrated locally around the wound (see below) and the remainder given intramuscularly. Wounds caused by animal bites should not be sutured.

B. Postexposure Immunization: The physician must reach a decision based on the recommendations of the USPHS Advisory Committee but should also be influenced by the circumstances of the bite, the extent and location of the wound, the presence of rabies in the region, the type of animal responsible for the bite, etc. (Consultation is provided by state and local health departments.) Treatment includes both passive antibody and vaccine.

The optimal form of passive immunization is rabies immune globulin (40 IU/kg). Up to 50% of the globulin should be used to infiltrate around the wound; the rest is administered intramuscularly. If immune globulin (human) is not available, equine rabies antiserum (20 IU/kg) can be used after appropriate tests for horse serum sensitivity. An inactivated human diploid cell rabies vaccine (HDCV) was licensed in the USA in 1989. It is given as five injections of 1 mL intramuscularly on days 0, 3, 7, 14, and 28 after exposure.

Rabies immune globulin and rabies vaccine (human diploid cell vaccine) should never be given in the same syringe or at the same site. Allergic reactions to the vaccine are rare, though local reactions (pruritus, erythema, tenderness) occur in about 25% and mild systemic reactions (headaches, myalgias, nausea) in about 20% of recipients. The vaccine is commercially available or can be obtained through health departments. Rabies immune globulin is not given if the patient has previously received pre- or postexposure vaccine.

In other countries, inactivated duck embryo vaccine or mouse brain vaccine may be available, but the method of administration is much more complex, the rate of allergic reactions is higher—particularly ascending paralysis—and the efficacy is less.

Preexposure prophylaxis with three injections of diploid cell vaccine is recommended for persons at high risk of exposure (veterinarians, animal handlers, etc). Simultaneous chloroquine prophylaxis for malaria may diminish the antibody response.

Treatment

This very severe illness with an almost universally fatal outcome requires skillful intensive care with attention to the airway, maintenance of oxygenation, and control of seizures. Universal blood and body fluid precautions are essential.

Prognosis

Once the symptoms have appeared, death almost inevitably occurs after 7 days, usually from respiratory failure.

Rabies prevention—United States 1991. Immunization Practices Advisory Committee (ACIP). MMWR Morb Mortal Wkly Rep 1991;40:1.

Warrell DA, Warrell MJ: Human rabies and its prevention: An overview. Rev Infect Dis 1988;10(Suppl 4):S726.

2. ARBOVIRUS ENCEPHALITIDES

Essentials of Diagnosis

- Fever, malaise, stiff neck, sore throat, and nausea and vomiting, progressing to stupor, coma, and convulsions.
- Signs of an upper motor neuron lesion (exaggerated deep tendon reflexes, absent superficial reflexes, pathologic reflexes, spastic paralysis).
- Cerebrospinal fluid protein and pressure often increased, with lymphocytic pleocytosis.

General Considerations

The arboviruses are mosquito- and tick-borne agents that produce clinical manifestations in humans. They include three alphaviruses (causing Western, Eastern, and Venezuelan equine encephalitis), four flaviviruses (causing St. Louis and Japanese B encephalitis, dengue, and yellow fever), and bunyaviruses (causing California [the LaCrosse agent] encephalitis and a series of viral hemorrhagic fevers [Rift Valley fever; hemorrhagic fever with renal syndrome from the Hantaan agent]). Only those agents causing primarily encephalitis will be discussed here (Table 31–3).

In the USA, the leading causes of arbovirus encephalitis are St. Louis and California encephalitis. Agent-specific reservoirs (typically small mammals or birds) are responsible for maintaining the encephalitis-producing viruses in nature; horses serve as sentinels for infection with the equine agents, though birds maintain the life cycle.

Clinical Findings

A. Symptoms and Signs: The symptoms are fever, malaise, sore throat, nausea and vomiting, lethargy, stupor, coma, and convulsions. Signs include stiff neck, signs of meningeal irritation, tremors, convulsions, cranial nerve palsies, paralysis of extremities, exaggerated deep tendon reflexes, absent superficial reflexes, and pathologic reflexes.

B. Laboratory Findings: The white blood cell count is variable. Cerebrospinal fluid pressure and protein content are often increased; glucose is normal; lymphocytic pleocytosis may be present (polymorphonuclears may predominate early in some forms). The virus may sometimes be isolated from blood or, rarely, from cerebrospinal fluid. Serologic tests of blood or cerebrospinal fluid may be diagnostic in specific types of encephalitis (by demonstrating virus-specific IgM in cerebrospinal fluid or a fourfold change in complement-fixing or neutralizing antibodies). A CT scan of the brain may reveal the temporal lobe lesions indicative of herpesvirus but is more important in excluding mass lesions.

Differential Diagnosis

Mild forms of encephalitis must be differentiated from aseptic meningitis, lymphocytic choriomeningitis, and nonparalytic poliomyelitis; severe forms from cerebrovascular accidents, brain tumors, brain abscess, and intoxications.

Arbovirus encephalitides (Table 31–3) must be differentiated from other causes of viral encephalitis (herpes simplex virus, mumps virus, poliovirus or other enteroviruses, HIV), encephalitis accompanying exanthematous diseases of childhood (measles, varicella, infectious mononucleosis, rubella), encephalitis following vaccination (a demyelinating type following rabies, measles, pertussis vaccination), toxic encephalitis (from drugs, poisons or bacterial

Table 31–3. Arbovirus (anthropod-borne) encephalitis.[1]

Disease	Geographic Distribution	Vector; Reservoir	Comment
California encephalitis	Throughout USA, especially Midwest	Mosquitoes; small mammals	Mainly in children
Eastern (equine) encephalitis	Eastern part of North, Central, and South America (coastal areas)	Mosquitoes; birds	Often occurs in horses in the area. High mortality rate; frequent sequelae (seizures, paresis), especially in children.
St. Louis encephalitis	Western and central USA, Florida	Mosquitoes; birds (including domestic fowl)	Frequent cranial nerve findings; prolonged convalescence
Venezuelan encephalitis	South America; Florida (rarely), Texas (rarely)	Mosquitoes; rodents	Rare in USA; low mortality rate; rare sequelae.
Western (equine) encephalitis	Throughout Western Hemisphere	Mosquitoes; birds	Often occurs in horses in this area; particularly affects infants and older adults
Japanese B encephalitis	Temperate East Asia, southern and southeastern Asia	Mosquitoes; pigs and birds	Vaccine available in Orient. High mortality rate (25%) and morbidity rate (50% with neuropsychiatric sequelae).

[1]Seasonal incidence varies with the mosquito season in different areas. It is mainly summer and fall (May through October) in the Northern Hemisphere.

toxins such as *Shigella dysenteriae* type 1), and Reye's syndrome.

Complications

Bronchial pneumonia, urinary retention and infection, and decubitus ulcers may occur. Late sequelae are mental deterioration, parkinsonism, and epilepsy.

Prevention

Effective measures include vigorous mosquito control (repellents, protective clothing, insecticides). A Japanese B vaccine is available in the Orient for summer travelers to rural areas of East Asia.

Treatment

Although specific therapy for the majority of causative entities is not available, vigorous supportive measures can be helpful. Such measures include reduction of intracranial pressure (mannitol), monitoring of intraventricular pressure, the control of convulsions, maintenance of the airway, administration of oxygen, and attention to adequate nutrition during periods of prolonged coma. Corticosteroids have not been shown to affect the outcome of Japanese B encephalitis.

Prevention or early treatment of decubitus ulcers, pneumonia, and urinary tract infections is important. Give anticonvulsants as needed.

No antiviral agent is effective for arboviral encephalitis; acyclovir is effective only for herpes simplex encephalitis (see above).

Prognosis

The prognosis is always guarded, especially in younger children. Sequelae may become apparent late in the course of what appears to be a successful recovery.

Hoke CH et al: Effect of high-dose dexamethasone: The outcome of acute encephalitis due to Japanese encephalitis virus. J Infect Dis 1992;165:631.

Rehle TM: Classification, distribution, and importance of arboviruses. Trop Med Parasitol 1989;40:391.

Tsai TF: Arboviral infections in the United States. Infect Dis Clin North Am 1991;5:73.

3. LYMPHOCYTIC CHORIOMENINGITIS

Essentials of Diagnosis

- "Influenza-like" prodrome of fever, chills, malaise, and cough, followed by meningitis with associated stiff neck.
- Kernig's sign, headache, nausea, vomiting, and lethargy.
- Cerebrospinal fluid: slight increase of protein, lymphocytic pleocytosis (500–3000/µL); low glucose (≥ 25%).
- Complement-fixing antibodies within 2 weeks.

General Considerations

Lymphocytic choriomeningitis is a viral (arenavirus) infection of the central nervous system. The reservoir of infection is the infected house mouse, although naturally infected guinea pigs, monkeys, dogs, and swine have been observed. Pet hamsters may be a source of infection. The virus is shed by the infected animal via oronasal secretions, urine, and feces, with transmission to humans probably through contaminated food and dust. The incubation period is probably 8–13 days to the appearance of systemic manifestations and 15–21 days to the appearance of meningeal symptoms. The disease is not communicable from person to person; outbreaks have occurred in laboratory workers exposed to rodents. Complications are rare.

This disease is principally confined to the eastern seaboard and northeastern states of the USA.

Clinical Findings

A. Symptoms and Signs: Symptoms are biphasic. The prodromal illness is characterized by fever, chills, headache, myalgia, cough, and vomiting, the meningeal phase by headache, nausea and vomiting, and lethargy. Signs of pneumonia are occasionally present during the prodromal phase. During the meningeal phase there may be neck and back stiffness and a positive Kernig sign (meningeal irritation). Severe meningitis may disturb deep tendon reflexes and may cause paralysis and anesthesia of the skin. Arthralgias can occur late.

The prodrome may terminate in complete recovery, or meningeal symptoms may appear after a few days of remission.

B. Laboratory Findings: Leukocytosis or leukopenia and thrombocytopenia may be present. Cerebrospinal fluid lymphocytic pleocytosis (total count is often 500–3000/µL) may occur, with slight increase in protein and normal to low glucose in at least 25%. Complement-fixing antibodies appear during or after the second week. The virus may be recovered from the blood and cerebrospinal fluid by mouse inoculation.

Differential Diagnosis

The influenza-like prodrome and latent period help distinguish this from other aseptic meningitides, and bacterial and granulomatous meningitis. A history of exposure to mice is an important diagnostic clue.

Treatment

Treat supportively as for encephalitis or aseptic meningitis.

Prognosis

Fatality is rare. The illness usually lasts 1–2 weeks, although convalescence may be prolonged.

Dykewicz CA et al: Lymphocytic choriomeningitis outbreak associated with nude mice in a research institute. JAMA 1992;267:1349.

4. VIRUS-LIKE AGENTS WITH LONG LATENCY (Including Prion Disease)

Several animal diseases (visna, scrapie) are caused by communicable agents with slow replication and long latent intervals in the host. Such agents have been called *pro*teinaceous *in*fectious particles resistant to most procedures that modify nucleic acid and are increasingly being referred to as "prions." Four such agents or related agents that cause human disease are discussed here.

Kuru and **Creutzfeldt-Jakob disease** are called spongiform encephalopathies, referring to the appearance of central nervous system tissue on pathologic examination. The agents are transmissible in brain or eye tissue to primates, including humans. On reactivation from the latent state after months to years, diseases ensue that are characterized by an inexorably progressively downhill course. Kuru—once prevalent in central New Guinea but no longer seen since the abandonment of cannibalism—was characterized by cerebellar ataxia, tremors, dysarthria, and emotional lability. Creutzfeldt-Jakob disease presents usually in mid life with progressive dementia, myoclonic fasciculations, ataxia, and somnolence and has an electroencephalographic pattern characterized by paroxysms with high voltages and slow waves. There is no specific treatment, and the only known means of prevention is avoidance of contamination by affected brain tissue, electrodes, or neurosurgical tools or by transplants of cornea or dura from infected donors. Disinfection of equipment requires autoclaving at 15 psi for 1 hour, and disinfection of contaminated surfaces requires 5% hypochlorite or 0.1-N sodium hydroxide solution.

Subacute sclerosing panencephalitis is also a slowly progressive disorder, but pathologic examination shows demyelination rather than spongiform lesions. The disease clinically presents in children (mean age at onset is 7 years) with seizures and dementia and is uniformly fatal. It has been associated with a defective measles virus; measles antibodies are elevated in the cerebrospinal fluid; and, inexplicably, the disease is more common among rural boys.

Progressive multifocal leukoencephalopathy is another progressive demyelinating central nervous system disorder with a propensity for immunosuppressed adults, including AIDS patients. The cause is probably JC virus (JCV), a papovavirus whose main central nervous system target is myelinating oligodendrocytes. JCV has also been identified—not necessarily associated with disease—in central nervous system tissue from HIV-infected and other individuals. Intrathecal cytarabine may be of benefit in AIDS-associated progressive multifocal leukoencephalopathy.

Berger JR, Mucke L: Progressive multifocal leukoencephalopathy associated with HIV infection: A review of the literature with a report of 16 cases. Ann Intern Med 1987;107:78.
Britton CB et al: Progressive multifocal leukoencephalopathy: Disease progression, stabilization, and response to intrathecal ara-C in 26 patients. Abstract Th.B.1512. VIII International Conference on AIDS, Amsterdam, 1992.
Johnson RT: Prion disease. N Engl J Med 1992;326:486.
Quinlivan EB et al: Subclinical central nervous system infection with JC virus in patients with AIDS. J Infect Dis 1992;166:80.

OTHER SYSTEMIC VIRAL DISEASES

1. DENGUE

Essentials of Diagnosis

- An incubation period of 2–7 days.
- Sudden onset of high fever, chills, severe aching, headache, sore throat, prostration, and depression.
- Biphasic fever curve: initial phase, 3–7 days; remission, few hours to 2 days; second phase, 1–2 days.
- The rash is biphasic: first evanescent, followed by maculopapular, scarlatiniform, morbilliform, or petechial changes from extremities to torso.
- Leukopenia.

General Considerations

Dengue is a viral (togavirus, flavivirus) disease transmitted by the bite of the *Aedes* mosquito. It may be caused by one of several serotypes widely distributed between latitudes 25 °N and 25 °S (eg, Thailand, India, Philippines; Caribbean, including Puerto Rico and Cuba; Central America; Africa). It occurs only in the active mosquito season (warm weather). The incubation period is 3–15 days (usually 5–8 days).

Clinical Findings

A. Symptoms and Signs: Dengue is usually a nonspecific, self-limited, febrile illness, but its presentation may range from asymptomatic infection through severe hemorrhage and sudden fatal shock. Severe dengue begins with a sudden onset of high fever, chilliness, and severe aching ("breakbone") of the head, back, and extremities, accompanied by sore throat, prostration, and depression. There may be conjunctival redness and flushing or blotching of the skin. The initial febrile phase lasts 3–7 days, typically but not inevitably followed by a remission of a few hours to 2 days. The skin eruption appears in 80% of cases during the remission or during the second febrile phase, which lasts 1–2 days and is accompanied by similar but usually milder symptoms than in the first phase. The rash may be scarlatiniform, morbilliform, maculopapular, or petechial. It appears first on the dorsum of the hands and feet and spreads to the arms, legs, trunk, and neck but rarely to the face. The rash lasts 2 hours to several days and may be followed by desquamation. Petechial rashes and gastrointestinal hemorrhages occur with dengue hemorrhagic fever, caused by variants of the same serotypes causing dengue and occurring in southeast Asia and the Caribbean. Some dengue virus envelope glycoproteins are homologous with segments of clotting factors, including plasminogen, and thus the hemorrhagic fever may represent an immunologic autoimmune reaction.

Before the rash appears, it is difficult to distinguish dengue from malaria, yellow fever, or influenza. With the appearance of the rash, the diagnosis is usually clear.

B. Laboratory Findings: Leukopenia is characteristic. Thrombocytopenia occurs in the hemorrhagic form of the disease. Virus may be recovered from the blood during the acute phase.

Complications

Depression, pneumonia, bone marrow failure, iritis, orchitis, and oophoritis are rare complications. Shock occurs in hemorrhagic dengue.

Prevention

Available prophylactic measures include control of mosquitoes by screening and insect repellents. An effective vaccine has been developed but has not been produced commercially.

Treatment

Treat shock by expanding circulating blood volume. Give acetaminophen as required for discomfort. Permit gradual restoration of activity during prolonged convalescence.

Prognosis

Fatalities are rare. Convalescence is slow.

Dengue and Kyasanur Forest disease: Part of symposium proceedings. Rev Infect Dis 1989;11(Suppl 4):S840.

Imported dengue—United States, 1991. MMWR Morb Mortal Wkly Rep 1992;41(39):725.

Markoff LJ et al: Development of cross-reactive antibodies to plasminogen during the immune response to dengue virus infection. J Infect Dis 1991;164:294.

Rosenfeld SJ, Young NS: Viruses and bone marrow failure. Blood Rev 1991;5:71.

2. COLORADO TICK FEVER

Essentials of Diagnosis

- Fever, chills, myalgia, headache, prostration.
- Leukopenia.
- Second attack of fever after remission lasting 2–3 days.
- Onset 1–19 days (average, 4 days) following tick bite.

General Considerations

Colorado tick fever is an acute viral (orbivirus) infection transmitted by *Dermacentor andersoni* bites. The disease is limited to the western USA and is most prevalent during the tick season (March to August). The incubation period is 3–6 days.

Clinical Findings

A. Symptoms and Signs: The onset of fever (to 38.9–40.6 °C [102–105 °F]) is abrupt, sometimes with chills. Severe myalgia, headache, photophobia, anorexia, nausea and vomiting, and generalized weakness are prominent symptoms. Abnormal physical findings are limited to an occasional faint rash. Fever continues for 3 days, followed by a remission of 1–3 days and then by a full recrudescence lasting 2–4 days. In an occasional case there may be three bouts of fever.

Influenza, Rocky Mountain spotted fever, and other acute leukopenic fevers must be differentiated.

B. Laboratory Findings: Leukopenia (2000–3000/μL) with a shift to the left occurs. Viremia may be demonstrated by inoculation of blood into mice or by fluorescent antibody staining of the patient's red cells (with adsorbed virus). Complement-fixing antibodies appear during the third week after onset of the disease.

Complications

Aseptic meningitis, encephalitis, and hemorrhagic fever occur rarely. Asthenia may follow, but fatalities are very rare.

Treatment

No specific treatment is available. Aspirin or another nonsteroidal anti-inflammatory agent—or codeine or hydrocodone—may be given for pain.

Prognosis

The disease is usually self-limited and benign.

Emmons RW: Ecology of Colorado tick fever. Annu Rev Microbiol 1988;42:49.

3. HEMORRHAGIC FEVERS

This is a diverse group of illnesses resulting from virus infections and perhaps immunologic responses to them. The common clinical features include high fever; hemorrhagic diathesis with petechiae or purpura; and bleeding from the nose, gastrointestinal tract, and genitourinary tract, with thrombocytopenia, leukopenia, and marked toxicity, often leading to shock and death. The viruses may be tick-borne (eg, Omsk hemorrhagic fever, Russia; Kyasanur Forest hemorrhagic fever, India), mosquito-borne (eg, Chikungunya hemorrhagic fever, yellow fever, dengue), or zoonotic (often derived from rodents, eg, hemorrhagic fever with renal syndrome secondary to Hantaan virus infection, Junin hemorrhagic fever, Argentina; Machupo hemorrhagic fever, Bolivia; Lassa hemorrhagic fever, West Africa; the newly described Puumala virus, Scandinavia, and Belgrade virus, Yugoslavia). The zoonotic group also includes Marburg hemorrhagic fever (from contact with African vervet monkeys) and Ebola hemorrhagic fever in central Africa.

Persons who present with symptoms compatible with those of hemorrhagic fever and who have traveled from a possible endemic area should be strictly isolated for diagnosis and symptomatic treatment. Conclusive diagnosis may be made by growing the virus from blood obtained early in the disease or by showing a significant specific antibody titer rise. Isolation is particularly important, because some of these infections are highly transmissible to close contacts, including medical personnel, and carry a mortality rate of 50–70%.

For most of these entities, no specific treatment is available. Lassa fever and hemorrhagic fever with renal syndrome can be effectively treated—if started early—with intravenous ribavirin (33 mg/kg as loading dose, followed by 16 mg/kg every 6 hours for 4 days and then 8 mg/kg every 8 hours for 3 days) (see Chapter 37). It is important to differentiate hemorrhagic fever from such easily treated entities as meningococcemia and Rocky Mountain spotted fever.

Hemorrhagic fevers: Symposium proceedings. Rev Infect Dis 1989;11(Suppl 4):S669.

Holmes GP et al: Lassa fever in the United States. N Engl J Med 1990;323:1120. (Discusses risk of importation and management of cases.)

Huggins JW et al: Prospective, double-blind, concurrent, placebo-controlled clinical trial of intravenous ribavirin therapy of hemorrhagic fever with renal syndrome. J Infect Dis 1991;164:1119.

4. YELLOW FEVER

Essentials of Diagnosis

- Sudden onset of severe headache, aching in legs, and tachycardia. After a brief (1 day) remission, bradycardia, hypotension, jaundice, hemorrhagic tendency.

- Proteinuria, leukopenia, bilirubinemia, bilirubinuria.
- Endemic area exposure (tropical South and Central America, Africa, but not Asia).

General Considerations

Yellow fever is a viral (group B arbovirus, togavirus) infection transmitted by the *Aedes* and jungle mosquitoes. It is endemic only in Africa and South America (tropical or subtropical), but epidemics have extended far into the temperate zone during warm seasons. The mosquito transmits the infection by first biting an individual having the disease and then biting a susceptible individual after the virus has multiplied within the mosquito's body. The incubation period in humans is 3–6 days. Adults and children are equally susceptible, though attack rates are highest among adult males because of their work habits.

Clinical Findings

A. Symptoms and Signs:

1. Mild form–Symptoms are malaise, headache, fever, retro-orbital pain, nausea, vomiting, and photophobia. Bradycardia may be present.

2. Severe form–Symptoms are the same as in the mild form, with sudden onset and then severe pains throughout the body, extreme prostration, bleeding into the skin and from the mucous membranes, oliguria, and jaundice. Signs include tachycardia, erythematous face, and conjunctival redness during the congestive phase, followed by a period of calm (on about the third day) with a normal temperature and then a return of fever, bradycardia, hypotension, jaundice, hemorrhages (gastrointestinal tract, bladder, nose, mouth, subcutaneous), and later delirium.

B. Laboratory Findings: Leukopenia occurs, although it may not be present at the onset. Proteinuria is present, sometimes as high as 5–6 g/L, and disappears completely with recovery. With jaundice there are bilirubinuria and bilirubinemia. The virus may be isolated from the blood by intracerebral mouse inoculation (first 3 days). Antibodies appear during and after the second week.

Differential Diagnosis

It may be difficult to distinguish yellow fever from hepatitis, malaria, leptospirosis, dengue, and other hemorrhagic fevers, and other forms of jaundice on clinical evidence alone.

Prevention

Transmission is prevented through mosquito control. Live virus vaccine is highly effective, safe, and should be provided for immunocompetent adults living in or traveling to endemic areas. Pregnant women should be immunized only if absolutely necessary. (See Chapter 29.)

Treatment

No specific antiviral therapy is available. Treatment is directed toward symptomatic relief and management of complications.

Prognosis

The mortality rate is high in the severe form, with death occurring most commonly between the sixth and the tenth days. In survivors, the temperature returns to normal by the seventh or eighth day. The prognosis in any individual case is guarded at the onset, since sudden changes for the worse are common. Intractable hiccup, copious black vomitus, melena, and anuria are unfavorable signs. Convalescence is prolonged, including 1–2 weeks of asthenia.

Monath TP: Yellow fever: A medically neglected disease. Rev Infect Dis 1987;9:165.

Yellow fever vaccine. Recommendations of the Immunization Practices Advisory Committee (ACIP). MMWR Morb Mortal Wkly Rep 1990;39(RR-6):1.

COMMON VIRAL RESPIRATORY INFECTIONS

Infections of the respiratory tract are perhaps the most common human ailments. While they are a source of discomfort, disability, and loss of time for most average adults, they are a substantial cause of morbidity and serious illness in young children and in the elderly. Specific associations of certain groups of viruses with certain disease syndromes have been established. Many of these viral infections run their natural course in older children and in adults without specific treatment and without great risk of bacterial complications. In young infants and in the elderly, or in persons with impaired respiratory tract reserves, bacterial superinfection increases morbidity and mortality rates.

Croup, epiglottitis, and the common cold are discussed in Chapter 8.

1. RESPIRATORY SYNCYTIAL VIRUS

Respiratory syncytial virus (RSV) causes annual outbreaks of pneumonia, bronchiolitis, and tracheobronchitis in the very young. Reinfection is common and manifests itself typically as a mild upper respiratory tract infection and tracheobronchitis in older children or adults. Serious pulmonary RSV infections have been described in elderly and immunocompromised adults, including outbreaks with a high mortality rate in bone marrow transplant and pediatric liver transplant patients. Infants with congenital heart disease are at high risk for severe or fatal RSV infection.

Annual epidemics occur in winter and spring. The average incubation period is 5 days. Inoculation may occur through the nose or the eyes.

In bronchiolitis, proliferation and necrosis of bronchiolar epithelium develops, producing obstruction from sloughed epithelium and increased mucus secretion. Signs include low-grade fever, severe tachypnea (up to 100/min in the very young), and expiratory wheezes. Hyperinflated lungs, decreased gas exchange, and increased work of breathing are present. Otitis media is a frequent complication.

RSV is the only respiratory pathogen that produces its most serious illness at a time when specific maternal antibody is invariably present.

In infants, diagnosis of lower respiratory tract disease may often be made on the basis of clinical and epidemiologic findings. Rapid diagnosis may be made by viral antigen identification of nasal washings using an ELISA or immunofluorescent assay.

Treatment consists of hydration, humidification of inspired air, and ventilatory support as needed. In infants, aerosolized ribavirin may help (1.1 g/d, diluted to 20 mg/mL, delivered as a particulate with oxygen over 12–18 hours per day for 3–7 days—although high-dose, short-duration therapy may be as effective). Pregnant women should avoid exposure to ribavirin. Patients with upper respiratory RSV infections probably do not need ribavirin. The role of intravenous immunoglobulin G prophylaxis or treatment is under study. No vaccine is available.

Englund JA et al: High dose, short duration ribavirin aerosol therapy in children with a suspected respiratory syncytial virus infection. J Pediatr 1990;117:313. (Up to 5 days with 60 mg/mL for three 2-hour periods was as effective as traditional therapy in children with RSV pneumonia.)

Groothuis JR et al: Use of intravenous gamma globulin to passively immunize high-risk children against respiratory syncytial virus: Safety and pharmacokinetics. The RSVIG Study Group. Antimicrob Agents Chemother 1991;35:1469.

Harrington RD et al: An outbreak of respiratory syncytial virus in a bone marrow transplant center. J Infect Dis 1992;165:987.

Takimoto CH, Cram DL, Root RK: Respiratory syncytial virus infections on an adult medical ward. Arch Intern Med 1991;151:706.

2. INFLUENZA

Essentials of Diagnosis

- Abrupt onset with fever, chills, malaise, cough, coryza, and muscle aches.
- Aching, fever, and prostration out of proportion to catarrhal symptoms.
- Leukopenia.
- Cases usually in epidemic pattern, not sporadic.

General Considerations

Influenza (an orthomyxovirus) is transmitted by

the respiratory route. Although sporadic cases occur, epidemics and pandemics appear at varying intervals, usually in the fall or winter. Antigenic types A and B produce clinically indistinguishable infections, whereas type C is usually a minor illness. The incubation period is 1–4 days.

It is difficult to diagnose influenza in the absence of a classic epidemic. The disease resembles many other mild febrile illnesses but is always accompanied by a cough.

Clinical Findings

A. Symptoms and Signs: The onset is usually abrupt, with fever, chills, malaise, muscular aching, substernal soreness, headache, nasal stuffiness, and occasionally nausea. Fever lasts 1–7 days (usually 3–5). Coryza, nonproductive cough, and sore throat are present. Signs include mild pharyngeal injection, flushed face, and conjunctival redness.

B. Laboratory Findings: Leukopenia is common. Proteinuria may be present. The virus may be isolated from the throat washings by inoculation of embryonated eggs or cell cultures. Complement-fixing and hemagglutination-inhibiting antibodies appear during the second week.

Complications

Influenza causes necrosis of the respiratory epithelium, which predisposes to secondary bacterial infections. The interactions between bacteria and influenza are bidirectional, with bacterial enzymes (eg, proteases, trypsin-like compounds, streptokinase, plasminogen) activating influenza viruses. Frequent complications are acute sinusitis, otitis media, purulent bronchitis, and pneumonia.

Pneumonia is commonly due to bacterial infection with pneumococci or staphylococci and rarely to the influenza virus itself. The circulatory system is not usually involved, but pericarditis, myocarditis, and thrombophlebitis sometimes occur.

Reye's syndrome is a rare and severe complication of influenza and other viral diseases (eg, varicella), particularly in young children. It consists of rapid development of hepatic failure and encephalopathy, and there is a 30% fatality rate. The pathogenesis is unknown, but the syndrome is associated with aspirin use. Hypoglycemia, elevation of serum transaminases and blood ammonia, prolonged prothrombin time, and change in mental status all occur within 2–3 weeks after onset of the virus infection. Histologically, the periphery of liver lobules shows striking fatty infiltration and glycogen depletion. Treatment is supportive and directed to the management of cerebral edema.

Prevention

Polyvalent influenza virus vaccine provides partial immunity (about 85% efficacy) for a few months to 1 year. The vaccine's antigenic configuration changes yearly and is based on prevalent strains of the preceding year. Vaccination (0.5 mL intramuscularly once during the fall) is recommended annually for persons over 65, children and teenagers receiving chronic aspirin therapy, nursing home residents, those with chronic lung or heart disease or other debilitating illnesses, and health care workers. Adequate immunity is achieved about 2 weeks after vaccination. Future vaccination may entail use of a live attenuated vaccine administered nasally.

Chemoprophylaxis for epidemiologically or virologically confirmed influenza A with amantadine hydrochloride, 200 mg/d orally (100 mg/d in the elderly, who may develop central nervous system side effects), will markedly reduce the attack rate among exposed unvaccinated individuals if begun immediately and continued for 10 days (Table 31–1). Amantadine may also be used during an outbreak while waiting for immunity to develop following vaccination.

Treatment

Many patients with influenza prefer to rest in bed. Analgesics and a cough mixture may be used. Amantadine may decrease the duration of signs and symptoms of clinical influenza by about 50%. Rimantadine (not licensed in the United States) is preferred in patients with renal failure. The clinical significance of resistance to antiviral agents is controversial. Ribavirin (1.1 g/d, diluted to 20 mg/mL and delivered as particulate aerosol with oxygen over 12–18 hours a day for 3–7 days [Table 31–1]) has helped severely ill patients with influenza A or B.

Antibacterial antibiotics should be reserved for treatment of bacterial complications. Acetaminophen rather than aspirin should be used for fever, especially in children.

Prognosis

The duration of the uncomplicated illness is 1–7 days, and the prognosis is excellent. Purulent bronchitis and bronchiectasis may result in chronic pulmonary disease and fibrosis that persist throughout life. Most fatalities are due to bacterial pneumonia. Influenzal pneumonia has a high mortality rate among pregnant women and persons with a history of rheumatic heart disease. In recent epidemics, the mortality rate has been low except in debilitated persons—especially those with severe heart disease.

If the fever persists for more than 4 days, if the cough becomes productive, or if the white blood cell count rises to about 12,000/μL, secondary bacterial infection should be ruled out or verified and treated. Pneumococcal pneumonia is most common, but staphylococcal pneumonia is most serious.

Monto AS, Arden NH: Implications of viral resistance to amantadine in control of influenza A. Clin Infect Dis 1992;15:362.

Prevention and control of influenza. Recommendations of the Immunization Practices Advisory Committee (ACIP). MMWR Morb Mortal Wkly Rep 1992;41(RR-9):1.

Schleiblaueer H et al: Interactions between bacteria and influenza A virus in the development of influenza pneumonia. J Infect Dis 1992;166:783.

Treanor JJ et al: Protective efficacy of combined live intranasal and inactivated influenza A virus vaccines in the elderly. Ann Intern Med 1992;117:625.

ADENOVIRUS INFECTIONS

Adenoviruses (there are more than 40 antigenic types) produce a variety of clinical syndromes. These infections are self-limited or clinically inapparent and most common among infants, young children, and military recruits. Outbreaks in liver, bone marrow, and renal transplant recipients have been reported, and dissemination may occur. The incubation period is 4–9 days.

Clinical types of adenovirus infection include the following: (1) The **common cold** (see Chapter 8) is characterized by rhinitis, pharyngitis, and mild malaise without fever. (2) **Acute undifferentiated respiratory disease, nonstreptococcal exudative pharyngitis** is characterized by fever lasting 2–12 days and accompanied by malaise and myalgia. Sore throat is often manifested by diffuse injection, a patchy exudate, and cervical lymphadenopathy. Cough is sometimes accompanied by rales and x-ray evidence of pneumonitis (primary atypical pneumonia). Conjunctivitis is often present. (3) **Pharyngoconjunctival fever** is manifested by fever and malaise, conjunctivitis (often unilateral), and mild pharyngitis. (4) **Epidemic keratoconjunctivitis** (often transmitted nosocomially) occurs in adults and is manifested by unilateral conjunctival redness, pain, tearing, and an enlarged preauricular lymph node. Keratitis leads to subepithelial opacities (especially with types 8, 19, or 37). (5) **Acute hemorrhagic cystitis** is a disorder of children that is often associated with adenovirus type 11. Adenoviruses also cause acute gastroenteritis (types 40 and 41) in infants.

Infected liver transplant recipients tend to develop hepatitis (type 5 adenovirus), whereas bone marrow and renal transplant recipients tend to develop pneumonia or hemorrhagic cystitis.

Vaccines are not available for general use. Live oral vaccines containing attenuated type 4 and type 7 have been used in military personnel.

Treatment is symptomatic.

Hierholzer JC: Adenoviruses in the immunocompromised host. Clin Microbiol Rev 1992;5:262.

OTHER EXANTHEMATOUS VIRUS INFECTIONS

1. ERYTHEMA INFECTIOSUM

This acute communicable viral illness occurs mainly in children 4–10 years old in focal and community-wide outbreaks. It is caused by a human parvovirus. Its initial manifestation is a fiery red appearance of the cheeks ("slapped cheeks"), with circumoral pallor, followed a few days later by a red, lacy, maculopapular rash on the trunk that may wax and wane for several days. Malaise, headache, and pruritus occur, but fever is rare. At the time of the rash, there may be arthralgias, synovitis, and arthritis (symmetric, involving mainly the hands, wrists, and knees, and particularly in women). The disease usually resolves in 4 weeks but may last for months. Human parvovirus B19 is also implicated in aplastic crisis, especially in sickle cell disease, and may cause disturbances in pregnancy (fetal loss, hydrops fetalis, but no evidence for birth defects).

The diagnosis is clinical (Table 31–2) but may be confirmed by an elevated titer of IgM anti-HPV antibodies in serum. Scarlet fever is the main differential diagnosis. The prognosis is excellent. Besides arthritis with hypocomplementemia, which is common in some outbreaks, encephalitis is a rare complication.

Treatment is symptomatic. Screening of donated blood could potentially prevent transfusion-related infection and is under investigation.

Kalish RA et al: Lupus-like presentation of human parvovirus B19 infection. J Rheumatol 1992;19:169.

McOmish PL et al: Detection of parvovirus B19 in donated blood: A model system for screening by polymerase chain reaction. J Clin Microbiol 1993;31:323. (A clever method for screening large samples of blood for parvovirus.)

Risks associated with human parvovirus B19 infection. MMWR Morb Mortal Wkly Rep 1989;38:81.

2. KAWASAKI SYNDROME

Kawasaki syndrome is a worldwide multisystemic disease also known as mucocutaneous lymph node syndrome. It occurs mainly in children but occasionally in adults, at times in epidemic fashion. It is an unexplained illness characterized by fever and four of the following: bilateral nonexudative conjunctivitis; mucous membrane changes of at least one type (injected pharynx, cracked lips, strawberry tongue); extremity changes of at least one type (edema, desquamation, erythema, a polymorphous rash); and cervical lymphadenopathy greater than 1.5 cm. Although the cause is unknown, a relationship has been noted to exposure to recently cleaned rugs or carpets.

A major complication is arteritis of the coronary vessels, occurring in 20% of untreated cases; arteritis of extremity vessels and peripheral gangrene have been reported also. The cause of these complications is likewise unknown.

Management is with aspirin (80–100 mg/kg/d in divided doses with subsequent tapering) and intravenous immune globulin in high doses. Corticosteroids are thought to increase the likelihood of development of coronary aneurysms.

Barron KS: Kawasaki disease: Epidemiology, late prognosis, and therapy. Rheum Dis Clin North Am 1991; 17:907.

Gersony WM: Diagnosis and management of Kawasaki disease. JAMA 1991;265:2699.

Tomita S et al: Peripheral gangrene associated with Kawasaki disease. Clin Infect Dis 1992;14:121.

Rauch AM et al: Outbreak of Kawasaki syndrome in Denver, Colorado: Association with rug and carpet cleaning. Pediatrics 1991;87:663.

3. POXVIRUS INFECTIONS

Among the nine poxviruses pathogenic for humans, five are clinically important: (1) **Variola:** Smallpox was a highly contagious disease characterized by severe headache, fever, and prostration and accompanied by a centrifugal rash developing in order of progression from macules to papules to vesicles to pustules. Immunization with vaccinia virus, culminating in a worldwide effort by WHO, apparently succeeded in eradicating smallpox from the world as of 1979. (2) **Molluscum contagiosum** may be transmitted sexually or by other close contact. It is manifested by pearly, raised, umbilicated skin nodules sparing the palms and soles. It tends to persist in AIDS patients. Treatment is nonspecific. (3) **Vaccinia:** The efficacy of vaccination with vaccinia was responsible for smallpox eradication. Since the world is free of smallpox, civilian vaccination is indicated only for laboratory workers who must handle variola or related viruses. Vaccination is still practiced among military forces. Smallpox vaccination is not required for any international travel. Any form of immunosuppression is an absolute contraindication to smallpox vaccination. Eczema (or a history of it) in a patient or family member, other forms of dermatitis, and burns also contraindicate vaccination. There is no indication for therapeutic use of smallpox vaccine. (4) **Orf** (contagious pustular dermatitis or ecthyma contagiosa) and (5) **paravaccinia** (milkers' nodules) are occupational diseases acquired by contact with sheep and cattle, respectively.

VIRAL GASTROENTERITIS

Viruses are responsible for probably 30–40% of cases of infectious diarrhea in the USA, and rotaviruses are a leading worldwide cause of dehydrating gastroenteritis in young children. The agents that can cause disease in adults include group B rotaviruses (responsible for outbreaks in China) and Norwalk agent (which causes epidemics of vomiting and diarrhea and is often transmitted by food—especially shellfish—and water).

Rotaviruses (four major serotypes) can also cause infections in adults exposed to infected infants and are ubiquitous in the environment of an outbreak. (Secondary rates are between 16% and 30%.) The disease is usually mild, but cases have also occurred among travelers, in epidemic fashion, and after waterborne exposure. Sensitive and specific immunoassays to detect viral RNA in fecal specimens are available. Treatment is symptomatic, with fluid and electrolyte replacement. Immunity does not appear to be serotype-specific, and lymphoproliferative responses are important. Vaccines are under development.

The **Norwalk agent** and **Norwalk-like agents** are responsible for about 40% of cases of group-related or institutional diarrhea, transmission usually being the fecal-oral route, though airborne transmission may also occur. Nausea and vomiting are especially common with Norwalk agent. An ELISA can detect the agent in stool samples. Treatment again is symptomatic.

Blacklow NR, Greenberg HB: Viral gastroenteritis. N Engl J Med 1991;325:252.

VIRUSES THAT PRODUCE SEVERAL SYNDROMES

1. COXSACKIEVIRUS INFECTIONS

Coxsackievirus infections cause several clinical syndromes. As with other enteroviruses, infections are most common during the summer. Two groups, A and B, are defined by their differing behavior after injection into suckling mice. There are more than 50 serotypes.

Clinical Findings
A. Symptoms and Signs: The clinical syndromes associated with coxsackievirus infection may be described briefly as follows:

1. Summer grippe (A and B)—A febrile illness, principally of children, which lasts 1–4 days; minor symptoms and respiratory tract infection are often present.

2. Herpangina (A2–6, 10)—Sudden onset of

fever, which may be as high as 40.6 °C (105 °F), sometimes with febrile convulsions; headache, myalgia, vomiting; and sore throat, characterized early by petechiae or papules on the soft palate that become shallow ulcers in about 3 days and then heal.

3. Epidemic pleurodynia (B1–5)–Sudden onset of recurrent pain in the area of diaphragmatic attachment (lower chest or upper abdomen); fever, often present during attacks of pain; headache, sore throat, malaise, nausea; tenderness, hyperesthesia, and muscle swelling of the involved area; orchitis, pleurisy, and aseptic meningitis may occur. Relapse may occur after recovery.

4. Aseptic meningitis (especially A7, 9; B types)–Fever, headache, nausea, vomiting, stiff neck, drowsiness, cerebrospinal fluid lymphocytosis without chemical abnormalities; rarely, muscle paralysis. A focal encephalitis has been reported with coxsackievirus group A.

5. Acute nonspecific pericarditis (B types)–Sudden onset of anterior chest pain, often worse with inspiration and in the supine position; fever, myalgia, headache; pericardial friction rub appearing early; pericardial effusion with paradoxic pulse, increased venous pressure, and increase in heart size; electrocardiographic and x-ray evidence of pericarditis are often present. One or more relapses may occur.

6. Myocarditis (B1–5)–Heart failure in the neonatal period may be the result of myocarditis associated with infection acquired in utero. Adult heart disease may be caused by coxsackievirus group B.

7. Hand, foot, and mouth disease (A5, 10, 16)–Sometimes occurring in epidemics, this illness is characterized by stomatitis and a vesicular rash on hands and feet.

B. Laboratory Findings: Routine laboratory studies show no characteristic abnormalities. Neutralizing antibodies appear during convalescence. The virus may be isolated from throat washings or stools inoculated into suckling mice.

Treatment & Prognosis

Treatment is symptomatic. With the exception of myocarditis, pericarditis, and rare illnesses such as pancreatitis or polio-like syndrome, all of the syndromes caused by coxsackieviruses are benign and self-limited.

Melnick JL: Enteroviruses: Polioviruses, coxsackieviruses, echoviruses, and newer enteroviruses. In: *Virology,* 2nd ed. Fields BN et al (editors). Raven Press, 1990.

2. ECHOVIRUS INFECTIONS

Echoviruses are enteroviruses that produce several clinical syndromes, particularly in children. Infection is most common during summer.

Over 30 serotypes have been demonstrated. Most cause aseptic meningitis, which may be associated with a rubelliform rash. Type 16 causes Boston exanthem, characterized by sudden onset of fever, nausea, and sore throat and a roseolous rash over the face and trunk that persists 1–10 days. Epidemic diarrhea, common respiratory diseases, and myocarditis have been associated with echoviruses.

As with other enterovirus infections, diagnosis is best established by correlation of clinical, epidemiologic, and laboratory evidence. Cytopathic effects are produced in tissue culture after recovery of virus from throat washings, blood, or cerebrospinal fluid. Fourfold or greater rises in antibody titer signify systemic infection.

Treatment is symptomatic. The prognosis is excellent, though there are reports of mild paralysis after central nervous system infection.

II. RICKETTSIAL DISEASES

The rickettsioses are febrile exanthematous diseases caused by rickettsiae, small gram-negative obligate intracellular bacterial parasites of arthropods. In arthropods, rickettsiae grow in the gut lining, often without harming the host. Human infection results from either an arthropod bite or contamination with its feces. In humans, rickettsiae grow principally in endothelial cells of small blood vessels, producing vasculitis, cell necrosis, thrombosis of vessels, skin rashes, and organ dysfunctions.

Different rickettsiae and their vectors are endemic in different parts of the world, but two or more types may coexist in the same geographic area. A summary of epidemiologic features is given in Table 31–4. The clinical picture is variable but usually includes a prodromal stage followed by fever, rash, and prostration. Isolation of rickettsiae from the patient is cumbersome and difficult and is best left to specialized laboratories; a promising new means of isolation is the centrifugation shell-vial technique. Laboratory diagnosis relies on the development of nonspecific antibodies to certain *Proteus* strains (Weil-Felix reaction based on shared rickettsial and *Proteus* antigens) and of specific antibodies detected by complement fixation (for diagnosis) or immunofluorescence or hemagglutination (for species identification) tests.

Prevention & Treatment

Preventive measures are directed at control of the vector, specific immunization when available, and (occasionally) drug chemoprophylaxis. All rickettsiae can be inhibited by tetracyclines or chloramphenicol. All early clinical infections respond in some degree to treatment with these drugs. Treatment

Table 31–4. Rickettsial diseases.[1]

Disease	Rickettsial Pathogen	Geographic Areas of Prevalence	Insect Vector	Mammalian Reservoir	Weil-Felix Agglutination		
					OX19	OX2	OXK
Typhus group							
Epidemic (louse-borne) typhus	*Rickettsia prowazekii*	South America, Africa, Asia, North America	Louse	Humans, flying squirrels	+	±	—
Endemic (murine) typhus	*Rickettsia typhi*	Worldwide; small foci (USA: Southeastern Gulf Coast)	Flea	Rodents	+	—	—
Scrub typhus	*Rickettsia tsutsugamushi*	Southeast Asia, Japan, Australia	Mite[2]	Rodents	—	—	+
Spotted fever group							
Rocky Mountain spotted fever	*Rickettsia rickettsii*	Western Hemisphere; USA (especially mid-Atlantic coastal region)	Tick[2]	Rodents, dogs	+	+	—
Boutonneuse fever, Kenya tick typhus, South African tick fever, Indian tick typhus	*Rickettsia conorii*	Africa, India, Mediterranean regions	Tick[2]	Rodents, dogs	+	+	—
Queensland tick typhus	*Rickettsia australis*	Australia	Tick[2]	Rodents, marsupials	+	+	—
North Asian tick typhus	*Rickettsia sibirica*	Siberia, Mongolia	Tick[2]	Rodents	+	+	—
Rickettsialpox	*Rickettsia akari*	USA, Korea, former USSR	Mite[2]	Mice	—	—	—
RMSF-like	*Rickettsia canada*	North America	Tick[2]	Rodents	?	?	—
Other							
Ehrlichiosis	*Ehrlichia canis*	Southeastern North America	Tick[2]	Dogs	?	?	?
Q fever	*Coxiella burnetii*	Worldwide	None[3]	Cattle, sheep, goats	—	—	—
Trench fever	*Rochalimaea quintana*	Europe, Africa, North America	Louse	Humans	?	?	?

[1]Modified from Brooks GF, Butel JS, Ornston LN: *Jawetz, Melnick & Adelberg's Medical Microbiology*, 19th ed. Appleton & Lange, 1991.
[2]Also serve as arthropod reservoir by maintaining rickettsiae through transovarian transmission.
[3]Human infection results from inhalation of dust.

usually consists of giving either tetracycline or chloramphenicol in the dosage schedules listed below. In seriously ill patients, initial treatment may consist of 1 g of tetracycline or chloramphenicol intravenously. The vector (louse, tick, mite) must be removed from patients. Supportive measures may include parenteral fluids, sedation, oxygen, and skin care.

TYPHUS GROUP

1. EPIDEMIC LOUSE-BORNE TYPHUS

Essentials of Diagnosis

* Prodrome of headache, then chills and fever.
* Severe, intractable headaches, prostration, persisting high fever.
* Macular rash appears on the fourth to seventh days

on the trunk and in the axillas, spreading to the rest of the body but sparing the face, palms, and soles.
* Laboratory confirmation by *Proteus* OX19 agglutination and specific serologic tests.

General Considerations

Epidemic louse-borne typhus is due to infection with *Rickettsia prowazekii,* a parasite of the body louse that ultimately kills the louse. Transmission is favored by crowded living conditions, famine, war, or any circumstances that predispose to heavy infestation with lice. When the louse sucks the blood of a person infected with *R prowazekii,* the organism becomes established in the gut of the louse and grows there. When the louse is transmitted to another person (through contact or clothing) and has a blood meal, it defecates simultaneously, and the infected feces are rubbed into the itching bite wound. Dry, infectious louse feces may also enter the respiratory tract and result in human infection. A deloused and bathed typhus patient is not infectious.

In a person who recovers from clinical or subclinical typhus infection, *R prowazekii* may survive in lymphoid tissues. Years later, there may be a recrudescence of disease (Brill's disease) without exposure to infected lice.

Mild and atypical cases of *R prowazekii* have rarely occurred in the USA after contact with flying squirrels or their ectoparasites or decades following exposure (eg, among concentration camp victims of World War II). Cases can be acquired by travel to pockets of infection (eg, central and northeastern Africa, including Somalia).

Clinical Findings

A. Symptoms and Signs: (Table 31–4.) Prodromal malaise, cough, headache, backache, arthralgia, and chest pain begin after an incubation period of 10–14 days. There is then an abrupt onset of chills, high fever, and prostration, with flu-like symptoms progressing to delirium and stupor. The headache is severe, with prolonged fever.

Other findings consist of conjunctivitis, flushed face, rales at the lung bases, and often splenomegaly. A macular rash (that may become confluent) appears first in the axillas and then over the trunk, spreading to the extremities but rarely involving the face, palms, or soles. In severely ill patients, the rash becomes hemorrhagic, and hypotension becomes marked. There may be renal insufficiency, stupor, and delirium. In spontaneous recovery, improvement begins 13–16 days after onset with rapid drop of fever.

B. Laboratory Findings: The white blood cell count is variable. Proteinuria and hematuria commonly occur. Serum obtained 5–12 days after onset of symptoms usually shows agglutinating antibodies for *Proteus* OX19 (rarely also OX2)—*R prowazekii* shares antigens with these *Proteus* strains—and specific antibodies for *R prowazekii* antigens demonstrated by complement fixation, microagglutination, or immunofluorescence. In primary rickettsial infection, early antibodies are IgM; in recrudescence (Brill's disease), early antibodies are predominantly IgG, and the Weil-Felix test is negative or low in titer.

C. Imaging: Radiographs of the chest may show patchy consolidation.

Differential Diagnosis

The prodromal symptoms and the early febrile stage are not specific enough to permit diagnosis in nonepidemic situations. The rash is usually sufficiently distinctive for diagnosis, but it may be missing in 5–10% of cases and may be difficult to observe in dark-skinned persons. A variety of other acute febrile diseases may have to be considered.

Brill's disease (recrudescent epidemic typhus) has a more gradual onset than primary *R prowazekii* infection, fever and rash are of shorter duration, and the disease is milder and rarely fatal.

Complications

Pneumonia, thromboses, vasculitis with major vessel obstruction and gangrene, circulatory collapse, myocarditis, and uremia may occur.

Prevention

Prevention consists of louse control with insecticides, particularly by applying chemicals to clothing or treating it with heat, and frequent bathing. Immunization with vaccines consisting of inactivated egg-grown *R prowazekii* gives some protection to laboratory personnel, physicians, or field workers who are exposed to the parasite. This vaccine is not currently available in the USA or Canada. An improved cell culture vaccine is being developed.

Treatment

Treatment consists of either tetracycline (25 mg/kg/d in four divided doses) or chloramphenicol (50–100 mg/kg/d in four divided doses) for 4–10 days.

Prognosis

The prognosis depends greatly upon age and immunization status. In children under age 10, the disease is usually mild. The mortality rate is 10% in the second and third decades but in the past reached 60% in the sixth decade. Effective vaccination can convert a potentially serious disease into a mild one.

Green CR, Gleiberman I: Brill-Zinsser: Still with us. JAMA 1990;264:1811.

Perine PL et al: A clinico-epidemiological study of epidemic typhus in Africa. Clin Infect Dis 1992;14:1149.

2. ENDEMIC FLEA-BORNE TYPHUS (Murine Typhus)

Rickettsia typhi (R mooseri) is transmitted from rat to rat through the rat flea (rarely, the rat louse). Humans acquire the infection (eg, in Central America, Texas) when bitten by an infected flea, which releases infected feces while sucking blood. Rare cases follow travel, usually to Southeast Asia.

Endemic typhus resembles recrudescent epidemic typhus in that it has a gradual onset and the fever and rash are of shorter duration (6–13 days). The symptoms are less severe than in endemic typhus and may mimic measles, rubella, or roseola. The rash is maculopapular and concentrated on the trunk and fades fairly rapidly. Pneumonia and gangrene are rare. Fatalities are rare and limited to the elderly.

Differentiation from Rocky Mountain spotted fever includes, besides laboratory criteria, the season of onset (earlier in the year for Rocky Mountain spotted fever), the character of the rash, and geography (urban or rural, versus rural for Rocky Mountain spotted fever).

Complement-fixing or immunofluorescent antibodies can be detected in the patient's serum with specific *R typhi* antigens. There is a rising titer of agglutinating antibodies to *Proteus* OX19.

Preventive measures are directed at control of rats and ectoparasites (rat fleas) with insecticides, rat poisons, and rat-proofing of buildings.. Antibiotic treatment with tetracycline (25–50 mg/kg/d in four divided doses) or chloramphenicol (50–75 mg/kg/d in four divided doses) is indicated through 3 full days of defervescence. An experimental vaccine was fairly effective, but it is not commercially available now.

Dumler JS et al: Clinical and laboratory features of murine typhus in South Texas, 1980 through 1987. JAMA 1991;266:1365.

3. SCRUB TYPHUS (Tsutsugamushi Disease)

Essentials of Diagnosis

- Exposure to mites in endemic area of Southeast Asia, the western Pacific, and Australia.
- Black eschar at site of bite, with regional and generalized lymphadenopathy.
- Conjunctivitis and a short-lived macular rash.
- Frequent pneumonitis, encephalitis, and cardiac failure.
- Laboratory confirmation with agglutinins to *Proteus* OXK and specific antibodies by immunofluorescence.

General Considerations

Scrub typhus is caused by *Rickettsia tsutsugamushi (R orientalis),* which is principally a parasite of rodents transmitted by mites in the endemic areas listed above. The mites live on vegetation but complete their maturation cycle by biting humans who come in contact with infested vegetation.

Clinical Findings

A. Symptoms and Signs: After a 1- to 3-week incubation period, malaise, chills, severe headache, and backache develop. At the site of the bite, a papule evolves into a flat black eschar. The regional lymph nodes are enlarged and tender, and there may be generalized adenopathy. Fever rises gradually, and a macular rash appears primarily on the trunk after a week of fever and may be fleeting or may last a week. The patient may become obtunded. During the second or third week, pneumonitis, myocarditis and cardiac failure, and, rarely, encephalitis may develop.

B. Laboratory Findings: Blood obtained during the first few days of illness may permit isolation of

the rickettsia by mouse inoculation. The Weil-Felix test usually shows a rising titer to *Proteus* OXK during the second week of clinical illness. The complement fixation test is often unsatisfactory, but fluorescein-labeled antirickettsial sera are diagnostic.

Differential Diagnosis

Leptospirosis, typhoid, dengue, malaria, and other rickettsial infections should be considered. When the rash is fleeting and the eschar not evident, laboratory results are the best guide to diagnosis.

Prevention

Repeated application of long-acting miticides can make endemic areas safe. When this is not possible, insect repellents on clothing and skin provide some protection. For short exposure, chemoprophylaxis with doxycycline (200 mg weekly) can prevent the disease but permits infection. No effective vaccines are available at present.

Treatment & Prognosis

Without treatment, fever may subside spontaneously after 2 weeks, but the mortality rate may be 10–30%. Treatment for 3–7 days with tetracycline, 25 mg/kg/d in four divided doses, or chloramphenicol, 50 mg/kg/d in four divided doses, virtually eliminates deaths.

Chayakul P, Panich V, Silpapojakul K: Scrub typhus pneumonitis: An entity which is frequently missed. Quart J Med 1988;68:595.

SPOTTED FEVERS

Tick-borne rickettsial infections occur in many different regions of the world and have been given regional or local names, eg, Rocky Mountain spotted fever in North America, Queensland tick typhus in Australia, boutonneuse fever in North Africa, Kenya tick typhus, etc. The causative agents (Table 31–4) are all antigenically related to *Rickettsia rickettsii,* and all are transmitted by hard (ixodid) ticks and have cycles in nature that involve dogs, rodents, or other animals. There is some similarity in the epidemiology and clinical presentation of spotted fevers and Lyme disease (see Chapter 33). Rickettsiae are often transmitted from one generation of ticks to the next (transovarian transmission) without passage through a vertebrate host. Patients infected with spotted fevers usually develop antibodies to *Proteus* OX19 and OX2 in low titer, in addition to specific rickettsial antibodies.

Control of spotted fevers involves prevention of tick bites, specific immunization when available, and antibiotic treatment of patients.

1. ROCKY MOUNTAIN SPOTTED FEVER

Essentials of Diagnosis

- Exposure to tick bite in endemic area.
- "Influenzal" prodrome followed by chills, fever, severe headache, widespread aches and pains, restlessness, and prostration; occasionally, delirium and coma.
- Red macular rash appears between the second and sixth days of fever, first on the wrists and ankles and then spreading centrally; it may become petechial.
- Laboratory confirmation by agglutination of *Proteus* OX19 and OX2 and by specific antibodies with complement fixation and immunofluorescence.

General Considerations

The causative agent, *R rickettsii*, is transmitted to humans by the bite of ticks, including the wood tick, *Dermacentor andersoni*, in the western USA and by the bite of the dog tick, *Dermacentor variabilis*, in the eastern USA. Other hard ticks transmit the organism in the southern USA and in Central and South America and are responsible for transmitting it among rodents, dogs, porcupines, and other animals. Most human cases occur in late spring and summer. In the USA, most cases occur in the eastern third of the country, with nearly 1000 reported per year.

Clinical Findings

A. Symptoms and Signs: Three to 10 days after the bite of an infectious tick, anorexia, malaise, nausea, headache, and sore throat occur. These progress, with chills, fever, aches in bones, joints, and muscles, abdominal pain, nausea and vomiting, restlessness, insomnia, and irritability. Cough and pneumonitis may develop. Delirium, lethargy, seizures, stupor, and coma may appear. The face is flushed and the conjunctiva injected. The rash (faint macules that progress to maculopapules and then petechiae) appears between days 2 and 6 of fever, first on the wrists and ankles, spreading centrally to the arms, legs, and trunk for 2–3 days. It is important to recognize that about 10% of cases occur without rash or with minimal rash. In some cases there is splenomegaly, hepatomegaly, jaundice, gangrene, myocarditis, or uremia. Other complications include suppurative otitis or parotitis, pneumonitis, and circulatory failure.

B. Laboratory Findings: Leukocytosis, thrombocytopenia, hyponatremia, proteinuria, and hematuria are common. Cerebrospinal fluid may show hypoglycorrhachia and mild pleocytosis. Owing to endothelial damage, there is activation of platelets, coagulation pathways, and fibrinolysis. Rickettsiae can sometimes be isolated in special laboratories from blood obtained in the first few days of illness. A rise in antibody titer during the second week of illness can be detected by specific complement fixation, immunofluorescence, and microagglutination tests or by the Weil-Felix reaction with *Proteus* OX19 and OX2. Antibody response may be suppressed if antimicrobial drugs are given very early.

Differential Diagnosis

The early signs and symptoms of Rocky Mountain spotted fever are shared with many other infections. The rash may be confused with that of measles, typhoid, or meningococcemia. The suspicion of the latter requires blood cultures and cerebrospinal fluid examination. Infection with *Ehrlichia canis* (ehrlichiosis), a leukocytic rickettsiosis resulting from a tick bite, may resemble Rocky Mountain spotted fever.

Prevention

Protective clothing, tick-repellent chemicals, and the removal of ticks at frequent intervals are helpful measures. Vaccines of inactivated *R rickettsii* grown in eggs or in cell culture have given moderate protection but were not commercially available in the USA or Canada in 1992.

Treatment & Prognosis

In mild, untreated cases, fever subsides at the end of the second week. The response to chloramphenicol (25–50 mg/kg/d orally or intravenously in four divided doses) or tetracycline (25–50 mg/kg/d orally in four divided doses) is prompt if the drugs are started early. Treatment is given for 7 days or through the third day of defervescence.

The mortality rate for Rocky Mountain spotted fever varies strikingly with age. In untreated elderly persons it may be 70%; in children, less than 20%, the usual cause of death being pneumonitis and respiratory or cardiac failure. Sequelae are rare but include seizures, encephalopathy, and motor deficits.

Kirk JL et al: Rocky Mountain spotted fever: A clinical review based on 48 confirmed cases, 1943–1986. Medicine 1990;69:35.

Sexton DJ, Corey RG: Rocky Mountain "spotless" and "almost spotless" fever: A wolf in sheep's clothing. Clin Infect Dis 1992;15:439.

Weber DJ, Walker DH: Rocky Mountain spotted fever. Infect Dis Clin North Am 1991;5:19.

2. RICKETTSIALPOX

Rickettsia akari is a parasite of mice, transmitted by mites (*Allodermanyssus sanguineus*). Upon close contact of mice with humans, infected mites may transmit the disease to humans. Rickettsialpox has an incubation period of 7–12 days. The onset is sudden, with chills, fever, headache, photophobia, and disseminated aches and pains. The primary lesion is a painless red papule that vesicates and forms a black eschar. Two to 4 days after onset of symptoms, a widespread papular eruption appears that becomes vesicular and forms crusts that are shed in about 10 days. Early lesions may resemble those of chickenpox.

Leukopenia and a rise in antibody titer with rickettsial antigen in complement fixation tests are often present. However, the Weil-Felix test is negative.

Treatment includes tetracycline, 15 mg/kg/d orally in four divided doses for 3–5 days.

Even without treatment, the disease is fairly mild and self-limited, treatment only hastening resolution. Control requires the elimination of mice from human habitations after insecticide has been applied to suppress the mite vectors.

Walker DH: Rickettsioses of the spotted fever group around the world. J Dermatol 1989;16:169.

3. TICK TYPHUS

Tick typhus is a term used to refer both to a variety of spotted rickettsial fevers (often named by geography: eg, Israel tick fever, Kenya tick fever, Mediterranean spotted fever) transmitted by ticks (under introduction above) by the rickettsial agents *R conori, R australis,* and *R sibirica.* The pathogens usually produce a black spot (tâche noire) at the site of the tick bite that may be useful in diagnosis. Endothelial injury produces perivascular edema and dermal necrosis; disseminated lesions and focal hepatic necrosis may occur. Rashless cases of Mediterranean spotted fever have been reported. The disease has occurred among travelers, and in the USA, 67 cases were recorded over a 10-year interval, largely among returnees from Africa. Diagnosis is clinical, with serologic confirmation (Weil-Felix antibodies are positive for *Proteus* OX19 and OX2). Prevention entails protective clothing, repellents, and inspection for and removal of ticks. Treatment is with the following drugs given for 7–10 days: tetracycline (25–50 mg/kg/d in four divided doses), chloramphenicol (50–75 mg/kg/d in four divided doses), or ciprofloxacin (500 mg twice daily).

Brouqui P et al: Spotless boutonneuse fever. Clin Infect Dis 1992;14:114.

OTHER RICKETTSIAL & RICKETTSIAL-LIKE DISEASES

1. EHRLICHIOSIS

Ehrlichiosis is due to *Ehrlichia canis,* a ubiquitous tick-borne pathogen mainly of dogs. It is an intracellular parasite of leukocytes and forms intracellular inclusion bodies evident on Giemsa-stained preparations.

Human ehrlichiosis has been diagnosed mainly in the Southeastern and South Central USA in patients exposed to ticks. Clinical disease ranges from mild to life-threatening. Typically, after a 12- to 14-day incubation period and a prodrome consisting of malaise, back pain and nausea, the patient develops sudden fever, relative bradycardia, and headache. Rashes are unusual. Leukopenia and absolute lymphopenia as well as thrombocytopenia occur frequently. Serious reported sequelae include acute respiratory failure, encephalopathy, and acute renal failure. An indirect fluorescent antibody assay that may be used to diagnose infection is available through CDC and requires acute and convalescent sera.

Tetracycline is given as 25 mg/kg/d in four divided doses.

Eng TR et al: Epidemiologic, clinical, and laboratory findings of human ehrlichiosis in the United States, 1988. JAMA 1990;264:2251.
McDade JE: Ehrlichiosis: A disease of animals and humans. J Infect Dis 1990;161:609.

2. TRENCH FEVER

Trench fever is a self-limited, louse-borne relapsing febrile disease caused by *Rochalimaea quintana,* a *Rickettsia*-like agent related to the causative agents of cat-scratch disease and bacillary angiomatosis (Chapter 32). This organism grows extracellularly in the louse intestine and is excreted in feces. Humans are infected when infected louse feces enter defects in skin. No animal reservoir except humans has been demonstrated.

This disease has occurred in epidemic forms in louse-infested troops and civilians during wars and in endemic form in Central America. Onset is abrupt, with fever lasting 3–5 days, often followed by relapses. The patient becomes weak and complains of severe pain behind the eyes and in the back and legs. Lymphadenopathy and splenomegaly may appear, as may a transient maculopapular rash. Subclinical infection is frequent, and a carrier state may occur. The differential diagnosis includes dengue, leptospirosis, malaria, relapsing fever, and typhus.

R quintana, unlike *Rickettsia,* grows on artificial media without living cells, can be cultivated on agar containing 10% fresh blood, and has been recovered from blood cultures of patients. The Weil-Felix test is negative, but a specific complement fixation test and a specific enzyme immunoassay are available.

The illness is self-limited, and recovery regularly occurs without treatment.

3. Q FEVER

Essentials of Diagnosis

- An acute or chronic febrile illness with severe headache, cough, prostration, and abdominal pain.
- Extensive pneumonitis, hepatitis, or encephalopathy; rarely endocarditis.
- Exposure to sheep, goats, cattle, or their products.

General Considerations

Coxiella burnetii is unique among rickettsiae in that it is usually transmitted to humans not by arthropods but by inhalation of infectious aerosols or ingestion of infected milk. It primarily infects cattle, sheep, and goats, in which it produces mild or subclinical infection. It is transmitted by cows and goats principally through the milk and placenta and by sheep through feces, placenta, and milk. Dry feces and milk, dust contaminated with them, and the tissues of these animals contain large numbers of infectious organisms that are spread by the airborne route. Inhalation of contaminated dust and of droplets from infected animal tissues is the main source of human infection. Outbreaks have been described in association with parturient cats. There is an occupational risk for animal handlers, slaughterhouse workers, veterinarians, etc. *Coxiella* is resistant to heat and drying, perhaps because the organism forms endospore-like structures. Thus, it survives in dust, on the fleece of infected animals, or in inadequately pasteurized milk. Spread from one human to another does not seem to occur even in the presence of florid pneumonitis, but fetal infection can occur.

Clinical Findings

A. Symptoms and Signs: After an incubation period of 1–3 weeks, a febrile illness develops with headache, prostration, and muscle pains, occasionally with a nonproductive cough, abdominal pains, or jaundice. Physical signs of pneumonitis are slight. Hepatitis may be severe. Endocarditis of the aortic valve occurs rarely but must always be considered when either culture-negative endocarditis or large vegetations exist with a suggestive epidemiologic background. At times, signs of encephalopathy are present. The clinical course may be acute or chronic and relapsing.

B. Laboratory Findings: Laboratory examination often shows leukopenia and a diagnostic rise in specific complement-fixing antibodies to *Coxiella* phase 2. The Weil-Felix test is negative. Liver function tests are often abnormal. In Q fever endocarditis, there is a titer of 1:200 or more by complement fixation or indirect immunofluorescence with phase 1 antigen of *C burnetii*. Isolation of the organism from blood or sputum in the future may be possible with the centrifugation shell-vial technique.

C. Imaging: Radiographs of the chest show variable pulmonary infiltration.

Differential Diagnosis

Viral, mycoplasmal, and bacterial pneumonias; viral hepatitis; brucellosis; tuberculosis; psittacosis; and other animal-borne diseases must be considered. The history of exposure to animals or animal dusts or tissues (eg, in slaughterhouses) should lead to appropriate specific serologic tests.

Prevention

Prevention must be based on detection of the infection in livestock, reduction of contact with infected animals or dusts contaminated by them, special care during contact with animal tissues, and effective pasteurization of milk. A vaccine of formalin-inactivated phase 1 *Coxiella* is being developed for persons at high risk of infection and appears to be protective.

Treatment & Prognosis

Treatment with tetracyclines (25 mg/kg/d in four divided doses) can suppress symptoms and shorten the clinical course but does not always eradicate the infection. Treatment should continue for 3 full days of defervescence. Even in untreated patients, the mortality rate is usually low, except with endocarditis.

Treatment of endocarditis consists of protracted—often for years—antibiotic therapy with doxycycline (200 mg/d) and either trimethoprim-sulfamethoxazole (320/1600 mg/d) or rifampin (900 mg/d, but may interact adversely with anticoagulant), or quinolones (ofloxacin, 400 mg/d, or equivalent); heart valves often need replacement, since the mainstays of antibiotic therapy (chloramphenicol, tetracycline) for rickettsial organisms are bacteriostatic.

Levy PY et al: Comparison of different antibiotic regimens for therapy of 32 cases of Q fever endocarditis. Antimicrob Agents Chemother 1991;35:533.

Pinsky RL et al: An outbreak of cat-associated Q fever in the United States. J Infect Dis 1991;164:202.

Raoult D et al: Acute and chronic Q fever in patients with cancer. Clin Infect Dis 1992;14:127.

Infectious Diseases: Bacterial & Chlamydial

32

Henry F. Chambers, MD

INFECTIONS CAUSED BY GRAM-POSITIVE BACTERIA

STREPTOCOCCAL INFECTIONS

1. PHARYNGITIS

Essentials of Diagnosis

- Abrupt onset of sore throat, fever, malaise, nausea, and headache.
- Throat red and edematous, with or without exudate; cervical nodes tender.
- Diagnosis confirmed by culture of throat.

General Considerations

Beta-hemolytic streptococci, classically group A, are the most common bacterial cause of exudative pharyngitis. *Mycoplasma* and *Chlamydia pneumoniae* (TWAR strain) have also been isolated from patients with pharyngitis, but their clinical significance remains to be clarified. Transmission is by droplets of infected secretions. Group A streptococci producing erythrogenic toxin may cause scarlet fever rashes in susceptible persons.

Clinical Findings

A. Symptoms and Signs: "Strep throat" is characterized by a sudden onset of fever, sore throat, pain on swallowing, tender cervical adenopathy, malaise, and nausea. The pharynx, soft palate, and tonsils are red and edematous, and there may be a purulent exudate. The rash of scarlet fever is diffusely erythematous, with superimposed fine red papules, and is most intense in the groin and axillas. It blanches on pressure, may become petechial, and fades in 2–5 days, leaving a fine desquamation. In scarlet fever, the face is flushed, with circumoral pallor; and the tongue is coated, with enlarged red papillae (strawberry tongue).

B. Laboratory Findings: Leukocytosis with an increase in polymorphonuclear neutrophils is a regular early finding. Throat culture onto a single blood agar plate has a sensitivity of 70–80%. A two-plate culture method (trimethoprim-sulfamethoxazole blood agar plate and a plain blood agar plate) detects an additional 20% of cases that are missed by the single-plate method. Rapid antigen detection methods are less sensitive than throat culture, with sensitivities as low as 40% or less.

Complications

The suppurative complications of streptococcal sore throat include sinusitis, otitis media, mastoiditis, peritonsillar abscess, and suppuration of cervical lymph nodes, among others.

Nonsuppurative complications are rheumatic fever (0.05–3%) and glomerulonephritis (0.2–20%). Rheumatic fever may follow recurrent episodes of pharyngitis with any type of group A streptococci and begins 1–4 weeks after the onset of symptoms. Glomerulonephritis follows a single infection with a nephritogenic strain of *Streptococcus* group A (eg, types 4, 12, 2, 49, and 60), more commonly on the skin than in the throat, and begins 1–3 weeks after the onset of the infection.

Differential Diagnosis

Streptococcal sore throat resembles (and cannot be reliably distinguished clinically from) pharyngitis caused by adenoviruses, Epstein-Barr virus, and other agents. Pharyngitis accompanied by generalized lymphadenopathy, splenomegaly, atypical lymphocytosis, and a positive serologic test (eg, Monospot) distinguishes mononucleosis from streptococcal pharyngitis. Diphtheria is characterized by a pseudomembrane; candidiasis shows white patches of exudate and less erythema; and necrotizing ulcerative gingivostomatitis (Vincent's fusospirochetal disease) presents with shallow ulcers in the mouth. Bacterial epiglottitis with odynophagia and difficulty handling secretions should be considered when severity of symptoms is disproportionate to findings on examination of the pharynx.

Treatment

Antimicrobial therapy has a minimal effect on resolution of symptoms. Because its main purpose is prevention of complications, therapy may be withheld pending results of culture. Because throat culture (especially if a single plate is used) and rapid detection methods may be falsely negative in 30% or more of cases, when clinical suspicion is high (eg, presence of exudative pharyngitis, tender adenopathy, high fever, and absence of cough and rhinorrhea) and the risk of therapy is low (eg, no drug allergy), antimicrobial therapy may be given without laboratory evaluation.

A. Benzathine penicillin G, 1.2 million units intramuscularly as a single dose, is optimal therapy and usually eradicates the streptococci.

B. Penicillin V potassium, 500 mg orally four times a day for 10 days, is effective, but this regimen is not easily completed, since the patient becomes asymptomatic in 2–4 days.

C. Patients allergic to penicillin may be treated with erythromycin, 0.5 g four times daily (40 mg/kg/d) for 10 days.

Prevention of Recurrent Rheumatic Fever

Effectively controlling rheumatic fever depends upon identification and treatment of primary streptococcal infection and secondary prevention of recurrences. Patients who have had rheumatic fever should be treated with a continuous course of antimicrobial prophylaxis for at least 5 years. Benzathine penicillin, 1.2 million units as a single intramuscular injection every 4 weeks, is the regimen of choice. Sulfadiazine, 1 g orally daily, or penicillin G, 500 mg orally daily, is also acceptable, but less reliable, as a prophylactic regimen.

Bisno AL: Group A streptococcal infections and acute rheumatic fever. New Engl J Med 1991;325:783. (Changing epidemiology and clinical features.)

Peter G: Streptococcal pharyngitis: Current therapy and criteria for evaluating new agents. Clin Infect Dis 1992;14(Suppl 2):S218.

Wegner DL, Witte DL, Schantz RD: Insensitivity of rapid antigen detection methods and single blood agar culture for diagnosing streptococcal pharyngitis. JAMA 1992; 267:695. (Evaluation of two-plate throat culture method versus routinely used culture and antigen detection tests.)

2. STREPTOCOCCAL SKIN INFECTIONS

Streptococci are not part of normal skin flora. Streptococcal skin infections usually result from colonization of normal skin by contact with other infected individuals or by preceding streptococcal respiratory infection.

Clinical Findings

A. Symptoms and Signs: Impetigo is a focal, vesicular, pustular lesion with a thick, amber-colored crust that has a "stuck-on" appearance.

Erysipelas is a painful superficial cellulitis that frequently involves the face. It is well demarcated from the surrounding normal skin. Erysipelas also affects skin with impaired lymphatic drainage, such as edematous lower extremities or wounds.

B. Laboratory Findings: Cultures obtained from a wound or pustule are likely to grow group A streptococci. Other cultures of the skin (eg, direct cultures or tissue fluid aspirated from an area of cellulitis or erysipelas) occasionally are positive if the specimen is obtained from the leading edge of the lesion. Blood cultures are occasionally positive.

Treatment

Parenteral antibiotics are indicated for patients with facial erysipelas or evidence of systemic infection. Penicillin, 1 million units intravenously every 4 hours, is the drug of choice.

Cutaneous infections caused by staphylococci may at times be difficult to differentiate from streptococcal infections. Co-infection with staphylococci also occurs. Therefore, initial therapy for severely ill patients or those who have risk factors for staphylococcal infection (eg, intravenous drug use, wound infection, diabetes) should include an agent—such as nafcillin, 1.5 g intravenously every 6 hours—that also is active against *Staphylococcus aureus*. In the patient with minor penicillin allergy, cefazolin, 500 mg intravenously or intramuscularly every 8 hours, may be used. In the patient with a serious penicillin allergy (ie, anaphylaxis), vancomycin, 1000 mg intravenously every 12 hours, should be used.

Patients who do not require parenteral therapy may be treated with penicillin V potassium, 500 mg orally, or erythromycin, 500 mg orally, four times daily for 7–10 days.

3. OTHER GROUP A STREPTOCOCCAL INFECTIONS

Arthritis, pneumonia, empyema, and endocarditis are relatively uncommon infections that may be caused by group A streptococci.

Arthritis generally occurs in association with cellulitis. In addition to intravenous therapy with penicillin G, 2 million units every 4 hours (or cefazolin or vancomycin in doses recommended above for penicillin-allergic patients), frequent percutaneous needle aspiration should be performed to remove joint effusions. Open surgical drainage usually is not necessary unless the hip or shoulder is infected, because these are less amenable to percutaneous drainage.

Pneumonia and **empyema** often are characterized by extensive tissue destruction and an aggressive, rapidly progressive clinical course associated with significant morbidity and mortality rates. High-dose penicillin and chest tube drainage are indicated for treatment of empyema. Vancomycin is an acceptable substitute in penicillin-allergic patients.

Group A streptococci can cause **endocarditis.** This complication should be suspected when bacteremia accompanies pneumonia, particularly if the patient abuses parenteral drugs. The tricuspid valve is most commonly involved. A patient with suspected endocarditis should be treated with 4 million units of penicillin G every 4 hours for 4 weeks. Vancomycin, 1000 mg every 12 hours, is recommended for persons allergic to penicillin.

4. NON-GROUP A STREPTOCOCCAL INFECTIONS

Non-group A streptococci produce a spectrum of disease similar to that of group A streptococci. Some non-group A streptococci are β-hemolytic (eg, groups B, C, and G). The treatment of infections caused by these strains is the same as for group A streptococci.

Group B streptococci are an important cause of sepsis, bacteremia, and meningitis in the neonate. This organism, which is part of the normal vaginal flora, may cause septic abortion, endometritis, or peripartum infections and, less commonly, cellulitis, bacteremia, and endocarditis in adults. Treatment of infections caused by group B streptococci is with either penicillin or vancomycin in doses recommended for group A streptococci. Because of in vitro synergism, some authorities recommend the addition of low-dose gentamicin, 1 mg/kg every 8 hours.

Viridans streptococci, which are nonhemolytic or α-hemolytic (ie, producing a green zone of hemolysis on blood agar), are part of the normal oral flora. Although these strains may produce focal pyogenic infection, they are most notable as the leading cause of native valve endocarditis (see Chapter 29).

Group D streptococci include *Streptococcus bovis* and the enterococci. *S bovis* is a cause of endocarditis in association with bowel neoplasia or cirrhosis. Endocarditis caused by *S bovis* is treated like viridans streptococci.

Enterococci have been classified into a genus separate from other streptococci. Two species, *Enterococcus faecalis* and *Enterococcus faecium,* are responsible for most human enterococcal infections. Enterococci cause wound infections, urinary tract infections, and endocarditis. Until recently, enterococci were uniformly susceptible to penicillin or vancomycin, with gentamicin added in endocarditis. Susceptibility to penicillin or vancomycin and gentamicin should be documented when treating serious enterococcal infections such as endocarditis and osteomyelitis. Except for endocarditis, enterococcal infec-

tions can still be treated with penicillin, 3 million units every 4 hours; ampicillin (which is slightly more active than penicillin in vitro), 2 g every 6 hours; or vancomycin, 1 g every 12 hours. Because these antibiotics are not bactericidal for enterococci, gentamicin in a dose of 1 mg/kg every 8 hours is added in endocarditis and considered in osteomyelitis.

Murray BE: The life and times of the enterococcus. Clin Microbiol Rev 1990;3:46.
Opal SM et al: Group B streptococcal sepsis in adults and infants: Contrasts and comparisons. Arch Intern Med 1988;148:641. (Descriptive study and association with underlying disease.)
Wells VD et al: Infections due to beta-lactamase-producing high-level gentamicin-resistant *Enterococcus faecalis.* Ann Intern Med 1992;116:285. (Clinical and molecular epidemiology of resistant enterococcal colonization and infection.)

PNEUMOCOCCAL INFECTIONS

1. PNEUMOCOCCAL PNEUMONIA

Essentials of Diagnosis

- Productive cough, fever, rigors, dyspnea, early pleuritic chest pain.
- Consolidating lobar pneumonia on chest x-ray.
- Lancet-shaped gram-positive diplococci on gram-stain of sputum.

General Considerations

The pneumococcus is the most common cause of community-acquired pyogenic bacterial pneumonia. Alcoholism, infection by HIV, sickle cell disease, splenectomy, and hematologic disorders are predisposing factors. The mortality rate remains high in the setting of advanced age, multilobar disease, severe hypoxemia, extrapulmonary complications, and bacteremia.

Clinical Findings

A. Symptoms and Signs: The illness typically evolves over a period of a few days. The patient presents with high fever, productive cough, occasionally hemoptysis, and pleuritic chest pain. Rigors occur within the first few hours of infection but are uncommon thereafter. Bronchial breathing is an early sign.

B. Laboratory Findings: Classically, pneumococcal pneumonia is a lobar pneumonia with radiographic signs of consolidation and occasionally effusion. Infiltrates may also be patchy.

Gram's stain of sputum always should be examined. Adequately collected samples (with < 10 epithelial cells and > 25 polymorphonuclear leukocytes per high power field) show gram-positive diplococci 80–90% of the time. Sputum culture alone is less sensitive than Gram's stain, and false positives are common as well. Blood cultures are positive in up to 25% of selected cases and much more commonly so in HIV-positive patients.

Complications

Parapneumonic (sympathetic) effusion is common and may cause recurrence or persistence of fever. These sterile fluid accumulations need no specific therapy. Empyema occurs in 5% or less of cases and is differentiated from sympathetic effusion by the presence of organisms on Gram-stained fluid or positive pleural fluid cultures.

Pneumococcal pericarditis is a rare complication that can cause tamponade. Pneumococcal arthritis also is uncommon. Pneumococcal endocarditis usually involves the aortic valve and often occurs in association with meningitis and pneumonia. Early heart failure and multiple embolic events are typical.

Treatment

A. Specific Measures: Although penicillin resistance does occur, pneumococcal strains usually are sensitive to penicillin. Uncomplicated pneumococcal pneumonia (ie, arterial PO_2 greater than 60 mm Hg, no coexisting medical problems, and single-lobe disease without signs of extrapulmonary infection) may be treated on an outpatient basis with penicillin V potassium, 500 mg orally four times a day for 7–10 days. For penicillin-allergic patients, either erythromycin, 500 mg orally four times a day, or trimethoprim-sulfamethoxazole, one double-strength tablet (320 mg trimethoprim and 1600 mg sulfamethoxazole) orally twice a day, may be used.

More seriously ill patients or those with other medical problems should be admitted and treated with procaine penicillin, 600,000 units intramuscularly every 12 hours, or aqueous penicillin G, 1 million units intravenously every 4 hours. For penicillin-allergic patients without anaphylaxis or other serious reactions, cefazolin, 500 mg either intravenously or intramuscularly every 8 hours, is effective. For serious penicillin or cephalosporin allergy, vancomycin, 30 mg/kg/d, up to 2000 mg total, in two divided doses, can be used. Trimethoprim-sulfamethoxazole given intravenously with doses of 10 mg/kg/d of the trimethoprim component divided into three doses also is effective. Intravenous erythromycin is effective, but it is generally less well tolerated because of phlebitis.

B. Treatment of Complications: Thoracentesis should be performed if pleural effusion develops. Chest tube drainage may be required if pneumococci are identified by culture or Gram stain.

Echocardiography should be done if pericardial effusion is suspected. Patients with pericardial effusion who are responding to therapy and have no signs of tamponade may be followed and treated with indomethacin, 50 mg three times daily, for pain. In patients with increasing effusion, unsatisfactory clinical response, or evidence of tamponade, pericardiocentesis will determine if the pericardial space is infected. Infected fluid must be drained either percutaneously (by tube placement or needle aspiration), by placement of a pericardial window, or by pericardiectomy. Pericardiectomy eventually may be required to prevent or treat constrictive pericarditis, a common sequela of bacterial pericarditis.

Endocarditis should be treated with 24 million units of penicillin G (or vancomycin for penicillin-allergic patients) daily for 4 weeks. Mild heart failure may respond to medical therapy alone, such as digoxin and diuretics, but moderate to severe heart failure is an indication for prosthetic valve implantation, as are systemic emboli or large friable vegetations as determined by echocardiography.

Janoff EN et al: Pneumococcal disease during HIV infection: Epidemiologic, clinical, and immunologic perspectives. Ann Intern Med 1992;117:314.

2. PNEUMOCOCCAL MENINGITIS

Essentials of Diagnosis

- Fever, headache, altered mental status.
- Meningismus.
- Gram-positive diplococci on Gram stain of cerebrospinal fluid; counterimmunoelectrophoresis may be positive in partially treated cases.

General Considerations

Streptococcus pneumoniae is the most common cause of meningitis in adults and the second most common cause of meningitis in children over the age of 6 years. Head trauma, cerebrospinal fluid leaks, and sinusitis may precede pneumococcal meningitis.

Clinical Findings

A. Symptoms and Signs: The onset is rapid, with fever, headache, and altered mentation. Pneumonia may be present. Compared to meningitis caused by the meningococcus, pneumococcal meningitis lacks a rash, and focal neurologic deficits, cranial nerve palsies, and obtundation are more prominent features.

B. Laboratory Findings: The cerebrospinal fluid typically has more than 1000 white blood cells per microliter, over 60% of which are polymorphonuclear leukocytes; the glucose concentration is less than 40 mg/dL, or less than 50% of the simultaneous serum concentration; the protein usually exceeds 150 mg/dL. Not all cases of meningitis will have these typical findings, and alterations in cerebrospinal fluid cell counts and chemistries may be surprisingly minimal, overlapping with those of aseptic meningitis.

Gram's stain of cerebrospinal fluid shows gram-positive cocci in 80–90% of cases, and in untreated cases blood or cerebrospinal fluid cultures are almost always positive. Tests such as counterimmuno-electrophoresis or latex agglutination to detect pneumococcal antigens in cerebrospinal fluid are less sensitive than culture and Gram's stain. Antigen detection tests may occasionally be helpful in establishing the diagnosis in the patient who has been partially treated and in whom cultures and stains are negative.

Treatment

Antibiotics should be given as soon as the diagnosis of meningitis is suspected. If lumbar puncture must be delayed (eg, while awaiting results of an imaging study to exclude a mass lesion), 4 million units of penicillin G intravenously is given after blood cultures (positive in 50% of cases) have been obtained. In the penicillin-allergic patient, chloramphenicol, 1.5 g, or ceftriaxone, 4 g/d, in one or two divided doses, is an effective alternative to penicillin. Penicillin, 24 million units daily in six divided doses, ceftriaxone, 4 g/d, or chloramphenicol, 6 g/d in four divided doses, is continued for 14 days in documented cases.

Penicillin-resistant pneumococci (MIC > 0.1 μg/mL) are rare, but their prevalence may be increasing. The best therapy for penicillin-resistant strains is not known. Ceftriaxone, 4 g/d, chloramphenicol, 100 mg/kg/d (provided the strain is susceptible), or vancomycin, 1 g every 12 hours, may be tried.

The role of steroids in adjunctive therapy of meningitis in the adult remains controversial. Some authorities suggest that dexamethasone, 0.15 mg/kg intravenously every 6 hours, be given when coma, focal deficits, and other signs of increased intracranial pressure are present.

Durand ML et al: Acute bacterial meningitis in adults: A review of 493 episodes. N Engl J Med 1993;328:21. (Analysis of microbiology, morbidity, mortality, and risk factors.)

Quadiarello V, Scheld WM: Bacterial meningitis: Pathogenesis, physiology, and progress. N Engl J Med 1992; 327:864.

STAPHYLOCOCCUS AUREUS INFECTIONS

1. SKIN & SOFT TISSUE INFECTIONS

Essentials of Diagnosis

- Localized erythema with induration.
- Tendency toward abscess formation.
- Folliculitis commonly observed.
- Gram's stain of pus with gram-positive cocci in clusters; cultures usually positive.

General Considerations

Most staphylococci found on cultures of normal skin belong to the *Staphylococcus epidermidis* group. *Staphylococcus aureus* is not normal skin flora. *S aureus* tends to cause more localized skin infections than streptococci, and abscess formation is common.

Clinical Findings

A. Symptoms and Signs: *S aureus* skin infections may begin around one or more hair follicles, causing folliculitis. These infections may localize to form boils (or furuncles) or spread to adjacent skin and deeper subcutaneous tissue (ie, a carbuncle). Myositis or fasciitis may occur, often in association with a deep wound or other inoculation or injection.

B. Laboratory Findings: Cultures of the wound or abscess material will almost always yield the organism. In patients with other systemic signs of infection, blood cultures should be obtained because of potential endocarditis, osteomyelitis, or metastatic seeding of other sites.

Treatment

Proper drainage of abscess fluid or other focal infections is the mainstay of therapy. Drainage may be all that is needed for cutaneous abscess. Antibiotic therapy alone is unlikely to be effective if collections of infected material are undrained.

For uncomplicated skin infections, oral therapy is satisfactory. An oral penicillinase-resistant penicillin or cephalosporin, such as dicloxacillin or cephalexin, 500 mg four times a day for 7–10 days, is the drug of choice. Erythromycin, 500 mg four times a day, may be used in the penicillin-allergic patient.

For more complicated infections with extensive cutaneous or deep tissue involvement or fever, parenteral therapy is indicated initially. A penicillinase-resistant penicillin such as nafcillin or oxacillin at a dose of 1.5 g every 6 hours intravenously is the drug of choice. In allergic patients without a serious reaction, cefazolin, 500 mg intravenously or intramuscularly every 8 hours, can be used. In patients with a serious allergy to β-lactam antibiotics or if the strain is methicillin-resistant, vancomycin, 1000 mg intravenously every 12 hours, is the drug of choice.

2. OSTEOMYELITIS

S aureus is the cause of approximately 60% of all cases of osteomyelitis. Osteomyelitis may be caused by direct inoculation, eg, from an open fracture or as a result of surgery; by extension from a contiguous focus of infection or open wound; or, more commonly, by hematogenous spread. Long bones and vertebrae are the usual sites. Epidural abscess with or without bone involvement is a common complication of vertebral osteomyelitis and should be suspected if fever and back pain are accompanied by radicular pain or neurologic signs or symptoms indicative of spinal cord compression (eg, incontinence).

Clinical Findings

A. Symptoms and Signs: The infection may be acute, with abrupt development of local symptoms and systemic toxicity; or indolent, with insidious onset of vague pain over the site of infection, progressing to local tenderness. Fever may be absent in up to a third of cases. Abscess formation is a late and unusual manifestation. Draining sinus tracts occur in chronic infections or infections of foreign body implants.

B. Laboratory Findings: The diagnosis is established by isolation of *S aureus* from the blood or bone of a patient with signs and symptoms of focal bone infection. Blood culture will be positive in approximately 60% of untreated cases of staphylococcal osteomyelitis. Bone biopsy and culture should be considered if blood cultures are sterile.

C. Imaging: Bone scan and gallium scan, each with a sensitivity of approximately 95% and a specificity of 60–70%, are useful in identifying or confirming the site of bone infection. Plain bone films early in the course of infection are often normal but will become abnormal in most cases even with effective therapy. Spinal infection (unlike malignancy) traverses the disk space to involve the contiguous vertebral body. CT is more sensitive than plain films and can be useful in localizing associated abscesses. MRI is somewhat less sensitive than bone scan but has a specificity of 90%. Myelography or MRI is indicated when epidural abscess is suspected in association with vertebral osteomyelitis.

Treatment

Prolonged therapy is required to cure staphylococcal osteomyelitis. Durations of 4–6 weeks or longer are recommended. Although oral regimens can be effective, parenteral regimens are advised for the first 2–4 weeks of therapy. Nafcillin or oxacillin, 9–12 g/d in six divided doses, is the drug of choice. Cefazolin, 1 g every 8 hours, also is effective. Vancomycin, 1 g every 12 hours, may be used for the penicillin-allergic patient.

Oral regimens are dicloxacillin or cephalexin, 1 g every 6 hours. Trimethoprim-sulfamethoxazole, 320/1600 mg, or ciprofloxacin, 750 mg twice a day, may be effective alternatives. Some authorities recommend that rifampin be added to the regimen for treatment of staphylococcal osteomyelitis. The dose is 300 mg twice a day.

Gupta NC, Prezio JA: Radionuclide imaging in osteomyelitis. Semin Nucl Med 1988;28:287.

Waldvogel FA, Vasey H: Osteomyelitis: The past decade. N Engl J Med 1980;303:360. (Still timely review.)

3. STAPHYLOCOCCAL BACTEREMIA

S aureus readily invades the bloodstream and infects sites distant from the primary site of infection, which may be relatively minor or even inapparent. Though commonly arising from skin lesions or intravenous lines, whenever *S aureus* is recovered from blood culture, the possibility of endocarditis, osteomyelitis, or other metastatic deep infection must be considered. The appropriate duration of therapy for uncomplicated bacteremia arising from a removable source (eg, intravenous device) or drainable focus (eg, skin abscess) has not been well defined. Although 2 weeks of parenteral therapy is commonly recommended, shorter courses and oral regimens may be successful. However, approximately 10% or more of patients still relapse, usually with endocarditis, even if treated for 2 weeks.

Because of this tendency—and based on the impression that longer courses of therapy reduce the relapse rate—10–14 days of nafcillin or oxacillin, 1.5 g intravenously every four to six hours, cefazolin, 500–1000 mg every 8 hours, or vancomycin, 1000 mg every 12 hours, is recommended for uncomplicated staphylococcal bacteremia. Vancomycin should be reserved for patients with serious penicillin allergy or with infections caused by methicillin-resistant strains because of data suggesting that it is less active than β-lactam antibiotics. Longer courses of either parenteral or oral therapy may be considered for patients (eg, those with diabetes, immunocompromised persons) at risk for late complications from bacteremia and for those in whom endocarditis is suspected (see Chapter 10).

Ehni WF, Reller B: Short-course therapy for catheter-associated *Staphylococcus aureus* bacteremia. Arch Intern Med 1989;149:533.

Karchmer AW: *Staphylococcus aureus* and vancomycin: The sequel. Ann Intern Med 1991;115:739. (Editorial review of data for vancomycin treatment of staphylococcal infection.)

4. TOXIC SHOCK SYNDROME

Some strains of staphylococci elaborate toxins that can cause three important entities: "scalded skin syndrome" in children, toxic shock syndrome in adults, and enterotoxin food poisoning. Toxic shock syndrome is characterized by abrupt onset of high fever, vomiting, and watery diarrhea. Sore throat, myalgias, and headache are often complaints. Hypotension with renal and cardiac failure is an ominous manifestation in severe cases. A diffuse macular erythematous rash and nonpurulent conjunctivitis are common, and desquamation, especially of palms and soles, is typical during recovery. Fatality rates may be as high as 15%. Although toxic shock syndrome has occurred in children and in males, the great majority of cases (90% or more) have been reported in women of child-bearing age. Of these, symptoms begin in nearly all patients within 5 days of the onset of a menstrual period in women who have used tampons. The syndrome is possible in any patient with a focus of toxin-producing *S aureus;* organisms from various sites, including the nasopharynx, vagina, or rectum or from wounds, have all been associated with the illness. Toxic shock syndrome is most often caused by toxic shock syndrome toxin-1 (TSST-1). Cases of toxic shock syndrome that are not tampon-associated are frequently caused by strains that do not produce TSST-1. Blood cultures are negative, because symptoms are due to the effects of the toxin and not to the invasive properties of the organism.

Important aspects of treatment include rapid rehydration, antistaphylococcal drugs, management of renal or cardiac insufficiency, and removal of sources of toxin, eg, removal of tampon, drainage of abscess.

Recently, a toxic shock-like syndrome has been reported in association with group A streptococcal infections. This syndrome is characterized by invasive skin or soft tissue infection, shock, myositis, adult respiratory distress syndrome, and renal failure. It differs from staphylococcal toxic shock syndrome in several respects. Bacteremia, which is uncommon in staphylococcal toxic shock, occurs in half or more of patients. Skin rashes and desquamation may be absent in the streptococcal syndrome. Exotoxin A, an erythrogenic exotoxin that produces scarlet fever, may mediate the systemic toxicity of the streptococcal syndrome.

Stevens DL et al: Severe group A streptococcal infections associated with toxic shock-like syndrome and scarlet fever toxin A. N Engl J Med 1989;321:1.

5. INFECTIONS CAUSED BY COAGULASE-NEGATIVE STAPHYLOCOCCI

Coagulase-negative staphylococci are an important cause of infections of intravascular devices and foreign bodies, though on rare occasions they cause infections such as endocarditis and osteomyelitis in the absence of predisposing factors. More than 20 species have been identified, but most human infections are caused by *Staphylococcus epidermidis, S haemolyticus, S hominis, S warnerii, S saprophyticus, S saccharolyticus,* and *S cohnii.* These common nosocomial pathogens are less virulent than *S aureus,* and infections caused by them tend to be more indolent.

Because coagulase-negative staphylococci are normal inhabitants of human skin, it can be difficult to determine whether their isolation is caused by infection or contamination. Infection is more likely if the patient has a foreign body (eg, sternal wires, pros-

thetic joint, prosthetic cardiac valve, intracranial pressure monitor, cerebrospinal fluid shunt, peritoneal dialysis catheter) or an intravascular device in place. Purulent or serosanguineous drainage, erythema, pain, or tenderness at the site of the foreign body or device suggests infection. Instability and pain are signs of prosthetic joint infection. Fever, a new murmur, instability of the prosthesis, or signs of systemic embolization are evidence of prosthetic valve infection. Immunosuppression and recent antimicrobial therapy also are risk factors for infection.

Infection is also more likely if the same strain is consistently isolated from two or more blood cultures (particularly if samples were obtained at different times) and from the foreign body site. Contamination rather than infection is favored by a single positive blood culture or if more than one strain is isolated from blood cultures. The antimicrobial susceptibility pattern and speciation—also called biotyping—is commonly used to determine whether one or more strains have been isolated. More sophisticated typing methods, such as plasmid pattern analysis or restriction endonuclease pattern analysis, may be required to identify distinct strains.

Whenever possible, the intravascular device or foreign body suspected of being infected by coagulase-negative staphylococci should be removed. However, removal and replacement of some devices (eg, prosthetic joint, prosthetic valve, cerebrospinal fluid shunt) can be a difficult or risky procedure, and it may sometimes be preferable to treat with antibiotics alone with the understanding that the probability of cure is low and that surgical management may eventually be necessary.

Coagulase-negative staphylococci are commonly resistant to methicillin and multiple other antibiotics. For patients with normal renal function, vancomycin, 1 g intravenously every 12 hours, is the treatment of choice for suspected or confirmed infection caused by these organisms until susceptibility to penicillinase-resistant penicillins or other agents has been confirmed. Duration of therapy has not been established for relatively uncomplicated infections, such as those secondary to intravenous devices, which may be eliminated by simply removing the infected device. Infection involving bone or a prosthetic valve should be treated for 6 weeks. A combination regimen of vancomycin plus rifampin, 300 mg orally twice daily, and gentamicin, 1 mg/kg intravenously every 8 hours, is recommended for treatment of prosthetic valve endocarditis caused by methicillin-resistant strains.

Nafziger DA, Wenzel RP: Coagulase-negative staphylococci: Epidemiology, evaluation, and therapy. Infect Dis Clin North Am 1989;3:915.

CLOSTRIDIAL DISEASES

1. CLOSTRIDIAL MYONECROSIS (Gas Gangrene)

Essentials of Diagnosis

- Sudden onset of pain and edema in an area of wound contamination.
- Prostration and systemic toxicity.
- Brown to blood-tinged watery exudate, with skin discoloration of surrounding area.
- Gas in the tissue by palpation or x-ray.
- Gram-positive rods in culture or smear of exudate.

General Considerations

Gas gangrene or clostridial myonecrosis is produced by entry of one of several clostridia (*Clostridium perfringens, Clostridium ramosum, Clostridium bifermentans, Clostridium histolyticum, Clostridium novyi,* etc) into devitalized tissues. Toxins produced under anaerobic conditions result in shock, hemolysis, and myonecrosis.

Clinical Findings

A. Symptoms and Signs: The onset of gas gangrene is usually sudden, with rapidly increasing pain in the affected area, fall in blood pressure, and tachycardia. Fever is present but is not proportionate to the severity of the infection. In the last stages of the disease, severe prostration, stupor, delirium, and coma occur.

The wound becomes swollen, and the surrounding skin is pale. Fluid accumulation beneath produces a foul-smelling brown, blood-tinged serous discharge. As the disease advances, the surrounding tissue changes from pale to dusky and finally becomes deeply discolored, with coalescent, red, fluid-filled vesicles. Gas may be palpable in the tissues. In clostridial sepsis, hemolysis and jaundice are common, often complicated by acute renal failure.

B. Laboratory Findings: Gas gangrene is a clinical diagnosis, and empiric therapy is indicated whenever the diagnosis is suspected. Radiographic studies may show gas within the soft tissues, but this is not sufficient to make the diagnosis because other organisms may produce gas. The smear, which typically shows a remarkable absence of neutrophils, is very suggestive if gram-positive rods are present. Anaerobic culture confirms the diagnosis.

Differential Diagnosis

Other types of infection can cause gas formation in the tissue, eg, *Enterobacter, Escherichia,* and mixed anaerobic infections including *Bacteroides* and peptostreptococci. Clostridia may produce serious puerperal infection with hemolysis.

Treatment

Penicillin, 2 million units every 3 hours intravenously, is effective. Although other agents (eg, tetracycline, clindamycin, metronidazole, chloramphenicol, cefoxitin) are active against *Clostridium* spp in vitro and probably in vivo as well, their clinical efficacy has not been demonstrated. Adequate surgical debridement and exposure of infected areas is essential, with radical surgical excision often necessary.

TETANUS

Essentials of Diagnosis

- History of wound and possible contamination.
- Jaw stiffness followed by spasms of jaw muscles (trismus).
- Stiffness of the neck and other muscles, dysphagia, irritability, hyperreflexia.
- Finally, painful convulsions precipitated by minimal stimuli.

General Considerations

Tetanus is caused by the neurotoxin elaborated by *Clostridium tetani.* Spores of this organism are ubiquitous in soil. When introduced into a wound, spores may germinate. The vegetative bacteria elaborate a toxin, tetanospasmin, that blocks the action of inhibitory mediators at spinal synapses and interferes with neuromuscular transmission. As a result, minor stimuli result in uncontrolled spasms, and reflexes are exaggerated. The incubation period is 5 days to 15 weeks, with the average being 8–12 days.

In the United States, most cases occur in unvaccinated individuals. Persons at risk are the elderly, migrant workers, newborns, and injection drug users, who may acquire the disease through subcutaneous injections.

Clinical Findings

A. Symptoms and Signs: The first symptom may be pain and tingling at the site of inoculation, followed by spasticity of the muscles nearby, and this may be all that happens. More frequently, however, the presenting symptoms are stiffness of the jaw, neck stiffness, dysphagia, and irritability. Hyperreflexia develops later, with spasms of the jaw muscles (trismus) or facial muscles and rigidity and spasm of the muscles of the abdomen, neck, and back. Painful tonic convulsions precipitated by minor stimuli are common. Spasms of the glottis and respiratory muscles may cause acute asphyxia. The patient is awake and alert throughout the illness. The temperature is normal or only slightly elevated.

B. Laboratory Findings: The diagnosis of tetanus is made clinically.

Differential Diagnosis

Tetanus must be differentiated from various acute

central nervous system infections. Trismus may occasionally develop with the use of phenothiazines. Strychnine poisoning should also be considered.

Complications

Airway obstruction is common. Urinary retention and constipation may result from spasm of the sphincters. Respiratory arrest and cardiac failure are late, life-threatening events.

Prevention

Tetanus is completely preventable by active immunization. Immunizations for children include tetanus toxoid, usually as DTP (see Table 29–4 for schedule). For primary immunization of adults, tetanus toxoid is administered as two doses 4–6 weeks apart, with a third dose 6–12 months later. Booster doses are given every 10 years or at the time of major injury if it occurs more than 5 years after a dose.

Passive immunization should be used in nonimmunized individuals and those whose immunization status is uncertain whenever a wound is contaminated or likely to have devitalized tissue. Tetanus immune globulin, 250 units, is given intramuscularly. Active immunization with tetanus toxoid should be started concurrently. Table 32–1 provides a guide to prophylactic management.

Treatment

A. Specific Measures: Give tetanus immune globulin, 5000 units intramuscularly.

B. General Measures: The patient is placed at bed rest with minimal stimulation. Sedation, paralysis with curare-like agents, and mechanical ventilation are often necessary. Penicillin, 20 million units daily, is administered to all patients—even those with mild illness—to eradicate toxin-producing organisms. Tetanic spasms can be controlled by treatment with chlorpromazine (50–100 mg four times daily) or diazepam combined with a sedative (amobarbital, phenobarbital, or meprobamate).

Table 32–1. Guide to tetanus prophylaxis in wound management (United States, 1985). (Modified from MMWR 1985;34:405).

History of Absorbed Tetanus Toxoid (Doses)	Clean, Minor Wounds[1]			
	Td	TIG	Td	TIG
Unknown or <3	Yes	No	Yes	Yes
≥3	No[2]	No	No[3]	No

Td = tetanus toxoid and diphtheria toxoid, adult form. Use only this preparation (Td-adult) in children older than 6 years. TIG = tetanus immune globulin.
[1]Such as, but not limited to, wounds contaminated with dirt, feces, soil, saliva, etc; puncture wounds; avulsions; and wounds resulting from missiles, crushing, burns, and frostbite.
[2]Yes, if more than 10 years since last dose.
[3]Yes, if more than 5 years since last dose. (More frequent boosters are not needed and can accentuate side effects.)

Prognosis

High mortality rates are associated with a short incubation period, early onset of convulsions, and delay in treatment. Contaminated lesions about the head and face are more dangerous than wounds on other parts of the body. The overall mortality rate historically is about 40%, but this can be considerably reduced with ventilator management as described.

Tetanus: United States 1987 and 1988. MMWR Morb Mortal Wkly Rep 1990;39:37. (Epidemiology of tetanus and occurrence in persons over age 50.)

BOTULISM

Essentials of Diagnosis

- History of recent ingestion of home-canned or smoked foods, and demonstration of toxin in serum or food.
- Sudden onset of diplopia, dry mouth, dysphagia, dysphonia, and muscle weakness progressing to respiratory paralysis.
- Pupils are fixed and dilated.

General Considerations

Botulism is food poisoning usually caused by ingestion of preformed toxin (usually type A, B, or E) of *Clostridium botulinum,* a ubiquitous, strictly anaerobic, spore-forming bacillus found in soil. Canned, smoked, or vacuum-packed anaerobic foods are involved—particularly home-canned vegetables, smoked meats, and vacuum-packed fish. Infant botulism and wound botulism differ in that organisms present in the gut or wound, respectively, elaborate toxin in vivo. Toxin blocks the release of acetylcholine from nerve endings. Clinically, early nervous system involvement leads to respiratory paralysis. The mortality rate in untreated cases is high.

Clinical Findings

A. Symptoms and Signs: Twelve to 36 hours after ingestion of the toxin, visual disturbances appear, particularly diplopia and loss of accommodation. Ptosis, cranial nerve palsies with impairment of extraocular muscles, and fixed dilated pupils are characteristic signs. Other symptoms are dry mouth, dysphagia, and dysphonia. Nausea and vomiting may be present, particularly with type E toxin. The sensorium remains clear and the temperature normal. Respiratory paralysis may lead to death unless mechanical assistance is provided.

Infants in the first few months of life may present with weakness, generalized hypotonicity, and electromyographic findings compatible with botulism. Toxin is found in the stool, not serum. Honey fed to infants under 1 year of age has been incriminated in this syndrome.

B. Laboratory Findings: Toxin in the patient's

serum and in suspected foods may be shown by mouse inoculation and identified with specific antiserum.

Differential Diagnosis

Cranial nerve involvement suggests vertebrobasilar insufficiency, the C. Miller Fisher variant of Guillain-Barré syndrome, myasthenia gravis, or any basilar meningitis, infectious or carcinomatous. Intestinal obstruction or other types of food poisoning are considered when nausea and vomiting are present.

Treatment

If botulism is suspected, the physician should contact the state health authorities or the Centers for Disease Control and Prevention for advice and help with procurement of botulinus antitoxin and for assistance in obtaining assays for toxin in serum, stool, or food. During off hours, the CDC provides assistance via a recorded message at (404) 639–2206.

Respiratory failure is managed with intubation and mechanical ventilation. Parenteral fluids or alimentation should be given while swallowing difficulty persists.

The removal of unabsorbed toxin from the gut may be attempted. Any remnants of suspected foods should be assayed for toxin. Persons who might have eaten the suspected food must be located and observed.

ANTHRAX

Anthrax is a disease of sheep, cattle, horses, goats, and swine caused by *Bacillus anthracis,* a gram-positive spore-forming aerobic rod. The organism is transmitted to humans by inoculation of broken skin or mucous membranes or by inhalation, causing either cutaneous or pulmonary infection. Human infection is rare. Anthrax is an occupational disease of farmers, veterinarians, and tannery and wool workers; prospective military use of the organism may result in future cases.

Clinical Findings

In cutaneous anthrax, an erythematous papule appears on an exposed area of skin and becomes vesicular, with a purple to black center. The area around the lesion is edematous and vesicular. The center of the lesion finally forms a necrotic eschar and sloughs. Regional adenopathy, fever, malaise, headache, and nausea and vomiting may be present. After the eschar sloughs, hematogenous spread and sepsis may occur, resulting in shock, cyanosis, sweating, and collapse. Hemorrhagic meningitis may also occur.

Pulmonary anthrax follows inhalation of spores from hides, bristles, or wool. It is characterized by fever, malaise, headache, dyspnea, and cough; con-

gestion of the nose, throat, and larynx; and evidence of pneumonia or mediastinitis.

Sputum or blood culture may be positive for *B anthracis.* Smears of skin lesions show gram-positive encapsulated rods, and cultures should be attempted.

Treatment

The mortality rate is high despite proper therapy, especially in pulmonary disease. Penicillin G, 2 million units intravenously every 4 hours, is the therapy of choice. Tetracycline, 500 mg orally every 6 hours, may be used for mild, localized cutaneous infection.

DIPHTHERIA

Essentials of Diagnosis

- Tenacious gray membrane at portal of entry in pharynx.
- Sore throat, nasal discharge, hoarseness, malaise, fever.
- Myocarditis, neuropathy.
- Culture confirms the diagnosis.

General Considerations

Diphtheria is an acute infection, caused by *Corynebacterium diphtheriae,* that usually attacks the respiratory tract but may involve any mucous membrane or skin wound. The organism is spread chiefly by respiratory secretions from patients with disease or healthy carriers. The incubation period is 2–7 days. Exotoxin produced by the organism is responsible for myocarditis and neuropathy. This exotoxin inhibits elongation factor, which is required for protein synthesis.

Clinical Findings

A. Symptoms and Signs: Nasal, laryngeal, pharyngeal, and cutaneous forms of diphtheria occur. Nasal infection produces few symptoms other than a nasal discharge. Laryngeal infection may lead to upper airway and bronchial obstruction. In pharyngeal diphtheria, the most common form, a tenacious gray membrane covers the tonsils and pharynx. Mild sore throat, fever, and malaise are followed by toxemia and prostration.

Myocarditis and neuropathy are the most common and most serious complications. Myocarditis causes cardiac arrhythmias, heart block, and heart failure. The neuropathy usually involves the cranial nerves first, producing diplopia, slurred speech, and difficulty in swallowing.

B. Laboratory Findings: The diagnosis is made clinically but can be confirmed by culture of the organism.

Differential Diagnosis

Diphtheria must be differentiated from streptococcal pharyngitis, infectious mononucleosis, adenovirus or herpes simplex infection, Vincent's angina, and candidiasis. A presumptive diagnosis of diphtheria must be made on clinical grounds without waiting for laboratory verification, since emergency treatment is needed.

Prevention

Active immunization with diphtheria toxoid is part of routine childhood immunization (usually as DTP) with appropriate booster injections. The immunization schedule for adults is the same as for tetanus. In order to avoid major allergic reactions, only the "adult type" toxoid (Td) should be used.

Susceptible persons exposed to diphtheria should receive a booster dose of toxoid plus active immunization if not previously immunized, as well as a course of penicillin.

Treatment

Antitoxin, which is prepared from horse serum, must be given in all cases when diphtheria is suspected. For mild early pharyngeal or laryngeal disease, the dose is 20,000–40,000 units; for moderate nasopharyngeal disease, 40,000–60,000 units; for severe, extensive, or late (3 days or more) disease, 80,000–100,000 units. Diphtheria equine antitoxin can be obtained from the Centers for Disease Control.

Antibiotics are a useful adjunct to antitoxin. Both penicillin and erythromycin are effective. The dosage of erythromycin is 500 mg orally four times daily for 7–10 days. Removal of membrane by direct laryngoscopy or bronchoscopy may be necessary to prevent or alleviate airway obstruction.

Rappuoli R, Perugini M, Falsen E: Molecular epidemiology of the 1984–1986 outbreak of diphtheria in Sweden. N Engl J Med 1988;318:12. (A virulence factor in addition to toxin is implicated.)

LISTERIOSIS

Listeria monocytogenes is a motile, gram-positive rod that is a facultative intracellular organism capable of invading several cell types. Most cases of infection caused by *L monocytogenes* are sporadic, but outbreaks have been traced to eating contaminated food, especially unpasteurized dairy products. Five types of infection are recognized:

(1) Infection during pregnancy, usually in the last trimester, is a mild febrile illness without an apparent primary focus. This is a relatively benign disease that may resolve without specific therapy.

(2) Granulomatosis infantisepticum is a neonatal infection acquired in utero and characterized by disseminated abscesses and granulomas and by a high mortality rate.

(3) Bacteremia with or without sepsis syndrome is an infection of neonates or immunocompromised adults. The presentation is that of a febrile illness without a recognized source.

(4) Meningitis caused by *L monocytogenes* affects infants under 2 months of age and adults, ranking third and fourth, respectively, among the common causes of bacterial meningitis. Adults with meningitis are usually immunocompromised, and cases have been associated with HIV infection. Cerebrospinal fluid shows a *neutrophilic* pleocytosis.

(5) Finally, focal infections, including adenitis, brain abscess, endocardiits, osteomyelitis, and arthritis, occur rarely.

Therapy of infections caused by *Listeria* is controversial with respect both to the most effective agent and the duration of treatment. The drug of choice is probably ampicillin, 8–12 g/d intravenously in four to six divided doses (the higher dose being recommended in cases of meningitis). It has relatively good penetration into cerebrospinal fluid, and, although there are few data, the response to ampicillin seems to be better than that to penicillin, erythromycin, or chloramphenicol. Gentamicin is synergistic with ampicillin against *Listeria* in vitro and in animal models, and the use of combination therapy may for that reason be considered during the first few days of treatment to enhance eradication of organisms. Mortality and morbidity rates still are high, and relapse does occur, perhaps related to poor penetration of ampicillin into cells where organisms reside. Anecdotal clinical data indicating efficacy of trimethoprim-sulfamethoxazole and its excellent penetration into cells and into the cerebrospinal fluid support its use for therapy of listeriosis. The dose is 10–20 mg/kg/d of the trimethoprim component. Therapy should be administered for at least 2–3 weeks. Longer durations—between 3 and 6 weeks—have been recommended for treatment of meningitis, especially in severely immunocompromised patients.

INFECTIONS CAUSED BY GRAM-NEGATIVE BACTERIA

BORDETELLA PERTUSSIS INFECTION (Whooping Cough)

Essentials of Diagnosis

- Predominantly in infants under age 2 years. Pertussis also affects adults, who may be an important reservoir of infection for children.
- Two-week prodromal catarrhal stage of malaise, cough, coryza, and anorexia.
- Paroxysmal cough ending in a high-pitched inspiratory "whoop."

- Absolute lymphocytosis, often striking; culture confirms diagnosis.

General Considerations

Pertussis is an acute infection of the respiratory tract caused by *Bordetella pertussis* that is transmitted by respiratory droplets. The incubation period is 7–17 days. Infants are most commonly infected; half of all cases occur before age 2 years.

Clinical Findings

A. Symptoms and Signs: The symptoms of classic pertussis last about 6 weeks and are divided into three consecutive stages. The catarrhal stage is characterized by its insidious onset, with lacrimation, sneezing, and coryza, anorexia and malaise, and a hacking night cough that tends to become diurnal. The paroxysmal stage is characterized by bursts of rapid, consecutive coughs followed by a deep, high-pitched inspiration (whoop). The convalescent stage usually begins 4 weeks after onset of the illness with a decrease in the frequency and severity of paroxysms of cough.

B. Laboratory Findings: The white blood cell count is usually 15,000–20,000/μL (rarely, as high as 50,000/μL or more), 60–80% of which are lymphocytes. The organism is recovered on special media in only about half of clinically diagnosed patients.

Prevention

Active immunization with pertussis vaccine is recommended for all infants, usually combined with diphtheria and tetanus toxoids (DTP). Because of the mildness of the disease in older individuals, neither primary nor booster immunization is recommended after age 6 years.

Infants and susceptible adults with significant exposure to pertussis should receive prophylaxis with erythromycin (40 mg/kg/d). Those previously immunized should receive a booster dose of vaccine.

Treatment

Erythromycin, 500 mg four times a day orally for 10 days, shortens the duration of carriage. It also may diminish the severity of coughing paroxysms.

Herwaldt LA: Pertussis in adults: What physicians need to know. Arch Intern Med 1991;151:1510. (Adults are an important reservoir for pertussis, which should be considered in adults with prolonged cough.)

Shapiro ED: Pertussis vaccines: Seeking a better mousetrap. JAMA 1992;267:2788. (Editorial reviewing pertussis vaccines.)

MENINGOCOCCAL MENINGITIS

Essentials of Diagnosis

- Fever, headache, vomiting, confusion, delirium, convulsions.
- Petechial rash of skin and mucous membranes in many.
- Neck and back stiffness with positive Kernig and Brudzinski signs is characteristic.
- Purulent spinal fluid with gram-negative intracellular and extracellular diplococci.
- Culture of cerebrospinal fluid, blood, or petechial aspiration confirms the diagnosis.

General Considerations

Meningococcal meningitis is caused by *Neisseria meningitidis* of groups A, B, C, Y, W-135, and others. Up to 40% of persons are nasopharyngeal carriers of meningococci, but relatively few develop disease. Infection is transmitted by droplets. The clinical illness may take the form of meningococcemia (a fulminant form of septicemia without meningitis), meningococcemia with meningitis, or predominantly meningitis. Chronic recurrent meningococcemia with fever, rash, and arthritis can occur, particular in those with terminal complement deficiencies (C7–C9).

Clinical Findings

A. Symptoms and Signs: High fever, chills, and headache; back, abdominal, and extremity pains; and nausea and vomiting are present. In severe cases, rapidly developing confusion, delirium, seizures, and coma occur.

On examination, nuchal and back rigidity are typical, with positive Kernig and Brudzinski signs. A petechial rash is found in most cases. Petechiae may vary from pinhead-sized to large ecchymoses or even areas of skin gangrene that may later slough if the patient survives.

B. Laboratory Findings: Lumbar puncture typically reveals a cloudy or purulent cerebrospinal fluid, with elevated pressure, increased protein, and decreased glucose content. The fluid usually contains more than 1000 cells/μL, with polymorphonuclear cells predominating and containing gram-negative intracellular diplococci. The absence of organisms in a gram-stained smear of the cerebrospinal fluid sediment does not rule out the diagnosis. The capsular polysaccharide can often be demonstrated in cerebrospinal fluid or urine by latex agglutination; this is especially useful in partially treated patients, though sensitivity is only 60–80%. The organism is usually demonstrated by smear or culture of the cerebrospinal fluid, oropharynx, blood, or aspirated petechiae.

Disseminated intravascular coagulation is an important complication of meningococcal infection. Prothrombin time and partial thromboplastin time are prolonged, fibrin dimers are elevated, fibrinogen is low, and the platelet count is depressed.

Differential Diagnosis

Meningococcal meningitis must be differentiated from other bacterial and viral meningitides. In small infants and in the elderly, the presentation may be atypical, without fever or stiff neck.

Rickettsial or echovirus infection and, rarely, other bacterial infections (eg, staphylococcal infections, scarlet fever) may also produce a petechial rash.

Complications

Arthritis, cranial nerve damage (especially the eighth nerve, with resulting deafness), and hydrocephalus may occur as complications.

Prevention

Effective polysaccharide vaccines for groups A, C, Y, and W-135 are available. A and C vaccine has reduced the incidence of infections with these meningococcus groups in military recruits. The vaccines are effective for control of epidemics in civilian populations.

Outbreaks in closed populations are best controlled by eliminating meningococcal carriage. Rifampin is the drug of choice in dosages as follows: 600 mg twice a day for 2 days for adults; 10 mg/kg twice a day for 2 days for children 1 month to 12 years; 5 mg/kg twice a day for 2 days for infants.

Household members exposed to a person with meningococcal meningitis are at increased risk and should be given rifampin prophylaxis. Day care center contacts are treated in the same manner. School and work contacts need not be treated. Hospital contacts need not be treated unless intense exposure has occurred (eg, mouth-to-mouth resuscitation).

Accidentally discovered carriers without known close contact with meningococcal disease do not require prophylactic antimicrobials.

Treatment

A. Specific Measures: Blood cultures must be obtained and intravenous antimicrobial therapy started immediately. This may be done prior to lumbar puncture in patients in whom the diagnosis is not straightforward and who therefore require CT scanning to exclude mass lesions. Aqueous penicillin G is the antibiotic of choice (24 million units/24 h) in divided doses every 4 hours. In penicillin-allergic patients or those in whom *Haemophilus influenzae* or gram-negative meningitis is a consideration, ceftriaxone, 4 g intravenously once a day, should be used. Chloramphenicol, 1 g every 6 hours, is an alternative in the severely penicillin- or cephalosporin-allergic patient.

Treatment should be continued in full doses by the intravenous route until the patient is afebrile for 5 days. In the past, the recommended duration of therapy has been 7–10 days. More recent studies suggest that shorter courses—as few as 4 days if ceftriaxone is used—are also effective.

B. General Measures: Shock is the most serious complication of meningococcal infections. Volume expansion and vasopressors (eg, dopamine) are initial therapy.

Obtundation or deterioration in mental status may result from cerebral edema and increased intracranial pressure. In critically ill patients with evidence of increased intracranial pressure, treatment with intravenous mannitol (2 g/kg), administration of dexamethasone (0.6 mg/kg/d in four divided doses), and hyperventilation should be considered as measures to lower the pressure, but data that morbidity and mortality rates are favorably influenced are lacking.

Heparinization is of theoretic value in disseminated intravascular coagulation and bleeding, but it does not influence prognosis.

INFECTIONS CAUSED BY *HAEMOPHILUS* SPECIES

Haemophilus influenzae type b is primarily a pathogen of children less than 5 years old. Meningitis and epiglottitis, which are almost always caused by type B strains, occur most often in this group. *H influenzae* and other *Haemophilus* species may cause sinusitis, otitis, bronchitis, epiglottis, pneumonitis, cellulitis, arthritis, meningitis, and endocarditis in adults at any age, however.

In adults, **pneumonia** is one of the more common infections caused by *H influenzae* type b. Nontypable strains of *H influenzae* actually are more common as a cause of pneumonia in HIV-infected patients, however. The presentation is that of a typical bacterial pneumonia, with purulent sputum containing a predominance of gram-negative, pleomorphic rods. Alcoholism, smoking, chronic lung disease, and HIV infection are important risk factors.

Although *Haemophilus* species and nontypable strains of *H influenzae* may cause pneumonia, they more frequently colonize the upper respiratory tract. Consequently, in the absence of positive pleural fluid or blood cultures, distinguishing pneumonia from colonization is difficult. Pneumonia from *Haemophilus* species probably is overdiagnosed for this reason.

Nontypable strains of *H influenzae* and other *Haemophilus* species cause **sinusitis, otitis, and respiratory tract infections.** Alcoholics, smokers, HIV-infected individuals, and patients with chronic lung disease are particularly at risk for respiratory infections with these organisms. *Haemophilus* species other than *H influenzae* (eg, *H parainfluenzae, H aphrophilus*) infrequently cause **endocarditis.**

Beta-lactamase-producing strains are less common in adults than in children. For most adult patients with sinusitis, otitis, or respiratory tract infection, oral amoxicillin, 500 mg every 8 hours, or parenteral ampicillin, 1–2 g every 6 hours, is adequate.

In the more seriously ill patient (eg, the toxic patient with multilobar pneumonia), use of a second- or third-generation cephalosporin—cefuroxime, 750–1500 mg every 8 hours, or ceftriaxone, 1 g/d—is advisable pending determination of whether the infecting strain is a β-lactamase producer. Trimethoprim-sulfamethoxazole, administered based on a dose of 10 mg/kg/d of trimethoprim, can be used for the penicillin-allergic patient.

Epiglottitis, which occasionally occurs in adults, is characterized by an abrupt onset of high fever, drooling, and inability to handle secretions. A foreign body sensation in the pharynx may precede these symptoms by several hours. Stridor and respiratory distress result from laryngeal obstruction. Early, elective intubation is recommended because airway obstruction may progress unpredictably and rapidly. The diagnosis is best made by direct visualization of the cherry-red, swollen epiglottis at laryngoscopy. Because laryngoscopy may provoke laryngospasm and obstruction, it should be performed in an intensive care unit or similar setting, and only at the time of intubation. Cefuroxime, 1.5 g every 8 hours, or ceftriaxone, 2 g every 24 hours, is the drug of choice. Trimethoprim-sulfamethoxazole (see above for dosage) or chloramphenicol, 4 g/d, may be used in the patient with serious penicillin allergy. Corticosteroids are often added to antibiotics.

Meningitis—also rare but still a possibility in adults—becomes a consideration in the patient who has meningitis associated with sinusitis or otitis. The presentation is the same as that of other bacterial meningitides. Initial therapy of suspected *H influenzae* meningitis should be with ceftriaxone, 4 g/d in one or two divided doses, until the strain is proved not to produce β-lactamase. Chloramphenicol, 100 mg/kg/d in four divided doses, can be used if the patient has a serious, life-threatening allergy to β-lactam antibiotics. Dexamethasone, 0.15 mg/kg intravenously every 6 hours, has been shown to be a valuable adjunctive agent in treatment of meningitis in infants and children, resulting in reduction in long-term sequelae, principally hearing loss. The role of steroids in adult meningitis is controversial.

Steinhart R et al: Invasive *Haemophilus influenzae* infections in men with HIV infection. JAMA 1992;268:3350.

Takala AK, Eskola J, Alphen L: Spectrum of invasive *Haemophilus influenzae* type b disease in adults. JAMA 1990;159:2573.

INFECTIONS CAUSED BY *MORAXELLA CATARRHALIS*

Moraxella catarrhalis is a gram-negative aerobic coccus that is morphologically and biochemically similar to *Neisseria*. This organism has recently been recognized as a cause of sinusitis, bronchitis, and pneumonia. Bacteremia and meningitis have also been reported in immunocompromised patients. The organism frequently colonizes the respiratory tract, and differentiation of colonization from infection can be difficult. If *M catarrhalis* is the predominant isolate, therapy should be directed against it. *M catarrhalis* typically produces beta-lactamase and therefore is usually resistant to ampicillin and amoxicillin. It is susceptible to amoxicillin-clavulanate, ampicillin-sulbactam, trimethoprim-sulfamethoxazole, ciprofloxacin, and second- and third-generation cephalosporins. Treatment is similar to that for *Haemophilus* infections.

Wallace MR, Oldfield EC: *Moraxella (Branhamella) catarrhalis* bacteremia: A case report and review of the literature. Arch Intern Med 1990;150:1332.

LEGIONNAIRES' DISEASE

Essentials of Diagnosis

- Patients are often immunocompromised, smokers, or have chronic lung disease.
- Scant sputum production, pleuritic chest pain, toxic appearance.
- Chest x-ray shows focal patchy infiltrates or consolidation.
- Gram's stain of sputum shows polymorphonuclear leukocytes and no organisms.

General Considerations

Legionella infection is a common cause of community-acquired pneumonia. In some series, 10% or more of community-acquired pneumonias and nosocomial pneumonias may be caused by *Legionella*. Legionnaires' disease is more common in immunocompromised persons, in smokers, and in those with chronic lung disease. Outbreaks of legionellosis have been associated with contaminated water sources, such as shower heads and faucets in patient rooms and air conditioning cooling towers.

Clinical Findings

A. Symptoms and Signs: Legionnaires' disease is one of the atypical pneumonias, so called because a Gram-stained smear of sputum does not show organisms. However, many features of legionnaires' disease are more like typical pneumonia, with high fevers, a "toxic" appearance of the patient, pleurisy, and purulent sputum (without predominant or identifiable organisms). Classically, this pneumonia is caused by *Legionella pneumophila,* though other species can cause disease that is clinically indistinguishable.

B. Laboratory Findings: Culture onto charcoal-yeast extract agar or similar enriched medium is the most sensitive method (80–90% sensitivity) for diagnosis of legionellosis and permits identification of infections caused by species and serotypes other than *L pneumophila* serotype 1. Dieterle's silver staining of tissue, pleural fluid, or other infected material is also a reliable method for detecting *Legionella* species. Direct fluorescent antibody stains and serologic testing are less sensitive because these will detect only infection caused by *L pneumophila* serotype 1.

Treatment

The drug of choice for treatment of legionellosis is erythromycin, 2–4 g daily for 14–21 days. Rifampin, 300 mg twice a day in combination with erythromycin, may be synergistic and may be considered for those with severe illness and in immunocompromised hosts, who tend to have more aggressive disease.

Tetracyclines and trimethoprim-sulfamethoxazole occasionally have been used to treat legionellosis, and ciprofloxacin is active in vitro. These agents are of unproved efficacy and should be considered for use only if erythromycin is contraindicated or cannot be tolerated.

GRAM-NEGATIVE BACTEREMIA & SEPSIS

There are several hundred thousand episodes of gram-negative sepsis annually. Patients with rapidly fatal underlying diseases (neutropenic patients or those immunosuppressed by virtue of an underlying disease or medication) have a mortality rate of 40–60%; patients with ultimately fatal underlying diseases (diseases likely to be fatal in 5 years, such as solid tumors, severe liver disease, and aplastic anemia) have a mortality rate of 15–20%; and patients with no underlying disease have a low mortality rate—5% or less. Gram-negative bacteremia can originate in a number of sites, the most common being the genitourinary system, hepatobiliary tract, gastrointestinal tract, and lungs. Less common sources include intravenous lines, infusion fluids, surgical wounds, surgical drains, and decubitus ulcers.

Clinical Findings

A. Symptoms and Signs: Most patients have fevers and chills, often with an abrupt onset. However, 15% of patients are hypothermic (temperature ≤ 36.4 °C [97.6 °F]) at the onset of sepsis, and 5% of patients never develop a temperature above 37.5 °C (99.6 °F). Hyperventilation with respiratory alkalosis and changes in mental status are important early manifestations. Hypotension and shock, which occur in 20–50% of patients, are unfavorable prognostic signs.

B. Laboratory Findings: Neutropenia or neutrophilia, often accompanied by increased numbers of immature forms of polymorphonuclear leukocytes, is the most common laboratory abnormality in septic

patients. Thrombocytopenia occurs in 50% of patients, laboratory evidence of coagulation abnormalities in 10%, and frank DIC in 2–3%. Both clinical manifestations and the laboratory abnormalities are nonspecific and insensitive, which accounts for the relatively low rate of blood culture positivity (approximately 20–40%) in patients with suspected gram-negative sepsis. If possible, three blood cultures should be obtained in rapid succession before starting antimicrobial therapy. The chance of recovering the organism from the blood of the septic patient with bacteremia in at least one of the three blood cultures is greater than 95%. The false-negative rate for a single culture of 5–10 mL of blood is 30%. This may be reduced to a 5–10% false-negative rate (albeit with a slight false-positive rate due to isolation of contaminants) if a single volume of 30 mL is inoculated into several blood culture bottles. Because blood cultures may be falsely negative, if the patient with presumed septic shock, negative blood cultures, and no other good explanation for the clinical course responds to antimicrobials, therapy should be continued for 10–14 days.

Treatment

Several factors are important in the management of patients with sepsis.

A. Removal of Predisposing Factors: This usually means decreasing or stopping immunosuppressive medications and in certain circumstances (eg, documented positive blood cultures) giving granulocyte colony-stimulating factor (filgastrim; G-CSF) to the neutropenic patient.

B. Identifying the Source of Bacteremia: A search for the source of bacteremia should be made. By simply finding the source and either removing it (intravenous line) or draining it (abscess), it is possible to transform what might be a fatal disease into one that is easily treatable.

C. Supportive Measures: The use of fluids and pressors for maintaining blood pressure is discussed in Chapter 12; management of disseminated intravascular coagulation is discussed in Chapter 13.

D. Antibiotics: Antibiotics should be given as soon as the diagnosis of sepsis is seriously considered, since delays in therapy have been associated with increased mortality rates. In general, bactericidal antibiotics should be used and should be given intravenously to ensure therapeutic serum levels. Penetration of antibiotics into the site of primary infection is critical for successful therapy—ie, if the infection originates in the central nervous system, antibiotics that penetrate the blood-brain barrier should be used—eg, penicillin, ampicillin, chloramphenicol, and third-generation cephalosporins—but not first-generation cephalosporins or aminoglycosides, which penetrate poorly. Since one cannot distinguish gram-positive from gram-negative bacteremia on clinical grounds, initial therapy should include antibiotics active against both types of organisms.

The number of antibiotics necessary to treat sepsis remains controversial and depends upon the underlying disease. Most authorities believe that for patients with rapidly fatal underlying diseases, a synergistic combination of antibiotics, including an aminoglycoside, should be used. For patients with nonfatal and ultimately fatal underlying diseases and who are not in shock, a single-drug regimen with any of several broad-spectrum antibiotics (eg, a third-generation cephalosporin, ticarcillin-clavulanate, imipenem) is adequate. Therapy can be altered once results of culture and sensitivity are known.

E. Corticosteroids: There is no role for corticosteroids in the therapy of sepsis or septic shock.

F. Immunotherapy: Administration of a human monoclonal antiendotoxin antibody within the first several hours after onset of sepsis syndrome may reduce short-term mortality in patients with gram-negative sepsis. The ultimate role and long-term benefits of what presently is a very expensive experimental therapy remain to be seen.

Bone RC et al: A controlled clinical trial of high-dose methylprednisolone in the treatment of severe sepsis and septic shock. N Engl J Med 1987;317:653.
Bone RC: The pathogenesis of sepsis. Ann Intern Med 1991;115:457. (Review of role of numerous bacterial and host mediators of sepsis.)
Ziegler EJ et al: Treatment of gram-negative bacteremia and septic shock with HA-1A human monoclonal antibody against endotoxin: A randomized, double-blind, placebo-controlled trial. N Engl J Med 1991;324:429. (HA-1A may reduce mortality in patients with gram-negative bacteremia.)

SALMONELLOSIS

Salmonellosis includes infection by any of approximately 2000 serotypes of salmonellae. The taxonomy of *Salmonella* species has been confusing. All *Salmonella* serotypes are considered members of a single species, *S enterica.* Human infections are caused almost exclusively by *S enterica* subsp *enterica,* of which three serotypes—typhi, typhimurium, and choleraesuis—are predominantly isolated. Three clinical patterns of infection are recognized: (1) enteric fever, the best example of which is typhoid fever, due to serotype typhi; (2) acute enterocolitis, caused by serotype typhimurium, among others; and (3) the "septicemic" type, characterized by bacteremia and focal lesions, exemplified by infection with serotype choleraesuis. All types are transmitted by ingestion of the organism in contaminated food or drink.

1. ENTERIC FEVER (Typhoid Fever)

Essentials of Diagnosis

- Gradual onset of malaise, headache, sore throat, cough, and finally "pea soup" diarrhea, though constipation is more typical.
- Rose spots, relative bradycardia, splenomegaly, and abdominal distention and tenderness.
- Slow (stepladder) rise of fever to maximum and then slow return to normal.
- Leukopenia; blood, stool, and urine culture positive for *S enterica* serotype typhi.

General Considerations

Enteric fever is a clinical syndrome characterized by constitutional and gastrointestinal symptoms and by headache. It can be caused by any *Salmonella* species. The term "typhoid fever" applies when serotype typhi is the cause of enteric fever accompanied by bacteremia. Infection is transmitted by consumption of contaminated food or drink. the incubation period is 5–14 days. Infection begins when organisms penetrate the intestinal wall and invade mesenteric lymph nodes and the spleen. Serotypes other than typhi usually do not cause invasive disease, presumably because they lack the necessary human-specific virulence factors. Bacteremia occurs, and the infection then localizes principally in the lymphoid tissue of the small intestine (particularly within 60 cm of the ileocecal valve). Peyer's patches become inflamed and may ulcerate, with involvement greatest during the third week of disease. The organism may disseminate to the lungs, gallbladder, kidneys, or central nervous system.

Clinical Findings

A. Symptoms and Signs: The onset is usually insidious but in children may be abrupt, with chills and high fever. During the prodromal stage, there is increasing malaise, headache, cough, and sore throat, often with abdominal pain and constipation, while the fever ascends in a stepwise fashion. After about 7–10 days, the fever reaches a plateau and the patient is much more ill, appearing exhausted and often prostrated. There may be marked constipation, or "pea soup" diarrhea; marked abdominal distention occurs as well. If there are no complications, the patient's condition will gradually improve over 7–10 days. However, relapse may occur for up to 2 weeks after defervescence.

During the early prodrome, physical findings are few. Later, splenomegaly, abdominal distention and tenderness, relative bradycardia, dicrotic pulse, and occasionally meningismus appear. The rash (rose spots) commonly appears during the second week of disease. The individual spot, found principally on the trunk, is a pink papule 2–3 mm in diameter that fades on pressure. It disappears in 3–4 days.

B. Laboratory Findings: Typhoid fever is best diagnosed by isolation of the organism from blood culture, which is positive in the first week of illness in 80% of patients who have not taken antimicrobials. The rate of blood culture positivity declines thereafter, but one-fourth or more of patients still have positive blood cultures in the third week. Culture of bone marrow occasionally are positive when blood cultures are not. Stool culture is not reliable because it may be positive in gastroenteritis without typhoid fever.

Differential Diagnosis

Enteric fever must be distinguished from other gastrointestinal illnesses and from other infections that have few localizing findings. Examples include tuberculosis, infective endocarditis, brucellosis, lymphoma, and Q fever. Often there is a history of recent travel to endemic areas, and viral hepatitis, malaria, or amebiasis may be in the differential diagnosis as well.

Complications

Complications occur in about 30% of untreated cases and account for 75% of all deaths. Intestinal hemorrhage, manifested by a sudden drop in temperature and signs of shock followed by dark or fresh blood in the stool, or intestinal perforation, accompanied by abdominal pain and tenderness, is most likely to occur during the third week. Less frequent complications are urinary retention, pneumonia, thrombophlebitis, myocarditis, psychosis, cholecystitis, nephritis, osteomyelitis, and meningitis.

Prevention

Immunization is not always effective but should be provided for household contacts of a typhoid carrier, for travelers to endemic areas, and during epidemic outbreaks. Both oral and parenteral vaccines are available. Their efficacies are similar, but oral vaccine causes fewer side effects. Boosters, when indicated, should be given every 5 years and 3 years for oral and parenteral preparations, respectively.

Adequate waste disposal and protection of food and water supplies from contamination are important public health measures to prevent salmonellosis. Carriers must not be permitted to work as food handlers.

Treatment

A. Specific Measures: Ampicillin, chloramphenicol, and trimethoprim-sulfamethoxazole may be effective. All can be given orally or intravenously depending on the patient's condition. Because resistance to ampicillin and chloramphenicol is common, trimethoprim-sulfamethoxazole, administered as 10 mg/kg/d of trimethoprim, is probably the first choice. Ceftriaxone, 2 g once a day, also is effective. Fluoroquinolones such as ciprofloxacin, 750 mg twice a day, also are effective, but their use is contraindicated in children and pregnant women.

B. Treatment of Carriers: Chemotherapy often is unsuccessful in eradicating the carrier state. While treatment of carriage with ampicillin, trimethoprim-sulfamethoxazole, or chloramphenicol may be successful, one recent study suggests that ciprofloxacin, 750 mg twice a day for 4 weeks, is highly effective. Cholecystectomy may also achieve this goal.

Prognosis

The mortality rate of typhoid fever is about 2% in treated cases. Elderly or debilitated persons are likely to do poorly. The course is milder in children.

With complications, the prognosis is poor. Relapses occur in up to 15% of cases. A residual carrier state frequently persists in spite of chemotherapy.

Ferreccio C: Efficacy of ciprofloxacin in the treatment of chronic typhoid carriers. J Infect Dis 1988;157:1235. (Carrier state eliminated in 11 of 12 patients.)

Keusch GT: Antimicrobial therapy for enteric fever and typhoid fever: State of the art. Rev Infect Dis 1988; 10(Suppl 1):S199. (Experience with quinolones.)

Woodruff BA, Pavia AT, Blake PA: A new look at typhoid vaccination. Information for the practicing physician. JAMA 1991;265:756. (Oral vaccine recommendations.)

2. *SALMONELLA* GASTROENTERITIS

By far the most common form of salmonellosis is acute enterocolitis. Numerous *Salmonella* serotypes may cause enterocolitis. The incubation period is 8–48 hours after ingestion of contaminated food or liquid.

Symptoms and signs consist of fever (often with chills), nausea and vomiting, cramping abdominal pain, and diarrhea, which may be bloody, lasting 3–5 days. Differentiation must be made from viral gastroenteritis, food poisoning, shigellosis, amebic dysentery, acute ulcerative colitis, and acute surgical abdominal conditions. The diagnosis is made by culturing the organism from the stool.

The disease is usually self-limited, but bacteremia with localization in joints or bones may occur, especially in young infants and in patients with sickle cell disease.

Treatment of uncomplicated enterocolitis is symptomatic only. Young, malnourished, or immunocompromised infants, severely ill patients, those with sickle cell disease, and those with suspected bacteremia should be treated for 3–5 days with trimethoprim-sulfamethoxazole (one double-strength tablet twice a day), ampicillin (100 mg/kg intravenously or orally), or ciprofloxacin (750 mg twice a day).

3. *SALMONELLA* BACTEREMIA

Rarely, *Salmonella* infection may be manifested by prolonged or recurrent fevers accompanied by bacteremia and local infection in bone, joints, pleura, pericardium, lungs, or other sites. Mycotic abdominal aortic aneurysms may also cause this problem. Serotypes other than typhi usually are isolated. This complication tends to occur in immunocompromised persons and is seen in HIV-infected individuals, who frequently have bacteremia without an obvious source. Treatment is the same as for typhoid fever, plus drainage of any abscesses. In HIV-infected patients, relapse is common, and lifelong suppressive therapy may be needed. Ciprofloxacin, 750 mg twice a day, is effective both for therapy and, at lower doses, for suppression.

SHIGELLOSIS

Essentials of Diagnosis

- Diarrhea, often with blood and mucus.
- Crampy abdominal pain and systemic toxicity.
- White blood cells in stools; organism isolated on stool culture.

General Considerations

Shigella dysentery is a common disease, often self-limited and mild but occasionally serious. *Shigella sonnei* is the leading cause in the USA, followed by *Shigella flexneri*. *Shigella dysenteriae* causes the most serious form of the illness. Shigellae are invasive organisms: The infective dose is 10^2–10^3 organisms. Recently, there has been a rise in strains resistant to multiple antibiotics.

Clinical Findings

A. Symptoms and Signs: The illness usually starts abruptly, with diarrhea, lower abdominal cramps, and tenesmus. The diarrheal stool often is mixed with blood and mucus. Systemic symptoms are fever, chills, anorexia and malaise, and headache. The patient becomes progressively weaker and more dehydrated. The abdomen is tender. Sigmoidoscopic examination reveals an inflamed, engorged mucosa with punctate, sometimes large areas of ulceration.

B. Laboratory Findings: The stool shows many leukocytes and red cells. Stool culture is positive for shigellae in most cases, but blood cultures grow the organism in less than 5% of cases.

Differential Diagnosis

Bacillary dysentery must be distinguished from *Salmonella* enterocolitis and from disease due to enterotoxigenic *E coli, Campylobacter enteritis,* and *Y enterocolitica.* Amebic dysentery may be similar clinically and is diagnosed by finding amebas in the fresh stool specimen. Ulcerative colitis in the adolescent and adult is an important cause of bloody diarrhea.

Complications

Temporary disaccharidase deficiency may follow the diarrhea. Reiter's syndrome is an uncommon complication, usually occurring in HLA-B27 individuals infected by *Shigella.*

Treatment

A. Specific Measures: Treatment of dehydration and hypotension is lifesaving in severe cases. The current antimicrobial treatment of choice is trimethoprim-sulfamethoxazole (one double-strength tablet twice a day), or ciprofloxacin (750 mg twice a day; contraindicated in children and pregnant women). Shigellae resistant to ampicillin are common, but if the isolate is susceptible, a dose of 500 mg four times a day is also effective. Amoxicillin, which is less effective, should not be used. A single dose of a quinolone (eg, norfloxacin, 400 mg, or ciprofloxacin, 750 mg) may be as effective as a 5-day courses of therapy with other drugs.

B. General Measures: Parenteral hydration and correction of acidosis and electrolyte disturbances are of primary importance. Antispasmodics (eg, tincture of belladonna) are helpful when cramps are severe. Drugs that inhibit intestinal peristalsis (paregoric, diphenoxylate with atropine) may ameliorate symptoms but prolong fever, diarrhea, and excretion of *Shigella* in feces. Appropriate precautions should be taken both in the hospital and in the home to limit spread of infection.

Bennish ML et al: Treatment of shigellosis: III. Comparison of one- or two-dose ciprofloxacin with standard 5-day therapy. Ann Intern Med 1992;117:727. (A single 1-g dose of ciprofloxacin is effective for all but *S dysenteriae* type I infections.)

CHOLERA

Essentials of Diagnosis

- Voluminous diarrhea.
- Stool is liquid, gray, turbid, and without fecal odor, blood, or pus ("rice water stool").
- Rapid development of marked dehydration.
- History of travel in endemic area or contact with infected person.
- Positive stool cultures and agglutination of vibrios with specific sera.

General Considerations

Cholera is an acute diarrheal illness caused by certain serotypes of *Vibrio cholerae.* The disease is toxin-mediated, and fever is unusual. The toxin activates adenylyl cyclase in intestinal epithelial cells of the small intestines. This produces hypersecretion of water and chloride ion and a massive diarrhea of up to 15 L per day. Death results from profound hypovolemia.

Cholera occurs in epidemics under conditions of crowding, war, and famine (eg, in refugee camps) and where sanitation is inadequate. Infection is acquired by ingestion of contaminated food or water. Cholera was rarely seen in the United States until 1991, when epidemic cholera returned to the Western Hemisphere, originating as an outbreak in coastal cities of Peru. The epidemic has spread to involve several countries in South and Central America as well as Mexico, and cases have been imported into the United States. Cholera should be considered in the differential diagnosis of severe watery diarrhea, especially in those who have traveled to affected countries.

Clinical Findings

A. Symptoms and Signs: Cholera is characterized by a sudden onset of severe, frequent watery diarrhea (up to 1 L per hour). The liquid stool is gray, turbid, and without fecal odor, blood, or pus ("rice water stool"). Dehydration and hypotension develop rapidly.

B. Laboratory Findings: Stool cultures are positive, and agglutination of vibrios with specific sera can be demonstrated.

Prevention

A vaccine is available that confers short-lived, limited protection and may be required for entry into or reentry after travel to some countries. It is administered in two doses 1–4 weeks apart. A booster dose every 6 months is recommended for persons remaining in areas where cholera is a hazard.

Vaccination programs are expensive and not particularly effective in managing outbreaks of cholera. When outbreaks occur, efforts should be directed toward establishing clean water and food sources and proper waste disposal.

Treatment

Treatment is by replacement of fluids. In mild or moderate illness, oral rehydration usually is adequate and has dramatically decreased the mortality rate in developing countries. A simple oral replacement fluid can be made from 1 teaspoon of table salt and 4 heaping teaspoons of sugar added to 1 L of water. Intravenous fluids are indicated for persons in shock or those with other signs of severe hypovolemia and those who cannot take adequate fluids orally. Either lactated Ringer's injection or an intravenous fluid containing 4 g of NaCl, 1 g of KCl, 5.4 g of sodium lactate, and 8 g of glucose per liter is satisfactory.

Antimicrobial therapy will shorten the course of illness. Several antimicrobials are active against *V cholerae,* including tetracycline, ampicillin, chloramphenicol, trimethoprim-sulfamethoxazole, and fluor-oquinolones. Multiple antibiotic resistance does occur, so susceptibility testing, if available, is advisable.

Glass RI et al: Epidemic cholera in the Americas. Science 1992;256:1524. (CDC report tracking the recent cholera epidemic.)

INFECTIONS CAUSED BY OTHER *VIBRIO* SPECIES

Vibrios other than *Vibrio cholerae* that cause human disease are *Vibrio parahaemolyticus, Vibrio vulnificus,* and *Vibrio alginolyticus.* All are halophilic marine organisms. Infection is acquired by exposure to organisms in contaminated, undercooked, or raw crustaceans or shellfish and warm (> 20 °C) ocean waters and estuaries. Infections are more common during the summer months from regions along the Atlantic coast and the Gulf of Mexico in the United States and from tropical waters around the world. Oysters are implicated in up to 90% of food-related cases. *V parahaemolyticus* causes an acute watery diarrhea with crampy abdominal pain and fever, typically occurring within 24 hours after ingestion of contaminated shellfish. The disease is self-limited, and antimicrobial therapy is usually not necessary. *V parahaemolyticus* may also cause cellulitis and sepsis, though these findings are more characteristic of *V vulnificus* infection.

V vulnificus and *V alginolyticus*—neither of which is associated with diarrheal illness—are important causes of cellulitis and primary bacteremia, which may follow ingestion of contaminated shellfish or exposure to sea water. Cellulitis with or without sepsis may be accompanied by bulla formation and necrosis with extensive soft tissue destruction, at times requiring debridement and amputation. The infection can be rapidly progressive and is particularly severe in immunocompromised individuals—especially those with cirrhosis—with death rates as high as 50%. Patients with chronic liver disease and those who are immunocompromised should be cautioned to avoid eating raw oysters.

Tetracycline at a dose of 500 mg four times a day is the drug of choice for treatment of suspected or documented primary bacteremia or cellulitis caused by *Vibrio* species. *V vulnificus* is susceptible in vitro to penicillin, ampicillin, cephalosporins, chloramphenicol, aminoglycosides, and fluoroquinolones, and these agents may also be effective. *V parahaemolyticus* and *V alginolyticus* produce beta-lactamase and therefore are resistant to penicillin and ampicillin, but susceptibilities otherwise are similar to those listed for *V vulnificus.*

Koenig KL, Mueller J, Rose T: *Vibrio vulnificus:* Hazard on the half shell. West J Med 1991;155:400.

INFECTIONS CAUSED BY *CAMPYLOBACTER* SPECIES

Campylobacters are microaerophilic, motile, gram-negative rods. Two species infect humans: *Campylobacter jejuni,* an important cause of diarrheal disease; and *Campylobacter fetus* subsp *fetus*, which typically causes systemic infection and not diarrhea. Dairy cattle are an important reservoir for campylobacters. Outbreaks of enteritis have been associated with consumption of raw milk. *Campylobacter* gastroenteritis is associated with fever, abdominal pain, and diarrhea characterized by loose, watery, or bloody stools. The differential diagnosis includes shigellosis, salmonella gastroenteritis, and enteritis caused by *Yersinia enterocolitica* or invasive *Escherichia coli.* The disease is self-limited, but its duration can be shortened with antimicrobial therapy. Both erythromycin, 250–500 mg four times daily for 5–7 days, and ciprofloxacin, 500 mg twice daily for 5–7 days, are effective regimens. Pending identification of the causative agent of suspected bacterial gastroenteritis, ciprofloxacin is a rational choice for empirical therapy because all of the common bacterial pathogens are susceptible.

C fetus causes systemic infections that can be fatal, including primary bacteremia, endocarditis, meningitis, and focal abscesses. It infrequently causes gastroenteritis. Patients infected with *C fetus* are often elderly, debilitated, or immunocompromised. Closely related species, collectively termed *Campylobacter*-like organisms, cause bacteremia in HIV-infected individuals. Systemic infections respond to therapy with gentamicin, chloramphenicol, or ceftriaxone. These organisms are also susceptible in vitro to ciprofloxacin. Ceftriaxone or chloramphenicol should be used to treat infections of the central nervous system because of their ability to penetrate the blood-brain barrier.

Wood RC, MacDonald KL, Osterholm MT: *Campylobacter* enteritis outbreaks associated with drinking raw milk during youth activities: A ten-year review of outbreaks in the United States. JAMA 1992;268:3228.

BRUCELLOSIS

Essentials of Diagnosis

- Insidious onset: easy fatigability, headache, arthralgia, anorexia, sweating, irritability.
- Intermittent fever, especially at night, which may become chronic and undulant.
- Cervical and axillary lymphadenopathy; hepatosplenomegaly.
- Lymphocytosis, positive blood culture, elevated agglutination titer.

General Considerations

The infection is transmitted from animals to humans. *Brucella abortus* (cattle), *Brucella suis,* (hogs), and *Brucella melitensis* (goats) are the main agents. Transmission to humans occurs by contact with infected meat (slaughterhouse workers), placentae of infected animals (farmers, veterinarians), or ingestion of infected unpasteurized milk or cheese. The incubation period varies from a few days to several weeks. The disorder may become chronic. In the USA, brucellosis is very rare except in the midwestern states (from *B suis*) and in visitors or immigrants from countries where brucellosis is endemic (eg, Mexico, Spain, South American countries).

Clinical Findings

A. Symptoms and Signs: The onset may be acute, with fever, chills, and sweats, but typically is insidious. It may be weeks before the patient seeks medical care for weakness, weight loss, low-grade fevers, sweats, and exhaustion upon minimal activity. Symptoms also include headache, abdominal or back pains with anorexia and constipation, and arthralgia. Epididymitis occurs in 10% of cases in men. The chronic form may assume an undulant nature, with periods of normal temperature between acute attacks; symptoms may persist for years, either continuously or intermittently.

Physical findings are minimal. Half of cases have peripheral lymph node enlargement and splenomegaly; hepatomegaly is less common.

B. Laboratory Findings: Early in the course of infection, the organism can be recovered from the blood, cerebrospinal fluid, urine, and bone marrow. Because the organism is slow-growing, cultures should be incubated for 21 days before being read as negative. Cultures are more likely to be negative in chronic cases. The diagnosis often is made not by culture but by serologic testing. Rising serologic titers or an absolute agglutination titer of greater than 1:100 supports the diagnosis. Occasionally, falsely negative agglutination studies are reported when antibodies are present in extremely high titer (prozone phenomenon). In such cases, it is necessary to ask the laboratory to repeat the study on a diluted serum specimen.

Differential Diagnosis

Brucellosis must be differentiated from any other acute febrile disease, especially influenza, tularemia, Q fever, mononucleosis, and enteric fever. In its chronic form it resembles Hodgkin's disease, tuberculosis, HIV infection, malaria, and disseminated fungal infections such as histoplasmosis and coccidioidomycosis.

Complications

The most frequent complications are bone and joint lesions such as spondylitis and suppurative arthritis (usually of a single joint), endocarditis, and meningoencephalitis. Less common complications are pneumonitis with pleural effusion, hepatitis, and cholecystitis.

Treatment

Single-drug regimens are not recommended because the relapse rate may be as high as 50%. Combination regimens of two or three drugs are more effective. Either (1) doxycycline plus rifampin or streptomycin (or both) (2) trimethoprim-sulfamethoxazole plus rifampin or streptomycin (or both) are effective in doses as follows for 21 days: (1) doxycycline, 100–200 mg/d in divided doses; trimethoprim 320 mg/d plus sulfamethoxazole 1600 mg/d in divided doses; rifampin, 600–1200 mg/d; and streptomycin, 500 mg intramuscularly twice a day. Longer courses of therapy (eg, several months) may be required to cure relapses, osteomyelitis, or meningitis.

Ariza J et al: Treatment of human brucellosis with doxycycline plus rifampin or doxycycline plus streptomycin. Ann Intern Med 1992;117:25. (Doxycycline plus rifampin is effective.)

TULAREMIA

Essentials of Diagnosis

- Fever, headache, nausea, and prostration.
- Papule progressing to ulcer at site of inoculation.
- Enlarged regional lymph nodes.
- History of contact with rabbits, other rodents, and biting arthropods (eg, ticks in summer) in endemic area.
- Serologic tests or culture of ulcer, lymph node aspirate, or blood confirm the diagnosis.

General Considerations

Tularemia is an infection of wild rodents—particularly rabbits and muskrats—with *Francisella (Pasteurella) tularensis*. Humans usually acquire the infection by contact with animal tissues (eg, trapping muskrats, skinning rabbits) or from ticks. Infection in humans often produces a local lesion and widespread organ involvement but may be entirely asymptomatic. The incubation period is 2–10 days.

Clinical Findings

A. Symptoms and Signs: Fever, headache, and nausea begin suddenly, and a local lesion—a papule at the site of inoculation—develops and soon ulcerates. Regional lymph nodes may become enlarged and tender and may suppurate. The local lesion may be on the skin of an extremity or in the eye. Pneumonia may develop from hematogenous spread of the organism or may be primary after inhalation of infected aerosols, which are responsible for human-to-human transmission. Following ingestion of infected meat or water, an enteric form may be manifested by

gastrointestinal symptoms, stupor, and delirium. In any type of involvement, the spleen may be enlarged and tender and there may be nonspecific rashes, myalgias, and prostration.

B. Laboratory Findings: Culture of blood, an ulcerated lesion, or lymph node aspirate usually is negative unless special media are used. For this reason and because cultures of *F tularensis* may be hazardous to laboratory personnel, the diagnosis is usually made serologically. A positive agglutination test (> 1:80) develops in the second week after infection and may persist for several years.

Differential Diagnosis

Tularemia must be differentiated from rickettsial and meningococcal infections, cat-scratch disease, infectious mononucleosis, and various bacterial and fungal diseases.

Complications

Hematogenous spread may produce meningitis, perisplenitis, pericarditis, pneumonia, and osteomyelitis.

Treatment

Streptomycin, 0.5 g intramuscularly every 6–8 hours, together with tetracycline 0.5 g orally every 6 hours, is administered until 4–5 days after the patient becomes afebrile. Chloramphenicol may be substituted for tetracycline in the same dosage.

Evans ME et al: Tularemia: A 30-year experience with 88 cases. Medicine 1985;64:251. (With photographs.)

PLAGUE

Essentials of Diagnosis

- History of exposure to rodents in endemic area.
- Sudden onset of high fever, malaise, muscular pains, and prostration.
- Axillary or inguinal lymphadenitis (bubo).
- Bacteremia, sepsis, and pneumonitis may occur.
- Positive smear and culture from bubo and positive blood culture.

General Considerations

Plague is an infection of wild rodents with *Yersinia pestis,* a small gram-negative coccobacillus. It is transmitted among rodents and to humans by the bites of fleas or from ingestion of feces of fleas. Persons usually acquire the infection by contact with rodents and fleas from a plague-endemic area. If a plague victim develops pneumonia, the infection can be transmitted by droplets to other persons and an epidemic may be started in this way. The incubation period is 2–10 days.

Following the flea bite, the organisms spread through the lymphatics to the lymph nodes, which become greatly enlarged (bubo). They may then reach the bloodstream to involve all organs. When pneumonia or meningitis develops, the outcome is often fatal.

Clinical Findings

A. Symptoms and Signs: The onset is sudden, with high fever, malaise, tachycardia, intense headache, and severe myalgias. The patient appears profoundly ill. Delirium may ensue. If pneumonia develops, tachypnea, productive cough, blood-tinged sputum, and cyanosis also occur. Signs of meningitis may develop. A pustule or ulcer at the site of inoculation and signs of lymphangitis may be observed. Axillary, inguinal, or cervical lymph nodes become enlarged and tender and may eventually suppurate and drain. With hematogenous spread, the patient may rapidly become toxic and comatose, with purpuric spots (black plague) appearing on the skin.

Primary plague pneumonia is a fulminant pneumonitis with bloody, frothy sputum and sepsis and is usually fatal unless treatment is started within a few hours after onset.

B. Laboratory Findings: The plague bacillus may be found in smears from aspirates of buboes examined with Gram's stain. Cultures from bubo aspirate or pus and blood are positive but may grow slowly. In convalescing patients, an antibody titer rise may be demonstrated by agglutination tests.

Differential Diagnosis

The lymphadenitis of plague is most commonly mistaken for the lymphadenitis accompanying staphylococcal or streptococcal infections of an extremity, sexually transmitted diseases such as lymphogranuloma venereum or syphilis, and tularemia. The systemic manifestations resemble those of enteric or rickettsial fevers, malaria, or influenza. The pneumonia resembles other bacterial pneumonias, and the meningitis is similar to those caused by other bacteria.

Prevention

Periodic surveys of rodents and their ectoparasites in endemic areas provide guidelines for control measures. Endemic areas in the United States areas include California, Nevada, Arizona, and particularly New Mexico.

Drug prophylaxis may provide temporary protection for persons exposed to the risk of plague infection, particularly by the respiratory route. Tetracycline hydrochloride, 500 mg orally 1–2 times daily for 5 days, can accomplish this.

Plague vaccines—both live and killed—have been used for many years, but their efficacy is not clearly established.

Treatment

Therapy must be started promptly when plague is suspected. Streptomycin, 1 g intramuscularly, is ad-

ministered immediately, and 0.5 g intramuscularly is then given every 6–8 hours. Tetracycline, 2 g daily orally (parenterally if necessary), is given at the same time. Intravenous fluids, pressor drugs, oxygen, and intubation and mechanical ventilation are used as required. Patients with plague pneumonia should be strictly isolated.

Crook LD, Tempest B: Plague: A review of 27 cases. Arch Intern Med 1992;152:1253.

GONOCOCCAL INFECTIONS

Essentials of Diagnosis

- Purulent and profuse urethral discharge, especially in men, with dysuria, yielding positive smear.
- Epididymitis, prostatitis, periurethral inflammation, proctitis in men.
- Cervicitis in women with purulent discharge, or asymptomatic, yielding positive culture; vaginitis, salpingitis, proctitis also occur.
- Fever, rash, tenosynovitis, and arthritis with disseminated disease.
- Gram-negative intracellular diplococci seen in a smear or cultured from any site, particularly the urethra, cervix, pharynx, and rectum.

General Considerations

Gonorrhea is the most prevalent reportable communicable disease in the USA, with an estimated 2.5 million or more cases annually. It is caused by *Neisseria gonorrhoeae*, a gram-negative diplococcus typically found inside polymorphonuclear cells. It is most commonly transmitted during sexual activity and has its greatest incidence in the 15- to 29-year-old age group. The incubation period is usually 2–8 days.

Anatomic Classification

A. Urethritis and Cervicitis: In men, there is initially burning on urination and a serous or milky discharge. One to 3 days later, the urethral pain is more pronounced and the discharge becomes yellow, creamy, and profuse, sometimes blood-tinged. Without treatment, the disorder may regress and become chronic or progress to involve the prostate, epididymis, and periurethral glands with acute, painful inflammation. This in turn becomes chronic, with prostatitis and urethral strictures. Rectal infection is common in homosexual men. Atypical sites of primary infection (eg, the pharynx) must always be considered. Systemic involvement also occurs. Asymptomatic infection is common and occurs in both sexes.

Women may have dysuria, urinary frequency, and urgency, with a purulent urethral discharge. Vaginitis and cervicitis with inflammation of Bartholin's glands are common. Infection may be asymptomatic, with only slightly increased vaginal discharge and moderate cervicitis on examination. Infection may remain as a chronic cervicitis—an important reservoir of gonococci. It may progress to involve the uterus and tubes with acute and chronic salpingitis and with ultimate scarring of tubes and sterility. In pelvic inflammatory disease, anaerobes and chlamydiae often accompany gonococci. Rectal infection is common both as spread of the organism from the genital tract and as a result of infection by anal coitus. Systemic involvement also occurs.

Smears of urethral discharge in men, especially during the first week after onset, typically show gram-negative diplococci in polymorphonuclear leukocytes. Smears are less often positive in women. Cultures are essential in all cases where gonorrhea is suspected and gonococci cannot be shown in gram-stained smears. This applies particularly to cervical, rectal, pharyngeal, and joint specimens. Specimens of pus or secretions are streaked on a selective medium such as Thayer-Martin or Transgrow. The latter is suitable for transport if a laboratory is not immediately available.

B. Disseminated Disease: Systemic complications follow the dissemination of gonococci from the primary site via the bloodstream. Gonococcal bacteremia is associated with intermittent fever, arthralgia, and skin lesions ranging from maculopapular to pustular or hemorrhagic, which tend to be few in number and peripherally located. Rarely, gonococcal endocarditis or meningitis develops. Arthritis and tenosynovitis are common complications, particularly involving the knees, ankles, and wrists. One or occasionally a few joints usually are involved. Gonococci can be isolated from less than half of patients with gonococcal arthritis.

C. Conjunctivitis: The most common form of eye involvement is direct inoculation of gonococci into the conjunctival sac. In adults, this occurs by autoinoculation of a person with genital infection. The purulent conjunctivitis may rapidly progress to panophthalmitis and loss of the eye unless treated promptly. A single 1-g dose of ceftriaxone is effective.

Differential Diagnosis

Gonococcal urethritis or cervicitis must be differentiated from nongonococcal urethritis; cervicitis or vaginitis due to *Chlamydia trachomatis, Gardnerella (Haemophilus) vaginalis, Trichomonas, Candida,* and many other agents associated with sexually transmitted diseases; pelvic inflammatory disease, arthritis, proctitis, and skin lesions. Often, several such agents coexist in a patient. Reiter's disease (urethritis, conjunctivitis, arthritis) may mimic gonorrhea or coexist with it.

Prevention

Prevention is based on education, mechanical or chemical prophylaxis, and early diagnosis and treatment. The condom, if properly used, can reduce the risk of infection. Effective drugs taken in therapeutic doses within 24 hours of exposure can abort an infection, but prophylaxis with penicillin is ineffective and contributes to the selection of penicillinase-producing gonococci.

Ophthalmic infection of the newborn is prevented by the instillation of 0.5% erythromycin ointment, 1% tetracycline ointment, or 1% silver nitrate solution into each conjunctival sac immediately after birth. Ceftriaxone, 125 mg intramuscularly once, is effective against both eye and systemic infections.

Treatment

Therapy typically is administered before antimicrobial susceptibilities are known. The choice of which regimen to use should be based on the prevalence of penicillin-resistant organisms. Recent data indicate a nationwide distribution of penicillin- and tetracycline-resistant gonococci. Consequently, penicillin should no longer be considered first-line therapy. All sexual partners should be treated.

A. Uncomplicated Gonorrhea: For urethritis or cervicitis, ceftriaxone, 250 mg intramuscularly, is the treatment of choice. Effective single-dose oral regimens are also available, such as cefixime, 400–800 mg, or one of the fluoroquinolones—ciprofloxacin, 500 mg, or ofloxacin, 400 mg. Amoxicillin, 3 g orally once, plus probenecid, 1 g orally once, is an alternative oral regimen but overall efficacy is less. Spectinomycin, 1 g intramuscularly once, may be used for the penicillin-allergic patient. Anal gonorrhea in women responds to the same drugs, but in males ceftriaxone is most effective. Pharyngeal gonorrhea responds to ceftriaxone in the same dosage or to trimethoprim-sulfamethoxazole, nine regular-strength tablets orally for 5 days.

Since coexistent chlamydial infection is common, the above courses should be followed by erythromycin or tetracycline, 500 mg four times daily orally, for 7 days. The latter is sometimes given concurrently.

B. Follow-Up: Urethral, rectal, or pharyngeal specimens should be obtained from men 1 week after treatment. Cervical, rectal, or pharyngeal specimens should be obtained from women 7–14 days after completion of treatment. Serologic tests for syphilis should also be obtained to exclude coexistent subclinical infection.

C. Treatment of Other Infections: Salpingitis, prostatitis, bacteremia, arthritis, and other complications due to susceptible strains in adults should be treated with penicillin G, 10 million units intravenously daily, for 5 days. Ceftriaxone, 2 g intravenously daily for 5 days, also is effective.

Postgonococcal urethritis or cervicitis, usually caused by chlamydiae, is treated with tetracycline or erythromycin, 0.5 g orally four times daily, for 7–10 days. Pelvic inflammatory disease requires cefoxitin,

2 g parenterally every 8 hours. Concurrent treatment for chlamydial infection also is indicated. Alternative drug choices exist.

Hansfield HH et al: A comparison of single-dose cefixime with ceftriaxone as treatment for uncomplicated gonorrhea. N Engl J Med 1991;325:1337.

Schwarcz SK et al: National surveillance of antimicrobial resistance in *Neisseria gonorrhoeae*. JAMA 1990; 264; 1413.

CHANCROID

Chancroid is a sexually transmitted disease caused by the short gram-negative bacillus *Haemophilus ducreyi*. Nonvenereal inoculation has occurred in medical personnel through contact with chancroid patients. The incubation period is 3–5 days.

The initial lesions at the site of inoculation is a vesicopustule that breaks down to form a painful, soft ulcer with a necrotic base, surrounding erythema, and undermined edges. Multiple lesions—started by autoinoculation—and inguinal adenitis often develop. The adenitis is usually unilateral and consists of tender, matted nodes of moderate size with overlying erythema. These may become fluctuant and rupture spontaneously. With lymph node involvement, fever, chills, and malaise may develop. Women may have no external signs of infection.

Swabs from lesions are best cultured on chocolate agar with 1% Isovitalex and vancomycin, 3 mg/mL, to yield *H ducreyi*. Mixed sexually transmitted disease is very common (including syphilis, herpes simplex, and HIV infection), as is infection of the ulcer with fusiforms, spirochetes, and other organisms.

Balanitis and phimosis are frequent complications.

Chancroid must be differentiated from other genital ulcers. The chancre of syphilis, by contrast, is clean and painless, with a hard base.

Treatment is with erythromycin, 0.5 g orally four times daily for 7 days; or trimethoprim-sulfamethoxazole, one double-strength tablet twice daily for 7 days. Single-dose regimens are also effective: trimethoprim-sulfamethoxazole, three double-strength tablets; ciprofloxacin, 500 mg; or ceftriaxone, 250 mg intramuscularly.

Bodhidatta L et al: Evaluation of 500 mg and 1000 mg doses of ciprofloxacin for the treatment of chancroid. Antimicrob Agents Chemother 1988;32:723. (Cure rates of 93–100%.)

GRANULOMA INGUINALE

Granuloma inguinale is a chronic, relapsing granulomatous anogenital infection due to *Calymmatobacterium (Donovania) granulomatis*. The pathogno-monic cell, found in tissue scrapings or secretions, is large (25–90 μm) and contains intracytoplasmic cysts filled with bodies (Donovan bodies) that stain deeply with Wright's stain.

The incubation period is 8 days to 12 weeks. The onset is insidious. The lesions occur on the skin or mucous membranes of the genitalia or perineal area. They are relatively painless infiltrated nodules that soon slough. A shallow, sharply demarcated ulcer forms, with a beefy-red friable base of granulation tissue. The lesion spreads by contiguity. The advancing border has a characteristic rolled edge of granulation tissue. Large ulcerations may advance onto the lower abdomen and thighs. Scar formation and healing may occur along one border while the opposite border advances.

Superinfection with spirochete-fusiform organisms is common. The ulcer then becomes purulent, painful, foul-smelling, and extremely difficult to treat.

Several therapies are available. Because of the indolent nature of the disease, duration of therapy tends to be relatively long. Erythromycin or tetracycline, 500 mg four times a day for 21 days is effective. Ampicillin, 500 mg four times a day, also is effective, but up to 12 weeks of therapy may be necessary.

Since other sexually transmitted diseases frequently coexist, cultures for these and a serologic test for syphilis must be performed.

Faro S: Lymphogranuloma venereum, chancroid, granuloma inguinale. Obstet Gynecol Clin North Am 1989; 16:517. (Presentation, diagnosis, and therapy.)

CAT-SCRATCH DISEASE

Essentials of Diagnosis

- A primary infected ulcer or papule-pustule at site of inoculation (30% of cases).
- Regional lymphadenopathy that often suppurates.
- History of scratch by cat at involved area.
- Positive intradermal test.

General Considerations

This is an acute infection that occurs worldwide and is more common in children and young adults in contact with cats and dogs. It may be transmitted by a scratch or other injury, but some cases lack such a history. The cause appears to be a small gram-negative bacterium, *Afipia felis*.

Clinical Findings

A. Symptoms and Signs: A few days after the scratch, about one-third of patients develop a primary lesion at the site of inoculation. This primary lesion appears as an infected, scabbed ulcer or a papule with a central vesicle or pustule. One to 3 weeks later, symptoms of generalized infection appear (fever, malaise, headache), and the regional lymph nodes become enlarged without evidence of lymphangitis. The nodes may be tender and fixed, with overlying inflammation; or nontender, discrete, and without evidence of surrounding inflammation. Suppuration may occur, with the discharge of sterile pus. While the course is usually benign, some adults have fever and severe systemic symptoms for weeks.

Lymph node enlargement must be differentiated from that of lymphoma or other malignancy, tuberculosis, lymphogranuloma venereum, and acute bacterial infection.

B. Laboratory Findings: The sedimentation rate is elevated, the white blood cell count is usually normal, and the pus from the nodes is sterile. Intradermal skin testing with antigen prepared from the pus is positive in most cases. Lymph node morphology is fairly characteristic; excisional biopsy, usually performed to exclude lymphoma, confirms the diagnosis.

Complications

Encephalitis occurs rarely. Macular or papular rashes and erythema nodosum are occasionally seen. A disseminated form of cat-scratch disease, recently renamed **bacillary angiomatosis,** has been reported in HIV-infected persons and other immunocompromised individuals. Clinically, the lesions—which can be cutaneous, lymphatic, or visceral—are vascular proliferative and histopathologically distinct from the granulomatous lesions of cat-scratch disease. Bacillary angiomatosis is caused by a bacillus that is closely related to rickettsiae and is probably not the agent of cat-scratch disease. Bacillary angiomatosis differs from cat-scratch disease in that it responds to treatment with erythromycin (the drug of choice) and tetracycline, which are inactive in cat scratch disease.

Treatment

Antimicrobial therapy of cat-scratch disease is ineffective. Symptoms resolve without treatment in one or two weeks.

English CK et al: Cat-scratch disease: Isolation and culture of the bacterial agent. JAMA 1988;259:1347. (Culture and susceptibility testing of an isolate that appeared to be derived from a cell wall-defective variant.)

Relman DA et al: The agent of bacillary angiomatosis: An approach to the identification of uncultured pathogens. N Engl J Med 1990;323:1573.

ANAEROBIC INFECTIONS

Anaerobic bacteria make up the majority of normal human flora. Prominent members of the normal microbial flora of the mouth (anaerobic spirochetes, *Bacteroides,* fusobacteria), the skin (anaerobic diph-theroids), the large bowel (*Bacteroides,* anaerobic streptococci, clostridia), and the female tract (*Bacteroides,* anaerobic streptococci, fusobacteria) may produce disease when displaced from their normal sites into tissues or closed body spaces.

Certain characteristics are suggestive of anaerobic infections: (1) They involve multiple organisms. (2) They produce closed-space infections, either in discrete abscesses (lung, brain, pleura, peritoneum) or by burrowing through tissue layers. (3) Pus from anaerobic infections often has a foul odor. (4) Septic thrombophlebitis and metastatic suppurative lesions are frequent and may require surgical drainage in addition to antimicrobial therapy. (Most of the important anaerobes except *Bacteroides fragilis* are highly sensitive to penicillin G, but the diminished blood supply that favors proliferation of anaerobes because of reduced tissue oxygenation also interferes with the delivery of antimicrobials to the site of anaerobic infection.) (5) Bacteriologic examination may yield negative results or only inconsequential aerobes unless rigorous culture conditions are used.

Important types of infections that are most commonly caused by anaerobic organisms are listed below. Treatment of all these infections consists of surgical exploration and judicious excision in conjunction with administration of antimicrobial drugs.

Upper Respiratory Tract

Bacteroides melaninogenicus together with anaerobic spirochetes is commonly involved in periodontal infections. These organisms, fusobacteria, and peptostreptococci are responsible for a substantial percentage of cases of chronic sinusitis and probably of peritonsillar abscess, chronic otitis media, and mastoiditis. Hygiene and drainage are as important in treatment as antimicrobials. Penicillin G is the drug of choice: 1–2 million units intravenously every 4 hours if parenteral therapy is required or 0.5 g orally four times daily for less severe infections. In the penicillin-allergic patient, clindamycin can be used (600 mg intravenously every 8 hours or 300 mg orally every 6 hours).

Chest Infections

Aspiration of saliva (which contains 10^8 anaerobic organisms per milliliter in addition to aerobes) may lead to necrotizing pneumonia, lung abscess, and empyema. While polymicrobial infection is the rule, anaerobes—particularly *B melaninogenicus,* fusobacteria, and peptostreptococci—are common etiologic agents. Most pulmonary infections respond to antimicrobial therapy alone. Percutaneous chest tube or surgical drainage is indicated for empyema.

Penicillin has long been considered the drug of choice for treatment of anaerobic lung infections. Although most oral anaerobes are susceptible to penicillin, penicillin-resistant *B fragilis* and *B melaninogenicus* are isolated in up to 25% of cases.

Clindamycin is more effective than penicillin for treatment of anaerobic lung infections. Penicillin failures have been associated with the presence of penicillin-resistant organisms. Clindamycin, 600 mg intravenously once, followed by 300 mg orally every 6–8 hours, is the treatment of choice for these infections. Penicillin, 2 million units intravenously every 4 hours, followed by amoxicillin, 500 mg every 8 hours orally, is a reasonable alternative. The second-generation cephalosporins cefoxitin, cefotetan, and cefmetazole are active in vitro against anaerobes, including those that are penicillin-resistant. Chloramphenicol is also effective, but it is used uncommonly given the numerous alternatives.

Gudiol F et al: Clindamycin vs penicillin for anaerobic lung infections: high rate of penicillin failures associated with penicillin-resistant *Bacteroides melaninogenicus.* Arch Intern Med 1990;150:2525.

Central Nervous System

Anaerobes are a common cause of brain abscess, subdural empyema, or septic central nervous system thrombophlebitis. The organisms reach the central nervous system by direct extension from sinusitis, otitis, or mastoiditis or by hematogenous spread from chronic lung infections. Antimicrobial therapy—eg, 20 million units intravenously in combination with chloramphenicol, 50 mg/kg/d in four divided doses, or metronidazole, 750 mg intravenously every 8 hours—is an important adjunct to surgical drainage. Some small multiple brain abscesses can be treated with antibiotics alone for 6–8 weeks and may heal without surgical drainage.

Intra-abdominal Infections

In the colon there are up to 10^{11} anaerobes per gram of content—predominantly *B fragilis,* clostridia, and peptostreptococci. These organisms play a central etiologic role in most intra-abdominal abscesses following trauma to the colon, diverticulitis, appendicitis, or perirectal abscess and may also participate in hepatic abscess and cholecystitis, often in association with aerobic coliform bacteria. The gallbladder wall may be infected with clostridia as well. The bacteriology includes anaerobes as well as enteric gram-negative rods and on occasion enterococci. Therapy should be directed primarily against anaerobes and gram-negative aerobes. Multiple antibiotics may be required. Antibiotics reliably active against *B fragilis* include metronidazole, chloramphenicol, imipenem, ampicillin-sulbactam, and ticarcillin-clavulanic acid. Cefoxitin, cefotetan, and clindamycin are active against 80–90% of strains, but third-generation cephalosporins have poor activity, inhibiting only 50% of isolates.

Several options are available for the treatment of these mixed infections. One common regimen includes ampicillin plus gentamicin to cover enteric gram-negative rods (and also enterococci, though their role is controversial) and metronidazole to cover anaerobes. Other examples might include imipenem alone (very expensive), ticarcillin-clavulanate, ampicillin-sulbactam alone or in combination with gentamicin, clindamycin with gentamicin, and cefoxitin or cefotetan alone or with gentamicin.

Although the upper intestinal tract contains far fewer organisms than the colon, anaerobes account for a major proportion of the normal flora. Consequently, the same antibiotic consideration apply to infections caused by flora originating there.

Female Genital Tract & Pelvic Infections

The normal flora of the vagina and cervix includes several species of *Bacteroides,* peptostreptococci, group B streptococci, lactobacilli, coliform bacteria, and, occasionally, spirochetes and clostridia. These organisms commonly cause genital tract infections and may disseminate from there.

While salpingitis is commonly caused by gonococci and chlamydiae, tubo-ovarian and pelvic abscesses are associated with anaerobes in a majority of cases. Postpartum infections may be caused by aerobic streptococci or staphylococci, but anaerobes are often found, and the most severe cases of postpartum or postabortion sepsis are associated with clostridia and *Bacteroides.* These have a high mortality rate, and treatment requires both antimicrobials directed against anaerobes and coliforms (see above) and abscess drainage or early hysterectomy.

Bacteremia & Endocarditis

Anaerobes are responsible for a small percentage of cases of bacteremia seen in general hospitals. Most of these originate from the gastrointestinal tract, the oropharynx, decubitus ulcers, and the female genital tract. Endocarditis due to anaerobic and microaerophilic streptococci and *Bacteroides* originates from the same sites. Rigorous anaerobic cultures are essential in patients whose "routine" blood cultures have remained negative but who are suspected clinically of having endocarditis. Most cases of aerobic streptococcal endocarditis can be effectively treated with 12–20 million units of penicillin G daily, but optimal therapy of other types of anaerobic bacterial endocarditis must rely on laboratory guidance. Anaerobic corynebacteria *(Propionibacterium),* clostridia, and *Bacteroides* occasionally cause endocarditis.

Skin & Soft Tissue Infections

Anaerobic infections in the skin and soft tissue usually follow trauma, inadequate blood supply, or surgery and are commonest in areas that are contaminated by oral or fecal flora. There may be progressive tissue necrosis and a putrid odor.

Several terms, such as bacterial synergistic gangrene, synergistic necrotizing cellulitis, necrotizing fasciitis, and nonclostridial crepitant cellulitis, have been used to classify these infections. Although there are some differences in microbiology among them, their differentiation on clinical grounds alone is difficult. All are mixed infections caused by aerobic and anaerobic organisms and require aggressive surgical debridement of necrotic tissue for cure. Surgical consultation is obligatory to assist in diagnosis and treatment.

Broad-spectrum antibiotics active against both anaerobes and gram-positive and gram-negative aerobes (eg, vancomycin plus metronidazole plus gentamicin or tobramycin) should be instituted empirically and modified by culture results. They are given for about a week after progressive tissue destruction has been controlled and the margins of the wound remain free of inflammation.

Brook I: Anaerobic bacterial bacteremia: 12-year experience in two military hospitals. J Infect Dis 1989;160: 1071.
Styrt B, Gorbach SL: Recent developments in the understanding of the pathogenesis and treatment of anaerobic infections. (Two parts.) N Engl J Med 1989;321:240, 298.

ACTINOMYCOSIS

Essentials of Diagnosis

- History of recent dental infection or abdominal trauma.
- Chronic pneumonia or indolent intra-abdominal or cervicofacial abscess.
- Sinus tract formation.

General Considerations

Actinomyces israelii and other species of *Actinomyces* occur in the normal flora of the mouth and tonsillar crypts. They are anaerobic, gram-positive, branching filamentous bacteria (1 μm in diameter) that may fragment into bacillary forms. When introduced into traumatized tissue and associated with other anaerobic bacteria, these actinomycetes become pathogens.

The most common site of infection is the cervicofacial area (about 60% of cases). Infection typically follows extraction of a tooth or other trauma. Lesions may develop in the gastrointestinal tract or lungs following ingestion or aspiration of the fungus from its endogenous source in the mouth.

Clinical Findings

A. Symptoms and Signs:

1. Cervicofacial actinomycosis–Cervicofacial actinomycosis develops slowly. The area becomes markedly indurated, and the overlying skin becomes reddish or cyanotic. Abscesses eventually draining to the surface persist for long periods. Sulfur granules—masses of filamentous organisms—may be found in the pus. There is usually little pain unless there is secondary infection. Trismus indicates that the muscles of mastication are involved. Radiography may reveal bony involvement.

2. Thoracic actinomycosis–Thoracic involvement begins with fever, cough, and sputum production with night sweats and weight loss. Pleuritic pain may be present. Multiple sinuses may extend through the chest wall, to the heart, or into the abdominal cavity. Ribs may be involved. Radiography shows areas of consolidation and in many cases pleural effusion. Cervicofacial or thoracic disease may occasionally result in central nervous system complications, most commonly brain abscess or meningitis.

3. Abdominal actinomycosis–Abdominal actinomycosis usually causes pain in the ileocecal region, spiking fever and chills, vomiting, and weight loss and may be confused with Crohn's disease. Irregular abdominal masses may be palpated. Pelvic inflammatory disease caused by actinomycetes has been associated with prolonged use of an intrauterine contraceptive device. Sinuses draining to the exterior may develop. CT scanning reveals an inflammatory mass that may extend to involve bone.

B. Laboratory Findings: The anaerobic, gram-positive organism may be demonstrated as a granule or as scattered branching gram-positive filaments in the pus. Anaerobic culture is necessary to distinguish *Actinomyces* from *Nocardia*, because specific therapy differs for the two infections.

Treatment

Penicillin G is the drug of choice. Ten to 20 million units are given via a parenteral route for 2–4 weeks, followed by oral penicillin V, 500 mg four times daily.

Sulfonamides such as sulfamethoxazole may be an alternative regimen at a total daily dosage of 2–4 g. Response to therapy is slow. Therapy should be continued for weeks to months after clinical manifestations have disappeared in order to ensure cure. Surgical procedures such as drainage and resection may be beneficial.

With penicillin and surgery, the prognosis is good. The difficulties of diagnosis, however, may permit extensive destruction of tissue before the diagnosis is identified and therapy is started.

NOCARDIOSIS

Nocardia asteroides and *Nocardia brasiliensis,* aerobic filamentous soil bacteria, cause pulmonary and systemic nocardiosis. Bronchopulmonary abnormalities (eg, alveolar proteinosis) predispose to colonization, but infection is unusual unless the patient is also receiving systemic corticosteroids or is otherwise immunosuppressed.

Pulmonary involvement usually begins with malaise, loss of weight, fever, and night sweats. Cough and production of purulent sputum are the chief complaints. Radiography may show infiltrates accompanied by pleural effusion. The lesions may penetrate to the exterior through the chest wall, invading the ribs.

Dissemination may involve any organ. Brain abscesses and subcutaneous nodules are most frequent. Dissemination is seen exclusively in immunocompromised patients.

N asteroides is usually found as delicate, branching, gram-positive filaments. It may be weakly acidfast, occasionally causing diagnostic confusion with tuberculosis. Identification is made by culture.

Therapy is initiated with intravenous trimethoprim-sulfamethoxazole and continued with oral trimethoprim-sulfamethoxazole, one double-strength tablet twice a day. Surgical procedures such as drainage and resection may be needed as adjunctive therapy.

Response may be slow, and therapy must be continued for at least 6 months. The prognosis in systemic nocardiosis is poor when diagnosis and therapy are delayed.

Wilson JP et al: *Nocardia* infections in renal transplant recipients. Medicine 1989;68:38. (Review of the literature.)

INFECTIONS CAUSED BY MYCOBACTERIA

NONTUBERCULOUS ATYPICAL MYCOBACTERIAL DISEASES

About 10% of mycobacterial infections seen in clinical practice are caused not by *Mycobacterium tuberculosis* but by atypical mycobacteria. Atypical mycobacterial infections are among the most common opportunistic infections in advanced HIV disease. These organisms have distinctive laboratory characteristics, occur ubiquitously in the environment, are not communicable from person to person, and are often strikingly resistant to antituberculous drugs.

Pulmonary Infections

Mycobacterium kansasii can produce clinical disease resembling tuberculosis, but the illness progresses more slowly. Most such infections occur in patients with preexisting lung disease, though 40% of patients have no known pulmonary disease. Microbiologically, *M kansasii* is similar to *M tuberculosis* and is sensitive to the same drugs. Therapy with isoniazid, ethambutol, and rifampin for 2 years (or 1 year after sputum conversion) has been highly successful.

The *Mycobacterium avium-intracellulare* complex (MAC) produces asymptomatic colonization or a wide spectrum of diseases, including coin lesions, bronchitis in patients with chronic lung disease, and invasive pulmonary disease that is often cavitary and occurs in patients with underlying lung disease. MAC is a common cause of disseminated disease in the late stages of HIV infection, when the CD4 cell count is less than $100/\mu L$. Persistent fever and weight loss are the most common symptoms. The organism can usually be cultured from multiple sites, including blood, liver, lymph node, or bone marrow; pulmonary disease is uncommon in immunoincompetent patients. Blood culture is the preferred means of establishing the diagnosis and has a sensitivity of 98%.

Agents that may be active against MAC include rifampin, rifabutin (formerly ansamycin, a rifampin analogue), cycloserine, ethionamide, clarithromycin, clofazimine, ethambutol, amikacin, and ciprofloxacin. However, combinations of four or more drugs (eg, ciprofloxacin, 750 mg twice a day; clofazimine, 100 mg once a day; ethambutol, 15 mg/kg once a day; and rifampin, 600 mg once a day) are necessary to control the infection. These regimens tend to be poorly tolerated; therefore, antimycobacterial therapy has been limited to patients with invasive pulmonary disease or AIDS patients with severe systemic symptoms such as disabling fever, fatigue, and weight loss. Clarithromycin, 500–1000 mg twice daily in combination with ethambutol, may be both effective and well-tolerated for treatment of MAC infections in AIDS patients. Single-agent therapy is generally not recommended because of rapid emergence of secondary resistance.

Less common causes of pulmonary disease include *Mycobacterium xenopi, Mycobacterium szulgai,* and *Mycobacterium gordonae.* These organisms have variable sensitivities, and treatment is based on results of sensitivity tests. *Mycobacterium fortuitum* and *Mycobacterium chelonei* also can cause pneumonia.

Lymphadenitis

Most cases of lymphadenitis (scrofula) in adults are caused by *Mycobacterium tuberculosis* and can be a manifestation of disseminated disease. In children, the majority of cases are due to nontuberculous mycobacterial species, with *Mycobacterium scrofulaceum* being the most common isolate. *Mycobacterium kansasii, Mycobacterium bovis, Mycobacterium chelonei,* and *Mycobacterium fortuitum* are less commonly observed. Unlike disease caused by *M tuberculosis,* which requires systemic therapy for 9 months, infection with nontuberculous mycobacteria can be successfully treated by surgical excision without antituberculous therapy.

Skin & Soft Tissues

Skin and soft tissue infections such as abscesses, septic arthritis, and osteomyelitis can result from direct inoculation or hematogenous dissemination or may occur as a complication of surgery.

M chelonei and *M fortuitum* are frequent causes of this type of infection. Most cases occur in the extremities and initially present as nodules. Ulceration with abscess formation often follows. The organisms are resistant to the usual antituberculous drugs but may be sensitive to a variety of antibiotics, including erythromycin, doxycycline, amikacin, cefoxitin, sulfonamides, imipenem, and ciprofloxacin. Therapy includes surgical debridement along with drug therapy. Initially, parenteral drugs are given for several weeks, and this is followed by an oral regimen to which the organism is sensitive. The duration of therapy is variable but usually continues for several months after the soft tissue lesions have healed.

Mycobacterium marinum infection ("swimming pool granuloma") presents as a nodular skin lesion following exposure to nonchlorinated water. The lesions respond to therapy with doxycycline, minocycline, or trimethoprim-sulfamethoxazole.

Mycobacterium ulcerans infection (Buruli ulcer) is seen mainly in Africa and Australia and produces a large ulcerative lesion. Therapy consists of surgical excision and skin grafting.

Horsburgh CR, Jr: Current concepts: *Mycobacterium avium* complex infection in acquired immunodeficiency syndrome. N Engl J Med 1991;324:1332.

Israel D, Polk RE: Focus on clarithromycin and azithromycin: Two new macrolide antibiotics. Hosp Formul 1992;27:115. (Use of these agents for infections caused by MAC and other bacteria.)

MYCOBACTERIUM TUBERCULOSIS INFECTIONS

The case rate of tuberculosis in the United States has been increasing since 1986, largely due to a dramatic increase in cases among HIV-infected individuals. Compared to a lifetime risk of developing active tuberculosis of approximately 10% in an infected immunocompetent person, the risk is up to 7% per year for the HIV-infected individual who is also infected with *M tuberculosis.* This greatly increased risk of developing active disease—as well as the recent occurrence in HIV-infected individuals of outbreaks of tuberculosis caused by strains of *M tuberculosis* resistant to multiple drugs—underscore the importance of early case identification and administration of effective antituberculous therapy. Accordingly, the principles of antituberculous therapy, the preferred treatment regimens, and the currently available antimicrobial agents are reviewed.

Except for the special case of tuberculous meningitis, which is discussed below, the clinical manifestations of tuberculous infection are discussed in the chapters pertaining to the organ system involved.

Treatment Considerations

Antimicrobial therapy of active tuberculosis is the same for HIV-infected and HIV-uninfected patients. Despite the HIV-infected patient's increased risk of developing active disease, the increased prevalence of extrapulmonary disease in HIV-infected individuals, and immunodeficiency caused by HIV infection, HIV-infected individuals respond well to therapy. The principles of therapy pertain mainly to the patient with pulmonary tuberculosis, but they also apply to those with extrapulmonary disease.

A. Initial Therapy: Patients with suspected or documented active tuberculosis should be treated with at least two drugs to which the strain is susceptible. Single-drug regimens are notoriously ineffective, with failure rates of 70% or more due to emergence of resistant mutants, which occurs at a frequency of one bacillus in 10^6. Because 10^7 to 10^9 acid-fast bacilli typically are present at the site of active infection, resistant mutants are invariably present when therapy is initiated. Therapy with two drugs, each possessing a different mechanism of action, is effective because the odds that a bacillus is resistant to both are $10^{-6} \times 10^{-6}$, or one in 10^{12}, which is at least three orders of magnitude less than the number of infecting organisms.

The results of susceptibility tests are not known when therapy is initiated. Therefore, drugs are chosen based on their relative potency and on prior susceptibility data obtained from within the community or within the relevant patient population. Isoniazid and rifampin are the two most potent antituberculous agents, and because clinical isolates from newly diagnosed cases were predictably susceptible to both (98% or more of strains), initial therapy with these two drugs was until recently considered appropriate for most cases. Three or four drug regimens were reserved for patients who had one or more risk factors for drug-resistant tuberculosis. Patients at risk for infection with resistant strains were those who had been previously treated for tuberculosis; those who failed to complete a prescribed course of therapy or were otherwise noncompliant; and patients or their close contacts who were from regions (eg, the Philippines, China, Southeast Asia, and Haiti) where the prevalence of primary drug-resistant strains is above 5%.

Recent outbreaks of multidrug-resistant tuberculosis in HIV-infected patients from Miami and New York have led to new recommendations for initial therapy of suspected tuberculosis. Initial therapy with an oral four-drug regimen consisting of isoniazid 300 mg, rifampin 600 mg, pyrazinamide 25 mg/kg, and ethambutol 15 mg/kg, each administered as a single daily dose, is recommended pending results of culture and susceptibility tests. Pyrazinamide is included for two reasons: (1) If the strain is susceptible to isoniazid, rifampin, and pyrazinamide (which is very likely the case), the patient is a candidate for treatment with a 6-month course of therapy; and (2) if the strain is resistant to either isoniazid or rifampin, the addition of pyrazinamide provides insurance against emergence of resistance to the other remaining most potent drug because the regimen still will contain two active drugs. The addition of ethambutol, the weakest of the four drugs in this regimen and the least toxic, is to provide additional insurance that the patient is being treated with two active agents even if the strain is resistant to both isoniazid and rifampin.

It may be reasonable to add or substitute other drugs (Table 32–2) depending on the epidemiologic data. For example, if a patient has had a relapse or has not responded to a particular regimen, two other drugs not used previously should be included in the regimen. If a strain is known to be resistant to a par-

ticular drug, another drug to which the strain is likely to be susceptible should be substituted. As a rule of thumb, two new drugs are always added to a failing regimen. Which drug or drugs eventually are selected will also depend upon their toxicities and the ability of the patient to tolerate them.

B. Definitive Therapy: Assuming that the four-drug regimen recommended above is used and that the strain is susceptible, ethambutol can be discontinued and the three-drug regimen of isoniazid, rifampin, and pyrazinamide administered for a total of 2 months. The pyrazinamide is then stopped, and isoniazid and rifampin are administered for at least four more months (total of 6 months). Treatment of pulmonary tuberculosis generally is continued for a total of 9–12 months if there is any evidence of noncompliance or slow bacteriologic response to treatment. Lifelong therapy is not indicated for HIV-infected patients who have successfully completed a prescribed course of therapy for tuberculosis caused by a susceptible strain.

If pyrazinamide is not used during the first 2 months of therapy, isoniazid and rifampin should be administered for a minimum of 9 months. If other drug combinations must be used because of toxicity or drug resistance, longer durations of therapy are required (Table 32–3).

Prognosis & Follow-Up

Response to therapy is monitored clinically and, if possible, bacteriologically. A qualitative decrease in numbers of acid-fast bacilli seen on sputum smears over the course of therapy is a reliable indicator of response. Most patients who are treated with the recommended four-drug regimen are culture-negative by 3 months. If sputum smears remain persistently positive, noncompliance should be suspected and institution of supervised daily therapy strongly considered. If noncompliance is unlikely, the possibility of drug resistance should be entertained and the regimen altered accordingly.

Barnes PF et al: Tuberculosis in patients with human immunodeficiency virus infection. (Current Concepts.) N Engl J Med 1991;324:1644.

Table 32–2. Antituberculous agents, ranked in order of preference, and usual daily doses.

Drug	Daily Dose and Route
Most potent; effectiveness proved	
Isoniazid	300 mg orally or IM
Rifampin	600 mg orally or IV
Moderately potent; effectiveness proved	
Ethambutol	15–25 mg/kg orally
Pyrazinamide	25 mg/kg orally
Streptomycin	15 mg/kg IM
Kanamycin	15 mg/kg IM
Amikacin	15 mg/kg IM
Capreomycin	15 mg/kg IM
Ethionamide	0.5–1 g orally
Cycloserine	0.5–1 g orally
Active; potency and efficacy unknown	
Ofloxacin	400 mg twice daily orally
Ciprofloxacin	750 mg twice daily orally

Table 32–3. Minimum recommended duration of antituberculous therapy.

Regimen	Duration (mo)
Isoniazid + rifampin + pyrazinamide[1]	6
Isoniazid + rifampin	9
Rifampin + ethambutol	12
Isoniazid + ethambutol	18–24

[1]Pyrazinamide for the first 2 months only.

Frieden TR et al: The emergence of drug-resistant tuberculosis in New York City. N Engl J Med 1993;328:521.

Goble M et al: Treatment of 171 patients with pulmonary tuberculosis resistant to isoniazid and rifampin. N Engl J Med 1993;328:527.

TUBERCULOUS MENINGITIS

Essentials of Diagnosis

- Gradual onset of listlessness, irritability, and anorexia.
- Headache, vomiting, and seizures common.
- Cranial nerve abnormalities typical.
- Tuberculosis focus may be evident elsewhere.
- Cerebrospinal fluid shows several hundred lymphocytes, low glucose, and high protein.

General Considerations

Tuberculous meningitis is caused by rupture of a meningeal tuberculoma resulting from earlier hematogenous seeding of tubercle bacillus from a pulmonary focus, or it may be a consequence of miliary spread.

Clinical Findings

A. Symptoms and Signs: The onset is usually gradual, with listlessness, irritability, anorexia, and fever, followed by headache, vomiting, convulsions, and coma. In older patients, headache and behavioral changes are prominent early symptoms. Nuchal rigidity and cranial nerve palsies occur as the meningitis progresses. Evidence of active tuberculosis elsewhere or a history of prior tuberculosis is present in up to 75% of patients.

B. Laboratory Findings: The spinal fluid is frequently yellowish, with increased pressure, 100–500 cells/μL (early, polymorphonuclear neutrophils; later, lymphocytes), increased protein, and decreased glucose. Acid-fast stains of cerebrospinal fluid usually are negative, and cultures also may be negative in at least 25% of cases. Chest x-ray often reveals abnormalities compatible with tuberculosis but may be normal.

Differential Diagnosis

Tuberculous meningitis may be confused with any other type of meningitis, but the gradual onset, the predominantly lymphocytic pleocytosis of the spinal fluid, and evidence of tuberculosis elsewhere often point to the diagnosis.

Fungal and other granulomatous meningitides, syphilis, and carcinomatous meningitis are in the differential diagnosis.

Treatment

Presumptive diagnosis followed by early, empiric antituberculous therapy is essential for survival and to minimize sequelae. Even if cultures are not positive, a full course of therapy is warranted if the clinical setting is suggestive of tuberculous meningitis.

Regimens that are effective for pulmonary tuberculosis are effective also for tuberculous meningitis. Rifampin, isoniazid, and pyrazinamide all penetrate into cerebrospinal fluid well. The penetration of ethambutol is more variable, but therapeutic concentrations can be achieved, and the drug has been successfully used for meningitis. Aminoglycosides penetrate less well. An effective four-drug short-course regimen consists of giving isoniazid and rifampin for 6 months plus pyrazinamide and ethambutol for the first 2 months. The same doses of isoniazid and rifampin may also be given as a two-drug regimen for 9 months. Other regimens may also be effective, but they are less reliable and generally must be given for longer periods.

Some authorities recommend the addition of corticosteroids for patients with focal deficits or altered mental status. Prednisone, 60 mg/d for 1–2 weeks, then discontinued in a tapering regimen over 4 weeks, may be used.

LEPROSY

Essentials of Diagnosis

- Pale, anesthetic macular—or nodular and erythematous—skin lesions.
- Superficial nerve thickening with associated anesthesia.
- History of residence in endemic area in childhood.
- Acid-fast bacilli in skin lesions or nasal scrapings, or characteristic histologic nerve changes.

General Considerations

Leprosy is a chronic infectious disease caused by the acid-fast rod *Mycobacterium leprae*. The mode of transmission probably is respiratory and involves prolonged exposure in childhood. Only rarely have adults become infected. The disease is endemic in tropical and subtropical Asia, Africa, Central and South America and the Pacific regions, and the southern USA.

Clinical Findings

A. Symptoms and Signs: The onset is insidious. The lesions involve the cooler body tissues: skin, superficial nerves, nose, pharynx, larynx, eyes, and testicles. Skin lesions may occur as pale, anesthetic macular lesions 1–10 cm in diameter; discrete erythematous, infiltrated nodules 1–5 cm in diameter; or a diffuse skin infiltration. Neurologic disturbances are manifested by nerve infiltration and thickening, with resultant anesthesia, neuritis, and paresthesia. Trophic ulcers and bone resorption and shortening of digits ensue. In untreated cases, disfigurement due to the skin infiltration and nerve involvement may be extreme.

The disease is divided clinically and by laboratory tests into two distinct types: lepromatous and tuberculoid. The lepromatous type occurs in persons with defective cellular immunity. The course is progressive and malignant, with nodular skin lesions; slow, symmetric nerve involvement; abundant acid-fast bacilli in the skin lesions; and a negative lepromin skin test. In the tuberculoid type, cellular immunity is intact and the course is more benign and less progressive, with macular skin lesions, severe asymmetric nerve involvement of sudden onset with few bacilli present in the lesions, and a positive lepromin skin test. Intermediate ("borderline") cases are frequent. Eye involvement (keratitis and iridocyclitis), nasal ulcers, epistaxis, anemia, and lymphadenopathy may occur.

B. Laboratory Findings: Laboratory confirmation of leprosy requires the demonstration of acid-fast bacilli in scrapings from slit skin smears or the nasal septum. Biopsy of skin or of a thickened involved nerve also gives a typical histologic picture. *M leprae* does not grow in artificial media.

Differential Diagnosis

The skin lesions of leprosy often resemble those of lupus erythematosus, sarcoidosis, syphilis, erythema nodosum, erythema multiforme, cutaneous tuberculosis, and vitiligo.

Complications

Renal failure and hepatomegaly from secondary amyloidosis may occur with long-standing disease.

Treatment

Combination therapy is recommended for treatment of all types of leprosy. Single-drug treatment is accompanied by emergence of resistance, and primary resistance to dapsone also occurs. For borderline and lepromatous cases, a three-drug regimen such as dapsone, 50–100 mg/d, clofazimine, 50 mg/d, and rifampin, 10 mg/kg/d (up to 600 mg/d), all given orally, should be used. Ethionamide, 250–375 mg/d, may be substituted for clofazimine. For indeterminate and tuberculoid leprosy, the dapsone-rifampin combination is recommended for at least 6 months, followed by a course of dapsone alone.

Because of the tendency for relapse, treatment must be continued for years—up to 5 years for the tuberculoid type. The large number of organisms that are present and defective immunity in lepromatous leprosy may require lifelong therapy. Isolation of patients under treatment is not necessary.

Two reactional states—erythema nodosum leprosum and reversal reactions—may occur as a consequence of therapy. The reversal reaction, typical of borderline lepromatous leprosy, probably results from enhanced host immunity. Skin lesions and nerves become swollen and tender, but systemic manifestations are not seen. Erythema nodosum

leprosum, typical of lepromatous leprosy, is a consequence of immune injury from antigen-antibody complex deposition in skin and other tissues; in addition to skin and nerve manifestations, fever and systemic involvement may be seen. High-dose corticosteroids or thalidomide, 300 mg/d (in the nonpregnant patient only), is effective for erythema nodosum leprosum. Corticosteroids are also indicated for treatment of reversal reactions. Therapy for leprosy should not be discontinued during treatment of reactional states.

Freerksen E, Rosenfeld M, Spannuth G: New forms of multidrug therapy for the treatment of leprosy. Chemotherapy 1989;35:133. (Promising new three-drug regimens.)

INFECTIONS CAUSED BY CHLAMYDIA

Chlamydiae are a large group of obligate intracellular parasites closely related to gram-negative bacteria. They are assigned to three species—*Chlamydia trachomatis*, *Chlamydia psittaci*, and *Chlamydia pneumoniae*—on the basis of intracellular inclusions, sulfonamide susceptibility, antigenic composition, and disease production. *C psittaci* causes psittacosis in humans and many animal diseases. *Chlamydia pneumoniae*, TWAR strain, is a newly identified species that caused respiratory tract infections. *C trachomatis* causes many different human infections involving the eye (trachoma, inclusion conjunctivitis), the genital tract (lymphogranuloma venereum, nongonococcal urethritis, cervicitis, salpingitis), or the respiratory tract (pneumonitis). A few specific diseases are described.

Schachter J: Chlamydial infection. West J Med 1990; 153:523. (Comprehensive review.)

CHLAMYDIA TRACHOMATIS INFECTIONS

1. LYMPHOGRANULOMA VENEREUM

Essentials of Diagnosis

- Evanescent primary genital lesion.
- Lymph node enlargement, softening, and suppuration, with draining sinuses.
- Proctitis and rectal stricture in women or homosexual men.
- Positive complement fixation test.

General Considerations

Lymphogranuloma venereum is an acute and chronic sexually transmitted disease caused by *Chlamydia trachomatis* types L1–L3. After the genital lesion disappears, the infection spreads to lymph channels and lymph nodes of the genital and rectal areas. The disease is acquired during intercourse or through contact with contaminated exudate from active lesions. The incubation period is 5–21 days. Inapparent infections and latent disease are not uncommon.

Clinical Findings

A. Symptoms and Signs: In men, the initial vesicular or ulcerative lesion (on the external genitalia) is evanescent and often goes unnoticed. Inguinal buboes appear 1–4 weeks after exposure, are often bilateral, and have a tendency to fuse, soften, and break down to form multiple draining sinuses, with extensive scarring. In women, the genital lymph drainage is to the perirectal glands. Early anorectal manifestations are proctitis with tenesmus and bloody purulent discharge; late manifestations are chronic cicatrizing inflammation of the rectal and perirectal tissue. These changes lead to obstipation and rectal stricture and, occasionally, rectovaginal and perianal fistulas. They are also seen in homosexual men.

B. Laboratory Findings: The complement fixation test may be positive, but cross-reaction with other chlamydiae occurs. Although a positive reaction may reflect remote infection, high titers usually indicate active disease. Specific immunofluorescence tests for IgM are more specific for acute infection.

Differential Diagnosis

The early lesion of lymphogranuloma venereum must be differentiated from the lesions of syphilis, genital herpes, and chancroid; lymph node involvement must be distinguished from that due to tularemia, tuberculosis, plague, neoplasm, or pyogenic infection; rectal stricture must be distinguished from that due to neoplasm and ulcerative colitis.

Treatment

The antibiotics of choice are the tetracyclines (contraindicated in pregnancy), 0.25–0.5 g orally four times daily, or doxycycline, 0.1 g twice daily for 10–20 days. Erythromycin, 500 mg four times a day, or trimethoprim-sulfamethoxazole, 160/800 mg twice a day for 14 days, also is effective.

2. CHLAMYDIAL URETHRITIS & CERVICITIS

Chlamydia trachomatis immunotypes D–K can be isolated in about 50% of cases of nongonococcal urethritis by appropriate techniques. In other cases, *Ureaplasma urealyticum* can be grown as a possible etiologic agent. *C trachomatis* is an important cause of postgonococcal urethritis. Co-infection with gonococci and chlamydiae is common, and postgonococcal (ie, chlamydial) urethritis may persist after successful treatment of the gonococcal component. Occasionally, epididymitis, prostatitis, or proctitis is caused by chlamydial infection.

Females infected with *Chlamydia* may be asymptomatic or may have signs and symptoms of cervicitis, salpingitis, or pelvic inflammatory disease. *Chlamydia* is probably the leading cause of infertility in females in the United States.

Diagnosis often is clinical and by exclusion, ie, failure to identify gonococci in a patient with urethritis or cervicitis. The urethral or cervical discharge tends to be less painful, less purulent, and more watery in chlamydial versus gonococcal infection. Absence of gram-negative intracellular diplococci in urethral discharge from a male is very suggestive of chlamydial infection. Culture is reliable but sometimes unavailable. Rapid monoclonal immunofluorescent antibody detection methods are about 75% sensitive.

Therapy often must be given presumptively. Sexual partners of infected patients should also be treated. Effective treatment regimens are tetracycline or erythromycin, 500 mg four times a day, or doxycycline, 100 mg twice daily, for 7–10 days. Trimethoprim-sulfamethoxazole, 160/800 mg twice a day, is acceptable but may be less effective than tetracyclines or erythromycin. Erythromycin is the drug of choice in the pregnant patient. A single 1-g dose of azithromycin, a new macrolide antibiotic, is effective for uncomplicated urethritis and cervicitis. Were it not so expensive, azithromycin could replace erythromycin and other agents as the treatment of choice because of improved patient compliance and minimal toxicity of single-dose therapy.

Martin DH et al: A controlled trial of a single dose of azithromycin for the treatment of chlamydial urethritis and cervicitis. N Engl J Med 1992;327:921.

CHLAMYDIA PSITTACI & PSITTACOSIS (Ornithosis)

Essentials of Diagnosis

- Fever, chills, and cough; headache common.
- Atypical pneumonia with slightly delayed appearance of signs of pneumonitis.
- Contact with infected bird (psittacine, pigeons, many others) 7–15 days previously.
- Isolation of chlamydiae or rising titer of complement-fixing antibodies.

General Considerations

Psittacosis is acquired from contact with birds (parrots, parakeets, pigeons, chickens, ducks, and many others). The history may be difficult to obtain if the patient acquired infection from a parrot, which may have been imported illegally.

Clinical Findings

A. Symptoms and Signs: In psittacosis, the onset is usually rapid, with fever, chills, myalgia, dry cough, and headache. Signs include temperature-pulse dissociation, dullness to percussion, and rales. Pulmonary findings may be absent early. Dyspnea and cyanosis may occur later. Endocarditis, which is culture-negative, may occur.

B. Laboratory Findings: The organism is rarely isolated from cultures. The diagnosis is usually made serologically; antibodies appear during the second week and can be demonstrated by complement fixation or immunofluorescence. Antibody response may be suppressed by early chemotherapy.

C. Imaging: The radiographic findings in typical psittacosis are those of atypical pneumonia, which tends to be interstitial and diffuse in appearance, though consolidation can occur. Psittacosis is indistinguishable from other bacterial or viral pneumonias by radiography.

Differential Diagnosis

This disease can be differentiated from acute viral, mycoplasmal, or rickettsial pneumonias only by the history of contact with potentially infected birds and by laboratory tests. Rose spots and leukopenia suggest typhoid fever. Psittacosis is in the differential diagnosis of culture-negative endocarditis.

Treatment

Treatment consists of giving tetracycline, 0.5 g orally every 6 hours or 0.5 g intravenously every 12 hours, for 14–21 days. Erythromycin may be effective as well.

McPhee SJ, Erb B, Harrington W: Psittacosis. West J Med 1987;146:91. (Microbiology, epidemiology, and clinical review.)

CHLAMYDIA PNEUMONIAE, TWAR STRAIN

Chlamydia pneumoniae is a newly recognized species that was initially thought to be related to *C psittaci*. Studies have shown that it is morphologically, serologically, and genetically unique.

C pneumoniae is more difficult to isolate in culture than *C trachomatis* or *C psittaci*, and diagnosis often has been based on serology. Difficulty in culturing the organism has hampered efforts to define precisely the clinical disease caused by it. Nevertheless, TWAR strains clearly can cause upper and lower respiratory tract infections that can be severe. The clinical presentation of pneumonia is that of an atypical pneumonia, resembling that caused by *Mycoplasma pneumoniae*. Up to 10% of pneumonias may be associated with TWAR strains. *C pneumoniae* may also be an important cause of bronchitis and new-onset asthma in adults.

Like *C psittaci*, TWAR strains are resistant to sulfonamides. Erythromycin or tetracycline, 500 mg four times a day for 10–14 days, appears to be effective therapy.

Grayston JT: *Chlamydia pneumoniae*, strain TWAR. Chest 1989;95:664. (Microbiology, epidemiology, clinical review.)

Hahn DL, Dodge RW, Golubjatnikov R: Association of *Chlamydia pneumoniae* (strain TWAR) infection with wheezing, asthmatic bronchitis, and adult-onset asthma. JAMA 1991;266:225. (*C pneumoniae* may be an important cause not only of acute respiratory tract infection but of more chronic bronchospastic lung disease as well.)

Infectious Diseases: Spirochetal

33

Richard A. Jacobs, MD, PhD

SYPHILIS

NATURAL HISTORY & PRINCIPLES OF DIAGNOSIS & TREATMENT

Syphilis is a complex infectious disease caused by *Treponema pallidum,* a spirochete capable of infecting almost any organ or tissue in the body and causing protean clinical manifestations (Table 33–1). Transmission occurs most frequently during sexual contact, through minor skin or mucosal lesions; sites of inoculation are usually genital but may be extragenital. The risk of developing syphilis after unprotected sex with an individual with early syphilis is approximately 30–50%. The organism is extremely sensitive to heat and drying but can survive for days in fluids; therefore, it can be transmitted in blood from infected persons. Syphilis can be transferred via the placenta from mother to fetus after the tenth week of pregnancy (congenital syphilis).

The immunologic response to infection is complex, but it provides the basis for most clinical diagnoses. The infection induces the synthesis of a number of antibodies, some of which react specifically with pathogenic treponemes and some with components of normal tissues (see below). If the disease is untreated, sufficient defenses develop to produce a relative resistance to reinfection; however, in most cases these immune reactions fail to eradicate existing infection and may contribute to tissue destruction in the late stages. Patients treated early in the disease are fully susceptible to reinfection.

The natural history of acquired syphilis is generally divided into two major clinical stages: early (infectious) syphilis and late syphilis. The two stages are separated by a symptom-free latent phase during the first part of which (early latency) the infectious stage is liable to recur. Infectious syphilis includes the primary lesions (chancre and regional lymphadenopathy); the secondary lesions (commonly involving skin and mucous membranes, occasionally bone, central nervous system, or liver); relapsing lesions during early latency; and congenital lesions. The hall-

mark of these lesions is an abundance of spirochetes; tissue reaction is usually minimal. Late syphilis consists of so-called benign (gummatous) lesions involving skin, bones, and viscera; cardiovascular disease (principally aortitis); and a variety of central nervous system and ocular syndromes. These forms of syphilis are not contagious. The lesions contain few demonstrable spirochetes, but tissue reactivity (vasculitis, necrosis) is severe and suggestive of hypersensitivity phenomena.

As a result of intensive public health efforts during and after World War II, there was a reduction in the incidence of infectious syphilis. With the marked increase in all sexually transmitted diseases since the 1970s, there has been a rise in the number of reported cases of syphilis. In the early 1980s, the incidence of infectious syphilis increased, with a particularly high rate among homosexual men. In the mid 1980s, there was a slight decrease in the incidence of syphilis, chiefly as a result of changes in sexual practices in response to the AIDS epidemic. Between 1985 and 1990, there was again a dramatic increase in infectious syphilis, with 50,223 cases of primary and secondary syphilis reported in 1990. Although much of the increase occurred in the inner city black population, higher rates were reported also in rural areas. There are several reasons for these epidemiologic trends, including limited access to health care in some rural and large urban areas, with delayed diagnosis of syphilis, and the increased use of illicit drugs (especially "crack cocaine"), which promotes the exchange of sex for drugs or money to buy drugs. Furthermore, because drug users tend to have multiple sexual partners, traditional contact tracing and prevention have become more difficult. Although most of the increase in syphilis has been in adolescents and young adults, no age group is exempt, and an increased incidence has been noted in adults over the age of 60 as well. Concomitantly with the increase in acquired syphilis, there has also been an increase in congenital syphilis, particularly in urban areas. Despite the complex epidemiology, intensive syphilis control programs targeting high-risk populations—women of childbearing age, sexually active teens, drug users, persons with multiple sexual partners or those who have sex with prostitutes—and emphasiz-

Table 33–1. Stages of syphilis and common clinical manifestations.

Primary syphilis
Genital ulcer: painless ulcer with clean base and firm indurated borders
Regional lymphadenopathy
Secondary syphilis
Skin and mucous membranes
Rash: diffuse (including palms and soles), macular, papular, pustular, and combinations
Condylomata lata
Mucous patches: painless, silvery ulcerations of mucous membrane with surrounding erythema.
Generalized lymphadenopathy
Constitutional symptoms
Fever, usually low-grade
Malaise
Anorexia
Arthralgias and myalgias
Central nervous system
Asymptomatic
Symptomatic
Headache
Meningitis
Cranial neuropathies (II–VIII)
Ocular
Iritis
Iridocyclitis
Other
Renal: glomerulonephritis, nephrotic syndrome
Liver: hepatitis
Bone and joint: arthritis, periostitis
Late syphilis
Late benign (gummatous): granulomatous lesion usually involving skin, mucous membranes and bones, but any organ can be involved.
Cardiovascular
Aortic insufficiency
Coronary ostial stenosis
Aortic aneurysm
Neurosyphilis
Asymptomatic
Meningovascular
Seizures
Hemiparesis or hemiplegia
Tabes dorsalis
Impaired proprioception and vibratory sensation
Argyll Robertson pupil
Shooting pains
Ataxia
Romberg's sign
Urinary and fecal incontinence
Charcot joint
Cranial nerve involvement (II–VIII)
General paresis
Personality changes
Hyperactive reflexes
Argyll Robertson pupil
Decreased memory
Slurred speech
Optic atrophy

ing screening, early treatment, contact tracing, and condom use have been successful in limiting the spread of this disease.

Laboratory Diagnosis

Since the infectious agent of syphilis cannot be cultured in vitro, diagnostic measures must rely mainly on serologic testing, microscopic detection of *T pallidum* in lesions, and other examinations (biopsies, lumbar puncture, x-rays) for evidence of tissue damage.

A. Serologic Tests for Syphilis: (Table 33–2.) There are two general categories of serologic tests for syphilis: (1) nontreponemal tests, which use a component of normal tissue (eg, beef heart cardiolipin) as an antigen to measure nonspecific antibodies (reagin) formed in the blood of patients with syphilis; and (2) treponemal tests, which employ live or killed *T pallidum* as antigen to detect antibodies specific for pathogenic treponemes.

1. Nontreponemal antigen tests–Commonly employed nontreponemal antigen tests are of two types: flocculation (VDRL, RPR) and complement fixation (Kolmer, Wassermann). The flocculation tests are easy, rapid, and inexpensive to perform and are therefore used primarily for routine (often automated) screening for syphilis. Quantitative expression of the reactivity of the serum, based upon titration of dilutions of serum, may be valuable in establishing the diagnosis and in evaluating the efficacy of treatment.

The VDRL test (the nontreponemal test in widest use) generally becomes positive 4–6 weeks after infection, or 1–3 weeks after the appearance of a primary lesion; it is almost invariably positive in the secondary stage. The VDRL titer is usually high (> 1:32) in secondary syphilis and tends to be lower (< 1:4) or even negative in late forms of syphilis. These serologic tests are not highly specific and must be closely correlated with other clinical and laboratory findings. The tests are positive in patients with non-sexually transmitted treponematoses (see below). More importantly, "false-positive" serologic reactions are frequently encountered in a wide variety of nontreponemal states, including connective tissue diseases, infectious mononucleosis, malaria, febrile diseases, leprosy, intravenous drug use, infective endocarditis, old age, and pregnancy. False-positive tests also occur more commonly in HIV-seropositive patients (4%) than in HIV-seronegative patients (0.8%). False-positive reactions are usually of low titer and transient and may be distinguished from true positives by specific treponemal antibody tests. The rapid plasma reagin (RPR) test is a simple, rapid, and

Table 33–2. Percentage of patients with positive serologic tests for syphilis.[1]

Test	Stage		
	Primary	**Secondary**	**Tertiary**
VDRL[2]	70–75%	99%	75%
FTA-ABS[3]	85–95%	100%	98%

[1]Based on untreated cases.
[2]VDRL = Venereal Disease Research Laboratory test.
[3]FTA-ABS = Fluorescent treponemal antibody test.

reliable substitute for the traditional VDRL test. RPR titers are often higher than VDRL titers and thus are not comparable. The RPR test is suitable for automated screening.

Nontreponemal antibody titers are used to assess adequacy of therapy. The time required for the VDRL or RPR to become negative depends on the stage of the disease, the height of the initial titer, and whether the infection is an initial or repeat episode. In general, individuals with repeat infections, higher initial titers, and more advanced stages of disease at the time of treatment have a slower seroconversion rate and are more likely to remain serofast (ie, titers do not become negative). Older data on which recommendations for re-treatment are based and which employed more intensive treatment regimens than are presently used (see below) indicate that in primary and secondary syphilis, the VDRL usually decreases fourfold by 3 months and eightfold by 6 months. Furthermore, seronegativity was seen in 97% of those with primary syphilis and 76% of those with secondary syphilis at 2 years. More recent data based on currently recommended treatment regimens (see below) suggest that decreases in titer may be slower, ie, in primary and secondary syphilis it may take 6 months to see a fourfold decrease in titer and 12 months to see an eightfold drop. In patients with early latent syphilis, response is even slower, with a fourfold drop in titer taking 12–24 months. Seronegativity was seen in 72% of patients with primary syphilis and only 56% of those with secondary syphilis after 3 years. Whether these recent data more accurately reflect response of nontreponemal serologies to current treatment regimens needs confirmation.

2. Treponemal antibody tests–The fluorescent treponemal antibody absorption (FTA-ABS) test is the most widely employed treponemal test. It measures antibodies capable of reacting with killed *T pallidum* after absorption of the patient's serum with extracts of nonpathogenic treponemes. The FTA-ABS test is of value principally in determining whether a positive nontreponemal antigen test is "false-positive" or is indicative of syphilis. Because of its great sensitivity, particularly in the late stages of the disease, the FTA-ABS test is also of value when there is clinical evidence of syphilis but the nontreponemal serologic test for syphilis is negative. The test is positive in most patients with primary syphilis and in virtually all with secondary syphilis. Like nontreponemal antigen tests, the specific treponemal antibody test may revert to negative with adequate therapy. This is seen almost exclusively in initial infections in individuals with primary syphilis. In one study, 11% of individuals with a first episode of primary syphilis were seronegative by the FTA-ABS test at 1 year posttreatment, and 24% were negative by 3 years. Immunologic status may also affect antibody titers. Seven percent of asymptomatic HIV-infected patients became seronegative after treat-

ment, as opposed to 38% of symptomatic HIV-infected individuals. The long-held belief that a positive FTA-ABS persists indefinitely is clearly not valid, and this test therefore cannot be used as a reliable marker of previous infection. False-positive FTA-ABS tests occur rarely in systemic lupus erythematosus and in other disorders associated with abnormal globulins. It is noteworthy that Lyme disease may cause a false-positive FTA-ABS test but rarely causes a false-positive reaginic test. A treponemal passive hemagglutination (TPHA) test is comparable in specificity and sensitivity to the FTA-ABS test but may become positive somewhat later in infection.

Final decisions about the significance of the results of serologic tests for syphilis must be based upon a total clinical appraisal.

B. Microscopic Examination: In infectious syphilis, *T pallidum* may be shown by darkfield microscopic examination of fresh exudate from lesions or material aspirated from regional lymph nodes. The darkfield examination requires considerable experience and care in the proper collection of specimens and in the identification of pathogenic spirochetes by observing characteristic features of morphology and motility. Repeated examinations may be necessary. Spirochetes usually are not found in late syphilitic lesions by this technique.

An immunofluorescent staining technique for demonstrating *T pallidum* in dried smears of fluid taken from early syphilitic lesions is available. Slides are fixed and treated with fluorescein-labeled antitreponemal antibody that has been preabsorbed with nonpathogenic treponemes. The slides are then examined for fluorescing spirochetes in an ultraviolet microscope. Because of its simplicity and convenience to physicians (slides can be mailed), this technique has replaced darkfield microscopy in most health departments and medical center laboratories.

C. Spinal Fluid Examination: Cerebrospinal fluid findings in neurosyphilis are variable. In "classic" cases there is an elevation of total protein, lymphocytic pleocytosis, and a positive cerebrospinal fluid reagin test (VDRL). However, cerebrospinal fluid may be completely normal in neurosyphilis, and the VDRL may be negative. In one recent study, 25% of patients with primary or secondary syphilis in whom *T pallidum* was isolated from cerebrospinal fluid had a normal cerebrospinal fluid examination. In later stages of syphilis, normal cerebrospinal fluid analysis in the presence of infection can occur, but it is unusual. Because false-positive reagin tests rarely occur in the cerebrospinal fluid, a positive test confirms the presence of neurosyphilis. Because the cerebrospinal fluid VDRL may be negative in 30–70% of cases of neurosyphilis, *a negative test does not exclude neurosyphilis.*

Cerebrospinal fluid examination is highly recommended in all cases of secondary syphilis or latent syphilis not previously adequately treated. Asymptomatic neurosyphilis (ie, positive cerebrospinal fluid findings without symptoms) requires prolonged penicillin treatment as given for symptomatic neurosyphilis. Adequate treatment is indicated by gradual decrease in cerebrospinal fluid cell count, protein concentration, and VDRL titer. Rarely, serologic tests of cerebrospinal fluid may remain positive for years after adequate treatment of neurosyphilis even though all other parameters have returned to normal. The use of FTA-ABS in the diagnosis of neurosyphilis is controversial and is not recommended by the CDC. Some feel that it is more sensitive than the VDRL, but this is not accepted uniformly, and a high serum titer of FTA-ABS may result in a positive cerebrospinal fluid titer in the absence of neurosyphilis.

Treatment

A. Specific Measures:

1. Penicillin, as benzathine penicillin G or aqueous procaine penicillin G, is the drug of choice for all forms of syphilis and other spirochetal infections. Effective tissue levels must be maintained for several days or weeks because of the spirochete's long generation time (about 30 hours). Penicillin is highly effective in early infections and variably effective in the late stages. The principal contraindication is hypersensitivity to the penicillins. The recommended treatment schedules are included below in the discussion of the various forms of syphilis.

2. Other antibiotic therapy—Oral tetracyclines are effective in the treatment of syphilis for patients who are sensitive to penicillin. Tetracycline, 500 mg orally four times daily for 14 days, or doxycycline, 100 mg orally twice daily for 14 days, is given for infectious syphilis. In syphilis of more than 1 year's duration or of unknown duration, treatment is continued for 28 days in the same doses. Erythromycin is less effective than penicillin, tetracycline, or doxycycline and should be avoided if possible. When it is given, the dose is 500 mg orally four times daily for 14 days (infectious syphilis) or 28 days (syphilis of > 1 year's duration or unknown duration). Close follow-up is required for all patients treated with erythromycin. Experience with these drugs in the treatment of syphilis is limited, and some failures have been reported.

Ceftriaxone is still an unproved drug for syphilis. A single dose of 125 mg (as used to treat gonorrhea) may cure incubating syphilis, but it is not currently recommended and should not be relied upon. A multiple-dose regimen of ceftriaxone (250 mg daily for 10 days or 500 mg every other day for five doses) may be effective for treating primary or secondary syphilis, but data are limited. Multiple doses of ceftriaxone are more costly than a single dose of benzathine penicillin and more inconvenient for the patient.

B. Local Measures (Mucocutaneous Le-sions): Local treatment is usually not necessary. No local antiseptics or other chemicals should be applied to a suspected syphilitic lesion until specimens for microscopy have been obtained.

C. Public Health Measures: Patients with infectious syphilis must abstain from sexual activity until rendered noninfectious by antibiotic therapy. All cases of syphilis must be reported to the appropriate public health agency for assistance in identifying, and treating contacts.

D. Epidemiologic Treatment: Patients who have been exposed to infectious syphilis within the preceding 3 months may be infected but seronegative and thus should be treated as for early syphilis. Others at high risk for infection—ie, those with other sexually transmitted diseases and those infected with HIV—should undergo serologic tests for syphilis. The present recommended therapy for gonorrhea (ceftriaxone and doxycycline) is probably effective against incubating syphilis. If alternative regimens are used to treat gonorrhea, follow-up serologic studies should be performed in 3 months.

Complications of Specific Therapy

The Jarisch-Herxheimer reaction is ascribed to the sudden massive destruction of spirochetes by drugs and release of toxic products and is manifested by fever and aggravation of the existing clinical picture. It is most likely to occur in early syphilis. Treatment should not be discontinued unless the symptoms become severe or threaten to be fatal or unless syphilitic laryngitis, auditory neuritis, or labyrinthitis is present, where the reaction may cause irreversible damage.

The reaction may be prevented or modified by simultaneous administration of antipyretics or corticosteroids. It usually begins within the first 24 hours and subsides spontaneously within the next 24 hours of penicillin treatment.

Follow-Up Care

Because treatment failures can occur and reinfection is always a possibility, patients treated for syphilis should be followed clinically and serologically. If nontreponemal antibody tests have not decreased fourfold by 3 months in primary and secondary syphilis or by 6 months in latent syphilis of less than one-year's duration, patients should have a cerebrospinal fluid examination and another course of treatment. In latent disease of more than 1 year's duration, nontreponemal tests should be repeated at 6 months and 12 months. If titers increase fourfold or if an initially high titer ($\geq$ 1:32) fails to decrease, the patient should be evaluated for neurosyphilis and should be retreated.

Prevention

Avoidance of sexual contact is the only completely

reliable method of prophylaxis but is an impractical public health measure for obvious reasons.

A. Mechanical: The standard latex condom is effective but protects covered parts only. The exposed parts should be washed with soap and water as soon after contact as possible. This applies to both sexes.

B. Antibiotic: If there is known exposure to infectious syphilis, abortive penicillin therapy may be used. Give 2.4 million units of procaine penicillin G intramuscularly. Treatment of gonococcal infection with penicillins, tetracyclines, and ceftriaxone is probably effective against incubating syphilis in most cases. However, other antimicrobial agents (eg, spectinomycin) may be ineffective in aborting preclinical syphilis. In view of the increasing use of antibiotics other than penicillin for gonococcal disease, patients treated for gonorrhea should have a serologic test for syphilis 3–6 months after treatment.

Course & Prognosis (See Table 33–3.)

The lesions associated with primary and secondary syphilis are self-limiting and resolve with few or no residua. Late syphilis may be highly destructive and permanently disabling and may lead to death. In broad terms, if no treatment is given, about one-third of people infected with syphilis will undergo spontaneous cure, about one-third will remain in the latent phase throughout life, and about one-third will develop serious late lesions.

Hook EW III, Marra CM: Acquired syphilis in adults. (Medical Progress.) N Engl J Med 1992;326:1060. (Epidemiology, diagnosis, clinical manifestations, and therapy.)

Hutchinson CM, Hook EW III: Syphilis in adults. Med Clin North Am 1990;74:1389.

Lukehart SA et al: Invasion of the central nervous system by *Treponema pallidum:* Implications for diagnosis and treatment. Ann Intern Med 1988;109:855. (Cerebrospi-

nal fluid abnormalities and isolation of *T pallidum* in untreated syphilis.)

Romanowski B et al: Serologic response to treatment of infectious syphilis. Ann Intern Med 1991;114:1005.

Sexually transmitted diseases: Treatment guidelines 1989. MMWR Morb Mortal Wkly Rep 1989;38(Suppl 8):1.

CLINICAL STAGES OF SYPHILIS

1. PRIMARY SYPHILIS

Essentials of Diagnosis

- History of sexual contact (often unreliable).
- Painless ulcer on genitalia, perianal area, rectum, pharynx, tongue, lip, or elsewhere 2–6 weeks after exposure.
- Nontender enlargement of regional lymph nodes.
- Fluid expressed from lesion contains *T pallidum* by immunofluorescence or darkfield microscopy.
- Serologic test for syphilis often positive.

General Considerations

This is the stage of invasion and may pass unrecognized. The typical lesion is the chancre at the site or sites of inoculation, most frequently located on the penis, labia, cervix, or anorectal region. Anorectal lesions are especially common among male homosexuals. The primary lesion occurs occasionally in the oropharynx (lip, tongue, or tonsil) and rarely on the breast or finger. The chancre starts as a small erosion 10–90 days (average, 3–4 weeks) after inoculation that rapidly develops into a painless superficial ulcer with a clean base and firm, indurated margins, associated with enlargement of regional lymph nodes, which are rubbery, discrete, and nontender. Bacterial infection of the chancre may occur and may lead to pain. Healing occurs without treatment, but a scar may form, especially with secondary bacterial infection.

Table 33–3. Natural course of untreated syphilis.

Stage of Disease	Likelihood of Developing Clinical Manifestations (%)	Comment
Latent	24%	90% of relapses occur in first year after infection.
Late		
Benign (gummatous)	15%	Many patients have more than one late manifestation. Skin, bone, and mucosa most frequently involved.
Cardiovascular	10%	Only seen in those who develop syphilis after 15 years of age. Pathologic findings more common, ie, 50–80%.
Neurosyphilis	6.5%	Asymptomatic neurosyphilis has been reported in 8–40%.

Laboratory Findings

The serologic test for syphilis is usually positive 1–2 weeks after the primary lesion is noted; rising titers are especially significant when there is a history of previous infection. Immunofluorescence or dark–field microscopy shows treponemes in at least 95% of chancres. Cerebrospinal fluid pleocytosis has been reported in 10–20% of patients with primary syphilis.

Differential Diagnosis

The syphilitic chancre may be confused with chancroid, lymphogranuloma venereum, genital herpes, or neoplasm. Any lesion on the genitalia should be considered a possible primary syphilitic lesion.

Treatment

Benzathine penicillin G, 2.4 million units intramuscularly in the gluteal area, is given once. For the penicillin-allergic patient (who is not pregnant), doxycycline, 100 mg orally twice daily for 2 weeks, or tetracycline, 500 mg orally four times a day for 2 weeks, can be used. If tetracyclines cannot be given, erythromycin, 500 mg orally four times a day for 2 weeks, can be substituted.

2. SECONDARY SYPHILIS

Essentials of Diagnosis

- Generalized maculopapular skin rash.
- Mucous membrane lesions, including patches and ulcers.
- Weeping papules (condylomas) in moist skin areas.
- Generalized nontender lymphadenopathy.
- Fever.
- Meningitis, hepatitis, osteitis, arthritis, iritis.
- Many treponemes in scrapings of mucous membrane or skin lesions by immunofluorescence or darkfield microscopy.
- Serologic tests for syphilis always positive.

General Considerations & Treatment

The secondary stage of syphilis usually appears a few weeks (or up to 6 months) after development of the chancre, when sufficient dissemination of *T pallidum* has occurred to produce systemic signs (fever, lymphadenopathy) or infectious lesions at sites distant from the site of inoculation. The most common manifestations are skin and mucosal lesions. The skin lesions are nonpruritic, macular, papular, pustular, or follicular (or combinations of any of these types), though the maculopapular rash is the most common. The skin lesions usually are generalized; involvement of the palms and soles is especially suspicious. Annular lesions simulating ringworm are observed in blacks. Mucous membrane lesions range from ulcers and papules of the lips, mouth, throat, genitalia, and anus ("mucous patches") to a diffuse redness of the pharynx. Both skin and mucous membrane lesions are highly infectious at this stage. Specific lesions—**condylomata lata**—are fused, weeping papules on the moist areas of the skin and mucous membranes.

Meningeal (aseptic meningitis or acute basilar meningitis), hepatic, renal, bone, and joint invasion, with resulting cranial nerve palsies, jaundice, nephrotic syndrome, and periostitis may occur. Alopecia (moth-eaten appearance), iritis, and iridocyclitis may also occur. A transient myocarditis may be manifested by temporary electrocardiographic changes.

All serologic tests for syphilis are positive in almost all cases. The cutaneous and mucous membrane lesions often show *T pallidum* on microscopic examination. A transient cerebrospinal fluid pleocytosis is seen in 30–70% of patients with secondary syphilis, though only 5% have positive serologic cerebrospinal fluid reactions. There may be evidence of hepatitis or nephritis (immune complex type). Circulating immune complexes exist in the blood and are deposited in blood vessel walls.

Skin lesions may be confused with the infectious exanthems, pityriasis rosea, and drug eruptions. Visceral lesions may suggest nephritis or hepatitis due to other causes. The diffusely red throat may mimic other forms of pharyngitis.

Treatment is as for primary syphilis unless central nervous system disease is present, in which case treatment is as for neurosyphilis (see below). Isolation of the patient is important.

3. RELAPSING SYPHILIS (Early Latent Syphilis)

The essentials of diagnosis are the same as in secondary syphilis.

The lesions of secondary syphilis heal spontaneously, but secondary syphilis may relapse if undiagnosed or inadequately treated. These relapses may include any of the findings noted under secondary syphilis: skin and mucous membrane, neurologic, ocular, bone, or visceral. Unlike the usual asymptomatic neurologic involvement of secondary syphilis, neurologic relapses may be fulminating, leading to death. Relapse is almost always accompanied by a rising titer in quantitative serologic tests; indeed, a rising titer may be the first or only evidence of relapse. About 90% of relapses occur during the first year after infection.

Treatment is as for primary syphilis unless central nervous system disease is present.

4. LATE LATENT ("HIDDEN") SYPHILIS

Essentials of Diagnosis
- No physical signs.
- History of syphilis with inadequate treatment.
- Positive serologic tests for syphilis.

General Considerations & Treatment

Latent syphilis is the clinically quiescent phase during the interval after disappearance of secondary lesions and before the appearance of tertiary symptoms. Early latency is defined as the first year after infection, during which time most infectious lesions recur ("relapsing syphilis"); after the first year, the patient is said to be in the late latent phase. Transmission to the fetus, however, can probably occur in any phase. There are (by definition) no clinical manifestations during the latent phase, and the only significant laboratory findings are positive serologic tests. A diagnosis of latent syphilis is justified only when the cerebrospinal fluid is entirely negative, x-ray and physical examination shows no evidence of cardiovascular involvement, and false-positive tests for syphilis have been ruled out. The latent phase may last from months to a lifetime.

It is important to differentiate latent syphilis from a false-positive serologic test for syphilis, which can be due to the many causes listed above.

Treatment is with benzathine penicillin G, 2.4 million units three times at 7-day intervals (total dose, 7.2 million units). In the penicillin-allergic patient, give tetracycline, 0.5 g orally four times a day for 28 days, or doxycycline, 100 mg orally twice daily for 28 days. If there is evidence of cerebrospinal fluid involvement, treat as for neurosyphilis. Only a small percentage of serologic tests will be appreciably altered by treatment with penicillin. The treatment of this stage of the disease is intended to prevent the late sequelae.

5. LATE (TERTIARY) SYPHILIS

Essentials of Diagnosis
- Infiltrative tumors of skin, bones, liver (gummas).
- Aortitis, aneurysms, aortic regurgitation.
- Central nervous system disorders, including meningovascular and degenerative changes, paresthesias, shooting pains, abnormal reflexes, dementia, or psychosis.

General Considerations

This stage may occur at any time after secondary syphilis, even after years of latency, and is seen in about one-third of untreated patients (Table 33–3). Late lesions probably represent, at least in part, a delayed hypersensitivity reaction of the tissue to the organism and are usually divided into two types: (1) a localized gummatous reaction, with a relatively rapid onset and generally prompt response to therapy ("benign late syphilis"); and (2) diffuse inflammation of a more insidious onset that characteristically involves the central nervous system and large arteries, is often fatal if untreated, and is at best arrested by treatment. Gummas may involve any area or organ of the body but most often the skin or long bones. Cardiovascular disease is usually manifested by aortic aneurysm, aortic regurgitation, or aortitis. Various forms of diffuse or localized central nervous system involvement may occur.

Late syphilis must be differentiated from neoplasms of the skin, liver, lung, stomach, or brain; other forms of meningitis; and primary neurologic lesions.

Although almost any tissue and organ may be involved in late syphilis, the following are the most common types of involvement.

Skin

Cutaneous lesions of late syphilis are of two varieties: (1) multiple nodular lesions that eventually ulcerate or resolve by forming atrophic, pigmented scars; and (2) solitary gummas that start as painless subcutaneous nodules, then enlarge, attach to the overlying skin, and eventually ulcerate.

Mucous Membranes

Late lesions of the mucous membranes are nodular gummas or leukoplakia, highly destructive to the involved tissue.

Skeletal

Bone lesions are destructive, causing periostitis, osteitis, and arthritis with little or no associated redness or swelling but often marked myalgia and myositis of the neighboring muscles. The pain is especially severe at night.

Eyes

Late ocular lesions are gummatous iritis, chorioretinitis, optic atrophy, and cranial nerve palsies, in addition to the lesions of central nervous system syphilis.

Respiratory System

Respiratory involvement by late syphilis is caused by gummatous infiltrates into the larynx, trachea, and pulmonary parenchyma, producing discrete pulmonary densities. There may be hoarseness, respiratory distress, and wheezing secondary to the gummatous lesion itself or to subsequent stenosis occurring with healing.

Gastrointestinal System

Gummas involving the liver produce the usually benign, asymptomatic hepar lobatum. Occasionally a picture resembling Laennec's cirrhosis is produced by liver involvement. Infiltration into the stomach wall causes "leather bottle" stomach with epigastric distress, inability to eat large meals, regurgitation, belching, and weight loss.

Cardiovascular System

Cardiovascular lesions (10–15% of late syphilitic lesions) are often progressive, disabling, and life-threatening. Central nervous system lesions are often present also. Involvement usually starts as an arteritis in the supracardiac portion of the aorta and progresses to cause one or more of the following: (1) Narrowing of the coronary ostia with resulting decreased coronary circulation, angina, cardiac insufficiency, and acute myocardial infarction. (2) Scarring of the aortic valves, producing aortic regurgitation with its water-hammer pulse, aortic diastolic murmur, frequent aortic systolic murmur, cardiac hypertrophy, and eventually congestive heart failure. (3) Weakness of the wall of the aorta, with saccular aneurysm formation and associated pressure symptoms of dysphagia, hoarseness, brassy cough, back pain (vertebral erosion), and occasionally rupture of the aneurysm. Recurrent respiratory infections are common as a result of pressure on the trachea and bronchi.

Treatment of tertiary syphilis (excluding neurosyphilis; see below) is as for latent syphilis. Reversal of positive serologic tests does not usually occur. A second course of penicillin therapy may be given if necessary. There is no known method for reliable eradication of the treponeme from humans in the late stages of syphilis. Viable spirochetes are occasionally found in the eyes, in cerebrospinal fluid, and elsewhere in patients with "adequately" treated syphilis, but claims for their capacity to cause progressive disease are speculative.

Neurosyphilis

Neurosyphilis (15–20% of late syphilitic lesions; often present with cardiovascular syphilis) is also a progressive, disabling, and life-threatening complication. It develops more commonly in men than in women and in whites than in blacks. There are four clinical types.

(1) Asymptomatic neurosyphilis: This form is characterized by spinal fluid abnormalities (positive spinal fluid serology, increased cell count, occasionally increased protein) without symptoms or signs of neurologic involvement.

(2) Meningovascular syphilis: This form is characterized by meningeal involvement or changes in the vascular structures of the brain (or both), producing symptoms of low-grade meningitis (headache, irritability); cranial nerve palsies (basilar meningitis); unequal reflexes; irregular pupils with poor light and accommodation reflexes; and, when large vessels are involved, cerebrovascular accidents. The cerebrospinal fluid shows increased cells (100–

1000/µL), elevated protein, and usually a positive serologic test for syphilis. The symptoms of acute meningitis are rare in late syphilis.

(3) Tabes dorsalis: This form is a chronic progressive degeneration of the parenchyma of the posterior columns of the spinal cord and of the posterior sensory ganglia and nerve roots. The symptoms and signs are impairment of proprioception and vibration sense, Argyll Robertson pupils (which react poorly to light but well to accommodation), and muscular hypotonia and hyporeflexia. Impairment of proprioception results in a wide-based gait and inability to walk in the dark. Paresthesias, analgesia, or sharp recurrent pains in the muscles of the leg ("shooting" or "lightning" pains) may occur. Crises are also common in tabes: gastric crises, consisting of sharp abdominal pains with nausea and vomiting (simulating an acute abdomen); laryngeal crises, with paroxysmal cough and dyspnea; urethral crises, with painful bladder spasms; and rectal and anal crises. Crises may begin suddenly, last for hours to days, and cease abruptly. Neurogenic bladder with overflow incontinence is also seen. Painless trophic ulcers may develop over pressure points on the feet. Joint damage may occur as a result of lack of sensory innervation (Charcot joint). The cerebrospinal fluid may have a normal or increased cell count (3–200/µL), elevated protein, and variable results of serologic tests.

(4) General paresis: This is generalized involvement of the cerebral cortex with insidious onset of symptoms. There is usually a decrease in concentrating power, memory loss, dysarthria, tremor of the fingers and lips, irritability, and mild headaches. Most striking is the change of personality; the patient becomes slovenly, irresponsible, confused, and psychotic. Combinations of the various forms of neurosyphilis (especially tabes and paresis) are not uncommon. The cerebrospinal fluid findings resemble those of tabes dorsalis.

Special considerations in treatment of neurosyphilis. It is most important to prevent neurosyphilis by prompt diagnosis, adequate treatment, and follow-up of early syphilis. Indications for lumbar puncture vary depending upon stage of the disease. In early syphilis (primary and secondary syphilis and early latent syphilis of less than 1 year's duration), cerebrospinal fluid abnormalities occur commonly, but neurosyphilis rarely develops in patients who have received the standard therapy outlined above. Thus, unless clinical signs and symptoms of neurosyphilis are present, a lumbar puncture in early syphilis is not recommended as part of the routine evaluation. In theory, all patients with syphilis of more than 1 year's duration should have a lumbar puncture. This is rarely strictly adhered to, and each case is usually individualized. Cerebrospinal fluid evaluation is strongly suggested in the later stages of syphilis if neurologic signs and symptoms are present; therapy other than with penicillin is to be given; if the patient is HIV-positive (see next section); if serum nontreponemal antibody titers are 1:32 or higher; or if there is evidence of active syphilis at other sites (aortitis, iritis, optic atrophy, etc). In the presence of definite cerebrospinal fluid or neurologic abnormalities, treat for neurosyphilis. The pretreatment clinical and laboratory evaluation should include neurologic, ocular, psychiatric, and cerebrospinal fluid examinations.

The regimen of 2.4 million units of benzathine penicillin intramuscularly weekly for three consecutive weeks results in low to undetectable cerebrospinal fluid levels of penicillin, and treatment failures have been described when this regimen has been used to treat neurosyphilis. For these reasons, present recommendations for the therapy of neurosyphilis employ higher doses of short-acting penicillin in order to achieve better penetration and higher levels of drug in the cerebrospinal fluid. Recommended regimens include 2–4 million units of aqueous crystalline penicillin G intravenously every 4 hours for 10–14 days. Alternatively, 2–4 million units of procaine penicillin can be given intramuscularly once daily along with 500 mg of probenecid orally four times daily, both for 10–14 days. Many experts recommend subsequent administration of 2.4 million units of benzathine penicillin intramuscularly once weekly for 3 weeks as additional therapy. Alternative therapy to penicillin has not been established for treatment of neurosyphilis, and patients with a history of penicillin allergy should be skin-tested and desensitized.

All patients should have spinal fluid examinations at 6-month intervals until the cell count is normal. Response may be gauged by clinical improvement and effective and persistent reversal of cerebrospinal fluid changes. A second course of penicillin therapy may be given if the cell count has not decreased at 6 months or is not normal at 2 years. Not infrequently, there is progression of neurologic symptoms and signs despite high and prolonged doses of penicillin. It has been postulated that these treatment failures are related to the unexplained persistence of viable *T pallidum* in central nervous system or ocular lesions in at least some cases.

6. SYPHILIS IN HIV-INFECTED PATIENTS

Because syphilis has variable clinical manifestations and an unpredictable course, evaluation of case reports of unusual clinical or laboratory manifestations of syphilis in HIV-infected patients is difficult. Nonetheless, recent reports have suggested that in this situation syphilis may have an accelerated course, serologic response to infection may be blunted or delayed, and treatment failures with benzathine penicillin may occur more commonly. Because of concern about false-negative serologic

tests or a delayed immunologic response, if the diagnosis of syphilis is suggested on clinical grounds but reagin tests are negative, alternative tests should be performed. These tests include darkfield examination of lesions and direct fluorescent antibody staining for *T pallidum* of lesion exudate or biopsy specimens. Treatment failures with presently recommended regimens of benzathine penicillin have been documented in HIV-infected patients. In one study, three of four patients treated with 2.4 million units of benzathine penicillin for secondary syphilis failed therapy, and all three were HIV-positive. In a review of 40 patients with neurosyphilis in HIV-infected patients, 16 had been previously treated with benzathine penicillin, usually a single dose of 2.4 million units. Because the number of patients who have failed standard treatment is small, no change in the therapy of early syphilis in patients coinfected with HIV is officially recommended. Instead, the emphasis has been placed on careful follow-up (see below). However, some feel that a more aggressive treatment regimen is indicated in this setting. The best treatment regimen—either three doses of 2.4 million units of benzathine penicillin at weekly intervals or 2.4 million units of procaine penicillin intramuscularly for 10 consecutive days, plus probenecid, 500 mg four times daily—is yet to be determined.

The diagnosis of neurosyphilis in HIV-infected patients is complicated by the fact that cerebrospinal fluid abnormalities are frequently seen and may be due to neurosyphilis or HIV infection itself. The exact prevalence of neurosyphilis in HIV-infected patients with positive serum nontreponemal tests is not precisely known. Retrospective studies have suggested that as many as 10–50% of asymptomatic patients with positive serum tests who have consented to lumbar puncture have neurosyphilis defined by a positive cerebrospinal fluid VDRL test. Because of the high potential for neurosyphilis and because neurosyphilis requires more aggressive therapy (either aqueous penicillin intravenously or procaine penicillin intramuscularly for 10 days, as described above), all HIV-infected patients who have syphilis should be strongly encouraged to have a lumbar puncture.

The role of ceftriaxone therapy in therapy of neurosyphilis is under investigation, but the drug cannot currently be recommended for this purpose.

Whether HIV-infected patients with syphilis have a different serologic response to penicillin therapy than noninfected individuals is unsettled. Nontreponemal titers tend to be higher in HIV-infected persons, and some studies have suggested a slower decline in these titers following treatment whereas others have not. Similarly, some studies have found that specific treponemal antibody tests (eg, FTA-ABS) are lost more frequently in HIV-infected patients, while others have found no difference in serologic response to therapy between HIV-positive and HIV-negative individuals. Despite the difficulties in interpretation of serologic test results, current recommendations are that in patients infected with HIV, nontreponemal quantitative tests should be repeated at 1, 2, and 3 months and thereafter at 3-month intervals until titers have stabilized. If titers have not fallen twofold by 3 months in primary syphilis or 6 months in secondary syphilis or if there is a fourfold or greater increase in titer, the patient should have a spinal fluid examination and be re-treated. In patients with neurosyphilis, cerebrospinal fluid examination is recommended at least every 6 months until serologic parameters have stabilized as described above.

Gourevitch MN et al: Effects of HIV infection on the serologic manifestations and responses to treatment of syphilis in intravenous drug users. Ann Intern Med 1993;118:350. (HIV infection did not affect clinical manifestations, clinical course, or response to treatment.)

Hook EW III, Marra CM: Acquired syphilis in adults. (Medical Progress.) N Engl J Med 1992;326:1060. (Includes a section on HIV-infected patients with syphilis.)

Musher DM: Syphilis, neurosyphilis, penicillin and AIDS. J Infect Dis 1991;163:1201. (How HIV infection has altered the clinical course of syphilis, with implications for diagnosis and therapy.)

Musher DM, Hamill RJ, Baughn RE: Effect of human immunodeficiency virus (HIV) infection on the course of syphilis and on the response to treatment. Ann Intern Med 1990;113:872. (Impact of HIV on manifestations of syphilis and implications for more aggressive therapy.)

Recommendations for diagnosing and treating syphilis in HIV-infected patients. MMWR 1988;37:600. (Official CDC recommendations.)

7. SYPHILIS IN PREGNANCY

All pregnant women should have a nontreponemal serologic test for syphilis at the time of the first prenatal visit. Seroreactive patients should be evaluated promptly. Such evaluation includes the history (including prior therapy), a physical examination, a quantitative nontreponemal test, and a confirmatory treponemal test. If the FTA-ABS test is nonreactive and there is no clinical evidence of syphilis, treatment may be withheld. Both the quantitative nontreponemal test and the FTA-ABS test should be repeated in 4 weeks. If the diagnosis of syphilis cannot be excluded with reasonable certainty, the patient should be treated as outlined below.

Patients for whom there is documentation of adequate treatment for syphilis in the past need not be re-treated unless there is clinical or serologic evidence of reinfection (eg, fourfold rise in titer of a quantitative nontreponemal test).

In women suspected of being at increased risk for syphilis, a second nontreponemal test should be performed during the third trimester.

The preferred treatment is with penicillin in dosage schedules appropriate for the stage of syphilis (see above). Penicillin prevents congenital syphilis in 90% of cases, even when treatment is given late in pregnancy. Tetracycline and doxycycline are contraindicated in pregnancy, and erythromycin is associated with a high risk of failure in the fetus. Women with a history of penicillin allergy should be skin-tested and desensitized if necessary.

The infant should be evaluated immediately, as noted below, and at 6–8 weeks of age.

McKown RR, Kapernick PS: Syphilis in pregnancy. South Med J 1988;81:447. (Follow-up of 356 pregnant patients who were serologically positive for syphilis.)

Sexually transmitted diseases: Treatment guidelines. MMWR Morb Mortal Wkly Rep 1989;38(Suppl 8):1. (Treatment of sexually transmitted diseases, including syphilis.)

8. CONGENITAL SYPHILIS

Congenital syphilis is a transplacentally transmitted infection that occurs in infants of untreated or inadequately treated mothers. The physical findings at birth are quite variable: The infant may have many or only minimal signs or even no signs until 6–8 weeks of life (delayed form). The most common findings are on the skin and mucous membranes—serous nasal discharge (snuffles), mucous membrane patches, maculopapular rash, condylomas. These lesions are infectious; T pallidum can easily be found microscopically, and the infant must be isolated. Other common findings are hepatosplenomegaly, anemia, or osteochondritis. These early active lesions subsequently heal, and if the disease is left untreated it produces the characteristic stigmas of syphilis—interstitial keratitis, Hutchinson's teeth, saddle nose, saber shins, deafness, and central nervous system involvement.

The presence of negative serologic tests at birth in both the mother and the infant usually means that the newborn is free of infection. However, recent infection near the time of delivery may result in negative tests because there has been insufficient time to develop a serologic response. Thus, one must maintain a high index of suspicion in infants who present with delayed onset of symptoms despite negative serologic tests at birth. The serologic evaluation for syphilis in newborn infants is complicated by the transplacental acquisition of maternal antibody (IgG). Evaluation of a newborn suspected of having congenital syphilis includes the history of maternal therapy, a careful physical examination, hematocrit (for possible anemia), a cerebrospinal fluid examination, and x-rays of long bones. It is particularly important to follow the infant every 2–3 weeks over a period of 4 months to watch for developing physical signs; a sustained rise or fall in VDRL titer during this time will reveal the need for treatment. If available, an FTA-ABS test on the purified 19S-IgM fraction of serum should be obtained. If positive, it is confirmatory of congenital syphilis.

Infants should be treated at birth if maternal treatment was inadequate, unknown, or done with drugs other than penicillin or if adequate follow-up of the infant cannot be ensured.

Therapy for congenital syphilis is 100,000–150,000 units/kg of aqueous crystalline penicillin G daily given in two or three divided doses intravenously, or 50,000 units/kg of procaine penicillin daily given as a single intramuscular injection for 10–14 days.

The quantitative nontreponemal test (VDRL) should be repeated 3, 6, and 12 months after therapy to establish falling titers. If titers fail to fall or increase at 6 months, the child should be re-treated.

Berry MC, Dajani AS: Resurgence of congenital syphilis. Infect Dis Clin North Am 1992;6:19. (Epidemiology, clinical manifestations, and therapy.)

Dorfman DH, Glasen JH: Congenital syphilis presenting in infants after the newborn period. N Engl J Med 1990;323:1299. (Congenital syphilis in infants of mothers with negative serologies.)

Lewis LL: Congenital syphilis: Serologic diagnosis in the young infant. Infect Dis Clin North Am 1992;6:31.

NON-SEXUALLY TRANSMITTED TREPONEMATOSES

A variety of treponemal diseases other than syphilis occur endemically in many tropical areas of the world. They are distinguished from disease caused by *T pallidum* by their nonsexual transmission, their relatively high incidence in certain geographic areas and among children, and their tendency to produce less severe visceral manifestations. As in syphilis, organisms can be demonstrated in infectious lesions with darkfield microscopy or immunofluorescence but cannot be cultured in artificial media; the serologic tests for syphilis are positive; the diseases have primary, secondary, and sometimes tertiary stages; and penicillin is the drug of choice. There is evidence that infection with these agents may provide partial resistance to syphilis and vice versa. Treatment with penicillin in doses appropriate to primary syphilis (eg, 2.4 million units of benzathine penicillin G intramuscularly) is generally curative in any stage of the non-sexually transmitted treponematoses. In cases of penicillin hypersensitivity, tetracycline is usually the recommended alternative.

YAWS
(Frambesia)

Yaws is a contagious disease largely limited to tropical regions that is caused by *Treponema pertenue*. It is characterized by granulomatous lesions of the skin, mucous membranes, and bone. Yaws is rarely fatal, though if untreated it may lead to chronic disability and disfigurement. Yaws is acquired by direct nonsexual contact, usually in childhood, although it may occur at any age. The "mother yaw," a painless papule that later ulcerates, appears 3–4 weeks after exposure. There is usually associated regional lymphadenopathy. Six to 12 weeks later, similar secondary lesions appear and last for several months or years. Painful ulcerated lesions on the soles are frequent and are called "crab yaws." Late gummatous lesions may occur, with associated tissue destruction involving large areas of skin and subcutaneous tissues. The late effects of yaws, with bone change, shortening of digits, and contractions, may be confused with similar changes occurring in leprosy. Central nervous system, cardiac, or other visceral involvement is rare.

PINTA

Pinta is a non-sexually transmitted spirochetal infection caused by *Treponema carateum*. It occurs endemically in rural areas of Latin America, especially in Mexico, Colombia, and Cuba, and in some areas of the Pacific. A nonulcerative, erythematous primary papule spreads slowly into a papulosquamous plaque showing a variety of color changes (slate, lilac, black). Secondary lesions resemble the primary one and appear within a year after it. These appear successively, new lesions together with older ones; are commonest on the extremities; and later show atrophy and depigmentation. Some cases show pigmentary changes and atrophic patches on the soles and palms, with or without hyperkeratosis, that are indistinguishable from "crab yaws." Very rarely, central nervous system or cardiovascular disease is observed late in the course of infection.

ENDEMIC SYPHILIS

Endemic syphilis is an acute or chronic infection caused by an organism indistinguishable from *T pallidum*. It has been reported in a number of countries, particularly in the eastern Mediterranean area, often with local names: bejel in Syria, Saudi Arabia, and Iraq; and dichuchwa, njovera, and siti in Africa. It also occurs in Southeast Asia. The local forms have distinctive features. Moist ulcerated lesions cf the skin or oral or nasopharyngeal mucosa are the most common manifestations. Generalized lymphadenopathy and secondary and tertiary bone and skin lesions are also common. Deep leg pain points to osteoperiostitis. Cardiovascular and central nervous system involvement is rare.

Chulay JD: *Treponema* species (yaws, pinta, bejel). In: *Principles and Practice of Infectious Diseases,* 3rd ed. Mandell GL, Douglas RG Jr, Bennett JE (editors). Churchill Livingstone, 1990. (A textbook review of non-sexually transmitted treponemal diseases.)

MISCELLANEOUS SPIROCHETAL DISEASES

RELAPSING FEVER

Relapsing fever is endemic in many parts of the world. The main reservoir is rodents, which serve as the source of infection for ticks (eg, *Ornithodoros*). The distribution and seasonal incidence of the disease are determined by the ecology of the ticks in different areas. In the USA, infected ticks are found throughout the West, especially in mountainous areas, but clinical cases are uncommon in humans.

The infectious organism is a spirochete, *Borrelia recurrentis*. It may be transmitted transovarially from one generation of ticks to the next. The spirochetes occur in all tissues of the tick, and humans can be infected by tick bites or by rubbing crushed tick tissues or feces into the bite wound. Tick-borne relapsing fever is endemic but is not transmitted from person to person. Different species (or strain) names have been given to *Borrelia* in different parts of the world where the organisms are transmitted by different ticks.

When an infected person harbors lice, the lice become infected with *Borrelia* by sucking blood. A few days later, the lice serve as a source of infection for other persons. Large epidemics may occur in louse-infested populations, and transmission is favored by crowding, malnutrition, and cold climate.

Clinical Findings

A. Symptoms and Signs: There is an abrupt onset of fever, chills, tachycardia, nausea and vomiting, arthralgia, and severe headache. Hepatomegaly and splenomegaly may develop, as well as various types of rashes. Delirium occurs with high fever, and there may be various neurologic and psychic abnormalities. The attack terminates, usually abruptly, after 3–10 days. After an interval of 1–2 weeks, relapse occurs, but often it is somewhat milder. Three to ten relapses may occur before recovery.

B. Laboratory Findings: During episodes of fever, large spirochetes are seen in blood smears stained with Wright's or Giemsa's stain. The organisms can be cultured in special media but rapidly lose pathogenicity. The spirochetes can multiply in injected rats or mice and can be seen in their blood.

A variety of anti-*Borrelia* antibodies develop during the illness; sometimes the Weil-Felix test for rickettsioses and nontreponemal serologic tests for syphilis may also be falsely positive. Cerebrospinal fluid abnormalities occur in patients with meningeal involvement. Mild anemia and thrombocytopenia are common, but the white blood cell count tends to be normal.

Differential Diagnosis

The manifestations of relapsing fever may be confused with malaria, leptospirosis, meningococcemia, yellow fever, typhus, or rat-bite fever.

Prevention

Prevention of tick bites (as described for rickettsial diseases) and delousing procedures applicable to large groups can prevent illness. Arthropod vectors should be controlled if possible.

An effective means of chemoprophylaxis has not been developed.

Treatment

A single dose of tetracycline or erythromycin, 0.5 g orally, or a single dose of procaine penicillin G, 600,000 units intramuscularly, probably constitutes adequate treatment for louse-borne relapsing fevers. Because of higher relapse rates, tick-borne disease is treated with 0.5 g of tetracycline or erythromycin given four times daily for 5–10 days. Jarisch-Herxheimer reactions may occur and respond to aspirin given every 4 hours. Pretreatment with steroids is not effective in preventing this reaction.

Prognosis

The overall mortality rate is usually about 5%. Fatalities are most common in old, debilitated, or very young patients. With treatment, the initial attack is shortened and relapses are largely prevented.

Flanigan TP et al: Relapsing fever in the US Virgin Islands: A previously unrecognized focus of infection. J Infect Dis 1991;163:1391. (Case report with review of epidemiology and diagnosis.)
Johnson WS Jr: *Borrelia* species: Relapsing fever. In: *Principles and Practice of Infectious Diseases,* 3rd ed. Mandell GL, Douglas RG Jr, Bennett JE (editors). Churchill Livingston, 1990.

RAT-BITE FEVER
(Spirillary Rat-Bite Fever, Sodoku)

Rat-bite fever is an uncommon acute infectious disease caused by *Spirillum minor*. It is transmitted to humans by the bite of a rat. Inhabitants of rat-infested slum dwellings and laboratory workers are at greatest risk.

Clinical Findings

A. Symptoms and Signs: The original rat bite, unless secondarily infected, heals promptly, but 1 to several weeks later the site becomes swollen, indurated, and painful; assumes a dusky purplish hue; and may ulcerate. Regional lymphangitis and lymphadenitis, fever, chills, malaise, myalgia, arthralgia, and headache are present. Splenomegaly may occur. A sparse, dusky-red maculopapular rash appears on the trunk and extremities in many cases, and there may be frank arthritis.

After a few days, both the local and systemic symptoms subside, only to reappear again in a few more days. This relapsing pattern of fever of 24–48 hours alternating with an equal afebrile period may persist for weeks. The other features, however, usually recur only during the first few relapses.

B. Laboratory Findings: Leukocytosis is often present, and the nontreponemal test for syphilis is often falsely positive. The organism may be identified in darkfield examination of the ulcer exudate or aspirated lymph node material; more commonly, it is observed after inoculation of a laboratory animal with the patient's exudate or blood. It has not been cultured in artificial media.

Differential Diagnosis

Rat-bite fever must be distinguished from the rat bite-induced lymphadenitis and rash of streptobacillary fever. Reliable differentiation requires an increasing titer of agglutinins against *Streptobacillus moniliformis* or identification of the causative organism. Rat-bite fever must also be distinguished from tularemia, rickettsial disease, *Pasteurella multocida* infections, and relapsing fever by identification of the causative organism.

Treatment

Treat with procaine penicillin G, 600,000 units intramuscularly every 12 hours; or tetracycline hydrochloride, 0.5 g every 6 hours for 10–14 days. Give supportive and symptomatic measures as indicated.

Prognosis

The reported mortality rate of about 10% should be markedly reduced by prompt diagnosis and antimicrobial treatment.

Washburn RG: *Spirillum minor* (rat-bite fever). In: *Principles and Practice of Infectious Diseases,* 3rd ed. Mandell GL, Douglas RG Jr, Bennett JE (editors). Churchill Livingstone, 1990.

LEPTOSPIROSIS

Leptospirosis is an acute and often severe infection that frequently affects the liver or other organs and is caused by serovars of *Leptospira interrogans*. The three most common serovars of infection are *Leptospira icterohaemorrhagiae* of rats, *Leptospira canicola* of dogs, and *Leptospira pomona* of cattle and swine. Several other varieties can also cause the disease, but *L icterohaemorrhagiae* causes the most severe illness. The disease is worldwide in distribution, and the incidence is higher than usually supposed. The leptospires are often transmitted to humans by the ingestion of food and drink contaminated by the urine of the reservoir animal. The organism may also enter through minor skin lesions and probably via the conjunctiva. Many infections have followed bathing in contaminated water. The disease is an occupational hazard among sewer workers, rice planters, abattoir workers, and farmers. The incubation period is 2–20 days.

Clinical Findings

A. Symptoms and Signs: Anicteric leptospirosis is the more common and milder form of the disease and is often biphasic. The initial or "septicemic" phase begins with abrupt fever to 39–40 °C (102.2–104 °F), chills, abdominal pain, severe headache, and myalgias, especially of the calf muscles. There is marked conjunctival suffusion. Leptospires can be isolated from blood, cerebrospinal fluid, and tissues. Following a 1- to 3-day period of improvement in symptoms and absence of fever, the second or "immune" phase begins. Leptospires are absent from blood and cerebrospinal fluid but are still present in the kidney, and specific antibodies appear. A recurrence of symptoms is seen as in the first phase of disease with the onset of meningitis. Uveitis, rash, and adenopathy may occur. The illness is usually self-limited, lasting 4–30 days, and complete recovery is the rule.

Icteric leptospirosis (Weil's syndrome) (usually caused by *L icterohaemorrhagiae*) is the most severe form of the disease, characterized by impaired renal and hepatic function, abnormal mental status, hypotension, and a 5–10% mortality rate. Signs and symptoms are continuous and not biphasic.

Pretibial fever, a mild form of leptospirosis caused by *Leptospira autumnalis,* occurred during World War II at Fort Bragg, USA. In pretibial fever, there is patchy erythema on the skin of the lower legs or generalized rash occurring with fever.

Leptospirosis with jaundice must be distinguished from hepatitis, yellow fever, and relapsing fever.

B. Laboratory Findings: The leukocyte count may be normal or as high as 50,000/µL, with neutrophils predominating. The urine may contain bile, protein, casts, and red cells. Oliguria is not uncommon, and in severe cases uremia may occur. In cases with meningeal involvement, organisms may be found in the cerebrospinal fluid during the first 10 days of illness. Early in the disease, the organism may be identified by darkfield examination of the patient's blood or by culture on a semisolid medium (eg, Fletcher's EMJH). Cultures take 1–6 weeks to become positive. The organism may also be grown from the urine from the tenth day to the sixth week. Specific agglutination titers develop after 7 days and may persist at high levels for many years; specific serologic tests are of particular value in diagnosis of the milder, anicteric forms and of aseptic meningitis. A rapid diagnosis can be made by the determination of specific IgM with the dot-ELISA method. Serum CK is usually elevated in leptospirosis patients and normal in hepatitis patients.

Complications

Myocarditis, aseptic meningitis, renal failure, and massive hemorrhage are not common but are the usual causes of death. Iridocyclitis may occur.

Treatment

Various antimicrobial drugs, including penicillin and tetracyclines, show antileptospiral activity. Penicillin (eg, 6 million units daily intravenously) is said to be beneficial in severe leptospirosis, especially if started within the first 4 days of illness. Jarisch-Herxheimer reactions may occur. Observe for evidence of renal failure, and treat as necessary. Effective prophylaxis consists of doxycycline, 200 mg orally, given once weekly during the risk of exposure. Doxycycline, 100 mg twice daily for 7 days, can also reduce the severity and duration of symptoms if given within 3 days after onset of disease.

Prognosis

Without jaundice, the disease is almost never fatal. With jaundice, the mortality rate is 5% for those under age 30 and 30% for those over age 60.

Sperber SJ, Schleupner CJ: Leptospirosis: A forgotten cause of aseptic meningitis and multisystem febrile illness. South Med J 1989;82:1285. (Case report and review of epidemiology, clinical manifestations, and treatment.)

Watt G et al: Placebo-controlled trial of intravenous penicillin for severe and late leptospirosis. Lancet 1988;1:433. (Value of early therapy.)

Watt G et al: The rapid diagnosis of leptospirosis: A prospective comparison of the dot enzyme-linked immunosorbent assay and the genus-specific microscopic agglutination test at different stages of illness. J Infect Dis 1988;157;840. (Equal sensitivity, specificity, and ease of performance.)

LYME DISEASE
(Lyme Borreliosis)

Essentials of Diagnosis

- Erythema migrans, a flat or slightly raised red lesion that expands with central clearing.
- Headache or stiff neck.
- Arthralgias, arthritis, and myalgias; arthritis is often chronic and recurrent.
- Wide geographic distribution, with most United States cases in the Northeast, Upper Midwest, and Pacific coastal regions.

General Considerations

This illness, named after the town of Old Lyme, Connecticut, is caused by the spirochete *Borrelia burgdorferi* and is transmitted to humans by ixodid ticks that are part of the *Ixodes ricinus* complex. Lyme disease is the most common vector-borne disease in the United States and is being reported with increasing frequency. It has been recognized in most regions of the USA, though most cases occur in the Northeast, Upper Midwest, and along the Pacific Coast. The vector is *Ixodes dammini* in the Northeast and Midwest, *Ixodes pacificus* on the West Coast of the USA, *Ixodes scapularis* in the southeastern United States, *Ixodes ricinus* in Europe, and *Ixodes persulcatus* in Asia. The disease also occurs in Australia (vector unknown). Mice and deer make up the major animal reservoir of *B burgdorferi,* but other rodents and birds may also be infected. Domestic animals such as dogs, cattle, and horses can also develop clinical illness, usually manifested as arthritis.

Ticks feed once during each of their three stages of life. Larval ticks feed in late summer, nymphs in the following spring and early summer, and adults during the fall. The preferred host for the nymphs and larvae is the white-footed mouse in the USA (the black-striped mouse in Europe). This animal is tolerant of infection—a fact that is critical in maintaining infection, since the mouse can remain spirochetemic and transmit the agent to the larvae the following spring after being infected by the nymphal form in early summer. Adult ticks prefer the white-tailed deer as host. Most infections occur in the summer, when tick exposure is high and nymphal ticks are active. Disease occurs less commonly in the cooler months (October to April), when adult ticks are active. This is due in part to the large size of the adult, making it easier to detect by the human host and allowing removal before disease transmission can occur. Any stage of the tick, however, can transmit disease.

The increased incidence of Lyme disease is due in part to the resurgence of the once-decimated deer population, the spread of tick vectors to new areas (perhaps by mammals or birds), and the encroachment of suburbs on once rural areas, bringing humans and ticks into closer proximity. Control of Lyme disease is best accomplished by avoiding tick-infested areas, wearing protective clothing, using repellents, and inspecting for ticks after possible exposures. Controlling ticks on residential property and in parks may also be helpful, but limiting the spread of ticks and deer control are not currently feasible.

Under experimental conditions, ticks must feed for 24–48 hours to transmit infections. In addition, the percentage of ticks infected varies on a regional basis. In the Northeast and Midwest, 15–50% of *I dammini* ticks are infected with the spirochete; in the Western United States, only 2% of *I pacificus* are infected. These are important epidemiologic features in assessing the likelihood that tick exposure will result in disease. Exposure to *I pacificus* is unlikely to result in disease, since so few ticks are infected, but this is not true of exposure to *I dammini*. Eliciting a history of brushing a tick off the skin (ie, the tick was not feeding) or removing a tick on the same day as exposure (ie, the tick did not feed long enough) decreases the likelihood that infection will develop, since ticks must feed for 24 hours to transmit disease.

Ixodes ticks are smaller than the more common dog ticks *(Dermacentor variabilis)*. Larvae are less than 1 mm in size, and the adult female is 2–3 mm in size, with a red body and black legs. After a blood meal, ticks can reach two to three times their unengorged size. Because the tick is so small, the bite is usually painless and goes unnoticed. After feeding, the tick drops off in 2–4 days. If a tick is found, it should be removed immediately. The best way to accomplish this is to grab the mouth part—not the body—where it enters the skin with a fine-tipped tweezers and pull firmly and repeatedly until the tick releases its hold. Saving the tick in a bottle of alcohol for future identification may be useful, especially if symptoms develop.

Congenital infection has been documented, but the exact frequency and manifestations have not been clearly defined. Similarly, because the organism can be latent, it is not known if women infected prior to becoming pregnant can activate the disease and transmit infection to the fetus. In one retrospective study, 5 of 19 pregnancies complicated by Lyme disease resulted in an adverse outcome, but all of the outcomes were different and could not be conclusively linked to infection.

Clinical Findings

The typical clinical description of Lyme disease divides the illness into three stages: stage 1, flu-like symptoms and a typical skin rash (**erythema migrans**); stage 2, weeks to months later, Bell's palsy or meningitis; and stage 3, months to years later, arthritis. The problem with this simplified scheme is that there is a great deal of overlap, and the skin, central nervous system, and musculoskeletal system can be involved early or late. A more accurate classification divides disease into early and late man-

ifestations and specifies whether disease is localized or disseminated.

A. Symptoms and Signs:

1. Stage 1, early localized infection–Stage 1 infection is characterized by erythema (erythema migrans). About 1 week after the tick bite (range, 3–30 days), a flat or slightly raised red lesion appears at the site, which is commonly in areas of tight clothing such as the groin, thigh, or axilla. This lesion expands over several days, with central clearing. About 20% of patients either do not have typical skin lesions or the lesions go unnoticed. A flu-like illness with fever, chills, and myalgia occurs in about half of patients. Even without treatment, the signs and symptoms of erythema migrans resolve in 3–4 weeks.

2. Stage 2, early disseminated infection–In stage 2, the spirochete may spread in the patient's blood or lymph to cause a wide variety of signs and symptoms. This usually occurs within days to weeks after inoculation of the organism. The most common manifestations involve the skin, central nervous system, and musculoskeletal system. In about half of patients, secondary lesions develop that are not associated with a tick bite. These lesions are similar in appearance to the primary lesion but are usually smaller. A rare skin lesion (1% of patients) seen primarily in Europe is *Borrelia* lymphocytoma. This presents as a small reddish nodule or plaque on the ear in children and on the nipple in adults. Headache and stiff neck can occur, as well as migratory pains in joints, muscles, and tendons. Fatigue and malaise are common. Generally, the neurologic and musculoskeletal symptoms are intermittent and last only hours, whereas fatigue is persistent. After hematogenous spread, the organism sequesters itself in certain areas and produces focal symptoms. Some patients experience cardiac (4–10% of patients) or neurologic (10–20% of patients) manifestations. Involvement of the heart includes myocarditis, with arrhythmias and heart block. Neurologic disease is most commonly manifested as aseptic meningitis, Bell's palsy, or encephalitis. Even in the absence of symptoms, seeding of the central nervous system can occur. Peripheral neuropathy (sensory or motor), transverse myelitis, and mononeuritis multiplex have also been described. Rarely, panophthalmitis can occur.

3. Stage 3, late persistent infection–Stage 3 infection occurs months to years after the initial infection and again primarily manifests itself as musculoskeletal, neurologic, and skin disease. Up to 60% of patients develop musculoskeletal complaints. Clinical manifestations are quite variable and include (1) joint and periarticular pain without objective findings (perhaps a manifestation of fibromyalgia that may be triggered by Lyme disease); (2) frank arthritis, mainly of large joints, that is chronic or recurrent over years (recurrences become less severe, less frequent, and shorter with time); and (3) chronic synovitis, which may result in permanent disability. Chronic arthritis has been associated with HLA-DR4 and HLA-DR2 histocompatibility genes, suggesting an immunogenetic predisposition. In addition, the patients who express HLA-DR4 respond poorly to therapy. Both the central and the peripheral nervous systems may be involved. Subacute encephalopathy, characterized by memory loss, mood changes, and sleep disturbance, is the most common chronic neurologic manifestation. An axonal polyneuropathy, manifested as distal sensory paresthesias or radicular pain, can occur either alone or, more commonly, in association with encephalopathy. Most of these patients have objective signs of disease when tested by electromyography. A rare form of chronic neurologic dysfunction—leukoencephalitis—presents with cognitive dysfunction, spastic paraparesis, ataxia, and bladder dysfunction. This form of the disease is seen more commonly in Europe than in the United States. The cutaneous manifestation of late infection, which can occur up to 10 years after infection, is **acrodermatitis chronicum atrophicans.** It has been described mainly in Europe and only rarely in the United States. There is usually bluish-red discoloration of a distal extremity with associated swelling. These lesions become atrophic and sclerotic with time and eventually resemble localized scleroderma.

B. Laboratory Findings: The diagnosis of Lyme disease is based on both clinical manifestations and laboratory findings. The National Surveillance Case Definition specifies a person with exposure to a potential tick habitat (within the 30 days just prior to developing erythema migrans) with (1) erythema migrans diagnosed by a physician or (2) at least one late manifestation of the disease and laboratory confirmation. Laboratory confirmation requires detection of specific antibodies to B burgdorferi in serum, either by indirect immunofluorescence assay (IFA) or enzyme-linked immunosorbent assay (ELISA); the latter is now preferred, because it is more sensitive and specific. A Western blot assay that can detect both IgM and IgG antibodies may be helpful in identifying false-positive ELISA tests. IgM antibody appears first 2–4 weeks after onset of erythema migrans, peaks at 6–8 weeks, and then declines to low levels after 4–6 months of illness. Persistence of IgM or reappearance of IgM late in the disease may be indicative of recurrent disease. IgG occurs later (6–8 weeks after onset of disease), peaks at 4–6 months, and remains elevated indefinitely despite appropriate therapy and resolution of symptoms. A fourfold rise or fall in IgG titer is required to confirm the diagnosis. In early disease, up to 50% of patients may be antibody-negative. In later stages, most patients are antibody-positive, but up to 5% may be seronegative. In this small subset of patients with seronegative late Lyme disease, a T cell-proliferative assay may be helpful in making the diagnosis. An antibody-capture ELISA appears to be the most sensitive—it is positive in 90% of patients with stage I

disease–and specific test, but it is difficult to perform and is available only in reference laboratories. Preparation of a purified flagellar protein to use as an antigen to detect IgM antibodies may improve our ability to detect early disease and is presently under investigation. Antibiotic therapy of early disease may abort seroconversion.

Caution should be exercised in basing the diagnosis of Lyme disease on serologic testing. In addition to the lack of sensitivity of the available tests as noted above, interlaboratory variation in test results is a major problem. In one study, aliquots of serum were sent to different laboratories, and there was a marked difference in reported test results, with known positive serum being identified in less than half of cases. When a second specimen of the same serum was sent 2 weeks later, 8 of 18 laboratories reported a fourfold difference in titers. These data demonstrate the difficulty in making the diagnosis of Lyme disease by serologic testing and emphasize the need for national standards. Lack of specificity is also a problem. Cross-reacting antibodies can occur in patients with syphilis, leptospirosis, relapsing fever, enteroviral and other viral illnesses, and autoimmune diseases and perhaps in patients with severe gingivitis caused by spirochetal organisms.

B burgdorferi has rarely been cultured from blood or cerebrospinal fluid. Aspiration of erythema migrans lesions has yielded positive cultures in up to 29% of cases, and cultures of biopsy specimens have been reported positive in 61%. Special silver staining of chronically inflamed synovial tissue demonstrates spirochetes in one-third of patients.

Treatment

Antibiotic sensitivity of B burgdorferi has been established in vitro. Tetracycline is effective against the spirochete, but penicillin is only moderately so. Erythromycin is effective in vitro but has been disappointing in clinical trials. Ampicillin, ceftriaxone, cefuroxime, and imipenem are also effective in vitro, but aminoglycosides, ciprofloxacin, and rifampin are not.

Present recommendations for therapy are outlined in Table 33–4. For early disease, oral antibiotic therapy shortens the duration of rash and usually prevents late sequelae. Either doxycycline, 100 mg twice daily for 10–30 days, or tetracycline, 250–500 mg four times daily for 10–30 days, is most commonly used. Amoxicillin is also effective and is recommended for children, for pregnant or lactating women, and for those who cannot tolerate doxycycline or tetracycline. Cefuroxime axetil, 500 mg twice daily, or azithromycin, 500 mg on day 1 followed by 250 mg daily for four days, has recently been shown to be as effective as doxycycline for early disease. Erythromycin is less effective. Although data are preliminary, in one small controlled study of patients with early disease without central nervous system involve-

Table 33–4. Treatment of Lyme disease.

Manifestation	Drug and Dosage	Pediatric Dosage
Erythema migrans	Doxycycline, 100 mg twice daily for 10–30 days; or tetracycline, 500 mg 4 times daily for 10–30 days; or amoxicillin, 250–500 mg 3 times daily for 10–30 days; or cefuroxime axetil, 500 mg twice daily for 10–30 days; or erythromycin, 250 mg 4 times daily for 10–30 days.	Amoxicillin, 20–40 mg/kg/d for 10–30 days; or erythromycin, 30 mg/kg/d for 10–30 days; or cefuroxime axetil, 250 mg twice daily for 10–30 days.
Neurologic disease Bell's palsy	Doxycycline, tetracycline, or amoxicillin as above for 1 month.	Amoxicillin, 20–40 mg/kg/d for 1 month
Other central nervous system disease	Ceftriaxone, 2 g IV once daily for 14 days; or penicillin G, 20 million units/d IV in 6 divided doses for 14 days.	Ceftriaxone, 50–80 mg/kg/ IV once daily for 14 days; penicillin, 250–400 units/kg/d IV in divided doses for 14 days
Cardiac disease First-degree block (PR < 0.3 s)	Doxycyline, tetracycline, or amoxicillin as above for 10–30 days.	Amoxicillin as above for 10–30 days
High-degree atrio ventricular block	Ceftriaxone or penicillin G as above for 14 days.	Penicillin G or ceftriaxone as above for 14 days
Arthritis Oral dosage	Doxycycline, tetracycline, or amoxicillin as above for 1 month.	Amoxicillin as above for 1 month
Parenteral dosage	Ceftriaxone or penicillin G as above for 14 days.	Penicillin G as above for 14 days
Acrodermatitis chronicum atrophicans	Doxycycline, tetracycline, or amoxicillin orally as above for 30 days.	Amoxicillin as above for 1 month

ment, azithromycin, 500 mg on day 1 followed by 250 mg daily for 4 more days, was as efficacious as doxycycline or amoxicillin given for 10 days. For disseminated stage 2 disease, oral medication—doxycycline or amoxicillin—can be used for Bell's palsy. If other central nervous system manifestations are present (meningitis), ceftriaxone is given intravenously. Intravenous penicillin is also effective for central nervous system disease, but ceftriaxone penetrates into the cerebrospinal fluid better and can be given once daily. Mild cardiac disease (PR < 0.3 s) can be treated with oral agents, but high-degree atrioventricular block should be treated with either intravenous ceftriaxone or penicillin. Therapy of arthritis is difficult because some patients fail to respond to any therapy and others who do respond do so slowly. Initial studies suggested that intravenous penicillin was superior to benzathine penicillin. In one small study, ceftriaxone appeared to be superior to intravenous penicillin. In a recent study, however, oral agents (doxycycline or amoxicillin) were just as effective as intravenous regimens (penicillin or ceftriaxone). A reasonable approach to the patient with Lyme arthritis is to start with oral therapy and if this fails to switch to an intravenous agent.

Unresolved issues with respect to therapy include the role of prophylaxis following tick bites and the role of therapy in pregnancy. Analysis of the cost-effectiveness of prophylactic therapy suggests that antibiotics administered for 2 weeks would be beneficial in preventing illness in endemic areas, where the risk of acquiring disease following a tick bite is 3.6% or greater. However, studies designed to examine the effect of prophylaxis have not shown any significant benefit. In one study of almost 400 patients in a highly endemic area, amoxicillin, 250 mg three times daily for 10 days, was no better than placebo in preventing disease in patients who had been bitten by a deer tick within the previous 72 hours. Since most patients who develop Lyme disease are symptomatic and since treatment of early disease successfully prevents late sequelae, it is reasonable to reserve treatment for patients who develop symptoms and not routinely administer prophylactic antibiotics. Data for treatment in pregnancy are limited. Because of the failure of oral agents to prevent fetal infection in one case, some have recommended intravenous penicillin in this setting.

Bakken LL et al: Performance of 45 laboratories participating in a proficiency testing program for Lyme disease serology. JAMA 1992;268:891. (Emphasizes inter- and intralaboratory variations in serologic testing.)

Buchstein SR, Garner P: Lyme disease. Infect Dis Clin North Am 1991;5:103.

Logigian EL, Kaplan RF, Steere AC: Chronic neurologic manifestations of Lyme disease. N Engl J Med 1991;323:1438. (Twenty-seven patients.)

Magid D et al: Prevention of Lyme disease after tick bites: A cost-effective analysis. N Engl J Med 1992;327:534.

Rahn DW, Malawista SE: Lyme disease: Recommendations for diagnosis and treatment. Ann Intern Med 1991; 114:472.

Rahn DW, Malawista SE: Lyme disease. West J Med 1991; 154:706.

Shapiro ED et al: A controlled trial of antimicrobial prophylaxis for Lyme disease after deer tick bites. N Engl J Med 1992;327:1769. (Comparison of amoxicillin versus placebo for prophylaxis, demonstrating no advantage for antimicrobial prophylaxis.)

Treatment of Lyme disease. Med Lett Drugs Ther 1992; 34:95. (Current therapeutic recommendations.)

34 | Infectious Diseases: Protozoal

Robert S. Goldsmith, MD, MPH, DTM&H

AFRICAN TRYPANOSOMIASIS (Sleeping Sickness)

Essentials of Diagnosis

- History of exposure to tsetse flies.

Hemolymphatic stage (usually absent or unnoticed in *T b gambiense* infections):

- Irregular fevers, headaches, joint pains, malaise, pruritus, papular skin rash, edemas.
- Posterior cervical or generalized lymphadenopathy.
- Anemia, weight loss.

Meningoencephalitic stage:

- Insomnia, motor and sensory disorders, abnormal reflexes, somnolence to coma.
- Trypanosomes and increased white cells and protein in cerebrospinal fluid.

General Considerations

African trypanosomiasis is caused by *Trypanosoma brucei rhodesiense* and *Trypanosoma brucei gambiense*, both hemoflagellates. The organisms are transmitted by bites of tsetse flies (*Glossina* species), which inhabit shaded areas along streams and rivers. Human disease occurs locally throughout tropical Africa from south of the Sahara to about 20° south latitude. *T b gambiense* infections are in the moist sub-Saharan savannah and riverine forests of West and Central Africa up to the eastern Rift Valley. *T b rhodesiense* occurs to the east of the Rift Valley in the savannah of East and Southeast Africa and along the shores of Lake Victoria. There are an estimated 10,000–20,000 new cases annually and 5000 deaths.

T b rhodesiense infection is primarily a zoonosis of game animals; humans are infected sporadically. Humans are the principal mammalian host for *T b gambiense*, but recent information suggests an animal reservoir as well.

Clinical Findings

A. Symptoms and Signs: *T b rhodesiense* infections go through the following three stages, are much more virulent, and untreated patients die within weeks to a year. In *T b gambiense* infections, however, chancres do not appear and the hemolymphatic stage is usually absent or goes unnoticed; when symptoms do become manifest after weeks to years,

they are initially so mild that they are often ignored by the patient.

1. The trypanosomal chancre–This is a local pruritic, painful inflammatory reaction (3–10 cm) with regional lymphadenopathy that appears about 48 hours after the tsetse fly bite and lasts 2–4 weeks.

2. The hemolymphatic stage–This stage usually begins 3–10 days later with invasion of the bloodstream and reticuloendothelial system. High fever, severe headache, joint pains, and malaise recur at irregular intervals corresponding to waves of parasitemia. Between febrile episodes there are symptom-free periods that last up to 2 weeks. Transient rashes may appear, often pruritic and papular or circinate. Examination reveals mild enlargement of the liver and spleen, and edema (peripheral, pleural, ascites, etc). Enlarged, rubbery, and painless lymph nodes occur in 75% of patients. In *T b gambiense,* only the posterior cervical group (Winterbottom's sign) may be enlarged. With progression of the disease, there is increasing weight loss and debilitation. Signs of myocardial involvement may appear early in Rhodesian infection, and the patient may succumb to myocarditis before signs of central nervous system invasion appear.

3. The meningoencephalitic stage–This stage appears within a few weeks or months of onset of Rhodesian infection but in Gambian sleeping sickness develops more insidiously, starting 6 months to several years after onset. Insomnia, anorexia, personality changes, apathy, and headaches are among the early findings. A variety of motor or tonus disorders may develop, including tremors and disturbances of speech, gait, and reflexes; somnolence appears late. The patient becomes severely emaciated and, finally, comatose. Death often results from secondary infection.

B. Laboratory Findings: Definitive diagnosis requires identifying the organism in the bite lesion (rare), blood, lymph node aspirate, or cerebrospinal fluid. Because the number of trypanosomes in the blood fluctuates in waves and because the organisms are undetectable about 3 out of 5 days, specimens should be examined daily for 15 days (1) for motile organisms in wet films, (2) after Giemsa staining of thick and thin films, and (3) after concentration by centrifugation of heparinized blood (trypanosomes are concentrated in the buffy coat). Other diagnostic techniques employing blood samples include intraperitoneal inoculation into laboratory rodents (most sensitive approach), culture, Millipore filtration, and DEAE-cellulose anion exchange. Lymph nodes selected for aspiration should still be soft (ie, not fibrosed). The cerebrospinal fluid contains increased numbers of cells (lymphocytes) and an increased protein concentration. Wet films and stained smears of centrifuged cerebrospinal fluid (double centrifugation is at least twice as sensitive as single centrifugation) may then show trypanosomes in advanced cases; the fluid should then be inoculated also into an experimental animal and culture medium. Serologic tests become positive about 12 days after onset of infection. Titers of circulating antibody fluctuate and, after high parasitemia, brief periods of excess antigen may depress antibody titers below detectable levels. In addition, in the late meningoencephalitic phase, both serologic titers and parasitemia may fall below demonstrable levels. ELISA and immunofluorescent tests of cerebrospinal fluid may prove useful in late disease.

Other findings include anemia, increased sedimentation rate, thrombocytopenia, reduced total serum protein, increased serum globulin, and an elevated IgM level. The latter begins to rise shortly after infection and may reach 10–20 times normal. However, normal or low levels of IgM in acute disease do not rule out the infection. In central nervous system involvement, an elevated IgM in the cerebrospinal fluid is pathognomonic for the meningoencephalitic stage of trypanosomiasis, except that false-negative results have been reported.

Differential Diagnosis

Trypanosomiasis may be mistaken for a variety of other diseases, including malaria, influenza, pneumonia, infectious mononucleosis, leukemia, lymphoma, the arbovirus encephalitides, cerebral tumor, and various psychoses. Serologic tests for syphilis may be falsely positive in trypanosomiasis.

Treatment

A. Hemolymphatic Stage: Drugs of choice are suramin for both parasites or eflornithine (DMFO) for *T b gambiense*. The alternative drug is pentamidine. Suramin and pentamidine frequently cause severe adverse reactions.

1. Late disease with central nervous system involvement–The drugs of choice are melarsoprol for both parasites or eflornithine for *T b gambiense*. An alternative treatment for both parasites is tryparsamide plus suramin.

Suramin and pentamidine, which do not penetrate the blood-brain barrier, cannot be used when the central nervous system is involved. Melarsoprol causes a reactive encephalopathy in up to 5% of patients; corticosteroids have been used by some workers to pre-

vent this. Eflornithine, which has proved highly effective with only mild toxicity in early and late *T b gambiense* infections, has recently been approved for use in the USA for this parasite. However, for the treatment of *T b rhodesiense* infection, the efficacy of eflornithine has been inconsistent. In the USA, suramin and melarsoprol are available only from the CDC Drug Service, Centers for Disease Control, Atlanta, GA 30333. Telephone: (404) 639–3670; (404) 639–2888 evenings, weekends, and holidays. See references for dosages.

Proper follow-up to ensure detection of the encephalitic stage requires initial cerebrospinal fluid examination, repeat studies at intervals during treatment, 3 months after treatment, and then at 6-month intervals for 2 years.

Prevention

Individual prevention in endemic areas should include wearing long sleeves and trousers, avoiding dark-colored clothing, and using mosquito nets while sleeping. Repellents have no effect. Pentamidine is used in chemoprophylaxis only against the Gambian type. In *T b rhodesiense* infection, pentamidine may suppress early symptoms, resulting in recognition of the disease too late in its course for effective treatment. Excretion of pentamidine is slow; therefore, one intramuscular injection (4 mg/kg, maximum 300 mg) protects for 3–6 months. The drug is potentially toxic and should only be used for persons at high risk (ie, those with constant, heavy exposure to tsetse flies in areas with known transmission of Gambian disease). Performing serologic tests every 6 months during exposure and for 3 years afterward is the safest method for detecting the disease at an early stage.

Prognosis

Most patients recover following treatment with eflornithine, suramin, or pentamidine for hemolymphatic disease. Generally, with early treatment of central nervous system disease, most patients treated with melarsoprol will recover, though relapses occur in about 2%; if therapy is started late, irreversible brain damage or death is common. If African trypanosomiasis is untreated, most persons will die.

Bailey JW, Smith DH: The use of the acridine orange QBC technique in the diagnosis of African trypanosomiasis. Trans R Soc Trop Med Hyg 1992;86:630.

Drugs for parasitic infections: Med Lett Drugs Ther 1992;34:17. (Important resource for dosages.)

Pepin J, Milord F: African trypanosomiasis and drug-induced encephalopathy: Risk factors and pathogenesis. Trans R Soc Trop Med Hyg 1991;85:222.

Zweygarth E, Kaminsky R: Evaluation of DL-α-difluoromethylornithine against susceptible and drug-resistant Trypanosoma brucei brucei. Acta Tropica 1991; 48:223. (Eflornithine [DFMO] usage in human trials.)

AMERICAN TRYPANOSOMIASIS
(Chagas' Disease)

Essentials of Diagnosis

Acute stage:
- Children principally affected.
- Inflammatory lesion at site of inoculation; prolonged fever, tachycardia, hepatosplenomegaly, lymphadenopathy, signs of myocarditis.
- Parasites in peripheral blood, positive serologic tests.

Chronic stage:
- Heart failure with cardiac arrhythmias; decreased intensity of heart sounds; episodes of thromboembolism.
- In some geographic regions, dysphagia, severe constipation, and radiologic evidence of megaesophagus or megacolon.
- Most important: Positive xenodiagnosis or hemoculture, positive serologic tests; abnormal ECG.

General Considerations

Chagas' disease is caused by *Trypanosoma cruzi*, a protozoan parasite of humans and wild and domestic animals. *T cruzi* occurs only in the Americas; it is found in wild animals and to a lesser extent in humans from southern South America to northern Mexico, Texas, and the southwestern USA. An estimated 12 million people are infected, mostly in rural areas, resulting in about 60,000 deaths yearly. In many countries of Latin America, particularly South America, Chagas' disease is the most important cause of heart disease. The infection is rare in the USA.

T cruzi is transmitted by many species of triatomine bugs that become infected by ingesting blood with circulating trypanosomes from infected animals or humans. Multiplication occurs in the digestive tract of the bug; infective forms are eliminated in feces. Infection in humans is through "contamination" with bug feces; the parasite penetrates the skin (generally through the bite wound) or the conjunctiva. Transmission can also occur by blood transfusion or in utero.

The trypanosomes first multiply close to the point of entry. They then enter the bloodstream as trypanosomes and later invade the heart and other tissues, where they assume a leishmanial form. Multiplication causes cellular destruction, inflammation, and fibrosis. Infection continues for many years, probably for life.

Clinical Findings

A. Symptoms and Signs: Most infected persons are asymptomatic. The **acute stage,** seen principally in children, lasts 2–4 months and leads to death in up to 10% of cases. The earliest findings are at the site of inoculation either in the eye—Romaña's sign (unilateral bipalpebral edema, conjunctivitis, local lymphadenopathy)—or in the skin—a chagoma (furuncle-like lesion with local lymphadenopathy). Subsequent findings include fever, malaise, headache, hepatomegaly, mild splenomegaly, and generalized lymphadenopathy. Acute myocarditis may lead to biventricular failure, but arrhythmias are rare. Meningoencephalitis is limited to young children and is often fatal.

A **latent period** may last from 10 to 30 years in which the patient is asymptomatic but in which serologic tests and sometimes parasitologic examination confirm the presence of the infection. Whether Chagas' disease may be reactivated by immunosuppression, especially that due to AIDS, is under study.

The **chronic stage** is usually manifested by cardiac disease in the third and fourth decades of life, characterized by arrhythmias, congestive heart failure (often with prominent right-sided findings), and systemic or pulmonary embolization originating from mural thrombi. Sudden cardiac arrest in young persons may occur and is attributed to ventricular fibrillation. Megacolon and megaesophagus, caused by damage to nerve plexuses in the bowel or esophageal wall, occur in some areas of Chile, Argentina, and Brazil; symptoms include dysphagia, regurgitation, and constipation.

B. Laboratory Findings: Appropriate selection of tests allows a definitive parasitologic diagnosis in most acute cases and in up to 40% of chronic ones. In the acute stage, trypanosomes should be looked for by examination of anticoagulated fresh blood for motile organisms and by examination of the following stained preparations: thick blood films, buffy coat (ie, interphase between red cells and leukocyte buffy coat), and the sediment after centrifuging (600 rpm) the supernatant of clotted blood. In the chronic stage, the parasite can only be detected by culture or xenodiagnosis. The latter consists of permitting uninfected laboratory-reared bugs of the local major vector to feed on the patients and then examining their intestinal contents for trypanosomes. In both acute and chronic infection, blood should also be cultured using Nicolle-Novy-MacNeal medium and inoculated into laboratory mice or rats 3–10 days old. *Trypanosoma rangeli*, a nonpathogenic blood trypanosome also found in humans in Central America and northern South America, must not be mistaken for *T cruzi*. Several serologic tests are routinely used and are of presumptive value when positive; when possible, more than one test should be used. Antibodies of the IgM class are usually elevated early in the acute stage but are replaced by IgG antibodies as the disease progresses. False-positive reactions can occur in the presence of leishmaniasis or *T rangeli* infection.. The most important electrocardiographic abnormalities are right bundle branch block, other conduction defects, and arrhythmias. In certain regions of South America, radiologic examination may show cardiac enlargement with characteristic apical aneurysms, megaesophagus, or megacolon.

Treatment

Therapy is unsatisfactory; the drugs used are toxic and often ineffective. In the acute phase, however, cure is usually possible. In the chronic phase, although parasitemia and xenodiagnosis become negative, treatment does not alter the serologic reaction, cardiac function, or progression of the disease.

Nifurtimox is given orally in daily doses of 10 mg/kg to adults and 15 mg/kg to children for 60–90 days. It generally produces anorexia, weight loss, tremors, and peripheral neuropathy. Hallucinations and convulsions are rare. In the USA, nifurtimox is available only from the Parasitic Disease Drug Service, Centers for Disease Control, Atlanta 30333 (call [404] 488–4240). Benznidazole, where available (not in the USA), is the alternative drug of choice at a dosage of 5–10 mg/kg/d for 30–60 days; it has side effects similar to those of nifurtimox. Clinical studies continue to evaluate allopurinol (600 mg/d for 30–60 days in treatment of chronic infection. Ketoconazole has resulted in parasitologic cure of mice and should be tried in humans. Treatment is not indicated during the latent period of infection.

In the chronic stage, diuretics are usually effective in cardiac failure, but digoxin is commonly not well tolerated. The most effective antiarrhythmic drug is amiodarone, but pulmonary and cardiac toxicity can be problems with its use.

Prognosis

Acute infections in infants and young children are often fatal, particularly when the central nervous system is involved. Adults with chronic cardiac infections also may ultimately succumb to the disease.

Ferreira MS et al: Acute fatal *Trypanosoma cruzi* meningoencephalitis in a human immunodeficiency virus-positive hemophiliac patient. Am J Trop Med Hyg 1991;45:723.

Gallerano RH, Marr JJ, Sosa RR: Therapeutic efficacy of allopurinol in patients with chronic Chagas' disease. Am J Trop Med Hyg 1990;43:159.

Morris SA et al: Pathophysiologic insights into the cardiomyopathy of Chagas' disease. Circulation 1990;82:1900.

Pan AA et al: Clinical evaluation of an EIA for the sensitive and specific detection of serum antibody to *Trypanosoma cruzi* (Chagas' disease). J Infect Dis 1992;165:585.

AMEBIASIS

Essentials of Diagnosis

- Mild to moderate colitis: recurrent diarrhea and abdominal cramps, sometimes alternating with constipation; mucus may be present; blood is usually absent.
- Severe colitis: semiformed to liquid stools streaked with blood and mucus, fever, colic, prostration. In fulminant cases, ileus, perforation, peritonitis, and hemorrhage occur.
- Hepatic amebiasis: fever, hepatomegaly, pain, localized tenderness.
- Laboratory findings: amebas in stools or in abscess aspirate; serologic tests positive with severe colitis or hepatic abscess, which is readily imaged by ultrasonography or CT scan.

General Considerations

Amebiasis is caused by the protozoan parasite *Entamoeba histolytica.* The organisms either live as commensals in the lumen of the large intestine without causing disease (the asymptomatic chronic carrier) or invade the colon wall causing acute dysentery or chronic diarrhea of variable severity. The organisms may also be carried by the blood to the liver, where they may produce hepatic abscesses. Rarely, they are carried to the lungs, brain, or other organs or invade the perianal skin.

The infection is present worldwide but is most prevalent and severe in tropical areas, where rates may exceed 40% under conditions of crowding, poor sanitation, and poor nutrition. It is estimated that there are about 50 million cases of invasive amebiasis and 40,000–100,000 deaths annually worldwide. In temperate areas, however, amebiasis tends to be asymptomatic or a mild, chronic infection that often remains undiagnosed. In the USA, seropositive rates up to 2–5% have been reported in some populations.

E histolytica exists as two forms in the lumen and mucosal crypts of the large bowel: cysts (10–14 μm) and motile trophozoites (12–50 μm). In the absence of diarrhea, trophozoites encyst in the large bowel. Trophozoites passed into the environment die rapidly, but cysts remain viable in soil and water for several weeks to months at appropriate temperature and humidity.

Humans are the only established host and are universally susceptible. Only cysts are infectious, since after ingestion they survive gastric acidity whereas trophozoites are destroyed.

Transmission generally occurs through ingestion of cysts from fecally contaminated food or water. Flies and other arthropods also serve as mechanical vectors; to an undetermined degree, transmission results from contamination of food by the hands of food handlers. Where human excrement is used as fertilizer, it is often a source of food and water contamination. Person-to-person contact is also important in transmission; therefore, all household members as well as an infected person's sexual partner should have their stools examined. Sexual transmission of *E histolytica* among male homosexuals in some temperate urban areas is predominantly of nonpathogenic strains. In closed institutions such as mental hospitals, prevalence rates as high as 50% have been reported. Amebiasis is rarely epidemic, but urban outbreaks have occurred because of common-source water contamination.

Culture of organisms followed by isoenzyme analysis (not a convenient laboratory method) has resulted in 22 zymodeme isolates from different parts of the world, of which nine have been associated with pathogenicity. Although the matter is controversial, evidence is increasing that the pathogenic and nonpathogenic strains of *E histolytica* are stable. If this is fully confirmed, nonpathogenic strains would not need to be treated, including infections in AIDS patients. Malnutrition and alcoholism probably predispose to enhanced virulence. Corticosteroids and other immunosuppressive drugs often convert a commensal infection to an invasive one. Women in late pregnancy and the puerperium are especially susceptible. Tissue invasion elicits both humoral (IgM and IgG) antibodies and a cellular immune response, but humoral antibody titers do not correlate with protective immunity.

The characteristic intestinal lesion is the amebic ulcer, which can occur anywhere in the large bowel (including the appendix) and sometimes in the terminal ileum but predominates in the cecum, descending colon, and the rectosigmoid colon—areas of greatest fecal stasis. Trophozoites invade the colonic mucosa by means of their ameboid movement and proteolytic secretions and induce necrosis to form the characteristic flask-shaped ulcers. Ulcers are usually limited to the muscularis, but if penetration to the serous layer occurs, bowel perforation, local abscess, or generalized peritonitis may result. In fulminating cases, ulceration may be extensive, and the bowel becomes thin and friable. Hepatic abscesses range from a few millimeters to 15 cm or larger, usually are single, occur more often in the right lobe (particularly the upper portion), and are more common in men.

Clinical Findings

A. Symptoms and Signs: Amebiasis can be classified into intestinal and extraintestinal disease and further subdivided into the clinical syndromes described below. Some patients have an acute onset of severe diarrhea as early as 8 days (commonly 2–4 weeks) after infection. Others may have an asymptomatic or mild intestinal infection for months to several years before either intestinal symptoms or liver abscess appears. Transition may occur from one type of intestinal infection to another, and each may give rise to hepatic abscess, or the intestinal infection may clear spontaneously.

1. Intestinal amebiasis–
a. Asymptomatic infection–In most infected persons, the organism lives as a commensal, and the patient is without symptoms.

b. Mild to moderate colitis (nondysenteric colitis)–A few stools a day are passed that are semiformed and have mucus but no blood. There may be abdominal cramps, flatulence, fatigue, and weight loss. Periods of remission and recurrence may last days to weeks or longer; during remissions, the patient may have constipation. Abdominal examination may show distention, hyperperistalsis, and tenderness. In some patients with chronic infection, the colon is thick and palpable, particularly over the cecum and descending colon.

c. Severe colitis (dysenteric colitis)–As the severity of intestinal infection increases, the number of stools increases, and they change from semiformed to liquid with streaks of blood beginning to appear. With larger numbers of stools, 10–20 or more, little fecal material is present, but blood (fresh or dark) and bits of necrotic tissue become increasingly evident. With increasing severity, the patient may become prostrate and toxic, with fever up to 40.5 °C (104.9 °F), and have colic, tenesmus, vomiting, generalized abdominal tenderness, and nonspecific hepatic enlargement and tenderness. Rare complications include appendicitis, bowel perforation (followed by peritonitis, pericolonic abscess, retroperitoneal fecal cellulitis, fistula to the abdominal surface), and fulminating colitis (with paralytic ileus, hypotension, massive mucosal sloughing, and hemorrhage). Death may follow.

d. Localized ulcerative lesions of the colon–Bowel ulcerations limited to the rectal area may result in passage of formed stools with bloody exudate. Ulcerations limited to the cecum may induce mild diarrhea and simulate acute appendicitis. Amebic appendicitis, in which the appendix is extensively involved but not the remainder of the large bowel, is rare.

e. Localized granulomatous lesions of the colon (ameboma)–This occurs as a result of excessive production of granulation tissue in response to amebic infection, either in the course of dysentery or slowly in chronic intestinal infection. These masses may present as an irregular tumor (single or multiple) that projects into the bowel or as an annular constricting mass up to several centimeters in length. Clinical findings (pain, obstructive symptoms, and hemorrhage) and x-ray findings may simulate bowel carcinoma, inflammatory bowel disease, tuberculosis, or lymphogranuloma venereum. At endoscopy, the mass is deep red and bleeds easily, and biopsy specimens show granulation tissue and *E histolytica,* though the number of organisms may be relatively few. Antiamebic drugs are usually adequate in treatment; surgical removal of the lesion without prior or immediate postoperative drug therapy is likely to result in death of the patient.

2. Extraintestinal amebiasis–
a. Hepatic amebiasis–Amebic liver abscess, although a relatively infrequent consequence of intestinal amebiasis, is not uncommon given the large number of intestinal infections. A large proportion of patients with liver abscess do not have concurrent intestinal symptoms, nor can they recall having had chronic intestinal symptoms. The onset of symptoms can be sudden or gradual, ranging from a few days to many months. Cardinal manifestations are fever

(often high), pain (continuous, stabbing, or pleuritic, and sometimes severe), and an enlarged and tender liver. Patients may also experience malaise or prostration, sweating, chills, anorexia, and weight loss. The liver enlargement may present subcostally, in the epigastrium, as a localized bulging of the rib cage, or, as a result of enlargement against the dome of the diaphragm, it may produce coughing and findings at the right lung base (dullness to percussion, rales, and diminished breath sounds). Intercostal tenderness is common. Localizing signs on the skin may be an area of edema or a point of maximum tenderness. Without prompt treatment, the hepatic abscess may rupture into the pleural, peritoneal, or pericardial space or other contiguous organs, and death may follow.

b. Nonspecific hepatic enlargement–A low-grade, nonspecific enlargement of the liver—in which amebic liver infection is not present—may accompany invasive amebic bowel disease. It disappears with eradication of the amebic bowel infection and without use of specific drugs required to eradicate an amebic liver infection.

3. Other extraintestinal infections–Skin infections may develop in the perianal area. Metastatic infection may rarely occur throughout the body, particularly the lungs, brain, and genitalia.

B. Laboratory Findings:

1. Intestinal amebiasis–Three specimens obtained under optimal conditions will generally detect only 80% of amebic infections, and three additional tests will raise the diagnostic rate to about 90%. Trophozoites predominate in liquid stools, cysts in formed stools.

A standard procedure is to collect three specimens at 2-day intervals or longer, with one of the three obtained after a laxative such as (1) sodium sulfate or phosphate (Fleet's Phospho-Soda), 30–60 g in a glass of water; or (2) bisacodyl 5–15 mL). Oil laxatives such as mineral oil should not be used. Specimens should be collected in a clean container. Because trophozoites rapidly autolyze, specimens should be examined within about 30 minutes or should immediately be mixed with a preservative.

If the patient has received specific therapy, antibiotics, antimalarials, antidiarrheal preparations (containing bismuth, kaolin, or magnesium hydroxide), barium, or mineral oil, specimen collection should be delayed 10–14 days.

On sigmoidoscopic examination, no findings are typical in mild intestinal disease; in severe disease, ulcers may be found that are 1 mm to 2 cm across, with intact intervening mucosa. If present, exudate should be collected with a glass pipette (not with cotton, to which trophozoites may adhere) or by scraping with a metal curette and examined immediately. The colon should not be cleansed before sigmoidoscopy, since this washes exudate from ulcers and destroys trophozoites. In some centers, rectal biopsy has enhanced diagnosis; the specimens are best ex-

amined by immunofluorescence methods. Where possible, in vitro culture of amebas can be attempted.

Finding trophozoites that contain ingested red blood cells is diagnostic for invasive *E histolytica*, but they may be confused with the occasional macrophage that also contains red blood cells. *E histolytica* cysts and trophozoites must be differentiated from the other pathogenic and nonpathogenic intestinal protozoa.

In dysentery, the white blood cell count can reach 20,000 or higher, but it is not elevated in mild colitis. A low-grade eosinophilia is occasionally present.

Serologic testing for amebiasis is specific and usually positive if there has been substantial tissue invasion (as occurs in severe intestinal infection); in mild or asymptomatic intestinal infection, few patients are positive. The indirect hemagglutination test is sensitive and apparently produces no false-positive reactions. Positive titers persist for several years after successful treatment. The agar gel methods, though less sensitive, are rapidly conducted laboratory tests that measure current invasion; the tests become negative within about 3–6 months after eradication of infection. ELISA, DNA probes, and other methods continue to be evaluated for detection of the organism or its antigen in stool or liver abscess aspirate.

2. Hepatic abscess–The size and location of abscess can be determined by ultrasonography (usually round or oval lesions, abrupt transition from normal liver to the lesion, hypoechoic center with diffuse echoes throughout the abscess), CT (well-defined, round, low-density lesions with an internal, nonhomogeneous structure), and radioisotope scanning. After intravenous injection of contrast material, CT may show a hyperdense halo around the periphery of the abscess. Elevation of the right dome of the diaphragm, with diminished motility, is well demonstrated by chest x-ray, fluoroscopy, and ultrasound. Serologic tests are usually positive, but stools often no longer contain the parasite. The white count ranges from 15,000 to 25,000/μL. Eosinophilia is not present. Liver function test abnormalities, when present, are usually minimal. In many patients, aspiration is indicated for diagnosis and, if the abscess is large, for therapy as well to prevent rupture. Aspiration risks are hemorrhage and bacterial infection; therefore, aspiration should be done under aseptic conditions. The aspirate is divided into serial 30- to 50-mL aliquots, but only the last sample is examined, as organisms are found only at the edge of the abscess.

Differential Diagnosis

Amebiasis should be considered in patients with acute or chronic diarrhea (including cases associated with only mild changes in bowel habits in patients who have an exposure history), liver abscess, and annular lesions of the colon. The infection is more likely to occur in persons residing in or travelers returning from endemic areas, in individuals intimately associated with known cases, and in homosexual men. All patients with presumed inflammatory bowel disease should be tested serologically and by multiple stool examinations because of the risk of overwhelming amebic disease if corticosteroid therapy were to be given in the presence of amebiasis.

Treatment

The choice of drug depends on the type of clinical presentation and the site of drug action. Treatment may require the concurrent or sequential use of several drugs. Table 34–1 outlines a preferred and an alternative method of treatment for each clinical type of amebiasis.

The **tissue amebicides** dehydroemetine and emetine act on organisms in the bowel wall and in other tissues but not on amebas in the bowel lumen. Chloroquine is active principally against amebas in the liver. The **luminal amebicides** diloxanide furoate, iodoquinol, and paromomycin act on organisms in the bowel lumen but are ineffective against amebas in the bowel wall or other tissues. Oral tetracycline inhibits the bacterial associates of *E histolytica* and thus has an indirect effect on amebas in the bowel lumen and bowel wall but not in other tissues. Given parenterally, antibiotics have little antiamebic activity at any site. Metronidazole is unique in that it is effective both in the bowel lumen and in the bowel wall and other tissues. However, metronidazole when used alone for bowel infections is not sufficient as a luminal amebicide, for it fails to cure up to 50% of infections. Metronidazole also reaches the central nervous system.

A. Asymptomatic Intestinal Infection: Cure rates with a single course of diloxanide furoate or iodoquinol are 80–85%. Usually in asymptomatic infection, a tissue amebicidal drug is not given to prevent liver infection. Other alternatives for treatment or re-treatment are paromomycin or metronidazole plus iodoquinol or diloxanide furoate.

B. Mild to Moderate Intestinal Infection: When iodoquinol is used, concomitant use of tetracycline probably increases intestinal cure rates. It is less well established that adding a tetracycline to diloxanide furoate therapy increases effectiveness. Chloroquine is used to destroy trophozoites carried to the liver or to eradicate an undetected early-stage amebic liver abscess; the minimum dose needed to accomplish this is not known. In endemic areas where intestinal infection and reinfection are common yet hepatic abscess is rare (eg, in urban communities where intestinal amebiasis is sexually transmitted among male homosexuals but hepatic amebiasis is uncommon), it is probably unnecessary to use chloroquine in the treatment of mild intestinal disease.

C. Severe Intestinal Infection: Fluid and electrolyte therapy and opiates to control bowel motility are necessary adjuncts to specific therapy. Though opiates relieve symptoms, they should be used cautiously because of the potential risk of toxic megacolon.

D. Hepatic Abscess: Hospitalization and bed rest are necessary. When metronidazole is given for 10 days, early or late treatment failure occurs rarely. If a satisfactory clinical response has not occurred within 2–3 days, especially if the abscess has been adequately drained, therapy should be changed to the alternative mode of treatment: dehydroemetine (or emetine) plus chloroquine. When the clinical response to metronidazole is adequate, it is suggested that a 2-week course of chloroquine follow to prevent rare late failures. The need for adding this course of chloroquine remains to be evaluated. Either mode of treatment also requires a luminal amebicide (diloxanide furoate or iodoquinol), whether or not the organism is found in the stool. Antibiotics are added only when there is concomitant bacterial liver abscess, which is rare. However, metronidazole itself is highly effective against anaerobic bacteria, a major cause of bacterial liver abscesses. After successful treatment, imaging defects in the liver disappear slowly (range: 3–130 months); some calcify.

The indications for therapeutic aspiration are still controversial. Aspiration is clearly indicated, however, when the diagnosis is in doubt, if a large abscess is present that may rupture, or if there is a lack of response to therapy. A preferred method by many workers is percutaneous drainage under ultrasound guidance, followed by intralesional administration of metronidazole.

E. Adverse Drug Reactions: Metronidazole often induces transient nausea or vomiting; if alcohol is taken during or shortly after treatment, a disulfiram-like reaction may occur. Metronidazole increases the rate of naturally occurring tumors in mice but not in nonrodent species. However, some authorities consider the drug to be essentially free of cancer risk in humans. Nevertheless, prudence requires that metronidazole be given to pregnant or nursing mothers or to young children only if other drugs cannot be used.

Dehydroemetine and emetine cause nausea, vomiting, and pain at the injection site. They are general protoplasmic poisons that have adverse effects on many tissues (particularly the heart) and a narrow range between therapeutic and toxic effects; dehydroemetine may be the safer of the two drugs. The tetracyclines should not be used for children under age 8 years or for pregnant women; use erythromycin stearate instead, even though it is less effective. Iodoquinol may cause mild, transient diarrhea; neurotoxicity has not been reported at standard doses. Flatulence is common with diloxanide furoate. Paromomycin may cause mild gastrointestinal symptoms, infrequently intense diarrhea, and rarely overgrowth of nonsusceptible organisms.

Table 34–1. Treatment of amebiasis.

	Drug(s) of Choice	Alternative Drug(s)
Asymptomatic intestinal infection	Diloxanide furoate[1,2]	Iodoquinol (diiodohydroxyquin)[3] or paromomycin[4]
Mild to moderate intestinal infection (non-dysenteric colitis)	(1) Metronidazole[5] **plus** (2) Diloxanide furoate[2] or iodoquinol[3]	(1) Diloxanide furoate[2] or iodoquinol[3] **plus** (2) A tetracycline[6] **followed by** (3) Chloroquine[7] **or** (1) Paromomycin[4] **followed by** (2) Chloroqune[7]
Severe intestinal infection (dysentery)	(1) Metronidazole[8] **plus** (2) Diloxanide furoate[2] or iodoquinol[3] **If parenteral therapy is needed initially:** (1) Intravenous metronidazole[9] until oral therapy can be started; (2) Then give oral metronidazole[8] plus diloxanide furoate[2] or iodoquinol[3]	(1) A tetracycline[6] **plus** (2) Diloxanide furoate[2] or iodoquinol[3] **followed by** (3) Chloroquine[10] **or** (1) Dehydroemetine[1,11] or emetine[11] **followed by** (2) A tetracycline[6] plus diloxanide furoate[2] or iodoquinol[3] **followed by** (3) Chloroquine[10]
Hepatic abscess	(1) Metronidazole[8,9] **plus** (2) Diloxanide furoate[2] or iodoquinol[3] **followed by** (3) Chloroquine[10]	(1) Dehydroemetine[1,12] or emetine[12] **followed by** (2) Chloroquine[13] **plus** (3) Diloxanide furoate[2] or iodoquinol[3]
Ameboma or extraintestinal infection	As for hepatic abscess, but not including chloroquine	As for hepatic abscess, but not including chloroquine

[1]Available in the USA only from the Parasitic Disease Drug Service, Centers for Disease Control and Prevention, Atlanta 30333. Telephone requests may be made by calling the central number: (404) 639-3356 days; 329-2888 nights, weekends, and holidays (emergencies only).

[2]Diloxanide furoate, 500 mg three times daily with meals for 10 days (for children, 20 mg/kg in three divided doses daily for 10 days).

[3]Iodoquinol (diiodohydroxyquin), 650 mg three times daily for 21 days (for children, 30–40 mg/kg [maximum 2 g] in three divided doses daily for 21 days).

[4]Paromomycin, 25–35 mg/kg (base) (maximum 3 g) in three divided doses after meals daily for 7 days (for children, the same dosage).

[5]Metronidazole, 750 mg three times daily for 10 days (for children, 35 mg/kg in three divided doses daily for 10 days).

[6]A tetracycline, 250 mg four times daily for 10 days; in severe dysentery, give 500 mg 4 times daily for the first 5 days, then 250 mg four times daily for 5 days. Tetracycline should not be used during pregnancy or in children under 8 years of age; in older children, give 20 mg/kg in four divided doses daily for 10 days).

[7]Chloroquine, 500 mg (salt) daily for 7 days (for children, 16 mg/kg (salt) daily for 7 days.

[8]Metronidazole, 750 mg three times daily for 10 days (for children, 35–40 mg/kg in three divided doses daily for 10 days).

[9]An intravenous metronidazole formulation is available; change to oral medication as soon as possible. See manufacturer's recommendation for dosage.

[10]Chloroquine, 500 mg (salt) daily for 14 days (for children, 16 mg/kg [salt] daily for 14 days.

[11]Dehydroemetine or emetine, 1 mg/kg subcutaneously (preferred) or intramuscularly daily for the least number of days necessary to control severe symptoms (usually 3–5 days) (maximum daily dose for dehydroemetine is 90 mg; for emetine, 65 mg). For children, the daily dose is divided into two parts.

[12]Use dosage recommended in footnote 11 for 8–10 days.

[13]Chloroquine, 500 mg (salt) orally twice daily for 2 days then 500 mg orally daily for 19 days (for children, 16 mg/kg [salt] daily for 21 days).

Follow-Up Care

In follow-up, examine at least three stools at 2- to 3-day intervals, starting 2–4 weeks after the end of treatment. For some patients, sigmoidoscopy and re-examination of stools within 3 months may be indicated.

Postdysenteric colitis is an uncommon sequela of severe amebic colitis. Following adequate treatment, diarrhea continues and the mucosa may be reddened and edematous, but no ulcers or organisms are found. Most such cases are self-limited, with permanent remission in weeks to months. Uncommonly, the diarrhea may be profound and unremitting and in some instances probably represents ulcerative colitis triggered by the amebic infection.

Prevention & Control

Prevention requires safe water supplies, sanitary disposal of human feces, adequate cooking of foods to destroy cysts, protection of foods from fly contamination, washing hands after defecation and before preparing or eating foods, and, in endemic areas, avoidance of foods that cannot be cooked or peeled. Water supplies can be boiled (briefly) or treated with iodine (0.5 mL tincture of iodine per liter for 20 minutes, or longer if the water is cold). Filters are also available to purify drinking water. Disinfection dips for fruits and vegetables are not advised, and no drug is safe or effective in prophylaxis.

Prognosis

The mortality rate from untreated amebic dysentery, hepatic abscess, or ameboma may be high. With modern chemotherapy instituted early in the course of the disease, the prognosis is good.

Barreda R, Ros PR: Diagnostic imaging of liver abscess. Crit Rev Diagn Imaging 1992;33:29.

Filice C et al. Outcome of hepatic amebic abscesses managed with three different therapeutic strategies. Dig Dis Sci 1992;37:240.

McAuley JB et al: Diloxanide furoate for treating asymptomatic *Entamoeba histolytica* cyst passers: 14 years' experience in the United States. Clin Infect Dis 1992; 15:464.

Reed S: Amebiasis: An update. Clin Infect Dis 1992;14: 385.

Reitano M, Masci JR, Bottone EJ: Amebiasis: Clinical and laboratory perspectives. Clin Rev Clin Lab Sci 1991; 28:357.

PATHOGENIC FREE-LIVING AMEBAS

Primary Amebic Meningoencephalitis

Primary amebic meningoencephalitis is a fulminating, purulent meningoencephalitis that resembles bacterial meningitis and is rapidly fatal. Most infections have been recognized in children and young adults. The usual responsible organisms are free-living ameboflagellates of the genus *Naegleria;* most cases are due to *Naegleria fowleri.* Other causative agents include *Acanthamoeba* species (see below) and the leptomyxid ameba, which has caused rare infections in immunosuppressed persons, including one AIDS patient.

N fowleri is a thermophilic organism found in fresh and polluted warm lake water, domestic water supplies, swimming pools, thermal water, and sewers. Most patients give a history of exposure to fresh water; dust is also a possible source of infection. Nasal and throat swabs have shown that there is a human carrier state, and serologic surveys suggest that inapparent infections occur.

The organism apparently invades the central nervous system through the cribriform plate. The incubation period varies from 1 to 14 days. Early symptoms include headache, fever, and lethargy, often associated with rhinitis and pharyngitis. Vomiting, disorientation, and other signs of meningoencephalitis develop within 1 or 2 days, followed by coma and then death on the fifth or sixth day. At autopsy, some victims have a nonspecific myocarditis.

Lumbar or ventricular cerebrospinal fluid contains several hundred to 25,000 leukocytes/μL (50–100% neutrophils) and erythrocytes (up to several thousand/μL). Protein is usually somewhat elevated and glucose moderately reduced. If conventional examinations for bacteria and fungi are negative, the fluid must then be examined for free-living amebas to make the specific diagnosis. A wet mount examined by an ordinary optical microscope with the aperture restricted or condenser down will enhance contrast and refractility; a warm stage is not needed. The fluid should not be centrifuged or refrigerated, as this tends to immobilize the amebas. Their brisk motility distinguishes them from leukocytes of various types, which they closely resemble. Culture and mouse inoculation studies should also be performed. Serologic testing for antibody and circulating antigen is experimental.

Precise species identification is based on morphology, demonstration of flagellate transformation (*Naegleria* only), and various immunologic studies.

Only two well-documented survivors have been reported. One was treated with intravenous and intrathecal amphotericin B and the other with a combination of amphotericin B, miconazole, and rifampin. Experimental studies have shown a marked synergistic effect between amphotericin B and either tetracycline or rifampin.

Acanthamoeba Infections

Free-living amebas of the genus *Acanthamoeba* are found in soil and in fresh, brackish, and thermal water as trophozoites (15–45 μm) or cysts (10–25 μm). Several species have been recognized only recently as human pathogens that cause a number of poorly defined syndromes: (1) a subacute and chronic focal granulomatous necrotizing meningoencephalitis that invariably has led to death in weeks to months, (2) skin lesions that resemble deep fungal infections, (3) granulomatous dissemination to many tissues, and (4) uveitis or chronic keratitis that may lead to blindness. Portals of entry may include the skin, eyes, or respiratory tract. A commensal nasal carrier state is established. Immunocompromised patients, including HIV-infected persons, may have increased susceptibility.

In the encephalitis syndrome, cerebrospinal fluid lymphocytosis has been described. Antemortem diagnosis has been made via biopsy specimens. The presence of distinctive cysts or mitotic division in tissue section may be pathognomonic of *Acanthamoeba* infection. Serology may be helpful. No treatment has been effective, but ketoconazole, miconazole, sulfonamides, clotrimazole, pentamidine, paromomycin, or flucytosine can be tried.

More than 200 cases of *Acanthamoeba* keratitis have been identified in the USA since 1981, most associated with wearing contact lenses, penetrating corneal trauma, or exposure to contaminated water. The clinical features suggestive of *Acanthamoeba* keratitis are (1) severe ocular pain, (2) partial or 360-degree paracentral stromal ring infiltrate on ophthalmologic examination, (3) recurrent corneal epithelial breakdown, and (4) a corneal lesion refractory to the usual medications. Typically, the keratitis progresses slowly over months. The diagnosis can be confirmed by vigorously scraping the cornea with a swab or platinum-tipped scapula. The material is microscopically examined after staining with Giemsa's or trichrome stain or by immunofluorescent techniques and is also placed in culture on nonnutrient agar seeded with *Escherichia coli*.

Although there is no established treatment for *Acanthamoeba* keratitis, a number of antimicrobials have been effective. One approach employs systemic ketoconazole and topical propamidine isethionate, miconazole, clotrimazole, and neomycin-polymyxin. Oral itraconazole with topical miconazole has shown promise. In spite of medical treatment, penetrating keratoplasty is often necessary to excise diseased tissue. Corticosteroid therapy is controversial.

Prevention requires use of disinfectant solutions to clean contact lenses; a recent report, however, showed that they were inadequate in destroying *Acanthamoeba* cysts when used for less than 6 hours.

Anzil AP et al: Amebic meningoencephalitis in a patient with AIDS caused by a newly recognized opportunistic pathogen, leptomyxid ameba. Arch Pathol Lab Med 1991;115:21.
Larkin DF: *Acanthamoeba* keratitis: Int Ophthalmol Clin 1991;31:163.
Ma P et al: *Naegleria* and *Acanthamoeba* infections: Review. Rev Infect Dis 1990;12:490.
Martinez AJ: Infection of the central nervous system due to *Acanthamoeba*. Rev Infect Dis 1991:13(Suppl 5):S399.
May LP, Sidhu GS, Buchness MR: Diagnosis of *Acanthamoeba* infection by cutaneous manifestations in a man seropositive to HIV. J Am Acad Dermatol 1992;26:352.

BABESIOSIS
(Piroplasmosis)

Babesia are tick-borne protozoal parasites of wild and domestic animals worldwide. Babesiosis in humans is a rare intraerythrocytic infection caused by two *Babesia* species. The infection has been recognized only in Europe *(Babesia divergens)* and North America *(Babesia microti),* but it has the potential to occur worldwide.

In the USA, B microti has been found in coastal and island areas of northeast and mid-Atlantic states as well as in Wisconsin, Minnesota, and California. Natural hosts for B microti are various wild and domestic animals, particularly the white-footed mouse and white-tailed deer. With extension of the deer's habitat, the range of human infection appears to be increasing as well. Serosurveys show frequent subclinical B microti infections. Humans are infected as a result of *Ixodes dammini* tick bites, but transmission from blood transfusion has also been reported. Without passing through an exoerythrocytic stage, the parasite enters the red blood cell and multiplies, resulting in cell rupture followed by infection of other cells. Splenectomized, elderly, or immunosuppressed persons are the most likely to have severe manifestations.

The incubation period is 1–4 weeks, but patients usually do not recall the tick bite. B microti infection lasts a few weeks to a month; the illness is characterized by irregular fever, chills, headache, diaphoresis, myalgia, and fatigue but is without malaria-like periodicity of symptoms. Most patients have a moderate hemolytic anemia, and some have hemoglobinuria or hepatosplenomegaly. Although parasitemia may continue for months, with or without symptoms, the disease is self-limited and most patients recover without sequelae.

Only a few B divergens infections have been reported, all in splenectomized patients. These infections progress rapidly with high fever, severe hemolytic anemia, jaundice, hemoglobinuria, and renal failure; death usually follows.

Diagnosis is by identification of the intraerythrocytic parasite (2–3 μm) on Giemsa-stained thick or thin blood smears; no gametocytes and no intracellular pigment are seen. A single red cell may contain different stages of the parasite. Repeated smears may be necessary. The organism must be differentiated from malarial parasites, particularly *Plasmodium falciparum*. Isolation of the parasite can be attempted by inoculating patient blood into hamsters or gerbils.

Serologic tests are available; serologic cross-reactions occur between *Babesia* and malaria parasites, but antibody titers are generally highest to the infecting organism.

No drug treatment is satisfactory. As *B microti* infections in patients with intact spleen are usually self-limiting, most infections can be treated symptomatically. In splenectomized patients, however, limited experience suggests that quinine (650 mg three times a day for 7 days) plus clindamycin (1.2 g twice daily parenterally or 600 mg three times a day orally for 7 days) may be useful; exchange transfusion has also been successful in several splenectomized patients. The only patients who have recovered from *B divergens* infections have been managed with transfusions and renal dialysis. Combined pentamidine and trimethoprim-sulfamethoxazole were reported to be curative for one patient.

Persing DH et al: Detection of *Babesia microti* by polymerase chain reaction. J Clin Microbiol 1992;30:2079.

Ruebush TK II: Babesiosis. In: *Tropical Medicine and Parasitology.* Goldsmith R, Heyneman D (editors). Appleton & Lange, 1989.

BALANTIDIASIS

Balantidium coli is a large ciliated intestinal protozoan found worldwide, but particularly in the tropics. Infection results from ingestion of cysts passed in stools of humans or swine, the reservoir hosts. In the new host, the cyst wall dissolves and the trophozoite may invade the mucosa and submucosa of the terminal ileum and large bowel, causing abscesses and irregularly rounded ulcerations. Many infections are asymptomatic and probably need not be treated. Chronic recurrent diarrhea, alternating with constipation, is most common, but severe dysentery with bloody mucoid stools, tenesmus, and colic may occur intermittently.

Diagnosis is established by finding trophozoites in liquid stools, cysts in formed stools, or the trophozoite in scrapings or biopsy of ulcers of the large bowel. Specimens must be examined rapidly or placed in preservative.

The treatment of choice is tetracycline hydrochloride, 500 mg four times daily for 10 days. The alternative drug is iodoquinol (diiodohydroxyquin), 650 mg three times daily for 21 days. Occasional success has also been reported with metronidazole (750 mg three times daily for 5 days) or paromomycin (25–30 mg/kg [base] in three divided doses for 5–10 days).

In properly treated mild to moderate symptomatic cases, the prognosis is good, but in spite of treatment, fatalities have occurred in severe infections as a result of intestinal perforation or hemorrhage.

Knight R: Giardiasis, isosporiasis and balantidiasis. Clin Gastroenterol 1978;7:31.

COCCIDIOSIS: ISOSPORIASIS, CRYPTOSPORIDIOSIS, SARCOCYSTOSIS

Coccidiosis is an intestinal infection usually accompanied by diarrhea and abdominal discomfort and caused by coccidia of three genera: *Isospora, Cryptosporidium,* and *Sarcocystis.* These infections occur worldwide but except for *Cryptosporidium* are recognized only sporadically.

General Considerations

A. Isosporiasis: Isosporiasis, caused by *Isospora belli,* is considered host-specific for humans, with transmission directly from person to person. Infection is by the fecal-oral route following ingestion of oocysts. Sporozoites excyst and invade jejunal and duodenal epithelial cells, in which they undergo both a sexual and an asexual cycle, resulting in the liberation of unsporulated oocysts, $20–30 \times 10–20 \ \mu m$, into the feces. Forty-eight hours are usually required for the oocyst to mature to infectivity.

The incubation period is 7–11 days. Some patients remain asymptomatic. Most symptomatic infections follow a benign, self-limited course lasting a few weeks or months. The principal findings are diarrhea, vague abdominal pain, flatulence, low-grade fever, vomiting, malaise, and anorexia. Infrequently, the disease is protracted (months to years) or recurrent; when severe, there may be intense diarrhea, steatorrhea, malabsorption, and weight loss. Several deaths have been reported. Isosporiasis, sometimes severe, is seen as an opportunistic infection in AIDS.

The diagnosis is made by finding the parasite in feces or duodenal aspirates or by duodenal biopsy. Diagnosis by stool examination is often difficult, for the organisms may be scanty even in the presence of significant symptoms. The laboratory should be notified of the need to search for the organisms, so that special concentration techniques (zinc sulfate or sugar flotation) will be used. Because of their buoyancy, oocysts must be looked for just beneath the coverslip of the preparation. Although the peroral duodenal string test or duodenal aspiration may also assist in diagnosis, frequently diagnosis can be made only after duodenal biopsy and search of multiple serial sections. Up to 50% of patients with isosporiasis have eosinophilia. Serologic tests are not available.

B. Cryptosporidiosis: *Cryptosporidium,* which causes diarrhea and respiratory infections in many animal species, has only recently been recognized in humans worldwide as a cause of sporadic mild diarrhea in all ages, acute childhood diarrhea (particularly in developing countries), traveler's diarrhea, and severe diarrhea in immunocompromised persons, particularly those with AIDS. Outbreaks in day care centers, clustering in families, and water-borne outbreaks have been reported. Stool surveys and duodenal aspiration in immunocompetent persons show an asymptomatic carrier state. It remains unsettled whether more than one species exists; *C parvum* is currently considered the agent responsible for infection in humans.

Fecal-oral transmission is from animals to humans or humans to humans; water-borne transmission is also important. Oocysts (about 4 μm in diameter) passed in stool are fully sporulated and infectious; infection occurs as a result of their ingestion. The incubation period appears to be 2–10 days. In humans as well as in animals, the full life cycle of *Cryptosporidium* occurs within a single host—asexual and sexual proliferation and parasite amplification. The organisms attach to the microvillous borders of enterocytes of the small bowel and also are found free in mucosal crypts. The host cell membrane deteriorates, leaving the parasitic membrane in direct contact with epithelial cell cytoplasm. The organisms do not, however, invade the tissues. Voluminous secretory or malabsorptive diarrhea results, but the mechanism has not been elucidated. *Cryptosporidium* infection has been associated with malnutrition; in some malnourished patients, the organism has been implicated in respiratory tract disease.

In immunocompetent persons, infection varies from no symptoms to mild enteritis to marked watery diarrhea (up to ten stools daily) without mucus or gross or microscopic blood. Accompanying findings may include low-grade fever, malaise, nausea, vomiting, abdominal cramps, and, sometimes, anorexia and weight loss. The infection is generally self-limited and lasts a few days to about 2 weeks. Occasionally observed are a malabsorption state with failure to thrive in children.

In immunologically deficient patients—especially those with AIDS—the illness is characterized by profuse (up to 15 L daily has been reported), cholera-like watery diarrhea and by severe malabsorption, electrolyte imbalance, marked weight loss, and lymphadenopathy; fever is uncommon. The diarrhea may recur or persist for months and contribute to death. In AIDS, infection may involve any part of the gastrointestinal tract, including the biliary tract; and multisystem involvement has also been described.

Diagnosis is by detection of oocysts in stool by a variety of flotation or concentration methods or by finding developomental stages in small bowel mucosal biopsies. Special stains are required that use a modified acid-fast stain (routine fecal staining methods do not detect the organism). Three stools submitted fresh or in preservative should be examined over 5–7 days, and—as for *Isospora*—the laboratory should be notified that *Cryptosporidium* is being sought. Current methods may lack sensitivity; the threshold of detection may be as high as 50,000 cysts per gram of feces. Stools are free of white or red blood cells. Peripheral blood leukocytosis and eosinophilia are uncommon. Serodiagnostic tests have been developed, including ELISA and immunofluorescent tests that detect IgG and IgM antibody, but they are not yet useful in diagnosing acute disease. Radiologic changes have been reported in the stomach, intestines, and bile ducts in severe disease. In AIDS patients with unexplained diarrhea, the organism should also be looked for in sputum and specimens obtained from lung tissue if stool specimens are negative.

C. Sarcocystosis: *Sarcocystis* is a two-host coccidian. Human disease occurs as two syndromes, both rare: (1) an enteric infection in which humans are the definitive host and (2) a muscle infection in which humans are an intermediate host. In the enteric form, sporocysts passed in human feces are not infective for humans but must be ingested by cattle or pigs. Humans become infected by eating poorly cooked beef or pork containing oocysts of *Sarcocystis bovihominis* or *Sarcocystis suihominis,* respectively. (Formerly, the causative agent was known as *Isospora hominis.*) Organisms enter intestinal epithelial cells and are transformed into oocysts that release sporocysts into the feces. Clinically, the intestinal infection is often asymptomatic or causes mild but protracted diarrhea. Diagnosis is by stool examination using a fecal flotation method.

The muscle form of sarcocystosis results when humans ingest sporocysts in feces from an infected carnivore that has eaten prey which harbored sarcocysts. The sporocysts liberate sporozoites that invade the intestinal wall and are disseminated to skeletal muscle. This results in subcutaneous and muscular inflammation lasting several days to 2 weeks and the finding of swellings at these sites, sometimes associated with eosinophilia. Sarcocysts are often asymptomatic, however, such as those found incidentally at autopsy in cardiac muscle.

Treatment

In **isosporiasis,** instances of effective treatment have been described using (1) sulfadiazine, 4 g, and pyrimethamine, 35–75 mg, in four divided doses daily for 3–7 weeks; or (2) trimethoprim (160 mg) and sulfamethoxazole (800 mg) four times daily for 10 days and then twice daily for 3 weeks. Efficacy in primary infection has also been reported for furazolidone (400 mg/d for 10 days), nitrofurantoin, metronidazole, and quinacrine.

No treatment has been successful for **sarcocystosis** or **cryptosporidiosis.** Cryptosporidiosis in immunologically competent persons is a self-limiting disease, though nonspecific supportive measures may be needed. In cryptosporidiosis in immunologically incompetent persons, spiramycin (1 g three times daily for 2 weeks or longer), zidovudine (AZT), paromomycin, octreotide, and eflornithine have sometimes been reported to be of value. Supportive treatment includes fluid and electrolyte replacement and, in chronic cases, parenteral nutrition.

Clezy K et al: Paromomycin for the treatment of crypto-sporidial diarrhoea in AIDS patients. AIDS 1991;5:1146.

Gellin BG, Soave R: Coccidian infections in AIDS: Toxo-plasmosis, cryptosporidiosis, and isosporiasis. Med Clin North Am 1992;76:205.

Kreinik G et al: Successful management of intractable cryptosporidial diarrhea with intravenous octreotide, a somatostatin analogue. AIDS 1991;5:765.

GIARDIASIS

Essentials of Diagnosis

- Most infections are asymptomatic.
- In some cases, acute or chronic diarrhea, mild to severe, with bulky, greasy, frothy, malodorous stools, free of blood and pus.
- Upper abdominal discomfort, cramps, distention, excessive flatus, and lassitude.
- Cysts and occasionally trophozoites in stools.
- Trophozoites in duodenal fluid.

General Considerations

Giardiasis is a protozoal infection of the upper small intestine caused by the flagellate *Giardia lamblia.* The parasite occurs worldwide and is nearly universal in children in developing countries. In the USA and Europe, the infection is considered the most common intestinal protozoal pathogen. Persons of all ages are affected, but occurrence is particularly high among children.

The organism occurs in feces as a symmetric, heart-shaped flagellated trophozoite measuring 10–25 × 6–12 μm and as a cyst measuring 8–13 × 6–11 μm. Only the cyst form is infectious by the oral route; trophozoites are destroyed by gastric acidity. Humans are the reservoir for *Giardia,* but dogs and beavers have been implicated as a zoonotic source of infection.

Most infections are sporadic, resulting from cysts transmitted as a result of fecal contamination of water or food, by person-to-person contact, or by anal-oral sexual contact. Multiple infections are common in households, and outbreaks occur in nursery schools and mental institutions and as a result of contamination of water supplies. Giardiasis is a well-recognized problem in special groups including travelers, campers, male homosexuals, and persons with impaired immune states.

After the cysts are ingested, trophozoites emerge in the duodenum and jejunum. They can cause epithelial damage, atrophy of villi, hypertrophic crypts, and extensive cellular infiltration of the lamina propria by lymphocytes, plasma cells, and neutrophils. It is likely that hypogammaglobulinemia, low secretory IgA levels in the gut, achlorhydria, and malnutrition favor the development of infection. Giardiasis does not appear to be an opportunistic infection in AIDS.

Clinical Findings

A. Symptoms and Signs: A large proportion of infected persons remain asymptomatic cyst carriers, and their infection clears spontaneously. The clinical forms of giardiasis are (1) acute diarrhea, (2) chronic diarrhea, and (3) malabsorption syndrome. The incubation period is usually 1–3 weeks but may be longer. The illness may begin gradually or suddenly. The acute phase may last days or weeks, but it is usually self-limited, although cyst excretion may continue. In a few patients, the disorder may become chronic and last for years, but it does not appear to last indefinitely.

In both the acute and chronic forms, diarrhea ranges from mild to severe; most often it is mild. There may be no complaints other than of one bulky, loose bowel movement a day, often after breakfast. With larger numbers of movements, the stools become increasingly watery and may contain mucus but are usually free of blood and pus; they are copious, frothy, malodorous, and greasy. The diarrhea may be daily or recurrent; if recurrent, stools may be normal to mushy during intervening days, or the patient may be constipated. Weight loss and weakness may occur. Less common are anorexia, nausea and vomiting, midepigastric discomfort and cramps (often after meals), belching, flatulence, borborygmi, and abdominal distention. Low-grade fever is infrequent, and headache, urticaria, and myalgia are rare.

A malabsorption syndrome occasionally develops in the acute or chronic stage that may result in marked weight loss and debility. Findings may include fat- and protein-losing enteropathy and vitamin B_{12}, and disaccharidase deficiency. The latter may persist for a long time in persons apparently cured after specific treatment.

B. Laboratory Tests: Diagnosis is by identifying cysts or trophozoites in feces or duodenal fluid. Detection can be difficult, because the number of cysts passed varies considerably from day to day, and at the onset of infection, patients may have symptoms for about a week before organisms can be detected.

If clinically warranted, diagnostic accuracy can be increased by proceeding as follows: (1) routine stool examinations {aro} (2) examination of upper intestinal fluid by the duodenal string test (Entero-Test) or by duodenal aspiration {aro} (3) duodenal biopsy examined after permanent staining. Three stool specimens should be examined at intervals of 2 days or longer. Since the first specimen is positive in about 75% of patients with giardiasis, it is sometimes preferable to await negative reports before testing second or third specimens. Unless they can be submitted within an hour, specimens should be preserved immediately in a fixative. Purges do not increase the likelihood of finding the organism. Use of barium, antibiotics, antacids, kaolin products, or oily laxatives may temporarily reduce the number of parasites or interfere with detection, requiring a delay in further examination for about 10 days. Duodenal aspirate should be concentrated by centrifugation at 500 rpm for 5 minutes and be examined by wet mount and after permanent staining. Duodenal biopsy specimens should first be pressed onto a slide to obtain a mucosal imprint for staining and then be sectioned for histologic examination. Biopsy is rarely done, however; most workers prefer instead an empiric course of treatment after presumptive diagnosis.

Stool ELISAs to detect coproantigen are reported to have sensitivities and specificities between 90% and 95%. Commercial kits are available but as yet should be reservedfor situations where stool specimens are negative for *Giardia* and other pathogens. An ELISA developed for serum IgG antibody does not distinguish present from past infection; however, an IgM test appears to be more promising. Radiologic examination of the small bowel is usually normal in mildly ill persons but may show nonspecific findings of altered motility, thickened mucosal folds, and barium column segmentation in patients with marked symptoms.

Treatment

Symptomatic patients should be treated. Although controversial, treatment of asymptomatic patients should be considered since they can transmit the infection to others and may occasionally become symptomatic themselves. In selected instances of asymptomatic infection, it may be best to wait a few weeks before starting treatment, as some infections will clear spontaneously in the absence of treatment.

Treatment can be conducted effectively with tinidazole, metronidazole, quinacrine, or furazolidone. Occasional treatment failures require re-treatment with an alternative drug. Tinidazole, where available, is the drug of choice, based on reports that it is effective as a single dose. In follow-up, one should wait about 2 weeks before rechecking two or more stools at weekly intervals.

All of these drugs occasionally have unpleasant side effects. Drug resistance can occur, but is rare. The potential carcinogenicity of furazolidone, metronidazole, and tinidazole appears to be negligible based on 2 decades of use. None of the agents cure more than about 90% of cases.

A. Metronidazole: Adults receive 250 mg three times daily for 5–10 days; children receive 5 mg/kg three times daily for 5 days. Metronidazole may cause gastrointestinal symptoms, headache, a metallic taste, and candidal overgrowth. Patients must be warned that alcohol may cause a disulfiram-like reaction. Liquid suspensions for pediatric use are available only outside the USA.

B. Quinacrine (Mepacrine): For adults, the dose is 100 mg three times daily after meals for 5–7 days; for children, 2 mg/kg three times daily (maximum, 300 mg/d) for 5–7 days. The drug has a bitter taste. Gastrointestinal symptoms, headache, and dizziness are common; harmless yellowing of the skin is infrequent. Toxic psychosis and exfoliative dermatitis, which are rare, may be severe and long-lasting. Young children tend to tolerate the drug poorly. Quinacrine is contraindicated in psoriasis or in persons with a history of psychosis.

C. Furazolidone: This is the most convenient pediatric drug, dispensed as a suspension. Adults receive 100 mg (children, 1.25 mg/kg) four times daily for 7–10 days. Gastrointestinal symptoms, fever, headache, rash, and a disulfiram-like reaction with alcohol occur. Furazolidone can cause mild hemolysis in glucose-6-phosphate dehydrogenase-deficient persons and rarely causes hypersensitivity reactions.

D. Tinidazole: (not available in the USA), 2 g (children, 35 mg/kg) given once, has had reported cure rates of 90–100%. Adverse reactions consist of mild gastrointestinal side effects in about 10% of patients; headache and vertigo are less common.

E. Others–Albendazole continues under evaluation; in one study, young children treated with albendazole (400 mg/d) and metronidazole for 5 days had equivalent cure rates (over 95%). Reports with paromomycin have been mixed.

Prevention

There is no effective chemoprophylaxis for giardiasis. Prevention is as for amebiasis (above).

Prognosis

With treatment and successful eradication of the infection, there are no sequelae. Without treatment, severe malabsorption may rarely contribute to death from other causes.

Flanagan PA: Giardia: Diagnosis, clinical course and epidemiology. A review. Epidemiol Infect 1992;109:1.
Meyer EA (editor): *Giardiasis.* In: *Human Parasitic Diseases,* vol 3. Elsevier. 1990.
Wolfe M: Giardiasis. Clin Microbiol Rev 1992;5:93.

LEISHMANIASIS

Leishmaniasis is infection by species of the genus *Leishmania.* The disease is a zoonosis transmitted by bites of sandflies (*Phlebotomus* [Old World leishmaniasis] and *Lutzomyia* [New World leishmaniasis] species) from wild or domestic animal reservoirs to humans—except in the case of Indian kala azar, which is transmitted from human to human. Leishmaniae have two distinct forms in their life cycle: (1) In mammalian hosts, the parasite is found in its amastigote form (Leishman-Donovan bodies, 2–3 μm in length) within mononuclear phagocytes. When sandflies feed on an infected host, the parasitized cells are ingested with a blood meal. (2) In the sandfly vector, the parasite converts to and is then transmitted during feeding as a flagellated extracellular promastigote.

The taxonomy of leishmaniasis is complex and unsettled. One simplified clinical formulation is as follows:

(1) Visceral leishmaniasis (kala azar), caused by the *L donovani* group of agents and characterized by hepatosplenomegaly and anemia. Other species that principally cause visceral leishmaniasis are *L chagasi* (New World) and *L infantum* (Old World).

(2) Cutaneous leishmaniasis: (a) Old World moist, dry, or diffuse cutaneous leishmaniasis, caused by the *L tropica* complex; (b) New World cutaneous or diffuse cutaneous leishmaniasis, caused by the *L mexicana* complex.

(3) Mucocutaneous leishmaniasis (espundia), caused by the *L braziliensis* complex. Espundia is characterized by an initial cutaneous ulcer that is followed in months to years by destructive nasopharyngeal lesions.

Over 1 million cases of leishmaniasis and 5000 deaths are estimated to occur each year in tropical and temperate zones. Severity of infection ranges from subclinical or minimally pathogenic (self-healing or easily treated) to severely incapacitating, metastasizing, mutilating, and fatal.

Laboratory Tests

Laboratory methods for diagnosis of leishmaniasis vary by species of infecting organism. Definitive diagnosis is achieved by finding the parasite—either the amastigote in stained smears or biopsies, or the motile promastigote in culture. Serologic and skin tests provide only indirect evidence of infection.

Treatment

Treatment is less than adequate because of drug toxicity, long courses required, and frequent need for hospitalization. The drug of choice is sodium stibogluconate. Alternative drugs for some forms of infection—but generally more toxic—are amphotericin B and pentamidine.

A. Sodium Stibogluconate: Treatment is started with a 200-mg test dose, followed by 20 mg/kg/d. Although the drug can be administered as a 5% solution intramuscularly (may be locally painful), intravenous administration is preferred (cough may occur) when the volume is high, as is the case for most adults. The drug is provided as a solution that contains 100 mg of antimony per milliliter; only fresh solutions should be used. The appropriate volume of drug is mixed with 50 mL of 5% dextrose in water and infused over at least a 10-minute interval. The drug is given on consecutive days: 30 days for visceral and mucocutaneous leishmaniasis and 20 days for cutaneous leishmaniasis. Although few side effects occur initially, they are more likely to appear

with cumulative doses. Most common are gastrointestinal symptoms, fever, and rash; hemolytic anemia and liver, renal, and heart damage are rare. Patients should be monitored weekly for the first 3 weeks and twice weekly thereafter by serum chemistries, complete blood counts, and electrocardiography. Discontinue therapy if the following occur: aminotransferases three to four times normal levels or significant arrhythmias, corrected QT intervals greater than 0.50 s, or concave ST segments. Relapses should be treated at the same dosage level for at least twice the previous duration. In the USA, the drug is available only from the Parasitic Drug Service, Centers for Disease Control and Prevention, Atlanta 30333 ([404]) 639–3670).

B. Pentamidine Isethionate: Pentamidine isethionate, 2–4 mg/kg intramuscularly (preferable) or intravenously, is given daily or on alternate days (up to 15 injections).For some forms of visceral leishmaniasis, it may be necessary to treat for a longer period or to repeat treatment. For adverse reactions, see Pneumocystosis (below).

C. Amphotericin B: Amphotericin B is dissolved in 500 mL of 5% dextrose and injected slowly intravenously over 6 hours on alternate days. The initial dose of 0.25 mg/kg/d is gradually increased to 1 mg/kg/d (0.25 {aro} 0.5 {aro} 1) until a total of about 30 mg/kg is given.

Goldsmith R, Heyneman D (editors): Leishmaniases. In: *Tropical Medicine and Parasitology*. Appleton & Lange, 1989.

Grogl M, Thomason TN, Franke ED: Drug resistance in leishmaniasis: Its implications in systemic chemotherapy of cutaneous and mucocutaneous disease. Am J Trop Med Hyg 1992;47:117.

Herwaldt BL, Berman JD: Recommendations for treating leishmaniasis with sodium stibogluconate (Pentostam) and review of pertinent clinical studies. Am J Trop Med Hyg 1992; 46:296.

Mukherjee A, Seth M, Bhaduri AP: Present status of leishmaniasis. Prog Drug Res 1990;34:447.

1. VISCERAL LEISHMANIASIS (Kala azar)

Visceral leishmaniasis is caused mainly by the *Leishmania donovani* complex: (1) *L d donovani* (eastern India, Bangladesh, Southeast Asia, Sudan, Ethiopia, Kenya, scattered foci in central Africa, Soviet Central Asia, and China), (2) *L d infantum* (Mediterranean littoral, Middle East, Iran, Saudi Arabia, Afghanistan, Pakistan), and (3) *L d chagasi* (South America, Central America, Mexico). In each locale, the disease has its own peculiar clinical and epidemiologic features; India, China, and East Africa have had epidemics. Both *L tropica* in Africa and Saudi Arabia and *L mexicana amazonensis* in Brazil have also been shown to cause visceral leishmaniasis in a few patients. Although humans are the major reservoir, animal reservoirs such as the dog, other canids, and rodents are important. The incubation period is usually 4–6 months (range, 10 days to 24 months).

A local nonulcerating nodule at the site of the bite may precede systemic manifestations but usually is inapparent. The onset may be acute or insidious. Fever often peaks twice daily, with chills and sweats, weakness, weight loss, cough, and diarrhea. The spleen progressively becomes huge, hard, and nontender. The liver is somewhat enlarged, and generalized lymphadenopathy is common. Hyperpigmentation of skin, especially on the hands, feet, abdomen, and forehead, is marked in light-skinned patients. In blacks, there may be warty eruptions or skin ulcers. Petechiae, bleeding from the nose and gums, jaundice, and ascites may occur. In some regions, oral and nasopharyngeal or cutaneous manifestations occur with or without visceral involvement. Wasting is progressive; death, often due to intercurrent infection, occurs within months to 1–2 years.

Although the *L donovani* complex of species are primarily viscerotropic, they sometimes cause cutaneous lesions without visceral involvement.

Post-kala azar dermal leishmaniasis may appear 1–2 years after apparent cure (up to 10 years in India and China). It may simulate leprosy, as multiple hypopigmented macules or nodules develop on pre-existing lesions. Erythematous patches may appear on the face. Leishmaniae are present in the skin. Antimony treatment should be tried but is often ineffective.

In HIV-infected persons—with or without AIDS—visceral leishmaniasis can be an opportunistic infection. These patients may have a shorter duration of symptoms, no fever or splenomegaly, and a poor response to treatment.

The diagnosis is made by demonstrating the organism in buffy coat preparations of blood; on stained smears of aspirates of sternal marrow or iliac crest, liver, lymph nodes, or spleen; and by culture. Because of the hazard of splenic aspiration, it should only be performed by experienced persons; contraindications are a soft spleen in the acute phase, a prolonged prothrombin time, and platelet counts under 40,000/µL. The direct agglutination IgM test is positive early in the disease. In most patients, the immunofluorescent IgG antibody test is positive at titers of 1:256 or higher. The leishmanin skin test is always negative during active disease and becomes positive months to years after recovery. Other characteristic findings are progressive leukopenia (seldom over 3000/µL after the first 1–2 months), with lymphocytosis and monocytosis, normochromic anemia, and thrombocytopenia. There is a marked increase in total protein up to or greater than 10 g/dL owing to an elevated IgG fraction; serum albumin is 3 g/dL or less. Liver function tests show hepatocellular damage. Proteinuria may be present.

The differential diagnosis includes leukemia, lymphoma, tuberculosis, brucellosis, malaria, typhoid, schistosomiasis, African trypanosomiasis, infective endocarditis, cirrhosis, and other entities.

Sodium stibogluconate (20 mg/kg/d for 30 days) is the drug of choice. Whereas Mediterranean kala azar responds to 10–15 daily doses, the disease in Kenya, Sudan, and India requires at least 30 days of treatment. With incomplete response or relapse, the treatment should be repeated for up to 60 days. However, the incidence of side effects when therapy continues over 30 days remains to be determined. Failure should lead to use of pentamidine or amphotericin B. Combined treatment with sodium stibogluconate and allopurinol, paromomycin, or γ-interferon is being evaluated.

Without treatment, the case-fatality rate can reach 90%. Early diagnosis and treatment reduces the mortality rate to 2–5%. Relapses (up to 10% in India and 30% in Kenya) are most likely to occur within 6 months after completion of treatment.

Magill AJ et al: Viscerotropic leishmaniasis in persons returning from Operation Desert Storm, 1990–1991. MMWR 1992;41:131.

Montalban C et al: Visceral leishmaniasis in patients infected with human immunodeficiency virus. Co-operative Group for the Study of Leishmaniasis in AIDS. J Infect 1990;21:261.

Thakur CP, Kumar M, Pandey AK: Comparison of regimes of treatment of antimony-resistant kala azar patients: A randomized study. Am J Trop Med Hyg 1991;45:453.

2. CUTANEOUS LEISHMANIASIS

Lesions can be single or multiple. Cutaneous swellings appear 2 to several months after sandfly bites. Depending on the leishmanial species and host immune response, lesions vary from small papules to nonulcerated dry plaques to large encrusted ulcers with well-demarcated raised and indurated margins. Satellite lesions may be present. The lesions are painless unless secondarily infected. Systemic symptoms are rare, but a low-grade fever of short duration may be present at the onset. Healing usually occurs spontaneously in months to 1–3 years, starting with central granulation tissue that spreads peripherally. Contraction of scars can cause deformities and disfigurement, especially if lesions are on the face.

Definitive diagnosis depends on demonstrating organisms by staining smears or biopsy sections or by isolating the organism in culture or in hamsters. *Leishmania* cannot be detected in pus but may be seen in scrapings from the cleaned edge of the ulcer or in material aspirated after injection of saline under the margin of the ulcer. The skin test becomes positive within about 3 months after the appearance of the skin lesions. Serologic tests are unreliable and generally of little use.

Old World Cutaneous Leishmaniasis

Agents of Old World cutaneous leishmaniasis are as follows:

(1) *L tropica* is the agent responsible for an urban infection of dogs and humans. It is found in the Middle East, northwestern India, southern USSR, Afghanistan, Pakistan, Armenia, Greece, and southern France and Italy. The lesions of *L tropica* infection tend to be single and dry, to ulcerate slowly or not at all, and to persist for a year or longer. Leishmaniasis recidivans is a relapsing form of *L tropica* infection in which slow spread of ulcers and scarring can be extensive; it is associated with hypersensitivity and a strongly positive skin test but scarce amastigotes.

(2) *L major* infection causes lesions in dry or desert rural areas and is primarily a disease of desert rodents. Human disease occurs in the Middle East, southern USSR, Arabian peninsula, Afghanistan, and Africa (North, East, and sub-Saharan Africa from Senegal to Sudan and Kenya). The lesions are characterized by multiple, wet, rapidly ulcerating sores with crusting.

(3) *L aethiopica* infection occurs in the Ethiopian and Kenyan highlands. Spontaneous healing is slow, and the lesions last for several years. An uncommon complication is diffuse cutaneous leishmaniasis, in which multiple nonulcerating lesions (that resemble lepromatous leprosy) occur over the entire body; this condition is associated with anergy and a negative leishmanial skin test, but amastigotes are abundant.

Old World leishmaniasis, especially in the Middle East, is generally self-healing in about 6 months and does not metastasize to the mucosa. Thus, it may be justified to withhold treatment if the lesions are small, in an unobtrusive place, and appear to be healing. Pentavalent antimony (20 days) should be used to treat patients with large or multiple lesions or if the lesions are on cosmetically or functionally important areas (eg, the wrist). Complete healing may not be evident until weeks after the course of treatment has been completed. Pentamidine or amphotericin B is used for failures. Other treatments for less severe disease are physical measures (local cryotherapy or heat therapy, electrocoagulation, surgical removal) and intralesional injection of sodium stibogluconate. Lesions should be kept clean and antibiotics used if secondary infection occurs.

New World Cutaneous Leishmaniasis

Agents of New World cutaneous leishmaniasis are (1) *L mexicana mexicana* (Mexico [Yucatan], Belize, Guatemala, rarely in southern USA), (2) *L m amazonensis* (Brazil [Amazon basin], Venezuela), (3) other members of the *L m mexicana* complex (South America), and (4) the *L braziliensis* complex (Central and South America).

Most New World cutaneous lesions are ulcers, but vegetative, verrucous, or nodular lesions may occur also. *L m mexicana* ("chiclero's ulcer") in the Yucatan and Central America produces destructive lesions on the ear cartilage. Up to 80% of *L b braziliensis* cutaneous lesions progress to espundia (see below); some *L braziliensis* complex strains also show a chain of palpable local lymph nodes and some *L m mexicana* and South American strains can cause diffuse cutaneous leishmaniasis.

In New World *L mexicana* infections from Mexico and Central America, solitary nodules or ulcers in inconspicuous sites generally will heal spontaneously, but metronidazole, 750 mg three times daily for 10 days, can be tried. Lesions on the ear, face, or hands should be treated with sodium antimony gluconate but usually require only a 12- to 14-day course. Under evaluation are ketoconazole, liposome-encapsulated compounds, combined sodium stibogluconate and allopurinol, and topically applied paromomycin. Cutaneous lesions acquired in regions of mucocutaneous leishmaniasis may be due to *L braziliensis* and should be treated with a full course of sodium stibogluconate. For treatment of diffuse cutaneous leishmaniasis, see references.

Davidson RN et al: Liposomal amphotericin B in drug-resistant visceral leishmaniasis. Lancet 1991;337:1061

Dogra J: Current therapies for treatment of cutaneous leishmaniasis in India. Infection 1992;20:189.

Harms G et al: A randomized trial comparing a pentavalent antimonial drug and recombinant interferon in the local treatment of cutaneous leishmaniasis. Trans R Soc Trop Med Hyg 1991;85:214.

Martinez S, Marr JJ: Allopurinol in the treatment of American cutaneous leishmaniasis. N Engl J Med 1992; 326:741.

Navin TR et al: Placebo-controlled clinical trial of sodium stibogluconate (Pentostam) versus ketoconazole for treating cutaneous leishmaniasis in Guatemala. J Infect Dis 1992;165:528.

3. MUCOCUTANEOUS LEISHMANIASIS (Espundia)

Leishmania b braziliensis causes severe naso-oral lesions in lowland forest areas of South America and Central America north to Belize. The initial lesion, single or multiple, is on exposed skin; at first it is papular (can be pruriginous or painful), then nodular, and later may ulcerate or become wart-like or papillomatous. Local healing follows, with scarring within several months to a year. Subsequent naso-oral involvement occurs in a small proportion of patients either by direct extension or, more often, metastatically to the mucosa. It may appear concurrently with the initial lesion, shortly after healing, or after many years. The mucosa of the anterior part of the nasal septum is generally the first area to be involved. Extensive destruction of the soft tissues and cartilage of the nose, oral cavity, and lips may follow and may extend to the larynx and pharynx. Gross and hideous destruction and marked suffering can result. Secondary bacterial infection is common. Regional lymphangitis, lymphadenitis, fever, weight loss, keratitis, and anemia may be present.

Diagnosis is by finding amastigotes in scrapings, biopsy specimens, or aspirated tissue fluid; the organism grows with difficulty in culture or after inoculation of hamsters. The leishmanin skin test is useful if it produces a fully developed papule in 2–3 days that disappears after a week. The direct agglutination test for IgM antibodies becomes positive in 4–6 weeks. IgG antibodies are detectable in most cases and disappear with cure. The main considerations in the differential diagnosis are paracoccidioidomycosis, polymorphic reticulosis, Wegener's granulomatosis, lymphoma, and nasopharyngeal carcinoma, which are distinguishable by biopsy.

In treatment, at least one full course of sodium stibogluconate is given. However, extended observation (several years) in severe disease shows that failure rates are high. Corticosteroids may be needed to control local inflammation due to release of antigens. If repeated and extended antimony treatment fails, amphotericin B is used. Antibiotics are usually needed to treat associated bacterial or fungal infection.

Franke ED et al: Efficacy and toxicity of sodium stibogluconate for mucosal leishmaniasis. Ann Intern Med 1990;113:934.

MALARIA

Essentials of Diagnosis

- History of exposure in a malaria-endemic area.
- Periodic attacks of sequential chills, fever, and sweating.
- Headache, myalgia, splenomegaly; anemia, leukopenia.
- Characteristic parasites in erythrocytes, identified in thick or thin blood films.
- Complications of falciparum malaria: Cerebral findings (mental disturbances, neurologic signs, convulsions), hemolytic anemia, hyperpyrexia, dysenteric or cholera-like stools, dark urine, anuria.

General Considerations

Four species of the genus *Plasmodium* are responsible for human malaria: *Plasmodium vivax, Plasmodium malariae, Plasmodium ovale,* and *Plasmodium falciparum.* Although the disease has been eradicated from most temperate zone countries, it continues to be endemic in many parts of the tropics and subtropics, and imported cases occur in the USA and other countries free of transmission. Malaria is present in parts of Mexico, Haiti, Central and South America, Africa, the Middle East, the Indian subcontinent, Southeast Asia, China, and Oceania. *P vivax* and *P falciparum* are responsible for most infections and are found throughout the malaria belt. *P malariae* is widely distributed but is less common. *P ovale* is rare, but in West Africa it seems to replace *P vivax*. Worldwide, there are an estimated 110 million cases (90 million in tropical Africa) and 1.2 million deaths yearly, with the greatest impact on children. In the USA, over the past 3 decades, an average of 2–3 deaths have occurred each year in travelers; most of these infections were acquired in tropical Africa.

Malaria is transmitted from human to human by the bite of infected female *Anopheles* mosquitoes. Congenital transmission and transmission by blood transfusion also occur. There are no animal reservoirs for human malaria.

The mosquito becomes infected by taking blood containing the sexual forms of the parasite (micro- and macrogametocytes). After a developmental phase in the mosquito, sporozoites in the salivary glands are inoculated into humans when the mosquito next feeds. The first stage of development in humans, the exoerythrocytic stage, takes place in the liver. Subsequently, parasites escape from the liver into the bloodstream, invade red blood cells, multiply, and 48 hours later (or 72 with *P malariae*) cause the red cells to rupture, releasing a new crop of parasites (merozoites). Within the bloodstream, this cycle of invasion, multiplication, and red cell rupture may be repeated many times. Symptoms do not appear until several of these erythrocytic cycles have been completed.

P falciparum and *P malariae* have only one cycle of liver cell invasion and multiplication. Liver infection ceases spontaneously in less than 4 weeks; thereafter, multiplication is confined to the red cells. Thus, 4 weeks after departure from an endemic area, treatment that eliminates these species from the red cells will cure the infection. *P vivax* (and presumably *P ovale*) have, however, a dormant hepatic stage (the hypnozoite) that is responsible for subsequent relapses. Cure of *P vivax* and *P ovale* infections, therefore, requires treatment to eradicate parasites both from the red cells and from the liver.

The incubation period for *P falciparum* is approximately 12 days (range, 9–60 days); for *P vivax* and *P ovale,* 14 days (range, 8–27 days [initial attacks for some temperate strains may not occur for up to 8 months]); and for *P malariae,* 30 days (range, 16–60 days). If untreated, *P falciparum* infections usually terminate spontaneously in 6–8 months but can persist for up to 1½ years; *P vivax* and *P ovale* infections can persist without treatment for as long as 5 years; and *P malariae* infections have lasted for as long as 50 years.

Clinical Findings

A. Symptoms and Signs: Typical malarial attacks show sequential shaking chills (the cold stage); fever (the hot stage) to 41 °C (105.8 °F) or higher; and marked diaphoresis (the sweating stage). A full attack lasts 4–8 hours. Associated symptoms may include fatigue, headache, dizziness, gastrointestinal symptoms (anorexia, nausea, slight diarrhea, vomiting, abdominal cramps), myalgia, arthralgia, backache, and dry cough.

Either from the onset of symptoms or with progression of the disease, the attacks may show an every-other-day (tertian) periodicity in vivax, ovale, or falciparum malaria or an every-third-day (quartan) periodicity in malariae malaria. Regular periodicity reflects synchronous parasite maturation, red cell rupture, and release of merozoites. Splenomegaly usually appears when acute symptoms have continued for 4 or more days; the liver is frequently mildly enlarged. The patient may be tired between attacks but otherwise feels well. After this primary episode, there is often a latent period followed by a recurrence.

P falciparum infection is more serious than the others because of the high frequency of severe or fatal complications, which sometimes occur within 24 hours. In severe falciparum malaria, red blood cell parasitemia is higher than 3–5%. Complications include (1) cerebral malaria with edema (headache, mental disturbances, neurologic signs, convulsions, delirium, coma); (2) hyperpyrexia; (3) hemolytic anemia; (4) noncardiogenic pulmonary edema; (5) acute tubular necrosis and renal failure, with production of dark urine (blackwater fever); (6) acute hepatopathy, with centrilobular necrosis and marked jaundice; (7) hypoglycemia; (8) adrenal insufficiency-like syndrome; (9) cardiac dysrhythmias; (10) gastrointestinal syndromes (including secretory diarrhea and dysentery); and (11) water and electrolyte imbalance. Nephrotic syndrome may occur in chronic *P malariae* infection. Tropical splenomegaly is an immunologic disorder related to chronic malaria. Current findings suggest that *P falciparum* does not act as an opportunistic infection in AIDS patients.

B. Laboratory Findings: The thick and thin blood film, dehemoglobinized and Giemsa-stained, is the mainstay of diagnosis. The much less sensitive thin film is used primarily for species differentiation after the presence of an infection is detected on a thick film. Because the level of parasitemia varies from hour to hour—especially for *P falciparum* infections, in which parasites may not be found—blood should be examined at 8-hour intervals for 2–3 days, during and between febrile spikes. The newly described quantitative buffy coat method to detect parasitemia is slightly more sensitive than thick smears, but it is expensive and requires fluorescent microscopy..

In all but *P falciparum* infections, the number of red cells infected seldom exceeds 2% of the total cells. In severe parasitemia in falciparum malaria, however, levels may reach 20–30% or more. During paroxysms, there may be transient leukocytosis; leukopenia develops subsequently, with a relative increase in large mononuclear cells. Hepatic function tests often become abnormal, but the tests revert to normal with treatment or spontaneous recovery. Hemolytic jaundice and thrombocytopenia may develop in severe infections.

Serologic tests are not used in the diagnosis of acute malaria but may be of value occasionally in investigation of recurrent febrile illness and in recognition of infection in persons returning from a malarious area. A titer of 1:64 in the indirect immunofluorescence test indicates that the patient has acquired malaria at some time in the past.

Differential Diagnosis

Uncomplicated malaria must be distinguished from a variety of other causes of fever, splenomegaly, anemia, or hepatomegaly. Often considered are influenza, urinary tract infections, typhoid fever, infectious hepatitis, dengue, kala azar, amebic liver abscess, leptospirosis, and relapsing fever. Malaria complications can mimic many diseases.

Drugs Used in Treatment & Chemoprophylaxis (Tables 34–2 and 34–3)

Consultation with a center working on malaria may be necessary to obtain up-to-date information on malaria prophylaxis and treatment. A source of information and advice in the USA is the Malarial Branch, Centers for Disease Control, in Atlanta, Georgia: For recorded information on prophylaxis, (404) 332–4555; for questions about management of acute attacks or on prophylaxis, (404) 488–4046 (emergencies, [404] 639–2888).

A. Drug Classification: By chemical groups, some of the major antimalarial drugs are as follows: **4-aminoquinolines**—chloroquine, hydroxychloroquine, amodiaquine;* **diaminopyrimidines**—pyrimethamine, trimethoprim; **biguanides**—proguanil* (chlorguanide, chlorproguanil); **8-aminoquinolines**—primaquine; **cinchona** alkaloids—quinine, quinidine; **sulfonamides**—sulfadoxine, sulfadiazine, sulfamethoxazole; **sulfones**—dapsone; **4-quinoline-carbinolamines**—mefloquine; and **antibiotics**—tetracycline, doxycycline, clindamycin; and **others**—halofantrine, qinghaosu and its derivatives. Pyrimethamine and proguanil are known as **antifolates,** since they inhibit dihydrofolate reductase of plasmodia. Drug combinations used to treat *P falciparum* malaria resistant to chloroquine include Fansidar (pyrimethamine plus sulfadoxine) and Maloprim (pyrimethamine plus dapsone).

---

*Not available in the USA but available in some other countries.

Table 34–2. Prevention of malaria in travelers.[1]

TO PREVENT ATTACKS OF ALL FORMS OF MALARIA AND TO ERADICATE *P FALCIPARUM* AND *P MALARIAE* INFECTIONS[2]

REGIONS WITH CHLOROQUINE-SENSITIVE *P FALCIPARUM* MALARIA: Central America west of the Panama Canal, the Caribbean, North Africa, and parts of the Middle East

Chloroquine[3]

Adult dose: Chloroquine phosphate, 500 mg salt (300 mg base); pediatric dose: 8.3 mg/kg salt (5 mg/kg base) up to the adult dose. Give a single dose of chloroquine weekly starting 2 weeks before entering the endemic area, while there, and for 4 weeks after leaving.

REGIONS WITH CHLOROQUINE-RESISTANT *P FALCIPARUM* MALARIA: All other regions of the world

Mefloquine (preferred method)[4]

Adult dose: one 250-mg tablet salt (228 mg base); pediatric dose: 15–19 kg, ¼ tablet; 20–30 kg, ½ tablet; 31–45 kg, ¾ tablet; >45 kg, one 250-mg tablet. Give a single dose of mefloquine weekly starting 1 week before entering the endemic area, while there, and for 4 weeks after leaving.

Doxycycline (alternative method)[5]

Adult dose: 100 mg daily; pediatric dose is 2 mg/kg (maximum, 100 mg) daily. Give the daily dose for 2 days before departure as a test dose. While in the endemic area, give the daily dose; continue doxycycline daily for 4 weeks after leaving endemic area.

Chloroquine (second alternative method)

Give chloroquine weekly at the above schedule.

plus

Proguanil[6] (when available)

Adult dose: 200 mg once daily. Pediatric doses: <2 years, 50 mg/d; 2–6 years, 100 mg/d; 7–10 years, 150 mg/d; >10 years, 200 mg/d

plus

Pyrimethamine-sulfadoxine (Fansidar)[7] (for one-time self-treatment of presumptive infections)

One dose only: Adult dose: 3 tablets; pediatric dose: 5–10 kg, ½ tablet; 11–20 kg, 1 tablet; 21–30 kg, 1½ tablets; 31–45 kg, 2 tablets; >45 kg, 3 tablets.

TO ERADICATE *P VIVAX* OR *P OVALE* INFECTIONS[2]

Primaquine[8]

Primaquine is indicated only for persons who have had a high probability of exposure to *P vivax* or *P ovale*. Start primaquine only after returning home, during the last 2 weeks of chemoprophylaxis. Adult dose: 26.3 mg salt (15 mg base) daily for 14 days; pediatric dose: 0.5 mg salt/kg (0.3 mg base/kg) daily for 14 days.

[1]For additional recommendations for prophylaxis, see the references or call the Centers for Disease Control and Prevention, Atlanta, GA 30333. Telephone (404) 488–4046 during the day for advice; (404) 332–4555 for recorded announcements.

[2]The blood schizonticides (chloroquine, mefloquine, and doxycycline), when taken for 4 weeks after leaving the endemic area, are curative for sensitive *P falciparum* and *P malariae* infections; primaquine, however, is needed to eradicate the persistent liver stages of *P vivax* and *P ovale*.

[3]Chloroquine can be used by pregnant women and by young children.

[4]Mefloquine is not recommended for use in pregnant women or in children who weigh less than 15 kg, or under certain other conditions (see text). Take with water and after eating.

[5]Doxycycline is contraindicated in pregnant women or in children under 8 years of age. The drug should be taken with the evening meal. Side effects include photosensitivity (preventive measures include the use of sunscreens that absorb ultraviolet radiation and avoidance of exposure to direct sunlight as much as possible), gastrointestinal symptoms, and candidal vaginitis.

[6]Proguanil (Paludrine), when taken in conjunction with chloroquine, is useful in East Africa and possibly in other regions of chloroquine resistance (but not in West Africa). The drug is not available in the USA but can be purchased in other countries.

[7]The drug should not be used for prophylaxis. It is used only for self-treatment of fever when a physician is not immediately available to make the diagnosis; but it is imperative that the patient see a physician promptly. Each tablet of Fansidar contains 25 mg of pyrimethamine and 500 mg of sulfadoxine. The drug is contraindicated in pregnancy at term, in known cases of sulfonamide sensitivity, and in children under 2 months of age. The drug is not effective in Thailand or adjacent countries.

[8]Before taking primaquine, patients should be screened to detect glucose-6-phosphate dehydrogenase deficiency. Primaquine is contraindicated in pregnancy. An alternative regimen in regions where cholorquine can be taken for prophylaxis is chloroquine phosphate, 500 mg (salt), plus primaquine phosphate, 78.9 mg (salt), weekly for 8 weeks.

The effectiveness of antimalarial drugs differs with different species of the parasite and with different stages of the life cycle. Drugs that act in the liver to eliminate developing exoerythrocytic schizonts or latent hypnozoites are called **tissue schizonticides** (primaquine). Those that act on blood schizonts are **blood schizonticides** or **suppressive agents** (eg, chloroquine, amodiaquine, proguanil, pyrimeth-amine, mefloquine, quinine, quinidine, halofantrine, and qinghaosu and its derivatives). **Gametocides** are drugs that prevent infection of mosquitoes by destroying gametocytes in the blood (eg, primaquine for *P falciparum* and chloroquine for *P vivax*, *P malariae*, and *P ovale*). **Sporonticidal** agents are drugs that render gametocytes noninfective in the mosquito (eg, pyrimethamine, proguanil).

Table 34–3. Treatment of malaria in nonimmune adult populations.

Treatment[1] of Infection With All Species (Except Chloroquine-Resistant *P falciparum*)	Treatment[1] of Infection With Chloroquine-Resistant *P falciparum* Strains
Oral treatment of *P falciparum*[2] or *P malariae* infection Chloroquine phosphate, 1 g (salt)[3,4] as initial dose, then 0.5 g at 6, 24, and 48 hours. **Oral treatment of *P vivax* or *P ovale* infection** Chloroquine[3,4] as above followed by 0.5 g on days 10 and 17 plus primaquine phosphate, 26.3 mg (salt)[5] daily for 14 days starting about day 4. **Parenteral treatment of severe attacks** Quinine dihydrochloride[6] or quinidine gluconate.[7] Start oral chloroquine therapy as soon as possible; follow with primaquine if the infection is due to *P vivax* or *P ovale*– or Chloroquine hydrochloride, 250 mg (salt) IM;[12] repeat every 6 hours. Start oral therapy as soon as possble; follow with primaquine if infection is due to *P vivax* or *P ovale*.	**Oral treatment** Quinine sulfate, 10 mg/kg 3 times daily for 3–7 days,[8] plus one of the following: (1) once only, pyrimethamine, 75 mg, and sulfadoxine, 1500 mg (= 3 tablets of Fansidar); (2) pyrimethamine, 25 mg twice daily for 3 days, and sulfadiazine, 500 mg 4 times daily for 5 days; (3) tetracycline,[9] 250–500 mg 4 times daily for 7 days; (4) doxycycline,[9] 100 mg twice daily for 7 days, or clindamycine,[9] 900 mg 3 times daily for 3 days. or Mefloquine,[10] 15–25 mg/kg (salt) once or in two divided doses 6 hours apart. or Halofantrine[11] **Parenteral treatment of severe attacks** Quinine dihydrochloride[6] or quinidine gluconate.[7] Start oral therapy with quinine sulfate plus a second drug (as above) as soon as possible.

[1]See text for cautions and contraindications for each drug.

[2]In falciparum malaria, if the patient has not shown a clinical response to chloroquine (48–72 hours for mild infections, 24 hours for severe ones), parasitic resistance to chloroquine should be considered. Chloroquine should be stopped and oral quinine or mefloquine started.

[3]500 mg chloroquine phosphate = 300 mg base.

[4]Chloroquine alone is curative for infection with sensitive strains of *P falciparum* and for *P malariae*, but primaquine is needed to eradicate the persistent liver stages of *P vivax* and *P ovale*. Start primaquine after the patient has recovered from the acute illness; continue chloroquine weekly during primaquine therapy. Patients should be screened for glucose-6-phosphate dehydrogenase deficiency before use of primaquine . An alternative mode for primaquine therapy is combined primaquine, 78.9 mg (salt), and chloroquine, 0.5 g (salt), weekly for 8 weeks.

[5]26.3 mg of primaquine phosphate = 15 mg primaquine base.

[6]Quinine dihydrochloride. Give 10 mg/kg (salt) in 500 mL of normal saline or 5% glucose solution IV slowly over 4 hours; repeat every 8 hours until oral therapy is possible (maximum, 1800 mg/d). Blood pressure and ECG should be monitored constantly to detect arrhythmias or hypotension. A higher initial loading dose of quinine is given (20 mg/kg) to patients who acquired infections in Southeast Asia if it is known with certainty that they have not already taken the medication. Extreme caution is required in treating patients with quinine who previously have been taking mefloquine in prophylaxis. In the USA, quinine dihydrochloride is no longer available from the CDC.

[7]When parenteral quinine is unavailable, quinidine gluconate can be used, administered as a continuous infusion. A loading dose of 10 mg/kg (salt) (maximum, 600 mg) is diluted in 300 mL of normal saline and administered over 1–2 hours, followed by 0.02 mg/kg/min (maximum, 10 mg/kg every 8 hours) until oral quinine therapy is possible. Blood pressure and ECG should be monitored constantly; widening of the QRS interval or lengthening of the QT interval requires discontinuation. Quinidine gluconate is available in the USA from the Centers for Disease Control and Prevention (CDC), Atlanta, GA 30333. Telephone (404) 488–4046 during the day; (404) 639–2888 nights, weekends, and holidays (emergencies only).

[8]Although quinine sulfate is usually given for 3 days, it should be continued for 7 days in patients who acquired infections in Thailand, where diminished sensitivity to quinine has been noted.

[9]Contraindicated in children under the age of 8 years and in pregnant women.

[10]The higher dose is used in Thailand and other areas with increasing resistance and in children, as they metabolize the drug more rapidly than adults. Serious side effects are rare. See text for cautions and contraindications. Mefloquine must not be given with quinine or quinidine.

[11]The adult dosage is 1 tablet (500 mg) every 6 hours for three doses; children under 40 kg, 8 mg/kg (suspension) every 6 hours for three doses.

[12]To avoid potential severe toxicity, give parenteral chloroquine by low-dose intramuscular injection (maximum, 3.5 mg/kg [salt] every 6 hours)

None of the drugs prevent infection (ie, are true **causal prophylactic drugs**.) However, proguanil and chlorproguanil—and to some extent the antibiotics and primaquine—prevent maturation of the early *P falciparum* and *P vivax* hepatic schizonts but do not eradicate the hypnozoites. Blood schizonticides destroy circulating plasmodia and thus prevent malarial attacks (**suppressive prophylaxis**) and, when given weekly for 4 weeks after departure from the endemic area, result in cure of *P falciparum* and *P malariae* infections. Primaquine destroys the hypnozoites of *P vivax* and *P ovale* and, when given with a blood schizonticide, prevents relapse from infection with these parasites and thus effects **radical cure (terminal prophylaxis).**

B. Parasite Resistance to Drugs:

1. *P falciparum* resistance–

a. Chloroquine-resistant strains of *P falciparum* have been confirmed or are probably present in all malarious areas except in the Caribbean, Central America west of the Panama Canal, North Africa, and parts of the Middle East, including Egypt. In regions of resistance, some strains of *P falciparum* are only partially resistant to the drug, as manifested by temporary subsidence of symptoms and transient decrease in asexual parasitemia, followed by return of both after several days to weeks.

b. Resistance to pyrimethamine-sulfadoxine (Fansidar) is present at low levels (5–30%) in parts of the Amazon basin of South America, sub-Saharan Africa, and Southeast Asia. In Thailand, Burma, and Cambodia, however, resistance is now too widespread for the drug to be used.

c. Resistance to pyrimethamine or proguanil when used alone is common in most endemic areas, but the degree and distribution are not accurately known.

d. Mefloquine–Sporadic or low (5–20%) levels of mefloquine resistance have been reported from Southeast Asia and parts of Africa. Along the Thai-Burmese and Thai-Cambodian borders, however, the frequency reaches 75%.

e. Quinine–Rarely, strains in Southeast Asia and East and West Africa have shown decreased sensitivity.

2. *P vivax* resistance–

a. Resistance of *P vivax* blood schizonts to pyrimethamine and proguanil, including the pyrimethamine-containing drugs Fansidar and Maloprim, has been reported in many areas of the world, particularly Southeast Asia.

b. Partial resistance of some strains of *P vivax* hepatic schizonts to primaquine in areas of the southwest Pacific and Thailand may require for cure a larger dose (15 mg of base/d for 21 days).

c. Several recent reports from Indonesia (Irian Jaya, Sumatra) and Papua New Guinea suggest for the first time possible *P vivax* blood schizonts resistant to chloroquine.

3. *P ovale* and *P malariae*–These forms have not shown resistance.

C. Indications, Limitations, and Adverse Side Effects of Selected Drugs:

1. Chloroquine phosphate–Chloroquine (Aralen) is used in chemoprophylaxis to prevent attacks (to suppress symptoms) of all forms of malaria except for infections due to resistant strains of *P falciparum*. However, in *P vivax* and *P ovale* infections, which have a persistent liver phase, initial attacks may be delayed or relapses may occur after chloroquine is stopped. Use of primaquine eradicates the persistent liver phases.

Chloroquine is also the drug of choice for treating acute attacks of malaria, but cure occurs only with *P falciparum* and *P malariae*. Cure for *P vivax* and *P ovale* requires primaquine.

Chloroquine is usually well tolerated when used for malaria prophylaxis or treatment and is safe to use in pregnancy and for young children. Gastrointestinal symptoms, mild headache, pruritus (especially in blacks), dizziness, blurred vision, anorexia, malaise, and urticaria may occur; taking the drug after meals or in divided twice-weekly doses may reduce these side effects.

If neither quinine nor quinidine is available—the preferred drugs for parenteral treatment of severely ill patients—chloroquine can be given intramuscularly or intravenously. However, chloroquine can be severely toxic unless it is given in small amounts (3.5 mg/kg) intramuscularly every 6 hours or by slow intravenous infusion. For some persons, the related compound hydroxychloroquine sulfate may be better tolerated in prophylaxis at a dosage of 400 mg of the salt weekly and for 4 weeks after leaving the endemic area.

Rare reactions from oral chloroquine include impaired hearing, psychosis, convulsions, blood dyscrasias, skin reactions, and hypotension. When given in large doses for prolonged periods as an anti-inflammatory agent in autoimmune diseases, chloroquine has caused ocular damage. Theoretically, a total cumulative dosage of 100 g (base) may be critical in the development of ocular, ototoxic, and myopathic effects. However, weekly administration of chloroquine beyond 6 years of age may be safe in most people if baseline and periodic follow-up ophthalmologic examinations are done. Chloroquine should be used with caution in patients who have histories of liver damage, alcoholism, or neurologic or hematologic disorders. It is contraindicated in patients with psoriasis.

Certain antacids and antidiarrheal agents (kaolin, calcium carbonate, and magnesium trisilicate) should not be taken within about 4 hours before or after chloroquine administration, since they interfere with its absorption.

2. Mefloquine hydrochloride–Mefloquine, a quinoline methanol derivative, recently was approved for use in the USA for oral prophylaxis and treatment of chloroquine-resistant and multidrug-resistant *P falciparum* malaria. In treatment, it is used only for mildly to moderately ill patients but not for severely ill patients, who require parenteral (quinine or quinidine) treatment. Mefloquine has strong schizonticidal activity against *P falciparum* (most but not all strains) and *P vivax*—and presumably against *P ovale* and *P malariae*—but it is not active against *P falciparum* gametocytes or the hepatic stages of *P vivax*, which require a course of primaquine.

Mefloquine is rapidly absorbed but has a long (13–26 days) elimination half-life.

In the lower doses used in prophylaxis, minor and transient side effects include nausea, vomiting, epigastric pain, diarrhea, headache, dizziness, syncope, and extrasystoles. With treatment doses—particularly over 1000 mg—gastrointestinal symptoms and fatigue are more likely to occur, and the frequency of neuropsychiatric symptoms (dizziness, headache, visual disturbances, vertigo, tinnitus, insomnia, restlessness, anxiety, depression, confusion, disorientation, acute psychosis, or seizures) may be of the order of 1%. In experimental animals, the drug affects fertility and is teratogenic; it also causes degenerative changes in the epididymis in rats and in the lens and retina of some species. In human males, however, no deleterious effects on spermatozoa were found, and no effects have been noted in the human retina or lens.

Mefloquine is contraindicated if there is a history of epilepsy or psychiatric disorder, and the drug should not be used for children weighing less than 15 kg or under 2 years of age. Also contraindicated is concurrent administration of mefloquine with quinine, quinidine, β-adrenergic or calcium channel-blocking agents, or other agents that may prolong or otherwise alter cardiac conduction. If quinine or quinidine precedes use of mefloquine, 12 hours should elapse before mefloquine is started. However, because of the long half-life of mefloquine, extreme caution is required if quinine or quinidine is used to treat malaria after mefloquine has been taken.

The development of neuropsychiatric symptoms during prophylaxis is an indication for stopping the drug. Patients should be instructed to use caution when driving or operating machinery. Mefloquine should not be taken by persons whose work requires fine coordination and spatial discrimination. Patients taking anticonvulsant drugs (particularly valproic acid and divalproex sodium) may have breakthrough seizures. The drug is best not used in pregnancy, especially the first trimester; it should be considered only if its anticipated benefit justifies the fetal risk. Women of childbearing potential who take mefloquine for antimalarial prophylaxis should avoid conception for the duration of mefloquine usage and for 2 months after the last dose. The safety of mefloquine administration beyond 1 year has not been established.

Note: The tablet formulation in the USA contains 250 mg of the salt (= 228 mg of base). However, in Canada and many other countries, the tablets contain 274 mg of the salt (= 250 mg of base).

3. Primaquine phosphate–Primaquine is used (1) to prevent relapse by eliminating persistent liver forms of *P vivax* or *P ovale* ("radical cure") in patients who have had an acute attack and (2) for prophylactic use against these parasites for individuals returning from an endemic area who have probably been exposed to malaria. In persons with a low probability of exposure, it is preferable to avoid primaquine's potential toxicity by not giving the drug. Instead, patients are advised to seek medical evaluation in the event of malaria-like symptoms, which usually occur within 2 years after infection but can occur up to 4 years after. Primaquine is sometimes given as a single 45 mg (base) dose to eliminate *P falciparum* gametocytes.

Primaquine is generally well tolerated. Occasional side effects of the drug are gastrointestinal disturbances, headache, dizziness, or neutropenia. Primaquine should not be used in pregnancy, in autoimmune disorders, or concurrently with quinine.

All patients should be tested for glucose-6-phosphate dehydrogenase (G6PD) deficiency before therapy is begun and followed carefully during treatment; this is because primaquine may cause mild, self-limited hemolysis or marked hemolysis or methemoglobinemia. G6PD deficiency is most common among persons of Mediterranean extraction, blacks, and certain Oriental groups. For individuals deficient in G6PD, it is safe, however, to give primaquine phosphate, 78.9 mg (45 mg base) weekly, and chloroquine phosphate, 0.5 g (0.3 g base) weekly, for 8 weeks. However, for persons suspected of having the Mediterranean or Canton forms of G6PD deficiency, it may be preferable not to give primaquine but to treat attacks of malaria with chloroquine as they occur.

4. Quinine–Oral quinine sulfate is used to treat malaria due to chloroquine-resistant strains of *P falciparum.* Although the drug alone will control acute attacks, in many infections—particularly with strains from Southeast Asia—it fails to prevent recurrence. Addition of one of several drugs (Table 34–3) lowers the rate of recurrence. For treatment of acute attacks of *P vivax, P ovale,* and *P malariae* malaria, however, chloroquine is more effective than quinine and is the drug of choice.

Because quinine is an irritant to the gastric mucosa, it should be taken with food. Mild to moderate quinine toxicity (cinchonism) is manifested by headache, nausea, slight visual disturbances, dizziness, and mild tinnitus. These symptoms may abate as treatment continues and usually do not require discontinuation of treatment. Where available, quinine blood levels can be monitored; desired plasma levels are 5–10 μg/mL. Severe cinchonism requiring temporary or permanent discontinuation of therapy is rare and begins to appear at plasma levels greater than 7 μg/mL; findings include fever, skin eruptions, deafness, marked visual abnormalities (scotomas, diplopia, contracted visual fields, retinal vessel spasticity, optic atrophy, blindness), other central nervous system abnormalities (vertigo, somnolence, confusion, seizures), disturbances in cardiac rhythm or conduction, massive intravascular hemolysis with renal failure (blackwater fever), agranulocytosis, and thrombocytopenia.

Parenteral quinine (dihydrochloride) is used in the treatment of severe attacks of malaria due to *P falciparum* strains sensitive or resistant to chloroquine. The drug is given only intravenously at a slow rate (Table 34–3); rapid infusions may be severely toxic. The drug should be used with extreme caution and only for patients who cannot take the medication orally; appropriate oral therapy should be started as soon as possible. Infusions may cause thrombophlebitis. In the USA, parenteral quinine is no longer available and quinidine gluconate is used instead.

See references and manufacturers' recommendations for drug interactions (including aluminum-containing antacids, digoxin, anticoagulants, and cimetidine); relative contraindications include pregnancy and a history of tinnitus or optic neuritis.

5. Quinidine gluconate–Quinidine is the dextrorotatory diasterioisomer of quinine. The two drugs are equally efficacious and safe in parenteral treatment of severe malaria. If quinidine gluconate is not locally available, it can be obtained on an emergency basis from the CDC ([404] 639–2888).

6. Pyrimethamine-sulfadoxine (Fansidar)–Fansidar is supplied as tablets that contain pyrimethamine (25 mg) and sulfadoxine (500 mg). Fansidar's limitations are (1) that it is effective only against susceptible strains of *P falciparum* (see above for regions with resistance) and not against *P vivax, P ovale,* or *P malariae;* (2) that it is slow-acting; and (3) that it may cause severe toxicity when used in weekly prophylaxis.

Current indications for the drug are (1) as a single dose (slow-acting) in conjunction with quinine (rapid-acting) in treatment of sensitive strains of acute chloroquine-resistant falciparum malaria and (2) in presumptive self-treatment of malaria—ie, in the event of malaria-like symptoms that cannot be immediately diagnosed and managed by a local physician, the patient decides when to self-treat with a single dose (3 tablets for adults). *It is imperative, however, that medical follow-up be sought promptly.* Fansidar is no longer used for continuing prophylaxis because of its rare potential for severe toxicity (eg, Stevens-Johnson syndrome) and death.

Fansidar is contraindicated for individuals with known sulfonamide sensitivity, in pregnancy at term, and in infants under 2 months of age. It should be used with caution in the presence of impaired renal or hepatic function, in patients with G6PD deficiency (hemolysis occurs in some), and in those with severe allergic disorders or bronchial asthma.

Preventing Mosquito Bites

Travelers should be told of the need to use protective measures when outdoors at times when mosquitoes are biting (chiefly between dusk and dawn). Clothing should cover most of the body, and deet (N,N-diethyl-3-methylbenzamide) should be applied to exposed areas and reapplied at frequent intervals

(1–2 hours). Mosquito bed nets (impregnated with permethrin, if available) and window screens should be used, and living and sleeping quarters should be sprayed with a pyrethrum-containing flying-insect spray to kill mosquitoes. Permethrin may also be sprayed on clothing.

Toxic encephalopathy after deet exposure has recently been recognized as a very rare complication in some persons, especially children. To minimize this risk, one should apply repellent sparingly and only to exposed skin or clothing; avoid applying high concentrations (over 35%) to the skin; avoid inhalation and contamination of the eyes, mouth, wounds, or irritated skin; and wash the skin after coming indoors.

Chemoprophylaxis for Nonimmune Populations (See Table 34–2 for methods and dosages.)

The decision to use chemoprophylaxis depends on the risk of exposure to infected mosquitoes, which may be difficult to estimate since it varies depending upon the region, rainy season, and altitude and on urban versus rural exposure; on whether exposure will occur during mosquito biting times; and on whether medical care will be readily available during travel. For those at risk, if safe and effective drugs are available, adults and children of all ages—including breast-feeding infants—should receive prophylaxis. The drug selected—except for Fansidar—should be given in a test dose before departure to evaluate possible side effects.

Travelers to malarious areas must be warned that malaria is a possible diagnosis if they develop fever and symptoms as early as 6 days after exposure (even when taking prophylaxis regularly) or as late as 6–12 months after departure.

Note: Schizonticides *not recognized for use in chemoprophylaxis* are halofantrine (erratic absorption and variable bioavailability), Fansidar (hypersensitivity reactions), amodiaquine (agranulocytosis and toxic hepatitis), and pyrimethamine (widespread resistance of both *P falciparum* and *P vivax*).

A. Chemoprophylaxis in Regions Where P falciparum Is Sensitive to 4-Aminoquinolines:

1. Drug of choice–Chloroquine prevents attacks for all forms of malaria and is curative for *P falciparum* and *P malariae* when taken for 4 weeks after leaving the endemic area. Primaquine is needed to provide cure of *P vivax* and *P ovale* (ie, to eliminate the continuing liver stages of these parasites). Pregnant women should take chloroquine throughout their pregnancy and only start primaquine after parturition.

2. Alternative drugs–For persons who cannot take chloroquine, hydroxychloroquine sulfate can be tried (see above under chloroquine). Other alternatives are **mefloquine** and **doxycycline.**

3. Proguanil* (chlorguanide,* paludrine*)– Some evidence suggests that proguanil remains effective against pre-erythrocytic stages when effectiveness is lost against blood forms. Rarely reported side effects from proguanil are nausea, vomiting, and mouth ulcers. In sub-Saharan Africa, the combination of chloroquine (0.5 g weekly) and proguanil (200 mg daily) while exposed and for 4 weeks afterward has been in use. However, the recent increase in failures of the combined drug against *P falciparum* make it too unreliable to be used in prophylaxis.

4. Primaquine (see above) may be indicated on returning home to eradicate *P vivax* or *P ovale* infections.

5. Prophylaxis for children and pregnant women–Children of all ages and pregnant women should be protected; malaria infection during pregnancy may be particularly severe. Drugs contraindicated in pregnancy are doxycycline, mefloquine, and primaquine. Doxycycline is also contraindicated in children under 8 years of age, mefloquine in those under 15 kg, and Fansidar in children under 2 months. Therefore, in children and pregnant women, the proper course is weekly chloroquine (or hydroxychloroquine) with Fansidar to be carried and taken in self-treatment as described above.

6. Chemoprophylaxis for natives in holo-endemic areas–Chemoprophylaxis is recommended for semi-immune pregnant women. However, for children under 5 years of age, surveillance and individual treatment are often recommended rather than mass prophylaxis.

B. Chemoprophylaxis in Regions Where *P falciparum* Is Resistant to Chloroquine: Prophylaxis is taken weekly while in the endemic area and for 4 weeks afterward. On returning home, primaquine is given to eradicate persistent liver stages of *P vivax* or *P ovale* if there has been significant exposure to these parasites. For additional details on the following drugs and on primaquine, see Table 34–2 and under the individual drugs (above).

1. Drug of choice–Mefloquine is the drug of choice. Note its cautions and contraindications (see under Mefloquine, above).

2. First alternative–Doxycycline is effective against chloroquine-resistant and chloroquine-sensitive *P falciparum* strains, *P vivax,* and (apparently) against *P ovale* and *P malariae*. However, doxycycline's side effects can be a problem for some persons (see Table 34–2). FDA considers use of doxycycline investigative for this indication.

3. Second alternative–Proguanil is taken daily and chloroquine weekly. Although the combination is useful in East Africa, effectiveness drops to about 65% in West Africa, and data for other parts of the world are not available.

If chloroquine is taken alone or in combination

with proguanil, a single dose of Fansidar (three tablets) is carried and is only taken as self-treatment for a febrile illness when medical care is not immediately available (see above under Fansidar for appropriate usage). Because of the high level of Fansidar and chloroquine resistance in Thailand, Burma, and Cambodia, these two drugs cannot be used in those areas.

**Treatment of Acute Attacks
(See Table 34–3 for dosages.)**
A. General Considerations: It is important to determine whether a patient has already been treated with antimalarials in the previous 24–36 hours (3 weeks for mefloquine) to avoid the risk of overdose and adverse drug reactions.

In monitoring the therapeutic response, it is essential also to determine the density of parasites on the blood smear (as a measure of the severity of infection) and to recheck at least daily. Within 48–72 hours, patients usually become afebrile and improve clinically; within 48 hours, parasitemia is generally reduced by about 75% (though there may be an initial increase during the first 6–12 hours). In falciparum malaria treated with chloroquine, if there is no improvement within 48–72 hours for mild infections or 24 hours for severe ones or if there is increasing asexual parasitemia after 1–2 days (in the presence of adequate drug ingestion and retention), parasite resistance to the drug must be assumed and treatment changed to oral quinine sulfate and another drug (Table 34–3).

B. Treatment of All Forms of Malaria Except *P falciparum* Strains Resistant to Chloroquine:
1. Elimination of asexual erythrocytic parasites–Infection by all four species of malaria is generally treated with oral chloroquine (Table 34–3). Alternative drugs if chloroquine cannot be tolerated are mefloquine (Table 34–3), Fansidar (single dose), quinine (650 mg three times daily for 7 days), or halofantrine (not yet available in the USA).

Patients with malaria should be treated parenterally if (1) vomiting is prominent and oral fluids and medication are not retained, (2) there are signs or symptoms of neurologic dysfunction, or (3) the peripheral asexual parasitemia is 5% (> 250,000/μL) or higher. Quinine dihydrochloride or quinidine gluconate is administered intravenously (Table 34–3) and oral treatment with chloroquine is begun as soon as possible. Chloroquine hydrochloride intramuscularly (contraindicated in young children) is a more toxic alternative parenteral drug.

2. Eradication of *P vivax* or *P ovale* infections–This is accomplished with a standard course of primaquine.

3. Elimination of persistent gametocytemia–Gametocytes of *P vivax*, *P ovale*, and *P malariae* can be eliminated by chloroquine. Gametocytes of *P falciparum* are eliminated by a single dose of 26.3 mg of primaquine salt.

---

*Not available in the USA but available in some other countries.

4. Treatment of semi-immunes–Treatment of attacks in semi-immune patients generally requires shorter courses of drug treatment.

C. Treatment of Falciparum Malaria Acquired in Areas Where *P falciparum* Is Resistant to Chloroquine: Start treatment with oral quinine sulfate and a second drug (Table 34–3). Quinine is a rapidly acting blood schizonticide, whereas the other drugs are slower-acting. Fansidar should not be used in areas of Southeast Asia where resistance is common. Alternative drugs are mefloquine (see Table 34–3) or halofantrine (not available in the USA). Available in some countries are investigational qinghaosu derivatives.

If the patient is severely ill, begin with parenteral quinine dihydrochloride or quinidine gluconate and start oral quinine sulfate as soon as possible (see Table 34–3). In emergencies requiring parenteral treatment, if parenteral quinidine is not available in hospital pharmacies, the CDC will provide the drug on an emergency basis ([404] 639–2888).

Special Measures for Treatment of Severe *P falciparum* Malaria

Severe and complicated falciparum malaria is a medical emergency that requires intensive care and the initiation of chemotherapy as rapidly as possible with a rapidly acting blood schizonticide (quinine dihydrochloride or quinidine gluconate) given intravenously. Rehydration of the patient should be carried out with caution, particularly in the first 24 hours, since overhydration may precipitate noncardiogenic pulmonary edema. Fluid, electrolyte, and acid-base balance must be monitored. In general, 2–3 L of fluid is required the first day, followed by 10–20 mL/kg/d; intake and output should be carefully recorded. Dialysis may be necessary for renal failure. Blood glucose levels should be monitored every 6 hours during the acute and early convalescent period, since hypoglycemia may be severe, especially during quinine therapy. Treatment is with 50% dextrose (1–2 mL/kg) followed by a 4-hour infusion of 10% dextrose. Patients with clinically significant disseminated intravascular coagulation should be treated with fresh whole blood. Anticonvulsants (eg, diazepam) are used for seizures; the temperature is maintained below 38.5 °C (101.3 °F). Exchange transfusions (5–10 L for adults) are indicated if more than 15% of red blood cells are parasitized (5% if severe dysfunction of other organs is present). Corticosteroids have been shown to be deleterious in cerebral malaria and should not be used. Heparin, dextran, epinephrine, and hyperimmune immunoglobulin have not proved useful.

Follow-Up for *P falciparum* Malaria

Blood films should be checked daily until parasi-temia clears; check weekly thereafter for 4 weeks to observe for recrudescence of infection.

Prognosis

The uncomplicated and untreated primary attack of *P vivax, P ovale,* or *P falciparum* malaria usually lasts 2–4 weeks; that of *P malariae* about twice as long. Attacks of each type of infection may subsequently occur (once or many times) before the infection terminates spontaneously. With modern antimalarial drugs, the prognosis is good for most malaria infections, but in *P falciparum* infections, when severe complications such as cerebral malaria develop, the prognosis is poor even with treatment.

Gilles HM: Malaria: An overview. J Infect 1989;18:11.

Hoffman SL: Diagnosis, treatment, and prevention of malaria. Med Clin North Am 1992;76:1327.

Miller KD, Greenberg AE, Campbell VCR: Treatment of severe malaria in the United States with a continuous infusion of quinidine gluconate and exchange transfusion. N Engl J Med 1989;321:65.

Recommendations for the prevention of malaria among travelers. MMWR Morb Mortal Wkly Rep 1990;39:1.

Schwartz IK: Prevention of malaria. Infect Dis Clin North Am 1992;6:313.

White NJ: Antimalarial pharmacokinetics and treatment regimens. Br J Clin Pharmacol 1992;34:1.

WHO Malaria Action Programme: Severe and complicated malaria. Trans Roy Soc Trop Med Hyg 1986;80 (Suppl):1.

WHO: Practical chemotherapy of malaria. Tech Report Ser 1990a;No. 805.

WHO: Severe and complicated malaria. Trans R Soc Trop Med Hyg 1990b;84(Suppl 2):1.

PNEUMOCYSTOSIS
(*Pneumocystis carinii* Pneumonia)

Essentials of Diagnosis

- Fever, dyspnea, nonproductive cough.
- Bilateral diffuse interstitial disease without hilar adenopathy by chest x-ray.
- Bibasilar crackles on auscultation in many cases; others have no findings.
- Reduced partial pressure of oxygen.
- *Pneumocystis carinii* in lung tissue or fluid.

General Considerations

P carinii is of uncertain taxonomic status. It was originally thought to be a protozoan, but recent phylogenetic analysis suggests that it is a fungus. The organism has been found in the lungs of a variety of domesticated and wild mammals and is distributed worldwide in humans. Although the disease is rare in the general population, serologic evidence indicates that asymptomatic infections have occurred in most persons by a young age. The overt infection (pneumocystosis) is an acute interstitial plasma cell pneumonia that occurs with high frequency among two groups: (1) as epidemics of primary infections among prematures or debilitated or marasmic infants on hospital wards, and (2) as sporadic cases among older children and adults who have an abnormal or altered immune status. Infection in the latter group is assumed to be due to reactivation of latent infection in the presence of immunosuppression. Cases occur generally in patients with cancer or severe malnutrition and debility, in patients treated with immunosuppressive or cytotoxic drugs or irradiation for the management of organ transplants and cancer, and, most commonly, in patients with AIDS (see Chapter 30).

The organism has three developmental forms: cysts, sporozoites, and trophozoites. The thick-walled cyst is 5–8 µm in diameter and contains eight sporozoites; when released from the cyst, these sporozoites become pleomorphic trophozoites, which are 1–4 µm in diameter. Not confirmed is that the life cycle includes both an asexual and a sexual phase. The mode of transmission in primary infection is unknown, but the evidence suggests airborne transmission. Following asymptomatic primary infection, latent and presumably inactive organisms are sparsely distributed in the alveoli.

In AIDS, *Pneumocystis* pneumonia occurs in up to 80% of patients and is a major cause of death. Its incidence increases in direct proportion to the fall in CD4 cells, with most cases occurring when the cells are below 200/µL. Dissemination of the infection to tissues other than the lung is rare. In non-AIDS patients receiving immunosuppressive therapy, symptoms frequently begin after corticosteroids have been tapered or discontinued.

Clinical Findings

A. Symptoms and Signs: With rare exceptions, findings are limited to the pulmonary parenchyma. In the sporadic form of the disease associated with deficient cell-mediated immunity, the onset is abrupt, with fever, tachypnea, shortness of breath, and mild and usually nonproductive cough. Pulmonary physical findings may be slight and disproportionate to the degree of illness and to the radiologic findings; many patients have bibasilar crackles, but others do not. Without treatment, the course is usually one of rapid deterioration and death. In adult disease, patients may present also with spontaneous pneumothorax. In the infantile form of the disease, the patient is generally free of fever and may show eosinophilia. Patients with AIDS will usually have other evidence of HIV-associated disease, including fever, fatigue, and weight loss, for weeks or months preceding the illness.

B. Laboratory Findings: In screening, chest radiographs most often show diffuse "interstitial" infiltration, which may be heterogeneous or miliary or patchy early in infection. There may also be diffuse or focal consolidation, cystic changes, nodules, or cavitation within nodules; 5–10% of patients with *P carinii* pneumonia have normal chest films. Chest films are more often atypical in patients who have received prophylaxis with aerosolized pentamidine.

Typically, there is reduction in vital and total lung capacity, and the single-breath diffusing capacity for carbon monoxide shows impaired diffusion. The blood gases usually show severe hypoxemia with hypocapnia. Gallium lung scanning (sensitivity > 95%, specificity 20–40%) shows diffuse uptake; the test should be reserved for those with normal chest films and normal pulmonary function. There may be increased clearance of inhaled ^{99m}Tc diethylenetriamine acetate, a marker of alveolar-capillary permeability. Isolated elevation or rising levels of serum LDH are characteristic. Lymphopenia with depleted CD4 lymphocytes is common. Serologic tests, including tests to detect antigenemia, are not helpful in diagnosis. Recently, however, some AIDS patients were shown to develop IgM antibodies with recurrent episodes of pneumocystosis.

Specific diagnosis depends on morphologic demonstration of the organisms in clinical specimens using specific stains. The organism cannot be cultured. Although patients rarely spontaneously produce sufficient sputum for examination, adequate specimens can usually be obtained with induced sputum by having patients inhale an aerosol of hypertonic saline (3%) produced by an ultrasonic nebulizer. Additional techniques for obtaining specimens include bronchoalveolar lavage (sensitivity 86–97%) followed by transbronchial lung biopsy (85–97%). Open lung biopsy and needle lung biopsy are less frequently done.

Treatment

Treatment should be based on a proved diagnosis. Trimethoprim-sulfamethoxazole (TMP-SMZ) and pentamidine isethionate are equally effective, but severe adverse reactions can occur in up to 50% of patients receiving either drug. In non-AIDS patients, the former drug is preferred because of its lower incidence of side effects. In AIDS patients, however, side effects are equivalent, and the choice of agent therefore depends on other factors (eg, in mild to moderately severe infection, TMP-SMZ but not pentamidine can be given orally; TMP-SMZ is used in preexisting renal disease; pentamidine is used if fluid must be restricted or if there is a history of sulfonamide drug sensitivity). Therapy should be continued with the selected drug for at least 5–10 days before one considers changing agents, as fever, tachypnea, and pulmonary infiltrates persist for 4–6 days after starting treatment; some patients have a transient worsening of their disease during the first 3–5 days, which may be related to an inflammatory response secondary to the presence of dead or dying organisms. Most clinicians prefer to treat episodes of AIDS-associated pneumocystis pneumonia for 21 days rather than the usual 14 days recommended for non-AIDS cases, though clinical data to support this view are not available.

A. Trimethoprim-Sulfamethoxazole: The dosage is TMP 20 mg/kg (12–15 mg/kg may decrease side effects without decreasing efficacy) and SMZ 100 mg/kg given orally or intravenously daily in four divided doses at 6-hour intervals for 14–21 days. Sulfonamide precautions must be observed; adverse reactions are generally those of sulfonamides. Patients with AIDS have a high frequency of hypersensitivity reactions—fever, rashes (sometimes severe), malaise, neutropenia, hepatitis, nephritis, thrombocytopenia, and hyperbilirubinemia.

B. Pentamidine Isethionate: This drug is administered intravenously (preferred) or intramuscularly as a single dose of 4 mg (salt)/kg/d (3 mg/kg/d may decrease side effects without decreasing efficacy) for 14–21 days. To avoid injection site pain or sterile abscesses, most workers administer the drug only intravenously by diluting it in 250 mL of 5% dextrose in water and giving it slowly over 1 hour. Pentamidine causes side effects in nearly 50% of patients. Occasional reactions include rash, neutropenia, abnormal liver function tests, serum folate depression, hyperkalemia, and hypocalcemia. Hypoglycemia (often clinically inapparent), hyperglycemia, hyponatremia, and delayed nephrotoxicity with azotemia may occur. Rarely, a variety of other severe adverse reactions may occur, including anemia, thrombocytopenia, ventricular arrhythmias, and fatal pancreatitis. Blood glucose levels should be monitored. Inadvertent rapid intravenous infusion may cause precipitous hypotension.

Aerosolized pentamidine continues to be used in treatment trials. However, the aerosol should not be used alone but in conjunction with oral or parenteral medication. When aerosolized, pentamidine is minimally absorbed and, for the most part, systemic toxicity is avoided; infrequent side effects are cough, bronchospasm, and bronchial bleeding; hypersensitivity reactions are rare. Pretreatment with bronchodilators such as albuterol may be useful.

C. Atovaquone, a hydroxynaphthoquinone, was recently FDA-approved for patients with mild to moderate disease who can not tolerate TMP-SMZ or pentamidine. One dosage regimen is 750 mg two to four times daily for 21 days.

D. Other Drugs: Eflornithine, trimetrexate with or without sulfadiazine, clindamycin with primaquine, and dapsone with trimethoprim are investigational therapies. Corticosteroids in conjunction with antimicrobials are being given commonly when PaO_2 on admission is less than 60 mm Hg or when the patient appears especially distressed; most clinicians believe their use improves the prognosis in severe *P carinii* pneumonia.

E. Supportive Care: Because of the hypoxia usually associated with this disease, oxygen therapy is indicated to maintain the oxygen saturation over 90% by pulse oximeter.

Prevention

The recommendation from the Centers for Disease Control is that prophylaxis be provided for all HIV-infected adults who have had an episode of pneumocystosis. Prophylaxis should also be initiated for those who have never had an episode if their T-helper lymphocytes are less than 200/µL or less than 20% of total lymphocytes. The treatment IND approved for use in the USA for aerosol pentamidine is a 300 mg dose every 4 weeks, with delivery recommended via the Respirgard II jet nebulizer. The dose is diluted in 6 mL of sterile water and delivered at 6 L/min from a 50-psi compressed air source until the reservoir is dry. Inhalation should be in a recumbent position and periodically to full lung capacity. Further information is available from (800) 727–7003.

Although less extensively studied, prophylaxis is also possible with oral TMP (160 mg) and SMZ (800 mg) twice daily plus 5 mg of leucovorin once daily. A high incidence of adverse reactions can be anticipated (granulocytopenia, fever, rash, pruritus, aminotransferase elevations, Stevens-Johnson syndrome). Regimens using lower doses—eg, one double-strength TMP-SMZ tablet daily or even twice weekly—may be just as effective with less toxicity. Oral dapsone is also useful and is inexpensive; it is instituted if the other regimens prove too toxic or impractical.

Chemoprophylaxis for high-risk non-AIDS immunocompromised patients consists of oral TMP (5 mg/kg) and SMZ (25 mg/kg) in two divided doses daily or on 3 consecutive days a week. Persons with G6PD deficiency should not receive such prophylaxis.

Prognosis

In the absence of early and adequate treatment, the fatality rate for the endemic infantile form of pneumocystosis is 20–50%; for the sporadic form in immunodeficient persons, the fatality rate is nearly 100%. Early treatment reduces the mortality rate to about 3% in the former and 25% in the latter forms of infection. In immunodeficient patients who do not receive prophylaxis, recurrences are common (30% in AIDS).

Abouya YL et al: *Pneumocystis carinii* pneumonia. An uncommon cause of death in African patients with acquired immunodeficiency syndrome. Am Rev Respir Dis 1992;145:617.

Atovaquone for *Pneumocystis carinii* pneumonia. Med Lett Drugs Ther 1993;35:28

Kovacs JA, Masur H: Prophylaxis for *Pneumocystis carinii* pneumonia in patients infected with human immunodeficiency virus. Clin Infect Dis 1992;14:1005.

Smulian AG, Walzer PD: The biology of *Pneumocystis carinii*. Crit Rev Microbiol 1992;18:191.

White DA, Zaman MK: Medical management of AIDS patients. Pulmonary disease. Med Clin North Am 1992; 76:19.

TOXOPLASMOSIS

Essentials of Diagnosis

Acute primary infection:

- Fever, malaise, headache, lymphadenopathy (especially cervical), myalgia, arthralgia, stiff neck, sore throat; occasionally, rash, hepatosplenomegaly, retinochoroiditis, confusion; in various combinations.
- Positive serologic tests with high and rising IgG and IgM.
- Isolation of *Toxoplasma gondii* from blood or body fluids; tachyzoites in histologic sections of tissue or cytologic preparations of body fluids.

Acute primary or recrudescent infection in immunocompromised patients:

- Central nervous system mass lesions; retinochoroiditis, pneumonitis, myocarditis less common; sometimes other findings as above.
- Positive IgG titers moderately high; IgM antibody usually absent.
- Tissue diagnosis as above.

General Considerations

T gondii, an obligate intracellular protozoan, is found worldwide in humans and in many species of animals and birds. The parasite is a coccidian of cats, the definitive host, and exists in three forms: The trophozoite (tachyzoite) is the rapidly proliferating form seen in the tissues and body fluids in the acute stage. The trophozoites can enter and multiply in most mammalian nucleated cells. The cyst (bradyzoite), containing viable trophozoites, is the latent form that can persist indefinitely in the host in the chronic stage and is found particularly in muscle and nerve tissue. The oocyst is the form passed only in the feces of the cat family. In the intestinal epithelium of cats, a sexual cycle occurs, with subsequent release of oocysts. Human infection results from (1) ingestion of oocysts (from soil by soil-eating children or by careless handling of cat litter), (2) ingestion of cysts in raw or undercooked meat, (3) transplacental transmission, or, rarely, (4) direct inoculation of trophozoites, as in blood transfusion. Antibody prevalence rates range from less than 5% in some parts of the world (absence of cats, minimal ingestion of meat) to about 55% in the USA and over 80% in France.

Clinical Findings

A. Symptoms and Signs: Over 80% of primary infections are asymptomatic. The incubation period for symptomatic persons is 1–2 weeks.

The clinical manifestations of toxoplasmosis may be grouped into four syndromes:

1. Primary infection in the normal host– Most infections are acute, mild, febrile multisystem illnesses that resemble infectious mononucleosis. Lymphadenopathy, particularly of the head and neck, is the most common finding. Other features in various combinations are malaise, myalgia, arthralgia, headache, sore throat, and maculopapular or urticarial rash. Hepatomegaly may occur. Rarely, severe cases are complicated by pneumonitis, meningoencephalitis, hepatitis, myocarditis, and retinochoroiditis. Symptoms may fluctuate, but most patients recover spontaneously over 1–2 months. Generally, on recovery, both asymptomatic and symptomatic infections persist as chronic infections.

2. Congenital infection–Congenital transmission occurs only as a result of infection (generally asymptomatic) in a nonimmune woman during pregnancy. Infection has been detected in up to 1% of women during pregnancy; 15–60% of such infections, varying by trimester, are transmitted to the fetus, but only a small percentage result in abortions or stillbirths or in active disease in premature or full-term, live-born infants. Though fetal infection may occur in any trimester, it is more severe early in pregnancy.

Signs of congenital toxoplasmosis may be present at birth or may develop during the first months of life: central nervous system disorders (microcephaly, internal hydrocephalus, seizures, retinochoroiditis, cerebral calcifications), hepatosplenomegaly, pneumonitis, rash, fever, jaundice, anemia, and thrombocytopenia. Psychomotor and learning disorders, hearing loss, mental retardation, and retinochoroiditis may not be apparent for years.

3. Retinochoroiditis–This develops gradually weeks to years after congenital infection (the preponderant form, which is generally bilateral) or rarely after an acquired infection in a young child (generally unilateral). Primary infections in older children and adults rarely progress to retinochoroiditis. The inflammatory process persists for weeks to months as focally necrotic retinal lesions with blurred margins. Visual defects include blurring, central defects, and scotomas. Rarely, progression may result in glaucoma and blindness. With healing, white or dark-pigmented scars may result.

4. Primary infection or reactivated disease in the immunologically compromised host–Primary or reactivated toxoplasmosis occurs in patients with AIDS, cancer, or those given immunosuppressive drugs. The infection may present in specific organs (brain most commonly, but also lung, heart, and liver) or as disseminated disease. In AIDS, depletion of CD4 T cell lymphocytes and macrophage dysfunction predispose to reactivation of latent *Toxoplasma* infection. In AIDS patients seropositive for *Toxoplasma,* up to 30% will develop focal or (less often) diffuse intracerebral toxoplasma lesions appear associated with clinical findings of fever, headache, altered mental status, seizures, and focal (or, infrequently, nonfocal) neurologic deficits.

B. Laboratory Findings: Diagnosis depends principally on serologic tests, which are sensitive and reliable. However, toxoplasmosis can be diagnosed occasionally by histologic examination of tissue or isolation of the parasite in mice or tissue culture (1–6 weeks may be required). Cysts or trophozoites may be directly identified by staining blood (buffy coat from centrifuged heparinized blood), bone marrow aspirates, cerebrospinal fluid sediment, sputum, and other tissue or body fluids or placental tissue. The demonstration of cysts does not establish a causal relationship to clinical illness, since cysts may be found in both acute and chronic infections. However, only finding tachyzoites in blood or body fluids confirms active infection. In the placenta, fetus, or newborn, the presence of cysts indicates congenital infection. Leukocyte counts are normal or reduced, often with lymphocytosis or monocytosis with rare atypical cells, but there is no heterophil antibody. Chest radiographs may show interstitial pneumonia.

Serologic tests—the Sabin-Feldman dye test and the indirect hemagglutination, indirect immunofluorescence (IFA), ELISA, and other tests—can be done on blood, cerebrospinal fluid, aqueous humor, and other body fluids. The dye test, which is extremely sensitive and specific, is the standard, but it is rarely used because of laboratory safety factors. The ELISA and IFA tests permit separation of IgM and IgG antibody. In the IFA test for IgM, antibody appears 1–2 weeks after start of infection, reaches a peak at 6–8 weeks, and then gradually declines; low titers persist for life in most patients, but in some, high titers persist. False-positive and false-negative tests can occur with the IFA test; the former can be avoided by use of IgM capture tests. Using various body fluids, diagnosis by detection of antigen or of nucleic acid sequences specific for *T gondii* is experimental.

The following are selected serologic findings in specific toxoplasmosis syndromes:

1. Acute infection in immunocompetent persons–The diagnosis is established by seroconversion from negative to positive, by a fourfold rise in serologic titers by any test, or by a single high titer (1:160) of IgM antibody. A presumptive diagnosis is based on a single IgM titer of over 1:64 and a very high IgG titer (> 1:1000). A negative dye or comparable test for IgG virtually excludes the diagnosis of acute toxoplasmosis.

2. Recrudescent infection in immunosuppressed patients–In AIDS patients with focal brain lesions, *Toxoplasma* can sometimes be isolated from the blood. Alternatively, definitive diagnosis is only by finding *Toxoplasma* organisms in cerebrospinal fluid (Wright-Giemsa stain) or by brain biopsy. To avoid the latter, empiric antibiotic treatment is generally started after presumptive evidence is obtained by MRI (the more sensitive test) or CT scan (typically:

multiple, isodense or hypodense, ring-enhancing mass lesions). Antibody titers cannot be depended on, since most patients have IgG titers that reflect past infection, significant rises are infrequent, and IgM antibody is rare. However, absence of IgG is strong evidence against the diagnosis of central nervous system toxoplasmosis. The cerebrospinal fluid may show mild pleocytosis (predominantly lymphocytes and monocytes), elevated protein, and normal glucose; rarely seen is a rise in antibody titers.

3. Toxoplasmic retinochoroiditis–This is usually associated with stable, usually low IgG titers and no IgM antibody. If IgG antibody in aqueous humor is higher than in the serum, the diagnosis is supported.

4. Congenital toxoplasmosis–An IgG titer in excess of 1:1000 or rising titers are presumptively diagnostic, but low titers are sometimes found. Confirmation is by a test for IgM and finally the isolation of *Toxoplasma.* IgG but not IgM is transferred across the intact placenta; if a leak occurs in the placenta, the IgM transferred has a half-life of 3–5 days.

Where available, testing for antigenemia has been used to demonstrate acute infection, and lymphocyte transformation to *Toxoplasma* antigens has provided a specific and sensitive indicator of prior infection.

Differential Diagnosis

In acute febrile disease, consider cytomegalovirus infection, infectious mononucleosis, and other causes of pneumonitis, myocarditis, myositis, hepatitis, and splenomegaly. With lymphadenopathy, possibilities include sarcoidosis, tuberculosis, tularemia, lymphoma, and metastatic carcinoma. With brain lesions in the immunosuppressed host, herpes simplex, cytomegalovirus infection, other viral encephalitides, multifocal leukoencephalopathy, fungal encephalitis, vascular stroke, tuberculosis, psychosis, and, in particular, central nervous system lymphoma.

Treatment

A. Approach to Treatment: Asymptomatic infections in normal hosts are not treated except in children under 5 years of age, who receive therapy to avoid possible occurrence of retinochoroiditis.

Symptomatic patients should be treated until manifestations of the illness have subsided and there is serologic evidence that immunity has been acquired.

Since most episodes of **retinochoroiditis** are self-limited, opinions vary on indications for treatment. See reference by Engstrom et al for details on indications and management.

Immunocompromised patients with active infection (primary or recrudescent) must be treated. Therapy should continue for 4–6 weeks after cessation of symptoms—which may require up to a 6-month course, to be followed by drug prophylaxis as long as immunosuppression persists. In AIDS patients, treatment should be continued indefinitely. Chronic asymptomatic infection in these patients usually need not be treated, but prophylaxis may be started if significant increase in antibody titer is noted.

Treatment is also indicated in **congenitally infected infants** with or without symptoms. Treatment of women who become infected during **pregnancy** is controversial because of possible toxic effects on the fetus. Because early treatment reduces (but does not eliminate) the incidence of fetal infection, most workers feel that treatment is justified. For details on management of congenital infections and those occurring during pregnancy, see specialized texts.

B. Choice of Drugs: The treatment of choice is pyrimethamine, 75 mg/d for 3 days, then 25 mg daily, plus either trisulfapyrimidines (2–6 g/d in four divided doses) or sulfadiazine (100 mg/kg/d [maximum 6 g/d] in four divided doses); continue this treatment for 3–4 weeks. Folinic acid (calcium leucovorin), 10 mg/d in two to four divided doses, is given to avoid the hematologic effects of pyrimethamine-induced folate deficiency. Platelet and white blood cell counts should be performed at least twice weekly. Patients should be screened for a history of sulfonamide sensitivity.

In the treatment of toxoplasmosis encephalitis in AIDS, higher dosages are used. Primary therapy (for 6 weeks or longer if necessary) is as follows: pyrimethamine, 200 mg as loading dose in two divided doses, then 1–1.5 mg/kg/d; sulfadiazine or trisulfapyrimidines, 4–6 g/d in four divided doses; folinic acid, 10–50 mg/d in two divided doses. Maintenance therapy is as follows: pyrimethamine, 25–50 mg/d; sulfadiazine or trisulfapyrimidines, 2 g/d in two divided doses; folinic acid, 5–20 mg/d in two divided doses. Corticosteroids are often added to reduce increased intracranial pressure.

Spiramycin is in use in Europe at a dosage of 2–4 g in four divided doses. Although safe and effective in pregnancy, the drug does not reach the fetus. It is not effective in encephalitis. In the USA, the drug is available from the manufacturer. Clindamycin (300 mg [450–600 mg in AIDS] four times daily) may be a useful alternative therapy; because it concentrates in the choroid, it is used in the treatment of ocular disease. Trimethoprim-sulfamethoxazole is being used but with unreliable results.

Prevention

Freezing of meat to –20 °C for 2 days or heating to 60 °C kills cysts in tissues. Under appropriate environmental conditions, oocysts passed in cat feces can remain infective for a year or more. Thus, children's play areas, including sandboxes, should be protected from cat and dog feces; hand washing is indicated after contact with soil potentially contaminated by animal feces. Indoor cats should be fed only dry, canned, or cooked meat. Litter boxes should be changed daily, as freshly deposited oocysts are not infective for 48 hours.

Pregnant women should have their serum examined for *Toxoplasma* antibody. If the IgM test is negative but an IgG titer is present and less than 1:1000, no further evaluation is necessary. Those with negative titers should take measures to prevent infection—preferably by having no further contact with cats and by thoroughly cooking meat. Hands should be washed after handling raw meat and before eating or touching the face.

Optimal regimens for primary or secondary prophylaxis for AIDS patients have not been established.

Prognosis

The outlook for acute toxoplasmosis in adults is excellent as long as the patient is immunocompetent. Acute infection in young children, however, may be followed by one or more attacks of retinochoroiditis; treatment appears to reduce the frequency of attacks. Treatment of immunosuppressed patients usually results in improvement if begun early, but recrudescence is common. Chronic asymptomatic infection, as indicated by a persistent antibody titer, is usually benign.

Ades AE: Evaluating the sensitivity and predictive value of tests of recent infection: Toxoplasmosis in pregnancy. Epidemiol Infect 1991;107:527.

Daffos F et al: Prenatal management of 746 pregnancies at risk for congenital toxoplasmosis. N Engl J Med 1988;318:271.

Dannemann B et al: Treatment of toxoplasmic encephalitis in patients with AIDS: A randomized trial comparing pyrimethamine plus clindamycin to pyrimethamine plus sulfadiazine. Ann Intern Med 1992;116:33.

Engstrom RE et al: Current practices in the management of ocular toxoplasmosis. Am J Ophthalmol 1991;111:601.

Luft BJ, Remington JS: Toxoplasmic encephalitis in AIDS. Clin Infect Dis 1992;15:211.

Pomeroy C, Filice GA: Pulmonary toxoplasmosis: A review. Clin Infect Dis 1992;14:863.

Renold C et al: *Toxoplasma* encephalitis in patients with the acquired immunodeficiency syndrome. Medicine 1992; 71:224.

REFERENCES

Drugs for Parasitic Infections. Med Lett Drugs Ther 1992;34:17.

Goldsmith RS: Clinical pharmacology of the anthelmintic drugs. In: *Basic & Clinical Pharmacology,* 5th ed. Katzung BG (editor). Appleton & Lange, 1991.

Goldsmith RS, Heyneman D (editors): *Tropical Medicine and Parasitology.* Appleton & Lange, 1989.

Health Information for International Travel. HHS Publication No. (CDC) 92–8280. Superintendent of Documents, Washington, DC 20402, 1992.

Maddison SE: Serodiagnosis of parasitic diseases. Clin Microbiol Rev 1991;4:457.

Markell EK, Voge M, John DT (editors): *Medical Parasitology,* 7th ed. Saunders, 1991.

Rosenblatt JE: Antiparasitic agents. Mayo Clin Proc 1992;67:276.

Strickland GT: *Hunter's Tropical Medicine,* 7th ed. Saunders, 1991.

Van Voorhis WC: Therapy and prophylaxis of systemic protozoan infections. Drugs 1990;40:176.

Warren KS, Mahmoud AAF: *Tropical and Geographic Medicine,* 2nd ed. McGraw-Hill, 1990.

Webster LT Jr: Chemotherapy of parasitic infections. In: *Goodman and Gilman's The Pharmacological Basis of Therapeutics,* 8th ed. Gilman AG et al (editors). Pergamon, 1990.

White NJ: Antiparasitic drugs in children. Clin Pharmacokinet 1989;17:138.

WHO Model Prescribing Information: Drugs Used in Parasitic Diseases. WHO, 1990.

35 Infectious Diseases: Helminthic

Robert S. Goldsmith, MD, MPH, DTM&H

TREMATODE (FLUKE) INFECTIONS

SCHISTOSOMIASIS (Bilharziasis)

Essentials of Diagnosis

- Acute phase: Abrupt onset (2–6 weeks' postexposure) of abdominal pain, weight loss, headache, malaise, chills, fever, myalgia, diarrhea (sometimes bloody), dry cough, hepatomegaly, and eosinophilia.
- Chronic phase: Either (1) diarrhea, abdominal pain, blood in stool, hepatomegaly or hepatosplenomegaly, and bleeding from esophageal varices (*Schistosoma mansoni* or *Schistosoma japonicum* infection); or (2) terminal hematuria, urinary frequency, and urethral and bladder pain (*Schistosoma haematobium* infection).
- Depending on species, characteristic eggs in feces, urine, or scrapings or biopsy of rectal or bladder mucosa.

General Considerations

Schistosomiasis, which infects more than 200 million persons worldwide, is caused mainly by three blood flukes (trematodes). *S mansoni*, which causes intestinal schistosomiasis, is widespread in Africa and occurs in the Arabian peninsula, northern and eastern South America, and the Caribbean (including Puerto Rico but not Cuba). Vesical (urinary) schistosomiasis, caused by *S haematobium*, is found throughout the Middle East and Africa. Asiatic intestinal schistosomiasis, due to *S japonicum*, is important in China and the Philippines, and a small focus is present in Sulawesi, Indonesia, but transmission in Japan has been interrupted. A number of schistosome species of animals sometimes infect humans, including *Schistosoma intercalatum* in central Africa and *Schistosoma mekongi* in the Mekong delta in Thailand, Cambodia, and Laos.

Mammals are important reservoirs for *S ja-* *ponicum.* Humans are the main reservoir for *S mansoni* and *S haematobium;* the few animal species infected with *S mansoni* are not epidemiologically important.

In the life cycle involving humans, the adult worms live in terminal venules of the bowel (*S mansoni*, *S japonicum*) or bladder (*S haematobium*). When eggs passed in feces or urine reach fresh water, a larval form is released that subsequently infects snails, the intermediate host. After development, infective larvae (cercariae) leave the snails, enter water, and infect exposed persons through the skin or mucous membranes. After penetration, the cercariae become schistosomula larvae that reach the portal circulation in the liver, where they rapidly mature. After a few weeks, adult worms pair, mate, and migrate mainly to terminal venules of specific veins, where females deposit their eggs. By means of their lytic secretions, some eggs reach the lumen of the bowel or bladder and are passed with feces or urine. Others are retained in the bowel or bladder wall, while still others are carried in the circulation to the liver, lung, and (less often) to other tissues. Except for the allergic response in the acute syndrome (see below), disease is primarily due to delayed hypersensitivity. Antigens released by the eggs stimulate a local T cell-dependent granulomatous response, followed by a strong fibrotic reaction. Live worms produce no lesions and rarely cause symptoms. The type or degree of tissue damage and symptoms varies with the intensity of infection (worm burden), degree of host reaction, site of egg deposition, and duration of infection.

S mansoni adults migrate to the inferior mesenteric veins of the large bowel and *S japonicum* to the superior and inferior mesenteric veins in the large and small bowel. Ulcers and polyps (common only in Egypt) result from granuloma formation and fibrosis in the bowel wall. Egg accumulation in the liver may result in periportal fibrosis and portal hypertension of the presinusoidal type, but liver function typically remains intact even in advanced disease. Collateralization due to portal hypertension results in embolization of eggs to the lungs, with subsequent endarteritis, pulmonary hypertension, and cor pulmonale. Because greater numbers of eggs are produced by *S japonicum,* the resulting disease is often more severe.

Adult *S haematobium* mature in the venous plexus of the bladder, rectum, prostate, and uterus. Ulcers and polyps result from granuloma formation and fibrosis in the bladder wall, and eggshell remnants may calcify. Stricture or distortion of the ureteral orifices of terminal ureters may result in hydroureter, hydronephrosis, and ascending infection. Lesions in the pelvic organs rarely progress to extensive fibrosis and infection. Eggs are carried to the liver or lungs, but severe pathologic changes in these organs are less frequent than in *S mansoni* infections.

In size, adult *S mansoni* are 6–13 × 1 mm. The prepatent period—from cercarial penetration until appearance of eggs in feces—is about 50 days. The life span of the worms ranges from 5 to 30 years or more.

Clinical Findings

A. Symptoms and Signs: The great majority of infected persons have light infections and are asymptomatic.

1. Cercarial dermatitis—Following cercarial penetration, clinical findings progress from an itchy erythematous or petechial rash to macules and papules that last up to 5 days. This syndrome is uncommon with human schistosome infections. Instead, most recognized cases occur worldwide in fresh or marine water and are due to skin invasion by bird cercariae, schistosomes that do not mature in humans and do not cause systemic symptoms.

2. Acute schistosomiasis (Katayama fever)—This syndrome, primarily an allergic response to the developing schistosomes, may occur with the three schistosomes (rare with *S haematobium*) and usually is not seen in natives. The incubation period ranges from 2 to 7 weeks and the severity of illness from mild to (rarely) life-threatening. In addition to fever, malaise, urticaria, diarrhea (sometimes bloody), myalgia, dry cough, and marked eosinophilia, the liver and spleen may be temporarily enlarged. The patient again becomes asymptomatic in 2–8 weeks. It is not established that drug treatment (praziquantel and, if the patient is severely ill, a corticosteroid) is safe during the acute stage because release of antigens from dying immature worms may severely exacerbate symptoms. An ELISA to detect antibody to antihemocyanin may prove useful in early diagnosis.

3. Chronic schistosomiasis—This stage begins 6 months to several years after infection. In *S mansoni* and *S japonicum* infections, findings include diarrhea, abdominal pain, blood in stool, a hard enlarged liver, and splenomegaly. With subsequent slow progression over 5–15 years or longer, the following may appear: anorexia, weight loss, weakness, polypoid intestinal tumors, and features of portal and pulmonary hypertension. Immune complex glomerulonephritis may also occur.

Early symptoms of urinary tract disease caused by *S haematobium* are frequency and dysuria, followed by terminal hematuria and proteinuria. Frank hematuria may be recurrent; obstruction of the ureteral orifices may lead to hydronephrosis. Sequelae may include bladder polyp formation, cystitis, chronic *Salmonella* infection and associated glomerulonephritis, pyelitis, pyelonephritis, urolithiasis, renal failure, and death. Severe liver, lung, genital, or neurologic disease is rare. Bladder cancer has been associated with vesicular schistosomiasis.

4. Other complications—

a. Portal hypertension may result in a contracted liver, splenomegaly, pancytopenia, esophageal varices, and variceal bleeding. Abnormal liver function, jaundice, ascites, and hepatic coma are end-stage findings.

b. Pulmonary hypertension with cor pulmonale is characterized by a parasternal lift and loud S_2; neck vein distention and edema due to right heart failure may supervene.

c. Colonic polyposis is manifested by bloody diarrhea, anemia, hypoalbuminemia, and clubbing.

d. Other large bowel complications include stricture, granulomatous masses, and *Salmonella* infection.

e. Collateral circulation of eggs and ectopic worms may cause transverse myelitis, epilepsy, or optic neuritis.

B. Laboratory Findings:

1. Eggs—Definitive diagnosis is made by finding characteristic eggs in excreta or by mucosal or (rarely) liver biopsy.

In *S haematobium* infection, eggs may be found in the urine or, less frequently, in the stools. Eggs are sought in urine specimens collected between 9 AM and 2 PM or in 24-hour collections. They are processed either by examination of the sediment or preferably by membrane filtration. Occasionally, eggs are sought by vesical mucosa biopsy.

In *S mansoni* and *S japonicum* infections, eggs may be found in stool specimens by direct examination, but some form of concentration is usually necessary; repeated examinations are often needed to find eggs in light infections. If results are negative, rectal mucosal biopsy of suspicious lesions or random biopsy specimens at two or three sites of normal mucosa may yield the diagnosis. Biopsy specimens should be examined as crush preparations between two glass slides.

2. Serologic tests—Screening for infection—which is possible by skin (to be discouraged) or serologic tests (ELISA and others)—may detect rare egg-negative or ectopic infection but does not distinguish between active and past infection. An immunoblot test (Western) can differentiate schistosome species. Detection of circulating antigen is under evaluation.

3. Other tests—Anemia is common. Eosinophilia, common during the acute stage, usually is absent in the chronic stage. In S mansoni and S japonicum infections, barium swallow, esophagoscopy, barium enema and colonoscopy, chest x-ray, and an ECG may be indicated. Ultrasound examination of the liver, which may show the pathognomonic pattern of periportal fibrosis, replaces the need for liver biopsy.

In schistosomiasis due to *S haematobium*, microscopic hematuria may be present. In advanced disease, cystoscopy may show "sandy patches," ulcers, and areas of squamous metaplasia; lower abdominal plain films may show calcification of the bladder wall or ureters. Sonography is considered the imaging technique of choice. Intravenous pyelography, retrograde cystography and pyelography, and CT may be useful.

Differential Diagnosis

Early intestinal schistosomiasis may be mistaken for amebiasis, bacillary dysentery, or other causes of diarrhea and dysentery. Later, the various causes of portal hypertension or of bowel polyps must be considered. In endemic areas, vesical schistosomiasis must be differentiated from other causes of urinary symptoms such as genitourinary tract cancer, bacterial infections of the urinary tract, nephrolithiasis, and the like.

Treatment

A. Medical Treatment: (Table 35–1.) Treatment should be given only if live ova are identified. The safety and effectiveness of current drugs make it possible to treat all infections orally, including advanced disease, and without concern for serious side effects. Praziquantel can be used to treat all species; alternative drugs of choice are oxamniquine for *S mansoni* and metrifonate for *S haematobium*.

After treatment, periodic laboratory follow-up for continued passage of eggs is essential, starting at 3 months and continuing at intervals for 1 year. If eggs are found, their viability should be determined, since dead eggs are passed for some months.

1. Praziquantel–Cure rates at 6 months for *S haematobium, S mansoni,* and *S japonicum* infections are 87%, 80%, and 84%, respectively, with marked reduction in egg counts in those not cured.

The dosage for treatment of all forms of schistosomiasis is 20 mg/kg three times daily at 4- to 6-hour intervals for 1 day. Lower dosages have been reported to be highly effective in some parts of the world for *S haematobium* (40 mg/kg once) or *S mansoni* (20 mg/kg twice in 1 day). Tablets are taken with water after a meal and should not be chewed.

Mild and transient side effects persisting for hours to 1 day are common and include malaise, headache, dizziness, and anorexia. Less frequent are fatigue, drowsiness, nausea, vomiting, generalized abdominal pain, loose stools, pruritus, urticaria, arthralgia and myalgia, and low-grade fever. Although minimal elevations of liver enzymes have occasionally been reported, the drug is well tolerated by patients who have hepatosplenomegaly with advanced schistosomiasis. It should not be used in pregnancy, and because of drug-induced dizziness, patients should not drive and should be cautioned if their work requires physical coordination or alertness. In areas where cysticercosis may coexist with a schistosomal infection being treated with praziquantel, treatment is best conducted in a hospital to monitor for death of cysticerci, which may be followed by neurologic complications.

2. Metrifonate–Metrifonate is a highly effective alternative drug for the treatment of *S haematobium* infections only. The dosage is 7.5–10 mg/kg (maximum 600 mg) once and then repeated twice at 2-week intervals. Cure rates range from 44% to 93%. Those not cured show marked reduction in egg counts. Side effects range from none to mild and transient findings, including gastrointestinal symptoms, headache, bronchospasm, weakness, and vertigo. Metrifonate is not available in the USA.

3. Oxamniquine is highly effective in *S mansoni* infections. For strains in the western hemisphere and western Africa, a dose of 12–15 mg/kg is given once (for children under 30 kg, 10 mg/kg twice daily for 1 day). In northern and southern Africa, give 15 mg/kg twice daily for 2 days (children under 30 kg, twice daily for 2–3 days). In eastern Africa and the Arabian peninsula, give 15–20 mg/kg twice daily for 1 day (children under 30 kg, twice daily for 1 day). The drug is administered with food; when divided doses are needed, they are separated by 6–8 hours. Cure rates are 70–95%, with marked reduction in those not cured. Side effects occur within hours: dizziness is most common; less frequent are drowsiness, nausea and vomiting, diarrhea, abdominal pain, and headache. An orange or red discoloration of the urine may occur. Rarely reported is central nervous system stimulation with behavioral changes, hallucinations, or seizures; patients should be observed for 2 hours after ingestion of the drug for appearance of these findings. Since the drug makes some patients dizzy or drowsy, it should be used with caution in patients whose work or activity requires mental alertness. The drug has shown mutagenic and embryocidal effects and is contraindicated in pregnancy.

B. Surgical Measures: In selected instances, surgery may be indicated for removal of polyps. For bleeding esophageal varices, sclerotherapy is the treatment of choice. As a last resort in patients who have repeated bleeding, splenorenal anastomosis is done rather than portacaval shunts, which are associated with a high level of chronic portal systemic encephalopathy. Distal splenorenal shunt and esophagogastric devascularization with splenectomy may be a more successful procedure. Severe pancytopenia is an indication for splenectomy. Filtering of *S mansoni* adults from the portal system should be con-

Table 35–1. Drugs for the treatment of helminthic infections.

Infecting Organism	Drug of Choice	Alternative Drugs
Roundworms (nematodes)		
Ascaris lumbricoides (roundworm)	Pyrantel pamoate or mebendazole	Piperazine, levamisole,[3] or albendazole[1]
Trichuris trichiura (whipworm)	Mebendazole	Albendazole[1] or oxantel/pyrantel pamoate[1]
Necator americanus (hookworm); *Ancylostoma duodenale* (hookworm)	Pyrantel pamoate[3] or mebendazole	Albendazole[1] or levamisole[3]
Combined infection with *Ascaris*, *Trichuris*, and hookworm	Mebendazole or albendazole[1]	Oxantel/pyrantel pamoate[1]
Combined infection with *Ascaris* and hookworm	Mebendazole or pyrantel pamoate	Albendazole[1]
Strongyloides stercoralis (threadworm)	Thiabendazole or ivermectin[4,6]	Albendazole,[1,4] mebendazole,[3,4]
Enterobius vermicularis (pinworm)	Mebendazole or pyrantel pamoate	Albendazole[1]
Trichinella spiralis (trichinosis)	Mebendazole[3,4] or thiabendazole.[4] Add corticosteroids for severe infection	Albendazole.[1,4,8] Add corticosteroids for severe infection.
Trichostrongylus species	Pyrantel pamoate[3] or mebendazole[3]	Albendazole[1,8] or levamisole[3]
Cutaneous larva migrans (creeping eruption)	Albendazole[1,4]	Thiabendazole
Visceral larva migrans	Thiabendazole or albendazole,[1,4,8]	Mebendazole[3,4] or ivermectin[4,6]
Angiostrongylus cantonensis	Levamisole[3,4]	Albendazole[1,4,8] or mebendazole[3,4]
Wuchereria bancrofti (filariasis); *Brugia malayi* (filariasis); tropical eosinophilia; *Loa loa* (loiasis)	Diethylcarbamazine[5]	Ivermectin[4,6]
Onchocerca volvulus (onchocerciasis)	Ivermectin[7]	Diethylcarbamazine[5] plus suramin[7]
Dracunculus medinensis (guinea worm)	Metronidazole[3]	Thiabendazole[3] or mebendazole[3,4]
Capilllaria philippinensis (intestinal capillariasis)	Albendazole[1,8]	Mebendazole[3] or thiabendazole[3]
Flukes (trematodes)		
Schistosoma haematobium (bilharziasis)	Praziquantel	Metrifonate[1]
Schistosoma mansoni	Praziquantel	Oxamniquine
Schistosoma japonicum	Praziquantel	None
Clonorchis sinensis (liver fluke); *Opisthorchis* species	Praziquantel[3]	Mebendazole[3,4] or albendazole[1,4,8]
Paragonimus westermani (lung fluke)	Praziquantel[3]	Bithionol[7]
Fascioloa hepatica (sheep liver fluke)	Bithionol[7] or triclabendazole[1,4]	Praziquantel[2,3] or emetine, or dehydroemetine[7]
Fasciolopsis buski (large intestinal fluke)	Praziquantel[3] or niclosamide[3]	Tetrachloroethylene[1]
Heterophyes heterophyes; *Metagonimus yokogawai* (small intestinal flukes)	Praziquantel[3] or niclosamide[3]	Tetrachloroethylene[1]
Tapeworms (cestodes)		
Taenia saginata (beef tapeworm)	Niclosamide or praziquantel[3]	Mebendazole[3,4]
Diphyllobothrium latum (fish tapeworm)	Niclosamide or praziquantel[3]	
Taenia solium (pork tapeworm)	Niclosamide[3] or praziquantel[3]	
Cysticercosis (pork tapeworm larval stage)	Albendazole[1,8]	Praziquantel[3]
Hymenolepis nana (dwarf tapeworm)	Praziquantel[3]	Niclosamide
Hymenolepis diminuta (rat tapeworm); *Dipylidium caninum*	Niclosamide[3] or praziquantel[3]	
Echinococcus granulosus (hydatid disease); *Echinococcus multilocularis*	Albendazole[1,8]	Mebendazole[3,4]

[1] Not available in the USA; available in some other countries.
[2] Effectiveness not high.
[3] Available in the USA but not labeled for this indication.
[4] Effectiveness not established.
[5] Available in the USA from Lederle Laboratories. Telephone (914) 735–5000.
[6] Available in the USA from Merck Sharpe & Dohme. Telephone (215) 397–2454.
[7] Available in the USA only from the Parasitic Disease Drug Service, Parasitic Diseases Branch, Centers for Disease Control and Prevention, Atlanta 30333. Telephone (404) 639–3670 during the day; (404) 639–2888 nights, weekends, and holidays (emergencies only).
[8] Available in the USA only from SmithKline Beecham. Telephone (800) 366–8700, Ext 5206.

sidered whenever splenectomy is contemplated. Surgery may be required for obstructive uropathy.

Prognosis

With treatment, as long as reinfection does not occur, the prognosis is excellent in early and light infections. There may be shrinkage or elimination of bladder and bowel ulcerations, granulomas, and polyps and reduction in detectable fibrosis by sonography. In advanced disease with extensive involvement of the intestines, liver, bladder, or other organs, the outlook is poor even with treatment.

Capron A, Dessaint JP: Immunologic aspects of schistosomiasis. Annu Rev Med 1992;43:209.

Da Silva LC, Carrilho FJ. Hepatosplenic schistosomiasis: Pathophysiology and treatment. Gastroenterol Clin North Am 1992;21:163.

Ghen MG, Mott KE: Progress in assessment of morbidity due to Schistosoma haematobium infection. Trop Dis Bull 1989;86:R2. (For S mansoni infections, see Trop Dis Bull 1988;85:R2.)

Hatz C, Jenkin JM, Tanner M: Ultrasound in schistosomiasis. Acta Tropica 1992;51:1. (Special issue with 8 articles.)

Homeida MA et al: Association of the therapeutic activity of praziquantel with the reversal of Symmers' fibrosis induced by Schistosoma mansoni. Am J Trop Med Hyg 1991;45:360.

Raia S et al. Portal hypertension in mansonic schistosomiasis. World J Surg 1991;15:176.

Shekhar KC: Schistosomiasis drug therapy and treatment considerations. Drugs 1991;42:379.

FASCIOLOPSIASIS

The large intestinal fluke, *Fasciolopis buski,* is a common parasite of humans and pigs in central and South China, Taiwan, Southeast Asia, Indonesia, eastern India, and Bangladesh. When eggs shed in stools reach water, they hatch to produce free-swimming larvae that penetrate and develop in the flesh of snails. Cercariae subsequently escape from the snails and encyst on various water plants. Humans are infected by eating these plants uncooked (usually water chestnuts, bamboo shoots, or caltrops). Adult flukes (length 2–7.5 cm) mature in about 3 months and live in the small intestine attached to the mucosa or buried in mucous secretions. The number of parasites ranges from a few to several thousand.

After an incubation period of 2–3 months, manifestations of gastrointestinal irritation appear in all but light infections. Symptoms in severe infections include nausea, anorexia, upper abdominal pain, and diarrhea, sometimes alternating with constipation. Ascites and edema of the face and lower extremities may occur later. Ileus, cachexia, and extreme prostration have been described.

Diagnosis depends on finding characteristic eggs or, occasionally, flukes in the stools. Leukocytosis with moderate eosinophilia is common. No serologic test is available. Because the adult worms live for only 6 months, absence from the endemic area for a longer period makes the diagnosis unlikely.

The drug of first choice is praziquantel as a single 25 mg/kg dose. The alternative drug is niclosamide, administered as for taeniasis but given every other day for three doses.

In light infections—even without treatment—the prognosis is good; generally, spontaneous cure occurs within 1 year. In rare cases—particularly in children—heavy infections with severe toxemia have resulted in death from cachexia or intercurrent infection.

Taraschewski H et al: Effects of praziquantel on human intestinal flukes (Fasciolopsis buski and Heterophyes heterophyes). Zbl Bakt Hyg A 1986;262:542.

FASCIOLIASIS

Infection by *Fasciola hepatica,* the sheep liver fluke, results from ingestion of encysted metacercariae on watercress or other aquatic vegetables or in water. A wide range of herbivorous mammals are reservoir hosts. The disease in humans probably occurs worldwide but is most prevalent in sheep-raising countries, particularly where raw salads are eaten. The infection has been reported from Europe, mainland USA, Hawaii, the West Indies, the Middle East, China, Siberia, and North, East and South Africa. Eggs of the worm, passed in host feces into fresh water, release a miracidium that infects snails; the snails subsequently release cercariae that in turn encyst as metacercariae on vegetation (some cercariae become metacercariae directly in the water) to complete their life cycle. The leaf-shaped adult flukes measure 3 × 1.5 cm.

In infection in humans, metacercariae excyst, penetrate and migrate through the liver, and mature in the bile ducts, where they cause local parenchymal necrosis and abscess formation. Although the infection is usually mild, three clinical syndromes can develop: acute, chronic latent, and chronic obstructive. The acute illness, associated with migration of immature larvae through the liver, shows an enlarged and tender liver, high fever, leukocytosis, and marked eosinophilia (to 90%). Pain may be present in the epigastrium or right upper quadrant, and the patient may experience headache, anorexia, and vomiting. Myalgia, urticaria, and other allergic reaction to the helminth may occur. In severe acute illness, the examination may show jaundice, cachexia, and prostration. Anemia and hypergammaglobulinemia are common; other liver function tests may be abnormal. Early diagnosis is difficult in the acute phase, because eggs are not found in the feces for 3–4 months.

In the chronic latent phase, many persons are free of symptoms. Others have variable degrees of hepatomegaly and other findings as seen in the acute phase.

The chronic obstructive phase takes place if the extrahepatic bile ducts are occluded, producing a clinical picture similar to that of choledocholithiasis. Occasionally, adult flukes migrate and produce lesions and symptoms in ectopic sites.

Diagnosis is established by detecting characteristic eggs in the feces; repeated examinations may be necessary. Sometimes the diagnosis can only be made by finding eggs in biliary drainage and, in rare instances, only after liver biopsy or at surgical exploration. Exogenous transient infection can occur as a result of ingestion of egg-containing cow or sheep liver. Eosinophilia is characteristic. Liver imaging may be useful. Serologic tests are often useful in presumptive diagnosis, particularly in the acute phase. Cross-reactions occur with other helminths.

In acutely ill children, fever and toxemia can be controlled with prednisone, 5–10 mg/d, before antiparasitic therapy is started. Bithionol, given as for paragonimiasis, is the drug of choice but is only moderately effective. Side effects occur in up to 40% of patients. Five recent studies suggest that triclabendazole, a veterinary fasciolicide, is curative; however, its safety, effectiveness, and dosage (12 mg/kg every other day for two doses) need further evaluation.

Reports on the effectiveness of praziquantel have been variable; generally, it is ineffective when used for 2–7 days at a dose of 25 mg/kg three times daily with a 4- to 6-hour interval between doses. If bithionol or praziquantel are not effective, give dehydroemetine or emetine hydrochloride in dosages used for amebic liver abscess may help (see Table 31–1); both drugs are potentially toxic, but dehydroemetine may be less so. For any of the drugs, the destruction of parasites followed by release of antigen in sensitized patients may evoke symptoms.

Bithionol and dehydroemetine are available in the USA only from the Parasitic Disease Drug Service, Centers for Disease Control, Atlanta 30333.

In endemic areas, aquatic plants should not be eaten raw; washing does not destroy the metacercariae, but cooking will. Drinking water must be boiled or purified.

Bacq Y et al: Successful treatment of acute fascioliasis with bithionol. Hepatology 1991;14:1066.

Laird PP, Boray JC: Human fascioliasis successfully treated with triclabendazole. Aust N Z J Med 1992;22:45.

Pulpeiro JR et al: Fascioliasis: Findings in 15 patients. Br J Radiol 1991;64:798.

CLONORCHIASIS & OPISTHORCHIASIS

Infection by *Clonorchis sinensis,* the Chinese liver fluke, is endemic in areas of Japan, Korea, China, Taiwan, and Southeast Asia. Over 20 million people are affected. Opisthorchiasis is caused by worms of the genus *Opisthorchis,* generally either *O felineus* (central, eastern, and southern Europe, eastern Asia, Southeast Asia, India) or *O viverrini* (Thailand, Laos, Vietnam). Clinically and epidemiologically, opisthorchiasis and clonorchiasis are identical.

Certain snails are infected when they ingest eggs shed into water in human or animal feces. Larval forms escape from the snails, penetrate the flesh of various freshwater fish, and encyst as metacercariae. Fish-eating mammals, including dogs and cats, are of great importance in maintaining the natural cycle. Human infection results from eating such fish, either raw or undercooked. Pickling, smoking, or drying may not suffice to kill the metacercariae. In humans, the ingested parasites excyst in the duodenum and ascend the bile ducts into the medium and small biliary radicals, where they mature and remain throughout their lives, shedding eggs in the bile. In the chronic stage of infection, there is progressive bile duct thickening, periductal fibrosis, dilatation, biliary stasis, and secondary infection. Little fibrosis occurs in the portal tracts.

Most patients harbor few parasites and are asymptomatic. Among symptomatic patients, an acute and chronic syndrome occurs. Acute symptoms follow entry of immature worms into the biliary ducts and may persist for several months. Findings include malaise, low-grade fever, an enlarged, tender liver, and pain in the hepatic area or epigastrium, with leukocytosis and eosinophilia. The acute syndrome is difficult to diagnose, since ova may not appear in the feces until 3–4 weeks after onset of symptoms.

In chronic infections, findings include weakness, anorexia, epigastric pain, diarrhea, prolonged low-grade fever, intermittent episodes of right upper quadrant pain, localized hepatic area tenderness, and progressive hepatomegaly.

Complications include intrahepatic bile duct calculi that may lead to recurrent pyogenic cholangitis, biliary abscess, or endophlebitis of the portal-venous branches. Although focal initially, this may gradually result in destruction of the liver parenchyma, fibrosis, and, in a few patients, cirrhoses with jaundice and ascites. Flukes may also enter the pancreatic duct, causing acute pancreatitis or cholelithiasis. Cholangiocarcinoma has been linked with prolonged *Clonorchis* and *Opisthorchis* infection.

Diagnosis is made by finding characteristic eggs in stools or duodenal aspirate. During the chronic stage, leukocytosis varies according to intensity of infection; eosinophilia may be present. In severe infection, the number of eggs per gram of feces may not reflect the heavy worm burden. In advanced disease, (1) liver function tests will indicate parenchymal damage; (2) CT and sonography may show diffuse dilatation of small intrahepatic bile ducts with no or minimal dilatation of the large intra- and extrahepatic ducts; and (3) transhepatic cholangiograms may show alternating stricture and dilatation of the biliary tree. Serologic tests are sometimes available.

The drug of choice is praziquantel. With a dosage of 25 mg/kg three times daily for 2 days (with a 4- to 6-hour interval between doses), cure rates over 95% can be anticipated for *Clonorchis* infections. One day of treatment may be sufficient for *Opisthorchis* infections. (For side effects, see Schistosomiasis, above.) Albendazole, undergoing early clinical trials, may prove to be a useful alternative drug; a dosage of 400 mg twice daily for 7 days can be tried.

The disease is rarely fatal, but patients with advanced infections and impaired liver function may succumb more readily to other diseases. The prognosis is good for light to moderate infections.

Haswell-Elkins MR, Sithithaworn P, Elkins D: *Opisthorchis viverrini* and cholangiocarcinoma in northeast Thailand. Parasitology Today 1992;8:86.

Lim JH et al: Clonorchiasis: Sonographic findings in 59 proven cases. AJR 1989;152:761.

PARAGONIMIASIS

Paragonimus westermani, the lung fluke, commonly infects humans throughout the Far East; foci are also present in West Africa, South and Southeast Asia, the Pacific Islands, Indonesia, and New Guinea. Many carnivores and omnivores in addition to humans serve as reservoir hosts for the adult fluke ($8-16 \times 4-8 \times 3-5$ mm). A number of other *Paragonimus* species also infect humans in China, Japan, and Central and South America.

Eggs reaching water, either in sputum or feces, hatch in 3–6 weeks. Released miracidia penetrate and develop in snails. Emergent cercariae encyst as metacercariae in the tissues of crabs and crayfish. When these crustaceans are eaten raw or pickled, or when crabs are crushed, food, vessels, or fingers are contaminated by metacercariae that are later ingested. Similarly, when drinking water is contaminated by metacercariae, immature flukes excyst in the small intestine and penetrate the peritoneal cavity. Most migrate through the diaphragm and enter the peripheral lung parenchyma; some may lodge in the peritoneum, the intestinal wall, the liver, the skin, or other tissues but most often they lodge in the brain. In the lungs, the parasite becomes encapsulated by granulomatous fibrous tissue, reaching up to 2 cm in diameter. The lesion, which usually opens into a bronchiole, may subsequently rupture, resulting in expectoration of eggs, blood, and inflammatory cells. Eggs from lung cysts may also enter the general circulation and be carried throughout the body, where they produce granulomas in the tissues.

The incubation period ranges from 1 month to 2 years. The majority of light and moderate infections are asymptomatic. In symptomatic patients, there is low-grade fever and dry cough, initially; subsequently, a rusty, blood-flecked viscous sputum may be produced, or frank hemoptysis may occur. Pleuritic chest pain is common. The condition is chronic and slowly progressive. Dyspnea, signs of bronchitis and bronchiectasis, weakness, malaise, and weight loss may be seen in heavy infections. Parasites in the peritoneal cavity or intestinal wall may cause abdominal pain, diarrhea, or dysentery. Those in the central nervous system, depending on their location, may provoke seizures, cranial neuropathies, or meningoencephalitis. Migratory subcutaneous nodules (a few millimeters to 10 cm in diameter) occur with about 10% of *P westermani* infections and up to 60% of *Paragonimus skrjabini* infections.

Pulmonary disease is diagnosed by finding characteristic eggs in sputum, feces, or pleural fluid or adult flukes in subcutaneous nodules or other surgical specimens. Serologic tests (ELISA and immunoblot) are available. Eosinophilia and low-grade leukocytosis are common. Chest x-rays may show a patchy consolidation, nodular shadows, pleural thickening or effusion, or calcifications. By CT, round, low-attenuation cystic lesions (5–15 mm) filled with fluid or gas are seen within the consolidation. In acute cerebral disease, CT shows multilocular, ring-like enhancement with surrounding low-density areas. In the chronic stage, round or oval-shaped calcifications appear, sometimes surrounded by low density areas.

In pulmonary paragonimiasis, praziquantel is the drug of choice (25 mg/kg after meals three times daily for 3 days, with a 4- to 6-hour interval between doses). (For side effects, see above under Schistosomiasis.) Bithionol is the alternative drug (30–50 mg/kg, given on alternate days for 10–15 doses [20–30 days]; the daily dose should be divided into a morning and evening dose). Side effects are frequent but generally mild and transient. Gastrointestinal symptoms, particularly diarrhea, occur in most patients. Liver function should be tested serially. Bithionol is available in the USA only from the Parasitic Disease Drug Service, Centers for Disease Control, Atlanta 30333. Antibiotics may be necessary for secondary pulmonary infection. Cure rates of over 90% can be anticipated for both praziquantel and bithionol.

In the acute stage of cerebral paragonimiasis, particularly meningitis, praziquantel or bithionol may be effective. Following administration of a drug and death of parasites, severe local reactions may occur. Therefore, corticosteroids should be given as in cerebral cysticercosis. In the chronic stage, both surgical removal of the parasites and drug usage are likely to be ineffective in diminishing neurologic symptoms.

Im JG et al: Pleuropulmonary paragonimiasis: Radiologic findings in 71 patients. Am J Radiol 1992;159:39.

Razaque MA, Mutum SS, Singh TS: Recurrent haemoptysis? Think of paragonimiasis. Trop Doct 1991;21:153.

Toyonaga S et al: Cerebral paragonimiasis: Report of five cases. Neurol Med Chir 1992;32:157.

CESTODE INFECTIONS

TAPEWORM INFECTIONS
(See also Cysticercosis and Echinococcosis, below.)

Classification

Six tapeworms infect humans frequently. The large tapeworms are *Taenia saginata* (the beef tapeworm, up to 25 m in length), *Taenia solium* (the pork tapeworm, 7 m), and *Diphyllobothrium latum* (the fish tapeworm, 10 m). The small tapeworms are *Hymenolepis nana* (the dwarf tapeworm, 25–40 mm), *Hymenolepis diminuta* (the rodent tapeworm, 20–60 cm), and *Dipylidium caninum* (the dog tapeworm, 10–70 cm). Four of the six tapeworms occur worldwide; the pork and fish tapeworms have more limited distribution. Humans are the only definitive host of *T saginata*, *T solium,* and *H nana*.

An adult tapeworm consists of a head (scolex), a neck, and a chain of individual segments (proglottids) in which eggs form in mature segments. The scolex is the attachment organ and generally lodges in the upper part of the small intestine.

Multiple infections are the rule for small tapeworms and may occur for *D latum;* however, it is rare for a person to harbor more than one or two of the taeniae.

A. Beef Tapeworm: The infection occurs in most countries with animal husbandry but is highly endemic in parts of the Far East, central and eastern Africa, and southern USSR. Gravid segments of *T saginata* detach themselves from the chain and are passed in feces to soil. When proglottids or eggs are ingested by grazing cattle, the eggs hatch to release embryos that encyst in muscle as cysticerci. Humans are infected by eating undercooked beef containing viable cysticerci. In the human intestines, the cysticercus develops into an adult worm.

B. Pork Tapeworm: This tapeworm is particularly prevalent in Mexico, Latin America, the Iberian Peninsula, the Slavic countries, Africa, Southeast Asia, India, and China. In the USA and Canada, the infection is rare, usually encountered in persons infected abroad, especially in visits to Latin America. The infection is no longer found in northwestern Europe. The life cycle of *T solium* is similar to that of

T saginata except that the pig is the host of the larval stage. Humans become infected when they eat undercooked pork. Humans are also the intermediate host when they become infected with the larval stage (see Cysticercosis, below) by accidentally ingesting eggs in human feces; the eggs are immediately infectious. Transmission of eggs may occur as a result of autoinfection (hand to mouth), direct person-to-person transfer, ingestion of food or drink contaminated by eggs, or (rarely) regurgitation of proglottids into the stomach.

C. Fish Tapeworm: *D latum* is found in temperate and subarctic lake regions in many areas of the world, including Europe, the USA, Alaska and Canada, Japan, the Middle East, central and southern Africa, and southern South America. Eggs passed in human feces that reach water are taken up first by crustaceans that in turn are eaten by fish, both of which are intermediate hosts. Human infection results from eating raw or inadequately cooked brackish or freshwater fish, including salmon. Nonhuman reservoir hosts include dogs, bears, and other fish-eating mammals.

D. Dwarf Tapeworm: The *H nana* life cycle is unusual in that both larval and adult stages are found in the human intestine and there is no intermediate host. Eggs passed in the feces are immediately infective. Egg transmission occurs in most cases directly from person to person and only infrequently involves fomites, water, or food. Internal autoinfection occurs when larvae hatch within the intestine, invade the mucosa, develop for a time, and then return to the lumen to mature.

E. Rodent Tapeworm: *H diminuta* is a common parasite of rodents. Many arthropods (eg, rat fleas, beetles, and cockroaches) serve as intermediate hosts. Humans are infected by accidentally swallowing the infected arthropods, usually in cereals or stored products.

F. Dog Tapeworm: *D caninum* infection generally occurs in young children in close association with infected dogs or cats. Transmission results from swallowing the infected intermediate hosts, ie, fleas or lice.

Clinical Findings
A. Signs and Symptoms:
1. Large tapeworms–Large tapeworm infections are generally asymptomatic. Occasionally, vague gastrointestinal symptoms (eg, nausea, diarrhea, abdominal pain) and systemic symptoms (eg, fatigue, hunger, dizziness) have been attributed to the infections. Vomiting of proglottid segments or obstruction of the bile duct, pancreatic duct, or appendix is rare.

Some persons (mostly Scandinavian residents) who harbor the fish tapeworm develop a macrocytic megaloblastic anemia accompanied by thrombocytopenia and mild leukopenia. Gastric acidity is normal. The anemia is a result of the worm's competing with the host for vitamin B_{12}. Clinical findings are indistinguishable from those of pernicious anemia and include glossitis, dyspnea, tachycardia, and neurologic findings (numbness, paresthesias, disturbances of coordination, impairment of vibration and position sense, and dementia).

2. Small tapeworms–Light infections are generally asymptomatic. Heavy infections, particularly with *H nana*, may cause diarrhea, abdominal pain, anorexia, vomiting, weight loss, and irritability, particularly in young children.

B. Laboratory Findings: Infection by a beef or pork tapeworm is often discovered by the patient finding segments in stool, clothing, or bedding. To determine the species, proglottid segments are either flattened between glass slides and examined microscopically for anatomic detail or differentiated by enzyme electrophoresis of glucose phosphate isomerase. Eggs are only infrequently present in stools, but the perianal cellophane tape test, as used to diagnose pinworm, is sometimes useful in detecting *T saginata* eggs. However, *Taenia* eggs look alike and do not permit species differentiation.

Fish tapeworm is diagnosed by finding characteristic operculated eggs in stool; repeat examinations may be necessary. Proglottids are passed occasionally, and their internal morphology is also diagnostic. The presence of hydrochloric acid in the stomach differentiates the anemia from pernicious anemia; in both conditions, the Schilling test is abnormal. However, addition of intrinsic factor or repeat testing after antibiotics does not correct the abnormality with fish tapeworm infection.

H nana and *H diminuta* infections are diagnosed by finding characteristic eggs in feces; proglottids are usually not seen. *D caninum* infection is diagnosed by detection of proglottids (the size of melon seeds) in feces or after their active migration through the anus.

Serologic tests are not available for tapeworm infections.

Treatment

A. Specific Measures: Although niclosamide and praziquantel are both drugs of choice for most tapeworm infections, praziquantel is more effective in hymenolepiasis, and some workers consider it to be somewhat more effective in taeniasis. In areas endemic for neurocysticercosis, a dose of praziquantel of 5 mg/kg or higher carries a small risk of activating the lesions.

1. *T saginata* and *D latum*– With a single dose of niclosamide, cure rates over 95% can be anticipated with the following dosages: adults, four tablets (2 g); children weighing more than 34 kg, three tablets; children 11–34 kg, two tablets. The drug is given in the morning before the patient has eaten. The tablets *must be chewed thoroughly* and swallowed with water. Eating may be resumed in 2 hours. Niclosamide usually produces no side effects.

Praziquantel in a single dose of 10 mg/kg achieves cure rates of about 99%. At this dose, side effects (see under Schistosomiasis, above) are minimal. For mass treatment, lower doses are also effective.

Pre- and posttreatment purges are not used for either drug. The anemia and neurologic manifestations of *D latum* respond to vitamin B_{12} as used in treatment of pernicious anemia.

2. *T solium*–The choice of drugs and methods of treatment are as above. For both drugs, it may be useful to give a moderate purgative 2–3 hours after treatment to rapidly eliminate segments from the bowel. The patient must be instructed about the need after defecation for careful washing of the hands and perianal area and for safe disposal of feces for 4 days following therapy.

3. *H nana*–Praziquantel, the drug of choice, produces 95% cure rates with a single 25 mg/kg dose. Niclosamide, the alternative drug, produces cure rates of 75% when given at the above dosage for 5–7 days; some workers repeat the course 5 days later.

4. *H diminuta* and *D caninum*–Treatment is with niclosamide or praziquantel in dosages as for *H nana*. Cure rates are not established.

B. Follow-Up Care: In treatment of large tapeworm infections, a disintegrating worm is usually passed within 24–48 hours of treatment. Since efforts are not generally made to recover and identify the scolex, cure can be presumed only if regenerated segments have not reappeared 3–5 months later. If it is preferred that parasitic cure be established immediately, the head (scolex) must be found in posttreatment stools; a laxative is given 2 hours after treatment, and stools must be collected in a preservative for 24 hours. To facilitate examination, toilet paper must be disposed of separately.

Prognosis

Because the prognosis is often poor in cerebral cysticercosis (see below), *T solium* infections must be immediately eradicated.

Chappell CL, Enos JP, Penn HM: *Dipylidium caninum,* an underrecognized infection in infants and children. Pediatr Infect Dis 1990;9:745.

Despommier DD: Tapeworm infection: The long and short of it. N Eng J Med 1992;327:727.

Pawlowski ZS: Efficacy of low doses of praziquantel in taeniasis. Acta Tropica 1990;48:83. (Also reviews risk of use when cysticercosis is present concurrently.)

CYSTICERCOSIS

Essentials of Diagnosis

• History of exposure in an endemic region; concomitant or past intestinal infection by *Taenia solium*.

- Seizures, symptoms and signs of a focal space-occupying central nervous system lesion, intracranial hypertension.
- Subcutaneous or muscular nodules (5–10 mm); calcified lesions on x-rays of soft tissues.
- Calcified or uncalcified cysts by CT scan or MRI; positive serologic tests.

General Considerations

Human cysticercosis is infection by the larval (cysticercus) stage of the tapeworm *T solium* (see above), which can form cysts in any tissue. Cysticercosis occurs mainly wherever pork is eaten raw or undercooked and human fecal sanitation is inadequate. Prevalence rates to 4% are recognized in some endemic areas. Although swine-to-human transmission of the tapeworm infection is nearly unknown in the USA, recent immigration of persons from endemic areas has resulted in frequent recognition of cysticercosis cases and, rarely, of human-to-human transmission of eggs from persons who had imported tapeworm infections.

Locations of cysts in order of frequency are the central nervous system, the subcutaneous tissues and striated muscle, the globe of the eye, and, rarely, other tissues. Cysts reach 5–10 mm in soft tissues but may be larger (up to 5 cm) in the central nervous system. Attached to the inner wall of the cyst is an invaginated protoscolex with four suckers and a crown of hooks.

The natural history of the infection in incompletely known, including whether the parasite causes little or no local inflammatory reaction until it dies or if the host inflammatory response results in death of the parasite. Cysticerci complete their development within 2–4 months after larval entry and live for months to years. Cyst death is followed by vesicular enlargement or by pericyst inflammatory edema that may be associated vasculitis. Subsequently, the cyst degenerates and may disappear or be replaced by fibrous tissue and sometimes may calcify. Cysts at different stages of their life cycle may be present in the same organ.

Clinical Findings

A. Signs and Symptoms: In many patients, cysts remain asymptomatic. When symptomatic, the incubation period is highly variable (usually from 1 to 5 years but sometimes shorter). Manifestations are due to mass effect, inflammatory response, or obstruction of the brain foramina and ventricular systems. Neurologic findings are varied and nonspecific, in large part determined by the number and location of the cysts.

1. Neurocysticercosis–

a. Acute invasive stage–This rare event, occurring shortly after invasion, results from extensive spread of cysticerci to the brain parenchyma. Fever, headache, myalgia, marked eosinophilia, and coma may occur.

b. Parenchymal cysts–Cysticerci can present singly or multiply and may be scattered or in clumps. Findings include epilepsy (focal or generalized), focal neurologic deficits, intracranial hypertension (intense headache, vomiting, papilledema, visual loss), and altered mental status.

c. Meningeal cysts–The basilar membranes, principally the arachnoid are affected. Adhesive arachnoiditis may result in obstructive hydrocephalus, intracranial hypertension, arterial thrombosis leading to transient ischemia or stroke, and cranial nerve dysfunction (most often of the optic nerve).

d. Ventricular cysts may float freely (usually singly) within the ventricles or cerebral aqueduct or may be attached to the ventricular wall. They are usually asymptomatic but can cause increased intracranial pressure as a result of intermittent or total blockage.

e. Racemose cysts are rare aberrant forms that are multiple-branched, nonencysted, and lack a scolex; they present as grape-like irregular clusters and may reach over 10 cm in diameter. They generally are found in the ventricular and basal subarachnoid spaces, where they cause marked adhesive arachnoiditis and often obstructive hydrocephalus.

f. Spinal cord cysts can be extraspinal or intraspinal and cause arachnoiditis (meningitis, radiculopathy) or pressure symptoms.

2. Ophthalmocysticercosis–Usually there is a single cyst, free-floating in the vitreous or under the retina. Presenting symptoms include periorbital pain, scotomas, and progressive deterioration of visual acuity. Findings may include disk hemorrhage and edema, retinal detachment, iridocyclitis, and chorioretinitis.

3. Subcutaneous and muscular cysticercosis–These cysts present as nodules that tend to appear, collapse and disappear, and then reappear in other sites after variable periods of time. They are usually asymptomatic.

B. Laboratory Tests: Definitive diagnosis of neurocysticercosis requires finding the parasite on histologic section of specimens removed by excisional biopsy of skin or subcutaneous tissues (not of brain tissue). Patients should be thoroughly examined by palpation for pea-sized nodules. Presumptive diagnosis may be made by the following tests.

1. Imaging–Plain radiographs of soft tissues may detect oval or linear calcified lesions ($4–10 \times 2–5$ mm). The lesions are usually multiple, sometimes in the hundreds, and the long axes of the cysts are nearly always in the plane of the surrounding muscle fibers. Plain skull films may demonstrate one or more cerebral calcifications (generally 5–10 mm; sometimes 1–2 mm when only the scolex is calcified).

The most useful procedures for examining the skull are imaging by CT and MRI. Although MRI has superior resolution and is relatively artifact-free, its cost and availability dictate that evaluation usually begin with CT. CT patterns include (1) rounded areas of low density that show no enhancement after contrast medium (viable cysts), (2) hypodense or isodense lesions surrounded by edema that show ring-like or nodular enhancement (host inflammatory response), and (3) small calcifications or granulomas (dead cysts). Signs of increased intracranial pressure may also be seen. Often a combination of CT images is found, owing to different stages of development among cysticerci. Intraventricular cysts, which are isodense with cerebrospinal fluid, are not demonstrated on routine CT but require intraventricular CT contrast medium. MRI, by which calcified cysts can be recognized only with difficulty, may detect 2- to 4-mm nodules (protoscoleces) within cyst fluid. Spinal cysticercosis is evaluated by CT myelography or MRI.

2. Immunologic tests–With serum, the new immunoelectrotransfer blot test appears to reach nearly 100% specificity and 95% sensitivity, whereas the ELISA showed, respectively, 63% and 65%. Hydatid disease and *H nana* infections cross-react in the ELISA. Sensitivity using cerebrospinal fluid was 86% by immunoblot and 62% by ELISA. Older tests—eg, complement fixation—are insufficiently sensitive or specific. Patients presenting with only calcified lesions are generally serologically negative.

3. Other tests–The cerebrospinal fluid in neurocysticercosis typically shows increased protein, decreased glucose, and a cellular reaction consisting mainly of lymphocytes and eosinophils; eosinophilia over 20% is diagnostically important. The EEG may be abnormal. Though the patient usually no longer harbors a tapeworm at the time cysticercosis is diagnosed, stools from both the patient and family members should be examined over several days by each individual for the passage of proglottids and by the laboratory for proglottids and eggs.

Differential Diagnosis

The differential diagnosis includes tuberculoma, tumor, hydatid disease, vasculitis, chronic fungal disorders, and neurosyphilis.

Treatment

Medical treatment with albendazole or praziquantel is usually preferable to surgical removal of lesions. Drug treatment is most effective for parenchymal cysts; is less effective for intraventricular, subarachnoid, or racemose cysts; and has no effect on calcified parasites. Patients with only calcified cysts, granulomas, or cysts that show enhancement probably do not need specific therapy.

Short-term (for 3–6 months) follow-up of comparative studies indicate that albendazole may be more effective than praziquantel. Long-term follow-up, however, for local recurrence or appearance of new cysts has not yet been reported. Other potential advantages of albendazole over praziquantel are that it is less expensive; that it achieves better penetration of cerebrospinal fluid; and that when corticosteroids are given concomitantly, the plasma concentration of albendazole increases but that of praziquantel decreases. A suggested approach is a course of albendazole plus steroid; if the response is inadequate, a trial of praziquantel should be given. For selected patients, some clinicians wait 3 months to see if cysts will spontaneously disappear. Treatment should be conducted in hospital.

Within less than a week after the start of treatment with either drug, inflammatory reactions around dying parasites may be manifested by meningismus, headache (analgesics may be sufficient for mild symptoms), vomiting, hyperthermia, mental changes, and convulsions; decompensation with death is very rare. It remains controversial whether to give steroids concomitantly to avoid or diminish this reaction or to use them only if marked symptoms appear or increase. Even when steroids are given prospectively, the inflammatory reaction may occur. Prednisone, 30 mg/d in two or three divided doses, starting 1–2 days before use of the drug and continuing at diminishing doses for about 14 days afterward, is one regimen. The reaction usually subsides in 48–72 hours, but continuing severity may require steroids in higher dosage and mannitol. Use of anticonvulsants must be continued during drug treatment and probably for an indefinite time afterward.

Following treatment, 50% cure rates (disappearance of cysts and clearing of symptoms) have been reported both for albendazole and praziquantel. Of the remaining patients, many have amelioration of symptoms, including intracranial hypertension and seizures.

A. Specific Measures:
1. Albendazole–15 mg/kg/d in divided doses with meals for 8 days has been shown to be as effective as a 30-day course. The drug is not yet available in the USA but can be obtained for compassionate use from the manufacturer (SmithKline Beecham, 1-800-366-8900).

2. Praziquantel–Give 50 mg/kg/d for 15 days in three divided doses.

3. Surgery–Surgery has successfully removed orbital, cisternal, and ventricular cysts and, if accessible, cerebral, meningeal, or spinal cord cysts. When hydrocephalus is present, surgical shunt is required even when the parasites have been destroyed. Ocular cysticercosis is treated by surgical removal of cysts; drug therapy is not effective and is contraindicated.

B. General Measures: Symptomatic treatment of neurocysticercosis is based on the use of steroids and mannitol for cerebral edema and anticonvulsants for seizures.

Prognosis

The fatality rate for untreated neurocysticercosis is about 50%; survival time from onset of symptoms ranges from days to many years. Drug treatment has reduced the mortality rate to about 5–15%. Surgical procedures to relieve intracranial hypertension along with use of steroids to reduce edema improve the prognosis for those not effectively treated by praziquantel.

Centers for Disease Control: Locally acquired neurocysticercosis. JAMA 1992;267:1183.

Davis LE, Kornfeld M: Neurocysticercosis: Neurologic, pathogenic, diagnostic and therapeutic aspects. Eur Neurol 1991;31:229.

Del Brutto OH, Sotelo J: Neurocysticercosis: An update. Rev Infect Dis 1988;10:1075.

Takayanagui OM, Jardim E: Therapy for neurocysticercosis: Comparison between albendazole and praziquantel. Arch Neurol 1992;49:290.

ECHINOCOCCOSIS & HYDATIDOSIS (Hydatid Disease)

Human echinococcosis results from parasitism by the larval stage of two *Echinococcus* species: *Echinococcus granulosus* (cystic hydatid disease) and *Echinococcus multilocularis* (alveolar hydatid disease). Very rarely, *Echinococcus vogeli* (polycystic hydatid disease) has been reported from northern South America and Panama. Echinococcosis is a zoonosis in which humans are an intermediate host of the larval stage of the parasite. The definitive host is a carnivore (all of which, except for the lion, are Canidae) that harbors the adult tapeworm in the small intestine; the carnivore becomes infected by ingesting the larval form in tissue of the intermediate host. The intermediate hosts, chiefly herbivorous mammals but also humans, become infected by ingesting tapeworm eggs passed in carnivore feces. The larval stage is referred to as a hydatid cyst.

1. CYSTIC HYDATID DISEASE (Unilocular Hydatid Disease)

Essentials of Diagnosis

- History of exposure to dogs associated with livestock in a hydatid-endemic region.
- Avascular cystic tumor of liver, lung, or, infrequently, bone, brain, or other organs as detected by imaging procedures.
- Symptoms and signs vary, depending upon size and location of cysts.
- Positive serologic tests.

General Considerations

Human infection with *E granulosus* occurs principally where dogs are used to herd grazing animals, particularly sheep. The disease is common throughout southern South America, the Mediterranean littoral and the Middle East, central Asia, and East Africa. Foci of endemicity are in eastern Europe, Russia, Australasia, India, and the United Kingdom. In North America, endemic foci have been reported from the western USA, the lower Mississippi valley, Alaska, and northwestern Canada.

There are at least two geographic strains of the parasite. The pastoral strain—which is more pathogenic to humans—has a transmission cycle in which dogs are the definitive host, and sheep (usually) but also cattle, hogs, and other domestic livestock are intermediate hosts. The sylvatic, or northern, strain is maintained in wolves and wild ungulates (moose and reindeer) in northern Alaska, Canada, Scandinavia, and Eurasia.

Human infection occurs when eggs passed in dog feces are accidentally swallowed. Embryos liberated from the eggs penetrate the intestinal mucosa, enter the portal bloodstream, and are carried to the liver where they are trapped and become hydatid cysts (65% of all cysts). Some larvae reach the lung (25%) and develop into pulmonary hydatids. Infrequently, cysts form in the brain, bones, skeletal muscles, kidneys, spleen, or other tissues. Cysts of the sylvatic strain tend to localize in the lungs.

The cyst wall has three layers: an inner germinal layer that gives rise within the cyst to germinal elements, a supporting intermediate layer, and an outer layer produced by the host. In the liver, cysts may increase in size 1–5 cm in diameter per year and become enormous, but symptoms generally do not develop until they reach about 10 cm. Some cysts die spontaneously. Part or all of the inner layer of some hepatic or splenic cysts may calcify, which does not necessarily mean cyst death.

Clinical Findings

A. Symptoms and Signs: A liver cyst may remain silent for 10–20 or more years until it becomes large enough to be palpable, to be visible as an abdominal swelling, to produce pressure effects, or (rarely) to produce symptoms due to leakage or rupture. There may be right upper quadrant pain, nausea, and vomiting. The effects of pressure may result in biliary obstruction, with secondary bacterial cholangitis, cirrhosis, and portal hypertension. If a cyst ruptures suddenly, anaphylaxis and death may occur. If fluid and hydatid particles escape slowly, allergic manifestations may result, including a rise in the eosinophil count. Rupture can occur into the pleural, pericardial, or peritoneal space or into the duodenum, colon, or renal pelvis. Dissemination of germinal elements may be followed by the development of multiple secondary cysts. A characteristic clinical syndrome may follow intrabiliary extrusion of cyst contents—jaundice, biliary colic, and urticaria.

Pulmonary cysts cause no symptoms until they leak; become large enough to obstruct a bronchus, causing segmental collapse; or erode into bronchus and rupture. Brain cysts produce symptoms earlier and may cause seizures or symptoms of increased intracranial pressure. Cysts in the bone marrow or spongiosa do not have a host layer, are irregular in shape, erode osseous tissue, and may present as pain or as spontaneous fracture. The bones most often affected are the vertebrae; many of these patients develop epidural extension with compression of the spinal cord and paraplegia. Because 20% of patients have multiple cysts, upon diagnosis each patient should be screened for cysts in the liver, spleen, kidneys, lungs, brain, bones, skin, tongue, vitreous, and other tissues.

B. Imaging: Sonography and CT scan are most commonly used to detect a cystic mass in the liver. Nearly pathognomonic is the presence within a hydatid cyst of daughter cysts; they must be distinguished, however, from blood clots within the cavity of simple cysts. The mass can also be defined by MR imaging, scintillation scan, or by angiography (rarely used). Spotty calcified densities or a calcified cyst wall may be seen in the liver or spleen. Chest films and thoracic CT scans may show a pulmonary lesion, but calcification of the wall does not occur. An intravenous urogram or bone scan may detect cysts at other sites.

C. Laboratory Findings: Several serologic tests (indirect hemagglutination, indirect immunofluorescence, ELISA) are useful for screening for serum antibody. False-negative reactions may occur in 5–10% of liver cysts and up to 50% of lung cysts. In addition, false-positive cross-reactions may occur with other helminthic infections, liver cirrhosis, and cancer. Persons positive in the screening test should be tested by one of several methods to detect arc 5; its presence is considered diagnostic except for cross-reactions with *T solium* infections. A new test by immunoblot assay was reported to be 100% specific and 91% sensitive. Persons from whom cysts have been completely removed and carriers of dead cysts may become seronegative. The Casoni intracutaneous skin test has been abandoned because of poor specificity.

Eosinophilia is uncommon except after cyst rupture. Liver function tests are usually normal. Confirmation of the diagnosis is possible only by examination of cyst contents after surgical removal.

Heretofore, percutaneous aspiration of hydatid cysts for diagnostic and therapeutic (injection of a scolicidal agent) purposes until recently had been contraindicated because of risk of leakage at the aspiration site (viable cysts are usually under pressure), with potential for anaphylaxis and dissemination of infection. Several workers have recently reported safe results achieved with the aid of sonographic monitoring, but the number of patients so treated is small and the duration of follow-up is short.

Differential Diagnosis

Noninfected hydatid cysts of the liver need to be differentiated from simple (epithelial cysts); infected cysts, from bacterial and amebic abscesses. Hydatid cysts in any site may be mistaken for a variety of malignant and nonmalignant tumors and cysts. In the lung, a cyst may be confused with cavitary tuberculosis. Allergic symptoms arising from cyst leakage may resemble those associated with many other diseases.

Treatment & Prevention

A. Surgical Treatment: The current definitive treatment is surgical removal of cysts if their location and the patient's general condition permit. All lung cysts should be removed but not all liver cysts. Newly available chemotherapy may alter this position. Decision-making must take into account that surgical mortality rates range from 1% to 4%, and recurrence rates after surgery are 10% or higher. Operative treatment of liver cysts involves two major problems: (1) selection of a method to sterilize and remove cyst contents without spillage, and (2) management of the remaining cavity. Germicidal solutions, which include cetrimide (5%), hypertonic saline (20%), silver nitrate (0.5%), and sodium hypochlorite (3.75%), have come under criticism because of their potential for direct and indirect toxicity (an estimated 20% of cysts are thought to communicate with the biliary tract). To reduce the risk of recurrence due to operative spillage, the use pre- or postoperatively (or both) of albendazole or postoperatively of praziquantel continues to be evaluated. For the treatment of bone cysts, curettage, lavage, and instillation of chemical sterilization substances and chemotherapy are indicated.

B. Drug Treatment:

1. Albendazole–Albendazole is much more readily absorbed than mebendazole; this permits a substantially lower dosage of albendazole to be used, yet its active metabolite, the sulfoxide, reaches effective concentrations in cyst wall and fluid. A current regimen is four tablets (800 mg) daily for three 28-day courses, with 2-week rest periods between courses. Among 253 patients treated in multiple studies, the outcomes for liver and lung cysts were, respectively, as follows: cured (33%, 40%), improved (44%, 37%), no change (21%, 22%), and worse (2%, 1%). However, most patients were not followed long enough to permit evaluation for recurrences (4 occurred among the 29 persons followed over 2 years). Bone cysts may prove more refractory to treatment. In the 3-month courses, drug side effects include reversible low-grade transaminase elevations (17%), leukopenia to 2900/μL (2%), and rare gastrointestinal symptoms, dizziness or headache, alopecia, rash, and pruritus. Anaphylaxis has been reported once and eosinophilia twice, probably related to cyst fluid leakage.

2. Mebendazole–When mebendazole was used

at high doses for several months, marked regression and apparent death of cysts occurred in some patients. In others, cysts were either stable or continued to grow and if removed were viable. The dosage is 50 mg/kg/d in three divided doses for 3 months, with many patients requiring repeated courses. When possible, mebendazole levels should be monitored; serum levels in excess of 100 mg/L 1–2 hours after an oral dose may be necessary for parasite killing. In unresponsive cases, it is possible that plasma levels of mebendazole are insufficient; some researchers, therefore, give up to 200 mg/kg/d. Occasional side effects with treatment include pruritus, rash, alopecia, reversible leukopenia, gastric irritation, musculoskeletal pain, fever, and acute pain in the cyst area; six cases of glomerulonephritis and three of agranulocytosis (with one death) have been reported.

C. Prevention: In endemic areas, prevention is by prophylactic treatment of pet dogs with 5 mg/kg of praziquantel at monthly intervals to remove adult tapeworms and by health education to prevent feeding of offal to dogs.

Prognosis

Most liver and lung cysts can be removed surgically without great difficulty, but in patients with cysts in less accessible sites the prognosis is less favorable. The prognosis is always grave when there has been spillage and the development of secondary cysts. About 15% of untreated patients eventually die because of the disease or its complications.

2. ALVEOLAR HYDATID DISEASE (Multilocular Hydatid Disease)

Alveolar hydatid disease results from infection by the larval form of *Echinococcus multilocularis*. The life cycle involves foxes as definitive host and microtine rodents as intermediate host. Domestic dogs and cats can also become infected with the adult tapeworm when they eat infected wild rodents. Human infection is by accidental ingestion of tapeworm eggs passed in fox or dog feces. The disease in humans has been reported in parts of central Europe, much of Siberia, northwestern Canada, and western Alaska. A single case has been reported in Minnesota. The primary localization of alveolar cysts is in the liver, where they may extend locally or metastasize to other tissues. The larval mass has poorly defined borders and behaves like a neoplasm; it infiltrates and proliferates indefinitely by exogenous budding of the germinative membrane, producing an alveolus-like pattern of microvesicles. X-rays show hepatomegaly and characteristic scattered areas of radiolucency often outlined by 2- to 4-mm calcific rings. Serologic tests are the same as for cystic hydatid disease and cannot distinguish between the species. Treatment is by surgical removal of the entire larval mass, when possible. Ninety percent of patients with nonresectable masses die within 10 years. Long-term mebendazole therapy (40 mg/kg/d) inhibits growth of the parasite and has extended patient survival, but larval tissue is not completely destroyed.

Awar GN et al: Monitored medico-surgical approach to the treatment of cystic hydatidosis. Bull World Health Organ 1991;69:477.
Todorov T et al: Chemotherapy of human cystic echinococcosis: comparative efficacy of mebendazole and albendazole. Ann Trop Med Parasitol 1992;86:59.
Tompkins RK: Management of echinococcal cysts of the liver. Mayo Clin Proc 1991;66:1281.

NEMATODE (ROUNDWORM) INFECTIONS

ANISAKIASIS

Anisakiasis is larval invasion of the stomach or intestinal wall by anisakid nematodes. In the acute form, the infection may mimic surgical abdomen; in the chronic form, mild symptoms may persist for weeks to years.

Definitive hosts are marine mammals, including whales, seals, and dolphins. Eggs discharged with feces are ingested by crustaceans, in which larvae develop that are infective for squids, mackerel, herring, cod, halibut, rockfish, salmon, tuna, and other marine fish. In the fish, the larvae pass to the musculature and are able to transfer from fish to fish along the food chain, eventually reaching a marine mammal, where they mature into the adult stage.

Humans are infected when they ingest larvae in marine fish or squid eaten raw, undercooked, salted, or lightly pickled. Larvae liberated in the stomach attach to or partially penetrate the gastric or intestinal mucosa (small bowel is more common; colon is rare), resulting in localized ulceration, edema, and eosinophilic granuloma formation; eventually, the parasite dies. Rarely, worms are coughed up and expectorated or penetrate the gut wall, enter the peritoneal cavity, and migrate. Most larvae, however, probably fail to cause infection and are passed in feces. Although the larvae sometimes develop to the adult stages, gravid females are not found in humans.

The infection occurs worldwide, but most cases have been reported in Japan and the Netherlands, with a few in the United States, Scandinavia, Chile, and other fish-eating countries. Regional foods eaten raw such as sashimi in Japan, pickled herring in the Netherlands, and seviche in Latin America are common vehicles of infection.

Clinical Findings

A. Symptoms and Signs: The majority of acute cases present as gastric anisakiasis; occasionally, acute infection is followed by a chronic course.

1. Acute gastric anisakiasis–Within hours after larval ingestion, the patient experiences nausea, vomiting, and epigastric pain that progressively becomes more severe. Urticaria has been reported; hematemesis is rare.

2. Acute intestinal anisakiasis–Within 1–7 days, colicky pain appears in the lower abdomen, often localized at the ileocecal region, accompanied by diarrhea, nausea, vomiting, diffuse abdominal tenderness, and mild fever.

3. Chronic disease–For weeks to several years, symptoms may continue that mimic gastric ulcer, gastritis, gastric tumor, bowel obstruction, or inflammatory bowel disease.

B. Laboratory Findings: Stools may show occult blood. Mild leukocytosis and eosinophilia may be present. ELISA and RAST serologic tests may be tried but are not reliable in chronic disease.

C. Imaging and Endoscopy: In acute infection, the larvae sometimes can be seen and removed endoscopically from the stomach. X-rays of the stomach may show a localized edematous, ulcerated area with an irregularly thickened wall, decreased peristalsis, and rigidity. Double contrast technique may show the threadlike larvae. Small bowel x-rays may show thickened mucosa and segments of stenosis with proximal dilatation.

In the chronic stage, x-rays and endoscopy of the stomach—but not of the bowel—may be helpful. The diagnosis is often made only at laparotomy with surgical removal of the parasite.

Prevention & Treatment

Prevention is by avoidance of ingestion of raw or incompletely cooked squid or marine fish, especially salmon, rockfish, herring, and mackerel. Larvae within fish may with difficulty be seen as colorless, tightly coiled or spiraled worms in 3-mm whorls or as reddish or pigmented larvae lying open in muscles or viscera. The larvae are killed by temperatures about 60 °C or by freezing at –20 °C for 24 hours (7 days is advised by some workers). Smoking procedures that do not bring the temperature to 60 °C and salt-curing are not reliable.

There is no drug treatment. Except where larvae can be removed by fiberoptic gastroscopy or colonoscopy, treatment of acute and chronic lesions is limited to symptomatic measures; symptoms generally improve in 1–2 weeks. Surgical excision of the worm may be necessary in severe cases.

Ikeda K, Kumashiro R, Kifune T: Nine cases with acute gastric anisakiasis. Gastrointest Endosc 1989;35:304.

Matsumoto T et al: Anisakiasis of the colon: Radiologic and endoscopic features in six patients. Radiology 1992;183:97.

Schantz PM: The dangers of eating raw fish. N Engl J Med 1989;320:1143.

ANGIOSTRONGYLIASIS

1. ANGIOSTRONGYLIASIS CANTONENSIS (Eosinophilic Meningoencephalitis)

A nematode of rats, *Angiostrongylus cantonensis,* is the causative agent of a form of eosinophilic meningoencephalitis. It has been reported from Hawaii and other Pacific islands, Southeast Asia, Japan, China, Taiwan, Hong Kong, Australia, Egypt, Madagascar, Nigeria, Bombay, Cuba, Puerto Rico, Bahamas, Brazil, and New Orleans.

Human infection results from the ingestion of infected larvae contained in uncooked food—either infected mollusks (snails, slugs, or land planarians, the intermediate hosts) or transport hosts (crabs, shrimp, fish) that have ingested mollusks. Leafy vegetables containing small mollusks may also be the source of infection, as can fingers during the collection and preparation of snails for cooking. The mollusks become infected by ingesting larvae excreted in feces of infected rodents, the definitive host.

The incubation period in humans is 1–3 weeks. Ingested larvae (0.5 × 0.025 mm) invade the central nervous system, where, during migration, they may cause extensive tissue damage; at their death, a local inflammatory reaction ensues. The usual clinical findings are those of meningoencephalitis, including severe headache, fever, neck stiffness, nausea and vomiting, and multiple neurologic findings, particularly asymmetric transient cranial neuropathies. Worms in the spinal cord may result in sensory abnormalities in the trunk or extremities; worms have also been seen in the eye.

The spinal fluid characteristically shows elevated protein and an eosinophilic pleocytosis. Occasionally, the parasite can be recovered from spinal fluid. Peripheral eosinophilia with a low-grade leukocytosis is common. A serologic test is available from the Centers for Disease Control and Prevention; its sensitivity and specificity are not established. CT and MRI may show a central nervous system lesion.

The differential diagnosis includes tuberculosis, coccidioidal or aseptic meningitis, syphilis, lymphoma, gnathostomiasis, cysticercosis, paragonimiasis, echinococcosis, and schistosomiasis japonicum.

No specific treatment is available; however, levamisole, albendazole, thiabendazole, or mebendazole can be tried. Symptomatic treatment with analgesics or corticosteroids may be necessary. The illness usually persists for weeks to months, the parasite dies, and the patient then recovers spontaneously, usually without sequelae. However, fatalities have been recorded.

Prevention is by rat control; cooking of snails, prawns, fish, and crabs for 3–5 minutes, or their freezing (–15 °C for 24 hours); and examining vegetables for mollusks before eating. Washing contaminated vegetables to eliminate larvae contained in mollusk mucus is not always successful.

2. ANGIOSTRONGYLIASIS COSTARICENSIS

Angiostrongylus costaricensis has been identified in humans (predominantly children) in Mexico, Central America, Venezuela, Brazil, and the USA (Texas). The known geographic range of the parasite in rats (the definitive host) extends from northern South America to Texas. Infection occurs from ingestion of the intermediate host, a slug, or from food contaminated by larvae in slug mucus. In humans, the larvae mature in the mesenteric vessels, where they cause thrombosis, and ischemic necrosis of the intestine. Eggs lodging in capillaries give rise to eosinophilic granulomas, most commonly in the appendix but also in the terminal ileum, the cecum, the first part of the ascending colon, and the regional lymph nodes. Findings include fever, right lower quadrant abdominal pain and a mass, leukocytosis, and eosinophilia. Bowel complications consist of incomplete or complete obstruction and infarction. No serologic test is available; neither eggs nor larvae are passed in stool. The disease usually simulates acute appendicitis, which can in fact be caused by the parasite. Intraabdominal mass can mimic tumor. There is no specific treatment; albendazole, thiabendazole, or mebendazole can be tried.. Operative treatment is frequently necessary.

Hulbert TV, Larsen RA, Chandrasoma PT: Abdominal angiostrongyliasis mimicking acute appendicitis and Meckel's diverticulum: Report of a case in the United States and review. Clin Infect Dis 1992;14:836.

Koo J, Pien F, Kliks MM: *Angiostrongylus (Parastrongylus)* eosinophilic meningitis. Rev Infect Dis 1988;10:1155.

Noskin GA, McMenamin MB, Grohmann SM: Eosinophilic meningitis due to *Angiostrongylus cantonensis* Neurology 1992;42:1423.

ASCARIASIS

Essentials of Diagnosis

- Pulmonary phase: Transient cough, dyspnea, wheezing, urticaria, with eosinophilia and transient pulmonary infiltrates.
- Intestinal phase: Vague upper abdominal discomfort; occasional vomiting, abdominal distention.
- Eggs in stools; worms passed per rectum, nose, or mouth.

General Considerations

Ascaris lumbricoides is the most common of the intestinal helminths; an estimated 1 billion people are infected worldwide. It is cosmopolitan in distribution and is found in high prevalence wherever there are low standards of hygiene and sanitation or where human feces are used as fertilizer. The infection is specific for humans and occurs in all age groups. Heavy worm burdens, however, are usually seen only in children; there is evidence of resistance to superinfection in adults. Whether ascariasis impacts on the nutritional status of children is being evaluated.

Adult worms live in the upper small intestine. After fertilization, the female produces enormous numbers of eggs that pass in feces. Direct transmission between humans does not occur, as the eggs must remain on the soil for 2–3 weeks before they become infective. Thereafter, they can survive for years. Infection occurs through ingestion of mature eggs in fecally contaminated food and drink. The eggs hatch in the small intestine, releasing motile larvae that penetrate the wall of the small intestine and reach the right heart via the mesenteric venules and lymphatics. From the heart they move to the lung, burrow through the alveolar walls, and migrate up the bronchial tree into the pharynx, down the esophagus, and back to the small intestine. Egg production begins 60–75 days after ingestion of infective eggs. Adult worms (20–40 cm × 3–6 mm) live for 1 year or more.

Clinical Findings

A. Symptoms and Signs: Migrating larvae in the lung cause capillary and alveolar damage, which may result in low-grade fever, cough, blood-tinged sputum, wheezing, dyspnea, and substernal pain. There may be localized rales, and urticaria on skin examination. Eosinophilia is common during this phase. Rarely, larvae lodge ectopically in the brain, kidney, eye, spinal cord, etc, and may cause symptoms referable to those organs.

Small numbers of adult worms in the intestine usually produce no symptoms. With heavy infection, colic may be seen in children, peptic ulcer-like symptoms in adults, or vague pre- or postprandial abdominal discomfort in either group. Adult worms may also migrate with heavy infections; they may be coughed up, vomited, or emerge through the nose or anus. They may also force themselves into the common bile duct, pancreatic duct, appendix, diverticula, and other sites, which may lead to cholangitis, cholecystitis, pyogenic liver abscess, or pancreatitis. With very heavy infestations, masses of worms may cause intestinal obstruction, volvulus, or intussusception. During typhoid fever, worms may penetrate the weakened bowel wall. Rare cases of lung abscess or laryngeal obstruction with suffocation have been described.

B. Imaging: During the larval migratory phase, chest radiographs may show scattered, patchy, ill-defined asymmetric infiltrations. Intestinal infection is sometimes established by chance, when radiologic examination of the abdomen (with or without barium) shows the presence of worms.

C. Laboratory Findings: Diagnosis usually depends upon finding the characteristic eggs in feces. Occasionally, an adult worm spontaneously passed per rectum or orally reveals an unsuspected infection. Serologic tests are not useful. During the pulmonary phase, eosinophils may reach 30–50% and remain high for about a month; larvae are occasionally found in sputum. During the intestinal phase, there is no eosinophilia.

Differential Diagnosis

Pulmonary ascariasis with eosinophilia must be differentiated from nonparasitic causes (asthma, Löffler's syndrome, eosinophilic pneumonia, allergic bronchopulmonary aspergillosis), and parasitic causes (tropical pulmonary eosinophilia, toxocariasis, strongyloidiasis, hookworm, paragonimiasis). *Ascaris*-induced pancreatitis, appendicitis, diverticulitis, etc, must be differentiated from other causes of inflammation of these tissues. Postprandial dyspepsia may simulate duodenal ulcer, hiatal hernia, gallbladder disease, or pancreatic disease.

Treatment

Pyrantel pamoate is the treatment of choice. None of the drugs listed below require pre- or posttreatment purges. Stools should be rechecked at 2 weeks and patients re-treated until all ascarids are removed. Ascariasis, hookworm, and trichuriasis infections, which often occur together, may be treated simultaneously by mebendazole, albendazole, or oxantelpyrantel pamoate.

Because anesthesia stimulates the worms to become hypermotile, they should be removed in advance in infected patients undergoing elective surgery. In pregnancy, ascariasis should be treated after the first trimester.

Drug treatment should not be used in the migratory phase. In the treatment of biliary ascariasis, endoscopic removal of the worm under ultrasonographic guidance is often successful. In intestinal obstruction, surgery may be avoided by nasogastric suction followed by piperazine given via the tube in standard dosages every 12–24 hours for six doses.

A. Pyrantel Pamoate: Pyrantel pamoate as a single oral dose of 10 mg base/kg (maximum, 1 g) results in 85–100% cure rates. It may be given before or after meals. Infrequent and mild side effects include vomiting, diarrhea, headache, dizziness, and drowsiness.

B. Piperazine: The dosage for piperazine (as the hexahydrate) is 75 mg/kg body weight (maximum, 3.5 g) for 2 days in succession, giving the drug orally before or after breakfast. For heavy infestations, treatment should be continued for 4 days in succession or the 2-day course should be repeated after 1 week.

Gastrointestinal symptoms and headache occur occasionally; central nervous system symptoms (temporary ataxia and exacerbation of seizures) are rare. Allergic symptoms have been attributed to piperazine. The drug should not be used for patients with hepatic or renal insufficiency or in those with a history of seizures or chronic neurologic disease.

C. Mebendazole: Mebendazole is highly effective when given in a dosage of 100 mg twice daily before or after meals for 3 days. Gastrointestinal side effects are infrequent, but worms may appear occasionally at the nose or mouth of children under age 5. The drug is contraindicated in pregnancy.

D. Other Drugs: In light infections, a single dose of albendazole (400 mg) results in cure rates over 95%; in heavy infections, however, a 2- to 3-day course is indicated. Side effects are rare. Albendazole is not available in the USA.

Levamisole, available in the USA but not approved for this indication, is highly effective as a single oral dose of 150 mg (children, 3 mg/kg). Occasional mild and transient side effects are nausea, vomiting, abdominal pain, headache, and dizziness.

Prognosis

The complications caused by wandering adult worms require that all *Ascaris* infections be treated and eradicated.

Khuroo MS, Zargar SA, Mahajan R: Hepatobiliary and pancreatic ascariasis in India. Lancet 1990;335:1503.

Ochoa B: Surgical complications of ascariasis. World J Surg 1991;15:222.

Thein-Hlaing et al: A controlled chemotherapeutic intervention trial on the relationship between *Ascaris lumbricoides* infection and malnutrition. Trans R Soc Trop Med Hyg 1991;85:523.

Tietze PE, Tietze PH: The roundworm, *Ascaris lumbricoides*. Primary Care 1991;18:25.

CUTANEOUS LARVA MIGRANS (Creeping Eruption)

Cutaneous larva migrans, prevalent throughout the tropics and subtropics, is caused by larvae of the dog and cat hookworms, *Ancylostoma braziliense* and *Ancylostoma caninum*. A number of other animal hookworms, gnathostomiasis, and strongyloidiasis are rarely also causative agents. Human infection is common in southeastern USA, particularly where people come in contact with moist sandy soil (eg, beaches, children's sand piles) contaminated by dog or cat feces.

At the site of larval entry, particularly on the hands or feet, up to several hundred minute, intensely pruritic erythematous papules appear. Two to 3 days later, serpiginous eruptions appear as the larvae migrate at a rate of several millimeters a day; the parasite lies slightly ahead of the advancing border. The process continues for weeks to a year, and the lesions may remain severely pruritic, vesiculate, and become encrusted and secondarily infected. Without treatment, the larvae eventually die and are absorbed.

The diagnosis is based on the characteristic appearance of the lesions and the frequent presence of eosinophilia. Biopsy is usually not indicated. The differential diagnosis includes strongyloidiasis and gnathostomiasis.

Simple transient cases may not require treatment. Where available, albendazole, which is nearly free of side effects, is the drug of choice. The dosage is 400 mg daily or twice daily for 3 days. The alternative drug, thiabendazole, given as for strongyloidiasis, has significant side effects in about one-third of patients. Progression of the lesions and itching are usually stopped within 48 hours, but if active lesions are still present at that time, treatment is repeated. Thiabendazole cream (15% in a hygroscopic base) applied topically daily for 5 days may also be effective. Antihistamines are helpful in controlling pruritus, and antibiotic ointments may be necessary to treat secondary infections. Ivermectin (under evaluation) shows promise in treatment.

Jones SK et al: Oral albdendazole for the treatment of cutaneous larva migrans. Brit J Dermatol 1990;122:99.
Sanguigini S et al: Albendazole in the therapy of cutaneous larva migrans. Trans R Soc Trop Med Hyg 1990;84:831.

DRACUNCULIASIS
(Guinea Worm Infection, Dracunculosis, Dracontiasis)

Dracunculiasis is an infection of connective and subcutaneous tissues by the nematode *Dracunculus medinensis*. It occurs only in humans and is one of the major causes of disability among people in endemic areas. An estimated 3 million persons are infected in the Indian subcontinent; West and Central Africa north of the equator (Cameroon to Mauritania, Uganda, and southern Sudan); and Saudi Arabia, Iran, and Yemen. All ages are affected, and the prevalence may reach 60% in some areas.

Infection occurs by swallowing water containing the infected intermediate host, the crustacean *Cyclops* (copepods, water fleas). In the stomach, larvae escape from the crustacean and mature in subcutaneous connective tissue. After mating, the male worm dies and the gravid female (60–80 cm × 1.7–2.0 mm)

moves to the surface of the body, where its head reaches the dermis and provokes a blister that ruptures on contact with water. Intermittently over 2–3 weeks, whenever the ulcer comes in contact with water, the uterus discharges great numbers of larvae. The life cycle is completed when larvae are ingested by copepods. Most adult worms are gradually extruded; some worms retract and reemerge; and others die in the tissues, disintegrate, and may provoke a severe inflammatory reaction. Infection does not induce protective immunity.

Clinical Findings

A. Symptoms and Signs: The incubation period is 9–14 months. Infection may be at one or several sites. Several hours before the head appears at the skin surface, local erythema, burning, pruritus, and tenderness often develop at the site of emergence. There may also be a 24-hour systemic allergic reaction (pruritus, fever, nausea and vomiting, dyspnea, and generalized urticaria). After rupture, the tissues surrounding the ulceration frequently become indurated, reddened, and tender. Because most lesions appear on the leg or foot, patients often must give up walking and working. Uninfected ulcers heal in 4–6 weeks. The worm rarely reaches ectopic sites.

Secondary infections, including tetanus, are common. Deep "cold" abscesses may result at the sites of dying worms. Ankle and knee joint infections with resultant deformity are common complications.

B. Laboratory Findings: When an emerging adult worm is not visible in the ulcer or under the skin, the diagnosis may be made by detection of larvae in smears from discharging sinuses. Immersion of an ulcer in cold water stimulates larval expulsion. Eosinophilia is usually present. Skin and serologic tests are not useful. Calcified worms can be recognized on radiographs.

Treatment

All persons in an endemic area should be actively immunized against tetanus.

A. General Measures: The patient should be at bed rest with the affected part elevated. Cleanse the lesion, control secondary infection with antibiotics, and change dressings daily.

B. Manual Extraction: Traditional extraction of emerging worms by gradually rolling them out a few centimeters each day on a small stick is still useful, especially when done along with chemotherapy and use of aseptic dressings. The process appears to be facilitated by placing the affected part in water several times a day. If the worm is broken during removal, however, secondary infection almost always results, leading to cellulitis, abscess formation, or septicemia.

C. Anthelmintic Therapy: Metronidazole and thiabendazole are sometimes useful in alleviating symptoms and in reducing the duration of infection (by expediting spontaneous extrusion of worms or facilitating their manual extraction). The drugs have an anti-inflammatory effect but do not kill the adult or larvae.

1. Metronidazole, 250 mg three times daily for 10 days, causes only minimal toxicity. (See under Amebiasis).

2. Thiabendazole, 25 mg/kg twice daily for 2–3 days after meals, frequently causes side effects, sometimes severe (see under Strongyloidiasis, below).

3. Mebendazole, 400—800 mg daily for 6 days, can be tried.

D. Surgical Removal: Preemergent female worms can be surgically removed intact under local anesthesia if not firmly embedded in deep fascia or around tendons.

Prevention & Control

The disease is readily prevented by use of only noncontaminated drinking water. This can be accomplished either (1) by preventing contamination of community water supplies through use of tube wells, hand pumps, or cisterns or treating water sources with temephos; or (2) by household action to filter water through nets (eg, nylon nets of 100 μm pore size) or by boiling water. The potential exists for eradication of the disease; such programs are currently in progress.

Muller R. Guinea worm eradication: Four more years to go. Parasitology Today. 1992;8:387.

Sullivan JJ, Long EG: Synthetic-fibre filters for preventing dracunculiasis: 100 versus 200 micrometres pore size. Trans R Soc Trop Med Hyg 1988;82:465.

ENTEROBIASIS
(Pinworm Infection)

Essentials of Diagnosis

- Nocturnal perianal and vulvar pruritus, insomnia, irritability, restlessness.
- Vague gastrointestinal symptoms.
- Eggs demonstrable by cellulose tape test; worms visible on perianal skin or in stool.

General Considerations

Enterobius vermicularis (8–13 mm) is common worldwide. Humans are the only host. Young children are affected more often than adults, and multiple infections occur frequently in households with young children.

The adult worms inhabit the cecum and adjacent bowel areas, lying loosely attached to the mucosa. Gravid females migrate through the anus to the perianal skin and deposit eggs in large numbers. The eggs become infective in a few hours and may then infect others or be autoinfective if transferred to the mouth by contaminated food, drink, fomites, or hands. After being swallowed, the eggs hatch in the duodenum, and the larvae migrate down to the cecum. Retroinfection occasionally occurs when the eggs hatch on the perianal skin and the larvae migrate through the anus into the large intestine. The development of a mature ovipositing female from an ingested egg requires about 3–4 weeks. Eggs remain viable for 2–3 weeks outside the host. The life span of the worm is 30–45 days.

Clinical Findings

A. Symptoms and Signs: Many patients are asymptomatic. The most common and important symptom is perianal pruritus (particularly at night), due to the presence of the female worms or deposited eggs. Insomnia, restlessness, enuresis, and irritability are common symptoms, particularly in children. Many mild gastrointestinal symptoms have also been attributed to enterobiasis, but the association is difficult to prove. At night, worms may occasionally be seen near the anus. Perianal scratching may result in excoriation and impetigo. Adults sometimes report a "crawling" sensation in the anal area. Rarely, worm migration results in ectopic inflammation or granulomatous reaction in various organs, including the appendix; or, in young girls, vulvovaginitis, urethritis, endometritis, salpingitis, and pelvic granuloma may occur. Recurrent urinary tract infections have also been associated with the infection.

B. Laboratory Findings: Diagnosis is made by finding eggs on the perianal skin (eggs are seldom found on stool examination). The most reliable method is by applying a short strip of sealing cellulose pressure-sensitive tape (eg, Scotch Tape) to the perianal skin and then spreading the tape on a slide for low-power microscopic study; toluene is used to clear the preparation. Three such preparations made on consecutive mornings before bathing or defecation will establish the diagnosis in about 90% of cases. Before the diagnosis can be ruled out, five to seven such examinations are necessary. Nocturnal examination of the perianal area or gross examination of stools may reveal adult worms, which should be placed in preservative, alcohol, or saline for laboratory examination. The worms can sometimes be seen on anoscopy. Eosinophilia is rare.

Differential Diagnosis

Pinworm pruritus must be distinguished from similar pruritus due to mycotic infections, allergies, hemorrhoids, proctitis, fissures, strongyloidiasis, and other conditions.

Treatment

A. General Measures: Symptomatic patients should be treated, and in some situations all members of the patient's household should be treated concurrently, since for each overt case there are usually several inapparent cases. Generally, however, treatment of all nonsymptomatic cases is not necessary. Careful washing of hands with soap and water after defecation and again before meals is important. Fingernails should be kept trimmed close and clean and scratching of the perianal area avoided. Ordinary washing of bedding will usually kill pinworm eggs.

B. Specific Measures: Treatment with the following drugs should be repeated at 2 and 4 weeks. The drugs should not be used in pregnancy.

1. Pyrantel pamoate is a highly effective oral drug (with cure rates of over 95%) and a drug of choice. It is administered as a 10 mg (base)/kg (maximum, 1 g) dose. It may be given before or after meals. Infrequent side effects include vomiting, diarrhea, headache, dizziness, and drowsiness.

2. Mebendazole is highly effective and also a drug of choice. It is administered as a 100 mg oral dose, irrespective of body weight. It may be given with or without food and should be chewed for best effect. Gastrointestinal side effects are infrequent.

3. Other drugs–Albendazole (not available in the USA) achieves 100% cure rates when given as a 400 mg dose. Piperazine is less favored, because treatment requires 1 week. Thiabendazole is not recommended, because it causes frequent side effects which rarely are severe and life-threatening.

Prognosis

Although annoying, the infection is benign. Cure is readily attainable with one of several effective drugs, but reinfection is common. Recurrence is frequent in children, however, because of continued exposure outside the home.

Russel LJ: The pinworm, *Enterobius vermicularis.* Prim Care 1991;18:13.

Sinniah B et al. Enterobiasis: A histopathologic study of 259 patients. Ann Trop Med Parasitol 1991;85:625.

FILARIASIS

More than 80 million people are infected with lymphatic filariasis, which is caused by three filiarial nematodes: *Wuchereria bancrofti, Brugia malayi,* or *Brugia timori. W bancrofti* is widely distributed in the tropics and subtropics of both hemispheres and on Pacific islands and is transmitted by *Culex, Aedes,* and *Anopheles* mosquitoes. *B malayi* is transmitted by *Mansonia* and *Anopheles* mosquitoes of South India, Sri Lanka, Southeast Asia, South China, the northern coastal areas of China, and South Korea. *B timori* is found on the southeastern islands of Indonesia.

No animal reservoir hosts are known for *W bancrofti* or *B timori*; cats, monkeys, and other animals may harbor *B malayi.* Mosquitoes become infected by ingesting microfilariae with a blood meal;

at subsequent feedings, they can infect new susceptible hosts. Over months, adult worms (females, 8–9 cm × 0.2–0.3 mm) mature and live in or near superficial and deep lymphatics and lymph nodes and produce large numbers of viviparous circulating microfilariae, which may be seen in the blood starting 6–12 months after infection.

Pathologic changes in lymph vessels are due to host immunologic reactions to developing and mature worms. Living microfilariae generally cause no lesions, with the exception of tropical pulmonary eosinophilia. Rapid death of microfilariae, however, does produce findings, and an abscess may form at the site of a dying adult worm.

Dirofilariasis, infection by *Dirofilaria immitis,* the dog heartworm, has been reported in the USA, Japan, and Australia. Nodules have been found in the skin or as solitary 1–2 cm "coin" lesions in the periphery of the lungs. The serologic test for filariasis is positive.

Other filiarial worms. Several other species infect humans—*Mansonella perstans, Mansonella streptocerca,* and *Mansonella ozzardi*—but usually without causing important findings.

Clinical Findings

A. Symptoms and Signs: Many infections remain asymptomatic, with or without microfilariae. The incubation period is generally 8–16 months in expatriates but may be longer in indigenous persons.

1. Acute disease–Episodes of fever, with or without inflammation of lymphatics and nodes, occur at irregular intervals and last for several days. Characteristically, the adenolymphangitis presents as retrograde extension from the affected node. With disease progression, epididymitis and orchitis as well as involvement of pelvic, abdominal, or retroperitoneal lymphatics may also occur intermittently. Lymph node enlargement may persist.

2. Chronic disease–Obstructive phenomena occur as a result of interference with normal lymphatic flow and include hydrocele, scrotal lymphedema, lymphatic varices, and elephantiasis, particularly of the extremities, genitals, and breasts. Chyluria may result from rupture of distended lymphatics into the urinary tract.

3. Occult disease–A small proportion of the population develops the occult form of the disease, in which classic clinical manifestations and microfilaremia are not present but microfilariae are present in the tissues. Extrapulmonary manifestations seen in some patients include lymphadenopathy or moderate hepatomegaly or splenomegaly.

In tropical pulmonary eosinophilia, microfilariae of *W bancrofti* or *B malayi* are sequestered in the lungs. The condition is characterized by episodic nocturnal coughing or wheezing, hypereosinophilia, high filarial antibody titers and IgE levels, diffuse miliary lesions or increased bronchovascular markings on chest films, fever (sometimes), and a response to diethylcarbamazine treatment (6 mg/kg daily for 21 days). Relapses (in 20%) require re-treatment with up to 12 mg/kg daily for up to 30 days. If untreated, the condition progresses to chronic pulmonary fibrosis.

B. Laboratory Findings: Diagnosis is established by finding microfilariae in the blood. In indigenous persons, they are rare in the first 2–3 years, abundant as the disease progresses, and again rare in the obstructive stage. In persons from nonendemic areas, inflammatory reactions may be prominent in the absence of microfilariae. Microfiliariae of *W bancrofti* are found in the blood chiefly at night (nocturnal periodicity 10 PM to 2 AM), except for a nonperiodic variety in the South Pacific. *B malayi* microfilariae are usually nocturnally periodic but in Southeast Asia may be present at all times, with a slight nocturnal rise. Anticoagulated blood specimens are collected at times related to the periodicity of the local strain. Specimens may be stored at ambient temperatures until examined in the morning by wet film for motile larvae and by Giemsa-stained thin smears for specific morphology. A formalin-anionic detergent preservative can also be used. If these are negative, the blood specimens should be concentrated by the Knott concentration or membrane filtration technique. If all are negative, oral administration of 50 mg of diethylcarbamazine often results in positive blood specimens or a systemic reaction (itching, papular rash, myalgia) in 1–24 hours. If negative, repeat with 200 mg. When onchocerciasis or loiasis may be present, this test must be done with extreme caution.

Serologic tests may be helpful in diagnostic screening, but false-positive and false-negative reactions occur. An indirect hemagglutination titer of 1:128 and a bentonite flocculation titer of 1:5 in combination are considered minimum significant titers. Lymphangiography and lymphoscintigraphy are helpful in differential diagnosis. Testing for antigenemia, now experimental, may prove useful in diagnosis when examining daytime blood specimens and in monitoring efficacy of treatment. In amicrofilaremic subjects there is no antigenemia.

Treatment, Prevention, & Prognosis

Diethylcarbamazine, the drug of choice, rapidly kills blood microfilariae but only slowly kills or injures adult worms. Cure may require multiple 3-week courses (2 mg/kg three times a day after meals, starting with small doses, and gradually increasing over 3–4 days). At this dose, the drug rarely produces direct toxicity. However, adverse immunologic reactions to dying microfilariae and adult worms are common—more so with brugian than with bancroftian filariasis. Reactions are local (lymphadenitis, abscess, ulceration) and systemic (fever, headache, myalgia, dizziness, malaise, and other allergic re-

sponses). Antipyretics and analgesics may be helpful. In areas where onchocerciasis or loiasis is also prevalent, special care must be taken not to provoke reactions to dying microfilariae of these parasites. Diethylcarbamazine has also been used extensively used in mass treatment programs and is being evaluated for prophylaxis. In the USA, the drug is available only from the manufacturer, Lederle Laboratories, (914) 735–5000.

During acute inflammatory episodes, it is controversial whether to treat and whether drug usage will shorten the attack. General measures include bed rest, antibiotics for secondary infections, use of elastic stockings and pressure bandages for leg edema, and suspensory bandaging for orchitis and epididymitis.

Small hydroceles may benefit from a locally injected sclerosing agent, or surgery may be indicated. To manage elephantiasis, lymphovenous shunt procedures may be useful, combined with removal of excess subcutaneous fatty and fibrous tissue, postural drainage, and physiotherapy.

Ivermectin, a microfilaricide, is under evaluation as a convenient single-dose or two-dose schedule (possibly a clearing dose of 20 μg/kg followed by 400 μg/kg). Diethylcarbamazine is still needed to kill the adult worms. Both drugs appear to be equally efficacious in reducing microfilarial burdens; mild side effects (myalgia, headache, fever) are similar in some studies but less so for ivermectin in others.

The prognosis is good with treatment of early and mild cases (including low-grade lymphedema, chyluria, small hydrocele), but in advanced infection the prognosis is poor.

Addiss DG et al: Tolerance of single high-dose ivermectin for treatment of lymphatic filariasis. Trans R Soc Trop Med Hyg 1991;85:265.

Asimacopoulos PJ, Katras A, Christie B: Pulmonary dirofilariasis. The largest single-hospital experience. Chest 1992;102:851.

Ottesen EA: Filariasis now. Am J Trop Med Hyg 1989;41:9.

Otteson EA, Nutman TB: Tropical pulmonary eosinophilia. Annu Rev Med 1992;43:417.

WHO Expert Committee on Filariasis: *Lymphatic Filariasis: The Disease and Its Control.* WHO Technical Report Series No. 821, 1992.

GNATHOSTOMIASIS

Gnathostomiasis is due to infection by the larval stage of the nematode *Gnathostoma spinigerum.* Eggs passed in feces of the definitive hosts, wild and domestic dogs and cats, are infective for copepods. Ingestion of copepods by secondary hosts results in encysted larvae in their tissues. Humans are infected when larvae are ingested in raw, marinated, or inadequately cooked freshwater fish, chicken or other fowl, frogs, or pork. Infection has also been attributed to ingestion of infected copepods in water. Human infection is most common in Thailand and Japan but is also reported from Southeast Asia, China, India, Mexico, and Israel.

Within 24–48 hours, larval migration through the intestinal wall can cause acute epigastric pain, vomiting, urticaria, and eosinophilia. The worm then migrates to subcutaneous and other tissues but is unable to mature. Most common is a pruritic subcutaneous swelling up to 25 cm across, occasionally accompanied by stabbing pain. The swelling may remain in one area for days or weeks, or move continuously. Occasionally the worm becomes visible under the skin.

Internal organs and the eye may also be invaded. Spontaneous pneumothorax, leukorrhea, hematemesis, hematuria, hemoptysis, paroxysmal coughing, and edema of the pharynx with dyspnea have been reported as complications. Invasion of the brain can result in encephalitis, or subarachnoid hemorrhage with cerebrospinal fluid eosinophilia. Spinal cord invasion can lead to myelitis or radiculopathy.

Definitive diagnosis is sometime possible by surgical removal of the worm when it appears close to the skin. Marked eosinophilia is common, except for parasites in the central nervous system. Serodiagnosis by immunoblot assay or ELISA is promising. Skin and other serologic tests are unsatisfactory.

A recent report suggests that treatment with albendazole may be effective. Among presumptively diagnosed cases, 94 of 100 persons were apparently cured after a dosage of 400 mg or 800 mg (in divided doses) of the drug daily for 21 days. Larval death appeared to occur slowly over 1–2 weeks. Alternatively, chemotherapy with diethylcarbamazine (as for filariasis) or with thiabendazole can be tried but has not been very successful. Courses of prednisolone have provided temporary relief of symptoms.

Punyagupta S, Bunnag T, Juttijudata P: Eosinophilic meningitis in Thailand. J Neurol Sci 1990;96:241.

Kraivichian P et al: Albendazole in the treatment of human gnathostomiasis. Trans R Soc Trop Med Hyg 1992; 86:418.

Tapchaisri P et al: Specific antigen to *Gnathostoma spinigerum* for immunodiagnosis of human gnathostomiasis. Int J Parasitol 1991;21:315.

HOOKWORM DISEASE

Essentials of Diagnosis

Early findings (not commonly recognized):

- Dermatitis: pruritic, erythematous, papulovesicular eruption at site of larval invasion.
- Pulmonary migration of larvae: transient episodes of coughing, asthma, fever, blood-tinged sputum, marked eosinophilia.

Later findings:

- Intestinal symptoms: anorexia, diarrhea, abdominal discomfort.
- Anemia (iron deficiency): fatigue, pallor, dyspnea on exertion, poikilonychia, heart failure.
- Characteristic eggs and occult blood in the stool.

General Considerations

Hookworm disease, widespread in the moist tropics and subtropics, is caused by *Ancylostoma duodenale* and *Necator americanus.* Probably a quarter of the world's population is infected, and in many areas hookworms are a major cause of general debility, retardation of growth of children, and increased susceptibility to infections. About 50,000 deaths yearly are attributed directly to hookworm infection. Deaths of many young, infested children occur from other infections that could normally be tolerated, such as malaria, measles, and those that cause diarrhea.

In the Western Hemisphere and tropical Africa, *Necator* was the prevailing species, and in the Far East, India, China, and the Mediterranean area, *Ancylostoma* was prevalent, but both species have now become widely distributed. Infection is rare in regions with less than 40 inches of rainfall annually. Humans are the only host for both species.

The adult worms are approximately 1 cm long. Eggs produced by female worms are passed in the stool and must fall on warm, moist soil if hatching followed by larval development is to take place. Larvae remain infective for hours to about a week, depending on environmental conditions. Following skin penetration, the larvae migrate in the bloodstream to the pulmonary capillaries, break into alveoli, and then are carried by ciliary action upward to the bronchi, trachea, and mouth. After being swallowed, they reach and attach to the mucosa of the upper small bowel, where they develop into adult worms. *Ancylostoma* infection can probably also be acquired by ingestion of the larvae in food or water. Adult *Ancylostoma* survive about a year; *Necator,* about 3–5 years.

Worms suck blood at their attachment sites. The estimated hookworm load for 1000 eggs per gram of feces (light infection) is 11 for *Ancylostoma* and 32 for *Necator;* the daily blood loss per worm is estimated, respectively, to be 0.2 mL and 0.04 mL. Over a period of years, even small hookworm loads can significantly deplete iron reserves: Depending on the host's dietary intake of iron, severe anemia may result if 30 or more *Ancylostoma* or 100 or more *Necator* worms are present. A moderate worm load is 2000–8000 eggs per gram of feces.

Clinical Findings

A. Symptoms and Signs: Ground itch, the first manifestation of infection, is a pruritic erythematous dermatitis, either maculopapular or vesicular, that follows skin penetration of the infective larvae. Severity is a function of the number of invading larvae and the sensitivity of the host. Scratching may result in secondary infection. Strongyloidiasis and cutaneous larva migrans must be considered in the differential diagnosis at this stage.

The pulmonary stage, in which there is larval migration through the lungs, may show dry cough, wheezing, blood-tinged sputum, and low-grade fever.

After two or more weeks, maturing worms attach to the mucosa of the duodenum and upper jejunum. In heavy infections, worms may reach the ileum. Patients who have light infections and adequate iron intake often remain asymptomatic. In heavy infections, however, there may be anorexia, diarrhea, vague abdominal pain, and ulcer-like epigastric symptoms. Severe anemia may result in pallor, deformed nails, pica, and cardiac decompensation. Marked protein loss may also occur, resulting in hypoalbuminemia, with edema and ascites. There are conflicting reports of malabsorption in some severe infections.

Reduction in worm loads and symptoms after the first decade of life suggests that a moderate degree of immunity develops.

B. Laboratory Findings: Diagnosis depends upon demonstration of characteristic eggs in feces. The stool usually contains occult blood. Hypochromic microcytic anemia can be severe, with hemoglobin levels as low as 2 g/dL, a low serum iron and a high iron-binding capacity, and low serum ferritin. Eosinophilia (as high as 30–60% of a total white blood count reaching 17,000/μL) is usually present in the pulmonary migratory stage of infection but is not marked in the chronic intestinal stage.

Treatment

A. General Measures: The availability of safe anthelmintics makes it possible to treat all patients initially, irrespective of the intensity of infection; nevertheless, it may not be necessary or beneficial to treat light infections. Re-treatment is often necessary at 2-week intervals until the worm burden is reduced to a low level as estimated by semiquantitative egg counts. Eradication of infection is not essential, since light infections do not injure the well-nourished patient and iron loss is replaced if the patient is receiving adequate dietary iron.

If anemia is present, oral ferrous sulfate and a diet high in protein and vitamins are required for at least 3 months after the anemia has been corrected in order to replace iron stores. A dosage schedule for ferrous sulfate tablets (200 mg) for adults is one tablet three times daily for 2 months followed by one tablet daily for 4 months. Parenteral iron is rarely indicated. Blood transfusion may be necessary if anemia is severe.

B. Specific Measures: Mebendazole, pyrantel, and albendazole are highly effective drugs for treatment of hookworm infections; mebendazole or albendazole can be used to treat concurrent trichuriasis,

and all three drugs can be used to treat concurrent ascariasis. The drugs are given before or after meals, without purges. For the three drugs, mild gastrointestinal side effects are rare; none should be used in pregnancy. Albendazole and mebendazole should not be given to children under 2 years of age, and pyrantel should not be given to children under 1 year of age.

1. Pyrantel pamoate–In *A duodenale* infections, pyrantel given as a single dose, 10 mg (base)/kg (maximum 1 g), produces cures in 76–98% of cases and a marked reduction in the worm burden in the remainder. For *N americanus* infections, a single dose may give a satisfactory cure rate in light infection, but for moderate or heavy infection a 3-day course is necessary. If the species is unknown, treat as for necatoriasis. Mild and transient drowsiness and headache may occur.

2. Mebendazole–When mebendazole is given at a dosage of 100 mg twice daily for 3 days, reported cure rates for both hookworm species range from 35% to 95%.

3. Albendazole, given orally once only at a dosage of 400 mg, results in the cure of 85–95% of patients with *Ancylostoma* infection and markedly reduces the worm burden in those not cured. Because cure rates for single-dose treatments of *Necator* infection were 33–90%, treatment should be continued for 2–3 days, especially in heavy infections.

Prognosis

If the disease is recognized before serious secondary complications appear, complete recovery is the rule following treatment.

Crompton DWT: Hookworm disease: Current status and new directions. Parasitol Today 1989;5:1.

Pawlowski ZS, Schad GA, Stott GJ: *Hookworm Infection and Anemia. Approaches to Prevention and Control.* WHO, 1991.

Schad GA, Warren KS (editors): *Hookworm Disease: Current Status and New Directions.* Taylor & Francis, 1990.

LOIASIS

Loiasis is a chronic filarial disease caused by infection with *Loa loa*. The infection occurs in humans and monkeys in rain and swamp forest areas of West Africa from Nigeria to Angola and throughout the Congo river watershed of central Africa eastward to Southwest Sudan and western Uganda.

The adult worms live in the subcutaneous tissues. Gravid females release microfilariae into the bloodstream which subsequently are ingested in a blood meal by the vector-intermediate host, female *Chrysops* spp, day-biting flies. When the fly feeds again, the larval stage can infect a new host or cause superinfection. The time to worm maturity and detection of new microfilariae is 6 months to several years.

Clinical Findings

A. Symptoms and Signs: Many infected persons are asymptomatic. In symptomatic persons, the worms (females, 4–7 cm × 0.5 mm) are evidenced by their temporary appearance beneath the skin or conjunctiva, by unilateral edema of an extremity, or by Calabar swellings. The latter are subcutaneous edematous reactions, 3–10 cm in diameter, nonpitting and nonerythematous, and at times associated with low-grade fever, local pain, and pruritus. The swellings may migrate a few centimeters for 2–3 days or stay in place before they subside. At irregular intervals, they recur at the same or different sites, but only one appears at a time. When near joints, they may be temporarily disabling. Migration across the eye may be asymptomatic or may produce pain, intense conjunctivitis, and eyelid edema. Dying adult worms may elicit small nodules or local sterile abscesses, and dead worms may result in radiologically detectable calcification.

Microfilariae in the blood do not induce symptoms. Rarely, however, they enter the central nervous system and may cause encephalitis, myelitis, or jacksonian seizures; the larvae can also induce lesions and complications in the retina, heart, lungs, and other tissues.

Natives generally have a mild form of the infection, often showing only microfilaremia and being otherwise asymptomatic. The disease among visitors, however, is more often characterized by more pronounced allergic symptoms (frequent and debilitating Calabar swellings, high peripheral eosinophilia, hypergammaglobulinemia, increased serum IgE), frequently without detectable microfilaremia.

B. Laboratory Findings: Specific diagnosis is made by finding characteristic microfilariae in daytime (10 AM to 4 PM) blood specimens by concentration methods; in order of increasing sensitivity, they are (1) thick films, (2) Knott's concentration, and (3) Nuclepore filtration. Presumptive diagnosis that permits treatment is based on Calabar swellings, a history of residence in an endemic area, and marked eosinophilia (40% or greater). Serologic tests may be helpful, but cross-reactions occur with other filarial diseases.

Treatment & Prognosis

See references for details on proper use of diethylcarbamazine (drug of choice as a micro- and macrofilaricide), since side effects to dying microfilariae may be severe, and life-threatening encephalitis can occur. Reactions are more likely with pretreatment microfilaria counts greater than 25/μL. Cytapheresis has been used to reduce parasite loads before starting diethycarbamazine. Prednisone, 60 mg daily for 3 days, is sometimes indicated to mini-mize reactions. Ivermectin, a microfilaricide, is being evaluated for initial treatment of patients with high microfilaria loads. Surgical removal of adult worms from the eye or skin is not recommended.

Individual protection is facilitated by daytime use of insect repellent and by wearing light-colored clothing with long sleeves and trousers. Diethylcarbamazine prophylaxis, 300 mg weekly, may be useful if the risk of exposure is high. It is not indicated, however, for the casual traveler or for persons who might previously have acquired any of the filarial infections.

Most infections run a benign course, but some are accompanied by severe and temporarily disabling symptoms. The prognosis is excellent with treatment.

Klion AD et al: Pulmonary involvement in loiasis. Am Rev Respir Dis 1992;145:961.
Markell EK: Loiasis. In: *Tropical Medicine and Parasitology.* Goldsmith R, Heyneman D (editors). Appleton & Lange, 1989.
Noireau F et al: Clinical manifestations of loiasis in an endemic area of the Congo. Trop Med Parasitol 1990; 41:37.

ONCHOCERCIASIS

Onchocerciasis is a chronic filarial disease caused by *Onchocerca volvulus.* The advent of the safe and effective drug ivermectin has led to the effective treatment and control of the disease. Primary findings are subcutaneous nodules that contain adult worms and skin and eye changes that result from dead or dying microfilariae. Heavy infection leads to chronic pruritus, disfiguring skin lesions, visual impairment, and debility. An estimated 20 million persons are infected, of whom 0.3 million are blinded by the condition. In hyperendemic areas, more than 40% of inhabitants over 40 years of age are blind. The infection, predominant in West Africa, also occurs in many other parts of tropical Africa and in localized areas of the southwestern Arabian peninsula, southern Mexico, Guatemala, Venezuela, Colombia, and northwestern Brazil.

Humans are the only important host. The vector and intermediate host are *Simulium* flies, day biters that breed in rivers and fast-flowing streams and become infected by ingesting microfilariae with a blood meal; at subsequent feedings, they can infect new susceptible hosts.

Clinical Findings

A. Symptoms and Signs: Adult worms, which live for years, typically are in fibrous subcutaneous nodules that are painless, freely movable, and 0.5–1 cm in diameter. Within 10–20 months after infection (range, 7–24 months), female worms begin to release motile microfilariae into the skin, subcutaneous tissues, lymphatics, and eyes; microfilariae are occasionally seen in the urine but rarely in blood or cerebrospinal fluid. Skin manifestations are localized or cover large areas. Pruritus may be severe, leading to skin excoriation and lichenification; other findings include pigmentary changes, papules, scaling, atrophy, pendulous skin, and acute inflammation. There may be marked enlargement of femoral and inguinal nodes and generalized lymph node enlargement. Microfilariae in the eye may lead to visual impairment and blindness; findings include itching, photophobia, corneal opacities (punctate keratitis), sclerosing keratitis, anterior uveitis (with secondary glaucoma), cataract, chorioretinitis, and optic neuritis.

B. Laboratory Findings: Diagnosis is by demonstrating microfilariae in skin snips (usually obtained with a punch biopsy instrument), identifying them in the cornea or anterior chamber by slitlamp examination, or by nodule aspiration or excision. Skin snips are placed in saline and incubated overnight before examination. When microfilariae are absent, a small challenge dose of diethylcarbamazine may facilitate the diagnosis (see references for method). Adult worms may be recovered in excised nodules, whereas ultrasound has been used to detect nonpalpable onchocercomas. Skin and serologic tests are usually positive, but cross-reactions occur with other forms of filariasis. Immunoblot analysis of IgG4 antibodies appears to be more sensitive than skin snips earlier in infection. Eosinophilia (15–50%) is common. Eosinophilia (15–50%) is common.

Treatment & Prognosis

Nodules on or near the head should be removed surgically. Nodules on or hear the head should be removed surgically. Ivermectin, a microfilaricide, is the drug of choice. A single oral dose of 150 µg/kg is given with water on an empty stomach and repeated at 4- to 12-month intervals, based on skin microfilarial levels and symptoms. This results in a rapid, prolonged (up to 12 months), and marked reduction in skin microfilariae and slow clearance (over months) of microfilariae from the anterior chamber. In addition to stopping progression of the disease, there may be improvement in the dermatitis and anterior segment eye disease. The effect of ivermectin on posterior segment disease is unknown. In comparison studies, ivermectin was as effective as diethylcarbamazine in reducing the number of microfilariae but did so with significantly fewer systemic and ocular adverse reactions. Recent reports suggest that serial treatments at intervals of 6 months or longer result in slow death of some adult worms. Ivermectin is not marketed but is available on a compassionate use basis from the manufacturer (Merck Sharp & Dohme). Alternative treatment, only if ivermectin is not available, is the combined use of diethylcarbamazine to kill the microfilariae and suramin to kill the adult worms; however, these drugs frequently induce severe adverse reactions and, therefore, should be administered only by experts.

With treatment, some skin and ocular lesions improve, and ocular progression is prevented. The prognosis is unfavorable only for those patients who are seen for the first time with already far-advanced ocular onchocerciasis.

Awadzi K: Onchocerciasis. In: *Tropical Medicine and Parasitology.* Goldsmith R, Heyneman D (editors). Appleton & Lange, 1989.
Duke BOL et al: Effects of three-month doses of ivermectin on adult *Onchocerca volvulus* Am J Trop Med Hyg 1992;46:189.
Green BM,:Modern medicine versus an ancient scourge: Progress toward control of onchocerciasis. J Infect Dis 1992;166:15. (Also a review of treatment.)
Whitworth J: Treatment of onchocerciasis with ivermectin in Sierra Leone. Parasitology Today 1992;8:138.

STRONGYLOIDIASIS

Essentials of Diagnosis

- Pruritic dermatitis at sites of larval penetration.
- Diarrhea, epigastric pain, nausea, malaise, weight loss.
- Cough, rales, transient pulmonary infiltrates.
- Eosinophilia; characteristic larvae in stool specimens, duodenal aspirate, or sputum.
- Hyperinfection syndrome: Severe diarrhea, bronchopneumonia, ileus.

General Considerations

Strongyloidiasis is caused by infection with *Strongyloides stercoralis* (2–2.5 × 30–50 mm). Major symptoms result from adult parasitism, principally in the duodenum and jejunum, or from larval migration through pulmonary and cutaneous tissues.

The condition is an infection of humans, but dogs, cats, and primates have been found naturally infected with strains indistinguishable from those of humans. The disease is endemic in tropical and subtropical regions; although the prevalence is generally low, in some areas disease rates exceed 25%. In temperate areas, the disease occurs sporadically. In the USA, the disease is endemic in southern wet areas. Multiple infections in households are common, and prevalence in institutions, particularly mental institutions, may be high. Hospital staff should be protected from contact with feces and sputum from infected patients.

The parasite is uniquely capable of maintaining its life cycle both within the human host and in soil. Infection occurs when filariform larvae in soil penetrate the skin, enter the bloodstream, and are carried to the lungs, where they escape from capillaries into alveoli and ascend the bronchial tree to the glottis. The larvae are then swallowed and carried to the duodenum and upper jejunum, where maturation to the adult stage takes place. The parasitic female, generally held to be parthenogenetic, matures and lives embedded in the mucosa, where its eggs are laid and hatch. Rhabditiform larvae, which are noninfective, emerge, and most migrate into the intestinal lumen to leave the host via the feces. The life span of the adult worm may be as long as 5 years.

In the soil, the rhabditiform larvae metamorphose into the infective (filariform) larvae. However, the parasite also has a free-living cycle in soil, in which some rhabditiform larvae develop into adults that produce eggs from which rhabditiform larvae emerge to continue the life cycle.

Autoinfection in humans, which probably occurs at a low rate in most infections, is an important factor in determining worm burden and is responsible for the persistence of asymptomatic or symptomatic infections for many years. Internal autoinfection takes place in the lower bowel when some rhabditiform larvae, instead of passing with the feces, develop into filariform larvae that penetrate the intestinal mucosa, enter the intestinal lymphatic and portal circulation, are carried to the lungs, and return to the small bowel to complete the cycle. This process is accelerated by achlorhydria, constipation, diverticula, and other conditions that reduce bowel motility. In addition, an external autoinfection cycle can occur as a result of fecal contamination of the perianal area. Homosexual men may be at increased risk.

In the hyperinfection syndrome, autoinfection is greatly increased, resulting in a marked increase in the intestinal worm burden and in massive dissemination of filariform larvae to the lungs and most other tissues, where they can cause local inflammatory reactions and granuloma formation. Occasionally, in the lungs and elsewhere, larvae metamorphose into adults. Hyperinfection is generally initiated under conditions of depressed host cellular immunity, especially in debilitated, malnourished persons and in patients receiving immunosuppressive therapy, particularly corticosteroids. It is rare, however, in AIDS. The syndrome can also occur in individuals who show no obvious predisposing cause. Penetration of the bowel wall by filariform larvae can result in polymicrobial gram-negative septicemia.

Clinical Findings

A. Signs and Symptoms: The time from larval penetration of the skin by filariform larvae until their appearance in the feces is 3–4 weeks. An acute syndrome can sometimes be recognized in which cutaneous symptoms are followed by pulmonary and then intestinal symptoms. Patients usually present, however, with chronic symptoms (continuous or with irregular exacerbations) that can persist for years or for life.

1. Cutaneous manifestations–Skin invasion is usually of the feet. The reaction in unsensitized patients may be minimal, with only a macule or papule, but in sensitized patients there may be focal edema, inflammation, petechiae, serpiginous or urticarial tracts, and intense itching. In chronic infections, there may be both stationary urticaria and larva currens, the latter characterized by transient eruptions that migrate in serpiginous tracts.

2. Intestinal manifestations–Symptoms range from mild to severe, the most common being diarrhea, abdominal pain, and flatulence. Anorexia, nausea, vomiting, and epigastric tenderness may be present. The diarrhea may alternate with constipation, and in severe cases the feces contain mucus and blood. The pain is often epigastric in location and may mimic duodenal ulcer. Malabsorption or a protein-losing enteropathy can result from a large intestinal worm burden.

3. Pulmonary manifestations–With migration of larvae through the lungs, bronchi, and trachea, symptoms may be limited to a dry cough and throat irritation or low-grade fever, bronchitis, dyspnea, wheezing, and hemoptysis may occur. Bronchopneumonia, pleural effusion, progressive dyspnea, and miliary abscesses can develop; the cough may become productive of an odorless, mucopurulent sputum.

4. Other findings–Severe infection may present with fever, malaise, and weakness leading to prostration and emaciation.

5. Hyperinfection syndrome–Massive increase in the intestinal worm burden with intense dissemination of larvae to the lungs and other tissues can result in the following complications: severe diarrhea with generalized abdominal pain and distention, malabsorption, bronchopneumonia, pleural effusion, pericarditis and myocarditis, hepatic granulomas, cholecystitis, purpura, ulcerating lesions at all levels of the gastrointestinal tract, paralytic ileus, perforation and peritonitis, gram-negative septicemia, meningitis, cachexia, shock, and death.

B. Laboratory Findings:

1. Detection of eggs and larvae–Eggs are seldom found in feces. Diagnosis requires finding the larval stages in feces or duodenal fluid. Rhabditiform larvae may be found in recently passed stool specimens; filariform larvae will be present in specimens held in the laboratory for some hours. Three specimens, preserved or unpreserved, should be collected at 2-day intervals or longer, since the number of larvae in feces may vary considerably from day to day. Each specimen should be examined by direct microscopy, and one or more should be processed by the Baermann concentration method to increase sensitivity of testing. Stool specimens used in the Baermann procedure must be unpreserved; they can be received in the laboratory up to 48 hours after passage if held at refrigerated but nonfreezing temperatures. An agar plate method appears to result in high detection rates.

Although larvae cannot be found in the stools of 25% or more of infected patients, the diagnosis can often be made by examination of duodenal mucus for rhabditiform larvae or ova. Mucus is obtained by means of the duodenal string test or by duodenal intubation and aspiration. Duodenal biopsy is seldom indicated but will confirm the diagnosis in most patients. Occasionally, filariform or rhabditiform larvae can be detected in sputum during the pulmonary phase of the disease.

2. Serologic and hematologic findings—In chronic low-grade intestinal strongyloidiasis, the white blood cell count is often normal, with a slightly elevated percentage of eosinophils. However, with increasing larval migration, eosinophilia may reach 50% and leukocytosis 20,000/µL. Mild anemia may be present. Serum IgE immunoglobulins may be elevated. An ELISA is sensitive and specific.

3. Imaging—Small bowel x-rays may show inflammation, irritability, and prominent mucosal folds; there may also be bowel dilatation, delayed emptying, and ulcerative duodenitis. In chronic infections, the findings can resemble those in nontropical and tropical sprue, or there may be narrowing, rigidity, and diminished peristalsis. During pulmonary migration of larvae, fine nodularity or irregular patches of pneumonitis may be seen.

4. Hyperinfection—In the hyperinfection syndrome, there may also be findings of hypoproteinemia, malabsorption, and abnormal liver function. Ova and rhabditiform and filariform larvae may be present in sputum, and filariform larvae in the urine; eosinopenia, when present, is thought to be an unfavorable prognostic sign.

Differential Diagnosis

Because of varied signs and symptoms, the diagnosis of strongyloidiasis is often difficult, especially in nonendemic areas. The disease should always be considered in patients with unexplained eosinophilia. Eosinophilia plus one or more of the following factors should further enhance consideration of the diagnosis: endemic area exposure, duodenal ulcer-like pain, persistent or recurrent diarrhea, recurrent coughing or wheezing, and transient pulmonary infiltrates. The duodenitis and jejunitis of strongyloidiasis can also mimic giardiasis, cholecystitis, and pancreatitis. Transient pulmonary infiltrates must be differentiated from tropical pulmonary eosinophilia and Löffler's syndrome. The diagnosis should be considered among the many causes of malabsorption in the tropics.

Treatment

Since *Strongyloides* can multiply in humans, treatment should continue until the parasite is eradicated. Patients receiving immunosuppressive therapy should be examined for the presence of the infection before and probably at intervals during treatment. In concurrent infection with *Strongyloides* and *Ascaris*

or hookworm (which is common), eradicate *Ascaris* and hookworms first and *Strongyloides* subsequently.

A. Thiabendazole: Thiabendazole is the drug of choice. An oral dose of 25 mg/kg (maximum, 1.5 g per dose) is given after meals twice daily for 2–3 days. A 5- to 7-day course is needed for disseminated infections. Tablet and liquid formulations are available; tablets should be chewed. Side effects, including headache, weakness, vomiting, vertigo, and decreased mental alertness, occur in as many as 30% of patients and may be severe. These symptoms are lessened if the drug is taken after meals. Other potentially serious side effects occur rarely. Erythema multiforme and the Stevens-Johnson syndrome have been associated with thiabendazole therapy; several fatalities have occurred in children.

B. Alternative Drugs: Albendazole is undergoing clinical trials. At a dosage of 400 mg twice daily for 3–7 days and repeated in 1 week, cure rates in several studies reached about 80%. Ivermectin shows promise; with a single dose of 200 µg/kg, cure rates were 90%. Cambendazole, where available, can be tried, as can mebendazole (500 mg three times daily for 14 days), but efficacy is not established.

Prognosis

The prognosis is favorable except in the hyperinfection syndrome. Infections associated with emaciation, advanced liver disease, cancer, immunologic disorders, or the use of immunosuppressive drugs may be difficult to treat. In selected instances, a 2-day course of treatment with thiabendazole once monthly can be tried to control infections that cannot be eradicated.

Chanthavanich P et al: Repeated doses of albendazole against strongyloidiasis in Thai children. Southeast Asian J Trop Med Public Health 1989;20:221.

DeVault GA et al: Opportunistic infections with *Strongyloides stercoralis* in renal transplantation. Rev Infect Dis 1990;12:653.

Gompels MM et al: Disseminated strongyloidiasis in AIDS: Uncommon but important. AIDS 1991;5:329.

Grove DI (editor): Strongyloidiasis: A major roundworm infection in man. Taylor & Francis, 1989.

Koga K et al: A modified agar plate method for detection of *Strongyloides stercoralis*. Am J Trop Med Hyg 1991;45:518.

Wijesundera MS, Sanmuganathan PS: Ivermectin therapy in chronic strongyloidiasis. Trans R Soc Trop Med Hyg 1992;86:291.

TRICHINOSIS
(Trichinelliosis, Trichinellosis)

Essentials of Diagnosis

- History of ingestion of raw or inadequately cooked pork, boar, or bear.
- First week: diarrhea, cramps, malaise.

- Second week to 1–2 months: muscle pain and tenderness, fever, periorbital and facial edema, conjunctivitis.
- Eosinophilia and elevated serum enzymes; positive serologic tests; larvae in muscle biopsy.

General Considerations

Trichinosis is caused by *Trichinella spiralis*. The disease is present wherever pork is eaten but is a greater problem in many temperate areas than in the tropics. In the USA, there has been a marked reduction in the prevalence of trichinosis both in humans and in pigs; prevalence in commercial pork now ranges from nil to 0.7%. Fewer than 100 human cases are reported per year, but many mild or asymptomatic infections are undetected or misdiagnosed.

Human infections occur sporadically or in outbreaks. Infection is usually acquired by eating viable encysted larvae in raw or uncooked pork or pork products. Ground beef has also been a source of infection when adulterated with pork or inadvertently contaminated in a common meat grinder. In some cases, the source of infection is the flesh of wild animals, particularly bear, walrus, or bush pigs.

Gastric juices liberate the encysted larvae. They rapidly mature and mate, and the adult female then burrows into the mucosa of the small intestine. Within 4–5 days, the female begins to discharge viviparous larvae (100 × 6 μm) that are disseminated via the lymphatics and bloodstream to most body tissues. Larvae that reach striated muscle encyst and remain viable for months to years; those that reach other tissues are rapidly destroyed. Adult worms (2–3.6 mm × 75–90 μm) survive for up to about 6 weeks.

In the natural cycle, larvae develop into adult worms in the intestines when a carnivore ingests parasitized muscle. Reservoir hosts include swine, dogs, cats, rats, and many wild animals, including the wolf, bear, and boar; marine animals in the Arctic; and the hyena, jackal, and lion in the tropics. Pigs generally become infected by feeding on uncooked food scraps or, less often, by eating infected rats.

Clinical Findings

A. Symptoms and Signs: The incubation period is generally from 2 to 7 days (range, 12 hours to 28 days). Severity depends upon intensity of infection, tissues invaded, immune status of the host, age of the host (children have less severe infections), and perhaps the strain of the parasite. Infection ranges from asymptomatic to a mild febrile illness with one or more mild, short-lasting symptoms to a severe progressive illness with multiple system involvement that in rare cases is fatal.

1. Intestinal stage–When present, intestinal symptoms persist for 1–7 days: diarrhea, abdominal cramps, and malaise are the major findings; nausea and vomiting occur less frequently; and constipation is uncommon. Fever and leukocytosis are rare during the first week.

2. Muscle invasion stage–This begins at the end of the first week and lasts about 6 weeks. Parasitized muscles show an intense inflammatory reaction. Clinical findings include fever (low-grade to marked); muscle pain (especially upon movement) and muscle tenderness, edema, and spasm; periorbital and facial edema; sweating; photophobia and conjunctivitis; weakness or prostration; pain on swallowing; dyspnea, coughing, and hoarseness; subconjunctival, retinal, and nail splinter hemorrhages; and rashes and formication. The most frequently parasitized muscles and sites of findings are the masseters, the tongue, the diaphragm, the intercostal muscles, and the extraocular, laryngeal, paravertebral, nuchal, deltoid, pectoral, gluteus, biceps, and gastrocnemius muscles. Inflammatory reactions around larvae that reach tissues other than muscle may result in a broad range of findings, including the development of meningitis, encephalitis, myocarditis, bronchopneumonia, nephritis, and peripheral and cranial nerve disorders.

3. Convalescent stage–This generally begins in the second month but in severe infections may not begin before 3 months or longer. Vague muscle pains and malaise may persist for several more months. Permanent muscular atrophy has been reported.

B. Laboratory Findings: The diagnosis is supported by findings of eosinophilia, elevated serum muscle enzymes (CK, AST), and positive serologic tests; confirmation is by detection of larvae in muscle biopsy specimens.

Leukocytosis and eosinophilia appear during the second week after ingestion of infected meat. The proportion of eosinophils rises to a maximum of 20–90% in the third or fourth week and then slowly declines to normal over the next few months.

Serologic tests can detect most clinically manifest cases but are not sufficiently sensitive to detect low-level infections (ie, a few larvae per gram of ingested muscle). More than one test should be used and then repeated to observe for seroconversion or for a rising titer. The bentonite flocculation (BF) test (positive titer, ≥ 1:5) is highly sensitive and is considered nearly 100% specific. It becomes positive in the third or fourth week, and reaches a maximum titer at about 2 months, and generally reverts to negative in 2–3 years. The immunofluorescence test (positive titer > 16) is also highly sensitive, though less specific than the BF test; it may become positive in the second week. The ELISA is also showing high sensitivity and specificity for antibody and detecting circulating antigens. The intradermal test is no longer recommended, as it may remain positive for years and batches of antigen vary in potency.

Adult worms may be looked for in feces, though they are seldom found. In the second week, there are occasional larvae in blood, duodenal washings, and, rarely, in centrifuged spinal fluid. In the third to fourth weeks, biopsy of skeletal muscle may be definitive (particularly gastrocnemius and pectoralis), preferably at a site of swelling or tenderness. Portions of the specimen should be examined microscopically by compression between glass slides, by digestion, and by preparation of multiple histologic sections. If the biopsy is done too early, larvae may not be detectable. Myositis even in the absence of larvae is a significant finding.

Nonspecific laboratory findings include elevation of serum enzymes (creatinine phosphokinase, lactate dehydrogenase, serum aspartate aminotransferase [AST], and serum aldolase). Absence of an elevated sedimentation rate is a useful diagnostic clue. There may be a marked hypergammaglobulinemia with reversal of the albumin-globulin ratio.

C. Imaging: Chest films during the acute phase may show disseminated or localized infiltrates. Late calcification of muscle cysts cannot be detected radiologically.

Complications

The more important complications are granulomatous pneumonitis, encephalitis, and cardiac failure.

Differential Diagnosis

Because of its protean manifestations, trichinosis may resemble many other diseases. Eosinophilia, muscle pain and tenderness, and fever should lead the physician to consider collagen vascular disorders such as dermatomyositis or polyarteritis nodosa.

Prevention

The frequency and intensity of infection in the USA and other countries have been significantly reduced by public health measures to prevent feeding of uncooked garbage to hogs and by animal inspection (not in the USA). The chief safeguard against trichinosis is adequate cooking of pork at the newly recommended temperature of 77 °C. Alternatively, larvae can be made nonviable by freezing meat at –15 °C for 30 days (longer if meat is over 15 cm thick). *T spiralis* in game is often relatively resistant to freezing. Low doses of gamma irradiation are also effective in killing larvae.

Treatment

Treatment is principally supportive, since in most cases recovery is spontaneous without sequelae.

A. Intestinal Phase: Mebendazole is the drug of choice at a dosage of 200–400 mg three times daily for 3 days, followed by 400–500 mg three times daily for 10 days. The alternative drug is thiabendazole at a dosage of 25 mg/kg (maximum, 1.5 g per dose) twice daily after meals for 3–7 days; side effects, sometimes severe, are common (see Strongyloidiasis, above). Albendazole, 400 mg twice daily for 15 days,

is undergoing clinical trials. Corticosteroids are contraindicated in the intestinal phase.

B. Muscle Invasion Phase: In this stage, severe infections require hospitalization and high doses of corticosteroids for 24–48 hours, followed by lower doses for several days or weeks to control symptoms. However, because corticosteroids may suppress the inflammatory response to adults worms, they should be used only when symptoms are severe. Thiabendazole has been tried in the muscle stage with equivocal relief of muscle pain or tenderness or lysis of fever; further trials are recommended.Mebendazole and albendazole may also be tried.

Prognosis

Death is rare—sometimes within 2–3 weeks in overwhelming infections, more often in 4–8 weeks from a major complication such as cardiac failure or pneumonia.

Bailey TM, Schantz PM: Trends in the incidence and transmission patterns of trichinosis in humans in the United States: Comparisons of the periods 1975–1981 and 1982–1986. Rev Infect Dis 1990;12:5.

Campbell WC (editor): *Trichinella and Trichinosis.* Plenum Press, 1983.

Fröscher W et al: Chronic trichinosis: Clinical, bioptic, serological, and electromyographic observations. Eur Neurol 1988;28:221.

McAuley JB et al: A trichinosis outbreak among Southeast Asian refugees. Am J Epidemiol 1992;135:1404.

Olaison L, Ljungstrom I: An outbreak of trichinosis in Lebanon. Trans R Soc Trop Med Hyg 1992;86:658.

TRICHURIASIS
(Trichocephaliasis, Whipworm)

Essentials of Diagnosis

- Most infections are silent; heavy infections may cause chronic diarrhea, lower abdominal cramps, flatulence, hematochezia, tenesmus, and rectal prolapse.
- Characteristic barrel-shaped eggs and (less commonly) adult worms are found in the stool.

General Considerations

Trichuris trichiura is a common intestinal parasite of humans throughout the world, particularly in the subtropics and tropics. Persons of all ages are affected, but infection is heaviest and most frequent in children. The slender worms, 30–50 mm in length, attach by means of their anterior whip-like end to the mucosa of the large intestine, particularly to the cecum. Eggs are passed in the feces but require 2–4 weeks for larval development after reaching the soil before becoming infective; thus, person-to-person transmission is not possible. Infections are acquired by ingestion of the infective egg. The larvae hatch in the small intestine and mature in the large bowel but do not migrate through the tissues.

Clinical Findings

A. Symptoms and Signs: Light (fewer than 10,000 eggs per gram of feces) to moderate infections rarely cause symptoms. Heavy infections (30,000 or more eggs per gram of feces) may be accompanied by abdominal cramps, tenesmus, diarrhea, distention, flatulence, nausea, vomiting, and weight loss. Rectal prolapse and hematochezia or chronic occult blood loss may also occur, most often in malnourished young children. Sometimes, adult worms are seen in stools. Invasion of the appendix, with resulting appendicitis, is rare.

B. Laboratory Findings: Diagnosis is by identification of characteristic eggs and, sometimes, adult worms in stools. Eosinophilia (5–20%) is common with all but light infections. Severe iron deficiency anemia may be present with heavy infections.

Treatment

Patients with asymptomatic light infections do not require treatment. For those with heavier or symptomatic infections, give mebendazole, albendazole, or oxantel.

A. Mebendazole: The dosage is 100 mg twice daily before or after meals for 3 days. It may be therapeutically advantageous for the tablets to be chewed before swallowing. Cure rates of 60–80% and higher are reported after one course of treatment, with marked reduction in ova counts in the remaining patients. For severe trichuriasis, a longer course of treatment (up to 6 days) or a repeat course will often be necessary. Gastrointestinal side effects from the drug are rare. The drug is contraindicated in pregnancy, and experience with it is limited in children under age 2.

B. Albendazole: Albendazole, given orally at a single dose of 400 mg, has resulted in cure rates of 33–90%, with marked reduction in egg counts in those not cured. An appropriate dosage to achieve higher cure rates in moderate to heavy infections remains to be determined, but daily treatment for 2–3 days can be tried. Albendazole (not available in the USA) should not be used in pregnancy or in children under 2 years of age.

C. Oxantel Pamoate: Oxantel pamoate is an analogue of pyrantel pamoate and acts only on *T trichiura*. Cure rates of 57–100% have been reported in various trials. One treatment schedule is 15 mg/kg (base) daily for 2 days for patients with mild to moderate intensity of infection. For patients with severe infection, give 10 mg/kg (base) daily for 5 days. Oxantel is not available in the USA. Safety in pregnancy and young children is not established.

D. Thiabendazole: Thiabendazole should *not* be used, because it is not effective and is potentially toxic.

Bundy DA, Cooper ES: *Trichuris* and trichuriasis in humans. Adv Parasitol 1989;28:107.

Nokes C et al: Moderate to heavy infections of *Trichuris trichiura* affect cognitive function in Jamaican school children. Parasitology 1992;104:539.

VISCERAL LARVA MIGRANS (Toxocariasis)

Most cases of visceral larva migrans are due to *Toxocara canis,* an ascarid of dogs and other canids, but in a few cases *Toxocara cati* in domestic cats has been implicated and rarely *Belascaris procyonis* of raccoons. The adult worms live in the intestinal tracts of their respective hosts and release large numbers of eggs in the stool.

The reservoir mechanism for *T canis* is latent infections in female dogs which are reactivated during pregnancy. Transmission from mother to puppies is via the placenta and milk. Most eggs passed to the environment are from puppies (2 weeks to 6 months) and lactating bitches (up to 6 months after parturition). The life cycle of *T cati* is similar, but transplacental transmission does not occur.

Human infections are sporadic and probably occur worldwide. Infection is generally in dirt-eating young children who ingest *T canis* or *T cati* eggs from soil or sand contaminated with animal feces, most often from puppies. Direct contact with infected animals does not produce infection, as the eggs require a 3- to 4-week extrinsic incubation period to become infective; thereafter, eggs in soil remain infective for months to years.

In humans, hatched larvae are unable to mature and continue to migrate through the tissues for up to 6 months. Eventually they lodge in various organs, particularly the lungs and liver and less often the brain, eyes, and other tissues, where they produce eosinophilic granulomas up to 1 cm in diameter.

Clinical Findings

A. Acute Infection: Migrating larvae induce fever, cough, wheezing; hepatomegaly, and sometimes splenomegaly and lymphadenopathy are present. A variety of other findings may occur when other organs are invaded. The acute phase may last 2–3 weeks, but resolution of all physical and laboratory findings may take up to 18 months.

Leukocytosis is marked (may exceed 100,000/μL), with 30–80% due to eosinophils. Hyperglobulinemia occurs when the liver is extensively invaded and is a useful clue in diagnosis. An ELISA test is the most specific (92%) and sensitive (78%) serologic test and permits a presumptive diagnosis. Nonspecific isohemagglutinin titers (anti-A and anti-B) are usually greater than 1:1024. Chest radiographs may show infiltrates. With central nervous system involvement, the cerebrospinal fluid may show eosinophils. No parasitic forms can be found by stool examination.

Ultrasonography has been used to detect 1-cm hypoechoic lesions in the liver, each with a threadlike hyperechoic line. Specific diagnosis can only be made by liver biopsy or by direct biopsy of a granuloma at laparoscopy, but these procedures are seldom justified.

B. Ocular Toxocariasis: Most cases occur in children, most commonly 5–10 years old, who present with visual impairment in one eye. The principal pathologic entity is eosinophilic granuloma of the retina that resembles retinoblastoma. Until the recent development of the ELISA test, this resulted in the enucleation of many eyes. The most common clinical findings are a diffuse, painless endophthalmitis; posterior pole granuloma; and a peripheral inflammatory mass. Uncommonly seen are an iris nodule, optic nerve granuloma, uniocular pars planitis, and a migrating retinal nematode. Ocular toxocariasis is generally not associated with peripheral eosinophilia, hypergammaglobulinemia, or isohemagglutinin elevation. Serum ELISA tests may be positive, but a negative test does not rule out the diagnosis. If doubt exists about whether a patient with a positive serum ELISA test has retinoblastoma, examination of the vitreous humor for ELISA antibody and eosinophils can be helpful. High-resolution CT scanning of the orbit should be done.

Prevention, Treatment, & Prognosis

Disease in humans is best prevented by periodic treatment of puppies, kittens, and nursing dog and cat mothers, starting at 2 weeks postpartum, repeating at weekly intervals for 3 weeks and then every 6 months. Children should be supervised to prevent dirt-eating; their hands should be washed after playing in soil and sand; and play areas should be protected from animal feces.

A. Acute Infection: There is no specific treatment, but thiabendazole (as used in strongyloidiasis), mebendazole (200–400 mg in divided doses for 5 days), albendazole, or ivermectin should be tried. Corticosteroids, antibiotics, antihistamines, and analgesics may be needed to provide symptomatic relief. Symptoms may persist for months but generally clear within 1–2 years, and the ultimate prognosis is usually good.

B. Ocular Toxocariasis: Treatment includes corticosteroids (subconjunctival applications may be preferable to oral usage), vitrectomy for vitreous traction, laser photocoagulation, and an anthelmintic drug. Partial or total permanent visual impairment is rare.

Dinning WJ et al: Toxocariasis: A practical approach to management of ocular disease. Eye 1988;2:580.

Ishibashi H et al: Hepatic granuloma in toxocaral infection: Role of ultrasonography in hypereosinophilia. J Clin Ultrasound 1992;20:204.

Roig J et al: Acute eosinophilic pneumonia due to toxocariasis with bronchoalveolar lavage findings. Chest 1992;102:294.

Schantz PM: *Toxocara* larva migrans now. Am J Trop Med Hyg 1989;41:21

REFERENCES
(See also Chapter 34 references.)

Benenson AS (editor): *Control of Communicable Diseases in Man: An Official Report of the American Public Health Association,* 15th ed. The Association, 1990.

Cook GC. Anthelmintic agents: Some recent developments and their clinical application. Postgrad Med J 1991;67:16.

Goldsmith R, Heyneman D (editors): *Tropical Medicine and Parasitology.* Appleton & Lange, 1989.

Gutierrez Y: *Diagnostic Pathology of Parasitic Infections With Clinical Correlations.* Lea & Febiger, 1990.

MacLeod C: *Parasitic Infections in Pregnancy and the Newborn.* Oxford Medical, 1988.

Macpherson, CNL: Ultrasound in the diagnosis of parasitic disease. Tropical doctor 1992;22:14.

Maddison SE. Serodiagnosis of parasitic diseases. Clin Microbiol Rev 1991;4:457.

Reeder MM, Palmer PE (editors): *The Radiology of Tropical Disease With Epidemiological, Pathological, and Clinical Correlation.* Williams & Wilkins, 1980.

Rosenblatt JE. Antiparasitic agents. Mayo Clin Proc 1992;67:276.

WHO Model Prescribing Information: *Drugs Used in Parasitic Diseases.* WHO, 1990.

Infectious Diseases: Mycotic* **36**

Harry Hollander, MD

Fungal infections have assumed an increasingly important role as use of broad-spectrum antimicrobial agents has increased and the number of immunodeficient patients has risen. Some pathogens (eg, *Cryptococcus, Candida, Fusarium*) virtually never cause serious disease in normal hosts. Other endemic fungi (eg, *Histoplasma, Coccidioides, Paracoccidioides*) commonly cause disease in normal hosts but tend to be more aggressive in immunocompromised ones.

The major fungal diseases are discussed in this chapter.

CANDIDIASIS

Essentials of Diagnosis

- Common normal flora but opportunistic pathogen.
- Gastrointestinal mucosal disease, particularly esophagitis, most common, but catheter-associated fungemia frequent in hospitals.
- Diagnosis of invasive systemic disease requires tissue biopsy or evidence of retinal disease.

General Considerations

Candida albicans can be cultured from the mouth, vagina, and feces of most people. Cutaneous and oral lesions are discussed in Chapters 6 and 8, respectively. The risk factors for invasive candidiasis include prolonged neutropenia, diabetes mellitus, broad-spectrum antibiotic therapy, the presence of intravascular catheters (especially when providing total parenteral nutrition), and intravenous drug use. Cellular immunodeficiency predisposes to mucocutaneous disease. When no other underlying cause is found, persistent oral candidiasis should arouse a suspicion of HIV infection; over the course of their disease, AIDS patients will almost without exception have candidiasis as a complication.

Clinical Findings & Treatment

Esophageal involvement is the most frequent type of invasive mucosal disease. Individuals present with substernal odynophagia, gastroesophageal reflux, or

nausea without substernal pain. Oral candidiasis, though often associated, is not invariably present. Diagnosis is best confirmed by endoscopy with biopsy and culture, since radiographically the condition may be difficult to distinguish from esophagitis caused by infection with cytomegalovirus or herpes simplex virus. Therapy depends upon the severity of disease. If patients are able to swallow and take adequate amounts of fluid orally, ketoconazole, 200–400 mg/d, or fluconazole, 100–200 mg/d, will usually suffice. In the individual who is more ill, a 10- to 14-day course of amphotericin B at a dose of 0.3 mg/kg/d usually results in resolution.

Candidal funguria usually resolves with discontinuance of antibiotics or removal of bladder catheters. When funguria persists, oral fluconazole, 50 mg/d for 3 days, can be used if renal function is normal. If creatinine clearance is less than 10 mL/min, irrigation with 5 mg/d of amphotericin B may be necessary. Rare complications of candidal funguria are ureteral obstruction and dissemination.

Candidal fungemia may represent a benign, self-limited process, but until proved otherwise it should be considered a sign of serious disseminated disease. If fungemia resolves with removal of intravascular catheters, there are often no further complications. The incidence of endophthalmitis may be higher than previously recognized, and a short course of intravenous amphotericin B to a total dose of 200 mg appears to lower this incidence. Such an approach is strongly recommended for all immunocompromised patients with candidal fungemia.

If fungemia is documented repeatedly or if *Candida* is isolated from other sites, the patient is considered to have disseminated disease. Important clinical findings in disseminated candidiasis are fluffy white retinal infiltrates that extend into the vitreous and raised, erythematous skin lesions that may be painful. However, though characteristic, these are seen in less than 50% of cases. Other organ system involvement in disseminated disease may include the brain, meninges, and myocardium. Amphotericin B to a total dose of 1 g is the agent of choice. Flucytosine, 150 mg/kg/d orally in four divided doses, is added if central nervous system involvement occurs. Culture of skin lesions, when present, has a good diagnostic yield, even when blood cultures are negative. Unfor-

---

*Superficial mycoses are discussed in Chapter 6.

tunately, serologic tests for *Candida* have not proved helpful in differentiating transient fungemia from disseminated disease.

Candidal endocarditis rarely is a complication of transient fungemia. It usually results from direct inoculation at the time of open heart surgery or repeated inoculation with intravenous drug use. Splenomegaly and petechiae are common, and there is a predilection for large-vessel embolization. Non-albicans species such as *Candida parapsilosis* and *Candida tropicalis* are more often important etiologic agents than in fungemia, when *C albicans* is usual. Blood cultures are more often positive than in other types of endocarditis. The diagnosis is established definitively by culturing *Candida* from emboli or from large vegetations at the time of valve replacement. Valve destruction (usually aortic or mitral) is common, and surgical therapy is necessary in addition to a prolonged course of amphotericin therapy, usually to a total dose of 1–1.5 g intravenously. In addition, *Candida* endocarditis occurs with increased frequency on prosthetic valves in the first few months following surgery.

It is important to note that non-*albicans* species of *Candida* are often resistant to imidazole antibiotics such as fluconazole. The widespread use of these agents for prophylaxis in immunocompromised patients can lead to the emergence of pathogens such as *Candida krusei*. Dissemination of this organism has been reported in patients undergoing bone marrow transplantation for leukemia.

Another form of disseminated disease is hepatosplenic candidiasis. This results from aggressive chemotherapy and prolonged neutropenia in patients with underlying hematologic cancers. Patients typically present with fever and variable abdominal pain weeks after chemotherapy, when neutrophil counts have recovered. Blood cultures are generally negative. Liver function tests reveal an alkaline phosphatase elevation that may be marked. CT scanning of the abdomen shows hepatosplenomegaly, most often with multiple low-density defects in the liver. Diagnosis is established by liver biopsy and culture. Amphotericin B is given to a total dose of 1 g intravenously but often works poorly; fluconazole or liposomal amphotericin B may be better.

In all forms of invasive candidiasis, an important element of therapy is reversal of the underlying predisposing factor when possible.

Bross J et al: Risk factors for nosocomial candidemia: A case-control study in adults without leukemia. Am J Med 1989;87:614. (Role of antibiotics and central venous catheters.)

Wingard JR et al: Increase in *Candida krusei* infection among patients with bone marrow transplantation and neutropenia treated prophylactically with fluconazole. N Engl J Med 1991;325:1274.

HISTOPLASMOSIS

Essentials of Diagnosis

- Epidemiologically linked to bird droppings and bat exposure; common along river valleys.
- Most patients asymptomatic; respiratory illness most common clinical problem.
- Rare patients with normal immune function develop dissemination, with hepatosplenomegaly, lymphadenopathy, and oral ulcers.
- Widespread disease especially common in AIDS or other immunosuppressed states, with poor prognosis.
- Skin test and serology seldom diagnostic; biopsy of affected organs with culture, urinary capsular antigen most useful.

General Considerations

Histoplasmosis is caused by *Histoplasma capsulatum,* a mold that has been isolated from soil in endemic areas (central and eastern USA, eastern Canada, Mexico, Central America, South America, Africa, and southeast Asia). Infection presumably takes place by inhalation of spores. These convert into small budding cells that are engulfed by phagocytic cells in the lungs. The organism proliferates and is carried hematogenously to other organs.

Clinical Findings

A. Symptoms and Signs: Most cases of histoplasmosis are asymptomatic or mild and so are unrecognized. Past infection is recognized by the development of a positive histoplasmin skin test and occasionally by pulmonary and splenic calcification noted on x-rays taken to investigate unrelated problems. Signs and symptoms of pulmonary involvement are usually absent even in patients who subsequently show areas of calcification on chest x-ray. Symptomatic infection may present with mild influenza-like illness, often lasting 1–4 days. Moderately severe infections are frequently diagnosed as atypical pneumonia. These patients have fever, cough, and mild chest pain lasting 5–15 days. Physical examination is usually negative. Radiographic findings during acute illness are variable and nonspecific.

Clinically evident infections occur also in several other forms: (1) Acute histoplasmosis frequently occurs in epidemics. It is a severe disease manifested by marked prostration, fever, and relatively few pulmonary complaints even when x-rays show pneumonia. The illness may last from 1 week to 6 months but is almost never fatal. (2) Progressive disseminated histoplasmosis is usually fatal within 6 weeks or less. Symptoms usually consist of fever, dyspnea, cough, loss of weight, and prostration. Diarrhea is usually present in children. Ulcers of the mucous membranes of the oropharynx may be present. The liver and spleen are nearly always enlarged, and all the organs of the body are involved. (3) Chronic progressive histoplasmosis is usually seen in older patients with chronic obstructive lung disease and in mildly immunocompromised patients. The lungs show chronic progressive changes, often with cavities. Clinically, chronic histoplasmosis appears to be primarily confined to the lungs, though any organ may be involved in the terminal stage. (In each of these three, symptomatic illness directly follows exposure to the organism.) (4) In contrast, disseminated disease in the profoundly immunocompromised host often represents reactivation of prior infectious foci. This form is commonly seen in patients with underlying HIV infection and is characterized by fever and multiple organ system involvement. Chest x-rays may show a miliary pattern. Presentation may be fulminant, with death ensuing rapidly unless treatment is provided.

B. Laboratory Findings: In the moderately to severely ill patient, the sedimentation rate is elevated. Leukopenia may be present, with normal differential count or neutropenia. Most patients with progressive disease show anemia of chronic disease. Bone marrow involvement may be prominent in disseminated forms with occurrence of pancytopenia. Alkaline phosphatase elevation is also common.

In pulmonary disease, sputum culture is rarely positive except in chronic disease; in contrast, blood or bone marrow cultures from immunocompromised patients with acute disseminated disease are positive more than 80% of the time. An antigen assay has a sensitivity of greater than 90% for disseminated disease in AIDS patients and can be used to diagnose relapse. The sensitivity of screening immunodiffusion is 50% in acute pulmonary histoplasmosis, and complement fixation titers are positive in about 80% of cases. Combined results in immunodeficient patients approach 80%. Since skin test reactivity may persist for years following infection, it is generally not useful for establishing the diagnosis. Skin testing may also interfere with subsequent serologic diagnosis.

Treatment

For severe or progressive localized disease and for nonmeningeal disseminated disease in immunocompetent patients, itraconazole, 100–200 mg/d orally is the treatment of choice with an overall response rate of approximately 80%. Duration of therapy ranges from 2 weeks to several months depending upon the severity of illness. Amphotericin B is reserved for individuals who cannot take oral medications, failure of itraconazole therapy, meningitis, or disseminated disease in an immunocompromised host. Up to 2.5 g total may need to be given in the latter two situations. Patients with AIDS-related histoplasmosis require lifelong suppressive therapy with itraconazole, 100–200 mg/d orally.

Dismukes WE et al: Itraconazole therapy for blastomycosis and histoplasmosis. Am J Med 1992;93:489.
Sarosi GA, Johnson PC: Disseminated histoplasmosis in patients infected with human immunodeficiency virus. Clin Infect Dis 1992;14(Suppl 1):S60.
Wheat LJ: Histoplasmosis in Indianapolis. Clin Infect Dis 1992;15(Suppl 1):S91.

COCCIDIOIDOMYCOSIS

Essentials of Diagnosis

- Influenza-like illness with malaise, fever, backache, headache, and cough.
- Arthralgia and periarticular swelling of knees and ankles.
- Erythema nodosum common.
- Dissemination may result in meningitis, bony lesions, or skin findings.
- X-ray findings vary widely from pneumonitis to cavitation.
- Serologic tests useful; sporangia containing endospores demonstrable in sputum or tissues.

General Considerations

Coccidioidomycosis should be considered in the diagnosis of any obscure illness in a patient who has lived in or visited an endemic area.

Infection results from the inhalation of arthroconidia of *Coccidioides immitis,* a mold that grows in soil in certain arid regions of the southwestern USA, in Mexico, and in Central and South America.

About 60% of infections are subclinical and unrecognized other than by the subsequent development of a positive coccidioidin skin test. In the remaining cases, symptoms may be of severity warranting medical attention. Fewer than 1% of immunocompetent hosts show dissemination, but among these patients the mortality rate is high.

In HIV-infected people in endemic areas, coccidioidomycosis is now a common opportunistic infection.

Clinical Findings

A. Symptoms and Signs: Symptoms of primary coccidioidomycosis occur in about 40% of infections. The onset (after an incubation period of 10–30 days) is usually that of a respiratory tract illness with fever and occasionally chills. Pleuritic pain is common. Nasopharyngitis may be followed by bronchitis accompanied by a dry or slightly productive cough. A morbilliform rash may appear 1–2 days after the onset of symptoms.

Arthralgia accompanied by periarticular swellings, often of the knees and ankles, is common. Erythema nodosum may appear 2–20 days after onset of symptoms. Erythema multiforme may also occur rarely. Persistent pulmonary lesions, varying from cavities and abscesses to parenchymal nodular densities or bronchiectasis, occur in about 5% of diagnosed cases.

About 0.1% of white and 1% of nonwhite patients are unable to localize or control infection caused by *C immitis*. Filipinos are especially susceptible, as are pregnant women. Symptoms in progressive coccidioidomycosis depend upon the site of dissemination. Any organ may be involved. Pulmonary findings usually become more pronounced, with mediastinal lymph node enlargement, cough, and increased sputum production. Lung abscesses may rupture into the pleural space, producing an empyema. Extension to bones and skin may take place, and pericardial and myocardial extension has been occasionally observed. Dissemination may be associated with fungemia, characterized clinically by a diffuse miliary pattern on chest x-ray and by early death. The course may be particularly rapid in immunosuppressed patients. HIV-infected persons with disseminated disease have a higher incidence of miliary infiltrates, inguinal adenopathy, and meningitis, but skin lesions are uncommon.

Bone lesions most often occur at bony prominences. Meningitis occurs in 30–50% of cases of dissemination. Subcutaneous abscesses and verrucous skin lesions are especially common in fulminating cases. Lymphadenitis may occur and may progress to suppuration. Mediastinal and retroperitoneal abscesses are not uncommon.

B. Laboratory Findings: In primary coccidioidomycosis, there may be moderate leukocytosis and eosinophilia and an elevated sedimentation rate. A persisting elevated or increasing sedimentation rate is a sign of progressive disease. The coccidioidin skin test becomes positive early after localized infection and may remain positive for years; however, it is typically negative with disseminated disease. Serologic testing is useful for both diagnosis and prognosis. The immunodiffusion test (CIE) and the tube precipitin test are useful for screening, and IgG and IgM by immunodiffusion are also adequate for diagnosis. Historically, a persistent risking complement fixation titer (≥ 1:16) has been considered suggestive of disseminated disease. Serum complement fixation titer may be low when there is meningitis but no other disseminated disease. A false-negative rate up to 30% is seen in patients with HIV-related coccidioidomycosis. Demonstrable antibodies in spinal fluid are diagnostic of coccidioidal meningitis. These are found in over 90% of cases. Spinal fluid findings include increased cell count with lymphocytosis and reduced glucose. Sporangia filled with endospores may be found in biopsy specimens; though they are not infectious, they convert to the highly contagious arthroconidia when grown in culture media. Exoantigen testing is in widespread use and substantially reduces the risk to laboratory personnel. Blood cultures in appropriate media are only uncommonly positive in disseminated disease. Spinal fluid culture is positive in approximately 30% of meningitis cases.

C. Imaging: Radiographic findings vary, but patchy, nodular pulmonary infiltrates and thin-walled cavities are most common. Hilar lymphadenopathy may be visible and is seen in localized disease; mediastinal lymphadenopathy suggests dissemination. There may be pleural effusions and lytic lesions in bone.

Treatment

General symptomatic therapy is given as needed for disease limited to the chest with no evidence of progression. For progressive pulmonary or extrapulmonary disease, amphotericin B intravenously has proved effective in some patients (see Chapter 37). Therapy should be continued to a total dose of 2.5–3 g. For meningitis, systemic maintenance amphotericin B may be required for the lifetime of the individual as guided by symptoms and spinal fluid complement fixation titers. Intrathecal amphotericin B, 1–5 mg, is generally given weekly until the disease has been controlled and monthly for at least several years thereafter.

Preliminary results with fluconazole suggest that it may be possible to treat approximately half of selected patients with mild coccidioidal meningitis with oral fluconazole. Such therapy is not yet standard care, however.

Oral ketoconazole, 200–800 mg daily 1–2 hours before breakfast, is an alternative for disease limited to the chest; however, therapy must be continued for 6 months or longer in order to prevent relapse. Itraconazole also has potent activity against this organism; preliminary results are promising for nonmeningeal disease.

Thoracic surgery is occasionally indicated for giant, infected, or ruptured cavities. Surgical drainage is also useful for subcutaneous abscesses. Amphotericin B is advisable following extensive surgical manipulation of infected tissue.

Prognosis

The prognosis in the case of limited disease is good, but persistent pulmonary cavities may cause complications. Nodules, cavities, and fibrotic residuals may rarely progress after long periods of stability or regression. Disseminated and meningeal forms still have significant mortality rates.

Catanzaro A, Fierer J, Friedman PJ: Fluconazole in the treatment of persistent coccidioidomycosis. Chest 1990; 97:666.

Galgiani JN: Coccidioidomycosis: Changes in clinical expression, serologic diagnosis, and therapeutic options. Clin Infect Dis 1992;14(Suppl 1):S100.

Graybill JR et al: NIAID mycoses study group: Itraconazole treatment of coccidioidomycosis. Am J Med 1990; 89:282.

CRYPTOCOCCOSIS

Essentials of Diagnosis

- Most common cause of fungal meningitis.
- Predisposing factors: Hodgkin's disease, corticosteroids, HIV infection.
- Symptoms of headache, abnormal mental states; meningismus seen occasionally, though rarely in HIV-infected patients.
- Demonstration of capsular antigen diagnostic; 95% of HIV-infected patients also show it in serum.

General Considerations

Cryptococcosis is caused by *Cryptococcus neoformans,* an encapsulated budding yeast that has been found worldwide in soil and on dried pigeon dung.

Infections are acquired by inhalation. In the lung, the infection may remain localized, heal, or disseminate. Immunocompetent hosts rarely develop clinically apparent cryptococcal pneumonia. Progressive lung disease and dissemination most often occur in the setting of cellular immunodeficiency, including underlying hematologic cancer under treatment, Hodgkin's disease, long-term corticosteroid therapy, or HIV infection.

Clinical Findings

A. Symptoms and Signs: Disseminated disease may involve any organ, but central nervous system disease usually predominates. Headache is usually the first symptom of meningitis. Confusion and other mental status changes as well as cranial nerve abnormalities may be seen as the disease progresses. Nuchal rigidity and meningeal signs occur about 50% of the time but are uncommon in HIV-infected patients with this complication. Intracerebral mass lesions (cryptococcomas) are rarely seen. Obstructive hydrocephalus may complicate the course.

B. Laboratory Findings: Abnormalities of the central nervous system are common but more often reflect the predisposing conditions. Spinal fluid findings include increased pressure, variable pleocytosis, budding encapsulated fungus cells, increased protein, and decreased glucose. Cryptococcal antigen in cerebrospinal fluid and culture establish the diagnosis 90% of the time, though as many as 50% of AIDS patients have no pleocytosis. These patients often have the antigen in both cerebrospinal fluid and serum, and extrameningeal disease is common.

Treatment

There has been a trend away from amphotericin B-based regimens, particularly in HIV-infected patients. However, this agent remains important, especially in severe disease. A combination of amphotericin B (0.3 mg/kg/d administered as for coccidioidomycosis) and flucytosine, 150 mg/kg/d orally or intravenously divided into four equal doses and given every 6 hours, is as effective as higher doses of amphotericin B alone and may cause less toxicity. However, flucytosine may not be tolerated, particularly in AIDS patients, because of diarrhea and leukopenia. Ventricular shunting may be important if hydrocephalus is a complication. In non-HIV-related cryptococcal meningitis, amphotericin B therapy is usually continued to a total dose of 1.5–2 g. Therapy is generally continued if cerebrospinal fluid cultures remain positive or cerebrospinal fluid antigen titers remain greater than 1:8. In AIDS patients, it may be very difficult to achieve such a low cerebrospinal fluid titer. Thus, the end points for amphotericin B therapy are clinical response and culture negativity of the cerebrospinal fluid.

In AIDS-related cryptococcal meningitis, oral fluconazole, 400 mg/d, has efficacy comparable to that of amphotericin B. The best candidates for initial fluconazole therapy are patients with an intact level of consciousness and a spinal fluid antigen titer of less than 1:128. Higher risk patients should receive amphotericin B initially, but it may be possible to shorten the course and change to fluconazole once they are clinically stable.

A preliminary study suggests that fluconazole plus flucytosine is efficacious for mild cases, but this regimen has not been compared with fluconazole alone.

Maintenance antifungal therapy is important after treatment of an acute episode in HIV-related cases, since otherwise the rate of relapse is greater than 50%. Fluconazole, 200 mg/d, is the maintenance therapy of choice, decreasing the relapse rate approximately tenfold compared with placebo and threefold compared with weekly amphotericin B.

Prognosis

Factors that indicate a poor prognosis include the activity of the predisposing conditions, lack of spinal fluid pleocytosis, high initial antigen titer in either serum or cerebrospinal fluid, and the presence of disease outside the nervous system. In AIDS-related cryptococcal meningitis, decreased mental status, hyponatremia, and age less than 35 years also portend a poorer outcome.

Bozzette SA et al: A placebo-controlled trial of maintenance therapy with fluconazole after treatment of cryptococcal meningitis in the acquired immunodeficiency syndrome. N Engl J Med 1991;324:580.

Powderly WG et al: A controlled trial of fluconazole or amphotericin B to prevent relapse of cryptococcal meningitis in patients with the acquired immunodeficiency syndrome. N Engl J Med 1992;326:793.

Saag MS et al: Comparison of amphotericin B with fluconazole in the treatment of acute AIDS-associated cryptococcal meningitis. N Engl J Med 1992;326:83.

ASPERGILLOSIS

Aspergillus fumigatus is the usual cause of aspergillosis, though many species may cause a wide spectrum of disease. Burn eschar and detritus in the external ear canal are often colonized by these fungi. Clinical illness results either from an aberrant immunologic response or tissue invasion.

Allergic bronchopulmonary aspergillosis leads to wheezing and transient pulmonary infiltrates. This diagnosis should be considered when patients with a history of asthma develop worsening bronchospasm and fleeting infiltrates accompanied by eosinophilia, high levels of IgE, and *Aspergillus* precipitins in the blood. It also may complicate cystic fibrosis. The disease characteristically has a waxing and waning course with gradual improvement over time. For acute exacerbations, oral prednisone is begun at a dose of 1 mg/kg/d and then tapered slowly over several months. Antifungal agents do not have a role in the management of allergic aspergillosis, since clinical symptoms appear to be due to an immunologic reaction to the fungus and not related to tissue invasion.

Invasive manifestations may be seen in immunocompetent adults. These include chronic sinusitis and colonization of preexisting pulmonary cavities (aspergilloma). Sinus disease may require long courses of antibiotics as well as surgical debridement. Aspergillomas of the lung may be found by incidental radiographic studies but may also present with significant hemoptysis. Intracavitary instillation of amphotericin B and bronchoscopic removal have been tried with little success; but the most effective therapy for symptomatic aspergilloma remains surgical resection.

Life-threatening invasive disease most commonly occurs in profoundly immunodeficient patients, particularly those with prolonged severe neutropenia. It has been recently recognized that patients with advanced HIV disease may also be at risk for invasive aspergillosis, particularly if they have other risk factors for the disease.

Pulmonary disease is most common, with patchy infiltration leading to a severe necrotizing pneumonia. There is often tissue infarction as the organism grows into blood vessels; clues to this are the development of pleuritic chest pain and elevation of serum LDH. At any time, there may be hematogenous dissemination to the central nervous system, skin, and other organs. Early diagnosis and reversal of any correctable immunosuppression are essential. Blood cultures have very low yield. In contrast to allergic aspergillosis, serologic tests and antigen detection have low sensitivities for invasive disease. Isolation of *Aspergillus* from pulmonary secretions does not necessarily imply invasive disease. Therefore, the mainstay of diagnosis is demonstration of *Aspergillus* in tissue. Histologically, one sees branched septate hyphae. Biopsy specimens will not invariably grow the organism.

When severe invasive aspergillosis is considered clinically likely or is demonstrable by biopsy, rapid institution of high doses of amphotericin B may be life-saving (see Chapter 37). The total daily dose is rapidly increased to 0.8–1 mg/kg/d intravenously as tolerated for the first several weeks of therapy. Thereafter, more traditional doses of 0.6 mg/kg/d are continued until a total dose of at least 2 g has been reached. The addition of flucytosine is of unclear benefit. Itraconazole has activity against *Aspergillus*, and initial clinical experience is favorable. Until more data accumulate, amphotericin B should remain the first-line drug for invasive disease. The mortality rate of pulmonary or disseminated disease in the immunocompromised patient remains well above 50%, however.

Denning DA et al: Pulmonary aspergillosis in the acquired immunodeficiency syndrome. N Engl J Med 1991;324; 654. (Thirteen patients with late HIV disease. Most had invasive disease, but three had a novel bronchial obstructive form.)

Denning DW et al: Treatment of invasive aspergillosis with itraconazole. Am J Med 1989;86:791. (Excellent responses in 12 of 20 patients.)

MUCORMYCOSIS

The term "mucormycosis" (zygomycosis, phycomycosis) is applied to opportunistic infections caused by members of the genera *Rhizopus, Mucor, Absidia,* and *Cunninghamella.* Predisposing conditions include diabetic ketoacidosis, chronic renal failure, and treatment with steroids or cytotoxic drugs. These organisms appear in tissues as broad, branching nonseptate hyphae. Biopsy is almost always required for diagnosis. Invasive disease of the sinuses, orbits, and the lungs may be noted. Widely disseminated disease has been more commonly seen recently in patients who have received aggressive chemotherapy. The diagnosis should be considered in acidotic diabetic patients with black necrotic lesions of the nose or sinuses or with new cranial nerve abnormalities. Without treatment, meningeal invasion may ensue. High-dosage amphotericin B therapy initiated early, control of diabetes or other underlying conditions, and extensive surgical removal of necrotic, nonperfused tissue are essential. Even when these measures are introduced in a time fashion, the prognosis is poor, with a 30–50% mortality rate for localized disease and higher rates in disseminated cases.

Ingram CW et al: Disseminated zygomycosis: Report of four cases and review. Rev Infect Dis 1989;2:741. (Must be considered in immunocompromised patients. Prognosis very poor.)

BLASTOMYCOSIS

Blastomycosis occurs more often in men and in a geographically delimited area of the south central and midwestern USA and Canada. A few cases have been found in Mexico and Africa.

Pulmonary infection may be asymptomatic. When dissemination takes place, lesions are most frequently seen on the skin, in bones, and in the urogenital system.

Cough, moderate fever, dyspnea, and chest pain are evident in symptomatic patients. These may resolve or progress, with bloody and purulent sputum production, pleurisy, fever, chills, loss of weight, and prostration. Radiologic studies usually reveal infiltrates and enlarged regional lymph nodes, though less commonly than in histoplasmosis or coccidioidomycosis. Raised, verrucous cutaneous lesions that have an abrupt downward sloping border are usually present in disseminated blastomycosis. The border extends slowly, leaving a central atrophic scar. These lesions persist untreated for long periods, mimicking skin cancer. Bones—often the ribs and vertebrae—are frequently involved. Lesions appear to be both destructive and proliferative on radiography. Epididymitis, prostatitis, and other involvement of the male urogenital system may occur. Central nervous system involvement is uncommon. Cases in HIV-infected persons may progress rapidly, with dissemination common.

Laboratory findings usually include leukocytosis, anemia, and elevated sedimentation rate, though these are not specific. The organism is found in clinical specimens as a thick-walled cell 5–20 mm in diameter that may have a single bud. It grows readily on culture. Serologic tests are not well standardized.

Itraconazole, 100-200 mg/d orally, is now the therapy of choice for nonmeningeal disease, with a response rate of over 70%. Amphotericin B is given for treatment failures or cases with central nervous system involvement.

Follow-up for relapse should be regularly made for several years so that therapy may be resumed or another drug instituted.

Bradshur RW: Systemic fungal infections: Diagnosis and treatment: 1. Blastomycosis. Rev Infect Dis 1989;2:741.
Pappas PG et al: Itraconazole therapy for blastomycosis and histoplasmosis. Am J Med 1992;93:489.

PARACOCCIDIOIDOMYCOSIS
(South American Blastomycosis)

Paracoccidioides brasiliensis infections have been found only in patients who have resided in South or Central America or Mexico. Long asymptomatic periods enable patients to travel far from the endemic areas before developing clinical problems. Ulceration of the naso- and oropharynx is usually the first symptom. Papules ulcerate and enlarge both peripherally and deeper into the subcutaneous tissue. Differential diagnosis includes mucocutaneous leishmaniasis and syphilis. Extensive coalescent ulcerations may eventually result in destruction of the epiglottis, vocal cords, and uvula. Extension to the lips and face may occur. Eating and drinking are extremely painful. Skin lesions may occur, usually on the face. Variable in appearance, they may have a necrotic central crater with a hard hyperkeratotic border. Lymph node enlargement may follow mucocutaneous lesions, eventually ulcerating and forming draining sinuses; in some patients, it is the presenting symptom. Hepatosplenomegaly may be present as well. Cough, sometimes with sputum, indicates pulmonary involvement, but the signs and symptoms are often mild, even though radiographic findings indicate severe parenchymatous changes in the lungs. The extensive ulceration of the upper gastrointestinal tract may prevent caloric intake and result in cachexia.

Laboratory findings are nonspecific. Serology by immunodiffusion is positive in 98% of cases. Complement fixation titers correlate with progressive disease and fall with effective therapy. The fungus is found in clinical specimens as a spherical cell that may have many buds arising from it. If direct examination does not reveal the organism, biopsy with Gomori staining may be helpful.

Oral ketoconazole, 200–400 mg daily 1–2 hours before breakfast, generally results in a clinical response within 1 month and effective control after 6 months. The rare relapse responds to resumed ketoconazole therapy. Itraconazole, 100 mg orally daily, also is effective. Finally, fluconazole, 200–400 mg daily, resulted in a response rate of better than 90% and may ultimately be the drug of choice.

Diaz M et al: A pan-American 5-year study of fluconazole therapy for deep mycoses in the immunocompetent host. Clin Infect Dis 1992;14(Suppl 1):S23.

SPOROTRICHOSIS

Sporotrichosis is a chronic fungal infection caused by *Sporothrix schenckii*. It is worldwide in distribution; most patients have had contact with soil, plants, or decaying wood. Infection takes place when the organism is inoculated into the skin—usually on the hand, arm, or foot.

The most common form of sporotrichosis begins with a hard, nontender subcutaneous nodule. This later becomes adherent to the overlying skin and ulcerates. Within a few days to weeks, similar nodules usually develop along the lymphatics draining this area, and these may ulcerate as well. The lymphatic vessels become indurated and are easily palpable.

Blood-borne dissemination is rare, and the general health of the patient is not affected.

Disseminated sporotrichosis is rare in the immunocompetent host but may present with lung, bone, joint, and central nervous system involvement in immunocompromised patients.

Cultures are needed to establish diagnosis. Antigen tests may be useful for diagnosis of disseminated disease.

Potassium iodide taken orally in increasing dosage has been the treatment of choice for cutaneous disease. It is administered as the saturated solution, 5 drops three times a day after meals, increasing by 1 drop per dose until 40 drops three times a day are being given. It is continued until signs of the active disease have disappeared. The dosage is then decreased by 1 drop per dose until 5 drops are being given, and then is discontinued. Care must be taken to reduce the dosage if signs of iodism appear; either hypothyroidism or hyperthyroidism may result when pharmacologic doses of iodine are given.Amphotericin B intravenously, 1.5–2 g (see Chapter 37), is tried in systemic infection, but its role is uncertain. As experience with itraconazole for this infection has increased, it seems likely that this drug will become the agent of choice for localized disease and some cases of disseminated disease.

Surgery is usually contraindicated except for simple aspiration of secondary nodules.

The prognosis is good for all forms of sporotrichosis except the disseminated type.

Calhoun DL et al: Treatment of systemic sporotrichosis with ketoconazole. Rev Inf Dis 1991;13:47.

CHROMOMYCOSIS

Chromomycosis is a chronic, principally tropical cutaneous infection caused by several species of closely related black molds (*Fonsecaea* sp and *Phialophora* sp).

Lesions are slowly progressive and occur most frequently on a lower extremity. The lesion begins as a papule or ulcer. Over months to years, papules enlarge to become vegetating, papillomatous, verrucous elevated nodules. Satellite lesions may appear along the lymphatics. There may be secondary bacterial infection. Elephantiasis may result.

The fungus is seen as brown, thick-walled, spherical, sometimes septate cells in pus. The type of reproduction found in culture determines the species.

Surgical excision is the treatment of choice for early lesions. Medical therapy is generally disappointing, but flucytosine, 150 mg/kg/d, alone or in combination with ketoconazole, 200–400 mg orally, has been successful in some cases. Itraconazole, 100–400 mg/d orally, has also resulted in some clinical responses.

MYCETOMA
(Maduromycosis & Actinomycetoma)

Maduromycosis is the term used to describe mycetoma caused by the true fungi. Actinomycotic mycetoma is caused by *Nocardia* and *Actinomadura* spp. The disease begins as a papule, nodule, or abscess that over months to years progresses slowly to form multiple abscesses and sinus tracts ramifying deep into the tissue. Secondary bacterial infection may result in large open ulcers. Radiographs may show destructive changes in the underlying bone. The agents occur as white, yellow, red, or black granules in tissue or pus. Microscopic examination assists in the diagnosis.

The prognosis is good for patients with actinomycetoma, since they usually respond well to sulfonamides and sulfones, especially if treated early. Trimethoprim-sulfamethoxazole, 160/800 mg orally twice a day, or dapsone, 100 mg twice daily after meals, has also been reported to be effective. Streptomycin, 14 mg/kg/d intramuscularly, may be useful during the first month of therapy. All other medications must be taken for months and continued for several months after clinical cure to prevent relapse. Debridement assists healing.

The prognosis for maduromycosis is poor. Early trials indicate that itraconazole may be useful. Surgical excision of early lesions may prevent spread. Amputation is necessary in far-advanced cases.

MYCOTIC KERATITIS

Candida albicans, Fusarium, and *Aspergillus* are most often responsible for mycotic keratitis. Trauma to the cornea followed by corticosteroid and antibiotic therapy is often a predisposing factor. Prompt withdrawal of corticosteroids, removal of the infected necrotic tissue, and application of natamycin or ketoconazole are useful in management. Amphotericin B and flucytosine are used for fungal endophthalmitis.

OTHER OPPORTUNISTIC
MOLD INFECTIONS

Fungi previously considered to be harmless colonizers are emerging as significant pathogens in immunocompromised patients. This occurs most often in patients being treated for hematopoietic malignancies. Infection may be localized in the skin, lungs, or sinuses, or widespread disease may appear with lesions in multiple organs. Colonization of old cavitary disease may cause minimal symptoms or may precede dissemination with meningitis or brain abscesses. Endocarditis occurs more commonly in intravenous drug abusers. Sinus infection may cause

Table 36–1. Agents for systemic mycoses.

Drug	Dosing	Renal Clearance?	CSF Penetration?	Toxicities	Spectrum of Activity
Amphotericin B	0.3–1 mg/kg/d IV[1]	No	Poor	Rigors, fever, azotemia, hypokalemia, renal tubular acidosis, anemia	All major pathogens except *Pseudallescheria*
Flucytosine (5-FC)	150 mg/kg/d orally in 4 divided doses	Yes	Yes	Leukopenia,[2] rash, diarrhea, hepatitis	Cryptococcosis,[3] candidiasis,[3] chromomycosis
Ketoconazole	200–800 mg/d orally in 1 or 2 doses	No	Poor	Anorexia, nausea, suppression of testosterone and cortisol, rash, hepatitis	Nonmeningeal histoplasmosis and coccidioidomycosis, blastomycosis, paracoccidioidomycosis, mucosal candidiasis (except urinary)
Fluconazole	100–400 mg/d as single dose IV or orally	Yes	Yes	Nausea	Mucosal candidiasis (including urinary tract), cryptococcosis, histoplasmosis, perhaps coccidioidomycosis
Itraconazole	100–400 mg/d orally as single dose	No	Variable	Nausea	Same as ketoconazole plus sporotrichosis, aspergillosis, chromomycosis

[1]Trials of higher doses encapsulated in liposomes are in progress.
[2]Use should be monitored with blood levels to prevent this.
[3]In combination with amphotericin B.

bony erosion. Infection in subcutaneous tissues following traumatic implantation may develop as a well-circumscribed cyst or as an ulcer.

Nonpigmented septate hyphae are seen in tissue and are indistinguishable from those of *Aspergillus* when infections are due to *Pseudallescheria boydii* or species of *Fusarium, Paecilomyces, Penicillium,* or other hyaline molds. Spores or mycetoma-like granules are rarely present in tissue.

Infection by any of a number of black molds is designated as phaeohyphomycosis. These black molds are common in the environment, especially on decaying vegetation, and do not cause infection in the normal host, although some black molds, as well as some hyaline molds, are allergens. In tissues of patients with phaeohyphomycosis, the mold is seen as black or faintly brown hyphae, yeast cells, or both. Culture on appropriate medium is needed to identify the agent. Histologic demonstration of these organisms is definitive evidence of invasive infection; positive cultures must be interpreted cautiously and not assumed to be contaminants in immunocompromised hosts.

Some isolates are sensitive to antifungal antibiotics. The differentiation of *Pseudallescheria boydii* and *Aspergillus* is particularly important, since the former is uniformly resistant to amphotericin B but may be sensitive to imidazole antibiotics.

Anaissie E et al: New spectrum of fungal infections in patients with cancer. Rev Infect Dis 1989;11:369.

ANTIFUNGAL THERAPY

With recent advances in drug development, the field of antifungal chemotherapy is changing rapidly. In addition to the newer imidazoles, novel classes of agents are beginning to undergo clinical trials. Table 36–1 summarizes the major properties of currently available antifungal agents.

Antifungal drugs are discussed in Chapter 37.

REFERENCES

Bodey GP: Azole antifungal agents. Clin Infect Dis 1992; 14(Suppl 1):S161.
Kaufman L: Laboratory methods for the diagnosis and confirmation of systemic mycoses. Clin Infect Dis 1992; 14(Suppl 1):S23.

Myer RD: Current role of therapy with amphotericin B. Clin Infect Dis 1992;14(Suppl 1):S154.

37

Anti-infective Chemotherapeutic & Antibiotic Agents

Richard A. Jacobs, MD, PhD

Some Rules for Antimicrobial Therapy

Antimicrobial drugs are used on a very large scale, and their proper use gives striking therapeutic results. On the other hand, they can create serious untoward reactions and should therefore be administered only upon proper indication.

Drugs of first choice and alternative drugs are presented in Table 37–1.

The following steps are required in each patient considered for antibiotic therapy.

A. Etiologic Diagnosis: Formulate an etiologic diagnosis based on clinical observations. Microbial infections are best treated early. The physician must decide on clinical grounds (1) whether the patient has a microbial infection that can be favorably influenced by antimicrobial drugs and (2) the kind of pathogen most probably causing such infection ("best guess").

B. "Best Guess": (Tables 37–2 and 37–3.) Select a specific antimicrobial drug on the basis of past experience for empiric therapy. Based on a "best guess," the physician should choose a drug or combination of drugs that is likely to be effective against the suspected pathogens.

C. Laboratory Control: In most cases, specimens for laboratory examination are obtained before antimicrobial therapy is started to determine the causative infectious organism and, if desirable, susceptibility to antimicrobial drugs.

D. Clinical Response: Based on the clinical response of the patient, evaluate the laboratory reports and consider the desirability of changing the antimicrobial drug regimen. Laboratory results should not overrule clinical judgment. Isolation of an organism that confirms the initial clinical impression is useful. Conversely, laboratory results may contradict the initial clinical impression and compel its reconsideration. If the specimen was obtained from a site that is normally devoid of bacterial flora and not exposed to the external environment (eg, blood, cerebrospinal fluid, pleural fluid, joint fluid), the recovery of a microorganism is a significant finding even if the organism recovered is different from the clinically suspected etiologic agent, and this may force a change in treatment. On the other hand, isolation of unexpected microorganisms from the respiratory tract, gut, or surface lesions (sites that have a complex flora) must be critically evaluated before drugs are abandoned that were judiciously selected on the basis of an initial "best guess" for empiric treatment.

E. Drug Susceptibility Tests: Some microorganisms are fairly uniformly susceptible to certain drugs; if such organisms are isolated from the patient, they need not be tested for drug susceptibility. For example, group A hemolytic streptococci and most pneumococci and clostridia respond predictably well to penicillin. On the other hand, some organisms (eg, enteric gram-negative rods) are variably susceptible to antimicrobial agents and require drug susceptibility testing whenever they are isolated from a significant specimen.

Antimicrobial drug susceptibility tests may be done on solid media as "disk tests," in broth in tubes, or in wells of microdilution plates. The latter method yields results expressed as MIC (minimal inhibitory concentration), and the technique can be modified to give MBC (minimal bactericidal concentration) results. In some infections, the MIC or MBC permits a better estimate of the amount of drug required for therapeutic effect in vivo.

Disk tests usually indicate whether an isolate is susceptible or resistant to serum concentrations of drug achieved in vivo with conventional dosage regimens, thus providing valuable guidance in selecting therapy. When there appear to be marked discrepancies between test results and clinical response of the patient, the following possibilities must be considered:

1. Selection of an inappropriate drug, dosage, or route of administration.

2. Failure to drain a collection of pus or to remove a foreign body.

3. Failure of a poorly diffusing drug to reach the site of infection (eg, central nervous system) or to reach intracellular phagocytosed bacteria.

4. Superinfection in the course of prolonged chemotherapy. After suppression of the original infection or of normal flora, a second type of microorganism may establish itself against which the originally selected drug is ineffective.

Table 37–1. Drugs of choice for suspected or proved microbial pathogens, 1994. (± = alone or combined with)

Suspected or Proved Etiologic Agent	Drug(s) of First Choice	Alternative Drug(s)
Gram-negative cocci		
Moraxella catarrhalis	TMP-SMZ[1]	Newer cephalosporins,[2] erythromycin,[3] tetracycline,[4] azithromycin, amoxicillin-clavulanic acid
Niesseria gonorrhoeae (gonococcus)	Ceftriaxone	Cefixime, ciprofloxacin, spectinomycin, ofloxacin, cefpodoxime proxetil
Neisseria meningitidis	Penicillin[5]	Newer cephalosporins,[2] ampicillin, chloramphenicol
Gram-positive cocci		
Pneumococcus *(Streptococcus pneumoniae)*	Penicillin[5]	Erythromycin,[3] cephalosporin,[6] vancomycin
Streptococcus, hemolytic, groups A, B, C, G	Penicillin[5]	Erythromycin,[3] cephalosporin,[6] vancomycin, clindamycin, azithromycin, clarithromycin
Streptococcus viridans	Penicillin[5] ± aminoglycosides[7]	Cephalosporin,[6] vancomycin
Staphylococcus, methicillin-resistant	Vancomycin ± gentamicin or rifampin (or both)	TMP-SMZ
Staphylococcus, non-penicillinase-producing	Penicillin	Cephalosporin,[6] vancomycin
Staphylococcus, penicillinase-producing	Penicillinase-resistant penicillin[8]	Vancomycin, cephalosporin,[6] clindamycin, amoxicillin-clavulanic acid, ticarcillin-clavulanic acid, ampicillin-sulbactam
Streptococcus faecalis (enterococcus)	Ampicillin + gentamicin	Vancomycin + gentamicin
Gram-negative rods		
Acinetobacter	Imipenem	Minocycline, TMP-SMZ,[1] doxycycline, aminoglycosides,[7] pipericillin
Bacteroides, oropharyngeal strains	Penicillin,[5] clindamycin	Metronidazole, cefoxitin, cefotetan
Bacteroides, gastrointestinal strains	Metronidazole	Cefoxitin, chloramphenicol, clindamycin, cefotetan, cefmetazole, imipenem, ticarcillin-clavulanic acid, ampicillin-sulbactam
Brucella	Tetracycline[4] + gentamicin	TMP-SMZ[1]
Campylobacter	Erythromycin[3]	Tetracycline,[4] ciprofloxacin, ofloxacin,
Enterobacter	TMP-SMZ,[1] imipenem	Newer cephalosporins,[2] aminoglycoside,[7] ciprofloxacin, ofloxacin
Escherichia coli (sepsis)	Newer cephalosporins[2]	Ampicillin, TMP-SMZ,[1] ciprofloxacin, imipenem, aminoglycosides
Escherichia coli (first urinary infection)	Sulfonamide,[9] TMP-SMZ[1]	Ampicillin, cephalosporin,[6] ciprofloxacin, ofloxacin
Haemophilus (meningitis, respiratory infections)	Newer cephalosporins[2]	Ampicillin and chloramphenicol[1]
Klebsiella	Newer cephalosporins[2]	TMP-SMZ,[1] aminoglycoside,[7] imipenem, ciprofloxacin, ofloxacin
Legionella sp (pneumonia)	Erythromycin[3] + rifampin	TMP-SMZ,[1] clarithromycin, azithromycin, ciprofloxacin
Pasteurella (Yersinia) (plague, tularemia)	Streptomycin	Chloramphenicol, a tetracycline,[4] gentamicin
Proteus mirabilis	Ampicillin	Newer cephalosporins,[2] aminoglycoside,[7] TMP-SMZ,[1] ciprofloxacin, ofloxacin
Proteus vulgaris and other species	Newer cephalosporins[2]	Aminoglycoside,[7] imipenem, TMP-SMZ, ciprofloxacin, ofloxacin
Pseudomonas aeruginosa	Aminoglycoside[7] + antipseudomonal penicillin[10]	Ceftazidime ± aminoglycoside; imipenem ± aminoglycoside; aztreonam ± aminoglycoside; ciprofloxacin
Pseudomonas pseudomallei (melioidosis)	Ceftazidime	Chloramphenicol, tetracycline,[4] TMP-SMZ,[1] amoxicillin-clavulanic acid
Pseudomonas mallei (glanders)	Streptomycin + tetracycline[4]	Chloramphenicol + streptomycin
Salmonella	Ceftriaxone	TMP-SMZ,[1] ciprofloxacin, ampicillin, ofloxacin, chloramphenicol
Serratia, Providencia	Newer cephalosporins,[2] ciprofloxacin ofloxacin	TMP-SMZ,[1] aminoglycosides,[7] ciprofloxacin, ofloxacin
Shigella	Ciprofloxacin, ofloxacin	Ampicillin, TMP-SMZ,[1]
Vibrio (cholera, sepsis)	Tetracycline[4]	TMP-SMZ,[1] ciprofloxacin
Gram-positive rods		
Actinomyces	Penicillin[5]	Tetracycline[4]
Bacillus (eg, anthrax)	Penicillin[5]	Erythromycin,[3] tetracycline[4]
Clostridium (eg, gas gangrene, tetanus)	Penicillin[5]	Metronidazole, chloramphenicol, clindamycin
Corynebacterium diphtheriae	Erythromycin,[3]	Penicillin[5]
Corynebacterium jeikeium	Vancomycin	Ciprofloxacin, penicillin and gentamicin
Listeria	TMP-SMZ[1]	Ampicillin ± aminoglycoside[7]

Table 37–1. Drugs of choice for suspected or proved microbial pathogens, 1994. (± = alone or combined with)

Suspected or Proved Etiologic Agent	Drug(s) of First Choice	Alternative Drug(s)
Acid-fast rods		
Mycobacterium tuberculosis	INH + rifampin + pyrazinamide + ethambutol	Other antituberculous drugs
Mycobacterium leprae	Dapsone + rifampin ± clofazimine	Minocycline, ofloxacin
Mycobacterium kansasii	INH + rifampin ± ethambutol	Ethionamide, cycloserine
Mycobacterium avium-intracellulare	Clarithromycin + ethambutol + rifampin + clofazimine ± ciprofloxacin ± amikacin	Other anittuberculous drugs
Mycobacterium fortuitum-chelonei	Amikacin + doxycycline	Cefoxitin, erythromycin, sulfonamide
Nocardia	TMP-SMZ[1]	Minocycline, imipenem, sulfonamide[9]
Spirochetes		
Borrelia burgdorferi (Lyme disease)	Tetracycline[4]	Amoxicillin, ceftriaxone, erythromycin, cefuroxime axetil, azithromycin
Borrelia recurrentis (relapsing fever)	Tetracycline[4]	Penicillin
Leptospira	Penicillin[5]	Tetracycline[4]
Treponema pallidum (syphilis)	Penicillin[5]	Tetracycline,[4] ceftriaxone
Treponema pertenue (yaws)	Penicillin[5]	Tetracycline[4]
Mycoplasmas	Erychromycin[3] or tetracycline[4]	Clarithromycin
Chlamydiae		
C psittaci	Tetracycline[4]	Chloramphenicol
C trachomatis (urethritis or pelvic inflammatory disease)	Doxycycline or erythromycin[3]	Ofloxacin or azithromycin
C pneumoniae)	Tetracycline[4]	Erythromycin,[3] clarithromycin
Rickettsiae	Tetracycline[4]	Chloramphenicol

[1]TMP-SMZ is a mixture of 1 part trimethoprim and 5 parts sulfamethoxazole.

[2]Newer cephalosporins (1994) include cefotaxime, cefuroxime, ceftriaxone, ceftazidime, ceftizoxime, cefuroxime axetil, cefixime, and others.

[3]Erythromycin estolate is best absorbed orally but carries the highest risk of hepatitis; erythromycin stearate and erythromycin ethylsuccinate are also available.

[4]All tetracyclines have similar activity against microorganisms. Dosage is determined by rates of absorption and excretion of various preparations.

[5]Penicillin G is preferred for parenteral injection; penicillin V for oral administration—to be used only in treating infections due to highly sensitive organisms.

[6]Older cephalosporins are cephalothin, cefazolin, cephapirin, and cefoxitin for parenteral injection; cephalexin and cephradine can be given orally.

[7]Aminoglycosides—gentamicin, tobramycin, amikacin, netilmicin—should be chosen on the basis of local patterns of susceptibility.

[8]Parenteral nafcillin or oxacillin; oral dicloxacillin, cloxacillin, or oxacillin.

[9]Oral sulfisoxazole and trisulfapyrimidines are highly soluble in urine; parenteral sodium sulfadiazine can be injected intravenously in treating severely ill patients.

[10]Antipseudomonal penicillins: ticarcillin, carbenicillin, mezlocillin, azlocillin, pipericillin.

[11]First choice for previously untreated urinary tract infection is a highly soluble sulfonamide (see Note 9). TMP-SMZ (see Note 1) is acceptable.

5. Emergence of drug-resistant or tolerant organisms.

6. Participation of two or more microorganisms in the infectious process, of which only one was originally detected and used for drug selection.

F. Adequate Dosage: Adequacy of therapy is usually assessed by a favorable clinical response. In most infections, either a bacteriostatic or a bactericidal agent can be used. In some infections (eg, infective endocarditis and meningitis), it is mandatory to kill the infecting organism to achieve a cure. In the therapy of endocarditis, proper choice of drug and dose can be judged by "serum assay." Two days after initiation of a drug regimen, serum is obtained from the patient 1–2 hours after a drug dose. Dilutions of this serum are inoculated with the organism originally isolated from the patient, and antibacterial activity is estimated. If an adequate dose of a proper drug is being given, the serum will be bactericidal in a dilution of 1:4 or more. When potentially toxic drugs (eg, aminoglycosides, vancomycin) are used, the serum levels of the drug should be measured to avoid toxicity and ensure appropriate dosage. In patients with altered clearance of drugs, the dose or frequency of administration must be adjusted. This can sometimes be done by reference to dosage nomograms or formulas, but it is best to measure levels directly and adjust therapy accordingly.

In renal or hepatic failure, the dosage must be adjusted as shown in Table 37–4.

G. Duration of Antimicrobial Therapy: Generally, effective antimicrobial treatment results in reversal of the clinical and laboratory parameters of active infection and marked clinical improvement. However, varying periods of treatment may be required for cure. This is influenced by such factors as

Table 37–2. Examples of initial antimicrobial therapy for acutely ill adults pending identification of causative organism.

	Suspected Clinical Diagnosis	Likely Etiologic Diagnosis	Drugs of Choice	Alternative Drugs
(a)	Meningitis, bacterial	Pneumococcus, meningo-coccus	Penicillin G, 4 million units IV every 4 hours	Cefotaxime,[1] 3 g IV every 6 hours, or ceftriaxone, 2 g IV every 12 hours.
(b)	Meningitis, postoperative (or posttraumatic)	S aureus, gram-negative bacteria (pneumococcus, posttraumatic)	Penicillin G as in (a) + nafcillin, 1.5 g every 4 hours, + gentamicin,[2] 1.7 mg/kg IV every 8 hours, + gentami-cin,[2] 8 mg intrathecally once daily.	Vancomycin, 10 mg/kg every 8 hours, + cefotaxime,[1] 3 g IV every 6 hours (ceftazidime, 3 g every 8 hours, if Pseudomonas suspected).
(c)	Brain abscess	Mixed anaerobes, pneumo-cocci, streptococci	Penicillin G as in (a) + cefotaxime or ceftriaxone as in (a).	Metronidazole, 500 mg IV every 8 hours, + penicillin G as in (a).
(d)	Pneumonia, acute, commu-nity-acquired, severe	Pneumococci, M pneu-moniae, Legionella, C pneu-moniae	Erythromycin, 0.5 g orally or IV 4 times daily.	TMP-SMZ,[3] 5–8 mg TMP and 25–40 mg SMZ IV every 12 hours.
(e)	Pneumonia, postoperative	S aureus, Klebsiella, mixed anaerobes	Nafcillin as in (b) + gentami-cin[2] as in (b) + penicillin G as in (d).	Cefotaxime,[1] 2 g IV every 8–12 hours.
(f)	Pneumonia in chronic lung disease, aspiration	Pneumococci, H influenzae, S aureus, mixed anaerobes	Cefotaxime as in (e).	Clindamycin, 900 mg IV every 8 hours, + TMP-SMZ as in (d).
(g)	Endocarditis, acute (including prosthetic or IV drug user)	S aureus, S faecalis, gram-negative aerobic bacteria	Penicillin G as in (a) + nafcillin as in (b) + gentami-cin[2] as in (b).	Gentamicin[2] as in (b) + vancomycin as in (b).
(h)	Septic thrombophlebitis (eg, IV tubing, IV shunts)	Pneumcocci, gram-negative aerobic bacteria	Nafcillin as in (b) + gentami-cin[2] as in (b).	Vancomysin, 20–30 mg/kg/d in 2 or 3 divided doses, + cefotaxime as in (e).
(i)	Osteomyelitis	S aureus	Nafcillin as in (b).	Vancomycin as in (b).
(j)	Septic arthritis	S aureus, N gonorrhoeae	Ceftriaxone, 2 g IV	Nafcillin as in (b) + penicillin G as in (a).
(k)	Urinary tract infection, first episode, community-ac-quired	E coli	TMP-SMZ, 1 tablet double-strength twice daily for 3 days.	Ampicillin, 0.5 g orally 4 times daily for 3 days.
(l)	Pyelonephritis with flank pain and fever (recurrent UTI)	E coli, Klebsiella, Enterobac-ter, Pseudomonas	Gentamicin[2] as in (b).	Cefotaxime[1] as in (e).
(m)	Suspected sepsis in neu-tropenic patient receiving cancer chemotherapy	S aureus, Pseudomonas, Klebsiella, E coli	Ticarcillin, 18 g IV daily, + tobramycin,[2] 1.7 mg/kg every 8 hours.	Ceftazidime, 2 g IV every 8 hours, + vancomycin as in (b) + tobramycin
(n)	Intra-abdominal sepsis (eg, postoperative, peritonitis, cholecystitis)	Gram-negative bacteria, Bacteroides, anaerobic bac-teria, streptococci, clostridia	Ampicillin as in (f) + gentami-cin[2] as in (b) + metronida-zole as in (c).	Clindamycin, 600 mg IV every 8 hours, + gentamicin[2] as in (b).

[1]Cefotaxime, ceftriaxone, ceftazidime, or ceftizoxime can be used. Most studies on meningitis have been done with cefotaxime or ceftriaxone (see text).
[2]Depending on local drug susceptibility pattern, use tobramycin, 5–7 mg/kg/d, or amikacin, 15 mg/kg/d, in place of gentamicin.
[3]TMP-SMZ is a fixed combination of one part trimethoprim and five parts sulfamethoxazole. Single-strength tablets: 80 mg TMP, 400 mg SMZ; double-strength tablets: 160 mg TMP, 800 mg SMZ.

(1) the type of infecting organism (bacterial infections can be cured more rapidly than fungal or myco-bacterial ones), (2) the location of the process (eg, endocarditis and osteomyelitis require prolonged therapy), and (3) the immunocompetence of the patient.

The following examples are illustrative: Strepto-coccal pharyngitis requires 10 days of effective peni-cillin levels to eradicate the organism and prevent the noninfectious complication of rheumatic fever. Acute

uncomplicated gonococcal urethritis can be cured in males in 24 hours. Endocarditis due to viridans strep-tococci is curable in 2–4 weeks; that caused by staph-ylococci requires 4–6 weeks of treatment. Acute un-complicated cystitis in women often responds to 3 days of therapy.

To minimize untoward reactions from drugs and the risk of superinfection, treatment should be contin-ued only as long as needed to eradicate the infection.

H. Adverse Reactions: All antimicrobials can

Table 37–3. Examples of empirical choices of antimicrobials for adult outpatient infections.

Suspected Clinical Diagnosis	Likely Etiologic Agents	Drug(s) of Choice	Alternative Drug(s)
Erysipelas, impetigo, cellulitis, ascending lymphangitis	Group A streptococcus	Phenoxymethyl penicillin, 0.5 g orally 4 times daily	Erythromycin, 0.5 g orally 4 times daily, or cephalexin, 0.5 g orally 4 times daily for 7–10 days.
Furuncle with surrounding cellulitis	*Staphylococcus aureus*	Dicloxacillin, 0.5 g orally 4 times daily for 7–10 days.	Cephalexin, 0.5 g orally 4 times daily for 7–10 days.
Pharyngitis	Group A streptococcus	Phenoxymethyl penicillin, 0.5 g orally 4 times daily for 10 days.	Erythromycin, 0.5 g orally 4 times daily for 10 days.
Otitis media	*Streptococcus pnuemoniae, Haemophilus influenzae, Moraxella catarrhalis*	Ampicillin, 0.5 g orally 4 times daily; amoxicillin, 0.5 g orally 3 times daily; or TMP-SMZ,[1] 1 double-strength tablet twice daily for 10 days.	Augmentin,[2] 0.5 g orally 3 times daily; cefuroxime, 0.5 g orally twice daily; cefixime, 0.2–0.4 g daily for 10 days.
Acute sinusitis	*S pneumonaiae, H influenzae, M catarrhalis*	Ampicillin, 0.5 g orally 4 times daily; amoxicillin, 0.5 g orally 3 times daily; or TMP-SMZ,[1] 1 double-strength tablet twice daily for 10 days.	Augmentin,[2] 0.5 g orally 3 times daily; cefuroxime, 0.5 g orally twice daily; cefixime, 0.2–0.4 g daily for 10 days.
Acute bronchitis	*S pneumoniae, H influenzae*	Tetracycline, 0.5 g orally 4 times daily; erythromycin, 0.5 g orally 4 times daily; ampicillin, 0.5 g orally 4 times daily.	TMP-SMZ[1] 1 double-strength tablet twice daily for 10 days.
Aspiration pneumonia	Mixed oropharyngeal flora, including anaerobes	Clindamycin, 0.3 g orally 4 times daily for 10–14 days.	Phenoxymethyl penicillin, 0.5 g orally 4 times daily for 10–14 days.
Pneumonia	*S pneumoniae, Mycoplasma pneumoniae, Legionella pneumophila, Chlamydia pneumoniae*	Erythromycin, 0.5 g orally 4 times daily for 10–14 days.	Phenoxymethyl penicillin, 0.5 g orally 4 times daily for 10 days.
Cystitis	*Escherichia coli, Klebsiella pneumoniae, Proteus* spp, *Staphylococcus saprophyticus*	TMP-SMZ,[1] 1 double-strength tablet twice daily for 3 days.	Ampicillin, 0.5 g orally 4 times daily for 3 days.
Pyelonephritis	*E coli, K pneumoniae, Proteus* spp, *S saprophyticus*	TMP-SMZ,[1] 1 double-strength tablet twice daily for 10 days.	Ampicillin, 0.5 g orally 4 times daily for 10 days.
Gastroenteritis	*Salmonella, Shigella, Campylobacter, Entamoeba histolytica*	see Note 3.	
Urethritis	*Neisseria gonorrhoeae, Chlamydia trachomatis*	Ceftriaxone, 250 mg IM once for *N gonorrhoeae*; doxycycline, 100 mg twice daily for 7 days for *C trachomatis*.	Cefixime, 400 mg once, or ciprofloxacin, 500 mg once, for *N gonorrhoeae*; erythromycin, 0.5 g orally 4 times daily for 7 days, or azithromycin, 1 g orally once, for *C trachomatis*.
Pelvic inflammatory disease	*N gonorrhoeae, C trachomatis,* anaerobes, gram-negative rods	Ceftriaxone, 250 mg IM once, followed by doxycycline, 100 mg orally twice daily for 10–14 days.	Cefoxitin, 2 g IM, with probenecid, 1 g orally, followed by doxycycline, 100 mg orally twice daily for 10–14 days.
Syphilis Early syphilis (primary, secondary, or latent of less than 1 year's duration)	*Treponema pallidum*	Benzathine penicillin G, 2.4 million units IM once.	Doxycycline, 100 mg orally twice daily; or tetracycline, 0.5 g orally 4 times daily; or erythromycin, 0.5 g orally 4 times daily for 15 days.
Latent of more than 1 year's duration or cardiovascular syphilis		Benzathine penicillin G, 2.4 million units IM per week for 3 weeks.	Tetracycline, 0.5 g orally 4 times daily; or doxycycline, 100 mg orally twice daily for 4 weeks.
Neurosyphilis		Aqueous penicillin G, 12–24 million units/d IV for 10 days.	Procaine penicillin G, 2–4 million units/d IM, plus probenecid, 500 mg orally 4 times daily, both for 10 days.

[1]TMP-SMZ is a fixed combination of 1 part trimethoprim and 5 parts sulfamethoxazole. Single-strength tablets: 80 mg TMP, 400 mg SMZ; double-strength tablets: 160 mg TMP, 800 mg SMZ.

[2]Augmentin is a combination of amoxicillin, 250 mg or 500 mg, plus 125 mg of clavulanic acid.

[3]The diagnosis should be confirmed by culture before therapy. *Salmonella* gastroenteritis does not require therapy. For *Shigella*, give TMP-SMZ double-strength tablets twice daily for 5 days; or ampicillin, 0.5 g orally 4 times daily for 5 days; or ciprofloxacin, 0.5 g orally 4 times daily for 5 days. For *Campylobacter*, give erythromycin, 0.5 g orally 4 times daily for 5 days; or ciprofloxacin, 0.5 g orally 4 times daily for 5 days. For *E histolytica*, give metronidazole, 750 mg orally 3 times daily for 5–10 days, followed by diiodohydroxyquin, 600 mg 3 times daily for 3 weeks.

Table 37–4. Use of antimicrobials in patients with renal failure[1] and hepatic failure.

	Principal Mode of Excretion or Detoxification	Approximate Half-Life in Serum		Proposed Dosage Regimen in End-Stage Renal Failure		Removal of Drug by Hemodialysis	Dose After Hemodialysis	Dosage in Hepatic Failure
		Normal	Renal Failure	Initial Dose	Maintenance Dose			
Acyclovir	Renal	2.5–3.5 hours	20 hours	2.5 mg/kg	2.5 mg/kg q24h	Yes	2.5 mg/kg	No change
Amphotericin B	Unknown	360 hours	360 hours	No change	No change	No	None	No change
Ampicillin	Tubular secretion	0.5–1 hour	8–12 hours	1 g	1 g q8–12h	Yes	1 g	No change
Azithromycin	Renal 20%; hepatic 35%	3–4 hours	Not known	500 mg	250 mg q24h	No	None	Not known[4]
Azlocillin	Renal 50–70%; biliary 20–30%	1 hour	3–6 hours	3 g	2 g q6–8h	Yes	1 g	1–2 g q8h
Aztreonam	Renal	1.7 hours	6 hours	1–2 g	0.5–1 g q6–8h	Yes	0.5–1 g	No change
Carbenicillin	Tubular secretion	1 hour	16 hours	4 g	2 g q12h	Yes	2 g	No change
Chloramphenicol	Mainly liver	3 hours	4 hours	0.5 g	0.5 g q6h	Yes	0.5 g	0.25–0.5 g q12h
Ciprofloxacin	Renal and liver	4 hours	8.5 hours	0.5 g	0.25–0.75 g q24h	No	None	No change
Clarithromycin	Renal 30%; hepatic >50%	3–4 hours	15 hours	500 mg	250 mg q12h	No	None	Not known[4]
Clindamycin	Liver	2–4 hours	2–4 hours	0.6 g IV	0.6 g q8h	No	None	0.3–0.6 g q8h
Doxycycline	Renal	15–24 hours	15–24 hours	100 mg	100 mg q12h	No	None	Not Known[4]
Erythromycin	Mainly liver	1.5 hours	1.5 hours	0.5–1 g	0.5–1 g q6h	No	None	0.25–0.5 g q6h
Fluconazole	Renal	30 hours	98 hours	0.2 g	0.1 g q24h	Yes	Give q24h dose	No change
Foscarnet	Renal	3–8 hours	Not known	90–120 mg	Not known[5]	No	None	No change
Flucytosine	Renal	3–6 hours	60–80 hours	30 mg/kg	25 mg/kg q24h	Yes	15 mg/kg	No change
Ganciclovir	Renal	3 hours	11–28 hours	1.25 mg/kg	1.25 mg/kg q24h	Yes	Give q24h dose	No change
Imipenem	Glomerular filtration	1 hour	3 hours	0.5 g	0.25–0.5 g q12h	Yes	0.25–0.5 g	No change
Isoniazid	Renal	1–5 hours	2.5 hours	300 mg	300 mg q24h	Yes	None	Not known[4]
Itraconazole	Hepatic	21 hours	25 hours	50–200 mg	50–200 mg q24h	No	None	Not known[4]
Ketoconazole	Hepatic	8 hours	8 hours	200 mg	200–400 mg q24h	No	None	Not known[4]
Lomefloxacin	Renal	10–12 hours	25 hours	400 mg	200 mg q24h	No	None	No change
Metronidazole	Liver	6–10 hours	6–10 hours	0.5 g IV	0.5 g q8h	Yes	0.25 g	0.25 g q12h
Mezlocillin	Renal 50–70%; biliary 20–30%	1 hour	3–6 hours	3 g	2 g q6–8h	Yes	1 g	1–2 g q8h

(continued)

Table 37–4. Use of antimicrobials in patients with renal failure[1] and hepatic failure. (continued)

	Principal Mode of Excretion or Detoxification	Approximate Half-Life in Serum		Proposed Dosage Regimen in End-Stage Renal Failure		Removal of Drug by Hemodialysis	Dose After Hemodialysis	Dosage in Hepatic Failure
		Normal	Renal Failure	Initial Dose	Maintenance Dose			
Nafcillin	Liver 80%; kidney 20%	0.75 hours	1.5 hours	1.5 g	1.5 g q4h	No	None	2–3 g q12h
Ofloxacin	Renal	6–8 hours	36 hours	400 mg	200 mg q24h	Not known	Not known	No change
Penicillin G	Tubular secretion	0.5 hours	7–10 hours	1–2 million units	1 million units q8h	Yes	500,000 units	No change
Piperacillin	Renal 50–70%; biliary 20–30%	1 hour	3–6 hours	3 g	2 g q6–8h	Yes	1 g	1–2 g q8h
Rifampin	Hepatic	2–3 hours	3–5 hours	600 mg	600 mg q24h	No	None	Not known[4]
Ticarcillin	Tubular secretion	1.1 hour	15–20 hours	3 g	2 g q6–8h	Yes	1 g	No change
Trimethoprim-sulfamethoxazole	Some liver	TMP 10–12 hours; SMZ 8–10 hours	TMP 24–48 hours; SMZ 18–24 hours	320 mg TMP + 1600 mg SMZ	80 mg TMP + 400 mg SMZ every 12 hours	Yes	80 mg TMP + 400 mg SMZ	No change
Vancomycin	Glomerular filtration	6 hours	6–10 days	1 g	1 g q6–10d based on serum levels[6]	No	None	No change

[1]For cephalosporins, see text and Table 37–7; for aminoglycosides, see Table 37–8.
[2]Considered here to be marked by creatinine clearance of 10 mL/min or less.
[3]For a 70-kg adult with a serious systemic infection.
[4]Dose adjustment in hepatic failure has not been studied, but because clearance of the drug is principally hepatic, dose reduction may be required.
[5]When creatinine clearance is 30 mL/min, a dose of 60 mg/kg is given once daily. For clearances less than 30 mL/min, the dose has not been established.
[6]When serum levels reach 5–10 μg/mL, another dose should be given.

cause adverse effects. Most commonly these are (1) hypersensitivity reactions (eg, fever, rashes, anaphylaxis), (2) direct toxicity (eg, diarrhea, vomiting, impairment of renal or hepatic function, neurotoxicity), or (3) superinfection by drug-resistant microorganisms. Physicians prescribing antimicrobials must be familiar with the adverse effects associated with specific drugs.

When an adverse reaction develops, the physician must assess its severity and prognosis in the context of the infection being treated. If the infection is life-threatening and treatment cannot be stopped, the reactions may be managed symptomatically (especially if mild) or another drug may be chosen that does not cross-react with the offending one (Table 37–1). If the infection is less severe, it may be possible to stop all antimicrobials and follow the patient carefully.

I. Oral Antibiotics: Food does not significantly influence the bioavailability of most oral antibiotics. Exceptions include tetracycline and the quinolones, which are chelated by heavy metals and thus should be given between meals. Ketoconazole and azithromycin also have decreased bioavailability with food and should be given 1 hour before or 2 hours after meals.

J. Intravenous Antibiotics: When an antibiotic must be administered intravenously (eg, for serious or life-threatening infection or to sustain very high blood levels), the following cautions should be observed:

(1) Give in neutral solution (pH 7.0–7.2) of sodium chloride (0.9%) or dextrose (5%) in water.

(2) Give alone without admixture of any other substance in order to avoid chemical and physical incompatibilities (which are frequent). Help from the clinical pharmacist will avoid physiologic incompatibilities, a few of which are mentioned in the discussions of individual drugs.

(3) Administer by intermittent addition to the intravenous infusion ("bolus injection") to avoid inactivation (by temperature, changing pH, etc) and prolonged vein irritation from high drug concentration, which favors thrombophlebitis.

(4) Peripheral Teflon catheters and steel needles must be routinely changed every 48–72 hours to prevent phlebitis—or sooner if the catheter is thought to be infected. Most catheter-related infections present with local signs of infection (erythema, tenderness) at the insertion site. However, "occult" catheter infections can occur in which the catheter is the cause of fever or bacteremia despite a normal-appearing insertion site. In the evaluation of a patient with fever who is receiving intravenous therapy, the catheter must always be considered as a potential source. Some small-gauge (20–23F) peripherally inserted silicone or polyurethane catheters (Per Q Cath, A-Cath, Ven-A-Cath, and others) are associated with a very low infection rate and can be maintained for 3–6 months without replacement. Such catheters are ideal for long-term outpatient antibiotic therapy.

K. Cost of Antibiotics: Because of the widespread use of antibiotics, the cost of these agents can be substantial both to institutions and to individuals. Cost should not be the only determinant in choosing antibiotics, but if several drugs with equal efficacy and toxicity are available, one should choose the least expensive. Table 37–5 lists the cost of commonly used antibiotics.

The Choice of Antimicrobial Drugs. Med Lett Drugs Ther 1992;34:49.
Handbook of Antimicrobial Therapy: The Medical Letter on Drugs and Therapeutics, 1990.
Mills J, Barriere SL, Jawetz E: Clinical use of antimicrobials. In: *Basic & Clinical Pharmacology,* 5th ed. Katzung BG (editor). Appleton & Lange, 1992.
Moellering RC Jr: Principles of anti-infective therapy. In: *Principles and Practice of Infectious Diseases,* 3rd ed. Mandell GL, Douglas RG, Bennett JE (editors). Wiley, 1990. (General discussion of antibiotic choice.)
Wilkowske CJ: General principles of antimicrobial therapy. Mayo Clin Proc 1991;66:931.

PENICILLINS

The penicillins are a large group of antimicrobial substances, all of which share a common chemical nucleus (6-aminopenicillanic acid) that contains a β-lactam ring essential to their biologic activity. All β-lactam antibiotics inhibit formation of microbial cell walls.

Penicillins fall into four major categories, discussed below.

Antimicrobial Action & Resistance

The initial step in penicillin action is the binding of the drug to receptors—penicillin-binding proteins—some of which are transpeptidation enzymes. The penicillin-binding proteins of different organisms differ in number and in affinity for a given drug. After penicillins have attached to receptors, peptidoglycan synthesis is inhibited because the activity of transpeptidation enzymes is blocked. The final bactericidal action is the removal of an inhibitor of the autolytic enzymes in the cell wall, which activates the enzymes and results in cell lysis. Organisms that are defective in autolysin function are inhibited but not killed by β-lactam antibiotics ("tolerance"). Organisms that produce β-lactamases (penicillinases) are resistant to some penicillins because the β-lactam ring is broken and the drug inactivated. Only organisms that are actively synthesizing peptidoglycan (in the process of multiplication) are susceptible to β-lactam antibiotics. Nonmultiplying organisms or those lacking cell walls (L forms) are not susceptible but may act as "persisters."

Table 37–5. Costs of antimicrobials. (Based on costs at the University of California, San Francisco, 1993.)

	Unit Cost	Dose per Day[1]	Daily Cost of Therapy
INTRAVENOUS PREPARATIONS			
Acyclovir (0.5 g)	$36.47	15 mg/kg (mucocutaneous herpes)	$109.41
Acyclovir (1 g)	$72.93	30 mg/kg (CNS herpes)	$218.79
Amikacin (0.5 g)	$42.34	15 mg/kg	$84.68
Ampicillin (2 g)	$0.79	100 mg/kg	$3.16
Aztreonam (1 g)	$10.98	50 mg/kg	$32.94
Cefazolin (1 g)	$1.38	50 mg/kg	$4.14
Cefoxitin (1 g)	$4.65	80 mg/kg	$27.90
Ceftazidime (1 g)	$11.01	50 mg/kg	$33.03
Ceftizoxime (1 g)	$5.50	50 mg/kg	$16.50
Ceftriaxone (1 g)	$23.76	30 mg/kg	$47.52
Cefuroxime (1.5 g)	$10.43	60 mg/kg	$31.29
Ciprofloxacin (0.2 g)	$11.93	0.8 g	$47.72
Clindamycin (0.6 g)	$2.04	2400 mg	$8.16
Fluconazole (0.2 g)	$64.61	0.2–0.4 g daily	$64.61–94.93
Fluconazole (0.4 g)	$94.43		
Foscarnet (1 g)	$9.81	180 mg/kg (induction) 90–120 mg/kg (maintenance)	$117.72 $68.17
Gentamicin (80 mg)	$0.25	4.5 mg/kg	$1.50
Imipenem (0.5 g)	$14.45	50 mg/kg	$115.60
Metronidazole (0.5 g)	$1.34	1500 mg	$4.02
Mezlocillin (3 g)	$7.91	250 mg/kg	$47.46
Nafcillin (2 g)	$1.70	100 mg/kg	$6.80
Penicillin (1million units)	$0.60	12 million units	$7.20
Pipericillin (3 g)	$8.25	250 mg/kg	$49.50
Ticarcillin (3 g)	$7.39	250 mg/kg	$44.34
Tobramycin (80 mg)	$3.38	4.5 mg/kg	$20.28
Trimethoprim-sulfamethoxazole (0.32 g TMP in 20 mL)	$1.62	7.5–10 mg/kg TMP	$3.24
Vancomycin (0.5 g)	$3.06	20 mg/kg	$9.18
ORAL PREPARATIONS			
Acyclovir (0.2 g)	$0.69	1000 mg (therapy of herpes)	$3.45
Acyclovir (0.8 g)	$2.75	600 mg (herpes suppression)	$2.07
Amoxicillin (0.5 g)	$0.09	30 mg/kg	$0.36
Ampicillin (0.5 g)	$0.07	30 mg/kg	$0.28
Augmentin (0.5 g amoxicillin plus 0.125 g clavulanic acid)	$1.90	30 mg/kg	$5.70
Azithromycin (0.25 g)	$6.59	500 mg as loading dose, then 250 mg/d	$6.59
Azithromycin (1 g)	$26.36	1 g as single dose for C trachomatis	$26.36
Cefaclor (0.5 g)	$3.11	20–30 mg/kg	$9.33
Cefixime (0.4 g)	$4.11	400 mg	$4.11
Cefpodoxime proxetil (0.2 g)	$2.56	400 mg	$5.12
Cefprozil (0.5 g)	$4.35	15 mg/kg	$8.70
Cefuroxime axetil (0.5 g)	$3.93	15 mg/kg	$7.86
Cephalexin (0.5 g)	$0.13	30 mg/kg	$0.52
Ciprofloxacin (0.5 g)	$2.42	0.5–0.75 g twice daily	$4.84–8.40
Ciprofloxacin (0.75 g)	$4.20		
Clarithromycin (0.25 or 0.5 g)	$2.09	250–500 mg twice daily	$4.18
Clindamycin (0.3 g)	$1.70	15 mg/kg	

(continued)

Table 37–5. Costs of antimicrobials. (Based on costs at the University of California, San Francisco, 1993.) (continued)

	Unit Cost	Dose per Day[1]	Daily Cost of Therapy
Doxycycline (0.1 g)	$0.06	3 mg/kg	$0.12
Erythromycin (0.5 g)	$0.06	30 mg/kg	$0.24
Fluconazole (0.1 g)	$5.47	0.1–0.2 g daily	$5.47–8.95
Fluconazole (0.2 g)	$8.95		
Flucytosine (0.5 g)	$1.57	150 mg/kg	$31.40
Itraconazole (0.1 g)	$4.08	200–400 mg	$8.16–16.32
Ketoconazole (0.2 g)	$1.92	0.2–0.4 g daily	$1.92–3.84
Lomefloxacin (0.4 g)	$4.72	400 mg	$4.72
Loracarbef (0.4 mg)	$2.56	800 mg	$5.12
Metronidazole (0.5 g)	$0.04	2 g (*Trichomonas*) 20 mg/kg	$0.16 $0.12
Ofloxacin (0.4 g)	$2.58	400 mg twice daily	$5.16
Phenoxymethyl penicillin (0.5 g)	$0.04	30 mg/kg	0.16
Tetracycline (0.5 g)	$0.03	30 mg/kg	$0.12
Trimethoprim-sulfamethoxazole (80 mg TMP and 400 mg SMZ)	$0.03	5 mg/kg TMP	$0.12

[1]Dose based on a 70-kg individual with normal renal function.
[2]Daily cost for intravenous antibiotics includes acquisition cost only and not preparation and administration costs.

Microbial resistance to penicillins is caused by four factors:

1. Production of β-lactamases, eg, by staphylococci, gonococci, *Haemophilus* species, and coliform organisms.

2. Lack of penicillin receptors (eg, resistant pneumococci) or impermeability of cell envelope, so that penicillins cannot reach receptors (eg, metabolically inactive bacteria).

3. Failure of activation of autolytic enzymes in the cell wall; "tolerance," eg, in staphylococci, group B streptococci.

4. The presence of cell wall-deficient (L) forms or mycoplasmas, which do not synthesize peptidoglycans.

1. NATURAL PENICILLINS

The natural penicillins include forms of penicillin G for parenteral administration (aqueous crystalline, procaine, and benzathine penicillin G) or for oral administration (penicillin G and phenoxymethyl penicillin [penicillin V]). They are most active against gram-positive organisms, less active against gram-negatives, and susceptible to hydrolysis by β-lactamases. They are used for infections caused by pneumococci, streptococci, meningococci, non-β-lactamase-producing staphylococci and gonococci, *Treponema pallidum* and other spirochetes, *Bacillus anthracis* and other gram-positive rods, clostridia, *Actinomyces,* and most anaerobes except β-lactamase-producing strains, eg, *Bacteroides fragilis* (Table 37–1).

Pharmacokinetics & Administration

While aqueous crystalline penicillin G can be given intramuscularly or intravenously, the intravenous route, by intermittent bolus injection or continuous infusion, is often preferred to avoid local pain. After parenteral administration, penicillin is widely distributed in tissues. An intravenous dose of 1 million units of penicillin G produces a peak serum level of 10 μg/mL. (One million units of penicillin G equals 0.6 g.) Levels equal to those in serum occur in many tissues, but lower levels prevail in the eye, prostate, and central nervous system. However, with acute inflammation of the meninges (eg, in bacterial meningitis), penicillin G levels in the cerebrospinal fluid exceed 0.2 μg/mL with a daily parenteral dose of 20 million units. This level is more than is required to kill sensitive pneumococci and meningococci. Consequently, systemically administered penicillin G is adequate to treat meningitis caused by these organisms.

Special dosage forms of penicillin permit delayed absorption to yield low blood and tissue levels for long periods, eg, benzathine penicillin G. After a single intramuscular injection of 1.2 million units (0.9 g), serum levels in excess of 0.02 μg/mL are maintained for 10 days and levels in excess of 0.004 μg/mL for 3 weeks. The latter is sufficient to protect against β-hemolytic streptococcal infection; the former, to treat an established infection with these organisms. Procaine penicillin also has delayed absorption. After intramuscular injection of 1–2 million units (1–2 g), serum levels of 0.1 μg/mL persist for 18–24 hours.

Phenoxymethyl penicillin (penicillin V) is the oral

penicillin of choice. It is more acid-stable than oral penicillin G, is better absorbed, and gives higher serum levels. A 250 mg dose results in serum levels of 2–3 μg/mL.

Most of the absorbed penicillin is rapidly excreted by the kidneys into the urine; small amounts are excreted by other routes. About 10% of renal excretion is by glomerular filtration and 90% by tubular secretion. Tubular secretion can be partially blocked by probenecid, 0.5 g (10 mg/kg) every 6 hours orally, to achieve higher systemic levels. Individuals with impaired renal function likewise tend to maintain higher penicillin levels longer, and the dose should be reduced in moderate to severe renal failure. One commonly used formula for calculating the maximum daily dose of penicillin in millions of units in patients with a creatinine clearance of less than 40 mL/min is as follows (see also Table 37–4):

$$\text{Dosage} = 3.2 + \frac{\text{Creatinine clearance}}{7}$$

Renal excretion of penicillin results in very high levels in the urine. Thus, systemic daily doses of 10 million units (6 g) of penicillin may yield urine levels of 500–3000 μg/mL; this is enough to suppress not only gram-positive but also many gram-negative bacteria in the urine (provided they produce little β-lactamase).

Penicillin is also excreted into sputum and milk to levels of 3–15% of those present in the serum. This is the case in both humans and cattle. The presence of penicillin in the milk of cows treated for mastitis presents a problem for those who drink milk and are allergic to penicillin.

Clinical Uses

Most infections caused by organisms sensitive to penicillin will respond to aqueous penicillin G in daily doses of 0.6–5 million units (0.36–3 g) administered intramuscularly or intravenously in divided doses every 4–6 hours. For severe or life-threatening infections (meningitis, endocarditis), much larger daily doses (10–24 million units) should be given by intermittent intravenous infusion every 2–4 hours in equally divided doses.

Penicillin V is indicated only in minor infections such as mild respiratory infections, pharyngitis, and skin and soft tissue infections. The usual dose is 1–2 g/d in four equally divided doses.

A single injection of 1.2 million units of benzathine penicillin intramuscularly is satisfactory for treatment of β-hemolytic streptococcal pharyngitis. An injection of 1.2–2.4 million units every 3–4 weeks provides satisfactory prophylaxis for rheumatics against reinfection with group A streptococci. Syphilis can be treated with benzathine penicillin, 2.4 million units intramuscularly weekly for 1–3 weeks, depending on the stage of the disease (see Table 37–3).

Procaine penicillin is used primarily for treatment of uncomplicated pneumococcal pneumonia in a dose of 600,000 units twice a day.

Penicillins should not be given intrathecally because they are neurotoxic and can cause seizures. Penicillins are highly sensitizing and should not be applied to the skin.

2. EXTENDED-SPECTRUM PENICILLINS

The extended-spectrum group of penicillins includes the aminopenicillins ampicillin and amoxicillin; the carboxypenicillins carbenicillin and ticarcillin; and the ureidopenicillins piperacillin, azlocillin, and mezlocillin. These drugs are all susceptible to destruction by staphylococcal (and other) β-lactamases. They tend to be active against many gram-negative rods but less active against gram-positive bacteria than the natural penicillins.

Antimicrobial Activity

Ampicillin and amoxicillin are active against most strains of *Escherichia coli*, *Proteus mirabilis*, *Salmonella*, *Listeria*, and non-β-lactamase-producing strains of *Haemophilus influenzae* but inactive against most strains of *Klebsiella*, *Pseudomonas*, *Serratia*, *Enterobacter*, and indole-positive *Proteus*. While these drugs are less active than penicillin in vitro against pneumococci and streptococci, they are clinically effective in treating infections caused by these organisms. They are more active than penicillin G against enterococci.

Carbenicillin extends the activity of ampicillin to include many strains of *Pseudomonas*, *Enterobacter*, *Serratia*, and indole-positive *Proteus*, but it has poor activity against most strains of *Klebsiella*. Ticarcillin is similar to carbenicillin but is 2–4 times more active against *Pseudomonas*. Neither drug is effective against enterococci.

The ureidopenicillins are similar to carbenicillin and ticarcillin but exhibit slight differences in activity against gram-negative organisms. Piperacillin is more active than ticarcillin against *Pseudomonas aeruginosa* and *Klebsiella*, but otherwise its spectrum of activity is similar to that of ticarcillin. Mezlocillin is similar in activity to piperacillin but slightly less active against *P aeruginosa*. Azlocillin is as active as piperacillin against *P aeruginosa* but less active than the other ureidopenicillins against most other gram-negative organisms.

The extended-spectrum penicillins are active against most anaerobes. Ampicillin and amoxicillin are not active against β-lactamase-producing strains of *B fragilis*—in contrast to the other drugs in this class at high concentrations.

Pharmacokinetics & Administration

Ampicillin can be given orally or parenterally. The usual oral dose is 1–2 g/d (15–50 mg/kg/d), resulting in serum levels of 4–6 μg/mL. Intravenous doses range from 20 to 200 mg/kg/d (the higher doses required in meningitis), resulting in serum levels of up to 40 μg/mL. Amoxicillin is given orally only, in doses of 25–100 mg/kg/d, usually as 250 or 500 mg tablets three times daily, and is absorbed better than ampicillin, resulting in serum levels twice as high as those achieved with ampicillin. Bacampicillin, an esterified form of ampicillin that is hydrolyzed to release ampicillin, is well absorbed and can be given twice daily in a dose of 400–800 mg.

Carbenicillin is given intravenously (400–500 mg/kg/d) in doses of 5 g every 4 hours. The other carboxy- and ureidopenicillins are given intravenously (200–300 mg/kg/d) in doses of 3–4 g every 4–6 hours, resulting in serum levels of 250–300 μg/mL. Oral indanyl sodium carbenicillin is suitable only for treatment of urinary tract infections in a dose of 1–2 tablets (382 mg per tablet) every 6 hours.

Dosage adjustments in renal failure are required for the extended-spectrum penicillins and are summarized in Table 37–4.

Clinical Uses

Ampicillin and amoxicillin are given orally for minor infections, such as bronchitis, sinusitis, otitis, or urinary tract infections. Ampicillin is given intravenously for pneumonia, meningitis, bacteremia, or endocarditis. In meningitis in the neonate or elderly, ampicillin is given concurrently with a second- or third-generation cephalosporin to cover *Listeria.* Typhoid or paratyphoid fever caused by susceptible *Salmonella* is treated with ampicillin, 6–12 g/d intravenously. *Shigella* dysentery can be treated with oral ampicillin.

Amoxicillin is frequently used for urinary tract infections, sinusitis, otitis, and bronchitis and as antibacterial prophylaxis to prevent endocarditis (see section on Antimicrobial Chemoprophylaxis). It has also been used in combination with metronidazole and H₂ blockers to treat recurrent gastric and duodenal ulcers caused by *Helicobacter pylori.* Because of its better absorption from the intestinal tract, less drug remains in the intestine, and amoxicillin is thus less effective than ampicillin for shigellosis. Carbenicillin is rarely used because of its large sodium load and the coagulation abnormalities that have been associated with its use. Although ticarcillin, mezlocillin, azlocillin, and piperacillin have been used as single drugs, they are commonly used in combination with an aminoglycoside to treat serious *Pseudomonas* infections and as empiric therapy in the febrile neutropenic patient.

3. PENICILLINS COMBINED WITH BETA-LACTAMASE INHIBITORS

The addition of β-lactamase inhibitors (clavulanic acid, sulbactam) can prevent inactivation of the parent penicillin by bacterial β-lactamases. Augmentin (amoxicillin, 250 mg or 500 mg, plus 125 mg of clavulanic acid), Timentin (ticarcillin, 3 g, plus 100 mg of clavulanic acid), and Unasyn (ampicillin, 1 g, plus 500 mg of sulbactam) are available. Augmentin is given orally and the others intravenously. In general, the β-lactamase inhibitors effectively inactivate β-lactamases produced by anaerobes, *Staphylococcus aureus, H influenzae, Moraxella catarrhalis,* and *Neisseria gonorrhoeae.* thus making Augmentin, Timentin, and Unasyn effective agents for these organisms. In contrast the β-lactamase inhibitors are variably and unpredictably effective against β-lactamases produced by aerobic enteric gram-negative rods and pseudomonads and thus cannot be relied upon to treat these organisms unless specific sensitivity testing is done.

Augmentin, because of its high cost, is limited to the treatment of refractory cases of sinusitis and otitis that have not responded to less costly agents and is used for therapy and prophylaxis of infections resulting from animal and human bites. The roles of Timentin and Unasyn are not well defined at present. One possible application of these agents would be to use them alone or in combination with an aminoglycoside to treat polymicrobial infections such as peritonitis from a ruptured viscus, osteomyelitis in a diabetic patient, or traumatic osteomyelitis.

The dosage regimens of these drugs are the same as those of the parent drugs.

4. PENICILLINASE-RESISTANT PENICILLINS

Methicillin, oxacillin, cloxacillin, dicloxacillin, nafcillin, and others are relatively resistant to destruction by β-lactamases produced by staphylococci and are limited to the treatment of infections with such organisms. They are less active than natural penicillins against gram-positives and inactive against gram-negatives.

Oxacillin, cloxacillin, and dicloxacillin are given orally in doses of 0.25–0.5 g every 4–6 hours in mild or localized staphylococcal infections (50–100 mg/kg/d for children).

For serious systemic staphylococcal infections, nafcillin, 6–12 g/d, is given intravenously in four to six divided doses (50–100 mg/kg/d for children). Eighty percent of administered nafcillin is excreted into the biliary tract and only 20% by tubular secretion. Thus, the action and dose of nafcillin are little affected by renal failure.

5. ADVERSE EFFECTS OF PENICILLINS

The penicillins undoubtedly possess less direct toxicity than other antibiotics. Most of the serious side effects are due to hypersensitivity.

Allergy

All penicillins are cross-sensitizing and cross-reacting. Any preparation containing penicillin may induce sensitization, including foods or cosmetics. In general, sensitization occurs in proportion to the duration and total dose of penicillin received in the past. The responsible antigenic determinants appear to be degradation products of penicillins, particularly penicilloic acid and products of alkaline hydrolysis (minor antigenic determinants) bound to host protein. Skin tests with penicilloyl-polylysine, with minor antigenic determinants, and with undegraded penicillin can identify most hypersensitive individuals. Among positive reactors to skin tests, the incidence of subsequent immediate severe penicillin reactions is high. Although many persons develop IgG antibodies to antigenic determinants of penicillin, the presence of such antibodies is not correlated with allergic reactivity (except for rare instances of hemolytic anemia), and serologic tests have little predictive value. A history of a penicillin reaction in the past is not reliable. Only one-fourth of patients with a history of penicillin allergy have an adverse reaction when challenged with the drug. The decision to administer penicillin or related drugs (other β-lactams) to patients with an allergic history depends upon the severity of the reported reaction, the severity of the infection being treated, and the availability of alternative drugs. For patients with a history of severe reaction (anaphylaxis), alternative drugs should be used. In the rare situations when there is a strong indication for using penicillin (eg, syphilis in pregnancy) despite a history of severe reaction, desensitization can be attempted. If the history is unclear or the reaction mild (rash), the patient may be rechallenged with penicillin or may be given another β-lactam antibiotic. (See Chapter 29 for discussion and methods of desensitization.)

Allergic reactions may occur as typical anaphylactic shock, typical serum sickness type reactions (urticaria, fever, joint swelling, angioneurotic edema, intense pruritus, and respiratory embarrassment occurring 7–12 days after exposure), and a variety of skin rashes, oral lesions, fever, interstitial nephritis, eosinophilia, hemolytic anemia, other hematologic disturbances, and vasculitis. The incidence of hypersensitivity to penicillin is estimated to be 1–5% among adults in the USA but is negligible in small children. Acute anaphylactic life-threatening reactions are fortunately very rare (0.05%). Ampicillin produces maculopapular skin rashes more frequently than other penicillins, but some ampicillin rashes are not allergic in origin. The nonallergic ampicillin rash usually occurs after 3–4 days of therapy, is maculopapular, is more common in patients with coexisting viral illness (especially Epstein-Barr infection), and resolves with continued therapy. Methicillin and other penicillins can induce nephritis with primary tubular lesions associated with anti-basement membrane antibodies. Nafcillin is less nephrotoxic than methicillin.

Individuals known to be hypersensitive to penicillin can at times tolerate the drug during corticosteroid administration.

Toxicity

Since the action of penicillin is directed against a unique bacterial structure, the cell wall, it is virtually without effect on animal cells. The toxic effects of penicillin G are due to the direct irritation caused by intramuscular or intravenous injection of exceedingly high concentrations (eg, 1 g/mL). Such concentrations may cause local pain, induration, thrombophlebitis, or degeneration of an accidentally injected nerve. All penicillins are irritating to the central nervous system and can cause seizures. There is no indication for intrathecal administration at present. In rare cases, a patient with renal insufficiency receiving large doses may exhibit signs of cerebrocortical irritation as a result of passage of unusually large amounts of penicillin into the central nervous system. With doses of this magnitude, direct cation toxicity (Na^+, K^+) can also occur. Potassium penicillin G contains 1.7 meq of K^+ per million units (2.8 meq/g), and potassium may accumulate in renal failure. Carbenicillin contains 4.7 meq of Na^+ per gram—a risk in heart failure.

Large doses of penicillins given orally may lead to gastrointestinal upset, particularly nausea and diarrhea. This is most pronounced with the broad-spectrum penicillins—ampicillin or amoxicillin—and Augmentin and may be due to overgrowth of staphylococci, *Pseudomonas,* clostridia, or yeasts or to toxin production by *Clostridium difficile.* Superinfections in other organ systems may occur with penicillins as with any other antibiotic. Methicillin, nafcillin, and carbenicillin can cause granulocytopenia. Carbenicillin and ticarcillin can produce hypokalemic alkalosis and elevation of serum transaminases and can damage platelets or induce hemostatic defects leading to bleeding tendency.

Dever LA, Dermody TS: Mechanisms of bacterial resistance to antibiotics. Arch Intern Med 1991;151:886. (Molecular basis of antibiotic resistance.)

Donowitz GR, Mandell GL: Beta-lactam antibiotics. (Two parts.) N Engl J Med 1988;318:419, 490. (Activity and clinical indications.)

Wright AJ, Wilkowske CJ: The penicillins. Mayo Clin Proc 1991;66:1047. (Pharmacology, activity, and clinical indications.)

CEPHALOSPORINS
(Tables 37–6 and 37–7)

The cephalosporins are structurally related to the penicillins. They consist of a β-lactam ring attached to a dihydrothiazoline ring. Substitutions of chemical groups at various positions on the basic structure have resulted in a proliferation of drugs with varying pharmacologic properties and antimicrobial activities.

The mechanism of action of cephalosporins is analogous to that of the penicillins: (1) binding to specific penicillin-binding proteins that serve as drug receptors on bacteria, (2) inhibition of cell wall synthesis, and (3) activation of autolytic enzymes in the cell wall that result in bacterial death. Resistance to cephalosporins may be due to poor permeability of the drug into bacteria, lack of penicillin-binding proteins, or degradation by β-lactamases.

Cephalosporins have been divided into three major groups or "generations" (Table 37–6) based mainly on their antibacterial activity: First-generation cephalosporins have good activity against aerobic gram-positive organisms and many community-acquired gram-negative organisms; second-generation drugs have a slightly extended spectrum against gram-negative bacteria, and some are active against anaerobes; and third-generation cephalosporins have less activity against gram-positives but are extremely active against most gram-negative bacteria. Not all cephalosporins fit neatly into this grouping, and there are exceptions to the general characterization of the drugs in the individual classes; however, the generational classification of cephalosporins is useful for discussion purposes.

Both parenteral and oral cephalosporins—especially second- and third-generation agents—are quite costly (Table 37–5). Because of their broad spectrum of activity and low toxicity, these drugs are used to treat many infections. As discussed below, cephalosporins are infrequently the drug of first choice (see Tables 37–2 and 37–3), but they are useful in certain specific clinical settings. Because of their cost, their broad spectrum of activity, and concerns about se-

lecting for resistant organisms, the use of cephalosporins should be limited to those situations in which clear-cut superiority over less expensive drugs with more narrow spectrums of activity has been demonstrated.

1. FIRST-GENERATION CEPHALOSPORINS

Antimicrobial Activity

These drugs are very active against gram-positive cocci, including pneumococci, viridans streptococci, group A hemolytic streptococci, and *S aureus*. Like all cephalosporins, they are inactive against enterococci and methicillin-resistant staphylococci. Among gram-negative bacteria, *E coli*, *Klebsiella pneumoniae*, and *P mirabilis* are usually sensitive except for some hospital-acquired strains. There is very little activity against such gram-negatives as *P aeruginosa*, indole-positive *Proteus*, *Enterobacter*, *Serratia marcescens*, *Citrobacter*, and *Acinetobacter*. Anaerobic cocci are usually sensitive, but *B fragilis* is not.

Pharmacokinetics & Administration

A. Oral: Cephalexin, cephradine, and cefadroxil are variably absorbed from the gut. Urine levels of these drugs are several hundred times higher than serum levels, but concentrations in other tissues are variable and usually lower than in the serum. Cefadroxil, because of its longer half-life, can be given twice daily. Dosage adjustment is required in renal insufficiency.

B. Intravenous: Cefazolin is preferred over cephalothin and cephapirin because it has a longer half-life, requires less frequent dosing, and achieves higher serum levels. In renal insufficiency, all of these agents require dosage adjustments.

C. Intramuscular: Both cephapirin and cefazolin can be given intramuscularly, but pain on injection is less with cefazolin.

Clinical Uses

Although the first-generation cephalosporins have a broad spectrum of activity and are relatively nontoxic, they are rarely the drugs of choice. Oral drugs are indicated for treatment of urogenital infections in patients who are allergic to sulfonamides or penicillins, and they can be used for minor staphylococcal infections in penicillin-allergic patients. Oral cephalosporins may also be preferred for minor polymicrobial infections (eg, cellulitis, soft tissue abscess). Oral cephalosporins should not be relied on in serious systemic infections.

Intravenous first-generation cephalosporins penetrate most tissues well and are the drugs of choice for surgical prophylaxis, particularly surgery undertaken for placement of a prosthesis. More expensive sec-

Table 37–6. Major groups of cephalosporins.

First Generation	Second Generation	Third Generation
Cephalothin	Cefamandole	Cefotaxime
Cephapirin	Cefuroxime	Ceftizoxime
Cefazolin	Cefonicid	Ceftriaxone
Cefalexin[1]	Ceforanide	Ceftazidime
Cephadrine[1]	Cefaclor[1]	Cefoperazone
Cefadroxil[1]	Cefoxitin	Moxalactam
	Cefotetan	Cefixime[1]
	Cefprozil[1]	Cefpodoxime
	Cefuroxime axetil[1]	proxetil[1]
	Cefmetazole	

[1]Oral agents

Table 37–7. Pharmacology of the cephalosporins.

Drug	Peak Serum Level (μg/mL) After 1 g IV	Serum Half-Life (min)	Total Daily Dose (mg/kg)	Dosage Interval (hours)	Dosage Adjustments in Renal Failure		
					Moderate (Cl$_{cr}$ 10–50 mL/min)	Severe (Cl$_{cr}$ <10 mL/min)	Post-hemodialysis Dose
Cephalothin, cephapirin	40–60	40	50–200	4–6	1–2 g every 6–12 hours	1 g every 12 hours	1 g
Cefazolin	90–120	90	25–100	8	0.5–1 g every 12 hours	0.5 g daily	0.5 g
Cephalexin, cephradine[1]	15–20	50–60	15–30	6	0.25–0.5 g every 8–12 hours	0.25–0.5 g daily	0.5 g
Cefadroxil[1]	15	75	15–30	12–24	1 g daily	0.5 g daily	0.5 g
Cefamandole	60–80	45	75–200	6–8	1 g every 12 hours	1–2 g daily	0.5 g
Cefuroxime	80–100	80	50	6–12	1 g every 12 hours	1–2 g daily	0.5 g
Cefuroxime ax-etil[1]	6–8	75	5–15	12	0.5 g every 24 hours	0.25 g daily	0.25 g
Cefonicid	200–250	240	15–30	24	0.5 g daily	1 g every 72 hours	0.25 g
Ceforanide	125	180	15–30	12	1 g daily	1 g every 48 hours	0.25 g
Cefaclor[1]	15–20	50	20–40 children, 10–15 adults	6–8	0.5 g every 8–12 hours	0.25–0.5 g every 12–24 hours	0.25–0.5 g
Cefixime[1]	3–5	180–240	8 (with maximum of 0.4 g/d total)	12–24	0.4 g daily	0.1 g daily	None
Cefpodoxime proxetil[1]	2	150	5	12	0.2 g every 24 hours	0.2 g 3 times per week after dialysis	0.2 g
Cefprozil[1]	10	90	10–15	12	0.5 g every 12–24 hours	0.25–0.5 g every 12–24 hours	0.5 g
Cefotetan	60–80	150	50–100	8–12	1 g every 8–12 hours	0.5–1 g daily	0.5 g
Cefotaxime	40–60	60	50–75	6–8	1–2 g every 6–8 hours	1–2 g every 12 hours	1–2 g
Cefoxitin	60–80	60	50–100	6–8	1 g every 12 hours	1–2 g daily	0.5 g
Cefmetazole	70–100	60–80	50–100	6–8	1 g every 12–24 hours	1–2 g every 24–48 hours	1 g
Ceftizoxime	80–100	100	50–75	8–12	0.5–1 g every 8–12 hours	0.25–0.5 g every 12–24 hours	0.5 g
Ceftriaxone	150	480	30–50	12–24	1–2 g daily	1–2 g daily	None
Ceftazidime	100–120	120	50–75	8–12	1 g every 12 hours	0.5–1 g daily	0.5 g
Cefoperazone	150	120	30–200	8–12	1–2 g every 12 hours	1–2 g every 12 hours	None
Loracarbef[1]	10	60	10–15	12	0.2 g every 24 hours	0.2 g 3 times per week after dialysis	0.2 g
Moxalactam	60–100	120	50–200	6–12	0.5–1 g every 12 hours	0.25–0.5 g every 12 hours	0.5 g

[1]Oral agents. Serum levels based on 0.5 g oral dose.

ond- and third-generation cephalosporins offer no advantage over the first-generation drugs for surgical prophylaxis and should not be used for that purpose.

Other major uses of intravenous first-generation cephalosporins include infections for which they are the least toxic drugs (eg, *Klebsiella* infections) and infections in persons with a history of *mild* penicillin allergy (not anaphylaxis).

First-generation cephalosporins do not penetrate the cerebrospinal fluid and cannot be used to treat meningitis.

2. SECOND-GENERATION CEPHALOSPORINS

Second-generation cephalosporins are a heterogeneous group with marked individual differences in activity, pharmacokinetics, and toxicity. In general, all are active against organisms also covered by first-generation drugs, but they have an extended gram-negative coverage. *Enterobacter,* indole-positive *Proteus,* and *Klebsiella* (including cephalothin-resistant strains) are usually sensitive. Cefamandole, cefuroxime, cefonicid, ceforanide, cefuroxime axetil, cefprozil, and cefaclor are active against *H influenzae,* including β-lactamase-producing strains, but have little activity against *Serratia* and *B fragilis.* In contrast, cefoxitin and cefotetan are active against 80–90% of strains of *B fragilis* and some strains of *Serratia* but have poor activity against *Enterobacter* and *H influenzae.* Cefmetazole is similar in activity to cefoxitin and cefotetan but has more activity against *H influenzae.* Against gram-positive organisms, these drugs are less active than the first-generation cephalosporins. Like the latter, second-generation drugs have no activity against *P aeruginosa* or enterococci.

Pharmacokinetics & Administration

A. Oral: Only cefaclor, cefuroxime axetil, and cefprozil can be given orally. Cefaclor and cefprozil are available as capsules (0.25 or 0.5 g) and in suspension (0.125 or 0.25 g/5 mL). Cefuroxime axetil releases cefuroxime after absorption. Its longer half-life permits twice-daily dosing. It is available only in tablet form, and absorption is enhanced when it is taken with food (as is not the case with many other oral antibiotics).

B. Intravenous and Intramuscular: Because of differences in drug half-life and protein binding, peak serum levels achieved and dosing intervals vary greatly for this group of drugs (Table 37–7). Drugs with shorter half-lives (cefoxitin, cefamandole) require higher doses and more frequent dosing than drugs with longer half-lives (cefuroxime, cefonicid, ceforanide, cefotetan). Dosage adjustments are required with renal impairment.

Clinical Uses

Because of their activity against β-lactamase-producing *H influenzae* and *M catarrhalis,* cefaclor, cefprozil, and cefuroxime axetil can be used to treat sinusitis and otitis media in patients who are allergic to ampicillin or amoxicillin or have not responded to treatment with those drugs. Cefuroxime is the only second-generation cephalosporin that crosses the blood-brain barrier in sufficient amounts to be useful for treatment of meningitis, but treatment failures have been described, and this drug should be used with caution in this setting.

Because of their activity against *B fragilis,* cefoxitin, cefmetazole, and cefotetan can be used to treat mixed anaerobic infections, eg, peritonitis and diverticulitis. Ceftriaxone is indicated for the therapy of gonorrhea, chancroid, and certain more serious forms of Lyme disease (see Chapter 33). Because of its long half-life and once-daily dosing requirement, ceftriaxone is also an ideal drug for use for outpatient parenteral therapy of infections due to susceptible organisms. Cefonicid and ceforanide have been promoted for use in surgical prophylaxis, but there is no evidence that they are more effective than first-generation cephalosporins, and they tend to be more expensive. Cefamandole, like cefuroxime, may be useful for the treatment of community-acquired pneumonia, but it has few other uses.

3. THIRD-GENERATION CEPHALOSPORINS

Antimicrobial Activity

These drugs are active against staphylococci (not methicillin-resistant strains) but less so than first-generation cephalosporins. They have no activity against enterococci but do inhibit nonenterococcal streptococci. A major advantage of these cephalosporins is their expanded gram-negative coverage. In addition to organisms inhibited by other cephalosporins, they are consistently active against *Citrobacter freundii, S marcescens, Providencia, Haemophilus,* and *Neisseria,* including β-lactamase-producing strains. Two drugs—ceftazidime and cefoperazone—have good activity against *P aeruginosa,* whereas the others inhibit only 40–60% of strains. *Acinetobacter, Enterobacter,* and non-*aeruginosa* strains of *Pseudomonas* are variably sensitive to third-generation cephalosporins, and *Listeria* is resistant. Activity against *B fragilis* is variable, and these agents should not be relied upon to treat serious infections with this organism.

Cefixime and cefpodoxime proxetil, the only oral agents in this group, are more active than cefuroxime axetil but are not as active as parenteral third-generation cephalosporins against gram-negative organisms such as *Pseudomonas, Enterobacter, Morganella,* and *S marcescens.* Cefpodoxime proxetil has greater activity than cefixime against methicillin-sensitive *S aureus* and *Staphylococcus epidermidis* (neither is active against methicillin-resistant strain), and, like other members of this class, both drugs are inactive against enterococci and *Listeria monocytogenes.*

Pharmacokinetics & Administration

These agents penetrate well into body fluids and tissues and—except for cefoperazone—reach levels in the cerebrospinal fluid that exceed those needed to inhibit most pathogens, including gram-negative rods. The half-lives of these drugs are variable, which accounts for the differences in dosing intervals (Table 37–7). Cefoperazone and ceftriaxone are eliminated primarily by biliary excretion, and no dosage adjustment is required in renal insufficiency. The other drugs are eliminated by the kidney and thus require dosage adjustments in renal insufficiency.

Clinical Uses

Because of their penetration into the cerebrospinal fluid, third-generation cephalosporins—except cefoperazone—can be used to treat meningitis. Meningitis due to pneumococci, meningococci, *H influenzae,* and susceptible enteric gram-negative rods has been successfully treated. In meningitis in the elderly, third-generation cephalosporins should be combined with ampicillin until *L monocytogenes* has been excluded as the etiologic agent. Ceftazidime has been used to treat *Pseudomonas* meningitis. The dosage for meningitis should be near the top of the recommended range, because cerebrospinal fluid levels of these drugs are only 10–20% of serum levels. However, since 10–20% of *B fragilis* and many enteric gram-negative organisms are resistant to these drugs, for severe life-threatening intra-abdominal infections metronidazole plus an aminoglycoside or third-generation cephalosporin is preferred.

Other potential indications include (1) infections in which cephalosporins are the least toxic agent available; (2) sepsis of unknown cause in the immunocompetent patient; and (3) fever in the immunocompromised neutropenic patient, in which case the drug should be given in combination with an aminoglycoside.

Cefixime, because of its long half-life, can be given once daily. For improved compliance, this may be advantageous in treating sinusitis and otitis in children. Cefixime (400 mg as a single dose) and cefpodoxime proxetil (200 mg as a single dose) are as effective as ceftriaxone (250 mg intramuscularly) for the therapy of genital and pharyngeal gonorrhea.

Because of the high cost of third-generation cephalosporins, their use should be limited. When they are used empirically, therapy can be changed to the most efficacious, least toxic, and least expensive drug once the etiologic agent has been identified.

4. ADVERSE EFFECTS OF CEPHALOSPORINS

Allergy

Cephalosporins are sensitizing, and a variety of hypersensitivity reactions occur, including anaphylaxis, fever, skin rashes, nephritis, granulocytopenia, and hemolytic anemia. The frequency of cross-allergy between cephalosporins and penicillins is not known but is estimated to be about 6–10%. Persons with a history of anaphylaxis to penicillins should not receive cephalosporins.

Toxicity

Local pain can occur after intramuscular injection, or thrombophlebitis after intravenous injection. Hypoprothrombinemia is a frequent adverse effect (40–68%) of cephalosporins that have a methylthiotetrazole group (eg, cefamandole, moxalactam, cefmetazole, cefoperazone, cefotetan). Prophylactic administration of vitamin K, 10 mg twice weekly, can prevent this complication. Moxalactam interferes with platelet function and has been associated with severe bleeding. Drugs containing the methylthiotetrazole ring can also cause severe disulfiram-like reactions, and use of alcohol or medications containing alcohol (eg, theophylline elixir) must be avoided. Ceftriaxone has been associated with cholelithiasis due to precipitation of drug when its solubility in bile is exceeded.

Superinfection

Many newer cephalosporins have little activity against gram-positive organisms, particularly staphylococci and enterococci. Superinfection with these organisms—as well as with fungi—may occur.

Donowitz GR, Mandell GL: Beta-lactam antibiotics. (Two parts.) N Engl J Med 1988;318:419, 490.

Gustaferro CA, Steckelberg JM: Cephalosporin antimicrobial agents and related compounds. Mayo Clin Proc 1991;66:1064. (Activity, pharmacology, toxicity, and clinical uses.)

OTHER BETA-LACTAM DRUGS

Monobactams

These are drugs with a monocyclic β-lactam ring that are resistant to β-lactamases and active against gram-negative organisms (including *Pseudomonas*) but have no activity against gram-positive organisms or anaerobes. Aztreonam resembles aminoglycosides in activity. The usual dose is 1–2 g intravenously every 6–8 hours, providing peak serum levels of 100 µg/mL. Clinical uses of aztreonam are limited because of the availability of third-generation cephalosporins with a broader spectrum of activity and minimal toxicity. When administered orally, aztreonam is poorly absorbed and reaches very high levels in the gastrointestinal tract. This property, along with its activity against most bacterial enteropathogens, has made it a useful agent for the therapy of traveler's diarrhea. Despite the structural similarity of aztreonam to other β-lactam drugs, cross-reactivity with them is limited and it can be used in most patients with penicillin allergy.

Carbapenems

This class of drugs is structurally related to β-lactam antibiotics. Imipenem, the first drug of this type, has a wide spectrum of activity that includes most gram-negative rods (including *P aeruginosa*) and gram-positive organisms and anaerobes, with the exception of *Pseudomonas cepacia, Pseudomonas maltophilia, Streptococcus faecium,* and most methicillin-resistant *S aureus* and *S epidermidis.* It is resistant to β-lactamases but is inactivated by dipeptidases in renal tubules. Consequently, it must be combined with cilastatin, a dipeptidase inhibitor, for clinical use.

The half-life of imipenem is 1 hour. Penetration into body tissues and fluids, including the cerebrospinal fluid, is good. The usual dose is 0.5–1 g intravenously every 6 hours. Dosage adjustment is required in renal insufficiency. For patients with creatinine clearances of 10–30 mL/min, one-half the usual dose is given; for those with clearances of 10 mL/min, 0.5 g is given every 12 hours. An additional dose is given after hemodialysis.

The role of imipenem in therapy has not been defined. Because of its high cost and broad spectrum of activity, it should not be routinely used as first-line therapy unless the organism causing infection is multidrug-resistant and is known to be sensitive to imipenem. In patients hospitalized for a prolonged period who may have infection with a multi-drug-resistant organism, empiric use of imipenem while awaiting culture results is reasonable. *Pseudomonas* may rapidly develop resistance to imipenem. The use of imipenem alone appears to be as effective as combination therapy in the febrile neutropenic patient.

The most common adverse effects of imipenem are nausea, vomiting, diarrhea, reactions at the infusion site, and skin rashes. Seizures can occur, especially in patients with impaired renal function. Patients allergic to penicillins may be allergic to imipenem as well.

Carbacephems

Loracarbef is a beta-lactam antibiotic that is structurally similar to cefaclor except that a methylene group has replaced the sulfur in the dihydrothiazine ring. This structural change adds chemical stability to the drug but does not greatly enhance antibacterial activity, which is essentially the same as that of cefaclor, cefuroxime axetil, and cefprozil. The high cost of loracarbef precludes its use as a first-line

agent, and it should be reserved for the therapy of sinusitis, otitis media, bronchitis, and urinary tract infections in patients who have failed therapy with less familiar agents (eg, ampicillin, amoxicillin, trimethoprim-sulfamethoxazole). The usual dose is 200–400 mg orally every 12 hours.

Aztreonam: The expanding clinical profile. Rev Inf Dis 1991;13:(Suppl 7):1. (Summary of clinical trials.)
Hellinger WC, Brewer NS: Imipenem. Mayo Clin Proc 1991;66:1074. (Activity, pharmacology, and clinical indications.)

ERYTHROMYCIN GROUP (Macrolides)

The erythromycins are a group of closely related compounds characterized by a macrocyclic lactone ring to which various sugars are attached.

Antimicrobial Activity

Erythromycins inhibit protein synthesis by binding to the 50S subunit of bacterial ribosomes. They are bacteriostatic or bactericidal for gram-positive organisms, including pneumococci, streptococci, and corynebacteria in a concentration of 0.02–2 μg/mL. Chlamydiae, mycoplasmas, *Legionella,* and *Campylobacter* are also susceptible. There is complete cross-resistance among all members of the group. Activity is enhanced at alkaline pH.

Pharmacokinetics & Administration

Preparations for oral use include erythromycin base, erythromycin stearate, estolate, and ethyl succinate. The base is most acid-stable and the estolate is the best-absorbed of the oral forms. Clinically, however, none of the oral preparations have any advantage over others. The usual adult oral dose is 250–500 mg four times daily, resulting in serum levels of 1–2 μg/mL. Erythromycins are excreted largely in the bile; only 5% is excreted in the urine, and no adjustment is therefore required in renal failure.

Erythromycin lactobionate and gluceptate are available for intravenous use. The usual dose is 250–500 mg every 6 hours, but larger doses (1 g every 6 hours) are used initially in the treatment of legionnaires' disease.

Clinical Uses

Erythromycins are drugs of choice for infections caused by *Legionella, Mycoplasma, Corynebacterium* (including diphtheria and bacteremia), and *Chlamydia* (including ocular, respiratory, and genital infections). They are effective in streptococcal and pneumococcal disease and for endocarditis prophylaxis in dental procedures in penicillin-allergic patients. They can also be used in combination with sulfisoxazole for acute otitis media; with neomycin in prophylaxis for bowel surgery; and for therapy of syphilis in penicillin-allergic patients. When administered early, erythromycin may shorten the course of *Campylobacter* enteritis. Spiramycin may be useful in treating acute toxoplasmosis in pregnant women in the first trimester and congenital toxoplasmosis.

Adverse Effects

Nausea, vomiting, and diarrhea may occur after oral intake. Erythromycins—particularly the estolate—can produce acute cholestatic hepatitis (fever, jaundice, impaired liver function), probably as a hypersensitivity reaction. Most patients recover, but hepatitis recurs if the drug is readministered. Reversible auditory impairment can occur when large doses (4 g/d or more) are given to patients with impaired renal or hepatic function. Erythromycins can increase the effects of oral anticoagulants, digoxin, theophylline, and cyclosporine by competition for protein-binding sites in serum. Patients taking these medications who are treated with erythromycin should have levels monitored and dosages adjusted appropriately. Erythromycin can also result in accumulation of terfenadine, resulting in prolongation of the QT interval and ventricular arrhythmias. This drug combination should be avoided.

Smilack JD, Wilson WR, Cockerill FR III: Tetracyclines, chloramphenicol, erythromycin, clindamycin and metronidazole. Mayo Clin Proc 1991;66:1270. (Activity, adverse effects, and clinical indications.)

AZALIDES

Azalides (azithromycin, clarithromycin, and others) are a group of antibiotics closely related structurally to the macrolides. Like erythromycin, they are active against *Streptococcus pneumoniae,* group A streptococcus, viridans streptococci, *M catarrhalis, Legionella, Mycoplasma pneumoniae,* and *Chlamydia pneumoniae* and are slightly more active than erythromycin against *H influenzae* (with azithromycin having better activity than clarithromycin against the latter pathogen). They are also active against *Chlamydia trachomatis* and *Haemophilus ducreyi.* In addition, these drugs have in vitro activity against a number of unusual pathogens. including atypical mycobacteria *(Mycobacterium avium-intracellulare, Mycobacterium chelonei, Mycobacterium fortuitum, Mycobacterium marinum), Toxoplasma gondii,* and *Borrelia burgdorferi.*

The azalides are more acid-stable than erythromycin, penetrate tissues well, and have a long terminal half-life, with high tissue concentrations that persist for days. Azithromycin and clarithromycin are approved for treatment of streptococcal pharyngitis, uncomplicated skin infections, and acute bacterial exacerbations of chronic bronchitis. Because of the long half-life, treatment with azithromycin is with once-daily dosing for a total of 5 days (500 mg on day 1 and then 250 mg on days 2–5). Clarithromycin is usually administered in a dose of 250–500 mg twice daily.

The azalides are more expensive than erythromycin. Whether the decreased gastrointestinal distress, shorter course of therapy, and once-daily administration needed with these drugs outweighs the increased cost is yet to be determined.

Azithromycin has also been approved as single-dose therapy (1 g) for chlamydial genital infections. This is much more expensive than 7 days of treatment with doxycycline (Table 37–5), but the assurance of adequate supervised therapy for this infection makes azithromycin preferred therapy in some patients. Azithromycin is as effective as amoxicillin or doxycycline for the therapy of early Lyme disease but is much more costly and offers little advantage. Clarithromycin has been used for the therapy of *Mycobacterium avium-intracellulare* infections, usually in combination with other drugs (eg, rifabutin, clofazimine, ethambutol). The role of these agents in the therapy of toxoplasmal encephalitis is under investigation.

Neu HC: New macrolide antibiotics: Azithromycin and clarithromycin. Ann Intern Med 1992;116:517. (Editorial summarizing activity and potential uses.)

TETRACYCLINE GROUP

The tetracyclines are a large group of drugs with common basic chemical structures, antimicrobial activity, and pharmacologic properties. Microorganisms resistant to this group show extensive cross-resistance to all tetracyclines.

Antimicrobial Activity

Tetracyclines are inhibitors of protein synthesis and are bacteriostatic for many gram-positive and gram-negative bacteria. They are strongly inhibitory for the growth of mycoplasmas, rickettsiae, chlamydiae, spirochetes, and some protozoa (eg, amebas). Equal concentrations of all tetracyclines in blood or tissue have approximately equal antimicrobial activity. However, there are great differences in the susceptibility of different strains of a given species of microorganism, and laboratory tests are therefore important. Because of the emergence of resistant strains, tetracyclines have lost some of their former usefulness. *Proteus* and *Pseudomonas* are regularly resistant; resistant *Bacteroides,* pneumococci, staphylococci, streptococci, shigellae, and vibrios are increasingly common.

Pharmacokinetics & Administration

Tetracyclines are absorbed irregularly from the

gut. Absorption is impaired by dairy products, aluminum hydroxide gels (antacids), and chelation with divalent cations, eg, Ca^{2+} or Fe^{2+}. Absorption is least with chlortetracycline (30%); intermediate with tetracycline, oxytetracycline, and demeclocycline (60–80%); and highest with doxycycline and minocycline (95% or more). An oral dose of 250 mg of tetracycline hydrochloride gives serum levels of 2–3 μg/mL, and 100 mg of doxycycline gives serum levels of 1–2 μg/mL. Tetracyclines are widely distributed in tissues, but levels in the central nervous system, cerebrospinal fluid, and joint fluid are only 5–15% of serum levels.

The usual dose of tetracyclines is 250–500 mg four times daily. Doxycycline and minocycline are given as 100 mg twice daily and demeclocycline and methacycline as 150 mg four times daily or 300 mg twice daily.

Tetracyclines are metabolized in the liver and concentrated in bile. Excretion is mainly through bile and urine. All tetracyclines—except doxycycline—accumulate in renal insufficiency and are antianabolic in high doses. Doxycycline requires no dosage adjustment in renal failure; the other tetracyclines should be avoided or given in reduced dosage.

For patients unable to take oral medication, some tetracyclines are formulated for parenteral administration in doses similar to the oral ones. A 1% topical tetracycline ointment is available for conjunctival infections.

Clinical Uses

Tetracyclines are the drugs of choice for chlamydial, rickettsial, and *Vibrio* infections and some spirochetal infections. Sexually transmitted diseases in which chlamydiae often play a role—endocervicitis, urethritis, proctitis, and epididymitis—should be treated with a tetracycline for 7–14 days. Pelvic inflammatory disease is often treated with doxycycline plus cefoxitin. Other chlamydial infections (psittacosis, lymphogranuloma venereum, trachoma) and sexually transmitted diseases (granuloma inguinale) also respond to tetracyclines. Other uses include treatment of acne, urinary tract infections, exacerbations of bronchitis, Lyme disease and relapsing fever, brucellosis and tularemia (often in combination with streptomycin), cholera, mycoplasmal pneumonia, and infections caused by *M marinum* and *Pasteurella multocida* (often after an animal bite). Tetracycline has also been used in combination with other drugs for amebiasis, falciparum malaria, and recurrent ulcers due to *H pylori*.

Minocycline achieves a high concentration in the saliva and can be used for eradication of meningococci in carriers who cannot tolerate rifampin.

Adverse Effects

A. Allergy: Hypersensitivity reactions with fever or skin rashes are uncommon.

B. Gastrointestinal Side Effects: Gastrointestinal side effects, especially diarrhea, nausea, and anorexia, are common. These can be diminished by reducing the dose, but sometimes they force discontinuance of the drug. After a few days of oral use, the gut flora is modified so that drug-resistant bacteria and yeasts become prominent. This may cause functional gut disturbances, anal pruritus, and even enterocolitis with shock and death.

C. Bones and Teeth: Tetracyclines are bound to calcium deposited in growing bones and teeth, causing fluorescence, discoloration, enamel dysplasia, deformity, or growth inhibition. Therefore, tetracyclines should not be given to pregnant women or children under 6 years of age.

D. Liver Damage: Tetracyclines can impair hepatic function or even cause liver necrosis, particularly during pregnancy, in the presence of preexisting liver damage, or with doses of more than 3 g intravenously.

E. Kidney Damage: Outdated tetracycline preparations have been implicated in renal tubular acidosis and other forms of renal damage. Tetracyclines may increase blood urea nitrogen when diuretics are administered.

F. Other: Vaginal candidiasis is a common complication of tetracycline therapy. Tetracyclines—principally demeclocycline—may induce photosensitization, especially in fair-skinned individuals. Intravenous injection may cause thrombophlebitis, and intramuscular injection may induce local inflammation with pain. Minocycline induces vestibular reactions (dizziness, vertigo, nausea, vomiting), with a frequency of 35–70% after doses of 200 mg daily. Demeclocycline inhibits antidiuretic hormone.

CHLORAMPHENICOL

Antimicrobial Activity

Chloramphenicol is active against many gram-positive and gram-negative bacteria and rickettsiae. It binds to the 50S subunit of ribosomes and inhibits protein synthesis. It is bacteriostatic for most organisms but bactericidal for *S pneumoniae*, *H influenzae*, and *Neisseria meningitidis*. This bactericidal activity accounts for the efficacy of chloramphenicol in the treatment of meningitis caused by these organisms.

Pharmacokinetics & Administration

For most systemic infections, chloramphenicol, 30 mg/kg/d, is given intravenously, but meningitis in adults may require 50 mg/kg/d in four divided doses. With a dose of 1 g intravenously, serum levels reach 15–20 μg/mL. Since the intravenous preparation chloramphenicol sodium succinate must be hydrolyzed to active drug by nonspecific plasma esterases, it yields somewhat lower levels than the oral form. A 1 g oral dose gives serum levels of 20–25 μg/mL.

Chloramphenicol is widely distributed in tissues, including the eye and central nervous system. Cerebrospinal fluid levels are 70–80% of serum levels, and the levels in brain tissue may even exceed those in serum.

Chloramphenicol is metabolized in the liver, and less than 10% is excreted unchanged in the urine. Thus, no dosage adjustment is needed in renal insufficiency. Patients with liver disease may accumulate the drug, and levels should be monitored.

Clinical Uses

Because of potential toxicity and the availability of other effective drugs (eg, cephalosporins), chloramphenicol is a possible choice only in the following circumstances: (1) Symptomatic *Salmonella* infections, eg, typhoid fever. Many strains of *Salmonella* are resistant to chloramphenicol, and trimethoprim-sulfamethoxazole, ceftriaxone, or ciprofloxacin is often used. (2) Serious infections with *H influenzae*, eg, meningitis, epiglottitis, pneumonia. However, cefotaxime or ceftriaxone may be considered drugs of choice. (3) Meningococcal or pneumococcal infections of the central nervous system in patients hypersensitive to β-lactam drugs. (4) Anaerobic or mixed infections in the central nervous system, eg, brain abscess. (5) Topical chloramphenicol is occasionally used in ophthalmic infections. Rarely, chloramphenicol is used as an alternative to tetracyclines in rickettsial infections, especially in pregnant women, in whom tetracycline is contraindicated.

Adverse Effects

Nausea, vomiting, and diarrhea occur infrequently. The most serious adverse effects pertain to the hematopoietic system. Adults taking chloramphenicol in excess of 50 mg/kg/d regularly exhibit disturbances in red cell maturation within 1–2 weeks. There is anemia, rise in serum iron concentration, reticulocytopenia, and the appearance of vacuolated nucleated red cells in the bone marrow. These changes regress when the drug is stopped and are not related to the rare aplastic anemia.

Serious aplastic anemia is a rare consequence of chloramphenicol administration and represents a specific, probably genetically determined individual defect. It is seen more frequently with prolonged or repeated use. It tends to be irreversible. It has been estimated that fatal aplastic anemia occurs in one of 25–40 thousand courses of chloramphenicol treatment. Hypoplastic anemia may be followed by the development of leukemia.

Chloramphenicol inhibits the metabolism of certain drugs. Thus, it may prolong the action and raise the blood concentration of tolbutamide, phenytoin, chlorpropamide, and warfarin sodium.

Chloramphenicol is specifically toxic for newborns, particularly premature infants. Because they lack the mechanism for detoxification of the drug in the liver, the drug may accumulate, producing the highly fatal "gray syndrome," with vomiting, flaccidity, hypothermia, and collapse.

Smilack JD, Wilson WR, Cockerill FR III: Tetracyclines, chloramphenicol, erythromycin, clindamycin and metronidazole. Mayo Clin Proc 1991;66:1270. (Activity, adverse effects, and clinical indications.)

AMINOGLYCOSIDES

Aminoglycosides are a group of bactericidal drugs sharing chemical, antimicrobial, pharmacologic, and toxic characteristics. At present, the group includes streptomycin, neomycin, kanamycin, amikacin, gentamicin, tobramycin, sisomicin, netilmicin, and others. All these agents inhibit protein synthesis in bacteria by attaching to and inhibiting the function of the 30S subunit of the bacterial ribosome. Resistance is based on (1) a deficiency of the ribosomal receptor (chromosomal mutant); (2) the enzymatic destruction of the drug (plasmid-mediated transmissible resistance of clinical importance) by acetylation, phosphorylation, or adenylylation; or (3) a lack of permeability to the drug molecule or failure of active transport across cell membranes. (This can be chromosomal, eg, streptococci are relatively impermeable to aminoglycosides; or plasmid-mediated, eg, in gram-negative enteric bacteria.) Anaerobic bacteria are resistant to aminoglycosides because transport across the cell membrane is an oxygen-dependent energy-requiring process.

All aminoglycosides are more active at alkaline than at acid pH. All are potentially ototoxic and nephrotoxic, though to different degrees. All can accumulate in renal insufficiency; therefore, dosage adjustments must be made in patients with renal dysfunction (see Table 37–8).

Aminoglycosides are used most widely against gram-negative enteric bacteria or when there is a suspicion of sepsis. Although aminoglycosides demonstrate in vitro activity against many gram-positive bacteria, they should never be used alone to treat infections caused by these organisms—both because there is no clinical experience with the treatment of such infections and because less toxic alternatives are available. In the treatment of bacteremia or endocarditis caused by fecal enterococci or by some gram-negative bacteria, the aminoglycoside is given together with a β-lactam drug to enhance permeability and facilitate the entry of the aminoglycoside. Aminoglycosides are selected according to recent susceptibility patterns in a given area or hospital until susceptibility tests become available on a specific isolate.

Table 37–8. Dosing of aminoglycosides.[1]

1. Select loading dose in mg/kg (ideal weight) to provide peak serum levels in range listed below for desired aminoglycoside.

Aminoglycoside	Usual Loading Doses	Expected Peak Serum Levels
Tobramycin		
	1.5–2 mg/kg	4–10 µg/mL
Gentamicin		
Amikacin		
	5–7.5 mg/kg	15–30 µg/mL
Kanamycin		

2. Select maintenance dose (as percentage of chosen loading dose) to continue peak serum levels indicated above according to desired dosing interval and the patient's corrected creatinine clearance.[2]

		Percentage of Loading Dose Required for Dosage Interval Selected		
C(c)cr (mL/min)	Half-Life[3] (hours)	8 hours	12 hours	24 hours
90	3.1	84%	. . .	. . .
80	3.4	80	91%	. . .
70	3.9	76	88	. . .
60	4.5	71	84	. . .
50	5.3	65	79	. . .
40	6.5	57	72	92%
30	8.4	48	63	86
25	9.9	43	57	81
20	11.9	37	50	75
17	13.6	33	46	70
15	15.1	31	42	67
12	17.9	27	37	61
10[4]	20.4	24	34	56
7	25.9	19	28	47
5	31.5	16	23	41
2	46.8	11	16	30
0	69.3	8	11	21

[1]Reproduced, with permission, from Sarubbi FA, Hull JH: Amikacin serum concentrations: Prediction of levels and dosage guidelines. Ann Intern Med 1978;89(Part 1):612.
[2]Calculate corrected creatinine clearance [C(c)cr] as follows:

$$C(c)cr \text{ male} = 140 - \text{Age} \div \text{Serum creatinine}$$
$$C(c)cr \text{ female} = 0.85 \times C(c)cr \text{ male}$$

[3]Alternatively, one-half of the chosen loading dose may be given at an interval approximately equal to the estimated half-life.
[4]Dosing for patients with C(c)cr $\leq$ 10 mL/min should be assisted by measured serum levels.

General Properties of Aminoglycosides

Because of the similarities of the aminoglycosides, a summary of properties is presented briefly.

A. Physical Properties: Aminoglycosides are water-soluble and stable in solution. If they are mixed in solution with β-lactam antibiotics, they may form complexes and lose some activity.

B. Absorption, Distribution, Metabolism, and Excretion: Aminoglycosides are well absorbed after intramuscular or intravenous injection, but they are not absorbed from the gut. They are distributed widely in tissues and penetrate into pleural, peritoneal, or joint fluid in the presence of inflammation. They diffuse poorly into the eye, prostate, bile, central nervous system, or spinal fluid after parenteral injection.

There is no significant metabolic breakdown of aminoglycosides. The serum half-life is 2–3 hours. Excretion is almost entirely by glomerular filtration.

Urine levels usually are 10–50 times higher. Aminoglycosides are removed fairly effectively by hemodialysis but irregularly by peritoneal dialysis.

C. Dose and Effect of Impaired Renal Function: In persons with normal renal function, the dose of kanamycin or amikacin is 15 mg/kg/d in two divided doses; that for gentamicin or tobramycin is 4.5–6 mg/kg/d, usually injected in three equal amounts every 8 hours. Studies in patients with normal renal function employing a single large daily dose of gentamicin or tobramycin (5–6 mg/kg) have indicated that this dosing regimen is just as efficacious as and no more toxic than smaller amounts administered every 8 hours.

In persons with impaired renal function, excretion is diminished and there is the danger of drug accumulation with increased side effects. Therefore, if the interval is kept constant, the dose has to be reduced, or the interval must be increased if the dose is kept constant. Nomograms have been constructed relating creatinine clearance to adjustments of treatment regimens. One widely used nomogram is shown in Table 37–8. Because aminoglycoside levels vary considerably in different patients with similar creatinine values, serum drug levels should be monitored to avoid severe toxicity, especially when renal function is rapidly changing.

D. Adverse Effects: All aminoglycosides can cause varying degrees of ototoxicity and nephrotoxicity. Ototoxicity, though rare, is worrisome because it is often irreversible and is cumulative with repeated use of the drug. Ototoxicity can present either as hearing loss (cochlear damage) that is noted first with high-frequency tones, or as vestibular damage, manifested by vertigo, ataxia, and loss of balance. Of the commonly used aminoglycosides, amikacin appears to be more ototoxic than gentamicin, tobramycin, or netilmicin. Nephrotoxicity, which occurs more frequently than ototoxicity, is evident with rising serum creatinine levels or reduced creatinine clearance. Nephrotoxicity is usually reversible and occurs with similar frequency with gentamicin, tobramycin, amikacin, and netilmycin.

In very high doses, aminoglycosides can be neurotoxic, producing a curare-like effect with neuromuscular blockade that results in respiratory paralysis. Calcium gluconate or neostigmine can serve as an antidote to this reaction. Rarely, aminoglycosides cause hypersensitivity and local reactions.

1. STREPTOMYCIN

Streptomycin is bactericidal for both gram-positive and gram-negative bacteria. The usual dose is 15–25 mg/kg/d (about 1 g/d) injected in one or two divided doses intramuscularly. Streptomycin exhibits all the adverse effects typically associated with the aminoglycosides. It should not be given concurrently with other aminoglycosides, because excessive ototoxicity may occur.

Resistance emerges so rapidly and has become so widespread that only a few specific indications for this drug remain:

(1) Plague and tularemia.

(2) Endocarditis caused by *Enterococcus faecalis* or *Streptococcus viridans* (use in conjunction with a penicillin) in strains that are susceptible to high levels of streptomycin (ie, ≤ 2000 μg/mL). Gentamicin is often substituted for streptomycin in this setting.

(3) Serious active tuberculosis (use with other antituberculosis drugs).

(4) Acute brucellosis (use with tetracycline).

2. NEOMYCIN & KANAMYCIN

These aminoglycosides are closely related, with similar activity and complete cross-resistance. The related drug paromomycin is used in amebiasis. Systemic use has been abandoned because of oto- and nephrotoxicity.

Ointments containing 1–5 mg/g neomycin, often combined with bacitracin and polymyxin, can be applied to infected superficial skin lesions. The drug mixture covers most staphylococci and gram-negative bacteria likely to be present, but the efficacy of such topical treatment is in doubt. Solutions of neomycin, 2.5–5 mg/mL, have been used for irrigation of infected joints or wounds. The total amount of drug must be kept below 15 mg/kg/d, because absorption can lead to systemic toxicity.

In preparation for elective bowel surgery, 1 g of neomycin is given orally every 6–8 hours for 1–2 days (often combined with erythromycin, 1 g) to reduce aerobic bowel flora. Action on gram-negative anaerobes is negligible. In hepatic coma, the coliform bacteria can be suppressed for prolonged periods by oral neomycin or kanamycin, 1 g every 6–8 hours, during reduced protein intake. This results in diminished ammonia production and intoxication.

Kanamycin is somewhat less toxic than neomycin. It is used for the same indications and in the same doses as neomycin for topical application and oral intake.

In addition to oto- and nephrotoxicity, which can result from systemic absorption, neomycin or kanamycin can give rise to allergic reactions when applied topically to skin or eye. Respiratory arrest has followed the instillation of 3–5 g of kanamycin into the peritoneal cavity after colonic surgery; this can be overcome by neostigmine.

3. AMIKACIN

Amikacin is a semisynthetic derivative of kanamycin. It is relatively resistant to several of the enzymes that inactivate gentamicin and tobramycin, and bacterial resistance is increasing only slowly. Many gram-negative enteric bacteria—including many strains of *Proteus, Pseudomonas, Enterobacter,* and *Serratia*—are inhibited by 1–20 μg/mL of amikacin in vitro. After injection of 500 mg of amikacin intramuscularly every 12 hours (15 mg/kg/d), peak levels in serum are 10–30 μg/mL. Some infections caused by gram-negative bacteria resistant to gentamicin respond to amikacin. Central nervous system infections require intrathecal or intraventricular injection of 5–10 mg daily. In addition to therapy for serious gram-negative infections, amikacin is often included with other drugs for therapy of *M avium-intracellulare* infections.

Like all aminoglycosides, amikacin is nephrotoxic

and ototoxic (particularly for the auditory portion of the eighth nerve). Its levels should be monitored in patients with renal failure.

4. GENTAMICIN

With doses of 4.5–6 mg/kg/d of this aminoglycoside, serum levels reach 3–8 µg/mL—sufficient for bactericidal effect against many strains of staphylococci, coliforms, and other gram-negative organisms. Enterococci are resistant unless a penicillin is also given. Gentamicin may be synergistic with penicillins active against *Pseudomonas, Proteus, Enterobacter, Klebsiella,* and other gram-negatives. Sisomicin resembles the C1a component of gentamicin.

Indications, Dosages, & Routes of Administration

Gentamicin is used in severe infections caused by gram-negative bacteria. Included are sepsis, infected burns, pneumonia, and other serious infections. The dosage is 4.5–6 mg/kg/d intramuscularly (or intravenously) in three equal doses. In endocarditis due to viridans streptococci or *E faecalis,* gentamicin in lower doses (3 mg/kg/d in two or three divided doses) is combined with penicillin or ampicillin. In renal insufficiency, the dose should be adjusted according to Table 37–8. About 2–3% of patients develop vestibular dysfunction and loss of hearing when peak serum levels exceed 10 µg/mL. For infected burns or skin lesions, creams containing 0.1% gentamicin are used. Such topical use should be restricted to avoid favoring the development of resistant bacteria in hospitals. In meningitis due to gram-negative bacteria, 5–10 mg of gentamicin has been injected daily intrathecally or intraventricularly in adults.

5. TOBRAMYCIN

Tobramycin closely resembles gentamicin in antibacterial activity and pharmacologic properties and exhibits partial cross-resistance. Tobramycin may be effective against some gentamicin-resistant gram-negative bacteria. A daily dose of 4.5–6 mg/kg is given in three equal amounts intramuscularly or intravenously at intervals of 8 hours. In renal insufficiency, dosage adjustment is necessary (Table 37–8). Tobramycin and gentamicin are potentially ototoxic and nephrotoxic. The frequency of these adverse effects is similar for both drugs.

Netilmicin shares many characteristics with gentamicin and tobramycin and can be given in a dose of 5–7 mg/kg/d. It may be less ototoxic and less nephrotoxic than the other aminoglycosides.

Edson RS, Terrell CL: The aminoglycosides: Mayo Clin Proc 1991;66:1158. (Spectrum of activity, pharmacology, toxicity, and clinical indications.)

6. SPECTINOMYCIN

Spectinomycin is an aminocyclitol antibiotic (related to aminoglycosides) for intramuscular administration. Its sole application is in the treatment of gonococci producing β-lactamase in persons with gonorrhea who are hypersensitive to penicillin. (It is not effective for pharyngeal gonorrhea.) One injection of 2 g (40 mg/kg) is given. About 5–10% of gonococci are probably resistant. There is usually pain at the injection site, and there may be nausea and fever.

POLYMYXINS

The polymyxins are basic polypeptides that are bactericidal for most gram-negative aerobic rods, including *Pseudomonas.* Because of their poor distribution to tissues and substantial toxicity—and in view of the availability of better drugs—they are now rarely considered for systemic administration but are used topically.

Solutions of polymyxin B sulfate, 1 mg/mL, can be applied to infected surfaces; injected into joint spaces, the pleural cavity, or subconjunctivally; or inhaled as aerosols. Ointments containing 0.5 mg/g of polymyxin B sulfate in a mixture with neomycin or bacitracin (or both) are often applied to superficial infected skin lesions. Polymyxins are inactivated by purulent exudates. They rarely cause local sensitization.

ANTITUBERCULOUS DRUGS

Singular problems exist in the treatment of tuberculosis and other mycobacterial infections, which tend to be exceedingly chronic but may give rise to hyperacute lethal complications. The organisms are frequently intracellular, have long periods of metabolic inactivity, and tend to develop resistance to any one drug. Therefore, combined drug therapy is employed to delay the emergence of this resistance. "First-line" drugs, often employed together in tuberculous meningitis, miliary dissemination, or severe pulmonary disease, are isoniazid, ethambutol, rifampin, and pyrazinamide. A series of "second-line" drugs will be mentioned only briefly. Most patients become noninfectious within 2–4 weeks after effective drug therapy is instituted. In active pulmonary tuberculosis without complications, treatment schedules including isoniazid and rifampin for 6–9 months are satisfactory. Multidrug-resistant strains of *Myco-*

bacterium tuberculosis have been isolated with increasing frequency, comprising 20% of all isolates in some geographic areas. These strains occur most commonly in patients who have previously received antituberculous therapy and in HIV-infected individuals. Nosocomial spread has been documented, and therapy is difficult. Despite using drugs active against these isolates, progression to extrapulmonary infection is common; ability to eradicate the organism from sputum is difficult; and the mortality rate is high even with prolonged therapy. The emergence of these multidrug-resistant organisms emphasizes the urgent need for development of new antimycobacterial drugs as well as the need for aggressive public health measures to control the spread of this disease.

1. ISONIAZID

Isoniazid is the hydrazide of isonicotinic acid (INH), the most active antituberculosis drug. Isoniazid in a concentration of 0.2 μg/mL or less inhibits and kills most tubercle bacilli. However, some "atypical" mycobacteria as well as some strains of *M tuberculosis* are resistant (see above). In susceptible large populations of *M tuberculosis,* isoniazid-resistant mutants occur. Their emergence is delayed in the presence of a second drug. There is no cross-resistance between isoniazid and other antituberculosis drugs.

Isoniazid is well absorbed from the gut and diffuses readily into all tissues, including the central nervous system. The inactivation of isoniazid—particularly its acetylation—is under genetic control. However, the speed of isoniazid acetylation has little influence over the selection of drug regimens. Isoniazid and its conjugates are excreted mainly in the urine.

Indications, Dosages, & Routes of Administration

Isoniazid is the most widely used drug in tuberculosis. It should not be given as the sole drug in active tuberculosis. This favors emergence of resistance (up to 30% in some countries). In active, clinically manifest disease, it is given in conjunction with one or more drugs. The usual oral adult dose is 300 mg/d. In noncompliant patients, it can be given twice weekly in a dose of 15 mg/kg/dose (maximum, 900 mg/dose). In anephric patients, the dose is reduced to 200 mg/d.

Individuals who convert from a negative to a positive tuberculin test (defined as a > 10 mm increase within a 2-year period for individuals under 35 years of age and > 15 mm increase in individuals over 35) but who have no evidence of active disease may be given 10 mg/kg/d (maximum: 300 mg/d) for 6–12 months as prophylaxis against the 5–15% risk of meningitis or miliary dissemination. For this "prophylaxis," isoniazid is given as the sole drug. Other indications for prophylaxis are discussed in Chapter 9.

Toxic reactions to isoniazid include insomnia, restlessness, fever, myalgia, hyperreflexia, and even convulsions and psychotic episodes. Some of these are attributable to a relative pyridoxine deficiency and peripheral neuritis and can be prevented by the administration of pyridoxine, 100 mg/d. Isoniazid can induce hepatitis. Progressive liver damage occurs rarely in patients under age 20; in 1.5% of persons between 30 and 50 years of age; and in 2.5% of older individuals. The risk of hepatitis is greater in alcoholics. Mild elevations (2–3 times normal) of transaminases are common, occurring in 10–20% of patients taking isoniazid. Most physicians do not discontinue the drug unless there is more definite hepatic impairment, with transaminases three to five times normal values. Isoniazid can reduce the metabolism of phenytoin, increasing its blood level and toxicity.

2. ETHAMBUTOL

Ethambutol is a synthetic, water-soluble, heat-stable compound, dispensed as the hydrochloride.

Many strains of *M tuberculosis* and of "atypical" mycobacteria are inhibited in vitro by ethambutol, 1–5 μg/mL. The mechanism of action is not known.

Ethambutol is well absorbed from the gut. About 20% of the drug is excreted in feces and 50% in the urine, in unchanged form. Excretion is delayed and dosage adjustment is required in renal insufficiency; with creatinine clearance of 10–30 mL/min, one-half the usual dose is given, and with clearance of less than 10 mL/min, 35% of the usual dose. In meningitis, ethambutol appears in the cerebrospinal fluid.

Resistance to ethambutol emerges fairly rapidly among mycobacteria when the drug is used alone. Therefore, ethambutol, 15 mg/kg, is usually given as a single daily dose in combination with other antituberculosis drugs.

Hypersensitivity to ethambutol occurs infrequently. It may cause a rise in the serum uric acid. The commonest side effects are visual disturbances: reduction in visual acuity, optic neuritis, and perhaps retinal damage occur in some patients receiving ethambutol, 25 mg/kg/d for several months. Most changes are reversible, but periodic visual acuity testing is mandatory when doses above 15 mg/kg/d are used. At lower doses, side effects are rare.

3. RIFAMPIN & RIFABUTIN

Rifampin is a semisynthetic derivative of rifamycin. Rifampin, 1 μg/mL or less, inhibits many gram-positive cocci, meningococci, and mycobacteria in vitro. Gram-negative organisms are often more resistant. Highly resistant mutants occur frequently in susceptible microbial populations (one in 10^6–10^8 bacteria).

Rifampin binds strongly to DNA-dependent bacterial RNA polymerase and thus inhibits RNA synthesis in bacteria. Rifampin penetrates well into phagocytic cells and can kill intracellular organisms. Rifampin sometimes enhances the activity of amphotericin B against various fungi in vitro.

Rifampin given orally is well absorbed and widely distributed in tissues, including the central nervous system. Levels in cerebrospinal fluid are 50% of those in serum. The drug is excreted mainly through the liver and to a lesser extent in the urine. With oral doses of 600 mg, serum levels exceed 5 μg/mL for 4–6 hours, and urine levels may be 3–20 times higher. No adjustment is needed in renal insufficiency.

In the treatment of tuberculosis, a single oral dose of 600 mg (10–20 mg/kg) is given daily or, in noncompliant patients, 600 mg twice weekly. In order to delay the rapid emergence of resistant microorganisms, combined treatment with other antituberculous drugs is required. Rifampin is effective for treatment of leprosy (see below). Rifampin, 600 mg twice daily for 2 days, can terminate the meningococcal carrier state, but rifampin-resistant strains emerge in 10% of subjects. Close contacts of children with manifest *H influenzae* infection (eg, in the family or in day care centers) can receive rifampin, 20 mg/kg/d for 4 days, as prophylaxis. Rifampin combined with trimethoprim-sulfamethoxazole can eradicate staphylococcal carriage in the nasopharynx. Combination of rifampin with either penicillin or clindamycin is effective in eradication of group A β-hemolytic streptococci from the pharynx of chronic carriers. Synergistic action of rifampin with nafcillin and vancomycin against staphylococci in vitro is of uncertain clinical significance. However, in patients with *S aureus* or *S epidermidis* prosthetic valve endocarditis, rifampin at a dose of 300 mg every 8 hours for 6 weeks is recommended along with nafcillin or vancomycin for 6 weeks and gentamicin for 2 weeks. With the exception of prophylaxis, rifampin should never be used alone.

Rifampin imparts an orange color to urine, sweat, and contact lenses. Occasional adverse effects include rashes, thrombocytopenia, impaired liver function, light-chain proteinuria, and some impairment of immune response. In intermittent administration, rifampin must be given at least twice weekly to avoid a "flu syndrome," anemia, and other adverse affects. Rifampin increases the metabolism of oral anticoagulants and contraceptives and lowers serum levels of methadone, ketoconazole, and chloramphenicol.

Rifabutin is structurally similar to rifampin but is 10–20 times more active against *M aviumintracellulare*. Rifabutin, 0.3 g/d, is effective for prophylaxis against *M avium-intracellulare* in HIV-infected patients with CD4 counts less than 100/μL. Adverse effects and drug interactions are the same as those associated with rifampin.

4. STREPTOMYCIN

The general pharmacologic features and toxicity of streptomycin are described above. Streptomycin, 1–10 μg/mL, is inhibitory and bactericidal for most tubercle bacilli, whereas most "atypical" mycobacteria are resistant. All large populations of tubercle bacilli contain some streptomycin-resistant mutants. Therefore, streptomycin is employed only in combination with another antituberculosis drug.

Streptomycin penetrates poorly into cells and exerts its action mainly on extracellular tubercle bacilli. Since at any moment 90% of tubercle bacilli are intracellular and thus unaffected by streptomycin, treatment for many months is required.

For combination therapy in tuberculous meningitis, miliary dissemination, and severe organ tuberculosis, streptomycin is given intramuscularly, 0.5–1 g daily (30 mg/kg/d for children) for weeks or months. This is followed by streptomycin, 1 g intramuscularly 2–3 times a week for months.

Prolonged streptomycin treatment may impair vestibular function and result in inability to maintain equilibrium. Later, some compensation usually occurs, so that patients can function fairly well.

5. PYRAZINAMIDE

Pyrazinamide is bactericidal for most *M tuberculosis* strains and also for "atypical" mycobacteria. It is well absorbed after oral administration and is widely distributed in tissues. It penetrates well into the cerebrospinal fluid and achieves levels equal to those in serum. The usual oral dose is 20–30 mg/kg (1.5–2 g) given once daily. In noncompliant patients, 50–70 mg/kg can be given twice weekly. Pyrazinamide is commonly used in the therapy of tuberculosis because of its demonstrated efficacy in short-course therapy regimens (see below).

The major adverse effect is hepatotoxicity, seen in 1–5% of patients. Nausea, vomiting, drug fever, and hyperuricemia can occur.

6. SHORT-COURSE THERAPY

For uncomplicated pulmonary tuberculosis due to sensitive organisms (and perhaps extrapulmonary disease), treatment for only 6–9 months can be satisfactory *provided that* both isoniazid and rifampin are administered (see Chapter 9). In adults, isoniazid, 300 mg, and rifampin, 600 mg, are given daily for 9 months. Alternatively, isoniazid, rifampin, and pyrazinamide (30 mg/kg/d) can be given for 2 months followed by 4 additional months of isoniazid and rifampin. Ethambutol (15 mg/kg/d) or streptomycin should be included in the regimen if the patient resides in or has come from an area with a high level of drug resistance. In noncompliant patients, twice-weekly administration of drug has been shown to be effective. One such regimen is the use of isoniazid 300 mg and rifampin 600 mg daily for 2 months, followed by twice-weekly administration of isoniazid (15 mg/kg or a maximum dose of 900 mg) and rifampin (10 mg/kg or a maximum of 600 mg), to complete a total of 9 months of therapy. If isoniazid and rifampin cannot be used (ie, when resistant strains are isolated), short course therapy should not be used. If the organism is isoniazid-resistant, 12 months of treatment with ethambutol and rifampin is given. For infections caused by multidrug-resistant strains, even longer therapy (ie, 18 months or more) is indicated and should be continued at least 6 months after the last positive culture.

7. ALTERNATIVE DRUGS IN TUBERCULOSIS TREATMENT

The drugs listed alphabetically below are usually considered only in cases of drug resistance (clinical or laboratory) to "first-line" drugs and when expert guidance is available to deal with toxic side effects.

Aminosalicylic acid (PAS), closely related to p-aminobenzoic acid, inhibits most tubercle bacilli in concentrations of 1–5 µg/mL but has no effect on other bacteria.

Aminosalicylic acid is readily absorbed from the gut. Doses of 8–12 g/d orally give blood levels of 10 µg/mL. The drug is widely distributed in tissues (except the central nervous system) and rapidly excreted into the urine.

Common side effects include anorexia, nausea, diarrhea, and epigastric pain. Sodium aminosalicylate may be given parenterally. Hypersensitivity reactions include fever, skin rashes, granulocytopenia, lymphadenopathy, and arthralgias.

Clofazimine is a phenazine dye used in the treatment of leprosy and is active in vitro against *M avium-intracellulare*. It is given orally as a single daily dose of 100 mg for treatment of *M avium-intracellulare* disease. Adverse effects include nausea, vomiting, abdominal pain, and skin discoloration from red-brown to black.

Cycloserine, 0.5–1 g/d orally, has been used in retreatment regimens and for primary therapy of highly resistant *M tuberculosis*. It can induce a variety of central nervous system dysfunctions and psychotic reactions. These may be controlled by phenytoin, 100 mg/d orally. In smaller doses (15–20 mg/kg/d), cycloserine has been used in urinary tract infections.

Ethionamide, 0.5–1 g/d orally, has been used in combination therapy but produces marked gastric irritation.

Drugs for tuberculosis. Med Lett Drugs Ther 1992;34:10. (Recommendations for therapy and description of commonly used drugs.)

Van Scoy RE, Wilkowske CJ: Antituberculous agents. Mayo Clin Proc 1992;67:179. (Summary of drugs and regimens.)

SULFONAMIDES & ANTIFOLATE DRUGS

Since the demonstration in 1935 of the striking antibacterial activity of sulfanilamide, the molecule has been drastically altered in many ways. More than 150 different sulfonamides have been marketed at one time or another, the modifications being designed principally to achieve greater antibacterial activity, a wider antibacterial spectrum, greater solubility, or more prolonged action. Because of their low cost and their relative efficacy in some common bacterial infections, sulfonamides are still used widely.

Antimicrobial Activity

Sulfonamides are structural analogues of p-aminobenzoic acid (PABA) and compete with PABA to block its conversion to dihydrofolic acid. Organisms that require exogenous PABA in the synthesis of folates and pyrimidines are inhibited. Animal cells and some resistant microorganisms can utilize exogenous folate and thus are not affected by sulfonamides.

Trimethoprim, a substituted pyrimidine, inhibits the conversion of dihydrofolic to tetrahydrofolic acid by blocking the enzyme dihydrofolate reductase. It inhibits this enzyme of bacteria 50,000 times more efficiently than the same enzyme of mammalian cells.

Sulfonamides inhibit many gram-positive (including *Nocardia*) and gram-negative organisms. Emerging resistance, particularly among streptococci, gonococci, meningococci, and enteric gram-negative organisms, has limited their use somewhat. Sulfonamides are also active against chlamydiae and such parasites as *Toxoplasma* and *Plasmodium*.

The combination of trimethoprim (TMP) (one part) plus sulfamethoxazole (SMZ) (five parts) is bactericidal for such gram-negative rods as *E coli*, *Klebsiella*, *Enterobacter*, *Salmonella*, and *Shigella*. It is also active against many strains of *Serratia*, *Providencia*, *P maltophilia*, *P cepacia*, *Pseudomonas pseudomallei*, and *Pseudomonas mallei* but not against *P aeruginosa*. It is inactive against anaerobes, enterococci, and group A streptococci but inhibits *S aureus* and *S epidermidis*, *M catarrhalis*, *H influenzae*, *H ducreyi*, and some atypical mycobacteria, eg, *M marinum*.

Pharmacokinetics & Administration

Sulfisoxazole is widely used because of its low cost and high solubility. Like other soluble sulfonamides (sulfadiazine, sulfamethoxazole), it is well absorbed from the gut and widely distributed in tissues. For mild infections (eg, urinary tract infections), the usual dose is 0.5–1 g four times daily (30–60 mg/kg/d), while for systemic infections, 100 mg/kg/d is appropriate. A 1 g oral dose of sulfisoxazole yields serum levels of 50–100 μg/mL.

One-half the dose of sulfisoxazole is excreted unchanged in the urine. In mild renal insufficiency, no dosage adjustment is needed; in severe renal failure (creatinine clearance < 5 mL/min), one-third to one-half the usual dose is given.

Insoluble sulfonamides, eg, phthalylsulfathiazole and salicylazosulfapyridine (sulfasalazine), are little absorbed from the gut and are largely excreted in the feces. Phthalylsulfathiazole has been used in the past for preparation of the bowel for surgery (8–15 g/d for 5–7 days). Sulfasalazine is used for ulcerative colitis (6 g/d in four doses); it is broken down to sulfapyridine and salicylate in the bowel, and the latter is anti-inflammatory.

For patients who are unable to take oral drugs, some intravenous sulfonamide preparations are available. Most widely used is trimethoprim-sulfamethoxazole. Each vial contains 80 mg TMP + 400 mg SMZ in a volume of 5 mL, which must be diluted in 125 mL of 5% dextrose in water. For many bacterial infections, the dose is 10 mg TMP + 50 mg SMZ/kg/d in two doses; for pneumocystis infections, 15 mg TMP + 75 mg SMZ/kg/d is given in four doses. This dose is suitable for patients with creatinine clearances above 50 mL/min. Half to three-fourths of that dose is given for patients with creatinine clearances of 10–50 mL/min and one-quarter of the dose for clearances under 5 mL/min.

The topical application of sulfonamides to skin, wounds, or mucous membranes is undesirable because of the high risk of allergic sensitization or reaction. Exceptions are the application of sodium sulfacetamide solution (30%) or ointment (10%) to the conjunctiva and mafenide acetate cream (Sulfamylon) or silver sulfadiazine (Silvadene) to burn wounds.

Clinical Uses

Present indications for sulfonamides include the following:

A. Urinary Tract Infections: Coliform bacteria, the commonest cause of urinary tract infections, often remain susceptible to sulfonamides. "Single-dose" therapy with TMP-SMZ (two double strength tablets of 160 mg TMP + 800 mg SMZ) is effective in many patients with symptoms of less than a week's duration. One such tablet given twice daily for 3 days is slightly more effective than single-dose therapy and equally as efficacious as 7–10 days of treatment.

Since TMP is concentrated in the prostate, TMP-SMZ, one double-strength tablet twice daily for 14–21 days, is effective in acute prostatitis. In chronic prostatitis, treatment for 6–12 weeks is indicated.

B. Parasitic Infections: TMP-SMZ is effective for prophylaxis and treatment of *Pneumocystis carinii* pneumonia and *Isospora belli* infection. For therapy of pneumocystis pneumonia, 15 mg/kg/d of trimethoprim and 75 mg/kg/d of sulfamethoxazole in four divided doses is administered intravenously or orally—depending upon the severity of disease—for 3 weeks. The dose for prophylaxis is 160 mg TMP + 800 mg SMZ once daily or every other day. *I belli* infection in AIDS has been successfully treated with 160 mg TMP + 800 mg SMZ orally four times daily for 10 days followed by twice-daily administration for 3 weeks. Treatment with 160 mg TMP + 800 mg SMZ three times a week or 500 mg sulfadoxine with 25 mg pyrimethamine once a week has prevented recurrences. Sulfadiazine with pyrimethamine is also used to treat toxoplasmosis and chloroquine-resistant falciparum malaria. Low-dose TMP-SMZ (160 mg TMP + 800 mg SMZ twice daily, 2 days per week) may be effective prophylaxis against toxoplasmal encephalitis.

C. Bacterial Infections: Sulfonamides are the drugs of choice for *Nocardia* infections. TMP-SMZ has a wide spectrum in therapy. It penetrates into the cerebrospinal fluid and has been used to treat meningitis caused by gram-negative rods, though third-generation cephalosporins are now preferred. TMP-SMZ is a frequent choice for management of acute sinusitis, otitis media, acute bronchitis, and shigellosis. The usual dose for adults is 160 mg TMP + 800 mg SMZ twice daily for 10 days. Other uses of TMP-SMZ include treatment of melioidosis (*P pseudomallei*) and infections by *P maltophilia* or *P cepacia;* of chancroid (*H ducreyi*); in combination with rifampin for eradication of nasopharyngeal carriage of *S aureus;* for prophylaxis of meningococcal disease when susceptible *N meningitidis* strains prevail; for prophylaxis in chronic granulomatous disease to prevent bacterial infections; as prophylaxis (320 mg TMP + 1600 mg SMZ daily) in organ transplant patients to prevent bacterial infections and pneumocystis pneumonia; and for therapy of legionellosis in patients who cannot tolerate or fail to respond to erythromycin; for *Listeria monocytogenes* meningitis in patients who cannot tolerate ampicillin; and as possible therapy for Wegener's granulomatosis.

D. Chlamydial Infections: Sulfonamides effectively suppress trachoma, urethritis, inclusion conjunctivitis, and other manifestations, but erythromycin or tetracyclines are preferred.

E. Leprosy: Certain sulfones are widely used (see below).

Adverse Effects

Adverse reactions to sulfonamides occur in 10–15% of non-AIDS patients (usually a minor rash or gastrointestinal disturbance) and in up to 50% of patients with AIDS (predominantly rash, fever, neutropenia, and thrombocytopenia, often severe enough to require discontinuation of therapy). These drugs are capable of producing a wide variety of side effects—due partly to hypersensitivity, partly to direct toxicity—that must be considered whenever unexplained symptoms or signs occur in a patient who may have received these drugs. Except in the mildest reactions, fluids should be forced, and—if symptoms and signs progressively increase—the drugs should be discontinued. Precautions to prevent complications (below) are important.

A. Systemic Side Effects: Fever, skin rashes, urticaria; nausea, vomiting, or diarrhea; stomatitis, conjunctivitis, arthritis, exfoliative dermatitis; bone marrow depression, thrombocytopenia, hemolytic (in G6PD deficiency) or aplastic anemia, granulocytopenia, leukemoid reactions; hepatitis, polyarteritis nodosa, vasculitis, Stevens-Johnson syndrome; psychosis; and many others.

Trimethoprim can evoke similar side effects. It may precipitate folate deficiency.

Application of mafenide to burns may cause severe pain.

B. Urinary Tract Disturbances: Sulfonamides may precipitate in urine, especially at neutral or acid pH, producing hematuria, crystalluria, or even obstruction. They have also been implicated in various types of nephritis and nephrosis. Sulfonamides and methenamine salts should not be given together.

Precautions in the Use of Sulfonamides

(1) There is cross-allergenicity among all sulfonamides. Obtain a history of past administration or reaction. Observe for possible allergic responses.

(2) Keep the urine volume above 1500 mL/d by forcing fluids.

(3) Check hemoglobin, white blood cell count, and differential count once weekly to detect possible disturbances early in high-risk patients.

Cockerill FR III, Edson RS: Trimethoprim-sulfamethoxazole. Mayo Clin Proc 1991;66:1260. (Pharmacokinetics, spectrum of activity, and clinical use.)

SULFONES USED IN THE TREATMENT OF LEPROSY

A number of drugs closely related to the sulfonamides (eg, dapsone; diaminodiphenylsulfone, DDS) have been used effectively in the long-term treatment of leprosy. Dapsone, 100 mg daily, may also be effective for pneumocystis pneumonia in AIDS when combined with trimethoprim, 20 mg/kg/d in four divided doses. Dapsone, 50–100 mg daily, is effective prophylaxis for recurrent *P carinii* infection. The clinical manifestations of both lepromatous and tuberculoid leprosy can often be suppressed by treatment extending over several years. It appears that 5–30% of *Mycobacterium leprae* organisms were resistant to dapsone in 1990. Consequently, initial combined treatment with rifampin is advocated.

Absorption, Metabolism, & Excretion

All sulfones are well absorbed from the intestinal tract, are distributed widely in all tissues, and tend to be retained in skin, muscle, liver, and kidney. Skin involved by leprosy contains ten times more drug than normal skin. Sulfones are excreted into the bile and reabsorbed by the intestine. Consequently, blood levels are prolonged. Excretion into the urine is variable, and the drug occurs in urine mostly as a glucuronic acid conjugate. Some persons acetylate sulfones slowly and others rapidly; this requires dosage adjustment.

Dosages & Routes of Administration

See Leprosy, Chapter 32, for recommendations.

Adverse Effects

The sulfones may cause any of the side effects listed above for sulfonamides. Anorexia, nausea, and vomiting are common. Hemolysis, methemoglobinemia, or agranulocytosis may occur. If sulfones are not tolerated, clofazimine can be substituted.

SPECIALIZED DRUGS AGAINST BACTERIA

1. BACITRACIN

This polypeptide is selectively active against gram-positive bacteria. Because of severe nephrotoxicity upon systemic administration, its use has been limited to topical application on surface lesions, usually in combination with polymyxin or neomycin. Occasionally it is given orally for pseudomembranous colitis caused by toxin-producing *C difficile* (see below).

2. MUPIROCIN

Mupirocin (formerly pseudomonic acid) is a naturally occurring antibiotic produced by *Pseudomonas fluorescens* that is active against most gram-positive cocci, including methicillin-sensitive and methicillin-resistant *S aureus*. It is used topically. It is effective in eliminating staphylococcal nasal carriage in the majority of patients for up to 3 months after application to the anterior nares twice daily for 5 days. Whether this drug is more effective than alternative treatments (trimethoprim-sulfamethoxazole or dicloxacillin plus rifampin) for eradication of staphylococcal nasal carriage is unknown.

3. LINCOMYCIN & CLINDAMYCIN

These drugs resemble erythromycin (although different in structure) and are active against gram-posi-

tive organisms (except enterococci). Lincomycin, 0.5 g orally every 6 hours, or clindamycin, 0.15–0.3 g orally every 6 hours, yields serum concentrations of 2–5 μg/mL. The drugs are widely distributed in tissues. Excretion is through the bile and urine. The drugs are alternatives to erythromycin as substitutes for penicillin. Clindamycin is currently recommended as the alternative drug for prophylaxis against endocarditis following oral procedures in patients allergic to amoxicillin (see Table 37–9). Clindamycin, 300 mg orally twice daily for 7 days, can be used as an alternative to metronidazole for the therapy of bacterial vaginosis. Topical application of

Table 37–9. Endocarditis prophylaxis.[1,2]

DENTAL AND UPPER RESPIRATORY TRACT PROCEDURES[3]	
Oral[4]	
Amoxicillin[5]	3 g 1 hour before procedure and 1.5 g 6 hours later
Penicillin allergy:	
Erythromycin	1 g 2 hours before procedure and 0.5 g 6 hours later
or	
Clindamycin	300 mg orally 1 hour before procedure and 150 mg 6 hours later
Parenteral[4,6]	
Ampicillin	2 mg IM or IV 30 minutes before procedure
plus	
Gentamicin	15 mg/kg IM or IV 30 minutes before procedure
Penicillin allergy	
Vancomycin	1 g IV infused *slowly over 1 hour* beginning 1 hour before procedure
or	
Clindamycin	200 mg IV 30 minutes before procedure and an intravenous or oral dose of 150 mg 6 hours later
GASTROINTESTINAL AND GENITOURINARY PROCEDURES	
Oral[4]	
Amoxicillin[5]	3 g 1 hour before procedure and 1.5 g 6 hours later
Parenteral[4,6]	
Ampicillin	2 g IM or IV 30 minutes before procedure
plus	
Gentamicin	1.5 mg/kg IM or IV 30 minutes before procedure
Penicillin allergy:	
Vancomycin	1 g IV infused *slowly over 1 hour* beginning 1 hour before procedure
plus	
Gentamicin	1.5 mg/kg IM or IV 30 minutes before procedure

[1]Modified from *Handbook of Antimicrobial Therapy*, rev ed. The Medical Letter on Drugs and Therapeutics, 1990.
[2]For patients with previous endocarditis, valvular heart disease, prosthetic heart valves, most forms of congenital heart disease (but not uncomplicated secundum atrial septal defect), idiopathic hypertrophic subaortic stenosis, and mitral valve prolapse with regurgitation. Viridans streptococci are the most common cause of endocarditis after dental or upper respiratory procedures; enterococci are the most common cause of endocarditis after gastrointestinal or genitourinary procedures.
[3]For a review of the risk of bacteremia and endocarditis with various procedures, see Durack D in: *Principles and Practice of Infectious Disease*, 3rd ed. Mandell GL et al (editors). Churchill Livingstone, 1990.
[4]Oral regimens are more convenient and safer. Parenteral regimens are more likely to be effective; they are recommended especially for patients with prosthetic heart valves, those who have had endocarditis previously, or those taking continuous oral penicillin for rheumatic fever prophylaxis.
[5]Amoxicillin is recommended because of its excellent bioavailability and good activity against streptococci and enterococci.
[6]A single dose of parenteral drug is probably adequate, because bacteremia after most dental and diagnostic procedures is of short duration. An additional dose may be given 8 hours later in patients judged to be at higher risk.

a 2% vaginal cream once or twice daily for 7 days is also effective. Clindamycin is active against most anaerobes, including *Bacteroides*. It is frequently used to treat infections in which anaerobes are significant pathogens (eg, aspiration pneumonia in penicillin-allergic patients; pelvic and abdominal infections), sometimes in combination with an aminoglycoside. In patients with necrotizing pneumonia or lung abscess following aspiration, clindamycin appears to be superior to penicillin. Seriously ill patients are given clindamycin, 600–900 mg (20–30 mg/kg/d) intravenously, during a 1-hour period every 8 hours. Success has also been reported in staphylococcal osteomyelitis. In the sulfonamide-allergic patient, high-dose clindamycin therapy (600–1200 mg intravenously every 6 hours or 600 mg orally every 6 hours) in conjunction with pyrimethamine has been used to treat toxoplasmosis of the central nervous system and appears to be as effective as pyrimethamine and sulfadiazine. Clindamycin in combination with primaquine has been reported to be effective in the therapy of pneumocystis pneumonia in patients with AIDS. These drugs are ineffective in meningitis.

Common side effects are diarrhea, nausea, and skin rashes. Impaired liver function and neutropenia have been noted. If 3–4 g is given rapidly intravenously, cardiorespiratory arrest may occur. Bloody diarrhea with pseudomembranous colitis has been associated with the administration of clindamycin and other antibiotics. This antibiotic-associated colitis is due to a necrotizing toxin produced by *C difficile*. The organism is resistant to the antimicrobial, is selected out by its presence, and is favored in its growth and toxin production. *C difficile* is usually susceptible to—and can be treated with—vancomycin (see below), bacitracin, or metronidazole given orally.

4. METRONIDAZOLE

Metronidazole is an antiprotozoal drug (see Chapter 34) that also has striking antibacterial effects against most anaerobes, including *Bacteroides*. It is well absorbed after oral administration, is widely distributed in tissues, and yields serum levels of 4–6 μg/mL after a 250 mg dose. It penetrates well into the cerebrospinal fluid, yielding levels similar to those in serum. The drug is metabolized in the liver, and dosage reduction is required in severe hepatic insufficiency. Metronidazole can be given intravenously.

Metronidazole is employed in amebiasis and giardiasis (see Chapter 34) and in the following circumstances:

(1) *Trichomonas* vaginitis responds to either a single dose (2 g) or to 250 mg orally three times daily for 7–10 days. Bacterial vaginosis responds to a single 2 g dose or to 500 mg twice daily for 7 days. Metronidazole vaginal cream (0.75%) applied twice daily for 5 days is also effective.

(2) In anaerobic or mixed infections, metronidazole can be given orally or intravenously, 500 mg three times daily (30 mg/kg/d).

(3) As an alternative to oral vancomycin for antibiotic-associated colitis due to *C difficile,* give 500 mg three times daily orally. If oral medication is impractical, it is given intravenously. Metronidazole is less expensive than clindamycin or vancomycin.

(4) Preparation of the colon before bowel surgery.

(5) Therapy of brain abscess, often in combination with penicillin or a third-generation cephalosporin.

(6) In combination with tetracycline, bismuth subsalicylate (Pepto-Bismol), or amoxicillin for therapy of some *H pylori* infections.

Adverse effects include stomatitis, nausea, and diarrhea. Ingestion of alcohol while taking metronidazole can result in flushing, hypotension, nausea, and vomiting. With prolonged use at high doses, reversible peripheral neuropathy can develop. Metronidazole has been shown to be carcinogenic in animals and mutagenic for certain bacteria. To date, human studies have not confirmed an increased incidence of malignancy after treatment.

Smilack JD, Wilson WR, Cockerill FR III: Tetracyclines, chloramphenicol, erythromycin, clindamycin and metronidazole. Mayo Clin Proc 1991;66:1270. (Activity, adverse effects, and clinical indications.)

5. VANCOMYCIN

This drug is bactericidal for most gram-positive organisms, particularly staphylococci and streptococci—and is bacteriostatic for most enterococci—in concentrations of 0.5–10 μg/mL. Resistant mutants are very rare, and there is no cross-resistance with other antimicrobial drugs. Vancomycin is not absorbed from the gut. It is given orally only for the treatment of antibiotic-associated enterocolitis. For systemic effect the drug must be administered intravenously (20–30 mg/kg/d in 2–3 divided doses). An intravenous injection of 10 mg/kg over a period of 20 minutes yields blood levels of 20–30 μg/mL. Vancomycin is excreted mainly via the kidneys but may accumulate also in liver failure. In renal insufficiency, the half-life may be up to 8 days. Thus, only one dose of 0.5–1 g may be given every 4–8 days to a uremic individual undergoing hemodialysis.

Indications for parenteral vancomycin include the following: (1) Severe staphylococcal infections in penicillin-allergic patients; it is the drug of choice for methicillin-resistant *S aureus* and *S epidermidis* infections. (2) Severe enterococcal infections in the penicillin-allergic patient, usually in combination with an aminoglycoside. (3) Other gram-positive infections in penicillin-allergic patients, eg, viridans streptococcal endocarditis. (4) Surgical prophylaxis in penicillin-allergic patients. (5) For gram-positive infections due to organisms that are multi-drug-resistant, ie, *Corynebacterium jeikeium*. (6). Endocarditis prophylaxis in the penicillin-allergic patient undergoing certain genitourinary and gastrointestinal procedures (in combination with an aminoglycoside). (See Table 37–9.)

In antibiotic-associated enterocolitis, vancomycin, 0.125–0.5 g, is given orally four times daily.

Vancomycin is irritating to tissues; chills, fever, and thrombophlebitis sometimes follow intravenous injection. The drug is somewhat ototoxic and perhaps nephrotoxic. Rapid infusion may induce diffuse hyperemia ("red man syndrome") and can be avoided by extending infusions over 1–2 hours or by pretreating with a histamine antagonist such as hydroxyzine.

Wilhelm MP: Vancomycin. Mayo Clin Proc 1991;66:1165. (Activity, toxicity, and clinical indications.)

Sahai J et al: Influence of antihistamine pretreatment on vancomycin-induced red-man syndrome. J Inf Dis 1989;160:876. (Prevention of "red man syndrome" with pretreatment with antihistamines.)

QUINOLONES

The quinolones are synthetic analogues of nalidixic acid that have an exceedingly broad spectrum of activity against many bacteria. The mode of action of all quinolones involves inhibition of bacterial DNA synthesis by blocking the enzyme DNA gyrase.

The earlier quinolones (nalidixic acid, oxolinic acid, cinoxacin) did not achieve systemic antibacterial levels after oral intake and thus were useful only as urinary antiseptics. The newer fluorinated derivatives (norfloxacin, ciprofloxacin, enoxacin, pefloxacin, ofloxacin, and lomefloxacin) have greater antibacterial activity, achieve clinically useful levels in blood and tissues, and have low toxicity.

Antimicrobial Activity

A number of fluoroquinolones are currently available. Most have quite similar spectrums of activity. In general, these drugs have superb activity against Enterobacteriaceae but are also active against other gram-negative bacteria such as *Haemophilus, Neisseria, Moraxella, Brucella, Legionella, Salmonella, Shigella, Campylobacter, Yersinia, Vibrio,* and *Aeromonas.* Ciprofloxacin has slightly better activity against *P aeruginosa* than the other fluoroquinolones, and none of these agents have reliable activity against *P maltophilia* or *P cepacia.* Against genital tract pathogens such as *Mycoplasma hominis, Ureaplasma urealyticum,* and *C pneumoniae,* ofloxacin possesses more activity than the others, and against *Gardnerella vaginalis* ciprofloxacin and ofloxacin are the most active. *M tuberculosis* is sensitive to the quinolones, as is *M fortuitum* and *Mycobacterium kansasii.* Although *M avium-intracellulare* is resistant to fluoroquinolones when combined with other agents (ethambutol, rifampin, clofazimine, and amikacin), ciprofloxacin appears to be effective in treating infections caused by this organism.

In general, the fluoroquinolones are less active against gram-positive than gram-negative organisms, with norfloxacin, enoxacin, and lomefloxacin having less activity than ciprofloxacin and ofloxacin. Ciprofloxacin and ofloxacin are active against *S aureus* and *S epidermidis,* including methicillin-resistant strains. However, recent reports of the emergence of ciprofloxacin-resistant strains of staphylococci developing during therapy may severely limit the use of quinolones to treat infections caused by these organisms. *M pneumoniae* and enterococci, including *E faecalis, S pneumoniae,* group A, B, and D streptococci, and viridans streptococci are only moderately sensitive to the quinolones. Anaerobic bacteria, *T pallidum,* and *Nocardia* are resistant to the fluoroquinolones.

Pharmacokinetics & Administration

After oral administration, the fluoroquinolones are well-absorbed and widely distributed in body fluids and tissues. Fluoroquinolones are bound by some heavy metals, and absorption is inhibited when they are given with food, antacids, or milk. Highest serum levels are achieved if they are given 1 hour before or 2 hours after meals. Ofloxacin and pefloxacin appear to penetrate into the cerebrospinal fluid better than other fluoroquinolones. The serum half-life ranges from 4 hours (ciprofloxacin) to 8–12 hours (pefloxacin, lomefloxacin), with ofloxacin and enoxacin having a half-life of 6–8 hours. After ingestion of 400–600 mg, the peak serum level of ciprofloxacin is 2.5 μg/mL and is lower than that of the other quinolones (4–6 μg/mL), but this is offset by ciprofloxacin's slightly greater in vitro activity against most organisms. Ciprofloxacin and ofloxacin can be administered intravenously. The usual dose is 400 mg given every 12 hours, which results in peak serum levels of 4–5 μg/mL. The fluoroquinolones are excreted mainly through the kidney by tubular secretion (which can be blocked by probenecid) and by glomerular filtration. Up to 20% of the dose is metabolized by the liver. In renal insufficiency, half-lives are prolonged, but only slight dosage adjustment is needed with the exception of ofloxacin, in which the half-life increases from 8 to 35 hours. These drugs are not removed by hemodialysis or peritoneal dialysis.

Clinical Uses

Because of their high cost, broad spectrum of activity, and tendency for some organisms (eg, *P aeruginosa,* staphylococcal species) to develop resistance, these agents should not be routinely used as first-line therapy when less expensive and less toxic agents are available. Despite their extensive in vitro activity, the exact role of quinolones in therapy has not been clearly defined.

Urinary tract infections caused by multidrug-resistant gram-negative organisms that are sensitive to quinolones can be treated with norfloxacin, 400 mg twice daily; ciprofloxacin, 500 mg twice daily; ofloxacin, 200 mg twice daily; enoxacin, 400 mg twice daily; or lomefloxacin, 400 mg once daily.

Because of good penetration into prostatic tissue, quinolones are effective in treating bacterial prostatitis and are alternatives when less expensive drugs cannot be used or have been used without success (doses for prostatitis are the same as for urinary tract infection, but the duration should be 6–12 weeks).

Quinolones have been approved for use in therapy of certain sexually transmitted diseases. Ofloxacin, 400 mg twice daily for 7 days, is as effective as doxycycline, 100 mg twice daily for 7 days, for the therapy of *C pneumoniae* cervicitis, urethritis, and proctitis. It is also effective for nongonococcal urethritis caused by *U urealyticum.* Ciprofloxacin and norfloxacin are not effective for the therapy of chlamydial infections or nongonococcal urethritis. In general, the use of quinolones for the therapy of any sexually transmitted disease will be limited by their lack of efficacy in syphilis and the need to exclude that disease. Although ceftriaxone, 125–250 mg intramuscularly as a single injection, remains the treatment of choice for uncomplicated gonococcal urethritis, cervicitis, pharyngitis, and proctitis, these infections can also be treated with a single dose of 500 mg of ciprofloxacin, 400 mg of ofloxacin, or 400 mg of enoxacin.

The use of these drugs in salpingitis and disseminated infection has not been studied. *H ducreyi,* the agent that causes chancroid, is sensitive to quinolones, and ciprofloxacin, 500 mg twice daily, or enoxacin, 400 mg daily for 3 days, can be used as an alternative to erythromycin or ceftriaxone as therapy for this disease.

Ciprofloxacin and ofloxacin have been successfully used to treat complicated skin and soft tissue infections and osteomyelitis caused by gram-negative organisms. Ciprofloxacin, 500–750 mg twice daily for at least 6 weeks, has been effective therapy for malignant otitis externa.

Because quinolones are the only available oral agents active against *Campylobacter* and the other major bacterial pathogens associated with diarrhea (*Salmonella, Shigella,* toxigenic *E coli*), they have been used for the therapy of traveler's diarrhea as well as domestically acquired acute diarrhea. Norfloxacin, ciprofloxacin, and ofloxacin are effective in eradicating the chronic carrier state of *Salmonella* when therapy is continued for 4–6 weeks.

Ciprofloxacin has been used to eradicate meningococci from the nasopharynx of carriers.

Norfloxacin, ciprofloxacin, and ofloxacin are effective for prophylaxis against gram-negative infections in the neutropenic patient, and intravenous ciprofloxacin in combination with aminoglycosides or β-lactam antibiotics has been used successfully to treat the febrile neutropenic patient.

Although some clinical studies have suggested that ciprofloxacin and ofloxacin are efficacious in the therapy of lower respiratory tract infections, caution should be exercised since the drug has only marginal activity against *S pneumoniae* and *M pneumoniae,* and failures in treating pneumococcal pneumonia have been reported. One setting in which ciprofloxacin and ofloxacin are indicated for the therapy of lower respiratory tract infections is in cystic fibrosis, where *P aeruginosa* is the predominant pathogen.

Further controlled studies comparing fluoroquinolones with other available agents are needed to define their role. As noted above, ciprofloxacin in combination with other agents has been used to treat *M avium-intracellular* infections.

Adverse Effects

The most prominent adverse effects of the quinolones are nausea, vomiting, and diarrhea. Occasionally, headache, dizziness, insomnia, impaired liver function, and skin rashes have been observed as well as more serious reactions such as acute renal failure and anaphylaxis. Superinfections with enterococci and yeasts can develop. Clearance of theophylline may be inhibited by fluoroquinolones (especially enoxacin), and drug levels should be monitored in patients receiving both drugs. Prolongation of the prothrombin time has been observed in some patients receiving stable doses of warfarin after ciprofloxacin has been given. Because fluoroquinolones cause joint damage in young animals, they are not recommended for children or pregnant women. While fluoroquinolones appear in general to be well tolerated, their role—as compared with other drugs—needs to be established.

Grieden TR, Mangi RJ: Inappropriate use of oral ciprofloxacin. JAMA 1990;264:1438. (Case reports of inappropriate use.)

Hooper DC, Wolfson JS: Fluoroquinolone antimicrobial agents. N Engl J Med 1991;324:384. (Activity and clinical indications.)

Walker RC, Wright AJP: The fluoroquinolones. Mayo Clin Proc 1991;66:1249. (Activity, pharmacology, and clinical indications.)

PENTAMIDINE & ATOVAQUONE

Pentamidine and atovaquone are antiprotozoal agents that are primarily used to treat pneumocystis pneumonia. Pentamidine is discussed in Chapters 30 and 34. Atovaquone inhibits mitochondrial electron transport and probably also folate metabolism. It is poorly absorbed and should be given with food to maximize bioavailability. It has moderate activity against *P carinii*. In comparative trials with trimethoprim-sulfamethoxazole and pentamidine in the therapy of pneumocystis pneumonia in AIDS, atovaquone was less effective than both agents but better tolerated. Major adverse effects include rash, nausea, vomiting, diarrhea, fever, and abnormal liver function tests. The use of atovaquone is limited to patients with pneumocystis infections who have failed other therapies.

URINARY ANTISEPTICS

These drugs exert antimicrobial activity in the urine but have little or no systemic antibacterial effect. Their usefulness is limited to urinary tract infections.

1. NITROFURANTOIN

Nitrofurantoin is bacteriostatic and bactericidal for both gram-positive (including enterococci and staphylococci) and many gram-negative bacteria (not *S marcescens* or *P aeruginosa*) in concentrations of 10–500 µg/mL. Microbial resistance does not emerge rapidly. The activity of nitrofurantoin is greatly enhanced at pH 6.5 or less.

Nitrofurantoin is rapidly absorbed from the gut, but levels in serum and tissues are negligible. Thus, there is no systemic antibacterial effect. Use of the drug is limited to lower urinary tract infections. It is rapidly excreted in urine, where concentrations may be 200–400 µg/mL. In renal failure, there is virtually no excretion into the urine and no therapeutic effect.

The average daily dose in urinary tract infections is 100 mg orally four times daily, taken with food. A single daily dose of 50–100 mg can prevent recurrent urinary tract infections in women.

Oral nitrofurantoin often causes nausea and vomiting. Hemolytic anemia occurs in G6PD deficiency. Hypersensitivity may produce skin rashes and pulmonary infiltration.

2. NALIDIXIC ACID & CINOXACIN

Nalidixic acid is a synthetic urinary antiseptic that inhibits many gram-negative bacteria in concentrations of 1–50 µg/mL but has no effect on *Pseudomonas* or gram-positive organisms. In susceptible bacterial populations, resistant mutants emerge fairly rapidly.

Nalidixic acid is readily absorbed from the gut. In the blood, virtually all drug is firmly bound to protein. Thus, there is no systemic antibacterial action. About 20% of the absorbed drug is excreted in the urine in active form to give urine levels of 20–200

µg/mL, which may produce false-positive tests for glucose.

The dose in urinary tract infections is 1 g orally four times daily (for children, 30–60 mg/kg/d). Adverse reactions include nausea, vomiting, rash, drowsiness, visual hallucinations, excitement, and, rarely, increased intracranial pressure with convulsions.

Cinoxacin, a drug related to nalidixic acid, can be effective in urinary tract infections in oral doses of 250 mg four times daily or 500 mg twice daily. Because it is more expensive than nalidixic acid and has similar activity, its use is limited.

3. METHENAMINE MANDELATE & METHENAMINE HIPPURATE

These are salts of methenamine and mandelic acid or hippuric acid. The action of the drug depends on the liberation of formaldehyde from methenamine in the presence of acid. Almost all bacteria are inhibited by formaldehyde, which reaches levels of 200–800 µg/mL after an oral dose of 1 g. Little drug is excreted into the urine in renal insufficiency. Ammonia-producing organisms (eg, *Proteus*) produce an alkaline urine and may be resistant to these drugs. Sulfonamides and methenamine must not be given simultaneously. The usual dose is 2–6 g orally daily.

4. ACIDIFYING AGENTS

Urine with a pH below 5.5 tends to be antibacterial. Many substances can acidify urine and thus produce antibacterial activity. Ammonium chloride, ascorbic acid, methionine, and mandelic acid are sometimes used. The dose must be established for each patient by testing the urine for acid pH with test paper at frequent intervals.

SYSTEMICALLY ACTIVE DRUGS IN URINARY TRACT INFECTIONS

Many antimicrobial drugs are excreted in the urine in very high concentration. For this reason, low and relatively nontoxic amounts of many different antimicrobials can produce effective urine levels. Many penicillins, cephalosporins, aminoglycosides, quinolones, and trimethoprim-sulfamethoxazole can reach very high urine levels and can thus be effective in urinary tract infections.

ANTIFUNGAL DRUGS

Most antibacterial substances have no effect on pathogenic fungi. Only a few drugs are known to be therapeutically useful in mycotic infections (see Table 36–1).

1. AMPHOTERICIN B

Amphotericin B, 0.1–0.8 μg/mL, inhibits in vitro several organisms producing systemic mycotic disease in humans, including *Histoplasma, Cryptococcus, Coccidioides, Candida, Blastomyces, Sporothrix,* and others. This drug can be used for treatment of these systemic fungal infections. Intrathecal administration is necessary for the treatment of *Coccidioides* meningitis and may be required in meningitis caused by other fungi if systemic therapy fails (eg, *Cryptococcus, Candida*). *Pseudallescheria boydii* and *Fusarium* are often resistant to amphotericin B.

There is no absolute consensus on how amphotericin B should be administered or on the proper dosage and duration of therapy. Rarely, anaphylactic reactions to amphotericin B have been reported, and some clinicians prefer to give a test dose before starting therapy while others do not feel this is necessary. If a test dose is administered, 1 mg is given intravenously in 200 mL of 5% dextrose in water over 2–4 hours. If no adverse effects occur and the patient is not critically ill, 5 mg is given in 500 mL of 5% dextrose in water over 4–6 hours. Thereafter, the dose is increased by 5–10 mg daily until a final dosage of 0.4–0.75 mg/kg/d is reached. In critically ill patients, the dose is boosted more rapidly, eg, a test dose of 1 mg followed by 0.25 mg/kg; on day 2, 0.5 mg/kg; and on day 3, 0.75 mg/kg. The final dose is usually continued daily (or in double doses on alternate days) for many weeks. The usual infusion period has been 4–6 hours, though some advocate infusion over a shorter period (1–2 hours).

In fungal meningitis, amphotericin B, 0.5 mg, is injected intrathecally three times weekly; continuous treatment (many weeks) with an Ommaya reservoir is sometimes employed. Relapses of fungal meningitis (especially *Coccidioides* meningitis) occur commonly and can be seen years after completion of therapy. Thus, when treating meningitis due to *Coccidioides immitis,* intrathecal therapy is given three times a week for 8–10 weeks initially, and the frequency is then decreased to once-weekly doses for 6 months. Subsequent therapy is dictated by cerebrospinal fluid titers. In meningitis due to other fungi, long-term therapy beyond the initial 8–10 weeks is rarely needed. Combined treatment with flucytosine is beneficial in systemic candidiasis and cryptococcal meningitis. Amphotericin B can also be effective in *Naegleria* meningoencephalitis.

Amphotericin B has been used prophylactically to prevent invasive fungal infections in bone marrow transplant recipients and may be beneficial in this setting. Whether prophylactic administration is better than early empiric therapy in febrile patients who have not responded to broad-spectrum antibiotics has not been determined.

In patients with Foley catheters in place who have candiduria, amphotericin B bladder irrigations have been used to decrease colony counts. Twenty-five to 50 milligrams of drug is added to 500–1000 mL of sterile water . This solution is used for continuous (30–50 mL/h) or intermittent irrigation (200 mL four or five times daily with clamping of the catheter for ½ to 1 hour).

In impaired renal function, the dose of amphotericin B need not be reduced initially. However, if the serum creatinine reaches 2.5–3 mg/dL, the dose is temporarily lowered (or even stopped for a few days) until renal function recovers. Amphotericin B is then resumed at about one-half the previous dose and increased in 5 mg daily increments as tolerated. The drug is not removed by hemodialysis, and no additional drug is needed after dialysis.

The intravenous administration of amphotericin B usually produces chills, fever, vomiting, and headache. Tolerance may be enhanced by temporary lowering of the dose or by administration of aspirin, diphenhydramine, phenothiazines, meperidine, and corticosteroids. Therapeutically active amounts of amphotericin B commonly impair kidney and liver function and produce anemia (impaired iron utilization by bone marrow). Electrolyte disturbances (hypokalemia, distal renal tubular acidosis), shock, and a variety of neurologic symptoms also occur.

Liposomal amphotericin B, a water-soluble preparation, permits the administration of larger doses over a shorter period (30–60 minutes) with fewer adverse effects. Preliminary results suggest that this formulation may be beneficial for treatment of systemic fungal infections in the neutropenic patient—particularly hepatosplenic candidiasis that has not responded to conventional therapy with amphotericin B.

Galles HA, Drew RH, Pickard WW: Amphotericin B: 30 years of clinical experiences. Rev Inf Dis 1990;12:308. (Extensive review of clinical use and toxicity.)

2. GRISEOFULVIN

Griseofulvin is an antibiotic that can inhibit the growth of some dermatophytes but has no effect on bacteria or on the fungi that cause deep mycoses. Absorption of griseofulvin microsize, 1 g/d, gives blood levels of 0.5–1.5 μg/mL. The absorbed drug has an affinity for skin and is deposited there, bound to keratin. Thus, it makes keratin resistant to fungal growth, and the new growth of hair or nails is free of infection. As keratinized structures are shed, they are replaced by uninfected ones. The bulk of ingested griseofulvin is excreted in the feces. Topical application of griseofulvin has little effect.

Oral doses of 0.5–1 g/d for 3–5 weeks are given if only the skin is involved and for 3–6 months or longer if the hair and nails are involved. Griseofulvin is most successful in severe dermatophytosis, particularly if caused by *Trichophyton rubrum,* though some strains are resistant.

An ultramicrosize particle formulation (Gris-PEG) is better absorbed. The dose is 0.33–0.66 g orally daily.

Griseofulvin is relatively nontoxic and has a long history of clinical safety. Headache, nausea, vomiting, diarrhea, photosensitivity, and leukopenia have all been reported but are reversible and often will resolve without interruption of therapy. Routine monitoring for adverse effects is not required.

Major indications for use of this drug include tinea capitis, widespread tinea corporis, and tinea unguium (onychomycosis), though success rates in the latter are only 25–30%.

3. NYSTATIN

Nystatin has a wide spectrum of antifungal activity but is used almost exclusively to treat superficial candidal infections. It is too toxic for systemic administration, and the drug is not absorbed from mucous membranes or the gastrointestinal tract. Several preparations are available, including oral suspension (100,000 units/mL) and ointments, gels, and creams (100,000 units g). For oral candidiasis, 500,000 units of suspension is used to rinse the mouth and is retained in the mouth as long as possible before it is swallowed. This is repeated four times a day for at least 2 days after resolution of the infection. Infections of skin are treated with cream or ointment, 100,000 units applied to the affected area twice daily until resolution of the infection. Nystatin is less effective than miconazole and clotrimazole for therapy of vaginal candidiasis.

4. FLUCYTOSINE

Flucytosine inhibits some strains of *Candida, Cryptococcus, Aspergillus, Torulopsis,* and other fungi. Dosages of 3–8 g daily (150 mg/kg/d) orally produce good levels in serum and cerebrospinal fluid. Clinical remissions of meningitis or sepsis due to yeasts have occurred. However, resistant organisms are selected out rapidly, and flucytosine is therefore not employed as a single drug except in urinary tract infections.

In renal insufficiency, flucytosine may accumulate to toxic levels, and dosage adjustments are needed.

With normal renal function, the usual dose is 37.5 mg/kg every 6 hours; for creatinine clearance of 26–50 mL/min, 37.5 mg/kg every 12 hours is given; for creatinine clearance of 10–25 mL/min, 37.5 mg/kg once daily is given; and for clearance less than 10 mL/min, 12–25 mg/kg once daily is given. The drug is effectively removed by hemodialysis. Toxic effects include bone marrow depression, abnormal liver function, loss of hair, and others. The side effects may be caused by conversion of flucytosine to fluorouracil in the body. Combined use of flucytosine and amphotericin B in systemic candidiasis and cryptococcal meningitis has been shown to be of value. Flucytosine is effective for therapy of urinary tract infections caused by sensitive organisms.

Francis P Walsh TJ: Evolving role of Flucytosine in immunocompromised patients: New insights into safety, pharmacokinetics and antifungal therapy. Clin Infect Dis 1992;15:1003. (Uses and toxicities.)

5. NATAMYCIN

Natamycin is a polyene antifungal drug effective against many different fungi in vitro. When it is combined with appropriate surgical measures, topical application of 5% ophthalmic suspension may be beneficial in the treatment of keratitis caused by *Fusarium, Cephalosporium,* or other fungi. The drug may also be effective in the treatment of oral or vaginal candidiasis. The toxicity after topical application appears to be low.

6. ANTIFUNGAL IMIDAZOLES

These antifungal drugs increase membrane permeability and inhibit lipid and enzyme synthesis.

Clotrimazole, taken orally in 10 mg troches five times daily, can suppress oral candidiasis. Vaginal tablets (200 mg) inserted daily for 3 days are effective for vaginal candidiasis. Toxicity precludes systemic use.

Miconazole is active in vitro against *Coccidioides, Candida, Histoplasma, Cryptococcus, Paracoccidioides, Pseudallescheria,* and other fungi. However, it has substantial toxicity and little clinical activity and is rarely used intravenously. It is a drug of choice only for *P boydii* infections in a dose of 30 mg/kg/d in three doses. Its major use is as a 2% cream for dermatophytosis and as a 200 mg vaginal suppository for vaginal candidiasis.

Ketoconazole inhibits synthesis of sterols in fungal cell membranes. It can be given orally as a single dose, 200–600 mg daily, preferably with food. It is well absorbed and reaches serum levels of 2–4 μg/mL. The dose remains the same in renal or hepatic failure. Absorption is impaired by antacid, cimetidine, or rifampin administration.

Ketoconazole is primarily used to treat superficial infections caused by *Candida,* including oral, vaginal, and esophageal candidiasis. It dramatically improves lesions of chronic mucocutaneous candidiasis. Ketoconazole is also effective therapy for some deep-seated fungal infections such as blastomycosis, paracoccidioidomycosis, and nonmeningeal, localized histoplasmosis. However, this drug has been disappointing in the treatment of deep-seated candidal and coccidioidal infections (other than cutaneous lesions) and cryptococcal meningitis, where amphotericin B remains the drug of choice.

Adverse effects include nausea, vomiting, skin rashes, and occasional elevations in transaminase levels. Ketoconazole blocks the synthesis of adrenal steroids and testosterone and can cause gynecomastia and impotence. Ketoconazole also inhibits metabolism of terfenadine, causing accumulation of drug, prolongation of the QT interval, and ventricular arrhythmias. This combination should be avoided.

Fluconazole, a *bis*-triazole with activity similar to that of miconazole, is water-soluble and can be given both orally and intravenously. It penetrates well into the cerebrospinal fluid and eye and reaches therapeutically significant levels in the urine, making it an attractive agent for the therapy of fungal urinary tract infections due to susceptible organisms. The drug has been shown to be effective in therapy of infections with *Candida, Aspergillus, Cryptococcus, Blastomyces,* and other fungi in animal models, but experience in treating human disease is limited. Fluconazole (50–100 mg) appears to be as efficacious as ketoconazole (200 mg/d) and clotrimazole troches in the therapy of oropharyngeal candidiasis and is superior to ketoconazole for therapy of candidal esophagitis in immunosuppressed patients. It is also effective therapy for vaginal candidiasis and chronic mucocutaneous candidiasis. Fluconazole for therapy of invasive candidal infections has not been adequately studied. Encouraging reports have been published of clinical responses to fluconazole in leukemic patients with hepatosplenic candidiasis. These patients either failed to respond to amphotericin B or had severe reactions to it. A direct comparison of amphotericin B with fluconazole as initial therapy for invasive candidiasis has not been done and fluconazole thus cannot be recommended as initial therapy. Fluconazole (200 mg/d) is effective as chronic suppressive therapy of cryptococcal meningitis in patients with AIDS and is the drug of choice in this setting. Its use as initial therapy for cryptococcal meningitis in patients with AIDS is unclear. At a dose of 200 mg/d, response rates and overall mortality rates were the same in patients treated with oral fluconazole and with amphotericin B. However, the mortality rate in the first 2 weeks of therapy was higher in the fluconazole-treated group, and it took longer to sterilize the cere-

bral spinal fluid in the group. It is possible that higher doses (400–800 mg daily) may be more effective, but data are lacking. Based on the above findings, a reasonable approach to the AIDS patient with cryptococcal meningitis would be to initiate therapy with amphotericin B for 2 weeks and then switch to oral fluconazole. Experience with fluconazole in treatment of coccidioidomycosis is preliminary, and no recommendations can be made. Fluconazole, 400 mg daily, appears to be effective as prophylaxis against superficial and invasive fungal infections in bone marrow transplant recipients, but concern about superinfection with resistant organisms *(Candida krusei)* has been raised.

Although pharmacologic properties of the drug and early reports indicating fewer drug interactions than ketoconazole (ie, it may have less of an effect in cyclosporine levels) make fluconazole an attractive agent, it should be emphasized that controlled trials comparing it to existing agents have not been reported, and compared to ketoconazole it is expensive. (One 200 mg tablet of ketoconazole costs $1.68, versus $8.97 for one 200 mg tablet of fluconazole.)

Itraconazole is another oral imidazole with antifungal and pharmacologic properties similar to those of ketoconazole. It is well absorbed from the gastrointestinal tract (food increases absorption) and widely distributed in tissues with the notable of exception of the central nervous system, where levels in spinal fluid are undetectable. The drug is metabolized by the liver, and no dosage adjustment is needed in renal insufficiency. Itraconazole is very active against most strains of *Histoplasma capsulatum, Blastomyces dermatitidis, Cryptococcus neoformans, Sporotrichum schenkii,* and various dermatophytes. It is also active, though less so, against *Candida* and *Aspergillus* species and is inactive against *Fusarium* and zygomycetes. Itraconazole in doses of 200–400 mg/d is effective and approved therapy for localized or disseminated histoplasmosis and blastomycosis and is effective prophylaxis against recurrent histoplasmosis in patients with AIDS. It is also effective in sporotrichosis, dermatophytic infections, and oral and esophageal candidiasis. Noncomparative clinical trials indicate efficacy in therapy of invasive aspergillosis (55–80%) and coccidioidomycosis (57–94%). In the absence of comparative trials with other agents active against *C immitis* and *Aspergillus,* it is difficult to know if itraconazole should be used as a first-line drug against these organisms. Certainly the oral route of administration makes the drug attractive, particularly in patients who are not critically ill.

Adverse effects are similar to those of ketoconazole and fluconazole, with anorexia, nausea, vomiting, and abdominal pain occurring most commonly. Skin rash has been reported in up to 8% of patients. Hepatitis and hypokalemia occur uncommonly. Drugs that increase hepatic drug-metabolizing enzymes (isoniazid, rifampin, phenytoin, phenobarbital) may increase itraconazole metabolism, and higher doses may be needed when these drugs are administered concurrently with itraconazole. Itraconazole also impairs the metabolism of cyclosporine and can result in toxic levels unless the dose is adjusted.

The usual dose is 200 mg once or twice daily with meals, the latter dose being preferred in immunosuppressed patients and those with invasive aspergillosis. In patients with life-threatening infections, a 600-mg loading dose is given for 3 or 4 days.

Goodman JL et al: A controlled trial of fluconazole to prevent fungal infections in patients undergoing bone marrow transplantation. N Engl J Med 1992;326:845. (Superiority of fluconazole to placebo.)
Saaj MS et al: Comparison of amphotericin B with fluconazole in the treatment of acute AIDS-associated cryptococcal meningitis. N Engl J Med 1992;326:83. (Comparable response and mortality rates.)
Terrell CL, Hughes CE: Antifungal agents used for deep-seated mycotic infections. Mayo Clin Proc 1992; 67:69. (Available agents, clinical use, and toxicity.)

ANTIVIRAL CHEMOTHERAPY

Several compounds can influence viral replication and the development of viral disease.

Amantadine is active against influenza A (but not influenza B) and has efficacy both in prophylaxis and therapy of this infection. Yearly immunization against influenza is recommended (see Chapter 29) for disease prevention, but in certain select situations amantadine can be used for this purpose. Amantadine prophylaxis is 70–90% effective and is suggested for the influenza season (6–8 weeks) in patients who cannot be immunized who are at increased risk of developing complications of influenza (those with chronic pulmonary and cardiac diseases, persons over 65 years of age, persons with chronic metabolic diseases such as diabetes mellitus, and chronic renal failure); in medical personnel who cannot receive vaccine but are capable of transmitting influenza to high-risk patients; if vaccine is not available; and if vaccine strains differ from the strain causing an epidemic. Short-term prophylaxis (2 weeks) is indicated if an outbreak occurs before vaccination has been given. In this setting, amantadine will protect against disease while antibody production is induced and will not interfere with antibody production. Because of its modest therapeutic benefit, high-risk patients and others with influenza A may benefit from treatment with amantadine if it is instituted within 48 hours after the onset of symptoms and continued for 1 week. The usual adult dose is 200 mg orally per day (in persons over 65 years of age, 100 mg). The most marked untoward effects are insomnia, nightmares, and ataxia, especially in the elderly. Amantadine may accumulate and be more toxic in patients with renal insufficiency, and the dosage should be reduced.

Rimantadine, an analogue of amantadine, is as effective as amantadine and perhaps less toxic. It is marketed in Europe but is investigational in the USA.

Idoxuridine, 0.1% solution or 0.5% ointment, can be applied topically every 2 hours to the lesions of acute dendritic herpetic keratitis to enhance healing. It is also used, with corticosteroids, for stromal disciform lesions of the cornea to reduce the chance of acute epithelial herpes. Because of its toxicity for the cornea, it must not be used for more than 2–3 weeks.

Trifluridine ointment (1%) is more effective than idoxuridine in herpetic keratitis but also more expensive.

Vidarabine (adenine arabinoside), 3% administered topically, is very effective in herpetic keratitis. Vidarabine, 15 mg/kg/d intravenously, provides systemic treatment for some herpesvirus infections. It is effective in the therapy of herpes zoster infections in immunocompromised patients, for herpes encephalitis, and for neonatal herpes infections. Its use is limited, however, since acyclovir has equal or greater efficacy in these infections and is less toxic. The incidence of cytomegalovirus pneumonia in recipients of bone marrow transplants or kidney transplants has not been reduced by prophylactic vidarabine. Vidarabine is not effective for acyclovir-resistant mucocutaneous infections. (Foscarnet is the drug of choice; see below.) Topical vidarabine likewise has no effect on herpetic lesions of skin or mucous membranes.

The untoward effects of vidarabine include rashes, gastrointestinal disturbances, and neurologic abnormalities, including tremors, ataxia, abnormal electroencephalogram, paresthesias, and encephalopathy. All of these are enhanced in renal failure.

Methisazone, 2–4 g orally given within 2 days after exposure to smallpox, protects against clinical disease. The drug is also effective against complications of vaccinia, which continue to occur in military personnel in the USA. The most serious adverse effect is profuse vomiting.

Acyclovir is the least toxic antiviral drug, with therapeutic effects in infections due to herpes simplex and in herpes zoster-varicella infections. In herpes-infected cells, it is selectively active against viral DNA polymerase and thus inhibits virus proliferation. Given intravenously (15 mg/kg/d or 250–500 mg/m^2 every 8 hours), it can prevent and promote healing of mucocutaneous herpes simplex in immunocompromised patients. It can reduce pain, accelerate healing, and prevent dissemination of herpes zoster and varicella in immunocompromised patients. The usual dose for varicella-zoster infections is 30 mg/kg/d in three equal doses intravenously. The drug has no effect on establishment of latency, frequency of recurrence, or incidence of postherpetic neuralgia. Acyclovir (30 mg/kg/d in three equal doses intravenously) is the drug of choice for herpes encephalitis. Intravenous or oral acyclovir is effective prophylaxis against recurrent mucocutaneous and visceral herpes infections in transplant and other severely immunosuppressed patients. Intravenous acyclovir may also help in reducing cytomegalovirus infections in seropositive bone marrow and renal transplant patients.

Oral acyclovir, 200 mg five times daily, has therapeutic effects similar to those achieved with intravenous acyclovir, particularly in primary genital herpes simplex infections. Oral acyclovir for recurrent genital herpes has marginal effects on symptoms or viral shedding and is generally not used in this setting. When taken prophylactically (200 mg three times daily or 400 mg twice daily) for 4–6 months, oral acyclovir can reduce the frequency and severity of recurrent genital herpetic lesions during this period. Acyclovir minimally affects symptoms or viral shedding in recurrent herpes labialis and should not be used for this disease. However, in a dose of 400 mg twice daily, it is effective in preventing recurrent herpes labialis in those with frequent relapses and in preventing sun-induced relapses.

Other possible uses of oral acyclovir include (1) therapy of herpetic keratitis, (2) prevention and treatment of herpetic whitlow, (3) perhaps acceleration of healing of herpes zoster in immunocompetent patients if initiated within 48 hours after onset (600–800 mg five times daily for 10 days), (4) more rapid healing of rash and lessened clinical symptoms of primary varicella in adults and children if instituted within 24 hours after onset of rash and continued for 5–7 days, and (5) therapy of herpes proctitis (400 mg five times daily for 10 days).

Topical 5% acyclovir ointment can shorten the period of pain and viral shedding in herpes simplex mucocutaneous oral lesions in immunosuppressed patients but not in patients with normal immunity. Topical acyclovir has largely been replaced by the oral form of the drug.

Serum levels of 2.5 μg/mL are achieved after a 200 mg oral dose, and levels of 35–50 μg/mL are seen after an intravenous infusion of 5 mg/kg. Dosage reduction in renal insufficiency is required. For most infections except encephalitis, the usual dose is 5 mg/kg every 8 hours. For patients with creatinine clearances of 25–50 mL/min, give 5 mg/kg every 12 hours; for clearances of 10–24 mL/min, give 5 mg/kg every 24 hours; and for clearances of 0–10 mL/min, give 2.5 mg/kg every 24 hours. Since hemodialysis reduces serum levels significantly, the daily dose should be given after hemodialysis.

Acyclovir is relatively nontoxic. Precipitation of drug in renal tubules has been described and can best be avoided by maintaining adequate hydration and urine flow. Central nervous system toxicity manifested by confusion, agitation, tremors, and hallucinations has been described. Resistance has been described, usually in immunosuppressed patients who have received multiple courses of therapy.

Foscarnet (trisodium phosphonoformate) is a pyrophosphate analogue that inhibits viral DNA polymerase of human herpesviruses (CMV, herpes simplex, varicella-zoster) and the reverse transcriptase of human immunodeficiency virus. The drug is more expensive than ganciclovir, less well tolerated, and more difficult to administer. Therefore, its use is largely limited to patients who do not respond to ganciclovir or cannot tolerate it. Isolates of CMV resistant to ganciclovir and herpes simplex and varicella-zoster resistant to acyclovir are sensitive to foscarnet. Although studies are limited, foscarnet appears to be effective for CMV retinitis and has been used successfully in patients who have failed to respond to ganciclovir. Once therapy is stopped, recurrences develop, and lifelong suppressive therapy is required. In one study comparing foscarnet with ganciclovir for CMV retinitis in AIDS, the mortality rate was significantly lower in the foscarnet-treated group (34% versus 51%). It is not clear whether this result was due to the antiretroviral activity of foscarnet or to the lower dosage of zidovudine in the ganciclovir-treated group because of bone marrow suppression. Foscarnet has also been used to treat acyclovir-resistant mucocutaneous herpes simplex in AIDS patients (and is more effective than vidarabine in this setting) as well as varicella cutaneous lesions in AIDS patients who failed to respond to acyclovir. Uncontrolled trials suggest efficacy in CMV gastrointestinal disease, therapy of CMV infection following bone marrow and renal transplantation, and prevention of CMV disease when the drug is given prophylactically to seropositive bone marrow transplant recipients. Oral absorption is poor, and the drug must be given intravenously. The half-life is 3–5 hours, and this is prolonged with renal insufficiency. The usual induction dose is 60 mg/kg every 8 hours, and doses for maintenance therapy are 90–120 mg/kg once daily. Adjustments are required for even minimal impairment in renal function (see package insert).

Toxicity is a major drawback to widespread use of foscarnet. The drug can cause severe phlebitis and must be diluted to a concentration of 12 mg/mL to be given peripherally. At higher concentrations, it must be given centrally. Nephrotoxicity, which is dose-dependent and reversible, is its major toxicity. Uncontrolled studies have suggested that prehydration with 2.5 L of normal saline may protect against nephrotoxicity. Foscarnet binds divalent cations and hypocalcemia with peripheral neuropathy, seizures and arrhythmias, hypomagnesemia, hypophosphatemia, and hypocalcemia can occur. Monitoring of electrolytes and renal function is required during therapy. Anemia (20–50%), and nausea and vomiting (20–30%) are other common adverse effects.

Ribavirin aerosols sprayed into the respiratory tract early in influenza A and B infection of young adults or respiratory syncytial virus infections of small children resulted in a reduction of symptoms and more rapid recovery. Intravenous ribavirin can significantly lower the fatality rate of Lassa fever. The drug is teratogenic in animals, and pregnant women should not take care of patients receiving the aerosol.

Zidovudine (Retrovir; formerly azidothymidine [AZT]) is a synthetic thymidine analogue that can be incorporated into DNA by the DNA polymerase (reverse transcriptase) of retroviruses. This terminates chain synthesis of viral DNA. HIV reverse transcriptase is about 100 times more susceptible to inhibition by zidovudine than the DNA polymerase of mammalian cells.

Zidovudine, didanosine (dideoxyinosine, ddI), and **zalcitabine** (dideoxycytidine, ddC) inhibit reverse transcriptase of the HIV virus. They are used exclusively in the therapy of HIV-infected individuals and are discussed in detail in Chapter 30.

Ganciclovir is an analogue of acyclovir that has broad antiviral activity, including activity against CMV. Most information about its potential usefulness for the therapy of CMV infections comes from uncontrolled open trials. The drug appears to be efficacious in the therapy of CMV retinitis in AIDS patients, but once therapy is stopped, the relapse rate is high, and long-term maintenance suppressive therapy is required. Ganciclovir has a modest effect on CMV colitis in AIDS patient. In one of the few prospective, double-blinded, controlled, randomized studies performed, ganciclovir at a dosage of 5 mg/kg every 12 hours for 14 days decreased the incidence of positive cultures and improved the appearance of the colon on colonoscopy compared with placebo, but diarrhea, weight loss, and fever were unaffected. In another controlled study of bone marrow transplant recipients with CMV gastroenteritis (esophagitis, gastritis, duodenitis), ganciclovir was no better than placebo in relief of symptoms. Therapy of CMV pneumonitis with this agent has been disappointing. Uncontrolled studies of small numbers of patients have suggested that the addition of intravenous immunoglobulin to ganciclovir may improve therapy of CMV pneumonitis. CMV viremia and hepatitis are often self-limited diseases, and the role of ganciclovir in treating these syndromes awaits clarification. Ganciclovir appears to be most efficacious as a prophylactic agent. Several studies have shown that administration of ganciclovir prophylactically for 100–120 days to seropositive bone marrow transplant recipients decreases the incidence of CMV disease. Similar results have been demonstrated in heart transplant recipients treated for 28 days. As noted above, although ganciclovir alone is not effective in the therapy of CMV pneumonia, if the drug is initiated when asymptomatic viral excretion occurs (as determined by a positive culture in bronchoalveolar lavage), there is a marked reduction in the subsequent development of pneumonia. This again emphasizes

ganciclovir's efficacy as a prophylactic agent. It should be emphasized that regimens employing high-dose intravenous and oral acyclovir have also been shown to be effective in preventing CMV disease following bone marrow and renal transplants. Whether ganciclovir is more or less effective than acyclovir has not yet been determined.

The initial dose of ganciclovir is usually 2.5 mg/kg every 8 hours or 5 mg/kg every 12 hours, resulting in peak serum levels of 18–24 µg/mL and cerebrospinal fluid levels of 2–2.7 µg/mL. The drug is cleared by the kidneys, and dosage adjustments are required for creatinine clearances less than 50 mL/min. For clearances of 30–50 mL/min, 2.5 mg/kg every 12 hours should be given; for clearances of 10–29 mL/min, 2.5 mg/kg once daily should be given; and for a clearance of less than 10 mL/min, a single daily dose of 1.25 mg/kg is given. Usual maintenance therapy in a patient with normal renal function is 5 mg/kg/d for 5 days a week.

The major adverse effect is neutropenia, which is reversible but requires dosage reduction. Thrombocytopenia, disorientation, nausea, rash, and phlebitis occur less commonly.

Human interferons. Interferons have been prepared from stimulated lymphocytes and more recently by DNA recombinant technology. These agents have antiviral, antitumor, and immunoregulatory properties and are currently approved in the USA for treatment of hairy cell leukemia, condyloma acuminatum, Kaposi's sarcoma in AIDS, and chronic hepatitis C virus infection and as prophylaxis against infection in patients with chronic granulomatous disease. Approval is pending for therapy of basal cell carcinoma. Usefulness against a number of other diseases (chronic myelogenous leukemia, cutaneous squamous cell carcinoma, hepatitis B, laryngeal papillomatosis, life-threatening hemangioma in infancy) is under investigation. Relapse of the underlying disease after cessation of therapy is common but usually responds to reinstitution of drug. Adverse effects are common and include an influenza-like illness with fever, chills, nausea, vomiting, headache, arthralgia, and myalgias. Bone marrow suppression, especially with high-dose therapy, has also been reported.

Baron S et al: The interferons: Mechanism of action and clinical applications. JAMA 1991;266:1375. (Mechanism of action, toxicity, and approved and potential uses.)

Drugs for viral infections. Med Lett Drugs Ther 1990; 32:73.

Goodrich JM et al: Ganciclovir prophylaxis to prevent cytomegalovirus disease after allogenic marrow transplant. Ann Intern Med 1993;118:173. (A double-blind placebo controlled study demonstrating efficacy of ganciclovir in prophylaxis.)

Keating MR: Viral agents. Mayo Clin Proc 1992;67:160.

(Mechanisms, toxicity, and clinical uses of approved and some investigational agents.)

Whitley RJ, Gnann JW: Acyclovir: A decade later. N Engl J Med 1992;327:782. (Clinical uses and adverse effects.)

IMMUNOGLOBULINS

Immunoglobulins are proteins that are produced by B lymphocytes. Originally only available for intramuscular injection, several preparations now available for intravenous administration are safe, effective, and not associated with the discomfort experienced with intramuscular preparations. Immune globulin intravenous (IGIV) is well-preserved structurally and functionally and has a half-life similar to that of native immunoglobulin G (IgG), ie, 18–23 days. It has been used in a wide variety of diseases, including primary and secondary immune deficiency states and immune regulatory disorders (eg, idiopathic thrombocytopenic purpura) and for prophylaxis and treatment of bacterial and viral infections. Potential uses of IGIV include the following.

(1) Primary immunodeficiencies: IGIV reduces the rate of infection in patients with primary immunodeficiencies such as X-linked agammaglobulinemia and common variable immunodeficiency and is routinely used in these diseases.

(2) Bone marrow transplantation: IGIV reduces local infections and septicemia and may reduce graft-versus-host disease in these patients. IGIV does not prevent CMV pneumonia in the posttransplant period. Small uncontrolled studies have suggested that the addition of IGIV to ganciclovir improves the outcome of documented CMV pneumonia.

(3) Chronic lymphocytic leukemia: Serious bacterial infections can be prevented by use of IGIV in patients with chronic lymphocytic leukemia.

(4) Idiopathic thrombocytopenic purpura (ITP): IGIV has been used in both children and adults to increase platelet counts in patients with life-threatening hemorrhage. IGIV has also been used in patients with steroid-refractory ITP and in chronic ITP to delay the need for splenectomy.

(5) Kawasaki syndrome: A single large dose of IGIV (2 g/kg) with or without aspirin reduces the inflammatory response and decreases the incidence of coronary artery aneurysm formation.

(6) Pediatric AIDS: eh6 Children with symptomatic HIV infection and greater than 200 CD4 lymphocytes per microliter who are treated with 400 mg/kg of IGIV every 28 days have fewer serious bacterial infections (primarily pneumonia and bacteremia), a reduced rate of hospitalization for acute care, and a longer time free from serious infection than similar patients who do not receive IGIV. Treatment with IGIV does not affect mortality rate. Most of the patients who benefited from IGIV were not receiving zidovudine or prophylaxis for pneumocystis pneumo-

nia. Whether patients receiving such prophylaxis will also benefit from IGIV is under investigation.

(7) Other potential uses: IGIV has been used in a number of other clinical settings, including prophylaxis in high-risk postoperative patients to reduce the risk of infection (primarily gram-negative pneumonia and bacteremia), infection prevention in low-birth-weight infants, as adjunctive therapy in neonatal infections, for chronic inflammatory demyelinating polyneuropathies, in Guillain-Barré syndrome, and for intractable seizures in children. At present, large controlled studies have not been done in patients with these entities, and the routine use of IGIV for these purposes cannot be recommended.

Adverse effects occur in about 5% of patients, but they are usually mild and do not prevent repeated use. Pyrogenic reactions with high fevers and minor systemic reactions manifested by myalgias, nausea, vomiting, headache, and tachycardia are among the most common adverse effects. More serious anaphylactic reactions have been described but are rare.

The adverse reactions can be prevented by reducing the rate of infusion or by premedicating with hydrocortisone. Hepatitis B virus and HIV are not transmitted by these preparations.

The doses of IGIV vary depending on the disease state being treated. The manufacturers' recommendations or the two comprehensive reviews cited below should be consulted for specific dosages.

Berkman SA, Lee ML, Gale RP: Clinical uses of intravenous immunoglobulins. Ann Intern Med 1990;112:278. (Based on extensive review of the literature.)

NIH Consensus Conference: Intravenous immunoglobulin: Prevention and treatment of disease. JAMA 1990; 264:3189. (Indications and risks, future research.)

ANTIMICROBIAL DRUGS USED IN COMBINATION

Indications

Possible reasons for employing two or more antimicrobials simultaneously instead of a single drug are as follows:

(1) Prompt broad-spectrum treatment in desperately ill patients suspected of having a serious microbial infection. A good guess about the most probable two or three pathogens is made, and drugs with activity against these organisms are given. Before such treatment is started, adequate specimens must be obtained for identifying the etiologic agent in the laboratory. Examples include suspected gram-negative or staphylococcal sepsis and bacterial meningitis.

(2) To delay the emergence of microbial mutants resistant to one drug in chronic infections by the use of a second or third non-cross-reacting drug. The most prominent example is the use of multiple drugs to treat active tuberculosis.

(3) Mixed infections, particularly those following massive trauma or peritonitis following rupture of a viscus where multiple organisms may be involved. Each drug is aimed at an important pathogenic microorganism.

(4) To achieve bactericidal synergism (see below). In some infections (endocarditis and meningitis), bactericidal drugs are needed for a successful outcome. Most enterococci are inhibited—but not killed—by ampicillin or vancomycin. Thus, when treating endocarditis due to this organism, a bactericidal combination of drugs (ampicillin or vancomycin in combination with gentamicin) is needed for a successful outcome. Unfortunately, such synergism is unpredictable. A given drug pair may be synergistic for only one microbial strain. Occasionally, simultaneous use of two drugs permits significant reduction in dose and thus avoids toxicity but still provides satisfactory antimicrobial action. Finally, use of synergistic combinations of drugs may allow for a shorter course of therapy—eg, endocarditis due to penicillin-sensitive viridans streptococci can be treated with 2 weeks of penicillin plus gentamicin or 4 weeks of penicillin alone.

Disadvantages

The following disadvantages of using antimicrobial drugs in combinations must always be considered:

(1) The doctor may feel that since several drugs are already being given, everything possible has been done for the patient. This attitude leads to relaxation of the effort to establish a specific diagnosis. It may also give a false sense of security.

(2) The more drugs are administered, the greater the chance for drug reactions to occur or for the patient to become sensitized to drugs.

(3) The cost is unnecessarily high.

(4) Antimicrobial combinations often accomplish no more than an effective single drug.

(5) On rare occasions, one drug may antagonize a second drug given simultaneously. Antagonism resulting in higher morbidity and mortality rates has been observed mainly in bacterial meningitis when a bacteriostatic drug (eg, tetracycline or chloramphenicol) was given prior to or with a bactericidal drug (eg, a penicillin or aminoglycoside). However, antagonism is usually limited by time-dose relationships and is overcome by an excess dose of one of the drugs in the pair and is therefore a very infrequent problem in clinical therapy.

(6) Combination therapy with broad-spectrum antibiotics may promote superinfection with resistant organisms.

Synergism

Antimicrobial synergism can occur in several types of situations. Synergistic drug combinations must be selected by complex laboratory procedures.

(1) Sequential block of a microbial metabolic pathway by two drugs. Sulfonamides inhibit the use of extracellular p-aminobenzoic acid by some microbes for the synthesis of folic acid. Trimethoprim or pyrimethamine inhibits the next metabolic step, the reduction of dihydrofolic to tetrahydrofolic acid. The simultaneous use of a sulfonamide plus trimethoprim is effective in some bacterial infections (eg, urinary tract, enteric) and in some parasitic infections (*Pneumocystis* infection). Pyrimethamine plus a sulfonamide is used in toxoplasmosis and malaria.

(2) One drug may greatly enhance the uptake of a second drug and thereby greatly increase the overall bactericidal effect. Penicillins enhance the uptake of aminoglycosides by enterococci. Thus, a penicillin plus an aminoglycoside may be essential for the eradication of *E faecalis,* particularly in sepsis or endocarditis. Similarly, ticarcillin (and other antipseudomonal β-lactams) plus gentamicin may be synergistic against some strains of *Pseudomonas.* Cell wall inhibitors (penicillins and cephalosporins) may also enhance the entry of aminoglycosides into other gram-negative bacteria and thus produce synergistic effects.

(3) One drug may affect the cell membrane and facilitate the entry of the second drug. The combined effect may then be greater than the sum of its parts. Polymyxins have been synergistic with trimethoprim-sulfamethoxazole or rifampin against *Serratia,* and amphotericin B has been synergistic with flucytosine against *Candida* and *Cryptococcus.*

(4) One drug prevents the inactivation of a second drug by microbial enzymes. Thus, inhibitors of β-lactamase (eg, clavulanic acid) can protect amoxicillin or ticarcillin from inactivation by β-lactamase-producing *H influenzae* and other organisms.

ANTIMICROBIAL CHEMOPROPHYLAXIS

Anti-infective chemoprophylaxis implies the administration of antimicrobial drugs to prevent infection. In a broader sense, it also includes the use of antimicrobial drugs soon after the acquisition of pathogenic microorganisms (eg, after compound fracture) but before the development of signs of infection.

Useful chemoprophylaxis is limited to the action of a specific drug on a specific organism. An effort to prevent all types of microorganisms in the environment from establishing themselves only selects the most drug-resistant organisms as the cause of a resulting infection. In all proposed uses of prophylactic antimicrobials, the risk of the patient's acquiring an infection must be weighed against the toxicity, cost, inconvenience, and enhanced risk of superinfection resulting from the "prophylactic" drug.

Prophylaxis in Persons of Normal Susceptibility Exposed to a Specific Pathogen

In this category, a specific drug is administered to prevent one specific infection (prophylaxis). Outstanding examples are the injection of benzathine penicillin G, 1.2 million units intramuscularly once every 3–4 weeks, to prevent reinfection with group A hemolytic streptococci in patients who have had rheumatic fever; prevention of meningitis by eradicating the meningococcal carrier state with rifampin, 600 mg orally twice daily for 2 days, or minocycline, 100 mg every 12 hours for 5 days; prevention of *H influenzae* disease in contacts of patients with rifampin, 20 mg/kg/d for 4 days; prevention of syphilis by the injection of benzathine penicillin G, 2.4 million units intramuscularly, within 24 hours of exposure; and prevention of plague pneumonia in contacts of plague victims with tetracycline, 0.5 g twice daily for 5 days.

Early treatment of an asymptomatic infection is sometimes called "prophylaxis." Thus, administration of isoniazid, 6–10 mg/kg/d (maximum, 300 mg daily) orally for 6 months, to an asymptomatic person who converts from a negative to a positive tuberculin skin test may prevent later clinically active tuberculosis.

Prophylaxis in Persons of Increased Susceptibility

Certain anatomic or functional abnormalities predispose to serious infections. It may be feasible to prevent or abort such infections by giving a specific drug for short periods. Some important examples are listed below:

A. Heart Disease: Persons with abnormalities of heart valves or with prosthetic valves are unusually susceptible to implantation of microorganisms circulating in the bloodstream. Thus, bacterial endocarditis can sometimes be prevented if the proper drug can be used during periods of bacteremia. Large numbers of viridans streptococci are introduced into the circulation during dental procedures and operations on the mouth or throat. At such times, the increased risk warrants the use of a prophylactic antimicrobial drug aimed at viridans streptococci, eg, amoxicillin, 3 g orally 1 hour before and 1.5 g 6 hours after the procedure. In high-risk patients such as those with prosthetic valves or a history of endocarditis, parenteral therapy may be given (ampicillin plus gentamicin followed by oral amoxicillin), though recent recommendations indicate that oral prophylaxis is satisfactory even in these patients. (See Table 37–9 for prophylactic regimens in dental, oral, or upper respiratory tract procedures.) In persons hypersensitive to penicillin or those receiving daily doses of penicillin for prolonged periods (for rheumatic fever prophy-

laxis), either erythromycin or clindamycin can be given.

Enterococci cause 5–15% of cases of bacterial endocarditis. They reach the bloodstream from the urinary or gastrointestinal tract or from the female genital tract. During surgical procedures in these areas, persons with heart valve abnormalities can be given prophylaxis directed against enterococci, eg, ampicillin, 2 g intramuscularly or intravenously, plus gentamicin, 1.5 mg/kg intramuscularly, 30 minutes prior to the procedure followed by amoxicillin, 1.5 g orally 6 hours after the initial dose or followed by the parenteral regimen 8 hours after the initial dose (See Table 37–9).

The risk of developing an infection of a prosthetic joint following invasive procedures is thought to be very low, and the role of prophylactic antibiotics in preventing these infections has not been studied. Nonetheless, most physicians do administer prophylactic antibiotics to persons with prosthetic joints, and the regimens followed are the same as those for endocarditis prophylaxis (Table 37–9).

During and after cardiac catheterization, blood cultures may be positive in 10–20% of patients. Many of these persons also have fever, but very few acquire endocarditis. Prophylactic antimicrobials do not appear to influence these events.

B. Respiratory Tract Disease: Persons with functional and anatomic abnormalities of the respiratory tract—eg, emphysema or bronchiectasis—are subject to attacks of "recurrent chronic bronchitis." This is a recurrent bacterial infection, often precipitated by acute viral infections and resulting in respiratory decompensation. The most common organisms are pneumococci and *H influenzae*. Chemoprophylaxis consists of giving tetracycline or ampicillin, 1 g daily orally, during the "respiratory disease season." This is successful only in patients who are not hospitalized; otherwise, superinfection with *Pseudomonas, Proteus,* or yeasts is common. Similar prophylaxis of bacterial infection has been applied to children with cystic fibrosis who are not hospitalized. In spite of this, such children contract complicating infections caused by *Pseudomonas* and staphylococci. The efficacy of aerosolized aminoglycosides in preventing recurrences of infection in cystic fibrosis has not been conclusively demonstrated. Trimethoprim-sulfamethoxazole is effective as a prophylactic against pneumocystis pneumonia in immunocompromised persons.

C. Recurrent Urinary Tract Infection: In certain women who are subject to frequently recurring urinary tract infections, oral intake of nitrofurantoin, 100 mg, or trimethoprim (40 mg)-sulfamethoxazole (200 mg), daily or three times weekly; trimethoprim, 100 mg daily; and others may markedly reduce the frequency of symptomatic recurrences.

Some women frequently develop symptoms of cystitis after sexual intercourse. The ingestion of a single dose of antimicrobial drug —trimethoprim, 40 mg, plus sulfamethoxazole, 200 mg; or 100 mg of nitrofurantoin or 250 mg of cephalexin— can prevent postcoital cystitis by early inhibition of growth of bacteria moved into the proximal urethra or bladder from the introitus during intercourse.

D. Opportunistic Infections in Immunocompromised Patients: Patients with leukemia or neoplasm develop profound leukopenia while being given antineoplastic chemotherapy or when undergoing bone marrow transplantation. When the neutrophil count falls below 500/µL, they become unusually susceptible to opportunistic infections, most often gram-negative sepsis. In some cancer centers, such individuals are given a drug combination (antipseudomonal penicillin, aminoglycoside, cephalosporin) directed at the most prevalent opportunists at the earliest sign (eg, fever) of infection. This is continued until the granulocyte count rises again. Studies indicate that early institution of antibiotics to these highly susceptible individuals decreases morbidity and mortality. Fluconazole and amphotericin B may prevent fungal infections in these patients.

In some centers, neutropenic patients are given drugs to suppress the bowel flora such as oral insoluble antimicrobials (neomycin + polymyxin + nystatin, trimethoprim-sulfamethoxazole, norfloxacin, or ciprofloxacin) during the period of granulopenia to reduce the incidence of gram-negative sepsis. Some benefit has been reported from this approach.

Ganciclovir can prevent CMV infection in bone marrow transplant patients, and acyclovir appears to be effective in prevention of CMV disease in renal transplant recipients.

Prophylaxis in Surgery

A major portion of all antimicrobial drugs used in hospitals is employed on surgical services with the stated intent of "prophylaxis." The administration of antimicrobials before and after surgical procedures is sometimes viewed as "banning the microbial world" both from the site of the operation and from other organ systems that suffer postoperative complications. Regrettably, the provable benefit of antimicrobial prophylaxis in surgery is much more limited.

Several general features of "surgical prophylaxis" merit consideration.

(1) In clean elective surgical procedures (ie, procedures during which no tissue bearing normal flora is traversed, other than the prepared skin), the disadvantages of "routine" antibiotic prophylaxis (allergy, toxicity, superinfection) generally outweigh the possible benefits.

(2) Prophylactic administration of antibiotics should generally be considered only if the expected rate of infectious complications approaches or exceeds 5%. An exception to this rule is the elective insertion of prostheses (cardiovascular, orthopedic),

where a possible infection would have a catastrophic effect.

(3) If prophylactic antimicrobials are to be effective, a sufficient concentration of drug must be present at the operative site to inhibit or kill bacteria that might settle there. Thus, it is essential that drug administration begin 2 hours before operation.

(4) Prolonged administration of antimicrobial drugs tends to alter the normal flora of organ systems, suppressing the susceptible microorganisms and favoring the implantation of drug-resistant ones. Thus, antimicrobial prophylaxis should be continued for no longer than 24 hours after the procedure to prevent superinfection, and in most cases single-dose therapy is as effective as multiple doses.

(5) Systemic antimicrobial levels usually do not prevent wound infection, pneumonia, or urinary tract infection if physiologic abnormalities or foreign bodies are present.

In major surgical procedures, the administration of a "broad-spectrum" bactericidal drug just before the procedure has been found effective. First-generation cephalosporins have been most extensively studied and are usually employed for prophylaxis. They are as effective as second- and third-generation cephalosporins for prophylaxis and are much less expensive (see Table 37–5). Thus, cefazolin, 1 g intramuscularly or intravenously given 2 hours before gastrointestinal, pelvic, or orthopedic procedures, reduces the risk of deep infections at the operative site. Similarly, in cardiovascular surgery, antimicrobials directed at the commonest organisms producing infection are begun just prior to the procedure. While this prevents drug-susceptible organisms from producing endocarditis, pericarditis, or similar complications, it may favor the implantation of drug-resistant bacteria or fungi.

Other forms of surgical prophylaxis attempt to reduce normal flora or existing bacterial contamination at the site. Thus, the colon is routinely prepared not only by mechanical cleansing through cathartics and enemas but also by the oral administration of insoluble drugs (eg, neomycin, 1 g, plus erythromycin base, 1 g, every 6 hours) for 1 day before operation. In the case of a perforated viscus resulting in peritoneal contamination, there is little doubt that immediate treatment with an aminoglycoside, a penicillin, or clindamycin reduces the impact of seeded infection. Similarly, grossly infected compound fractures or war wounds benefit from a penicillin or cephalosporin plus an aminoglycoside. In all these instances, the antimicrobials tend to reduce the likelihood of rapid and early invasion of the bloodstream and tend to help localize the infectious process—though they generally are incapable of preventing it altogether. The surgeon must be watchful for the selection of the most resistant members of the flora, which tend to manifest themselves 2 or 3 days after the beginning of such "prophylaxis"—which is really an attempt at very early treatment.

In all situations where antimicrobials are administered with the hope that they may have a "prophylactic" effect, the risk from these same drugs (allergy, toxicity, selection of superinfecting microorganisms) must be evaluated daily, and the course of prophylaxis must be kept as brief as possible.

Topical antimicrobials (intravenous tube site catheter, closed urinary drainage, within a surgical wound, acrylic bone cement, etc) may have limited usefulness but must always be viewed with suspicion.

Certain procedures such as cardiac catheterization, thoracentesis, gastrointestinal endoscopy, and line placement do not require prophylaxis.

Antimicrobial prophylaxis in surgery. Med Lett Drugs Ther 1992;34:6.

Conte JE Jr: Antibiotic prophylaxis: Nonabdominal surgery. In: *Current Clinical Topics in Infectious Diseases,* vol 10. Remington JS, Swartz MN (editors). Blackwell, 1989. (Review of literature and recommendations for prophylaxis.)

Dajani AS et al: Prevention of bacterial endocarditis: Recommendations by the American Heart Association. JAMA 1990;264:2919. (Recent review of standard and alternative prophylactic regimens, including listings of dental or surgical procedures for which prophylaxis is and is not recommended. Also includes clindamycin oral and intravenous alternatives.)

Disorders Due to Physical Agents

38

Richard Cohen, MD, MPH

DISORDERS DUE TO COLD

Cold tolerance varies considerably among individuals. Factors that increase the likelihood of injury from exposure to cold include poor general physical conditioning, nonacclimatization, advanced age, systemic illness, poor tissue oxygenation, and the use of alcohol or other sedative drugs. High wind velocity ("wind-chill factor") increases the severity of cold injury at low temperatures.

Cold Urticaria

Some persons have a familial or acquired hypersensitivity to cold and may develop urticaria upon even limited exposure to a cold wind. The urticaria usually occurs only on exposed areas, but in markedly sensitive individuals the response can be generalized. Immersion in cold water may result in severe systemic symptoms, including shock. Recognition of the disorder is important because it has been responsible for deaths from swimming in cold water. Familial cold urticaria, manifested as a burning sensation of the skin occurring about 30 minutes after exposure to cold, does not seem to be a true urticarial disorder. In some patients with acquired cold urticaria, the disorder may be associated with the administration of drugs such as griseofulvin or with infections such as infectious mononucleosis. Cold urticaria may occur secondarily to cryoglobulinemia. Cold urticaria may be associated with cold hemoglobinuria as a complication of syphilis. In most cases of acquired cold urticaria, the cause is not known. For diagnosis, an ice cube is usually applied to the skin of the forearm for 4–5 minutes, then removed, and the area is observed for 10 minutes. As the skin rewarms, an urticarial wheal appears at the site and may be accompanied by itching. Histamine and other mediators released in the cold urticaria response are similar to those found in allergic reactions. Cyproheptadine in divided doses of 16–32 mg/d is the drug of choice for cold urticaria.

Raynaud's Phenomenon

See Chapter 12.

SYSTEMIC HYPOTHERMIA

Systemic hypothermia may result from exposure (atmospheric or immersion) to prolonged or extreme cold. The condition may arise in otherwise healthy individuals in the course of occupational or recreational exposure or in victims of accidents.

Systemic hypothermia may follow exposure even to comparatively ordinary temperatures when there is altered homeostasis due to debility or disease. In colder climates, elderly and inactive individuals living in inadequately heated housing are particularly susceptible. Acute alcoholism is commonly a predisposing cause. Patients with cardiovascular or cerebrovascular disease, mental retardation, malnutrition, myxedema, and hypopituitarism are more vulnerable to accidental hypothermia. The use of sedative and tranquilizing drugs may be a contributing factor. Prolonged postoperative hypothermia with increased mortality rates after surgery has been reported, especially in elderly patients. Administration of large amounts of refrigerated stored blood (without rewarming) can cause systemic hypothermia.

Pathogenesis

Systemic hypothermia is a reduction of core (rectal) body temperature below 35 °C (95 °F). It causes reduced physiologic function—with decreased oxygen consumption and slowed myocardial repolarization, peripheral nerve conduction, gastrointestinal motility, and respirations—as well as hemoconcentration and pancreatitis. The body defends itself against cold exposure by superficial blood vessel constriction and increased metabolic heat production.

Clinical Findings

Early manifestations of hypothermia are not specific. There may be weakness, drowsiness, lethargy, irritability, confusion, and impaired coordination. A lowered body temperature may be the sole finding.

The internal (core) body temperature in accidental hypothermia may range from 25 to 35 °C (77–95 °F).

Oral temperatures are useless, so an esophageal or rectal probe that reads as low as 25 °C is required. At core temperatures below 35 °C, the patient may become delirious, drowsy, or comatose and may stop breathing. Indeed, the pulse and blood pressure may be unobtainable, leading clinicians to believe the patient is dead. Metabolic acidosis, pneumonia, pancreatitis, ventricular fibrillation, hypoglycemia or hyperglycemia, coagulopathy, and renal failure may occur. Abnormalities in cardiac rhythm are directly related to the lowering of core temperature; cardiac arrhythmias may occur, especially during the rewarming process. Progression of electrocardiographic abnormalities can also occur, including the pathognomonic J wave of Osborn—a second upward wave immediately following the S wave, which has been well described in lead II. Death in systemic hypothermia usually results from cardiac arrest or ventricular fibrillation.

Treatment

Patients with mild hypothermia (rectal temperature > 33 °C [91.4 °F]) who have been otherwise physically healthy usually respond well to a warm bed or to rapid rewarming with a warm bath or warm packs and blankets. A conservative approach is also usually employed in treating elderly or debilitated patients, using an electric blanket kept at 37 °C (98.6 °F).

Patients with moderate or severe hypothermia (core temperatures of < 33 °C [91.4 °F]) do not have the thermoregulatory shivering mechanism and so require active rewarming with individualized supportive care. Adequate cardiovascular support, acid-base balance, arterial oxygenation, and adequate intravascular volume should be established prior to rewarming to minimize the risk of organ infarction. The methods and rate of active rewarming are controversial. Successful treatment usually includes a combination of active external and internal methods (see below). Aggressive rewarming should be attempted only by those experienced in the methods. *Once begun, CPR should continue until the patient has been rewarmed to at least 32 °C (89.6 °F).* The need for oxygen therapy, endotracheal intubation, controlled ventilation, warmed intravenous fluids, and treatment of metabolic acidosis should be dictated by careful clinical and laboratory monitoring during the rapid rewarming process. Essential laboratory tests include serum amylase, electrolytes, pH, hemoglobin, glucose, blood gases, and urine volume. Cardiac rhythm should be monitored, and cardiac, central vascular, or chest trauma or stimulation (catheter, cannulas, etc) should be avoided unless essential because of the risk of inducing ventricular fibrillation. The patient should be evaluated for trauma and peripheral cold injury (eg, frostbite). Steroids and antibiotics are not routinely given and should be used only if indicated. Core temperature (esophageal preferred over rectal) should be monitored frequently during and after initial rewarming because of reports of delayed (repeated) hypothermia.

Active external rewarming methods. Although relatively simple and generally available, active external warming methods may cause marked peripheral dilation that predisposes to ventricular fibrillation and hypovolemic shock. Either heated blankets or warm baths may be used for active external rewarming. Rewarming by a warm bath is best carried out in a tub of stirred water at 40–42 °C (104–107.6 °F), with a rate of rewarming of about 1–2 °C/h. It is easier, however, to monitor the patient and to carry out diagnostic and therapeutic procedures when heated blankets are used for active rewarming. Selective (external) thoracic rewarming has been recommended as a means of reducing the risk of peripheral vasodilation and resulting hypotension.

Active internal (core) rewarming methods. Internal rewarming is recommended for patients with severe hypothermia; extracorporeal blood rewarming (femorofemoral bypass) is the treatment of choice. Repeated peritoneal dialysis may be employed with 2 L of warm (43 °C [109.4 °F]) potassium-free dialysate solution exchanged at intervals of 10–12 minutes until the core temperature is raised to about 35 °C (95 °F). Parenteral fluids should be warmed to 40 °C (104 °F) prior to administration. The administration of heated, humidified air through a face mask or endotracheal tube may be useful, either alone or as an adjunct to other rewarming techniques. Warm colonic and gastrointestinal irrigations are of less value.

Prognosis

With proper early care, more than 75% of otherwise healthy patients may survive moderate or severe systemic hypothermia. The risk of aspiration pneumonia is great in comatose patients. The prognosis is grave if there are underlying predisposing causes or treatment is delayed.

HYPOTHERMIA OF THE EXTREMITIES

Exposure of the extremities to cold produces immediate localized vasoconstriction followed by generalized vasoconstriction. When the skin temperature falls to 25 °C (77 °F), tissue metabolism is slowed, but the demand for oxygen is greater than the slowed circulation can supply, and the area becomes cyanotic. At 15 °C (59 °F), tissue metabolism is markedly decreased and the dissociation of oxyhemoglobin is reduced; this gives a deceptive pink, well-oxygenated appearance to the skin. Tissue damage occurs at this temperature. Tissue death may be caused by ischemia and thromboses in the smaller vessels or by actual freezing. Freezing (frostbite) does not occur until the skin temperature drops to –10 to –4 °C (14–24.8 °F) or even lower, depending on such factors as wind, mobility, venous stasis, malnutrition, and occlusive arterial disease. Neuropathic sequelae such as pain, numbness, tingling, hyperhidrosis, cold sensitivity of the extremities, and nerve conduction abnormalities may persist for many years after the cold injury.

Prevention

"Keep warm, keep moving, and keep dry." Individuals should wear warm, dry clothing, preferably several layers, with a windproof outer garment. Wet clothing, socks, and shoes should be replaced with dry ones. Extra socks, mittens, and insoles should always be carried in a pack when a person is in cold or icy areas. Cramped positions, constricting clothing, and prolonged dependency of the feet are to be avoided. Arms, legs, fingers, and toes should be exercised to maintain circulation. Wet and muddy ground and exposure to wind should be avoided. Tobacco and alcohol should be avoided when the danger of frostbite is present.

CHILBLAIN
(Pernio)

Chilblains are red, itching skin lesions, usually on the extremities, caused by exposure to cold without actual freezing of the tissues. They may be associated with edema or blistering and are aggravated by warmth. With continued exposure, ulcerative or hemorrhagic lesions may appear and progress to scarring, fibrosis, and atrophy.

Treatment consists of elevating the affected part slightly and allowing it to warm gradually at room temperature. Do not rub or massage injured tissues or apply ice or heat. Protect the area from trauma and secondary infection.

FROSTBITE

Frostbite is injury of the tissues due to freezing. In mild cases, only the skin and subcutaneous tissues are involved; the symptoms are numbness, prickling, and itching. With increasing severity, deep frostbite involves deeper structures, and there may be paresthesia and stiffness. Thawing causes tenderness and burning pain. The skin is white or yellow, loses its elasticity, and becomes immobile. Edema, blisters, necrosis, and gangrene may appear. Scintigraphy has been used to assess the degree of involvement in severe frostbite and to distinguish viable from nonviable tissue.

Treatment

A. Immediate Treatment: Treat the patient for associated systemic hypothermia.

1. Rewarming–Superficial frostbite (frostnip) of extremities in the field can be treated by firm steady pressure with the warm hand (without rubbing), by placing fingers in the armpits, and, in the case of the toes or heels, by removing footwear, drying feet, rewarming, and covering with adequate dry socks or other protective footwear.

Rapid thawing at temperatures slightly above body heat may significantly decrease tissue necrosis. If there is any possibility of refreezing, the frostbitten part should not be thawed, even if this might mean prolonged walking on frozen feet. Refreezing results in increased tissue necrosis. Rewarming is best accomplished by immersing the frozen portion of the body for several minutes in a moving water bath heated to 40–42 °C (104–107.6 °F) *(not warmer)*. Water in this temperature range feels warm but not hot to the normal hand. Dry heat (eg, stove or open fire) is more difficult to regulate and is not recommended. After thawing has occurred and the part has returned to normal temperature (usually in about 30 minutes), discontinue external heat. Victims and rescue workers should be cautioned not to attempt rewarming by exercise or thawing of frozen tissues by rubbing with snow or ice water.

A protocol for treatment of frostbite is presented in Table 38–1.

2. Protection of the part–Pressure or friction is avoided and physical therapy contraindicated in the early stage. The patient is kept at bed rest with the affected parts elevated and uncovered at room temperature. Casts, dressings, or bandages are not applied. A combination of ibuprofen and aloe vera has been used to prevent dermal ischemia.

3. Anti-infective measures–It is very important to prevent infection after the rewarming process. Protect skin blebs from physical contact. Local infections may be treated with mild soaks of soapy water

---

Table 38–1. Modified Heggers/Robson protocol for treatment of frostbite.[1]

1. Patients with frostbite injuries are admitted to the hospital.
2. On admission, the affected areas are rapidly rewarmed in circulating warm water (104–105 °F) for 15–30 minutes. (Patients presenting 24 hours after injury are not rewarmed.)
3. On completion of rewarming, the affected parts are treated as follows:
   a. Blisters are debrided, and topical treatment with aloe vera gel every 6 hours is instituted.
   b. The affected parts are elevated, with splinting as indicated.
4. Tetanus prophylaxis.
5. Analgesia with IV or IM morphine or meperidine as indicated.
6. Unless contraindicated by the medical history, ibuprofen, 12 mg/kg PO per day for 1 week.
7. Penicillin, 500,000 units every 6 hours IM if signs of infection are present.
8. Daily hydrotherapy.
9. Physical therapy once edema resolves.

[1]From Heggers JP et al: Experimental and clinical observations on frostbite. Ann Emerg Med 1987;16:1956.

or povidone-iodine. Whirlpool therapy at temperatures slightly below body temperature twice daily for 15–20 minutes for a period of 3 or more weeks helps cleanse the skin and debrides superficial sloughing tissue. Antibiotics may be required for deep infections.

B. Follow-Up Care: Gentle, progressive physical therapy to promote circulation should be instituted as soon as tolerated.

C. Surgery: Early regional sympathectomy (within 36–72 hours) has been reported to protect against the sequelae of frostbite, but the value of this measure is controversial. In general, other surgical intervention is to be avoided. *Amputation should not be considered until it is definitely established that the tissues are dead.* Tissue necrosis (even with black eschar formation) may be quite superficial, and *the underlying skin may sometimes heal spontaneously even after a period of months.*

Prognosis

Recovery from frostbite is most often complete, but there may be increased susceptibility to discomfort in the involved extremity upon reexposure to cold.

IMMERSION SYNDROME
(Immersion Foot or Trench Foot)

Immersion foot (or hand) is caused by prolonged immersion in cool or cold water or mud, usually less than 10 °C (50 °F). The affected parts are first cold and anesthetic. They become hot with intense burning and shooting pains during the hyperemic period and pale or cyanotic with diminished pulsations during the vasospastic period; blistering, swelling, redness, heat, ecchymoses, hemorrhage, or gangrene and secondary complications such as lymphangitis, cellulitis, and thrombophlebitis follow later.

Treatment is best instituted during the stage of reactive hyperemia. Immediate treatment consists of protecting the extremities from trauma and secondary infection and gradual rewarming by exposure to cool air (not ice or heat) without massaging or moistening the skin or immersing it in water. Bed rest is required until all ulcers have healed. Affected parts are elevated to aid in removal of edema fluid, and pressure sites (eg, heels) are protected with pillows. Later treatment is as for Buerger's disease (see Chapter 12).

Bolgiano E et al: Accidental hypothermia with cardiac arrest: Recovery following rewarming by cardiopulmonary bypass. J Emerg Med 1992;10:427. (Use of femorofemoral bypass for treatment of severe hypothermia.)

Britt LD, Dascombe WH, Rodriguez A: New horizons in the management of hypothermia and frostbite injury. Surg Clin North Am 1991;71:345. (Pathophysiology, assessment, and clinical management of systemic hypothermia and frostbite.)

Jolly BT, Ghezzi KT: Accidental hypothermia. Emerg Med Clin North Am 1992;10:311. (Evaluation and emergency therapy of systemic hypothermia.)

DISORDERS DUE TO HEAT

Four medical disorders comprise a spectrum of illness that can result from excessive exposure to hot environments (in order of increasing severity): heat syncope, heat cramps, heat exhaustion, and heat stroke. A stable internal temperature requires a balance between heat production and heat loss, which the hypothalamus regulates by initiating changes in muscle tone, vascular tone, and sweat gland function.

Etiology

Sweat production and evaporation is a major mechanism of heat removal. Conduction (convection)—the direct transfer of heat from the skin to the surrounding air—also occurs, but with diminished efficiency as the ambient temperature rises. The passive transfer of heat from a warmer to a cooler object by radiation accounts for 65% of body heat loss under normal conditions. Radiant heat loss decreases as the temperature of the surrounding environment increases up to 37.2 °C (99 °F), the point at which heat transfer reverses direction. At normal temperatures, evaporation accounts for approximately 20% of the body's heat loss, but at high temperatures it becomes the major mechanism for dissipation of heat. This mechanism is also limited as humidity increases.

Health conditions that inhibit sweat production or evaporation and increase susceptibility to heat disorders include obesity, generalized skin diseases (miliaria), diminished cutaneous blood flow, dehydration, malnutrition, hypotension, and reduced cardiac output. Medications that impair the sweating mechanism are the anticholinergics, antihistamines, phenothiazines, tricyclic antidepressants, monoamine oxidase inhibitors, and diuretics; reduced cutaneous blood flow results from use of vasoconstrictors and β-adrenergic blocking agents; and dehydration results from use of alcohol. Illicit drugs—eg, phencyclidine, LSD, amphetamines, and cocaine—can cause increased muscle activity and thus generate increased body heat. Drug withdrawal syndrome may have the same effect, as may prolonged seizures.

Prevention

Medical evaluation and monitoring should be used to identify individuals at increased risk of heat disorders. The exposed public should be made aware of the early signs and symptoms of heat disorders. It is not recommended to make salt tablets available for use without medical supervision; close monitoring of fluid and electrolyte intake may be necessary in situations necessitating activity in hot environments. Athletic events should be organized and managed with attention to thermoregulation: the WBGT (wet bulb globe temperature) Index should be monitored, fluid consumption should be encouraged, and medical support should be immediately accessible. Workers should not begin work in hot temperatures without proper acclimatization and should be encouraged to take water frequently.

Protective air-cooled suits have been used successfully in the nuclear power industry for prolonged work in environments up to 60 °C (140 °F).

Acclimatization is achieved by scheduled regulated exposure to hot environments and by gradually increasing the duration of exposure and the work load, until the body adjusts by starting to produce sweat of lower salt content in greater amounts at lower ambient temperatures. Acclimatization is accompanied by increased plasma volume, cardiac output, and cardiac stroke volume and a slower heart rate.

SPECIFIC SYNDROMES DUE TO HEAT EXPOSURE

1. HEAT SYNCOPE

Sudden unconsciousness can result from cutaneous vasodilation with consequent systemic and cerebral hypotension. Systolic blood pressure is usually less than 100 mm Hg, and there is typically a history of vigorous physical activity for 2 hours or more just preceding the episode. The skin is typically cool and moist, and the pulse is weak.

Treatment consists of rest and recumbency in a cool place, with fluids by mouth (or intravenously if necessary).

2. HEAT CRAMPS

Fluid and electrolyte depletion can result in slow, painful skeletal muscle contractions ("cramps") and even severe muscle spasms lasting 1–3 minutes, usually of the muscles most heavily used. Cramping results from salt depletion as sweat losses are replaced with water alone. The skin is moist and cool, and the muscles are tender. There may be muscle twitching. The victim is alert, with stable vital signs, but may be agitated and complaining of pain. The body temperature may be normal or slightly increased. Involved muscle groups are hard and lumpy. There is almost always a history of vigorous activity just preceding

the onset of symptoms. Laboratory evaluation may show low serum sodium and hemoconcentration.

The patient should be moved to a cool environment and given oral saline solution (4 tsp of salt per gallon of water) to replace both salt and water. *Because of their slower absorption, salt tablets are not recommended.* The victim may have to rest for 1–3 days with continued dietary salt supplementation before returning to work or resuming heavy activity in the heat.

3. HEAT EXHAUSTION

Heat exhaustion results from prolonged heavy activity with inadequate salt intake in a hot environment and is characterized by dehydration, sodium depletion, or isotonic fluid loss with accompanying cardiovascular changes.

The diagnosis is based on prolonged symptoms and a rectal temperature over 37.8 °C (100 °F), increased pulse rate—usually more than half again the patient's normal rate—and moist skin. Symptoms associated with heat syncope and heat cramps may also be present. The patient may be quite thirsty and weak, with central nervous system symptoms such as headache, fatigue, and, in cases due chiefly to water depletion, anxiety paresthesias, impaired judgment, hysteria, and in some cases psychosis. Hyperventilation secondary to heat exhaustion can lead to respiratory alkalosis. Heat exhaustion may progress to heat stroke if sweating ceases.

Treatment consists of placing the patient in a shaded, cool environment and providing adequate hydration and salt replenishment—orally, if possible. Physiologic saline or isotonic glucose solution can be administered intravenously in severe cases or when oral administration is not appropriate. Intravenous 3% (hypertonic) saline may be necessary if sodium depletion is severe. At least 24 hours of rest is recommended.

4. HEAT STROKE

Heat stroke is a life-threatening medical emergency resulting from failure of the thermoregulatory mechanism. Heat stroke is imminent when the core (rectal) temperature approaches 41 °C (106 °F). It presents in one of two forms: classic heat stroke occurs in patients with compromised homeostatic mechanisms; exertional heat stroke occurs in previously healthy persons undergoing strenuous exertion in a thermally stressful environment. Morbidity or even death can result from cerebral, cardiovascular, hepatic, or renal damage.

Classic heat stroke is manifested by cerebral dysfunction with impaired consciousness, high fever, and absence of sweating. Persons at greatest risk are the elderly or chronically infirm or those receiving medications (eg, anticholinergics, antihistamines, phenothiazines) that interfere with heat-dissipating mechanisms.

Exertional heat stroke and exertion-related illnesses, including rhabdomyolysis, are appearing more frequently as complications of participation by unconditioned amateurs in strenuous athletic activities such as marathon running and triathlon competition.

Clinical Findings

A. Symptoms and Signs: Failure of the heat dissipation mechanism for any reason results in dizziness, weakness, emotional lability, nausea and vomiting, confusion, delirium, blurred vision, convulsions, collapse, and unconsciousness. The skin is hot and initially covered with perspiration. Later it dries. The pulse is strong initially. Blood pressure may be slightly elevated at first, but hypotension develops later. The core temperature is usually over 41 °C (106 °F). As with heat exhaustion, hyperventilation can occur, leading to respiratory alkalosis. Metabolic (lactic) acidosis may also develop.

Exertional heat stroke may present with sudden collapse and loss of consciousness followed by irrational behavior. Anhidrosis may not be present.

B. Laboratory Findings: Laboratory evaluation reveals dehydration, leukocytosis, elevated BUN, hyperuricemia, hemoconcentration, and decreased serum potassium, calcium, and phosphorus; urine is concentrated, with elevated protein, tubular casts, and myoglobinuria. Thrombocytopenia, increased bleeding and clotting times, fibrinolysis, and consumption coagulopathy may also be present. Rhabdomyolysis and myocardial, hepatic, or renal damage may be identified by appropriate tests.

Treatment

Treatment is aimed at reducing the core temperature rapidly (within 1 hour) and controlling the secondary effects. Evaporative cooling is rapid and effective and is easily performed in most emergency settings. The patient's clothing should be removed and the entire body sprayed with water (15 °C [59 °F]) while cooled or ambient air is passed across the patient's body with large fans or other means at high velocity (100 ft/min). The patient should be in the lateral recumbent position or supported in a hands-and-knees position to expose as much skin surface as possible to the air. Other alternatives include use of cold wet sheets accompanied by fanning or isopropyl alcohol instead of water. Cardiopulmonary bypass provides rapid cooling but is often not practical.

Immersion in an ice-water bath as initial treatment is no longer preferred because of its greater potential for complications of hypotension and shivering. However, it should be considered if core temperature is not decreased rapidly in response to other treatment. Alternatives include ice packs (groin, axillas, neck) and iced gastric lavage, though these are much less effective than evaporative cooling.

Treatment should be continued until the rectal temperature drops to 39 °C (102.2 °F). The temperature remains stable in most cases, but it should continue to be monitored for 24 hours. Chlorpromazine (25–50 mg intravenously) can be given initially and every 4 hours to control shivering and other muscular activity associated with increased heat load. Aspirin should not be given because of its antiplatelet effect; additionally, it has no effect on the hyperthermia.

Hypovolemic and cardiogenic shock must be carefully distinguished, as either or both may occur. Central venous or pulmonary artery wedge pressure should be monitored. Five percent dextrose in saline (500–1000 mL) may be given without overloading the circulation if hypovolemic shock is present.

The patient should also be observed for renal failure due to rhabdomyolysis, hypokalemia, cardiac arrhythmias, disseminated intravascular coagulation, and hepatic failure. Corticosteroids have not been shown to be of value.

Fluid output should be monitored through the use of an indwelling urinary catheter.

Because sensitivity to high environmental temperature continues in some patients for prolonged periods following an episode of heat stroke, immediate reexposure should be avoided.

Knochel JP: Heat stroke and related heat stress disorders. DM (May) 1989;35:303. (Predisposition, pathology, diagnosis, treatment, complications.)

Tek D, Olshaker JS: Heat illness. Emerg Med Clin North Am 1992;10:299. (Emergency diagnosis and treatment options.)

BURNS

Over 2 million injuries, 100,000 hospitalizations, and 12,000 deaths occur from burns each year in the USA. Burns are the leading cause of accidental death in children and are largely preventable.

Scalds are a common form of thermal injury to children and the elderly that can be partially prevented by regulating water temperatures. Enforcement of the Flammable Fabric Act in the USA has reduced the incidence of flame injury to children. However, loose-fitting clothing of the elderly is a hazard near an open flame. Carelessness with burning cigarettes is a common cause of dwelling fires.

...

CLASSIFICATION

Burns are classified by extent, depth, patient age, and associated illness or injury.

Extent

The "rule of nines" (Figure 38–1) is useful for rapidly assessing the extent of a burn. More detailed charts based on age are available when the patient reaches the burn unit. Therefore, it is important to view the entire patient after cleaning soot to make an accurate assessment, both initially and on subsequent examinations. Only second- and third-degree burns are included in calculating the total burn surface area (TBSA), since first-degree burns usually do not represent significant injury in terms of prognosis or fluid and electrolyte management.

Depth

Judgment of depth of injury is difficult. The **first-degree burn** may be red or gray but will demonstrate excellent capillary refill. First-degree burns are not blistered initially. If the wound is blistered, this represents a partial-thickness injury to the dermis, or a **second-degree burn**. However, a deep second-degree burn may have lost its blister and may actually appear hyperemic from fixed hemoglobin in the tissue. This redness will not have good refill and will not be as exquisitely sensitive as the hyperemia of the first-degree burn. The line between the partial- and full-thickness injury, or **third-degree burn,** may be

indefinite. The initial vasoconstriction of a second-degree burn may make it appear more severe at first. Concerning healing properties of any second- or third-degree burn, the critical factors are blood supply and appendage population. In areas rich in vascularity, hair follicles, and sweat glands, the prospects for reepithelialization are good. Otherwise, even when the dermis is healthy, epithelization may be slow and more scarring will result. Secondary infection may convert a burn from partial to full-thickness.

Age of the Patient

As much as extent and depth of the burn, age of the victim plays a critical part. Even a relatively small burn in an elderly patient or infant may be fatal, as demonstrated in Figure 38–2.

Associated Injuries & Illnesses

An injury commonly associated with burns is smoke inhalation (see Chapter 9). The products of combustion, not heat, are responsible for lower airway injury. Burning plastic products can produce both hydrochloric acid and hydrocyanic acid. Electrical injury that causes burns may also produce cardiac arrhythmias that require immediate attention. Premorbid physical and psychosocial disorders that complicate recovery from burn injury include cardiac or pulmonary disease, diabetes, alcoholism, drug abuse, and psychiatric illness.

Special Burn Care Units & Facilities

The American Burn Association and the American College of Surgeons have recommended that major burns be treated in specialized burn care facilities. They also advocate that even moderately severe burns be treated in a specialized facility or hospital where personnel have expertise in burn care. The American Burn Association has classified burn injuries as follows:

A. Major Burn Injuries:

1. Partial-thickness burns over more than 25% of body surface area in adults or 20% in children or the elderly.

2. Full-thickness burns over more than 10% of surface area in any age group.

3. Deep burns involving the hands, face, eyes, ears, feet, or perineum.

4. Burns complicated by inhalation injury.

5. Electrical and chemical burns.

6. Burns complicated by fractures and other major trauma.

7. Burns in poor-risk patients (extremes of age or intercurrent disease).

B. Moderate Uncomplicated Burn Injuries:

1. Partial-thickness burns over 15–25% of body surface area in adults or 10–20% of body surface area in children.

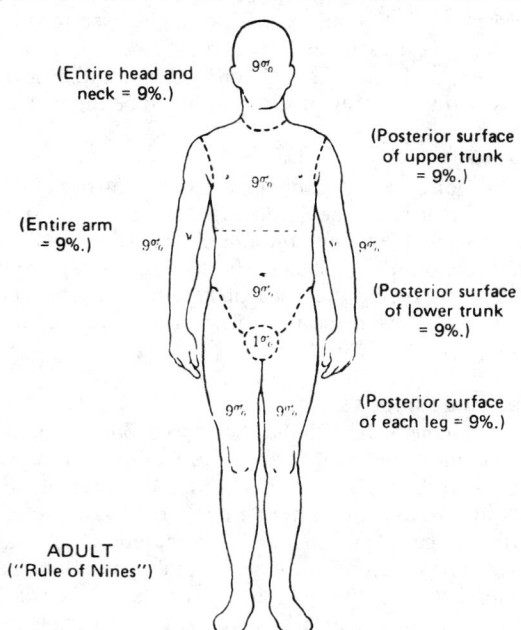

(Entire head and neck = 9%.)

9%

(Posterior surface of upper trunk = 9%.)

9%

(Entire arm = 9%.)

9% 9% 9%

(Posterior surface of lower trunk = 9%.)

9%

1%

(Posterior surface of each leg = 9%.)

9% 9%

ADULT
("Rule of Nines")

Figure 38–1. Estimation of body surface area in burns.

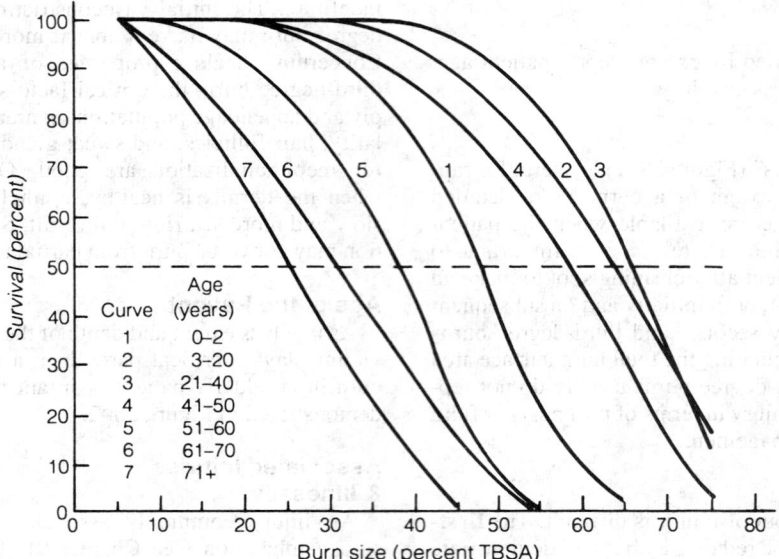

Figure 38–2. Patient survival and burn size according to patient age. (TBSA, total body surface area.) (Reproduced, with permission, from Merrell SW et al: Increased survival after major thermal injury. Am J Surg 1987;154:623.)

2. Full-thickness burns over 2–10% of body surface area.

3. Burns not involving the specific conditions listed above.

C. Minor Burn Injuries:

1. Partial-thickness burns over less than 15% of body surface area in adults or 10% in children or the elderly.

2. Full-thickness burns over less than 2% of body surface area.

INITIAL MANAGEMENT

Airway

The physician or emergency medical technician should proceed as with any other trauma. The first priority is to establish an airway, then to evaluate the cervical spine and head injuries, and then to stabilize fractures. *The burn wound itself has a lower priority.* Endotracheal intubation should be considered for major burn cases, regardless of the area of the body involved, for as fluid resuscitation proceeds, generalized edema develops, including the soft tissues of the upper airway and perhaps the lungs as well. *Tracheostomy is rarely indicated for the burn victim,* unless dictated by other circumstances. Supplemental oxygen should be administered. Inhalation injuries should be followed by serial blood gas determination and bronchoscopy. The use of corticosteroids is contraindicated because of the potential for immunosuppression.

Cooling the Wound

Cooling the victim for up to 20 minutes following the burn has been shown to reduce the depth of injury. Avoid prolonged application of cold water or ice packs to large surfaces, however, since they can cause systemic hypothermia and arrhythmias. Saline soaks at room temperature or cooler should be used. At the scene of an injury, a hose can be used for this purpose. Fire extinguishers and ice are not recommended, as further tissue injury may result. Hot or constricting clothing or jewelry should be removed.

History

As soon as possible, obtain a detailed history of the circumstances of the injury, including locale, substances involved, and duration of exposure; medications, mental disturbances, confusion resulting from the injury, or the presence of an endotracheal tube may later prevent the recording of an accurate history.

Vascular Access

Simultaneously with the above procedures, venous access must be sought, since the victim of a major burn is in hypovolemic shock. Ideally, a percutaneous intravenous line through nonburned skin is preferred. A peripheral line in an antecubital or subclavian vein is preferable to the femoral vein unless the femoral area is the only nonburned area. The last choice is to perform a well-secured peripheral cutdown. A burn eschar, since it has been flame-sterilized, is an acceptable location for cutdown. An arterial line may also be useful for monitoring mean arterial pressure. The line may be placed initially in the femoral artery and later changed (as peripheral resistance decreases) to a safer site such as the dorsalis pedis, temporal, or radial arteries.

FLUID RESUSCITATION

Crystalloids

Generalized capillary leak results from burn injury over more than 25% of the total body surface area. This often necessitates replacement of a large volume of fluid. An intravenous line is recommended in the management of deep partial-thickness and full-thickness burns that cover more than 20% of total body surface area.

There are many guidelines for fluid resuscitation, eg, those of Evans, Brooke, Monafo (3% hypertonic saline), and Parkland (Baxter). In the first 24 hours, all of these fluids deliver approximately 0.5–0.6 meq of sodium per kilogram of body weight per percent of body surface area burned. The total amount of fluid in all but the hypertonic saline formula is roughly the same but differs in distribution. The Parkland formula relies upon the use of lactated Ringer's injection. The fluid requirement in the first 24 hours is estimated as 3–5 mL/kg body weight per percent of body surface area burned (Figure 38–3). The smaller amounts would be used in the elderly or those with less severe burns; the larger amounts would be used in children (who have a larger relative surface-to-volume ratio) and for treatment of deep electrical burns. Four mL/kg body weight per percent of body surface area burned is begun, and this amount is varied according to the patient's response. *Remember that a formula is only a guideline.* Inhalation injury increases the fluid requirement.

Half the calculated fluid is given in the first 8-hour period. The remaining fluid, divided into two equal parts, is delivered over the next 16 hours. An extremely large volume of fluid may be required. For example, an injury over 40% of the total body surface area in a 70-kg victim may require 13 L *in the first 24 hours.* The first 8-hour period is calculated from the hour of injury.

Colloids

After 24 hours, capillary leaks have sealed in the majority of cases, and plasma volume may be restored with colloids (plasma or albumin). The Parkland formula calls for 0.3–0.5 mL/kg body weight per percent of body surface area burned to be given over the first 8-hour period of the second 24 hours. Fluids given in the following 16 hours consist of dextrose in water in quantities sufficient to maintain adequate urine output (Figure 38–4). It is hoped that during the second 24-hour period the vascular system will hold colloids and draw off edema fluid, resulting in diuresis.

Adequacy of Resuscitation

Mental alertness, urinary output, and the vital signs reflect the adequacy of fluid resuscitation. Mental alertness is important because it is the best indicator of adequate cerebral perfusion. Overmedication may cloud the sensorium during the resuscitation phase. For pain and anxiety, intravenous opioids and benzodiazepines can be used judiciously so as not to interfere with diagnosis or cause hypotension. Renal perfusion is judged by urinary output, which is the prime indicator of adequacy of resuscitation. Adequate urinary output is 30–50 mL/h in adults and 1 mL/kg body weight/h in children. A smaller output represents inadequate renal perfusion. However, a

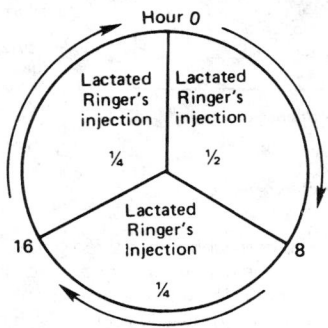

Figure 38–3. Half of the calculated crystalloid formula (lactated Ringer's injection [4 mL/kg wt per percent total body surface area]) is given in the first 8 hours, beginning at the time of the injury. The remainder is given evenly over the ensuing 16 hours.

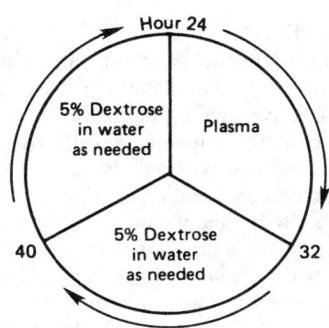

Figure 38–4. The colloid formula (aged plasma or 5% normal serum albumin) [0.3–0.5 mL/kg wt per percent total body surface area]) is given as calculated between hours 24 and 32. In the remaining 16-hour period, 5% dextrose in water is given as needed to maintain a urine output of no less than 30 mL/h.

larger output is unnecessary, and overloading results in edema in every organ.

Monitoring Fluid Resuscitation

A Foley catheter is essential for monitoring urinary output. *Diuretics have no role in this phase of patient management.*

Escharotomy

As edema fluid accumulates, ischemia may develop under any constricting eschar of an extremity. Similarly, an eschar of the thorax or abdomen may limit respiratory excursion. Escharotomy incisions through the anesthetic eschar can save life and limb.

Griglak MJ: Thermal injury. Emerg Med Clin North Am 1992;10:369. (Emergency assessment and management of burns.)

Purdue GF, Hunt JL: Inhalation injuries and burns in the inner city. Surg Clin North Am 1991;71:385. (Initial management, fluid resuscitation, and treatment of inhalation injuries.)

THE BURN WOUND

Treatment of the burn wound is based on several principles: (1) Prevention or delay of infection. (2) Protection from desiccation and further injury of those burned areas that will spontaneously reepithelialize in 7–10 days. (3) Early excision and grafting of burned areas that are infected or which cannot spontaneously reepithelialize during this period.

Systemic Prophylactic Antibiotics

Regardless of the severity of the burn, prophylactic systemic antibiotics are usually not recommended. Their effectiveness is unproved, and they have the disadvantage of favoring the growth of resistant organisms.

Topical Antibiotics

Topical antibiotics delay or prevent infection. An ideal agent would readily penetrate the burn wound eschar, be effective against both gram-negative and gram-positive microorganisms as well as *Candida,* be painless and inexpensive, and have no deleterious side effects. Such an ideal agent does not currently exist. Silver sulfadiazine is currently the most popular topical agent. It is painless, easy to apply, effective against most *Pseudomonas,* and a fairly good penetrator of eschar, but some microorganisms are resistant to it, and it may cause leukopenia or fever and delay epithelization.

Mafenide penetrates eschars better than silver sulfadiazine and is more effective against *Pseudomonas.* Mafenide inhibits carbonic anhydrase when used as a 10% solution and results in metabolic acidosis. It also delays epithelization and may be painful. When it is diluted to a 5% solution, pain and metabolic side effects are lessened. Mafenide is especially recommended for burns over cartilage (nose, ears), as it penetrates well. (Infections of the nose or ears result in chondritis, which can have catastrophic consequences.) It is useful also for deep burns, eg, electrical burns, and when silver sulfadiazine is ineffective. It is best to limit the use of mafenide to no more than 10% of the total body surface area at any given time because of its metabolic effect.

Povidone-iodine is especially useful against *Candida* and both gram-positive and gram-negative microorganisms. However, it penetrates eschar poorly, is very desiccating to the wound surface, and is painful. Also, significantly high blood iodine levels have been demonstrated in patients receiving this agent.

Wound Closure

The goal of therapy after fluid resuscitation is closure of the wound. Nature's own blister is the best cover to protect wounds that spontaneously epithelialize in 7–10 days (ie, superficial second-degree burns). The serum in the blister nurses the surface of the **zone of stasis** until epithelization takes place (Figure 38–5). Where the blister has been disrupted, human amnion, porcine heterografts (preferably fresh, or frozen and meshed), or collagen composite dressings (Biobrane) can substitute. Cadaver homografts can also serve this purpose if available.

Wounds that will not heal spontaneously in 7–10 days (ie, deep second-degree or third-degree burns)

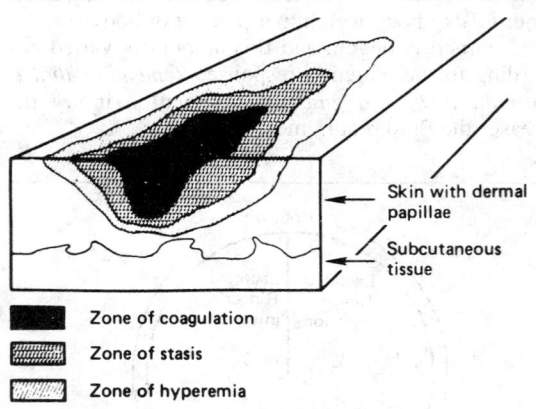

Zone of coagulation

Zone of stasis

Zone of hyperemia

Skin with dermal papillae

Subcutaneous tissue

Figure 38–5. The burn wound has three general zones of tissue death. The zone of necrosis or coagulation involves irreversible skin death. The intermediate zone of capillary stasis is vulnerable to desiccation and infection that can convert potentially salvageable tissue to full-thickness destruction and irreversible skin death. There is minimal cell involvement in the outermost hyperemic zone. (Modified from Zawacki BE: Reversal of capillary stasis and prevention of necrosis in burns. Ann Surg 1974;180:98. Redrawn, with permission, from Artz CP, Moncrief JA, Pruitt BA: *A Team Approach.* Saunders, 1979.)

are best treated by excision and autograft; otherwise, granulation and infection may develop. Granulation is nature's signal that attempts to close the wound have failed. A "skin equivalent"—a patient's own skin cells grown in culture into multilayered sheets of epithelium—is currently being tested in some burn centers. Wounds that do heal spontaneously after 10–14 days result in hypertrophic scars, which increase morbidity from disfigurement and functional loss.

Deitch EA: The management of burns. (Current concepts.) N Engl J Med 1990;323:1249.
Dodd D, Stutman HR: Current issues in burn wound infections. Adv Pediatr Infect Dis 1991;6:137. (Systemic and topical use of antibiotics in burns.)

PATIENT SUPPORT

During the wound closure phase, the patient must be supported in many ways. Most important is adequate nutrition. Enteral feedings may begin once the ileus of the resuscitation period is relieved, which usually coincides with the subsidence of edema. The large nasogastric sump tube used to decompress stomach contents during resuscitation may now be replaced with a smaller, preferably soft Silastic tube. This will aid in delivering large quantities (4000–6000 kcal/d) that may be required during the wound closure period. The metabolic demands are immense. A useful guide is to provide 25 kcal/kg body weight plus 40 kcal per percent of burn surface area. Fat emulsions (Intralipid) given intravenously are useful during the resuscitation period to span the period of ileus.

Many enteral formulas are available. The diet should be rich in carbohydrates (to decrease proteolysis), calories, and protein. Some fat supplementation is also necessary, but immune-suppressive fats such as omega-3 fatty acids should be avoided. Early enteral feedings reduce the need for antacids and lessen the likelihood of development of Curling's ulcer, a life-threatening complication of burn injury. Gastric pH and hourly antacid delivery should be monitored during the resuscitation phase. H_2 receptor blockers may be used to reduce acid production; however, undesirable side effects such as leukopenia and confusion in the elderly may result.

Pain plays a major role during the wound closure phase. The patient is more aware of pain during dressing changes and postsurgical periods. Hydrotherapy aids in dressing removal and joint range of motion, but it can be a source of wound contamination. Analgesics are essential, but overuse or underuse may be harmful.

The Burn Team
The burn team consists of a group of highly skilled professionals—nurses, dietitians, physical therapists, occupational therapists, and counselors—who work closely with the physician in providing comprehensive services for the victim from the period of intensive care through recovery and rehabilitation. Careful attention is given to the complex problems encountered during the intensive care and recovery periods, including fluid and electrolyte abnormalities, infection, physical discomfort, malnutrition, immobility, and psychologic suffering.

The residual physical and emotional problems in burn patients, eg, body disfigurement, impaired mobility, persistent itching, decreased ability to perspire, decreased skin sensitivity, and impairment of sexual enjoyment, require long-term committed care.

Becker WK, Pruitt BA: Parenteral nutrition in thermally injured patient. Compr Ther 1991;17:47.
Van Way CW III: Nutritional support in the injured patient. Surg Clin North Am 1991;71:537. (Enteral nutrition guidelines.)

ELECTRIC SHOCK

The possibility of life-threatening electrical injury exists wherever there is electric power or lightning. The amount and type of current, the duration and area of exposure, and the pathway of the current through the body determine the degree of damage. If the current passes through the heart or brain stem, death may occur immediately owing to ventricular fibrillation or apnea. Current passing through skeletal muscle can cause contractions severe enough to result in bone fracture. Current traversing peripheral nerves can cause acute or delayed neuropathy. Delayed effects can include damage to the spinal cord, peripheral nerves, bone, kidneys, and gastrointestinal tract as well as cataracts.

Direct current is much less dangerous than alternating current. Alternating current of high voltage with a very high number of cycles per second (hertz, Hz) may be less dangerous than a low voltage with fewer cycles per second. With alternating currents of 25–300 Hz, low voltages (< 220 Hz) tend to produce ventricular fibrillation; high voltages (> 1000 Hz), respiratory failure; intermediate voltages (220–1000 Hz), both. Domestic house current (AC) of 110 volts with low cycles (about 60 Hz) is, accordingly, dangerous to the heart, since it may cause ventricular fibrillation. DC current contact is more likely to cause asystole.

Lightning injuries differ from high-voltage electric shock injuries in that lightning usually involves higher voltage, briefer duration of contact, asystole rather than ventricular fibrillation, a shock wave characteristic, and multisystem pathologic involvement.

Electrical burns are of three distinct types: flash (arcing) burns, flame (clothing) burns, and the direct heating effect of tissues by the electric current. The latter lesions are usually sharply demarcated, round or oval, painless yellow-brown areas (Joule burn) with inflammatory reaction. There is usually a second burn mark where the current exits the body. The superficial appearance of many discrete burns is deceptive; operation frequently discloses more extensive destruction than anticipated. Little happens for several weeks; sloughing then occurs slowly over a fairly wide area.

Electric shock may produce loss of consciousness. With recovery there may be muscular pain, fatigue, headache, and nervous irritability. The physical signs vary according to the action of the current. Ventricular fibrillation or respiratory failure (or both) can occur; the patient may be unconscious, pulseless, hypotensive, cold and cyanotic, and without respirations.

Electric shock may be a hazard in equipment that is usually considered to be harmless (eg, home appliances and medical equipment). Proper installation, utilization, and maintenance of equipment by qualified personnel should minimize this hazard. Battery-operated devices provide the maximum protection from accidental electric shock. Electrochemical cutaneous burns have been reported with direct current voltages as low as 3 volts.

Treatment

A. Emergency Measures: The victim may be freed from the current in many ways, but the rescuer must be protected. Turn off the power, sever the wire with a dry wooden-handled axe, make a proper ground to divert the current, or drag the victim carefully away by means of dry clothing or a leather belt.

CPR is instituted if breathing and pulses are absent and continued according to the usual AHA protocol.

Lightning injury. Victims of lightning injury, in whom coma may last for a few minutes to several days, should receive prompt and sustained artificial resuscitation. This should be continued as long as there is no clinical evidence of brain death.

B. Hospital Measures: Lightning or unstable electroshock victims should be hospitalized when revived and observed for shock, arrhythmia, sudden cardiac dilatation, hemorrhage, or myoglobinuria. Electroshock injury cases should also be evaluated for blunt trauma, dehydration, skin burns, hypertension, posttraumatic stress, acid-base disturbances, and neurologic damage.

Aggressive hydration with Ringer's lactate should seek to achieve a urine output of 50–100 mL/h.

The unpredictable damage to deep tissues in electrical burns makes it difficult to assess the fluid requirements for patients who are in shock.

Prognosis

Complications may occur in almost any part of the body but most commonly include sepsis, limb amputation, or neurologic, cardiac, or psychiatric dysfunction.

Browne BJ, Gaasch LUR: Electrical injuries and lightning. Emerg Med Clin North Am 1992;10:211. (Emergency assessment and treatment.)
Patten BM: Lightning and electrical injuries. Neurol Clin 1992;10:1047.

IONIZING RADIATION REACTIONS

The effects of ionizing radiation on the body have been observed in clinical use of x-rays and radioactive agents, after occupational or accidental exposure, and following the use of atomic weaponry. The extent of damage due to radiation exposure depends on the quantity of radiation delivered to the body, the dose rate, the organs exposed, the type of radiation (x-rays, neutrons, gamma rays, alpha or beta particles), the duration of exposure, and the energy transfer from the radioactive wave or particle to the exposed tissue. The Chernobyl experience suggests that the best biologic indicators of dose are the duration of the asymptomatic latent period (particularly for nausea or emesis), the severity of early symptoms, the rate of decline of the lymphocyte count, and the number and distribution of dicentric chromosomes in peripheral lymphocytes.

The National Committee on Radiation Protection has set the maximum permissible radiation exposure for occupationally exposed workers over age 18 at 0.1 rem* per week for the whole body (but not to exceed 5 rem per year) and 1.5 rem per week for the hands. (For purposes of comparison, routine chest x-rays deliver from 0.1–0.2 rem.)

Death after acute lethal radiation exposure is usually due to hematopoietic failure, gastrointestinal mucosal damage, central nervous system damage, widespread vascular injury, or secondary infection. The

---

*In radiation terminology, a rad is the unit of absorbed dose and a rem is the unit of any radiation dose to body tissue in terms of its estimated biologic effect. Roentgen (R) refers to the amount of radiation dose delivered to the body. For x-ray or gamma ray radiation, rems, rads, and roentgens are virtually the same. For particulate radiation from radioactive materials, these terms may differ greatly (eg, for neutrons, 1 rad equals 10 rems). In the Système International (SI) nomenclature, the rad has been replaced by the gray (Gy), and 1 rad equals 0.01 Gy = 1 cGy. The SI replacement for the rem is the Sievert (Sv), and 1 rem equals 0.01 Sv.

acute radiation syndrome may be dominated by central nervous system, gastrointestinal, or hematologic manifestations depending on dose and survival. Four hundred to 600 cGy of x-ray or gamma radiation applied to the entire body at one time may be fatal within 60 days; death is usually due to hemorrhage, anemia, and infection secondary to hematopoietic injury. Levels of 1000–3000 cGy to the entire body destroy gastrointestinal mucosa; this leads to toxemia and death within 2 weeks. Total body doses above 3000 cGy cause widespread vascular damage, cerebral anoxia, hypotensive shock, and death within 48 hours.

ACUTE (IMMEDIATE) IONIZING RADIATION EFFECTS ON NORMAL TISSUES

Clinical Findings

A. Injury to Skin and Mucous Membranes: Irradiation may cause erythema, epilation, destruction of fingernails, or epidermolysis.

B. Injury to Deep Structures:

1. Hematopoietic tissues–Injury to the bone marrow may cause diminished production of blood elements. Lymphocytes are most sensitive, polymorphonuclear leukocytes next most sensitive, and erythrocytes least sensitive. Damage to the blood-forming organs may vary from transient depression of one or more blood elements to complete destruction.

2. Cardiovascular system–Pericarditis with effusion or constrictive carditis may occur after a period of months or even years. Myocarditis is less common. Smaller vessels (the capillaries and arterioles) are more readily damaged than larger blood vessels.

3. Gonads–In males, small single doses of radiation (200–300 R) cause temporary aspermatogenesis, and larger doses (600–800 R) may cause permanent sterility. In females, single doses of 200 R may cause temporary cessation of menses, and 500–800 R may cause permanent castration. Moderate to heavy irradiation of the embryo in utero results in injury to the fetus (eg, mental retardation) or in embryonic death and abortion.

4. Respiratory tract–High or repeated moderate doses of radiation may cause pneumonitis, often delayed for weeks or months.

5. Salivary glands–The salivary glands may be depressed by radiation, but relatively large doses may be required.

6. Mouth, pharynx, esophagus, and stomach–Mucositis with edema and painful swallowing of food may occur within hours or days after onset of irradiation. Gastric secretion may be temporarily (occasionally permanently) inhibited by moderately high doses of radiation.

7. Intestines–Inflammation and ulceration may follow moderately large doses of radiation.

8. Endocrine glands and viscera–Hepatitis and nephritis may be delayed effects of therapeutic radiation. The normal thyroid, pituitary, pancreas, adrenals, and bladder are relatively resistant to low or moderate doses of radiation; parathyroid glands are especially resistant.

9. Nervous system–The brain and spinal cord are much more sensitive to acute exposures than the peripheral nerves.

C. Systemic Reaction (Radiation Sickness): The basic mechanisms of radiation sickness are not known. Anorexia, nausea, vomiting, weakness, exhaustion, lassitude, and in some cases prostration may occur, singly or in combination. Dehydration, anemia, and infection may follow. Radiation sickness associated with x-ray therapy is most likely to occur when the therapy is given in large dosage to large areas over the abdomen, less often when given over the thorax, and rarely when therapy is given over the extremities.

Prevention

Persons handling radiation sources can minimize exposure to radiation by recognizing the importance of time, distance, and shielding. Areas housing x-ray and nuclear materials must be properly shielded. X-ray equipment should be periodically checked for reliability of output, and proper filters should be employed. When feasible, it is advisable to shield the gonads, especially of young persons. Fluoroscopic examination should be performed as rapidly as possible, using an optimal combination of beam characteristics and filtration and the beam size should be kept to a minimum required by the examination. Special protective clothing may be necessary to protect against contamination with radioisotopes. In the event of accidental contamination, all clothing should be removed and the body vigorously bathed with soap and water. This should be followed by careful instrument (Geiger counter) check to localize the ionizing radiation.

Emergency Treatment for Radiation Accident Victims

The proliferation of radiation equipment and nuclear energy plants and the increased transportation of radioactive materials necessitate hospital plans for managing patients who are accidentally exposed to ionizing radiation or contaminated with radioisotopes. The plans should provide for effective emergency care and disposition of victims and materials with the least possible risk of spreading radioactive contamination to personnel and facilities.

Treatment

The success of treatment of local radiation effects depends upon the extent, degree, and location of tissue injury. Particulate or radioisotope exposures should be decontaminated in designated confined areas. For many radioisotopes, chelation, blocking, or dilution therapy is indicated (see NCRP No. 65 reference, below). Treatment of systemic reactions is symptomatic and supportive. No truly effective anti-nauseant drug is available for the distressing nausea that frequently occurs. Chlorpromazine, 25–50 mg given deeply intramuscularly every 4–6 hours as necessary or 10–25 mg orally every 4–6 hours as necessary, may be of value. Dimenhydrate, 50–100 mg, or perphenazine, 4–8 mg, 1 hour before and 1 and 4 hours after radiation therapy has been recommended. Simple, palatable foods and emotional support may help.

When radiation dosage levels are sufficient to cause damage to gastrointestinal mucosa, bone marrow, and other important tissues, good medical and nursing care may be lifesaving. Blood and platelet transfusions, bone marrow transplants, antibiotics, fluid and electrolyte maintenance, and other supportive measures may be useful. Recombinant hematopoietic growth factors have been effective in accelerating hematopoietic recovery. Bone marrow transplantation should be considered following whole body exposures above 5–8 Gy.

CHRONIC (DELAYED) EFFECTS OF EXCESSIVE DOSES OF IONIZING RADIATION

Skin scarring, atrophy and telangiectasis, cataract, myelopathy, cerebral injury, obliterative endarteritis, pericarditis, hypothyroidism, pulmonary fibrosis, hepatitis, intestinal stenosis, and nephritis are known to occur following high-dose exposure. Neoplastic disease, including leukemia, is increased in persons exposed to excessive radiation. There is an increased incidence of thyroid cancer in patients who have received radiation exposure or therapy to the thymus. The latency period between radiation therapy and the development of cancer may be 30 years or longer. Prenatal irradiation may increase the risk of childhood cancer.

Microcephaly and other congenital abnormalities may occur in children exposed in utero, especially if the fetus was exposed during early pregnancy. Carcinogenesis from low-dose (< 10 rem) exposure to adults has not been demonstrated. However, because of age-related differences in sensitivity to radiation, carcinogenesis following childhood exposures has been observed.

Gale RP, Butturini A: Medical response to nuclear and radiation accidents. Occup Med 1991;6:581. (Treatment of acute radiation effects.)

Health Effects of Exposure to Low Levels of Ionizing Radiation. Committee on the Biological Effects of Ionizing Radiations, Board on Radiation Effects Research, Commission on Life Sciences, National Research Council. BEIR (Series); 5. National Academy Press, 1990. (Risk assessment based on animal and human data.)

National Council on Radiation Protection and Measurement (NCRP): *Management of Persons Accidentally Contaminated With Radionuclides.* Report No. 65. NCRP, 1985. (Treatment recommendations for exposure to specific isotopes.)

DROWNING

Drowning is the fourth leading cause of accidental death in the USA. The number of deaths due to drowning could undoubtedly be significantly reduced if adequate preventive and first aid instruction programs were instituted.

The asphyxia of drowning is usually due to aspiration of fluid, but it may result from airway obstruction caused by laryngeal spasm while the victim is gasping under water. About 10% of victims develop laryngospasms after the first gulp and never aspirate water ("dry drowning"). The rapid sequence of events after submersion—hypoxemia, laryngospasm, fluid aspiration, ineffective circulation, brain injury, and brain death—may take place within 5–10 minutes. This sequence may be delayed for longer periods if the victim, especially a child, has been submerged in very cold water or if the victim has ingested significant amounts of barbiturates. Immersion in cold water can also cause a rapid fall in the victim's core temperature, so that systemic hypothermia and death may occur before actual drowning.

The primary effect is hypoxia due to perfusion of poorly ventilated alveoli, intrapulmonary shunting, and decreased compliance. *Cardiopulmonary resuscitation is the immediate requirement of rescue.*

A number of circumstances or primary events may precede near drowning and must be taken into consideration in management: (1) use of alcohol or other drugs (a contributing factor in an estimated 25% of adult drownings), (2) extreme fatigue, (3) intentional hyperventilation, (4) sudden acute illness (eg, epilepsy, myocardial infarction), (5) head or spinal cord injury sustained in diving, (6) venomous stings by aquatic animals, and (7) decompression sickness in deep water diving.

When first seen, the near-drowning victim may present with a wide range of clinical manifestations. Spontaneous return of consciousness often occurs in otherwise healthy individuals when submersion is very brief. Many other patients respond promptly to immediate ventilation. Other patients, with more severe degrees of near drowning, may have frank pulmonary failure, pulmonary edema, shock, anoxic encephalopathy, cerebral edema, and cardiac arrest. A few patients may be deceptively asymptomatic during the recovery period, only to deteriorate or die as a result of acute respiratory failure within the following 12–24 hours.

Clinical Findings

A. Symptoms and Signs: The patient may be unconscious, semiconscious, or awake but apprehensive, restless, and complaining of headaches or chest pain. Vomiting is common. Examination may reveal cyanosis, trismus, apnea, tachypnea, and wheezing. A pink froth from the mouth and nose indicates pulmonary edema. Cardiovascular manifestations may include tachycardia, arrhythmias, hypotension, cardiac arrest, and circulatory shock. Hypothermia may be present.

B. Laboratory Findings: Urinalysis shows proteinuria, hemoglobinuria, and acetonuria. There is usually a leukocytosis. The PaO_2 is usually decreased and the $PaCO_2$ increased or decreased. The blood pH is decreased as a result of metabolic acidosis. Chest x-rays may show pneumonitis or pulmonary edema.

Treatment

A. First Aid: Immediate measures to combat hypoxemia at the scene of the incident—with sustained effective ventilation, oxygenation, and circulatory support—are critical to survival with complete recovery. Hypothermia and cervical spine injury should always be suspected.

1. Standard CPR is initiated if pulse and respirations are absent.

2. Do not waste time attempting to drain water from the victim's lungs, since this measure is most often of no value. The Heimlich maneuver (subdiaphragmatic pressure) should be used only if airway obstruction by a foreign body is suspected. The cervical spine should be immobilized if neck injury is possible.

3. Do not discontinue basic life support for seemingly "hopeless" patients until core temperature reaches 32 °C (89.6 °F). Complete recovery has been reported after prolonged resuscitation of hypothermic patients.

B. Hospital Care: Careful observation of the patient; continuous monitoring of cardiorespiratory function; serial determination of arterial blood gases, pH, and electrolytes; and measurement of urinary output are required. Pulmonary edema may not appear for 24 hours.

1. Ensure optimal ventilation and oxygenation—The danger of hypoxemia exists even in the alert, conscious patient who appears to be breathing normally. Oxygen should be immediately administered at the highest available concentration. Endotracheal intubation and mechanical ventilation are necessary for patients unable to maintain an open airway or normal blood gases and pH. If the victim does not have spontaneous respirations, intubation is required. Oxygen saturation should be maintained at 90% or higher. Positive end-expiratory pressure (PEEP) should be considered when the patient is unable to achieve a $PaO2$ greater than 55 mm Hg when receiving less than 50% oxygen. Serial physical examinations and chest x-rays should be carried out to detect possible pneumonitis, atelectasis, and pulmonary edema. Bronchospasm due to aspirated material may require use of bronchodilators. Antibiotics should be given only when there is clinical evidence of infection—not prophylactically.

2. Cardiovascular support—Central venous pressure (or, preferably, pulmonary artery wedge pressure) may be monitored as a guide to determining whether vascular fluid replacement and cardiac drug therapy are needed. If low cardiac output persists after adequate intravascular volume is achieved, pressors should be given. Otherwise, standard therapy for pulmonary edema, cardiogenic or not, is administered.

3. Correction of blood pH and electrolyte abnormalities—Metabolic acidosis is almost invariably present in near-drowning victims, but it is usually of minor importance and corrected through oxygenation. While controversial, bicarbonate administration (1 meq/kg) has been recommended for comatose patients.

4. Cerebral injury—Some near-drowning patients may progress to irreversible central nervous system damage despite apparently adequate treatment of hypoxia and shock. Several types of measures to prevent cerebral injury have been employed with varying degrees of success—hypothermia, barbiturates, corticosteroids, osmolar agents (eg, mannitol), and readjustment of ventilatory assistance.

5. Hypothermia—Core temperature should be measured and managed as appropriate (see Systemic Hypothermia, above).

Course & Prognosis

Victims of near drowning who have had prolonged hypoxemia should remain under close hospital observation for 2–3 days after all supportive measures have been withdrawn and clinical and laboratory findings have been stable. Residual complications of near drowning may include intellectual impairment, convulsive disorders, and pulmonary or cardiac disease.

Olshaker JS: Near drowning. Emerg Med Clin North Am 1992;10:339. (Epidemiology, pathophysiology, assessment, treatment, complications, and prognosis.)

OTHER DISORDERS DUE TO PHYSICAL AGENTS

DECOMPRESSION SICKNESS & DYSBARIC ILLNESS

Decompression sickness and other disorders related to rapid changes in environmental pressure are occupational hazards for fliers and professional divers who are involved in deep-water exploration, rescue, salvage, or construction. In recent years, the sport of scuba diving has exposed amateurs to the hazards of decompression sickness.

At low depths the greatly increased pressure (eg, at 30 meters [100 ft] the pressure is four times greater than at the surface) compresses the respiratory gases into the blood and other tissues. During ascent from depths greater than 9 meters, gases dissolved in the blood and other tissues escape as the external pressure decreases. The appearance of symptoms depends on the depth and duration of submersion; the degree of physical exertion; the age, weight, and physical condition of the diver; and the rate of ascent. The size and number of gas bubbles (notably nitrogen) escaping from the tissues depends on the difference between the atmospheric pressure and the partial pressure of the gas dissolved in the tissues. The release of gas bubbles and (particularly) the location of their release determine the symptoms.

Decompression sickness also occurs among fliers during rapid ascent from sea level to high altitudes when there is no adequate pressurizing protection. Deep-sea and scuba divers may be vulnerable to air embolism if airplane travel is attempted too soon (within a few hours) after diving.

The range of clinical manifestations includes gas bubble formation in the joints ("bends"), cerebral or pulmonary decompression sickness, arterial gas embolism (cerebral, pulmonary), ear and sinus barotrauma, and dysbaric osteonecrosis.

Predisposing factors include exercise, injury, obesity, dehydration, alcoholic excess, hypoxia, some medications (eg, narcotics, antihistamines), and cold. Reported sequelae include hemiparesis, neurologic dysfunction, and bone damage.

The onset of acute decompression symptoms occurs within 30 minutes in half of cases and almost invariably within 6 hours. Symptoms, which are highly variable, include pain (largely in the joints), headache, confusion, pruritic rash, visual disturbances, weakness or paralysis, dizziness or vertigo, dyspnea, paresthesias, aphasia, and coma.

Pulmonary decompression sickness ("chokes") presents with burning, pleuritic substernal pain, cough, and dyspnea.

Early recognition and prompt treatment are extremely important. Continuous administration of oxygen is indicated as a first aid measure, whether or not cyanosis is present. Aspirin may be given for pain, but narcotics should be used very cautiously, since they may obscure the patient's response to recompression. Rapid transportation to a treatment facility for recompression, hyperbaric oxygen, hydration treatment of plasma deficits, and supportive measures is necessary not only to relieve symptoms but also to prevent permanent impairment. It has been recommended, however, that decompression symptoms be treated whenever they are seen—even up to 2 weeks postinjury—since it is still possible to completely alleviate symptoms. The physician should be familiar with the nearest compression center. The local public health department or nearest naval facility should be able to provide such information. The National Divers Alert Network (DAN) ([919] 684–8111) provides assistance in the management of underwater diving accidents.

Jerrard DA: Diving medicine. Emerg Med Clin North Am 1992;10:329. (Diagnosis and treatment of dysbaric disorders.)

Melamed Y, Shupak A, Bitterman H: Current medical problems associated with underwater diving. N Engl J Med 1992;326:30. (Barotrauma and decompression sickness.)

MOUNTAIN SICKNESS

Lack of sufficient time for acclimatization, increased physical activity, and varying degrees of health may be responsible for the acute and chronic disturbances that result from hypoxia at altitudes greater than 2000 meters (6560 ft). Marked individual differences in tolerance to hypoxia exist. Patients with sickle cell disease are at high risk of painful crises from altitude-induced hypoxemia; if they have had no previous mountain exposure, they should be advised to avoid mountains.

Acute Mountain Sickness

Initial manifestations include dizziness, headache, lassitude, drowsiness, chilliness, nausea and vomiting, facial pallor, dyspnea, and cyanosis. Later, there is facial flushing, irritability, difficulty in concentrating, vertigo, tinnitus, visual (retinal hemorrhages may occur) and auditory disturbances, anorexia, insomnia, increased dyspnea and weakness on exertion, increased headaches (due to cerebral edema), palpitations, tachycardia, Cheyne-Stokes breathing, and weight loss. More severe manifestations include pulmonary edema and encephalopathy. Voluntary, periodic hyperventilation may relieve symptoms. In most individuals, symptoms clear within 24–48 hours, but in some instances, if the symptoms are sufficiently persistent or severe, the patient must be returned to lower altitudes. Administration of oxygen, 2–3 L/min, will often relieve acute symptoms. Acetazolamide, 250 mg every 8 hours, or dexamethasone, 4 mg every 8 hours, for as long as symptoms persist, is recommended therapy. Preventive measures include slow ascent (500–1000 ft/d), adequate rest and sleep the day before travel, reduced food intake, and avoidance of alcohol, tobacco, and unnecessary physical activity during travel. Acetazolamide, 250 mg every 8–12 hours, beginning the day before ascent and continuing for 48–72 hours at altitude, may be used as prophylaxis. Dexamethasone, 2–4 mg every 5 hours beginning on the day of ascent, continuing for 3 days at the higher altitude, and then tapering over 5 days, is an alternative, particularly for extreme situations.

Acute High-Altitude Pulmonary Edema

This serious complication usually occurs at levels above 3000 meters (9840 ft). Early symptoms of pulmonary edema may appear within 6–36 hours after arrival at a high-altitude area—dry, incessant cough, decreased exercise performance, fatigue, dyspnea at rest, and substernal oppression. Later, wheezing, orthopnea, and hemoptysis may occur. Recognition of the early symptoms may enable the patient to descend before incapacitating pulmonary edema develops, but strenuous exertion should be avoided. An early descent of even 500 or 1000 meters may result in improvement of symptoms. Physical findings include tachycardia, mild fever, tachypnea, cyanosis, prolonged respiration, and rales and rhonchi. The patient may become confused or even comatose, and the entire clinical picture may resemble severe pneumonia. The white count is often slightly elevated, but the blood sedimentation rate is usually normal. Chest x-ray findings vary from irregular patchy infiltration in one lung to nodular densities bilaterally or with transient prominence of the central pulmonary arteries. Transient, nonspecific electrocardiographic changes, occasionally showing right ventricular strain, may occur. Pulmonary arterial blood pressure is elevated, whereas pulmonary wedge pressure is normal.

Treatment, which must often be given under field conditions, consists of rest in the semi-Fowler position (head raised) and administration of 100% oxygen by mask at a rate of 6–8 L/min for 15–30 minutes. Sublingual nifedipine (5–10 mg) followed by 20 mg long-acting every 6 hours, may provide symptomatic relief. *Immediate descent is essential.* Recompression in a portable hyperbaric bag has also been successful if descent is not possible. To conserve oxygen, lower flow rates may be used for the next 24–48 hours until the victim recovers or can be evacuated to a lower altitude. Treatment for adult respiratory distress syndrome (see Chapter 9) may be required for some patients who have a prolonged course of pulmonary edema. Betamethasone, 5 mg every 6 hours, has been recommended if central nervous system symptoms are present. Acetazolamide, 250 mg every 8 hours, should be administered if acute mountain sickness is suspected. If bacterial pneumonia exists, appropriate antibiotic therapy should be given.

Preventive measures include education of prospective mountaineers regarding the possibility of serious pulmonary edema, optimal physical conditioning before travel, gradual ascent to permit acclimatization, and a period of rest and inactivity for 1–2 days after arrival at high altitudes. Prompt medical attention with rest and high-flow oxygen if respiratory symptoms develop may prevent progression to frank pulmonary edema. Persons with a history of high-altitude pulmonary edema should be hospitalized for further observation if possible. Pulmonary embolism and high-altitude bronchitis can also occur. Mountaineering parties at levels of 3000 meters or higher should carry a supply of oxygen and equipment sufficient for several days. Persons with symptomatic cardiac or pulmonary disease should avoid high altitudes.

Acute High-Altitude Encephalopathy

High-altitude encephalopathy appears to be an extension of the central nervous symptoms of acute mountain sickness (see above). It usually occurs at elevations above 2500 meters (8250 ft) and is more common in unacclimatized individuals. Clinical findings are due largely to hypoxemia and cerebral edema. Severe headaches, confusion, truncal ataxia, staggering gait, focal deficits, nausea and vomiting, and seizures may progress to obtundation and coma. Papilledema and retinal hemorrhages may be observed in about 50% of patients.

Early recognition of the encephalopathic symptoms is essential. Oxygen should be administered by mask. Betamethasone or dexamethasone, 4 mg every 6 hours, may be helpful if descent is impossible. If descent is accomplished as quickly as possible, recovery is usually rapid and complete.

Subacute Mountain Sickness

This occurs most frequently in unacclimatized individuals and at altitudes above 4500 meters. Symptoms, which are probably due to central nervous system anoxia without associated alveolar hyperventilation, are similar to but more persistent and severe than those of acute mountain sickness. There are additional problems of dehydration, skin dryness, and pruritus. The hematocrit may be elevated, and there may be electrocardiographic and chest x-ray evidence of right ventricular hypertrophy. Treatment consists of rest, oxygen administration, and return to lower altitudes.

Chronic Mountain Sickness (Monge's Disease)

This uncommon condition of chronic alveolar hypoventilation, which is encountered in residents of high-altitude communities who have lost their acclimatization to such an environment, is difficult to differentiate clinically from chronic pulmonary disease. The disorder is characterized by somnolence, mental depression, hypoxemia, cyanosis, clubbing of fingers, polycythemia (hematocrit often > 75%), signs of right ventricular failure, electrocardiographic evidence of right axis deviation and right atrial and ventricular hypertrophy, and x-ray evidence of right heart enlargement and central pulmonary vessel prominence. There is no x-ray evidence of structural pulmonary disease. Pulmonary function tests usually disclose alveolar hypoventilation and elevated CO_2 tension but fail to reveal defective oxygen transport. There is a diminished respiratory response to CO_2. Almost complete disappearance of all abnormalities eventually occurs when the patient returns to sea level.

Bezruchka S: High altitude medicine. Med Clin North Am 1992;76:1481. (Diagnosis, treatment, prevention.)

Sutton JR: Mountain sickness. Neurol Clin 1992;10:1015. (Pathophysiology, treatment, prevention.)

MEDICAL EFFECTS OF AIR TRAVEL & SELECTION OF PATIENTS FOR AIR TRAVEL

The decision about whether or not it is advisable for a patient to travel by air depends not only upon the nature and severity of the illness but also upon such factors as the duration of flight, the altitude to be flown, pressurization, the availability of supplementary oxygen and other medical supplies, the presence of attending physicians and trained nursing attendants, and other special considerations. Air carriers in the USA cannot legally allow the use of personal (passenger-supplied) oxygen containers, but most major airlines will supply oxygen upon advance written request from the passenger's physician. Airline policies, charges, and other details must be checked with each carrier. Medical hazards or complications of modern air travel are remarkably uncommon; unless there is some specific contraindication (Table 38–?), air transportation may actually be the best means of moving patients. The most common inflight emergencies are cardiovascular, syncopal, neuropsychiatric, and abdominal. The Air Transport Association of America defines an incapacitated passenger as "one who is suffering from a physical or mental disability and who, because of such disability or the effect of the flight on the disability, is incapable of self-care; would endanger the health or safety of such person or other passengers or airline employ-

Table 38–2. Contraindications to commercial air travel.[1]

Cardiovascular
  Within 4 weeks after myocardial infarction.[2]
  Within 2 weeks after cerebrovascular accident
  Severe hypertension
  Decompensated cardiovascular disease or restricted cardiac reserve[3]
Bronchopulmonary
  Pneumothorax
  Congenital pulmonary cysts
  Vital capacity less than 50%
Eye, ear, nose, and throat
  Recent eye surgery
  Acute sinusitis or otitis media
  Surgical mandibular fixation (permanent wiring of jaw)
Gastrointestinal tract
  Less than 10–14 days after abdominal surgery
  Acute diverticulitis or ulcerative colitis
  Acute esophageal varices
  Acute gastroenteritis
Neuropsychiatric
  Epilepsy (unless well controlled medically and cabin altitude does not exceed 2500 m [8000 ft])
  Previous violent or unpredictable behavior
  Recent skull fracture
  Brain tumor
Hematologic
  Anemia (hemoglobin <8.5 g/dL or red blood cell count of <3 million/μL in an adult)
  Sickle cell disease (except below 6800-m [22,500-foot] altitude)
  Blood dyscrasias with active bleeding (hemophilia, leukemia)
Pregnancy
  Beyond 240 days or with threatened miscarriage
Miscellaneous
  Need for intravenous fluids or special medical apparatus[2]

[1]Slightly modified and reproduced, with permission, from Mod Med (June) 1982;50:196. Based on recommendations of the American Medical Association in JAMA 1982;247:1009.
[2]Consultation with an airline flight surgeon is suggested.
[3]In some cases, low-altitude flights can be made without supplemental oxygen in accordance with recommendations of the American College of Chest Physicians.

ees; or would cause discomfort or annoyance of other passengers."

All commercial airlines retain medical consultants to assist their personnel in making decisions regarding the transportation of passengers with noticeable symptoms of sickness or injury. Physicians may contact these medical consultants by calling or writing the medical departments of major airlines.

Cardiovascular Disease

A. Cardiac Decompensation: Patients in congestive failure should not fly until they are compensated by appropriate treatment, or unless they are in a pressurized plane with 100% oxygen therapy available during the entire flight.

B. Compensated Valvular or Other Heart Disease: Patients should not fly above 2400–2800 m unless the aircraft is pressurized and oxygen is administered at altitudes of 2400 m or higher.

C. Acute Myocardial Infarction, Convalescent and Asymptomatic: At least 4 weeks of convalescence are recommended even for asymptomatic patients if flying is contemplated. Ambulatory, stabilized, and compensated patients tolerate air travel well. Oxygen should be available.

D. Angina Pectoris: Air travel is inadvisable for patients with severe angina. In mild to moderate cases of angina, air travel may be permitted, especially in pressurized planes. Oxygen should be available.

Respiratory Disease

A. Nasopharyngeal Disorders: Nasal allergies and infections predispose to development of aerotitis. Chewing gum, nasal decongestants, appropriate anti-infective treatment, and avoiding sleep on descent may prevent barotitis.

B. Asthma: Patients with mild asthma can travel without difficulty. Patients with status asthmaticus should not be permitted to fly.

C. Congenital Pulmonary Cysts: Patients should not travel unless cleared by a physician.

D. Tuberculosis: Patients with active, communicable tuberculosis or pneumothorax should not be permitted to travel by air.

E. Other Pulmonary Disorders: Patients may be flown safely unless vital capacity is less than 50% of predicted or unless pneumothorax is present.

Anemia

If hemoglobin is less than 8–9 g/dL, oxygen should be available. Patients with severe anemia (hemoglobin < 8.5 g/dL or red cell count < 3 million/μL) should not travel by air until hemoglobin has been raised to a reasonable level. Patients with sickle cell disease appear to be particularly vulnerable.

Diabetes Mellitus

Diabetics who do not need insulin or who can administer their own insulin during flight may fly safely. "Brittle" diabetics who are subject to frequent episodes of hypoglycemia should be in optimal control before flying and should carry sugar or candy in case hypoglycemic reactions occur.

Patients With Surgical Problems

Patients convalescing from thoracic or abdominal surgery should not fly until 10 days (abdominal) to 21 days (thoracic) after surgery, and then only if the wound is healed and there is no drainage.

Colostomy patients may be permitted to travel by air providing they are nonodorous and colostomy bags are emptied before flight.

Patients with large hernias unsupported by a truss or binder should not be permitted to fly in nonpressurized aircraft because of an increased danger of strangulation of the herniated bowel.

Postsurgical or posttraumatic eye cases require pressurized cabins and oxygen therapy to avoid retinal damage due to hypoxia and intraocular gas bubbles.

Long flights increase the risk of deep vein thrombosis and resulting embolic disease. Prevention includes avoidance of smoking and alcohol, low-dose aspirin, and leg exercises and walking during the flight.

Psychiatric Disorders

Severely psychotic, agitated, or disturbed patients should not be permitted to fly on scheduled airlines even when accompanied by a medical attendant.

Extremely nervous or apprehensive patients may travel by air if they receive adequate sedatives or tranquilizers before and during flight.

Motion Sickness

Patients subject to motion sickness should receive sedatives or antihistamines (eg, dimenhydrinate or meclizine), 50 mg four times daily, before and during the flight, or one transdermal scopolamine disk applied behind one ear at least 4 hours before the antiemetic effect is desired. Small meals of easily digested food before and during the flight may reduce the tendency to nausea and vomiting.

Pregnancy

Pregnant women may be permitted to fly during the first 8 months of pregnancy unless there is a history of habitual abortion or premature birth. During the ninth month of pregnancy, air travel is not recommended; if travel is essential, a physician's authorization is required. Infants less than 1 week old should not be flown at high altitudes or for long distances.

AMA Commission on Emergency Medical Services: Medical aspects of transportation aboard commercial aircraft. JAMA 1982;247:1007. (Recommendations re specified conditions.)

Bia FJ, Barry M: Special health considerations for travelers. Med Clin North Am 1992;76:1295. (Pathophysiology, travel recommendations, prevention.)

Gong H Jr: Air travel and oxygen therapy in cardiopulmonary patients. Chest 1992;101:1105. (Physiology, preflight patient evaluation, and use of inflight oxygen.)

39

Poisoning

Kent R. Olson, MD

INITIAL EVALUATION OF THE PATIENT WITH POISONING OR DRUG OVERDOSE

Patients with drug overdoses or poisoning may initially present with no symptoms or with varying degrees of overt intoxication. The asymptomatic patient may have been exposed to or may have ingested a lethal dose of a poison but not yet have any manifestations of toxicity. It is always important to (1) quickly assess the potential danger, (2) perform gut decontamination to prevent absorption, and (3) observe the patient for an appropriate interval.

Assess the Danger

If the toxin is known, the danger can be assessed by consulting a text or computerized information resource (eg, POISINDEX) or by calling a regional poison control center (Table 39–1). Assessment will usually take into account the dose ingested (in milligrams per kilogram of body weight), the time interval since ingestion, the presence of any clinical signs, and serum drug or toxin levels. Be aware that the history given by the patient or family may be unreliable.

Gut Decontamination

The choice of gut decontamination procedure depends on the toxin and the circumstances. (See below for more discussion of methods.)

Observation of the Patient

Asymptomatic or mildly symptomatic patients should generally be observed for at least 4–6 hours. After that time, the patient may be discharged if no symptoms have developed and adequate gastric decontamination has been assured (as shown by passage of a charcoal-laden stool). Before discharge, psychiatric evaluation should be performed to assess suicidal risk. Intentional ingestions in adolescent girls should raise the possibility of unwanted pregnancy or sexual abuse in the home.

THE SYMPTOMATIC PATIENT

In symptomatic patients, treatment of life-threatening complications takes precedence over gut decontamination or in-depth diagnostic evaluation. Patients with mild symptoms may deteriorate rapidly, which is why all potentially significant exposures should be observed in an acute care facility. The following complications may occur, depending on the type of poisoning.

COMA

Assessment & Complications

Coma is commonly due to ingestion of large doses of antihistamines and anticholinergics, barbiturates, benzodiazepines, ethanol, opioids, phenothiazines, and tricyclic antidepressants. The most common cause of death in comatose patients is respiratory failure (hypoventilation or apnea), which may occur abruptly. Pulmonary aspiration of gastric contents may also occur, especially in victims who are comatose or convulsing. Hypoxia and hypoventilation may aggravate or even cause other common complications such as arrhythmias, hypotension, and seizures. Thus, protection of the airway and assisted ventilation are the most important treatment measures for any poisoned patient.

Treatment

A. Emergency Management: The initial emergency management of coma can be remembered by the mnemonic *ABCD*, for *A*irway, *B*reathing, *C*irculation, and *D*extrose, thiamine, and naloxone or flumazenil, respectively (Table 39–2).

1. Airway–Establish a patent airway by positioning, suction, or insertion of an artificial nasal or oropharyngeal airway. If the patient is deeply comatose or if there is no gag or cough reflex, perform endotracheal intubation. These airway interventions may not

Table 39-1. AAPCC-certified regional poison control centers.[1]

The American Association of Regional Poison Control Centers has certified the following regional poison control centers as meeting their minimum operating criteria. Regional poison control centers operate 24 hours a day, utilizing specially trained and dedicated staff with access to a variety of texts, files, and computerized poison information resources. They can also provide immediate telephone consultation with a physician specializing in medical toxicology.

State	Poison Control Center	Phone Number	State	Poison Control Center	Phone Number
Alabama	Children's Hospital of Alabama, Birmingham	(800) 292–6678 (205) 939–9201	Nebraska	The Poison Center, Omaha	(800) 629–1123
Arizona	Arizona Poison and Drug Information Center, Tucson	(800) 362–0101 (602) 626–6016	New Jersey	New Jersey Poison Information and Education System, Newark	(800) 962–1253
	Samaritan Regional Poison Center, Phoenix	(602) 253–3334	New Mexico	New Mexico Poison and Drug Information Center, Albuquerque	(800) 432–6866 (505) 843–2551
California	Fresno Regional Poison Control Center, Fresno	(800) 346–5922 (209) 445–1222	New York	Hudson Valley Poison Center, Nyack	(800) 336–6997 (914) 353–1000
	San Diego Regional Poison Center, San Diego	(800) 876–4766 (619) 543–6000		Long Island Regional Poison Control Center, East Meadow	(516) 542–2323
	San Francisco Bay Area Regional Poison Center, San Francisco	(800) 523–2222		New York City Poison Control Center, New York City	(212) 340–4494 (212) 764–7667
	Santa Clara Valley Medical Center Regional Poison Control Center, San Jose	(800) 662–9886 (408) 299–5112	Ohio	Central Ohio Poison Center, Columbus	(800) 682–7625 (614) 228–1323
	UC Davis Medical Center, Regional Poison Center, Sacramento	(800) 342–9293 (916) 734–3692		Cincinnati Drug and Poison Information Center, Cincinnati	(800) 872–5111 (513) 558–5111
Colorado	Rocky Mountain Poison and Drug Center, Denver	(303) 629–1123	Oregon	Oregon Poison Center, Portland	(800) 452–7165 (503) 494–8968
Florida	Florida Poison Information Center, Tampa	(800) 282–3171 (813) 253–4444	Pennsylvania	Central Pennsylvania Poison Center, Hershey	(800) 521–6110
Georgia	Georgia Poison Control Center, Atlanta	(800) 282–5846 (404) 589–4400		The Poison Control Center, Philadelphia	(215) 386–2100
Indiana	Indiana Poison Center, Indianapolis	(800) 382–9097 (317) 929–2323		Pittsburgh Poison Center, Pittsburgh	(412) 681–6669
Maryland	Maryland Poison Center, Baltimore	(800) 492–2414 (410) 528–7701	Texas	North Texas Poison Center, Dallas	(800) 441–0040 (214) 590–5000
Massachusetts	Massachusetts Poison Control System, Boston	(800) 682–9211 (617) 232–2120		Texas State Poison Center, Galveston Houston	(409) 765–1420 (713) 654–1701
Michigan	Blodgett Regional Poison Center, Grand Rapids	(800) 632–2727	Utah	Intermountain Regional Poison Center, Salt Lake City	(800) 456–7707 (801) 581–2151
	Poison Control Center, Children's Hospital, Detroit	(313) 745–5711	Virginia	Blue Ridge Poison Center, Charlottesville	(804) 924–5543
Minnesota	Hennepin Regional Poison Center, Minneapolis	(612) 347–3141	Washington, DC	National Capitol Poison Center, Washington, DC	(202) 625–3333
	Minnesota Regional Poison Center, St. Paul	(612) 221–2113	West Virginia	West Virginia Poison Center, Charlestown	(800) 642–3625 (304) 348–4211
Missouri	Cardinal Glennon Children's Hospital Regional Poison Center, St. Louis	(800) 366–8888 (314) 772–5200	Wyoming	The Poison Center, Omaha, NE	(800) 955–9119 (402) 390–5555
Montana	Rocky Mountain Poison and Drug Center, Denver	(800) 629–1123			

[1]American Association of Poison Control Centers, 1993.

Table 39–2. Initial management of coma.

A	Airway control
B	Breathing
C	Circulation
D	Dextrose 50%, 50–100 mL IV; thiamine, 100 mg IM or IV; and naloxone, 0.4–2 mg IV

be necessary if the patient is intoxicated by an opioid or a benzodiazepine and responds rapidly to intravenous naloxone (see below).

2. Breathing–Clinically assess the quality and depth of respiration, and provide assistance if necessary with a bag-valve-mask device or mechanical ventilator. Provide supplemental oxygen. The arterial blood CO_2 tension is useful in determining the adequacy of ventilation. The arterial blood PO_2 determination may reveal hypoxemia, which may be caused by respiratory arrest, bronchospasm, pulmonary aspiration, or noncardiogenic pulmonary edema.

3. Circulation–Measure the pulse and blood pressure, and estimate tissue perfusion (eg, by measurement of urinary output, skin signs, blood pH). Insert an intravenous line, and draw blood for blood count, glucose, electrolytes, and possible toxicologic testing.

4. Dextrose and thiamine–Unless promptly treated, severe hypoglycemia can cause irreversible brain damage. Therefore, in all comatose or convulsing patients, give 50% dextrose, 50–100 mL by intravenous bolus, unless a rapid bedside blood sugar test is available and rules out hypoglycemia. In alcoholic or very malnourished patients who may have marginal thiamine stores, give thiamine, 100 mg intramuscularly or over 2–3 minutes intravenously.

B. Narcotic Antagonists: Naloxone, 0.4–2 mg intravenously, may reverse opioid-induced respiratory depression and coma. If opioid overdose is strongly suspected, give additional doses of naloxone (up to 5–10 mg may be required to reverse potent opioids). *Caution:* Naloxone has a much shorter duration of action (2–3 hours) than most common opioids; repeated doses may be required, and continuous observation for several hours is mandatory.

C. Flumazenil: Flumazenil, 0.2–0.5 mg intravenously, repeated every 30 seconds as needed up to a maximum of 3 mg, may reverse benzodiazepine-induced coma. *Caution:* Flumazenil has a short duration of effect (2–3 hours), and resedation requiring additional doses is common.

HYPOTHERMIA

Assessment & Complications

Hypothermia commonly accompanies coma due to opioids, ethanol, hypoglycemic agents, phenothi-azines, barbiturates, and other sedative-hypnotics and depressants.

Hypothermic patients may have a barely perceptible pulse and blood pressure and often appear to be dead. Hypothermia may cause or aggravate hypotension, and the hypotension will not reverse until the temperature is normalized.

Treatment

Hypothermia treatment is discussed in Chapter 35. Gradual rewarming is preferred unless the patient is in cardiac arrest.

HYPOTENSION

Assessment & Complications

Hypotension may be due to poisoning with antihypertensive drugs, beta-blockers, calcium channel blocking agents, iron, theophylline, opioids, phenothiazines, barbiturates, and tricyclic antidepressants.

Hypotension in the poisoned or drug-overdosed patient may be caused by venous or arteriolar vasodilatation, depressed cardiac contractility, or a combination of these effects. The only certain way to determine the cause of hypotension in any individual patient is to insert a pulmonary artery catheter and measure the left ventricular filling pressure and then calculate the cardiac output and peripheral vascular resistance. Alternatively, a central venous pressure monitor may indicate a need for further fluid therapy.

Treatment

If cardiac catheterization and CVP monitoring are not practical, keep in mind that most patients respond to empiric treatment (200 mL intravenous boluses of normal saline or other isotonic crystalloid up to total of 1–2 L). If fluid therapy is not successful, give dopamine, 5–15 µg/kg/min by intravenous infusion in a large peripheral or central line.

Hypotension caused by certain toxins may respond to specific treatment. For hypotension caused by overdoses of tricyclic antidepressants or related drugs, administer sodium bicarbonate, 1–2 meq/kg by intravenous bolus injection. For beta-blocker overdose, administer glucagon, 5–10 mg by intravenous bolus injection. For calcium antagonist overdose, administer calcium chloride, 15–20 mg/kg intravenously (repeated doses may be necessary).

HYPERTENSION

Assessment & Complications

Hypertension may be due to poisoning with amphetamines, anticholinergics, cocaine, phencyclidine (PCP), phenylpropanolamine, or monoamine oxidase inhibitors (interactions).

Severe hypertension (diastolic blood pressure

> 105–110 mm Hg) can result in acute intracranial hemorrhage, myocardial infarction, or aortic dissection. Patients often present with headache, chest pain, or encephalopathy.

Treatment

Treat hypertension if the patient is symptomatic or if the diastolic pressure is greater than 105–110 mm Hg—especially if there is no prior history of hypertension.

Administer phentolamine, 2–5 mg intravenously, or nitroprusside sodium, 0.25–8 µg/kg/min intravenously. If excessive tachycardia is present, add propranolol, 1–5 mg intravenously, or esmolol 25–100 µg/kg/min intravenously. *Caution:* Do not give beta-blockers alone, since doing so may paradoxically worsen hypertension.

ARRHYTHMIAS

Assessment & Complications

Arrhythmias may occur with a variety of drugs or toxins (Table 39–3). They may also occur as a result of hypoxia, metabolic acidosis, or electrolyte imbalance (eg, hyper- or hypokalemia, hypocalcemia).

Treatment

Arrhythmias are often caused by hypoxia or electrolyte imbalance, and these conditions should be sought and treated. If ventricular arrhythmias persist, administer lidocaine or phenytoin. *Caution:* avoid class Ia agents (quinidine, procainamide, disopyramide), which may aggravate arrhythmias caused by tricyclic antidepressants, calcium antagonists, or beta-blockers.

For tachyarrhythmias induced by sympathomimetic agents, use propranolol or esmolol (see doses given above in hypertension section). Wide QRS complex tachycardia in the setting of tricyclic antide-

pressant overdose (or quinidine and other class Ia drugs) should be treated with sodium bicarbonate, 50–100 meq intravenously by bolus injection. (See discussion of tricyclic antidepressant poisoning.)

CONVULSIONS

Assessment & Complications

Convulsions may be due to poisoning with amphetamines, antihistamines, camphor, cocaine, isoniazid, lindane, phencyclidine (PCP), phenothiazines, strychnine (rigidity), theophylline, tricyclic antidepressants, or withdrawal from alcohol or sedative-hypnotics.

Convulsions may also be caused by hypoxia, hypoglycemia, hyponatremia, head trauma, central nervous system infection, and idiopathic epilepsy.

Prolonged or repeated convulsions may lead to hypoxia, metabolic acidosis, hyperthermia, and rhabdomyolysis.

Treatment

Administer diazepam, 5–10 mg intravenously over 2–3 minutes, or lorazepam, 2–3 mg intravenously, or—if intravenous access is not immediately available—midazolam, 5–10 mg intramuscularly. If convulsions continue, administer phenobarbital, 15–20 mg/kg slowly intravenously over no less than 30 minutes; or phenytoin, 15 mg/kg intravenously over no less than 30 minutes (maximum infusion rate, 50 mg/min). Both drugs may be used if necessary. Maintenance doses may be required if drug toxicity is expected to last more than 18–24 hours.

Convulsions due to a few drugs and toxins may require antidotes or other specific therapies (as listed in Table 39–4).

Table 39–3. Common toxins or drugs causing arrhythmias.

Arrhythmia	Common Causes
Sinus bradycardia	Beta-blockers, verapamil, organophosphates, digitalis glycosides, opioids, clonidine, sedative-hypnotics.
Atrioventricular block	Beta-blockers, digitalis glycosides, calcium antagonists, tricyclic antidepressants, lithium.
Sinus tachycardia	Theophylline, caffeine, cocaine, amphetamines, phencyclidine, metaproterenol and beta-agonists, iron, anticholinergics, tricyclic antidepressants, antihistamines.
Wide QRS complex	Tricyclic antidepressants, quinidine and type Ia antiarrhythmics, type Ic antiarrhythmics, phenothiazines, hyperkalemia.

Table 39–4. Convulsions requiring special consideration (see text for doses).

Toxin or Drug	Comments
Isoniazid (INH)	Administer pyridoxine.
Lithium	May indicate need for hemodialysis.
Organophosphates	Administer pralidoxime (2-PAM) and atropine.
Strychnine	"Convulsions" are actually spinally mediated muscle spasms and usually require neuromuscular paralysis.
Theophylline	Convulsions indicate need for charcoal hemoperfusion.
Tricyclic antidepressants	Hyperthermia and cardiotoxicity are common complications of repeated convulsions; paralyze early with neuromuscular blockers.

HYPERTHERMIA

Assessment & Complications

Hyperthermia may be due to poisoning with amphetamines, atropine and other anticholinergic drugs, cocaine, dinitrophenol and pentachlorophenol, haloperidol and other neuroleptics, monoamine oxidase inhibitors, phencyclidine (PCP), salicylates, strychnine, tricyclic antidepressants, and various other medications.

Hyperthermia is a rapidly life-threatening complication. Severe hyperthermia (temperature > 40–41 °C [104–105.8 °F]) may rapidly cause brain damage and multiorgan failure, including rhabdomyolysis, renal failure, and coagulopathy.

Treatment

Treat hyperthermia aggressively by removing all clothing, spraying with tepid water, and fanning the patient. If this is not rapidly effective, as shown by a normal rectal temperature within 30–60 minutes or if there is significant muscle rigidity or hyperactivity, induce neuromuscular paralysis with pancuronium, 0.1 mg/kg intravenously. Once paralyzed, the patient must be intubated and mechanically ventilated; therefore, an anesthesiologist or other physician skilled in endotracheal intubation should be present. Absence of visible muscular convulsive movements may give the false impression that brain seizure activity has ceased; however, this must be confirmed by electroencephalography.

Dantrolene (2–5 mg/kg intravenously) may be effective for hyperthermia associated with muscle rigidity that does not respond to neuromuscular blockade (ie, malignant hyperthermia). Bromocriptine, 2.5–7.5 mg orally daily, has been recommended for neuroleptic malignant syndrome.

OTHER TREATMENT

ANTIDOTES

Give "specific" antidotes when there is reasonable certainty of a specific diagnosis (Table 39–5). To effectively negate the physiologic effects of the toxic agent, the antidote must be given promptly. Keep in mind, however, that antidotes frequently have serious side effects of their own. The indications and dosages for specific antidotes are discussed in the respective sections for specific toxins. See also Table 39–6.

Table 39–5. Some toxic agents for which there are "specific" antidotes.

Toxic Agent	Specific Antidote
Acetaminophen	Acetylcysteine
Anticholinergics (eg, atropine)	Physostigmine
Anticholinesterases (eg, organophosphate pesticides)	Atropine and pralidoxime (2-PAM)
Benzodiazepines	Flumazenil
Carbon monoxide	Oxygen
Cyanide	Sodium nitrite, sodium thiosulfate
Digitalis glycosides	Digoxin-specific Fab antibodies
Heavy metals (eg, lead, mercury, iron) and arsenic	Specific chelating agents
Isoniazid	Pyridoxine (vitamin B_6)
Methanol, ethylene glycol	Ethanol (ethyl alcohol)
Opioids	Naloxone
Snake venom	Specific venom anti-sera

DECONTAMINATION OF THE SKIN

Corrosive agents rapidly injure the skin and eyes and must be removed immediately. In addition, many toxins are readily absorbed through the skin, and systemic absorption can only be prevented by rapid action.

Wash the affected areas with copious quantities of lukewarm water or saline. Wash carefully behind the ears, under the nails, and in skin folds. For oily substances (eg, pesticides), wash the skin at least twice with plain soap and shampoo the hair.

Table 39–6. Examples of ineffective or dangerous "antidotes."[1]

"Antidote"	Application	Problems
Amphetamines, caffeine, or doxapram	Nonspecific arousal, eg, sedative overdose	Cardiac arrhythmias, seizures
Mineral oil	Petroleum distillate ingestion	Lipoid pneumonia
Physostigmine	Nonspecific arousal, eg, diazepam overdose, tricyclic antidepressants	Bradycardia, asystole, seizures
"Universal antidote" (burnt toast, tea)	Adsorbent in gut	Ineffective; aspiration; wastes time
Vinegar, other weak acids	Neutralization of alkali burns	Ineffective; may worsen injury

[1]Reproduced, with permission, from Saunders CE, Ho MT (editors): *Current Emergency Diagnosis & Treatment,* 4th ed. Appleton & Lange, 1992.

DECONTAMINATION OF THE EYES

Act quickly to prevent serious damage. Flush the eyes with copious amounts of water or saline. (If available, instill local anesthetic drops (eg, proparacaine) in the eye before beginning irrigation.) Remove contact lenses if present.) Place the victim supine under a tap or stream of water, and direct the stream so that it will flow across both eyes after running off the nasal bridge. Lift the tarsal conjunctiva to look for undissolved particles and to facilitate irrigation. Continue irrigation for 15 minutes by the clock or until each eye has been irrigated with at least 1 L of solution. If the toxin is an acid or a base, check the pH of the tears after irrigation, and continue irrigation if the pH is abnormal.

After irrigation is complete, perform fluorescein examination of the eye, using Wood's lamp to identify areas of corneal injury. Patients with serious conjunctival or corneal injury should be immediately referred to an ophthalmologist.

GASTROINTESTINAL DECONTAMINATION

Removal of ingested poisons is an essential part of emergency treatment. However, if more than 60 minutes has passed, induced emesis and gastric lavage are relatively ineffective. For small or moderate ingestions of most substances, toxicologists generally recommend activated charcoal alone without prior gastric emptying. Exceptions are large ingestions of anticholinergic compounds and salicylates, which often delay gastric emptying, and ingestion of sustained-release or enteric-coated tablets, which may remain intact for several hours.

Gastric emptying is not generally used for ingestion of corrosive agents or petroleum distillates, because further esophageal injury or pulmonary aspiration may result. However, in certain cases, removal of the toxin may be more important than concern over possible complications. Consult a medical toxicologist or regional poison control center (Table 39–1) for advice.

Emesis

Emesis using syrup of ipecac is a convenient and fairly effective way to evacuate gastric contents if given shortly after ingestion (eg, at work or at home). However, it may delay or prevent use of oral activated charcoal and is not generally used in the hospital management of ingestions.

A. Indications: For removal of poison in conscious, cooperative patients and for promptness, ipecac can be given in the home or at work in the first few minutes after poisoning.

B. Contraindications: Induced emesis is contraindicated for drowsy, unconscious, or convulsing patients and for patients who have ingested kerosene or other hydrocarbons (danger of aspiration of stomach contents), corrosive poisons, or rapidly acting convulsants (eg, cyclic antidepressants, strychnine, nicotine, camphor).

C. Technique: Give syrup of ipecac, 30 mL (15 mL in children), followed by an 8-oz glass of water. Repeat in 20 minutes if necessary.

Gastric Lavage

Gastric lavage is more effective for liquid poisons or small pill fragments and is most effective when started within 60 minutes after ingestion. The lavage procedure may delay administration of activated charcoal and may mechanically push pills and other toxic material into the small intestine.

A. Indications: Gastric lavage is indicated for removal of ingested poisons when emesis is refused, contraindicated, or unsuccessful; for collection and examination of gastric contents for identification of poison; and for convenient administration of charcoal and antidotes.

B. Contraindications: Do *not* use lavage for stuporous or comatose patients with absent gag reflexes unless they are endotracheally intubated beforehand. Some authorities advise against lavage when caustic material has been ingested; others regard it as essential to remove such material from the stomach.

C. Technique: In obtunded or comatose patients, the danger of aspiration pneumonia is reduced by first protecting the airway with endotracheal intubation. Gently insert a lubricated, soft but noncollapsible stomach tube (at least 37–40F) through the mouth or nose into the stomach. Aspirate and save the contents, and then lavage repeatedly with 50–100 mL of fluid until the return fluid is clear. Always remove excess lavage fluid. Use lukewarm tap water or saline.

Activated Charcoal

Activated charcoal effectively adsorbs almost all drugs and poisons. Note: Poorly absorbed substances include iron, lithium, potassium, sodium, cyanide, mineral acids, and alcohols.

A. Indications: Activated charcoal should be used for prompt adsorption of drugs or toxins in the stomach and intestine. Given alone, it may be as effective as or more effective than ipecac-induced emesis or gastric lavage.

B. Contraindications: Activated charcoal should not be used for stuporous, comatose, or convulsing patients unless it can be given by gastric tube and the airway is first protected by cuffed endotracheal tube. This substance is contraindicated also for patients with ileus or intestinal obstruction or those who have ingested corrosives for whom endoscopy is planned.

C. Technique: Administer activated charcoal, 60–100 g orally or via gastric tube, mixed in aqueous slurry. Repeated doses may be given to ensure gastrointestinal adsorption or to enhance elimination of some drugs (see below).

Catharsis

A. Indications: Catharsis is indicated for stimulation of peristalsis to hasten the elimination of unabsorbed drugs and poisons and the charcoal slurry.

B. Contraindications and Cautions: Do not use mineral oil or other oil-based cathartics. Avoid sodium-based cathartics in patients with hypertension, renal failure, and congestive heart failure and magnesium-based cathartics in those with renal failure.

C. Technique: Magnesium sulfate 10%, 2–3 mL/kg; or sorbitol 70%, 1–2 mL/kg. Sorbitol is commonly used in prepackaged charcoal slurry products.

Whole Bowel Irrigation

Whole bowel irrigation utilizes large volumes of balanced polyethylene glycol-electrolyte solution to push tablets through the intestinal tract. There is no net gain or loss of systemic fluids or electrolytes.

A. Indications: Whole bowel irrigation is particularly effective for massive iron ingestion in which intact tablets persist on abdominal x-ray despite emesis and lavage. It has also been reported to be useful for ingestions of sustained-release and enteric-coated tablets.

B. Contraindications: Same as for cathartics.

C. Technique: Administer the balanced polyethylene glycol-electrolyte solution (CoLyte, Go-LYTELY) into the stomach via gastric tube at a rate of 1–2 L/h until the rectal effluent is clear. Several hours of irrigation may be required.

Increased Drug Removal

A. Forced Diuresis: Forced diuresis is hazardous; the risk of complications (pulmonary edema, electrolyte imbalance) usually outweighs its benefits. Acidic drugs (eg, salicylates, phenobarbital) are more rapidly excreted with an alkaline urine. Acidification (sometimes promoted for amphetamines, phencyclidine) is *not* very effective and is contraindicated in the presence of rhabdomyolysis or myoglobinuria.

B. Dialysis (Hemodialysis or Hemoperfusion): The indications for dialysis are as follows: (1) Known or suspected potentially lethal amounts of a dialyzable drug (Table 39–7). (2) Poisoning with deep coma, apnea, severe hypotension, fluid and electrolyte or acid-base disturbance, or extreme body temperature changes which cannot be corrected by conventional measures. (3) Poisoning in patients with severe renal, cardiac, pulmonary, or hepatic disease who will not be able to eliminate the toxin by usual mechanisms.

Many of the substances that cannot be removed effectively by aqueous dialysis can be removed by hemoperfusion through specially designed coated

Table 39–7. Recommended use of hemodialysis (HD) and Hemoperfusion (HP) in poisoning.

Poison	Procedure	Indications[1]
Carbamazepine	HP	Seizures, severe cardiotoxicity.
Digitoxin[2]	HP	Severe toxicity, Fab not available.
Ethylene glycol	HD	Acidosis, serum level > 100 mg/dL.
Lithium	HD	Severe symptoms.
Methanol	HD	Acidosis, serum level > 50 mg/dL.
Paraquat	HP	Ingestion of known lethal dose.
Phenobarbital	HP	Intractable hypotension, acidosis despite maximal supportive care.
Salicylate	HD	Severe acidosis, CNS symptoms, level >100 mg/dL (acute) or >60 mg/dL (chronic).
Theophylline	HP	Serum level >90–100 mg/L (acute) or seizures and serum level >40–60 mg/L (chronic).

[1]Contact a regional poison control center or a clinical toxicologist before undertaking these procedures. See text for further discussion of indications.
[2]Digoxin and other cardiac glycosides are not removed by hemoperfusion.

charcoal columns. Indications are the same as for dialysis. Peritoneal dialysis may occasionally be employed for acute poisonings when hemodialysis is not available, but it is very inefficient. Dialysis should usually augment rather than replace well-established emergency and supportive measures.

C. Repeat-Dose Charcoal: Repeated doses of activated charcoal, 20–30 g every 3–4 hours, may hasten elimination of some drugs (eg, digitoxin, theophylline, phenobarbital) by adsorbing drug excreted into the gut lumen ("gut dialysis"). Sorbitol or other cathartics should *not* be used with each dose, or resulting large stool volumes may lead to in dehydration or hypernatremia.

DIAGNOSIS OF POISONING

The identity of the ingested substance is usually known, but occasionally a comatose patient is found with an unlabeled container or refuses or otherwise fails to give a coherent history. By performing a directed physical examination and ordering common clinical laboratory tests, the clinician can often make a tentative diagnosis that may allow empiric interventions or may suggest specific toxicologic tests.

PHYSICAL EXAMINATION

Important diagnostic variables in the physical examination include blood pressure, pulse rate, temperature, pupil size, sweating, and the presence or absence of peristaltic activity. Poisonings with many drugs fit into one of four common syndromes.

Sympathomimetic Syndrome

The blood pressure and pulse rate are elevated, though with severe hypertension reflex bradycardia may occur. The temperature is often elevated, pupils are dilated, and the skin is sweaty, though mucous membranes are dry. Patients are usually agitated, anxious, or even psychotic.

Examples: Amphetamines, cocaine, ephedrine and pseudoephedrine, phencyclidine (pupils normal or small), phenylpropanolamine (bradycardia common).

Sympatholytic Syndrome

The blood pressure and pulse rate are decreased and body temperature is low. The pupils are small or even pinpoint. Peristalsis is usually decreased. Patients are usually obtunded or comatose.

Examples: Barbiturates, benzodiazepines and other sedative hypnotics, clonidine and related antihypertensives, ethanol, opioids.

Cholinergic Syndrome

Stimulation of muscarinic receptors causes bradycardia, miosis, sweating, and hyperperistalsis as well as bronchorrhea, wheezing, excessive salivation, and urinary incontinence. Nicotinic receptor stimulation may produce initial hypertension and tachycardia as well as fasciculations and muscle weakness. Patients are usually agitated and anxious.

Examples: Carbamates, nicotine, organophosphates, physostigmine.

Anticholinergic Syndrome

Tachycardia with mild hypertension is common, and the body temperature is often elevated. Pupils are widely dilated. The skin is flushed, hot and dry. Peristalsis is decreased, and urinary retention is common. Patients may have myoclonic jerking or choreoathetoid movements. Agitated delirium is frequently seen, and severe hyperthermia may occur.

Examples: Atropine, scopolamine, other anticholinergics, amantadine, antihistamines, phenothiazines (hypotension, small pupils), tricyclic antidepressants.

CLINICAL LABORATORY TESTS IN MANAGEMENT OF POISONING

The following clinical laboratory tests are recommended for routine screening of the overdosed patient: serum osmolality and osmolar gap, serum electrolytes, serum glucose, serum creatinine, serum urea nitrogen, urinalysis (eg, oxalate crystals with ethylene glycol poisoning, myoglobinuria with rhabdomyolysis), and electrocardiography. In addition, it is recommended that serum acetaminophen and ethanol levels be determined in all patients with drug overdoses.

OSMOLAR GAP

The osmolar gap is defined and calculation of the gap is described in Table 39–8. It is increased in the presence of large quantities of low-molecular-weight substances, most commonly ethanol. Common poisons associated with increased osmolar gap are acetone, ethanol, ethylene glycol, isopropyl alcohol, methanol, and propylene glycol. The presence of a combined osmolar and elevated anion gap suggests poisoning by methanol or ethylene glycol.

ANION GAP

Metabolic acidosis associated with an elevated anion gap is usually due to an accumulation of lactic acid or other acids (see Chapter 18). Common causes of elevated anion gap in poisoning include carbon monoxide, cyanide, ethylene glycol, medicinal iron, isoniazid, methanol, phenformin, and salicylates.

One should also check the osmolar gap; combined elevated anion and osmolar gap suggests poisoning by methanol or ethylene glycol.

TOXICOLOGY LABORATORY EXAMINATION

The routine toxicology screen (Table 39–9) is of little value in the initial care of the poisoned patient—on the contrary, it is time-consuming, expensive, and frequently erroneous. Specific quantitative levels of certain drugs may be extremely helpful (Table 39–10), however, especially if specific antidotes or interventions (eg, dialysis, antidotes) would be indicated based upon the results.

If a toxicology screen is required, urine is the best specimen for broad qualitative screening. Blood samples may be saved for possible quantitative testing,

Table 39–8. Use of the osmolar gap in toxicology.[1]

The osmolar gap (Δosm) is determined by subtracting the calculated serum osmolality from the measured serum osmolality.

$$\text{Calculated osmolality (osm)} = 2[Na^+ \text{(meq/L)}] + \frac{\text{Glucose (mg/dL)}}{18} + \frac{\text{BUN (mg/dL)}}{2.8}$$

$$\Delta\text{osm} = \text{Measured osmolality} - \text{Calculated osmolality}$$

Serum osmolality may be increased by contributions of circulating alcohols and other low-molecular-weight substances. Since these substances are not included in the calculated osmolality, there will be a gap proportionate to their serum concentration and inversely proportional to their molecular weight:

$$\frac{\text{Serum concentration (mg/dL)}}{} = \Delta\text{osm} \times \frac{\text{Molecular weight}}{10}$$

For ethanol (the commonest cause of Δosm), a gap of 30 mosm/L indicates an ehtanol level of approximately

$$30 \times \frac{46}{10} = 138 \text{ mg/dL}$$

	Molecular Weight	Toxic Concentration	Appproximate Corresponding Δosm (mosm/L)
Ethanol	46	300	65
Methanol	32	50	16
Ethylene glycol	62	50	8
Ispropanol	60	150	25

[1]Modified from Saunders CE, Ho MT (editors): *Current Emergency Diagnosis & Treatment,* 4th ed. Appleton & Lange, 1992.
Note: Most laboratories use the freezing point method for calculating osmolality. If the vaporization point method is used, alcohols are driven off and their contribution to osmolality is lost.

but blood is not appropriate for screening purposes since it is relatively insensitive for many common drugs, including psychotropic agents, opioids, and stimulants.

ABDOMINAL X-RAYS

A plain film of the abdomen may reveal radiopaque iron tablets, drug-filled condoms, or other toxic material. Studies suggest that few tablets are predictably visible (eg, ferrous sulfate, sodium chloride, calcium carbonate, and potassium chloride). Thus, the x-ray is useful only if positive.

Table 39–9. Common drugs screened for in blood and urine in the toxicology laboratory.[1]

Blood
Acetaminophen, alcohols, barbiturates, benzodiazepines, carisoprodol, ethchlorvynol, glutethimide, meprobamate, methaqualone, phenytoin, salicylates.

Urine
Acetaminophen, alcohols, barbiturates, chlorpheniramine, cocaine, codeine, dextromethorphan, diphenhydramine, ethchlorvynol, lidocaine, meperidine, meprobamate, methadone, methyprylon, morphine, pentazocine, phencyclidine, phenothiazines, propoxyphene, salicylates, tricyclic antidepressants.

[1]**Note:** The urine screen is generally more comprehensive, detecting drugs of abuse (opiates, stimulants), antihistamines, and, in many cases, drugs also found in serum.

Table 39–10. Specific quantitative levels and potential therapeutic interventions.[1]

Drug or Toxin	Treatment
Acetaminophen	Use of specific antidote (acetylcysteine) based on serum level.
Carbon monoxide	High carboxyhemoglobin level indicates need for 100% oxygen.
Digitalis	On basis of serum digitalis and potassium levels, treatment with Fab antibody fragments may be indicated.
Ethanol	Low serum level may suggest nonalcoholic cause for coma (eg, trauma, other drugs, other alcohols). May also be used in monitoring ethanol therapy for methanol or ethylene glycol poisoning.
Ethylene glycol	High level of acidosis indicates need for hemodialysis and ethanol therapy.
Iron	Level may indicate need for chelation with deferoxamine.
Lithium	Serum levels and calculated half-life can guide decision to hemodialyze.
Methanol	Acidosis, high methanol level indicate need for hemodialysis, ethanol therapy.
Methemoglobin	Methemoglobinemia can be treated with methylene blue intravenously.
Salicylates	High level may indicate need for hemodialysis, alkaline diuresis.
Theophylline	Immediate hemoperfusion may be indicated based on serum level.

[1]Some drugs or toxins may have profound and irreversible toxicity unless rapid and specific management is provided outside of routine supportive care. For these agents, laboratory testing may provide the serum level or other evidence required for administering a specific antidote or arranging for hemodialysis.

TREATMENT OF COMMON SPECIFIC POISONINGS (Alphabetical Order)

ACETAMINOPHEN

Acetaminophen is a common analgesic found in many nonprescription and prescription products. After absorption, it is metabolized mainly by glucuronidation and sulfation, with a small fraction metabolized via the P-450 mixed-function oxidase system to a highly toxic reactive intermediate. This toxic intermediate is normally detoxified by cellular glutathione. With acute acetaminophen overdose (> 140 mg/kg, or 7 g in an average adult), hepatocellular glutathione is rapidly depleted and the reactive intermediate attacks other cell proteins, causing necrosis. Chronic alcohol abuse may increase the likelihood of toxicity by inducing cytochrome P450 activity and reducing hepatic glutathione stores. Alcoholics may develop hepatic toxicity after chronic accidental overuse of acetaminophen.

Clinical Findings

Shortly after ingestion, patients may have nausea or vomiting, but there are no other signs of toxicity until 24–48 hours after ingestion, when hepatic aminotransferase levels increase. With severe poisoning, massive hepatic necrosis may occur, resulting in jaundice, hepatic encephalopathy, renal failure, and death.

The diagnosis of severe poisoning after acute overdose is based on measurement of the serum acetaminophen level. Plot the serum level versus the time since ingestion on the acetaminophen nomogram shown in Figure 39–1.

Treatment

A. Emergency and Supportive Measures: Empty the stomach by emesis or gastric lavage, and administer activated charcoal (see p 1321). If more than 3–4 hours have passed since ingestion, do not induce emesis, because it is ineffective and may delay oral administration of the antidote acetylcysteine. Although charcoal may bind the oral antidote acetylcysteine, this is not considered clinically significant.

Provide supportive care for hepatic injury. Some patients who progress to massive hepatic failure with encephalopathy may require emergency liver transplantation.

B. Specific Treatment: If the serum acetaminophen level is higher than the toxic line on the nomogram (Figure 39–1), begin treatment with a loading dose of acetylcysteine, 140 mg/kg orally, followed by

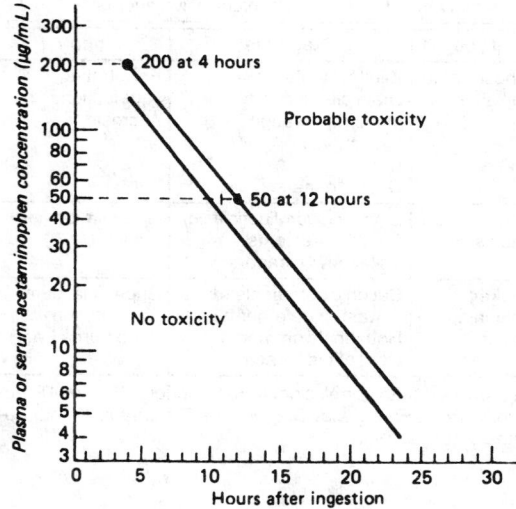

Figure 39–1. Nomogram for prediction of acetaminophen hepatotoxicity following acute overdosage. The upper line defines serum acetaminophen concentrations known to be associated with hepatotoxicity; the lower line defines serum levels 25% below those expected to cause hepatotoxicity. To give a margin for error, the lower line should be used as a guide to treatment. (Modified and reproduced, with permission, from Rumack BH, Matthew H: Acetaminophen poisoning and toxicity. Pediatrics 1975;55:871.)

70 mg/kg every 4 hours for 17 doses or until the serum acetaminophen level is zero. Treatment with acetylcysteine is most effective if started within 8–10 hours after ingestion.

Acetylcysteine may also be given intravenously; this is the preferred method in Europe and Canada, but there is no approved parenteral formulation or dosing schedule in the United States.

Ashbourne JF et al: Value of rapid screening for acetaminophen in all patients with intentional overdose. Ann Emerg Med 1989;18:1035. (Although the incidence of missed acetaminophen overdose is small, the authors recommend a stat screening test for acetaminophen in all patients with drug overdose.)

Smilkstein MJ et al: Efficacy of oral N-acetylcysteine in the treatment of acetaminophen overdose. N Engl J Med 1988;319:1557. (A major multicenter study confirming the efficacy of oral N-acetylcysteine.)

ACIDS, CORROSIVE (Table 39–11)

The strong mineral acids exert primarily a local corrosive effect on the skin and mucous membranes. In severe burns, circulatory collapse may result. Symptoms include severe pain in the throat and upper

Table 39–11. Common corrosive agents.[1]

Type	Examples	Injury
Concentrated alkalies	Clinitest tablets Drain cleaners Industrial-strength ammonia Lye Oven cleaners	Penetrating liquefaction necrosis
Concentrated acids	Etchers (hydrofluoric acid) Pool disinfectants Toilet bowl cleaners	Coagulation necrosis
Weaker cleaning agents	Cationic detergents (dishwasher detergents) Household ammonia Household bleach	Superficial burns and irritation; deep burns (rare)

[1]Reproduced, with permission, from Saunders CE, Ho MT (editors): *Current Emergency Diagnosis & Treatment,* 4th ed. Appleton & Lange, 1992.

gastrointestinal tract, marked thirst, bloody vomitus; difficulty in swallowing, breathing, and speaking; discoloration and destruction of skin and mucous membranes in and around the mouth; and shock. Severe systemic metabolic acidosis may occur.

Severe deep destructive tissue damage may occur after exposure to hydrofluoric acid because of the penetrating fluoride ion. Systemic hypocalcemia and hyperkalemia may occur.

Inhalation of volatile acids, fumes, or gases such as chlorine, fluorine, bromine, or iodine causes severe irritation of the throat and larynx and may cause upper airway obstruction and noncardiogenic pulmonary edema.

Treatment

A. Ingestion: Do *not* induce emesis. Dilute immediately by giving a glass (4–8 oz) of milk or water to drink. Do *not* give bicarbonate or other neutralizing agents. Some experts recommend immediate gastric lavage.

Perform flexible endoscopic esophagoscopy promptly to determine the presence and extent of injury but do not attempt to pass beyond the injury. Perforation, peritonitis, and major bleeding are indications for surgery.

B. Skin Contact: Flood with water for 15 minutes. Use no chemical antidotes; the heat of the reaction may cause additional injury. For hydrofluoric acid burns, soak the affected area in magnesium sulfate solution or apply 2.5% calcium gluconate gel (prepared by adding 3.5 g calcium gluconate to 5 oz of water-soluble surgical lubricant, eg, K-Y Jelly); then arrange immediate consultation with a plastic surgeon or other specialist. Binding of the fluoride ion may be achieved by injecting 0.5 mL of 5% calcium gluconate (*caution:* do not use calcium *chloride*) per square centimeter under the burned area.

C. Eye Contact: Anesthetize the conjunctiva and corneal surfaces with topical local anesthetic

drops. Flood with water for 15 minutes, holding the eyelids open. Check pH with pH 6.0–8.0 test paper, and repeat irrigation, using normal saline, until pH is 7.0. Check for corneal damage with fluorescein and slit-lamp examination; consult an ophthalmologist about further treatment.

D. Inhalation: Remove from further exposure to fumes or gas. Check skin and clothing. Treat pulmonary edema.

Caravati EM: Acute hydrofluoric acid exposure. J Emerg Med 1988;6:143. (Review of the pathophysiology, diagnosis, and treatment of burns from this unusual acid.)

Gumaste W, Dave PB: Ingestion of corrosive substances by adults. Am J Gastroenterol 1992;87:1. (A review of gastrointestinal injuries from corrosive acids and alkali.)

ALKALIES
(Table 39–11)

The strong alkalies are common ingredients of household cleaning compounds and may be suspected by their "soapy" texture. Those with alkalinity above pH 12.0 are particularly corrosive. Clinitest tablets and disk batteries are also a source. Alkalies cause liquefactive necrosis, which is deeply penetrating. Symptoms include burning pain in the upper gastrointestinal tract, nausea, vomiting, and difficulty in swallowing and breathing. Examination reveals destruction and edema of the affected skin and mucous membranes and bloody vomitus and stools. X-ray may reveal the presence of disk batteries in the esophagus or lower gastrointestinal tract.

Treatment

A. Ingested: Do *not* induce emesis. Dilute immediately with a glass of water. Some gastroenterologists recommend immediate gastric lavage after ingestion of liquid caustic substances to remove residual material.

Immediate endoscopy is recommended to evaluate the extent of damage. If x-ray reveals the location of ingested disk batteries in the esophagus, immediate endoscopic removal is mandatory.

The use of corticosteroids to prevent stricture formation is of no proved benefit and is definitely contraindicated if there is evidence of esophageal perforation.

B. Skin Contact: Wash with running water until the skin no longer feels soapy. Relieve pain and treat shock.

C. Eye Contact: Anesthetize the conjunctival and corneal surfaces with topical anesthetic. Irrigate with water or saline continuously for 20–30 minutes, holding the lids open. Check pH with pH test paper, and repeat irrigation, using normal saline, for additional 30-minute periods until the pH is 7.0. Check for corneal damage with fluorescein and slit-lamp examination; consult an ophthalmologist for further treatment.

Anderson KD et al: A controlled trial of corticosteroids in children with corrosive injury of the esophagus. N Engl J Med 1990;323:637. (Randomized prospective study proving no benefit from steroids to reduce stricture formation.)

Zargar SA et al: Ingestion of strong corrosive alkalis: Spectrum of injury. Am J Gastroenterol 1992;87:337. (Prospective study of 31 patients with alkali ingestion. In this series, there was a high incidence of major complications and death.)

AMPHETAMINES & COCAINE

Amphetamines and cocaine are widely abused for their euphorigenic and stimulant properties. Both drugs may be smoked, snorted, ingested, or injected. The forms most commonly used for smoking are "ice" (amphetamine base) and "crack" or "freebase" (cocaine base). Amphetamines and cocaine produce central nervous system stimulation and a generalized increase in central and peripheral sympathetic activity. The toxic dose of each drug is highly variable and depends on the route of administration and individual tolerance. The onset of effects is most rapid after intravenous injection or smoking.

Clinical Findings

Patients may present with anxiety, tremulousness, tachycardia, hypertension, diaphoresis, dilated pupils, agitation, muscular hyperactivity, and psychosis. In severe intoxication, seizures and hyperthermia may occur. Sustained or severe hypertension may result in intracranial hemorrhage, aortic dissection, or myocardial infarction.

The diagnosis is supported by finding amphetamines, cocaine, or the cocaine metabolite benzoylecgonine in the urine. Blood screening is not sensitive enough to detect these drugs.

Treatment

A. Emergency and Supportive Measures: Maintain a patent airway and assist ventilation, if necessary. Treat coma or seizures as described at the beginning of this chapter. Rapidly lower the body temperature in patients who are hyperthermic (40 °C). Treat agitation or psychosis with a benzodiazepine such as diazepam, 5–10 mg intravenously (repeated as needed up to 20 mg), or midazolam, 0.1–0.2 mg/kg intramuscularly.

For poisoning by ingestion, perform gastric lavage and administer activated charcoal, or administer activated charcoal alone without prior gut emptying (see p 1321). Do *not* induce emesis, because of the risk of seizures.

B. Specific Treatment: Treat hypertension with a vasodilator drug such as phentolamine (1–5 mg intravenously) or nifedipine (10–20 mg orally) or a combined α- and β-adrenergic blocker such as labetalol (10–20 mg intravenously). Do *not* administer a pure beta-blocker such as propranolol alone, as this may result paradoxic worsening of the hypertension as a result of unopposed α-adrenergic effects.

Treat tachycardia or tachyarrhythmias with a short-acting beta-blocker such as esmolol (25–100 µg/kg/min by intravenous infusion).

Derlet RW et al: Emergency department presentation of cocaine intoxication. Ann Emerg Med 1989;18:182. (Retrospective review of 137 patients. Presenting problems included chest pain, syncope, and seizures. Sixteen patients were admitted and one died.)

Kloner R et al: The effects of acute and chronic cocaine use on the heart. Circulation 1992;85:407. (The pharmacologic basis for cocaine cardiotoxicity, clinical manifestations, and proposed treatment.)

ANTICOAGULANTS

Warfarin and related compounds (including ingredients of many rodenticides) inhibit the clotting mechanism by blocking hepatic synthesis of vitamin K-dependent clotting factors.

Anticoagulants may cause hemoptysis, gross hematuria, bloody stools, hemorrhages into organs, widespread bruising, and bleeding into joint spaces. The prothrombin time is increased within 12–24 hours (peak 36–48 hours) after a single overdose. After ingestion of brodifacoum and indanedione rodenticides (so-called superwarfarins), inhibition of clotting factor synthesis may persist for several weeks after a single dose.

Treatment

A. Emergency and Supportive Measures: Discontinue the drug at the first sign of gross bleeding, and determine the prothrombin time. If the patient has ingested an acute overdose, empty the stomach by emesis or lavage and administer activated charcoal (see p 1321).

B. Specific Treatment: If the prothrombin time is elevated, give phytonadione (vitamin K), 5–10 mg subcutaneously, and give fresh-frozen plasma as needed to rapidly correct the coagulation factor deficit if there is serious bleeding. If the patient is chronically anticoagulated and has strong medical indications for being maintained in that status (eg, prosthetic heart valve), give much smaller doses of vitamin K (1 mg) and fresh-frozen plasma (or both) to titrate to the desired prothrombin time.

If the patient has ingested brodifacoum or related super-rodenticides, prolonged observation (over weeks) and repeated administration of vitamin K may be required.

Katona B et al: Superwarfarin poisoning. J Emerg Med 1989;7:627. (Review of the newer anticoagulants, emphasizing their prolonged duration of action and appropriate strategies for management.)

Smolinske SC et al: Superwarfarin poisoning in children: A prospective study. Pediatrics 1989;84:490. (Prospective study in 110 children determined that to exclude serious poisonings, prothrombin time should be measured at 24 and 48 hours after ingestion.)

ARSENIC

Arsenic is found in pesticides and industrial chemicals. Symptoms of poisoning usually appear within 1 hour after ingestion but may be delayed as long as 12 hours. They include abdominal pain, vomiting, watery diarrhea, and skeletal muscle cramps. Profound dehydration and shock may occur. In chronic poisoning, symptoms can be vague but often include those of peripheral sensory neuropathy. Urinary arsenic levels may be misleading and are falsely elevated after certain meals (eg, seafood) that contain large quantities of relatively nontoxic organic arsenic.

Treatment

A. Emergency Measures: Induce vomiting or perform gastric lavage, and administer 60–100 g of activated charcoal (see p 1321).

B. Antidote: For symptomatic patients or those with massive overdose, give dimercaprol injection (BAL), 10% solution in oil, 2.5–3 mg/kg dimercaprol intramuscularly, then 2–3 mg/kg intramuscularly every 4 hours for 2 days. The side effects include nausea, vomiting, headache, and hypertension. An antihistamine such as diphenhydramine, 25–50 mg orally, will reduce the side effects if given 30 minutes before dimercaprol. Follow dimercaprol with oral penicillamine, 100 mg/kg/d in four divided doses (maximum, 2 g/d) for 1 week. Consult a medical toxicologist or regional poison control center (Table 39–1) for advice regarding continued chelation.

Gorby MS: Arsenic poisoning. (Clinical Conference.) West J Med 1988;149:308. (Sources of exposure, pathophysiology, clinical manifestations. and treatment.)

ATROPINE & ANTICHOLINERGICS

Atropine, scopolamine, belladonna, diphenoxylate with atropine (Lomotil), *Datura stramonium, Hyoscyamus niger,* some mushrooms, tricyclic antidepressants, and antihistamines are antimuscarinic agents with variable central nervous system effects. The patient complains of dryness of the mouth, thirst, difficulty in swallowing, and blurring of vision. The physical signs include dilated pupils, flushed skin, tachycardia, fever (although hypothermia has been reported), delirium, myoclonus, ileus, and flushed appearance. Antidepressants and antihistamines may induce convulsions.

Antihistamines are commonly available with or without prescription. Diphenhydramine commonly causes delirium, tachycardia, and seizures. Massive overdose may mimic triglyceride antidepressant poisoning. Newer nonsedating antihistamines, eg, terfenadine and astemizole, have caused QT interval prolongation and torsade de pointes atypical ventricular tachycardia.

Treatment

A. Emergency and Supportive Measures: Induce vomiting or perform gastric lavage, and administer activated charcoal (see p 1321). Do *not* induce emesis in patients who have ingested antidepressants, because seizures may occur abruptly. Tepid sponge baths and sedation are indicated to control high temperatures.

B. Specific Treatment: For pure atropine or related anticholinergic syndrome, if symptoms are severe (eg, hyperthermia or excessively rapid tachycardia), give physostigmine salicylate, 0.5–1 mg slowly intravenously over 5 minutes, with electrocardiographic monitoring, until symptoms are controlled. Bradyarrhythmias and convulsions are a hazard with physostigmine administration, and it should not be used in patients with tricyclic antidepressant overdose.

Fahy P et al: Serial serum drug concentrations and prolonged anticholinergic toxicity after benztropine (Cogentin) overdose. Am J Emerg Med 1989;7:199. (Prolonged anticholinergic syndrome—9 days—apparently due to prolonged intermittent absorption of the drug.)

BETA-ADRENERGIC BLOCKERS

There are a wide variety of β-adrenergic blocking drugs, with varying pharmacologic and pharmacokinetic properties. The most commonly used and most toxic beta-blocker is propranolol. Propranolol competitively blocks β_1 and β_2 adrenoceptors and also has direct membrane-depressant and central nervous system effects.

Clinical Findings

The most common findings with mild or moderate intoxication are hypotension and bradycardia. With more severe poisoning, cardiac depression may occur that is often unresponsive to conventional therapy with β-adrenergic stimulants such as dopamine and norepinephrine. In addition, with propranolol and other lipid-soluble drugs, seizures and coma may occur.

The diagnosis is based on typical clinical findings.

Toxicology screening does not usually include beta-blockers.

Treatment

A. Emergency and Supportive Measures:
Maintain a patent airway and assist ventilation, if necessary. Treat coma, hypotension, and seizures as described at the beginning of this chapter. Initially, treat bradycardia or heart block with atropine (0.5–2 mg intravenously), isoproterenol (2–20 µg/min by intravenous infusion, titrated to the desired heart rate), or an external transcutaneous cardiac pacemaker. Specific antidotal treatment may be necessary (see below).

For ingested drugs, empty the stomach by gastric lavage and administer activated charcoal (see p 1321). Do *not* induce emesis because of the risk of seizures.

B. Specific Treatment: If the above measures are not successful in reversing bradycardia and hypotension, give glucagon, 5 mg intravenously, followed by an infusion of 1–5 mg/h. Glucagon is an inotropic agent that acts at a different receptor site and is therefore not affected by beta-blockade.

Tai YT et al: Successful resuscitation and survival following massive overdose of metoprolol. Br J Clin Pract 1990;44:746. (Case report of successful use of glucagon in a patient with shock and asystole after beta-blocker overdose.)

CALCIUM ANTAGONISTS

Calcium antagonists used in the United States include verapamil, diltiazem, nifedipine, nicardipine, and nimodipine. These drugs share the ability to cause arteriolar vasodilation and depression of cardiac contractility, especially after acute overdose. Patients may present with bradycardia, AV nodal block, hypotension, or a combination of these effects. With severe poisoning, cardiac arrest may occur. The diagnosis is made clinically; these drugs are not included in routine toxicology screening.

Treatment

A. Emergency and Supportive Measures:
Maintain a patent airway and assist ventilation, if necessary. Treat coma, hypotension, and seizures as described at the beginning of this chapter. Treat bradycardia with atropine (0.5–2 mg intravenously), isoproterenol (2–20 µg/min by intravenous infusion), or a transcutaneous or internal cardiac pacemaker.

For ingested drugs, perform gastric lavage and administer activated charcoal (see p 1321). Do *not* induce emesis because of the risk of seizures.

B. Specific Treatment: If bradycardia and hypotension are not reversed with these measures, administer calcium chloride 10%, 5–10 mL in-travenously, or calcium gluconate 10%, 10–15 mL intravenously. Calcium is most useful in reversing negative inotropic effects and is less effective for AV nodal blockade and bradycardia. The serum calcium should be raised by 2–3 mg/dL for maximum benefit. Epinephrine infusion (1–4 meq/min initially) and glucagon, 5–10 mg intravenously, have also been recommended.

Pearigen PD, Benowitz NL: Poisoning due to calcium antagonists: Experience with verapamil, diltiazem and nifedipine. Drug Safety 1991;6:408. (Overdose and its treatment, including use of calcium.)

CARBON MONOXIDE

Carbon monoxide is a colorless, odorless gas produced by the combustion of carbon-containing materials. Poisoning may occur as a result of suicidal or accidental exposure to automobile exhaust, smoke inhalation in a fire, or accidental exposure to an improperly vented gas heater or other appliance. Carbon monoxide avidly binds to hemoglobin, with an affinity approximately 250 times that of oxygen. This results in reduced oxygen-carrying capacity and altered delivery of oxygen to cells (see also Smoke Inhalation in Chapter 9).

Clinical Findings

At low carbon monoxide levels (carboxyhemoglobin saturation 10–20%), victims have may headache, dizziness, abdominal pain, and nausea. With higher levels, confusion, dyspnea, and syncope may occur. Hypotension, coma, and seizures are common with levels greater than 50–60%. Survivors of acute severe poisoning may develop permanent neurologic deficits. The fetus and newborn may be more susceptible because of high carbon monoxide affinity for fetal hemoglobin.

Carbon monoxide poisoning should be suspected in any person with severe headache or acutely altered mental status, especially in cold weather, when improper heating systems may have been used. Diagnosis depends on specific measurement of the arterial or venous carboxyhemoglobin saturation. Routine arterial blood gas testing and pulse oximetry are not useful because they give falsely normal calculated oxyhemoglobin saturation determinations.

Treatment

A. Emergency and Supportive Measures:
Maintain a patent airway and assist ventilation, if necessary. Remove the victim from exposure. Treat patients with coma, hypotension, or seizures, as described at the beginning of this chapter.

B. Specific Treatment: The half-life of the carboxyhemoglobin complex is about 4–5 hours in room air but is reduced dramatically by high concentrations of oxygen. Administer 100% oxygen by tight-fitting high-flow reservoir face mask or endotracheal tube. Hyperbaric oxygen can provide 100% oxygen under higher than atmospheric pressures, further shortening the half-life; it may be useful if immediately available for patients with coma or seizures and in pregnant women.

Caravati EM et al: Fetal toxicity associated with maternal carbon monoxide poisoning. Ann Emerg Med 1988; 17:714. (The fetus is especially susceptible because of the greater affinity of fetal hemoglobin for CO.)

Sloan EP et al: Complications and protocol considerations in carbon monoxide-poisoned patients who require hyperbaric oxygen therapy: Report from a ten-year experience. Ann Emerg Med 1989;18:629. (Patients requiring transfer to another facility for treatment with hyperbaric oxygen may suffer serious cardiorespiratory complications during transport.)

CHEMICAL WARFARE AGENTS

Nerve agents used in chemical warfare work by cholinesterase inhibition and are most commonly organophosphates. Agents such as **tabun** (dimethylphosphoramidocyanidic acid ethyl ether) and **sarin** (methylphosphonofluoridic acid 1-methylethyl ester) are similar to insecticides such as malathion but are vastly more potent. They may be inhaled or absorbed through the skin. Systemic effects due to unopposed action of acetylcholine include miosis, salivation, abdominal cramps, diarrhea, and muscle paralysis producing respiratory arrest. Inhalation also produces severe bronchoconstriction and copious nasal and tracheobronchial secretions.

Treatment
A. Emergency and Supportive Measures: Perform thorough decontamination of exposed areas with repeated soap and shampoo washing. Personnel caring for such patients must be wear protective clothing and gloves, since cutaneous absorption may occur through normal skin.

B. Specific Treatment: Give atropine in an initial dose of 2 mg intravenously, and repeat as needed to reverse signs of acetylcholine excess. (Some victims have required several hundred milligrams.) Treat also with pralidoxime, 1–2 g intravenously stat and then 200–400 mg/h. United States military personnel are equipped with autoinjectable units containing this dose plus 600 mg of the cholinesterase-reactivating agent pralidoxime. Repeated doses of atropine are occasionally necessary.

Dunn MA, Siddell FR: Progress in medical defense against nerve agents. JAMA 1989;262:649. (Battlefield prevention and treatment of poisoning by organophosphates.)

CHLORINATED INSECTICIDES (Chlorophenothane [DDT], Lindane, Toxaphene, Chlordane, Aldrin, Endrin)

DDT and other chlorinated insecticides are central nervous system stimulants that can cause poisoning by ingestion, inhalation, or direct contact. The estimated lethal dose is about 20 g for DDT, 3 g for lindane, 2 g for toxaphene, 1 g for chlordane, and less than 1 g for endrin and aldrin. The manifestations of poisoning are nervous irritability, muscle twitching, convulsions, and coma. Arrhythmias may occur. Hepatic and renal damage are reported.

Treatment
Do *not* induce emesis, since seizures may occur abruptly. Perform lavage, and give activated charcoal (see p 1321). Repeat-dose activated charcoal may be effective for large ingestions. For convulsions, give diazepam, 5–10 mg slowly intravenously, or other anticonvulsants.

Perform thorough decontamination of exposed areas with repeated soap and shampoo washing. Personnel caring for such patients must be wear protective clothing and gloves, since cutaneous absorption may occur through normal skin.

Prendergast T et al: Endrin poisoning associated with taquito ingestion—California. MMWR 1989;38:345. (Case report of poisoning by this highly toxic organochlorine insecticide.)

CLONIDINE & OTHER SYMPATHOLYTIC ANTIHYPERTENSIVES (Clonidine, Methyldopa, Prazosin)

Overdosage with these agents causes bradycardia, hypotension, miosis, respiratory depression, and coma. (Hypertension occasionally occurs after clonidine overdosage, a result of peripheral alpha effects of this drug in high doses.) Symptoms are usually resolved in less than 24 hours, and deaths are rare. Similar symptoms may occur after ingestion of topical nasal decongestants related to clonidine (oxymetazoline, tetrahydrozoline).

Treatment
A. Emergency and Supportive Measures: Empty the stomach by emesis or lavage. Give activated charcoal and a cathartic (see p 1321). Maintain the airway and support respiration if necessary. Symptomatic treatment is usually sufficient even in massive overdose. Maintain blood pressure with intravenous fluids. Dopamine can also be used. Atropine is usually effective for bradycardia.

B. Specific Treatment: There is no specific antidote. Although tolazoline has been recommended for clonidine overdose, its effect are unpredictable and it should not be used. Naloxone has been reported to be successful in a few anecdotal and poorly substantiated cases.

Wiley JF et al: Clonidine poisoning in young children. J Ped 1990;116:654.

CYANIDE

Cyanide is a highly toxic chemical used widely in research and commercial laboratories and many industries. Its gaseous form, hydrogen cyanide, is an important component of smoke in fires. Cyanide-generating glycosides are also found in the pits of apricots and other related plants. Cyanide is generated by the breakdown of nitroprusside and can cause poisoning with rapid high-dose infusions. Cyanide is also formed by metabolism of acetonitrile, found in over-the-counter fingernail glue removers. Cyanide is rapidly absorbed by inhalation, skin absorption, or ingestion. It disrupts cellular function by inhibiting cytochrome oxidase and preventing cellular oxygen utilization.

Clinical Findings

The onset of toxicity is nearly instantaneous after inhalation of hydrogen cyanide gas but may be delayed for minutes to hours after ingestion of cyanide salts or cyanogenic plants or chemicals. Symptoms of intoxication include headache, dizziness, nausea, abdominal pain, and anxiety, followed by confusion, syncope, shock, seizures, coma, and death. The odor of "bitter almonds" may be detected on the victim's breath or in vomitus, though this is not a reliable finding. The venous oxygen saturation may be elevated (> 90%) in severe poisonings because tissues have failed to take up arterial oxygen. There are no reliable rapid bedside laboratory tests for cyanide.

Treatment

A. Emergency and Supportive Measures: Maintain a patent airway and assist ventilation, if necessary. Remove the victim from exposure, taking care to avoid exposure to rescuers. Treat coma, hypotension, and seizures as described at the beginning of this chapter. For suspected cyanide poisoning due to nitroprusside infusion, stop or slow the rate of infusion. (Metabolic acidosis and other signs of cyanide poisoning usually clear rapidly.)

For cyanide ingestion, empty the stomach by gastric lavage with charcoal, or immediate oral administration of charcoal, or immediate emesis (if lavage or charcoal is not available) (see p 1321). Although charcoal has a low affinity for cyanide, the usual doses of 60–100 g are adequate to bind typically ingested lethal doses (100–200 mg).

B. Specific Treatment: In the United States, the cyanide antidote kit (Table 39–12) contains nitrites

Table 39–12. Currently available (prepackaged) cyanide antidotes.[1,2]

Antidote	How Supplied	Dose
Amyl nitrite	0.3 mL (aspirol inhalant)	Break 1–2 aspirols under patient's nose.
Sodium nitrite	3 g/dL (300 mg in 10 mL [vials])	6 mg/kg intravenously (0.2 mL/kg)
Sodium thio-sulfate	25 g/dL (12.5 g in 50 mL [vials])	250 mg/kg intravenously (1 mL/kg)

[1]Reproduced, with permission, from Saunders CE, Ho MT (editors): *Current Emergency Diagnosis & Treatment,* 4th ed. Appleton & Lange, 1992.
[2]In USA, manufactured by Eli Lilly & Co.

(to induce methemoglobinemia, which binds free cyanide) and thiosulfate (to promote conversion of cyanide to the less toxic thiocyanate). Administer amyl nitrite by crushing an ampule under the victim's nose or at the end of the endotracheal tube; and administer 3% sodium nitrite solution, 10 mL intravenously (300 mg; for children, 0.3 mg/kg to a maximum of 10 mL) over 3–5 minutes. *Caution:* Nitrites may induce hypotension and dangerous levels of methemoglobin, especially in children. Also administer 25% sodium thiosulfate solution, 50 mL intravenously (12.5 g; for children, 400 mg/kg, or 1.6 mL/kg to maximum 50 mL).

Caravati EM et al: Pediatric cyanide intoxication and death from an acetonitrile-containing cosmetic. JAMA 1988;260:3470. (Two children developed severe cyanide poisoning after ingesting artificial nail glue remover; one child died. Acetonitrile is metabolized to inorganic cyanide over a few hours after ingestion.)
Lambert RJ et al: The efficacy of superactivated charcoal in treating rats exposed to a lethal oral dose of potassium cyanide. Ann Emerg Med 1988;17:595. (Although cyanide binds poorly to activated charcoal, doses of about 100 g charcoal per gram of cyanide decreased lethality in rats.)

DIGITALIS & OTHER CARDIAC GLYCOSIDES

Cardiac glycosides are derived from a variety of plants and are widely used to treat heart failure and supraventricular arrhythmias. These drugs have potent vagotonic effects and also paralyze the Na^+/K^+-ATPase pump. Intracellular effects include enhancement of calcium-dependent contractility and shortening of the action potential duration. Digoxin and ouabain are highly tissue-bound, but digitoxin has a volume of distribution of just 0.6 L/kg, making it the only cardiac glycoside accessible to enhanced removal procedures such as hemoperfusion or repeated doses of activated charcoal.

Clinical Findings

Intoxication may result from acute single exposure or chronic accidental overmedication. After acute overdosage, patients frequently develop nausea and vomiting, bradycardia, hyperkalemia, and atrioventricular block. Patients who develop toxicity gradually during chronic therapy are often hypokalemic and hypomagnesemic owing to concurrent diuretic treatment and more commonly present with ventricular arrhythmias (eg, ectopy, bidirectional ventricular tachycardia, or ventricular fibrillation).

Treatment

A. Emergency and Supportive Measures: Maintain a patent airway and assist ventilation, if necessary. Monitor potassium levels and cardiac rhythm closely. Treat ventricular arrhythmias initially with lidocaine (2–3 mg/kg intravenously) or phenytoin (10–15 mg/kg intravenously slowly over 30 minutes) and treat bradycardia initially with atropine (0.5–2 mg intravenously), isoproterenol (1–5 μg/min initially), or a transcutaneous external cardiac pacemaker. Consider the use of digoxin-specific antibodies (see below).

After acute ingestion, perform gastric lavage and administer activated charcoal (see p 1321). Emesis is not recommended because it may enhance vagotonic effects such as bradycardia and AV block.

B. Specific Treatment: For patients with severe intoxication (eg, marked bradycardia or AV block unresponsive to atropine, or ventricular arrhythmias unresponsive to lidocaine or phenytoin), administer digoxin-specific antibodies (digoxin immune Fab [ovine]; Digibind). Estimation of the Digibind dose is based on the body burden of digoxin calculated from the ingested dose or the steady-state serum digoxin concentration:

1. From the ingested dose–Number of vials = approximately $1.5 \times$ ingested dose (mg).

2. From the serum concentration–Number of vials = approximately serum digoxin (ng/mL) × body weight kg × 10^{-2}.

Note: After administration of Digibind, serum digoxin levels are falsely elevated.

3. Emergency empiric dose–For life-threatening intoxication when ingested amount and serum level are not known: 10–20 vials.

Antman EM et al: Treatment of 150 cases of life-threatening digitalis intoxication with digoxin-specific Fab antibody fragments. Circulation 1990;81:1744. (Multicenter study of 150 pages aged 1 day to 94 years and serum digoxin levels ranging from 8 to 156 ng/mL. Eighty percent of patients improved, with majority better in less than 1 hour.)

Muaskopf JA, Wenger TL: Cost-effectiveness analysis of the use of digoxin immune Fab (ovine) for treatment of digoxin toxicity. Am J Cardiol 1991 68:1709. (When digoxin-specific antibodies are used to treat less seriously toxic patients, total medical costs decrease because of shorter stays in the intensive care unit.)

ETHANOL, BARBITURATES, BENZODIAZEPINES, & OTHER SEDATIVE-HYPNOTIC AGENTS

The group of agents known as sedative-hypnotic drugs include a variety of products used for the treatment of anxiety, depression, insomnia, and epilepsy. Ethanol and other selected agents are also popular recreational drugs. All of these drugs depress the central nervous system reticular activating system, cerebral cortex, and cerebellum. Some agents (eg, glutethimide) also have anticholinergic properties.

Clinical Findings

Mild intoxication produces euphoria, slurred speech, and ataxia. Ethanol intoxication may produce hypoglycemia, even at relatively low concentrations. With more severe intoxication, stupor, coma, and respiratory arrest may occur. Death or serious morbidity is usually the result of pulmonary aspiration of gastric contents. Bradycardia, hypotension, and hypothermia are common. Patients with massive intoxication may appear to be dead, with no reflex responses and even absent electroencephalographic activity. Diagnosis and assessment of severity of intoxication is usually based on clinical findings. Ethanol serum levels greater than 300 mg/dL (0.3 g/dL; 65 mmol/L) usually produce coma in persons who are not chronically abusing the drug, but regular users may remain awake at much higher levels. Phenobarbital levels greater than 80–100 mg/L usually cause coma.

Treatment

A. Emergency and Supportive Measures: Maintain a patent airway, and assist ventilation if necessary. Treat coma, hypotension, and hypothermia as described at the beginning of this chapter.

Empty the stomach by emesis or gastric lavage and administer activated charcoal (see p 1321). Repeat-dose charcoal may enhance elimination of phenobarbital, and hemoperfusion may be necessary for patients with severe phenobarbital intoxication, but these procedures are not effective for most other drugs in this group.

B. Specific Treatment: Flumazenil is a new benzodiazepine receptor-specific antagonist; it has no effect on ethanol, barbiturates, or other sedative-hypnotic agents. Flumazenil is given slowly intravenously, 0.2 mg over 30–60 seconds, repeated as needed up to a total dose of 3–5 mg. *Caution:* Flumazenil may induce seizures in patients with pre-existing seizure disorder, benzodiazepine addiction, or concomitant tricyclic antidepressant overdose. If seizures occur, diazepam and other benzodiazepine anticonvulsants will not be effective. As with naloxone, the duration of action of flumazenil is short (2–3 hours) and resedation may occur, requiring repeated doses.

Hojer J et al: Benzodiazepine poisoning: Experience of 702 admissions to an intensive care unit during a 14-year period. J Int Med 1989;226:117. (Nearly a third of the cases had coingested alcohol, and almost half required endotracheal intubation.)

Hojer J et al: Diagnostic utility of flumazenil in coma with suspected poisoning: A double-blind, randomised controlled study. Br Med J 1990;301:1308. (The benzodiazepine antagonist flumazenil was found to be safe and effective in this study, in many cases obviating the need for endotracheal intubation or diagnostic procedures.)

IRON

Iron is widely used therapeutically for the treatment of anemia and as a daily supplement in multiple vitamin preparations. Most children's preparations contain about 12–15 mg of elemental iron (as sulfate, gluconate, or fumarate salt) per dose, compared with 60–90 mg in most adult-strength preparations. Severe iron intoxications occur most often in children who ingest adult-strength preparations. Iron is corrosive to the gastrointestinal tract and, once absorbed, has depressant effects on the myocardium and on peripheral vascular resistance. Intracellular toxic effects of iron include disruption of Krebs cycle enzymes.

Clinical Findings

Ingestion of less than 30 mg/kg of elemental iron usually produces only mild gastrointestinal upset. Ingestion of more than 40–60 mg/kg usually causes vomiting (sometimes with hematemesis), diarrhea, hypotension, and acidosis. Death may occur as a result of profound hypotension due to massive fluid losses and bleeding, metabolic acidosis, peritonitis from intestinal perforation, or sepsis. Survivors of the acute ingestion may suffer permanent gastrointestinal scarring.

Serum iron levels greater than 350–500 µg/dL are considered toxic, and levels over 1000 µg/dL are usually associated with severe poisoning. A plain abdominal x-ray may reveal radiopaque tablets.

Treatment

A. Emergency and Supportive Measures: Maintain a patent airway and assist ventilation if necessary. Treat hypotension aggressively with intravenous crystalloid solutions (normal saline or lactated Ringer's injection). Fluid losses may be massive owing to vomiting and diarrhea as well as third-spacing into injured intestine.

Empty the stomach by emesis or gastric lavage if more than 30 mg/kg of elemental iron has been ingested (see p 1321). Activated charcoal is not effective but may be used if other ingestants are suspected. If many tablets remain visible on abdominal x-ray, perform whole bowel irrigation—and consider endoscopy or surgical removal.

B. Specific Treatment: Deferoxamine is a selective iron chelator. It may be given intramuscularly or intravenously but is not useful as an oral binding agent. For patients with established manifestations of toxicity—and particularly those with markedly elevated serum iron levels (eg, greater than 500–600 µg/dL)—administer 10–15 mg/kg/h by constant intravenous infusion; higher doses (up to 40–50 mg/kg/h) have been used in massive poisonings. Hypotension may occur. The presence of iron-deferoxamine complex in the urine may give it a "vin rosé" appearance. Continue the infusion until the iron level is less than 350 µg/dL. Deferoxamine is safe for use in pregnant women with acute iron overdose.

Schauben JL et al: Iron poisoning: Report of three cases and a review of therapeutic intervention. J Emerg Med 1990;8:309. (Emphasis on gastrointestinal decontamination techniques.)

Vernon DD et al: Hemodynamic effects of experimental iron poisoning. Ann Emerg Med 1989;18:863. (Experimental study showing profound hemodynamic effects of acute iron poisoning and suggesting importance of aggressive intravenous fluid administration to treat shock.)

ISONIAZID

Isoniazid (INH) is an antibacterial drug used mainly in the treatment and prevention of tuberculosis. It may cause hepatitis in certain patients with chronic use. It produces acute toxic effects by competing with pyridoxal 5-phosphate, resulting in lowered brain γ-aminobutyric acid (GABA) levels. Acute ingestion of as little as 1.5–2 g of isoniazid can cause toxicity, and severe poisoning is likely to occur after ingestion of more than 80–100 mg/kg.

Clinical Findings

Confusion, slurred speech, and seizures may occur abruptly after acute overdose. Severe lactic acidosis—out of proportion to the severity of seizures—is probably due to inhibited metabolism of lactate.

Diagnosis is based on a history of ingestion and the presence of severe acidosis associated with seizures. Isoniazid is not usually included in routine toxicologic screening, and serum levels are not readily available.

Treatment

A. Emergency and Supportive Measures: Maintain a patent airway and assist ventilation if necessary. Treat coma, hypotension, and seizures as described at the beginning of this chapter. Seizures may require higher doses of diazepam (15–20 mg intravenously) or administration of pyridoxine as antidote (see below).

Empty the stomach by gastric lavage and administer activated charcoal (see p 1321). Do *not* induce emesis, because of the risk of abrupt onset of seizures.

B. Specific Treatment: Pyridoxine (vitamin B_6) is a specific antagonist of the acute toxic effects of isoniazid and is usually successful in controlling convulsions that do not respond to diazepam. Give 5 g intravenously over 1–2 minutes or, if the amount is known, give a gram-for-gram equivalent amount of pyridoxine.

Brent J et al: Reversal of isoniazid-induced coma by pyridoxine. Arch Intern Med 1990;150:1751. (Three patients awakened after receiving pyridoxine; in two cases, seizures had been controlled with initial pyridoxine but the patients remained comatose until additional doses were given.)

LEAD

Lead is used in a variety of industrial and commercial products, such as storage batteries, solders, paints, pottery, plumbing, and gasoline. Children are susceptible to lead poisoning by repeatedly ingesting lead-containing paints or dusts. Lead toxicity is rare after a single exposure. Lead produces a variety of adverse effects on cellular function and primarily affects the nervous system, gastrointestinal tract, and hematopoietic system.

Clinical Findings

Lead poisoning often goes undiagnosed initially because presenting symptoms and signs are nonspecific and exposure is not suspected. Common symptoms include colicky abdominal pain, constipation, headache, and irritability. Severe poisoning may cause coma and convulsions. Chronic intoxication can cause learning disorders (in children) and motor neuropathy (eg, wrist drop).

Diagnosis is based on measurement of the blood lead level. Whole blood lead levels less than 25 μg/dL are usually considered nontoxic. Levels of 50–70 μg/dL are associated with moderate toxicity, and levels greater than 70–100 μg/dL are often associated with severe poisoning. Other laboratory findings of lead poisoning include microcytic anemia with basophilic stippling and elevated free erythrocyte protoporphyrin.

Treatment

A. Emergency and Supportive Measures: For patients with encephalopathy, maintain a patent airway and treat coma and convulsions as described at the beginning of this chapter.

For recent acute ingestion, give activated charcoal and a cathartic (see p 1321). If a large lead-containing object (eg, fishing weight) is still visible in the stomach on abdominal x-ray, repeated cathartics, whole bowel irrigation, endoscopy, or even surgical removal may be necessary to prevent subacute lead poisoning.

Conduct an investigation into the source of the lead exposure. Workers with lead levels greater than 60 μg/dL must by federal law be removed from the site of exposure.

B. Specific Treatment: Lead may be chelated parenterally with edetate calcium disodium (EDTA) or dimercaprol (BAL). The indications for chelation depend on the blood lead level and the patient's clinical state. A medical toxicologist or regional poison control center (Table 39–1) should be consulted for advice about selection and use of these antidotes.

1. Severe toxicity–Patients with severe intoxication (encephalopathy or levels greater than 70–100 μg/dL) should receive dimercaprol, 4–5 mg/kg intramuscularly every 4 hours for 5 days; and edetate calcium disodium, 1500 mg/m^2/kg/d (approximately 50 mg/kg/d) in four to six divided doses or as a continuous intravenous infusion.

2. Less severe toxicity–Patients with less severe symptoms and asymptomatic patients with blood lead levels between 55 and 69 μg/dL may be treated with edetate calcium disodium alone in dosages as above. A new chelator, dimercaptosuccinic acid (DMSA; succimer), is now available for oral use in patients with mild to moderate intoxication.

3. Challenge test–Edetate calcium disodium may also be used in patients with lower lead levels as a mobilization or "challenge" test to determine if there is a pool of chelatable lead. Administer 20–25 mg/kg (1 g maximum) in 100 mL of 5% dextrose intravenously over 1 hour, and then collect urine in a lead-free container over the next 24 hours. If the number of micrograms of lead excreted is greater than the number of milligrams of edetate calcium disodium given, the test is considered positive.

Rempel D: The lead-exposed worker. JAMA 1989;262:532. (Federal law provides specific guidelines for monitoring and treating lead-exposed workers; this article makes recommendations for physicians managing such patients.)

Schneitzer L et al: Lead poisoning in adults from renovation of an older home. Ann Emerg Med 1990;19:415. (Three cases from a group exposure during renovation. One case required chelation treatment.)

MERCURY

Acute mercury poisoning usually occurs by ingestion of inorganic mercuric salts or inhalation of metallic mercury vapor. Ingestion of the mercuric salts causes a metallic taste, salivation, thirst, a burning sensation in the throat, discoloration and edema of oral mucous membranes, abdominal pain, vomiting, bloody diarrhea, and shock. Direct nephrotoxicity causes acute renal failure. Inhalation of high concentrations of metallic mercury vapor may cause acute fulminant chemical pneumonia. Chronic mercury poisoning causes weakness, ataxia, intention tremors, irritability, and depression. Chronic intoxication in children may be a cause of acrodynia. Exposure to alkyl (organic) mercury derivatives from contaminated fish or fungicides used on seeds has caused ataxia, tremors, and convulsions and catastrophic birth defects.

Treatment

A. Acute Poisoning: There is no effective specific treatment for mercury vapor pneumonitis. Remove ingested mercuric salts by emesis and lavage, and administer activated charcoal and a cathartic (see p 1321). For acute ingestion of mercuric salts, given dimercaprol (BAL) at once, as for arsenic poisoning. Penicillamine, 100 mg/kg orally in divided doses (maximum, 2 g/d), is also effective. Maintain urine output. Treat oliguria and anuria if they occur.

B. Chronic Poisoning: Remove from exposure. Neurologic toxicity is not considered reversible with chelation, although some authors recommend a trial of penicillamine.

Aronow R et al: Mercury exposure from interior latex paint—Michigan. MMWR 1990;39:125. (Mercury intoxication resulted from exposure to off-gassing vapors of organic mercury used as a preservative in paint.)

METHANOL & ETHYLENE GLYCOL

Methanol (wood alcohol) is commonly found in a variety of products, including solvents, duplicating fluids, record cleaning solutions, and paint removers. It is sometimes ingested intentionally by alcoholics as a substitute for ethanol and may also be found as a contaminant in bootleg whiskey. Ethylene glycol is the most common constituent in antifreeze. The toxicity of both agents is caused by metabolism to highly toxic organic acids—methanol to formic acid; ethylene glycol to glycolic and oxalic acids.

Clinical Findings

Shortly after ingestion of either of these agents, patients usually appear "drunk." The serum osmolality (measured with the freezing point device) is usually elevated, but acidosis is often absent early. After several hours, metabolism to toxic organic acids leads to a severe anion gap metabolic acidosis, tachypnea, confusion, convulsions, and coma. Methanol intoxication frequently causes visual disturbances, while ethylene glycol often produces oxalate crystalluria and renal failure. The urine may fluoresce under a Wood (UV) lamp if fluorescein was added to the commercial ethylene glycol product (eg, antifreeze).

Treatment

A. Emergency and Supportive Measures: Maintain a patent airway, and assist ventilation if necessary. Treat coma, hypotension, and seizures as described at the beginning of this chapter. Treat metabolic acidosis with sodium bicarbonate by intravenous infusion because it enhance excretion of toxic acids.

For patients presenting within 30–60 minutes after ingestion, empty the stomach by emesis or gastric lavage and administer activated charcoal (see p 1321). (*Note:* Charcoal is not very effective.)

Patients with significant toxicity (manifested by severe acidosis, altered mental status, serum methanol or ethylene glycol level > 50 mg/dL) should undergo hemodialysis as soon as possible to remove the parent compound and the toxic metabolites.

B. Specific Treatment: Ethanol blocks metabolism of the parent compounds by competing for the enzyme alcohol dehydrogenase. The desired serum ethanol concentration is 100 mg/dL. To achieve this, administer a loading dose of approximately 750 mg/kg orally or in a dilute intravenous solution (available from the pharmacy in 5% and 10% solution), and then provide a maintenance infusion of 100–150 mg/kg/h. The infusion will have to be increased to about 175–250 mg/kg/h during hemodialysis to replace dialysis elimination of ethanol.

Burkhart KK, Kulig KW: The other alcohols: Methanol, ethylene glycol, and isopropanol. Emerg Med Clin North Am 1990;8:913. (Pathophysiology and clinical presentation of poisoning by ethanol substitutes.)

Eisen TF et al: Serum osmolality in alcohol ingestions: Differences in availability among laboratories of teaching hospital, nonteaching hospital, and commercial facilities. Am J Emerg Med 1989;7:256. (If the vapor point osmometer is used instead of the freezing point device, volatile alcohols may evaporate, giving a falsely normal serum osmolality.)

METHEMOGLOBINEMIA-INDUCING AGENTS

A large number of chemical agents are capable of oxidizing ferrous hemoglobin to its ferric state (methemoglobin), a form that cannot carry oxygen. Drugs and chemicals known to cause methemoglobinemia include benzocaine (a local anesthetic), aniline, nitrites, nitrogen oxide gases, nitrobenzene, dapsone, pyridium, and many others. Dapsone has a long elimination half-life and may produce prolonged or recurrent methemoglobinemia after initial treatment.

Clinical Findings

Methemoglobinemia reduces oxygen-carrying capacity and may cause dizziness, nausea, headache, dyspnea, confusion, seizures, and coma. The severity of symptoms depends on the percentage of hemoglobin oxidized to methemoglobin; severe poisoning is usually present with methemoglobin fractions of greater than 40–50%. Even at low levels (15–20%), victims appear cyanotic because of the "chocolate brown" color of methemoglobin, but they have normal PO_2 results on arterial blood gas determinations. Pulse oximetry gives inaccurate oxygen saturation measurements. Hemolysis may occur, especially in patients susceptible to oxidant stress (ie, those with glucose-6-phosphate dehydrogenase deficiency).

Treatment

A. Emergency and Supportive Measures: Maintain a patent airway, and assist ventilation if necessary. Administer high-flow supplemental oxygen. Treat coma, hypotension, and seizures as described at the beginning of this chapter.

If the causative agent was recently ingested, empty the stomach by emesis or gastric lavage and administer activated charcoal (see p 1321). For dapsone ingestion, give repeat-dose activated charcoal to enhance dapsone elimination (see p 1322).

B. Specific Treatment: Methylene blue is a commonly used dye that enhances the conversion of methemoglobin to hemoglobin by increasing the activity of the enzyme methemoglobin reductase. For symptomatic patients, administer 1–2 mg/kg (0.1–0.2 mL/kg of 1% solution) intravenously. The dose may be repeated once in 15–20 minutes if necessary. Patients with hereditary methemoglobin reductase deficiency or glucose-6-phosphate dehydrogenase deficiency may not respond to methylene blue treatment.

Dawson AH, Whyte IM: Management of dapsone poisoning complicated by methaemoglobinemia. Med Toxicol Adv Drug Exper (now called Drug Safety) 1989;4:387. (Dapsone has a long half-life, and repeated doses of methylene blue may be required because of continuing oxidative stress.)

MONOAMINE OXIDASE INHIBITORS (Isocarboxazid, Phenelzine)

Overdoses cause ataxia, excitement, hypertension, and tachycardia, followed several hours later by hypotension, convulsions, and hyperthermia.

Ingestion of tyramine-containing foods may cause a severe hypertensive reaction. These foods include aged cheese and red wines. Hypertensive reactions may also occur with any sympathomimetic drug. Fatal hyperthermia may occur if patients receiving monoamine oxidase inhibitors are given meperidine, fluoxetine, or other serotonin-enhancing drugs.

Treatment

Remove ingested drug by gastric lavage, and administer activated charcoal and a cathartic (see p 1321). Treat severe hypertension with nitroprusside, phentolamine, or other rapid-acting vasodilator (see p 1319). Treat hypotension with fluids and positioning, but avoid use of pressor agents. Observe patients for at least 24 hours, since hyperthermic reactions may be delayed. Treat hyperthermia with aggressive cooling; neuromuscular paralysis may be required (see p 1320).

Lippman SB, Nash K: Monoamine oxidase inhibitor update: Potential adverse food and drug interactions. Med Toxicol 1990;5:195. (A variety of foods and medications may cause life-threatening reactions in patients taking these drugs.)

MUSHROOMS

There are thousands of mushroom species that cause a variety of toxic effects. The most dangerous species of mushrooms are *Amanita phalloides, Amanita verna, Amanita virosa, Gyromitra esculenta,* and the *Galerina* species, all of which contain amatoxin, a potent cytotoxin. Ingestion of part of one mushroom of a dangerous species may be sufficient to cause death.

The pathologic finding in fatalities from amatoxin-containing mushroom poisoning is acute necrosis of the liver, kidneys, heart, and skeletal muscles.

Clinical Findings
(Table 39–13)

A. Symptoms and Signs:

1. Amatoxin-type cyclopeptides (*Amanita phalloides, Amanita verna, Amanita virosa,* and *Galerina* species)–After a latent interval of 8–12 hours, severe abdominal cramps and vomiting begin and progress to profuse diarrhea, bloody vomitus and stools, followed by hepatic necrosis, hepatic encephalopathy, and frequently renal failure. The fatality rate is about 20%. Cooking the mushrooms does not prevent poisoning.

2. Gyromitrin type (*Gyromitra* and *Helvella* species)–Toxicity is more common following ingestion of uncooked mushrooms. Vomiting, diarrhea, hepatic necrosis, convulsions, coma, and hemolysis may occur after a latent period of 8–12 hours. The fatality rate is probably less than 10%.

3. Muscarinic type (*Inocybe* and *Clitocybe* species)–Vomiting, diarrhea, bradycardia, hypotension, salivation, miosis, bronchospasm, and lacrimation occur shortly after ingestion. Cardiac arrhythmias may occur. Fatalities are rare.

Table 39–13. Poisonous mushrooms.[1]

Toxin	Genus	Symptoms and Signs	Onset	Treatment
Amanitin	*Amanita (A phalloides, A verna, A virosa)*	Severe gastroenteritis, followed by delayed hepatic and renal failure after 48–72 hours.	6–24 hours.	Supportive. Correct dehydration. Thioctic acid is of unproved benefit.
Muscarine	*Inocybe, Clitocybe*	Muscarinic (salivation, miosis, bradycardia, diarrhea).	30 minutes to 1 hour.	Supportive. Give atropine, 0.5–2 mg intravenously, for severe cholinergic symptoms and signs.
Ibotenic acid, muscimol	*Amanita muscaria* ("fly agaric")	Anticholinergic (mydriasis, tachycardia, hyperpyrexia, delirium).	30 minutes to 2 hours.	Supportive. Give physostigmine, 0.5–2 mg intravenously, for severe anticholinergic symptoms and signs.
Coprine	*Coprinus*	Disulfiram-like effect occurs with ingestion of ethanol.	30 minutes to 2 days.	Supportive. Abstain from ethanol for 3–4 days.
Monomethylhydrazine	*Gyromitra*	Gastroenteritis; occasionally hemolysis, hepatic and renal failure.	6–12 hours.	Supportive. Correct dehydration. Pyridoxine, 2.5 mg/kg intravenously, may be helpful.
Orellanine	*Cortinarius*	Nausea, vomiting; renal failure after 1–3 weeks.	2–14 days.	Supportive.
Psilocybin	*Psilocybe*	Hallucinations.	15–30 minutes.	Supportive.
Gastrointestinal irritants	Many species	Nausea and vomiting, diarrhea.	30 minutes to 2 hours.	Supportive. Correct dehydration.

[1]Modified and reproduced, with permission, from Becker CE et al: West J Med 1976;125:100.

4. Anticholinergic type (eg, *Amanita muscaria, Amanita pantherina*)–This type causes a variety of symptoms that may be atropine-like, including excitement, delirium, flushed skin, dilated pupils, and muscular jerking tremors, beginning 1–2 hours after ingestion. Fatalities are rare.

5. Gastrointestinal irritant type (eg, *Boletus, Cantharellus*)–Nausea, vomiting, and diarrhea occur shortly after ingestion. Fatalities are rare.

6. Disulfiram type (*Coprinus* species)–Disulfiram-like sensitivity to alcohol may persist for several days. Toxicity is characterized by flushing, hypotension, and vomiting after coingestion of alcohol.

7. Hallucinogenic type (*Psilocybe* and *Panaeolus* species)–Mydriasis, nausea and vomiting, and intense visual hallucinations occur 1–2 hours after ingestion. Fatalities are rare.

8. *Cortinarius orellanus*–This mushroom may cause acute renal failure due to tubulointerstitial nephritis.

B. Laboratory Findings: (Type 1 [amatoxin] or 2 [gyromitrin] mushrooms.) Creatinine and blood urea nitrogen may be elevated. Effects on the liver are revealed by increased aminotransferase and bilirubin levels and prothrombin time. The blood glucose should be monitored frequently when hepatotoxicity is present.

Treatment

A. Emergency Measures: After the onset of symptoms, efforts to remove the toxic agent are probably useless, especially in cases of amatoxin or gyromitrin poisoning, where there is a delay of 12 hours or more before symptoms occur. However, induction of vomiting is recommended for any recent ingestion of an unidentified or potentially toxic mushroom. Activated charcoal and a cathartic should also be given (see p 1321).

B. General Measures:

1. Amatoxin-type cyclopeptides–A variety of unproved antidotes (eg, thioctic acid, silibinin, penicillin, corticosteroids) have been suggested for amatoxin-type mushroom poisoning, but experimental results are equivocal. Aggressive fluid replacement for diarrhea and intensive supportive care for hepatic failure are the mainstays of treatment.

Interruption of enterohepatic circulation of the amatoxin by the administration of activated charcoal and laxatives may be of value. However, by the time this method is employed, most of the amatoxin has already caused cellular damage and has already been excreted.

Liver function has been known to begin to return 6–8 days after exposure, followed by eventual complete recovery. Liver transplant may be the only hope for survival in gravely ill patients (encephalopathy, severe coagulopathy).

2. Gyromitrin type–For gyromitrin poisoning, give pyridoxine, 25 mg/kg intravenously.

3. Muscarinic type–For mushrooms producing predominantly muscarinic-cholinergic symptoms, give atropine, 0.005–0.01 mg/kg intravenously, and repeat as needed.

4. Anticholinergic type–For anticholinergic type, physostigmine, 0.5–1 mg intravenously, may calm extremely agitated patients and reverse peripheral anticholinergic manifestations, but it may also cause bradycardia, asystole, and seizures.

5. Gastrointestinal irritant type–Treat with antiemetics and intravenous or oral fluids.

6. Disulfiram type–For *Coprinus* ingestion, avoid alcohol. Treat alcohol reaction with fluids and supine position.

7. Hallucinogenic type–Provide a quiet, supportive atmosphere. Diazepam or haloperidol may be used for sedation.

8. *Cortinarius*–Provide supportive care and hemodialysis as needed for renal failure.

Klein AS et al: *Amanita* poisoning: Treatment and role of liver transplantation. Amer J Med 1989;86:187. (Two patients who received liver transplantation; the authors summarize the literature and provide a management protocol.)

OPIOIDS
(Morphine, Heroin, Codeine, Propoxyphene, etc)

Prescription and illicit opioids are popular drugs of abuse and the cause of frequent hospitalizations for overdose. These drugs have widely varying potencies and durations of action; for example, some of the illicit fentanyl derivatives are up to 2000 times more potent than morphine. All of these agents decrease central nervous system activity by acting on opiate receptors in the brain.

Clinical Findings

Mild intoxication is characterized by euphoria, drowsiness, and constricted pupils. More severe intoxication may cause hypotension, bradycardia, hypothermia, coma, and respiratory arrest. Pulmonary edema may occur. Death is usually due to apnea or pulmonary aspiration of gastric contents. While the duration of effect for heroin is usually 3–5 hours, methadone intoxication may last for 48–72 hours or longer. Most opioids, with the exception of illicit newer fentanyl derivatives, are detectable on urine toxicology screening.

Treatment

A. Emergency and Supportive Measures: Maintain a patent airway, and assist ventilation if necessary. Treat coma, hypothermia, and hypotension as described at the beginning of this chapter.

If the patient arrives for medical care shortly after ingestion, empty the stomach by emesis or gastric lavage and administer activated charcoal (see p 1321).

B. Specific Treatment: Naloxone is a specific opioid antagonist that can rapidly reverse signs of narcotic intoxication. Although it is structurally related to the opioids, it has no agonist effects of its own. Administer 0.4–2 mg intravenously, and repeat

as needed to awaken the patient and maintain airway protective reflexes and spontaneous breathing. Very large doses (10–20 mg) may be required for patients intoxicated by some opioids (eg, propoxyphene, codeine, fentanyl derivatives). ***Caution:*** The duration of effect of naloxone is only about 2–3 hours; repeated doses may be necessary for patients intoxicated by long-acting drugs such as methadone. Continuous observation for at least 3 hours after the last naloxone dose is mandatory.

Ford M et al: Opioids and designer drugs. Emerg Med Clin North Am 1990;8:495. (Emphasizes supportive care and use of naloxone.)

Hoffman JR et al: The empiric use of naloxone in patients with altered mental status: A reappraisal. Ann Emerg Med 1991;20:246. (Clinical criteria of opioid intoxication—decreased respirations, miotic pupils, and circumstantial evidence of opioid use—were effective predictors of response to naloxone in patients with altered mental status. The authors suggest limiting prehospital naloxone to patients with these criteria.)

PARAQUAT

Paraquat is used as a herbicide. Concentrated solutions of paraquat are highly corrosive to the oropharynx, esophagus, and stomach. The fatal dose after absorption may be as small as 4 mg/kg. If not rapidly fatal because of its corrosive effects, paraquat causes pulmonary edema and fibrosis with respiratory insufficiency, and renal damage with anuria. Patients with plasma paraquat levels above 2 mg/L at 6 hours or 0.2 mg/L at 24 hours are likely to die.

Treatment

Remove ingested paraquat by immediate emesis, or by gastric lavage if the patient is already in a health care facility. Clay (bentonite or fuller's earth) and activated charcoal are effective adsorbents. Administer repeated doses of 60 g of activated charcoal by gastric tube every 2 hours for at least three or four doses. Charcoal hemoperfusion, 8 hours per day for 2–3 weeks, has been anecdotally reported to be lifesaving. Supplemental oxygen should be withheld unless the PO_2 is less than 70 mm Hg. For further information and for rapid determination of paraquat levels, call the nearest regional poison center or ICI America Inc ([800] 327–8633).

Hampson EC et al: Failure of haemoperfusion and haemodialysis to prevent death in pxxttxaraquat poisoning: A retrospective review of 42 patients. Med Toxicol 1988;3:64. (Despite previous studies and case reports suggesting efficacy of hemoperfusion for paraquat, the authors found no reduction in mortality.)

PESTICIDES: CHOLINESTERASE INHIBITORS
(Organophosphates: Parathion, TEPP, Malathion, Thimet, Phosdrin, Systox, HETP, EPN, OMPA, Etc; Carbamates: Carbaryl, Aldicarb, Benomyl)

Organophosphate and carbamate insecticides are widely used in commercial agriculture and home gardening and have largely replaced older, more environmentally persistent organochlorine compounds such as DDT and chlordane. The organophosphates and carbamates—also called anticholinesterases because they inhibit the enzyme acetylcholinesterase—cause an increase in acetylcholine activity at nicotinic and muscarinic receptors and in the central nervous system. There are a variety of chemical agents in this group, with widely varying potencies. Most of them are poorly water-soluble and are formulated with an aromatic hydrocarbon solvent such as xylene. Most of them are well absorbed through intact skin.

Clinical Findings

Inhibition of cholinesterase results in abdominal cramps, diarrhea, vomiting, excessive salivation, sweating, lacrimation, miosis (constricted pupils), wheezing and bronchorrhea, seizures, and skeletal muscle weakness. Initial tachycardia is usually followed by bradycardia. Profound skeletal muscle weakness, aggravated by excessive bronchial secretions and wheezing, may result in respiratory arrest and death. Signs and symptoms of poisoning may persist or recur over several days, especially with highly lipid-soluble agents such as fenthion.

The diagnosis is suspected in patients who present with miosis, sweating, and hyperperistalsis. Serum and red blood cell cholinesterase activity can be measured in the laboratory and is usually depressed at least 50% below baseline in those victims who have severe intoxication.

Treatment
A. Emergency and Supportive Measures: Maintain a patent airway, and assist ventilation if necessary. Administer supplemental oxygen. Suction excessive secretions from the airway.

If the agent was recently ingested, empty the stomach by emesis or gastric lavage and administer activated charcoal (see p 1321). Gastric lavage is preferred over emesis because of the risk of abrupt onset of seizures. If the agent is on the victim's skin or hair, wash repeatedly with soap or shampoo and water. Providers must take care to avoid skin exposure by wearing gloves and waterproof aprons.

B. Specific Treatment: Atropine reverses excessive muscarinic stimulation and is effective for treatment of salivation, wheezing, abdominal cramping, and sweating. However, it does not interact with nicotinic receptors and has no effect on muscle weakness. Administer 2 mg intravenously, and give repeated doses as needed to dry bronchial secretions and decrease wheezing; as much as several hundred milligrams of atropine have been given to treat severe poisoning.

Pralidoxime (2-PAM, Protopam) is a specific antidote that reverses organophosphate binding to the cholinesterase enzyme; therefore, it is effective at all sites. It should be started as soon as possible, to prevent permanent binding of the organophosphate to cholinesterase. Administer 1–2 g intravenously (20–40 mg/kg in children), and repeat every 3–4 hours as needed. A continuous infusion (200–400 mg/h) may be more effective because of the short duration of action of single doses. Continue to give pralidoxime as long as there is any evidence of acetylcholine excess. Pralidoxime is of questionable benefit for carbamate poisoning, because carbamates have only a transitory effect on the cholinesterase enzyme.

Clifford NJ et al: Organophosphate poisoning from wearing a laundered uniform previously contaminated with parathion. JAMA 1989;262:3035. (A pair of coveralls contaminated with parathion caused recurrent poisoning by skin absorption even after repeated laundering.)
Lotti M: Treatment of acute organophosphate poisoning. Med J Aust 1991;154:51. (General review of mechanism, diagnosis, and treatment.)

PETROLEUM DISTILLATES
(Petroleum Ether, Charcoal Lighter Fluid, Kerosene, Paint Thinner, Benzine, Gasoline, Etc)

Petroleum distillate toxicity occurs almost entirely as a result of pulmonary aspiration during or after ingestion. Acute manifestations of aspiration pneumonitis are vomiting, coughing, and bronchopneumonia. Some hydrocarbons—ie, those with aromatic or halogenated subunits—can also cause severe systemic poisoning after oral ingestion (Table 39–14). Most hydrocarbons can also cause systemic intoxication by inhalation, but only with very high concentrations of the vapors in an enclosed space. Vertigo, muscular incoordination, irregular pulse, myoclonus, and convulsions occur with serious poisoning and may be due to hypoxemia or the systemic effects of some agents (eg, camphor). Chlorinated and fluorinated hydrocarbons (trichloroethylene, freons, etc) can cause ventricular arrhythmias by a mechanism of myocardial sensitization after inhalation.

Treatment
(See Table 39–14.)
Remove the patient to fresh air. Since aspiration is the primary danger with many common products, use of lavage or emesis is controversial. Removal of in-

Table 39–14. Clinical features of hydrocarbon poisoning.[1]

Type	Examples	Risk of Pneumonia	Risk of Systemic Toxicity	Treatment
High-viscosity	Vaseline Motor oil	Low	Low	None.
Low-viscosity, nontoxic	Furniture polish Mineral seal oil Kerosene Lighter fluid	High	Low	Observe for pneumonia. *Do not* induce emesis.
Low-viscosity, unknown systemic toxicity	Turpentine Pine oil	High	Variable	Observe for pneumonia. *Do not* induce emesis if less than 1–2 mL/kg was ingested.
Low-viscosity, known systemic toxicity	Camphor Phenol Chlorinated insecticides Aromatic hydrocarbons (benzene, toluene, etc)	High	High	Perform lavage. Give activated charcoal.

[1]Reproduced, with permission, from Saunders CE, Ho MT (editors): *Current Emergency Diagnosis & Treatment,* 4th ed. Appleton & Lange, 1992.

gested hydrocarbon is usually suggested only if the preparation contains toxic solutes (eg, an insecticide) or is an aromatic or halogenated product. If lavage is done in an obtunded or comatose patient, prophylactic insertion of a cuffed endotracheal tube is recommended to prevent aspiration. Watch the victim closely for 6–8 hours for signs of aspiration pneumonitis (cough, localized rales or rhonchi, tachypnea, and infiltrates on chest radiograph). The use of corticosteroids to treat pneumonitis is controversial. If fever occurs, give a specific antibiotic after identification of pathogens by laboratory studies. Because of the risk of arrhythmias, use bronchodilators only with caution in patients with chlorinated or fluorinated solvent intoxication.

Machado B et al: Accidental hydrocarbon ingestion cases telephoned to a regional poison center. Ann Emerg Med 1988;17:804. (Review of 184 telephone calls to a poison control center after hydrocarbon ingestion. The authors conclude that patients who are asymptomatic or whose symptoms clear quickly can be safely managed at home without hospitalization.)

PHENCYCLIDINE

Phencyclidine (PCP) was until recently one of the most commonly abused street drugs—second only to alcohol as a cause of emergency room visits for drug intoxication in many cities. It occurs under a variety of names or is misrepresented as other psychotomimetic agents. The drug has a wide range of toxic manifestations. Doses under 5 mg (adults) cause hyperactivity, horizontal and vertical nystagmus, incoordination, diaphoresis, flushing, rigidity, dissociative anesthesia, rhabdomyolysis with myoglobinuria, and wild movements. Doses over 10 mg cause, in ad-

dition, seizures, coma, hyperthermia, rhabdomyolysis, and myoglobinuria. Symptoms may persist for several days.

Treatment

A. General Measures: Maintain a quiet, calm atmosphere. Sedate the agitated patient with diazepam, 5–10 mg intravenously, midazolam, 0.1 mg/kg intramuscularly, or haloperidol, 0.05–0.1 mg/kg intramuscularly. Endotracheal intubation and mechanical ventilation may be necessary. Restrict sensory input, prevent injuries, and monitor vital signs.

Control convulsions by giving diazepam, 5–10 mg intravenously. Hyperthermia should be treated aggressively, with control of muscular rigidity or hyperactivity by paralysis with neuromuscular blockers and endotracheal intubation (see p 1320).

If the patient is awake and cooperative, give activated charcoal orally. In obtunded patients, perform gastric lavage prior to charcoal administration (see p 1321). Repeated administration of activated charcoal may remove additional PCP secreted into the acidic stomach. However, repeated use of charcoal and cathartics may lead to dehydration and hypernatremia from massive fluid loss in stools. Lowering urine pH may slightly increase urinary elimination of phencyclidine by ion trapping but is hazardous and may promote myoglobinuric renal failure.

Leiken JB et al: Clinical features and management of intoxication due to hallucinogenic drugs. Med Toxicol Adv Drug Exper (now called Drug Safety) 1989;4:324. (Review article including discussion of LSD, PCP, psilocybin, mescaline, and designer drugs.)

PHENOTHIAZINE & RELATED TRANQUILIZERS
(Chlorpromazine, Promazine, Haloperidol, Prochlorperazine, Etc)

Chlorpromazine and related drugs are synthetic chemicals derived in most instances from phenothiazine. They are used as antiemetics and psychic inhibitors and as potentiators of analgesic and hypnotic drugs.

Minimum doses induce drowsiness and mild orthostatic hypotension in as many as 50% of patients. Larger doses cause obtundation, miosis, severe hypotension, tachycardia, convulsions, and coma with massive doses. Abnormal cardiac conduction may occur, resulting in prolongation of QRS or QT intervals (or both) and ventricular arrhythmias.

With therapeutic doses, some patients develop an acute extrapyramidal reaction similar to Parkinson's disease, with spasmodic contractions of the face and neck muscles, extensor rigidity of the back muscles, carpopedal spasm, and motor restlessness. Severe rigidity accompanied by hyperthermia and metabolic acidosis ("neuroleptic malignant syndrome") may occasionally occur and is life-threatening.

Treatment
A. Emergency and Supportive Measures: Remove ingested overdoses by emesis or gastric lavage (see p 1321). Follow with activated charcoal and cathartic. For severe hypotension, treatment with fluids and pressor agents may be necessary. Control convulsions cautiously with diazepam, 5–10 mg intravenously. Treat hyperthermia as outlined on p 1320. Maintain cardiac monitoring.

B. Specific Treatment: Hypotension and cardiac arrhythmias associated with widened QRS intervals on the ECG may respond to intravenous sodium bicarbonate as used for tricyclic antidepressants.

For extrapyramidal signs, give diphenhydramine, 0.5–1 mg/kg intravenously, or benztropine mesylate, 1–2 mg intramuscularly. Treatment with oral doses of these agents should be continued for 24–48 hours.

Bromocriptine (2.5–7.5 mg orally daily) may be effective for neuroleptic malignant syndrome.

Li C, Gefter WB: Acute pulmonary edema induced by overdosage of phenothiazines. Chest 1992;101:102. (Other manifestations included coma, miosis, and hypotension. The etiology of pulmonary edema is not clear but perhaps neurogenic.)

QUINIDINE & RELATED ANTIARRHYTHMICS

Quinidine, procainamide, and disopyramide are class Ia antiarrhythmic agents, and flecainide and encainide are class Ic agents. These drugs have membrane-depressant effects on the sodium-dependent channel responsible for cardiac cell depolarization. Manifestations of toxicity include diarrhea, arrhythmias, syncope, respiratory failure, and hypotension. The ECG may show widening of the QRS complex, a lengthened QT and PR interval, and atypical or polymorphous ventricular tachycardia (torsades de pointes). Associated toxicity due to digitalis may result from increased blood levels owing to concomitant quinidine administration.

Treatment
A. Emergency and Supportive Measures: Remove ingested drug by gastric lavage followed by activated charcoal and catharsis (see p 1321).

B. Specific Treatment: Treat cardiotoxicity (atrioventricular block, hypotension, QRS interval widening) with intravenous boluses of sodium bicarbonate, 50–100 meq. Ventricular tachycardia of the torsade de pointes variety may be treated with intravenous magnesium (1–2 g), isoproterenol (1–5 µg/min), or overdrive pacing.

Kim SY, Benowitz NL: Poisoning due to class IA antiarrhythmic drugs. Quinidine, procainamide, and disopyramide. Drug Saf 1990;5:393. (Pharmacology, pathophysiology of overdose, and treatment options, including use of bicarbonate and dialysis procedures.)

SALICYLATES

Salicylates (aspirin, methyl salicylate, etc) are found in a variety of over-the-counter and prescription medications. Salicylates uncouple cellular oxidative phosphorylation, resulting in anaerobic metabolism and excessive production of lactic acid and heat, and they also interfere with several Krebs cycle enzymes. A single ingestion of more than 200 mg/kg of salicylate is likely to produce significant acute intoxication. Poisoning may also occur as a result of chronic excessive dosing over several days. Although the half-life of salicylate is 2–3 hours after small doses, it may increase to 20 hours with intoxication.

Clinical Findings
Acute ingestion often causes nausea and vomiting, occasionally with gastritis. Mild to moderate intoxication is characterized by hyperpnea (deep and rapid breathing), tachycardia, tinnitus, and elevated anion gap metabolic acidosis. Serious intoxication may result in agitation, confusion, coma, seizures, cardiovascular collapse, pulmonary edema, hyperthermia, and death. The prothrombin time is often elevated owing to salicylate-induced hypoprothrombinemia.

Diagnosis is suspected in any patient with metabolic acidosis and is confirmed by measuring the serum salicylate level. Patients with levels greater than 100 mg/dL (1000 mg/L) after an acute overdose (see Figure 39–2) are more likely to have severe poisoning. On the other hand, patients with chronic intoxication may suffer severe symptoms with levels of only 60–70 mg/dL. The arterial blood gas typically reveals a respiratory alkalosis with an underlying metabolic acidosis.

Treatment

A. Emergency and Supportive Measures: Maintain a patent airway, and assist ventilation if necessary. Treat coma, hyperthermia, hypotension, and seizures as described at the beginning of this chapter. Treat metabolic acidosis with intravenous sodium bicarbonate.

After acute suicidal or accidental ingestion of more than 150–200 mg/kg salicylate, empty the stomach by emesis or gastric lavage and administer activated charcoal (see p 1321). Extra doses of activated charcoal may be needed in patients who ingest more than 10 g of aspirin.

B. Specific Treatment: Alkalinization of the urine enhances renal salicylate excretion by trapping the salicylate anion. Add 100 meq (two ampules) of sodium bicarbonate to 1 L of 5% dextrose in 0.25-N saline, and infuse this solution intravenously at a rate of about 150–200 mL/h. Unless the patient is oliguric, add 20–30 meq of potassium to each liter of intravenous fluid.

Hemodialysis may be lifesaving and is indicated

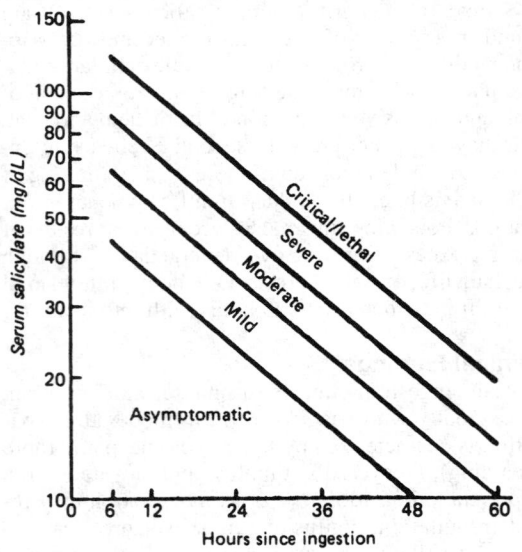

Figure 39–2. Nomogram for determining severity of salicylate intoxication. Absorption kinetics assume acute (one-time) ingestion of non-enteric-coated preparation. (Redrawn and reproduced, with permission, from Done AK: Salicylate intoxication: Significance of measurement of salicylate in blood in cases of acute ingestion. Pediatrics 1960;26:800.)

for patients with severe metabolic acidosis, markedly altered mental status, or significantly elevated salicylate levels (eg, > 100–120 mg/dL [1000–1200 mg/L] after acute overdose or > 60–70 mg/dL [600–700 mg/L] with chronic intoxication).

Dugandzic RM et al: Evaluation of the validity of the Done nomogram in the management of acute salicylate intoxication. Ann Emerg Med 1989;18:1186. (Retrospective study of 55 cases of acute salicylate overdose showed that the nomogram tends to overpredict severity of intoxication in the moderate to severe categories.)

SEAFOOD POISONINGS

A variety of intoxications may occur after eating certain types of fish or other seafood. These include scombroid, ciguatera, paralytic shellfish, and puffer fish poisoning. The mechanisms of toxicity and clinical presentations are described in Table 39–15. In the majority of cases, the seafood has a normal appearance and taste (scombroid may have a peppery taste).

Treatment

A. Emergency and Supportive Measures: *Caution*: Abrupt respiratory arrest may occur with paralytic shellfish and puffer fish poisoning. Observe symptomatic patients for at least 4–6 hours. Maintain a patent airway, administer supplemental oxygen, and assist ventilation if necessary. Replace fluid and electrolyte losses from gastroenteritis with intravenous saline or other crystalloid solution.

For recent ingestions, it may be possible to adsorb residual toxin in the gut with activated charcoal, 50–60 g orally.

B. Specific Treatment: There is no specific antidote for paralytic shellfish of puffer fish poisoning.

1. Ciguatera–There are anecdotal reports of successful treatment of severe neurologic symptoms with mannitol, 1 g/kg intravenously.

2. Scombroid–Antihistamines such as diphenhydramine, 25–50 mg intravenously, and the H_2 blocker cimetidine, 300 mg intravenously, are usually effective. For severe reactions, give also epinephrine, 0.3–0.5 mL of a 1:1000 solution subcutaneously.

Gellert GA et al: Scombroid fish poisoning: Underreporting and prevention among noncommercial recreational fishers. West J Med 1992;157:645.
Lange WR: Puffer fish poisoning. Am Fam Physician 1990;42:1029.
Swift AE, Swift TR: Ciguatera. J Toxicol Clin Toxicol 1993;31:1.

SNAKE BITES

The venom of poisonous snakes and lizards may be predominantly neurotoxic (coral snake) or predomi-

Table 39–15. Common seafood poisonings.

Type of Poisoning	Mechanism	Clinical Presentation
Ciguatera	Reef fish ingest toxic dinoflagellates, whose toxins accumulate in fish meat. Commonly implicated fish in the USA are barracuda, jack, snapper, and grouper.	1–6 hours after ingestion, victims develop abdominal pain, vomiting, and diarrhea accompanied by a variety of neurologic symptoms, including paresthesias, reversal of hot and cold sensation, vertigo, headache, and intense itching. Autonomic disturbances, including hypotension and bradycardia, may occur.
Scombroid	Improper preservation of large fish results in bacterial degradation of histidine to histamine. Commonly implicated fish include tuna, mahi mahi, bonita, mackerel, and kingfish.	Allergic-like (anaphylactoid) symptoms are due to histamine, usually begin within 15–90 minutes, and include skin flushing, itching, urticaria, angioedema, bronchospasm, and hypotension as well as abdominal pain, vomiting, and diarrhea.
Paralytic shellfish poisoning	Dinoflagellates produce saxitoxin, which is concentrated by filter-feeding mussels and clams. Saxitoxin blocks sodium conductance and neuronal transmission in skeletal muscles.	Onset is usually within 30–60 minutes. Initial symptoms include perioral and intraoral paresthesias. Other symptoms include nausea and vomiting, headache, dizziness, dysphagia, dysarthria, ataxia, and rapidly progressive muscle weakness that may result in respiratory arrest.
Puffer fish poisoning	Tetrodotoxin is concentrated in liver, gonads, intestine, and skin. Toxic effects are similar to those of saxitoxin. Tetrodotoxin is also found in some North American newts and Central American frogs.	Onset is usually within 30–40 minutes but may be as short as 10 minutes. Initial perioral paresthesias are followed by headache, diaphoresis, nausea, vomiting, ataxia, and rapidly progressive muscle weakness that may result in respiratory arrest.

nantly cytolytic (pit viper). Neurotoxins cause respiratory paralysis; cytolytic venoms cause tissue destruction by digestion and hemorrhage due to hemolysis and destruction of the endothelial lining of the blood vessels. The manifestations of cytolytic envenomation (eg, rattlesnake venom) are local pain, redness, swelling, and extravasation of blood. Perioral tingling, metallic taste, nausea and vomiting, hypotension, and coagulopathy may also occur. Neurotoxic envenomation may cause ptosis, dysphagia, diplopia, and respiratory arrest.

Treatment

A. Emergency Measures: Immobilize the patient and the bitten part in a horizontal position. Avoid manipulation of the bitten area. Transport the patient to a medical facility for definitive treatment. Do *not* give alcoholic beverages or stimulants; do *not* apply ice; do *not* apply a tourniquet. The trauma to underlying structures resulting from incision and suction performed by unskilled people is probably not justified in view of the small amount of venom that can be recovered.

B. Specific Antidote and General Measures:

1. Pit viper (eg, rattlesnake) envenomation– With local signs such as swelling, pain, and ecchymosis but no systemic symptoms, give four or five vials of polyvalent crotalid antivenin by intravenous drip in 250–500 mL saline. (This should be preceded by skin testing for horse serum sensitivity with the kit supplied.) For more serious envenomation with marked local effects and systemic toxicity (eg, hypotension, coagulopathy), 10–20 vials may be required. Epinephrine should be available for immediate use in the event of an allergic reaction. Specific antiserum

therapy is more effective if given soon after the bite. Monitor vital signs and the blood coagulation profile. Type and cross-match blood. The adequacy of venom neutralization is indicated by improvement in signs and symptoms, and the rate of swelling slows. Serum sickness reactions are common after antivenin use, usually occur 5–10 days after antivenin administration, and may be treated with prednisone, 45–60 mg daily with tapering doses.

2. Elapid (coral snake) envenomation–Give 1–2 vials of specific antivenom as soon as possible.

To locate antisera for exotic snakes, call the Arizona Poison and Drug Information Center, Tucson ([602] 626–6016).

Nelson BK: Snake envenomation: Incidence, clinical presentation and management. Med Toxicol 1989;4:17. (Efficacy of first-aid measures and use of antivenins.)

SPIDER BITES & SCORPION STINGS

The toxin of most species of spiders causes only local pain, redness, and swelling. That of the more venomous black widow spiders (*Latrodectus mactans*) causes generalized muscular pains, muscle spasms, and rigidity. The brown recluse spider (*Loxosceles reclusa*) causes progressive local necrosis as well as hemolytic reactions (rare). Stings by most scorpions cause only local pain. Stings by the more toxic *Centruroides* species (found in the southwestern USA) may cause muscle cramps, twitching and jerking, and occasionally hypertension, convulsions, and pulmonary edema.

Treatment

A. Black Widow Spider Bites: Pain may be relieved with parenteral narcotics or muscle relaxants (eg, methocarbamol, 15 mg/kg). Calcium gluconate 10%, 0.1–0.2 mL/kg intravenously, may relieve muscle rigidity. Antivenin is rarely indicated, usually only for very young or elderly patients who do not respond to the above measures. Horse serum sensitivity testing is required. (Instruction and testing materials are included in the antivenin kit.)

B. Brown Recluse Spider Bites: Because bites occasionally progress to extensive local necrosis, some authorities recommend early excision of the bite site, whereas others use oral corticosteroids. Recently, interest has focused on the use of dapsone and colchicine and an antivenin is being developed. All of these treatments remain of unproved value.

C. Scorpion Stings: No specific treatment is available. For *Centruroides* stings, some toxicologists use a specific antivenom, but this is neither FDA-approved nor widely available.

Banner W Jr: Bites and stings in the pediatrics patient. Curr Probl Pediatr 1988;18(1):1.

Moss HS, Binder LS: A retrospective review of black widow spider envenomation. Ann Emerg Med 1987; 16:188. (Severe regional pain and muscle cramping may be delayed in onset and persist for 1–2 days.)

THEOPHYLLINE

Theophylline is commonly used in the treatment of bronchospasm due to asthma, chronic lung disease, and congestive heart failure. Its toxicity may be caused by several of its pharmacologic effects, including inhibition of phosphodiesterase and adenosine and release of catecholamines. Theophylline may cause intoxication after an acute single overdose or as a result of chronic accidental repeated overmedication or reduced elimination caused by hepatic dysfunction or interacting drug (eg, cimetidine, erythromycin). The usual serum half-life of theophylline is 4–6 hours, but this may increase to more than 20 hours after overdose.

Clinical Findings

Mild intoxication causes nausea, vomiting, tachycardia, and tremulousness. Severe intoxication is characterized by ventricular and supraventricular tachyarrhythmias, hypotension, and seizures. Status epilepticus is common and often intractable to usual anticonvulsants. After acute overdose (but not chronic intoxication), hypokalemia, hyperglycemia, and metabolic acidosis are common. Seizures and other manifestations of toxicity may be delayed for several hours after acute ingestion, especially if a sustained-release preparation such as Theo-Dur was taken.

Diagnosis is based on measurement of the serum theophylline concentration. Acute overdose patients with serum levels greater than 100 mg/L are likely to develop seizures and hypotension. Patients with chronic intoxication may develop serious toxicity at lower levels (ie, 60 mg/L).

Treatment

A. Emergency and Supportive Measures: Maintain a patent airway, and assist ventilation if necessary. Administer supplemental oxygen. Treat seizures with diazepam and phenobarbital as described on p 1319.

After acute ingestion, empty the stomach by emesis or gastric lavage and administer activated charcoal and a cathartic (see p 1321). Repeated doses of activated charcoal may enhance theophylline elimination by "gut dialysis" (see p 1322).

Hemoperfusion is effective in removing theophylline and is indicated for patients with status epilepticus or markedly elevated serum theophylline levels (eg, > 100 mg/L after acute overdose or > 60 mg/L with chronic intoxication).

B. Specific Treatment: There is no antidote for seizures, but hypotension and tachycardia—which are mediated through excessive β_2-adrenergic stimulation—may respond dramatically to beta-blocker therapy. Administer esmolol, 25–50 µg/kg/min by intravenous infusion, or propranolol, 0.5–1 mg intravenously.

Gaar GG et al: The effects of esmolol on the hemodynamics of acute theophylline toxicity. Ann Emerg Med 1987;16:1334. (Animal study demonstrating effectiveness of low-dose esmolol (25 µg/kg/min) on reversal of tachycardia and hypotension associated with theophylline intoxication.)

Shannon M, Lovejoy FH Jr: The influence of age vs peak serum concentration on life-threatening events after chronic theophylline intoxication. Arch Intern Med 1990;150:2045. (Elderly patients are more likely to have serious complications with chronic theophylline intoxication, and the serum concentration is a poor predictor of who will have a life-threatening event.)

TRICYCLIC ANTIDEPRESSANTS

Tricyclic antidepressants are among the most commonly implicated products in suicidal overdose. These drugs have anticholinergic and cardiac depressant properties. Tricyclic antidepressants produce more marked membrane-depressant cardiotoxic effects than the phenothiazines. All of these drugs are highly tissue-bound and are not effectively removed by hemodialysis procedures.

Newer antidepressants such as trazodone, fluoxetine, and buspirone are not chemically relted to the tricyclic antidepressant agents and do not generally produce cardiotoxic effects.

Clinical Findings

Signs of severe intoxication may occur abruptly and without warning within 30–60 minutes after acute overdose. Anticholinergic effects include dilated pupils, tachycardia, dry mouth, flushed skin, muscle twitching, and decreased peristalsis. Membrane-depressant cardiotoxic effects include QRS interval widening (> 0.12 s; see Figure 39–3), ventricular arrhythmias, atrioventricular block, and hypotension. Seizures and coma are common with severe intoxication. Life-threatening hyperthermia may result from status epilepticus and anticholinergic-induced impairment of sweating.

The diagnosis should be suspected in any overdose patient with anticholinergic side effects, especially if there is widening of the QRS interval. For intoxication by most tricyclics, the QRS interval correlates with the severity of intoxication more reliably than the serum drug level. However, newer antidepressants such as amoxapine and fluoxetine may cause seizures without QRS interval prolongation.

Treatment

A. Emergency and Supportive Measures: Maintain a patent airway, and assist ventilation if necessary. Treat coma, hypotension, and seizures as described at the beginning of this chapter. Observe patients for at least 6 hours, and admit all patients with evidence of anticholinergic effects (eg, delirium, dilated pupils, tachycardia, etc) or signs of cardiotoxicity.

Perform gastric lavage and administer activated charcoal. Do *not* induce emesis because of the risk of seizures (see p 1321).

B. Specific Treatment: Cardiotoxic membrane-depressant effects may respond to boluses of sodium bicarbonate (50–100 meq intravenously). Sodium bicarbonate provides a large sodium load that alleviates depression of the sodium-dependent channel. Rever-

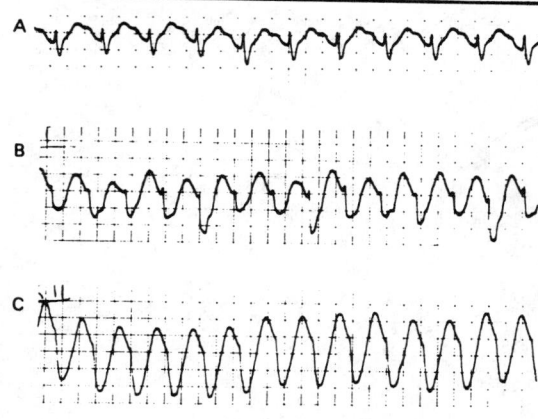

Figure 39–3. Cardiac arrhythmias resulting from tricyclic antidepressant overdose. **A:** Delayed intraventricular conduction results in prolonged QRS interval (0.18 s). **B and C:** Supraventricular tachycardia with progressive widening of QRS complexes mimics ventricular tachycardia. (Reproduced, with permission, from Benowitz NL, Goldschlager N: Cardiac disturbances in the toxicologic patient. In: *Clinical Management of Poisoning and Drug Overdose,* 2nd ed. Haddad LM, Winchester JF [editors]. Saunders, 1990.)

sal of acidosis may also have beneficial effects at this site. Maintain the pH between 7.45 and 7.5.

Caravati EM, Bossart PJ: Demographic and electrocardiographic factors associated with severe tricyclic antidepressant toxicity. J Toxicol Clin Toxicol 1991;29:31. (Retrospective review found predictors of major toxicity included heart rate > 120/min, serum TCA level > 800 ng/mL, QRS interval > 100 ms, and terminal 40 ms axis > 135 degrees.)

Pentel PR, Benowitz NL: Tricyclic antidepressant poisoning: Management of arrhythmias. J Med Toxicol 1986; 1:101.

REFERENCES

Bryson P: *Critical Review in Toxicology.* Aspens Systems, 1989.

Ellenhorn M, Barceloux D: *Medical Toxicology: Diagnosis and Treatment of Human Poisoning.* Elsevier, 1988.

Goldfrank LR et al (editors): *Goldfrank's Toxicologic Emergencies,* 4th ed. Appleton & Lange, 1990.

Haddad LM, Winchester JF: *Clinical Management of Poisoning and Drug Overdose,* 2nd ed. Saunders, 1990.

Olson KR et al: *Poisoning & Drug Overdose.* Appleton & Lange, 1990.

Rumack BH (editor): POISINDEX. National Center for Poison Information, Denver, CO 80204. A computerized and microfiche information system. Revised quarterly.

Other Sources of Information

The manufacturer or the local representative. Another way to identify the contents of a substance is to telephone the manufacturer or the local distributor, who will be able to provide information concerning the type of toxic hazard to be expected from the material in question and what treatment should be given.

Poisoning hotlines to manufacturers. Call the poison control center for the telephone number (Table 39–1).

Appendix: Laboratory Reference Ranges

Diana Nicoll, MD, PhD

Reference Ranges for Commonly Used Tests[1,2]

Test	Specimen	Reference Ranges Conventional Units	Reference Ranges SI Units[2]	Collection
Acetaminophen (Tylenol, others)	Serum	10–20 mg/L **Panic:** >50 mg/L	66–132 µmol/L	Marbled
Acetoacetate	Serum or urine	Negative	Negative	Marbled or urine container
Acid phosphatase (prostatic)	Serum	0.1–0.9 IU/L (method-dependent)	<15 nkat/L (method-dependent)	Marbled
Adrenocorticotropic hormone (ACTH)	Plasma	20–100 pg/mL	4–22 pmol/L	Heparinized plastic container
Alanine aminotransferase (ALT, SGPT, GPT)	Serum	0–35 units/L (laboratory-specific)	0–0.58 µkat/L (laboratory-specific)	Marbled
Albumin	Serum	3.4–4.7 g/dL	34–47 g/L	Marbled
Aldosterone	Plasma	Salt-loaded (120 meq Na⁺/d): Supine: 3–10 ng/dL Upright: 5–30 ng/dL Salt-depleted (20 meq Na⁺/d): Supine: 12–36 ng/dL Upright: 17–137 ng/dL	83–277 pmol/L 139–831 pmol/L 332–997 pmol/L 471–3795 pmol/L	Lavender or green
Alkaline phosphatase	Serum	41–133 IU/L (method- and age-dependent)	0.7–2.2 µkat/L (method- and age-dependent)	Marbled
Ammonia (NH_3)	Plasma	18–60 µg/dL	11–35 µmol/L	Green
Amylase	Serum	20–110 units/L (laboratory-specific)	0.33–1.83 µkat/L (laboratory-specific)	Marbled
Angiotensin-converting enzyme (ACE)	Serum	12–35 units/L (method-dependent)	<590 nkat/L (method-dependent)	Marbled
α_1-Antiprotease	Serum	110–270 mg/dL	1.1–2.7 g/L	Marbled
Antithrombin III (AT III)	Plasma	84–123% (qualitative) 22–39 mg/dL (quantitative)		Blue
Aspartate aminotransferase (AST, SGOT, GOT)	Serum	0–35 IU/L (laboratory-specific)	0–0.58 µkat/L (laboratory-specific)	Marbled
Bilirubin	Serum	Total: 0.1–1.2 mg/dL Direct (conjugated to glucuronide): 0.1–0.4 mg/dL Indirect (unconjugated): 0.1–0.7 mg/dL	2–21 µmol/L <7 µmol/L <12 µmol/L	Marbled
Blood urea nitrogen (BUN)	Serum	8–20 mg/dL	2.9–7.1 mmol/L	Marbled
C-peptide	Serum	0.8–4.0 ng/mL	0.8–4.0 µg/L	Marbled (fasting)
Calcitonin	Plasma	Male: <90 pg/mL Female: <70 pg/mL	Male: <90 ng/L Female: <70 ng/L	Green
Calcium (Ca^{2+})	Serum	8.5–10.5 mg/dL **Panic:** <6.5 or >13.5 mg/dL	2.1–2.6 mmol/L	Marbled

(continued)

Reference Ranges for Commonly Used Tests[1,2] (continued)

Test	Specimen	Reference Ranges		Collection
		Conventional Units	**SI Units[2]**	**Collection**
Calcium (U_{Ca})	Urine	100–300 mg/d	2.5–7.5 mmol/d	Urine bottle containing hydrochloric acid
Carbon dioxide (CO_2), total (bicarbonate)	Serum	22–28 meq/L **Panic:** <15 or >40 meq/L	22–28 mmol/L **Panic:** <15 or >40 mmol/L	Marbled
Carboxyhemoglobin (HbCO)	Whole blood	<9% of total hemoglobin (Hb)	<0.09 fraction of total hemoglobin	Lavender
Carcinoembryonic antigen (CEA)	Serum	0–2.5 ng/mL	0–2.5 µg/L	Marbled
Ceruloplasmin	Serum	20–35 mg/dL	200–350 mg/L	Marbled
Chloride (Cl^-)	Serum	98–107 meq/L	98–107 mmol/L	Marbled
Cholesterol	Serum	Desirable: <200 mg/dL Borderline: 200–239 mg/dL High risk: >240 mg/dL	Desirable: <5.2 mmol/L Borderline: 5.2–6.1 mmol/L High risk: >6.2 mmol/L	Marbled
Chorionic gonadotropin, β-subunit (β-hCG), quantitative	Serum	Males and nonpregnant females: undetectable or <2 mIU/mL	Males and nonpregnant females: undetectable or <2 IU/L	Marbled
Complement C3	Serum	64–166 mg/dL	640–1660 mg/L	Marbled
Complement C4	Serum	15–45 mg/dL	150–450 mg/L	Marbled
Complement CH50	Plasma or serum	22–40 units/mL (laboratory-specific)		Marbled
Cortisol	Plasma or serum	8:00 AM.: 5–20 µg/dL	140–550 nmol/L	Marbled, lavender, or green
Cortisol (urinary free)	Urine	10–110 µg/24 h	30–300 nmol/d	Urine bottle containing boric acid
Creatine kinase (CK)	Serum	32–267 IU/L (method-dependent)	0.53–4.45 µkat/L (method-dependent)	Marbled
Creatine kinase MB (CKMB)	Serum	<16 IU/L or <4% of total CK (laboratory-specific)	<0.27 µkat/L or <4% of total CK (laboratory-specific)	Marbled
Creatinine (Cr)	Serum	0.6–1.2 mg/dL	50–100 µmol/L	Marbled
Creatinine clearance (Cl_{Cr})	See Collection	Adults: 90–130 mL/min/1.73 m^2 BSA	1.5–2.2 mL/s	Carefully timed 24-hour urine and simultaneous serum or plasma creatinine sample
Cryoglobulins	Serum	<0.12 mg/dL		Marbled at 37°C
Erythrocyte count (RBC count)	Whole blood	$4.2–5.6 \times 10^6/\mu L$	$4.2–5.6 \times 10^{12}/L$	Lavender
Erythrocyte sedimentation rate (ESR)	Whole blood	Male: <10 mm/h Female: <15 mm/h (laboratory-specific)	Same	Lavender
Erythropoietin (EPO)	Serum	5–20 mIU/mL	5–20 IU/L	Marbled
Factor VIII assay	Plasma	40–150% of normal (varies with age)		Blue
Fecal fat	Stool	Random: <60 droplets of fat per high-power field 72-hour: <7 g/d		Qualitative: Random stool sample Quantitative: 72-hour collection following 2-day dietary fat regimen
Ferritin	Serum	Male: 16–300 ng/mL Female: 4–161 ng/mL	Male: 16–300 µg/L Female: 4–161 µg/L	Marbled
α-Fetoprotein (AFP)	Serum	0–15 ng/mL	0–15 µg/L	Marbled
Fibrin D-dimers	Plasma	Negative		Blue

(continued)

Reference Ranges for Commonly Used Tests[1,2] (continued)

Test	Specimen	Reference Ranges		Collection
		Conventional Units	SI Units[2]	
Fibrinogen (functional)	Plasma	175–433 mg/dL **Panic:** <75 mg/dL	1.75–4.3 g/L	Blue
Folic acid (red cells)	Whole blood	165–760 ng/mL	370–1720 nmol/L	Lavender
Follicle-stimulating hormone (FSH)	Serum	Female: 2–15 mIU/mL Peak production: 20–50 mIU/mL Male: 1–10 mIU/mL (laboratory-specific)	Female: 2–15 IU/L Peak production: 20–50 IU/L Male: 1–10 IU/L (laboratory-specific)	Marbled
Free erythrocyte protoporphyrin (FEP)	Whole blood	<35 µg/dL (method-dependent)		Lavender
Gamma-glutamyl transpeptidase (GGT)	Serum	9–85 units/L (laboratory-specific)	0.15–1.42 µkat/L (laboratory-specific)	Marbled
Gastrin	Serum	<300 pg/mL	<300 ng/L	Marbled
Glucose	Serum	60–115 mg/dL **Panic:** <40 or >500 mg/dL	3.3–6.3 mmol/L	Marbled (fasting)
Glucose-6-phosphate dehydrogenase (G6PD) screen	Whole blood	4–8 units/g Hb	0.07–0.14 µkat/L	Green or blue
Glutamine	CSF	6–16 mg/dL **Panic:** >40 mg/dL	0.41–1.10 mmol/L	Collect CSF in a plastic tube
Glycated (glycosylated) hemoglobin (HbA$_{Ic}$)	Serum	3.9–6.9% (method-dependent)		Lavender
Growth hormone (GH)	Serum	0–5 ng/mL	0–5 µg/L	Marbled
Haptoglobin	Serum	46–316 mg/dL	0.5–3.2 g/L	Marbled
Hematocrit (Hct)	Whole blood	Male: 39–49% Female: 35–45% (age-dependent)	Male: 0.39–0.49 Female: 0.35–0.45	Lavender
Hemoglobin A$_2$ (HbA$_2$)	Whole blood	1.5–3.5% of total hemoglobin	0.015–0.035	Lavender
Hemoglobin electrophoresis	Whole blood	HbA: >95% HbA$_2$: 1.5–3.5%		Lavender, blue, or green
Hemoglobin, fetal (HbF)	Whole blood	Adult: <2% (varies with age)		Lavender, blue, or green
Hemoglobin, total (Hb)	Whole blood	Male: 13.6–17.5 g/dL Female 12.0–15.5 g/dL **Panic:** ≤ 7 g/dL (age-dependent)	Male: 136–175 g/L Female 120–155 g/L	Lavender
Hemosiderin	Urine	Negative		Urine container
5-Hydroxyindoleacetic acid (5-HIAA)	Urine	2–8 mg/24 h	20–40 µmol/d	Urine bottle containing hydrochloric acid
IgG index	Serum and CSF	0.29–0.59 ratio		Marbled and glass or plastic tube for CSF
Immunoglobulins (Ig)	Serum	IgA: 78–367 mg/dL IgG: 583–1761 mg/dL IgM: 52–335 mg/dL	IgA: 0.78–3.67 g/L IgG: 5.83–17.6 g/L IgM: 0.52–3.35 g/L	Marbled
Insulin, immunoreactive	Serum	6–35 µU/dL	42–243 pmol/L	Marbled
Iron (Fe^{2+})	Serum	50–175 µg/dL	9–31 µmol/L	Marbled
Iron-binding capacity, total (TIBC)	Serum	250–460 µg/dL	45–82 µmol/L	Marbled
Lactate dehydrogenase (LDH)	Serum	88–230 units/L (laboratory-specific)	1.46–3.82 µkat/L (laboratory-specific)	Marbled
Lactate dehydrogenase (LDH) isoenzymes	Serum	LDH$_1$/LDH$_2$: <0.85		Marbled

(continued)

Reference Ranges for Commonly Used Tests[1,2] (continued)

Test	Specimen	Reference Ranges		Collection
		Conventional Units	SI Units[2]	
Lactic acid	Venous blood	0.5–2.0 meq/L	0.5–2.0 mmol/L	Gray
Lead (Pb)	Whole blood	Child: <25 µg/dL Adult: <40 µg/dL	Child: <1.21 µmol/L Adult: <1.93 µmol/L	Navy
Lecithin/sphingomyelin (L/S) ratio	Amniotic fluid	>2.0 (method-dependent)		Collect in a plastic tube
Leukocyte alkaline phosphatase (LAP)	Whole blood	40–130 Based on 0–4+ rating of 100 PMNs stained for alkaline phosphatase		Green
Leukocyte (white blood cell) count, total (WBC count)	Whole blood	3.4–10 × 10³/µL **Panic:** <1.5 × 10³/µL	3.4–10 × 10⁹/L	Lavender
Lipase	Serum	0–160 units/L (laboratory-specific)	0–2.66 µkat/L (laboratory-specific)	Marbled
Luteinizing hormone (LH)	Serum	Premenopausal: <30 mIU/mL Postmenopausal: >35 mIU/mL Male: 6–30 mIU/mL (laboratory-specific)	Premenopausal: <30 IU/L Postmenopausal: >35 IU/L Male: 6–30 IU/L (laboratory-specific)	Marbled
Magnesium (Mg²⁺)	Serum	1.8–3.0 mg/dL **Panic:** <0.5 or >4.5 mg/dL	0.75–1.25 mmol/L	Marbled
Mean corpuscular hemoglobin (MCH)	Whole blood	26–34 pg		Lavender
Mean corpuscular hemoglobin concentration (MCHC)	Whole blood	31–36 g/dL	310–360 g/L	Lavender
Mean corpuscular volume (MCV)	Whole blood	80–100 fL		Lavender
Metanephrines	Urine	0.3–0.9 mg/24 h	1.6–4.9 µmol/d	Urine bottle containing hydrochloric acid
Methemoglobin (MetHb)	Whole blood	<1% of total hemoglobin	<0.01 fraction of total hemoglobin	Lavender
β₂-Microglobulin (β₂M)	Serum	<0.2 mg/dL	<2.0 mg/L	Marbled
Osmolality	Serum	285–293 mosm/kg H₂O **Panic:** <240 or >320 mosm/kg H₂O	285–293 mmol/kg H₂O	Marbled
	Urine	Random: 100–900 mosm/kg H₂O	Random: 100–900 mmol/kg H₂O	Urine container
Oxygen, partial pressure (PO₂)	Whole blood	83–108 mm Hg	11.04–14.36 kPa	Heparinized syringe
Parathyroid hormone (PTH)	Serum	Intact PTH: 11–54 pg/mL (laboratory-specific)	Intact PTH: 1.2–5.7 pmol/L (laboratory-specific)	Marbled
Partial thromboplastin time, activated (PTT)	Plasma	25–35 seconds (range varies) **Panic:** ≥60 seconds		Blue
pH	Whole blood	Arterial: 7.35–7.45 Venous: 7.31–7.41		Heparinized syringe
Phosphorus	Serum	2.5–4.5 mg/dL **Panic:** <1.0 mg/dL	0.8–1.45 mmol/L	Marbled
Platelet count (Plt)	Whole blood	150–450 × 10³/µL **Panic:** <25 × 10³/µL	150–450 × 10⁹/L	Lavender
Platelet-associated IgG	Whole blood	Negative		Yellow (17 mL of blood)
Porphobilinogen (PBG)	Urine	Negative		
Potassium (K⁺)	Serum	3.5–5.0 meq/L **Panic:** <3.0 or >6.0 mq/L	3.5–5.0 mmol/L	Marbled

(continued)

Reference Ranges for Commonly Used Tests[1,2] (continued)

Test	Specimen	Reference Ranges		Collection
		Conventional Units	SI Units[2]	
Prolactin (PRL)	Serum	<20 ng/mL	<20 µg/L	Marbled
Prostate-specific antigen (PSA)	Serum	0–4 ng/mL	0–4 µg/L	Marbled
Protein C	Plasma	71–176%		Blue
Protein electrophoresis	Serum	Adults: Albumin: 3.3–4.7 g/dL α_1: 0.1–0.4 g/dL α_2: 0.3–0.9 g/dL β_2: 0.7–1.5 g/dL γ: 0.5–1.4 g/dL		Marbled
Protein S (antigen)	Plasma	76–178%		Blue
Protein, total	Plasma or serum	6.0–8.0 g/dL	60–80 g/L	Marbled
Prothrombin time (PT)	Whole blood	11–15 seconds **Panic:** ≥30 seconds		Blue
Renin activity (PRA)	Plasma	High-sodium diet (75–150 meq Na$^+$/d): Supine: 0.2–2.3 ng/mL/h Standing: 1.3–4.0 ng/mL/h Low-sodium diet (30–75 meq Na$^+$/d): Standing: 4.0–7.7 ng/mL/h		Lavender
Reptilase clotting time	Plasma	13–19 seconds		Blue
Reticulocyte count	Whole blood	$33–137 \times 10^3/\mu L$	$33–137 \times 10^9/L$	Lavender
Russell's viper venom clotting time (dilute) (RVVT)	Plasma	24–37 seconds		Blue
Salicylate (aspirin, others)	Serum	20–30 mg/dL **Panic:** >35 mg/dL	200–300 mg/L	Marbled
Sodium (Na$^+$)	Serum	135–145 meq/L **Panic:** <125 or >155 meq/L	135–145 mmol/L	Marbled
Somatomedin C	Plasma	123–463 ng/mL (age- and sex-dependent)		Lavender
Testosterone	Serum	Male: 3.0–10.9 ng/mL Female: 0.3–0.7 ng/mL	Male: 10–35 nmol/L Female: 1.0–2.4 nmol/L	Marbled
Thrombin time	Plasma	24–35 seconds (laboratory-specific)		Blue
Thyroglobulin	Serum	3–42 ng/mL	3–42 µg/L	Marbled
Thyroid-stimulating hormone (TSH)	Serum	0.4–6 µU/mL	0.4–6 mU/L	Marbled
Thyroid-stimulating immunoglobulin (TSI)	Serum	<130% of basal activity of adenylyl cyclase		Marbled
Thyroxine (T$_4$), total	Serum	5.0–11.0 µg/dL	64–142 nmol/L	Marbled
Thyroxine, free (FT$_4$)	Serum	Varies with method		Marbled
Thyroxine index, free (FT$_4$I)	Serum	6.5–12.5		Marbled
Triglycerides	Serum	<165 mg/dL	<1.65 g/L	Marbled (fasting)
Triiodothyronine (T$_3$), total	Serum	95–190 ng/dL	1.5–2.9 nmol/L	Marbled
Uric acid	Serum	Male: 2.4–7.4 mg/dL Female: 1.4–5.8 mg/dL	Male: 140–440 µmol/L Female: 80–350 µmol/L	Marbled

(continued)

Reference Ranges for Commonly Used Tests[1,2] (continued)

Test	Specimen	Reference Ranges		Collection
		Conventional Units	SI Units[2]	
Vanillylmandelic acid (VMA)	Urine	2–7 mg/24 h	10–35 μmol/d	Urine bottle containing hydrochloric acid
Vitamin B$_{12}$	Serum	140–820 pg/mL	100–600 pmol/L	Marbled
Vitamin B$_{12}$ absorption test (Schilling's test)	24-hour urine	Excretion of >8% of administered dose		
Vitamin D, 25-hydroxy (25[OH]D)	Serum or plasma	10–50 ng/mL	25–125 nmol/L	Marbled or green
Vitamin D, 1,25-dihydroxy (1,25[OH]$_2$D)	Serum or plasma	20–76 pg/mL		Marbled or green

[1]The reference ranges given here in conventional units and in SI units are from several large medical centers. Always use the reference ranges provided by your clinical laboratory, since ranges may be method-dependent.

[2]Reference: Young DS: Implementation of SI units for clinical laboratory data. Ann Intern Med 1987;106:114.

Index

of aorta and iliac arteries, 390
of femoral and popliteal arteries, 391
of lower leg and foot arteries, 392
neurogenic, 849
Claustrophobia, 876
Clavulanic acid, with penicillin, 1263
Clear cell carcinoma, of vagina, diethylstilbestrol exposure and, 592, 593
Clear liquid diet, 1044
Clemastine, for IgE-mediated allergy, 661*t*
Clicks, 282
in hypertension, 372
Clindamycin, **1281–1282**
for acne, 117
for bacterial vaginosis, 591
cost of, 1260*t*
for endocarditis prophylaxis, 1281*t*
for malaria treatment, 1200*t*
for pelvic inflammatory disease, 601
in renal/hepatic failure, 1257*t*
Clinoril. *See* Sulindac
Clitocybe mushrooms, poisoning caused
by, 1336, 1337*t*
CLL. *See* Leukemias, chronic lymphocytic
Clofazimine
for leprosy, 1160
for tuberculosis, 1278
Clofibrate
for cholesterol lowering, 1023
nutrient absorption and metabolism affected by, 1030*t*
Clomiphene, for ovulation induction,
607–608
Clomipramine, 865*t*
Clonazepam, 868
for manic episodes, 891
for seizures, 802*t*
Clonidine
for diarrhea, 473
for hypertension, 375*t*
for hypertensive crisis, 380*t*, 384
for migraine, 799*t*
overdose of, **1330–1331**
Clonorchis sinensis (clonorchiasis),
1217–1218
drugs for infection with, 1215*t*
Clorazepate, 868*t*
Clostridium, **1136–1138**
bifermentans, 1136
botulinum
botulism caused by, 852, 1137
diarrhea and food poisoning caused
by, 1065*t*
difficile
in antibiotic-associated colitis, 513–
514 metronidazole for, 1282
diarrhea and food poisoning caused
by, 1065*t*
diseases caused by, **1136–1138**
drugs for, 1253*t*
histolyticum, 1136
novyi, 1136
perfringens
diarrhea and food poisoning caused
by, 1065*t*
myonecrosis caused by, 1136
ramosum, 1136
tetani, 1136
Clotrimazole, 1287
Cloxacillin, 1263
Clozapine, 859*t*
agranulocytosis caused by, 860

Clozaril. *See* Clozapine
Clubbed digits, 144, 208
Cluster of differentiation, lymphocyte
types identified by, 644. *See also
under* CD
Cluster headaches, 800
CMF regimen, 73
CMFP regimen, 73
CMML. *See* Leukemias, chronic
myelomonocytic
CMV. *See* Continuous mechanical ventilation
CO₂. *See* Carbon dioxide
Coagulation
disorders of. *See* specific type and
Coagulopathies
disseminated intravascular, **460–461**
vitamin K in, 459
Coagulation factors
deficiency of
in hemophilia A, 456–457
in hemophilia B, 458
miscellaneous, 458
in von Willebrand's disease, 453–454
synthesis of in liver, 458
Coagulation studies, in upper gastrointestinal bleeding, 474
Coagulopathies, **449–462**. *See also specific type*
in cirrhosis, 543
of liver disease, **458–459**
lower gastrointestinal bleeding and, 475
miscellaneous, 458
in renal failure, 769–770
Coal worker's pneumoconiosis, 263
Coarctation of aorta, **287**
Cobalamin (vitamin B₁₂), **1042**
deficiency of, **421–422**
neuropathy in, 842
in pernicious anemia, 421, 491
subacute combined degeneration of
spinal cord caused by, 833–834
laboratory reference range for, 1351*t*
recommended dietary allowances for,
1026*t*
Cocaine
cardiotoxicity of, 353
myocardial ischemia caused by, 309
nursing infant affected by, 637*t*
overdose of, **1327**
Cocaine abuse, 902
Coccidioides immitis (coccidioidomycosis), **1245–1246**
bone and joint involvement in, **705**, 1245
Coccidiosis, **1190–1192**
Cochlea, diseases of, hearing loss and, 183
Codeine, 9
for diarrhea, 473
overdose of, **1338**
Codominant phenotype, 784
Codons, 782
Coffee-ground emesis, in upper gastrointestinal bleeding, 473
in peptic ulcer disease, 497
Cogentin. *See* Benztropine
Cognitive therapy, 871
Colchicine
for gout, 670, 671
nutrient absorption and metabolism af-
fected by, 1030*t*
Cold, disorders caused by, **1297–1300**.
See also specific type

Cold agglutinin disease, **431**
Cold (common), **188**, 1120
Cold sore, **109–110**
Cold therapy, in arthritis management,
666–667
Cold urticaria, 1297
Colectomy, in ulcerative colitis, 518
Colestipol, for cholesterol lowering,
1021*t*, 1022–1023
Colic, in urinary stone disease, 747
Colitis. *See also* Diarrhea
in amebiasis, 1184, 1185, 1186, 1187*t*
antibiotic-associated, **513–514**
metronidazole for, 1282
cathartic, 512
dysenteric, 1184
fulminant, 517
functional, 512
infectious, **513**
ischemic, 395
laxative, 512
left-sided, 515
mucous, 512
postdysenteric, 1188
pseudomembranous, 513–514
metronidazole for, 1282
spastic, 512
ulcerative, **515–518**
arthritis and, 700
Collagen diseases, **681–694**. *See also specific type and* Autoimmune dis-
eases
organic mental syndromes and, 904
Colloids
for fluid resuscitation in burns, 1305
for volume replacement in shock, 413
Colon
angiodysplasia of, **522**
cancer of, **523–524**. *See also* Colorectal
cancer
chemotherapy of, 67*t*
lower gastrointestinal bleeding and, 475
polyps and, 522
ulcerative colitis and, 517–518, 519
diseases of, **512–524**. *See also specific
type and* Colitis
constipation and, 469
dementia in elderly and, 50
diverticular disease of, **521–522**
irritable, 512
motor activity of, in irritable bowel syndrome, 512
polyps of, **522–523**
in schistosomiasis, 1213
"Colon cutoff sign," in acute pancreatitis,
558
Colonoscopy, in angiodysplasia of colon,
522
Color Doppler, 283
Color perception, loss of in occipital lobe
lesions, 820
Colorado tick fever, **1116**
Colorectal cancer. *See also* Colon, cancer
of
chemotherapy of, 67*t*
incidence of, 62*t*
polyps and, 522
regional enteritis and, 502
ulcerative colitis and, 517–518, 519
Colostomy, air travel in patients with, 1315
Colposcopy, 588*t*, 593–594
for biopsy, 594

Thiamin (vitamin B₁), **1040**
for coma caused by poisoning or overdose, 1318
deficiency of, 1040
neuropathy in, 842
Wernicke's encephalopathy caused
by, 834
recommended dietary allowances for,
1026t
toxicity of, 1040
Thiazide diuretics
adverse ocular effects of, 173t
for heart failure, 347
for hypertension, 374t, 377–379
in combination product, 374t, 377
Thiethylperazine, for chemotherapy-in-
duced nausea and vomiting, 76
Thimet poisoning, **1339**
Thioguanine, 69t
Thioridazine, 859t
Thiosulfate, sodium, for cyanide poison-
ing, 1331
Thiothixene, 859t
Thiouracil, nursing infant affected by, 637t
Thiourea, for Graves' disease, 935
Thioxanthenes, 859t
Third-degree burn, 1303
Third heart sound, 282
Third nerve paralysis, 169
Third-trimester bleeding, **628–629**
Thoracentesis
in pneumonia, 231
in pulmonary effusion, 274–276
Thoracic actinomycosis, 1155
Thoracic aortic aneurysm, **386–387**
Thoracic outlet syndrome, **676–677**
Thoracostomy, tube
for parapneumonic effusion, 277
for pneumothorax, 278
Thorazine. See Chlorpromazine
Threadworm infection, drugs for, 1215t
Threatened abortion, 622, 623
Thrills, 282
Throat cultures, 197
Thrombasthenia, Glanzmann's, 455
Thrombin time, laboratory reference
range for, 1350t
Thromboangiitis obliterans, **397–398**
Thrombocytopenia
causes of, 450t
chemotherapy and, 74
in hemolytic-uremic syndrome, 452
in idiopathic thrombocytopenic purpura, 450
immune, autoimmune hemolytic anemia and, 430
in thrombotic thrombocytopenic purpura, 451
Thrombocytosis, essential, 435t
Thromboembolism
oral contraceptive use and, 609–610
pulmonary, **252–258**
Thromboendarterectomy
for atherosclerotic occlusive disease
of aorta and iliac arteries, 390
of femoral and popliteal arteries, 391
carotid, for transient ischemic attacks,
810
Thrombolytic therapy
for myocardial infarction, 317–319
for pulmonary embolism, 257
for unstable angina, 314

Thrombophlebitis (venous thrombosis),
403–406. See also Thrombosis
anticoagulation therapy for, 255–257
cancer-related, 87t
deep vein. See Deep vein thrombosis
intracranial, **817**
pulmonary embolism and, 252–253,
254–255
septic
central nervous system anaerobic,
1154
drugs for, 1255t
superficial vein, **406**
suppurative, in perforated appendicitis,
511
in varicosities, 403
Thromboplastin time, partial. See Partial
thromboplastin time
Thrombosis, **462–463**
arterial, acute, **396–397**
catheter, in central vein parenteral nutrition, 1051–1052
in disseminated intravascular coagulation, 460
"effort," in thoracic outlet syndrome,
677
in polycythemia vera, 435
sigmoid sinus, otitis media and, 181
venous. See Thrombophlebitis
Thrombotic thrombocytopenic purpura,
451–452
Thrush, **195**, 1243
in AIDS/HIV infection, 205, 1078, 1084
Thymoma
paraneoplastic syndromes associated
with, 87t
pure red cell aplasia and, 424, 425
Thyroglobulin
laboratory reference range for, 1350t
serum, 928
Thyroglossal duct cyst, **204**
Thyroid antibodies, 928
Thyroid function tests, **925–929**
Thyroid gland
cancer of, **938–941**
chemotherapy for, 68t
diseases of, **924–942**. See also Hyperthyroidism; Hypothyroidism
in AIDS/HIV infection, 1086
fine-needle biopsy of, 928, 939
ultrasonography of, 928
Thyroid hormone
deficiency of, **929–933**
for hypopituitarism, 919
Thyroid nodules
cold vs. hot, 939, 940t
toxic solitary, 936–937
Thyroid-stimulating hormone
immunoassay for, 927–928
laboratory reference range (normal values) for, 927, 1350t
Thyroid-stimulating immunoglobulin, laboratory reference range for,
1350t
Thyroid "storm," 934, 937
Thyroid surgery (thyroidectomy)
for goiter, 929
for Graves' disease, 936
for thyroid cancer, 940–941
for toxic nodular goiter, 936
Thyroid uptake and scan, **38–39**, **927**
resin, 926–927

Thyroiditis, **941–942**
Hashimoto's, 934, 937, 941, 942
Riedel's, 942
subacute, 933, 937, 941–942
suppurative, 942
Thyrotoxicosis, **933–938**
factitia, 933
during pregnancy, 633
Thyrotropin, cancer-related, 87t
Thyrotropin-releasing hormone test, in
psychiatric evaluation, 857
Thyroxine
free
immunoassay for, 925–926
index for, 927
laboratory reference range (normal
values) for, 927, 1350t
laboratory reference range (normal
values) for, 925, 1350t
immunoassay for, 926
total, laboratory reference range for,
1350t
uptake of, 926–927
TIAs. See Transient ischemic attacks
TIBC. See Iron-binding capacity, total
Tibial artery, atherosclerotic occlusive disease of, 392
Tibial nerve, compression of, 846
Tic douloureux, 801–802
vertigo and, 187
Ticarcillin, 1262–1263
cost of, 1260t
in renal/hepatic failure, 1258t
Tick bites, 135
Lyme disease transmission and, 1176
Tick typhus, 1123t, **1127**
Tics, in Gilles de la Tourette's syndrome,
830
Tietze's syndrome, 310
Timentin, 1263
Timolol
for glaucoma, 160
for hypertension, 376t
Tinea
capitis, **101–102**
circinata, **102–103**
corporis, **102–103**
cruris, **103–104**
manuum, **104–105**
pedis, **104–105**
unguium, 145
versicolor, 104, **105–106**
Tinel's sign, in carpal tunnel syndrome,
679
Tinidazole, for giardiasis, 1193
Tinnitus, **184**
TIPS. See Transjugular intrahepatic
portosystemic shunt
Tissue plasminogen activator
for myocardial infarction, 318
for pulmonary embolism, 257
TLC. See Total lung capacity
TMP-SMZ. See Trimethoprim-sulfamethoxazole
TNM system, for cancer staging, 64
in bladder cancer, 761t
in breast cancer, 570, 571t
in kidney cancer, 763
in prostate cancer, 758t
in testicular cancer, 765t
Tobacco use, 903
cessation of, in disease prevention, 4–5

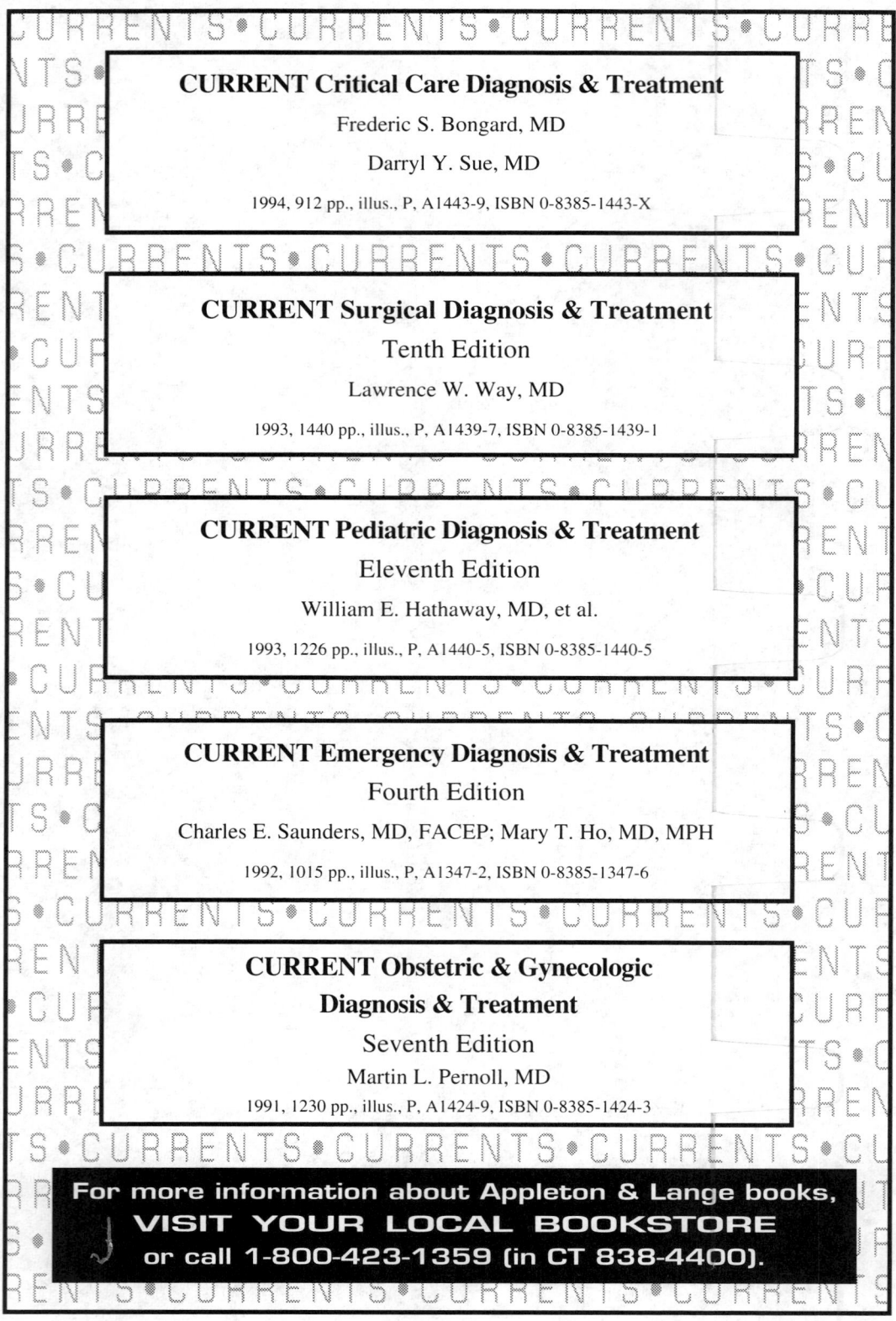

CURRENT Critical Care Diagnosis & Treatment

Frederic S. Bongard, MD

Darryl Y. Sue, MD

1994, 912 pp., illus., P, A1443-9, ISBN 0-8385-1443-X

CURRENT Surgical Diagnosis & Treatment

Tenth Edition

Lawrence W. Way, MD

1993, 1440 pp., illus., P, A1439-7, ISBN 0-8385-1439-1

CURRENT Pediatric Diagnosis & Treatment

Eleventh Edition

William E. Hathaway, MD, et al.

1993, 1226 pp., illus., P, A1440-5, ISBN 0-8385-1440-5

CURRENT Emergency Diagnosis & Treatment

Fourth Edition

Charles E. Saunders, MD, FACEP; Mary T. Ho, MD, MPH

1992, 1015 pp., illus., P, A1347-2, ISBN 0-8385-1347-6

CURRENT Obstetric & Gynecologic Diagnosis & Treatment

Seventh Edition

Martin L. Pernoll, MD

1991, 1230 pp., illus., P, A1424-9, ISBN 0-8385-1424-3